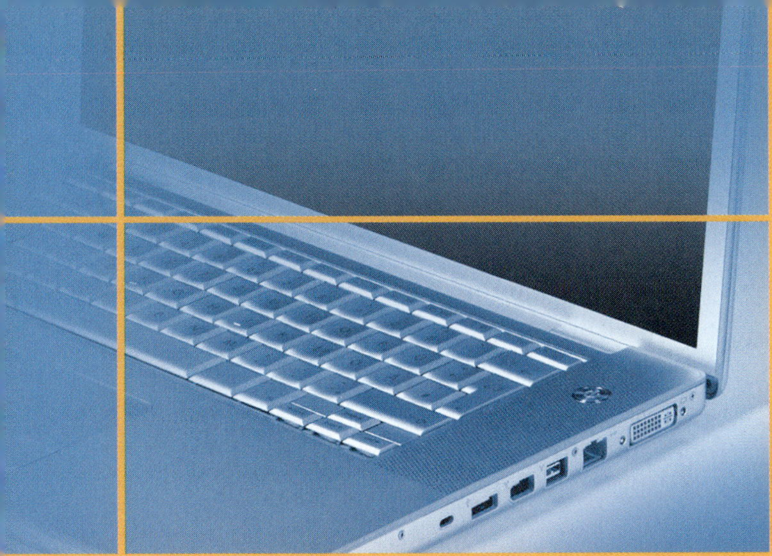

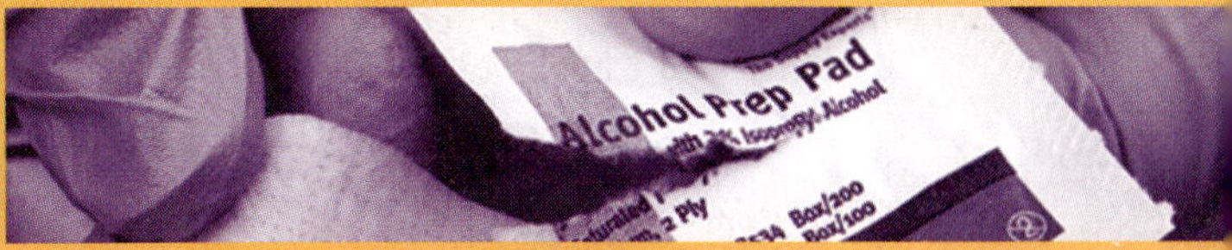

Delmar's

Clinical Medical Assisting

4th Edition

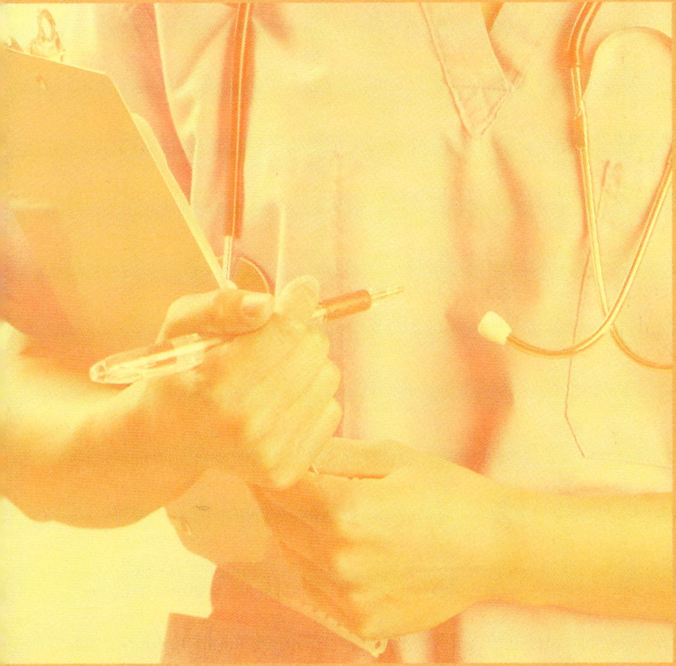

Wilburta Q. Lindh
CMA (AAMA)

Marilyn S. Pooler
RN, MEd

Carol D. Tamparo
CMA (AAMA), PhD

Barbara M. Dahl
CMA (AAMA), CPC

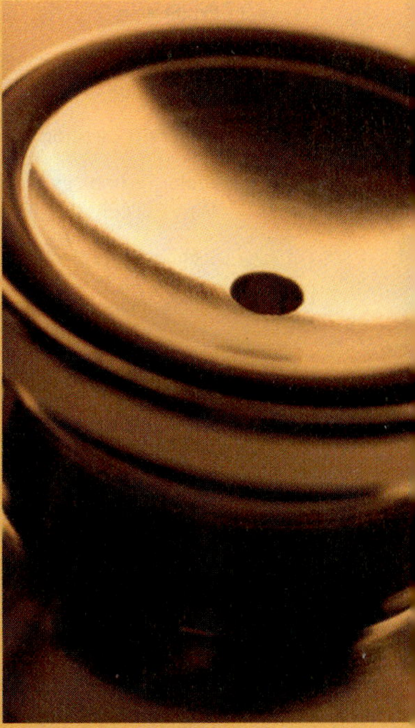

DELMAR
CENGAGE Learning™

Australia • Brazil • Japan • Korea • Mexico • Singapore • Spain • United Kingdom • United States

DELMAR
CENGAGE Learning™

Delmar's Clinical Medical Assisting, Fourth Edition

Wilburta Q. Lindh, Marilyn S. Pooler, Carol D. Tamparo, Barbara M. Dahl

Vice President, Career and Professional Editorial: Dave Garza

Director of Learning Solutions: Matthew Kane

Senior Acquisitions Editor: Rhonda Dearborn

Managing Editor: Marah Bellegarde

Senior Product Manager: Sarah Prime

Editorial Assistant: Chiara Astriab

Vice President, Career and Professional Marketing: Jennifer McAvey

Marketing Director: Wendy Mapstone

Senior Marketing Manager: Nancy Bradshaw

Marketing Coordinator: Erica Ropitzky

Production Director: Carolyn Miller

Content Project Manager: Anne Sherman

Senior Art Director: Jack Pendleton

Senior Technology Product Manager: Mary Colleen Liburdi

Technology Project Manager: Ben Knapp

Technology Project Manager: Erin Zeggert

Library of Congress Control Number: 2008930399

ISBN-13: 978-1-4354-1925-4

ISBN-10: 1-4354-1925-1

Delmar
5 Maxwell Drive
Clifton Park, NY 12065-2919
USA

Cengage Learning is a leading provider of customized learning solutions with office locations around the globe, including Singapore, the United Kingdom, Australia, Mexico, Brazil, and Japan. Locate your local office at: **international.cengage.com/region**

Cengage Learning products are represented in Canada by Nelson Education, Ltd.

To learn more about Delmar, visit **www.cengage.com/delmar**
Purchase any of our products at your local college store or at our preferred online store **www.ichapters.com**

Printed in the United States of America
1 2 3 4 5 6 7 12 11 10 09

Table of Contents

Chapter 6: The Therapeutic Approach to the Patient with a Life-Threatening Illness 81

Unit 3: Responsible Medical Practice 92

Chapter 7: Legal Considerations 93

Chapter 8: Ethical Considerations 120

Chapter 9: Emergency Procedures and First Aid 137

SECTION II: CLINICAL PROCEDURES 167

Unit 4: Integrated Clinical Procedures 168

Chapter 10: Infection Control and Medical Asepsis 169

Unit 7: Laboratory Procedures 791

Unit 9: Entry into the Profession 1057

List of Procedures

Preface

The world of health care continues to change rapidly, and, as medical assistants, you will be called on to do more and respond to an increasing number of responsibilities. Now is the time to equip yourself with the skills you will need to excel in the field. Now is the time to maximize your potential, expand your base of knowledge, and dedicate yourself to becoming the best multifaceted, multiskilled medical assistant that you can be.

The new edition of *Delmar's Clinical Medical Assisting* will guide you on this journey. This text is part of a dynamic learning system that includes software, workbook, and online materials. Together, this learning package includes coverage of the entry-level competencies identified by the Accrediting Bureau of Health Education Schools (ABHES) and the Commission on Accreditation of Allied Health Education Programs (CAAHEP). It will also help you prepare for certification examinations from the American Association of Medical Assistants (AAMA), the American Medical Technologists (AMT), and the National Healthcareer Association (NHA).

You will find this edition continues to provide you with opportunities to use your critical thinking skills, through case studies, critical thinking boxes, question boxes, scenarios, and features that tie directly to *Delmar's Skills and Procedures and Critical Thinking for Medical Assistants DVD Series*. You will also see that the text addresses topics that will make you workplace-ready, including electronic health records (EHRs), Total Practice Management System (TPMS) software, professionalism, and confidentiality and privacy issues.

Some of the special new features and updates to this edition include:

- Emphasis on EHRs and TPMS software; where appropriate, each chapter includes a figure illustrating how the chapter content relates to TPMS
- More than 200 new photos illustrating a greater number of procedures and showing the latest equipment
- More than 30 new procedures
- English and Spanish glossary of terms included in the book, with free downloadable Spanish terms for mp3 players at Delmar's Mobile Download Web site
- Broadening of cultural diversity in the text and the workbook
- Updated certification and examination information for AAMA, AMT, and NHA
- Updated to 2008 CAAHEP curriculum standards, including safety and emergency practices
- New technology initiatives that focus on assessment, interactivity, and competency mapping

HOW THE TEXT IS ORGANIZED

Section I, General Procedures (Chapters 1 through 9), provides the groundwork for understanding the role and responsibilities of the medical assistant. Topics include the medical assisting profession, the health care team, the history of medicine, communication skills, legal and ethical issues, and emergency and first aid procedures.

New material in this section includes:

- Information on National Healthcare Association (NHA)
- Expanded information about AMT, ABHES, RMA, CMAS, and CMA (AAMA)
- New Advanced Directives and forms
- New section on Safety and Emergency Practices
- Summary of layperson and provider-level CPR
- New topics in Section I: Boutique or concierge medical care; communication barriers caused by cultural and religious diversity; burnout prevention; five stages of grief and the acronym TEAR; intimate partner violence; treating a culturally diverse clientele

Section II, Clinical Procedures (Chapters 10 through 32), gives you a thorough understanding of clinical, diagnostic, and laboratory procedures you will be performing and assisting with in the medical office. Topics include asepsis, patient history, vital signs, body system examinations, specialty examinations, minor surgery, diagnostic imaging, nutrition, ECG, pharmacology, dosage calculation, venipuncture, urinalysis, and laboratory tests.

New material in this section includes:

- Information on new charting methodology—SOAPER and CHEDDAR
- The Joint Commission's goals for Patient Safety Solutions and updated Joint Commission dangerous abbreviations
- Laboratory procedure documentation samples that include both patient chart documentation and laboratory report documentation
- Moved surgical asepsis to Chapter 19 (Assisting with Ambulatory/Office Surgery)
- Information and procedure on using a temporal artery thermometer
- New American Cancer Society Guidelines on Pap smear and BSE
- Expanded information on CLIA, including criteria for PPMP and updated waived lab test criteria
- Applications for EHR and TPMS in the medical laboratory
- New photo series for each venipuncture method (syringe, vacuum tube, butterfly)
- Information and new procedures on protime/prothrombin time (PT) and International Normalized Ratio (INR)
- Photos of casts, crystals, and miscellaneous structures found in urine sediment
- New topics in Section III: MRSA, SARS, and avian flu; HPV; massage therapy; nutrition in childhood; proper disposal of expired medication; e-prescribing; digital Holter monitors

Section III, Professional Procedures (Chapters 33 through 36), examines the role of the medical assistant as office manager and human resources manager and provides tools and techniques to use when preparing for practicums, medical assistant credentials, and employment.

New material in this section includes:

- Updated certification and examination information
- Information on the NHA and CCMA and CMAA examinations
- Updated W-4 and W-2 forms
- Expanded typical questions asked during an interview
- Expanded discussion on employment separations
- New procedures on processing employee payroll, performing an inventory of equipment and supplies, and performing routine maintenance or calibration of administrative and clinical equipment.
- New topics in Section IV: Harassment in the workplace; EHRs and the office manager; common errors found in resumes; importance of interviewing the employer; follow-up suggestions for after you are employed

The Complete Learning Package

The new **Critical Thinking Challenge 2.0** *(CD-ROM in the back of the book)* simulates a 3-month practicum in a medical office. You will be confronted with a series of situations in which you must use your critical thinking skills to choose the most appropriate action in response to the situation. Your decisions will be evaluated in three categories: how your decisions affect the practice, the patient, and your career. The 2.0 version includes 10 all-new video-based scenarios with more branching options. After successfully completing the program, print out a Certification of Completion. *See Appendix E for more information about the Critical Thinking Challenge 2.0.*

The **StudyWARE Software CD-ROM** *(CD-ROM in the back of the book)* launches two programs:

1. **StudyWARE** is interactive software with learning activities and quizzes to help study key concepts and test your comprehension. The activity and quiz content corresponds with each chapter in the book:
    - Multiple choice, true/false, and fill-in-the-blank quizzes
    - Flash cards, concentration, hangman, case studies
    - Championship game
    - Visual instrument flash cards
    - Visual instrument concentration
    - Animations library
2. **Audio Library:** Practice pronouncing and recognizing medical terminology using the Audio Library. Search for terms by word or body system. Once a word is selected, it is pronounced correctly and defined on the screen.

The **Workbook** *(Print)* has been fully revised to map closely to the book. Designed to reinforce and apply concepts and develop critical thinking, the workbook helps strengthen the knowledge and skills presented in the book. Competency Assessment Checklists for each procedure track all of the entry-level competencies designated by ABHES and CAAHEP.

- Assignment Sheets:
    - Incorporate a mix of review exercises and application activities in the chapter assignment sheets
    - Feature more hands-on application activities, case studies, and forms practice and certification exam practice
- Competency Assessment Checklists:
    - New source materials, scenarios, and forms accompanying the competency assessment checklists
    - Streamlined competency assessment checklists, with competency mapping and Work Documentation areas

The **Instructor's Manual** *(Print)* has been revised to be one comprehensive tool for instructors. Features include:

- Instructor Tips and Strategies for teaching, lesson planning, and evaluation
- Chapter Overviews, Outlines, and Activities
- Answers to Critical Thinking Boxes in the text

Instructor Resources *(CD-ROM)* is a tool to help prepare for class, deliver effective presentations, and monitor student progress throughout the course. Create a total lesson plan, which includes visual examples, computer-generated tests, and more. Tools include:

- A Computerized Test Bank in ExamView with more than 1,200 questions and answers, organized by chapter
- Instructor slides created in PowerPoint for each chapter, which cover key concepts presented in the text and includes graphics, animations, and video clips
- An Image Library of more than 700 images from the text
- Complete, customizable Instructor's Manual files

The **Online Companion** offers extra content for both instructors and students.

1. **Instructors**—Log on to www.delmar.cengage.com/companions to get these resources and more:
    - CourseForward curriculum and curriculum mapping tools
    - Customizable Competency Assessment Checklists
    - Crossover and conversion guides
    - Support documentation for software programs
2. **Students**—Log on to www.delmarlearning.com/dl_login.aspx and register your *Access Code* (located on the tear-out card in the front of the book) to get these resources and more:
    - The Competency Challenge 2.0
    - Spelling Bee and Image Labeling games to practice anatomy and physiology
    - Link to Mobile Download Web site, to access the free mp3 downloads of Spanish terms

CourseForward Curriculum *(on the Online Companion)* is a modular curriculum solution that breaks down content into topics for ease of learning and serves as a road map for course material. CourseForward is designed for instructors to spend less time planning and more time teaching. Some of the features of CourseForward include:

- Equipment lists
- Homework assignments
- In-class discussion topics and suggested responses, individual and group activities
- Key Concepts table mapped to activities and assignments

The **Competency Challenge 2.0** *(on the Online Companion)* features interactive activities, better assessment, and a new concluding capstone element. To help practice the competencies necessary to become a medical assistant, you are "virtually" externing at a local medical office.

- Days 1 through 4 focus on 26 video-based case studies with interactive exercises.
- Day 5 is a "day in the life" capstone event that applies the competencies practiced to a realistic patient case study. In the case study, you will follow a new patient through an office visit for a physical exam.
- Features printable quiz scoring and competency checklists

Web Tutor Advantage on Blackboard or WebCT platforms *(Online)* is an online classroom management tool that takes your course beyond the classroom wall. Web Tutor provides rich communication and course management tools, including a Course Calendar, Chat, email, Threaded Discussions, Web Links, and a White Board. It also contains additional content to reinforce and enhance learning and test student learning, including:

- Learning Links explore health care topics through research on the Internet
- Critical thinking questions and case studies with video clips
- Discussion questions and quizzes for each chapter
- Quizzes by chapter, unit, and section
- A comprehensive terminal examination
- PowerPoint presentations which include animations and video clips

Web Tutor Toolbox on Blackboard or WebCT platforms *(Online)* is an online classroom management tool that takes your course beyond the classroom wall. Web Tutor provides rich communication and course management tools, including a Course Calendar, Chat, email, Threaded Discussions, Web Links, and a White Board. Preloaded content includes objectives, advance preparation, and FAQs.

SUPPLEMENTS AT-A-GLANCE

SUPPLEMENT:	WHAT IT IS:	WHAT'S IN IT:
Critical Thinking Challenge 2.0	Software program (CD-ROM in the back of the book)	10 all-new video scenarios, with several follow-on scenarios Scoring, outcomes, and feedback for each decision selected Printable Certification of Completion at the end of the program
StudyWARE Software CD-ROM	Software program (CD-ROM in the back of the book)	StudyWARE software with games, visual instrument flash cards, and quizzes Audio Library of medical terms
Competency Challenge 2.0	Software program, web access (on Online Companion)	26 video-based case studies with interactive exercises New capstone patient case study Printable quiz scores and Competency Checklists
Workbook	Print	Streamlined Competency Assessment Checklists More hands-on application activities, case studies, and forms practice Maps more closely to the text
Instructor's Manual	Print	Answer Keys to the book and Workbook Chapter outlines, overviews, and activities
Instructor Resources	CD-ROM	PowerPoint presentations Computerized Test Bank Image library Electronic Instructor's Manual files
Student Online Companion	Web site (tear-out access card located in front of book)	http://www.delmarlearning.com/dl_login.aspx The Competency Challenge 2.0, StudyWARE games, and much more
Instructor Online Companion	Web site	http://www.delmar.cengage.com/companions Customizable Competency Assessment Checklists CourseForward Curriculum, mapping tools, and more
CourseForward Curriculum	Web access (on Online Companion)	Modular curriculum solution that breaks down content into smaller topics Key Concepts outline mapped to suggested activities and homework assignments
Web Tutor Advantage	Web access	On Blackboard and WebCT platforms Comprehensive terminal examination Content and quizzes corresponding to each chapter Video case studies and critical thinking activities
Web Tutor Toolbox	Web access	On Blackboard and WebCT platforms

About the Authors

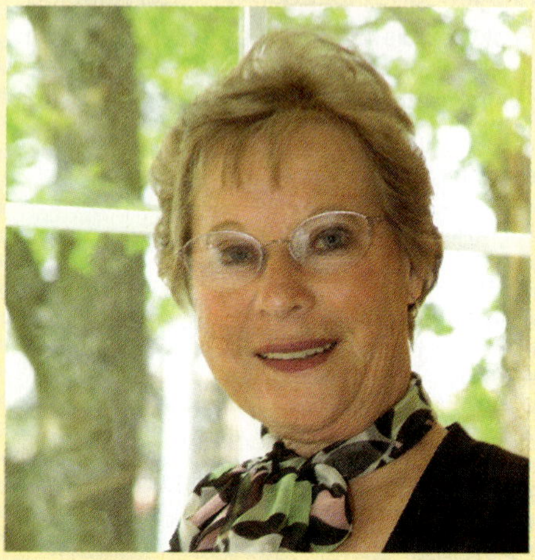

Wilburta (Billie) Q. Lindh, CMA (AAMA), holds professor emerita status at Highline Community College, Des Moines, Washington. She is the former program director and consultant to the medical assistant program at Highline Community College and recipient of the 2000 Outstanding Faculty Member of the year award. She is coauthor of *Therapeutic Communications for Health Care* published by Delmar Cengage Learning. She also coauthored *The Radiology Word Book* and *The Ophthalmology Word Book,* texts frequently used by transcriptionists, and is the medical assistant chapter author for *Guide to Careers in the Health Professions.* Lindh is a member of the SeaTac Chapter of the American Association of Medical Assistants (AAMA) and has lectured at AAMA seminars on the national level and at Washington and Oregon State meetings. She resides in Federal Way, Washington, with her husband DeVere.

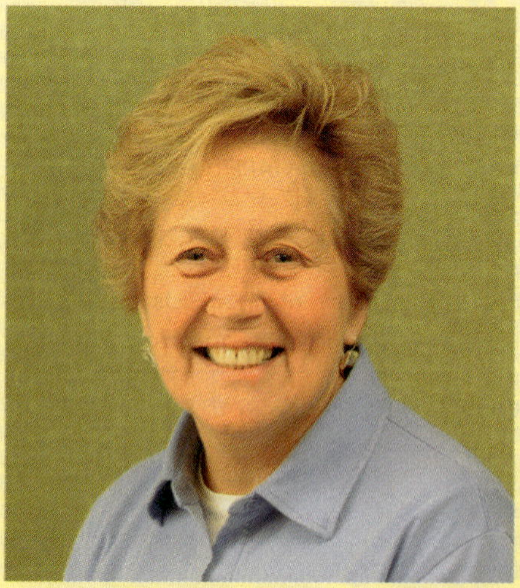

Marilyn S. Pooler, RN, MEd, served as a professor in medical assisting and taught for more than 25 years at Springfield Technical Community College in Springfield, Massachusetts, where she served as the medical assisting department chairperson for several years. Marilyn also served on the Certifying Board of the AAMA Task Force for test construction and was a site surveyor for the AAMA for many years. Pooler is a member of the Hampden District chapter of the American Association of Medical Assistants (AAMA), and she has been a speaker at local and state medical assisting meetings and seminars, emphasizing the importance of education, certification, and recertification of medical assistants. For a number of years, she was a member of the Executive Board of the Northeast Association of Allied Health Educators. Presently, she works in health services at Baypath College, in Longmeadow, Massachusetts; at Baystate Health Systems in Springfield, Massachusetts, in their ambulatory/clinic areas; and for the Center of Business and Technology at Springfield Technical Community College, where she teaches review courses to medical assistants.

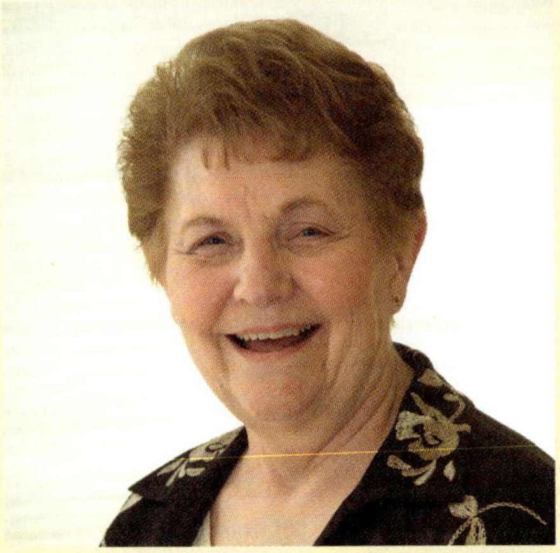

Carol D. Tamparo, CMA (AAMA), PhD, served as a medical assistant instructor for 24 years and as program director for medical assisting for 15 years at Highline Community College, Des Moines, Washington. She was the Dean of Business and Allied Health programs at Lake Washington Technical College in Kirkland, Washington, for 4 years. She is the coauthor of *Therapeutic Communications for Health Care; Medical Law, Ethics, & Bioethics for Ambulatory Care;* and *Diseases of the Human Body*. She is a member of the SeaTac Chapter of AAMA and is a frequent speaker for medical assistants in the Northwest.

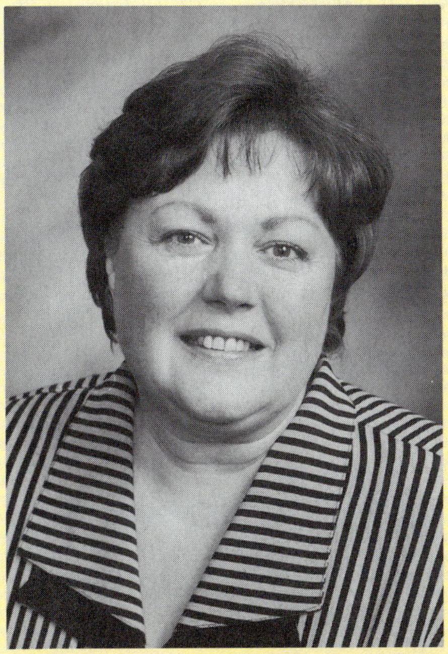

Barbara M. Dahl, CMA (AAMA), CPC, has dedicated her professional life to the recognition, education, and advancement of medical assistants through quality education, increased public awareness, legislative compliance, and positive professional development. She is a tenured faculty member of Whatcom Community College in Bellingham, Washington and has been the Medical Assisting Program Coordinator since 1991. She is an active member of the Whatcom County Chapter of Medical Assistants, Washington State Society of Medical Assistants, the AAMA, and the Washington State Medical Assisting Educators. She is a former chapter and state president and has served on and chaired many committees on the chapter, state, and national levels. She was instrumental in developing and designing the AAMA Excel award-winning WSSMA website and continues to serve as the state co-webmaster. Barbara is currently serving as the state parliamentarian and on the Coalition for the Medical Assisting Scope of Practice for Washington state. Through the years she has acquired a wealth of knowledge and understanding about the professional and legal aspects of medical assisting, particularly in regards to the Washington State HCA Law. As a Certified Professional Coder she has been a member of the AAPC for many years. She has served as a presenter for many conferences and seminars both on the local and state levels in many clinical, administrative, legal, and leadership topics.

Acknowledgments

A special thank you to my husband, DeVere, who continually supports, encourages, and assists me in so many ways. Thank you to my family and friends who also understood when I was not available for activities, but still encouraged and accepted my commitment to excellence. I also want to thank the great team I worked with: Carol, Marilyn, Barbara, and all at Delmar, Cengage Learning. This has truly been an enriching experience.

Billie Q. Lindh

Thanks to my husband, Jud, and to my family for their patience and understanding during the writing of this edition. Thanks also to Billie, Carol, and Barbara, a great team of authors who together made this text a tremendous learning tool for medical assistants. A special thank you to Sarah Prime for her expertise, patience, and kindness.

Marilyn S. Pooler

Writing a textbook, even the revision of a textbook, requires the input and dedication of many individuals, especially in the field of health care where changes occur almost daily. Collaborating with Billie, Marilyn, and Barbara has ensured that the most recent information is included in this text. Thank you, Sarah Prime, for your vision and guidance. My special thanks to Cecile Favreau, subject matter expert on MOSS, who provided electronic procedures as appropriate. Thanks to Tom, my husband, who assumed many household chores and took us out to dinner at just the right times.

Carol D. Tamparo

First and foremost I would like to thank my husband, Ed, for his support and encouragement during this 4th edition revision. It has been a very exciting experience—making sure our textbook is the best and most current representation of what today's medical assistant student needs to know to enter the profession; covering the cognitive, psychomotor, and affective domains; as well as adding current technology and new clinical diagnostics and equipment. I appreciate the opportunity to continue working with my diversely talented team members, Billie, Carol, and Marilyn, to create this nationally respected resource. Special thanks to Whatcom Community College and my students for supporting me in this phase of my professional development; to Sarah Prime, Jack Pendleton, and the Cengage Learning team; Dan Fitzgerald; and Ferndale Family Medical Clinic, especially Mary Kilmer, CMA (AAMA), for helping with our photo opportunities.

Barbara M. Dahl

The Authors and Publisher would like to thank the following people and locations for assisting with our photo shoots:

Eastside Community Health, Tacoma, WA

Gregory Plancich, DDS, Tacoma, WA

Kathy Bonavita, Springfield Technical Community College, Springfield, MA

Mary Kilmer, CMA (AAMA)

Joanne Kindle, Clinic Manager, Eastside Community Health, Tacoma, WA

Sharon at the Uniform Station in Auburn, WA, for providing scrubs

Connie Pettingill, Springfield Technical Community College, Springfield, WA

Tom Stock, Stock Studios Photography, Saratoga Springs, NY

Springfield Technical Community College, Springfield, MA

Whatcom Community College, Bellingham, WA

Ferndale Family Medical Center, Ferndale, WA

Contributors

Gerry A. Brasin, AS, CMA (AAMA), CPC
Corporate Education Coordinator
Premier Education Group
Springfield, MA
Subject Matter Expert for the Critical Thinking Challenge 2.0

Cecile Favreau, MBA, CPC
Professional Relations Specialist UMass Memorial Medical Group
Faculty at The Salter School
Worcester, MA
Administrative Procedures for Medical Office Simulation Software 2.0
Subject Matter Expert for Medical Office Simulation Software 2.0

Helen J. Houser, RN, MSHA, RMA
Director, Medical Assisting and Patient Care Technician Programs
Phoenix College
Phoenix, AZ
Subject Matter Expert for the Competency Challenge 2.0

Cathy Kelley-Arney, CMA (AAMA), MLTC, BSHS
Subject Matter Expert for the Critical Thinking Challenge 2.0

Melinda Parker, MA
Developing Administrative StudyWARE Content

Lisa Wright, CMA (AAMA), MT (ASCP), SH
Medical Assisting Program Coordinator
Medical Support Programs Department Chair
Bristol Community College
Fall River, MA
Developing Clinical StudyWARE Content

Reviewers

Diane Alagna, RN, AHI, CPT
Branford Hall Career Institute
Southington, CT

Ana T. Alvarez-Calonge, MLT, RMA, AHI
Medical Assisting Program Director
Keiser Career College
Miami Lakes, FL

Michelle Blesi, CMA (AAMA), AA, BA
Medical Assistant Program Director
Century College—East Campus
White Bear Lake, MN

George Fakhoury, MD, DORCP, CMA (AAMA)

Jeanette Goodwin, BSN, CMA (AAMA)
Program Chair
Southeast Community College
Lincoln, NE

Cynthia Harms, MEd, CMA (AAMA), CPC, CPC-H
Mildred Elley School
Latham, NY

Shirley Jelmo, CMA (AAMA), RMA
Medical Assisting Lead Instructor
PIMA Medical Institute
Colorado Springs, CO

Robin Kern, RN, BSN
Medical Assisting Instructor
Moultrie Technical College
Moultrie, GA

Claire E. Maday-Travis, MA, MBA, CPHQ
Allied Health Program Director
The Salter School
West Boylston, MA

Lori Malone, CMA (AAMA)
Medical Assistant Program Clinical Lab Assistant
Century College—East Campus
White Bear Lake, MN

Sharon McSain, BS, MA Edu, CMA (AAMA)
Academic Dean
Medical Assisting Program Director
Elmira Business Institute
Elmira, NY

Pat Gallagher Moeck, PhD, MBA, CMA (AAMA)
Director, Medical Assisting Program
El Centro College
Dallas, TX

Patricia Moseley, BS, MEd
Academic Dean
Concorde Career Institute
Arlington, TX

Cornelia Mutts, RN, BSN, CMA (AAMA), MBA, PhD
Program Director of Allied Health
Bryant & Stratton College
Virginia Beach, VA

Bev Philpott, BSc, CMA (AAMA)
Kirkwood Community College
Davenport, IA

Lynn G. Slack, BS, CMA (AAMA)
Medical Programs Director
Kaplan Career Institute—ICM Campus
Pittsburgh, PA

Lori Starnes, CMA (AAMA), AAS
Medical Assisting Program Director
South Piedmont Community College
Monroe, NC

Tracy Thomas, BS
St. Louis College of Health Careers
St. Louis, MO

Lisa Wright, CMA (AAMA), MT (ASCP), SH
Medical Assisting Program Coordinator
Medical Support Programs Department Chair
Bristol Community College
Fall River, MA

How to Use the Book

Icons

Icons appear throughout the book to highlight chapter material on topics important to today's medical assistant:

- Using Computers in the Medical Office
- Cultural Diversity
- Electronic Health Records (EHR)
- HIPAA Compliance
- Legal Issues
- Professionalism
- Safety and Security

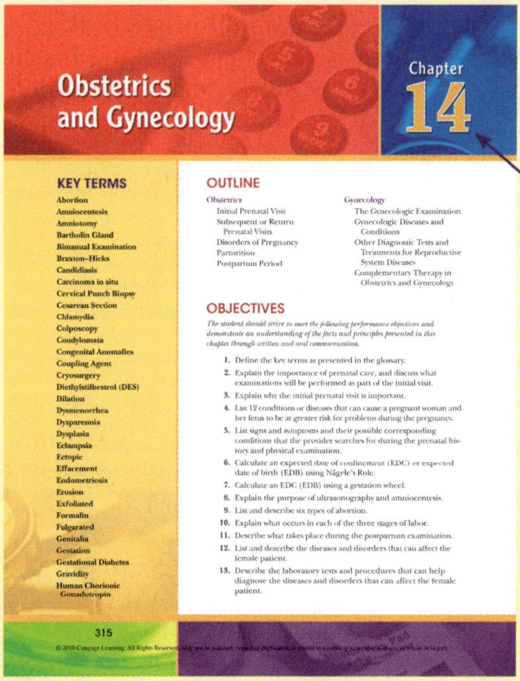

Obstetrics and Gynecology

Chapter 14

KEY TERMS

Abortion
Amniocentesis
Amniotomy
Bartholin Gland
Bimanual Examination
Braxton–Hicks
Candidiasis
Carcinoma in situ
Cervical Punch Biopsy
Cesarean Section
Chlamydia
Colposcopy
Condylomata
Congenital Anomalies
Coupling Agent
Cryosurgery
Diethylstilbestrol (DES)
Dilation
Dysmenorrhea
Dyspareunia
Dysplasia
Eclampsia
Ectopic
Effacement
Endometriosis
Erosion
Exfoliated
Formalin
Fulgarated
Genitalia
Gestation
Gestational Diabetes
Gravidity
Human Chorionic Gonadotropin

OUTLINE

Obstetrics
- Initial Prenatal Visit
- Subsequent or Return Prenatal Visits
- Disorders of Pregnancy
- Parturition
- Postpartum Period

Gynecology
- The Gynecologic Examination
- Gynecologic Diseases and Conditions
- Other Diagnostic Tests and Treatments for Reproductive System Diseases
- Complementary Therapy in Obstetrics and Gynecology

OBJECTIVES

The student should strive to meet the following performance objectives and demonstrate an understanding of the facts and principles presented in this chapter through written and oral communication.

1. Define the key terms as presented in the glossary.
2. Explain the importance of prenatal care, and discuss what examinations will be performed as part of the initial visit.
3. Explain why the initial prenatal visit is important.
4. List 12 conditions or diseases that can cause a pregnant woman and her fetus to be at greater risk for problems during the pregnancy.
5. List signs and symptoms and their possible corresponding conditions that the provider searches for during the prenatal history and physical examination.
6. Calculate an expected date of confinement (EDC) or expected date of birth (EDB) using Nägele's Rule.
7. Calculate an EDC (EDB) using a gestation wheel.
8. Explain the purpose of ultrasonography and amniocentesis.
9. List and describe six types of abortion.
10. Explain what occurs in each of the three stages of labor.
11. Describe what takes place during the postpartum examination.
12. List and describe the diseases and disorders that can affect the female patient.
13. Describe the laboratory tests and procedures that can help diagnose the diseases and disorders that can affect the female patient.

315

© 2010 Cengage Learning. All Rights Reserved.

Chapter Openers

At the beginning of each chapter, you will find an **Outline, Objectives,** and a list of **Key Terms.** Use these as a road map to understand the chapter content.

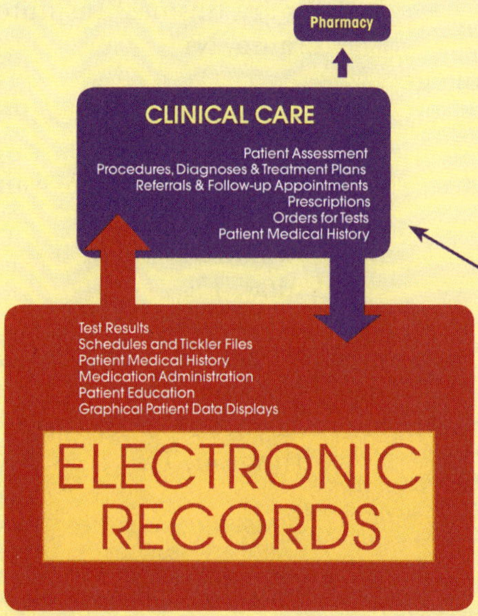

Figure 24-1 In a total practice management system, the patient's vital signs are often entered by the medical assistant during clinical care. Many programs have the ability to output vital signs data in a graph format, so a provider can easily note fluctuations in a patient's weight, blood pressure, normal temperature, etc.

Total Practice Management Figures

Special figures illustrate how each chapter's content fits in to the overall total practice management data flow.

Spotlight on Certification

RMA Exam Outline
- Vital signs and Measurements

CMA (AAMA) Content Outline
- Equipment preparation and operation
- Principles of operations
- Vital signs

CMAS Exam Outline
- Vital signs and measurements

Spotlight on Certification

This feature maps the chapter material to the content outlines for the RMA, CMA (AAMA), and CMAS exams to help you prepare to obtain medical assistant credentials.

Patient Education

Sensitive medical assistants will encourage patients to verbalize their concerns. The ability to ask questions in a nonprobing way and to elicit patient responses is an important function in any ambulatory care setting, because it is critical to know a patient's history, current medications, and other relevant data.

Critical Thinking

What is your opinion of the concierge type of medical practice? Would you feel comfortable working in such an environment? Why or why not?

Patient Education, HIPAA, and Critical Thinking Boxes

These boxes give you specific guidance on how to be prepared to provide Patient Education instructions and suggestions as well as comply with HIPAA regulations. Critical thinking boxes help you think about and deal with issues you may face on the job.

Procedures

Step-by-step procedures, grouped together at the end of each chapter, give instruction on all important administrative, clinical, and general competencies. They feature graphical illustration of the steps to be performed as well as rationales and correct documentation.

CHAPTER 24 Vital Signs and Measurements 585

Procedure 24-2

Measuring an Aural Temperature Using a Tympanic Thermometer

STANDARD PRECAUTIONS:

PURPOSE:
To obtain an aural temperature using a tympanic thermometer.

EQUIPMENT/SUPPLIES:
Tympanic thermometer (Figure 24-21)
Probe covers or ear speculum
Waste container

PROCEDURE STEPS:
1. Wash hands following Standard Precautions.
2. Assemble equipment.
3. Identify the patient.
4. Explain procedure. RATIONALE: This will help gain patient's cooperation and consent.
5. Place cover on thermometer (Figure 24-22).
6. Set thermometer to start.
7. Gently straighten ear canal up and back for adults and place probe into ear canal to seal the area and activate the system (Figure 24-23). RATIONALE: Air leaks will occur if the ear canal is not sealed.
8. Wait until the temperature is displayed on the screen.
9. Remove from the ear.
10. Discard cover into waste container by pressing the release button.
11. Wash hands.

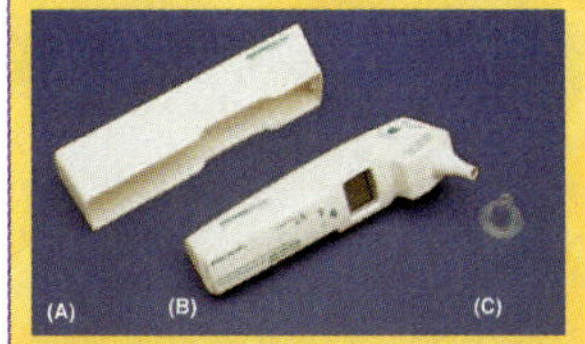

Figure 24-21 Tympanic thermometer: (A) Holder. (B) Tympanic thermometer. (C) Disposable speculum or cover.

12. Replace thermometer.
13. Record temperature in patient's chart or electronic medical record.

DOCUMENTATION
5/26/20XX 4:00 PM T 99.6° (Tym) F, P 100, R 20.
C. McInnis, RMA

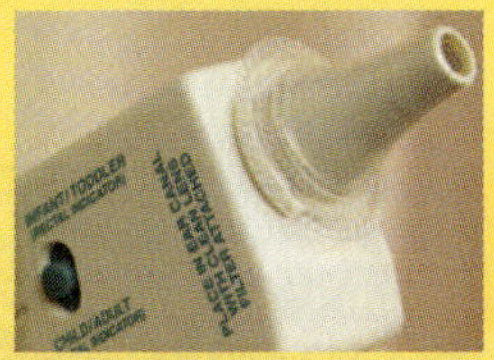

Figure 24-22 Attach the disposable speculum or cover to the tympanic thermometer to prevent spread of microorganisms between patients.

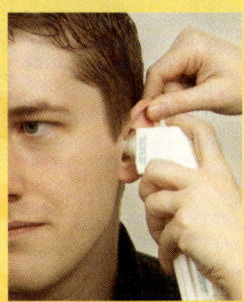

Figure 24-23 Pull up on the ear to straighten the auditory canal for an accurate reading.

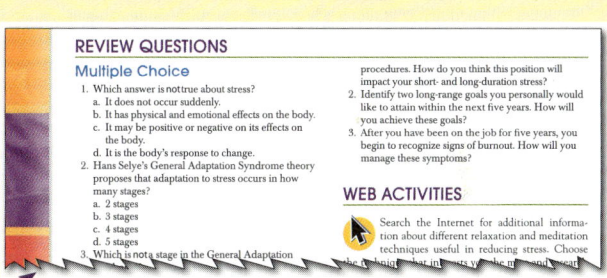

REVIEW QUESTIONS

Multiple Choice

1. Which answer is **not** true about stress?
   a. It does not occur suddenly.
   b. It has physical and emotional effects on the body.
   c. It may be positive or negative on its effects on the body.
   d. It is the body's response to change.
2. Hans Selye's General Adaptation Syndrome theory proposes that adaptation to stress occurs in how many stages?
   a. 2 stages
   b. 3 stages
   c. 4 stages
   d. 5 stages
3. Which is **not** a stage in the General Adaptation

procedures. How do you think this position will impact your short- and long-duration stress?

2. Identify two long-range goals you personally would like to attain within the next five years. How will you achieve these goals?
3. After you have been on the job for five years, you begin to recognize signs of burnout. How will you manage these symptoms?

WEB ACTIVITIES

Search the Internet for additional information about different relaxation and meditation techniques useful in reducing stress. Choose

End of Chapter Review

Test your comprehension of the chapter through structured multiple choice questions and open-ended critical thinking questions. Web activities give you practice researching on the Internet.

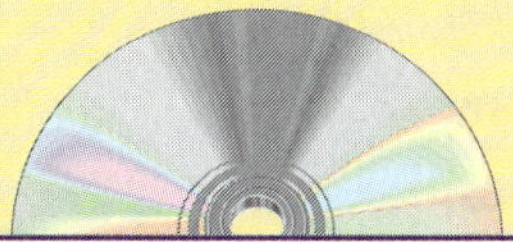

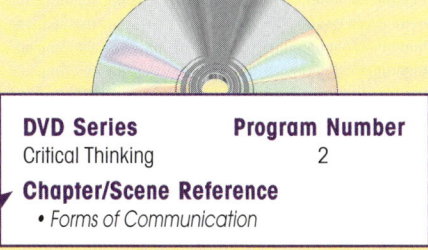

DVD Series	**Program Number**
Critical Thinking	2

Chapter/Scene Reference
- *Forms of Communication*

The DVD Hook-Up

Scene references to *Delmar's Skills and Procedures and Critical Thinking for Medical Assistants DVD Series* show the real-world application of the chapter material. Use the questions to facilitate thought-provoking discussion and the journal summary to share the ideas learned.

How to Use the StudyWARE Software CD

Quizzes

StudyWARE is interactive software with activity and quiz content corresponding to each chapter in the book. Quizzes can be taken in test mode or in practice mode, which gives immediate feedback after each question.

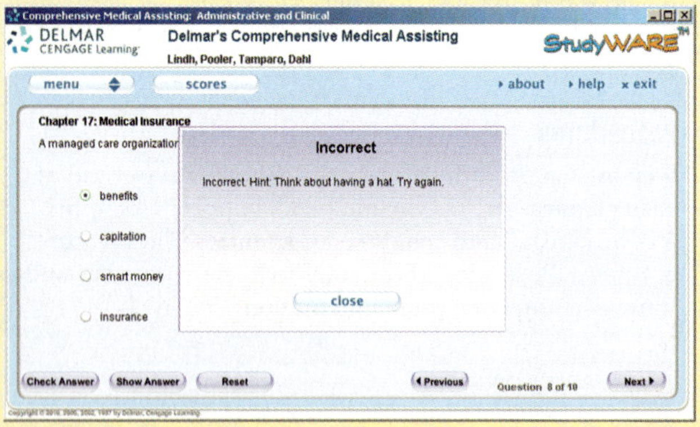

Activities

Activities include concentration, hangman, case studies, a championship game, and key term flash cards.

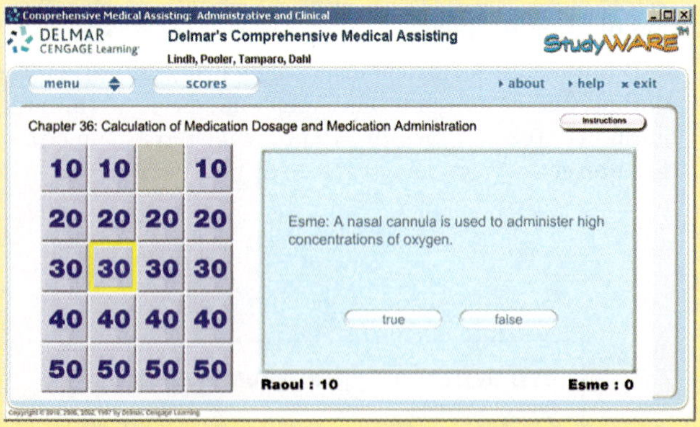

StudyWARE Instruments Review

Practice and expand your knowledge of instrument identification through the visual instrument flash card and concentration activities.

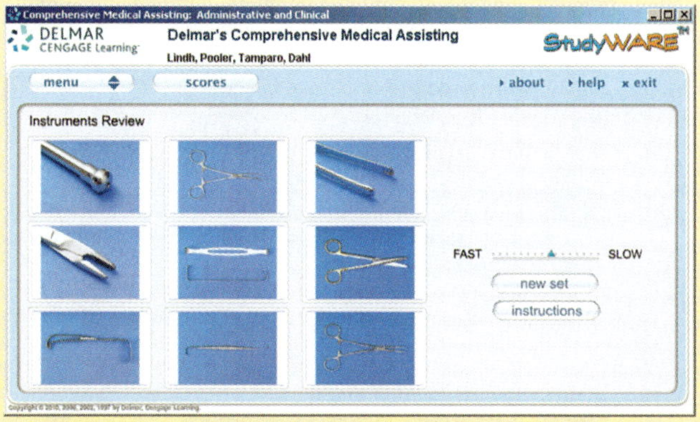

Audio Library

Practice pronouncing and recognizing medical terminology using the Audio Library. Search for terms by word or body system. Once a word is selected, it is pronounced correctly and defined on the screen.

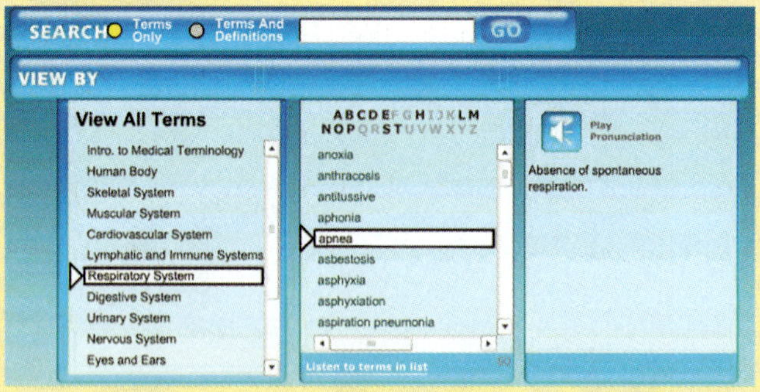

How to Use the Critical Thinking Challenge 2.0

About the Game

You are on a 3-month externship in a medical office. You will be confronted with a series of situations in which you must use your critical thinking skills to choose the most appropriate action in response to the situation. Your decisions will be evaluated in three categories: how they affect the practice, the patient, and your career.

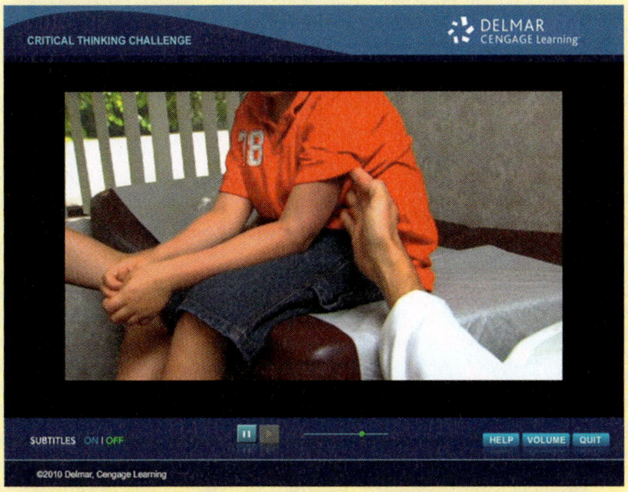

Completing the Game

If you make good decisions and actions, you will be hired by the office as a full-time medical assistant. However, if you show a lack of critical thinking skills that threatens the well-being of the patients and the practice, your practicum will be terminated and you will have to start over.

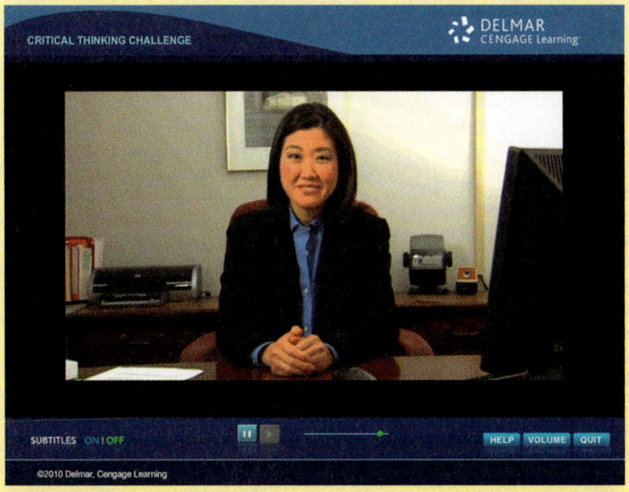

Resources

To help you determine the best action to take, you may consult with members of the office staff and document resources. Keep in mind that, just as in real life, not all of these resources will always be available to you or helpful to you.

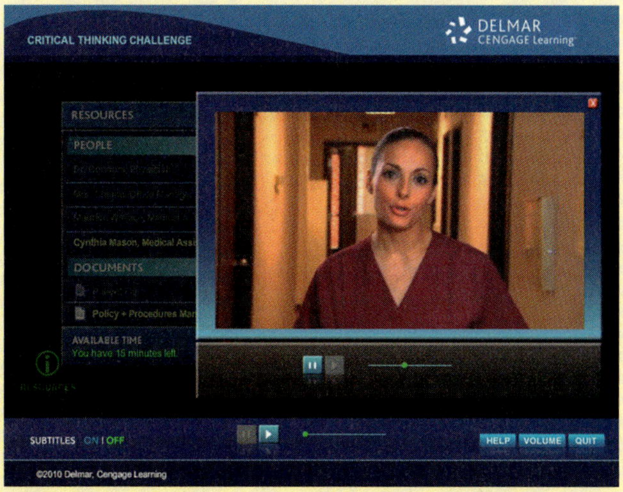

Appendix E contains additional information and support material for the Critical Thinking Challenge 2.0.

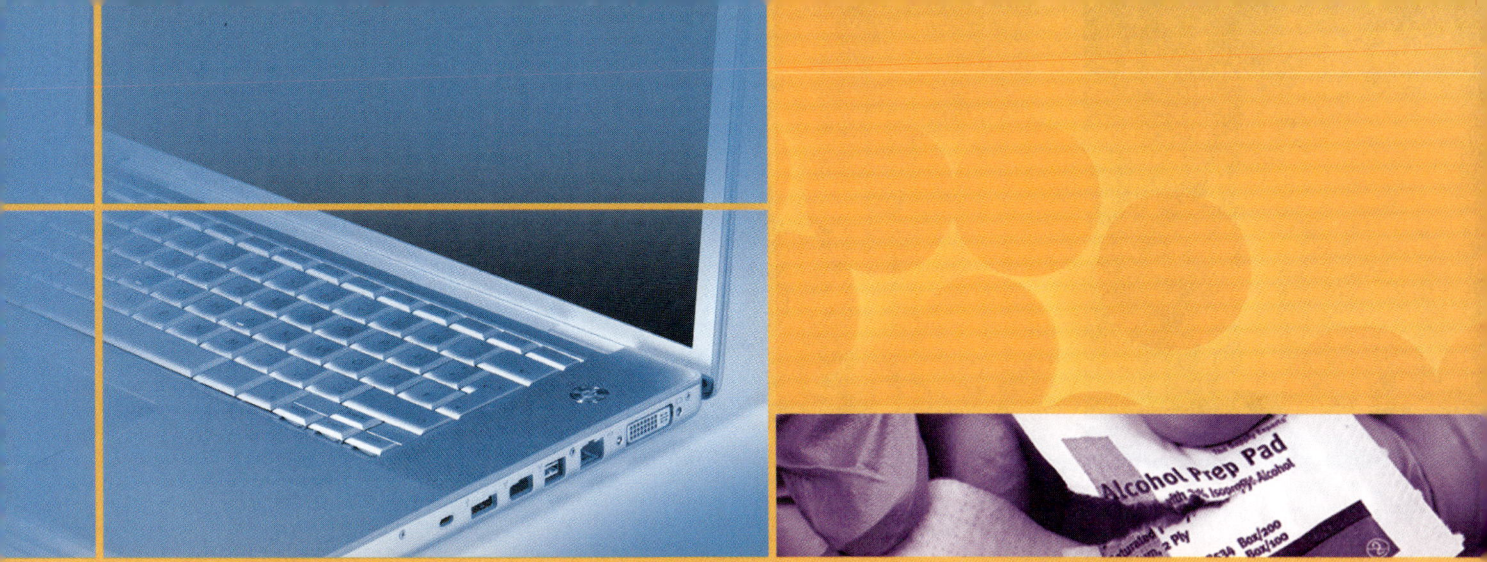

SECTION I

General Procedures

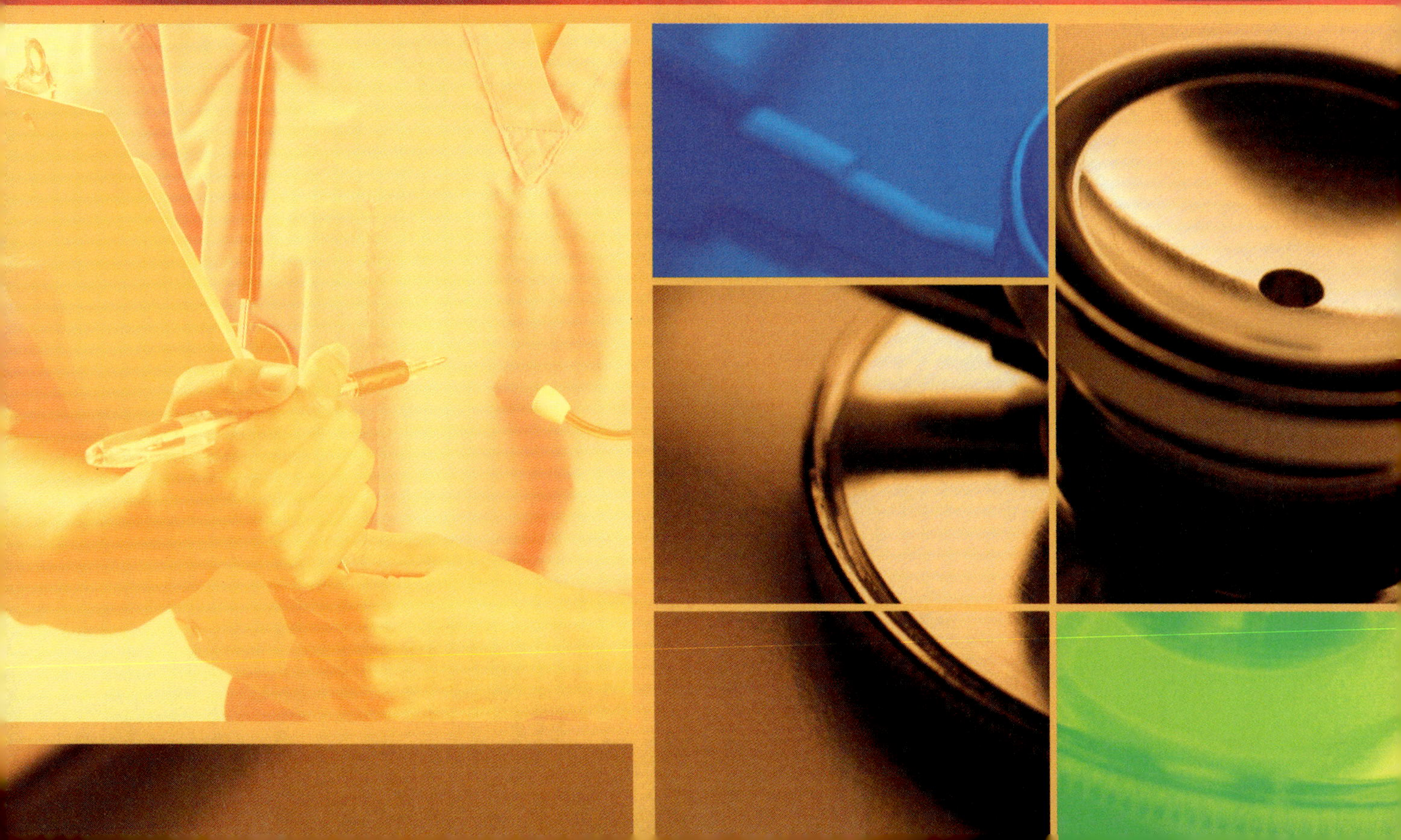

UNIT 1

Introduction to Medical Assisting and Health Professions

The Medical Assisting Profession

Chapter 1

KEY TERMS

Accreditation
Ambulatory Care Setting
Attribute
Bachelor's Degree
Certification
Certified Medical Assistant (CMA [AAMA])
Competency
Compliance
Credentialed
Dexterity
Diploma
Disposition
Empathy
Facilitate
Improvise
Integrate
License
Licensure
Litigious
Practicum
Professionalism
Proprietary
Registered Medical Assistant (RMA)
Scope of Practice

OUTLINE

- Historical Perspective of the Profession
- Career Opportunities
- Education of the Medical Assistant
  - Courses in a Medical Assisting Program
  - Practicum
  - Associate and Bachelor Degrees
- Accreditation of Medical Assisting Programs
  - CAAHEP
  - ABHES
- Attributes of a Medical Assistant Professional
  - Empathy
  - Attitude
  - Dependability
  - Initiative
  - Flexibility
  - Desire to Learn
  - Physical Attributes
  - Ability to Communicate
  - Ethical Behavior
- American Association of Medical Assistants
  - Certification
  - Continuing Education
- American Medical Technologists
  - Registered Medical Assistant
  - Certified Medical Administrative Specialist
  - Continuing Education
- National Healthcareer Association
  - Certification
  - Continuing Education
- Regulation of Health Care Providers
  - Scope of Practice

OBJECTIVES

The student should strive to meet the following performance objectives and demonstrate an understanding of the facts and principles presented in this chapter through written and oral communication.

1. Define the key terms as presented in the glossary.
2. Discuss the history of medical assisting.
3. Describe the practicum experience.
4. Recall two criteria for the selection of practicum sites.
5. List three benefits of the practicum to student and site.
6. Describe the profession of medical assisting and analyze its career opportunities in relationship to your interests.
7. Identify and discuss nine attributes that are important for a professional medical assistant to have.

OBJECTIVES (continued)

8. Describe the American Association of Medical Assistants and discuss its major functions.
9. Discuss the role of the American Medical Technologists in the credentialing of medical assistants.
10. Explain the purpose of the National Healthcareer Association.
11. Explain accreditation, certification, and continuing education as they pertain to the professional medical assistant.
12. Identify the importance of the accreditation process to an educational institution.
13. Recall at least two methods available to obtain recertification.
14. List five means of obtaining continuing education units.
15. Differentiate among certification, licensure, and registration.
16. State the importance of understanding the scope of practice for the medical assistant.

Scenario

A group of high school freshmen have come to tour the medical assisting class and laboratory areas. The Program Director of Medical Assisting is showing the students around the department. The Program Director then takes them into the medical assisting laboratory, where the senior medical assistant students are practicing their clinical skills. Each senior student pairs up with a high school freshman, and each pair talks about medical assisting, with the medical assistant students answering questions the others may have. The medical assistant students are in uniform as part of their preparation to go into various health care agencies to do their externship or practicum. The medical assistant students look professional, clean, fresh, and motivated. They tell the high school students about medical assisting and describe the personal and physical attributes desirable for those who want to become medical assistants. They explain the importance of these attributes, as well as what duties a professional medical assistant performs and what education is needed to pursue a career in medical assisting.

Throughout the question and answer discussions, the senior medical assistant students and the program director stress the importance of ethics, empathy, attitude, dependability, and teamwork as favorable attributes. Individuals seeking a career in medical assisting should develop and maintain these characteristics.

INTRODUCTION

Historically, medical science has been fascinating to most people. Perhaps you have been drawn to medical assisting because you too are intrigued by medicine and want to learn about advances in health care and become involved in providing care to patients. More than likely you have a desire to help others.

Medical assistants have always played an integral role in providers' offices and **ambulatory care settings** *such as clinics and urgent care facilities, where health care services are offered on an outpatient basis. And now more than ever, because of the explosion of knowledge and high technology in medicine, medical assistants are involved in an ever-widening scope of clinical and administrative duties. With the medical assistant's expanded role has come the responsibility to become a well-educated and highly competent professional dedicated to providing the highest quality of health care.*

Consumers of health care have become increasingly aware, primarily through the media, of the availability of the latest advances, techniques, and discoveries in

Spotlight on Certification

RMA Content Outline

- Medical ethics
- Human relations

CMA (AAMA) Outline

- Legal concepts

CMAS Content Outline

- Professionalism

medicine. They realize that they have a right to have health care provided to them by educated, skilled, and competent professionals.

As you study to become a medical assistant, it is important for you to understand what a professional is. According to Merriam-Webster's Collegiate Dictionary, 10th edition, it is "one who has acquired a specialized body of knowledge, skills, and attitudes." You will practice **professionalism** *as you learn the technical and ethical standards of this profession.*

You will learn to **integrate**, *or unify, your desire and need to help others with the knowledge, skills, and attitudes you acquire through your studies. By blending all of these, you will be able to provide patients with the best health care possible and will learn what it means to be a professional medical assistant.*

HISTORICAL PERSPECTIVE OF THE PROFESSION

Historically, when health care providers began their practices, it was common for them to hire individuals and train them on the job. Originally they hired nurses, but eventually they came to realize that nurses alone could not perform the variety of duties that are required in medical offices and ambulatory care centers. The nurse's role was limited to assisting the provider with clinical procedures, whereas the medical assistant's role was and is much broader and includes a large number of activities, procedures, and responsibilities, both administrative and clinical.

Today, with a much more informed patient comes the need for educated and credentialed medical assistants. In addition, in today's **litigious** atmosphere, which makes health care providers vulnerable to malpractice suits, most employers recognize the importance of employing medical assistants who are professionally prepared through formal education. Providers want knowledgeable and dependable medical assistants so they can focus their time and attention on the medical decisions, treatments, and techniques for which they have been educated and trained. This leaves the medical assistant to assist the provider in the operation and management of the practice.

In 1978, the profession of medical assisting was formally recognized by the United States Department of Education. In 1991, the board of trustees of the American Association of Medical Assistants (AAMA) approved the current definition of medical assisting:

> Medical Assisting is an allied health profession whose practitioners function as members of the health care delivery team and perform administrative and clinical procedures.

Medical assisting has become well respected among the professions in allied health.

CAREER OPPORTUNITIES

Medical assistants have been described as health care's most versatile, multifaceted professionals.

That medical assistants possess a broad scope of knowledge and skills makes them ideal professionals for any ambulatory care setting. Indeed, because of such versatility, medical assistants find employment in a variety of settings: offices, clinics, medical laboratories, insurance companies, government agencies, pharmaceutical companies, educational institutions, surgical centers, urgent care, and electrocardiography (ECG or EKG) departments in hospitals. Although the range of employment opportunities continues to grow, in the past decade, about four of five medical assistants were employed in providers' offices and clinics. About one in five worked in offices of other health care practitioners, such as chiropractors, optometrists, and podiatrists. Other career opportunities are available to the medical assistant. Some

Critical Thinking

Patients and providers prefer to have working for them professional medical assistants who have had the benefit of a formal education. Discuss the impact of this education on patients and employers. Why is it important to both groups?

medical assistants work as phlebotomists, coding specialists, medical laboratory assistants, and medical administrative specialists. The outlook for employment of medical assistants is promising.

According to the AAMA, there are more than one million medical assistants in the work force. The United States Department of Labor Bureau of Statistics listed medical assisting as one of the fastest growing allied health professions for the years 1998 to 2012. Increased employment opportunities for medical assistants result from the increased medical needs of an aging population, growth in the number of health care practitioners and their desire to hire the most qualified person for the task, increased diagnostic testing, greater volume and complexity of paperwork and computer information, managed care's emphasis on ambulatory care, and the insurance-mandated shorter stay of patients in hospitals.

EDUCATION OF THE MEDICAL ASSISTANT

Formal education of medical assistants takes place in community and junior colleges, as well as in **proprietary** schools. Educational requirements are based on current entry-level responsibilities that medical assistants perform in the medical office. These requirements were previously known as the Developing A CUrriculuM (DACUM) Analysis. In 1997, in coordination with the National Board of Medical Examiners, educators, and practicing Certified Medical Assistants (CMAs), the AAMA developed the Medical Assistant Role Delineation Chart, now known as Occupational Analysis of the CMA (AAMA) (see Appendix C to review this chart). Entry-level competencies must be mastered by students in academic programs.

Classroom instruction takes place in community colleges, proprietary schools, and junior colleges that offer courses in medical assisting. The lecture portion of classes takes place in a classroom setting. The skills portion take place in a laboratory setting in which supplies and equipment similar to those in the medical office/ambulatory care setting are available for practice.

An important new mode of education is online education. Some schools offer medical assistant courses online, and, if the school is accredited, many students who cannot or desire not to take traditional classroom courses can work toward becoming certified or registered through this method. On graduation, the student will receive a **diploma** or certificate of completion. If a student decides to pursue additional courses, it could take another year to complete (a total of 2 years) for an associate's degree or longer for a bachelor's degree.

Courses in a Medical Assisting Program

Some of the administrative, general, and clinical courses are listed in Table 1-1. Another aspect of an educational medical assisting program is the **practicum**, a period when students participate in an on the job training. This provides an excellent opportunity to apply theory to practices (see Chapter 36).

Practicum

Practicum, externship, and **internship** are all terms used to define the transition period between the classroom and actual employment. A practicum

Table 1-1 Some Typical Administrative, General, and Clinical Courses in an Accredited Medical Assisting Program

Administrative Courses	Electronic medical records (EMRs) and electronic health records (EHRs) Word processing Appointments and scheduling Insurance claims/coding Billing, collections, patients' accounts
General Courses	Anatomy and physiology Medical terminology Diseases Law and ethics Patient education
Clinical Courses	Infection control Disease prevention Medical prevention Pharmacology Temperature, pulse, respirations, and blood pressure Assisting the provider with physical exams Assisting the provider with minor surgery Drawing blood samples Urine and blood testing in the laboratory CPR (provider-level certification), first aid

is planned and supervised by a coordinator from the medical assisting program and the health care facility that agrees to become a partner in the education and employability of the student.

Practicum Sites. Sites for practicum are chosen carefully to ensure that a variety of experiences is available for the student. The sites should provide the student with adequate administrative, clinical, and general experiences. The staff at the various sites must be willing to make a commitment to the medical assistant's education by spending appropriate time observing and instructing the student.

Students at their practicum site are expected to be:

- Professional in appearance and demeanor
- Punctual
- Willing to learn
- Open to criticism
- Accepting of assignments
- Helpful to coworkers
- Working to the best of their ability
- Mindful of patient confidentiality

Students at their practicum site are expected *not* to:

- Consider asking for or taking medication samples without permission
- Feel entitled to any special treatment
- Anticipate free treatment for self, family, or friends
- Expect to be paid (this is part of the requirements of the accrediting body)

Benefits of Practicum. The practicum experience is mutually beneficial to the student and staff at the health care facility that is providing the educational experiences. Some of the benefits to the student are the opportunity to:

- Apply classroom knowledge and skill in a real-world medical setting
- Obtain references for employment
- Use externship experience as part of a resume
- Recognize improvement in performance and knowledge
- Understand that there may be more than one acceptable method of performance
- Begin to establish a network of support through colleagues

Some of the benefits to the practicum site are:

- Greater alertness of staff because of their educational responsibilities to the student
- Opportunity for staff to observe students who will soon be seeking employment
- Possibility that staff will learn more about the profession of medical assisting

Associate and Bachelor Degrees

Educational institutions that confer associate or bachelor degrees require general education courses for graduation in addition to the administration and clinical courses.

Some four-year institutions of higher learning offer a **bachelor's degree** to medical assistants who have graduated with an associate's degree from a community or junior college. The graduate is accepted as a third-year student and can obtain a bachelor's degree in areas such as health care management or health care facility administrator.

Because of the demand for medical assistant educators, some experienced medical assistants take education courses to become allied health educators.

ACCREDITATION OF MEDICAL ASSISTING PROGRAMS

Educational institutions seeking accreditation for a medical assisting program must develop the curricula to meet the *Standards and Guidelines* set by the Commission on Accreditation for Allied Health Education Programs (CAAHEP), or the standards set by the Accrediting Bureau of Health Education Schools (ABHES) to ensure the highest quality medical assistant education and employment preparedness.

CAAHEP

The Commission on Accreditation for Allied Health Education Programs (CAAHEP) is an accrediting body for medical assisting programs in private and public postsecondary institutions and programs that prepare individuals for entry into the profession.

A medical assisting program that is accredited by CAAHEP meets the standards as outlined in the *Standards and Guidelines for an Accredited Education Program for the Medical Assistant.* Standards are the minimum standards of quality used in accrediting programs that prepare individuals to enter the medical assisting profession.

On-site review teams evaluate the program's **compliance** with, or adherence to, the standards. All aspects of programs seeking accreditation status undergo scrutiny to ascertain the program's quality and to ensure continued compliance with the standards.

For more information, see the CAAHEP Web site at http://www.caahep.org.

ABHES

The Accrediting Bureau of Health Education Schools (ABHES) is the agency that also grants accreditation to medical assisting programs. ABHES is recognized by the United States Department of Education (USDE) as an accrediting agency of public and private schools and colleges that primarily offer health education. This includes medical assisting, medical laboratory technology, and surgical technology programs. Besides being recognized by the USDE, recognition for ABHES comes from the AAMA, AMT, National League for Nursing Accrediting (NLNA), and National Board of Surgical Technology and Surgical Assisting (NBSTSA).

More information about ABHES can be obtained through the ABHES Web site at http://www.abhes.org.

ATTRIBUTES OF A MEDICAL ASSISTANT PROFESSIONAL

Medical assistants should strive to cultivate certain characteristics or personal qualities. These are the **attributes** that identify a true professional; when caring for patients, these qualities should be sincere. They will enable the patient to trust you, the caregiver.

Empathy

To have **empathy** means to consider the patient's welfare and to be kind. It means stepping into the patient's place, discovering what the patient is experiencing, and then recognizing and identifying with those feelings.

Medical assistants should treat patients as they themselves would want to be treated. A visit to the providers' office is often a time of fear and anxiety. Patients can feel vulnerable. Apprehension can be allayed tremendously when patients realize that their caregiver understands their feelings and desires to make their lives more pleasant and comfortable (Figure 1-1).

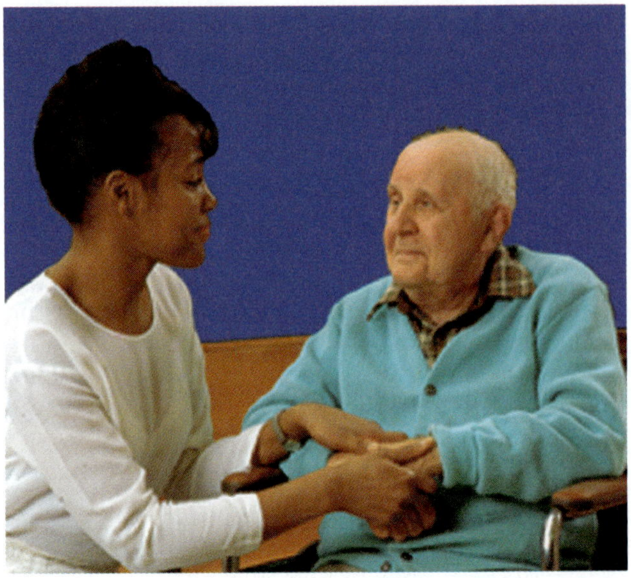

Figure 1-1 The medical assistant should have a friendly disposition and communicate empathy for the patient.

It is important to realize that patients' health problems can have a profound effect on you, the medical assistant. By maintaining a balanced outlook, medical assistants can safeguard themselves from becoming too emotionally involved with patients' problems. Empathy is extremely important in the health care profession; however, emotionalism can cloud one's judgment.

Attitude

A friendly, warm **disposition** and a sense of humor will help patients feel more at ease. A sincere affection for people can be conveyed by actions that **facilitate** open and honest communication. Your attitude should radiate genuine interest. Be sure all contact with patients is positive.

On occasion, difficult patients can test the tolerance level of the most experienced medical assistant because they seldom seem to be content with the care or services received. But no matter what the circumstances, patients should never be treated with disinterest or in an unfriendly manner. The medical assistant should always be pleasant and courteous.

Patients should be treated equally, with no reservations about their disease, race, religion, economic status, or sexual orientation.

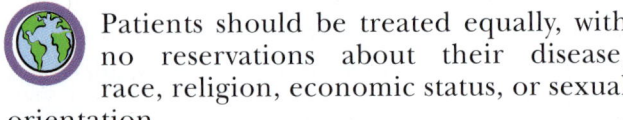

HIPAA As a member of the health care delivery team, the medical assistant needs to be cooperative and supportive of all other members, working with the team in an honest, open manner while keeping in mind the patient's right to privacy and confidentiality.

Dependability

When providing for a patient's well-being, it is important to focus attention on activities in the office or clinic environment that will demonstrate that you are well organized, accurate, and responsive to patients' needs.

Being dependable means that employer and coworkers rely on the medical assistant to be respectful of them, of patients, and of equipment and materials. Other members of the health care team will expect you to be accountable for the duties and responsibilities you undertake. A dependable person interacts with coworkers in a supportive manner, is punctual, and limits absences from work.

Initiative

The willingness and ability to work independently shows initiative. A person with initiative is observant, notices work that needs to be done, and then takes action to complete those tasks without being told to do them. Employers and coworkers must be able to count on one another to anticipate patients' needs and be attentive to work that needs to be accomplished. The successful medical assistant will be ready to pitch in and recognize when others need assistance. Team work and a positive work ethic are valuable characteristics.

By asking appropriate questions and seeking information that will improve performance, medical assistants will demonstrate that they have the foresight and the "get up and go" needed to complete the numerous and varied tasks of the ambulatory care environment.

Flexibility

The ability to be adaptable is a trait that serves all professionals well. When caring for ill people, unexpected situations arise daily, and medical assistants must be able to respond to a variety of situations (many of them emergencies and unanticipated) without losing a sense of equilibrium. Finding solutions to problems and developing alternative action plans demonstrates flexibility. To **improvise,** or solve problems that arise either routinely or spontaneously, is a characteristic worth nurturing. Willingness to help with various aspects of the office offers opportunities to adjust to various situations. It shows your adaptability and willingness to respond to new circumstances.

Desire to Learn

A willingness to continually learn and grow is the mark of a true professional. With the growing technology in medicine, there is an ongoing necessity for constant learning. Medical assistants must be dedicated to high standards of performance, which can be accomplished by showing a desire to acquire information and by constantly updating their knowledge and skills. Keeping abreast of the latest diseases, treatments, procedures, and techniques can be achieved in a variety of ways, such as college courses, seminars, workshops, reading, and simply by being observant. The sharper the power of observation, the more the medical assistant will learn from the provider-employer and coworkers.

The gaining and maintaining of **competency** through participation in continuing education is the responsibility of every medical assistant. Active involvement and membership in the medical assistant professional organizations allows students and CMAs (AAMA) and RMAs to participate in meetings and events that can increase professional skills. This benefits medical assistant skills as well as future careers. Students can attend medical assisting meetings (usually free of charge), enjoy student discounts, and network at the meetings.

Physical Attributes

Appearance is important in patients' perceptions of the delivery of their care. Imparting the look of a professional requires an appearance that is clean, fresh, and wholesome—in general, an appearance that reflects good health habits (Figure 1-2). Good personal hygiene practices (daily shower, deodorant), weight control, and healthy-looking skin, hair, teeth, and nails all contribute to a professional appearance. Rest, good nutrition, regular exercise, and recreation all promote good health. A smile can help alleviate some of the anxiety a patient may be experiencing. Your smile gives a pleasant and encouraging appearance to the patient.

Female medical assistants should wear only appropriate light daytime makeup. For the safety of both the professional and the patient, no necklaces or dangling earrings should be worn. The only jewelry worn should be single earposts or wedding rings. Hair should be neat and off the collar. Fingernails should be short and manicured. Male medical assistants should be clean-shaven and have short hair. Colognes, perfumes,

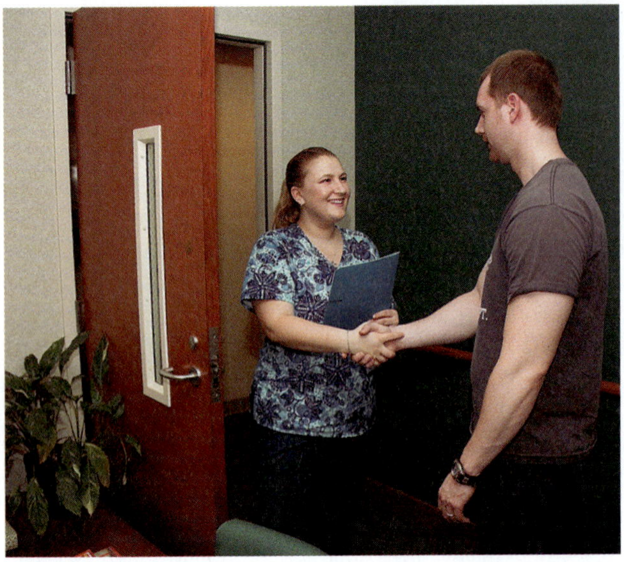

Figure 1-2 A professional, neat appearance makes patients feel at ease with their health care provider.

and aftershave should not be worn at work. Body piercings and tattoos should not be visible. Proper appearance has a positive effect on the patient.

It is important to know and follow the appropriate dress code for your facility. The Centers for Disease Control and Prevention (CDC) recommends that artificial nails and nail extenders not be worn when caring for "high-risk" patients (intensive care, surgery, dialysis). Many ambulatory facilities have more stringent rules about artificial nails and extenders.

Patient care can place physical demands on medical assistants. Lifting and moving patients is often required, and the use of correct body mechanics will help minimize injuries to the back. Although every reasonable accommodation is made for physically challenged medical assistants, to be mobile without assistance is important because medical assistants move about throughout the day while performing tasks and procedures. It is frequently necessary to bend, stoop, kneel, and crouch, especially when filing and retrieving patients' records and for other tasks as well. Most procedures require that medical assistants have the ability to hear and see well for the accurate completion of tasks (Figure 1-3). Listening to blood pressures, taking a medical history, observing patients, performing phlebotomy, and identifying microorganisms under a microscope are some of the routine tasks and procedures performed daily in a medical facility.

Manual **dexterity** is also needed for manipulating certain instruments and for entering data using a computer.

Critical Thinking

Of all the personal attributes that your text describes, which do you think is your most developed attribute? Give an example of that attribute that comes from your daily life.

Ability to Communicate

It is important that medical assistants learn to develop the ability to communicate well verbally and nonverbally with patients, staff, and other professionals.

Compliance with the provider's treatment plan is important for a positive outcome of patients' illnesses (Figure 1-4). Also, patients will feel more comfortable and less threatened in a medical office or ambulatory center that encourages staff to keep them informed. Consistent kindness and concern help patients develop trust in you.

Ethical Behavior

No discussion about personal attributes is complete without the mention of ethics. Ethics is a system of values each individual has that determines perceptions of right and wrong. Our life experiences mold this set of values, which is considered a personal code of ethics.

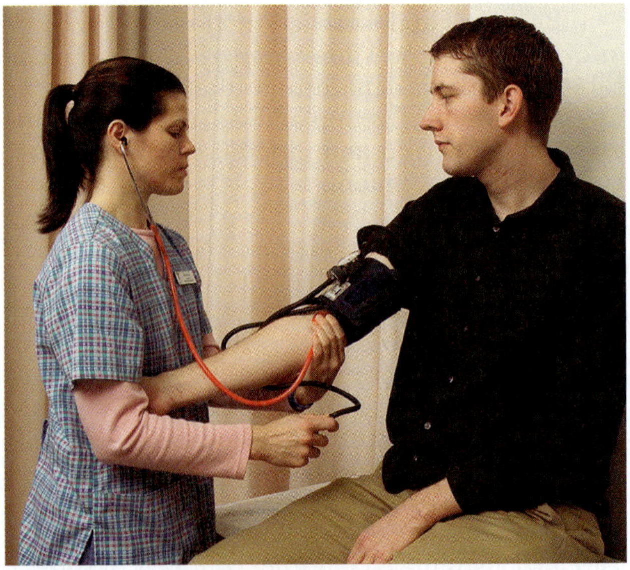

Figure 1-3 Measuring blood pressure is a task that requires the medical assistant to see and hear well.

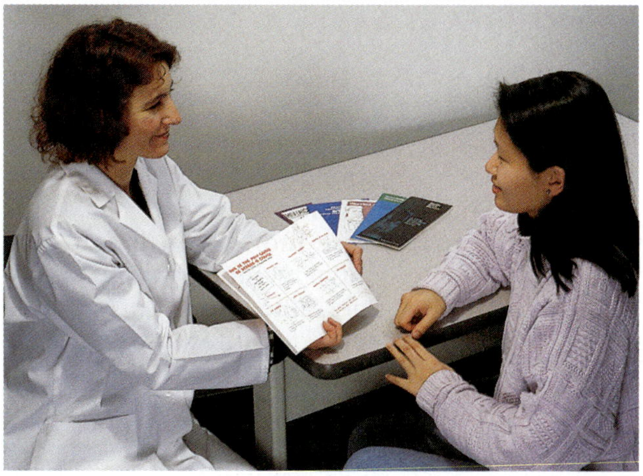

Figure 1-4 Patient education requires skill in communicating instructions to patients in language appropriate to their needs.

Medical ethics govern medical conduct or that behavior practiced as health care providers. These ethics involve relationships with patients, their families, fellow professionals, and society in general. Good ethical behavior will have a positive impact on the profession of medical assisting and on the medical community as well. By adhering to the medical assistants' Code of Ethics, we endeavor to elevate the profession to a position of dignity and respect. Medical assistants interact on a daily basis with patients and are entrusted with information about their medical and personal histories. Such information must, by law, be kept confidential. (A more in-depth discussion of ethics and the Code of Ethics can be found in Chapter 8.)

The personal qualities of empathy, healthy attitude, dependability, initiative, flexibility, the desire to learn, a wholesome physical presence, the ability to communicate well, and ethical behavior are some of the characteristics that most professionals have and that medical assistants should strive to develop. When entering into the profession of medical assisting, it is important to learn more about these and other qualities and to begin to use and refine them. Skills and knowledge alone do not guarantee success. There are personal characteristics that must go along with them.

Professional attitudes, attributes, and values are important for beginning medical assistant students to understand. Students' behaviors can impact the public's opinion of the provider and the medical assistant profession.

The public has a right to expect that the medical assistant will be competent to practice medical assisting in accordance with the medical assistants' Code of Ethics (see Chapter 8) and with the standards and guidelines set by their professional organizations (AMT, AAMA).

AMERICAN ASSOCIATION OF MEDICAL ASSISTANTS

Twenty-four years before the official recognition of the medical assisting profession in 1978, a group of medical assistants gathered to establish a professional organization. With support, encouragement, and guidance from the American Medical Association (AMA), the American Association of Medical Assistants (AAMA) was founded in 1956 (Figure 1-5). The first president of the organization was Maxine Williams.

Certification

As the profession grew and developed, some states came to require special licensure or certification to perform certain tasks; in other states, health professionals were challenged by the skill and broad spectrum of the medical assistant's ability. To defend medical assistants whose right to practice clinical procedures was being challenged, the AAMA responded at their 1995 convention with the following policy:

> that any candidate for the AAMA Certification Examination be a graduate of a CAAHEP-accredited medical assisting program or a graduate of an ABHES accredited program with one year of documented work experience. Anticipated benefits of the recommendation are to: (1) safeguard the quality of care to the consumer; (2) ensure the CMA's role in the rapidly evolving health care delivery system; and (3) continue to promote the identity and stature of the profession.

AFFILIATE OF THE AMERICAN ASSOCIATION OF MEDICAL ASSISTANTS

CERTIFIED MEDICAL ASSISTANTS: HEALTHCARE'S MOST VERSATILE PROFESSIONALS

Figure 1-5 Logo of the AAMA, a professional organization founded in 1956. (Courtesy of the American Association of Medical Assistants.)

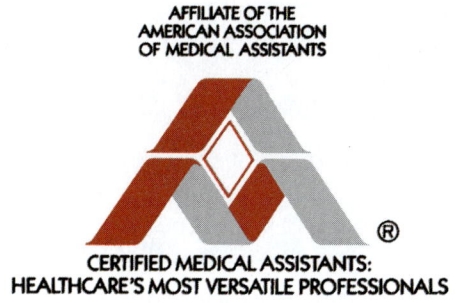

Certified Medical Assistant. **Certification** is voluntary, not mandatory, for medical assistants to practice, although an increasing number of employers are preferring (or even insisting) that their medical assistants be CMA (AAMA) certified. The examination measures professional knowledge at job entry level. Successful completion of the examination earns the individual the CMA (AAMA) credential (Figure 1-6). The initials follow the individual's name. Conferring of the CMA (AAMA) status is referred to as being **credentialed**. The Certification Program of the Certifying Board of the American Association of Medical Assistants is accredited by the National Commission for Certifying Agencies (NCCA) as a result of demonstrating compliance with the *NCCA Standards for the Accreditation of Certification Programs*.

Continuing Education

The AAMA vigorously encourages continuing education for all medical assistants. This can be accomplished through various means such as educational meetings, seminars, workshops, conventions, and the AAMA's self-study publications, a series of study courses for continuing education credit.

Membership in the AAMA is trilevel: local, state, and national. Educational meetings are held regularly at local and state meetings and conventions. The annual AAMA national convention provides an excellent forum for attaining knowledge through its educational offerings and for networking with other medical assistants.

Continuing an education is a lifelong process and serves as testimony to a commitment to professionalism (see the AAMA Web site at http://www.aama-ntl.org).

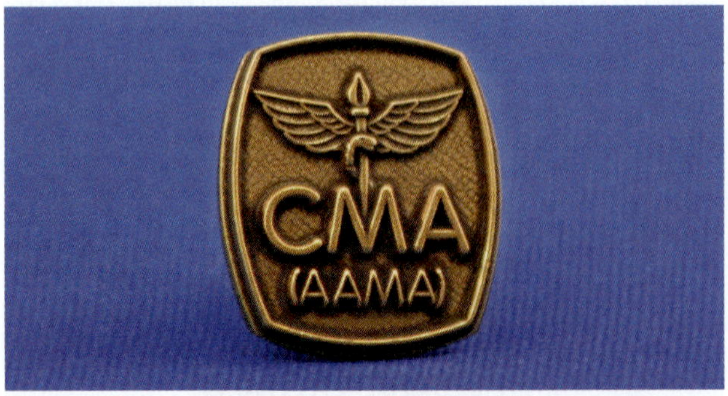

Figure 1-6 Certified medical assistant (CMA) pin awarded by the American Association of Medical Assistants on successful completion of the national certification examination.

AMERICAN MEDICAL TECHNOLOGISTS

Founded in 1939, the American Medical Technologists (AMT) is a national certification and professional membership association that represents 38,000 allied health care individuals. Its purpose is to certify and credential medical assistants, clinical laboratory personnel, allied health instructors, dental assistants, medical administrative specialists, and others. The AMT has its own bylaws, conventions, committees, state chapters, officers, and registration and certification examinations.

Registered Medical Assistant

In 1972, the AMT established the certification examination for medical assistants. The designation of **registered medical assistant (RMA)** is conferred on those individuals who successfully pass the examination (Figure 1-7).

RMA is a voluntary credential for the profession of medical assisting. RMA credentials are national, and examinations are given throughout the United States in both computerized and paper and pencil format. Voluntary means that neither the federal government nor most states require a medical assistant to be registered or certified to practice the profession. Most employers, however, prefer to employ credentialed medical assistants. Most providers want to hire employees with credentials because they recognize that doing so safeguards the quality of patient care and reduces the risk for liability issues for themselves. Some providers will not hire unless the person is credentialed.

The RMA certification examination includes general medical assisting topics, medical terminology, clinical medical assisting, medical law and ethics, human relations, administrative medical assisting,

(A) AMT American Medical Technologists
Allied Health Professionals

(B) RMA®

Figure 1-7 (A) Logo of the American Medical Technologists. (B) Logo of Registered Medical Assistant. (Courtesy of American Medical Technologists.)

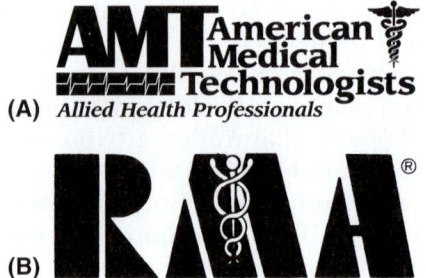

pharmacology, therapeutic modalities, laboratory procedures, electrocardiography, and first aid.

RMAs have been active in legislation to protect medical assistants, ensuring improvement in medical assistant education.

Certified Medical Administrative Specialist

Another profession that the AMT certifies is the Medical Administrative Specialist (MAS). Individuals who successfully pass the AMT certification examination are conferred with the credential of Certified Medical Administrative Specialist (CMAS). The CMAS exam is given in both computerized and paper and pencil format.

The CMAS serves an important role in the hospital, clinic, or medical office. The CMAS is competent in a multitude of skills such as medical records management, coding and billing for insurance, practice finance management, information processing, and fundamental management practices. The CMAS also is familiar with the clinical and administrative concepts that are required to coordinate office functions in the health care setting.

Graduating from a program accredited by either CAAHEP or ABHES has significant benefits, such as proof that the student has completed a program that meets national standards, recognition of his or her education by professional peers, and eligibility for AMT or AAMA credentialing exams.

Some medical assistants choose to attain both RMA and CMA (AAMA) credentials. Neither credential is higher than the other.

It is important for graduates to know what the employment market is when choosing a professional credential and that personal preference may also be a factor.

It is important to remember that credentialing, whether through the AAMA (CMA) or AMT (RMA), is evidence to employers and patients alike that you want the profession of medical assisting to be recognized and promoted. Also, credentials safeguard patients because you will deliver health care at the highest quality with the most current techniques and procedures. Credentials help secure the medical assistant's role in the health care field. (See Chapter 35 for more information about credentialing for medical assisting).

Continuing Education

AMT encourages and promotes continuing education. The Certification Continuation Program (CCP) requires members to document activities that attest to their continued effort to carry the competencies needed to maintain certification. Proof of compliance is required every three years. To maintain the RMA credential, you must obtain 30 points in a three-year period. The points can be earned through professional education, authoring textbooks, presentations, seminars, workshops, and conventions. Another avenue for RMAs to earn continuing education credit is through the American Medical Technologists Institute for Education (AMTIE). AMTIE awards certificates of compliance and certificates of excellence to RMAs. It is a continuing education recording system. Yearly compliance with AMTIE is sufficient to support CCP compliance. According to AMT, the CCP program does not change the AMTIE program. (For more information, call 1-800-275-1268; write to AMT, 10700 West Higgins Road, Rosemont, IL 60018; or access the Web site at http://www.amt1.com).

NATIONAL HEALTHCAREER ASSOCIATION

The National Healthcareer Association (NHA) is a certifying body for health care professionals (Figure 1-8). Its main goals are to certify and to offer continuing education course development, membership services for professionals, and a registry for certified professionals.

Certification

NHA offers two ways to attain certification. The first is by successful completion of the national certification exam. The criteria to sit for the exam is to be a graduate of a health care training program or have one or more years of full-time employment in the profession in which certification is being sought. The second way to achieve certification is through the NHA home study courses for experienced professionals. The courses cover the skills and competencies of the profession and are followed by an assessment.

National Healthcareer Association

"The Benchmark In Allied Healthcare Certification"

Figure 1-8 Logo of the National Healthcareer Association. (Courtesy of the National Healthcareer Association.)

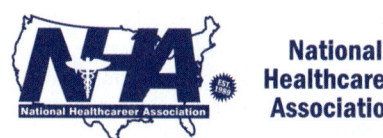

NHA offers certification to the following professions as well as others:

- Phlebotomy Technician (CPT)
- Electrocardiogram Technician (CET)
- Certified Clinical Medical Assistant (CCMA)
- Billing and Coding Specialist (CBCS)
- Medical Transcription (CMT)
- Patient Care Technician (PCT)
- Patient Care Associate (PCA)
- Nurse Technician (NT)
- Pharmacy Technician (CPhT)
- Medical Laboratory Assistant (MLA)

Continuing Education

Continuing education is another goal of NHA. Courses are offered online and are worth from 1.0 to 2.0 credits, for a total of 5.0 credits yearly. By doing so, the certification remains current. Once the online topics are completed, they are assessed by NHA, and, if successfully completed, the individual receives a "CREDITS COMPLETED" sticker to affix to the certification ID card.

NHA has been recognized by and has won approval of many organizations, including the following:

- City University of New York (several campuses)
- Elsevier Publishing
- Florida Department of Education
- Massachusetts Career Vocational Technical Education
- Massachusetts Department of Education
- Mosby Publishing
- New Jersey Department of Education
- U.S. Department of Labor National Office of Job Corps
- U.S. Department of Veterans Affairs

There are several more organizations as well. A complete list can be found at the NHA Web site (http://www.nhanow.com). See Chapter 35 for more about medical assisting credentials.

REGULATION OF HEALTH CARE PROVIDERS

One way health care providers can be regulated is through the process of credentialing. Credentialing recognizes health care providers who are professionally and technically competent. Recognition comes from professional associations, certifying agencies, and the state or federal government. Regulation ensures:

- Competence of health care providers
- A minimum standard of knowledge, training, and skill
- The limiting of the performance of certain procedures to a specific occupation

Licensure, certification, and registration are three kinds of regulations/credentialing (Table 1-2).

Scope of Practice

Medical assisting is not licensed as a profession; however, some states require that medical assistants be graduates of an accredited medical assisting program and be certified to work as medical assistants.

Table 1-2 Comparison of Requirements for Certification, Licensure, and Registration

	Certification	Licensure	Registration
Practice Requirement	Voluntary	Mandatory	Voluntary
Conferred By	Nongovernmental agency or professional association If qualified and meets requirements Must pass national examination	Legislated by each state If qualified and meets requirements Must pass state examination	Professional association If qualified and meets requirements Listed on an official roster Passing examination not always required
How Restrictive	Used by most professionals	Most restrictive	Least restrictive

Two examples of licensed professions are medicine and nursing. A **license** regulates the activities of these professions by enacting laws that specify educational requirements and by defining the **scope of practice.** A license is conferred on an individual who successfully completes specialized educational requirements and successfully passes an examination administered by the state in which the individual resides. The state grants a license to that individual to practice medicine or nursing. Licensure is mandatory and forbids anyone who is not licensed from performing activities that are designated by that particular license. For example, the law states that the medical license allows diagnosing and prescribing treatment. If someone were to diagnose or prescribe without a medical license, that individual would be committing an illegal act and would be practicing medicine without a license, which is considered a felony.

There are state laws that govern the practice of medicine and nursing (medical practice acts, nursing practice acts), and many states have acts that give providers the right to delegate certain clinical procedures to qualified allied health professionals. Because medical assistants are not required to be licensed, they can become certified voluntarily. They are allowed to perform clinical procedures only under the supervision of the provider or other licensed health care professional who is granted the right and who delegates the specific clinical procedures to them.

In some states, including California, Washington, and others, unlicensed health care providers are required to have authorization from the state to perform allergy testing and venipuncture and to give injections. A registration fee and mandatory training are required. In such circumstances, medical assistants or other health care providers would be breaking the law if they performed these procedures without registration and training.

In some states, authorization is required for unlicensed health care providers to expose patients to X-rays.

On March 30, 2007 a bill called the CARE bill (Consistency, Accuracy, Responsibility and Excellence in Medical Imaging and Radiation Therapy) was introduced before the U.S. Senate. If passed, it would require all persons who perform medical imaging (including X-rays) and radiation therapy (excluding ultrasound) procedures to meet specific federal education and credentialing standards in order to participate in Medicare and Medicaid. Presently, the law in some states requires only voluntary basic training standards. This situation allows individuals without formal education to perform imaging procedures.

The AAMA supports the legislation that would require specific educational and certification standards for individuals performing medical imaging. Medical assistants do not perform procedures for which they have not been educated and in which they are not proficient. The AAMA's Occupational Analysis for the CMA (AAMA) in Appendix C, and the AMT's Medical Assisting Task List in Appendix D are excellent reference sources that identify the clinical, administrative, and general procedures medical assistants are educated to perform. However, because of the variability of state statutes, the medical assistant would be wise to check with the AAMA or AMT if in doubt about the legality of certain clinical procedures.

The AMT and the AAMA (the two leading organizations that certify medical assistants) agreed on a model state law outlining the medical assistant's scope of practice. Both the AMT and AAMA took from existing state laws regarding medical assistants' right to practice the most important aspects of these and developed the model. Both organizations agreed to require a medical assistant to graduate from an accredited medical assistant program and to obtain certification from AMT, AAMA, or other approved agencies that certify. A nonexclusive list of functions that a supervised medical assistant may perform was developed. The purpose of the Model State Legislation is to protect the medical assistant's right to practice. A copy of the model legislation is available at state medical assistant societies.

Critical Thinking

A medical assistant relates to a patient on the telephone that her symptoms are "probably the flu" and to "take over-the-counter cough syrup" for her cough. Is this an appropriate or inappropriate action for the medical assistant to take? Discuss your answer and explain why you came to your decision.

Case Study 1-1

Review the scenario at the beginning of the chapter.

CASE STUDY REVIEW

1. If you were a freshman in high school and interested in medical assisting, would you like to have an opportunity to visit a program and tour the classroom and laboratories? Why or why not?
2. List 3 or 4 questions you might ask of the senior medical assistant students while you are touring the medical assisting department that would help to clarify what the profession is, the course requirements, etc.

SUMMARY

Progress has been made in the advancement of the profession of medical assisting since the first group of medical assistants gathered to become organized and formed the AAMA and the AMT. For example, the number of certified medical assistants has exceeded 47,500 and continues to grow since certification began in 1963. The total number of medical assistants in the work force is approximately 387,000, and employment opportunities continue to grow. Educational requirements have become increasingly important. The AAMA, the AMT, and the NHA continue to promote standards of excellence for its members, encouraging continuing education and awarding continuing education credits to members of AAMA, AMT, and the NHA via various means.

All of these factors are evidence of a strong professional perspective and should offer encouragement and support to any student or graduate of medical assisting.

Becoming a professional is a gradual process and cannot be learned in its entirety from a textbook. The challenge of becoming a professional medical assistant will require open-mindedness and a desire for continued learning and education, certification and recertification of the CMA (AAMA) or RMA credential, and professional involvement through organizational participation.

As the scope of work done by medical assistants broadens and medical assistants seek and require formal education, the professional medical assistant will gain additional respect and be in even greater demand. Medical assistants must continuously pursue excellence, which is the hallmark of all professional behavior.

STUDY FOR SUCCESS

To reinforce your knowledge and skills of information presented in this chapter:

- Review the Key Terms
- Answer the Review Questions
  - Multiple Choice
  - Critical Thinking
- Navigate the Internet and complete the Web Activities
- Practice the StudyWARE activities on the textbook CD
- Apply your knowledge in the Student Workbook activities
- Complete the Web Tutor sections
- View and discuss the DVD situations

REVIEW QUESTIONS

Multiple Choice

1. The designation CMAS is awarded by the:
   a. AAMA
   b. ABHES
   c. AMA
   d. AMT
2. Increased employment opportunities for medical assistants result from:
   a. regulation of diagnostic testing
   b. the volume of paperwork
   c. managed care's emphasis on ambulatory care
   d. "baby boomers" beginning to retire
   e. all of the above
3. Ethics is:
   a. a system of values each individual has that determines perceptions of right and wrong
   b. a code established by an agency that has nothing to do with the medical assistant's belief in right or wrong
   c. making patients more comfortable
   d. willingness to work as a team member
4. Accreditation means:
   a. meeting appropriate standards
   b. obtaining the CMA (AAMA) or RMA credential
   c. being listed on an official roster
   d. having a curriculum with courses that are unrestricted
5. Licensure is:
   a. voluntary and up to the individual practitioner
   b. unrestrictive in scope
   c. conferred on an individual through a non-government agency
   d. mandatory and legislated by states

Critical Thinking

1. Describe two benefits for medical assistants who join their professional organization.
2. Explain what opportunities are available for medical assistants to improve their skills while on practicum.
3. Describe how certification or registration can enhance the medical assistant's career.
4. What is the primary difference between the CMA (AAMA) and the RMA credentials?
5. Compare the content of the CMA (AAMA) and RMA certification examination. Explain six similarities. Are there any significant differences?
6. Many employers require credentialed medical assistants. Give two specific reasons why they do.
7. Explain two ways in which a certified or registered medical assistant can remain current with changes in health care and technology.
8. Research which of the credentials is most widely accepted in your geographical area. How would pursuing a different professional credential affect your ability to be employed?
9. Contact the AAMA, AMT, or NHA in the state in which you live. Review newsletters and other periodicals about medical assisting that have been published recently. What did you find that promoted

WEB ACTIVITIES

1. Visit the American Medical Technologists (AMT) Web site at http://www. amt1.com
   - What allied health professions other than medical assistants and medical laboratory technicians are credentialed by AMT?
   - Does AMT have a code of ethics for the medical assistant?
   - What are the eligibility requirements for individuals to take the RMA examination?
2. Visit the American Association of Medical Assistants Web site at http://www.aama-ntl.org
   - What allied health profession(s) does the AAMA sponsor?
   - What are the eligibility requirements for individuals to take the CMA (AAMA) examination?
   - What resources are available on the Web for medical assistants interested in continuing education?
3. Visit the National Healthcareer Association Web site at http:// www.nhanow.com
   - What are five functions of the association?
   - What is NHA's goal?
   - Describe NHA's continuing education program.

REFERENCES/BIBLIOGRAPHY

American Association of Medical Assistants, Executive Office, 20 N. Wacker Dr., Chicago, IL 60606.

American Medical Technologists, Allied Health Professions, 10700 West Higgins Rd., Rosemont, IL 60018.

Balasa, D. (2000). Securing the future for medical assistants to practice. *Professional medical assistant,* January/February 2000, 6–7.

Balasa, D. (2003). Vigilance is key to protecting practice rights. *CMA Today,* 36(4). Retrieved April 15, 2007, from http://www.aama-ntl.org/cmatoday/archives.

Balasa, D. (2004). Model legislation designed to protect practice rights. *CMA Today,* 37(2). Retrieved April 15, 2007, from http://www. aama-ntl.org/cmatoday/archives.

Balasa, D. (2005). CARE bill gains momentum in Congress. *CMA Today,* 38(4). Retrieved April 15, 2007, from http://www.aama-ntl.org/cmatoday/archives.

McCarty, M. (2003). The lawful scope of a medical assistant's practice. *AMT Events,* March 2003.

Merriam-Webster (2002). *Merriam-Webster's Collegiate Dictionary* (11th ed.). Springfield, MA: Author.

National Healthcareer Association, 7 Ridgedale Ave., Suite 203, Cedar Knolls, NJ 07927.

THE DVD HOOK-UP

As you can see from reading Chapter 1, your character is important when working as a medical assistant. Taking on a professional demeanor is hard work and takes lots of practice. You must start now, while you are in training, to develop the characteristics of a true professional.

In the first scene of program 1, we observe Dee walking into class late. Dee's appearance is in total disarray and her attitude is poor. Even though Dee promised her teacher that she would work on her professional characteristics, Dee enters her externship with the same attitude that she possessed in school. After Dee speaks with her externship supervisor, she starts to realize that her teacher is right, and that she does need to develop her professional skills if she is going to succeed as a medical assistant.

1. This chapter lists characteristics that are important to possess as a professional. Using that list, write down all the characteristics of a professional that Dee was lacking in the first three scenes of program 1.
2. What kind of verbal and nonverbal messages did Dee send to her teacher, classmates, and externship personnel?
3. Do you see any similarities between Dee and yourself?

DVD Journal Summary

After watching the designated scenes from program 1, write a paragraph in your journal that summarizes what you learned from watching these scenes. What kind of verbal and nonverbal messages do you typically send to your classmates? What will you do to improve other people's impressions of your professional characteristics?

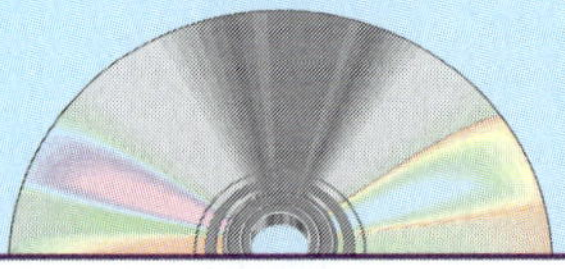

DVD Series	**Program Number**
Critical Thinking	1

Chapter/Scene Reference
- *Classroom Performance*
- *Externship*
- *Learning from Supervisors*
- *Growing from Experience*

Health Care Settings and the Health Care Team

Chapter 2

KEY TERMS

Acupuncture
Ambulatory Care Setting
Fringe Benefits
Health Maintenance Organization (HMO)
Homeopathy
Independent Physician Association (IPA)
Integrative Medicine
Managed Care Operation
Preferred Provider Organization (PPO)

OUTLINE

OBJECTIVES

The student should strive to meet the following performance objectives and demonstrate an understanding of the facts and principles presented in this chapter through written and oral communication.

1. Define the key terms as presented in the glossary.
2. Identify and describe the three primary medical management models.
3. Analyze the benefits and limitations of working in the different ambulatory health care settings.
4. Assess the role of managed care in the health care environment.
5. Describe the function of the health care team.
6. List and describe a minimum of 12 providers.
7. List and describe a minimum of three alternative health care specialists.
8. List and describe a minimum of 12 allied health professionals.
9. Discuss the role of the medical assistant in ambulatory health care.
10. Critique alternative therapies and discuss their role in today's health care setting.
11. Identity the value of the medical assistant to the health care team.

Scenario

You always had thought you wanted to be a medical assistant and work in a clinic where you would see a variety of patients. But after discussing this chapter in class, you are really intrigued with becoming a physical therapy assistant. What kind of research can you do to make certain you have chosen the right path? Consider working hours, rate of pay, patient contact, required schooling, and job availability.

INTRODUCTION

There are few professions in our society as rich and complex as the health care profession. Particularly in recent years, the health care environment has been very much in flux as the profession seeks ways to provide quality care while containing costs. This effort to curtail costs has resulted in the rise of managed care, which, in turn, has spawned a number of medical models such as health maintenance organizations (HMOs) and preferred provider organizations (PPOs), two well-known managed care entities.

Many other types of networks and alliances are also being established as providers merge to give patients the best of care while controlling their costs. Ambulatory care settings, where services are provided on an outpatient basis, have become increasingly pivotal to consumer health care as insurers direct dollars away from hospitals and toward outpatient care.

Just as the medical setting continues to evolve to meet new societal needs, health care technology is ever-changing. Health care is a dynamic, stimulating industry that requires the medical assistant and other professionals to constantly develop new skills if they are to contribute to the team effort. The range of skills within the health care team is astonishing and includes providers in more than 25 specialties, an increasing number of nontraditional alternative practitioners licensed to practice, and more than 20 kinds of allied health professionals.

AMBULATORY HEALTH CARE SETTINGS

Although medical assistants work in a number of different environments, including laboratories or hospitals, most are employed in an **ambulatory care setting** such as a medical office or clinic (either a solo-provider or group practice), an urgent or primary care center, or a managed care organization.

Often, the medical assistant chooses to work in one setting rather than another based on interests, personality, and work preferences. For instance, the individual practice may provide medical assistants with the opportunity to use their full array of skills, whereas in urgent care centers, the work of the medical assistant is often more specialized in nature.

Medical assistants should also recognize the three major forms of medical practice management and how they affect salary, benefits, and liability issues (Figure 2-1).

Individual and Group Medical Practices

For years, the most common form of ambulatory health care was the individual provider or group practice. This model competes with a variety of other models such as urgent and managed care centers, but many medical assistants find the individual or group practice the most challenging place of employment.

Individual Practices. In the individual practice, also called the solo practice, one primary provider sees and treats all patients. Although this type of arrangement is limited in the number of people it can serve, many patients feel secure in this kind of health care setting because they come to know and trust their provider. Because they always see the same provider, they feel their health care is being managed in a personal way. The solo-provider practice, however, can be an expensive arrangement, because one provider must undertake the costs of office space, equipment, and personnel.

Group Practices. Group practices are attractive arrangements where two or more providers can share the costs of space, equipment, and personnel. The advantages of a group practice are not solely economic, however; providers learn from and consult one another, and patients

FORMS OF MEDICAL PRACTICE MANAGEMENT

Medical assistants employed in ambulatory care settings or medical offices and clinics are likely to see three major forms of medical practice management: sole proprietorships, partnerships, and corporations.

Whatever form of management is chosen by providers, they are responsible for the employees that serve with them. (Refer to the discussion of *respondeat superior* in Chapter 7.) Employers and their medical assistants must have the kind of healthy working relationship where mutual trust and respect are apparent. The provider must understand the skill level of the medical assistant, and the medical assistant must feel secure enough to ask any necessary questions or admit any errors. Critical errors are often made when this trust does not exist between employer and employee. This causes a breakdown in the delivery of the best health care for patients.

Sole Proprietorships

In the past, many providers preferred a solo practice. A solo practice entitles the sole proprietor to hold exclusive right to all aspects of the medical practice or sole proprietorship, including profits and debts. If the business fails, the sole proprietor's personal property may also be attached.

A sole proprietorship may employ other providers to participate in the practice. The employed provider(s) is entitled to any employee **fringe benefits** such as health insurance and paid vacation, but the solo practitioner is not so entitled.

Partnerships

When two or more providers join together under a legal agreement to share in the total business operations of the practice, a partnership is formed. Several providers who share a facility and practice medicine are often referred to as a group. Partners share income, expenses, debt, equipment, records, and personnel according to a predetermined agreement. Partners are liable for only their own actions but may be liable for the whole amount of the partnership debts.

Corporations

Providers may form a corporation, usually referred to as a professional service corporation. The shareholders are considered employees of the corporation. A corporation allows income and tax advantages to all employees. A variety of fringe benefits can be offered to the employees, which may include pension; profit-sharing plans; medical expense reimbursement; and life, health, and disability insurance. These benefits are separate from salary. Another advantage is that professional employees of a corporation are liable only for their own acts, and personal property cannot be attached in litigation. A sole proprietor may incorporate if the practice is large enough.

The health maintenance organization (HMO) is one type of corporation in which providers often practice. Basically, providers are employees of the HMO and are paid by various methods; providers in the HMO usually serve as the primary care provider (PCP). In this situation, a referral from the PCP may be necessary before a patient can see a specialist or allied health professional.

Figure 2-1 Different forms of medical practice management.

receive the benefit of this exchange of information and knowledge. Often, a group practice has more than one office or clinic and some employees are asked to travel between sites to cut overhead. Group practices may be formed to offer specialized care, such as oncology or women's health care.

In most group practices, patients may request that they see the same provider for all appointments, although sometimes patients are assigned to the next available provider. For emergencies, group practices have the staff and flexibility to ensure that there is always a provider on call.

Most medical practices are still groups of three or four providers, but in the most recent past a trend shows a return to one- and two-provider practices. Merritt, Hawkins, and Associates, a staffing and recruiting firm in Texas, reports that providers in two-person partnerships increased from 9% in 1998 to 22% in 2002. In a 2006 survey the same firm reported that over 60% of primary care providers practice in groups of three or more, 10% practice in two-provider clinics, and 29% give medical care as solo practitioners.

Many providers in small groups allowed large practice management firms to acquire their assets and manage the business side of their practice. In some cases, these practice management firms were sold to even larger practice management companies that eventually went bankrupt, forcing them to shed all their practices. This dilemma left providers with no recourse except to start over. Therefore, a number of providers are returning to the **preferred provider organization (PPO),** where providers network to offer discounts to employers and other purchasers of health insurance and agree to discounted fees for services.

Urgent Care Centers

Urgent care centers are usually private, for-profit centers that provide services for primary care, routine injuries and illnesses, and minor surgery. Sometimes laboratory services and a radiology department are located on the premises. Providers and other health care professionals in the center are often salaried employees, not owners who share in the profits, and often are associated with other medical facilities.

The pace in most urgent care centers is brisk, and typically a number of providers are working at one time. Patients are usually encouraged to make appointments, but drop-ins are accepted, especially for emergencies.

Because these centers often see a higher volume of patients during expanded hours, usually for a lower cost than a hospital emergency room, experts predict that urgent care centers will continue to grow in popularity.

Managed Care Operations

Health maintenance organizations, or **HMOs,** are probably the most familiar **managed care operation.** Originally, HMOs were designed to provide a full range of health care services under one roof. More recently, the HMO without walls has become established, which is typically a network of participating providers within a defined geographic area.

Originally, the HMO with walls was conceived to provide patients with comprehensive health care services at one facility. Today, as managed care and managed competition sweep the health care industry, other arrangements include the preferred provider organization (PPO), where providers network to offer discounts to employers and other purchasers of health insurance, and the **Independent Provider Association (IPA)**, the members of which agree to treat patients for an agreed-upon fee.

"Boutique" or "Concierge" Medical Practice

According to the American Academy of Family Physicians, there are several hundred "boutique" or "concierge" practices emerging and growing in popularity with both patients and providers. Providers who are discouraged by their shrinking insurance reimbursement and managed care plans dictating what procedures and tests will be performed have turned to another avenue for providing health care. Patients who are disappointed in the quality of care received and frustrated by being bounced from one insurer to another as employers seek a cost reduction in their health care benefits are willing to pay the extra amount for the "concierge" care.

Concierge care generally offers patients the following services:

- Immediate access to their provider by phone 24 hours a day, 7 days a week
- Convenient and unhurried appointments
- Unlimited email, fax, or phone consultation with their provider
- Home or work visits as needed
- Coordination of specialist referrals
- Friendly staff who understand a patient's unique health needs
- Free parking

Patients who choose this type of service pay a set fee per year from $2,000 to $3,000 for one individual and up to $5,000 to include a spouse or $6,000 to include children. Patients are expected to carry a major medical plan to cover referrals to specialists, hospitalization, and emergency care.

Ethical concerns have been raised regarding concierge services. Some say the "extra" services should be available to everyone; others believe the extra fees make the service very exclusive. Some providers follow a "retainer" model for concierge services where patients pay a monthly fee for priority access to their provider, unlimited office visits, annual physicals, preventive care, and wellness

Critical Thinking

What is your opinion of the concierge type of medical practice? Would you feel comfortable working in such an environment? Why or why not?

screenings and compare the cost of the services to less than a pack of cigarettes a day.

Providers practicing in a concierge service report a greater satisfaction with their chosen profession, enjoy really getting to know their patients, and serve a few hundred patients rather than a few thousand in a traditional practice. Patients report satisfaction in receiving more time and personal care from a provider who determines the best options for maintaining their health.

THE HEALTH CARE TEAM

In every kind of health care setting, the team concept is critical to the quality of patient care. A primary care provider is most likely the main source of health care for patients. From time to time, however, a specialist is sought or recommended. A number of different allied health professionals, including the medical assistant, supply additional health care as ordered by the provider. Increasingly, patients are looking outside traditional medicine for portions of their health care. The Centers for Disease Control and Prevention's (CDC) 2002 National Health Interview Survey revealed that 36% of adults in the United States use some form of complementary and/or alternative medical (CAM) care. The survey also indicated greater use of a CAM among women and individuals with higher education. In 2001, the World Health Organization (WHO) estimated that between 65% and 80% of the world's population relied on alternative medicine as their primary health care source. One third of all medical schools in the United States now have courses in alternative medicine, and many people in the United States seem to desire a more "natural" approach to health care whenever possible. Although alternative care is not always covered by medical insurance, traditional and nontraditional health care practices are nonetheless blending in many areas.

In whatever manner health care is sought, all members of the health care team must communicate, sometimes in person and sometimes just through the medical history and record, with one another to ensure quality patient care. The Patient Education box on page 25 discusses another major member of the health care team.

The Title "Doctor"

The public is often confused by the title *doctor.* The term implies an earned academic degree of the highest level in a particular area of study. Physicians have earned the MD, or Doctor of Medicine, degree. Other medical degrees include the Doctor of Osteopathy (DO), Doctor of Dentistry (DDS), Doctor of Optometry (OD), Doctor of Podiatric Medicine (DPM), Doctor of Chiropracty (DC), and Doctor of Naturopathy (ND). In the medical field, the abbreviation *Dr.* is used and the title *doctor* is addressed to these individuals qualified by education, training, and licensure to practice medicine.

In nonmedical disciplines, persons who have achieved a doctorate conferred by a college or university include the Doctor of Education (EdD), the Doctor of Philosophy (PhD), and the Doctor of Psychology (PSYD). All three have several areas of specialty and are referred to as *doctor.*

Health Care Professionals and Their Roles

Doctor of Medicine. A doctorate degree in medicine and a license to practice allows a person to diagnose and treat medical conditions. The doctor of medicine candidate attends four years of medical school after receiving a bachelor's degree. Newly graduated MDs enter into a residency program that consists of three to seven years of additional training and education depending on the specialty chosen. This residency comes under the direct supervision of senior medical doctor educators. Family practice, internal medicine, and pediatrics require a three-year residency; general surgery requires a five-year residency. Some refer to the first year of residency as an internship; the American Medical Association (AMA) no longer uses this term, however. At this point, many medical doctors choose to be board certified, which is optional and voluntary. Certification assures the public that the doctor's knowledge, experience, and skills in a particular specialty have been tested and deemed qualified to provide care in that specialty. Doctors of medicine can be certified through 24 specialty medical boards and in 88 subspecialty fields. Table 2-1 gives a partial listing of these fields.

Medical doctors must still obtain a license to practice medicine from a state or jurisdiction of the United States in which they are planning to practice. They apply for the permanent license after completing a series of examinations and completing a minimum number of years of graduate medical education. Medical doctors must continue to receive a certain number of continuing medical education (CME) requirements each year to ensure that their knowledge and skills are current. CME requirements vary by state, professional organizations, and hospital staff organizations.

Table 2-1 Selected Medical and Surgical Specialties

Specialties	Title of Doctor	Description
Allergy and Immunology	Allergist and Immunologist	Evaluates diseases/disorders of the immune system and problems related to asthma and allergy
Cardiology	Cardiologist	Evaluates and treats medical conditions of the heart
Dermatology	Dermatologist	Evaluates disorders/diseases of skin, hair, nails, and related tissues
Emergency Medicine	Emergency Medical Doctor	Evaluates and treats medical conditions that result from trauma or sudden illness; manages emergency department
Family Practice	Family Practitioner	Treats the whole family from infancy to death
Internal Medicine	Internist	Provides comprehensive care, practices preventive care, treats long-term and chronic conditions
Obstetrics and Gynecology	Obstetrician and Gynecologist	Provides care to pregnant women, delivers babies, treats disorders/diseases of reproductive system
Ophthalmology	Ophthalmologist	Provides comprehensive care of the eye and its structures and offers vision services
Orthopedic Surgeon	Orthopedist	Examines, diagnoses, and treats diseases and injuries of the musculoskeletal system
Otolaryngology	Otolaryngologist	Treats diseases/disorders of the ears, nose, and throat
Pediatrics	Pediatrician	Treats diseases/disorders of children and adolescents; monitors growth and development of children
Psychiatry and Neurology	Psychiatrist and Neurologist	Diagnoses and treats patients with mental, emotional, or behavioral disorders
General Surgery	Surgeon	Operates to repair or remove diseased or injured parts of the body
Colon and Rectal	Colorectal Surgeon	Operates to remove or repair diseased colon and rectal areas of the body
Neurological	Neurosurgeon	Treats conditions of the nervous systems, often through surgery
Plastic	Plastic Surgeon	Repairs and reconstructs physical defects; provides cosmetic enhancements
Thoracic	Thoracic Surgeon	Performs surgery on the respiratory system, chest, heart, and cardiovascular system
Radiology	Radiologist	Interprets diagnostic images, performs special procedures, manages radiological services
Urology	Urologist	Treats diseases/disorders of the urinary tract

Patient Education

Continually remind your patients of the important role they carry in their own health care. *Only your patients* know exactly what happens to their bodies and minds in any particular illness. *Only your patients* know if their pain is too much to bear. *Only your patients* know whether they will remain on any treatment regimen established. *Only your patients* know if they are already embracing some alternative form of treatment. *Only your patients* know how much financial burden they can handle for health care. In initial interviews and pre-provider preparations, ask your patients questions that encourage them to tell you what is happening, whether they are coping, and how their particular problem affects their daily lives. Listen to them carefully. Do not rush or second-guess their responses. Be mindful of the special needs of elderly patients and individuals for whom English is their second language. They are likely unfamiliar with taking a major role in their own health care. Always remember to be therapeutic and observe nonverbal cues. Empower your patients to be a member of their own health care team.

Doctor of Osteopathy. Osteopaths are generally recognized as equal to medical doctors in all respects. The Doctor of Osteopathy, or DO, is a fully qualified provider licensed to perform surgery and prescribe medication. The training and education are quite similar to that of the MD. Osteopathic medicine was established in 1874 by Dr. Andrew Taylor Still, who was one of the first practitioners to study the attributes of good health to better understand the process of disease. He identified the musculoskeletal system as a key element of health and encouraged preventive medicine, eating properly, and keeping fit. The education of an osteopath includes a four-year undergraduate degree plus four years of medical school. After graduation from medical school, a DO can choose to practice in any of the 18 American Osteopathic Association specialty areas, requiring from two to six years of additional training. Approximately 65% of all osteopaths practice in primary care areas such as family practice, pediatrics, obstetrics/gynecology, and internal medicine. DOs must pass a state licensure examination and maintain currency in their education. Most patients find little difference between an MD and a DO. However, doctors of osteopathy can incorporate osteopathic manipulative treatment (OMT) in their treatment of patients as deemed helpful.

Critical Thinking

Discuss with a peer what action might be taken when patients refuse all opportunities to be a member of their own health care team. How might you encourage patients to take even a small part in their own health care? How would major decisions be made?

Integrative Medicine and Alternative Health Care Practitioners

Many **integrative medicine** and alternative health care practitioners also carry the title *doctor,* but they have a different training regimen than required for the MD or DO. The training is highly specialized and specific; when licensed, these professionals are allowed to diagnose and treat medical conditions.

As mentioned earlier, alternative therapies are increasingly being perceived as complements to traditional health care in a form of integrative medicine. In this text, three broad disciplines are identified: chiropractic, naturopathy, and Oriental medicine/acupuncture.

Doctor of Chiropractic. Chiropractic is a branch of the healing arts that gives special attention to the physiological and biochemical aspects of the body's structure and includes procedures for the adjustment and manipulation of the articulations and adjacent tissues of the human body, particularly of the spinal column. Chiropractic is a nonsurgical science that does not include pharmaceuticals or surgery.

The roots of chiropractic care can be traced back to the beginning of recorded time. Writings from China and Greece written in 2700 B.C. and 1500 B.C. mention spinal manipulation and maneuvering of the lower extremities to ease lower back pain. Daniel David Palmer founded the chiropractic profession in the United States in 1895. Throughout the twentieth century, doctors of chiropractic gained legal recognition and licensure in all 50 states.

Doctors of chiropractic (DC) complete four to five years of study at an accredited chiropractic college. The curriculum includes a minimum of 4,200 hours of classroom, laboratory, and clinical experience. About 555 hours are devoted to adjustive techniques and spinal analysis. This specialized education must be preceded by a minimum of 90 hours of undergraduate courses focusing on science. On successful completion of their education and training, doctors of chiropractic must also pass the national board examination and all examinations or licensure requirements identified by the particular state in which the individual wishes to practice.

Doctors of chiropractic frequently treat patients with neuromusculoskeletal conditions, such as headaches, joint pain, neck pain, lower back pain, and sciatica. Chiropractors also treat patients with osteoarthritis, spinal disk conditions, carpal tunnel syndrome, tendonitis, sprains, and strains. Chiropractors also may treat a variety of other conditions, such as allergies, asthma, and digestive disorders. There are obstacles to chiropractors in some areas, however, because states vary in what they authorize chiropractors to practice and may limit their ability to practice **homeopathy** or **acupuncture** or to dispense or sell dietary supplements.

Doctor of Naturopathy. Naturopathy, often referred to as "natural medicine," is based on the belief that the cause of disease is violation of nature's laws. The goal of the naturopath is to remove the underlying causes of disease and to stimulate the body's natural healing processes. Naturopathic treatments may include fasting; adhering to natural food diets; taking vitamins and herbs; tissue minerals; counseling; homeopathic remedies; manipulation of the spine and extremities; massage; exercise; naturopathic hygienic remedies; acupuncture; and applications of water, heat, cold, air, sunlight, and electricity. Most of these treatment methods are used to detoxify the body and strengthen the immune system.

In the United States, a Doctor of Naturopathy (ND) or Doctor of Naturopathic Medicine (NMD) receives education, training, and credentials from a full-time naturopathy college. Full-time education includes two years of science courses and two years of clinical work. Naturopaths are currently licensed to practice in 13 states, four Canadian provinces, and Puerto Rico and the Virgin Islands. The number of states licensing NDs is expected to increase. In many states, naturopaths practice independently and unlicensed, or they practice under the direction of a physician.

Oriental Medicine and Acupuncture. Oriental medicine is a comprehensive system of health care with a history of more than 3,000 years. Oriental medicine includes acupuncture, Chinese herbology and bodywork, dietary therapy, and exercise based on traditional Oriental medicine principles. This form of health care is used extensively in Asia and is rapidly growing in popularity in the West.

Oriental medicine is based on an energetic model rather than the biochemical model of Western medicine. The ancient Chinese recognized a vital energy behind all life-forms and processes called *qi* (pronounced "chee"). Oriental healing practitioners believe that energy flows along specific pathways called *meridians.* Each pathway is associated with a particular physiological system and internal organ. Disease is the result of deficiency or imbalance of energy in the meridians and their associated physiological systems. Acupuncture points are specific sites along the meridians. Each point has a predictable effect on the vital energy passing through it. Modern science has measured the electrical charge at these points, corroborating the locations of the meridians. Traditional Oriental medicine uses an intricate system of pulse and tongue diagnosis, palpation of points and meridians, medical history, and other signs and symptoms to create a composite diagnosis. A treatment plan then is formulated to induce the body to a balanced state of health.

The WHO recognizes acupuncture and traditional Oriental medicine's ability to treat many common disorders, including the following:

- *Gastrointestinal disorders:* food allergies, peptic ulcer, chronic diarrhea, constipation, indigestion, anorexia, gastritis
- *Urogenital disorders:* stress incontinence, urinary tract infections, sexual dysfunction
- *Gynecological disorders:* irregular, heavy, or painful menstruation; premenstrual syndrome (PMS); infertility
- *Respiratory disorders:* emphysema, sinusitis, asthma, allergies, bronchitis
- *Neuromusculoskeletal disorders:* arthritis; migraine headaches; neuralgia; insomnia; dizziness; low back, neck, and shoulder pain
- *Circulatory disorders:* hypertension, angina pectoris, arteriosclerosis, anemia
- *Eye, ear, nose, and throat disorders:* otitis media, sinusitis, sore throats
- *Emotional and psychological disorders:* depression; anxiety; addictions to alcohol, nicotine, and drugs
- *Pain:* elimination or control of pain for chronic and painful debilitating disorders

In the hands of a comprehensively trained acupuncturist, patients do not find acupuncture painful. Sterile, very fine, flexible needles about the diameter of a human hair are used in treatment. Practitioners may also recommend herbs, dietary changes, and exercise together with lifestyle changes.

Training for acupuncture and Oriental medicine can be obtained in schools and colleges accredited by the Accreditation Commission for Acupuncture and Oriental Medicine. A minimum of two years of undergraduate study is required, and some colleges prefer applicants to have a bachelor's degree. Most of these specialized programs are three years, and on completion graduates are conferred with a Masters in Acupuncture and Oriental Medicine (MAOM) or a Masters in Acupuncture (MA) degree. Nearly all states regulate the practice of acupuncture and Oriental medicine, either through licensure or a ruling by the Board of Medical Examiners. It is likely that passing a national certification examination or other testing procedure is required before licensure. Many doctors (MDs, DOs, DCs, and NDs) have become qualified to perform acupuncture and to use Oriental medicine in their practices through additional education and training.

Future of Integrative Medicine

There was a time when osteopaths and chiropractors were not accepted by the medical establishment and had difficulty with licensure. Naturopaths, acupuncturists, and Oriental medicine practitioners face similar challenges, and states vary greatly in their regulations of any form of alternative medicine.

The road may be bumpy for alternative practitioners, but their numbers are increasing rapidly. By 2010, the number of chiropractors, naturopaths, and Oriental medicine practitioners will increase by 88%. Managed care health plans are offering increased access to alternative medicine practitioners, mostly because of the ability to expand patient choices at a lower cost. It is expected that states will broaden their licensure to increased numbers of well-educated and trained alternative practitioners.

Neither the growth in the number of alternative medicine practitioners nor the laws and insurance practices that facilitate their access by patients likely would have occurred without broad public acceptance of alternative and complementary medicine. Americans seem quite willing to pay out-of-pocket expenses for alternative forms of treatment, such as massage therapy, aromatherapy, biofeedback, guided imagery, hydrotherapy, hypnotherapy, and homeopathy. Furthermore, many patients are seeking the more integrated form of medicine that occurs when primary care providers are willing to refer to an alternative practitioner and vice versa. Table 2-2 gives a brief description of a few alternative modalities that integrate fairly easily with traditional medical practices.

ALLIED HEALTH PROFESSIONALS AND THEIR ROLES

In the health care team, allied health professionals bring specific educational backgrounds and a broad array of skills to the medical environment. Medical assistants are considered allied health professionals.

The Role of the Medical Assistant

In the ambulatory care setting, a critical allied health professional is the medical assistant. The medical assistant, performing both administrative and clinical tasks under the direction of the provider, is an important link between patient and provider. The medical assistant serves in many capacities—receptionist, secretary, office manager, bookkeeper, insurance coder and biller, sometimes transcriptionist, patient educator, and clinical assistant. The latter requires the medical assistant to be able to administer injections and perform venipuncture, prepare patients for examinations, assist with examinations and special procedures, and perform electrocardiography and various laboratory tests. Medical assistants screen and assess patient needs when scheduling appointments and tests. However, although medical assistants have a broad range of responsibilities, it is critical that they perform only within the scope of their training and personal capabilities and always function within ethical and legal boundaries and state statutes.

Because medical assistants are often the patient's first contact with the facility and its providers, a positive attitude is important. They must be excellent communicators, both verbally and nonverbally, and project a professional image of themselves and their employer. Medical assistants who believe in their work, who are proud of their career, and who convey compassion and caring provide a positive experience for patients who are ill or in a great deal of discomfort.

Table 2-2 Selected Alternative Medicine Modalities

Acupressure: A massage technique that applies pressure to specific acupuncture-like points on the body; pressure encourages the flow of vital energy *(qi)* along the meridian pathways. It is used to control chronic pain, migraine headaches, and backaches.
Aromatherapy: The inhalation and bodily application of essential oils from aromatic plants to relax, balance, rejuvenate, restore, or enhance the body's mind and spirit. It strengthens the self-healing process by indirect stimulation of the immune system.
Biofeedback: Biofeedback machines gauge internal bodily functions and help patients tune in to these functions and identify the triggers that evoke symptoms. Relaxation can be taught to relieve the symptoms.
Guided Imagery: Uses images or symbols to train the mind to create a definitive physiological or psychological effect; relieves stress and anxiety and reduces pain.
Homeopathy: Healing that claims highly diluted doses of certain substances can leave an energy imprint in the body and bring about a cure. Homeopathic remedies are made from naturally occurring plant, animal, or mineral substances and are manufactured by pharmaceutical companies under strict guidelines.
Hydrotherapy: Hydrotherapy uses the buoyancy, warmth, and effects of water and its turbulence to speed recovery after surgery and to reduce pain and stress, spasm and discomfort. It is especially beneficial for work- or sports-related injuries and arthritis.
Hypnotherapy: Hypnotherapy facilitates communication between the right and left sides of the brain with the patient in a state of focused relaxation when the subconscious mind is open to suggestions. It is currently used to help people lose weight; stop smoking; reduce stress; and relieve pain, anxiety, and phobias.
Massage: Massage reduces stress, manages chronic pain, promotes relaxation, and increases circulation of the blood and lymph. Hand stroking on the body helps patients become more familiar with their pain.

Table 2-3 (see page 29) lists some of the allied health professionals recognized by the Commission on Accreditation of Allied Health Education Programs (CAAHEP) and the Accrediting Bureau of Health Education Schools (ABHES).

As a medical assistant, you may not work directly with all the identified allied health care professionals, but you likely will have contact with many of them by telephone and written or electronic communication. Knowledge of the roles these health professionals play enables you to interact more intelligently with all members of the health care team.

In addition to the professionals listed in Table 2-3, you may encounter some or all of the following health care professionals in daily patient care.

Health Unit Coordinator

Health unit coordinators (HUCs) perform nonclinical patient care tasks for the nursing unit of a hospital. HUCs maintain patients' charts, schedule tests, order supplies, screen new patients, and give directions to visitors. This profession requires a self-motivated, mature individual who can handle the stress and hectic pace of coordinating personnel and their duties at the nurses' station. Also called unit secretary, administrative specialist, ward clerk, or ward secretary, a health unit coordinator receives on-the-job training or completes a six-month to one-year certificate program.

Medical Laboratory Technologist

Medical laboratory technologists (MLTs) physically and chemically analyze, as well as culture, urine, blood, and other body fluids and tissues. They work closely with specialists such as oncologists, pathologists, and hematologists. Knowledge of specimen collection, anatomy and physiology, biochemistry, laboratory equipment, asepsis, and quality control is essential. The American Society of Clinical Pathology (ASCP) is a professional organization that oversees credentialing and education in the medical laboratory professions (Figure 2-2 on page 30).

Registered Dietitian

Registered dietitians (RDs) have specialized training in the nutritional care of groups and individuals and have successfully completed an examination of

Table 2-3 Selected Allied Health Professions

Occupation	Abbreviations	Job Description
Anesthesiologist Assistant	AA	Performs preoperative tasks, performs airway management and drug administration for induction and maintenance of anesthesia during surgery under direction of a licensed and qualified anesthesiologist
Athletic Trainer	AT	Provides a variety of services including injury prevention, recognition, immediate care, treatment, and rehabilitation after athletic trauma
Clinical Laboratory Technician *Associate Degree*	CLT	Performs all routine tests in a medical laboratory and is able to discriminate and recognize factors that directly affect procedures and results. Works under direction of pathologist, provider medical technologist, or scientist
Diagnostic Medical Sonographer	DMS	Provides patient services using medical ultrasound under the supervision of a provider
Electroneurodiagnostic Technologist	EEG-T	Possesses the knowledge, attributes, and skills to obtain interpretable recordings of a patient's nervous system functions
Emergency Medical Technician—Paramedic	EMT-P	Recognizes, assesses, and manages medical emergencies of acutely ill or injured patients in prehospital care settings, working under the direction of a provider (often through radio communication)
Medical Assistant	MA	Functions under the supervision of licensed medical professionals and is competent in both administrative/office and clinical/laboratory procedures
Medical Illustrator	MI	Creates visual material designed to facilitate the recording and dissemination of medical, biological, and related knowledge through communication media
Occupational Therapist	OT	Educates and trains individuals in the application of purposeful, goal-oriented activity in the evaluation, diagnosis, and treatment of loss of ability to cope with the tasks of daily living and impairment caused by physical injury, illness, or emotional disorder; congenital or developmental disability; or the aging process
Ophthalmic Medical Technician or Technologist	OMT	Assists ophthalmologists to perform diagnostic and therapeutic procedures
Personal Fitness Trainer	PFT	Develops activity plans for each individual that integrates a complete approach to fitness and wellness through exercise, strength training, and proper diet
Radiographer	RT(R)	Provides patient services using imaging modalities, as directed by providers qualified to order and perform radiologic procedures
Registered Health Information Administrator	RHIA	Manages health information systems consistent with the medical, administrative, ethical, and legal requirements of the health care delivery system
Registered Health Information Technician	RHIT	Possesses the technical knowledge and skills necessary to process, maintain, compile, and report patient data
Respiratory Therapist	RRT	Applies scientific knowledge and theory to practical clinical problems of respiratory care
Surgical Technologist	ST	Works as an integral member of the surgical team, which includes surgeons, anesthesiologists, registered nurses, and other surgical personnel delivering patient care and assuming appropriate responsibilities before, during, and after surgery

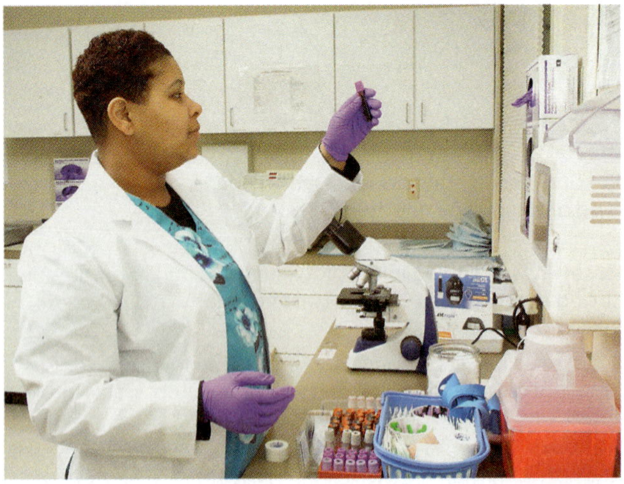

Figure 2-2 Medical laboratory personnel performing blood analysis.

the Commission on Dietetic Registration. Dietitians assist patients in regulating their diets. Although they are typically employed in hospitals and clinics, they can also be found working with the public in personal nutritional counseling. Education includes a bachlor's degree with a major in dietetics, food and nutrition, or food service systems management in addition to completion of an approved internship.

Pharmacist

Pharmacists (RPh) are licensed by each state to prepare and dispense all types of medications as well as medical supplies related to medication administration. They can practice in hospitals, medical centers, and pharmacies. The minimum training for a pharmacist is a five-year bachelor's degree; some pharmacists pursue a Doctor of Pharmacy degree (PharmD), which is offered by major universities in the United States.

Pharmacy Technician

Pharmacy technicians assist the pharmacist with preparation and administration of medications; they also perform receptionist and billing duties. In hospitals, nursing homes, and assisted living facilities, their responsibilities may include reading patient charts and preparing and delivering medications to patients. Pharmacists must check all orders before delivery. The technician can copy the information about the prescribed medication onto the patient's profile. Professional certification of pharmacy technicians varies from state to state and is administered by state pharmacy associations (Figure 2-3).

Phlebotomist

Phlebotomists are trained in the art of drawing blood for diagnostic laboratory testing. Phlebotomists are also referred to as laboratory liaison technicians. Phlebotomists may be nationally certified and are employed in medical clinics, hospitals, and laboratories. Training consists of one to two semesters in a community college program or on-the-job training.

Physical Therapist

Physical therapists (PTs) are licensed professionals who assist in the examination, testing, and treatment of physically disabled or challenged people. They also assist in physical rehabilitation of patients after an accident, injury, or serious illness using special exercises, application of heat or cold, *ultrasound* therapy, and other techniques. Educational requirements for a PT are a minimum of a four-year bachelor's degree (Bachelor of Science) or a special certificate course after obtaining the Bachelor of Science in a related field. PTs must also successfully complete a state licensure examination (Figure 2-4).

Physical Therapy Assistant

Physical therapy assistants (PTAs) are trained to use and apply physical therapy procedures, such as exercise, and physical agents under the supervision of a physical therapist. The PTA has earned

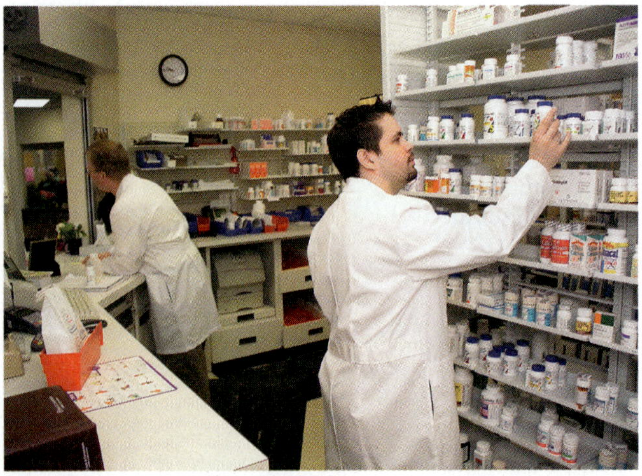

Figure 2-3 Pharmacy technician working with pharmacist preparing medications.

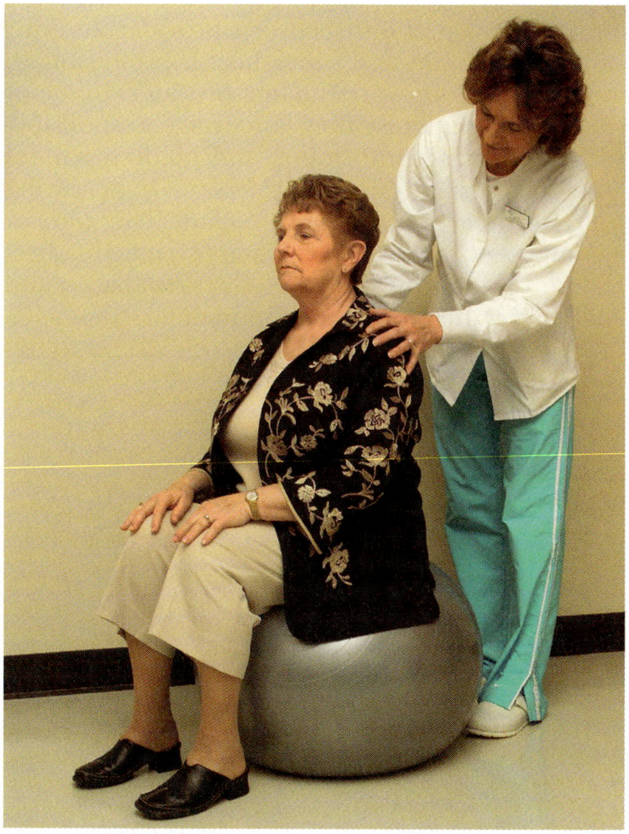

Figure 2-4 Physical therapist working with a patient requiring physical rehabilitation.

an Associate of Science degree from an accredited program and must pass a licensure or registry examination in selected states.

Nurse

Neither ABHES nor CAAHEP is responsible for nurse education or accreditation, but they are listed here as a major participant in health care. Nurses are licensed by the state in which they practice. Although nurses' education and training are oriented to bedside care, some are employed in medical offices as clinical assistants, especially in offices where surgery is performed. Nurses play a number of roles on the health care team.

Registered Nurse. In the United States, registered nurses (RNs) are professionals who have completed, at a minimum, a two-year course of study at a state-approved school of nursing and passed the National Council Licensure Examination (NCLEX-RN). Employment settings most often include hospitals, convalescent homes, clinics, and home health care.

Licensed Practical Nurse. A licensed practical nurse (LPN) is a professional trained in basic nursing techniques and direct patient care. LPNs practice under the direct supervision of an RN or provider and are employed in similar settings to RNs. Training includes completion of a state-approved program in practical nursing and successful completion of a national licensure examination.

Nurse Practitioner. Sometimes referred to as an Advanced Registered Nurse Practitioner (ARNP), a nurse practitioner (NP) is an RN who, by advanced education (usually a master's degree) and clinical experience in a branch of nursing, has acquired expert knowledge in a specific medical specialty. Nurse practitioners are employed by providers in private practice or in clinics and sometimes practice independently, especially in rural areas. ARNPs may or may not be licensed to prescribe medications.

Physician Assistant

Physician assistants (PAs) receive formal education and training to provide diagnostic, therapeutic, and preventive health care services delegated by and under the supervision of providers and surgeons. PAs take medical histories, examine and treat patients, order and interpret laboratory tests and X-rays, and make diagnoses. They also treat minor injuries by suturing, splinting, and casting. PAs write progress notes, instruct and counsel patients, and order tests and therapy. In 48 states and the District of Columbia, PAs may prescribe some medications. They can supervise technicians and medical assistants. PAs may be primary care providers in areas where the supervising physician is not present all the time but is always available for conferring as necessary and required by law.

Most PA programs are two years in length with the added requirement of at least two years of college and some health care experience. For licensure, all states require PAs to complete an accredited, formal education program and to pass the Physician Assistant National Certifying Examination administered by the National Commission on Certification of Physician Assistants (NCCPA). The examination is available only to graduates of an accredited PA education program. Upon successful completion of the examination, the credential "Physician Assistant-Certified" can be used.

THE VALUE OF THE MEDICAL ASSISTANT TO THE HEALTH CARE TEAM

With their broad range of competencies in both administrative and clinical areas, medical assistants are increasingly valued as health care team members. Medical assistants are the great communicators, serving as liaison between provider and hospital staff and between provider and any number of allied and other health professionals. Because they often are the first providers to see or speak with patients, they undertake responsibility for directing, informing, and guiding patient care while establishing a professional and caring tone for the entire health care team. The value of a competent, professional, compassionate medical assistant is immeasurable in today's fast-paced and challenging health care environment.

Case Study 2-1

Review the scenario at the beginning of the chapter.

CASE STUDY REVIEW

1. Where will you research additional information on being a physical therapy assistant?
2. Compare the working hours, rate of pay, contact with patients, required schooling, and job availability to those of the medical assistant.
3. If other health professions discussed in the chapter are of special interest to you, answer the same questions. This review helps to clarify the position of the medical assistant for you.

Case Study 2-2

You are the medical assistant for a family practice provider, Bill Claredon, who is close to retirement. He is much adored by all his patients, but he thinks alternative medicine is outright quackery. Marjorie Johns, a patient with debilitating back pain, tells you she is seeing an acupuncturist and is taking less and less of her prescribed medications. You quietly mention that to Dr. Claredon before he enters the examination room to see Marjorie. He glares at you with disgust at the information and is quite agitated when he enters the examination room.

CASE STUDY REVIEW

1. Describe the discussion that you think will occur between Dr. Claredon and Marjorie.
2. If Marjorie is unhappy when she is ready to leave the facility, what can you do or say to help her?
3. What can you do to help Dr. Claredon?

SUMMARY

The health care environment is a dynamic service that changes rapidly in response to new technology and societal needs. In an effort to provide quality care to the most individuals at a reasonable cost, some form of managed care likely will dominate the health care industry for years to come. A strong health care team is critical in the health care setting, as primary care providers, specialists of all disciplines, alternative care practitioners, and allied and other health professionals collaborate on the best way to provide integrative medicine and quality patient care. In almost any health care environment, but especially the ambulatory care setting, the medical assistant is a vital link in the team and is responsible for a range of responsibilities, both clinical and administrative.

STUDY FOR SUCCESS

To reinforce your knowledge and skills of information presented in this chapter:

- Review the Key Terms
- Consider the Case Studies and discuss your conclusions
- Answer the Review Questions
  - Multiple Choice
  - Critical Thinking
- Navigate the Internet and complete the Web Activities
- Practice the StudyWARE activities on the textbook CD
- Apply your knowledge in the Student Workbook activities
- Complete the Web Tutor sections
- View and discuss the DVD situations

REVIEW QUESTIONS

Multiple Choice

1. Medical assistants are mostly employed in:
   a. hospitals
   b. nursing facilities
   c. ambulatory care settings
   d. insurance companies
2. A health maintenance organization is one kind of:
   a. managed care operation
   b. individual practice
   c. sole proprietorship
   d. hospital
3. With its emphasis on controlling costs, managed care is likely to affect:
   a. only hospitals
   b. all health care settings
   c. only providers in private practice
   d. only patients
4. The health care team:
   a. should exclude the patient as part of the team
   b. is only important in the hospital setting
   c. is made up of physicians and nurses
   d. includes physicians, nurses, allied health care professionals, patients, and integrative medicine practitioners
5. Integrative health care approaches:
   a. are increasingly accepted as complementary to traditional health care
   b. are always covered by insurance
   c. are seldom approved for licensure
   d. are not important to understand
6. A medical assistant permitted by law to draw blood for diagnostic laboratory testing performs a procedure similar to those performed by a:
   a. health unit coordinator
   b. health information technician
   c. phlebotomist
   d. respiratory therapist
7. The "boutique" or "concierge" medical practice:
   a. is another form of managed care
   b. allows patients special privileges in their health care
   c. is covered by all major insurance plans
   d. does not require special fees for services

8. Providers just establishing their practice often seek to work with another provider in the same field. When expenses and profits are shared, this form of management is called a/an:
   a. HMO
   b. corporation
   c. sole proprietor
   d. group or partnership
9. Which of the following will the medical assistant *not* do in health care?
   a. code and bill insurance, bookkeeping
   b. diagnose and treat ailments
   c. screen when making appointments
   d. assist provider, perform clinical and laboratory procedures
10. An alternative approach to medicine that treats patients using thin, flexible needles is called:
    a. acupuncture
    b. naturopathy
    c. chiropractic
    d. homeopathy

Critical Thinking

1. Evaluate the different health care settings and discuss the pros and cons of working in each setting.
2. From a patient's point of view, which health care setting do you think offers the most benefits? Why?
3. Review the three forms of medical management models. Which is probably the most advantageous from the provider's point of view? From the medical assistant's point of view? Justify your responses.
4. Recall a few types of allied health professionals and, working in small groups, create scenarios in which the medical assistant needs to coordinate patient care with two or three allied professionals.
5. Identify as many reasons as you can for why patients might be seeking alternative approaches to traditional medicine. Explain your choices.
6. Compare Doctors of Osteopathy and Chiropractic. When and why might one be selected over the other?
7. Discuss the validity of licensure or national certification for health care practitioners.

WEB ACTIVITIES

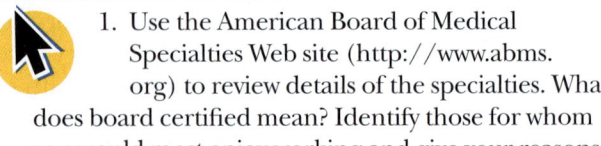

1. Use the American Board of Medical Specialties Web site (http://www.abms.org) to review details of the specialties. What does board certified mean? Identify those for whom you would most enjoy working and give your reasons.
2. Scan the Natural Healers Web site (http://www.naturalhealers.com) for a listing of alternative therapy modalities. Select one modality and identify the schools/colleges where education is available and what kind of credentialing is necessary to practice the modality.
3. American Osteopathic Association (http://www.osteopathic.org): After you visit this Web site, discuss the role of the osteopath as a primary care provider in today's health care structure.
4. If you have doubts about alternative medicine, you might want to view the following Web site: http://www.quackwatch.org. Click on "Whats new?" It is helpful to research as many thoughts on a subject as possible. Examine the validity of the Web site and whether any biases are evident.

REFERENCES/BIBLIOGRAPHY

American Board of Medical Specialties. (2006). *Approved ABMS specialty boards & certificate categories.* Evanston, IL: Author.

Bondurant, S. (2005). Mainstream and alternative medicine: Converging paths require common standards. *Annals of Internal Medicine, 142*(2), 149–150.

Eisenberg, D. M., Cohen, M. H., Hrbek, A., Grayzel, J., Van Rompay, M. I., & Cooper, R. A. (2002). Credentialing complementary and alternative medical providers. *Annals of Internal Medicine, 137*(12), 965–973.

Frenkel, M. A., & Borkan, J. M. (2003). An approach for integrating complementary-alternative medicine into primary care. *Family Practice, 20*(3), 324–332.

Health professions career & education directory (2007–2008). Chicago, IL: American Medical Association.

Sansweet, J. B. (2005). Choosing the right practice entity. *Family Practice Management, 12*(10), 42–49.

Tamparo, C. D., & Lewis, M. A. (2005). *Diseases of the human body* (4th ed.). Philadelphia: F. A. Davis Publishers.

THE DVD HOOK-UP

This chapter discusses various types of medical specialties and the importance of choosing a career path that is right for you. You also learned about the role of the medical assistant and the importance of being a team player.

In the scene "Preparing for a Job Interview," we observe Dee writing to her teacher and sharing her accomplishments after graduation. Dee determined that certification was essential to climbing the ladder of success as a medical assistant. Dee also used good critical thinking skills in establishing what specialty area would work best for her individual circumstances.

1. What are some of the individual circumstances that influenced Dee to accept a position in pediatrics?
2. We can see that Dee has really made progress in taking the necessary steps toward becoming a professional. Would you say that Dee is perfect at this point? Are you perfect? Will you ever be perfect? Why is it important to work on your professional skills while you are still in school?

DVD Journal Summary

After watching the designated scene from program 1, write a paragraph in your journal that summarizes what you learned from watching this scene. Are you interested in any specialty areas? What are some short- and long-term goals that you are interested in achieving after graduation?

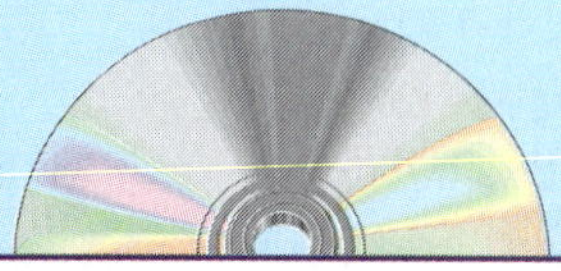

DVD Series	**Program Number**
Critical Thinking	1

Chapter/Scene Reference
- *Preparing for a Job Interview*

Chapter

3

History of Medicine

OUTLINE

OBJECTIVES

The student should strive to meet the following performance objectives and demonstrate an understanding of the facts and principles presented in this chapter through written and oral communication.

1. Define the key terms as presented in the glossary.
2. Discuss the effects of culture on medicine.
3. Identify the role of religion, magic, and science in medicine's history.
4. Describe how attitudes toward illness are manifested today.
5. Identify a minimum of three previously used common medical treatments.
6. Recall a minimum of three theories/practices of ancient medicine that are still prevalent today.
7. Name and describe the historical roles of medical specialists.
8. Describe three major epidemics and their impact on medical care.
9. Discuss the role of women in medicine.
10. Trace the progression of medical education.
11. Name at least five significant contributions to medicine.
12. Identify a minimum of three recent developments in medicine.

KEY TERMS

Allopathic
Asepsis
Bubonic Plague
Malaria
Moxibustion
Opiates
Pharmacopoeia
Pluralistic (Pluralism)
Septicemia
Trephination
Typhus (Typhoid)
Yellow Fever

Scenario

You may recall your mom putting a mentholated salve on your chest when you had a cold. Your cousins had to take a spoonful of cod-liver oil each night before they went to bed. Grandma made chicken soup with homemade noodles when you had the flu. An apple a day, mustard plaster for the chest, hot or cold steam in a room, and many more are medical practices of years gone by. Many still stand, however, and from them others have developed. Interestingly, medicine has a rich history, and every culture exhibits that history differently. The more you know and understand of that history and its various cultural influences, the more effective and therapeutic will be your communication with patients.

INTRODUCTION

The historical development of medicine has been driven by many and varied events. These include the presence of illness and injury, plagues and widespread epidemics, the dissection first of animals and then of human bodies, the discovery of bacteria, and the experimentation with herbs and potions for medicinal purposes. Medicine as it is known today is the result of multiple revolutions of thought throughout the world. The history of medicine must remind us that more than one discipline and more than one philosophy have contributed to medicine. This is perhaps more true now than ever as our world becomes smaller and our society becomes increasingly **pluralistic,** *ethnically, culturally, and religiously.*

CULTURAL HERITAGE IN MEDICINE

Today's health professional will give care to individuals of varied cultures who hold differing philosophical beliefs toward medicine. The informed and caring health professional will recognize that a person's culture and ethnic heritage play an enormous role in any kind of health care. For example, if the patient's culture and history lean toward a more natural, nonmedical form of health care, treating the patient with prescription drugs will necessitate a careful explanation and rationale for the use of medications. Otherwise, the patient may refuse to take all or part of the medications, thus hindering recovery. It would be better to seek a treatment for the patient that embraces both the health care professional's desire to heal and the individual's wish to respect cultural tradition.

In every society, medicine has been an important element for its people. From the earliest time, culture was an important influence on medicine, and modern day medicine is in many ways a reflection of this diverse and rich heritage.

It is certain that religion, magic, and science all played a vital part in the history of medicine. Religion was important because it was perceived that certain gods were to be called on for a cure through ceremonies, prayers, and sacrifices. Magic was practiced because it was such an important part of many societies and was seen as an essential ingredient to chase away evil spirits. The importance of science was demonstrated in the use of plants and minerals for medicinal purposes that is found throughout medicine's history. Unearthed clay tablets reveal hundreds of plants, minerals, and animal substances used for medicinal purposes in ancient Mesopotamia and Babylon. The Chinese **pharmacopoeia** was rich in the use of herbs.

Skeletal remains of prehistoric cultures show advanced stages of arthritis, a nearly toothless jaw, and only a 20- to 40-year life span for humans. Skull bones reveal round holes referred to as **trephination,** believed necessary to release the evil spirits thought to be causing a person's illness. Mesopotamian cultures believed that illness was a punishment by the gods for violation of a moral code. Ancient Egyptians believed the body was a system of channels for air, tears, blood, urine, sperm, and feces. All the channels were thought to come together in the rectum and were believed to become easily clogged. Thus, emetics, enemas, and purges of the anus were common treatments. In ancient India, punishment for adultery was cutting off the nose, therefore allowing practitioners many opportunities to practice and refine the art of nose reconstruction or plastic surgery.

The ancient Chinese cultures examined and carefully monitored the pulse in each wrist. It was believed that the pulse had hundreds of characteristics important in medical treatment. There were five methods of treatment to bring a person back to the right track. They were:

1. Cure the spirit.
2. Nourish the body.
3. Give medications.
4. Treat the whole body.
5. Use acupuncture and moxibustion.

Acupuncture is the piercing of the skin by very thin, sterile, flexible needles into any of 365 points along 12 meridians that transverse the body and transmit the active life force called "qi" (pronounced "chee") (Figure 3-1). Each of these spots is related to a particular organ. **Moxibustion** requires the use of a powdered plant substance that is made into a small mound on the person's skin and then burned, usually raising a blister.

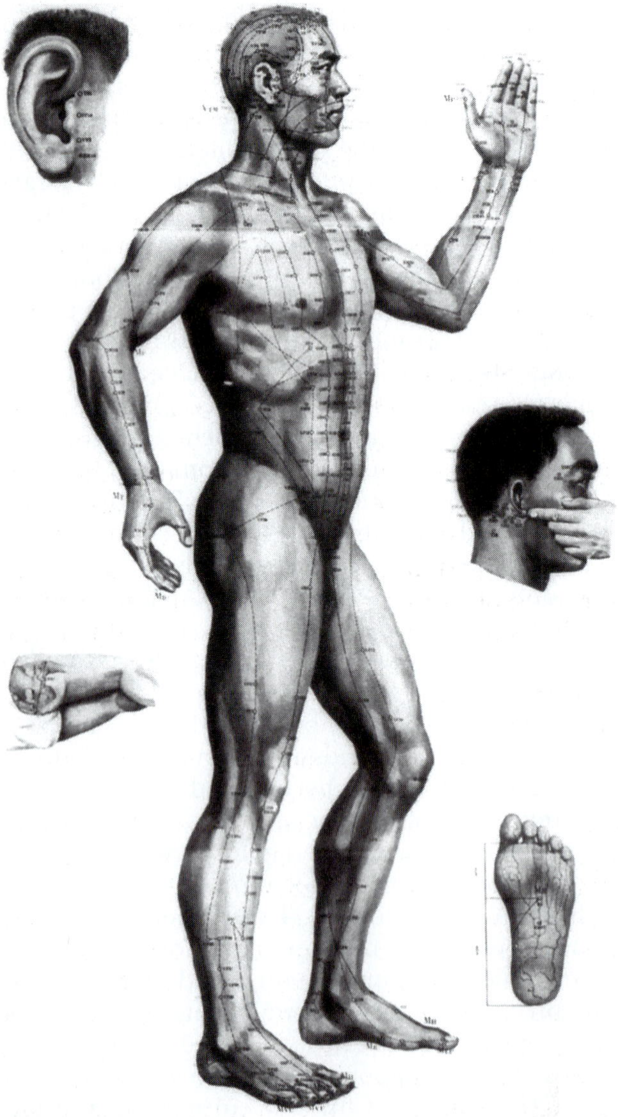

Figure 3-1 Chinese acupuncture points and meridians. (Courtesy of the World Health Organization.)

Even today's **allopathic,** or traditional, practitioners would agree that the first four methods of treatment from Chinese culture are excellent guidelines for health care. There also is new awareness that acupuncture has a valid place in allopathic medicine, not only for the control of some types of pain but for treating some illnesses. A type of moxibustion can be used today with acupuncture treatment. There are many different techniques for moxibustion in which varying substances are used to apply heat to a broad area of the skin. The intense direct heating of points is used to treat some diseases, to relax tense muscles, and to gently relieve aching and mild pain without making skin blisters.

MEDICAL SPECIALISTS IN HISTORY

Medicine's history gives early evidence of many "specialists" in the healing arts. They were known by various names—witch doctors, medicine men and women, shamans or healing priests, and physicians. These healers were more than ancestors of the modern practitioner, however, for they performed many functions that involved the welfare of the entire community or village. By today's standards, they were considered to be equivalent to spiritual advisers, social workers, counselors, and teachers.

These medical specialists were among the world's earliest professionals. They were present at important "rites of passage," such as births and deaths, puberty initiations, and marriages. The role of the healers varied among cultures, but central to all cultures was the belief that the healers had the ability to draw upon some power beyond themselves. Their goal was to help others live and work in harmony with nature and each other.

Evidence also suggests that many ancient healers used a variety of mind-altering drugs. A mythical drug called "soma" is reported in India's religious literature. Primitive tribes of Central, South, and North America used "yage" and "peyote" to induce trance-like experiences. Many ancient healers also practiced certain types of what today might be called yoga and meditation.

These healers were given special status in their culture. Sometimes they were recognized by their dress and the pouch or satchel they carried. They were not expected to work, and their needs were supplied by the members of their tribe. Much later, when medical education was available, a healer was called "physician" if a university degree was held. Surgeons were part of a lower class because they usually had only apprentice training and included the group of barbering surgeons who used their razors to cut into blood vessels to relieve infection and fever.

Today the more common term "provider" or "practitioner" is often used because there are so many health professionals who are a part of the patient's health care team.

From the earliest times, it appears that some payment was expected for medical services rendered. In many instances, the payment was dependent on the status of the practitioner, as well as the patient. At the same time, some cultures punished a practitioner who was not successful in treatment by forcing that practitioner to treat only those too poor to pay.

HISTORY OF MEDICAL EDUCATION

During the rise of Christianity, emphasis was placed on the soul rather than the body; therefore, early Christian monks held great control over medicine. This is evidenced by St. Benedict of Nursia (480–554), who forbade the study of medicine. The care of the sick was encouraged, but only through prayer and divine intervention. Thus, Christ's healing mission was institutionalized in a fashion that was to control medical care almost completely for the next 500 years, until the seventh century.

At that time the religion of Islam moved to preserve the classical learning that had been achieved in medicine, and practitioners were not only able to return to the same methods as those practiced by earlier Greek and Roman cultures, but medical study was now encouraged.

Medical education in established universities began in the ninth century. These universities included Salerno in southern Italy, the University of Montpelier in southern France, and the University of Paris. By the time the Renaissance was at its height in the midfifteenth century, the practitioner had become licensed, was receiving great status, and was attending the ill in a velvet bonnet and fur-trimmed cloak.

Art and science were more closely related during the Renaissance than at any other period. Michelangelo (1475–1564) spent years on careful human dissection, and this anatomical detail is evident in his paintings in the Sistine Chapel in the Vatican in Rome. Leonardo da Vinci (1452–1519) made anatomical preparations from which he produced drawings representing the skeletal, muscular, nervous, and vascular systems. His accurate sketch of the spinal vertebrae went undiscovered for more than 100 years.

HISTORY OF ATTITUDES TOWARD ILLNESS

Various attitudes prevailed toward the ill person. A sick person might be excused from daily activity but was likely to be shunned if the disease was believed to be a punishment by the gods for mortal sin. This forced isolation may well have been beneficial to the community. In contrast, touching by Jesus was an important component of healing, as was the faith of the individual involved. The New Testament parable of the Good Samaritan helped establish a nexus between the early church and a concern for the sick. It was believed that though the body might be wasted and foul with disease, the purity of the soul guaranteed life everlasting. This was unlike the pagan religions that tended to abandon individuals thought to be ill because they were in disfavor with the gods.

Native Americans had various feelings about illness. The ill were treated with kindness among the Navaho and Cherokee, and some who recovered from serious illness were considered to have extraordinary powers. However, if a tribe was faced with famine, suicide by the aged and infirm was considered the highest form of bravery. The Eskimos put their older adults unprotected onto ice floes. Neither the Romans nor the Greeks treated the hopelessly ill or deformed, and unwanted infants were disposed of quickly or left to die.

Some of these attitudes are seen even today. The Western medical community and the consumers it serves are heatedly debating the right to choose life or death and the ethics and legality of physician-assisted death, which is acceptable in many other cultures. Even with our vast knowledge of medicine and the disease process, many individuals are still fearful of any illness they do not understand or that they perceive as threatening their health—AIDS is a good example. This fear is often accompanied by public ill treatment of the individuals suffering from certain diseases. For example, until 1993, Cuba quarantined everyone who tested positive for human immunodeficiency

Critical Thinking

What steps are taken today in hospitals and in ambulatory care settings to prevent the spread of harmful bacteria and viruses? Name the antibiotic-resistant bacteria that plagues hospitals today. What steps do you personally take?

virus (HIV) infection, even if they showed no signs of illness. Since that time, Cuba requires individuals who test positive for HIV to spend at least 3 months in one of Cuba's 17 AIDS sanitariums, where they learn how to live with HIV and protect others from infection. The sanitarium model places emphasis on preventive care rather than acute care and on early diagnosis and treatment. It is reported that HIV infection in Cuba affects only 0.1% of adults aged 15 to 49 years. According to *HIV/AIDS in the Caribbean: Issues and Options,* that incidence is very low compared to other Caribbean cultures reported to have an HIV infection rate of 2%, or as high as 12% in Haiti.

HISTORICAL MEDICAL TREATMENTS

The writings of ancient Egypt reveal that when a woman suspected she was pregnant, she urinated over a mixture of wheat and barley seeds combined with dates and sand. If any of the grains sprouted, she was surely pregnant. If the wheat grew, she would have a boy. If the barley grew, it would be a girl. Urine is still used in modern tests to determine pregnancy.

During the Ming dynasty (1368–1644), Chinese medicine seemed to reach its peak. This is the time that Li Shih-chen wrote his Pen ts'ao kang mu, "The Great Herbal." This pharmacopoeia summarizes what was known of herbal medicine up to the late sixteenth century, describing in detail more than 1,800 plants, animal substances, minerals, and metals, together with their medicinal properties and applications.

Early medical treatments were often crude. For a sore throat, a practitioner might mix barley water, vinegar, and mulberry syrup for a gargle. Someone suffering with rheumatism might be given a prescription of chopped mice, lynx claws, and elk hooves. Rhubarb, senna, bitter apple, turpentine, camphor, and mercury were among the practitioners' staples. Some practitioners washed the instruments used in treating the ill; others scoffed at such a practice. **Malaria,** diphtheria, tuberculosis, **typhoid,** and dysentery were commonplace. Leprosy was prevalent, and venereal diseases were rife. Smallpox was frequent in villages; sometimes the sufferer would be placed in a meat pickling vat and fumigated. The death toll from such diseases was particularly high among children. Finally, in the eighteenth century, Edward Jenner made a great contribution to the prevention of disease by discovering a method of vaccination against smallpox.

Medicine progressed rapidly during the nineteenth century. Two important discoveries occurred: anesthesia to alleviate pain during surgery, and the realization that some bacteria cause disease. Once it had been proved that certain bacteria were causes of diseases and were transmissible agents responsible for contagion, greater care was taken to prevent that transmission. **Asepsis** became important to reduce the risk for infection. The Hungarian physician and obstetrician Ignaz Philipp Semmelweis (1818–1865) was able to prove that physicians who came from an autopsy directly to the care of postpartum women, without scrubbing their hands and washing instruments, carried infection with them that often caused puerperal fever (**septicemia** after childbirth) and death to the new mothers.

The names of Louis Pasteur (1822–1895), Joseph Lister (1827–1912), and Robert Koch (1843–1910) are familiar to all bacteriologists. Louis Pasteur has sometimes been referred to as the father of preventive medicine as the result of his work in recognizing the relationship between bacteria and infectious disease (Figure 3-2). Joseph Lister revolutionized surgery because of his belief in Pasteur's theory of using carbolic acid as an antiseptic spray. He insisted that all instruments and physicians' hands be washed with the solution. Robert Koch used the culture-plate method for isolating bacteria and demonstrated how cholera was transmitted by food and water. His discovery changed the way health departments cared for persons with infectious disease.

Fortunately, early in the twentieth century, society was finally liberated from many of the infectious and epidemic diseases that had scourged the human race for millennia. Smallpox vaccinations became common, causes of **yellow fever, typhus,** and **bubonic plague** were determined, and appropriate measures were taken to eradicate the diseases. Life expectancy increased. Tuberculosis became less frequent. In 1922, Frederick G. Banting and a medical student, Charles Best, were able to isolate and inject insulin into a 14-year-old boy who was dying of diabetes. Two weeks later, the boy was

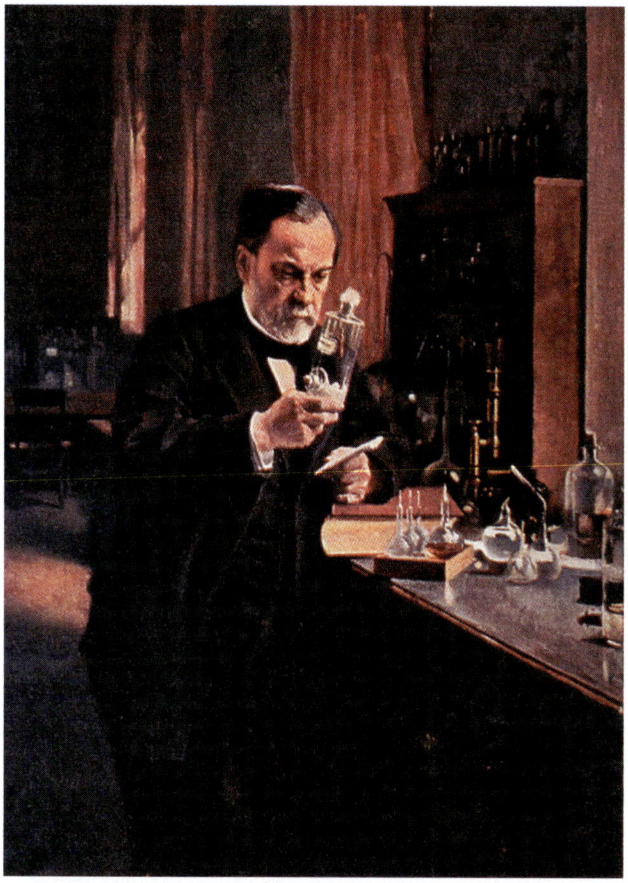

Figure 3-2 Louis Pasteur, known for his recognition of the relationship between bacteria and infectious disease.

alive and alert. By 1923, insulin was available for general sale in pharmacies throughout the world. Antibiotics were discovered and the Salk and Sabin vaccines were found for poliomyelitis.

The first electrocardiogram machine was invented in 1903. George Papanicolaou discovered cancer cells in 1928, the same year penicillin was discovered by Alexander Fleming. Penicillin, however, required further development, which was accomplished by Howard Florey and Ernst Chain, and was finally brought into production in 1945. C. Walton Lillehei performed the first successful open-heart surgery in 1952. Dr. Christian Barnard performed the first human heart transplant in 1967. Advancing technology enabled medicine to march steadily forward.

The Scourge of Epidemics

There is a saying, "Two steps forward—one step back." At the same time giant strides are made in medicine for one disease, the battle rages for eradication of another. What follows is a discussion of three diseases that have caused much fear in our world, are still a great concern throughout the world, and are still a challenge for medical research.

Paralytic Poliomyelitis. Paralytic poliomyelitis, a virus spread through the fecal–oral route, multiplies in the intestine and invades the nervous system. It is often referred to as infantile paralysis. It mostly affects children under the age of 5 years, and there is no cure.

A 3,000-year-old Egyptian stone carving indicates the presence of the virus in ancient times. There is evidence of polio outbreaks occurring during the summer months in the late 1890s in the U.S. During the Great Depression of the 1930s and into the 1950s, infantile paralysis was greatly feared. It struck mostly children, resulted in crippling paralysis within hours, and sometimes caused death. Children were hospitalized and isolated in polio wards. Children were kept from swimming pools and public playgrounds and were reminded not to get too tired or chilled. A practitioner was called if headache, fever, sore throat, stiff neck, or aching muscles occurred.

Those individuals with bulbar polio, a poliomyelitis that affected nerve cells in the medulla oblongata or the lowest portion of the brainstem responsible for regulating heart rate, breathing, and blood pressure, were placed in iron lungs. Iron lungs worked by creating an airtight seal around individuals placed on their backs so that only their heads were visible. A pump alternately raised and lowered the air pressure inside to fill and deflate the lungs, forcing the body to simulate breathing (Figure 3-3). Lying in the iron lung,

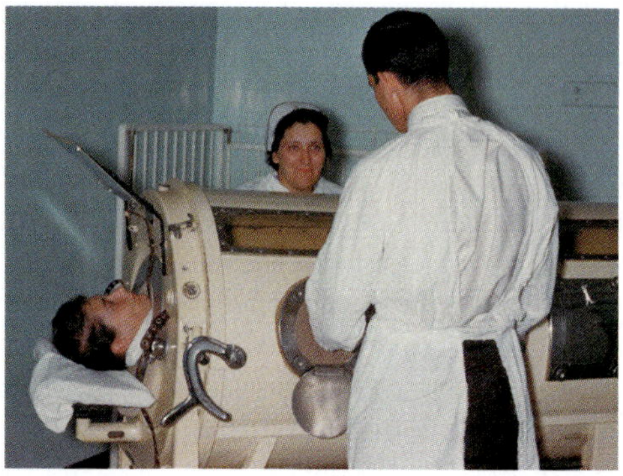

Figure 3-3 A doctor and nurse with a patient in an iron lung during the Rhode Island polio epidemic, 1960. (Courtesy of the Centers for Disease Control and Prevention.)

individuals were fully dependent on their caregivers, relying entirely for their view of the world on a mirror suspended above their face and angled toward the rest of the room.

President Franklin D. Roosevelt, diagnosed with polio in 1921, waged war on the disease. He funded polio research that eventually led to a vaccine. Roosevelt founded the National Foundation for Infantile Paralysis, which later became known as the March of Dimes. Children throughout the U.S. placed dimes in card folders to take to school to donate to a cure for polio. Dr. Jonas Salk developed the first polio vaccine in 1952, and Dr. Albert Sabin developed an oral polio vaccine in 1961. In 1979 the last case of polio in the United States was reported. Scientists knew that children could have lifelong protection from polio with the polio vaccine given multiple times.

Worldwide, however, polio was still a major problem. Many agencies, including Rotary International, the World Health Organization (WHO), United Nations International Children's Emergency Fund (UNICEF), and the U.S. Centers for Disease Control and Prevention (CDC), established programs to vaccinate the world's children. For 20 years, the incidences of polio decreased all around the world. The WHO had hoped to announce in 2005 that polio had disappeared from the world. Instead, out of fear and superstition, leaders of a few nations began to counsel against the polio vaccine. They told mothers the vaccine would make their children infertile and infect them with HIV. Unfortunately, in December 2007, there were still 992 cases of polio diagnosed in the world.

Cancer. Cancer was an affliction long before polio was first evidenced. The earliest specimen of cancer was noted in the remains of a skull dated in the Bronze Age (1900–1600 B.C.). The writings of Hippocrates describe cancers of many body sites. In the nineteenth century, the pathology of cancer was viewed with a microscope, and metastasis was first understood. It was believed that cancer growth was like planting seeds to be carried through the bloodstream into another organ that was hospitable.

Researchers first believed that cancer resulted from excess bile collecting in various body sites. Some believed cancer was the result of fermenting and deteriorating lymph fluid. Today, trauma, chronic irritation, and viral and cellular derivations are considered the primary causes of cancer.

Cancer is often removed through surgery. Radiation and/or chemotherapy may also be used to rid the body of the disease. Today an individual's DNA structure is considered in treatment. Chemotherapy drugs are matched to the specific genetic code of an individual, can be designed to prevent blood vessel growth from surrounding tissue to a solid tumor, or can prevent cancer cells from multiplying and invading other tissues. Recently it was discovered that cancers contain stem cells that produce other cancer cells. Research now turns to identifying markers specific to these stem cells and to creating therapies that can eliminate the reproducing stem cells.

Even with the many years of research and the millions of dollars spent to cure cancer, nearly 1.5 million new cancers are diagnosed every year in the U.S., and more than half a million people will die of cancer each year.

HIV Infection/AIDS. In 1981, a rare cancer outbreak known as Kaposi sarcoma was seen in young gay men in New York and California. In addition, increased cases of a pneumonia called pneumocystitis were reported among the same demographic group. The CDC later coined the term AIDS (acquired immune deficiency syndrome). In 1981, 1,600 cases of AIDS were reported, with close to 700 deaths. As the death rate soared in the next few years, researchers sought the cause of and a cure for the disease. In 1984 the human immunodeficiency virus (HIV) was discovered to be the cause of AIDS.

HIV is a virus that slowly destroys the body's immune system, thus making an individual much more susceptible to infection and other illnesses. There is no cure for AIDS, but with prompt and aggressive treatment, individuals with HIV are living long and productive lives. HIV can be transmitted through bodily fluids during sexual contact; by sharing contaminated needles to inject drugs; by accidental sticks or pokes from HIV-contaminated needles; by transfusion of infected blood products (rare since 1992); and from mother to baby during pregnancy, delivery, and breast-feeding (greatly reduced in the last few years).

Any life-altering, life-threatening disease is a challenge, but HIV infection and AIDS come with awareness that some in society will condemn and shun those infected. Education in the United States has done much to calm the nerves and erase some of the fear infected individuals face from those who would condemn.

In 2006, the CDC reported that HIV and AIDS had claimed the lives of more than 22 million persons worldwide, including more than 500,000 persons in the United States. In 2007, more than 1 million persons were living with HIV/AIDS in the United States, and an estimated 40,000 new HIV infections were expected to occur. Although HIV infection and AIDS cases show decline in the

U.S., there are still serious challenges to be met. A large majority of infected persons are unaware they are infected and are passing the virus on to others. Three quarters of new infections in women in the U.S. are heterosexually transmitted. Cultural differences sometimes create difficulty in preventing the disease if condoms are frowned upon or men have multiple heterosexual partners at the same time they are having sex with other men. Of the 33 million people currently living with HIV/AIDS, 74% live in sub-Saharan Africa. It is estimated that by the year 2010, Ethiopia, Nigeria, China, India, and Russia will add 50 to 75 million new cases of HIV/AIDS to the statistics.

AIDS causes serious and debilitating physical and mental difficulties. The United Nations estimates that by the year 2010, 25 million children will be orphaned due to the death of both parents from AIDS.

Early in the twenty-first century, we are still quite aware of the limitations of modern medicine. In developing countries torn with war and strife, cholera causes the deaths of thousands simply because there is no proper sanitation. In the microbial world, new, drug-resistant strains of malaria, tuberculosis, and other diseases are not responding to known treatments. Health professionals in hospitals and health care facilities, especially nursing homes and dialysis centers, are very much aware of a new type of bacteria known as methicillin-resistant staphylococcus aureus (MRSA), which is resistant to many antibiotics. This infection is especially dangerous to individuals with weakened immune systems. It can come from medical facilities or be community based. The latter can be found in athletic locker rooms and in other areas where large numbers of individuals congregate. The use of antibiotics completely changed medicine by providing the ability to cure bacterial-related disease. However, bacteria have now evolved to be resistant to those antibiotics. This is another example of the earlier statement, "Two steps forward—one step back." The challenge of medicine is as strong today as it was 100 years ago.

SIGNIFICANT CONTRIBUTIONS TO MEDICINE

Hippocrates (c. 460–c. 377 B.C.) is the physician most frequently recalled from the Greek culture. It is not known why his name surfaces above all other Greek physicians, for some were surely just as prominent. His writings, however, have contributed much to today's medical culture. Hippocrates is remembered by many for his well-known Hippocratic Oath, which established guidelines for a physician's practice of medicine (Figure 3-4). Although few physicians swear to this oath today when they embark on their medical career, it is still recognized for its validity and wisdom. There are various translations of the Hippocratic Oath, but all communicate the same fundamental message.

It would be impossible to identify all the other individuals who made significant contributions to medicine in this text. However, Table 3-1 lists several notable individuals in the history of medicine.

THE OATH OF HIPPOCRATES

I swear by Apollo Physician and Aesculapius and Hygeia and Panacea and all the gods and goddesses, making them my witnesses, that I will fulfill according to my ability and judgment this oath and this covenant:

To hold him who has taught me this art as equal to my parents and to live my life in partnership with him, and if he is in need of money to give him a share of mine, and to regard his offspring as equal to my brothers in male lineage and to teach them this art—if they desire to learn it—without fee and covenant; to give a share of precepts and oral instruction and all the other learning to my sons and to the sons of him who has instructed me and to pupils who have signed the covenant and have taken an oath according to the medical law, but to no one else.

I will apply dietetic measures for the benefit of the sick according to my ability and judgment; I will keep them from harm and injustice.

I will neither give a deadly drug to anybody if asked for it nor will I make a suggestion to this effect. Similarly, I will not give to a woman an abortive remedy. In purity and holiness I will guard my life and my art.

I will not use the knife, not even on sufferers from stone, but will withdraw in favor of such men as are engaged in this work.

Whatever houses I may visit, I will come for the benefit of the sick, remaining free of all intentional injustice, of all mischief, and in particular of sexual relations with both female and male persons, be they free or slaves.

Figure 3-4 The Hippocratic Oath.

Table 3-1 Important Persons And Events In The History Of Medicine

Moses (1205 B.C.)	Advocate of health rules in Hebrew religion
1000 B.C.	Beginnings of ancient Chinese medicine
Hippocrates (460–377 B.C.)	Greek physician; "father of medicine"
Chang Chung-ching (168–196)	Chinese physician; called the Hippocrates of China
1368–1644	Chinese medicine reaches its peak
Andreas Vesalius (1514–1564)	Brussels physician; wrote first anatomical studies
Anton van Leeuwenhoek (1632–1723)	Dutch lens grinder; discovered lens magnification
John Hunter (1728–1793)	Founder of scientific surgery
Edward Jenner (1749–1823)	Developed smallpox vaccine
Rene Laennec (1781–1826)	Invented the stethoscope
Samuel Hahnemann (1755–1843)	German physician; established homeopathy
Ignaz Semmelweis (1818–1865)	Introduced hand washing to prevent childbed fever
W. T. G. Morton (1819–1868)	U.S. physician; introduced ether as anesthetic
Louis Pasteur (1822–1895)	"Father of bacteriology"
Florence Nightingale (1820–1910)	Founder of modern nursing
Elizabeth Blackwell (1821–1910)	First female physician in the United States
Clara Barton (1821–1912)	Started the American Red Cross in 1881
Joseph Lister (1827–1912)	Laid the groundwork on asepsis
Andrew Taylor (1828–1917)	Established the first school of osteopathy in 1892
Daniel David Palmer (1845–1913)	Founded chiropractic profession in Iowa in 1895
Elizabeth G. Anderson (1836–1917)	First female physician in Great Britain
Frederick G. Banting (1891–1941)	Isolated and injected insulin for diabetes treatment in 1922
1903	First electrocardiogram machine invented
Robert Koch (1843–1910)	Bacteriologist; developed culture-plate method
Wilhelm Roentgen (1845–1923)	Discovered X-rays (roentgenograms)

(continues)

Table 3-1 (continued)

George Papanicolaou (1883–1962)	Discovered cancer cells in 1928
Sir Alexander Fleming (1881–1955)	Discovered penicillin in 1928
Albert Schatz (1920–2005)	Discovered streptomycin in 1943; cure for tuberculosis
1945	Penicillin brought into production
Paul Zoll (1911–1999)	Created the first heart pacemaker in 1952
C. Walton Lillehei (1918–1999)	Performed first successful open-heart surgery in 1952
John Gibbon (1903–1973)	First heart–lung machine used for surgery (1953)
Joseph Murray (1919–)	Performed first person-to-person kidney transplant in 1954
Christian Barnard (1922–2001)	Performed first human heart transplant in 1967
Ian Wilmut (1944–)	Cloned a Finn Dorset sheep called Dolly in 1996
1953	Three-dimensional structure of DNA discovered First human heart–lung bypass machine used on human
1950–1960	Vaccines against polio, measles, and rubella developed
1978	First baby born from in vitro fertilization
1982	Hepatitis B vaccine available
1990–2000	Human genome map created by team of scientists
1991	Women's Health Initiative begins 15-year research on cardiovascular disease, cancer, and osteoporosis
1995	Varicella (chickenpox) and hepatitis A vaccines available
2005	Combination vaccine for measles-mumps-rubella and varicella (MMRV) available
2006	Vaccine for adult shingles approved
2007	Diabetics using stem-cell therapy stop taking insulin Minimally invasive procedures performed • Surgeons at University of California/San Diego Medical Center remove diseased gallbladder through vagina • Surgeons at University of Texas Southwestern Medical Center remove diseased kidney through belly button

Note that only a few entries are made in the most recent years, not because no major medical discoveries are occurring, but because so many are occuring that they cannot all be listed.

Women in Medicine

Whereas women were accepted as healers in primitive societies, later cultures reduced their status to that of being allowed to care only for women and to assist in childbirth. In any culture that granted women only secondary status, women were also considered unqualified to become physicians. In Chinese culture, the first reference to a female physician mentioned by name is in documents from the Han dynasty (206 B.C.–A.D. 220). In Muslim society, the reluctance of Arabic physicians to violate social taboo and touch the genitals of female strangers further encouraged relegating the practice of obstetrics and gynecology to midwives.

Women were not accepted as medical physicians in Western culture until the nineteenth and twentieth centuries. Italy granted women the status earlier than other cultures. In the United States, the first female physician was Elizabeth Blackwell, who was awarded her degree in 1849. Although she was snubbed by the public, she soon earned the respect of her colleagues. When she refused to be absent from class when the male reproductive system was discussed, her fellow male students supported her actions.

In 1860 there were nearly 200 female practitioners in the U.S. In 2004, 26.8% of U.S. physicians were women, and there were ten female deans in U.S. medical schools. Today women are represented in all areas of medicine; however, the majority work in internal medicine, family practice, pediatrics, obstetrics/gynecology, psychiatry, and anesthesiology.

FRONTIERS IN MEDICINE

There has been phenomenal growth in medicine in the past two decades. Only a few advances are mentioned here. Much better imaging leading to much better diagnosis is now available. Where exploratory surgery might have been performed in the past to determine a diagnosis, noninvasive ultrasound, CT scans, and MRIs assist in diagnosis now. A 64-slice cardiac CT scan developed in 2004 can capture images of a human heart in just five heartbeats. In a technique known as volume computed tomography (VCT), the VCT system can perform a whole-body trauma scan in less than 10 seconds. People who have worn glasses or contact lenses for many years are turning to laser eye surgery and implantable lenses.

Surgeons have performed the first successful human larynx transplant. Consider the implications of the AIDS saliva test that creates a needle-free way to test for HIV. Needleless injections are now possible. There is a flu prevention inhaler and an osteoporosis pill.

Since 2000 there has been successful use of adult stem cells in the treatment of some diseases. Adult bone marrow stem cells are able to produce multiple tissues, and adult stem cells from various organs of the body have shown amazing abilities to develop into healthy tissue. Adult stem cells can be stimulated to form insulin-secreting pancreatic cells, to repair eye retinal damage, and to stimulate growth in children with bone disease. There is the possibility that adult stem cells will also be able to treat Parkinson's disease and other degenerating neural disorders. In the meantime, the political debate continues over the use of human embryonic stem cells.

A smooth plastic capsule with a tiny camera at each end, known as the PillCam ESO, is able to take as many as 2,600 pictures of the esophagus in less that 20 minutes. This marvel makes it easier to diagnose diseases of the esophagus without sedating a patient as is normally done in traditional endoscopy. Scientists are developing spider silk for extraordinarily fine sutures to be used in nerves and eyes. The combination of the all-encompassing broadband technology and new cellular infrastructure makes it easier for health professionals to stay in touch with patients. Medical Bluetooth makes an easy path for connection of medical devices. For example, remote heart-care diagnostics can be transmitted from a cell phone to providers who can determine if a patient needs to travel to the clinic for further care. Computer chips are being used to create bionic eyes for patients with advanced retinal degeneration, with implanted image sensors taking over the functions of damaged retinal cells.

Experimentation with aromatherapy indicates that some aromas actually improve brain function. Research has shown that individuals suffering from dementia often respond favorably to the odor of freshly roasted coffee and bread baking. Inhaling the scents of green apple, banana, and peppermint stimulates positive feelings. It is thought that with aromatherapy we will soon accelerate learning and speed up rehabilitation for people who have had a stroke.

The *British Journal of Psychiatry* recently reported that music therapy can be of value in individuals with schizophrenic illnesses. There also is evidence that music therapy can help to:

- Relieve treatment-related distress in individuals with cancer
- Calm individuals undergoing cardiac catheterization procedures
- Provide pain relief
- Decrease apathy in people with dementia

The American Music Therapy Association notes that extensive use of specifically chosen music during massage, acupuncture, yoga, and t'ai chi ch'uan enhances each type of practice. Some surgeons report better concentration and more relaxed patients when certain music is played during surgery.

Who can possibly predict what the future will bring in medicine?

Case Study 3-1

Refer to the scenario at the beginning of the chapter and recall two or three medical treatments or practices used in your family and culture.

CASE STUDY REVIEW

1. Were these medical treatments helpful? If so, how?
2. Is any part of these treatments still used today? If so, describe.
3. Discuss this case study with a friend or classmate.

Case Study 3-2

You are a male practitioner on call in your hospital's emergency department when a woman, 5 months pregnant, is brought in. She is hemorrhaging. Her husband shuns you and requests a female practitioner. You quickly realize this couple is Muslim. Role-play this scenario with a classmate.

CASE STUDY REVIEW

1. How can you solve the dilemma?
2. Consider the possibility that your only female practitioner is out of the country on vacation.

Case Study 3-3

Your employer, Dr. Anne Shea, an internist in Southern California, is considering renting office space to an acupuncturist and a naturopath because many of her patients often seek treatment from both. Dr. Shea believes her practice can be integrated, therefore allowing patients one-stop treatment for their illnesses. As the CMA (AAMA) and office manager, you are asked to participate in a meeting of all three practitioners to discuss guidelines for the clinic.

CASE STUDY REVIEW

1. What questions will you ask the group?
2. What will be necessary to get the word out to patients?

SUMMARY

Medicine's history leaves us with a rich heritage and a sound basis for the future of health care. Medical history continues to be in the making today. For example, research in gene manipulation has the potential benefit of being able to reverse the progression of many debilitating diseases. One day we will look on medical discoveries of this decade and be impressed by how much further medicine has advanced.

STUDY FOR SUCCESS

To reinforce your knowledge and skills of information presented in this chapter:

- Review the Key Terms
- Consider the Case Studies and discuss your conclusions
- Answer the Review Questions
  - Multiple Choice
  - Critical Thinking
- Navigate the Internet and complete the Web Activities
- Practice the StudyWARE activities on the textbook CD
- Apply your knowledge in the Student Workbook activities
- Complete the Web Tutor sections

REVIEW QUESTIONS

Multiple Choice

1. A pharmacopoeia is:
   a. a book describing drugs and their preparation
   b. an ancient religious rite used in medicine
   c. a source of magic
   d. used only by twentieth-century physicians
2. At one time, women were typically allowed to use their health care skills to:
   a. cure everyone in society
   b. care only for women and to assist in childbirth
   c. become physicians
   d. care only for older adults
3. An accurate sketch of the spinal vertebrae was created during the Renaissance by:
   a. Leonardo da Vinci
   b. Michelangelo
   c. early Christian monks
   d. Louis Pasteur
4. Hippocrates is a Greek physician often called:
   a. the founder of scientific surgery
   b. the inventor of the smallpox vaccine
   c. the father of medicine
   d. the father of preventive medicine
5. The first woman physician in the United States was:
   a. Florence Nightingale
   b. Clara Barton
   c. Elizabeth Anderson
   d. Elizabeth Blackwell
6. The physician who introduced hand washing to prevent childbed fever was:
   a. Joseph Lister
   b. John Hunter
   c. Ignaz Semmelweis
   d. Edward Jenner
7. Medicine was greatly influenced by:
   a. Greek and Chinese physicians
   b. Culture and science
   c. Religion and magic
   d. b and c
8. Paralytic poliomyelitis
   a. was first evidenced during the summer of 1890
   b. is cured by childhood vaccinations
   c. caused great fear in the U.S. during the 1970s
   d. has been eradicated from the world
9. Cancer
   a. metastasis was first understood in the nineteenth century
   b. is only treated with chemotherapy
   c. deaths will total 1.5 million in 2007
   d. is the result of an inherited tendency
10. HIV/AIDS:
    a. was first known in the Bronze Age
    b. is decreasing in the U.S. but rages on in other parts of the world
    c. only infects gay men
    d. is caused by a bacteriaum transmitted through bodily fluids

Critical Thinking

1. With a group of peers, identify the effects of culture on today's medicine.
2. How does the role of a medical specialist today compare to the role of a medical specialist in the past? Consider both similarities and dissimilarities.
3. You are the medical assistant. Your practitioner–employer has just prescribed **opiates** for a young Asian woman suffering from migraine headaches. You overhear the young woman arguing with her

mother, who thinks that she should take non-addictive Chinese herbs. What, if anything, would you do?

4. Discuss with a peer the role of women in medicine today. What difficulties, if any, might a female practitioner face today? Compare today's difficulties with those of female health care practitioners 100 years ago.
5. Using the example of aromatherapy in Frontiers in Medicine, identify any new frontiers using integrative medicine that you know about or have seen used in patient treatment.

WEB ACTIVITIES

The Internet is an ideal place to seek evidence of new and emerging technologies in medicine. One such avenue is "Medical Breakthroughs" reported by Ivanhoe Broadcast News, Inc. Identify at least two or three recent discoveries you find particularly interesting from your research on the Internet.

1. Do an Internet search using the keywords "penicillin discovered" to find some interesting sites. Determine the reasons it took so long to put penicillin into production. What kind of hurdles do new medications face today before they are available on the market to consumers and patients?
2. Search the Internet for "Women in Medicine: An AMA Timeline 1800s." This publication compiled by the American Medical Association provides valuable and interesting information about women in medicine. What surprises you the most? Are female applicants to medical school increasing or decreasing? By what percent?
3. The U.S. National Library of Medicine and the National Institutes of Health have a Web site with a section on "Changing the Face of Medicine." This site enables the reader to discover how women have influenced the practice of medicine and to determine if the exhibition will be in your geographical region any time soon. Go to the Web site http://www.nlm.nih.gov/changingthefaceofmedicine/ to view pictures and historical information on women in medicine. The section on the greatest obstacles faced by these women is particularly interesting. Who inspires you the most? Explain.
4. Access the Internet to compare/contrast medical schools and universities in the United States with medical universities in China. What major differences do you note? Are there any similarities?

REFERENCES/BIBLIOGRAPHY

American Cancer Society. (2007). *Surveillance research.* Retrieved May 23, 2007, from http://www.rare-cancer.org/.

American Medical Association. (2004). *Women in medicine.* Retrieved May 20, 2007, from http://www.ama-assn.org/go/wpc.

Centers for Disease Control and Prevention (CDC). (2006). Twenty-five years of HIV/AIDS—United States, 1981–2006. *MMWR Weekly.* Retrieved April 24, 2007, from http://www.cdc.gov/mmwr/preview/.

D'Adesky, A. (2003). Cuba fights AIDS its own way. *The Gully Online Magazine.* Retrieved May 17, 2007, from http://www.thegully.com/.

David, M. (2006). Engineers work medical miracles every day. *Electronic design.* Retrieved May 18, 2007, from http://www.elecdesign.com/Articles.

Fenster, J. M. (2003). *Mavericks, miracles, and medicine.* New York: Carroll & Graf Publishers.

Lewis, M. A., & Tamparo, C. D. (2007). *Medical law, ethics, and bioethics for health professions* (6th ed.). Philadelphia: F. A. Davis.

Lyons, A. S., & Petrucelli II, J. R. (1978). *Medicine: An illustrated history.* New York: Harry N. Abrams.

McNeil, D. G. (2007). U.N. to say it overstated H.I.V. cases by millions. *The New York Times.* Retrieved January 11, 2008, from http://www.nytimes.com/2007/11/20/world/20aids.html/.

Sanofi Pasteur, SA. (2006). *Polio: The disease. Polio eradication.* Retrieved May 17, 2007, from http://www.polio.info/polio-eradication/.

Until There's A Cure. (2006). *Vital statistics.* Retrieved May 17, 2007, from http://www.until.org/statistics/shtm.

UNIT
2
The Therapeutic Approach

Therapeutic Communication Skills

Chapter 4

KEY TERMS

Active Listening
Bias
Body Language
Closed Questions
Clustering
Compensation
Congruency
Cultural Brokering
Culture
Decode
Defense Mechanism
Denial
Displacement
Encoding
Hierarchy of Needs
High-Context Communication
Indirect Statements
Interview Techniques
Kinesics
Low-Context Communication
Masking
Open-Ended Questions
Perception
Prejudice
Projection
Rationalization
Regression
Repression
Roadblocks
Sublimation
Therapeutic Communication
Time Focus
Undoing

OUTLINE

Importance of Communication
The Communication Cycle
- The Sender
- The Message
- The Receiver
- Feedback
- Listening Skills

Types of Communication
- Verbal Communication
- Nonverbal Communication
- Congruency in Communication

Factors Affecting Therapeutic Communication
- Age and Gender Barriers
- Economic Barriers
- Education and Life Experience Barriers
- Bias and Prejudice Barriers
- Verbal Roadblocks to Therapeutic Communication
- Defense Mechanisms as Barriers
- Barriers Caused by Cultural and Religious Diversity
- Human Needs as Barriers to Therapeutic Communication
- Maslow's Hierarchy of Needs

Establishing Multicultural Communication
- Cultural Brokering

Therapeutic Communication in Action
- Interview Techniques
- Point of Care Techniques

Community Resources

OBJECTIVES

The student should strive to meet the following performance objectives and demonstrate an understanding of the facts and principles presented in this chapter through written and oral communication.

1. Define the key terms as presented in the glossary.
2. Identify the importance of communication.
3. List and define the four basic elements of the communication cycle.
4. Identify the four modes or channels of communication most pertinent in our everyday exchange.
5. Discuss the importance of active listening in therapeutic communication.
6. Differentiate between the terms *verbal* and *nonverbal communication*.
7. Analyze the five Cs of communication and describe their effectiveness in the communication cycle.

OBJECTIVES (continued)

8. Demonstrate the following body language or nonverbal communication behaviors: facial expressions, personal space, position, posture, gestures/mannerisms, and touch.
9. Identify and explain congruency in communication.
10. Differentiate between low-context and high-context communication styles.
11. Discuss Table 4-2 and generalizations of cultural/religious effects on health care.
12. Discuss the use of Maslow's hierarchy of needs in therapeutic communication.
13. Recall at least four influences on therapeutic communication related to culture and describe four common biases/prejudices in today's society.
14. Recall at least three steps to building trust with culturally diverse patients.
15. Discuss cultural brokering and its use in medical facilities.
16. Recall eight significant roadblocks to therapeutic communication.
17. List and describe seven common defense mechanisms.
18. Compare/contrast closed questions, open-ended questions, and indirect statements.

Scenario

In the two-provider office of Drs. Lewis and King, four medical assistants constantly interact with patients, allaying their concerns, scheduling their appointments, instructing them on medications, and helping them understand their insurance coverage. On any given day, office manager Marilyn Johnson, CMA (AAMA), is greeting patients warmly as they arrive for their appointments. Some patients, such as Anna and Joseph Ortiz, are new to the practice. Marilyn's warm manner puts them at ease. Other patients, such as Martin Gordon, who has prostate cancer, may be depressed and anxious. Marilyn tries to create an environment where they feel free to share their concerns and anxieties.

Marilyn demonstrates therapeutic communication by acknowledging each patient as they arrive for appointments and puts them at ease by providing instructions. Medical assistants who project a warm, courteous presence while maintaining composure, even during difficult situations, and who ask the right questions in a nonthreatening manner will achieve therapeutic communication.

INTRODUCTION

Of all the tasks and skills required of the medical assistant in the ambulatory care setting, none is quite so important as communication. Communication is the foundation for every action taken by health care professionals in the care of their patients. Because medical assistants are often the liaison between patient and provider, it is critical to be aware of all the complexities of the communication process.

Everyday, Marilyn, Ellen, and the two clinical medical assistants at the offices of Drs. Lewis and King face many communication challenges. This chapter describes effective communication principles, applies those principles to face-to-face communication, and describes the basic roadblocks to communication. The key word to all communication in the medical setting is therapeutic. In all conversations with patients, the more therapeutic the conversation, the more satisfied the patient will be with the care provided.

IMPORTANCE OF COMMUNICATION

Therapeutic communication differs from normal communication in that it introduces an element of empathy into what can be a traumatic experience for the patient. It imparts a feeling of comfort in the face of even the most horrific news about the patient's prognosis. The patient is made to feel validated and respected. Therapeutic communication uses specific and well-defined professional skills.

Communication in the health care setting is the foundation of all patient care and is of the utmost importance. Communication must be in nontechnical language the patient can understand, delivered with feeling for the patient's emotional situation and state of mind, yet it still must be technically accurate. The medical staff must be alert to the patient's state of stress and whether defense mechanisms have taken over to the extent that the patient has "tuned out" and is no longer communicating with the staff.

Patients seeking an ambulatory care service look for medical professionals with technical skills and a clinical staff capable of communicating with them. Questions frequently asked by individuals seeking a new provider and clinic include: "Will the doctor talk with me so that I understand?" "Will the doctor listen to what I have to say?" and "Can I talk to the doctor honestly and openly?" The answer to all of these questions needs to be "yes." This chapter discusses these issues and presents specific techniques for therapeutic communication.

Spotlight on Certification

RMA Content Outline

- Patient relations
- Other interpersonal relations

CMA (AAMA) Content Outline

- Basic principles (psychology)
- Defense mechanisms
- Recognizing and responding to verbal and nonverbal communication
- Professional communication and behavior
- Evaluating and understanding communication
- Interviewing techniques
- Identifying community resources

CMAS Content Outline

- Professionalism
- Communication

THE COMMUNICATION CYCLE

All communication, whether social or therapeutic, involves two or more individuals participating in an exchange of information. The communication cycle involves sending and receiving messages even when not consciously aware of them.

Four basic elements are included in the communication cycle. They are (1) the sender, (2) the message and a channel or mode of communication, (3) the receiver, and (4) feedback (Figure 4-1).

The Sender

The sender begins the communication cycle by **encoding** or creating the message to be sent. This is an important step, and much care should be taken in formulating the message. Before creating the message, the sender must observe the receiver to determine the complexity of the words to be used within the message, the receiver's ability to interpret the message, and the best channel by which to send the message.

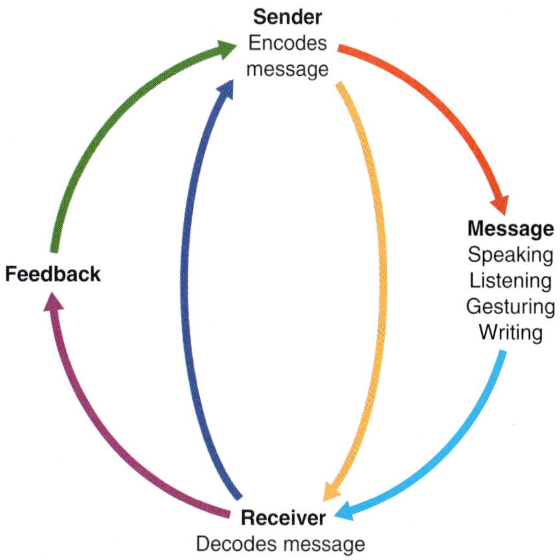

Figure 4-1 The communication cycle and channels of communication.

The Message

The message is the content being communicated. The message must be understood clearly by the receiver. Various levels of complexity in communication are used depending on the ability of the receiver to recognize and understand the words contained within the message. Children do not have the vocabulary base or the cognitive skills to communicate and understand at the same level as adults. The health of the receiver also must be considered. A patient who is experiencing stress or is in pain may find it difficult to concentrate on the message. If the patient is of a different nationality or culture from the sender, verbal communication may require special skill. When visual or hearing acuity is impaired, another challenge must be surmounted.

The four modes of communication, also called channels of communication, most pertinent in our everyday exchange are (1) speaking, (2) listening, (3) gestures or body language, and (4) writing. These modes or channels are affected by our physical and mental development, our culture, our education and life experiences, our impressions from models and mentors, and in general by how we feel and accept ourselves as individuals. Each mode or channel of communication has its appropriateness and must be considered when formulating the message.

The Receiver

The receiver is the recipient of the sender's message. The receiver must **decode,** or interpret, the meaning of the message. The primary sensory skill used in verbal communication is listening. It is hard work to concentrate and listen. When decoding the message, the receiver must be aware that not only the spoken word but the tone and pitch of the voice and the speed at which the words are spoken carry meaning and must be evaluated.

> **HIPAA**
>
> The idea of minimum necessary access to protected health information (PHI) is important to job performance. HIPAA requires that a reasonable effort be made to limit access to PHI to only what is necessary to accomplish the intended purposes of the use, disclosure, or request. The information accessed must fit the needs of the job description and nothing more. Employees must be careful to not discuss PHI with those outside the scope of their work. For example, a Certified Medical Administrative Specialist (CMAS) scheduling appointments does not need to know the diagnosis after the patient has been seen by the provider.

Feedback

Feedback takes place after the receiver has decoded the message sent by the sender. Feedback is the receiver's way of ensuring that the message that is understood is the same as the message that was sent. Feedback also provides an opportunity for the receiver to clarify any misunderstanding regarding the original message and to ask for additional information.

Listening Skills

A vital part of feedback in the communication cycle is listening. A good listener is alert to all aspects of the communication cycle—the verbal and nonverbal message, as well as verification of the message through appropriate feedback.

Active listening is one method used in therapeutic communication. In this technique, the received message is sent back to the sender, worded a little differently, for verification from the sender.

Sender: "How can I possibly pay this fee when I have no insurance?"
Receiver: "You're worried about paying your bill?"

The preceding example illustrates how the receiver is able to validate the sender's concerns at the same time the message is checked for accuracy. The door is then left open for a therapeutic response, such as:

Sender: "Our bookkeeper will be glad to work out a payment plan with you that will fit your resources."

Active listening involves listening with a "third ear," that is, being aware of what the patient is *not* saying or picking up on hints to the real message by observing body language. The health care professional should have three listening goals:

- To improve listening skills sufficiently so that patients are heard accurately
- To listen either for what is *not* being said or for information transmitted only by hints
- To determine how accurately the message has been received

So many health professionals try to "fix" everything with a recommendation, a prescription, even advice. Sometimes, none of those things is necessary. The patient simply needs someone to listen, to acknowledge the difficulty, and to remember that the patient is not helpless in finding a solution to the problem.

Skill in communication takes years of practice and frequent review. It will never become perfect; we can only hope that we will become better at it with each passing day. Communication is and always will be the basis for any therapeutic relationship (Tamparo & Lindh, 2008).

TYPES OF COMMUNICATION

We communicate by what we say, and also by our tone of voice, body movements, and facial expressions. The following paragraphs present the aspects of verbal and nonverbal communication. The importance of maintaining consistency between verbal and nonverbal messages also is stressed.

Verbal Communication

Verbal communication takes place when the message is spoken. However, one must keep in mind that unless the words have meaning, and unless the sender and the receiver apply the same meaning to the spoken words, verbal communication may be misunderstood. If, for example, you overhear a conversation in a language foreign to you, you are indeed a witness to verbal communication, but you may not understand the message. To have any meaning, the spoken word must be understood by all parties of the communication (Tamparo & Lindh, 2008).

The Five Cs of Communication. The book *Legal Nurse Consulting Principles and Practice*, edited by Patricia W. Iyer, identifies the five Cs of communication. They are (1) complete, (2) clear, (3) concise, (4) cohesive, and (5) courteous. These five Cs apply equally well in other health care professions.

Complete. The message must be complete, with all the necessary information given. The medical assistant cannot expect the patient to be compliant if all the instructions are not given and understood.

Clear. The information given in the message must also be clear. Health care professionals must be able to articulate by using good diction and by enunciating each word distinctly. The patient must be allowed time to process the message and verify its meaning. The message must also be heard to promote understanding.

Concise. A concise message is one that does not include any unnecessary information. It should be brief and to the point (Figure 4-2). Patients must not be overloaded with technical terms that may not be understood or that tend to distract them by diverting their attention away from the balance of the message.

Cohesive. A cohesive message is organized and logical in its progression. The cohesive message does not ramble and does not jump from one subject to another. The patient should be able to follow the message easily. The medical assistant should always allow time to summarize detailed messages and use responding skills to verify that the patient fully understands the message.

When communicating within the health professions, keep in mind the following:

1. Good communication skills are necessary in establishing rapport with patients.

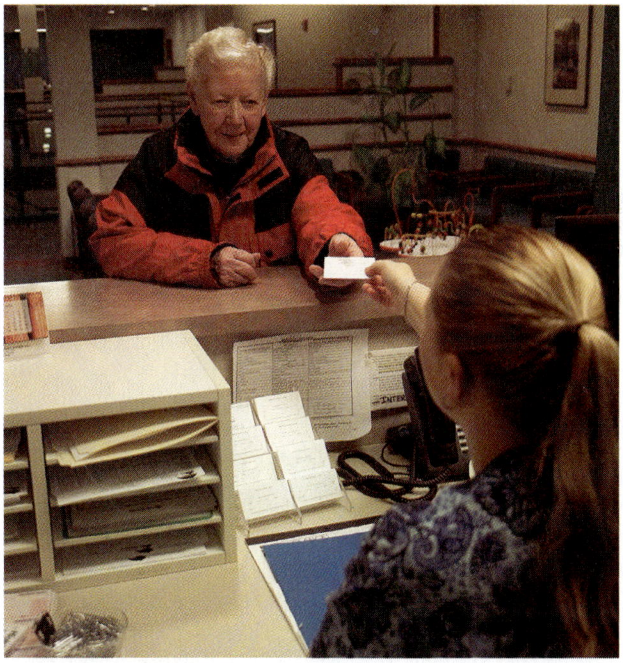

Figure 4-2 To say to the patient after greeting her by name, "I've completed an appointment card to remind you of your next appointment, Tuesday at 2:00 PM," is an example of a concise message that is brief and to the point.

2. Patients feel respected and validated when called by their full name, such as Mary O'Keefe or Mrs. O'Keefe.
3. Patients should be encouraged to verbalize their feelings and concerns.
4. Patients should be given technical information in a manner that they can understand.
5. Patients should be allowed to make practical application to their personal health needs.

Courteous. Courtesy is important in all aspects of communication. It only takes a moment to acknowledge a patient with a smile or by name. Knocking on the examination room door before entering validates the patient's right to privacy and builds self-esteem.

Remember to be courteous to colleagues in the office. Good working relationships and professionalism are always enhanced by simple courtesy.

Nonverbal Communication

Verbal communication alone is not always adequate in conveying the message being sent. In most instances, more than one mode or channel of communication is used. Nonverbal communication, often referred to as **body language,** includes the unconscious body movements, gestures, and facial expressions that accompany speech. The study of body language is known as **kinesics** (Figure 4-3).

Nonverbal communication is the language we learn first. It is learned seemingly automatically when infants learn to return a smile or respond to touches on the cheek. Much of our body language is a learned behavior and is greatly influenced by the primary caregivers and the culture in which we are raised.

Feelings and emotions are communicated most often through nonverbal means. The body expresses its true repressed feelings using body language. Most of the negative messages we communicate are also expressed nonverbally and usually are unintentional. Experts tell us that 70% of communication is nonverbal. The tone of voice communicates 23% of the message—only 7% of the message is actually communicated by the spoken word.

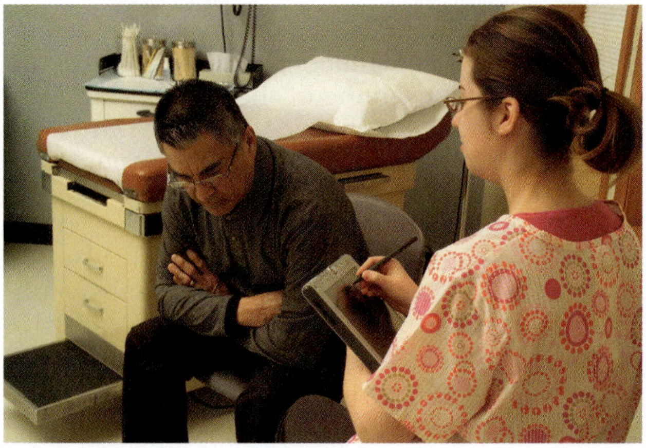

Figure 4-3 Body language can communicate more than spoken words.

Facial Expression. Facial expression is considered one of the most important and observed nonverbal communicators. Each facet or aspect of the anatomy of the face sends a nonverbal message.

Often expressions of joy and happiness or sorrow and grief are reflected through the eyes. The anatomy of the eyes does not change, but the movements of the structures surrounding the eyes enhance or magnify the message being communicated.

Children are told it is not polite to stare at people. It is acceptable to stare at animals in the zoo or art objects in the museum, but not at humans. Staring is dehumanizing and is often interpreted as an invasion of privacy.

The medical assistant must learn not to stare when patients present with ailments that make them "look" different. Patients such as these are individuals who have needs, who perhaps feel pain and discomfort, and who have decreased self-esteem and value. These feelings will only be amplified if the medical assistant and other health professionals are unable to "see" them as humans. A lack of eye contact may also be viewed as avoidance or disinterest in being involved.

The movements of the eyebrow indicate many nonverbal cues as well. Surprise, puzzlement, worry, amusement, and questioning are often nonverbal messages reflected by the position of the eyebrow. Wrinkling of the forehead sends similar messages.

Patient Education

Sensitive medical assistants will encourage patients to verbalize their concerns. The ability to ask questions in a nonprobing way and to elicit patient responses is an important function in any ambulatory care setting, because it is critical to know a patient's history, current medications, and other relevant data.

Cultural influences affect customs and different forms of facial expressions. It is important to remember that there are many cross-cultural similarities in body language, but there are also many differences. Various cultures denote different meanings to various gestures. If your patient is from another culture, never assume that gestures used hold the same meaning for the patient as they do for you. For example, some cultures believe that prolonged eye contact is rude and an invasion of privacy, whereas others consider it a sign of intimacy. Some people stare at the floor when concentrating or thinking through a process. Other cultures avoid eye contact to display modesty, whereas others feel eye contact expresses hostility or aggression. It is important to understand the cultures of the patients treated in the facility in which you are employed.

Personal Space. Personal space is the distance at which we feel comfortable with others while communicating. In the classroom, for example, students claim their personal space the first day of class. The area is well defined by using books and papers, or by placing the arm, hand, or chair on boundary lines. When another invades the personal space, a shift in body position or the use of eye contact sends the message, "This is my area." Individuals may feel threatened when others invade their personal space without permission. Some examples of comfortable personal space for U.S. culture are as follows:

- Intimate: touching to 1½ feet
- Personal: 1½ to 4 feet
- Social: 4 to 12 feet (most often observed)
- Public: 12 to 15 feet

As with facial expressions, personal space is handled differently by various cultures. For example, there is no word for privacy in the Japanese language. Population numbers require crowding together publicly, as well as privately. Public crowding is often viewed as a sign of warmth and pleasant intimacy in Japan. In the private home, several generations may live together; however, each considers this space to be his own and resents intrusion into it.

Arabs like to touch their companions, to feel and to smell them. To deny a friend your breath is to be ashamed. When two Arabs talk to each other, they look each other in the eyes with great intensity. U.S. businessmen often end a business arrangement with a handshake; however, American Indians may view a handshake as an act of aggression or an offensive behavior. Each culture has its own distinct nonverbal communication cues.

The medical assistant may perform many invasive tasks during the course of an office visit. Examples include taking vital signs or giving injections, both of which require touching the patient. It is beneficial to explain procedures that invade another's space before beginning the procedure so that it will not be perceived as threatening. This helps to empower the patient by involving the patient in the decision-making process and builds a sense of trust in the medical assistant.

Posture. Like personal space, posture is important to health care professionals. Posture relates to the position of the body or parts of the body. It is the manner in which we carry ourselves, or pose in situations. We tend to tighten up in threatening or unknown situations and to relax in nonthreatening environments. Those who study kinesics believe that a posture involves at least half the body, and that the position can last for nearly five minutes.

When the patient is seated with the arms and legs crossed, the message of closure or being opinionated may be relayed. In contrast, sitting in a chair relaxed with the hands clasped behind the head indicates an attitude of being open to suggestions. Slumped shoulders may signal depression, discouragement, or, in some cases, even pain.

Position. Position, the physical stance of two individuals while communicating, is a key factor to consider while communicating with the patient. Most provider–patient relationships use the face-to-face communication arrangement. When speaking with a patient, the provider or medical assistant will want to maintain a close but comfortable position, enabling observation of all cues being sent, both verbal and nonverbal (Figure 4-4).

Standing over a patient can convey a message of superiority, and too much distance between the two parties may be interpreted as avoidance or exclusivity. Generally, leaning toward the patient expresses warmth, caring, interest, acceptance, and trust. Moving away from the patient may be interpreted as dislike, disinterest, boredom, indifference, suspicion, or impatience.

Whenever possible, it is best to have a chair in the examination room and to have the patient seated comfortably in the chair to begin the communication cycle. The medical assistant or provider can sit on a stool that can be moved easily toward the patient. This arrangement aids the patient in

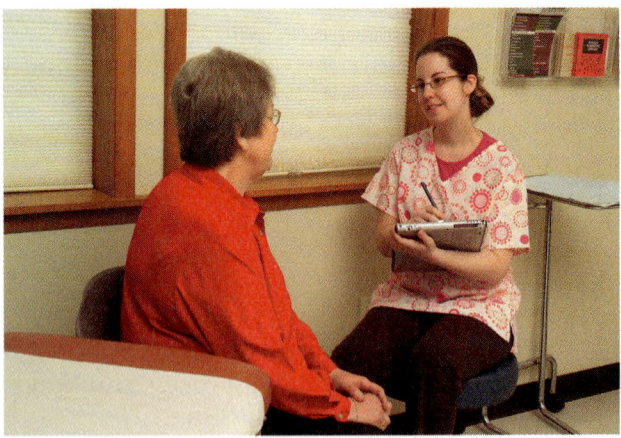

Figure 4-4 Positive posture and position encourage therapeutic communication.

feeling valued, listened to, and cared for as a fellow human being.

Gestures and Mannerisms. Most of us use gestures and mannerisms when we "talk" with our hands. This form of body language may be useful in enhancing the spoken word by emphasizing ideas, thus creating and holding the attention of others. Some common gestures and their possible meanings are as follows:

Finger-tapping	Impatience, nervousness
Shrugged shoulders	Indifference, discouragement
Rubbing the nose	Puzzlement
Whitened knuckles and clenched fists	Anger
Fidgeting	Nervousness

Touch. Touch is a powerful tool that communicates what cannot be expressed in words. Its appropriateness in the patient–health professional relationship has well-defined boundaries and requires the use of good judgment on the part of the professional. Infants who are not touched, cuddled, and loved do not grow and develop as those who receive these reassuring gestures. Touch is personal and is linked closely to personal space. Understanding touch as it relates to various cultures must be considered. For example, Vietnamese, Cambodian,

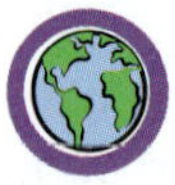

Hmong, or Thai families traditionally consider the head to be the site of the soul. During conversation and patient assessment, avoid touching the patient's head unless it is necessary for the examination. Southeast Asian clients may fear bodily intrusion; therefore, physical examination and treatment procedures should be explained carefully and completely before they are performed. The touch that communicates caring, sincerity, understanding, and reassurance is usually welcomed and considered to be a therapeutic response. Most patients will understand and accept the touching behavior as it relates to the medical setting; however, we must remember that not all patients are comfortable with touch. Whenever the patient is not comfortable with touch, ask permission and create as safe and reassuring an environment as possible.

Congruency in Communication

Using some keys to successful communication promotes effective communication. There must be **congruency** between the verbal and nonverbal communication. Shaking your head NO while saying YES verbally sends a mixed message. In most cases, the nonverbal messages will be accepted as the intended message.

It is also important to remember that most nonverbal messages are sent in groups of various forms of body language. The grouping of nonverbal messages into statements or conclusions is known as **clustering. Masking** involves an attempt to conceal or repress the true feeling or message. The perceptive professional will be aware of all these messages.

Perception as it relates to communication is the conscious awareness of one's own feelings and the feelings of others. To be most useful and therapeutic as health professionals, we must first explore our own feelings and appreciate and accept ourselves.

Learning to use perception involves the ability to sense another's attitudes, moods, and feelings. It takes practice and experience to develop and use this skill effectively. Being attentive to other professionals and observing their use of perception will yield insight into its usefulness and provide an example to emulate. A word of caution—the use of perception may easily be misinterpreted, especially when going with your feeling or assessment of what is happening regarding the patient. Always follow perceived assessments with verbal validation before assuming your perception of the circumstance is correct.

Nonverbal communication is easily misinterpreted. Careful observation for congruency between verbal and nonverbal communication, and clustering nonverbal cues being sent into nonverbal statements will strengthen your ability to interpret the message accurately.

FACTORS AFFECTING THERAPEUTIC COMMUNICATION

Anything that interferes with the patient's ability to focus has a negative impact on therapeutic communication. The following paragraphs discuss significant barriers. The medical assistant must recognize that until these barriers are dealt with or minimized, therapeutic communication will be significantly affected.

Age and Gender Barriers

Age and gender are factors with a strong influence on communication. How and when do you communicate with a young child? What do you communicate to that child? How do you impress upon an older gentleman who has taken few medications throughout his lifetime that he now must take his pill everyday? In a culture where the husband is the authority, how does the provider discuss with the female patient the inadvisability of another pregnancy at this time?

Economic Barriers

The influence of economics may reveal a discomfort if the office staff and patients have a different perception about how billing is managed and when and how payment is expected. A discussion of billing and payment procedures at the first office visit or before a major procedure will be beneficial to all concerned parties.

Education and Life Experience Barriers

Educational and life experiences will, in part, determine how patients react to their care. Patients with family members being treated for a chronic illness will have more knowledge and understanding of that illness in their own lives. Individuals who have already suffered a great deal of loss and grief in their lives may handle the information of a life-threatening illness more calmly than someone who has experienced little grief.

Bias and Prejudice Barriers

Personal preferences, biases, and prejudices will enter into many provider–patient relationships. Such biases affect the types of communication possible. When individuals are not aware of their biases or prejudices, hostile attitudes may prevail.

For therapeutic communication to take place, biases must be examined, a person's comfort level with each bias determined, and measures taken to ensure that a hostile attitude is not present. **Bias** is defined as a slant toward a particular belief. **Prejudice** is defined as an opinion or judgment that is formed before all the facts are known; prejudice is a preconceived and unfavorable concept. Common biases and prejudices in today's society include:

1. A preference for Western style medicine
2. Choosing providers according to gender
3. Prejudice related to a person's sexual preference
4. Discrimination based on race or religion
5. Hostile attitudes toward people with different value systems than one's own
6. A belief that people who cannot afford health care should receive less care than someone who can pay for full services

Medical assistants must recognize such biases and prejudices so that their own culture with its biases does not prevent them from responding therapeutically in communications with patients. Such recognition requires being aware of the differences among human beings and willingly accepting the uniqueness of each person.

> **Critical Thinking**
>
> Define in your own words the terms *bias* and *prejudice.* Now identify one bias and one prejudice that you have. How will these impact your ability to respond therapeutically in the medical setting? What steps can you take to become more accepting of the uniqueness of others, thereby improving therapeutic communication?

Verbal Roadblocks to Therapeutic Communication

Being sensitive to patients' unique personalities and needs will enable the health care professional to avoid **roadblocks** to communication (Table 4-1).

It must be the concern of each health care professional to facilitate communication by

Table 4-1 Roadblocks to Communication

Roadblock	Example
Reassuring clichés	"Don't worry about not having a job, Mr. McKay; you'll find another one really soon."
Moralizing/lecturing	"If you were smart, Mrs. Johnson, you'd lose fifty pounds and you wouldn't have such a problem with your diabetes and hypertension."
Requiring explanations	"Why would you not want to have chemotherapy, Mr. Gordon? Seeing your wife die of cancer should surely make you want to seek treatment."
Ridiculing/shaming	"Ha, ha, Mr. Gordon! It's not *prostrate*—it's prostate cancer."
Defending/contradicting	"Mr. Marshal, I assure you the physician is *very busy*. He will not see you until he has finished with his other patients."
Shifting subjects	"Yes, Mrs. Jover, your work is very interesting, but I must ask you to sign this permission form to test for HIV."
Criticizing	"Mrs. O'Keefe, why in the world would you stay with an abusive husband?"
Threatening	"There is no way you will get rid of this cough if you do not stop smoking, Mr. Fowler."

encouraging and enabling patients to express themselves honestly without fear. Roadblocks close communication and prevent quality care of the total person.

Defense Mechanisms as Barriers

Therapeutic communication becomes difficult if a patient is in a highly emotional state. A patient who is frightened, ashamed, guilty, or threatened often will resort to defense mechanisms as a means of avoiding injury to the ego. We all use defense mechanisms to some limited extent, but they become harmful when they result in a breakdown in therapeutic communication. Failure by the patient to face problems often results in inability to provide satisfactory treatment on the part of the medical practitioner. Recognizing common defense mechanisms enables the medical staff to minimize the triggering event and to communicate more effectively.

Defense mechanisms are defined as behavior that is used to protect the ego from guilt, anxiety, or loss of esteem. Use of defense mechanisms is most often subconscious to the person using them. It is the body's way of seeking relief from uncomfortable or painful reality. A mentally healthy person uses defense mechanisms to put a problem on hold until sufficient time has passed to permit him or her to address it without unacceptable emotional pain. Excessive use of defense mechanisms or failure to address a problem even after sufficient time has elapsed may be a sign of mental health issues.

Defense mechanisms are usually readily apparent to the disaffected observer; however, they are difficult to analyze without knowledge of the motive behind the behavior. The following paragraphs describe some commonly observed defense mechanisms.

Regression is an attempt to withdraw from an unpleasant circumstance by retreating to an earlier, more secure stage of life. It is usually used when the person feels powerless to affect the events causing the pain; it can be thought of as a desperation move. A toddler's regression to bedwetting or soiling himself or herself shortly after a new baby arrives in the family is an example of this defense mechanism. Use of a security blanket by an adult or child when faced with something that disrupts his or her life is another example.

Denial is refusal to accept painful information that is readily apparent to others. This defense mechanism commonly is encountered in the case of a person being diagnosed with a disease such as cancer or experiencing the death of a close family member or associate. Denial has a devastating effect on communication. The person will not hear what you say, but will quite frequently acknowledge what you are saying. Careful attention to what the person is saying will reveal that he or she does not accept his or her situation and is not mentally conscious that it is happening. Denial is often the first stage of an emotional response after a traumatic event. The next stage is anger toward the event, the medical staff, God, or others. The stage after anger is frequently depression. A mentally healthy person eventually reaches the final stage of acceptance.

Repression is similar to denial, but it is a totally subconscious reaction. In the case of repression, the person seems to experience temporary amnesia. It is the mind's way of defending itself from mental trauma by forgetting or wiping things out of the conscious memory. A child subconsciously forgetting to tell parents that he or she got into trouble at school is an example. The fear associated with the event becomes overwhelming, causing the mind to forget. Repression should not be confused with outright lying. In severe cases, repression can be related to mental illness.

Projection is attributing unacceptable desires, impulses, and thoughts falsely to others to avoid acknowledging they are actually the person's own experiences. It is a means of defending against feelings or urges the person does not want to admit they are experiencing. A mother who abuses her child might accuse the medical assistant of being rough with the child while performing patient assessment to conceal her feelings of wanting to throttle the child. Projection is an indication of mental illness.

Sublimation is the channeling of a socially unacceptable behavior into a socially acceptable behavior. An overly aggressive person directed to play football to relieve aggression is an example. Constructive behavior is substituted for destructive behavior.

Displacement is the subconscious transfer of unacceptable emotions, thoughts, or feelings from one's self to a more acceptable external substitute. A patient who is angry with the provider for some reason slams the door as he or she leaves the clinic.

Compensation is a conscious or subconscious overemphasizing of a characteristic to offset a real or imagined deficiency. This defense mechanism involves substituting strength for a weakness and may be viewed as healthy. An example is the young boy whose physical stature keeps him from being a football star, so he compensates by achieving an academic award.

Rationalization is the mind's way of making unacceptable behavior or events acceptable by devising a rational reason. The purpose of rationalization is to avoid embarrassment or guilt or to avoid obeying a directive. The rational reason is usually a stretch of the truth and can be quite apparent to disinterested individuals. An example is the patient who tells the provider that he or she did not take his or her blood pressure medication because he or she did not have enough time before leaving for work. The medication easily could have been taken at home or at work. Most people rationalize things to some extent, but excessive rationalization may be construed as unhealthy.

Undoing is actions designed to make amends or to cancel out inappropriate behavior. Showering the abused person with gifts to compensate for unacceptable actions that took place in the past is an example.

Barriers Caused by Cultural and Religious Diversity

True therapeutic communication cannot take place without taking into consideration the cultural and religious background of the patient. **Culture** is a pattern of many concepts, beliefs, values, habits, skills, instruments, and art of a given group of people in a given period. Culture and religion influence the patient's communication context, caregiving expectations, time focus, and attitude toward Western medicine practiced in the United States. Table 4-2 presents characteristics that are typical of different cultural and religious groups.

Communication Context. Communication context can be one of two styles: low-context or high-context. **Low-context communication** uses few environmental idioms to convey an idea. It relies on explicit and highly detailed language. **High-context communication** relies on body language, reference to environmental objects, and culturally relevant phraseology to communicate an idea. Neither communication style is superior to the other. It is important, however, that both the speaker and the listener be cognizant of the style being used in the conversation. In the medical office, the medical assistant should be aware of communication content and attempt to utilize the style used by the patient to the extent that it is practical.

Persons having different communication styles can easily develop an incorrect impression of the other person. Low-context communication is direct and in-your-face, whereas high-context communication is indirect and seems to take forever

TABLE 4-2 Generalization of Cultural/Religious Effects on Health Care

Culture or Religion	Medical Care Background	Caregiving Structure	Communication Traits	Time Focus*
Caucasian, Western Culture	**Western Medicine,** rely on prescription medications, practice preventive medicine, may rely on holistic medicine or folk medicine in some rural areas.	**Individual,** immediate family, close friends	**Low Context,** direct, eye contact expected, not adverse to therapeutic touching, may challenge medical opinions, basic English, speaks loudly.	**Future**
African American, Western Culture	**Western Medicine,** rely on prescription medications, practice preventive medicine, may rely on holistic medicine or folk medicine in some rural areas.	**Extended family,** relatives, close friends, neighbors, church family.	**Low Context,** direct, eye contact expected, not adverse to therapeutic touching, may challenge medical opinions and can distrust medical personnel, basic English sometimes mixed with street language (Ebonics).	**Present/** Future
Black, African, or Caribbean Culture	**Mixture** of Western and holistic medicine combined with spiritualism	**Extended family,** relatives, close friends, neighbors, church family, tribal affiliation	**Low Context,** eye contact expected, highly emotional, basic English strongly mixed with local dialect.	**Present**
Asian Culture Asian, Indian, Chinese, Filipino, Japanese, Korean, Thai, Laotian, Vietnamese	**Mixture** of Western and holistic medicine combined with Confucian principals, i.e., mind control of the body and maintaining a balance between natural forces and energy in the body, eating foods designated as having hot and cold properties to cure illness is common, mental illness is considered shameful and is denied.	**Immediate family,** opinions of family and particularly elders are important.	**High Context,** indirect, avoid eye contact, show little emotion, avoid therapeutic touching, youth speak basic English, elders may speak little English, may agree with what is said even when they do not understand in order to avoid conflict or to avoid losing face, speak softly.	**Present/** Past
Native American, South Sea Island Cultures	**Mixture** of Western and folk medicine combined with importance of a balance between the forces of nature.	**Extended family,** relatives, close friends, neighbors, tribal affiliation.	**High Context,** avoid eye contact, speak softly and slowly, basic English mixed with tribal dialects.	**Present**
Hispanic and Latino Cultures	**Mixture** of Western and folk medicine combined with a strong belief in intervention by God, eating foods designated as having hot and cold properties to cure illness is common.	**Extended family,** relatives, church family, collective community	**High Context,** be respectful and make direct eye contact, speak softly, some basic English, most speak Spanish.	**Present/** Past
Judaism	**Western Medicine,** religion does not allow eating pork and requires kosher food.	Culturally dependent	Culturally dependent	**Future/** Present
Hinduism/ Buddhism	**Western Medicine,** religions do not allow eating meat, modest regarding their body.	Culturally dependent	Culturally dependent	**Future/** Present

(continues)

TABLE 4-2 (continued)

Culture or Religion	Medical Care Background	Caregiving Structure	Communication Traits	Time Focus*
Islam	**Mixture** of Western and folk medicine combined with a strong belief in intervention by Allah, match gender of caregiver and client, women may not be permitted to be examined by male medical professional, mental illness denied, do not ingest alcohol, believe complete rest is proper for all illnesses, do not eat pork.	**Immediate family,** opinions of family and particularly male head of household are important.	**High Context,** touching between men and women is prohibited for strict believers, do not discuss sexual dysfunction, females do not make direct eye contact, will not discuss many taboo subjects (mental illness, birth defects, contraception, hospice, those from Middle East speak loudly to indicate the importance of what they are saying.	**Future/ Present**

*The bold term represents the predominant focus.

to reach a conclusion. The high-context speaker is often thought of as mentally slow or uneducated, and the low-context speaker is thought of as being rude or arrogant. Conclusions based on communication style usually are preconceived misconceptions and should be considered at all times when health care professionals are working with patients.

Caregiving Expectations. Caregiving expectations refer to the arrangements for taking responsibility for medical requirements. Most persons from the Western culture are individualistic and take personal responsibility for their medical care. However, many other cultures and religions do not share this philosophy. This can result in problems related to privacy requirements and patient compliance.

Time Focus. The cultural background as well as the socioeconomic environment of the patient have considerable impact on time focus. **Time focus** relates to whether the patient's attitude toward life is future, present, or past. Time focus is culture and religion related and is not necessarily related to current circumstances.

Future time focus is found in persons whose physical needs have been met and who can sacrifice immediate gratification to achieve perceived greater future returns. Future-oriented persons are time conscious and plan out their daily lives in considerable detail. Persons from affluent Western cultures usually are future oriented.

Present time focus is found in persons who are less assured of being able to meet their physical needs. It is difficult to plan for the future when basic items in the hierarchy of needs have not been met. Punctuality usually is not important to present-focus persons.

Past time focus is associated with persons from cultures having long-standing traditions. Tradition becomes the central focus of their life.

Human Needs as Barriers to Therapeutic Communication

Human needs, such as those discussed in Maslow's hierarchy of needs, are barriers to effective therapeutic communication if they are not met. A patient who does not know where he or she will find food or shelter or who feels rejected and unloved will frequently put these needs first and of primary concern in their mind. Communication regarding other concerns is nearly impossible to focus upon until the basic needs have been met. This section discusses human needs and how they can be satisfied by the medical assistant or by referrals provided by health care professionals.

Maslow's Hierarchy of Needs

Abraham Maslow is considered the founder of humanistic psychology and is most well known for his **hierarchy of needs** (Figure 4-5). *Webster's Dictionary* defines hierarchy as "a group of persons or things arranged in order of rank, grade, class etc." According to Maslow's theory, human needs could be grouped into five levels. He also theorized that each level of need must be satisfied before one could move on to the next level.

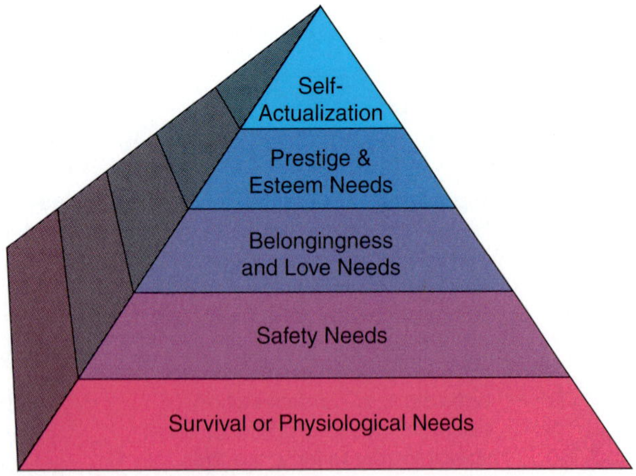

Figure 4-5 Maslow's hierarchy of needs (Adaptation based on Maslow's Hierarchy of Needs).

The needs in the first level include physiologic or survival needs. These needs include food, water, and air to breathe—homeostasis for the body. The second level includes needs of safety and security, that is, the need for security, stability, and protection. Everyone has the desire to be free from fear and anxiety. Safety needs also include the need for structure, law and order, and limits.

The third level involves belonging and love needs. This level of need involves both giving and receiving affection. Additional words that express our connectedness are roots, origins, peers, friends, family, neighborhood, territory, clan, class, and gang. We have a basic animal tendency to herd, flock, join, and belong.

The fourth level, prestige and esteem needs, comes from a basic need for a stable, healthy self-respect for ourselves and others. There is the desire for achievement, strength, and confidence. Also, there is the need for recognition, prestige, reputation, status, and even fame. Satisfaction of these needs leads to feelings of self-confidence and worth. The final level is self-actualization. In this stage, we are at our peak, doing what truly fits us. It is an achievement of potential.

Individuals may move back and forth from one need to another depending on circumstances.

Critical Thinking

An established patient arrives 20 minutes early for his appointment. He is in obvious pain and discomfort and tells the administrative medical assistant, "I can't sleep, I can't eat, and I can't go to work today." Which of Maslow's stages most accurately describes this patient? What actions should the medical assistant take to assist this patient?

ESTABLISHING MULTICULTURAL COMMUNICATION

Multicultural communication is the ability to communicate effectively with individuals of other cultures while recognizing one's own personal cultural biases and prejudices and putting them aside.

Approximately one third of the population of the United States comes from a culture other than mainstream American (i.e., Caucasian, English-speaking, Judeo-Christian). Figure 4-6 illustrates the percentage of various cultures living in the United States.

Medical professionals working within a specific cultural community should seek further information relating to that particular culture. In many instances, health care professionals can develop rapport with their ethnically diverse patients by simply demonstrating an interest in their culture and background.

Before multicultural or any therapeutic communication can begin, the patient must first be willing to discuss his or her health care issues, listen to the professional's questions, and give honest answers to those questions. The patient must trust the professional. Several steps to building trust include:

- *Risk/Trust:* The need for the helping professional to build an atmosphere of trust, making it easier

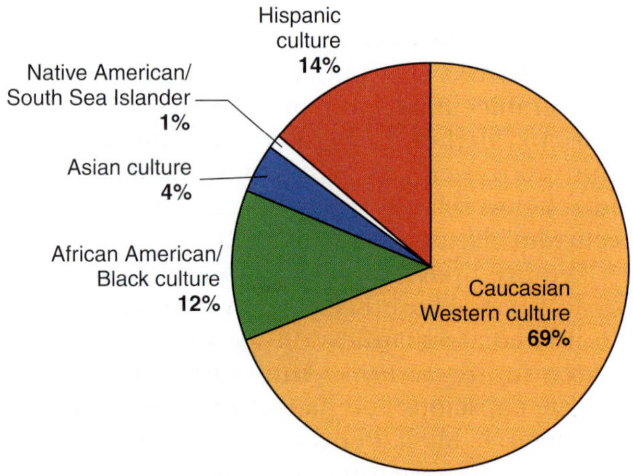

Figure 4-6 United States demographic make-up (2000 Census).

for the patient to risk expressing feelings and attitudes about the problem, is essential. Trust has to be earned. Remember to promise no more than you can deliver, be honest, and carefully and thoroughly explain procedures and policies. Answer all questions truthfully and honestly.

- *Empathy:* Empathy is the ability to accept another's private world as if it were your own. Empathy communicates identification with and understanding of another's situation. It states, "I'm available to walk this road with you."
- *Respect:* Respect values another person and considers him or her as a special individual. It is important to respect the patient's personal space, to provide privacy, and to use his or her full name and title when appropriate.
- *Genuineness:* This means being real and honest with others. The health care professional must be able to communicate honestly with others, while being careful not to blame or condemn.
- *Active listening:* Active listening involves verbal and nonverbal clues that send the message you are completely involved in the communication. Sit facing the patient with no barriers, such as a desk, between you. Lean toward the patient slightly to convey genuine concern and interest. Establish and maintain appropriate eye contact to elicit interest and concern. Maintain an open, relaxed posture to establish a nonthreatening environment for the patient. Listen carefully to the words the patient uses to describe problems, and use those terms rather than medical terminology when discussing symptoms.

Cultural Brokering

Cultural brokering is "the act of bridging, linking, or mediating between groups or persons through the process of reducing conflict or producing change" (National Center for Cultural Competence, Georgetown University Center for Child and Human Development, Georgetown University Medical Center, 2004). A cultural broker serves as a go-between, or one who advocates on behalf of another individual or group within the health care community. The 2000 Census indicates the projected demographic trends in the United States are more complex than ever measured previously. The belief systems related to health, healing, and wellness are diverse, with many cultural variations in the perception of illness and disease and their causes. Cultural brokers respect the values of diverse cultures and health care systems and are knowledgeable of both. They are able to overcome any existing language barriers, so that everyone understands each other clearly. The goal of cultural brokering is to increase the capacity of health care and mental health programs to design, implement, and evaluate culturally and linguistically competent service delivery systems. Cultural and linguistic competence have been determined to be fundamental in the goal of eliminating racial and ethnic disparities in health care.

Cultural brokers may assume the role of medical interpreter. An interpreter is one who takes the spoken message in one language and converts it to another language. Interpreters do not provide word-to-word equivalence, but rather focus on the accurate expression of equivalent meaning. They serve as communicators and liaisons between the patient and the provider in health care facilities. If an interpreter is necessary, it is important to remember to speak directly to the patient, not the interpreter. If English is the second language or a heavy accent is involved, speaking clearly and slowly can greatly enhance communication.

In some cases, a family member may serve as the interpreter. This may not be the best solution because the family member may not understand the medical terminology. It would also be difficult for a family member to be the one to share a life-threatening diagnosis or a poor prognosis report.

Understanding this hierarchy helps to assess a patient's needs. If the most basic of needs are not met, it is highly unlikely that a patient can be successful with any treatment protocol. Keeping this hierarchy in mind will help to facilitate therapeutic communication.

THERAPEUTIC COMMUNICATION IN ACTION

The following section identifies the proper communication techniques medical assistants should use as part of the most important communication function they perform: patient interview techniques.

Interview Techniques

All health professionals must be adept at **interview techniques**—knowing how to encourage the best communication between themselves and the patient. It is important to remember that an unequal relationship exists between the health professional and the patient. The health professional, whether it be the provider or the medical assistant, is in the power position and has a great deal of control over the patient. Therefore, it is important to equalize the relationship as much as possible. That is the reason why some professionals use the term *client* rather than *patient*.

Early in the interview, the patient must feel comfortable enough to risk being honest with the health professional. The health professional must build an atmosphere of trust by showing concern for the patient. A gentle touch and a warm, caring facial expression may be all that is necessary. Always be honest and genuine in your responses to patients. Be sympathetic and empathic and create an environment that is free of hypocrisy.

When the medical assistant is interviewing the patient for the presenting problem or chief complaint, it is important to listen with a "third" ear. Listen to what the patient is not saying but is apt to exhibit through nonverbal communication.

You might choose to share your observation of the nonverbal message with the patient, thus encouraging the patient to verbalize more freely. When feelings are shared, validate and acknowledge those feelings through such statements as "I understand your distress." You can verify the communication by reflecting or paraphrasing what the patient has said.

You will be asking **closed questions** during the interview. Closed questions can be answered with a simple yes or no.

> "Are you still taking your medication?"
> "Are you in pain now?"

You will also use **open-ended questions** with the patient. These questions encourage therapeutic communication because the patient is required to verbalize more information.

> "What kind of help will you have at home during your recovery?"
> "How are you coming along on this diet?"

Indirect statements will also prove helpful in facilitating therapeutic communication. An indirect statement will elicit a response from a patient without the patient feeling questioned.

> "Tell me what you've been doing since you retired."
> "I'd like to know more about your exercise program."

Refer to Chapter 11 for additional information related to patient interviewing.

Point of Care Techniques

Point of care refers to the location in which the patient and provider or patient and office personnel physically interact. This interaction may take place at the reception desk, in the laboratory, or in the examination room. The goal of therapeutic communication at the point of care is varied. It may be to determine the reason for the visit, collect a blood specimen, or explain a course of treatment to the patient. The principal barrier to communication at the point of care is emotional tension, that is, the patient is upset. The patient may be upset due to fear of the illness or diagnosis, pain, or anger as part of the loss of quality of life resulting from the illness. Other barriers to communication less frequently encountered are language, speech or hearing impairment, or mental conditions such as low IQ or old age and were discussed in other sections of this chapter.

If the patient is delivered unpleasant information skillfully, he or she can take in and process the material rather than reject it. Words and statements that promote anxiety or anger should be avoided. Examples are complex medical terminology that the patient may not understand and judgmental statements about lifestyle. Both can instill fear and anger in a patient. Every effort should be made to clarify the information being communicated to the patient. Patients should be encouraged to restate the information in their own words. Under no circumstance should the patient be given false reassurance. This can result in a lack of trust if the patient perceives that he or she is being deceived. The medical assistant should be alert to notice emotional reactions by the patient and be prepared to take appropriate corrective action.

Avoid familiar phrasings and mannerisms—for example, the type we use when unsure of what to say in an uncomfortable situation, such as saying "perhaps," rather than the more usual "maybe," or nervously clearing our throats. All of these are signs of self-protection on the part of the speaker, which the patient may notice. Good communication skills and forethought make such self-protective mechanisms less necessary.

Patient Education

Education of a patient or caregiver should consist of the following fundamentals regardless of the subject:

- Do not attempt to educate the client while he or she is emotionally upset or distressed. Under these conditions the individual will not be communicative; that is, they are listening but not hearing what is said to them. Make every effort to calm the client. If necessary, reschedule another time for the educational session.
- Use multiple methods, such as visual, verbal, and action, to convey the message. This approach ensures that your communication style will be versatile and meet the needs of the client. Convey information in a clear, concise manner using context that is relevant to the client.
- Limit the amount of material covered. If necessary, schedule additional sessions so that the client is not overwhelmed.
- Communicate in simple words, avoiding medical terminology that may not be understood by the client.

COMMUNITY RESOURCES

There may be circumstances in which a patient will need a referral to a community resource. These resources range from the more simple acts of arranging with Meals on Wheels to deliver a hot meal daily to making complex arrangements for skilled nursing facilities or hospice care. The medical assistant will need to know the patient's name, address, and telephone number, as well as the particular resource needed, the diagnosis, and the reason for the service.

It is helpful to have a list of community resources readily available. The list may be computerized, or hardcopy information may be filed in a notebook. The information should be put into categories for ease in locating it quickly. See Procedure 4-1 for steps in developing a Community Resource reference.

Procedure 4-1

Identifying Community Resources

PURPOSE:
To have a list of community resources readily available for referral to patients.

EQUIPMENT/SUPPLIES:
Computer and printer
Following is a list of information sources to consider when beginning to put together a Community Resource Reference:

- Local Public Health Department
- Internet
- Community service numbers in the local telephone directory
- State/federal agencies
- Visiting nurses
- Counselor/social workers at local hospitals
- Nursing home associations
- Local charities

PROCEDURE STEPS:

1. Determine the type of information to be in your database. RATIONALE: Only resources useful to your specific office should be maintained to save time and space.
2. Contact the sources listed previously and request any listings they may have. RATIONALE: This will save time.

continues

Procedure 4-1 (continued)

3. Search the Internet using your favorite search engine. Enter the city, state, and community resources. You may have to modify the subject of your search to obtain the desired resources. RATIONALE: This is an effective way to access information quickly.
4. Develop a database on your computer so you can search easily for the resource when needed by a patient and simply print it out. You may wish to have a notebook with the information printed and indexed so that other office staff can simply copy a page for a patient. Your data should include as many resources for assistance as you can find for each type of resource. RATIONALE: To have a listing of community resources readily available for office use.

Case Study 4-1

Review the scenario at the beginning of this chapter and respond to the following.

It is a typically active day at the offices of Drs. Lewis and King. Despite the three emergencies in the early afternoon and the full schedule of patients, everything is running smoothly with Dr. Lewis, and the entire staff is responding quickly but thoroughly to patient concerns.

At 4:00 PM, another emergency patient arrives; at the same time, Jim Marshal, an architect in a downtown firm, comes in early for a routine appointment and demands to be seen immediately. Jim, a regular patient, has a history of being difficult and impatient; being a bit arrogant, he tends to put his needs first. However, Dr. Lewis is occupied with another patient. It is critical to treat the patient with the emergency as soon as possible, and Jim is half an hour early.

Joe Guerrero, CMA (AAMA), the office's administrative and clinical medical assistant, calmly asks Mr. Marshal to please wait until his scheduled appointment time. When he threatens to leave, Joe explains to Mr. Marshal that there are two patients ahead of him, but that the provider will see him at his scheduled appointment time.

CASE STUDY REVIEW

1. What communication roadblocks did medical assistant Joe Guerrero avoid in reacting to Jim Marshal's demands to see the provider?
2. With another student, role-play the scenario, with one student taking the role of patient and one student the role of the medical assistant. Identify roadblocks to communication imposed by the patient. How is the medical assistant using the five Cs of communication to deal with the situation?
3. Do you think the medical assistant reacted appropriately? What else could he have done? What should he *not* do in this situation?

Case Study 4-2

You have learned in this chapter that communication has not been successful until the cycle is complete. Consider the following scenario.

An 82-year-old woman with moderate dementia and a hearing impairment is brought to the surgeon's office for a follow-up appointment after hip replacement surgery. The woman's daughter accompanies her. The goal of the appointment is to make certain the hip is healing nicely and to discuss precautions before the patient returns to her assisted-living apartment. Almost immediately, the conversation is directed toward the daughter because it is so much easier to explain to her what should be done.

CASE STUDY REVIEW

1. What might the staff do to help the patient understand the following?
   - Use the walker consistently.
   - Shoes must be leather tennis shoe type or uniform style; consider Velcro closure as opposed to laces that have to be tied.
   - Do not wear pantyhose.
   - You will not be able to walk your dog on a leash.
2. Should the patient be left out of the conversation? Should the daughter be included?
3. In cases such as these, is something other than verbal communication indicated?

SUMMARY

Throughout this text you are reminded of the importance of effective communication techniques. Good communication takes practice. Use the techniques identified in this chapter with your family and with your peers. Watch for roadblocks, be aware of defense mechanisms, and remember the five Cs of communication.

STUDY FOR SUCCESS

To reinforce your knowledge and skills of information presented in this chapter:

- Review the Key Terms
- Practice the Procedure
- Consider the Case Studies and discuss your conclusions
- Answer the Review Questions
    - Multiple Choice
    - Critical Thinking
- Navigate the Internet by completing the Web Activities
- Practice the StudyWARE activities on the textbook CD
- Apply your knowledge in the Student Workbook activities
- Complete the Web Tutor sections
- View and discuss the DVD situations

REVIEW QUESTIONS

Multiple Choice

1. Factors affecting therapeutic communication include which of the following?
    a. age and gender barriers
    b. education and experience barriers
    c. bias and prejudice barriers
    d. all of the above
2. In the cycle of communication, encoding means:
    a. deciphering a message
    b. creating the message to be sent
    c. sending the message
    d. receiving the message
3. Body language:
    a. is used to express feelings and emotions
    b. is not as important as verbal communication
    c. only makes up 7% of the message
    d. is only used in Eastern cultures
4. A comfortable social space is defined as:
    a. touching to 1½ feet
    b. 1½ feet to 4 feet
    c. 12 to 15 feet
    d. 4 to 12 feet
5. A reassuring cliché is:
    a. a way of calming down a patient
    b. a means of rationalizing a decision
    c. a roadblock to communication
    d. always useful in daily communications
6. Redirecting a socially unacceptable impulse into one that is socially acceptable is an example of which of these defense mechanisms?
    a. sublimation
    b. rationalization
    c. projection
    d. displacement
7. When using an open-ended question with a patient, we expect:
    a. a yes or no answer
    b. him or her to tell us the truth
    c. a response that permits the patient to elaborate
    d. only the right answers
8. High-context communication relies on all of the following *except*:
    a. body language
    b. reference to environmental objects
    c. explicit and highly detailed language
    d. culturally relevant phraseology

Critical Thinking

1. A 15-year-old girl awaiting a sports physical examination says that she is overweight and has pimples. How will you respond therapeutically?
2. Bill, who is 28 years old, comes for his annual checkup. When reviewing his social data sheet, you discover he is now living in an apartment and has a new phone number. He mumbles to you that his wife left him and won't let him see the kids. How will you respond therapeutically?
3. You try to be gentle and gracious with Edith. She is fragile and difficult to please. While positioning her for a radiograph, she sneers and says, "You are about the roughest person who ever cared for me." How will you respond therapeutically, and how will you control your body language?
4. When you report to Herb that his cholesterol is quite high and that the doctor wants to discuss medication and diet, he responds, "That is impossible; you must have made some mistake." Which defense mechanism is Herb using? How will you respond therapeutically?
5. How might the unequal relationship between provider and client/patient impact therapeutic communication?

WEB ACTIVITIES

Select three cultures of particular interest to you personally and search the Internet for information regarding these cultures and communicationt traditions. How might this new information be applied to the provider whose clientele is primarily made up of these cultures? How might this new knowledge benefit a medical assistant employed in this type of setting?

REFERENCES/BIBLIOGRAPHY

Blair, G. M. (January 23, 2000). *Conversation as communication.* Retrieved August 22, 2008, from http://www.see.ed.ac.uk/~gerard/Management/art7.html?see.ed.ac.uk/~gerard/Management/art7.html.

Iyer, P. W. (Ed.) (2002). *Legal nurse consulting principles and practice.* Boca Raton, FL: CRC Press.

Luckmann, J. (2000). *Transcultural communication in health care.* Clifton Park, NY: Delmar Cengage Learning.

National Center for Cultural Competence, Georgetown University Center for Child and Human Development, Georgetown University Medical Center. (Spring/Summer 2004). *Bridging the cultural divide in health care settings: The essential role of cultural broker programs.* Washington, DC: Author.

Taber's cyclopedic medical dictionary. (19th ed.). (2004). Philadelphia: F. A. Davis.

Tamparo, C. D., & Lindh, W. Q. (2008). *Therapeutic communications for health care.* Albany, NY: Delmar Cengage Learning.

THE DVD HOOK-UP

In this chapter, you learned the importance of positive communication and what distractions can impede the communication process. You also learned the importance of nonverbal communication and how it is not necessarily what you say, but rather how you say it, that leaves the strongest impression on others.

Program 2 of Critical Thinking deals with many of the same issues that are listed in this chapter. We observed the effects of body language in the communication process. Communicating with special populations also was addressed. We learned the office's responsibility in providing an interpreter for our deaf patients and how we can better serve our blind patients. We also learned about managing the angry patient.

1. What are some benefits to being bilingual?
2. What is one mistake that many people make when working with blind patients?
3. What is the best approach to take when dealing with an angry patient?

DVD Journal Summary

Write a paragraph that summarizes what you learned from watching the designated scenes from today's DVD program. How do you feel about working with patients from different cultures? Are you the type of person who gets angry when conversing with other people who are angry? What steps will you take to deal with an angry patient or coworker?

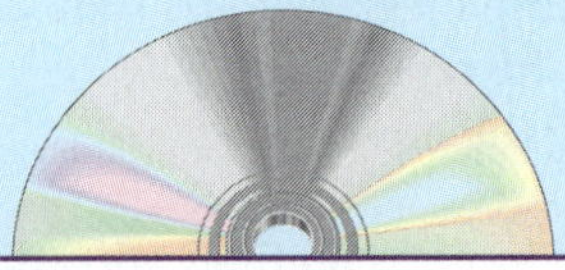

DVD Series Critical Thinking

Program Number 2

Chapter/Scene Reference

- *Introduction*
- *Forms of Communication*
- *Professional Communication*

(Skip: Communicating with Patients and Communication on the Telephone)

- *Communicating with Special Populations*

Chapter 5

Coping Skills for the Medical Assistant

KEY TERMS

Burnout
Goal
Inner-Directed People
Long-Range Goals
Outer-Directed People
Parasympathetic Nervous System
Self-Actualization
Short-Range Goals
Stress
Stressors
Sympathetic Nervous System

OUTLINE

What Is Stress?
- Adaptation to Stress

Management of Stress

What Is Burnout?
- Stages of Burnout
- Role of Personality and Work Environnment
- Burnout Prevention
- What to Do If You Are Burned Out

Goal Setting as a Stress Reliever

OBJECTIVES

The student should strive to meet the following performance objectives and demonstrate an understanding of the facts and principles presented in this chapter through written and oral communication.

1. Define the key terms as presented in the glossary.
2. Differentiate between stress and stressors.
3. Describe the three categories of stressors.
4. Differentiate between short-duration and long-duration stress.
5. Describe Hans Selye's General Adaptation Syndrome theory.
6. Identify several approaches to managing stress in the ambulatory care setting.
7. Identify three characteristics associated with burnout in the workplace.
8. Describe the four stages of burnout.
9. List a minimum of five ways to reduce the risk for burnout.
10. Differentiate between long-range and short-range goals.

Scenario

At the office of providers Lewis and King, there are four full-time medical assistants who collaborate to make the office run smoothly, both administratively and clinically. One day a month, though, office manager Marilyn Johnson, CMA (AAMA), is out of town, leaving Ellen Armstrong, CMA (AAMA) the administrative medical assistant, in charge of a busy reception area and an ever-ringing telephone.

On these days, Ellen is particularly careful to organize her work so that things run as they should. Although Ellen cannot anticipate every emergency, she does try to influence the situation rather than let events control her.

INTRODUCTION

Even in the most well-managed ambulatory care setting, medical assistants and other health providers are likely to feel the effects of stress from time to time. They may be overworked on certain days, they may face difficult patient situations, and they may find that the administrative and paperwork load is getting ahead of them.

This chapter helps today's busy, multifaceted medical assistant pinpoint the symptoms of stress and provides ideas for coping with stress as it occurs. The better equipped the medical assistant is to confront and solve the sources of stress, the less likely stressors will become so overwhelming as to lead to burnout on the job. Goal setting, recognizing one's limitations and potentials, setting priorities, and keeping a balanced perspective can work together to reduce stress and enable the medical assistant to take pleasure in working with patients and colleagues.

WHAT IS STRESS?

The body's response to mental and physical change is termed **stress.** What constitutes stress is highly individual and depends to a great extent on personality type. Events that may be stressful to one person may be enjoyable to another. A delayed airplane flight may be very stressful to a person who worries about making another connection or missing a meeting. Another person will simply look for an alternative flight or notify the people he or she was to meet and then take the time to enjoy a good book, experiencing little or no mental or physical change. Adaptive behavior patterns we assume in response to real physical threats or emotional effects result in either eustress (positive feelings) or distress (negative feelings). Moving to a new city or receiving a promotion usually are perceived as positive events, whereas going through a divorce or losing a job are conversely negative events; however, each of these events can result in inducing stress in the body. These events are called **stressors.** Stressors can be divided into three categories:

1. *Frustrations:* Circumstances that prevent us from doing what we want to do
2. *Conflicts:* Incompatibility between two important things or objectives equally important to us
3. *Pressure:* Demands of schedule, workload, or expectations placed on us by ourselves or others

According to Hans Selye, who first conceived the theory of nonspecific reaction as stress, the body does not differentiate positively and negatively induced stress. It is only the level of the stress and its duration that affect the body. Short-duration stress, sometimes called *acute stress,* can be beneficial. Short-duration stress adds anticipation and a feeling of "being alive," for example, when we experience a roller coaster ride or bungee jump off a cliff. The short-lived adrenaline rush brings the world into sharper focus and enhances our lives. It helps us focus on details, achieve difficult goals, and perform at our best. When we have a last-minute rush in the office or are hurrying to get an assignment finished for school, we are experiencing short-duration stress. Short-duration stress is experienced when the telephone rings, the examination rooms are full, and the provider is called to the hospital on an emergency. Immediately, the body's stress mode is activated and adrenaline is produced, enabling you to make quick judgements and decisions, to be organized and efficient, and to accomplish tasks within minimal time limits.

Longer-duration stress is sometimes called *episodic* or *chronic stress.* Episodic stress is the result of events over which we have control. Examples of episodic stress include taking on too many projects or needlessly worrying. Chronic stress is the result of events over which we have little control, such as long-term unemployment, dysfunctional relationships, or chronic illness. Longer duration stress, normally associated with negative events, can be harmful to the body, resulting in illnesses such as headaches, insomnia, allergies, cancer, acute indigestion, stomach ulcers, hypertension, blood clots, stroke, and immune system disorders. Psychologically, the body also is influenced by long-duration stress. Onsets of depression and anxiety, as well as eating problems resulting in weight loss or gain, are associated with the body's psychological response to stress. Anorexia and bulimia are common eating disorders attributed to long-duration stressful events. Long-duration stress can also affect our ability to think clearly, and objectivity may be impaired. Physical symptoms of these emotional effects include cigarette smoking, obesity, and lack of interest in or excessive sexual activity.

Adaptation to Stress

The body's response to stress goes back to early human development. That response was designed to help humans survive whatever they were experiencing that caused a fearful response. The **sympathetic nervous system** prepared the body for "fight or flight" to allow humans the best chance of survival. The brain inhibits short-term memory, promotes long-term memory, and releases hormones such as adrenaline into the bloodstream. The respiration rate becomes more rapid, blood flow increases, red and white blood cells are released by the spleen, and the immune system is altered to allow immune-boosting bodies to be sent to the body. Blood vessels in the skin contract to minimize blood loss from wounds, blood vessels in the muscles dilate to increase circulation, and fluids are diverted from nonessential locations; the metabolism rate is diminished to permit all available energy to be focused on the event that triggered the fight-or-flight response.

All of these caveman responses to stress are with us today. The symptoms of headache, stomach ache, diarrhea, cold clammy hands, heart palpitations, indigestion, and short-term memory loss that we experience are the result of our body's reaction to stressors that has been developed over millennia. Short term, these responses are not harmful, and the body's **parasympathetic nervous system** returns to normal after the stressor has been removed. Long term, these responses are harmful to the body. See Figure 5-1 for an illustration of the adaptive stages related to stress.

MANAGEMENT OF STRESS

Stress cannot be prevented; in fact, life would be dull without short-duration stress. Anticipating the birth of a child, planning an upcoming wedding, or graduating from school are all stressful changes, albeit pleasant ones, that make life interesting. Long-duration stressful situations are not desirable, but the situations leading to them can be managed if we understand the causes. Some causes of long-duration stress are:

- *Powerlessness:* Inability to control expectations, workload, and duties; feelings of frustration and panic because of schedules
- *Round peg in square hole:* Not suited for the position you hold
- *Traumatic events on the job:* Not emotionally prepared for trauma involved in the job
- *Environmental:* Physical conditions such as noise, lighting, or temperature influence work
- *Management style:* Your manager's style causes uproar or instability in work demands
- *Failure to satisfy needs:* Job conditions do not permit achievement of Maslow's needs (see Chapter 4 for information related to Maslow's hierarchy of needs)

Requesting that you have a written job description can control powerlessness. You will then know your duties and responsibilities, and you will not experience sudden change when you least expect it. A job description will also help to avoid some of the instability resulting from a manager who is too sanguine or manages from one

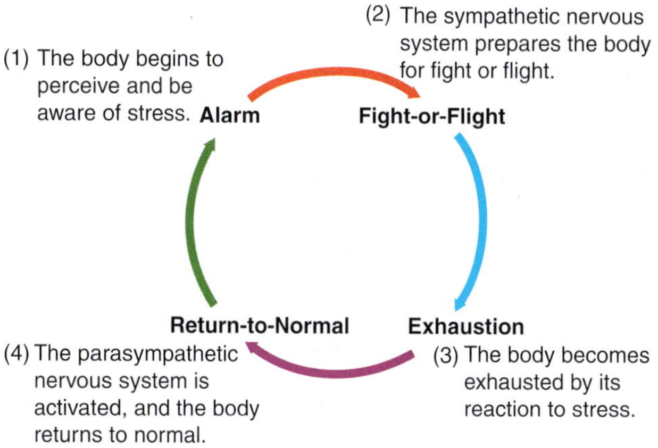

Figure 5-1 Hans Selye's General Adaptation Syndrome (GAS) theory proposes that four stages are involved in adapting to stress.

Critical Thinking

Practice in Time Management Analysis

List all of the tasks you do in a typical day. Beside each task write down how many minutes/hours you spend on each task. At the conclusion of the exercise, draw a histogram showing the percentage of each day spent on each task. This will quickly show where you spend most of your time. How could you save time? Develop a plan to reduce time spent in nonproductive, unessential activities.

crisis to another. If you know what your job entails, you can anticipate the events and take action to prevent a crisis.

Planning and prioritization can help to prevent panic and reduce stress when faced with the inevitable situation of too much work and too little time. A job that looks impossible can be broken down into elements that are manageable. Prioritization of the smaller elements and proceeding without wasting time procrastinating usually results in getting the job finished in the allotted time or at least with a minimum amount of stress.

Managing your lifestyle also becomes part of stress management. Finding time to relax and divert your mind from the worries of the job is an effective tool in managing stress. Instead of working during lunch to solve a problem, taking a break away from the problem will reduce the stress to the point that you will actually increase your productivity.

This is probably a good time to discuss worry. Worry is defined as undue concern for problems over which you have no control. Worry causes stress, yet it does nothing to resolve the problem causing your worry. Therefore, just remembering this definition and thinking about it every time you are inclined to worry will help you to stop worrying.

Mental attitude plays a role in tolerance to stress. Individuals who can focus on the positive can offset the depression often associated with stress. Identifying what is being accomplished versus focusing on what is not being accomplished or what does not meet your expectations is what is meant by focusing on the positive. Maintaining an active social network that allows you to discuss your problems is also quite helpful. The network should not include persons of negative self-attitude who have common problems. This situation is likely to have as its outcome a "complain session."

Physical condition affects your body's tolerance to stress. Maintaining a regular sleep cycle, eating a proper diet, and getting regular exercise

Critical Thinking

Checking Your Success-Oriented Attitude

Select three attitude attributes for which you are quite negative and develop a plan of action to make them more positive. Implement your plan; after two weeks, review whether your actions have impacted the stress level associated with that activity.

Negative Attributes	20%	40%	60%	80%	100%	Positive Attributes
Bored						Enthusiastic
Unhappy						Joyful
Never						Can do
Lethargic						Energetic
Cut corners						Honest
Out of control						Under control
Lack of confidence						Confident
Selfish						Selfless
Unyielding						Flexible
Loner						Part of a group
Know it all						Open to suggestion

contribute to improving your body's tolerance to stressors (Figure 5-2). Stress can affect sleep and appetite, but intentionally not getting enough sleep or not eating a balanced diet makes you more susceptible to stress in the first place. Anything that "bugs" you contributes to stress. Some people believe that soft background music will reduce stress, but for a job requiring intense concentration, any distraction contributes to stress. Clothes or shoes that are uncomfortable can "bug" you and contribute to stress. The color of the walls in your office can contribute to stress. If the color "bugs" you, it will contribute to stress. Telephone interruptions can result in a stressful situation. All of these "minor" things that contribute to stress are manageable and should be considered as part of a plan to manage stress. See Table 5-1 for suggested techniques for reducing stress at work.

Maintaining a good interpersonal relationship with fellow employees or fellow students and faculty is important to achieving a satisfying work or school experience. Before a strong interpersonal relationship is established with others, a positive self-attitude is needed. The choices we make affect our positive attitude. Making positive decisions will affect our school and work environment, and hence the level and duration of stress experienced. Following are choices we all make in our lives:

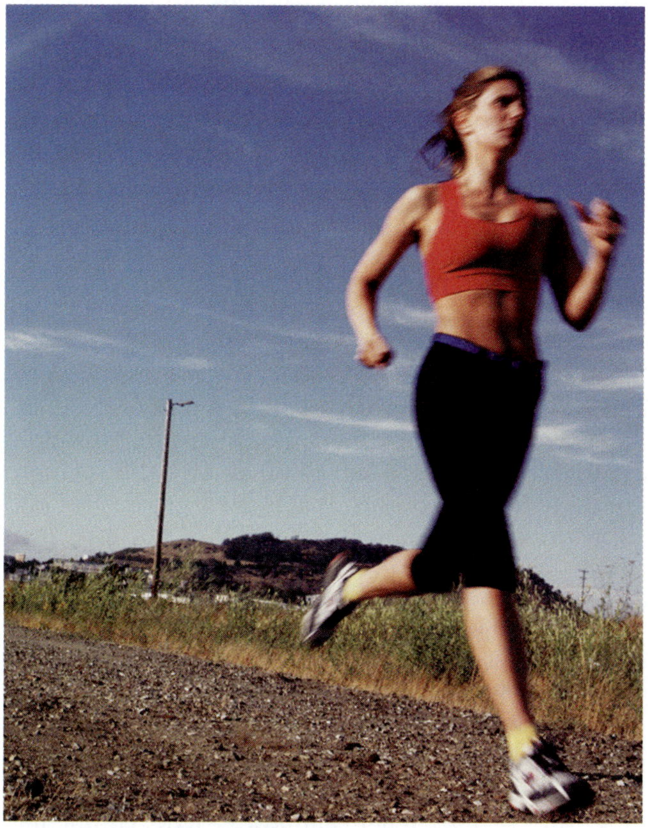

Figure 5-2 Regular exercise in some form improves the body's tolerance to stress.

Table 5-1 Techniques for Reducing Stress at Work

Stretch or change positions.
Slowly roll your head from side to side and forward and back.
Slowly rotate your shoulders forward and backward several times.
Turn away from the computer, or close your eyes for several seconds.
Walk around and deliver charts or laboratory specimens.
Stand or sit tall and take a few deep breaths.
Meditate for 30 seconds.
Know your limits and be aware of your body's needs.

- To be respectful of others
- To be a diligent worker
- To be willing to learn
- To be honest
- To be willing to assume responsibility for actions
- To express appropriate humor
- To have an attitude of humility
- To be goal directed
- To understand Maslow's hierarchy of needs

By anticipating how an organization can cause stress, we can be prepared and minimize its effects. Following are common causes of stress in an organization:

- *Low salary:* Salary plays an important role in our needs. It leads to frustration if we believe it is too low, and this contributes to a negative attitude. Positive job conditions can overshadow low salary; however, if combined with other negative feelings, it is an overpowering cause of stress.
- *Little opportunity for career growth:* This reason results in frustration and leads to stress and burnout.
- *Overspecialization:* This problem results in the employee never seeing the overall picture and receiving little or no satisfaction from his or her work.

Critical Thinking

Self-Evaluation

- List several situations in your life that are stressful. Select the one that is most stressful.
- List as many things as possible about the situation that make it stressful to you.
- How would you change each of the things you have listed to make them less stressful?
- List the things you "could do" to effect the changes you listed.
- Rank the items in your "could do" list in terms of achievability.
- Select one or two of the items that are achievable and discuss them with a classmate. Now attempt to put them into practice for a week. Report back to your classmate on how effective these items were in reducing stress in your life.

- *Workload:* Continual work level beyond your capability to complete it results in frustration, and ultimately burnout.
- *Job complexity versus skill level:* Expectation to perform beyond your skill level leads to long-duration stress but also can lead to personal growth and increased job satisfaction if the individual is a high achiever.
- *Responsibility delineation:* Lack of delineation of responsibility leads to continual questioning of whom is responsible for what job and ultimately to frustration.
- *Organization size:* Some individuals can get lost in a large organization.
- *Discrimination:* This illegal activity leads to bad feelings and frustration.
- *Poor time management skills:* The inability to prioritize and manage time effectively can lead to work overload.
- *Technological changes:* Change, even good changes, can cause stress.
- *Not being in control of your situation:* Lacking control leads to frustration.

WHAT IS BURNOUT?

Burnout is the result of stress and frustration, principally brought about by unrealistic expectations. Fatigue and exhaustion resulting from trying to meet unrealistic expectations compound it. Because burnout is so damaging, it needs to be discussed as a unique topic.

Stages of Burnout

Burnout has four stages:

- *Honeymoon:* Love your job and have unrealistic expectation placed on you either by your manager or by yourself if you are a perfectionist; take work home and look for all the work you can get, cannot say "no" to accepting additional work
- *Reality:* Begin to have doubts you can meet expectations; feel frustrated with your progress, work harder to meet expectations; begin to feel pulled in many directions; may not have a role model to follow, and established guidelines may not be defined
- *Dissatisfaction:* Loss of enthusiasm; try to escape frustrations by binges of one sort or another, drinking, partying, shopping, or excessive eating or sex; fatigue and exhaustion develop
- *Sad state:* Depression, work seems pointless, lethargic with little energy, consider quitting, and look on yourself as a failure; represents full-blown burnout

All of these stages are part of the process leading to burnout. The honeymoon stage might seem desirable, and it is pleasant, however, the seeds of the illness are present in the unrealistic expectations and the workaholic attitude of the employee. Unless these causes are eliminated, the progression to full burnout is ensured.

Role of Personality and Work Environment

Burnout happens to people who previously were enthusiastic and bursting with energy and new ideas when first hired on the job or beginning a new experience. When individuals with a high need to achieve do not reach their goals, they are apt to feel angry and frustrated and become negative toward their job. Failing to recognize these signs as symptoms of burnout, they may throw themselves even more fully into work-related goals. Unless there is some type of revitalization outside of the workplace, burnout occurs.

Four characteristics associated with burnout in the workplace include:

- *Role conflict:* When employees have conflicting responsibilities, they feel pulled in many directions. The perfectionist tries to do everything equally well without setting priorities. Fatigue and exhaustion associated with burnout begin to set in after time.

- *Role ambiguity:* The employee does not know what is expected and how to accomplish it because there may not be a role model to follow or ask, or established guidelines to follow.
- *Role overload:* If the employee cannot say no and continues to accept more responsibility than they can handle, burnout is sure to set in.
- *Role value:* If the employee feels the job is not worth doing or that he or she is not appreciated, dissatisfaction sets in and speeds up the burnout process initiated by other factors.

Burnout Prevention

Taking steps to prevent burnout before it occurs is the best path to follow if you find you have symptoms of burnout or if the characteristics leading to burnout are present in your job situation.

The following changes in your approach to your work environment and lifestyle will help to prevent burnout:

- Develop time management and prioritization techniques both at work and outside the work environment.
- Detach yourself from your work when you leave for the day and do not take work home.
- Develop outside interests that result in an active social life.
- Take steps to live a healthful life by getting enough sleep, eating a balanced diet, and getting physical exercise.
- Conduct a self-evaluation and set realistic goals for your life and your job.
- Obtain a written job description that defines your responsibilities and expectations.

What to Do If You Are Burned Out

If you recognize yourself in one of the stages of burnout, you have reached a turning point. It is imperative that you make some changes in your relationship with your job. All of the suggested changes given to prevent burnout are applicable and possibly more important once you have entered one of the stages of burnout. The following changes are in order once you have entered the burnout stage:

- Make a concerted effort to say "No" when asked to assume additional work. Job scope creep is a leading factor in burnout.

Critical Thinking

Negative attitudes combined with low pay are a formula for burnout. Why?

- If you have more work than you can realistically accomplish, either prioritize it with the approval of your superior or delegate it within the limit of your authority.
- Change your work-related environment by creating variations. Modify your work routine slightly, rearrange your workstation to make it more personal, or change the computer desktop picture or screensaver to something you find pleasant and which generates positive emotions.
- Evaluate the negative feelings you have regarding your job and attempt to replace them with more positive thoughts (i.e., instead of thinking the glass is half empty, think the glass is half full).
- Try to look on work as a "fun" experience.
- Establish some long- and short-term realistic goals and write them down along with a plan to make them happen.
- Attempt to develop friendships with coworkers and occasionally go to lunch together to laugh a little.
- Embark on a program of relaxation and meditation to reduce stress. Relaxation reduces muscle tension resulting from stress and can be achieved in a few minutes. Meditation requires about 20 minutes each day. Meditation affects body processes such as heart rate, blood pressure, metabolic rate, and brain activity and helps to obtain a feeling of "well-being."

GOAL SETTING AS A STRESS RELIEVER

Do you direct your life, or do you allow others to influence and make decisions for you? **Outer-directed people** let events, other people, or environmental factors dictate their behavior. By contrast, **inner-directed people** decide for themselves what they want to do with their lives. Laurence Peter, author of *The Peter Principle*, states, "If you don't know where you are going, you will end up somewhere else" (Wilkes & Crosswait, 1995).

Discoveries prove that goal-oriented employees are more effective and assertive than are colleagues with no goals or future objectives. Recognizing the value of goal planning, many employers arrange planning sessions or seminars to encourage goal setting as a practical application for coping with stress and burnout and to develop career objectives. If your employer does not offer these outlets, seek your own seminars for goal setting. Such an activity not only "centers" you in your current employment but helps you clearly picture your future plans and hopes.

What is a **goal**? According to *Merriam-Webster's Collegiate Dictionary,* a goal is "the result or achievement toward which effort is directed." To reach a desired goal, a person must implement planning together with a sincere desire to work hard. Skill in goal setting allows the medical assistant to clarify what must be accomplished and to develop a strategic plan to successfully achieve the goal.

A goal must be specific, challenging, realistic, attainable, and measurable. Specific goals are focused and have precise boundaries. A goal that is challenging creates enthusiasm and interest in achievement. Realistic goals are practical or beneficial for the present and for future **self-actualization**. An attainable goal refers to the fact that the goal is possible to fulfill. Measurable goals achieve some form of progress or success. By reflecting on the process, one is encouraged to establish additional goals.

Long-range goals are achievements that may take three to five years to accomplish. Long-range goals give direction and definition to our lives and serve to keep us "on track," so to speak. Much discipline, perseverance, determination, and hard work will be expended in accomplishing long-range goals. Some adjustment and readjustment to your goals may be necessary, however. The rewards of goal achievement include satisfaction, pride, a sense of accomplishment, and a job well done.

Short-range goals take apart long-range goals and reassemble the required activities into smaller, more manageable time segments. The time segments may be daily, weekly, monthly, quarterly, or yearly periods.

As a graduate and new employee, one of your long-range goals might be to become the office manager in the ambulatory care setting in which you are currently employed. You may wish to attain this goal within the next three to five years; by breaking it into three longer range goals and a series of short-range goals, you will be able to measure progress and feel a sense of accomplishment.

Examples of long- and short-range goals might include:

Long-range goal 1:

- To become proficient in all back-office clinical skills during the first year of employment.

Short-range goals necessary to achieve this:

- Practice accuracy and proficiency when performing tasks and skills.
- Practice efficiency by planning ahead for the equipment and supplies needed for each task performed.
- Evaluate your progress on a regular basis, and identify areas that need improvement.

Long-range goal 2:

- To add front-office administrative tasks and skills to your routine during the second year of employment.

Short-range goals necessary to achieve this:

- Practice accuracy and proficiency when performing all front-office tasks and skills.
- Practice efficiency by planning ahead for the equipment and supplies needed for each task performed.
- Evaluate your progress on a regular basis, and identify areas that need improvement.

Long-range goal 3:

- To begin to focus on office management during the third year of employment.

Short-range goals necessary to achieve this:

- Develop a procedure manual for all back- and front-office tasks and skills.
- Enroll in office management classes.
- Focus on team-building skills.

By the fourth year, you will be ready to move into the office manager position.

Long- and short-range goals work together to help make changes in our lives. Goals keep life interesting and give us something for which to strive. We can all reach goals successfully with some planning, hard work, discipline, and dedication.

Case Study 5-1

Review the scenario at the beginning of this chapter.

CASE STUDY REVIEW

1. What work can Ellen Armstrong, CMA (AAMA), organize the night before the office manager is out of town, leaving Ellen in charge of the reception area and ever-ringing telephone the next day?
2. How might Ellen relieve stress as the hectic day progresses?

Case Study 5-2

Ellen Armstrong, CMA (AAMA), has been employed for five years as an administrative medical assistant with providers Lewis and King. Ellen is a perfectionist and has pushed herself to achieve many of her short- and long-term goals. The office staff has become aware that Ellen does not have a sense of humor lately. She seems frustrated and irritable, and she is becoming critical of herself and others. Ellen has felt physically and emotionally exhausted, yet she continues to focus on her high standard of job performance; however, work is becoming a chore. At the end of the day, if everything has not been completed to her satisfaction, she feels like a failure.

CASE STUDY REVIEW

1. Do you feel Ellen is stressed or experiencing burnout? On what do you base your conclusions?
2. What might Ellen do to differentiate these two conditions?
3. What changes might Ellen implement to resolve this problem?

SUMMARY

Stress is very much a part of the medical profession. Each individual working in a medical career experiences consecutive days of demanding, emotionally and physically draining interactions with patients and staff members. This highly technical and ever-changing career requires its professionals to maintain a high level of skill and training and to be familiar with the newest technology.

Goal setting is one approach to reducing stress and burnout and promoting a sense of pride in the workplace, self-actualization, and possible employment promotion. Both long-range and short-range goal planning work together to help make changes in our lives.

STUDY FOR SUCCESS

To reinforce your knowledge and skills of information presented in this chapter:

- Review the Key Terms
- Consider the Case Studies and discuss your conclusions
- Answer the Review Questions
  - Multiple Choice
  - Critical Thinking
- Navigate the Internet by completing the Web Activities
- Practice the StudyWARE activities on the textbook CD
- Apply your knowledge in the Student Workbook activities
- Complete the Web Tutor sections

REVIEW QUESTIONS

Multiple Choice

1. Which answer is *not* true about stress?
   a. It does not occur suddenly.
   b. It has physical and emotional effects on the body.
   c. It may be positive or negative on its effects on the body.
   d. It is the body's response to change.
2. Hans Selye's General Adaptation Syndrome theory proposes that adaptation to stress occurs in how many stages?
   a. 2 stages
   b. 3 stages
   c. 4 stages
   d. 5 stages
3. Which is *not* a stage in the General Adaptation Syndrome?
   a. fight-or-flight
   b. exhaustion
   c. burnout
   d. alarm
4. Signs and symptoms of burnout include all of the following *except:*
   a. emotional and physical exhaustion
   b. hair-trigger display of emotion
   c. feelings of accomplishment and pride in work
   d. irritability and impatience
5. Long-range goals are easy to achieve if:
   a. they are not too challenging
   b. they are divided into a series of short-range goals
   c. they don't involve too much hard work
   d. you never change or adjust them

Critical Thinking

1. You have just graduated from a two-year medical assisting program and have been hired by a pediatric practice as an administrative medical assistant. The practice is busy with many telephone calls daily and many new patients who need charts created and information entered into the database. While in school you learned that you enjoyed the laboratory and clinical work much more than the front-office procedures. How do you think this position will impact your short- and long-duration stress?
2. Identify two long-range goals you personally would like to attain within the next five years. How will you achieve these goals?
3. After you have been on the job for five years, you begin to recognize signs of burnout. How will you manage these symptoms?

WEB ACTIVITIES

Search the Internet for additional information about different relaxation and meditation techniques useful in reducing stress. Choose the technique that interests you the most and research it completely. Compile your information into a report for your instructor. Be sure to include a bibliography identifying your Web sources.

REFERENCES/BIBLIOGRAPHY

Keir, L., Wise, B. A., Krebs, C., & Kelly-Arnex, C. (2008). *Medical assisting: Administrative and clinical competencies* (6th ed.). Clifton Park, NY: Delmar Cengage Learning.

Merriam-Webster's collegiate dictionary (11th ed.). (1998). Springfield, MA: Merriam-Webster.

Milliken, M.E., & Honeycutt, A. (2004). *Understanding human behavior: A guide for health care providers.* Clifton Park, NY: Delmar Cengage Learning.

Tamparo, C. D., & Lindh, W. Q. (2008). *Therapeutic communications for health care.* Clifton Park, NY: Delmar Cengage Learning.

What you need to know about stress management. (2004). Retrieved February 27, 2008, from http://stress.about.com.

Wilkes, M., & Crosswait, C. B. (1995). *Professional development: The dynamics of success.* San Diego: Harcourt Brace Jovanovich.

The Therapeutic Approach to the Patient with a Life-Threatening Illness

Chapter 6

KEY TERMS

Durable Power of Attorney for Health Care

Health Care Directive

Psychomotor Retardation

OUTLINE

- Life-Threatening Illness
  - Cultural Perspective on Life-Threatening Illness
- Choices in Life-Threatening Illness
- The Range of Psychological Suffering
- The Therapeutic Response to the Patient with HIV/AIDS
- The Therapeutic Response to the Patient with Cancer
- The Therapeutic Response to the Patient with End-Stage Renal Disease
- The Stages of Grief
  - Denial
  - Anger
  - Bargaining
  - Depression
  - Acceptance
- The Challenge for the Medical Assistant

OBJECTIVES

The student should strive to meet the following performance objectives and demonstrate an understanding of the facts and principles presented in this chapter through written and oral communication.

1. Define the key terms as presented in the glossary.
2. Describe possible patient perspectives when facing a life-threatening illness.
3. Define "life-threatening" illness.
4. Discuss cultural manifestations of life-threatening illness.
5. Identify the strongest cultural influence in the life of a patient.
6. List at least four choices to be made when facing a life-threatening illness.
7. Briefly describe the use of living wills and health care directives.
8. Explain how a durable power of attorney for health care is used.
9. Discuss the range of psychological suffering that accompanies life-threatening illnesses.
10. Discuss additional concerns/fears when the life-threatening illness is AIDS, cancer, or end-stage renal disease.
11. List the five stages of grief and the meaning of the acronym TEAR.
12. Recall a number of challenges faced by the medical assistant when caring for people with life-threatening illnesses.

Scenario

You have seen the medical reports and agonize with your employer who must tell Suzanne Markis, a long-time patient, when she comes in today that she has inoperable pancreatic cancer. When she arrives, you treat her as you normally would, making certain she suspects nothing from you. When she emerges from the physician's room, you make certain to meet her, take her arm, and ask if you can call someone for her. You do not present her with a bill or make another appointment at this time. You recognize that anything you say probably will not be remembered, so you focus entirely on this patient and her immediate needs. In a day or two, as instructed by your employer, you will make a phone call to set up an appointment for Suzanne and anyone she might want present at her visit with the physician so any questions can be answered.

INTRODUCTION

Everything you learned in Chapter 4 regarding therapeutic communications is heightened and considered more difficult when the patient has a life-threatening illness. If you were told today that your life probably would be shortened because of a serious illness, your perspective would likely change. What was important yesterday may mean little or nothing now. Something that meant nothing to you yesterday suddenly takes on great importance to you now. It is essential for the medical assistant to remember this difference in perspective and what is likely to be important to patients with a life-threatening illness.

It also must be remembered that no two individuals respond to a life-threatening illness in the same way. Some respond with denial and act as if the information had never been shared with them. Others alter their lives radically and drastically change their priorities. Still others quietly continue their lives, changing little outwardly, but recognize that their choices may now be limited (Figure 6-1).

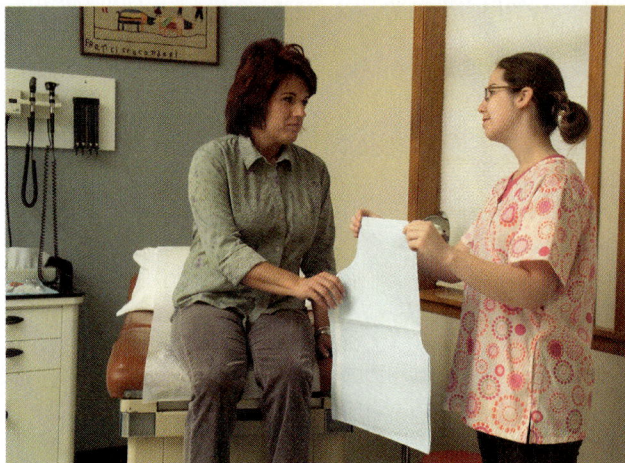

Figure 6-1 Establishing a caring and trusting relationship can help the patient come to terms with a life-threatening illness.

LIFE-THREATENING ILLNESS

A life-threatening illness is not easily defined. Some use the word *terminal;* others refuse to use that word because they believe it removes any hope from the situation. Still others believe even the term *life-threatening* is too hopeless and prefer to use the term *life-limiting.* Also, what is life-threatening for one individual may not be for another. For our purposes, life-threatening is used to imply a life that in all probability will be shortened because of a serious or debilitating illness or disease. It may be defined as death that is imminent; it may be defined in terms of a serious illness that a person will battle for many years but will ultimately shorten his or her life.

Cultural Perspective on Life-Threatening Illness

Strong cultural manifestations will be seen during the treatment of a life-threatening illness and in anyone facing death. Culture is defined as how we live our lives, how we think, how we speak, and how we behave. Cultures can be accepting, denying, or even defying of death. Death can be considered either as the end of existence or as a transition to another state of being or consciousness. Death can be considered as profane or sacred. In some cultures, a life-threatening illness may be viewed or referred to as a "slow-motion" death because of degenerative diseases that often exhaust the resources and emotions of patients and their families.

Some cultures prefer that the life-threatening illness not be shared with the patient in the beginning, but with the family who helps to prepare

Spotlight on Certification

RMA Content Outline

- Patient relations
- Interpersonal skills
- Develop, assemble, and maintain patient resource materials

CMA (AAMA) Content Outline

- Basic principles (psychology)
- Hereditary, cultural, and environmental influence on behavior
- Communication
- Patient instruction
- Professional communication and behavior
- Medicolegal guidelines and requirements
- Legislation

CMAS Content Outline

- Professionalism
- Patient information and community resources

the patient for the inevitable. A few cultures generally do not seek care for an illness until it is quite advanced; this practice can make pain management and treatment more difficult or impossible in some cases. Some cultures surround the person who is ill with great attention, never leaving the person alone. Other cultures view the illness as something that must be removed from the body, perhaps even believing that the individual has been given this illness because of some past sin or transgression.

Pain is viewed in the same manner. Some cultures believe it is to be endured quietly without complaint; others believe there is to be no pain, and family members will go to great lengths to have health care providers relieve the pain. When questioning a patient about the pain level, it must be within a cultural perspective. For example, cultures with an Asian influence are more likely to describe pain in general terms related to the imbalance of the body than in terms of "piercing, intermittent, or throbbing" or on a scale from 1 to 10.

The strongest influence in managing any life-threatening illness in the life of the patient is *not* the health care team; it is the family and those closest to the patient. Therefore, great care must be taken to determine and understand the patient's cultural perspective as much as possible, and the patient must be given great respect. Often, the cultural influence may contradict the standard of care preferred by the health care provider. It is better to understand the culture and work within it than to deny it and continually work against the patient's belief system and influence of family.

CHOICES IN LIFE-THREATENING ILLNESS

Many choices are available to a patient with a life-threatening illness, but many decisions are to be made, also. The urgency of the decisions will depend, in part, on possible life expectancy. Sometimes these decisions may seem contrary to recommended medical intervention.

Patients have the right to choose or to refuse treatment in most cases. Some rush into a treatment protocol only to discover later that their choices have brought them pain, disability, and expense far beyond what originally was assumed. Although it is the health care professional's goal to heal, if healing is not likely or possible, patients ought not to be "urged" into treatment protocols that are likely to be contrary to their personal wishes for the sake of treatment only.

Although health care professionals seem less comfortable with death than they are with saving life, there are some issues appropriate to discuss with patients especially when facing life-threatening illness. Those issues include the following:

1. Alternative methods of treatment should be discussed, as well as the outcome if no treatment is sought. At some point, many patients will want to know *all* the treatment protocols that are feasible. This is a logical time to discuss any alternative or integrative medicine therapies that have shown success. Explanations should be made in language that the patient can understand. Illustrations and diagrams can be beneficial. Referrals might be made to integrative medicine practitioners, and patients are to be encouraged to discuss any chosen alternative therapies with their primary care provider. Sometimes treatment alternatives the patient may consider are not within the realm of recognized medical acceptability, but it is better to have that discussion than to ignore the possibility. Patients may also ask what happens if no treatment is chosen. This question can be difficult for health care providers who are anxious to provide some form of treatment for patients,

but patients may have a number of reasons not to seek treatment. Remember the earlier statement indicating that family members and friends bring more influence to bear than does the health care professional.

2. Discussion of pain management and treatment is essential. The major fears patients have in facing life-threatening illness are pain and loss of independence. A frank discussion of pain control and how that can be accomplished can alleviate a fair amount of concern. Providers should be ready to discuss loss of independence related to any life-threatening illness or to make a referral to someone who can be helpful. Patients have concerns such as wanting to know how long before the disease takes its toll, how long can they drive, what kind of care or assistance will be necessary, whether they can remain in their own home, and how long before they must have someone make decisions for them.

3. A **durable power of attorney for health care** allows an individual to make decisions related to health care when the patient is no longer able to do so. In the best of circumstances, this document will carry out the decisions the patient has already made in a **health care directive** regarding terminal conditions and whether to prolong life. Advances in medicine allow patients' lives to be sustained even when they are unlikely to recover from a persistent and vegetative state. The health care directive and the durable power of attorney for health care allow patients to make decisions before becoming incapacitated on whether life-prolonging medical or surgical procedures are to be continued, withheld, or withdrawn, as well as if or when artificial feeding and fluids are to be used or withheld. These documents can help providers and patients talk about dying and open the door to a positive, caring approach to death. The health care directive and the durable power of attorney for health care documents are legal in all 50 states. Although states may vary somewhat in the wording of these documents, they provide the same overall benefit to patients (see Chapter 7 for more information.) The federal government passed the Patient Self-Determination Act in 1990 giving all patients receiving care in institutions receiving payments from Medicare and Medicaid written information about their right to accept or refuse medical or surgical treatment. The act also requires that patients be given information about their options to create living wills and to appoint someone to act on their behalf in making health care decisions (durable power of attorney for health care). Any documents of this nature that the patient has should be copied in the medical chart that goes with the patient when admitted to the hospital. At any time the patient makes a change in such a document, the old document is to be replaced with the new one.

4. Finances are to be considered. What will insurance cover (if there is insurance)? Who makes the decisions in a managed care environment? What family resources can or will be used? Finances are no one's favorite subject, especially for providers. However, such a discussion is important. Often, patients fear not being able to meet their financial obligations and leaving large debts to surviving family members almost as much as the life-threatening illness itself. As a medical assistant, you can help patients understand the parameters of their health insurance and any restrictions there might be on particular illnesses or treatments. Can medical insurance be canceled if employment pays a portion of the health insurance and the patient is no longer able to work? If there is a life insurance policy, help patients determine if any portion of the policy can be used for end-of-life expenses. Any services you can provide to the patient or family members in relieving the financial stress can bring great relief to everyone involved.

5. Emotional needs of the patient and family members are important. Emotional support is vital when dealing with a life-threatening illness. Health care professionals will want to determine the source of that support for the patient. Should a support group be suggested for the patient and family members? For some patients and families, an individual giving spiritual guidance is seen as a member of the family and a member of the health care team. For others, no spiritual influence is recognized or sought.

It is not the responsibility of the health care professionals treating the individual with life-threatening illness to provide all these services, but a health care professional who raises these issues for patients and families to deal with is more closely in tune with a patient's power in the illness.

Life-threatening illnesses are family illnesses. There are primary (the person suffering from the illness) and secondary (family and friends) patients. Stress on a spouse or partner is enormous as they think about taking over the other person's role and as they try to deal with their own feelings. Patients and their families and friends often feel angry. The situation is especially tragic if it might have been avoided (for example, a long-time smoker dying of lung cancer). There needs to be time to grieve. Depression is common among patients with life-threatening illness and warning signs should be reported to the provider. Remember that how patients live their last days is just as important as the numbers on the laboratory reports.

THE RANGE OF PSYCHOLOGICAL SUFFERING

The range of suffering associated with a life-threatening illness is extensive. Patients feel extreme distress. Anxiety and depression are common. At the time of diagnosis, patients' responses may include denial, numbness, and inability to face the facts. Sadness, hopelessness, helplessness, and withdrawal often are exhibited.

The range of psychological suffering leads to physical symptoms, such as tension, tachycardia, agitation, insomnia, anorexia, and panic attacks. The provider may be so intent on treating the physical ramifications of the illness that the psychological suffering is mostly ignored.

Relationships of individuals with a life-threatening illness often change. Close friends may feel uncomfortable with someone who is dying. Some fear touching or caressing the dying and become aloof and distant. However, new friendships can often be made if patients meet others with the same or similar life-threatening issues and help maintain each other's self-esteem. Relationships are important because they provide support and encouragement beyond any other source. Patients experience a loss of self-esteem when they are ill, are in pain, and have a body that is failing them. When self-image is lost, patients feel useless, see themselves as burdens, and have difficulty accepting help from anyone. The psychological effect of this "loss of self" can even hasten death.

It is often helpful to encourage patients to set goals for themselves. These can be small goals such as walking around the block, eating all their dinner, and connecting with a friend. The goals may also be much larger, such as staying alive until a son graduates from college, or putting all financial matters in order for surviving family members. Personal goals give the patient something other than the illness to plan for and work toward.

Careful listening to patients and seeking clues for what *may not* be said is essential for the medical assistant and support staff caring for patients. Putting yourself in their shoes and asking what would be helpful is often beneficial. Be ready with a list of community resources that may benefit patients at this time.

It is not the intention of this chapter to specifically identify the many life-threatening illnesses and their particular needs. However, three life-threatening illnesses are identified in the following sections with some specific information (see Chapter 3 for additional information on AIDS and cancer).

THE THERAPEUTIC RESPONSE TO THE PATIENT WITH HIV/AIDS

Patients testing positive for human immunodeficiency virus (HIV) and those with acquired immune deficiency syndrome (AIDS) feel great stress from the infection, the disease, and the fear of other life-threatening illnesses. Persons with HIV infection may have only a short time before the onset of AIDS; others may have a much longer period. AIDS is a disease that can have many periods of fairly good health and many periods of serious near-death illnesses. Recent developments in the treatment of HIV infection and AIDS help patients to live longer, but their lives are greatly compromised because of their suppressed immune system.

In some cases, guilt develops about past behavior and lifestyles or the possibility of having transmitted the disease to others. Individuals with HIV infection may feel added strain if this is the first

> Complex criteria determine whether a patient's illness is identified as AIDS rather than HIV infection. Some providers prefer not to use the term *AIDS;* rather, they discuss the illness as early or later stage HIV infection. Many providers in the United States and around the world use the term *AIDS* when patients' CD4 counts (healthy T4 lymphocytes) decline to less than 200. (The average healthy individual will have CD4 lymphocyte counts of 800–1,500.) Many developing countries in the world, however, are unable to measure the CD4 counts. AIDS is then diagnosed by the symptoms and any immunodeficient illnesses the patients have. Using only a CD4 count for diagnosis can be quite discouraging for patients who monitor those counts quite closely. Also, a patient's CD4 count can decrease dramatically into the "AIDS zone" one time, and then increase in sufficient numbers to move the patient back into HIV infection another time. Other criteria that may identify an illness as AIDS are a particular type of opportunistic infection or tumor, an AIDS-related brain or lung illness, and severe body wasting. Allied health professionals will need to take the lead from their employers.

knowledge their families have of any high-risk behaviors they have that are associated with the transmission of the disease. When the disease is contracted by individuals who feel they are protected or safe from the disease, anger is paramount. HIV affects mostly individuals who are relatively young. Thus, they are not as likely to have substantial financial resources or permanent housing. Treating HIV is expensive, and many patients have little or no insurance coverage.

Patients with HIV may experience central nervous system involvement. Forgetfulness and poor concentration may be followed by **psychomotor retardation,** or the slowing of physical and mental responses, decreased alertness, apathy, withdrawal, and diminished interest in work. Some patients later experience confusion and progressive impairment of intellectual function or dementia. When HIV-infected patients contract other opportunistic diseases, those symptoms are experienced as well.

THE THERAPEUTIC RESPONSE TO THE PATIENT WITH CANCER

The first reaction patients with cancer usually have is the fear of loss of life. Patients think, "Cancer equals death. Am I going to die?" After that, issues begin to differ for each person. A few may choose no treatment and allow life to take its course. Most, however, will wonder about what treatment to choose, how to make that choice, and how effective will it be. Many patients are empowered by taking a major role in the decision making related to their cancer. Research can be helpful in studying the many options that may be available in treatment. The fact is that many patients diagnosed with cancer will die, whereas others diagnosed will live many years after diagnosis and treatment.

The three most likely treatments of cancer are surgery, radiation, and chemotherapy. Often, treatment is a combination of the three. Patients can experience serious side effects from both radiation and chemotherapy. Alternative practitioners have shown that meditation or acupuncture can help relieve the side effects for some patients. Loss of hair, nausea, vomiting, and pain are quite disconcerting to patients trying to cope. The American Cancer Society (http://www.cancer.org) has a number of resources for patients.

The most common signs and symptoms of advanced cancer are weakness, loss of appetite and weight, pain, nausea, constipation, sleepiness or confusion, and shortness of breath. Make certain your patients understand your provider's willingness to relieve and treat these symptoms. Even when there is "nothing more to do" related to the cancer, there is still "much to do" to maintain comfort and to give patients the chance to do the things that are meaningful to them and their families.

Critical Thinking

Many individuals in the end stages of both AIDS and cancer have lost their image of themselves. Their bodies have been diminished; they may have lost a great deal of weight from the disease or gained much weight from medications taken. They may have no hair. They may have lost their ability to speak or to control bodily functions. What can you do or say to help them feel like a human being?

THE THERAPEUTIC RESPONSE TO THE PATIENT WITH END-STAGE RENAL DISEASE

Loss of kidney (renal) function leads to serious illness known as end-stage renal disease (ESRD). When the kidneys fail completely, patients cannot live for long unless they receive dialysis or a kidney transplant. A successful kidney transplant relieves the person of kidney failure. However, there are not enough transplants for every person who needs one, and not all transplants are appropriate or successful. Dialysis is the process of artificially replacing the main functions of the kidneys—filtering blood to remove wastes. Choosing dialysis as a treatment plan can sustain life for years and is covered by Medicare, but it does have complications that burden patients and their caregivers.

Depending on age, a patient's general health, and other circumstances, some patients will opt not to have dialysis and to let death come from kidney failure. The by-products of the body's chemistry accumulate in renal failure and cause an array of symptoms. Mild confusion and disorientation are common. Upsetting hallucinations or agitation can occur. Certain minerals concentrated in the blood can cause muscle twitching, tremors, and shakes. Some patients experience mild or severe itching. Appetite decreases early, and breathing can be rapid and shallow. Many patients with kidney failure pass little or no urine. Fluid overload results in edema, or swelling of the body, particularly of the legs and abdomen. Patients with some urine output may live for months even after stopping dialysis. People with no urine output are likely to die within a week or two. Patients will lose energy and become sleepy and lethargic. Typically, patients slip into a deeper sleep and gradually lose consciousness. Kidney failure has a reputation for being a gentle death.

THE STAGES OF GRIEF

There are a number of different philosophies on grief and the stages patients are apt to experience when they know their lives are about to end, but none is so widely known as that of Dr. Elisabeth Kübler-Ross, who was one of the first to conduct research and determine possible stages of grief. Those stages are as follows.

Denial

This is the stage where patients cannot believe that this is happening. They are likely to experience shock and dismay. If the grief is for the loss of a loved one, it is difficult for them to believe that the loved one is dead. If the grief is for themselves and some incident in their lives, they have a hard time accepting the reality of the loss. Words such as "I can't believe it is true," and "There must be some mistake" are common.

It is difficult to help someone in denial. You may be able to reaffirm the reality of the circumstances, but there is little you can do to move someone from the stage of denial.

Anger

Patients express anger, sometimes openly and assertively. Other times, the anger is turned inward and is difficult to accurately express. Patients ask the question "Why?" and often need explanations of what is occurring. Anger is often expressed to others who have no idea what is happening in patients' lives.

This type of anger should be realized for what it is when possible and never taken personally. Patients are angry at the event, not at you. Patients can be helped to express the anger in a realistic and nonhurtful manner.

Bargaining

In this stage, patients bargain with God or a higher being and even their providers and express their desire to make a certain milestone in their lives. "If you can just get me through this current crisis so I can make it to my 40th wedding anniversary, I can accept what is happening." Goals can be very helpful to patients, and they can be encouraged to continue to set realistic goals during their grieving.

Depression

Patients who reach this stage are sad, sometimes quiet and withdrawn. There is a feeling that they have given up. They often prefer not to be around anyone. The depression can be and often is treated so that patients' grief is eased somewhat. This is true especially when patients remain in this stage for a very long time.

Acceptance

This is the time that patients accept the loss. If it is death that is being faced, they often feel they are ready. Everything is in place, and peace has been made with the prognosis. If a loss is being suffered, it is the time when patients begin to move on and make other plans for their lives and their future.

Dr. Kübler-Ross reminds health care professionals that not all patients go through all five stages; some patients go through all five stages over and over again, each time with a little less stress. Others get stuck in one stage, usually denial. Grief and dying are very personal. No two patients will follow the same pattern. Family members suffering grief are often in different stages; therefore, communication and help for each other often are difficult. Remember that grief work is exhausting. So much energy is spent in the grief process that it is often difficult to carry on day-to-day tasks. Any help that can be made available is appreciated.

Critical Thinking

What steps would you personally take to make certain you do not burnout from caring for patients with a life-threatening illness?

The acronym TEAR is fairly popular and is often used to describe the grieving process. It has similarities to the five stages of grief:

T: To accept the reality of the loss

E: Experience the pain of the loss

A: Adjust to what was lost

R: Reinvest in a new reality

Although the five stages of grief and TEAR discussed in this chapter are directed toward patients with life-threatening illnesses, remember that family members and loved ones of patients also will experience grief. Both of these principles can be applied to any kind of serious loss that occurs in one's life—loss of a job, divorce, disaster, war, famine, loss of a limb or important body function, Alzheimer's disease, loss of a friend, even the death of a beloved pet. The stages of grief and the acronym TEAR can apply just as easily to these situations.

Dr. Kübler-Ross, in her final days before her own death in 2004, reminded her co-author to "Listen to the dying. They will tell you everything you need to know about when they are dying. And it is easy to miss."

THE CHALLENGE FOR THE MEDICAL ASSISTANT

As a medical assistant, you face the challenge of caring for people with a life-threatening illness; you can comfort those who face great suffering and death. You will become a source of information for patients and their support members. Be sensitive and respectful toward individuals who may be shunned by society. Examine your own beliefs, lifestyle, and biases so that you can be comfortable treating all patients, no matter what the illness is or how it was contracted.

As well as assisting your employer in providing the best possible medical care, many nonmedical forms of assistance may be required by patients suffering from a life-threatening illness. You may need to make referrals to community-based agencies or service groups. Health departments, social workers, trained hospice volunteers, and AIDS and cancer volunteers may also be helpful to you, your patients, and their families.

The best therapeutic response to the patient with a life-threatening illness will build on the person's own culture and coping abilities, capitalize on strengths, maintain hope, and show continued human care and concern. Patients may want up-to-date information on their disease, its causes, modes of transmission, treatments available, and sources of care and social support. Be prepared to recommend support groups where patients can discuss their feelings and express their concerns. Treat patients with concern and compassion and assure them everything will be done to provide continuity of care and relief from distress. Patients also may be encouraged to call on a spiritual advisor.

Case Study 6-1

Review the scenario at the beginning of the chapter. As you prepare for the second visit of Suzanne Markis, you make a mental note of what kind of information you will have available.

CASE STUDY REVIEW

1. What paperwork might be necessary?
2. What questions might you have for Suzanne?
3. What might family members who may accompany Suzanne want to know?
4. As the medical assistant, how does your role differ from that of your employer?

Case Study 6-2

The extended family of Wong Lee is concerned about his illness and his care. Chronic obstructive pulmonary disease (COPD) has ravaged his body. He is on oxygen all the time now. He wants to remain at home to die; his family wants that, too. The family has been with him and has been involved in his care plan all along. However, you are uncertain of how much information to give to members of his extended family when they call.

CASE STUDY REVIEW

1. Are the questions the extended family members raise intended to harm or help Mr. Lee?
2. Is there a durable power of attorney for health care in place?
3. Which, if any, of the family's desires are related to the culture?
4. What can you and your employer suggest to be of help to everyone involved?

Case Study 6-3

Jeff and Amy live in rural Tennessee. They are expecting their first baby and are excited beyond belief because they had so much trouble getting pregnant. You are the medical assistant for their family practice provider. Test results from their recent ultrasound have been returned to your clinic, and the news is not good. There appears to be some difficulty and one or more apparent birth defects in the developing fetus. You and your employer discuss possible resources.

CASE STUDY REVIEW

1. As the medical assistant, what is your first responsibility to these expectant parents?
2. Where might you look for possible resources?
3. Identify three to five possible resources.
4. If referral to a specialist is to be made, what role might you play in that referral?

SUMMARY

Medical assistants will want to remember that when caring for patients with a life-threatening illness, having even the slightest fear of death can undermine the ability to respond professionally, with empathy and support. If you feel yourself losing the ability to be helpful, it is time to briefly step aside. This does not mean withdrawal from your position or refusal to care for your patients. It means that you do whatever is necessary so that your perspective is not lost. It may mean taking a day off from work to "fill up your psyche" and to give yourself a rest. If the ambulatory care setting has an abundance of patients with life-threatening illnesses, it may require that you spend some time in a support group of your own so that you are better able to cope. Never be afraid to feel sad or weep with your patients. It is better to sense their pain and, at times, feel the pain with them, than it is to be so clinically objective that you miss their true needs.

STUDY FOR SUCCESS

To reinforce your knowledge and skills of information in this chapter:

- Review the Key Terms
- Consider the Case Studies and discuss your conclusions
- Answer the Review Questions
  - Multiple Choice
  - Critical Thinking
- Navigate the Internet and complete the Web Activities
- Practice the StudyWARE activities on the textbook CD
- Apply your knowledge in the Student Workbook activities
- Complete the Web Tutor sections
- View and discuss the DVD situations

REVIEW QUESTIONS

Multiple Choice

1. When a practice treats patients with HIV/AIDS, cancer, or ESRD, it is important for medical assistants to:
   a. warn other patients about the dangers of transmission
   b. segregate these patient reception areas from other patient areas
   c. be supportive and free of prejudice
   d. deny any information to patients regarding the seriousness of the illness
2. The Patient Self-Determination Act:
   a. allows a patient to have a choice of providers
   b. ensures a patient's right to accept or refuse treatment
   c. gives patients the right to formulate advance directives
   d. all of the above
   e. only b and c
3. The strongest influence on a patient with a life-threatening illness is:
   a. the provider
   b. the hospital
   c. the family
   d. the patient
4. Life-threatening illness may be defined as:
   a. a life shortened because of serious illness or disease
   b. death that is imminent
   c. serious illness to battle for many years but may shorten life
   d. all of the above
5. Culture may be defined in part as:
   a. how we choose a friend
   b. how we think and live our lives
   c. how we select a medication
   d. all of the above
6. Therapeutic communication with a patient with a life-threatening illness:
   a. is no different than communicating with any patient
   b. is heightened and considered more difficult
   c. is left to nonmedical support staff
   d. comes naturally and requires no special skill
7. Cultural influence may in part determine:
   a. when/how to involve family members
   b. whether spiritual support is sought
   c. how the illness and its pain is managed
   d. all of the above
8. Durable power of attorney for health care:
   a. enables someone other than the patient to make only health care decisions
   b. enables someone other than the patient to make any decisions for the patient
   c. makes certain that patients' financial responsibilities are met
   d. makes certain an attorney's wishes are followed
9. The confusion, disorientation, and mental deficiency sometimes seen in patients with life-threatening illness:
   a. may make communication difficult or impossible
   b. is a good reason for a durable power of attorney for health care
   c. is made easier if patients expressed earlier their desires in a health care directive
   d. all of the above
10. Effective pain management may depend on:
    a. patient's medical insurance
    b. family wishes and patient's needs
    c. professional nursing criteria
    d. all of the above

Critical Thinking

1. Discuss with a friend what cultural influences might affect each of you if you were facing a life-threatening illness. What choices would each of you make?
2. Discuss with a classmate your concerns in dealing with patients with a life-threatening illness. Would you choose to work where you seldom lost a patient to a life-threatening illness? If so, what are your reasons?
3. At Inner City Health Care, Dr. Ray Reynolds is known for his compassion and great warmth toward people. On difficult days at the center, this attitude holds him in good stead. Sometimes, he tends to take on the more challenging cases: patients with life-threatening diseases, often young people with AIDS who should be in the prime of their lives. Clinical medical assistant Wanda Slawson always tries to learn from Dr. Reynolds' example. Although she is quieter and not as outgoing as Dr. Reynolds, Wanda hopes to be both courteous and comforting to patients, especially those who are anxious. She makes it a point to help patients discover a new way to cope with debilitating diseases. What resources might she use?
4. Teri Montague, RMA, is the office manager for a pediatric oncologist. In the past several months there seem to have been more patient deaths than usual. She notices that the entire staff seems "low and a little depressed." She discusses this concern with her employer, Dr. Anita Glenn. The decision is made to close the office for a 2-hour lunch on

Wednesday. The lunch will be catered, and a very good friend of Dr. Glenn will be invited to join everyone. Dr. Penny Hein has a PhD in psychosocial nursing and years of experience in grief counseling. Teri and Dr. Glenn believe she can give everyone some helpful information. Is this a good plan? Why or why not?

5. A danger in having a fair amount of knowledge about life-threatening illnesses and the grief that accompanies them can be that we hope to be able to "fix" everything. With a friend, discuss the following statement made by Dr. Kübler-Ross: "Listen to the dying. They will tell you everything you need to know about when they are dying. And it is easy to miss." What does she mean? Why is it easy to miss?

WEB ACTIVITIES

1. Using your favorite search engine, key in American Cancer Society and look for statistics for the current year. Pay particular attention to the area reporting how long patients survive after diagnosis. What are the major changes in the last two years?
2. Search the Internet for sites on grieving or grief. Pay particular attention to sites that have resources for grieving children or teens. What particular help do you find? Do children and teens grieve differently than adults? If so, explain.
3. Using the Internet can be challenging, especially if you find more than a million sites to browse. That is what you will find if you key in "Helping the Dying." Choose a couple of the topics that are especially helpful to you or might help other students studying this chapter. Write a brief paragraph on each.

REFERENCES/BIBLIOGRAPHY

Kübler-Ross, E., & Kessler, D. (2005). *On grief and grieving*. New York: Scribner.

Lewis, M., & Tamparo, C. (2007). *Medical law, ethics, and bioethics for the health professions*. Philadelphia: F. A. Davis.

Purnell, L., & Paulanka, B. (1998). *Transcultural health care: A culturally competent approach*. Philadelphia: F. A. Davis.

Tamparo, C., & Lindh, W. (2007). *Therapeutic communications for health care*. Clifton Park, NY: Delmar Cengage Learning.

THE DVD HOOK-UP

This chapter introduces you to the concept of using a therapeutic approach when working with patients.

In the designated DVD clip, we observed Mrs. Smith become quite anxious about her abnormal mammogram results. We also observed how Gwen, the medical assistant, addressed Mrs. Smith's concerns.

1. Do you feel that Gwen demonstrated a therapeutic approach toward Mrs. Smith's concern over her abnormal mammogram results?
2. List some gestures that Gwen used that illustrated her concern and compassion toward the patient.
3. Did Gwen overstep her boundaries as a medical assistant when she discussed the mammogram results with Mrs. Smith, or do you think that Gwen was trying to help the patient understand what the provider had already explained?

DVD Journal Summary

Write a paragraph that summarizes what you learned from watching the designated scene from today's DVD program. Did you empathize with Mrs. Smith regarding her anxiety over her abnormal mammogram? What will you do when you are faced with similar challenges in the industry? Do you think that you could ever work in an oncology practice? Why or why not?

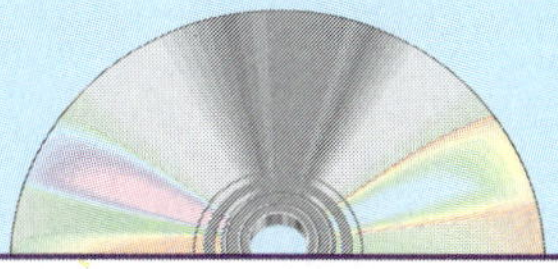

DVD Series	**Program Number**
Critical Thinking	2

Chapter/Scene Reference
- *Communicating with Patients*

UNIT 3

Responsible Medical Practice

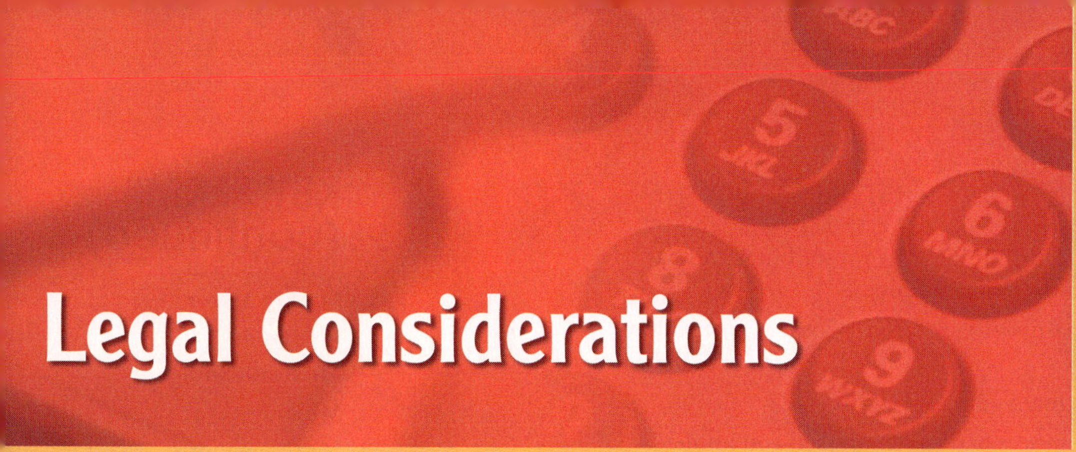

Chapter 7

Legal Considerations

KEY TERMS

Administer
Administrative Law
Agent
Alternative Dispute Resolution (ADR)
Arbitration
Civil Law
Common Law
Constitutional Law
Contract Law
Criminal Law
Defendant
Deposition
Discovery
Dispense
Durable Power of Attorney for Health Care
Emancipated Minor
Expert Witness
Expressed Contract
Felony
Health Insurance Portability and Accountability Act (HIPAA)
Implied Consent
Implied Contract
Incompetence
Informed Consent
Interrogatory
Intimate Partner Violence (IPV)
Libel
Litigation
Malfeasance
Malpractice

OUTLINE

Sources of Law
- Statutory Law
- Common Law
- Criminal Law
- Civil Law

Administrative Law
- Title VII of the Civil Rights Act
- Federal Age Discrimination Act
- Uniform Anatomical Gift Act
- Regulation Z of the Consumer Protection Act
- Occupational Safety and Health Act
- Controlled Substances Act
- Americans with Disabilities Act
- Family and Medical Leave Act
- Health Insurance Portability and Accountability Act

Contract Law
- Termination of Contracts

Tort Law
- Medical Practice Acts
- Standard of Care

Informed Consent
- Implied Consent
- Consent and Legal Incompetence

Risk Management

Civil Litigation Process
- Subpoenas
- Discovery
- Pretrial Conference
- Trial
- Statute of Limitations

Public Duties
- Reportable Diseases/Injuries
- Abuse
- Good Samaritan Laws

Advance Directives
- Living Wills/Advance Directives
- Durable Power of Attorney for Health Care
- Patient Self-Determination Act

OBJECTIVES

The student should strive to meet the following performance objectives and demonstrate an understanding of the facts and principles presented in this chapter through written and oral communication.

1. Define the key terms as presented in the glossary.
2. List and briefly describe the five sources of law.
3. Compare/contrast civil and criminal law.
4. Identify the three major areas of civil law that directly affect the medical profession.
5. Recall at least seven of the nine administrative law acts important to the medical profession.

OBJECTIVES (continued)

6. Compare/contrast administering, prescribing, and dispensing of controlled substances.
7. Describe the measures to take for disposal of controlled substances.
8. Recall the three main goals of HIPAA.
9. Explain the differences between expressed and implied contracts.
10. Identify the three main reasons for a provider/patient contract to be terminated.
11. Define and give examples of torts.
12. Compare/contrast intentional and negligent tort.
13. Discuss licensure renewal and revocation for physicians.
14. List and describe the 4Ds of negligence.
15. Discuss what constitutes battery in the ambulatory care setting.
16. Describe the two forms of defamation of character and how it might occur.
17. Recall how medical assistants can help to maintain a patient's privacy.
18. Discuss informed consent and its importance.
19. Compare/contrast the types of minors.
20. Identify at least 10 practices to help in risk management.
21. Outline the necessary steps in civil litigation and how a medical assistant might be involved.
22. Discuss how and when subpoenas are used.
23. Recall the special considerations for patients related to issues of confidentiality, the statute of limitations, and public duties.
24. Describe procedures to follow in reporting abuse.
25. Discuss Good Samaritan laws.
26. Identify various forms of advance directives.
27. Recall maintenance of advance directives in the ambulatory care setting.
28. Discuss the durable power of attorney for health care.

KEY TERMS (continued)

Mature Minor
Mediation
Medically Indigent
Minor
Misdemeanor
Misfeasance
Negligence
Noncompliant
Nonfeasance
Patient Self-Determination Act (PSDA)
Plaintiff
Precedents
Prescribe
Risk Management
Slander
Statutory Law
Subpoena
Tort
Tort Law

Scenario

Gwen, the office manager in Dr. Gold's office, is reviewing legal concerns in a staff meeting. Even though each employee is well aware of privacy, confidentiality, and the many ways their actions are legally binding, Gwen has noticed occasional carelessness creeping into their busy activities. Gwen has heard voices of staff from the hallway discussing confidential matters, notices an occasional medical chart in public view, and wants to review HIPAA compliance.

INTRODUCTION

The law as it relates to health care has grown increasingly complex in the last decade. The agendas of federal and state governments include an investigation of quality health care, a desire to control health care costs (while hoping to ensure equitable access to health care), and an interest in protecting the patient. A full discussion of health law requires several volumes; therefore, the aim of this chapter is awareness of the law and its implications and establishment of sound practices and procedures to both safeguard patient rights and protect the health care professional.

SOURCES OF LAW

Law is a binding custom or ruling for conduct that is enforceable by an agency assigned that authority. The highest authority in the United States is the U.S. Constitution. Adopted in 1787, this document provides the framework for the U.S. government. The Constitution includes 27 amendments, 10 of which are known as the Bill of Rights. This authority is sometimes referred to as **constitutional law.** The U.S. Constitution calls for three branches of the federal government:

- Executive branch: the President and Vice President (elected by U.S. citizens), Cabinet officers, and various other departments of the federal government
- Legislative branch: members of the U.S. Senate and the House of Representatives (elected by U.S. citizens) and the staffs of individual legislators and legislative committees.
- Judicial branch: the courts, including the U.S. Supreme Court, Courts of Appeals for the nine judicial regions, and District Courts

Laws enacted at the federal level are called acts or laws. An example is Title XIX of Public Law established in 1967 to provide health care for the **medically indigent.** This program is known as Medicaid.

Statutory Law

Constitutions in the 50 states identify the rights and responsibilities of their citizens and identify how their state is organized. States have a governor as the head and state legislatures (both elected by the state's citizens), as well as their own court systems with a number of levels. The body of laws made by states is known as **statutory law.** All powers that are not conferred specifically on the federal government are retained by the state, yet states vary widely in their interpretation of that power. State law cannot override the power of any laws defined in the U.S. Constitution or its amendments.

Common Law

Common law is not so easily defined but is essential to understanding law in the United States. Common law was developed by judges in England and France over many centuries and was brought to the United States with the early settlers. Common law is often called judge-made law. The law consists of rulings made by judges who base their decisions on a combination of a number of factors: (1) individual decisions of a court, (2) interpretation of the U.S. Constitution or a particular state constitution, and (3) statutory law. These decisions become known as **precedents** and often lay down the foundation for subsequent legal rulings.

Spotlight on Certification

RMA Content Outline

- Medical law
- Licensure, certification, registration
- Principles of medical ethics
- Ethical conduct
- Drugs
- Safety
- Legal responsibilities

CMA (AAMA) Content Outline

- Displaying professional attitude
- Performing within ethical boundaries
- Maintaining confidentiality
- Licenses and accreditation
- Legislative
- Documentation/reporting
- Releasing medical information
- Provider-patient relationship

CMAS Content Outline

- Legal and ethical considerations
- Professionalism
- Confidentiality
- Safety
- Risk management and quality assurance

Criminal Law

Criminal law addresses wrongs committed against the welfare and safety of society as a whole. Criminal law affects relationships between individuals and between individuals and the government. Another term that might be used to describe a criminal act is **malfeasance.** Malfeasance is conduct that is illegal or contrary to an official's obligation. Criminal offenses generally are classified into the basic categories of a **felony** or a **misdemeanor** that are specifically defined in statutes.

Felonies are more serious crimes and include murder, larceny or thefts of large amounts of money, assault, and rape. Punishment for a felony is more serious than for a misdemeanor. A convicted felon cannot vote, hold public office, or own any weapons. Felonies often are divided into groups such as first degree (most serious), second degree, and third degree. Sentences are generally for longer than one year and are served in a penitentiary. Misdemeanors are considered lesser offenses and vary from state to state. Punishment may include probation or a time of service to the community, a fine, or a jail sentence in a city or county facility. Misdemeanors also can be divided into groups or classifications, such as A, B, or C class misdemeanors, denoting the seriousness of the crime (Class A is the most serious).

For a person to be found guilty of a crime, a judge or jury must prove the evidence against the individual "beyond a reasonable doubt." In a criminal case, charges are brought against an individual by the state with the intent of preventing any further harm to society. For example, a physician practicing medicine without a proper license may be subject to criminal action by the courts for endangering a patient's life.

Civil Law

Civil law affects relationships between individuals, corporations, government bodies, and other organizations. Terms that may be used in civil law are **misfeasance,** referring to a lawful act that is improperly or unlawfully executed, and **nonfeasance,** referring to the failure to perform an act, official duty, or legal requirement. The punishment for a civil wrong is usually monetary in nature. When a charge is brought against a **defendant** in a civil case, the goal is to reimburse the **plaintiff** or the person bringing charges with a monetary amount for suffering, pain, and any loss of wages. Another goal might be to make certain the defendant is prevented from engaging in similar behavior again. In civil law, cases need to show that a "preponderance of the evidence" is more than likely true against the defendant. The most common forms of civil law that directly affect the medical profession are **administrative law, contract law,** and **tort law.**

ADMINISTRATIVE LAW

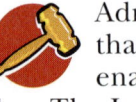

Administrative law establishes agencies that are given power to specialize and enact regulations that have the force of law. The Internal Revenue Service is an example of an administrative agency that enacts tax laws and regulations. Health care professionals are bound by federal administrative law through the Medicare and Medicaid program rules administered by the Social Security Administration.

There are a number of other regulations in administrative law governing health professionals and their employees. It is important that medical assistants be informed of legislation and any federal or state regulations that are critical to patients and the medical profession. Identified here with a brief description are additional administrative acts, some of which also are referred to in other chapters in this textbook.

Title VII of the Civil Rights Act

Title VII of the Civil Rights Act of 1964 protects employees from sexual harassment and a hostile work environment. The office of Equal Employment Opportunities Commission (EEOC) guidelines make the employer strictly liable for the acts of supervisory employees, as well as for some acts of harassment by coworkers and clients (see Chapter 34).

Harassment occurs when sexual favors are implied or requested by a supervisor in return for job advancement or special treatment on the job. Another form of harassment and a more common problem that may exist in the workplace is referred to as a "hostile work environment." When pervasive or severe sexual comments, jokes, or inappropriate touching create a workplace so negative that it interferes with an employee's work performance, a hostile work environment exists.

A written policy on sexual harassment detailing inappropriate behavior and stating specific steps to be taken to correct an inappropriate situation should be established. The policy should include (1) a statement that harassment is not tolerated, (2) a statement that an employee who feels harassed needs to bring the matter to the immediate attention of a person designated in the policy, (3) a statement about the confidentiality of any incidents and specific disciplinary action against the harasser, and

(4) the procedure to follow when harassment occurs. It is illegal for a supervisor or employer to ignore an employee's complaint. An employer or supervisor who does not take corrective action is liable.

Federal Age Discrimination Act

The Federal Age Discrimination Act of 1967 states that an employer with 15 or more employees must not discriminate in matters of employment related to age, sex, race, creed, marital status, national origin, color, or disabilities. Some states are more restrictive in their law and identify employers with eight or more employees. Valid reasons to decline applicants include (1) health issues that may interfere with the safe and efficient performance of the job, (2) unavailability for the work schedule of the particular job, (3) insufficient training or experience to perform the duties of the particular job, and (4) someone else is better qualified. Although some health care settings have fewer than 15 or even 8 employees, it is best to follow state and federal guidelines on all employment.

As of October 2008, 19 states have laws banning discrimination because of sexual orientation. Those states are California, Connecticut, Hawaii, Illinois, Iowa, Maine, Maryland, Massachusetts, Minnesota, Nevada, New Hampshire, New Jersey, New Mexico, New York, Oregon, Rhode Island, Vermont, Washington, and Wisconsin. The District of Columbia passed similar legislation.

Uniform Anatomical Gift Act

The Uniform Anatomical Gift Act of 1968 allows persons 18 years and older and of sound mind to make a gift of all or any part of their body (1) to any hospital, surgeon, or physician; (2) to any accredited medical or dental school, college, or university; (3) to any organ bank or storage facility; and (4) to any specified individual for education, research, advancement of medical/dental science, therapy, or transplantation. The gift may be noted in a will or by signing, in the presence of two witnesses, a donor's card. Some states allow these statements on the driver's license. There is no cost to donors or their families for gifts of all or part of the body.

Regulation Z of the Consumer Protection Act

Regulation Z of the Consumer Protection Act of 1967, referred to as the Truth in Lending Act, requires that an agreement by providers and their clients for payment of medical bills in more than four installments must be in writing and must provide information on any finance charge. This act is enforced by the Federal Trade Commission. These guidelines are often seen in prearrangements for surgery or prenatal care and delivery in fee-for-service plans, because patients may not be able to pay the entire fee in one payment.

Occupational Safety and Health Act

The Occupational Safety and Health Act (OSHA) of 1967 is a division of the U.S. Department of Labor. Its mission is to ensure that a workplace is safe and has a healthy environment. Penalties can be quite high for repeated and willful violations assessed by OSHA. These guidelines make certain that all employees know what chemicals they are handling, know how to reduce any health risks from hazardous chemicals that are labeled 1 to 4 for severity, and have Material Safety Data Sheets (MSDSs) listing every ingredient in the product. Other sections of this law protecting medical assistants and patients are detailed in additional chapters. They include Clinical Lab Improvement Amendments of 1988 (CLIA) (see Chapter 26), Blood-borne Pathogens Standard of July 1992 (see Chapter 10), and the Needle Stick Prevention Amendment of 2001 (see Chapter 10).

Controlled Substances Act

The Controlled Substances Act of 1970 became effective in 1971. The act is administered by the Drug Enforcement Administration (DEA) under the auspices of the U.S. Department of Justice. The Controlled Substances Act lists controlled drugs in five schedules (I, II, III, IV, and V) according to their potential for abuse and dependence, with Schedule I having the greatest abuse potential and no accepted medical use in the United States. This act and the U.S. Code of Federal Regulations regulate individuals who administer, prescribe, or dispense any drug listed in the five schedules. Any

Critical Thinking

Identify the type of providers or medical specialties most likely to administer and dispense controlled substances.

individual who **administers, prescribes,** or **dispenses** any controlled substance must be registered with the DEA. The DEA supplies a form for registration and mandates that renewal occurs every 3 years.

A provider who only prescribes Schedule II, III, IV, and V controlled substances in the lawful course of professional practice is not required to keep separate records of those transactions. The majority of all providers fall within this category. Providers who regularly administer controlled substances in Schedules II, III, IV, and V or who dispense controlled substances are required to keep records of each transaction.

An inventory must be taken every 2 years of all stocks of the substances on hand. The inventory must include (1) a list of the name, address, and DEA registration number of the provider; (2) the date and time of the inventory; and (3) the signatures of the individuals taking the inventory. This inventory must be kept at the location identified on the registration certificate for at least 2 years. All Schedule II drug records must be maintained separate from all other controlled substance records. These records must be made available for inspection and copying by duly authorized officials of the DEA. Some states are even more restrictive than the federal requirements.

Any necessary disposal of controlled substances, usually occurring when they become outdated or when a medical practice is closed, requires specific action. The provider's DEA number and registration certificate should be returned to the DEA. Specific guidelines for destruction of the controlled substances will need to be obtained from the nearest divisional office for the DEA. Using the Internet, search using the words "Controlled Substances Act of 1970" for a listing of sites providing more information. You will find a listing of drugs in each of the five schedules that change from time to time as new drugs come on the market and are classified.

Americans with Disabilities Act

The Americans with Disabilities Act (ADA) of 1990 prohibits discrimination preventing individuals who have physical or mental disabilities from accessing public services and accommodations, employment, and telecommunications. A disability implies that a physical or mental impairment substantially limits one or more of an individual's major life activities. ADA is identified in five titles. Title I, enforced by the EEOC, prohibits discrimination in employment (see Chapter 34 for further details). Essentially, Title I requires a potential employer to identify and prove that certain disabilities cannot be accommodated in performing the job requirements. Employers only have to provide reasonable accommodations rather than anything an employee demands or something that is extraordinarily expensive. Individuals who formerly abused drugs and alcohol and those who are undergoing rehabilitation also are covered by the ADA and cannot be denied employment because of their history of substance abuse.

Titles II, III, and IV mandate disabled individuals access to public services, public accommodations, and telecommunications. ADA protects persons with HIV infection or AIDS, making certain they cannot be refused treatment by health care professionals because of their health status. Generally speaking, health care professionals with HIV infection or AIDS cannot be kept from providing treatment either, unless that treatment could be found to be a significant risk to others. Title V covers a number of miscellaneous issues such as exclusions from the definition of "disability," retaliation, insurance, and other issues. The ADA applies to businesses with at least 15 employees, but some states have more stringent laws.

Family and Medical Leave Act

The Family and Medical Leave Act (FMLA) of 1993 is important for large ambulatory care centers and hospitals. FMLA requires all public employers and any private employer of 50 or more employees to provide up to 12 weeks of job-protected, unpaid leave each year for the following reasons: (1) birth and care of the employee's child, or placement for adoption or foster care of a child; (2) care of an immediate family member who has a serious health condition; and (3) care of the employee's own serious health issue. Employees must have been employed for at least 12 months and have worked at least 1,250 hours in the 12 months preceding the beginning of the FMLA leave.

Health Insurance Portability and Accountability Act

HIPAA

The **Health Insurance Portability and Accountability Act (HIPAA)** of 1996 requires the Department of Health and Human Services to adopt national standards for electronic health care transactions. The law also requires the adoption of privacy and security standards to protect an individual's identifiable health information. The goal of HIPAA is also to assist in making health insurance more affordable and accessible to individuals by protecting health insurance coverage for workers and their families when they change or lose their jobs.

HIPAA law is identified in seven titles. They are summarized briefly as follows:

I. Health Insurance Access, Portability, and Renewal: Increases the portability of health insurance, allows continuance and transfer of insurance even with preexisting conditions, and prohibits discrimination based on health status.

II. Preventing Health Care Fraud and Abuse: Establishes a fraud and abuse system and spells out penalty if either event is documented; improves the Medicare program through establishing standards; establishes standards for electronic transmission of health information.

III. Tax-Related Provisions: Promotes the use of medical savings accounts (MSAs) used for medical expenses only. Deposits are tax-deductible for self-employed individuals who are able to draw on the accounts for medical expenses.

IV. Group Health Plan Requirements: Identifies how group health care plans must plan for portability, access, and transferability of health insurance for its members.

V. Revenue Offsets: Details how HIPAA changed the Internal Revenue Code to generate more revenue for HIPAA expenses.

VI. General Provisions: Explains how coordination with Medicare-type plans must be carried out to prevent duplication of coverage.

VII. Assuring Portability: Ensures employee coverage from one plan to another; written specifically for health insurance plans to ensure portability of coverage.

As of April 21, 2006, all covered health care entities were to have been in compliance of HIPAA's regulations. These regulations caused concern among providers. However, once the electronic codes and transactions for electronic filing of health insurance claims were identified and put in place, the required security and privacy of all patient information was not so complex. Medical facilities and providers who were consistently diligent about protecting patient confidentiality found complying with HIPAA not too difficult. Many helpful Web sites are available simply by keying in HIPAA and having your favorite search engine identify sites. Look for a site that explains this public law and gives current updates. You will see mention of HIPAA throughout this text as identified by the HIPAA icon as shown on the left.

CONTRACT LAW

The contractual nature of the provider–patient relationship necessitates a discussion of contracts, which are an important part of any medical practice. A contract is a binding agreement between two or more persons. A provider has a legal obligation, or duty, to care for a patient under the principles of contract law. The agreement must be between competent persons to do or not to do something lawful in exchange for a payment.

A contract exists when the patient arrives for treatment and the provider accepts the patient by providing treatment. An example of a valid contract occurs when a patient calls the office or clinic to make an appointment for an annual physical examination. Assuming both provider and patient are competent, and that the provider performs the lawful act of the physical examination and the patient pays a fee, all aspects of the contract exist.

There are two types of contracts: expressed and implied. An **expressed contract** can be written or verbal and specifically describes what each party in the contract will do. A written contract requires that all necessary aspects of the agreement be in writing. An **implied contract** is indicated by actions rather than by words. The majority of provider–patient contracts are implied contracts. It is not required that the contract be written to be enforceable as long as all points of the contract exist. An implied contract can exist either by the circumstances of the situation or by the law. When a patient reports a sore throat and the provider takes a swab for a throat culture to diagnose and treat the ailment, an implied contract exists by the circumstances. An implied contract by law exists when a patient goes into anaphylactic shock and the provider administers epinephrine to counteract shock symptoms. The law says that the provider did what the patient would have requested had there been an expressed contract.

For a contract to be valid and binding, the parties who enter into it must be competent; therefore, the mentally incompetent, the legally insane, individuals under heavy drug or alcohol influences, infants, and some minors cannot enter into a binding contract.

Medical assistants are considered **agents** of the employers they serve, and as such must be cautious that their actions and words may become binding for their employers. For example, to say that the provider can cure the patient may cause serious legal problems when, in fact, a cure may not be possible.

Termination of Contracts

A broken contract or breach of contract occurs when one of the parties does not meet contractual obligations. A provider is legally bound to treat a patient until:

- The patient discharges the provider
- The provider formally withdraws from patient care
- The patient no longer needs treatment and is formally discharged by the provider

Patient Discharges Provider. When the patient discharges the provider, a letter should be sent to the patient to confirm and document the termination of the contract. The notice is sent by certified mail with return receipt requested. Keep a copy of the letter in the patient's record (Figure 7-1).

Provider Formally Withdraws from the Case. To avoid any charges of abandonment, the provider should formally withdraw from the case when, for example, the patient becomes **noncompliant** or the provider feels the patient can no longer be served. Again, notice should be sent to the patient by certified mail with return receipt requested, and a copy of the notice should be filed in the patient's record (Figures 7-2 and 7-3).

The Patient No Longer Needs Treatment. Unless a formal discharge or withdrawal has occurred, a provider is obligated to care for a patient until the patient's condition no longer requires treatment.

L&K LEWIS & KING, MD
2501 CENTER STREET
NORTHBOROUGH, OH 12345

January 6, 20XX

CERTIFIED MAIL

Jim Marshal
76 Georgia Avenue
Millerton, TX 43912

Dear Mr. Marshal:

This will confirm our telephone conversation today in which you discharged me as your attending physician in your present illness. In my opinion your condition requires continued medical supervision by a physician. If you have not already done so, I suggest that you employ another physician without delay.

You may be assured that after receiving a written request from you, I will furnish the physician of your choice with information regarding the diagnosis and treatment which you have received from me.

Very truly yours,

Winston Lewis

Winston Lewis, MD
WL:ea

Figure 7-1 Letter confirming a physician's discharge by the patient.

Inner City Health Care
222 S. First Avenue
Carlton, MI 11666

May 9, 20XX

CERTIFIED MAIL

Lenny Taylor
260 Second Street
Carlton, MI 11666

Dear Mr. Taylor:

You will recall that we discussed our professional relationship in my office on May 6, 20XX.

Your son, George Taylor, and Bruce Goldman, my medical assistant, were also present. As you know, the primary difficulty has been your failure to cooperate with the medical plan for your care.

While it is unfortunate that our relationship has reached this stage, I will no longer be able to serve as your physician. I will be available to you on an emergency basis only until June 10, 20XX. Meanwhile, you should immediately call or write the Medical Society, 123 Omega Drive, Carlton, MI 11666, Tel. 123-456-7899 and obtain a list of providers. Any delay could jeopardize your health, so please act quickly.

Your physical (and/or mental) problems include hypertensive heart disease, decreased kidney function, and arteriosclerosis. You could have additional medical problems that may also require professional care. Once you have found a new provider have him or her call my office. I will be happy to discuss your case with the provider assuming your care and will transfer a written summary of your case upon the receipt of a written request from you to do so.

Thank you for your anticipated cooperation and courtesy.

Very truly yours,

James Whitney

James Whitney, DO
JW:kr

Figure 7-2 Letter reiterating "for the record" the osteopath's decision to withdraw from the case discussed during a previous meeting with patient.

Inner City Health Care
222 S. First Avenue
Carlton, MI 11666

December 5, 20XX

CERTIFIED MAIL

Rhoda Au
41 Academy Road
Carlton, MI 11666

Dear Ms. Au:

I find it necessary to inform you that I am withdrawing further professional medical service to you because of your persistent refusal to follow my medical advice and treatment.

Because your condition requires medical attention, I suggest that you place yourself under the care of another provider without delay. If you so desire, I shall be available to attend you for a reasonable time after you have received this letter, but in no event later than January 7, 20XX. This should give you sufficient time to select someone from the many competent practitioners in this area.

You may be assured that, upon receiving your written request, I will make available to the provider of your choice your case history and information regarding the diagnosis and treatment that you have received from me.

Very truly yours,

Mark Woo

Mark Woo, MD
MW:kr

Figure 7-3 Letter notifying patient of provider's withdrawal from the case.

TORT LAW

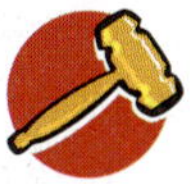

A **tort** is a wrongful act, other than a breach of contract, resulting in injury to one person by another.

Medical Practice Acts

Each state has medical practice acts that regulate the practice of medicine with the intent of protecting its citizens from harm. These statutes govern licensure, standards of care, professional liability and negligence, confidentiality, and torts. Table 7-1 summarizes medical doctor's licensure, renewal, and revocation. Medical assistants sometimes are asked to maintain their employer's records of continuing education for license renewal and to process the renewal at the proper time. In some states, the renewal may be done online if the license is active and in good standing.

States also may regulate personnel who are employed in the ambulatory care setting. Generally, medical assistants perform their duties and responsibilities under the direct supervision of the physician or doctor, and therefore are governed by Medical Practice Acts or the Board of Medical Examiners. Medical assistants employed and supervised by independent nurse practitioners are governed by the Nurse Practice Act and the Board of Nursing. Other health professionals, such as chiropractors and naturopaths, may have separate practice acts as well. Medical assistants employed by these practitioners will need to be knowledgeable of those laws. Some states require that medical assistants be licensed or certified to perform any invasive procedures. Other states require additional training in radiology for the medical assistant to be able to take radiographs. Furthermore, some states are so strict in their regulations that

Table 7-1 Licensure, Renewal, and Revocation for Medical Doctors

Licensure	Renewal	Revocation
Completion of medical education	Payment of a fee	Conviction of a crime
Completion of internship	Documentation of continuing medical education (CME)	Unprofessional conduct
Passing the U.S. Medical Licensing Examination (USMLE)	CMEs might include appropriate medical reading, teaching health professionals, attending conferences and workshops	Personal or professional incapacity

medical assistants mostly perform clerical functions and noninvasive clinical duties.

Certainly, medical assistants desiring to use their skills must be aware of state regulations and always perform only within the scope of those regulations. Medical assistants should be as diligent about maintaining their certification, registration, and licensure as any other health professional and should monitor any legislation that pertains to licensure or certification.

Standard of Care

To better understand torts, we must consider the standard of care and the four Ds of negligence. All health care providers have the responsibility and duty to perform within their scope of training and to always do what any reasonable and prudent health care professional in the same specialty or general field of practice would do. That is what is expected of every provider when a contact is made by a patient. Failure to do what any reasonable and prudent health care professional would do in the same set of circumstances can be seen as a breach of the standard of care.

Negligence is defined as the failure to exercise the standard of care that a reasonable person would exercise in similar circumstances. Negligence occurs when someone experiences injury because of another's failure to live up to a required duty of care. This is a primary cause of malpractice suits. **Malpractice** is professional negligence.

Four Ds of Negligence. The four elements of negligence, sometimes called the 4 Ds, are:

1. Duty: duty of care
2. Derelict: breach of the duty of care
3. Direct cause: a legally recognizable injury occurs as a result of the breach of duty of care
4. Damage: wrongful activity must have caused the injury or harm that occurred

If an individual has knowledge, skill, or intelligence superior to that of a layperson, that individual's conduct must be consistent with that status. Medical assistants are held to a high standard of care by virtue of their skills, knowledge, and intelligence. As professionals, medical assistants are required to have a standard minimum level of special knowledge and ability. This is what is known as duty of care.

The Medical Assistant's Role in Negligence. Medical assistants may commit a tort that may result in **litigation**. If it can be proven that the injury resulted from the medical assistant (or other health care professional) not meeting the standard of care governing their respective professions, then litigation is a possibility. If, however, the medical assistant (or other health care professional) commits a wrongful act but the patient experiences no injury or harm, then no tort exists. If, for example, the medical assistant changes a wound dressing, breaks sterile technique, and the patient suffers a severely infected wound, the medical assistant has committed a tort and can be held liable, and legal action can be taken. In contrast, if the medical assistant changes a wound dressing, breaks sterile technique, and the patient's wound does not become infected, no harm has occurred, and a tort does not exist. If a medical assistant fails to report to the provider an abnormal result on a blood test that causes the provider to fail to make an early diagnosis of a disease, the assistant's omission of an act has caused a breach in the standard of care.

There are two major classifications of torts: *intentional* and *negligent*. Intentional torts are deliberate acts of violation of another's rights. Negligent torts are not deliberate and are the result of omission and commission of an act. Malpractice is the unintentional tort of professional negligence; that is, a professional either failed to act in a reasonable and prudent manner and caused harm to the patient or did what a reasonable and prudent person would not have done and caused harm to a patient.

There are two Latin terms that can be used to describe aspects of negligence. These are known as doctrines. *Res ipsa loquitur*, or "the thing speaks for itself," is the term used in cases that involve situations such as a nick made in the bladder when the surgeon is performing a hysterectomy. The negligence is obvious. The other doctrine, *respondeat superior*, "let the master answer," expresses that providers are responsible for their employees' actions. If a medical assistant violates the standard of care, therein lies the basis for a suit of medical malpractice. For example, the medical assistant used the incorrect solution to clean the patient's wound and the patient sustained injuries to the wound. The provider–employer can be sued under the doctrine of *respondeat superior* because the provider–employer is responsible for the acts of employees committed in the scope of their employment. The medical assistant also can be sued because individuals are responsible for their own actions.

Some common areas of negligence may result in torts when adherence to the standard of care has not been carried out. Specific examples of common torts that can occur in the office or clinic are battery, defamation of character, and invasion of privacy.

Battery. The basis of the tort of battery is unprivileged touching of one person by another. A patient must consent to being touched. When a procedure is to be performed on a patient, the patient must give consent in full knowledge of all the facts. It does not matter whether the procedure that constitutes the battery improves the patient's health. Patients have the right to withdraw consent at any time.

One example of battery is when a medical assistant insists on giving the patient an injection that was ordered for the patient even though the patient refuses the injection. Another example can be seen when a surgeon performs additional surgery beyond the original procedure (the surgeon performed a hysterectomy, for which consent was given, but is liable for battery for removing an abdominal nevus from the patient's abdomen without consent). It does not matter that the surgeon does not charge for the additional procedure. It also does not matter if the patient would have given consent if asked in advance.

Defamation of Character. The tort of defamation of character consists of injury to another person's reputation, name, or character through spoken or written words for which damages can be recovered. Two kinds of defamation are **libel** and **slander**. Libel is false and malicious writing about another, such as in published materials, pictures, and media. An example can be seen when the medical assistant writes in the patient's record, "Mr. O'Keefe's wife and her negative attitude appear to be the cause of his ulcer." A copy of Mr. O'Keefe's records were later sent to a new provider, who reviewed the record and read the remarks quoted by the medical assistant.

Slander is false and malicious spoken words. Slander can be seen in the following comment directed by a patient to the provider, "Dr. Woo is incompetent. He should have his license revoked." The statement is overheard by the office administrative medical assistant and other patients waiting in the reception area.

For a tort of defamation of character (either libel or slander) to exist, a third party must see or hear the words and understand their meaning.

HIPAA **Invasion of Privacy.** Invasion of privacy is another kind of tort. It includes unauthorized publicity of patient information, medical records being released without the patient's knowledge and permission, and patients receiving unwanted publicity and exposure to public view. For example, if a minor unmarried girl has been examined for possible pregnancy, and the medical assistant telephones the girl's home and inadvertently gives the laboratory results to someone other than the patient, her privacy has been invaded. A second situation exists when persons other than those providing care and performing examinations and procedures (essential or nonessential personnel) are allowed to be present without the patient's consent. Yet another example of the patient's right to privacy being violated is when the patient is asked to walk from the examination room across the hall to a treatment room while wearing only a patient gown in full view of other patients and personnel.

Medical assistants and other health care professionals should:

- Close a door, pull a curtain, or provide a screen when looking at, handling, or examining the patient
- Expose only body parts necessary for treatment (drape the patient, exposing only the part that is being treated)
- Discuss patients with no one except those individuals involved in the patient's care, and then discuss only those aspects of care that relate to the needs of the patient

It is not an invasion of privacy to disclose information required by a court order, **subpoena,** or by statute to protect the public health and welfare, as in the reporting of violent crime.

INFORMED CONSENT

Documentation of **informed consent** becomes an important part of the patient care process. Every patient has a right to know and understand any procedure to be performed. The patient is to be told in language easily understood:

- The nature of any procedure and how it is to be performed
- Any possible risks involved, as well as expected outcomes of the procedure
- Any other methods of treatment and those risks
- Risks if no treatment is given

It is the responsibility of the health care provider to make certain the patient understands. If an interpreter is necessary, the provider must procure one.

Often, consent forms will be signed if there is to be a surgical or invasive procedure performed (Figure 7-4). The medical assistant may be asked to witness the patient's signature and may be expected to follow through on any of the provider's instructions or explanations but is not expected to explain

CONSENT TO
OPERATION, ADMINISTRATION OF ANESTHETICS AND
RENDERING OF OTHER MEDICAL SERVICES

1. I hereby authorize and direct Dr. ______________________________, my physician, and whomever he/she designates as his/her assistants (associates and/or resident physicians), to perform upon (state name of patient or myself) ______________________________

The following procedures: ______________________________

____

____

If any unforeseen condition arises in the course of this operation for the physician's judgment to perform procedures in addition to or different from those now contemplated, I further request and authorize him/her to do whatever he/she deems advisable and necessary in these circumstances. Such additional services may include, but are not limited to, the administration and maintenance of anesthesia and the performance of services involving pathology and radiology.

2. The following information has been explained to me to the degree that I wish to have it discussed:
   - The nature and character of the proposed treatment or procedure;
   - The anticipated results;
   - Possible recognized alternative methods of treatment, including non-treatment;
   - Recognized serious possible risks, complications, and anticipated benefits involved in proposed and alternative treatments, including non-treatment.

   My questions have been answered to my satisfaction. I acknowledge that no guarantee, warrantee, or assurance has been made as to the results or cure that may be obtained.

3. Federal Regulations (21 CFR Part 821) require manufacturers to track certain medical devices, and assist the U.S. Food and Drug Administration (FDA) with notification to individuals in the event that a certain medical device presents serious health risks. I authorize and agree to the release of my contact information to the manufacturer: ______________________________ for this tracking purpose only. I understand that the manufacturer may notify me, if necessary, of important safety information about my medical device, and may release my information to the FDA if ordered to do so. I understand that this consent is valid for the life of the medical device.

Any sections below that do not apply to the proposed treatment may be crossed out. The patient must initial any section crossed out.

4. I consent to the administration of blood and blood products if deemed medically necessary. I understand that all blood and blood products involve the risk of allergic reaction, fever, hives, and in rare circumstances infectious diseases such as hepatitis and HIV/AIDS. I understand that precautions are taken by the blood bank in screening donors and in matching blood for transfusion to minimize those risks.

5. I hereby consent to the disposal or use for research purposes any tissues, parts, or products of conception, which may be removed.

6. I authorize and agree to the presence of observers during my surgical procedure. These observers may include persons other than the medical staff that are considered appropriate by my health care provider during my care and treatment. The purpose of these individuals observing would be for instruction and medical study.

I certify that I have read this form and understand its contents.

PATIENT NAME & ID #

____
Signature of Patient or Legally Responsible Party

____
Relationship to patient, if not signed by patient

____
Signature of Witness

____
Printed Name of Witness

Date ______________ Time ______________ a.m. / p.m.

MRD: HOSP1
DISTRIBUTION: 1-**WHITE** – CHART 2-**CANARY** – PATIENT COPY

Figure 7-4 Model formal consent for treatment form.

the procedure to the patient. The signed consent form is kept in the medical chart, and a copy also is given to the patient.

Implied Consent

Two circumstances related to consent are worth mentioning at this point. **Implied consent** occurs when there is a life-threatening emergency, or the patient is unconscious or unable to respond. The provider, by law, is allowed to give treatment within his or her scope of practice without a signed consent. Implied consent also occurs in more subtle ways. The patient who rolls up a shirtsleeve for the medical assistant to take a blood pressure reading is implying consent to the procedure by the action taken.

Consent and Legal Incompetence

Consent for treatment is not valid if the patient is legally incompetent to give consent. Legal **incompetence** means that a patient is found by a court to be insane, inadequate, or to not be an adult. In such instances, consent must be obtained from a parent, a legal guardian, or the court on behalf of the patient. Consent for treatment can be given only by the natural parent or legal guardian as determined by the court for a **minor** child. A minor is a person who has not reached the age of majority (18–21 years old), depending on the laws of each state. Generally, a minor is considered unable to give effective consent for medical treatment; therefore, without proper consent from parents or guardians, medical professionals can be held liable for battery if medical treatment is given. Exceptions to this rule are in cases of emergency and for mature and **emancipated minors.** Emancipated minors are younger than 18 years who are free of parental care and are financially responsible, married, become parents, or join the Armed Forces. **Mature minors** are persons, usually younger than 18 years, who are able to understand and appreciate the nature and consequences of treatment despite their young age. Nearly every state allows minors to give consent for treatment for pregnancy, drug or alcohol addiction, and sexually transmitted disease. Some states have passed legislation that name minors as statutory adults at 14 years old for the purpose of receiving medical care. In these states, minors may consent and be protected by confidentiality and privacy even though their parents or legal guardians may still be financially responsible for their medical bills.

Questions of ability to give consent related to minors and emancipated minors often must be determined on a case-by-case basis because state statutes vary. Placing a telephone call to the state attorney general's office can help clarify issues, questions, and concerns that involve consent and treatment of minors.

RISK MANAGEMENT

Practicing good **risk management** makes the medical assistant and the provider–employer less vulnerable to litigation.

Following are some ways to avoid incidents that may lead to litigation:

- Perform only within the scope of your training and education.
- Comply with all state and federal regulations and statutes.
- Keep the office or clinic safe and equipment in readiness.
- Never leave a patient unattended; if you must leave, pass the responsibility for the patient's care on to another individual.
- Keep all patient information confidential.
- Follow all policies and procedures established for the office or clinic.
- Document fully only facts; formally document withdrawing from a case and discharging clients.
- Log telephone calls and return calls to clients within a reasonable time frame.
- Follow up on missed or canceled appointments.
- Never guarantee a cure or diagnosis, and never advise treatment without a provider's order.
- Secure informed consent as necessary.
- Do not criticize other practitioners.
- Explain any appointment delays.
- Be particularly watchful with patients who have special needs, such as the elderly, pediatric patients, and those with physical and emotional disabilities.
- Report any error that may have occurred to your employer.

Critical Thinking

Identify the suggestions in the previous risk management list that are most likely not performed if the staff in the ambulatory care setting find themselves overworked, overwhelmed, and behind. What might be done to prevent carelessness brought on by such circumstances?

CIVIL LITIGATION PROCESS

Despite all the best efforts of health care professionals and their employees, litigation can occur. Litigation is the process of taking a lawsuit or a criminal case through the courts. It is helpful to understand the steps taken for civil litigation to occur. The greatest amount of any litigation seen in the ambulatory care setting occurs when relationships between individuals break down for one reason or another. When this happens, the party, or plaintiff, bringing the action, usually a patient, seeks an attorney who agrees to bring the complaint to the courts. The provider, or defendant, is summoned to court. This summons or subpoena notifies the provider of the plaintiff's suit and allows the defendant to file an answer with the court.

Subpoenas

The subpoena is an order from the court naming the specific date, time, and reason to appear. A portion of a medical record or the entire medical record may be subpoenaed, the health care provider *(subpoena duces tecum)* may be subpoenaed to testify in court, or both may be subpoenaed. The staff in the ambulatory care setting usually will have ample time to make certain the record is current and complete before its inclusion in court. Out of courtesy, a provider will notify patients whose records have been subpoenaed. If, for any reason, the patient does not want the record released, the provider must call for legal advice on how to respond to the subpoena.

Certain records, because of their sensitive nature, may require more than a subpoena to be released. These include records related to sexually transmitted diseases, including AIDS and HIV testing; mental health records; substance abuse records; and sexual assault records. For the courts to have access to these records, a *court order* is required in some states.

HIPAA law requires clinics to identify in written policies and procedures what information they will release regarding patients. Before patient information is released, the following must be identified: (1) the purpose or need for the information, (2) the nature or extent of the information to be released, (3) the date of the authorization, and (4) the signature(s) of the person(s) authorized to give consent. Release only what the subpoena or court order specifically requests rather than releasing the entire medical record. Many practitioners keep a patient's consent information in a specific section of the medical record for quick referral and to demonstrate HIPAA compliance.

The care taken with subpoenas and court orders for certain information is to ensure patients of confidentiality. The information in the medical record, including the information a patient shared with the provider and medical assistant, is private.

No patient information can be given to another person or entity (provider, patient's attorney, insurance company, federal or state agency) without the expressed written consent of the patient. Care must be exercised at all times to ensure that the patient's right to confidentiality is not breached. For example, information given to unauthorized personnel associated with the provider's or clinic's practice in regard to the patient's condition or financial status regarding payment of bills violates the patient's right to confidentiality. Likewise, when discussing issues over the telephone that can be overheard, such as the patient's account being turned over to a collection agency, the patient's right to confidentiality has been violated.

Certain disclosures of information about a patient's conditions and suspected illnesses are required by law. Legally required disclosures are necessary when the public needs to know certain information for its safety and welfare. The disclosures supersede the patient's right to privacy and confidentiality (see section in Public Duties).

Discovery

In the litigation process, time of **discovery** follows the subpoenas. This is the time in which both parties are allowed access to all the information and evidence related to the case. Rules of discovery vary from state to state but may include the following:

1. An **interrogatory** is a written set of questions that can come from either the plaintiff or the defendant that must be answered, under oath, and within a specific time period.
2. A **deposition** is oral testimony taken with a court reporter present in a location agreed on by both parties. Both attorneys are usually present when depositions are taken.

Medical assistants may be asked to respond to an interrogatory or may be deposed by the plaintiff's attorney. The defendant's attorney will provide specific instructions in both situations. Because both are done under oath, honesty is an absolute. The medical assistant may be asked to refer to certain documents, recall specific information, or identify documentation in a medical record.

Expert Witnesses. Providers and members of their staff may be called to testify in court to the standard of care. In such a case, they are usually considered **expert witnesses.** An expert witness is one who has enough knowledge and experience in a field to be able to testify to what is the reasonable and expected standard of care. Expert witnesses are expected to tell what they know to be fact and are best counseled to use lay terms rather than complicated medical language. The goal is for jurors and judges to understand the nature of any medical information shared. Visual aids, charts, and computer simulations often are used to illustrate or clarify testimony given by expert witnesses.

Pretrial Conference

A pretrial conference is generally held close to the trial date to decide if there is just cause for the suit, to make certain that both parties are ready, and to determine if there might be an out-of-court settlement. If a trial seems imminent, **alternative dispute resolution (ADR)** may be suggested. ADR saves money, time, and adverse publicity that can come from a trial.

Mediation allows a neutral facilitator to help the two parties settle their differences and come to an acceptable solution. If no settlement is reached, the case can still look to the court for satisfaction. **Arbitration** allows the neutral party to settle the dispute. This arbitration can be binding or nonbinding. In binding arbitration, both parties agree at the outset to accept the neutral party's decision as final. In nonbinding arbitration, the case can look to the court for settlement.

Trial

A trial can be held before a judge or before a judge and a jury. When the trial begins, opening statements outlining the details of the case are made by both sides. The plaintiff's attorney calls witnesses to produce evidence first. This is known as direct examination. In cross examination, the defendant's attorney questions the witness. When the plaintiff's case is finished, the defendant presents the case in the same manner. When all the information has been presented, the case is turned over for judgment.

If the plaintiff's case is successful, the judge or jury may award a specific amount of money or damages. The judge will instruct a jury regarding the kinds of damages that can be considered in that state. A number of states have placed limits on monetary awards in malpractice cases. If the defendant's case is successful, the case is dismissed. After a court decision, the party that has lost the case can begin an appeal process. The appeal requests an opinion from higher courts that review cases usually on the basis of a faulty legal process or action.

Figure 7-5 outlines the civil case process.

Statute of Limitations

No discussion of negligence, malpractice, or medical records is complete without a brief statement regarding the statute of limitations that will, in part, determine how long medical records are kept. Generally, all records should be retained until after the statute has run, usually 3 to 6 years. Statutes of limitations most commonly begin at the time a negligent act was committed, when the act was discovered, or when the care of the patient and the provider–patient relationship ended. It is easy to understand why many providers choose to keep their records indefinitely, a plan made much easier with electronic files.

State and federal statutes set maximum time periods during which certain actions can be brought or rights enforced; there is a time limit for individuals to initiate legal action. The statute of limitations varies from one jurisdiction to another, and a lawsuit may not be brought after the statute of limitations has run. For example, in the Commonwealth of Massachusetts, the statute of limitations for an act of medical malpractice committed on an adult is 3 years. If harm to a patient resulted from a medical assistant administering the wrong dose of medication to a patient in Massachusetts, a lawsuit must be brought within 3 years from the time the medication error was made, with the 3 years commencing at the time the negligent act was committed.

PUBLIC DUTIES

Reportable Diseases/Injuries

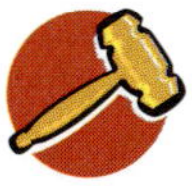

All medical providers have a duty to the public to report diseases and injuries that jeopardize public health and welfare. Transmittable or contagious diseases and injuries resulting from knife or gunshot are examples; these must be reported to the appropriate authorities. This is done without the patient's consent because it is required by law. When reporting, it is important to do so properly and according to the

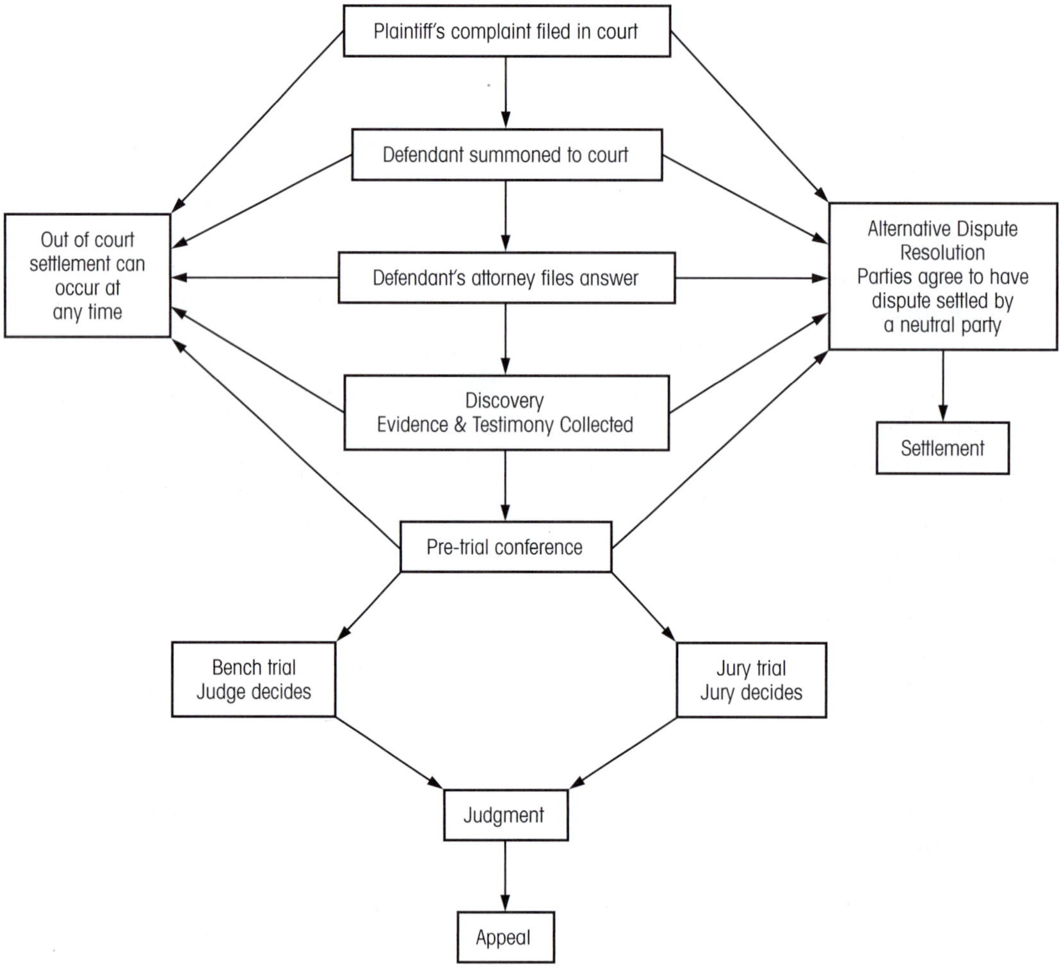

Figure 7-5 Civil litigation process.

laws of the state in which one is employed. Knowledge of which illnesses, injuries, and conditions to report, to whom to report, and the appropriate forms to submit is essential. Copies of all information must be kept for the office or clinic.

Medline Plus, a Web site sponsored by the U.S. National Library of Medicine and the National Institutes of Health, has an excellent site connected to the Medline Encyclopedia titled "Reportable Diseases" identifying guidelines for reportable diseases. Local, state, and national agencies such as the Centers for Disease Control and Prevention (CDC) require such diseases to be reported when diagnosed by providers or laboratories. States may vary in the diseases that require reporting, but their lists are likely to include the list of "Nationally Notifiable Infectious Diseases" listed on the CDC's Web site (http://www.cdc.gov). Some diseases require written reports. Others require reporting electronically or by telephone; they include rubeola (measles) and pertussis (whooping cough). Still others ask only for the number of cases to be reported. Such reporting is beneficial to society and all health care managers in tracking and preventing illness. The list changes as new diseases occur and are diagnosed.

Other generally required facts to report include births; deaths; childhood immunizations; rape; and abuse toward a child, elder, or intimate partner.

Some states have laws specific to the release of information relative to mental or psychological treatment, HIV testing, AIDS diagnosis and treatment, sexually transmitted diseases, and chemical substance abuse.

Local or state health departments can provide lists of diseases and injuries to report and will also provide the appropriate forms.

Abuse

Child abuse, **intimate partner violence**, and elder abuse are becoming more common in our society. As a result, patients experiencing such abuse may be seen in the ambulatory care setting. In all cases of abuse, medical records hold valuable information if a court procedure ensues. Careful documentation is critical. State laws are fairly specific in mandates to report child abuse, but laws related to elder abuse and domestic violence are not as detailed. In any case, the rights of victims must be protected. (See Table 8-1 for a summary.)

Child Abuse. All 50 states and the District of Columbia mandate, or require, that health care professionals, teachers, social workers, and certain others who suspect child abuse report the incident to the proper authorities. Confidentiality in the provider–patient relationship does not exist when children are abused. If a person has a reason to suspect abuse and reports the abuse to the police and, in the case of child abuse, to the child protective agency, this individual is protected against liability as a result of making the report. Failure to report could result in criminal or civil penalties. Usually, the Child Protective Unit of the State Department of Social Services is called to investigate suspected cases of child abuse. Some injuries that are commonly seen in child abuse are bruises, welts, burns, fractures, and head injuries. Evidence of neglect, intimidation, or sexual abuse also may be seen.

If a suspicion of abuse exists, the health care professional should:

- Treat the child's injuries
- Send the child to the hospital for further treatment when necessary
- Inform parents of the diagnosis and that it will be reported to the police and social services agency
- Notify the child protective agency (keep phone number posted)
- Document all information
- Provide court testimony if requested

Elder Abuse. Elder abuse may consist of neglect, physical abuse, punishment, physical restraint, or abandonment. Examples are seen when elders are overmedicated or undermedicated, physically restrained, intimidated by shouting or profanity, sexually abused, neglected or abandoned, or in any other way have their rights and dignity violated. The person reporting the abuse is generally a health care professional who observes or suspects the abuse, and the reporting agency is most likely one of a social service or welfare nature. The majority of states have laws protecting vulnerable adults and the elderly from abuse.

Intimate Partner Violence (IPV). The term "domestic violence" has been changed to be more encompassing of an escalating problem. "Intimate partner violence (IPV)" is now used and refers to violence or abuse between a spouse or former spouse; boyfriend, girlfriend, or former boyfriend/girlfriend; and same-sex or heterosexual intimate partner or former same-sex or heterosexual intimate partner. The abuse may include physical or sexual violence, threats of the same, and psychological or emotional violence. Physical violence is a criminal act, and failure to report it is considered a misdemeanor in some states. Victims of IPV should be treated as soon as possible after the assault so that evidence can be preserved for legal purposes. Some forms of IPV are considered acceptable behavior in many cultures, even in the United States. Some cultures believe the woman is chattel, or property, of her spouse, that she has no rights or authority, and that she must submit to her husband's, brother's, or father's demands.

An individual who manages to come to the ambulatory care setting with signs of IPV is courageous and probably is extremely frightened also, because reporting the violence may increase the risk for continued violence and even death in some instances.

Make certain that community resources are readily available for survivers of IPV, even if they choose to stay in the abusive situation. In many cases, the abused patient's options are so few that leaving is more frightening than staying in the abusive relationship. Do not pass judgment on these survivors; they desperately need your understanding and your compassion. Your understanding and compassion is perhaps the only door through which they might feel comfortable enough to enter to leave the abusive relationship.

Good Samaritan Laws

All 50 states have laws regarding the rendering of first aid by health care professionals at the scene of an accident or sudden injury. Good Samaritan laws, although not always clearly written, encourage health care professionals to provide medical care within the scope of their training without fear of being sued for negligence. In an emergency situation, medical assistants cannot be held liable should an injury result from some form of first aid rendered or from first aid they omitted to render as long as they acted in a reasonable way within the scope of their knowledge. Medical assistants and other health care professionals with skills in cardiopulmonary resuscitation (CPR) who are present when CPR is needed must perform the procedure on the victim or otherwise could be declared negligent. Emergencies that arise in the ambulatory care setting generally are not covered by Good Samaritan laws.

ADVANCE DIRECTIVES

Medical assistants in the ambulatory care setting will be asked to attach advance directives or living wills to patients' charts (Figure 7-6). These directives are legal documents in which patients indicate their wishes in the case of a life-threatening illness or serious injury. Health care providers in many states and cities have adopted the Physician Orders for Life-Sustaining Treatment (POLST) (Figure 7-7) form. This form is to be completed by a health care provider based on the patient's preferences on the type of life-sustaining treatment wanted and medical indications. POLST is most often brightly colored (neon pink or green). To be valid, the form must be signed by the proper authority. Some states may use another name than POLST, but the intent is quite similar. POLST is appropriate for seriously ill individuals with life-threatening or terminal illnesses. Some providers believe that even with an advance directive in place, it is advisable to complete a POLST form. This form goes with the patient when he or she is moved between care settings. For those in the home, it is recommended that the form be posted on the refrigerator where emergency responders can locate it easily. As of October 2008, 33 states had endorsed or are developing POLST documents (http://www.POLST.org). Such documents should always accompany the patients to the hospital for any treatment or care. They may be updated from time to time, and patients can ask to rescind such a document at any time. Medical assistants must remember that these documents reflect the choices of their patients and are to be respected as such.

Living Wills/Advance Directives

Patients' desire to make known in advance their choices related to health care, especially when death is near, will have living wills, advance directives, or a POLST order. The title of such a document is largely determined by the state in which the document is made. These documents are necessary because advances in medicine allow medical professionals to sustain life even if the individual will not recover from a persistent vegetative state. Persons who prefer not to remain in that state can use the living will or advance directive to make decisions about life support and to direct others to implement their wishes in that regard. Such a document allows individuals to indicate to family and health care professionals whether life-prolonging medical or surgical procedures are to be continued, withheld, or withdrawn, and if artificial feeding and fluids are to be used or withheld. The document allows individuals to make this decision before incapacitation.

To be valid, the proper and particular form, different in each state, must be used, and it must be lawfully executed. States vary in the number of witnesses required and whether a Notary Public is required for those signatures. The form goes into effect when provided to a patient's health care provider *and* when the patient is no longer capable of making health care decisions. Examples of incapacity include permanent unconsciousness, life-threatening illness in the latter stages, and inability to communicate. The U.S. Legal Forms Web site (http://USlegalforms.com) has samples of living wills for all 50 states and the District of Columbia under the heading "Living Will." A sample from each state is available without a fee.

Durable Power of Attorney for Health Care

Another document seen in the ambulatory care setting is the **durable power of attorney for health care** or Designation of Health Care Surrogate (Figure 7-8). This document allows a patient to name another person as the official spokesperson for the patient should the patient be unable to make health care decisions. The documents may allow another person to manage finances and personal matters (durable power of attorney) or just to make medical decisions.

Every state has a slightly different version of their living will, advance directive, durable power of attorney for health care, or POLST. Most forms and specific information can be found on the Internet by keying in a particular state and the title of the document wanted. Also, the Web site for Compassion and Choices (http://www.compassionandchoices.org/) located in Portland, Oregon, is quite helpful.

Patient Self-Determination Act

In 1991, the federal government passed the **Patient Self-Determination Act (PSDA),** which applies to all health care institutions receiving payments from

HEALTH CARE DIRECTIVE

Directive made this ______________________________ day of __________ , ______________ .
(Year)

I, ____ being of sound mind, willfully, and voluntarily make known my desire that my dying shall not be artificially prolonged under the circumstances set forth below, and do hereby declare that:

(A) If at any time I should have an incurable and irreversible condition certified to be a terminal condition by my attending physician, and where the application of life-sustaining treatment would serve only to artificially prolong the process of my dying, I direct that such treatment be withheld or withdrawn, and that I be permitted to die naturally. I understand "terminal condition" means an incurable and irreversible condition caused by injury, disease or illness that would, within reasonable medical judgment, cause death within a reasonable period of time in accordance with accepted medical standards.

(B) If I should be in an irreversible coma or persistent vegetative state, or other permanent unconscious condition as certified by two physicians, and from which those physicians believe that I have no reasonable probability of recovery, I direct that life-sustaining treatment be withheld or withdrawn.

(C) If I am diagnosed to be in a terminal or permanent unconscious condition, [*Choose one*]

I want __________ do not want __________

artificially administered nutrition and hydration to be withdrawn or withheld the same as other forms of life-sustaining treatment. I understand artificially administered nutrition and hydration is a form of life-sustaining treatment in certain circumstances. I request all health care providers who care for me to honor this directive.

(D) In the absence of my ability to give directions regarding the use of such life-sustaining procedures, it is my intention that this directive shall be honored by my family, physicians and other health care providers as the final expression of my fundamental right to refuse medical or surgical treatment, and also honored by any person appointed to make these decisions for me, whether by durable power of attorney or otherwise. I accept the consequences of such refusal.

(E) If I have been diagnosed as pregnant and that diagnosis is known to my physician, this directive shall have no force or effect during the course of my pregnancy.

(F) I understand the full import of this directive and I am emotionally and mentally competent to make this directive. I also understand that I may amend or revoke this directive at any time.

(G) I make the following additional directions regarding my care:

____

____

____

____

Signed: ____

The declarer has been personally known to me and I believe him or her to be of sound mind. In addition, I am not the attending physician, an employee of the attending physician or health care facility in which the declarer is a patient, or any person who has a claim against any portion of the estate of the declarer upon the declarer's decease at the time of the execution of the directive.

Witness: ________________________________

Witness: ________________________________

Figure 7-6 Sample health care directive (Reprinted by permission from WSMA, Seattle, Washington.)

HIPAA PERMITS DISCLOSURE OF POLST TO OTHER HEALTH CARE PROVIDERS AS NECESSARY

Physician Orders
for Life-Sustaining Treatment (POLST)

FIRST follow these orders, **THEN** contact physician, nurse practitioner or PA-C. This is a Physician Order Sheet based on the person's medical condition and wishes. Any section not completed implies full treatment for that section. Everyone shall be treated with dignity and respect.

Last Name

First/Middle Initial

Date of Birth

A Check One — **CARDIOPULMONARY RESUSCITATION (CPR):** Person has no pulse and is not breathing.

☐ CPR/Attempt Resuscitation ☐ DNR/Do Not Attempt Resuscitation (Allow Natural Death)

When not in cardiopulmonary arrest, follow orders in **B**, **C** and **D**.

B Check One — **MEDICAL INTERVENTIONS:** Person has pulse and/or is breathing.

☐ **COMFORT MEASURES ONLY** Use medication by any route, positioning, wound care and other measures to relieve pain and suffering. Use oxygen, oral suction and manual treatment of airway obstruction as needed for comfort. **Patient prefers no transfer:** *EMS contact medical control to determine if transport indicated.*

☐ **LIMITED ADDITIONAL INTERVENTIONS** Includes care described above. Use medical treatment, IV fluids and cardiac monitor as indicated. Do not use intubation, advanced airway interventions, or mechanical ventilation. **Transfer** *to hospital if indicated. Avoid intensive care if possible.*

☐ **FULL TREATMENT** Includes care described above. Use intubation, advanced airway interventions, mechanical ventilation, and cardioversion as indicated. **Transfer** *to hospital if indicated. Includes intensive care.*

Additional Orders: (e.g. dialysis, etc.) ____________________

C Check One — **ANTIBIOTICS:**

☐ No antibiotics. Use other measures to relieve symptoms.

☐ Determine use or limitation of antibiotics when infection occurs, with comfort as goal.

☐ Use antibiotics if life can be prolonged.

Additional Orders: ____________________

D Check One — **ARTIFICIALLY ADMINISTERED NUTRITION:** Always offer food and liquids by mouth if feasible.

☐ No artificial nutrition by tube.

☐ Trial period of artificial nutrition by tube. (Goal: ____________________)

☐ Long-term artificial nutrition by tube.

Additional Orders: ____________________

E — **SUMMARY OF GOALS AND SIGNATURES**

Discussed with:

☐ Patient ☐ Parent of Minor

☐ Health Care Representative

☐ Durable Power of Attorney for Health Care

☐ Court-Appointed Guardian

☐ Other: ____________________

Patient Goals/Medical Condition:

Print Physician/ARNP/PA-C Name	Phone Number	Patient/Resident or Legal Surrogate for Health Care Signature *(mandatory)*	Date
Physician/ARNP/PA-C Signature *(mandatory)*	Date		

SEND FORM WITH PERSON WHENEVER TRANSFERRED OR DISCHARGED

Use of original form is strongly encouraged. Photocopies and FAXes of signed POLST forms are legal and valid.

Figure 7-7 Physician Orders for Life-Sustaining Treatment (POLST) Form. (Reprinted by permission from WSMA, Seattle, Washington.)

HIPAA PERMITS DISCLOSURE OF POLST TO OTHER HEALTH CARE PROVIDERS AS NECESSARY

Other Contact Information (Optional)

Name of Guardian, Surrogate or other Contact Person	Relationship	Phone Number	
Name of Health Care Professional Preparing Form	Preparer Title	Phone Number	Date Prepared

Directions for Health Care Professionals

Completing POLST

- Must be completed by a health care professional based on patient preferences and medical indications.
- POLST must be signed by a physician, nurse practitioner or PA-C to be valid. Verbal orders are acceptable with follow-up signature by physician or nurse practitioner in accordance with facility/community policy.
- Use of original form is strongly encouraged. Photocopies and FAXes of signed POLST forms are legal and valid.

Using POLST

- Any section of POLST not completed implies full treatment for that section.
- A semi-automatic external defibrillator (AED) should not be used on a person who has chosen "Do Not Attempt Resuscitation."
- Oral fluids and nutrition must always be offered if medically feasible.
- When comfort cannot be achieved in the current setting, the person, including someone with "comfort measures only," should be transferred to a setting able to provide comfort (e.g., pinning of a hip fracture).
- A person who chooses either "comfort measures only" or "limited additional interventions" should not be entered into a Level I trauma system.
- An IV medication to enhance comfort may be appropriate for a person who has chosen "Comfort Measures Only."
- Treatment of dehydration is a measure which may prolong life. A person who desires IV fluids should indicate "Limited Interventions" or "Full Treatment."
- A person with capacity or the surrogate (if patient lacks capacity) can revoke the POLST at any time and request alternative treatment.

Reviewing POLST

This POLST should be reviewed periodically and a new POLST completed if necessary when:

(1) The person is transferred from one care setting or care level to another, or

(2) There is a substantial change in the person's health status, or

(3) The person's treatment preferences change.

To void this form, draw line through "Physician Orders" and write "VOID" in large letters.

Review of this POLST Form

Review Date	Reviewer	Location of Review	Review Outcome
			☐ No Change ☐ Form Voided ☐ New form completed
			☐ No Change ☐ Form Voided ☐ New form completed
			☐ No Change ☐ Form Voided ☐ New form completed

SEND FORM WITH PERSON WHENEVER TRANSFERRED OR DISCHARGED

Revised December 2006

Washington State Medical Association WSMA Physician Driven Patient Focused

Washington State Department of Health

Figure 7-7 (continued)

DURABLE POWER OF ATTORNEY FOR HEALTH CARE

Notice to Person Executing This Document

This is an important legal document. Before executing this document you should know these facts:

- This document gives the person you designate as your Health Care Agent the power to make MOST health care decisions for you if you lose the capability to make informed health care decisions for yourself. This power is effective only when you lose the capacity to make informed health care decisions for yourself. As long as you have the capacity to make informed health care decisions for yourself, you retain the right to make all medical and other health care decisions.
- You may include specific limitations in this document on the authority of the Health Care Agent to make health care decisions for you.
- Subject to any specific limitations you include in this document, if you do lose the capacity to make an informed decision on a health care matter, the Health Care Agent *GENERALLY* will be authorized by this document to make health care decisions for you to the same extent as you could make those decisions yourself, if you had the capacity to do so. The authority of the Health Care Agent to make health care decisions for you *GENERALLY* will include the authority to give informed consent, to refuse to give informed consent, or to withdraw informed consent to any care, treatment, service, or procedure to maintain, diagnose, or treat a physical or mental condition. You can limit that right in this document if you choose.
- A Health Care Agent can only act under state law. "Mercy killing" is not allowed under Washington state law. A Health Care Agent will **NEVER** be allowed to authorize "mercy killing," euthanasia or any procedure which would actually speed up the natural process of dying.
- When exercising his or her authority to make health care decisions for you when deciding on your behalf, the Health Care Agent will have to act consistent with your wishes, or if they are unknown, in your best interest. You may make your wishes known to the Health Care Agent by including them in this document or by making them known in another manner.
- When acting under this document the Health Care Agent *GENERALLY* will have the same rights that you have to receive information about proposed health care, to review health care records, and to consent to the disclosure of health care records.

1. Creation of Durable Power of Attorney for Health Care

I intend to create a power of attorney (Health Care Agent) by appointing the person or persons designated herein to make health care decisions for me to the same extent that I could make such decisions for myself if I was capable of doing so, as recognized by RCW 11.94.010. This designation becomes effective when I cannot make health care decisions for myself as determined by my attending physician or designee, such as if I am unconscious, or if I am otherwise temporarily or permanently incapable of making health care decisions. The Health Care Agent's power shall cease if and when I regain my capacity to make health care decisions.

2. Designation of Health Care Agent and Alternate Agents

If my attending physician or his or her designee determines that I am not capable of giving informed consent to health care, I ______________________________, designate and appoint:

Name ______________________________ Address ______________________________

City ____________________ State ________ Zip ________ Phone ______________

as my attorney-in-fact (Health Care Agent) by granting him or her the Durable Power of Attorney for Health Care recognized in RCW 11.94.010 and authorize her or him to consult with my physicians about the possibility of my regaining the capacity to make treatment decisions and to accept, plan, stop, and refuse treatment on my behalf with the treating physicians and health personnel.

In the event that ______________________________ is unable or unwilling to serve, I grant these powers to

Name ______________________________ Address ______________________________

City ____________________ State ________ Zip ________ Phone ______________

In the event that both ______________________________ and ______________________________

are unable or unwilling to serve, I grant these powers to

Name ______________________________ Address ______________________________

City ____________________ State ________ Zip ________ Phone ______________

Figure 7-8 Durable power of attorney for health care (Reprinted by permission from WSMA, Seattle, Washington.)

Your name (print)______________________________

3. General Statement of Authority Granted.

My Health Care Agent is specifically authorized to give informed consent for health care treatment when I am not capable of doing so. This includes but is not limited to consent to initiate, continue, discontinue, or forgo medical care and treatment including artificially supplied nutrition and hydration, following and interpreting my instructions for the provision, withholding, or withdrawing of life-sustaining treatment, which are contained in any Health Care Directive or other form of "living will" I may have executed or elsewhere, and to receive and consent to the release of medical information. When the Health Care Agent does not have any stated desires or instructions from me to follow, he or she shall act in my best interest in making health care decisions.

The above authorization to make health care decisions does not include the following absent a court order:

(1) Therapy or other procedure given for the purpose of inducing convulsion;
(2) Surgery solely for the purpose of psychosurgery;
(3) Commitment to or placement in a treatment facility for the mentally ill, except pursuant to the provisions of Chapter 71.05 RCW;
(4) Sterilization.

I hereby revoke any prior grants of durable power of attorney for health care.

4. Special Provisions

____

____

____

____

____

DATED this __________ day of __________, ________ .
(Year)

GRANTOR ____________________

STATE OF WASHINGTON)
)ss.
(COUNTY OF ____________)

I certify that I know or have satisfactory evidence that the GRANTOR, ____________________
signed this instrument and acknowledged it to be his or her free and voluntary act for the uses and purposes mentioned in the instrument.

DATED this __________ day of __________, ________ .
(Year)

____
NOTARY PUBLIC in and for the State of Washington,
residing at ____________________
My commission expires ____________________

Figure 7-8 (continued)

Patient Education

Because of increased awareness of confidentiality as a result of HIPAA, medical assistants can be helpful by suggesting that any family member(s) who might be involved and need to know about the patient's care be indicated in the patient's chart with a signed release from the patient. There have been examples recently of adult children of elder adults who were either not informed when their ailing parent was taken to emergency services in another state or were unable to get any information about their parent from a hospital or provider even though a durable power of attorney for health care was in place. If that directive does not go with the patient, no information can be given. For that reason, it is suggested that patients may want to keep a wallet card containing a notice of the advance directive, any appointed agent named, and any family member(s) who is allowed information.

Medicare and Medicaid. PSDA requires that all adults receiving health care from these institutions be given the opportunity to provide information about their wishes in an advance directive.

Copies of advance directives are to be provided to patients' providers so the documents can be transferred to a hospital or nursing facility as necessary. Any named agent should have a copy, and family members also may have a copy.

Case Study 7-1

Refer to the scenario at the beginning of the chapter. You realize that any breach of confidentiality is a serious matter, whether intentional or accidental.

CASE STUDY REVIEW

1. What corrective measures can you suggest to decrease voices heard in the hallway or from examination rooms?
2. How can medical charts or private patient information be kept out of public view?
3. What HIPAA regulations will you want to review?

Case Study 7-2

Three weeks ago, Dr. King treated a new patient, Boris Bolski, for lower back pain, which the patient believed was the result of consistent heavy lifting at his job. Medical assistant Joe Guerrero assisted Dr. King during the examination. Today, both Joe and Dr. King were served with subpoenas by Mr. Bolski's attorney. Mr. Bolski is alleging that unsafe conditions at his workplace caused severe strain on his back, and he is suing his employer for damages. Dr. King and Joe Guerrero were called as expert witnesses to a civil hearing; Joe, especially, is a bit nervous about this, because he has never been on the witness stand in court and is not sure what is expected of him.

CASE STUDY REVIEW

1. How will Mr. Bolski's medical record help Joe answer questions at the hearing?
2. What information should Joe gather so that he is prepared to testify?
3. As an expert witness, what is Joe expected to communicate to the judge in this case?

Case Study 7-3

Wanda Hanson is working on a part-time basis in Hudson, Florida, as an administrative medical assistant on the phone desk in the Emergency Department at Hudson Community Hospital when a frantic long-distance call is received. The caller is Larry Nelson from Cheyenne, Wyoming. He received a call from the nursing home where his 95-year-old mother was living informing him that she was taken by ambulance to your hospital. Larry wants to know if Muriel Nelson has arrived and what her condition is. Wanda is aware of a patient's right to privacy, confidentiality, and the new HIPAA regulations. Wanda observed Mrs. Nelson arrive at the emergency department quite incoherent and confused.

CASE STUDY REVIEW

1. What can Wanda tell Mr. Nelson, especially after noting that no records were with the elderly Mrs. Nelson when she arrived at the hospital?
2. What information would Wanda need from Mr. Nelson before complying with his request?
3. How can Wanda put Mr. Nelson at ease? What can Wanda do to help?

SUMMARY

Changing societal values have contributed to an increase of lawsuits in medical practice. Patients are more aware than ever of their rights, especially those of confidentiality and the right to privacy, consent, and records ownership. They are likely to seek redress when they perceive their rights have been violated.

A healthy relationship between all providers and patients and between medical assistants and patients, as well as respect for the patient's rights, reduces the likelihood of a lawsuit.

Additional knowledge of the laws that regulate medical and business practices in your state is necessary to be in compliance. Sources of information regarding state and federal laws can be obtained from the state medical society, the provider's liability insurance company, the state medical assistant society, the state attorney general's office, the Internet, or the public library.

STUDY FOR SUCCESS

To reinforce your knowledge and skills of information presented in this chapter:

- Review the Key Terms
- Consider the Case Studies and discuss your conclusions
- Answer the Review Questions
  - Multiple Choice
  - Critical Thinking
- Navigate the Internet and complete the Web Activities
- Practice the StudyWARE activities on the textbook CD
- Apply your knowledge in the Student Workbook activities
- Complete the Web Tutor sections
- View and discuss the DVD situations

REVIEW QUESTIONS

Multiple Choice

1. The type of contract that most often exists between provider and patient is:
   a. expressed
   b. implied
   c. privileged
   d. civil
2. The administrative law act that prohibits discrimination, has five sections, and is enforced by the EEOC is called the:
   a. Controlled Substances Act
   b. Federal Age Discrimination Act
   c. Americans with Disabilities Act
   d. Health Insurance Portability and Accountability Act
3. Slander is defamation through:
   a. spoken statements that damage an individual's reputation
   b. written statements that damage a person's reputation
   c. written falsehoods about an individual
   d. a, b, and c
4. Occasionally, a provider will be sued for the negligence of an employee, even though the provider is not guilty of any negligent act. This is done on the basis of the doctrine of:
   a. *res ipsa loquitur*
   b. *respondeat superior*
   c. proximate cause
   d. contract law
5. The standard of care expected of a provider is held by the courts to mean:
   a. on a par with all other providers engaged in the same medical specialty anywhere
   b. reasonable, attentive, diligent care comparable with other providers of the same specialty or general field of practice
   c. the best possible under the circumstances
   d. the same as the national norm
6. Advance directives:
   a. allow patients to direct how their billing is to be handled
   b. are designed to encourage providers to render first aid in an emergency
   c. indicate a patient's wishes in life-threatening circumstances
   d. are not considered legal documents
7. A subpoena:
   a. is a court order requesting data, an appearance in court, or both
   b. is sufficient to enforce a release of any type medical record or information
   c. may be ignored without consequences
   d. allows the person being served to select a specific date or time to appear
8. The 4 Ds of negligence are:
   a. duty, danger, damage, and disaster
   b. derelict, direct cause, damage, and danger
   c. danger, direct cause, damage, disaster
   d. duty, derelict, direct cause, damage
9. Emancipated minors:
   a. are considered adults and can consent to treatment
   b. live on their own and are self-supporting
   c. may be married or serve in the military
   d. all of the above
   e. only b and c
10. Torts:
    a. include battery, defamation of character, invasion of privacy
    b. are always intentional in nature
    c. do not require that harm has occurred
    d. do not include malpractice

Critical Thinking

1. Chris is a 6-year-old girl who Dr. King treated for a broken leg. Chris' parents fail to follow Dr. King's treatment plan for Chris. What, if any, action can Dr. King take? What is the legal term for this situation?
2. Jaime arrived in the clinic having sustained a serious laceration at his construction site. Dr. Woo determines surgery is required. Should a consent form be prepared? If so, by whom, and what should be included?
3. Do you have a living will or advance directive? Why or why not? Identify to a family member or a loved one what your wishes might be if you were seriously injured in an accident and were still in what appears to be an irreversible coma after 10 months.
4. Discuss the medical assistant's obligations in regard to public duties.
5. What is the Good Samaritan law? What must a medical assistant and any other health care professional remember when giving first aid at the scene of an accident?
6. Describe three types of abuse. Tell what your role as a medical assistant is when Juanita brings her 3-year-old son Henry to the clinic. Henry has bruises on his face and chest and appears quite frightened when you approach him. While you prepare Henry for the pediatrician's examination, Juanita's answers to your questions seem evasive.

WEB ACTIVITIES

1. Using the Internet, determine whether or when a medical clinic might be required to follow the federal guidelines of the Family and Medical Leave Act (FMLA). Identify reasons to follow the FMLA guidelines.
2. Using your favorite search engine, key in the words "Medical Malpractice Awards." A number of sites will appear. Has a national limit been set on malpractice awards? What makes this topic a political one? Identify those who favor malpractice award limits and also those who oppose these limits.
3. Research the Internet for the statute of limitations related to claims injuries. What is the time span in your state?

REFERENCES/BIBLIOGRAPHY

Balasa, D. A. (May/June 2004). Legal environment differs under independent nurse practitioners. *CMA TODAY,* 37(3), 24–25.

Compassion & Choices. Washington Durable Power of Attorney for Health Care. Retrieved June 26, 2007, from http://compassionindying.org.

Krager, D., & Krager, C. (2005). *HIPAA for medical office personnel.* Clifton Park, NY: Delmar Cengage Learning.

Lewis, M. A., & Tamparo, C. D. (2007). *Medical law, ethics, and bioethics for health professions* (6th ed.). Philadelphia: F. A. Davis.

Washington State Medical Association (WSMA). (2007). *Durable power of attorney for health care, health care directive, and POLST.* Retrieved June 2007, from http://www.wsma.org.

THE DVD HOOK-UP

This chapter deals with legal considerations that must be adhered to when working in the medical industry. One of the most important legal responsibilities that you have as a medical assistant is to stay within the boundaries of your scope and training as a medical assistant.

In one of the scenes listed above, Barb, the office manager, reprimands Eileen for administering a Demerol injection. Eileen states that the provider ordered her to give the injection, which is why she gave it. The office manager tells Eileen that medical assistants are not allowed to give controlled substances in that particular state. Eileen replies that she didn't know she could not give controlled substances, and that she gave controlled substances in the last office that she worked. Barb reminds Eileen that the information was posted in the office's procedures manual that she was suppose to have read at the time of orientation. Barb told Eileen that she had no other choice but to document this error in her personal record.

1. Why did Barb take such a hard approach with Eileen? What steps does Barb need to take in the future? What responsibility does the provider have?
2. How could Eileen have avoided this awkward situation?
3. What will you do if a provider orders you to perform a procedure that medical assistants are not allowed to perform?

DVD Journal Summary

Write a paragraph that summarizes what you learned from watching the designated scenes from today's DVD program. What steps will you take to make certain that you know what medical assistants can and cannot do in the state in which you practice?

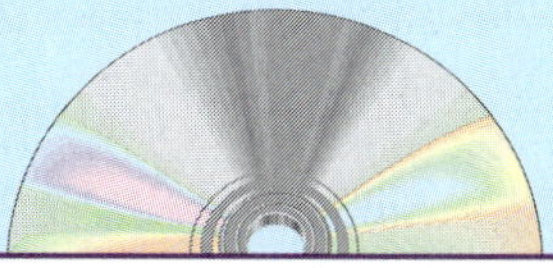

DVD Series	**Program Number**
Critical Thinking	3

Chapter/Scene Reference
- *Licensing and Scope of Practice*
- *Regulating Agencies OSHA, DEA, and CMS*

Chapter 8 Ethical Considerations

OUTLINE

KEY TERMS

Bioethics
Cryopreservation
Ethics
Genetic Engineering
In Vitro Fertilization (IVF)
Intimate Partner Violence (IPV)
Macroallocation
Microallocation
Surrogate

OBJECTIVES

The student should strive to meet the following performance objectives and demonstrate an understanding of the facts and principles presented in this chapter through written and oral communication.

1. Define the key terms as presented in the glossary.
2. Identify two reasons for Codes of Ethics.
3. Discuss the eight characteristics of principle-centered leadership.
4. Describe the five Ps of ethical power.
5. Recall the ethics check questions.
6. Relate the five principles of the AAMA code to patient care in the ambulatory care setting.
7. Discuss the ethical guidelines for health care providers, giving at least four examples.
8. Restate the dilemmas encountered by the following bioethical issues: (a) allocation of scarce medical resources; (b) abortion and fetal tissue research; (c) genetic engineering/manipulation; (d) artificial insemination/surrogacy; (e)in vitro fertilization; (f) dying and death; (g) HIV and AIDS.

Scenario

Harley Navarro is a new medical assistant in a busy internist's office. He finished school a few months ago and is awaiting the date to take his exam to become a certified medical assistant. He is nervous and scared. All the other medical assistants are female and have many years of experience. Harley wants so much to be accepted and recognized for his skills. Today, however, he twice had a rough time taking a blood pressure reading. In fact, the provider was ready for one of Harley's patients before he was finished with the reading, and the provider stepped in to take the reading. Harley was embarrassed. His current patient is obese. His first attempt at getting a blood pressure reading failed. He gets a larger cuff for his second reading. His patient complains, however, that her arm is hurting about halfway through the reading. Harley hurries the process and takes a guess at the diastolic pressure figure, but he knows it is close.

INTRODUCTION

It is impossible in today's world to function as a medical assistant without an awareness of the impact of ethics and bioethics on health care. Just as an understanding of the law and working within the law is vital information for the medical assistant, it is equally important to understand ethics and bioethics.

From Chapter 7, you have come to realize that there are many circumstances and situations that occur in health care that are guided and directed by state and federal laws. You, personally, are expected to be above reproach in all your actions in this regard. You must also work with your employer and other members of the health care team to ensure that each member of the staff functions within the law—protecting both patients and providers.

Spotlight on Certification

RMA Content Outline

- Principles of medical ethics
- Ethical conduct

CMA (AAMA) Content Outline

- Displaying professional attitude
- Performing within ethical boundaries
- Maintaining confidentiality
- Legislation
- Working as a team member to achieve goals

CMAS Content Outline

- Legal and ethical considerations
- Professionalism
- Confidentiality

Ethics plays a huge role in such an endeavor. To function ethically demands that you never function outside the law. Ethics, however, demands something more—ethics calls for honesty, trustworthiness, integrity, confidentiality, and fairness. To function ethically, you must know yourself well and understand weaknesses and any vulnerabilities that might prevent you from acting ethically.

The scenario described earlier is just one situation in which medical assistants may need to reflect on their actions and be sure that they are acting ethically and within the range of their skills. Medical assistants also need to recognize the warning signs that they, or some other staff member, may be about to breach a code of ethics. Often, this kind of breach occurs when one has, or seeks to have, too much power; when one attempts to take on too much authority; or when one has too little knowledge and experience or is afraid to ask for help. When a breach seems about to occur, the individuals involved should be encouraged to step back and review their actions and the likely consequences of those actions.

ETHICS

Traditionally, **ethics** is defined in terms of what is considered right or wrong. Sometimes ethics is referred to as "morals." However, morals refer to personal choices of conduct, whereas ethics is more of a philosophy related to making judgments about right and wrong. Professional organizations often identify their ethics in "codes," or a set of principles and guidelines. Providers, through the American Medical Association (AMA), have established such a code of ethics called the Principles of Medical Ethics. This code can be reviewed by accessing the AMA Web site (http://www.ama-assn.org). The Code of Medical Ethics Current

Opinions with Annotations is published every 2 years; this document provides up-to-date information on a number of ethical dilemmas. Medical assistants have a code of ethics and a creed. The AAMA Mission Statement, AAMA Medical Assistant Code of Ethics, and AAMA Medical Assistant Creed appear on the AAMA Web site (http://www.aama-ntl.org). Clicking on About AAMA will detail these statements for you.

There are more than 50 differing codes of ethics for professional organizations, and most are related to medicine. There are seven ethical codes that relate to the entire world. These include such famous codes as the Declaration of Geneva, Declaration of Helsinki, and the International Code of Medical Ethics. A listing of these codes is found by searching the Internet for "world medical ethics codes." Another fascinating Web site identifies the characteristics of Traditional Chinese Medical Ethics when you use the Internet to search for "Chinese Medical Ethics." Chinese medical ethics emphasizes self-cultivation and personal ethics of practitioners rather than a strict organizational code of ethics.

Codes of ethics bring standards of moral and ethical behavior together in one place. They assist organizations and individuals in putting words to their expected behaviors and actions. There is a benefit to such codes when they become reminders to everyone regarding their conduct. Codes also can have a limiting effect, however. For instance, if an organization does not have a code of ethics, is that organization viewed as unethical? When one answers that question, there also comes the understanding that having a code of ethics does not necessarily create an ethical organization.

Medical assistants and medical professionals are asked to balance personal and professional areas of their lives in the middle of constant pressure and crises. At the same time, the quality of one's personal life is going to be shown in the quality of their service to others in their professional life. To be effective in the medical profession, there needs to be maturity in both the personal and the professional selves that creates the utmost of ethical conduct and professionalism.

Principle-Centered Leadership

Stephen R. Covey, author of *The 7 Habits of Highly Effective People* and *Principle-Centered Leadership*, has identified eight characteristics of principle-centered leaders. Leaders who know themselves and understand their principles more easily abide by a code of ethics. Consider the following questions as guides to how you might perform ethically in a medical setting.

Are you continually learning? Do you seek training, take classes, listen to others, learn from your peers? Are you curious? Do you realize that developing new knowledge and skills is a lifelong endeavor?

Are you service-oriented? Do you see your life as a mission rather than a career? Are you generally a nurturing individual who seeks service in the medical field? Can you see yourself working alongside a coworker and pulling together with that person toward a goal? Can you put yourself in the place of others?

Do you radiate positive energy? Are you cheerful, pleasant, optimistic, and positive? Is your spirit hopeful? If it is, you carry a positive energy field that allows you to neutralize or sidestep a negative energy source. Do you see yourself as a peacemaker or one that can create harmony to undo negative energy?

Do you believe in other people? Can you keep from labeling, stereotyping, or prejudging other people? Can you believe in the unseen potential of others? Can you keep from overreacting to negative behaviors and criticism? Can you put aside any grudges?

The final characteristics of principle-centered leaders identified in Covey's *7 Habits of Highly Effective People* are more personal. They can help you understand yourself and how you might make ethical decisions in the medical field.

Do you lead a balanced life? Do you keep up with current affairs and events? Do you know what is happening in the medical field and how that affects you? Do you have at least one confidant with whom you can be transparent? Are you physically active within your limits of age and health? Do you enjoy yourself? Do you have a good sense of humor? Are you open to communication?

Do you see life as an adventure? Are you able to rediscover persons each time you meet them? Are you interested in others? Do you listen well? Are you flexible and unflappable? Does your security come from within rather than from without?

Are you synergistic? Synergy is what happens when the whole of something is greater than the sum of its parts. Do you know your weaknesses? Can you complement your weaknesses with the strength of others on the team? Can you work hard to improve most situations? Are you trusting? Can you separate the person from the problem?

Do you exercise for self-renewal? In this element, Mr. Covey identifies four dimensions of the human personality that need exercise: physical, mental, emotional, and spiritual dimensions. How do you keep your body in shape? How do you keep your mind alert? Do patience, unconditional love, and accepting responsibility for your own actions keep you emotionally healthy? Do you have a way to meditate, pray, or "draw away" for a period to "fill up your spirit"?

These questions and your responses to them can give you insight into your ability to function ethically and to be successful in the world of medicine.

Covey has another book entitled *The 8th Habit: From Effectiveness to Greatness* that discusses how individuals can be more excited about their lives and their work when they reach beyond effectiveness toward fulfillment, contribution, and greatness. Individuals who feel fulfilled and excited about their work are more apt to perform ethically than those who do not.

Five Ps of Ethical Power

Kenneth Blanchard and Norman Vincent Peale wrote a simple but powerful little book called *The Power of Ethical Management.* In it they discuss the "Five Ps of Ethical Power." The five Ps are as follows:

Purpose: Understand your objective or your purpose. Your purpose may change from time to time, but it is something that requires you to behave in a way that makes you feel good about yourself.

Pride: Have pride in what you do. Feel good about yourself and your accomplishments. Nurture your self-esteem while remaining humble. Be proud to be a medical assistant.

Patience: It takes time to create an atmosphere where your objective can be obtained. Strive to believe that no matter what happens, everything is going to work out. Expect results from yourself and your work, but refrain from demanding it "now."

Persistence: To act in an ethical manner means to strive to act in that manner all the time, not just when you want to or it seems easy to do. Winston Churchill said, "Never! Never! Never! Never! Give Up!" That is what persistence is. If you make a mistake, admit it, correct it, learn from the mistake, and move on, but never give up. An individual who is truly aware of his or her personal ethical power is able to admit an error, does not compromise any procedure or any technique, and does not ever put the patient at risk, even if it means facing reprimand from a supervisor.

Perspective: Keep your life and your purpose in perspective. Find time each day to maintain balance in your life (perhaps looking again at the eight characteristics of principle-centered individuals). Plan some quiet time, some fun time, but certainly some reflective time. The constant pressure and the crises will become overwhelming without keeping perspective.

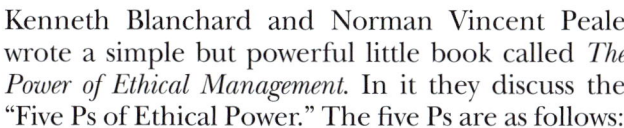

Critical Thinking

With a peer, identify one or more examples in your life when you truly did not give up on attaining your goals. Describe what you learned from that experience. How might "never giving up" help in your pursuit of a career?

Ethics Check Questions

Finally, those striving to act in an ethical manner can perform a little test each time they have a question about ethics. This, too, comes from Blanchard and Peale. The questions to ask are: (1) Is it legal? Is it against the law or any company policy? (2) Is it balanced? Is this the best possible approach for all concerned? Does it promote a win–win situation? (3) How will it make me feel about myself? Will I feel good if my decision is published in a newspaper? Will my family and coworkers be proud of my decision?

Ethics are not easy. Performing ethically is hard work. Being ethical means determining who you are and how you will act. Laws are more clearly defined than ethics, but acting in an unethical manner can cause as much pain and difficulty as can acting illegally. The ideas of Covey, Blanchard, and Peale give guidance, thoughts to ponder, and perhaps goals to reach. Keep them in mind as you review the next section.

BIOETHICS

Bioethics brings the entire focus of ethics into the field of health care and into those ethical issues dealing with life. Never before in the history of medical care has bioethics been such a topic of concern. In the past, most bioethical decisions were made by physicians and esteemed members of the medical or legal profession. However, advancing technology giving patients and consumers numerous choices regarding their health care leads everyone to take an active role in bioethics.

Medical assistants will encounter ethical and bioethical issues across the lifespan. In Figure 8-1,

ETHICAL ISSUES FOR CONTEMPLATION AND DISCUSSION

Infants

- Imperiled newborns (those who are severely disabled, deformed, often premature and have low birth weight) have a greater chance for survival with today's medical technology. However, this ability places parents and health care professionals in an uncomfortable position to determine when the costs of expensive intervention outweigh the benefits. Often medical insurance will not pay for these costs.
- Vulnerability of infants can lead to negligence, rejection, and even abuse. Parents also are vulnerable because they often are unable to cope with the needs of the entire family. How can families be helped in making a choice or in providing care for their family?

Children

- Children who are not well fed, housed, educated, and clothed exhibit great needs for preventive, curative, and rehabilitative health care. They likely do not have medical coverage, do not visit a health care provider regularly, and make more trips to the hospital emergency room than most children.
- Obesity in children is a serious health issue. Increasing numbers of children receive one or two free or low-cost meals at school, share few meals with their family members, and eat at fast-food restaurants. Sweets are often used as reward or to express love. How are children educated to make better choices?
- An increasing number of children live within very dysfunctional families where one or more parent is absent, is a substance abuser, has mental health issues, or has very little time to spend with their children. Many children have multiple parents or caregivers. Many spend large portions of the day in a daycare environment. Child abuse is a concern. Children must be protected, but they can be caught in a web of social services so overloaded and understaffed that only the most severe concerns receive attention. How do health professionals protect these children?

Adolescents

- The adolescent's growing autonomy, need for independence, changing values, and desire for peer acceptance often lead to the decision to become sexually active, use birth control, or experiment with drugs and alcohol.
- Adolescents as young as 14 to 18 years of age may seek treatment for substance abuse, birth control, even abortion without parental consent. Does this violate parents' right to medical information regarding their children? Should the adolescent, often fearful of parental reaction, have a right to treatment?

Adults

- A large number of men and women find that both must be employed in order to provide a home for their families. How is it possible to balance full-time employment, full-time parenting, full-time housekeeping, and full-time partnering, and still take care of oneself?
- Many low-income women lack sufficient access to prenatal care, even though it is a cost-saving medical measure that is critical to the health of both mother and infant.
- Adequate and quality health care is a problem. Some adults have no health care coverage; others are part of managed care programs that keep changing as employers seek lower health insurance premiums. Many adults do not have an ongoing provider–patient relationship.
- War, terrorist attacks, and an overburdened military place families in very stressful circumstances. Many who serve in the military are returning with horrendous lifelong and debilitating injuries. Lives are forever changed. How do they cope?
- Even with an advance directive or living will, a dying patient's wishes may not be followed. Technological advances in medicine have created situations where patients may not be able to exercise their wishes.

Senior Adults

- Elderly patients have the right to maintain dignity and privacy, but their dependency on others may deprive them of these basic rights.
- Many senior adults are finding that very few providers accept new Medicare patients. The problem is even more severe when senior adults must rely upon Medicaid for their medical care because of the few number of providers who accept Medicaid.
- Some elderly patients must choose between food on their tables or prescribed medications they cannot afford. Although Medicare Part D helped some, it did not help all.
- Dementia is a common problem that is physically and financially exhausting and heartbreaking to the caregiver who usually is a spouse, partner, or adult child. How do individuals cope in the "sandwich" arrangement of caring for themselves, their children, and elderly parents, some who may have dementia? What happens when there are insufficient funds for assisted living or long-term care?

Figure 8-1 Ethical issues across the life span. (Compiled by Carol D. Tamparo, CMA (AAMA), PhD, and Marilyn Pooler, RN, MEd.)

AAMA CODE OF ETHICS

The Code of Ethics of AAMA shall set forth principles of ethical and moral conduct as they relate to the medical profession and the particular practice of medical assisting.

Members of AAMA dedicated to the conscientious pursuit of their profession, and thus desiring to merit the high regard of the entire medical profession and the respect of the general public which they serve, do pledge themselves to strive always to:

A. render service with full respect for the dignity of humanity;
B. respect confidential information obtained through employment unless legally authorized or required by responsible performance of duty to divulge such information;
C. uphold the honor and high principles of the profession and accept its disciplines;
D. seek to continually improve the knowledge and skills of medical assistants for the benefit of patients and professional colleagues;
E. participate in additional service activities aimed toward improving the health and well-being of the community.

(A)

CREED

I believe in the principles and purposes of the Profession of Medical Assisting.
I endeavor to be more effective.
I aspire to render greater service.
I protect the confidence entrusted to me.
I am dedicated to the care and well-being of all people.
I am loyal to my employer.
I am true to the ethics of my profession.
I am strengthened by compassion, courage, and faith.

(B)

Figure 8-2 (A) American Association of Medical Assistants (AAMA) Code of Ethics. (B) AAMA Creed. (Copyright by the American Association of Medical Assistants, Inc. Revised October 1996.)

a few issues are identified for contemplation and discussion. Issues of bioethics common to every medical clinic are the allocation of scarce medical resources; abortion and fetal tissue research; genetic engineering or manipulation; and the many choices surrounding life, dying, and death.

For medical assistants to fully comprehend a discussion of ethics and bioethics, review of the Code of Ethics of AAMA (Figure 8-2) is beneficial.

KEYS TO THE AAMA CODE OF ETHICS

Medical assistants should consider the more salient points in the AAMA Code of Ethics and ask themselves the following questions:

A. *Render service with full respect for the dignity of humanity.*
- Will I respect every patient even if I do not approve of his or her morals or choices in health care?
- Will I honor each patient's request for information and explain unfamiliar procedures?
- Will I give my full attention to acknowledging the needs of every patient?
- Will I be able to accept the indigent, the physically and mentally challenged, the infirm, the physically disfigured, and the persons I simply do not like as equal and valid human beings with an equal right to service?

B. *Respect confidential information obtained through employment unless legally authorized or required by responsible performance of duty to divulge such information.*
- Will I refrain from needless comments to a colleague regarding a patient's problem?
- Will I refrain from discussing my day's encounters with patients with my family and friends?
- Will I always protect a patient's medical record and everything in it from unnecessary observation?
- Will I keep patients' names and the circumstances that bring them to my place of employment confidential?

C. *Uphold the honor and high principles of the profession and accept its disciplines.*
- Am I proud to serve as a medical assistant?
- Will I always perform within the scope of my profession, never exceeding the responsibility entrusted to me?
- Will I encourage others to enter the profession and always speak honorably of medical assistants?

D. *Seek to continually improve the knowledge and skills of medical assistants for the benefit of patients and professional colleagues.*
- Will I be willing to learn new skills, to update my skills, and seek improved methods for assisting the provider in the care of patients?
- Will I keep my credentials current and valid?
- Can I remember that I am a member of a group of broad-based health care professionals, and that my goal is to complement rather than to compete with that team?

E. *Participate in additional service activities aimed toward improving the health and well-being of the community.*
- Will I be able to serve in the community where I reside and work to further quality health care?
- Will I promote preventive medicine?
- Will I practice good health care management for myself, being a model for others to follow?

ETHICAL GUIDELINES FOR HEALTH CARE PROVIDERS

It is fairly common for each professional group of medical practitioners to have their own code of ethics. The AMA's Code of Medical Ethics and the "Current Opinions with Annotations of the Council on Ethical and Judicial Affairs" was mentioned earlier. The American Chiropractic Association has a Code of Ethics identified in six sections. The American Osteopathic Association has a Code of Ethics with 19 different sections. Other practitioners may consider their mission and policies to be their code of ethics. Some have no specific written code of ethics but rather call on their practitioners to refer to their culture as one based on ethics, mutual respect, and moral evaluation when ethical decisions are made. There are many similarities in these statements on ethics that are important for patients and medical employees. A few prominent statements are provided here.

Advertising

Health care providers and professional people traditionally have not advertised; however, it is not illegal or unethical to do so if claims made are truthful and not misleading. Advertisements may include credentials of providers and a description of the practice, kinds of services rendered, and how fees are determined. Managed care agencies may advertise their services and the names of participating providers.

Confidentiality

Providers must not reveal confidential information about patients without their consent unless the providers are otherwise required to do so by law. Confidentiality must be protected so that patients will feel comfortable and safe in revealing information about themselves that may be important to their health care. The following list contains examples of the kinds of reports that allow or require health professionals to report a confidence.

- A patient threatens another person and there is reason to believe that the threat may be carried out.
- Certain injuries and illnesses *must* be reported. These include injuries such as knife and gunshot wounds, wounds that may be from suspected child abuse, communicable diseases, and sexually transmitted diseases.
- Information that may have been subpoenaed for testimony in a court of law.

When in doubt, it is always recommended that a provider have the patient's permission to reveal any confidential information.

Extra caution must be taken to protect the confidentiality of any patient's data that are kept on a computer database. As few people as possible should have access to the computer data, and only authorized individuals should be permitted to add or alter data. Adequate security precautions must be used to protect information stored on a computer. HIPAA has specific guidelines for computer privacy.

Medical Records

Medical records and the information in them are the property of the provider and the patient. No information should be revealed without the patient's consent unless required by law. The record is confidential. Providers should not refuse to provide a copy of the record to another provider treating the patient so long as proper authorization has been received from the patient. Also, providers should provide a copy of the record or summary of its contents if a patient requests it. A record cannot be withheld because of an unpaid bill.

On a provider's retirement or death, or when a practice is sold, patients should be notified and given ample time to have their records transferred to another provider of their choice.

Professional Fees and Charges

Illegal or excessive fees should not be charged. Fees should be based on those customary to the locale and should reflect the difficulty of services and the quality of performance rendered. Fee splitting (a provider splits the fee with another provider for services rendered with or without the patient's knowledge) in any form is unethical. Providers may charge for missed appointments (if patients have first been notified of the practice) and may charge for multiple or complex insurance forms. Providers and their employees must be diligent to ensure that only the services actually rendered are charged or indicated on the insurance claim. Only what is documented in the patient's chart is to be billed.

Increasingly, a number of providers now refuse any insurance payments and operate strictly on a cash-only basis. Others charge a yearly fee to care for a family, providing all services necessary at that flat fee. Providers, upset by the rules and regulations of insurance, find this method of payment creates a simpler form of medical practice. Providers and patients alike will be discussing the ethics of such a move for some time. Although providers may choose whom they wish to serve, the cash-only basis is difficult for low-income families and the poor.

Professional Rights and Responsibilities

As stated earlier, providers may choose whom to serve, but they may not refuse a patient on the basis of race, color, religion, national origin, or any other illegal discrimination. It is unethical for providers to deny treatment to HIV-infected individuals on that basis alone if they are qualified to treat the patient's condition. Once a provider takes a case, the patient cannot be neglected or refused treatment unless official notice is given from the provider to withdraw from the case.

Patients have the right to know their diagnoses and the nature and purpose of their treatment and to have enough information to be able to make an informed choice about their treatment protocol. Providers should inform families of a patient's death and not delegate that responsibility to others.

Providers should expose incompetent, corrupt, dishonest, and unethical conduct by other providers to the disciplinary board. It is unethical for any provider to treat patients while under the influence of alcohol, controlled substances, or any other chemical that impairs the physician's ability.

Providers who know they are HIV positive should refrain from any activity that would risk the transmission of the virus to others.

Any activity that might be regarded as a "conflict of interest" (for example, a provider holding stock in a pharmaceutical company and prescribing medications only from that company) should be avoided. Financial interests are not to influence providers in prescribing medications, devices, or appliances.

Disaster Response

Medical professionals are essential at the time of any disaster, such as epidemics, floods, fires, weather-related disasters, and terrorist attacks. Care for the sick and injured is of primary concern when disaster strikes. Providers are encouraged to give their medical expertise not only to prepare for any type of disaster but to provide assistance when one occurs. Providers should consider seeking training in disaster preparedness and response and lend their knowledge where it is most beneficial and effective in making certain that medical care is available during such events.

Treatment for a Culturally Diverse Clientele

All providers are reminded to strive to provide the same quality of care to all their patients regardless of race or ethnicity. Providers must remember to eliminate biased behavior toward any group of patients deemed different from themselves. All patients have the right to participatory decision making with their providers based on mutual trust and understanding. Communication factors are to be considered and interpreters provided as necessary so that patients understand the medical information as well as any communication exchanged.

Diversity is to be encouraged in the medical profession and considered when hiring assistants. Ethnically diverse neighborhoods and clientele deserve an ethnically diverse group of medical professionals for their care. If it is not possible to employ an ethnically diverse group of medical professionals, then medical professionals who are keenly aware of and knowledgeable of the ethic group served is of primary importance.

Care of the Poor

From the earliest history of medical treatment, care for the poor has been a concern and a goal for medical practitioners. Today that obligation is still mentioned in most ethical codes and discussions. All medical providers have a responsibility to ensure that the needs of the poor in their communities are met. Caring for the poor should be a regular part of every provider's practice and can be accomplished in a number of ways. Providers can take a certain number of patients on a reduced-cost basis or provide free services. Providers can volunteer their time and efforts to treat patients in reduced-cost, freestanding clinics that treat the poor and/or provide services to those in homeless shelters for battered and abused individuals. Providers can volunteer their time to lobbying and being advocates for those without medical coverage.

Abuse

Abuse usually is described as neglect, physical, emotional/psychological/mental injury, or sexual. Child abuse also includes child molestation, sexual exploitation, and incest. Elder abuse includes the four basic types mentioned above and adds financial abuse. Stalking and rape are also forms of abuse.

All 50 states have legislation defining child abuse and mandate who is responsible for reporting such abuse. The majority of states have enacted legislation regarding the abuse of elder adults 60 years of age or older. Intimate partner (or domestic) violence is a criminal offense in some states, but whether a state requires that **intimate partner violence (IPV)** be reported depends in part upon whether a weapon is used.

Stalking is the repeated act of spying upon, following, or making contact with an individual or appearing at an individual's residence or place of employment after being asked not to. It is a crime in some states. *Rape,* also a crime of violence, is forced sexual intercourse or penetration of a body orifice with the penis or some other object. Gang rape involves several individuals. Rape is a reportable criminal act.

Medical assistants must know if their state specifically names them as a reporter for abuse. A discussion should be held with medical providers and employers regarding who, when, and how the abuse will be reported and documented. It is unethical for a medical assistant to fail to report abuse simply because an employer prefers "not to get too involved." For a clearer understanding of some of the factors that constitute abuse, review Table 8-1.

It is the responsibility of medical professionals and their employees to report all cases of suspected child abuse, to protect and care for the abused, and to treat the abuser (if known) as a victim also. This is not an easy task. Abuse is not easy to witness. Although there are specific laws regarding suspected child abuse, and in most states medical assistants are mandated to report abuse, the laws are vague or nonexistent for older adults or in cases of IPV. However, whatever form the abuse takes, it is best to treat all forms of abuse in the same manner by providing a safe environment for those abused and seeking treatment for the abused and the abuser.

BIOETHICAL DILEMMAS

Guidelines for bioethical issues are even harder to define than are guidelines for ethics, because each of the bioethical issues calls for decisions that directly affect a person's life. In some instances, the bioethical issue requires a choice about who lives and requires a definition of the quality of life. Such dilemmas are difficult, if not impossible, to approach from a neutral point of view even though medical professionals should strive not to impose their own moral values on patients or coworkers.

Allocation of Scarce Medical Resources

The issue faced daily by health care workers is the allocation of scarce medical resources. Even with the government's attempts at health care reform, medical resources still are not available to everyone. When the administrative medical assistant determines who receives the only available appointment in a day, when patients are turned away because they have no insurance or financial resources to pay for services, when Medicare/Medicaid patients are denied services because of low return from state and federal insurance programs, scarce medical resources are being denied.

The U.S. Census Bureau reported that 46.6 million people were without health insurance coverage in 2006. The number of uninsured is estimated to increase by one million each year. Adults were more likely to be uninsured than children because a number of state and federal programs cover children. However, more than 6% of children under age 18 years have no source of health care. Hispanic and non-Hispanic black children were more likely to have no health care than were non-Hispanic white children. Of note, the average waiting time by new patients for a medical

Table 8-1 Descriptions of Abuse

	Child Abuse	Elder Abuse	Intimate Partner Violence
Neglect	Failure to provide basic food, shelter, care; endangers health of child	Lack of attention that causes harm; withholding basic needs; abandonment; lack of help with hygiene or bathing	
Physical	Burns, unusual or severe bruising, lacerations, fractures, injury to internal organs; usually obvious	Assault, beating, whipping, hitting, punching, pushing, pinching, force-feeding, shaking, rough handling during caregiving, bodily harm or severe mental stress	Intent to harm; hitting, pushing, grabbing, biting, punching, slapping, restraining, burning; use of a weapon or one's own strength to harm
Emotional/ psychological	Harm to child's emotional and intellectual growth; not always obvious	Actions that dehumanize; social isolation, name calling, humiliating, insulting; threats to punish; yelling, screaming	Humiliating; controlling; isolating partner from friends/family, withholding funds or basic resources
Sexual	Using a child to engage in any sexual activity; not always obvious	Sexual contact without permission; fondling, touching, kissing, rape, coerced nudity; spying while in bathroom	Sexual contact without permission; abusive sexual contact; sex with one who is unable to say "no"
Financial		Exploitation of an elder's resources; forging signature on documents; withholding or cashing funds received	
Sexual exploitation	Pornography, prostitution; use of child's image in media		
Incest	Sexual activity between family members		

appointment was 14.5 days. Even the elderly, many of whom have both Medicare and supplemental health insurance, had difficulty finding providers who took new Medicare patients. This dilemma can be particularly problematic when the elderly move from their home and community to be closer to their children.

Weightier decisions might include who gets the surgery, a kidney transplant, or the experimental bone marrow transplant. These allocations are being made and will continue to require decisions on the part of the health care team. Rationing of health care may become more widespread as managed care operations try to achieve a balance between providing access to care while still curtailing costs.

Decisions made by Congress, health systems agencies, and insurance companies are termed **macroallocation** of scarce medical resources. Decisions made individually by providers and members of the health care team at the local level are termed **microallocation** of scarce resources. No matter what the level, medical assistants will be involved.

Abortion and Fetal Tissue Research

The issues associated with abortion and fetal tissue research will be with us for quite some time. Although the law as set forth in *Roe v. Wade* is specific on abortion guidelines, there is a continual challenge in the courts of its validity. Some states are more restrictive regarding whether and how abortions might be performed in the second and third trimesters of pregnancy. However, the current law stipulates that a woman has a right to an abortion in the first trimester without interference from regulations in any state.

Medical professionals must decide whether to perform abortions within the legal parameters and under what circumstances. Providers cannot be forced to perform abortions, nor can any employee be forced to participate or assist in an abortion. Employees not wishing to participate in abortions are advised to seek employment where they are not performed.

Many unanswered ethical questions related to abortion make the decision difficult for health care professionals. Should abortion be considered a form of birth control? If not, should birth control be readily available to all who seek it regardless of age? Should insurance pay for birth control? Is it ethical to deny an abortion to a woman on welfare but provide one to a woman who has money for the procedure or whose insurance pays? Should any abortion be legal? And, of course, the major unanswered question that must be considered by every individual is: When does life begin?

The abortion issue raises another bioethical issue—fetal tissue research and transplantation. As early as the 1950s, fetal tissue research led to the development of polio and rubella vaccines. Today, fetal cells hold promise for medical research into a variety of diseases and medical conditions, including Alzheimer's disease, Huntington's disease, spinal cord injury, diabetes, and multiple sclerosis. Some research indicates that fetal retinal transplants may be a successful treatment of macular degeneration, which is the leading cause of age-related blindness in the United States. This issue is political as well as bioethical, and it changes with each major political shift in our government. Fetal tissue research also gets caught up in the pro-life forces. About half of the states have laws regulating fetal research. Some ban research using aborted fetuses. Federal law prohibits the sale of fetal tissue and requires all federally funded fetal tissue research projects to comply with state and local laws. Fetal tissue research is not to be used to encourage women to have abortions; rather, the tissue would be available only after a decision had already been made regarding abortion.

While the debate related to the use of fetal tissues for research marches on, the door has opened for research using umbilical cord blood. The use of cord blood has not met with as much controversy as the use of fetal tissue. In 2005, President George W. Bush signed into legislation a federal program to collect and store cord blood and to expand the current bone marrow registry program to include cord blood. Stem cells in cord blood can help restore red blood cells in people with sickle cell anemia, and a small group of children newly diagnosed with type 1 diabetes who were transfused with their own stored cord blood showed reduced severity of the disease.

Genetic Engineering/ Manipulation

So much is possible today in the area of **genetic engineering,** and new discoveries increasingly are being made. This biotechnology can be used in the diagnosis of disease, in the production of medicines, for forensic documentation (DNA used in solving crimes), and for research. Some reasons for continuing study in this area include determining if anything can be done to prevent or cure some 4,000 recognized genetic disorders and major diseases that have large genetic components. Few individuals would not like to see a cure for certain illnesses, but there is a fear among many that genetic engineering may lead to choices that should not be made. Deciding what should be done when the unborn is determined to have a severe birth defect, manipulating genes to a more perfect offspring, and discarding defective embryos are just a few of those concerns.

If the United States moves past the dilemma related to the use of embryonic stem cells, then a number of significant medical advances might be made. Researchers may be able to create custom-made organs to replace those that are defective or diseased. Although it might be a wonderful thing to create a new pancreas or a semisynthethic liver to replace an organ that is no longer performing its necessary function, the greater fear of some individuals is that of cloning. Scientists already have cloned mice, sheep, rabbits, goats, pigs, and a dog. Where does cloning stop? Will human beings be cloned if science moves further into research with stem cells? Some countries with a different political arena than the one found in the United States are advancing further into this area. It is interesting to note, however, that the General Assembly of the United Nations voted to prohibit all forms of human cloning in August 2005.

Artificial Insemination/Surrogacy

For many individuals, artificial insemination is the only means by which they can conceive a child. Providers are called on to perform artificial insemination for couples, and women who want a child. If artificial insemination is performed, it is recommended that the signed consent of each party involved be obtained. It is also recommended that providers practicing artificial insemination by donor use many donors for semen and that meticulous screening be performed before the insemination.

Surrogacy is another bioethical issue. Men have been used as **surrogates,** or substitutes, for decades with the practice of artificial insemination, but society seems to have a more difficult time accepting surrogate mothers who are artificially inseminated by a donor and carry the fetus to term for another parent. Men seek surrogates who are able to provide them a child who represents half their genetic makeup. How should the rights of each individual in the exchange be protected? For many of these issues, there is little protection or guidance under the law; therefore, health professionals must make decisions on the basis of their own belief systems.

Ethical questions are sometimes raised regarding artificial insemination and surrogacy. Should artificial insemination be performed for individuals who do not fit the traditional family model? Who will be a fit mother or father for this infant? Some religious faiths consider artificial insemination by donor to be the same as adultery. Who or what agency carefully protects the selection and screening process of donors and surrogates? How are donors selected? Is there a responsibility to make certain that individuals with the same father through artificial insemination by donor do not marry? Some fertility specialists recommend that a donor be chosen from a city far from where the potential mother lives and that formal adoption occur immediately when the infant is born.

Artificial insemination and surrogacy were viewed as experimental and quite controversial just 20 years ago. Today, however, the procedures are widely practiced and available. Both artificial insemination and surrogacy are costly and can become legal tangles for all involved if careful steps are not taken.

In Vitro Fertilization

In vitro fertilization (IVF) is a process that has shown to be very successful in the past decade. In IVF, the ovum is fertilized in a culture dish, allowed to grow, and then implanted into the uterus. This procedure can be used for women with blocked fallopian tubes or oviducts. Ethically, this procedure faces little controversy when a husband's sperm is used to fertilize his wife's ovum, which is then implanted into her uterus. Other procedures raise ethical concerns for some and are not addressed in law.

A woman can have a donor's egg fertilized by her husband's sperm for implantation. A woman can receive donor embryos (embryo adoption) from successfully completed IVF from two unrelated individuals. Couples who have successfully had a baby through IVF are sometimes willing to donate their additional embryos. A woman can carry an embryo created from a donor egg and donor sperm that will have no genetic relationship to her.

It is possible to screen for genetic flaws among embryos created by IVF; however, the latest medical research indicates that such analysis sometimes causes abnormalities.

Medical assistants who work in fertility clinics must at all times respect the choices made by individuals seeking artificial insemination or IVF. These procedures are truly private and very personal. Anyone who feels uncomfortable with such procedures should seek employment elsewhere.

Dying and Death

The goal for all health professionals is to preserve and enhance life, thus, making death an event contrary to the goals of health care. Yet, death cannot be avoided. How death is faced can become both a legal and an ethical dilemma. Legally, individuals can make choices about their death and are encouraged to do so by health care professionals. When those wishes are indicated in documents such as advance directives and when health professionals disagree or refuse to honor those wishes, a legal problem exists.

The legal dilemma was made famous by the cases of Karen Ann Quinlan and Theresa (Terri) Schiavo. Both were young women, without any advance health care directives, whose deaths were caught up in battles between family members, the medical staff, and the courts. Quinlan lived for

Critical Thinking

When fertilization occurs outside the womb, additional embryos are stored and saved for future use. How long should they be stored? To whom do they belong? What happens if no one wants those embryos later? Should they be destroyed, given to some other hopeful parent, or used for research?

11 years in a vegetative state after much duress with health professionals and hospital staff who believed she should be kept on a respirator. The family members of Schiavo were in legal battles for 15 years before permission was received to remove her feeding tube; she died 14 days later. When there is conflict among family and those caring for someone near death, even a well-written and executed advance directive can be faced with challenges. Then a legal dilemma becomes an ethical dilemma as well.

Patients continue to make decisions expressing their choices in death. Oregon was the first state to pass legislation allowing physicians to assist patients in death. Washington state voters approved similar legislation November 2008. The Oregon law was voted upon and passed on two separate occasions and was challenged by the U.S. Attorney General before the U.S. Supreme Court determined that the law could stand. Many Oregonians find comfort in the law that allows them the right to choose the time and place for their own death; however, the number of individuals who choose physician-assisted death still is small—less that nine per 10,000 deaths. Some make the choice, receive the medications from their physician, and then do not use the medication. Others receive the medication and find much relief in their choice and do take the medication. Still others believe that any intervention that hastens death is criminal.

Choices available to patients who are dying create the question, what is "quality of life"? Although the answer to that question is different for everyone, it is a question often in conflict with today's medical technology that can, in many instances, keep a patient alive much longer than the patient might prefer. The benefits of advanced technology will continue to be weighed against what many consider the right to die with dignity and a minimum of medical intervention.

Hospice. Hospice is the term used to describe either a place of residence for those who are dying or an organization whose medical professionals and volunteers are in attendance of someone whose death is imminent. The main objective of hospice is to make patients comfortable and as free from pain as possible and to allow them dignity in their deaths. Cardiopulmonary resuscitation (CPR), intravenous therapy, and feeding tubes are discouraged. Death is treated as a natural end-of-life experience. Death is neither hastened nor prevented.

Hospice volunteers and trainers indicate that although most patients will choose hospice, some family members may not be as comfortable in that choice. Family members may not be ready to let go of a loved one; also, they may be uncomfortable if the hospice service is in the home rather than the hospital or a hospice facility. The latter is related to how comfortable family members are in observing or being a part of the death process. The expense of hospice is often covered by medical insurance and is less expensive than inpatient hospital care.

HIV and AIDS

The general public's fear of AIDS has caused some serious bioethical issues. Patients who suspect they have HIV or AIDS should be tested for the virus. In fact, the Centers for Disease Control and Prevention (CDC) recommend voluntary screening for HIV/AIDS to become a routine part of medical care for all patients ages 13 to 64 years. Confidentiality must be protected, however, because individuals with HIV/AIDS have been denied medical insurance, faced loss of employment and housing, and even suffered the loss of family members and friends. It is unethical to deny treatment to individuals because they test positive for HIV.

Although individuals with HIV/AIDS must be protected, so must the public. Therefore, if providers suspect that an HIV-seropositive patient is infecting an unsuspecting individual, every attempt should be made to protect the individual at risk. Health professionals must first encourage the infected person to cease endangering any person. Second, if the patient refuses to notify the person at risk or wishes the provider to notify the person, authorities can be contacted. Many states and cities have Partner Notification Programs that will anonymously notify any person at risk, keeping the source confidential. The program informs them that it has been brought to their attention that they are a "person at risk" and provides them with free testing. Third, the provider can notify the person at risk.

Case Study 8-1

Refer to the scenario at the beginning of the chapter.

Harley Navarro, the new medical assistant, is especially hesitant to ask for assistance or admit that he is having a problem. Twice today he was unable to get a good blood pressure reading on patients. One patient was very obese, and the other kept trying to carry on a conversation with him.

CASE STUDY REVIEW

1. If Harley's behavior does no harm to the patient, has he acted unethically? Illegally?
2. What might the office manager do if she senses Harley's lack of certainty?
3. Discuss the role of female and male medical assistants working together and how they might complement each other.

Case Study 8-2

Liz Corbin is a medical assistant in the fertility clinic of a large metropolitan medical clinic and hospital. Liz really likes her job and is delighted when parenthood is made possible for many of those seeking the clinic's advanced technology. The clinic also stores and maintains the unused frozen embryos that result from artificial insemination. She is a little alarmed when her provider–employer informs her that four of the embryos are to be destroyed. Her employer has been unable to contact the owners (now parents of more than one child from artificial insemination) for directions, and space for storage is limited. Liz is instructed to destroy the embryos.

CASE STUDY REVIEW

1. Liz is rather hesitant to comply with her employer's orders, so she does a little research. She discovers that most fertility clinics ask couples using **cryopreservation** to decide early in the process how to handle their excess embryos. The choices are: (1) discard the embryos, (2) donate anonymously to other infertile couples, and (3) donate to scientific research. What might Liz do to influence the clinic's policy?
2. Can anything be done to ensure that couples do not abandon their embryos?
3. If embryos are given to other infertile couples, how is a decision made on who should have them?

SUMMARY

As medical technology continues to advance, a greater need for ethical guidelines will be necessary. Providers and health care professionals at all levels must stay abreast of the issues and carefully consider all aspects before making any decision.

Medical assistants must, however, keep the following legal and ethical guidelines in mind: (1) always practice within the law; (2) preserve the patient's confidentiality; (3) maintain meticulous records; (4) obtain informed, written consent; (5) do not judge patients whose belief system differs from yours.

STUDY FOR SUCCESS

To reinforce your knowledge and skills of information in this chapter:

- Review the Key Terms
- Consider the Case Studies and discuss your conclusions
- Answer the Review Questions
    - Multiple Choice
    - Critical Thinking
- Navigate the Internet and complete the Web Activities
- Practice the StudyWARE activities on the textbook CD
- Apply your knowledge in the Student Workbook activities
- Complete the Web Tutor sections
- View and discuss the DVD situations

REVIEW QUESTIONS

Multiple Choice

1. Typically, ethics has been defined in terms of:
   a. what is right and wrong
   b. whether an action is legal
   c. the expedient thing to do
   d. professionalism in the workplace
2. Bioethics has to do with:
   a. biological reproduction
   b. the act of artificial insemination
   c. genetic engineering
   d. ethical issues that deal with life and health care
3. The AAMA Code of Ethics:
   a. is concerned with principles of ethical and moral conduct
   b. defines the duties the medical assistant can perform
   c. is intended for physicians only
   d. applies only to patient rights
4. When a provider or medical assistant suspects child abuse, they should:
   a. give the parent a warning
   b. report it to the proper authorities
   c. not impose their values on the parents
   d. give the child some hints on how to protect against abuse
5. When a patient has HIV:
   a. it is ethical for the provider not to provide treatment
   b. it is unethical for the provider not to provide treatment
   c. other patients should be warned of the possibility of infection
   d. all friends and family members of the patient should be notified
6. Macroallocation of scarce medical resources implies that
   a. the local health care team makes the decisions
   b. Congress, health systems agencies, and insurance companies make the decisions
   c. medical assistants will not be involved
   d. patients will get the benefit of the best medical care
7. The eight characteristics of principle-centered leaders originates from the following author:
   a. James R. Jones
   b. Stephen R. Covey
   c. Francis H. Ambrose
   d. Jason N. Diamond
8. The five Ps of ethical power are:
   a. Personality, performance, purpose, pride, patience
   b. Purpose, patience, perfection, personality, procrastination
   c. Patience, purpose, pride, persistence, perspective
   d. Purpose, pride, patience, perfection, perspective
9. Which of the following is true?
   a. A provider can choose whom to serve
   b. A provider may charge for completing multiple and complex insurance claims
   c. Providers and their employees cannot be forced to perform abortions
   d. All of the above
   e. None of the above
10. You are most likely to make ethical decisions correctly when:
    a. you have a clear picture of the situation
    b. you leave emotion out of the decision as much as possible

c. you understand your weaknesses and vulnerabilities
d. honesty and integrity are hallmarks of your entire life
e. all of the above

Critical Thinking

1. A provider observes another provider put a patient at risk while under the influence of alcohol and does nothing about it. What would constitute ethical behavior?
2. A provider refuses to accept any more Medicaid patients for medical care. Is this the provider's right? Is it ethical? Why or why not?
3. A clinical medical assistant whispers to the administrative medical assistant, "There goes the guy with AIDS." How should the administrative medical assistant view this behavior?
4. The services reported on the insurance claim are more complex than those actually rendered. Is this ethical or unethical? Legal or illegal? State your reasons.
5. A provider performs artificial insemination for a lesbian couple; however, the medical assistant refuses to participate or assist the provider. What are the ramifications of the medical assistant's behavior? Do you believe the medical assistant has a right to refuse?
6. Referring to Figure 8-1, select an ethical issue with which you may have had some personal experience. Now, form a small group, with each student leading a discussion on a different issue.

WEB ACTIVITIES

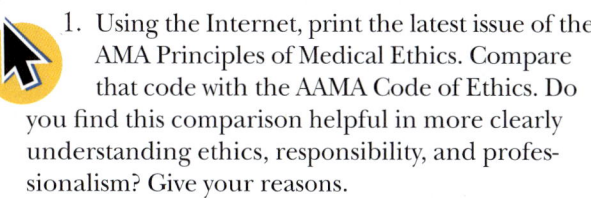

1. Using the Internet, print the latest issue of the AMA Principles of Medical Ethics. Compare that code with the AAMA Code of Ethics. Do you find this comparison helpful in more clearly understanding ethics, responsibility, and professionalism? Give your reasons.
2. Using the Web site given at the beginning of this chapter, select one additional code of ethics to compare with the AMA Principles and the AAMA Code. What are the similarities?
3. Using your favorite Internet search engine, key in two or three of the bioethical issues and do a small-scale review of items listed. From your research, identify at least three ethical/bioethical questions for your class to discuss.

REFERENCES/BIBLIOGRAPHY

American Diabetes Association. (2007). *First use of cord blood to alter course of type 1 diabetes.* Retrieved July 2007, from http://professional.diabetes.org/UserFiles/File/Scientific%20Sessions/Media/2007/Autologoos%20Cord%20Blood%20Final.doc.

American Medical Association. (2006–2007). Code of medical ethics. *Current opinions of the council on ethical and judicial affairs, 2006.* Chicago: American Medical Association.

Blanchard, K., & Peale, N. V. (1988). *The power of ethical management.* New York: William Morrow and Company, Inc.

Covey, S. R. (1991). *Principle-centered leadership.* New York: Simon & Schuster.

Lewis, M. A., & Tamparo, C. D., (2007). *Medical law, ethics, and bioethics for health professions* (6th ed.). Philadelphia: F. A. Davis.

THE DVD HOOK-UP

In this chapter, you learned about the importance of ethical behavior when working in the medical field. Ethics are not laws, but rather a set of morals or principles to which we adhere.

In the designated DVD clip, we observed Jen talking to Sarah about a patient who has diabetes. Jen feels that the patient has complications with her diabetes because she makes poor choices in her eating habits. Barb, the supervisor, overhears the conversation and talks to Jen and Sarah about the importance of being compassionate as health care providers. Even though this clip does not deal with some of the more noted ethical issues such as fetal tissue research or genetic engineering, judging the patient is a violation of ethical behavior and probably one of the more typical ethical issues that you will struggle with as a medical assistant.

1. As a medical assistant, you will make observations about your patients that can be helpful to the provider. What was inappropriate in the way Jen handled her observations?
2. Diseases such as emphysema, obesity, and diabetes can all be the result of unhealthy lifestyles. How will you as a medical assistant keep from judging a patient's actions or lifestyle that have resulted in illness?

DVD Journal Summary

Write a paragraph that summarizes what you learned from watching the designated scenes from today's DVD program. Ethical dilemmas may involve anyone in the medical office. For example, what would you do if you smelled alcohol on a coworker? What if you suspect the coworker is abusing alcohol? Are you obligated to say something? To whom? Why or why not?

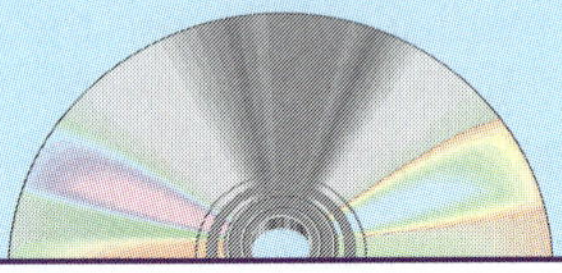

DVD Series	**Program Number**
Critical Thinking	3

Chapter/Scene Reference
- *Ethical Practice*

Emergency Procedures and First Aid

Chapter 9

KEY TERMS

Anaphylaxis
Automated External Defibrillator (AED)
Bandage
Cardiopulmonary Resuscitation (CPR)
Cardioversion
Cauterized
Constriction Band
Crash Tray or Cart
Crepitation
Dislocation
Dressing
Emergency Medical Services (EMS)
Explicit
First Aid
Fracture
Hypothermia
Implicit
Lackluster
Normal Saline
Occlusion
Rescue Breathing
Risk Management
Shock
Splint
Sprain
Standard Precautions
Strain
Syncope
Systemic
Universal Emergency Medical Identification Symbol
Vasovagal Syncope
Wound

OUTLINE

Recognizing an Emergency
- Responding to an Emergency
- Primary Survey
- Using the 911 or Emergency Medical Services System
- Good Samaritan Laws
- Blood, Body Fluids, and Disease Transmission

Preparing for an Emergency
- The Medical Crash Tray or Cart

Common Emergencies
- Shock
- Wounds
- Burns
- Musculoskeletal Injuries
- Heat- and Cold-Related Illnesses
- Poisoning
- Sudden Illness
- Cerebral Vascular Accident
- Heart Attack

Breathing Emergencies and Cardiac Arrest
- Rescue Breathing
- Cardiopulmonary Resuscitation

Safety and Emergency Practices

OBJECTIVES

The student should strive to meet the following performance objectives and demonstrate an understanding of the facts and principles presented in this chapter through written and oral communication.

1. Define the key terms as presented in the glossary.
2. Learn to recognize, prepare for, and respond to emergencies in the ambulatory care setting.
3. Understand the legal and disease transmission considerations in emergency caregiving.
4. Perform the primary assessment in emergency situations.
5. Identify and care for different types of wounds.
6. Understand the basics of bandage application.
7. Discriminate among first-, second-, and third-degree burns.
8. Assess injuries to muscles, bones, and joints.
9. Describe heat- and cold-related illnesses.
10. Describe how poisons may enter the body.
11. List the symptoms of a poisonous snake bite.
12. Recall the eight types of shock.
13. Define a cerebral vascular accident.
14. Describe the signs and symptoms of a heart attack.

Scenario

Inner City Health Care, which is located in Carlton, Michigan, has its share of cold, snowy winters, and when the temperature drops near freezing, that snow sometimes turns to ice. Last night, as Wanda Slawson, CMA (AAMA), was leaving for the evening, she noticed a woman from an adjacent office slip and fall in the parking lot. Wanda immediately went over to the woman to lend assistance and saw that, in falling, the woman had cut the palm of her hand. Apparently, the woman had tried to break her fall with her hand only to sustain a wound that was now bleeding moderately. Fortunately, Wanda knew that one of the providers was still in the office and she led the woman back to the building, reassuring her along the way. Once in the office, Wanda assisted Susan Rice, the provider, to examine the wound. After determining that sutures were not needed, Dr. Rice and Wanda cleansed the wound, applied a dry, sterile dressing, and covered it with an elastic bandage. The patient was instructed to call her own provider first thing in the morning.

INTRODUCTION

Although the ambulatory care setting is primarily designed to see patients under nonemergency conditions, occasionally the provider will need to administer emergency care, and the medical assistant will be called on to assist the provider in this care. For the medical assistant who may need to screen or assess the patient's condition, the first and most critical step in responding to an emergency is developing the skill to recognize when emergency measures should be taken.

Whereas some emergencies can be treated in the office, others cannot, and the medical assistant must know when to call for outside help. If the emergency occurs in the ambulatory care setting, the provider usually administers immediate care. It is possible, however, that the medical assistant may be the first emergency caregiver should the provider be out of the office. The medical assistant also may be called on to provide care in an emergency outside of the office environment.

This chapter acquaints the medical assistant with types of emergency situations that may occur either inside or outside of the office. However, this chapter is merely an introduction to emergency topics and does not substitute for first aid and cardiopulmonary resuscitation (CPR) instruction taught through the American Red Cross, the American Heart Association, the American Safety and Health Institute, or the National Safety Council. Medical assistants in CAAHEP- and ABHES-accredited programs must be certified to a provider-level in CPR and must be taught by instructors who are certified to teach CPR. These hands-on classes are vital teaching tools, and all medical assistants should take them on a regular basis to continually update their skills.

RECOGNIZING AN EMERGENCY

An emergency is considered any instance in which an individual becomes suddenly ill and requires immediate attention. Most emergencies develop quickly and usually without warning. They can occur unexpectedly at any time to anyone. Some may be gradual, as seen with dehydration or slow blood loss, and become an emergency over time.

Spotlight on Certification

RMA Content Outline

- Patient education
- Medical law
- Asepsis
- Vital signs and measurements
- Office safety
- First aid and emergency response

CMA (AAMA) Content Outline

- Principles of infection control (aseptic technique)
- Treatment area (safety precautions)
- Emergencies (preplanned action)
- First aid

CMAS Content Outline

- Vital signs and measurements
- Medical office emergencies (recognize and respond to medical emergencies)
- Safety

A common sign that an individual has an emergency is unusual noises, such as yelling, moaning, or crying. A person may appear to be behaving strangely when choking or if having difficulty breathing. To recognize when an emergency exists, it is important to have sharp senses of hearing, sight, and smell and be acutely sensitive to any unusual behaviors.

In the ambulatory care setting, medical assistants may encounter a range of emergency situations requiring first-aid techniques. **First aid** is designed to render immediate and temporary emergency care to persons injured or otherwise disabled before the arrival of a health care practitioner or transport to a hospital or other health care agency.

Emergency situations can be minor or severe and can include:

- Choking and breathing crises
- Chest pain
- Bleeding
- Shock
- Stroke
- Poisoning
- Burns
- Wounds
- Sudden illnesses such as fainting/falling
- Illnesses related to heat and cold
- Fractures

Some of these situations will be life threatening; all will require immediate care. In either case, it is critical to remain calm, to follow the emergency policies and procedures established by the ambulatory care setting, and to be well-versed in first-aid and be certified in CPR. The patient should not be further endangered.

Responding to an Emergency

Once it has been determined that an emergency exists, it is essential to act quickly. Before making any decisions about how to proceed, it is necessary to assess the nature of the situation. Does it include respiratory or circulatory failure, severe bleeding, burns, poisoning, or severe allergic reaction?

Sometimes, it is possible that more than one type of care must be administered. In this case, it is necessary to screen the situation so that treatment can be prioritized. When an individual experiences more than one illness or injury, care must be given according to the severity of the situation. When two or more patients present with emergencies simultaneously, screening helps determine which patient is treated first. The main principle of screening states that absence of heartbeat and breath and severe bleeding are immediate life threats. Table 9-1 lists the common ordering of screening situations.

To identify the nature of the emergency and respond effectively, it is critical that the patient be assessed. If the patient is conscious, ask for personal identification and identification of next of kin. Try to obtain information about symptoms being

Table 9-1 Examples of Emergency Categories

First Priority	Next Priority	Least Priority
Burns on face	Second-degree burns not on the neck and face	Fractures (simple)
Airway and breathing problems	Major or multiple fractures	Minor injuries
Cardiac arrest	Back injuries	Sprains, strains
Severe bleeding that is uncontrolled	Severe eye injuries	
Head injuries		
Poisoning		
Open chest or abdominal wounds		
Shock		
Second- and third-degree burns		

HIPAA

Patient confidentiality must be maintained during an emergency situation, as it must at all times. Sometimes, when a situationis urgent and the patient is having trouble breathing, is bleeding heavily, or is having a severe allergic reaction or any other kind of emergency, in your eagerness to assist the patient, your voice when talking to other health care providers may be overheard by other patients. Be certain other patients cannot hear any conversations. Privacy must be maintained when faxing information to the emergency department. Also be cautious when speaking on the telephone. Be cautious to keep the patient's anonymity protected.

experienced to identify the problem. Always check for a **universal emergency medical identification symbol** (Figure 9-1) and accompanying identification card, which will describe any serious or life-threatening health problems that the patient has. Quickly observe the patient's general appearance, including skin color and size and dilation of pupils. Check pulse and blood pressure.

Primary Survey

If the patient is unresponsive, it is critical to assess the ABCs, which include:

- Airway
- Breathing
- Circulation

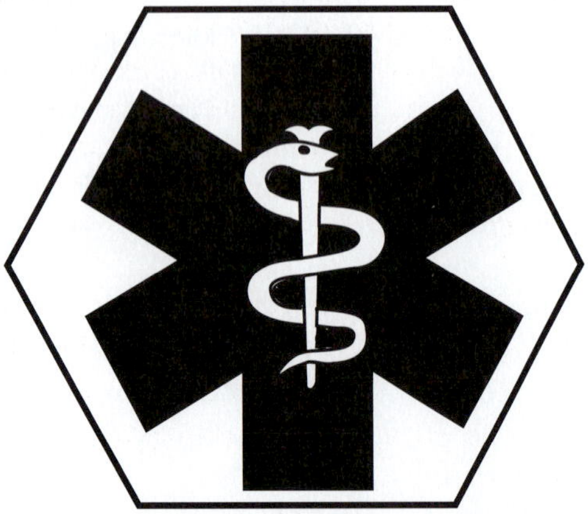

Figure 9-1 The universal emergency medical identification symbol.

Patient Education

Alert patients to the importance of carrying the universal emergency medical identification symbol and its accompanying identification card if the patient has severe heart disease, diabetes, or other life-threatening illnesses or allergies.

To assess whether the unresponsive patient is breathing and to determine if there is an open airway, place your face close to the patient's face and look, listen, and feel. Look at the patient's chest and notice whether the chest rises and falls with breathing. Listen for air entering and leaving the nose and mouth and feel for moving air.

If the individual is not breathing, first open the airway either by tilting the head and lifting the chin (Figure 9-2A) or by the jaw-thrust maneuver, which involves placing both thumbs on the patient's cheekbones and placing the index and middle fingers on both sides of the lower jaw (see Figure 9-2B). **CAUTION:** Do not attempt to tilt the head and lift the chin when the patient has a head, neck, or spinal cord injury.

If the patient still does not breathe after the airway has been opened, rescue breathing must be performed.

To assess circulation, check for the presence of a pulse at the carotid artery on the side of the neck below the ear. If no pulse is present, the patient may be in cardiac arrest and must be given CPR. Use of an **automated external defibrillator (AED)** may be necessary (see Chapter 25).

Using the 911 or Emergency Medical Services System

The **Emergency Medical Services (EMS)** system is a local network of police, fire, and medical personnel who are trained to respond to emergency situations. Other community experts and volunteers also act as resources in an EMS system. In many communities, the network is activated by calling 911. Even when preliminary emergency care is provided by the ambulatory care provider, the patient may still need to be transported to a hospital for follow-up care. It is also possible that the provider may not be equipped to deliver the type of emergency care required, in which case, one person should call for EMS help while another stays with the patient until help arrives.

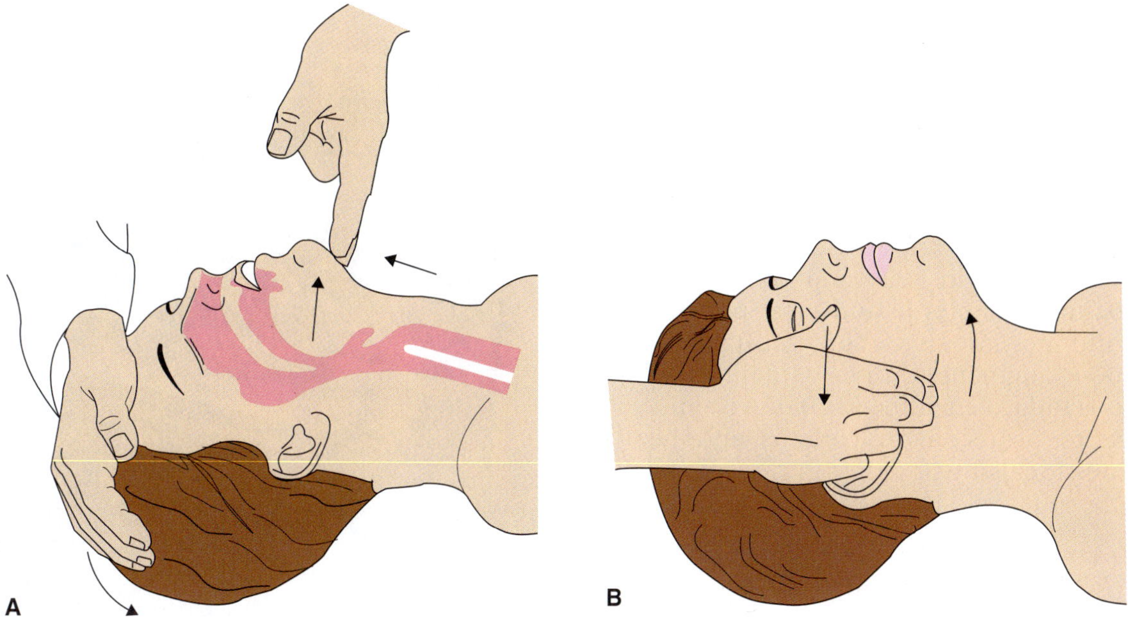

Figure 9-2 If the individual is not breathing, first open the airway (A) by tilting the head and lifting the chin, for victim without head or neck trauma, or (B) by the jaw-thrust maneuver, for victim with cervical spine injury. This involves placing both thumbs on the patient's cheekbones and placing the index and middle fingers on both sides of the lower jaw.

Never leave a seriously ill or unconscious patient unattended.

While waiting for EMS to arrive, continuously check the patient for the following signs: (1) degree of responsiveness, (2) airway/breathing ability, (3) heartbeat (rate and rhythm), (4) bleeding, and (5) signs of shock. Monitor vital signs. Keep patient warm and lying down. If there are no head injuries, the legs can be elevated on pillows.

Good Samaritan Laws

When delivering or assisting in delivering emergency care, the medical assistant may be concerned about professional liability. Most states have enacted Good Samaritan laws, which provide some degree of protection to the health care professional who offers first aid.

Most Good Samaritan laws provide some legal protection to those who provide emergency care to ill or injured persons. However, when medical assistants or any other individuals give care during an emergency, they must act as reasonable and prudent individuals and provide care only within the scope of their abilities. Remember that a primary principle of first aid is to prevent further injury.

Although Good Samaritan laws give some measure of protection against being sued for giving emergency aid, they generally protect *off-duty* health care professionals. Also, conditions of the law vary from state to state. As part of establishing emergency care guidelines, every ambulatory care setting should understand the **explicit** and **implicit** intent of the Good Samaritan law in its state (see Chapter 7 for more information on legal guidelines).

Blood, Body Fluids, and Disease Transmission

When providing emergency care, medical assistants should always protect themselves and the patient from infectious disease transmission. Serious infectious diseases, such as hepatitis B (HBV), hepatitis C (HCV), and HIV, can be transmitted through blood and body fluids (see Chapter 10 for more detailed information).

By establishing and following strict guidelines, the risk for contracting or transmitting an infectious disease while providing emergency care is greatly reduced.

- Always wash hands thoroughly before (if possible) and after every procedure or use hand sanitizer.
- Use protective clothing and other protective equipment (gloves, gown, mask, goggles) during the procedure.
- Avoid contact with blood and body fluids, if possible.

- Do not touch nose, mouth, or eyes with gloved hands.
- Carefully handle and safely dispose of soiled gloves and other objects.

Refer to Chapter 10 for more information on standard precautions. **Standard Precautions** were issued by the Centers for Disease Control and Prevention (CDC) in 1996 and combine many of the basic principles of universal precautions with techniques known as body substance isolation. These augmented 1996 guidelines represent the standard in infection control and are intended to protect both patients and health care professionals.

PREPARING FOR AN EMERGENCY

Emergencies are unexpected but can and should be anticipated and prepared for in the ambulatory care setting. Being properly prepared ensures that the office has the materials and resources needed to respond to emergencies.

An in-office handbook of policies and procedures should be developed and should be familiar to all staff members. Telephone numbers for the local emergency medical services (often this is 911) and the poison control center (1-800-222-1222) should be posted and kept in an established place so that there is no delay in calling for outside assistance. Materials and supplies should be maintained in proper inventory. All personnel should be trained in first aid and CPR so that every staff member can respond to or assist the provider in providing care. Proper documentation should be completed after any emergency situation. The office environment itself should be a safe one and as accident-proof as possible. Wipe up spills to prevent falls on a slippery floor, keep corridors free of clutter, and keep medications out of sight. These basic **risk management** techniques will help medical personnel focus on giving emergency care and also will protect the facility from possible litigation.

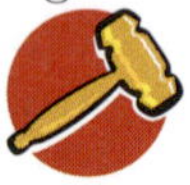

The Medical Crash Tray or Cart

Every health care facility should have a **crash tray or cart,** with a carefully controlled inventory of supplies and equipment (Figure 9-3). These first-aid supplies should be kept in an accessible place, and the inventory should be routinely monitored to ensure that all supplies are replaced. All medications should be up to date and have not reached their expiration dates.

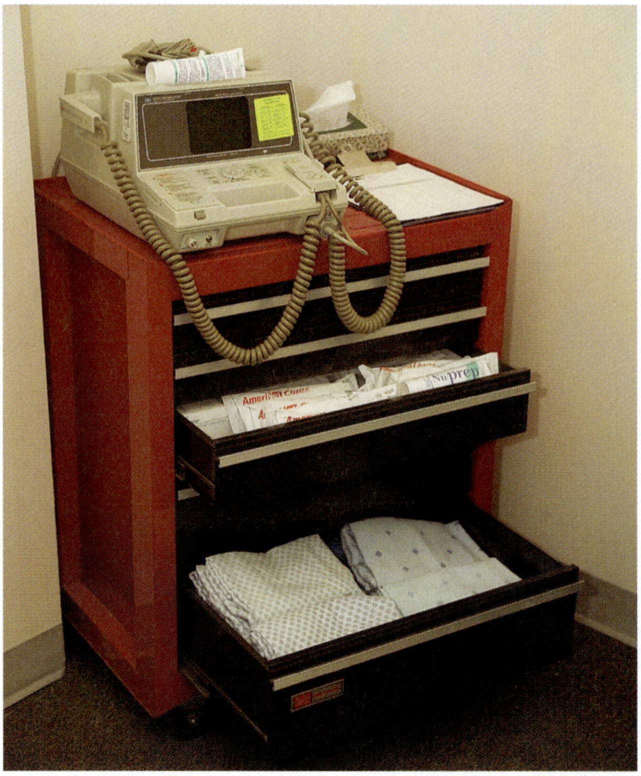

Figure 9-3 Medical crash cart with defibrillator.

A smaller practice may require only a portable tray for emergency and first-aid supplies. Larger urgent care centers may respond more frequently to emergencies and thus may need a cart that can hold a larger inventory and variety of supplies. Whether a tray or cart is used, supplies should be customized to the facility and the type of emergencies frequently encountered. Remember that only providers can order medications or treatment.

Following is a brief list of some common supplies found on most trays and carts (see Chapter 23 for more information on supplies and medications).

General supplies:

- Adhesive and hypoallergenic tape
- Alcohol wipes
- Bandage scissors
- Bandage material
- Blood pressure cuff (standard, pediatric, large)
- **Constriction band**
- Defibrillator
- Dressing material
- Gloves

- Hot/cold packs
- Intravenous (IV) tubing
- Needles and syringes for injection
- Glucose tabs or gel
- Penlight (with extra batteries)
- Personal protective equipment
- Stethoscope

Emergency medications	Uses
Activated charcoal	Poisonings
Aspirin	Fever, heart attack
Atropine	Slow heartbeat
Dextrose	Insulin reaction
Diazepam*	Antianxiety
Diphenhydramine	Antihistamine
Dopamine	Increases blood pressure
Epinephrine	Constricts blood vessels, increases blood pressure
Glucagon	Insulin reaction
Insulin	Hyperglycemia
Lidocaine	Local anesthetic, IV for cardiac arrhythmia
Nitroglycerin tablets, patches	Chest pain from angina pectoris
Phenobarbital*	Sedative
Verapamil	Hypertension, angina pectoris, irregular heartbeat, tachycardia
Xylocaine, Marcaine	Local anesthetics

*Controlled substance—must be kept in locked cabinet.

Respiratory supplies:

- Airways of all sizes for nasal and oral use
- Ambu bag™
- Bulb syringe for suction
- Oxygen mask
- Oxygen tank

This list represents just some of the supplies to be found on a well-stocked crash cart or tray. The type and list of supplies should always be overseen by facility providers and tailored to the emergency demands of the practice. The medical assistant should be familiar with the equipment and medication on the crash cart or tray. Practice "drills" simulating various emergency situations are helpful for preparing staff members for actual emergencies.

COMMON EMERGENCIES

Included in this discussion of common emergencies are shock, wounds, burns, musculoskeletal injuries, heat- and cold-related illnesses, poisoning, snake bite, sudden illness, cerebral vascular accident, and heart attack.

Shock

When a severe injury or illness occurs, shock is likely to develop. **Shock** is a condition in which the circulatory system is not providing enough blood to all parts of the body, causing the body's organs to fail to function properly.

Shock is always life threatening, and EMS should be activated. The body's attempt to compensate for a massive injury or illness, especially those involving the heart and lungs and severe bleeding, often lead to other problems. During shock, several things occur.

- The heart becomes unable to pump blood properly.
- Consequently, the body's cells, tissues, and organs do not get enough oxygen, which is carried by the blood.
- The body tries to compensate by sending blood to critical organs and reducing the flow of blood to arms, legs, and skin.

Signs and Symptoms of Shock. Learn to recognize the signs and symptoms of shock.

- Patient may be restless or feel irritable.
- Weakness, dizziness, thirst, or nausea may occur.
- Breathing may be shallow and rapid.
- Skin is cool, clammy, and pale.
- Pulse is weak and rapid.
- Blood pressure is low.
- Area around the lips, eyes, and fingernails may turn cyanotic (blue) from lack of oxygen.

- The patient may be confused or become suddenly unconscious, or both.
- Dilated pupils and **lackluster** eyes are obvious.

Types of Shock. The eight major types of shock are respiratory, neurogenic, cardiogenic, hemorrhagic, anaphylactic, metabolic, psychogenic, and septic. Table 9-2 lists a description of each.

Treatment for Shock. A person suffering from shock needs immediate medical attention. Call for outside emergency help first, then care for the patient until help arrives. **CAUTION:** Shock is progressive, and, if not treated immediately, most types can be life threatening. Once shock reaches a certain point, it is irreversible.

To care for a patient in shock (regardless of the type), follow these procedures:

- Lay the patient down. This minimizes pain and decreases stress on the body.
- Loosen the patient's clothing.
- Check for an open airway.
- Check breathing.
- Control any external bleeding.
- Help the patient maintain normal body temperature. A blanket over and under the patient can help avoid chilling. Do not overheat.
- Reassure the patient.
- Elevate the patients legs about 12 inches, unless you suspect head injury, spinal injuries, or broken bones involving the hips or legs.
- Do not give the patient anything to eat or drink.
- Ascertain that outside help has been called and stay with the patient until help arrives.
- Monitor vital signs.

Wounds

Typically, **wounds** are classified as open or closed. In the closed wound, there is no break in the skin; a bruise, contusion, and hematoma are common closed wounds. An open wound represents a break in the skin and can be classified as an abrasion, avulsion, incision, laceration, or puncture wound.

Table 9-2 Eight Types of Shock with Descriptions

Type of Shock	Description
Respiratory	Trauma to the respiratory tract (trachea, lungs) that causes a reduction of oxygen and carbon dioxide exchange. Body cells cannot receive enough oxygen.
Neurogenic	Injury or trauma to the nervous system (spinal cord, brain). Nerve impulse to blood vessels impaired. Blood vessels remain dilated and blood pressure decreases.
Cardiogenic	Myocardial infarction with damage to heart muscle; heart unable to pump effectively. Inadequate cardiac output. Body cells do not receive enough oxygen.
Hemorrhagic	Severe bleeding or loss of body fluid from trauma, burns, surgery, or dehydration from severe nausea and vomiting. Blood pressure decreases, thus blood flow is reduced to cells, tissues, and organs.
Anaphylactic	Results from reaction to substance to which patient is hypersensitive or allergic (allergen extracts, bee sting, medication, food). Outpouring of histamine results in dilation of blood vessels throughout the body, blood pressure decreases and blood flow is reduced to cells, tissue, and organs.
Metabolic	Body's homeostasis impaired; acid-base balance disturbed (diabetic coma or insulin shock); body fluids unbalanced.
Psychogenic	Shock caused by overwhelming emotional factors (e.g., fear, anger, grief). Sudden dilation of blood vessels results in fainting because of lack of blood supply to the brain. In most cases, not life threatening unless it leads to physical trauma as a result of a fall.
Septic	An acute infection, usually **systemic,** that overwhelms the body (e.g., toxic shock syndrome). Poisonous substances accumulate in bloodstream and blood pressure decreases, impairing blood flow to cells, tissues, and organs.

Closed Wounds. Most closed wounds do not present an emergency situation. If there is pain and swelling, the application of a cold compress can be effective. Protect the patient's skin by placing a cloth beneath the source of cold; apply the compress for 20 minutes, then remove for 20 minutes; continue for 24 hours. Then apply heat 20 minutes on and 20 minutes off for the next 24 hours. A common procedure for treating closed wounds is to RICE or MICE it.

RICE	MICE
• *R*est	• *M*otion or *M*ovement
• *I*ce	• *I*ce
• *C*ompression	• *C*ompression
• *E*levation	• *E*levation

Recently, some providers, especially those who treat sport injuries, advocate motion or movement as a means of treating a closed wound injury. They also advise ice, compression (elastic bandage), and elevation (MICE). Check for provider preference.

Some closed wounds, such as hematomas, can be dangerous and may cause internal bleeding. If the patient is in severe pain and was subject to an injury caused by high impact, call for help and keep the patient comfortable until the help arrives. Watch for symptoms of shock and monitor vital signs.

Open Wounds. Open wounds can be minor tears in the skin or more serious skin breaks, but all open wounds represent an opportunity for microorganisms to gain entry and cause an infection. Some major open wounds may involve heavy bleeding, which will need to be controlled, probably by suturing. A tetanus injection is indicated for an open wound if the patient has not had a booster in the last 7 to 10 years (see Chapter 10 for immunization information).

There are five common types of open wounds:

1. *Abrasions* are a superficial scraping of the epidermis. Because nerve endings are involved, they can be painful. However, they are not usually serious, unless they cover a large area of the body. Administer first aid by cleaning the area carefully with soap and water, apply an antiseptic ointment if prescribed by a provider, and cover with a dressing.
2. In an *avulsion,* the skin is torn off and bleeding is profuse. Avulsion wounds often occur at exposed parts: fingers, toes, ear. First, control bleeding (see Procedure 9-1). Then clean the wound. If there is a skin flap, reposition it. Apply a dressing, then bandage as necessary. Note that pieces of the body may be torn away. If possible, save the body part, keep moist, and transport with the patient.
3. *Incisions* are wounds that result from a sharp object, such as a knife or piece of glass. Incisions may need sutures. The wound must be cleaned with soap and water and a dressing applied.
4. *Lacerations* tear the body tissue and can be difficult to clean; therefore, care must be taken to avoid infection. If there is not severe bleeding, which in itself is a cleansing mechanism, these wounds may need to be soaked in antiseptic soap and water to remove debris. If there is severe bleeding, it must be controlled immediately (see Procedure 9-1). Lacerations with severe bleeding need suturing.
5. *Punctures* pierce and penetrate the skin and may be deep wounds while appearing insignificant. Usually, external bleeding is minimal, but the patient should be assessed for internal bleeding. Because a puncture wound is deep, the risk for infection is great and the patient should be advised to watch for signals of infection, such as pain, swelling, redness, throbbing, and warmth.

Use of Tourniquets in Emergency Care. In the past, tourniquets were regularly used in the field to control hemorrhaging from an extremity when all other attempts to control bleeding were unsuccessful. However, because tourniquet application was meant to completely stop blood flow, many times the complete lack of blood flow resulted in the death of the arm or leg. Often, the affected extremity needed to be amputated.

To remedy the situation, a "constriction band" was substituted for the tourniquet and is now widely used. The constriction band is made of a material similar to that used in the tourniquet. When the band is applied to an extremity to control bleeding, it is applied tightly enough to stem the rapid loss of blood but loosely enough to allow a small amount of blood to continue to flow. A pulse should be felt distally to the constriction band. The use of the constriction band applied in this manner allows a blood supply to the remainder of the extremity, unlike the tourniquet, which cuts off all blood flow. Chapter 19 provides information on wounds and minor surgery.

Dressings and Bandages. After the provider has treated an open wound, it is critical to dress and bandage it properly to curtail infection. Covering of the wound is accomplished by a series of **dressings** and **bandages.**

Typically, dressings are sterile gauze pads placed directly on the wound; they often have nonstick, sterile surfaces, but they are absorbent and will soak up blood and protect the wound from microorganisms. They are often made of a gauze-type material.

Bandages, which are nonsterile, are placed over the dressing. They hold the dressing in place and are made to conform to the area to be covered. Sometimes, as in a Band-Aid®, the dressing and bandage are combined. Roller bandages (sometimes called by their brand name, "Ace Bandages"), such as those made of elastic, can be placed over a dressing and used to help control bleeding or swelling.

Kling, a type of gauze that stretches and clings as it is applied, and roller bandages, long, soft, elastic material wound over itself, known by the brand name Ace Bandages, are other types of bandage materials.

Bandages and their applications can take many shapes and forms, depending on the type of injury and the injury site. In all cases, a bandage must be secure, but not constricting. Avoid too tight or too loose a wrap.

- Spiral bandages are useful for injuries to the arms or legs (Figure 9-4).
- A figure-eight bandage holds the dressing in place on a wound on the hand or wrist, knee, or ankle (Figure 9-5).
- Fingers, toes, arms, and legs can also be bandaged using a tubular gauze bandage (Figures 9-6, 9-7, and 9-8). Using a cylindrical applicator, a quantity of gauze is stretched over the wound site.
- Commercial arm slings are used to support injured or fractured arms (Figure 9-9). To apply, support the injured arm above and below the injury site while applying the sling.

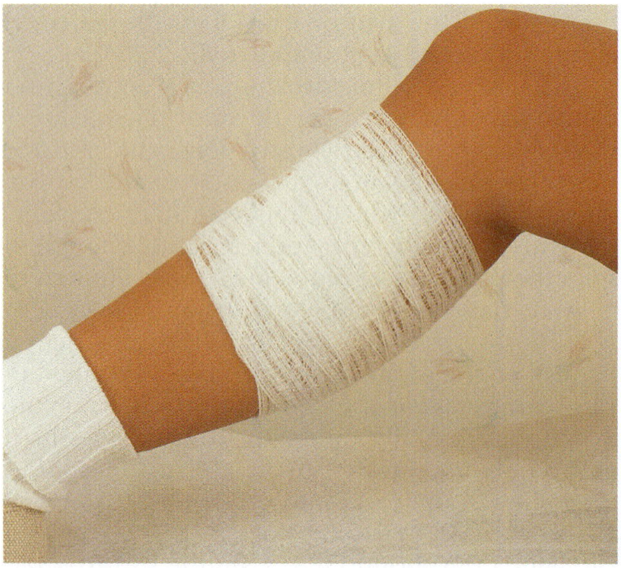

Figure 9-4 The spiral bandage is an option for arm and leg injuries.

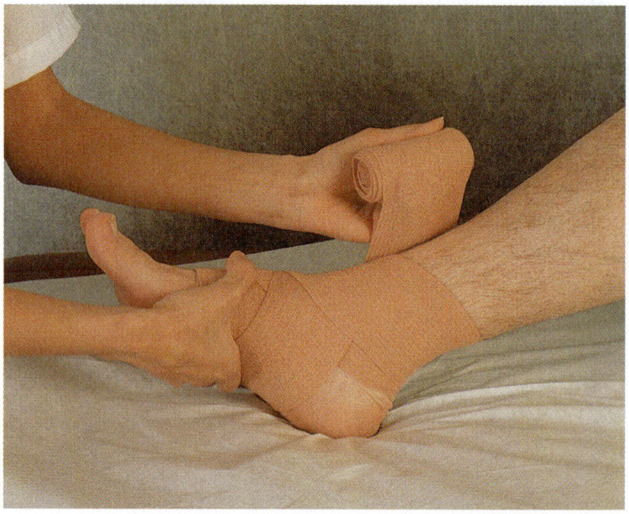

Figure 9-5 An elastic figure-eight bandage holds dressings in place or can be used for immobilization, as with an ankle sprain.

Burns

Most burns are caused by heat, chemicals, explosions, and electricity. Critical burns can be life threatening and require immediate medical care. According to the American Red Cross, critical burns have the following characteristics:

- Involve breathing difficulty
- Cover more than one body part
- Involve the head, neck, hands, feet, or genitals
- Involve any burns to a child or older adult (other than minor burns)

To distinguish critical from minor burns, it is important to understand the degrees of burns and what they mean.

First-, Second-, and Third-Degree Burns. First-degree burns are superficial burns that involve only the top layer of skin. The skin appears red, feels dry, is warm to the touch, and is painful. First-degree burns usually heal in a week or so with no permanent scarring.

In a second-degree burn, the skin is red and blisters are present. The healing process is slower, usually a month, and some scarring may occur. Second-degree burns affect the top layers of the skin and are very painful. Some scarring may occur.

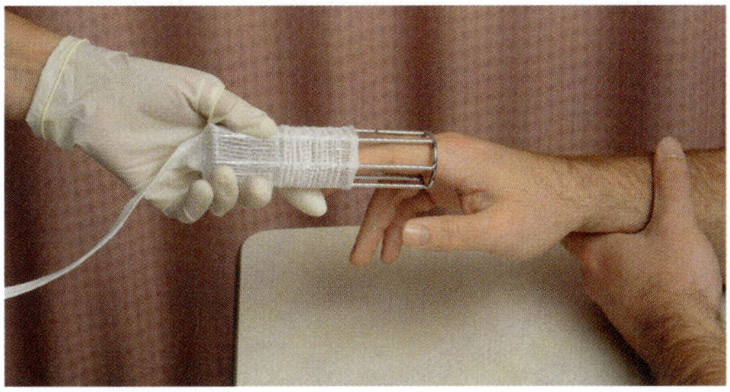

Figure 9-6 The cylindrical applicator is placed over the finger.

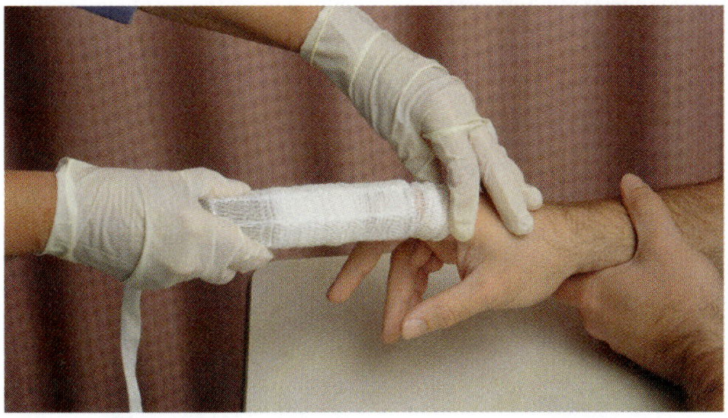

Figure 9-7 Gauze is stretched over the finger.

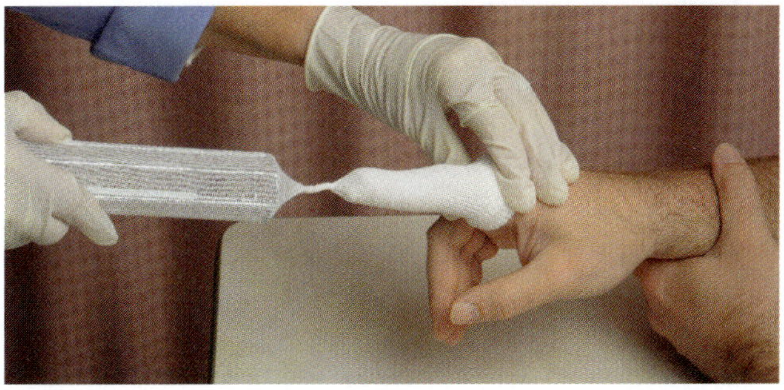

Figure 9-8 Applicator is pulled off, leaving the bandage.

Third-degree burns are the most serious, affecting or destroying all layers of tissue. It is not unusual for fat, muscles, bones, and nerves to be involved. These burns can look charred or brown. There may be great pain or, if nerve endings are destroyed, the burn may be painless. Victims of third-degree burns must receive immediate medical attention both for the burn and for shock. Of serious concern with a third-degree burn is the likelihood of infection and the amount of fluid loss. Scarring can result in loss of body function. Skin grafts may be necessary.

There is a formula for estimating the percent of body surface areas that have been burned (Figure 9-10A). In an adult, the head and each upper extremity are 9% each, the back of the trunk is 18%, as is the front (18%), each lower extremity is 18%, and the perineum is 1%.

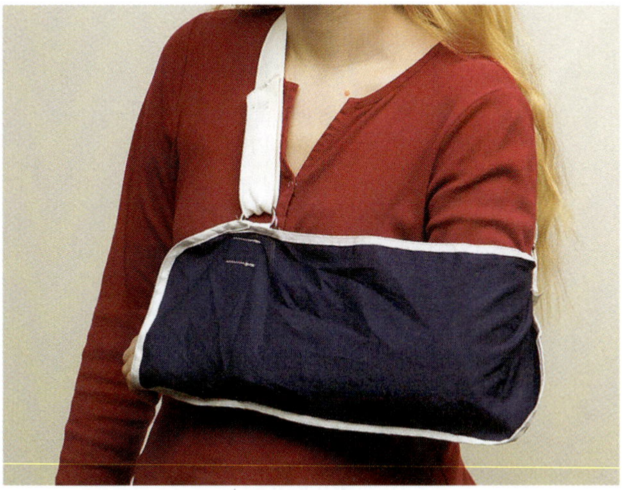

Figure 9-9 A commercial sling is used to support injured or fractured arms.

In a child, the head, back, and front of the torso are 18% each, each upper extremity is 9%, each lower extremity is 13.5%, and the perineum is 1%.

Providers use the formula to determine the amount of body surface area that has been burned. Together with the depth of the burn, it helps the provider determine the percent of the body burned and the degree of burn. The severity of a burn can be determined and appropriate treatment given.

Figure 9-10B shows the relative penetration level of each degree of burn into the skin and underlying structures.

General Guidelines for Caring for Burns. Treatment for burns depends on the type of agent causing the burn. General treatment strategies for any degree of burn include the following:

- Cool the burn with large amounts of cool normal saline, or water if saline is unavailable.
- Cover the burn with a sterile dressing if one is available and burn is minor. Otherwise, cover the burn with a sheet or other smooth textured cloth for a burn over a large area of the body.
- Be sure the patient is protected from being either chilled or overheated.

However, it is important to follow these guidelines:

- Do not apply ice or ice water to a burn.
- Do not touch a burn, except with a sterile dressing.
- Do not clean a severe burn, break blisters, or use any kind of ointment.

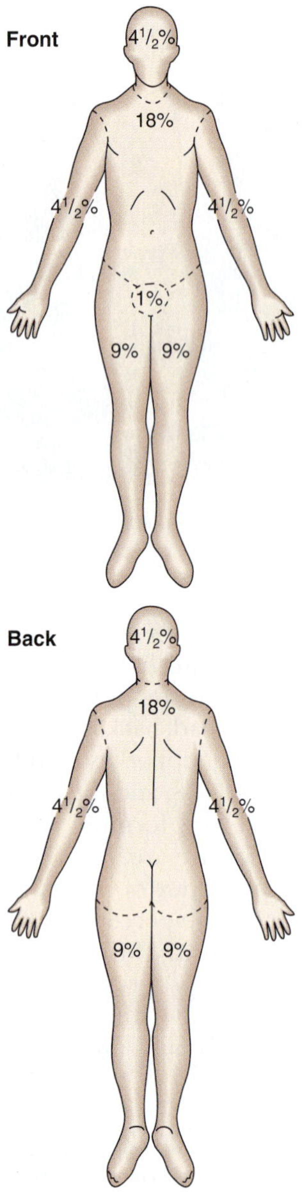

Figure 9-10A Diagram for use in calculating the extent of burns or other injuries in an adult.

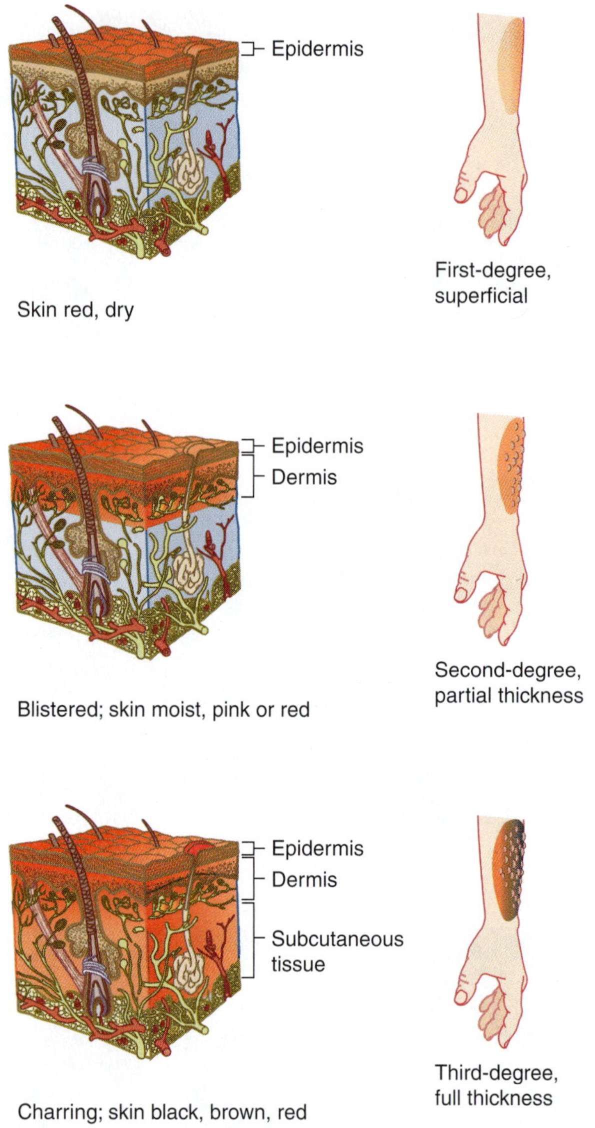

Figure 9-10B Classification of burn injuries.

- Do not remove pieces of clothing that may be sticking to the burn.

First Aid for Burns. First aid for burns is outlined in Table 9-3.

Types of Burns. Most burns are caused by heat; however, burns can also be caused by chemicals, electricity, and solar radiation.

Chemical Burns. Chemical burns can occur in the workplace or even in the home with "ordinary" household chemicals. To stop the burning process, you must remove the chemical from the skin. Have someone call EMS while you flush the skin or eyes

Patient Education

Some burns can be prevented. Advise patients who insist on sunbathing to protect themselves against harmful rays by using a sunscreen and avoiding the sun between 10 AM and 2 PM.

Patient Education

Advise patients not to run should their clothing catch on fire. They should fall to the ground or wrap themselves in a blanket or rug and roll on the ground to extinguish the flames.

Table 9-3 First Aid for Burns

First-Degree Burn Response Guide

Questions	Responses	Action to Take	Rationale
Is skin reddened without blisters? NO ⇩	YES ⇨	Submerge in cool normal saline or water 2–5 minutes. ⇨	Stops burning process.
Does area involve: • hands? • feet? • genitals? • face? NO ⇩	YES ⇨	Have patient come to office. ⇨	These are potential danger areas and require evaluation by the provider.
Is patient: • elderly? • very young? NO ⇩	YES ⇨	Have patient come to office. ⇨	These groups are susceptible to burn complications.
Consult provider.			Provider has final decision whether patient is seen.

Second-Degree Burn Response Guide

Questions	Responses	Action to Take	Rationale
Is skin reddened with blisters or splitting of the skin? NO ⇩	YES ⇨	Submerge in cool normal saline or water 10–15 minutes if skin is intact. Use compresses if skin is broken. Do not break blisters. Do not use anesthetic creams or sprays. ⇨	Stops burning process. If blisters are broken, can allow infection in burn. Creams or spray may slow healing process and increase severity of a burn.
Does area involve: • hands? • feet? • genitals? • face? NO ⇩	YES ⇨	Have patient come to office or go to the emergency department. ⇨	These are potentially dangerous areas and require medical attention.
Is the area involved larger than a child's hand? NO ⇩	YES ⇨	Have patient come to office or go to the emergency department. ⇨	Burns of this size are susceptible to complications.
Is patient experiencing trouble breathing? NO ⇩	YES ⇨	Patient should go to emergency department. ⇨	There may be swelling of the airways because of heat and noxious fumes.

(continues)

Table 9-3 First Aid for Burns (continued)

Second-Degree Burn Response Guide			
Questions	**Responses**	**Action to Take**	**Rationale**
Consult provider.			Provider has final decision whether patient is seen.

Third-Degree Burn Response Guide			
Questions	**Responses**	**Action to Take**	**Rationale**
Is skin gray, black, or charred appearing? Can muscle, fat, or bone be seen in wound? NO ⇩	YES ⇨	Tell patient or family to call EMS ⇨ immediately. Do not apply cold; do not remove burned clothing from burn area.	Life-threatening emergency that requires prompt attention.
Is patient experiencing: • pallor • loss of consciousness? • shivering? NO ⇩	YES ⇨	Patient in shock: ⇨ Tell family to call EMS and to: • maintain airway. • maintain body temperature. • elevate feet if appropriate. • monitor breathing. Patient may need oxygen and intravenous fluids while waiting for EMS to arrive.	Need to control shock caused by fluid loss.
Consult provider.			Provider has final decision whether patient is seen.

with cool water. Remove any clothing contaminated by the chemicals unless they adhere to the skin. If clothing clings to the skin, it can be cut with scissors. Do not attempt to pull clothing away from a burned area.

Electrical Burns. Electrical burns can be caused by power lines, lightning, or faulty electrical equipment in the home or work place. *It is important to remember never to go near a patient injured by electricity until you are sure the power has been shut off, because you could be injured.* If there is a downed line, call the power company and EMS.

A victim of an electricity burn may be suffering from two burns: one where the power entered the body, and one where it exited. Often, the burns themselves may be minor. Of more serious consequence are the possibilities of shock, breathing difficulties, and other injuries. CPR often is needed in this situation.

Solar Radiation. Most "sunburns," although not advisable or good for the skin, represent minor burns. If the patient has a severe burn, however, he or she should see a provider who will cover the burn area to reduce infection and protect the patient against chill.

Musculoskeletal Injuries

Most injuries to muscles, bones, and joints are not life threatening, but they are painful and, if not properly treated, can be disabling. Some injuries, such as those to the spinal cord, can be quite serious and can result in paralysis. These injuries are not typically seen in the ambulatory care setting.

Types of Injuries. A **sprain** is an injury to a joint, often an ankle, knee, or wrist, that involves a tearing of the ligaments. Some sprains are minor and heal quickly; others are more severe, include swelling, and may not heal properly if the patient continues to put stress on the sprained joint. Signs of a sprain are rapid swelling, discoloration at the site, and limited function. Many times it is difficult to determine whether the patient has sustained a sprain or a fracture because the degree of pain may not be a true indicator of the patient's injury. As with most closed wounds, treating the injury with the RICE or MICE method is beneficial and determined by the proivder's choice.

A **strain** results from the overuse or stretching of a muscle, tendons, or group of muscles, as with improper lifting or moving heavy objects. Applications of ice and heat (as described eariler in "Closed Wounds"), as well as rest, are indicated for treatment of strains. Surgery is not usually required for sprains and strains. Significant injuries (large tears) may need surgery. Slings, crutches, and removable splints help protect the injury from further damage and limit movement until a more specific diagnosis can be made.

Dislocations are painful and involve the separation of a bone from its normal position. These usually occur from the kind of wrenching motion that might result from a fall, automobile accident, or sports injury.

Fractures involve a break in a bone and can be caused by a fall, by a blow, from bone disease, or from sports injuries. There are several types of fractures, but all are classified as either open or closed fractures. An open fracture involves an open wound and is characterized by a protruding bone. In a closed fracture, the skin is not broken. Signs and symptoms that occur with a fracture may include swelling, discoloration, pain, deformity, and immobility of the body part. It is not unusual for patients to tell you that they heard the bone break or that they sensed a grating feeling. **Crepitation** is the term that describes the grating sensation experienced or heard when bone fragments rub together. Fractures are further defined as follows:

- *Incomplete or greenstick:* fracture in which the bone has cracked, but the break is not all the way through; frequently seen in children
- *Simple:* complete bone break in which there is no involvement with the skin surface
- *Compound:* fracture in which the bone protrudes though the skin surface, creating the possibility of infection
- *Impacted:* fracture in which the broken ends are jammed into each other
- *Comminuted:* more than one fracture line and several bone fragments are present
- *Spiral:* fracture that occurs with a severe twisting action, causing the break to wind around the bone
- *Depressed:* fracture that occurs with severe head injuries in which a broken piece of skull is driven inward
- *Colles:* fracture often caused by falling on an outstretched hand; involves the distal end of the radius and results in displacement, causing a bulge at the wrist

These fractures represent "major" types of fractures. Figure 9-11 shows examples of these fractures.

Assessing Injuries to Muscles, Bones, and Joints.

Sometimes it is difficult to determine the extent of an injury, especially in closed fractures. There are some assessment techniques to call on, however, to gauge the seriousness of an injury.

- Note the extent of bruising and swelling.
- Pain is a signal of injury.
- There may be noticeable deformity to the bone or joint.
- Use of the injured area is limited.
- Talk to the patient: What was the cause of the injury? What was the sound or sensation at the time of injury?

Caring for Muscle, Bone, and Joint Injuries. Most injuries to muscles, bones, and joints are treated in a similar way; some require rest, some motion, elevation of the injured part, immobilization, and the application of ice to the injury.

After calling EMS (always check for life-threatening symptoms, such as breathing difficulties; bleeding; or head, neck, or back injuries), it is important to immobilize the injured area if the patient must be moved. EMS personnel use a variety of **splints** to immobilize bones and joints. Some fractures must be treated in the hospital. Compound fractures and fractures with nerve or blood vessel involvement are some examples. Most often, a fracture can be treated with outpatient care. A splint and a cast may be applied to prevent movement and to hold the fracture steady. Procedure 9-2 gives instructions for splinting an arm in the ambulatory care setting.

Heat- and Cold-Related Illnesses

The condition of patients who have been subject to extreme heat and cold can deteriorate rapidly, and either a heat- or cold-related illness can result in death. Individuals especially vulnerable to extreme exposures include the very young and very old, individuals who must work outdoors, and people who suffer from poor circulation.

Heat-Related Illnesses. Illnesses related to heat, in increasing degree of severity, include heat cramps,

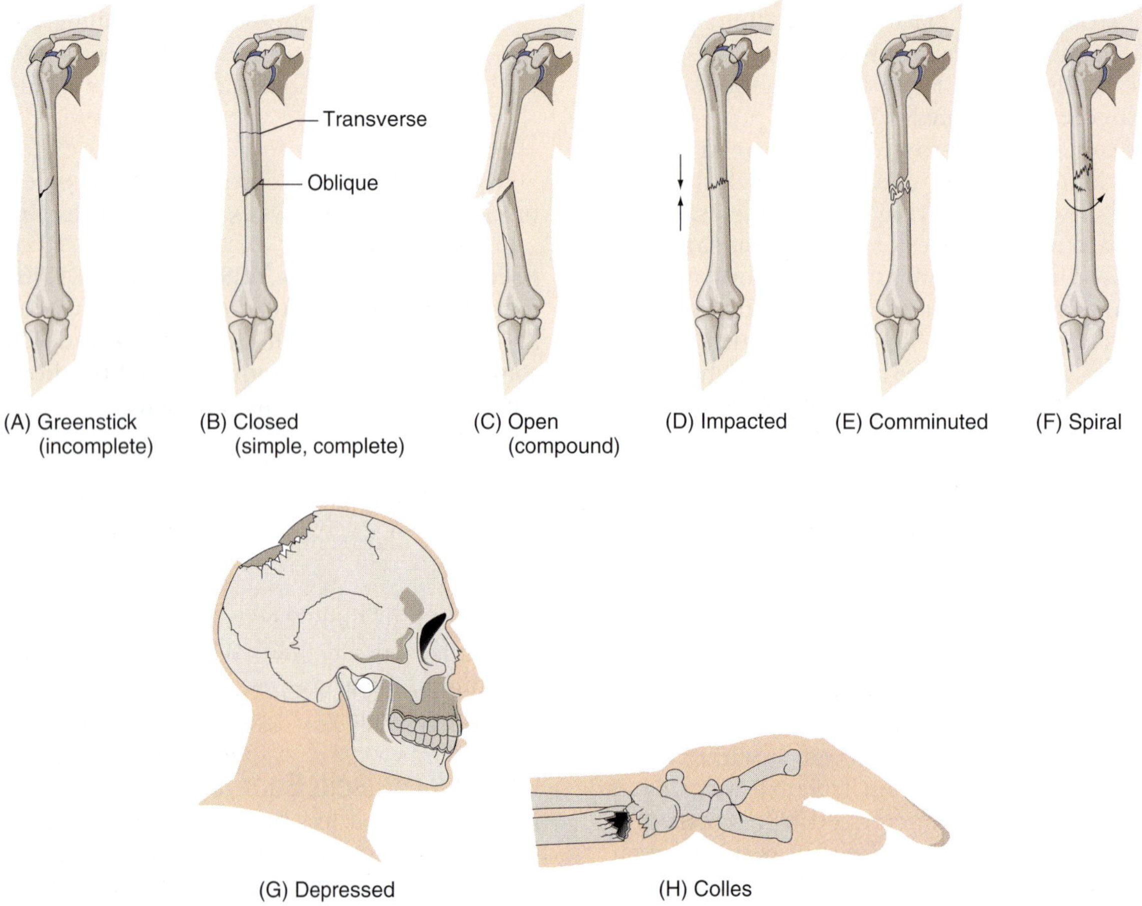

Figure 9-11 Types of fractures.

heat exhaustion, and heat stroke. Heat cramps, the least serious, involve cramping in the legs and abdomen caused by excessive body exposure or exercise in hot weather. Heat cramps should be considered a signal to stop, slow down, rest in a cool place, and drink plenty of water. Salt tablets should not be taken. The individual should lightly stretch the muscles. Heat cramps can progress to heat exhaustion or heat stroke, both of which are more serious conditions.

Heat exhaustion, often experienced by people who work or exercise in extreme heat, is a more serious reaction and is signaled by exhaustion, cold and clammy skin, profuse sweating, headache, and general weakness. The individual should come out of the heat immediately; apply cool, wet towels; and slowly drink cool water. The provider will advise the patient not to resume activity in the heat.

Heat stroke is the least common but the most dangerous of heat-related illnesses and requires immediate medical attention. Heat stroke is characterized by red, dry, hot skin; an abnormal, weak pulse; and breathing that is shallow and fast. In heat stroke, the body systems are extremely taxed. EMS should be alerted; until they arrive, stay with the patient, watch for breathing problems, and attempt to reduce body temperature by applying cool, wet towels or sheets.

Cold-Related Illnesses. Exposure to extreme cold for prolonged periods can lead to frostbite or hypothermia.

Frostbite, which typically affects the extremities such as fingers, toes, ears, and nose, involves the freezing of exposed body parts. Symptoms include skin that becomes off-color, is cold, or takes on a waxy appearance. Severity can range from the superficial (frostnip) to more penetrating stages, which may require amputation.

Individuals with frostbite need immediate medical attention. To care for frostbitten extremities, warm the area of injury by wrapping clothing or blankets around the affected body part. Be careful in handling the frozen part. It is best to have the patient transported as soon as possible to emergency care. This type of facility is better able to properly rewarm the frozen part, preventing further tissue damage.

Hypothermia is a serious illness in which the body temperature decreases to a perilously low level. It can result in death if the individual does not receive care and if the progression of hypothermia is not reversed. Hypothermia occurs when a person falls through the ice or is exposed to cold temperatures, for example, after getting lost in the woods while hiking. Symptoms include shivering, cold skin, and confusion.

After checking for breathing problems and alerting EMS, care for the patient. Make the individual comfortable, provide a source of warmth, such as a blanket, and *gradually* warm the body. If clothing is wet or cold, remove it and put on dry clothing. In extreme cases, it may be necessary to provide rescue breathing.

Poisoning

Poisons can enter the body in four ways:

- *Ingestion.* Ingested poisons enter the body by swallowing. Swallowed poisons may include medications, plant material, household chemicals, contaminated foods, and drugs.
- *Inhalation.* Poisons are inhaled into the body in poorly ventilated areas where cleaning fluids, paints and chemical cleaners, or carbon monoxide may be present.
- *Absorption.* Poisons absorbed through the skin include plant materials such as poison oak or ivy, lawn care products such as chemical pesticides, and other chemical powders or liquids.
- *Injection.* Drug abuse is the most common cause of injected poisons. The stingers of insects inject poisons into the body and can be extremely dangerous and can lead to anaphylactic shock in allergic individuals.

Patient Education

Remind patients who are parents of young children to remove any potential sources of poisoning from their homes or to keep them in locked cabinets. Also advise them to include the nearby poison control center in their list of emergency phone numbers. They should also keep activated charcoal on hand.

Some signs and symptoms of poisoning are dyspnea, nausea and vomiting, confusion, and convulsions. The Poison Control Center (1-800-222-1222) can advise if there is an antidote for the poison (if poison is known). For many years, the treatment of choice for ingested poison was to induce vomiting by using syrup of ipecac. This is no longer recommended. Activated charcoal given as soon as possible is the treatment of choice for ingested poison. It is quicker and more effective.

If a patient becomed unconscious, the provider will be concerned that the patient will vomit and aspirate vomitus into the lungs; therefore, the provider may insert a flexible tube into the larynx to alleviate that possibility.

In most poisoning cases, there are specific antidotes. They work either by reversing the effects of the poison or by preventing the poison from working.

On occasion, there is no specific treatment and just the symptoms will be treated. A ventilator may be needed if a patient has stopped breathing. Medications that control convulsions are available, and sedatives can be administered if the patient is disturbed and restless.

Whenever a patient calls regarding poisoning or there is a suspicion of poisoning, call the Poison Control Center (1-800-222-1222) or the local emergency number and ask for advice. Telephone numbers of the poison control center should be posted in a familiar and accessible place.

The treatment for poisoning will vary according to the source of the poisoning and must be tailored to the specific incident. The provider will have

Patient Education

Advise all patients with known allergic reactions to be particularly careful when working or playing outdoors. Insects are not usually aggressive until their nests are approached; however, often these nests are not easy to detect, and an individual may approach one without being aware of its presence. Patients with allergies to insects should always wear shoes when outside; wear light-colored clothing, preferably with long sleeves and pant legs; look before taking a sip from a beverage when outdoors; and inspect lawn areas, shrubbery, and building walls periodically for evidence of stinging insect nests.

advised staff regarding specific poisoning antidotes. Generally, do not give the patient anything to eat or drink; try to determine what poison the patient was exposed to and, if ingested, how much was taken; if the patient vomits, save some of the vomitus for analysis.

If prescribed by a provider or recommended by the poison control center, medication used to treat poisoning is activated charcoal, which is used to absorb certain swallowed poisons.

Insect Stings. The medical assistant in the ambulatory care setting is likely to receive calls every summer from patients who have been stung by insects, typically yellow jackets, hornets, honeybees, or wasps. In the nonallergic patient, the sting is likely to result in localized swelling, tenderness, and slight redness. The provider will recommend that these localized symptoms be managed with a topical cream and oral antihistamines. Swelling can be significant and cause for serious concern if the sting occurred in a vulnerable area of the body such as the mouth or tongue. Swelling in these locations can be frightening and dangerous because it can impair breathing. An antihistamine, administered as soon as possible after the sting, may help to curtail symptoms somewhat. Treatment of insect stings in nonallergic individuals consists of removing the stinger by scraping it off with the edge of something rigid such as a credit card or your fingernail. Tweezers can cause more venom to be dispersed into the patient's body tissues, so this method should not be used. Wash the area with soap and water, apply a cold pack to the site, and watch for a possible severe reaction.

The individual who experiences an allergic reaction or hypersensitivity to a sting needs to be seen immediately, because in severe cases a sting may induce an anaphylactic reaction that can lead to death. If allergic, individuals who have been stung are likely to experience symptoms within a half hour of the incident. Symptoms are generalized throughout the body and may include hives, itching, and lightheadedness and may progress to difficulty breathing, faintness, and eventual loss of consciousness.

For individuals with known allergic reactions, the provider will prescribe epinephrine, which patients should carry with them and self-inject should they not be able to get immediate emergency care. EPIPEN is a brand of epinephrine to self-inject. The patient should then seek immediate emergency treatment. For individuals who present at the ambulatory care setting with an apparent allergic reaction to a sting, the provider will prescribe epinephrine, an antihistamine, and corticosteroids if necessary.

Patient Education

Snake Bite

Most snakes are not poisonous, and snakes usually will not strike unless provoked. Some poisonous snakes are rattlesnake, copper snake, cottonmouth water moccasin, and coral snake. Individuals who live in snake-inhabited areas, campers, hikers, and other outdoor lovers need to be mindful and cautious when outdoors. To avoid a possible snake bite, wear thick high boots, stay on the hiking path, do not reach down to pick up something from the ground unless you have a clear view around the area, and be careful on rocks (snakes like to live in or around piles of rocks).

Common signs and symptoms of a snake bite are rapid pulse, nausea and vomiting, severe pain, swelling, blood and fang marks at wound site, convulsions, thirst, and diaphoresis.

Emergency treatment consists of the following:

- Call for emergency help immediately
- Wash wound with soap and water if possible
- Immobilize body part and keep below heart level if possible
- Apply a constriction band 4 inches above site
- Cover with clean cool cloth
- Monitor vital signs

Attempt to allay patient apprehension and monitor vital signs while waiting for EMS personnel to arrive.

Sudden Illness

Sudden illness is, by definition, an unexpected occurrence. Although the cause of the illness may be unexplainable, it is important to respond sensibly and responsibly within the parameters of knowledge and resources.

Sudden illnesses include, but are not limited to, fainting, seizures, diabetic reaction, and hemorrhage.

Fainting. Also known as **syncope,** fainting involves a loss of consciousness, caused by an insufficient supply of blood to the brain. Loss of consciousness may simply be the result of a fainting episode, or it may indicate a more serious medical problem such as diabetic coma or shock. A fall during a fainting incident may result in bodily harm.

If a patient in the office or clinic "feels faint," indicated by lightheadedness, weakness, nausea, or unsteadiness, have the individual lie down or sit down with head level with the knees. This may prevent a fainting episode.

The most common type of fainting episodes occur when the blood pressure drops quickly in response to a highly charged emotional or stressful situation. The name for this common fainting spell is **vasovagal syncope**. The individual's skin feels sweaty and clammy, and lightheadedness is common.

If a patient faints, gradually lower the patient to a flat surface, loosen any tight clothing, check breathing and for any life-threatening emergencies, and apply cool compresses to the forehead. Elevate the legs if there is no back or head injury. If vomiting occurs, place the patient on his or her side. Although fainting is typically not serious in itself, 911 or EMS may need to be called because the problem may be indicative of a more complex medical condition.

Seizures. Seizures or convulsions occur when normal brain functioning is disrupted, which can occur for a variety of reasons including fever, disease such as diabetes, infections, or injury to the brain. Epilepsy is a common cause of convulsions. Involuntary spasms or contractions of muscles characterize seizures.

To the onlooker, seizures look frightening and painful, which may lead inexperienced individuals to try to stop the seizure when they see it occurring in another individual. A patient experiencing a seizure should never be restrained; simply care for the victim with compassion and medical understanding. The goal is to protect the patient from self-injury during the episode. Do not force anything between the patient's clenched teeth—an individual experiencing seizures cannot "swallow" the tongue.

Most patients recover from a seizure in a few minutes. During the seizure, protect the patient from injury, cushion the patient's head, and roll the patient to the side if any fluid is in the mouth. After the seizure subsides, calm and comfort the patient.

If a patient is known to regularly have seizures and the patient's seizure subsides in a matter of minutes, EMS personnel usually do not need to be summoned. Repeated seizures during the same time frame, however, dictate a call to emergency services, as does any seizure if the patient is diabetic, pregnant, injured, or does not regain consciousness after the incident.

Diabetes. Diabetes is defined by the American Diabetes Society as the "inability of the body to properly convert sugar from food into energy."

Under normal functioning, the body produces a hormone called insulin, which transports sugars into body cells. In some cases, the body does not produce insulin at all or does not produce enough; this results in diabetes.

Diabetes occurs in two major types:

- Type 1, or insulin-dependent diabetes
- Type 2, or noninsulin-dependent diabetes, which usually occurs in adults; in type II, the body produces insulin in insufficient quantities

Complications from diabetes, which you may encounter in a medical office or clinic setting, include diabetic coma (acidosis) and insulin shock or reaction. The provider will prescribe either insulin or glucose before the patient is transported to the hospital. Both are serious emergencies that require immediate EMS assistance. Table 9-4 lists common causes and symptoms of diabetic coma or insulin shock (see Chapter 24 for calculation of medication dosage and medication administration).

Hemorrhage. The different sources of bleeding determine the seriousness of hemorrhage, or bleeding.

External Bleeding. External bleeding includes capillary, venous, and arterial bleeding. Capillary bleeding, often from cuts and scratches, usually clots without first-aid measures. Bleeding from a vein, which is characterized by dark red blood that flows steadily, needs to be controlled quickly (see Procedure 9-1) to prevent excessive blood loss. Bleeding from an artery produces bright red bleeding that spurts from the wound; this is the most serious type of bleeding and occurs when an artery is punctured or severed. Like venous bleeding, arterial bleeding requires immediate emergency care because serious loss of blood and profound irreversible shock can happen quickly.

Epistaxis, or nosebleed, may be the result of breathing dry air for a long period; result from injury or blowing the nose too hard; be caused by high altitudes; be caused by hypertension (high blood pressure); or result from overuse of medications such as aspirin and anticoagulants.

Table 9-4 Causes and Symptoms of Diabetic Coma and Insulin Shock

Diabetic Coma or Acidosis		**Insulin Shock or Reaction**	
Causes	Too little insulin, too much to eat, infections, fever, emotional stress	Causes	Too much insulin or oral hypoglycemic drug, too little to eat, an unusual amount of exercise
Symptoms	Skin: Dry and flushed Behavior: Drowsy Mouth: Dry Thirst: Intense Hunger: Absent Vomiting: Common Respiration: Exaggerated, air hungry Breath: Fruity odor of acetone Pulse: Weak and rapid Vision: Dim Blood glucose greater than 200 mg/100 mL	Symptoms	Skin: Moist and pale Behavior: Often excited Mouth: Drooling Thirst: Absent Hunger: Present Vomiting: Usually absent Respiration: Normal or shallow Breath: Usually normal Pulse: Full and pounding (gives patient feeling of heart pounding) Vision: Diplopia (double) Low blood glucose level (40–70 mg/100 mL or less)
First aid	Keep patient warm Obtain medical help immediately	First aid	If conscious, give patient sugar or any food containing sugar (fruit juice, candy, crackers) Obtain medical help immediately

To control nosebleeds, seat the patient, elevate the patient's head, and pinch the nostrils for at least 10 minutes. Assist the patient to sit with head tilted forward so blood running down the back of the throat will not be swallowed or aspirated. If bleeding cannot be controlled, the provider may request that you activate EMS. The patient's nostril may need to be **cauterized** or a gauze packing inserted (see Chapter 18).

Internal Bleeding. Internal bleeding may be minor or serious depending on the cause of the injury. A contusion, or bruise, will result in minor internal bleeding. A sharp blow may induce severe internal bleeding.

Because there is no visible blood flow, it is important to recognize other symptoms of internal bleeding. Symptoms are similar to those of shock and include a rapid and weak pulse, low blood pressure, shallow breathing, cold and clammy skin, dilated pupils, dizziness, faintness, thirst, restlessness, and a feeling of anxiety. There may be pain, tenderness, or swelling at the injury site. The abdomen may be boardlike (stiff and hard to the touch).

If internal bleeding is suspected, ask another staff member to call EMS; until they arrive, stay with the patient and take measures to prevent shock. Monitor vital signs.

Patient Education

Advise the patient not to blow the nose for several hours after an epistaxis.

Cerebral Vascular Accident

The common term for a cerebral vascular accident (CVA) is stroke. A stroke is the result of a ruptured blood vessel in the brain, or it can be caused by **occlusion** of a blood vessel by a clot. Both of these situations can result in the brain being deprived of oxygen, causing brain cells to die. Symptoms of a stroke include numbness in the face, arm, and leg on one side of the body; loss of vision; severe headache, mental confusion; slurred speech; nausea; vomiting; and difficulty in breathing and swallowing. Paralysis may be present. If a patient is suspected of having a stroke, call EMS, loosen tight clothing, lie the patient down, and keep him or her comfortable. Position the patient's head to facilitate the flow of secretion from the mouth to avoid choking and maintain an open airway. Do not give anything by mouth and monitor vital signs. Immediate emergency care is critical for all individuals experiencing strokes. If the stroke is caused by a clot that blocks blood flow, drugs may be able to protect the individual from permanent injury. Rapid transport to the hospital is important for treatment to be instituted as soon as possible. Treatment with the clot-dissolving drug must be given within 3 hours after onset of symptoms for it to be effective.

Heart Attack

Heart attack, also known as myocardial infarction, is usually caused by blockage of one or more of the coronary arteries. Symptoms include tightness of the chest, pain radiating down one or both arms, or pain radiating into the left shoulder and jaw. Other signs include rapid and weak pulse, excessive perspiration, agitation, nausea, and cold and clammy skin. Heart attack symptoms in a woman may or may not be similar to those experienced by a man. Women may have symptoms such as abdominal discomfort, burning sensation in the chest, discomfort or pain in the lower chest or back, unexplained sudden fatigue, sweating, and breathlessness.

If you suspect the patient is experiencing a heart attack, contact EMS immediately, loosen tight clothing, and keep the patient comfortable. Prepare to give oxygen and other medications such as aspirin, as directed by the provider. Monitor vital signs. If the patient experiences an episode of cardiac fibrillation, **cardioversion** or defibrillation may be necessary with an automatic external defibrillator. Prepare to begin CPR if necessary.

BREATHING EMERGENCIES AND CARDIAC ARREST

Breathing or respiratory emergencies occur for a variety of reasons, including choking, shock, allergies, and other illnesses or injuries such as drowning and electrical shock. When an individual stops breathing, artificial or rescue breathing must be given quickly, for without a constant supply of oxygen, brain damage or death will occur.

When the breathing problem is accompanied by cardiac arrest, the rescue breathing must be accompanied by chest compressions. This is known as **cardiopulmonary resuscitation (CPR).** Cardiac emergencies may occur in the medical office because of the large number of patients who have heart disease.

In order to graduate from a CAAHEP-accredited program, medical assistants must attain provider-level CPR certification and take first-aid training courses. Frequent refresher courses and recertification in CPR are necessary.

Patient Education

Lay Person CPR

- Do not need to be certified
- Chest compressions alone are sufficient
- Patients more likely to survive without brain damage with only chest compressions
- 30 compressions keeps blood moving to brain and heart
- Drowning victims and smoke inhalation victims are the exception. Both need rescue breathing and CPR

Rescue Breathing

Individuals in respiratory arrest require immediate emergency care. **Rescue breathing,** previously called mouth-to-mouth resuscitation, provides oxygen to the patient until emergency personnel arrive.

When performing rescue breathing procedures in the ambulatory care setting, it is recommended that resuscitation mouthpieces be used and that direct mouth-to-mouth (i.e., with no personal protective equipment) resuscitation never be used.

Cardiopulmonary Resuscitation

The combination of rescue breathing and chest compressions is known as CPR. Alone, CPR cannot save an individual from cardiac arrest—it represents preliminary care until advanced medical help is available to the heart attack victim.

In 2005, the American Heart Association (AHA) updated their emergency care guidelines for CPR and Emergency Cardiovascular Care (ECC) (http://www.americanheart.org/cpr.html). The new guidelines emphasize chest compressions being done "hard and fast." Studies have found that if bystanders act quickly and begin CPR, many more victims could be saved. It was determined that CPR plus a shock with an AED (Figure 9-12) is the treatment for cardiac arrest. The AHA says that early recognition of the emergency, calling EMS, and immediate CPR can double or triple a victim's chances of surviving. Furthermore, the AHA says that CPR plus defibrillation (AED) that is started

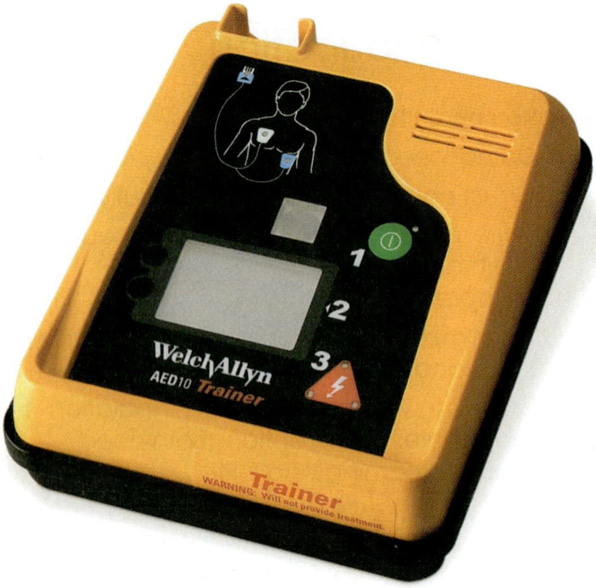

Figure 9-12 Automated external defibrillator (AED). (Courtesy of Welch-Allyn.)

within 3 to 5 minutes of collapse can boost survival significantly. Lay rescuer AEDs are available in airports, sports facilities, airplanes, casinos, and many other locations. The AED is becoming more readily available, is easy to use, and is very accurate.

The most significant change in the AHA's guidelines is the ratio of compressions to rescue breathing. The standard was 15 compressions and two breaths, but now the ratio is 30 compressions to two breaths. The 30:2 ratio is the same for adults, children, and infants. The study showed that blood circulation increases with each chest compression, and when compressions were interrupted to give rescue breaths, circulation drops and must be built back up again.

Another guideline change made by the AHA is the use of the AED. One shock is delivered followed by about 2 minutes of CPR beginning with chest compressions before reanalyzing the heart rhythm to determine if another shock is needed. Table 9-5 summarizes the AHA 2005 Guidelines for CPR, obstructed airway, and defibrillation.

More information is available from the following sources:

- American Heart Association (http://www.americanheart.org)

Table 9-5 Summary of American Heart Association 2005 CPR Guidelines

Airway	**Breathing**	**Circulation**
Adult—head tilt, chin lift Child—head tilt, chin lift Infant—head tilt, chin lift	Adult—2 breaths Child—2 breaths Infant—2 breaths	Adult—30 compressions center of chest between the nipples. Use 2 hands; heel of one hand on chest and other hand on top. Push hard and fast 1½–2 inches Child—30 compressions center of chest between the nipples. Hands same as adult or heel only of one hand. Push hard and fast ⅓ to ½ of the depth of the child's chest. Infant—30 compressions just below the nipples. Use 2 fingers. Push hard and fast ½–1 inch.
Obstructed Airway	**Use of Automatic External Defibrillator (AED)**	
Adult—5 abdominal thrusts Child—5 abdominal thrusts continuous Infant—5 back blows, 5 chest thrusts continuous	Adult Child—8 years or older Infant—under 8 years	Adult and child—one shock delivered followed by 2 minutes of CPR starting with compressions. Infant—same as adult. Use pediatric pads on AED.

- American Red Cross (http://www.redcross.org)
- National Safety Council (http://www.nsc.org)
- National Institutes of Health (http://www.health.nih.gov)

SAFETY AND EMERGENCY PRACTICES

The Commission on Accreditation of Allied Health Programs (CAAHEP) believes allied health students should understand how to respond in an emergency situation, as health care professionals and citizens. Medical assistant programs accredited by CAAHEP have within their Standards and Guidelines a new section requirement for safety and emergency practices. Provider-level CPR and basic first aid are part of these requirements for graduation.

Health professionals recognize an obligation to use their skills and knowledge in a disaster environment.

There are many kinds of mass disasters, natural and manmade. Some examples are floods, hurricanes, tornadoes, tsunamis, and earthquakes. Others are explosions, structural collapses (I-35W bridge collapse in Minneapolis in 2007), transportation accidents, and war or terrorism (see Chapter 10).

What would a large-scale disaster be like and how could we respond? Disaster threatens public health and safety; disrupts services (gas, water, electricity, transportation); destroys roads, bridges, homes, and other buildings; and makes food and water unsafe or impossible to obtain. Law enforcement, fire departments, hospitals, and military all could be affected. There is a need for collaboration between disaster experts and health professionals to plan for emergencies.

What can medical assistants do to help? How could you use your skills without technology (unavailable due to the disaster)? Some examples are assisting your neighbors at local shelters, using your first aid and CPR skills, helping out at a clinic, giving injections for mass immunizations, supporting overwhelmed providers, working with the American Red Cross, giving emotional support, and filling in at a hospital.

In addition to mass disasters, medical assistants should be prepared to respond to emergency situations in the medical office or a home environment. For instance, if a patient goes into shock, or if an elderly family member has a fall, or if the medical office needs to be evacuated for a fire, are examples of these emergency situations.

Medical assisting curriculum may include courses to be certain medical assisting graduates are prepared to help during an emergency situation.

In 2002, President Bush asked for teams of volunteers of medical and health professionals to contribute their skills during times of need in their communities. The Medical Reserve Corps (MRC) was established (http://www.medicalreservecorps.gov), and the teams of volunteers within the MRC work with Health and Human Services of the U.S. government and the American Red Cross. The MRC is community based. Its goal is to organize and use volunteers who want to donate their time and expertise to respond to emergencies and to promote healthy living throughout the year. The MRC supplements existing emergency and public health resources. Volunteers include providers, nurses, respiratory care therapists, massage therapists, pharmacists, dentists, and a whole array of allied health professionals such as medical assistants.

The MRC volunteer units are assigned to specific areas. They work with and support the country and state public health departments. The main office is in the Surgeon General's office in Washington, DC.

Procedure 9-1

Control of Bleeding

STANDARD PRECAUTIONS:

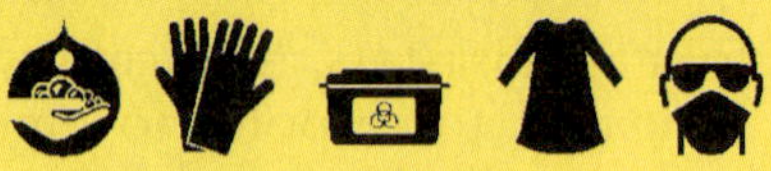

PURPOSE:

To control bleeding from an open wound.

EQUIPMENT/SUPPLIES:

Sterile dressings
Sterile gloves
Mask and eye protection
Gown
Biohazard waste container

PROCEDURE STEPS:

1. Wash hands.
2. Assemble equipment and supplies.
3. Apply eye and mask protection and gown if splashing is likely to occur.
4. Put on gloves.
5. Apply dressing and press firmly (Figure 9-13A).
6. If bleeding continues, elevate arm above heart level (Figure 9-13B). RATIONALE: Raising the arm above the heart level will slow the flow of blood because it is flowing against gravity.
7. If bleeding continues, press adjacent artery against bone (Figure 9-13C). Notify the provider if bleeding cannot be controlled. RATIONALE: Pressing the adjacent artery against a bone provides solid pressure to help control bleeding.
8. Apply pressure bandage over the dressing.
9. Dispose of waste in biohazard container.
10. Remove gloves and dispose in biohazard container.
11. Wash hands.
12. Document procedure in patient's chart or electronic medical record.

CAUTION: If wound is large and bleeding is not controlled, the patient may go into hemorrhagic shock. Be prepared to call EMS immediately.

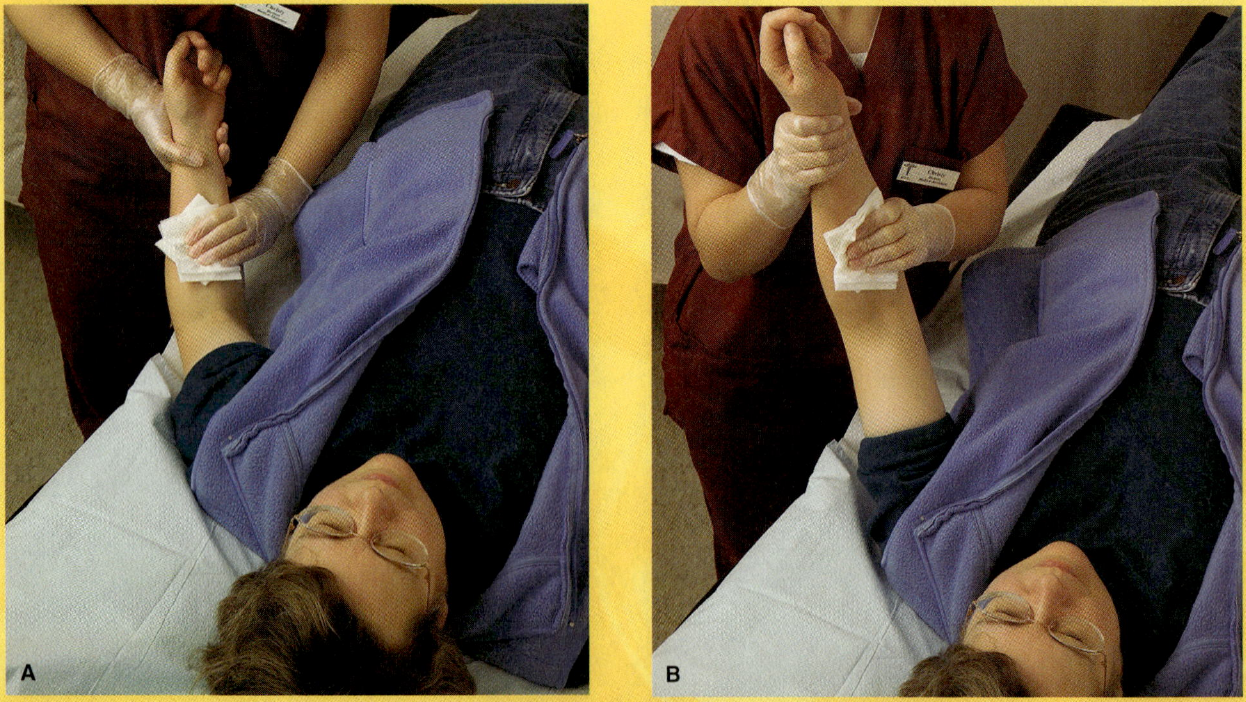

Figure 9-13 (A) Apply dressing and press firmly. (B) Elevate arm above heart level.

continues

Procedure 9-1 (continued)

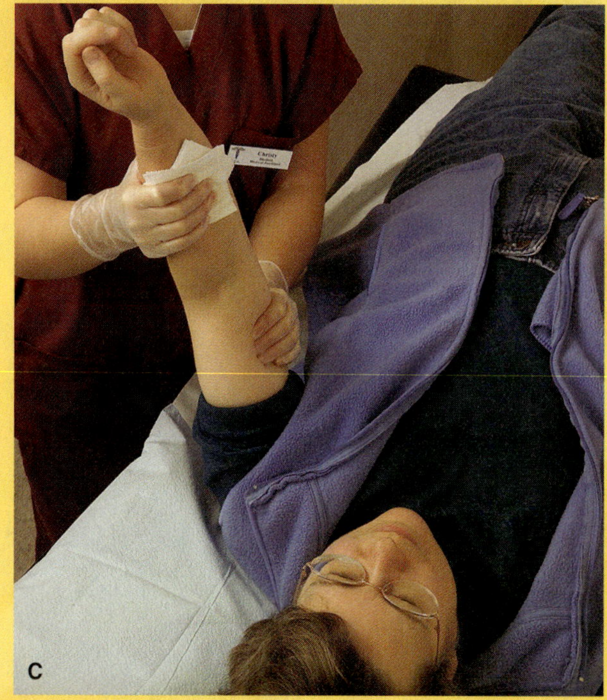

Figure 9-13 (continued) (C) Press artery against

DOCUMENTATION

4/4/20XX—10:00 AM Patient sustained small (1 cm) laceration on inside left forearm. Bleeding moderately. Pressure dressing applied to wound, left arm elevated above heart level. Bleeding continued. Pressure applied to brachial artery. Pressure bandage applied over dry sterile dressing. Bleeding seems to have subsided. BP 118/74, P 92. Seen by Dr. King. W. Slawson, CMA (AAMA) ————————

Procedure 9-2

Applying an Arm Splint

STANDARD PRECAUTIONS:

PURPOSE:

To immobilize the area above and below the injured part of the arm in order to reduce pain, immobilize, and prevent further injury.

EQUIPMENT/SUPPLIES:

Thin piece of rigid board; cardboard can be used if necessary
Gauze roller bandage

PROCEDURE STEPS:

1. Wash hands.
2. Place the padded splint under the injured area.
3. Hold the splint in place with gauze roller bandage. Pad gaps between arm and board (wrist) with gauze pads or other soft material. RATIONALE: More comfortable for patient.
4. After splinting, check circulation (note color and temperature of skin, note color of nails, check pulse) to ascertain that the splint is not too tightly applied. RATIONALE: Checks for impaired circulation.
5. A sling will be applied to keep the arm elevated, which increases comfort and reduces swelling.
6. Wash hands.
7. Document the procedure in patient's chart or electronic medical record.

DOCUMENTATION

4/4/20XX—2:00 PM Splint applied to right arm above and below injured area. Sling applied for comfort. Nail beds pink, hand warm, radial pulse easily palpated. Seen by Dr. Woo. J. Guerro, CMA (AAMA) ————————

Case Study 9-1

Refer to the scenario at the beginning of the chapter.

CASE STUDY REVIEW

1. Dr. Rice and Wanda cleansed the wound. How was it done?
2. There is another factor to consider with regard to treating the patient's wound and providing care for her. What could it be?

Case Study 9-2

Annette Samuels, a regular patient at Inner City Health Care, is walking her dog one morning, stops to rest on a grassy knoll, and notices a wasp on her arm. She brushes it away, unthinking and then realizes it has stung her. She receives two more stings and suddenly notices she is at a nest site. Annette is now a half-hour walk from home but is not really concerned because she has never had an allergic reaction to a wasp sting. However, a few minutes into her walk, her palms become itchy, her ears start to burn, and she feels lightheaded. She is not having difficulty breathing. She is determined to get home and she does, at which point she notices she is covered with hives. She calls Inner City Health Care to ask: Should she come in?

CASE STUDY REVIEW

1. Wanda Slawson, CMA (AAMA), is screening calls the morning Annette is stung. What questions should she ask Annette?
2. Because Annette obviously is having a hypersensitive or an allergic reaction, she is advised to seek emergency care immediately. What first-aid measures might be taken?
3. What advice about precautions against getting stung again should Wanda give Annette?

Case Study 9-3

Abigail Johnson has arrived at Inner City Health Care for her scheduled appointment with Dr. Lewis. As she checks in with Bruce Goldman, the medical assistant, she reports feeling nauseated, having some pressure in her chest, and being short of breath.

CASE STUDY REVIEW

1. What immediate actions should Bruce take to respond to Mrs. Johnson's complaints?
2. What equipment/supplies/medications should be ready and available for Dr. Lewis?
3. Because of the possibility of myocardial infarction, what action would Dr. Lewis direct Bruce to take after Mrs. Johnson has been stabilized?
4. What patient education can Bruce use in this situation?

SUMMARY

Although many of the emergencies covered in this chapter may never be seen by the medical assistant in the ambulatory care setting, it is nonetheless important to develop a broad base of information about the various types of potential emergency situations. This knowledge gives the medical assistant the confidence and the preparation to manage the emergencies that do occur with speed, accuracy, and understanding until outside emergency help arrives. Staff will need to assess their response to emergencies on a continual basis. Was protocol followed? Were there difficulties in the delivery of care? Were staff and equipment prepared and ready to deal with these potentially life-threatening situations? Staff meetings should be held to discuss these and other questions that may have arisen and to allow staff the opportunity to talk about any fears or concerns they might have. It must be stressed that this chapter is at best an introduction to the topic of emergency procedures and first aid; it is essential medical assistants in all ambulatory care settings, whether large or small, enroll in an American Red Cross, American Heart Association, American Safety and Health Institute, or National Heart Association first-aid and CPR program, attain provider-level CPR, and take refresher courses to update skills.

STUDY FOR SUCCESS

To reinforce your knowledge and skills of information presented in this chapter:

- Review the Key Terms
- Practice any Procedures
- Consider the Case Studies and discuss your conclusions
- Answer the Review Questions
  - Multiple Choice
  - Critical Thinking
- Navigate the Internet and complete the Web Activities
- Practice the StudyWARE activities on the textbook CD
- Apply your knowledge in the Student Workbook activities
- Complete the Web Tutor sections
- View and discuss the DVD situations

REVIEW QUESTIONS

Multiple Choice

1. Good Samaritan laws:
   a. are designed to protect the public
   b. protect non–health care professionals
   c. require that all individuals providing assistance act within the scope of their knowledge and training
   d. protect health care professionals on the job
2. First-degree burns:
   a. are the most serious and penetrate all layers of skin
   b. affect only the top layer of skin
   c. often leave scar tissue
   d. usually take more than a month to heal
3. A fracture in which the bone protrudes through the skin is called:
   a. greenstick fracture
   b. compound fracture
   c. depressed fracture
   d. comminuted fracture
4. To control a nosebleed, it is important to:
   a. have the patient lie down
   b. tilt the patient's head back
   c. tilt the patient's head forward
   d. call 911 immediately
5. Another name for a heart attack is:
   a. cerebral vascular accident
   b. cardiac arrest
   c. angina pectoris
   d. myocardial infarction

Critical Thinking

1. Sixteen-year-old Cindy Roland, a patient newly diagnosed with seizures caused by epilepsy, came into the office for a follow-up appointment today. She approached the reception desk and said she can see flashing bright lights in both eyes and that she feels "weird." The administrative medical assistant alerted the medical assistant, who immediately responded to the patient.
   a. What actions should the medical assistant take?
   b. Is there a significance to the flashing bright lights? Explain.
2. Mrs. Williams, a 75-year-old patient, came to the office today for a routine follow-up appointment for her diabetes. She suddenly collapsed onto the floor of the reception area. What immediate steps did the medical assistant take to provide care for this patient in distress?
3. Define the purpose of a crash cart or tray and compile a list of the major supplies and medications it should contain.
4. Describe shock and tell how and why it is important to prevent a patient from going into shock.
5. Recall three types of bandages and give examples of their use.
6. Describe the difference between first-, second-, and third-degree burns.
7. Recall and describe the four ways that poisons may enter the body.
8. What is a hemorrhage? What kinds of bleeding may the medical assistant encounter? What are the symptoms of each?
9. Explain when and why back blows and abdominal thrusts, rescue breathing, and CPR techniques are performed.
10. Explain steps to take if a patient has a laceration on the hand with moderate to heavy bleeding.

WEB ACTIVITIES

1. Search the Internet for sites and resources on the Emergency Medical Services (EMS) system. Are there any cities or towns within 100 miles of your place of residence that do not use the EMS system?
2. What sites can you recommend to patients and their families who are looking for first-aid information about diabetes and heart attack?
3. What organizations could you use to search for information that deals with first aid for convulsions?
4. Search the Internet for information regarding first aid for insect stings.
5. What sites are available for information about poisonings?

REFERENCES/BIBLIOGRAPHY

American Heart Association. (2005). Adult basic life support. *Circulation, 112,* IV19–IV34.

The American National Red Cross. (2001). *Staywell.* St. Louis, MO: Mosby-Year Book.

American Red Cross. (2005). *CPR and emergency cardiac care: New CPR guidelines for professionals and non-professionals.* Retrieved September 19, 2007, from http://www.redcross.org/cpr.html.

Consumer Reports on Health. (2008). *Consumer Unions, 20,* 7, 3.

Medical Reserve Corps. (2008). *Emergency medical care.* Retrieved September 17, 2007, from http://www.medicalreservecorps.gov.

National Institutes of Health. (2008). *New CPR guidelines.* Retrieved September 17, 2007, from http://www.health.nih.gov.

Taber's cyclopedic medical dictionary (21st ed.). (2003). Philadelphia: F. A. Davis.

THE DVD HOOK-UP

In this chapter, you learned about proper techniques to follow during emergency situations. In the designated DVD clip, we observed the medical assistant screening a call from a mother whose child was experiencing an asthma attack. The medical assistant used a triage manual to assist her in screening the call accurately. With the aid of the triage manual, the medical assistant instructs the mother to call the EMS. The mother refuses to call the EMS and decides to bring the child into the office. The mother hangs up the phone before the doctor gets a chance to speak with her. The next scene shows the mother bringing the child into the office in respiratory distress. The medical assistant and provider work together as a team to get the patient's breathing stabilized.

1. Do you think that it was wise of the medical assistant to take the extra time to ask screening questions once the mother stated that the child was having an asthma attack? Why or why not?
2. Why is it necessary for you to follow an approved triage manual if you are put into the role of screening patient calls?
3. Why was it important to get the patient's phone number at the beginning of the call?

DVD Journal Summary

Write a paragraph that summarizes what you learned from watching the designated scene from today's DVD program. What are some things you can do to help you know how to respond to emergencies before they happen?

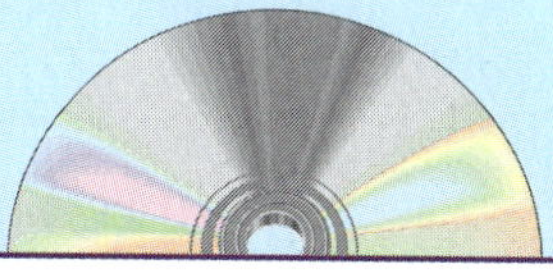

DVD Series	**Program Number**
Skills Based Series	8

Chapter/Scene Reference
- *Triaging Phone Emergencies*

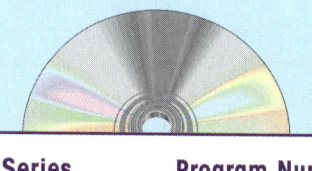

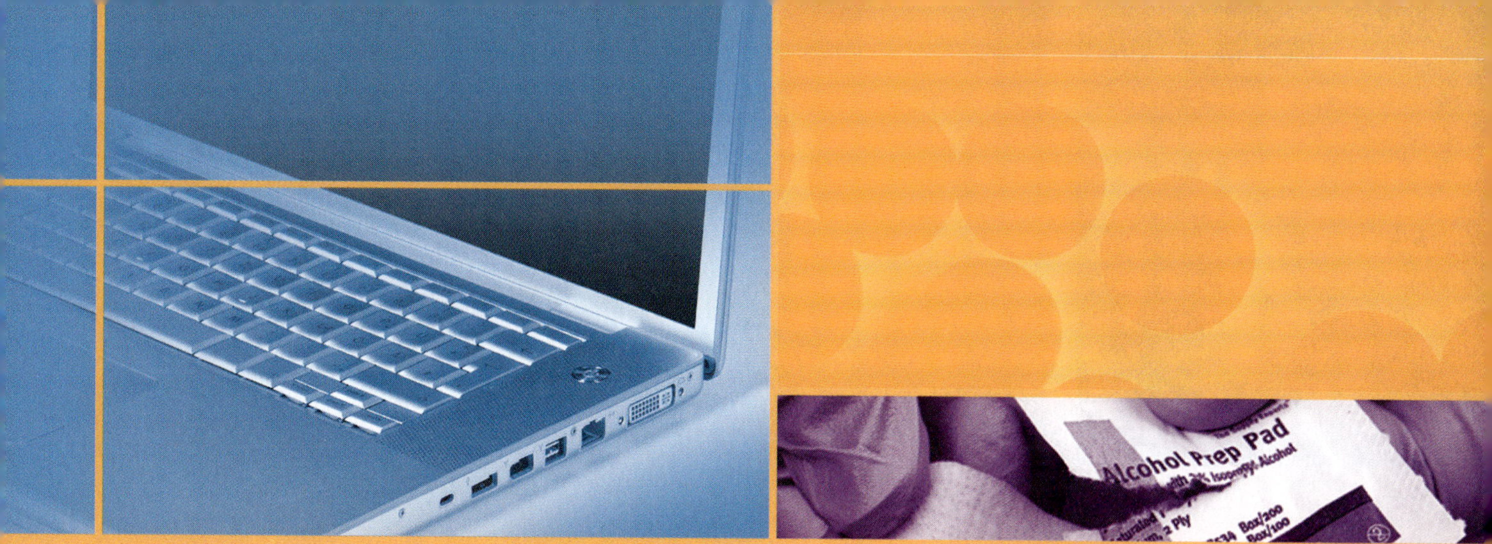

SECTION

II

Clinical Procedures

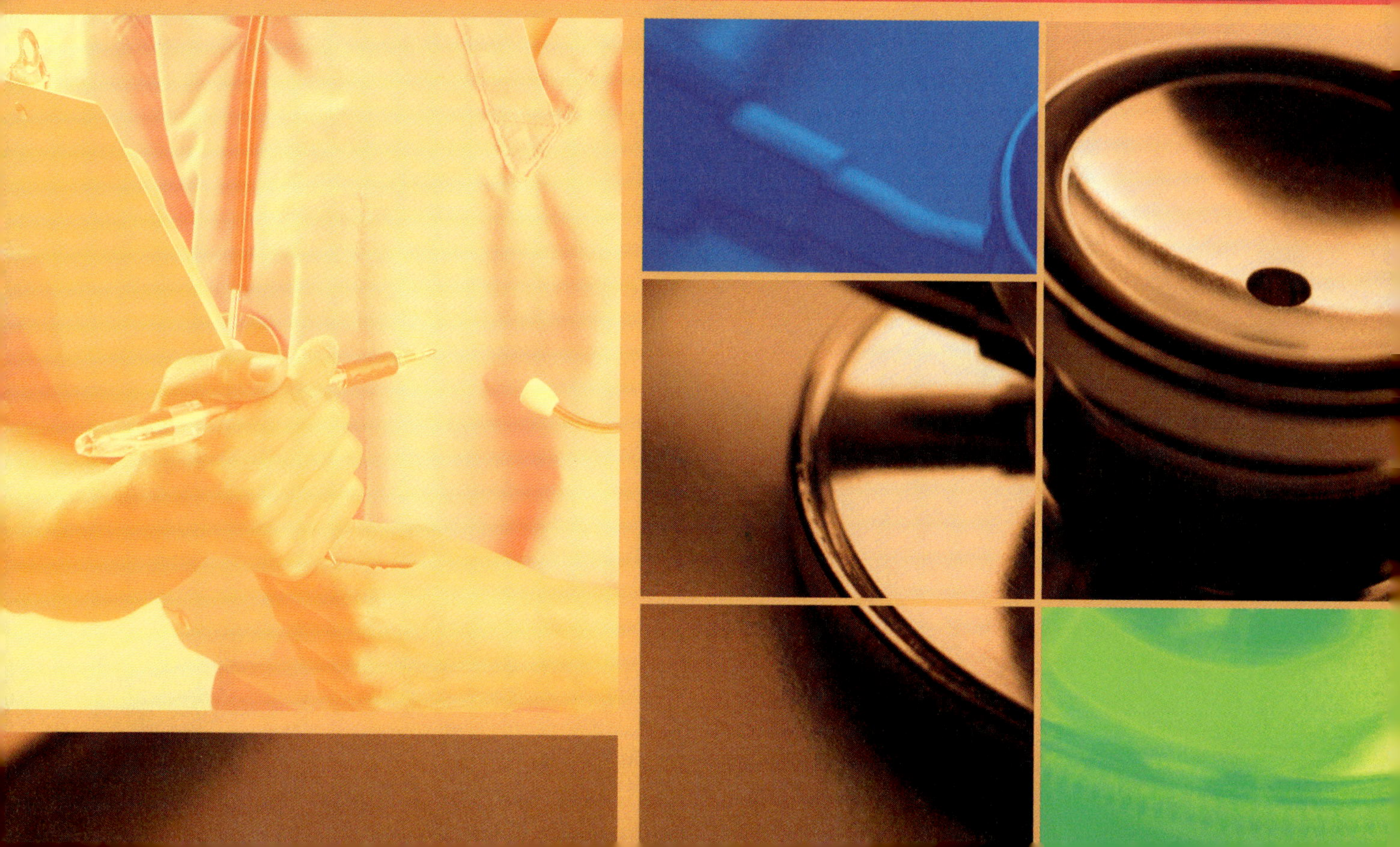

UNIT 4

Integrated Clinical Procedures

Infection Control and Medical Asepsis

Chapter 10

KEY TERMS

- Acquired Immunodeficiency Syndrome (AIDS)
- Acyclovir
- Airborne Transmission
- Amoebic Dysentery
- Antibodies
- Asepsis
- Barrier
- Bloodborne Pathogen
- Carrier
- Caustic
- Cell-Mediated Immunity
- Communicable
- Contact Transmission
- Contracting
- Coryza
- Cough Etiquette
- Debris
- Declination Form
- Droplet Transmission
- Epidemic
- Epidemiology
- Excoriated
- Excretion
- Expectorate
- Fomite
- Gross Contamination
- Human Immunodeficiency Virus (HIV)
- Humoral Immunity
- Immune System
- Immunoglobulins
- Immunomodulator
- Immunosuppressed

OUTLINE

- Impact of Infectious Diseases
- The Process of Infection
  - Growth Requirements for Microorganisms
- Chain of Infection
  - Infectious Agents
  - Reservoir
  - Portal of Exit
  - Means of Transmission
  - Portal of Entry
  - Susceptible Host
- The Body's Defense Mechanisms for Fighting Infection and Disease
  - The Body's Natural Barriers
  - Inflammatory Response
  - The Immune System and Immunity
- Stages of Infectious Diseases
  - Incubation Stage
  - Prodromal Stage
  - Acute Stage
  - Declining Stage
  - Convalescent Stage
- Disease Transmission
- Human Immunodeficiency Virus and Hepatitis B and C
  - HIV and AIDS
  - Acute Viral Hepatitis Diseases
- Reporting Infectious Disease
- Standard Precautions
  - Transmission-Based Precautions
  - Blood and Body Fluids
  - Personal Protective Equipment
  - Needlestick
  - Disposal of Infectious Waste
  - Federal Organizations and Infection Control
- OSHA Regulations
  - The Bloodborne Pathogen Standard
- OSHA Regulations and Students
  - Avoiding Exposure to Bloodborne Pathogens
- Principles of Infection Control
- Medical Asepsis
  - Hand Washing
  - Sanitization
  - Disinfection
- Bioterrorism

OBJECTIVES

The student should strive to meet the following performance objectives and demonstrate an understanding of the facts and principles presented in this chapter through written and oral communication.

1. Define the key terms as presented in the glossary.
2. Define and state the critical importance of infection control in the ambulatory care setting.
3. Outline the six links in the chain of infection.
4. Define the five classifications of infectious microorganisms.

OBJECTIVES (continued)

5. Recall and elaborate on the four phases the immune system uses to defend against infectious disease.
6. State the four stages of infectious diseases.
7. Recall at least five infectious diseases, their agents of transmission, and their symptoms.
8. Compare the routes of transmission of AIDS and hepatitis B and C and discuss the risk for infection from needlestick.
9. Describe the purpose of Standard Precautions and give six examples of ways health care providers should practice Standard Precautions.
10. Differentiate among the three types of Transmission-Based Precautions, defining what they are and how they are applied.
11. List eight types of body fluids and give an example of each.
12. Describe personal protective equipment.
13. Recognize five situations in which exposure to a patient's blood can occur, and discuss why Standard Precautions are important.
14. Describe proper disposal of infectious waste.
15. List human fluids that may contain HIV, HBV, and HCV.
16. Define medical asepsis.
17. Define bioterrorism and describe five agents that could be used in a bioterrorism attack.

KEY TERMS (continued)

Infection Control
Infectious Agent
Inflammatory Response
Inoculation
Isolation
Isolation Categories
Jet Injection
Lesion
Lymphadenopathy
Macular
Malaise
Malaria
Medical Asepsis
Microorganism
Morbidity
Mortality
Normal Flora
Nosocomial
Opportunistic Infections
Palliative
Papular
Parenteral
Pathogen
Pruritus
Regulated Waste
Resistance
Scabies
Scoop Technique
Secretion
Severe Acute Respiratory Syndrome (SARS)
Sharps
Solvent
Spill Kit
Sputum
Standard Precautions
Transmission-Based Precautions
Trichomoniasis
Ultrasonic Cleaner
Universal Precautions
Vaccine

KEY TERMS (continued)

Vector

Vesicular

Virulence

Scenario

At Inner City Health Care, a multiprovider urgent care center, medical assistant Bruce Goldman, CMA (AAMA), assumes responsibility for all infection control measures taken in the ambulatory care setting. In addition to his daily responsibilities related to medical and surgical asepsis, Bruce also makes it a point to stay current with infection control principles. Recently, Bruce attended a workshop about infection control. The Centers for Disease Control and Prevention (CDC) discussed that adults, just like children, need immunizations to stay well. The immunizations help prevent diseases that affect millions of adults per year. The diseases, according to the National Coalition for Adult Immunization and the CDC, can lead to hospitalization or death.

Joe learned that as many as 200,000 adults die yearly of flu-related illnesses; pneumonia causes 40,000 deaths per year; adults are 25 times more likely to die of chickenpox, and most adults with hepatitis B and C do not know that they are infected. These and other adult vaccines are available to prevent the flu, pneumonia, hepatitis A and B, measles, mumps, and rubella, tetanus, diphtheria, chickenpox, pertussis, herpes zoster, and human papillomavirus.

INTRODUCTION

Infectious diseases have plagued humans since the beginning of time. Recent scientific advances have changed our thoughts and behaviors regarding infectious disease. Advances such as antibiotic therapy and vaccination have significantly reduced risks for mortality from some previously fatal or debilitating infectious diseases. Infectious diseases that once were highly feared because of their likelihood of causing premature death are now preventable or treatable, causing us to forget the ***virulence*** *and destructive potential of epidemics of infectious disease. The presence of acquired immunodeficiency syndrome (AIDS) as an incurable and fatal infectious disease (although people are living with HIV and AIDS for many years), as well as* ***severe acute respiratory syndrome (SARS),*** *West Nile virus, avian flu, hepatitis C virus (HCV), and others, have caused the world to realize the enduring impact of pathogens on the human race.*

Although these medical advances have reduced the incidence of ***mortality*** *and* ***morbidity*** *from infectious diseases, humans must never underestimate the potential of resurgent infectious diseases. Tuberculosis has been the single leading cause of death in the history of humankind, yet was drastically reduced with the discovery of antituberculosis drugs. Today, however, the tuberculosis organism may be found that has adapted to the drugs, thereby becoming resistant to our only line of defense. Medical assistants must pay close attention to the prevention of infectious diseases.*

This chapter addresses the principles of the process of infection and control measures for use in ambulatory care settings. Because medical assistants deal directly with patients and other health care professionals, stringent adherence to the principles can greatly reduce transmission, or spread, of infectious disease. Continuous reliance on infection control measures ensures a clinical environment that is as safe as possible for employees, patients, and families. When infection control principles are not followed, infectious diseases may be transmitted to self, coworkers, or patients. The goals of infection control are to limit the presence of ***infectious agents,*** *to create barriers against transmission, and to decrease the risk to others for contracting infectious diseases. These goals can*

Spotlight on Certification

RMA Content Outline

- Asepsis
- Bloodborne pathogens and Universal (Standard) Precautions

CMA (AAMA) Content Outline

- Legislation
- Federal compliance
- Principles of infection control
- Medical asepsis
- Equipment preparation and operation
- Safety precautions

CMAS Content Outline

- Asepsis in the medical office

be achieved through medical asepsis and sterilization, by observation of all Standard Precautions and Transmission-Based Precautions set forth by the CDC, and by following the Occupational Safety and Health Administration (OSHA) guidelines.

IMPACT OF INFECTIOUS DISEASES

Since the discovery of the germ theory by Louis Pasteur and Robert Koch in the nineteenth century, we have seen dramatic changes in global mortality and morbidity statistics from infectious diseases. Many scientists devoted their professional lives to the quest for the prevention and cure of infectious diseases, which were the main cause of death in earlier centuries. In developed countries, deaths from diseases such as tuberculosis, pneumonia, and smallpox have been significantly reduced because of pharmacologic agents such as antibiotics and **vaccines.** Antibiotic agents were widely introduced during World War II, reducing deaths from traumatic wound infections. Edward Jenner is credited with the discovery of the first vaccine to protect against the deadly disease smallpox. Because of the vaccine, smallpox is considered to have been eradicated worldwide.

Epidemiology is the science that studies the history, cause, and patterns of infectious diseases. This field of medicine is credited to a Japanese bacteriologist in the late nineteenth century who recognized the connection between bubonic plague and rat infestation. Recent epidemiological studies have traced infectious diseases such as AIDS from the beginning of the epidemic. The future of studies in infectious diseases will focus on increasing the pharmacologic (drugs) war against infectious diseases.

Reliance only on treatment of infectious disease does not address the crucial step in the spread of infectious diseases, that is, of prevention, or **infection control.** Emerging issues related to infectious diseases involve microorganisms that are resistant to present technology, **bloodborne pathogen** transmission, increased **immunosuppressed** populations, and global access to infection control and treatment. Developed countries become accustomed to antiinfectious medications, clean water, and laws that protect the public from infectious agents found in food and other consumables. These safety measures may not be present in other countries where political or economic factors limit access to infection control measures.

In the future, drug-resistant infectious diseases will place greater emphasis on prevention because there may never be a safe and universally effective drug for all infectious diseases.

Study of the history of infectious diseases allows us to realize the impact these diseases have on the lifestyles of people in various cultures. Infectious diseases such as AIDS and other sexually transmitted diseases have differing levels of social or cultural impact. Medical assistants should be aware of facts regarding the infectious process of specific diseases to reduce cultural isolation for the patient and to dispel myths regarding infectious diseases (see Chapter 6).

THE PROCESS OF INFECTION

Infectious diseases are caused by pathogenic microorganisms that are capable of causing disease. **Microorganisms** are microscopic living creatures capable of reproduction and transmission in specific circumstances. **Pathogens** are microorganisms that can cause infectious disease. Although all pathogens are capable of causing disease, not all microorganisms cause disease. Many microorganisms are necessary for human, animal, and plant life survival. In the absence of microorganisms, life would not be possible. The term **normal flora** is used to recognize the beneficial role of microorganisms in certain parts of the body, in which microorganisms normally occupy space and use nutrients, thus retarding the potential of pathogenic growth in that specific body area. A fundamental concept in the study of infectious disease is that similar steps or phases occur in all infectious diseases; however, each specific microorganism causes unique characteristics and alterations in the process of infection. Medical assistants must apply the theoretical process of infectious disease growth and transmission to relate to specific pathogens. The goal is to reduce transmission and incidence of infectious diseases in patients, employees, and families.

Growth Requirements for Microorganisms

For microorganisms to survive and thrive, a suitable environment must be available to them. Following is a list of growth requirements for microorganisms:

- *Oxygen:* An aerobic microorganism needs oxygen to live; most pathogenic microorganisms need oxygen to survive: for example, *streptococcus* as in a "strep" throat
- *Lack of or no oxygen:* An anaerobic microorganism needs little or no oxygen to live; two examples are tetanus and gas gangrene
- *Moisture:* Microorganisms grow well in a moist environment; the body provides moisture
- *Nutrition:* The body supplies plenty of nutrients
- *Temperature:* The body's temperature of approximately 98.6°F is an optimum temperature for growth of microorganisms
- *Darkness:* The body's cavities and organs provide darkness
- *Neutral or slightly alkaline pH:* The body's fluids are neutral when in a healthy state

Through the understanding of the optimum growth requirements for microorganisms to grow and multiply, elimination of any or all of the factors helps keep microorganisms from growing and causing infection.

CHAIN OF INFECTION

For infectious diseases to spread, several necessary steps must occur. These steps, or links, are known as the "chain of infection." Each link or step in the infectious process must occur for the spread of infection to take place. Infection control is based on the fact that the transmission of infectious diseases will be prevented when any of the levels in the chain are broken or interrupted (Figure 10-1). The steps are:

1. Infectious agent
2. Reservoir
3. Portal of exit
4. Means of transmission
5. Portal of entry
6. Susceptible host

Infectious Agents

Infectious agents are microorganisms that can be grouped into five classifications: viruses, bacteria, fungi, parasites, and rickettsia. For an infection to occur, an infectious agent or microorganism must be present. When infectious diseases are identified according to the specific disease-causing microorganism, the disease may be prevented with the use of antiinfective drugs or infection control practices. Each of the five classifications of infectious microorganisms will be explored.

Viruses. Viruses are pathogens that require a living cell for reproduction and activity. These microorganisms are considered intracellular parasites, because they must live inside cells to multiply. They do so by altering particles of genetic material, such as DNA (deoxyribonucleic acid) or RNA (ribonucleic acid). Because viruses live inside cells, they are protected against agents such as chemical disinfectants and antibiotics. To survive, viruses have a notable characteristic of being able to change specific characteristics over time. For instance, viruses can adapt to their environment so they remain resistant to efforts to limit their growth. Viral infections have only a few pharmacologic treatment agents, and usually these agents are **palliative** because they only relieve symptoms of the disease instead of curing the infection. Some viral infections can be prevented by vaccination (Table 10-1). Figures 10-2A and B show the CDC's recommended adult immunization schedules.

Bacteria. Bacteria are single-celled microorganisms that live in tissues rather than in body cells and are identified by characteristic shapes, or morphology. Bacteria may also be grouped according to ability to accept laboratory staining agents. Gram-negative bacteria stain visibly red under the microscope, whereas gram-positive bacteria stain purple. The bacteria that do not accept stain are

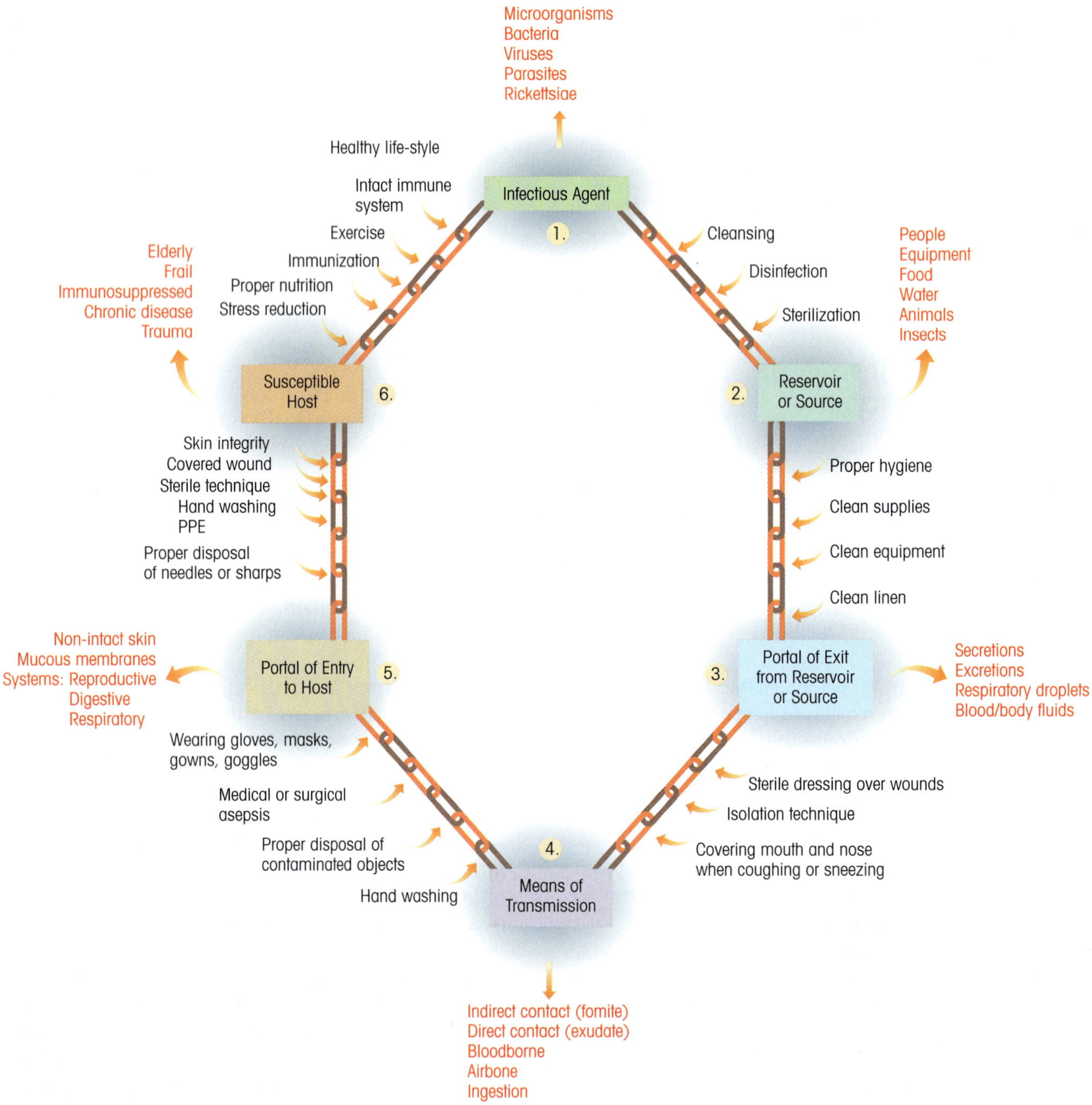

Figure 10-1 Health care worker's interventions used to break the chain of infection transmission.

considered spores, which are bacteria with a covering that protects them from many chemical disinfectants and higher levels of heat. The three classifications of bacteria are cocci (sphere or dot shaped), bacilli (rod shaped), and spirilla (spiral shaped). Bacteria are either pathogenic or nonpathogenic. Nonpathogenic bacteria normally reside on the skin of humans and in mucous membrane areas of the body. These are known as *normal flora.* Nonpathogenic bacteria use nutrients and occupy space, competing with the pathogenic bacteria. When nonpathogenic bacteria are reduced, the opportunity exists for pathogenic organisms to take over and cause infectious disease. A common cause of the reduction of nonpathogenic microorganisms is the use of antibiotic drugs. Examples of

Table 10-1 Common Viral Diseases

Disease/Agent	Type of Infection and Site	Vaccine Availability
Herpes groups		
Herpes Simplex Virus 1 (HSV-1) (Figure 10-3)	Cold sores/keratitis	No
Herpes Simplex Virus 2 (HSV-2) (Figure 10-3)	Genital herpes	No
Herpes zoster	Shingles (neurons)	Yes*
Rubeola	Measles	Yes
Rubella	German measles	Yes
Poliovirus	Poliomyelitis	Yes
Influenza (ABC)	Flu, pneumonia	Yes
Human papillomavirus	Genital warts, cervical cancer	Yes
Hepatitis (A, B, C, D, E)	Liver	A, B
Epstein-Barr	Infectious mononucleosis	No
Varicella zoster	Chickenpox (skin)	Yes

*The Advisory Council on Immunization Practice (ACIP) recommended to the CDC that adults over age 60 years receive the Zestavar vaccine. The CDC has given provisional approval.

some bacterial pathogens are listed in Table 10-2 and shown in Figure 10-4.

Fungi. Fungi are microorganisms that may be unicellular (single-cell) or multicellular (many cells). Mushrooms and molds are examples of fungi that are nonpathogenic. Pathogenic fungi cause athlete's foot, ringworm, and candida infections (Figure 10-5). Other pathogenic fungi include histoplasmosis and toxoplasmosis, which are fungal infections spread through the air from infected fowl and bird waste.

Parasites. Organisms that live in or on another organism are classified as parasites. They may be single-celled or multicelled. Examples include protozoa (single-cell microscopic organisms that cause **malaria, amoebic dysentery,** and **trichomoniasis** [Figure 10-6]); metazoa (multicellular organisms that cause pinworms, hookworms, and tapeworms); and ectoparasites (multicellular organisms that live superficially on another host, such as lice and **scabies**).

Rickettsiae. Rickettsiae are intracellular parasitic, small nonmotive bacteria. They are larger than viruses and can be seen under conventional microscopes after staining procedures. These microorganisms are susceptible to antibiotic therapy. Examples of rickettsial infections include typhus (transmitted by the body louse); Lyme disease (transmitted by ticks); and Rocky Mountain spotted fever (transmitted by ticks). Characteristic of rickettsia infections is a skin rash caused by the rickettsia invading the small blood vessels. This appears on the skin as a small hemorrhagic rash.

Reservoir

The second link in the chain of infection is the reservoir or location of the infectious agent. Reservoirs are people, equipment, supplies, water, food, and animals or insects (known as vectors). Methods of infection control in the reservoir link include hand washing, environmental hygiene, disinfection, sterilization, and maintenance of employee

Recommended Adult Immunization Schedule

UNITED STATES · 2009

Note: These recommendations *must* be read with the footnotes containing number of doses, intervals between doses, and other important information.

Figure 1. Recommended adult immunization schedule, by vaccine and age group

<table>
<tr><th>VACCINE ▼ / AGE GROUP ▶</th><th>19–26 years</th><th>27–49 years</th><th>50–59 years</th><th>60–64 years</th><th>≥65 years</th></tr>
<tr><td>Tetanus, diphtheria, pertussis (Td/Tdap)*</td><td colspan="4">Substitute 1-time dose of Tdap for Td booster; then boost with Td every 10 yrs</td><td>Td booster every 10 yrs</td></tr>
<tr><td>Human papillomavirus (HPV)*</td><td>3 doses (females)</td><td></td><td></td><td></td><td></td></tr>
<tr><td>Varicella*</td><td colspan="5">2 doses</td></tr>
<tr><td>Zoster</td><td></td><td></td><td></td><td colspan="2">1 dose</td></tr>
<tr><td>Measles, mumps, rubella (MMR)*</td><td colspan="2">1 or 2 doses</td><td colspan="3">1 dose</td></tr>
<tr><td>Influenza*</td><td colspan="5">1 dose annually</td></tr>
<tr><td>Pneumococcal (polysaccharide)</td><td colspan="4">1 or 2 doses</td><td>1 dose</td></tr>
<tr><td>Hepatitis A*</td><td colspan="5">2 doses</td></tr>
<tr><td>Hepatitis B*</td><td colspan="5">3 doses</td></tr>
<tr><td>Meningococcal*</td><td colspan="5">1 or more doses</td></tr>
</table>

*Covered by the Vaccine Injury Compensation Program.

- For all persons in this category who meet the age requirements and who lack evidence of immunity (e.g., lack documentation of vaccination or have no evidence of prior infection)
- Recommended if some other risk factor is present (e.g., on the basis of medical, occupational, lifestyle, or other indications)
- No recommendation

Report all clinically significant postvaccination reactions to the Vaccine Adverse Event Reporting System (VAERS). Reporting forms and instructions on filing a VAERS report are available at www.vaers.hhs.gov or by telephone, 800-822-7967. Information on how to file a Vaccine Injury Compensation Program claim is available at www.hrsa.gov/vaccinecompensation or by telephone, 800-338-2382. To file a claim for vaccine injury, contact the U.S. Court of Federal Claims, 717 Madison Place, N.W., Washington, D.C. 20005; telephone, 202-357-6400.

Additional information about the vaccines in this schedule, extent of available data, and contraindications for vaccination is also available at www.cdc.gov/vaccines or from the CDC-INFO Contact Center at 800-CDC-INFO (800-232-4636) in English and Spanish, 24 hours a day, 7 days a week. Use of trade names and commercial sources is for identification only and does not imply endorsement by the U.S. Department of Health and Human Services.

The recommendations in this schedule were approved by the:

Centers for Disease Control and Prevention's (CDC) Advisory Committee on Immunization Practices (ACIP)

American Academy of Family Physicians (AAFP)

American College of Obstetricians and Gynecologists (ACOG)

American College of Physicians (ACP)

CS124645

Figure 10-2A Recommended adult immunization schedule, by vaccine and age group. (Courtesy of the Centers for Disease Control and Prevention.)

Figure 2. Vaccines that might be indicated for adults based on medical and other indications

VACCINE ▼ / INDICATION ▶	Pregnancy	Immuno-compromising conditions (excluding human immunodeficiency virus [HIV])	HIV infection CD4+ T lymphocyte count <200 cells/μL	HIV infection CD4+ T lymphocyte count ≥200 cells/μL	Diabetes, heart disease, chronic lung disease, chronic alcoholism	Asplenia (including elective splenectomy and terminal complement component deficiencies)	Chronic liver disease	Kidney failure, end-stage renal disease, receipt of hemodialysis	Health-care personnel
Tetanus, diphtheria, pertussis (Td/Tdap)*	Td	Substitute 1-time dose of Tdap for Td booster; then boost with Td every 10 yrs							
Human papillomavirus (HPV)*		3 doses for females through age 26 yrs							
Varicella*	Contraindicated			2 doses					
Zoster	Contraindicated				1 dose				
Measles, mumps, rubella (MMR)*	Contraindicated			1 or 2 doses					
Influenza*	1 dose TIV annually								1 dose TIV or LAIV annually
Pneumococcal (polysaccharide)	1 or 2 doses								
Hepatitis A*	2 doses								
Hepatitis B*	3 doses								
Meningococcal*	1 or more doses								

*Covered by the Vaccine Injury Compensation Program.

- Yellow: For all persons in this category who meet the age requirements and who lack evidence of immunity (e.g., lack documentation of vaccination or have no evidence of prior infection)
- Purple: Recommended if some other risk factor is present (e.g., on the basis of medical, occupational, lifestyle, or other indications)
- White: No recommendation

These schedules indicate the recommended age groups and medical indications for which administration of currently licensed vaccines is commonly indicated for adults ages 19 years and older, as of January 1, 2009. Licensed combination vaccines may be used whenever any components of the combination are indicated and when the vaccine's other components are not contraindicated. For detailed recommendations on all vaccines, including those used primarily for travelers or that are issued during the year, consult the manufacturers' package inserts and the complete statements from the Advisory Committee on Immunization Practices (www.cdc.gov/vaccines/pubs/acip-list.htm).

DEPARTMENT OF HEALTH AND HUMAN SERVICES
CENTERS FOR DISEASE CONTROL AND PREVENTION

Figure 10-2B Recommended adult immunization schedule, by vaccine and medical and other indications. (Courtesy of the Centers for Disease Control and Prevention.)

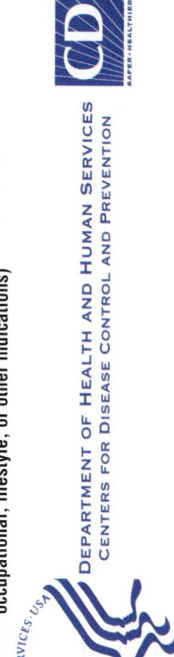

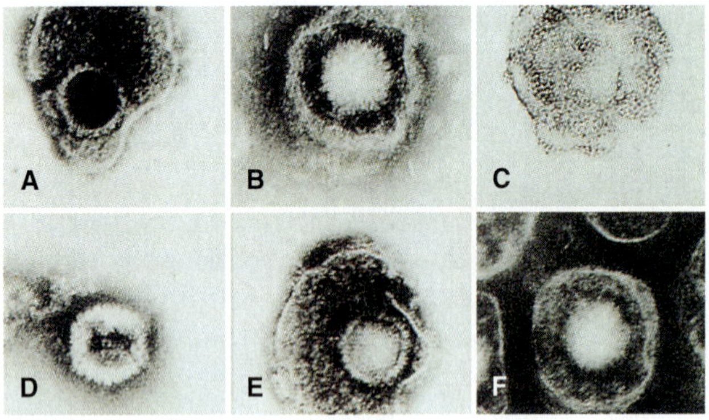

Figure 10-3 Electron micrographs of various types of herpes simplex virus. (Courtesy of the Centers for Disease Control and Prevention, Atlanta, GA)

health standards, such as annual tuberculosis skin testing.

Portal of Exit

Although the infectious agent is housed or living in the reservoir, it must leave the reservoir to infect another person. The portal of exit is the method by which an infectious agent leaves the reservoir. Microorganisms may leave the human body with normally occurring body fluids, such as **excretions, secretions,** skin cells, respiratory droplets, blood, or any body fluid. The portal of exit may be continuous, such as with respiratory droplets, or dependent on the body fluid exiting the body under unusual circumstances, such as when blood leaves the body during a surgical procedure or phlebotomy.

Table 10-2 Examples of Infectious Bacterial Diseases

Disease	Infectious Agent	Mode of Transmission
Anthrax	*Bacillus anthracis*	Inhalation
Chlamydia (sexually transmitted disease)	*Chlamydia trachomatis*	Sexual contact
Clostridial myonecrosis (gas gangrene)	Species of gram-positive clostridia	Wound entry
Escherichia coli	Gram-negative bacilli	Ingestion, wound entry
Gonorrhea (sexually transmitted disease)	*Neisseria gonorrhoeae*	Sexual contact
Legionnaire's disease (pneumonia)	*Legionella pneumophila*	Inhalation
Nosocomial (hospital-acquired) infection	Gram-negative bacteria	Normal flora transmitted during illness/procedures; opportunistic pathogens transmitted during debilitated condition
Pneumococci	*Streptococcus pneumoniae*	Respiratory (inhalation)
Staphylococcal infection (abscesses, food poisoning, urinary tract infections)	*Staphylococci*	Direct contact, ingestion, inhalation, bloodborne, vectors (animals)
Streptococcal infection (strep throat, otitis media, pneumonia)	Hemolytic *streptococci* (usually beta-hemolytic group A)	Inhalation
Syphilis (sexually transmitted disease)	*Treponema pallidum*	Sexual contact
Tetanus (lockjaw)	*Clostridium tetani*	Wound entry
Typhoid fever (enteric fever)	*Salmonella typhi*	Fecal-oral

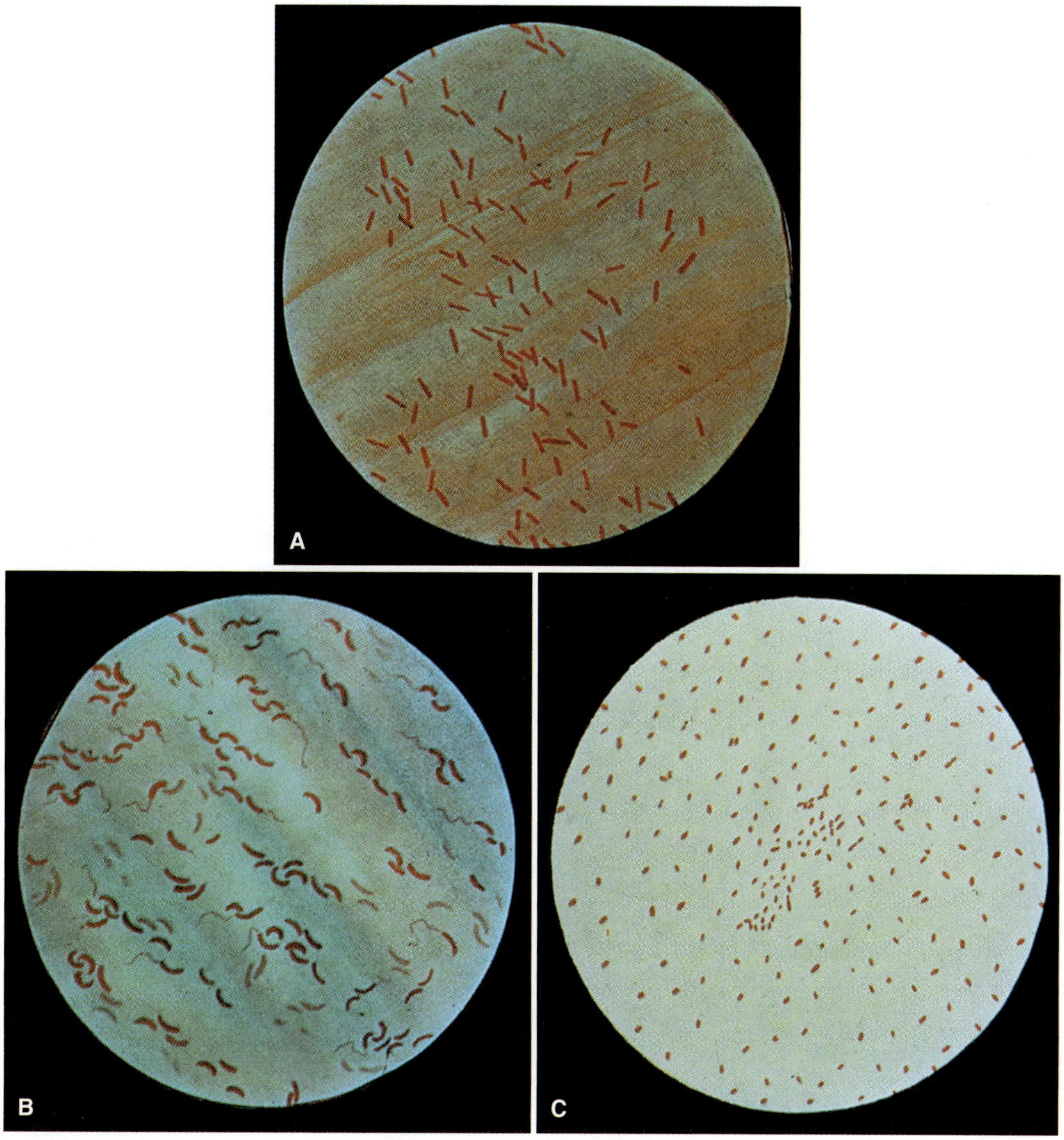

Figure 10-4 Bacterial forms: (A) *Escherichia coli,* (B) *Haemophilus pertussis,* (C) *Vibria cholerae.* (Courtesy of the Centers for Disease Control and Prevention, Atlanta, GA.)

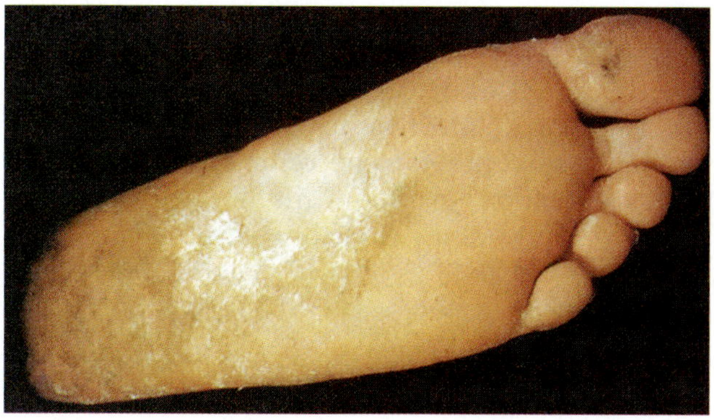

Figure 10-5 Ringworm of the foot (tinea pedis). (Courtesy of the Centers for Disease Control and Prevention, Atlanta, GA.)

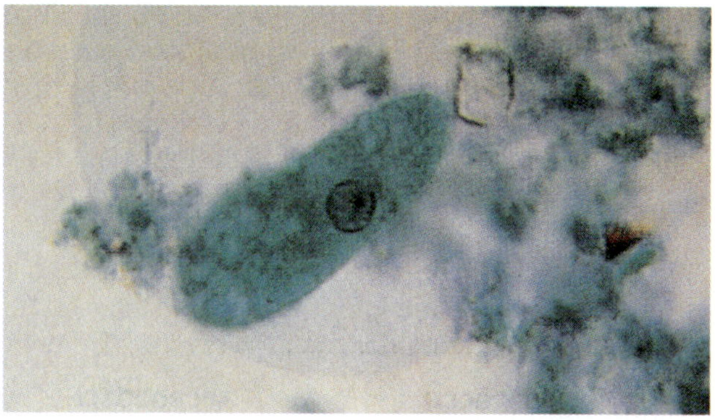

Figure 10-6 Intestinal protozoa, *Entamoeba coli.* (Courtesy of the Centers for Disease Control and Prevention, Atlanta, GA.)

Standard Precautions and **Transmission-Based Precautions** are infection control methods based on the knowledge that infectious diseases exiting the body can be spread to others. These precautions attempt to control the spread of infectious diseases as infectious agents leave or exit the reservoir.

Means of Transmission

The means of transmission are specific ways in which microorganisms travel from one place (reservoir) to another (susceptible host). Transmission depends on the characteristics of the microorganisms. Types of routes of transmission include:

- Direct contact (touching the exudate [drainage] from a person with an infected wound)
- Airborne transmission (inhaling the microorganism, such as mycobacterium tuberculosis [TB] into the susceptible host's respiratory system)
- Bloodborne transmission (infected blood enters susceptible host through blood or body fluids)
- Ingestion (eating or drinking contaminated items such as food or water)
- Indirect contact (microorganism, on a **fomite,** a nonliving object such as a table or piece of equipment that can retain and transmit infection, a doorknob or a fomite)
- **Vector** (a carrier of disease, usually an insect, such as a tick [Lyme disease] or mosquito [Eastern equine encephalitis])

Infection control measures in the ambulatory care area specifically address the transmission stage of the process of infection.

Methods that reduce the transmission of pathogens include adherence to Standard and Transmission-Based Precautions, hand washing, sanitization, disinfection, and sterilization. Methods of infection control are used in health care, food handling, water and sewage processing, and child care.

Portal of Entry

After being transmitted, the infectious agent must enter another person, or a susceptible host. The portal of entry allows the agent access to the next person. Common entrance sites to the human body include nonintact skin, mucous membranes, and systems of the body exposed to the external environment, such as the respiratory, gastrointestinal, and reproductive systems. Breathing in airborne microorganisms allows infectious diseases to be spread to the lungs. Eating or drinking contaminated water is a cause of gastrointestinal infectious diseases. Sexually transmitted diseases spread through vaginal, oral, and anal intercourse. Care of patients with infectious diseases includes careful consideration of infection control to limit further spread of the microorganism. Methods such as correct wound care, transmission-based precautions, and **aseptic** technique limit the transmission of infectious microorganisms. The portals of exit and entry need not be the same for infection to be transmitted.

Susceptible Host

Finally, for the infectious process to continue, microorganisms must enter another person who is susceptible. This means that the person is able to contract the pathogenic organism. The susceptible host is therefore not resistant or immune to the organism. Causes of susceptibility include the presence of other diseases, such as diabetes, immunosuppression (weakened immune system), HIV/AIDS, surgical procedures, trauma, or the absence of immunity to the specific microorganism. Susceptibility of a person depends on several factors, including:

1. Number and specific type of pathogen
2. Duration of exposure to the pathogen
3. General physical condition
4. Psychological health status
5. Occupation or lifestyle environment
6. Presence of underlying diseases or conditions
7. Youth or advanced age (young and old at greater risk)

The goal of infection control at this link in the chain of infection is to identify patients at risk for susceptibility, treat their underlying conditions if possible, and isolate them from those reservoirs that could be hazardous to the susceptible person.

Hospitalized patients are at risk for contracting a **nosocomial** infection. Surgical patients are especially susceptible to becoming infected. Nosocomial infections are found in all health care settings; nursing homes, and short-term care settings

Critical Thinking

Explain how to interrupt the transmission of infection.

such as clinics and ambulatory settings. These patients are at risk for being infected with the same pathogens as hospital patients.

A number of different pathogens are present in the hospital and other health care settings, and as new patients arrive, new pathogens are introduced to the facility. The overuse of antibiotics contributes to microorganisms becoming resistant to them. Some health care staff become carriers of these microorganisms. Table 10-3 provides information about methicillin-resistant *Staphylococcus aureus* (MRSA).

Patients have compromised immune systems for many reasons. Surgery opens the body to microorganisms, and radiation treatments, certain medications, catheters, and intravenous tubing all contribute to the means for infection to enter the body of a susceptible patient.

Nosocomial infections can occur from the hands of health care staff, equipment, and instruments. Hand washing and other methods of infection control and identification of vulnerable patients can help control nosocomial infections.

THE BODY'S DEFENSE MECHANISMS FOR FIGHTING INFECTION AND DISEASE

The Body's Natural Barriers

The body has many natural barriers and defenses in place to help us avoid exposure to pathogens and infection.

These barriers can be categorized under physical/mechanical, chemical, and cellular factors. Physical/mechanical factors include eyelashes and eyebrows, cilia (tiny hairs in the respiratory tract), and barriers such as eyelids and intact skin/mucous membranes. Chemical barriers include tears, sweat, mucus, saliva, gastrointestinal secretions, and vaginal secretions. Cellular barriers are also called body defenses and consist of white blood cells, which defend against infection in many ways in tissues, bloodstream, and lymphatic system. Cellular defenses are explained in more detail in the following two sections.

Inflammatory Response

Inflammation is the body's natural way of responding when invaded by a pathogen or physical trauma. Inflammation is a nonspecific response, meaning that it can occur with any threat to the body, not just in reaction to a particular pathogen. Inflammation can occur regardless of whether it is caused by an agent that is pathogenic, a trauma, a foreign body, or extremes in temperature. If a pathogen is present, the body goes through a distinct process in an attempt to destroy and eliminate the pathogenic microorganisms and their by-products and, if that is not possible, to restrict the amount of damage done.

The cardinal signs of inflammation are redness, heat, swelling, and pain. These symptoms may be slight, almost unnoticed, or quite evident. Remember, inflammation is a natural response and does not necessarily indicate infection. The two should not be confused. Inflammation can occur without infection, but infection does not occur without inflammation.

The steps in the inflammatory process are:

- Local dilation of blood vessels increases blood flow to injured (infected) area causing redness or heat.
- Plasma moves into the tissue causing swelling and pain due to pressure on nerve endings.
- White blood cells move into injured tissue to fight infection and phagocytes destroy invading pathogens.

After destruction of the pathogen, tissue repair can begin. If the **inflammatory response** is not effective, the specific immune response is necessary.

Indications that an inflammatory process is inadequate are: (1) the accumulation of purulent matter (pus) in the area (due to destroyed pathogens, white blood cells, and body cells); (2) lymph node enlargement (swollen glands); and (3) septicemia, which may result because pathogens have spread to the bloodstream.

Immediate antibiotic therapy is indicated in these circumstances because of the inadequacy of the inflammatory response.

The Immune System and Immunity

To fight infectious diseases, our bodies are equipped with several effective physical and chemical **barriers** such as the skin, mucous membranes, body excretions and secretions, and a complex, highly specific **immune system.** The immune system's purpose is to protect against pathogens and abnormal cell growth. The system is composed of various cells that collectively recognize, subdue, attack, and eliminate pathogens. The two types of immune responses include

Table 10-3 Examples of Infectious Diseases

Disease	Agent	Transmission	Symptoms	Diagnosis	Treatment	Comments	Patient Education
Acquired immunodeficiency syndrome (AIDS)	Human immunodeficiency virus (HIV)	• Bloodborne • Sexual contact • Intrauterine • Lactation	Opportunistic infections, **lymphadenopathy,** fatigue, malaise, fever	CD4 T-cell level less than 200/mm^3; Viral count Chest X-ray CBC	Palliative care and treatment for **opportunistic infections,** antiviral drugs	World Health Organization (WHO) estimates global statistics 40 million people living with HIV/AIDS (2006)	1. Careful infection control and asepsis to reduce contact with pathogens that cause opportunistic infections 2. Use of latex condoms in conjunction with effective spermicide 3. Support groups/education
**Avian influenza H5NI (bird flu)	Flu virus A found in birds	• Infected birds spread virus to susceptible birds through bird saliva, nasal secretions, and feces. • Direct human contact with infected birds (domesticated chickens, ducks, turkeys) or surfaces contaminated with secretions/excretions of infected birds has resulted in humans contracting H5NI. • Virus does not usually infect humans but can occur.	Flu-like cough, sore throat, fever, muscle aches, pneumonia, severe respiratory diseases, life-threatening and severe symptoms	Swab of nose and/or throat to check for avian flu using a molecular test; lab may attempt to grow the virus; these two laboratory tests are best performed within the first few days of illness.	H5NI is resistant to two antiviral medications now used for the flu; perhaps two other antiviral medications could help treat H5NI but more study is needed; symptomatic treatment	Virus does not usually affect humans, but confirmed human infections have been reported since 1997 and of those who have become infected, according to the CDC, more than 50% have died; influenza viruses have ability to change their form and there is concern that H5NI could infect humans and spread from person to person; because the viruses do not usually infect humans, there is little or no immune protection in humans; scientists are concerned about a worldwide outbreak and are closely watching and preparing for that possibility; the WHO and vaccine manufacturers are moving toward creating a global stockpile of H5NI avian flu vaccine; there is a ban on imported poultry from countries affected by avian flu viruses including H5NI.	Very rare disease in humans. Does not infect humans easily. Does not spread easily from person to person. 1. Seasonal flu vaccination does not protect against avian flu. 2. Wash hands before and after handling raw poultry and eggs. 3. Clean cutting board and utensils with soap and water to keep raw poultry from contaminating other foods. 4. Cook poultry to internal temperature of 165 degrees; egg yolks and whites should be firm. 5. Practice **cough etiquette**.

Foodborne illnesses	Bacteria or viruses (i.e., staphylococci, clostridium, botulinum, *E. coli*, shigella)	• Ingestion of contaminated food or water	Nausea, stomach pain, vomiting, bloody diarrhea, dehydration, respiratory failure, death	Culture of feces, vomitus, or suspected food or water	Fluid balance restoration, medications, emergency treatment as required	Report outbreaks to local authorities; especially dangerous in children and older adults; undercooked meat, vegetables and fruits washed in dirty water can carry *E.coli.*	1. Teach proper food handling. 2. Carefully wash hands before handling all food. 3. Report to provider all signs of dehydration. 4. Gastroenteritis usually communicable via feces for up to 7 weeks after exposure.
Impetigo	*Streptococcus*	• Direct contact with moist discharges of the lesions	Vesicles become pustular, rupture, and form crusts; **pruritus**	Culture of discharge	Antibiotics po or IV if severe; local antibiotic ointment	Good hygiene is necessary to help prevent transmission; gloves should be worn when cleaning lesions; expose lesions to air to help dry; can be fatal if not treated properly.	1. Good hygiene necessary to help prevent transmission. 2. Can be fatal to newborns if not treated promptly. 3. Wear gloves when touching lesions.
Influenza	Influenza viruses A, B, or C, *Haemophilus* (bacteria)	• Inhalation • Aerosolized • Mucous droplets	Acute upper/lower respiratory infection, severe cough, fever, malaise, sore throat, **coryza**	Tissue culture of nasal or pharyngeal secretions	Palliative therapy, active immunization (annual vaccine recommended for persons at risk [older adults, heart patients] for complications from infection)	Report cases to local health authority; may be fatal in older adults and children; may cause meningitis; may easily become epidemic; 80% of elderly who contract the flu die.	1. Bed rest for 2–3 days after fever declines. 2. Force fluids. 3. Report signs of secondary infections (pneumonia, otitis media). 4. Vaccine available. 5. Practice cough etiquette.
Lyme disease	Bacteria (*Borrelia burgdorferi*)	• Transmitted by the bite of infected tick	Rash, flu-like symptoms, headache, fatigue, joint pain	Presence of symptoms; laboratory tests may be inconclusive, taking 6 weeks or more for antibodies to appear in the blood; erythrocyte sedimentation rate; total serum; Ig M level; aspartate aminotransferase level	Antibiotics, po or IV	The tick is so small and bite so mild, patients may not realized they were bitten for a few days to weeks later; bacteria spread to other sites, causing symptoms to heart, joints, and nervous system; arthritis develops and may become chronic.	1. Use insect repellant. 2. Remove tick promptly (save for laboratory testing if possible). 3. Wear pants tucked into socks when in wooded areas or where ticks are present. 4. Complete recovery usually occurs if treated with antibiotics. 5. Disease has exacerbations and remissions.

(continues)

Table 10-3 Examples of Infectious Diseases (continued)

Disease	Agent	Transmission	Symptoms	Diagnosis	Treatment	Comments	Patient Education
Meningitis	***Bacteria (more severe); *Neisseria meningitides* is one type) Virus	• Bacterial through exchange of respiratory and throat secretions (coughing, sneezing, shared drinking glasses, bottles, cans, cigarettes)	High fever, severe headache, stiff neck, nausea, rash, vomiting, confusion, sleepiness, seizures	Culture and sensitivity of cerebral spinal fluid	Appropriate antibiotics, vaccine available for the bacteria responsible for 75% of the disease (vaccine lasts 3–5 years)	Rare but potentially fatal disease; there are two forms of meningitis: (1) inflammation of brain and spinal cord, and (2) meningococcemia (infection in the blood). Bacterial meningitis is contagious but not spread by casual contact or by breathing the air where an infected person is present; leading cause of meningitis in older children and young adults; cases have doubled since 1991.	1. Meningitis usually peaks in late winter and early spring and can be mistaken for the flu. 2. High-risk persons are college students living in dorms, immunosuppressed individuals, and persons traveling to areas of world where meningitis is prevalent (these people should get vaccine). 3. The CDC can advise travelers about areas for which they recommend the vaccine be given.
**Methicillin-resistant *Staphylococcus aureus* infections (MRSA skin infections)	Bacteria (*Staphylococcus aureus*—"Staph") commonly found on skin and in nose of healthy persons	• Direct skin-to-skin contact (e.g., shaking hands, wrestling, other direct skin contact) • Shared towels or shared athletic equipment • Bacteria gain entrance to the body through any break in the skin	Pus-filled boils, pimples, and rashes; same symptoms as other "Staph" infections	Culture and sensitivity of discharge from infected site; blood and other body fluids can be tested by culture and sensitivity	Good wound and skin care; keep area clean and dry; wear gloves and wash hands after caring for site; antibiotics, but MRSA is resistant to many common antibiotics	In the past MRSA was primarily seen in hospitalized patients; now, MRSA is seen in healthy younger people; these infections commonly are not acquired in a hospital but rather in the community; children in day care, athletes, prisoners, IV drug users, men who have sex with men are at higher risk; can cause surgical wound infections, septicemia, pneumonia; use Standard Precautions.	1. Regular hand washing helps prevent acquiring and spreading Staph, including MRSA. 2. Keep open sores and breaks in the skin covered until healed. 3. Avoid contact with other person's wounds or dressings. 4. Avoid sharing towels, toothbrushes, washcloths, razors. 5. Keep skin healthy to help avoid Staph on skin surface from causing an infection in nonintact skin and tissues. 6. Take all doses of antibiotic prescribed and do not share them with another person.

*Pertussis	*Bordetella pertussis* (bacteria)	• Direct contact with discharge from respiratory mucous membrane	Primarily seen in the pediatric population; severe coughing, whooping, and vomiting; apnea, pneumonia, seizures	Presence of whooping type cough; nasal pharyngeal culture PCR (polymer chain reaction) in patient younger than 11 years; serology in patient older than 11 years	DPT vaccine prevents disease; antibiotics may be given for secondary infection of pneumonia	High rate of morbidity and mortality in many countries; incidence in U.S. has increased steadily since the 1980s. In U.S. epidemics occur every 3–5 years; Increase seen in adolescents and adults.	1. Highly contagious 2. Adolescents and adults become susceptible when immunity wanes. 3. Practice cough hygiene****.
Pneumonia	****Bacteria ****Viruses Fungi Protozoa Rickettsia Aspirations of chemicals and dust	• Cough, sneeze, droplets in air	Cough with sputum, chills, fever, chest pain, dyspnea, fatigue	Chest X-ray, blood culture, sputum culture, CBC	Antibiotics if bacterial; treatment of symptoms if viral; oxygen therapy, bed rest	Elderly, immunosuppressed, and patients with chronic illness are more susceptible; vaccine available; practice cough hygiene.	1. Get vaccine. 2. Practice proper respiratory hygiene (cover nose and mouth when coughing or sneezing). 3. Use tissues to contain secretions and expectorations; dispose of used tissues in nearest waste receptacle. 4. If no tissues available, cover nose and mouth with bend of the elbow. 5. Practice proper hand hygiene.
Rubella (German measles)	Virus	• Spread by contact with infected person through coughing and sneezing	Rash, fever for 2–3 days, lymph node enlargement in head and neck	Rubella titer; presence of rubella antibodies in blood	None other than treatment of symptoms; pain and fever medications as needed; treat for shock; practice cough etiquette.	Rubella vaccine can prevent disease; part of the MMR vaccine; birth defects if a pregnant women acquires rubella (deafness, mental retardation, liver and spleen damage to fetus).	1. The following individuals should get the MMR vaccine: college students or any student beyond high school, people employed in a medical facility, people who travel internationally, people who are a passenger on a cruise ship, females of childbearing age. 2. Vaccine not given during pregnancy.

(continues)

Table 10-3 Examples of Infectious Diseases (continued)

Disease	Agent	Transmission	Symptoms	Diagnosis	Treatment	Comments	Patient Education
**Severe acute respiratory syndrome (SARS)	Virus	• Close person-to-person contact • Kissing • Sharing eating or drinking utensils • Perhaps respiratory droplets	High fever, headache, cough, shortness of breath, diarrhea	SARS serum antibodies validated by Centers for Disease Control and Prevention; blood culture; sputum culture	None; supportive only; may treat pneumonia with antibiotics but will not cure patient	Potentially serious illness; currently no known SARS transmissions; last transmission was in China, April 2004; because no one knows if SARS will recur, early recognition of cases and appropriate infection control are essential to control outbreaks; Transmission-Based Precautions (Isolation); airborne and direct contact	1. Travel to a previously SARS-affected area (China, Hong Kong, Taiwan) or close contact with an ill person who has such a travel history. 2. A diagnosis of pneumonia raises the suspicion of exposure to SARS. 3. Avoid close contact such as kissing, hugging, sharing of eating or drinking utensils. 4. Practice cough etiquette.
Toxic shock syndrome (TSS)	*Staphylococcus aureus Streptococcus*	• Associated with use of tampons and intravaginal contraceptive devices • Can occur post operationally with staphylococcal wound infections	Sudden onset of fever, chills, vomiting, muscle aches, and rash; progresses rapidly to hypotension and multisystem breakdown, shock, and death	Presence of symptoms, vaginal culture, CBC, blood culture	IV fluids and antibiotics; management of respiratory disease, renal impairment, gastrointestinal problems	CDS says TSS could be stopped if use of vaginal tampons ceases; menstruating women, women using barrier contraceptives, and persons with postoperative *Staphylococcus* infections are at risk	1. A woman who has had TSS is at risk for recurrence and should not use tampons at all. 2. Women should wash hands carefully before inserting a tampon. 3. Tampon should be changed every 6–8 hours.
*Tuberculosis (TB)	*Mycobacterium tuberculosis* bacillus	• Inhalation of contaminated airborne mucous droplets • Possibly ingestion	Productive cough, fatigue, fever, weight loss (behaviorial changes, anorexia, weight loss), night sweats	Sputum culture for *M. tuberculosis*, Mantoux skin test (PPD), chest X-ray, pleural needle biopsy	Antituberculosis agents, airborne transmission-based precautions until drug agents started	Increase in incidence of TB, especially among persons with AIDS and the homeless; may become drug resistant; health care professionals should have annual skin testing; report outbreaks.	1. Encourage hand washing, proper sputum tissue disposal. 2. Promote compliance with medications. 3. Encourage close contacts to have skin tests. 4. Encourage a well-balanced diet. 5. Practice cough etiquette.

**Vancomycin-resistant *Enterococcus* (VRE)	Bacteria (enterococci) normally found in intestines and female genital tract	• Direct contact with blood, urine, feces • Indirect contact with contaminated surfaces and from health care worker's hands	VRE can cause infections seen as: septicemia, pelvic, neonatal, and urinary disorders, otitis media	Culture and sensitivity of stool, urine, and/or blood	Antibiotics other than vancomycin	Spread directly by contact with feces, urine, or blood; spread indirectly from hands of health care workers or on contaminated surfaces; Standard Precautions used when caring for patients.	1. Wash hands thoroughly after using toilet and before touching food. 2. Wear gloves if handling body fluids containing VRE.
Varicella (chickenpox)	Varicella-zoster virus	• Direct and indirect contact with respiratory droplets	Sudden-onset fever, malaise, **maculo-papular-vesicular** skin rash	Vesicular fluid tissue culture during first 3 days after eruption; serology: increased antibodies 2 weeks after rash; **lesion** appearance characteristic of varicella	**Acyclovir** helpful to reduce severity of disease; zoster immunoglobulin (ZIG) for high-risk persons only within 96 hours of exposure; palliative therapy	Vaccine (varicella virus vaccine live) available in United States for children older than 12 months.	1. Communicable 1–2 days before rash until lesions crust. 2. Avoid scratching lesions to prevent secondary infection and scarring. 3. Benadryl and calamine lotion can be used for itch. 4. Acetaminophen can be used for fever. 5. Practice cough etiquette.
West Nile virus	Virus	• Infected mosquito	Central nervous system; fever, headache, coma, convulsions, paralysis; 80% of people infected show no signs or symptoms	West Nile virus, IgM capture, PRNT (plague reduction neutralization test)	None—supportive only; if hospitalized IV fluids, ventilator	Potentially serious illness; may have permanent neurologic effects.	1. Use insect repellent with DEET. 2. Wear long sleeves and pants when outside, especially at dawn and dusk. 3. Get rid of mosquito breeding sites by emptying standing water in flowerpots, buckets, and barrels. 4. Keep children's pools empty and on their sides when not in use. 5. A small number of cases are spread through blood transfusions, organ transplants, intrauterine, and breast feeding.

* Resurgent Diseases: Case rates of recent years have reversed and are now increasing.

** Emerging Diseases: Have become recognized in recent years.

*** Although meningitis can be bacterial or viral, the information in this table applies to bacterial meningitis because it is the more severe of the two.

**** Bacteria and viruses are the two main causes of pneumonia. Of the two, bacterial is more serious.

cell-mediated immunity and humoral immunity. **Cell-mediated immunity** is usually involved in attacks against viruses, fungi, organ transplants, or cancer cells. This type of immunity does not produce antibodies. **Humoral immunity** produces antibodies that are capable of killing microorganisms and of recognizing the pathogen in the future. Generally, both types of immune responses occur in four phases:

1. *Recognition of the invader.* The immune system is equipped with cells that identify agents, pathogens, and abnormal cell growth as foreign substances. Macrophages and helper T cells recognize foreign invaders, whether they are pathogens, cancer cells, or transplanted tissues.
2. *Growth of defenses, which allows for multiplication of helper T cells and B cells.* After foreign substance recognition, the immune system alerts T and B cells to multiply and move to the site of the foreign substance. In cell-mediated immunity, activation of helper T cells means that the T cells are specifically oriented to a unique antigen, a substance such as bacteria the body recognizes as foreign. Activated T cells divide, forming memory T cells and killer T cells. In humoral immunity, activated B cells are antigen specific and divide into memory B cells and plasma cells.
3. *Attack against the infection.* Cell-mediated immunity uses killer T cells and macrophages to phagocytize, or engulf and destroy the pathogens. Humoral plasma cells have the ability to produce specific **antibodies** that lock on to specific antigens, which prevents the disease-producing characteristics of the pathogen from forming. These antibodies are called **immunoglobulins** and they render the pathogen unable to reproduce or continue growth.
4. *Slowdown of the immune response after death of the infectious agent.* After the death of the foreign substance, the immune response is halted. T and B cells return to normal levels, and in the case of humoral immunity, the presence of antibody production causes the immune system to resist the specific infectious pathogen in future contacts with the pathogen.

Susceptibility to some infectious diseases is closely linked to the person's unique resistance, or immunity. Immunity is the ability of the body to resist specific pathogens and their toxins. **Resistance** occurs after an exposure to a pathogen, which is the antigen–antibody reaction. This natural body defense to fight infectious disease occurs gradually and over time as pathogens and other foreign substances such as antigens enter the human body. When the antigen enters the body, the immune system recognizes the antigen as foreign and attempts to contain and subdue the foreign invader. Specific chemical antibodies to the antigen are produced by B cells, which attempt to prevent the antigen from further growth. After the completion of the stages of that infectious disease, the body retains the ability to produce antibodies in response to that specific microorganism or antigen. Therefore, immunity can last for some length of time, possibly to provide lifetime protection against specific infectious microorganisms. Several forms of immunity can occur in response to specific antigens:

- Naturally acquired active immunity results from contracting an infectious agent and experiencing either an acute or subclinical infectious disease. This immunity is usually permanent.
- Artificially acquired active immunity is achieved after administration of vaccines. This immunity is semi-permanent to permanent.
- Naturally, congenitally acquired passive immunity occurs when antibodies pass to a fetus from the mother providing short-term immunity for the newborn. This immunity is temporary.
- Artificially acquired passive immunity may be achieved through administration of ready-made antibodies, such as gamma globulin, used to treat or prevent infectious diseases. This immunity is temporary.

Our defenses against diseases can be categorized as specific and nonspecific. Specific defenses include those things that protect us against a specific pathogen, whereas nonspecific defenses are not so particular. Some examples of specific defenses are:

- *Vaccines/immunizations:* Designed for specific pathogen
- *Antibodies:* Created against a specific pathogen
- *Tetanus shot:* Protects individuals from tetanus
- *Active immunities:* Created against a specific pathogen
- *Globulin:* Antibodies for exposure to a specific pathogen

Some examples of nonspecific defenses are:

- *Tears:* Contain chemical harmful to a variety of pathogens
- *Skin:* Creates a barrier against many different pathogens
- *Saliva:* Contains chemicals harmful to a variety of pathogens

- *Species resistance:* being human protects us from many diseases to which other animals are susceptible

Immunization. Immunizing individuals against specific infectious diseases provides immunity with active or passive vaccines. Most of the severe childhood communicable diseases can be prevented. The U.S. Department of Health and Human Services has estimated that about 80% of U.S. preschoolers younger than 2 years are fully vaccinated according to recommended schedules. Several factors influence vaccination compliance rates, such as access to health care, cost of vaccinations, and irregularity or confusion in maintaining young children on the recommended schedule. There are pockets within large cities of significant numbers of under-immunized children. A substantial number of these children are minority children. An outbreak could cause an **epidemic** of diseases that are preventable with vaccines (see Chapter 15).

There is a movement by parents and caregivers that is resisting the mandated childhood immunizations even though all states have immunization requirements for school admission. These groups want state laws changed and feel that they, as parents and caregivers, should be allowed to decide if they want their children immunized.

Exemptions from mandated immunizations are allowed in all states if there are medical reasons. Some states will exempt children for religious reasons and some on philosophical grounds.

In general, children would more likely suffer greater complications associated with childhood diseases than from the immunizations given to prevent them. Because most of the vaccinations are administered in ambulatory health care settings, medical assistants may have the responsibility to administer, document, and monitor immunizations (see Chapter 15).

There are various classifications of vaccines, depending on the method of immune stimulation:

1. *Live attenuated (changed) pathogens.* These pathogens stimulate the body's own antibody production. However, the patient does not contract the infectious disease (or only a mild or subclinical case) because the pathogen has been altered in some mechanical or chemical means by the manufacturer. Examples of live attenuated pathogens include measles and varicella.
2. *Pathogenic toxins.* Some pathogens produce toxins (poisonous substances) that can stimulate antibody production. Examples of toxin vaccines include tetanus and diphtheria.
3. *Killed pathogens.* Inactivated pathogens stimulate antibody production; however, several vaccines may be required to provide sustained protection. Examples include pertussis, rabies, and poliomyelitis.

STAGES OF INFECTIOUS DISEASES

Depending on the specific pathogen causing an infectious disease, several stages occur from the time of exposure until full recovery and the absence of infection. These stages are often predictable and offer guidelines for patient education and treatment opportunities.

Incubation Stage

The incubation stage is the interval of time between exposure to a pathogenic microorganism and the first appearance of signs and symptoms of the disease. Some infectious diseases have short incubation stages, whereas other infections have lengthy stages, lasting for years. If an exposure to an infectious agent occurs, the patient will manifest (reveal in an obvious why) the disease if the patient's immune system cannot contain the agent. If therapeutic medications are available, it can help to prevent disease progression. Not all infectious agents are treatable or preventable.

Prodromal Stage

The prodromal stage is the initial stage of the disease. It is characterized by common, general complaints of illness, such as **malaise** and fever. It is the interval between the earliest symptoms and the appearance of fever or rash that suggest an impending disease process is occurring.

Acute Stage

Disease processes reach their peak during the acute stage. Symptoms are fully developed and can often be differentiated from other specific symptoms. Treatment modalities are useful to reduce patient discomfort, to reduce possibilities of debilitation and adverse effects, and to promote healing and recovery.

The inflammatory process is the body's natural defensive reaction to the invasion by a foreign substance such as a pathogen, and it is in this acute state that the response is evident.

Patient Education

Drug-Resistant Bacteria

Antibiotic resistance occurs because bacteria can change their characteristics, thus reducing or eliminating the effectiveness of antibiotics. The resistant microorganisms survive, multiply, and cause a longer illness, necessitating more visits to the provider and more powerful and expensive antibiotics. Death can result from resistant bacteria. The number of antibiotic-resistant bacterial has increased significantly in the past 10 years. For example:

- MRSA (methicillin-resistant *Staphylococcus aureus*)
- Tuberculosis
- VRE (vancomycin-resistant *Enterococcus*)
- PRSP (penicillin-resistant streptococcus pneumonia)

These and other infectious diseases are becoming more resistant to standard antibiotic treatment. Drug options are increasingly limited, are expensive, or simply do not exist. An example of drug-resistant bacteria is the extensively drug-resistant tuberculosis (XDR TB). The bacteria are resistant to almost all antibiotics used to treat TB, including the two best first-line antibiotics, the second-line antibiotics, and at least one of three injectable antibiotics. Because XDR TB is resistant to several antibiotics, providers are left with much less effective treatment options that frequently have worse treatment outcomes.

- Antibiotics should be prescribed by a licensed provider and should be taken only when prescribed to treat a bacterial infection.
- Antibiotics should be taken exactly as directed for the entire course.
- Do not demand antibiotics from your provider. They do not cure a viral infection.

Declining Stage

Patient symptoms begin to subside or wane during the declining stage. The infectious disease remains, however, though the patient will demonstrate improving levels of health. It is often during the declining phase of an illness when patients begin to feel better that they prematurely discontinue taking the antibiotic that may have been prescribed. This premature discontinuance can result in microorganisms becoming resistant to antibiotics. It is important to educate patients in the proper use of antibiotics.

Convalescent Stage

Recovery and recuperation from the effects of a specific infectious disease are called the convalescent stage. The patient regains strength and stamina. The overall goal of this stage is returning the patient to as close as possible the original state of health.

DISEASE TRANSMISSION

When providing patients with health care, medical assistants run the risk for **contracting,** or acquiring, an infection from pathogens that are causing patients' illnesses. Such pathogens are viruses, bacteria, fungi, and others that can be found in patients' blood and body fluids. In medical offices, ambulatory care centers, and hospitals, many ill patients are seen everyday. Pathogens can be easily transmitted to another person if care is not taken to prevent such an occurrence.

Consistent use and adherence to infection control measures significantly reduce the risk for disease transmission. The CDC recommends that health care providers consider each patient to be potentially infectious for AIDS, hepatitis B and C, and other bloodborne pathogens and to routinely and conscientiously apply the techniques of Standard Precautions as a means of infection control.

Infectious diseases are caused by unique infectious agents, are characterized by various symptoms, are transmitted by differing means, and have unique treatments and prognoses. Medical assistants must recognize the unique characteristics of specific infectious diseases to prevent their transmission and help patients suffering from these infections. Table 10-3 classifies several common infectious diseases by critical components. When patients have contracted an infectious disease or are exposed to the risk for transmission, patient education plays an important role in infection control. Although a family member may have an infectious disease, proper training and education may protect other family members and close contacts.

Medical assistants are in a unique position to educate patients and the public about disease control. These measures become even more important with the increase in drug-resistant pathogens. All health care professionals must consistently and diligently use every infection control measure available, as well as teach our patients to do the same.

HUMAN IMMUNODEFICIENCY VIRUS AND HEPATITIS B AND C

A great deal of attention has been focused on the **human immunodeficiency virus (HIV)** that causes AIDS, and yet there remains no cure for the disease, although great advances have been made. With the focus on AIDS, other potentially life-threatening and fatal illnesses may seem less dangerous. In reality, hepatitis B and C are examples of other diseases that place health care providers at great risk for serious illness or death. Acute viral hepatitis deserves close attention.

HIV and AIDS

AIDS is caused by the bloodborne virus HIV. The viral infection directly affects the immune response. The HIV is responsible for T-cell destruction; T cells are the white blood cells that provide immunity.

HIV is carried in semen, blood, and other body fluids, and the virus can penetrate mucous membranes. Once inside the body, the reduced number of helper T cells leaves the patient vulnerable to a wide range of infections and malignancies. The infections that the patient contracts can be devastating. When people are positive for HIV infection, their T-cell counts must be regularly and closely monitored, and they must live their lives with careful consideration toward preventing opportunistic infections. If their T-cell count decreases to less than 200, they are considered to have AIDS. There is no curative treatment of HIV infections, but antiviral drugs such as lamivudine, azidothymidine, zidovudine, stavudine, and others are used to slow cell processes and weaken cell protein, which is important in the virus's reproduction. Many people are living for many years with HIV and AIDS. Table 10-4 provides information about HIV and AIDS.

Acute Viral Hepatitis Diseases

In any of the acute viral hepatitis diseases, the liver becomes inflamed, and hepatic cells can be destroyed. Healthy persons can regenerate cells, but older adult patients usually cannot. There are several types of viral hepatitis: hepatitis A (HAV), hepatitis B (HBV), hepatitis C (HCV), hepatitis D (HDV), and hepatitis E (HEV) and others. HAV, HBV, and HCV are the more common viruses; HDV and HEV are less common (see Table 10-5).

Despite the similarities among HIV, HBV, and HCV, the risk for contracting HBV and HCV is greater than for contracting HIV (Figure 10-7).

Medical assistants and all other health care providers must understand the importance of protecting themselves from the viruses that cause AIDS, HBV, HCV, and other pathogenic microorganisms. Through strict adherence to safety precautions and routine infectious disease control measures such as those found in **medical asepsis,** the risk for contracting an infectious disease can be minimized.

There is no vaccine to prevent HCV and no treatment after an exposure to prevent infection. Neither immunoglobulin nor antiviral drugs is recommended. It is a chronic disease, and patients carry the virus for the remainder of their lives. The

Table 10-4 Facts About HIV and AIDS

Signs and symptoms*	
Early (weeks to months after exposure)	• Flu-like illness • Swollen lymph nodes
Late (years after exposure)	• Persistent fevers • Night sweats • Prolonged diarrhea • Unexplained weight loss • Purple bumps on skin or inside mouth and nose • Chronic fatigue • Swollen lymph nodes • Recurrent respiratory infections

(continues)

Table 10-4 Facts About HIV and AIDS (continued)

Transmission	
HIV is spread by:	• Vaginal sex • Oral sex • Anal sex • Sharing needles to inject drugs, body piercing or tattooing • Contaminated blood products (rare) • Infected mother to newborn
HIV *cannot* be spread by:	• Shaking hands • A social kiss • Cups • Animals • Hugging • Swimming pools • Toilet seats • Food • Insects • Coughing
Complications/consequences	• Currently no cure available; most people eventually die of the disease (most live about 10 years after infection) • Spread to other sex partners and persons sharing needles
Pregnancy and HIV/AIDS	• HIV can be passed to unborn children from infected mother during pregnancy or childbirth. • Infected mother may infect infant through breast milk (rare)
Prevention	• Always use latex condoms during oral, vaginal, and anal sex. Latex condoms, when used consistently and correctly, are highly effective in preventing the transmission of HIV, the virus that causes AIDS. • Use a latex barrier (dental dam or condom cut in half) on a vagina or anus for oral sex. • Limit or avoid use of drugs and alcohol. • Do not share drug needles, cotton, or cookers. • Do not share needles for tattooing or body piercing. • Limit the number of sex partners. • Tests are available to detect antibodies for HIV through providers, STD clinics, and HIV counseling and testing sites. • Notify sex and needle-sharing partners immediately if HIV infected.
Treatment	• No treatment or medication available to cure HIV/AIDS. • Early diagnosis and treatment can prolong life for years. • Medications and treatments available to keep immune system working. • Antiviral drugs slow cell processes and weaken cell protein. • Medications available to treat AIDS-related illnesses. • Medications available for HIV-infected pregnant women to greatly reduce the chance of passing infection to newborn. • Experimental drug trials are testing new medications.

**NOTE:* These symptoms are not specific for HIV and may have other causes. Most persons with HIV have no symptoms at all for several years.

Table 10-5 Hepatitis Viruses A to C

	A	B	C
Causative agent	• Hepatitis A virus (HAV) • Fecal–oral; person to person	• Hepatitis B virus (HBV) • Blood; sexual contact; perinatal; breast milk; drug use (sharing needles); tattooing and body piercing	• Hepatitis C virus (HCV) • Blood or body fluids; intravenous drug use; mother to fetus; tattoo and body piercing; needle exchange
Risk groups	• Household/sexual contact with infected persons • International travelers • Men having sex with men • Drug users	• Injection drug users • Household/sexual contact with infected persons • Infants born to infected mothers • Health care workers • Multiple sex partners	• Recipients of blood transfusions or organ transplants before 1992 • People sharing needles • People exposed to blood and blood products • HBV- and HIV-infected persons
Incubation period	• 15–50 days	• 45–160 days	• 14–180 days
Infectious periods	• Usually less than 2 months	• Before symptoms appear; lifetime if carrier	• Before symptoms appear; lifetime if carrier
Diagnostic tests	• IgM anti-HAV	• HBsAg • HBeAg	• Anti-HCV • Serum ALT increased 10× • HCV RNA
Symptoms	• Flu-like • Jaundice • Dark yellow urine • Light-colored stools • Anorexia • Fatigue	• Flu-like • May have jaundice • Dark yellow urine • Light-colored stools • Malaise	• 80% have no symptoms • Flu-like • Jaundice • Anorexia
Prevention	• Hepatitis A vaccine (entire series) • Standard Precautions • Enteric precautions • Good personal hygiene, sanitization • Immunoglobulin (for short term)	• Hepatitis B vaccine (entire series) • Standard Precautions • Reduce risk behaviors • Good personal hygiene, sanitization • Immunoglobulin (for short term)	• Standard Precautions • Reduce risk behaviors • No vaccine
Treatment	• Immunoglobulin within 2 weeks of exposure	• Immunoglobulin (HBIg) • Alpha-interferon • Lamivudine	• Alpha-interferon • Ribavirin (Virazole)
Prognosis	• Rarely fatal • Not a carrier	• No cure • May become a carrier • Liver cancer may develop	• 85% or less have chronic infection • Chronic liver disease or cancer develop in 70%

ALT, alanine aminotransferase; HBeHg, hepatitis Be antigen; HBIg, hepatitis B immunoglobulin; HBsAg, hepatitis B surface antigen.

BLOODBORNE FACTS

WHAT IS HBV?

Hepatitis B virus (HBV) is a potentially life-threatening bloodborne pathogen. Centers for Disease Control estimates there are approximately 280,000 HBV infections each year in the United States.

Approximately 8,700 health care workers each year contract hepatitis B, and about 200 will die as a result. In addition, some who contract HBV will become carriers, passing the disease on to others. Carriers also face a significantly higher risk for other liver ailments which can be fatal, including cirrhosis of the liver and primary liver cancer.

HBV infection is transmitted through exposure to blood and other infectious body fluids and tissues. Anyone with occupational exposure to blood is at risk of contracting the infection.

Employers must provide engineering controls; workers must use work practices and protective clothing and equipment to prevent exposure to potentially infectious materials. However, the best defense against hepatitis B is vaccination.

WHO NEEDS VACCINATION?

The new OSHA standard covering bloodborne pathogens requires employers to offer the three-injection vaccination series free to all employees who are exposed to blood or other potentially infectious materials as part of their job duties. This includes health care workers, emergency responders, morticians, first-aid personnel, law enforcement officers, correctional facilities staff, launderers, as well as others.

The vaccination must be offered within 10 days of initial assignment to a job where exposure to blood or other potentially infectious materials can be "reasonably anticipated." The requirements for vaccinations of those already on the job took effect July 6, 1992.

WHAT DOES VACCINATION INVOLVE?

The hepatitis B vaccination is a noninfectious, yeast-based vaccine given in three injections in the arm. It is prepared from recombinant yeast cultures, rather than human blood or plasma. Thus, there is no risk of contamination from other bloodborne pathogens nor is there any chance of developing HBV from the vaccine.

The second injection should be given one month after the first, and the third injection six months after the initial dose. More than 90 percent of those vaccinated will develop immunity to the hepatitis B virus. To ensure immunity, it is important for individuals to receive all three injections. At this point it is unclear how long the immunity lasts, so booster shots may be required at some point in the future.

The vaccine causes no harm to those who are already immune or to those who may be HBV carriers. Although employees may opt to have their blood tested for antibodies to determine need for the vaccine, employers may not make such screening a condition of receiving vaccination nor are employers required to provide prescreening.

Each employee should receive counseling from a health care professional when vaccination is offered. This discussion will help an employee determine whether inoculation is necessary.

WHAT IF I DECLINE VACCINATION?

Workers who decide to decline vaccination must complete a declination form. Employers must keep these forms on file so that they know the vaccination status of everyone who is exposed to blood. At any time after a worker initially declines to receive the vaccine, he or she may opt to take it.

WHAT IF I AM EXPOSED BUT HAVE NOT YET BEEN VACCINATED?

If a worker experiences an exposure incident, such as a needlestick or a blood splash in the eye, he or she must receive confidential medical evaluation from a licensed health care professional with appropriate follow-up. To the extent possible by law, the employer is to determine the source individual for HBV as well as human immunodeficiency virus (HIV) infectivity. The worker's blood will also be screened if he or she agrees.

The health care professional is to follow the guidelines of the U.S. Public Health Service in providing treatment. This would include hepatitis B vaccination. The health care professional must give a written opinion on whether or not vaccination is recommended and whether the employee received it. Only this information is reported to the employer. Employee medical records must remain confidential. HIV or HBV status must NOT be reported to the employer.

U.S. Department of Labor
Occupational Safety and Health Administration

Single copies of fact sheets are available from OSHA Publications, Room N3101, 200 Constitution Ave. N.W., Washington, D.C. 20210 and from OSHA regional offices.

Figure 10-7 *Bloodborne Facts,* published by the U.S. Department of Labor, Occupational Safety and Health Administration (OSHA). This publication includes facts about hepatitis B virus, declination, and steps to be taken by the employer should exposure to blood, body fluids, or other potentially infectious material occur. (Courtesy of the U.S. Department of Labor.)

virus is spread through blood and body fluids, sharing needles, IV drug use, needlesticks or sharps exposure, or from mother to baby during delivery. HCV patients may be at risk for infection with HAV, HBV, and/or HIV. Patients with HCV should be vaccinated for HAV and HBV. Infection control practices (Standard Precautions) are necessary to prevent infection with HCV through blood and body fluids. Patients exposed to HCV should be tested for HCV antibodies and liver enzyme levels as soon as possible after exposure and again in 4 to 6 months.

Medication known as **immunomodulators,** (have the ability to change immune responses) are used to treat some patients who have chronic HCV. Two examples are peginterferon (Pegasys) and ribavirin (Copegus). Patients being treated with these medications must be closely monitored with periodic clinical and laboratory evaluations because the medications cause decreases in leukocyte and platelet counts. There are numerous side effects. The medications are used to prevent progressive liver destruction from the virus.

REPORTING INFECTIOUS DISEASE

Certain infectious diseases must be reported to the state and county health departments. The CDC requires that the information be reported to them. This helps the CDC control the spread of infection. Each state health department has forms for reportable diseases. Each disease has an identification number from the health department, and together with the appropriate form, the information is sent to the state health department and then to the CDC. Table 10-6 lists some of the diseases to be reported to the CDC's Notifiable Disease Surveillance System. Diseases reports can be sent via the computer to the appropriate agencies (Figure 10-8), which will reply with orders for tests and procedures and follow-up orders.

STANDARD PRECAUTIONS

The CDC spent several years researching, improving, and developing recommendations to protect health care providers, patients, and their visitors from infectious diseases. This intensive period of research resulted in Standard Precautions, a set of infection control guidelines that are now used by all health care professionals for all patients.

Table 10-6 Disease that Must Be Reported to the CDC

AIDS	Poliomyelitis
Anthrax	Rabies (animal and human)
Botulism	Rheumatic fever
Diphtheria	Rubella
Encephalitis	Salmonella
Hepatitis A, B, C	Sexually transmitted diseases
Lyme disease	Tetanus
Measles	Toxic shock syndrome
Meningitis	Tuberculosis
Pertussis	Tularemia

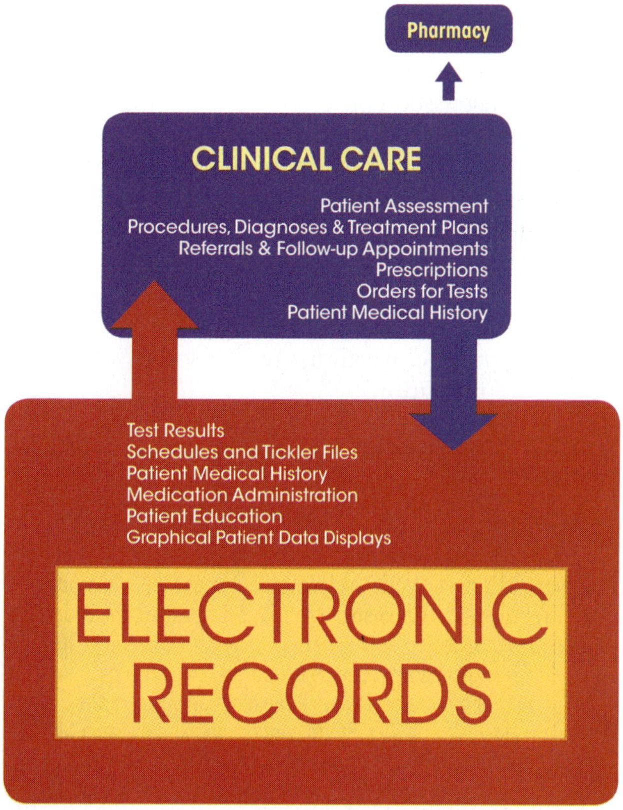

Figure 10-8 Diseases reportable to the local health department and CDC can be sent via computer to the appropriate agencies. They will reply with orders for tests and procedures and follow-up appointments.

According to the CDC, Standard Precautions are "designed to reduce the risk of transmission of microorganisms from both recognized and unrecognized sources of infection in hospitals." They apply to:

1. Blood
2. All body fluids, secretions, and excretions regardless of whether they contain visible blood
3. Nonintact skin
4. Mucous membranes

To be effective, Standard Precautions must be practiced conscientiously at all times. Although the Standard Precautions include many criteria specific to inpatient settings such as hospitals and skilled nursing facilities, they are absolutely applicable to any medical facility, including ambulatory care settings where medical assistants are more likely to work.

Figure 10-9 provides a comprehensive review of Standard Precautions.

Transmission-Based Precautions

When the CDC was in the process of developing a new guideline for isolation precautions in hospitals, the agency arrived at what it terms two tiers of precautions. The first tier is called the Standard Precautions, discussed earlier, designed for all patients regardless of their diagnosis or presumed infection status. The second tier of precautions is intended for patients diagnosed with or suspected of having specific highly transmissible diseases. These are known as Transmission-Based Precautions.

Transmission-Based Precautions reduce the risk for **airborne, droplet,** and **contact transmission** of pathogens and are always to be used *in addition to* Standard Precautions.

> **Latex Sensitivity**
>
> Health care providers should be aware that some people, including professionals and patients, can be allergic to latex products. Some personal protective equipment (PPE) is made from latex; medical and surgical products also are often made from this product.
>
> The allergic reaction can be a localized one such as dermatitis or a more severe systemic reaction such as anaphylaxis (see Chapter 9), a form of shock marked by vascular collapse, respiratory failure, hypotension, arrhythmia, and laryngeal edema. Vinyl gloves can be worn in place of latex for hypersensitive individuals. Any person with an allergy to latex should wear a bracelet or other form of identification indicating this fact because, in any emergency, medical personnel wear latex gloves (see Chapter 9).

These airborne, contact, and droplet precautions also list specific syndromes that can appear in adult and pediatric patients who are highly suspicious for infection. They identify the appropriate Transmission-Based Precautions to be used until a diagnosis can be made. Figures 10-10, 10-11, and 10-12 provide specific information on these three Transmission-Based Precautions. Remember that these precautions are for specific categories of patients and are to be used in addition to Standard Precautions, which are used for all patients.

Some medical assistants' externship experiences take place in a hospital setting. For example, the electrocardiography and clinical laboratory departments of the hospital are areas some students rotate through during their externships. It is important for medical assistants to know and understand how to protect themselves from infectious diseases. Transmission-Based Precautions (isolation) reduce the risk for airborne, droplet, and contact transmission of pathogens. Procedure 10-3 describes the use of barriers (gown, mask, goggles, gloves, and cap) that are used when entering an isolation room to perform an electrocardiogram or phlebotomy on a patient with an infectious disease such as tuberculosis (airborne contact), meningitis (respiratory droplets contact), and wound drainage (direct contact).

Blood and Body Fluids

In all infection control efforts, it is important to understand what is meant by blood and body fluids. Specifically, they are described as the blood, secretions, and excretions of a patient. Examples of blood and body fluids and some of the areas in which medical assistants may become exposed to them are:

Blood:

- Specimens drawn during venipuncture
- Open wounds or lesions of any kind
- Epistaxis, or nosebleeds
- Vaginal bleeding, including menses (menstruation), lochia (discharge after childbirth), and hemorrhage
- Feces and vomit or other body fluids with or without visible blood

Vaginal secretions:

- Physiologic leukorrhea (normal vaginal discharge)
- Vaginitis with discharge

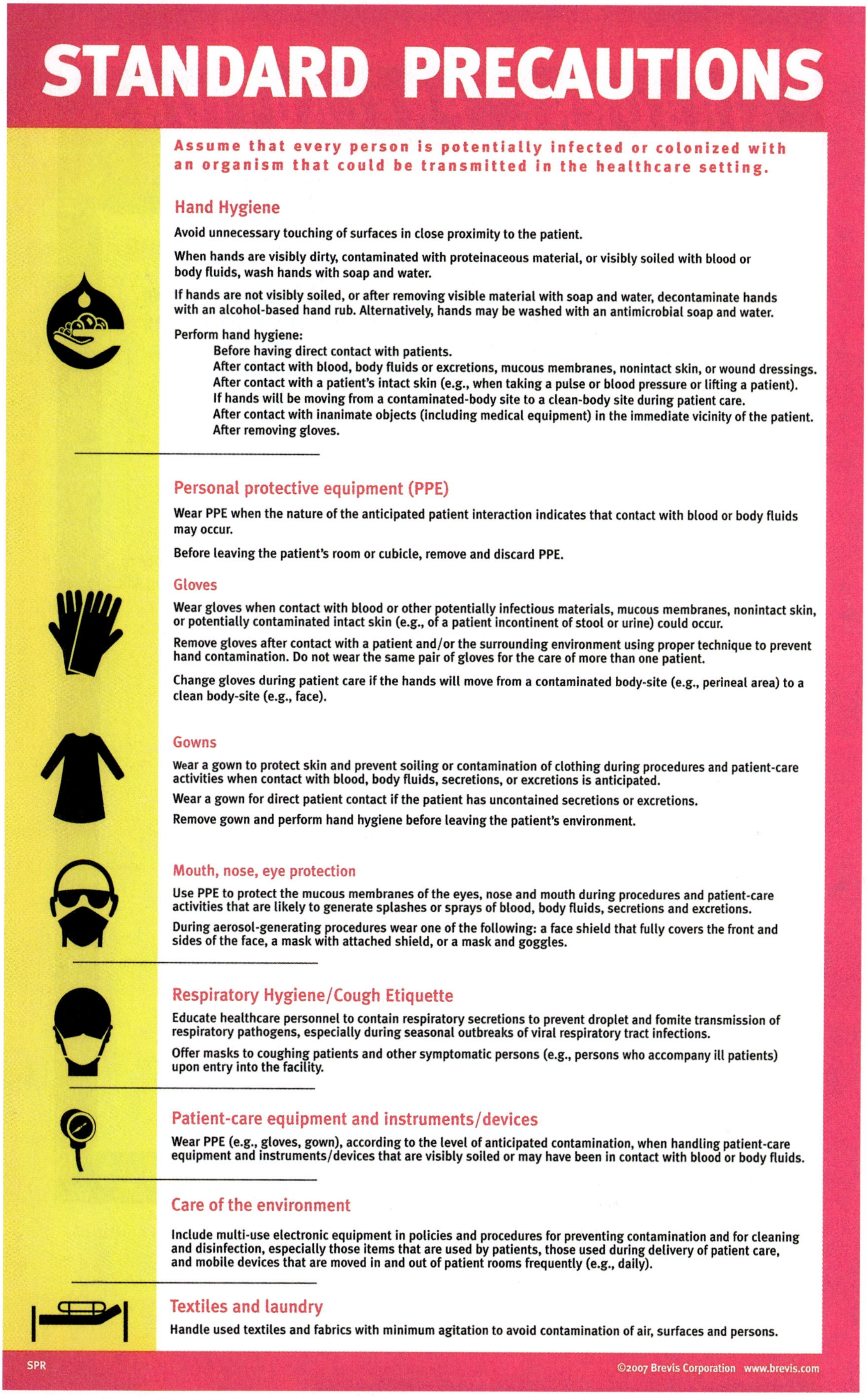

STANDARD PRECAUTIONS

Assume that every person is potentially infected or colonized with an organism that could be transmitted in the healthcare setting.

Hand Hygiene

Avoid unnecessary touching of surfaces in close proximity to the patient.

When hands are visibly dirty, contaminated with proteinaceous material, or visibly soiled with blood or body fluids, wash hands with soap and water.

If hands are not visibly soiled, or after removing visible material with soap and water, decontaminate hands with an alcohol-based hand rub. Alternatively, hands may be washed with an antimicrobial soap and water.

Perform hand hygiene:

- Before having direct contact with patients.
- After contact with blood, body fluids or excretions, mucous membranes, nonintact skin, or wound dressings.
- After contact with a patient's intact skin (e.g., when taking a pulse or blood pressure or lifting a patient).
- If hands will be moving from a contaminated-body site to a clean-body site during patient care.
- After contact with inanimate objects (including medical equipment) in the immediate vicinity of the patient.
- After removing gloves.

Personal protective equipment (PPE)

Wear PPE when the nature of the anticipated patient interaction indicates that contact with blood or body fluids may occur.

Before leaving the patient's room or cubicle, remove and discard PPE.

Gloves

Wear gloves when contact with blood or other potentially infectious materials, mucous membranes, nonintact skin, or potentially contaminated intact skin (e.g., of a patient incontinent of stool or urine) could occur.

Remove gloves after contact with a patient and/or the surrounding environment using proper technique to prevent hand contamination. Do not wear the same pair of gloves for the care of more than one patient.

Change gloves during patient care if the hands will move from a contaminated body-site (e.g., perineal area) to a clean body-site (e.g., face).

Gowns

Wear a gown to protect skin and prevent soiling or contamination of clothing during procedures and patient-care activities when contact with blood, body fluids, secretions, or excretions is anticipated.

Wear a gown for direct patient contact if the patient has uncontained secretions or excretions.

Remove gown and perform hand hygiene before leaving the patient's environment.

Mouth, nose, eye protection

Use PPE to protect the mucous membranes of the eyes, nose and mouth during procedures and patient-care activities that are likely to generate splashes or sprays of blood, body fluids, secretions and excretions.

During aerosol-generating procedures wear one of the following: a face shield that fully covers the front and sides of the face, a mask with attached shield, or a mask and goggles.

Respiratory Hygiene/Cough Etiquette

Educate healthcare personnel to contain respiratory secretions to prevent droplet and fomite transmission of respiratory pathogens, especially during seasonal outbreaks of viral respiratory tract infections.

Offer masks to coughing patients and other symptomatic persons (e.g., persons who accompany ill patients) upon entry into the facility.

Patient-care equipment and instruments/devices

Wear PPE (e.g., gloves, gown), according to the level of anticipated contamination, when handling patient-care equipment and instruments/devices that are visibly soiled or may have been in contact with blood or body fluids.

Care of the environment

Include multi-use electronic equipment in policies and procedures for preventing contamination and for cleaning and disinfection, especially those items that are used by patients, those used during delivery of patient care, and mobile devices that are moved in and out of patient rooms frequently (e.g., daily).

Textiles and laundry

Handle used textiles and fabrics with minimum agitation to avoid contamination of air, surfaces and persons.

SPR

Figure 10-9 Standard Precautions for Infection Control issued by the Centers for Disease Control and Prevention. (Courtesy Brevis Corp.)

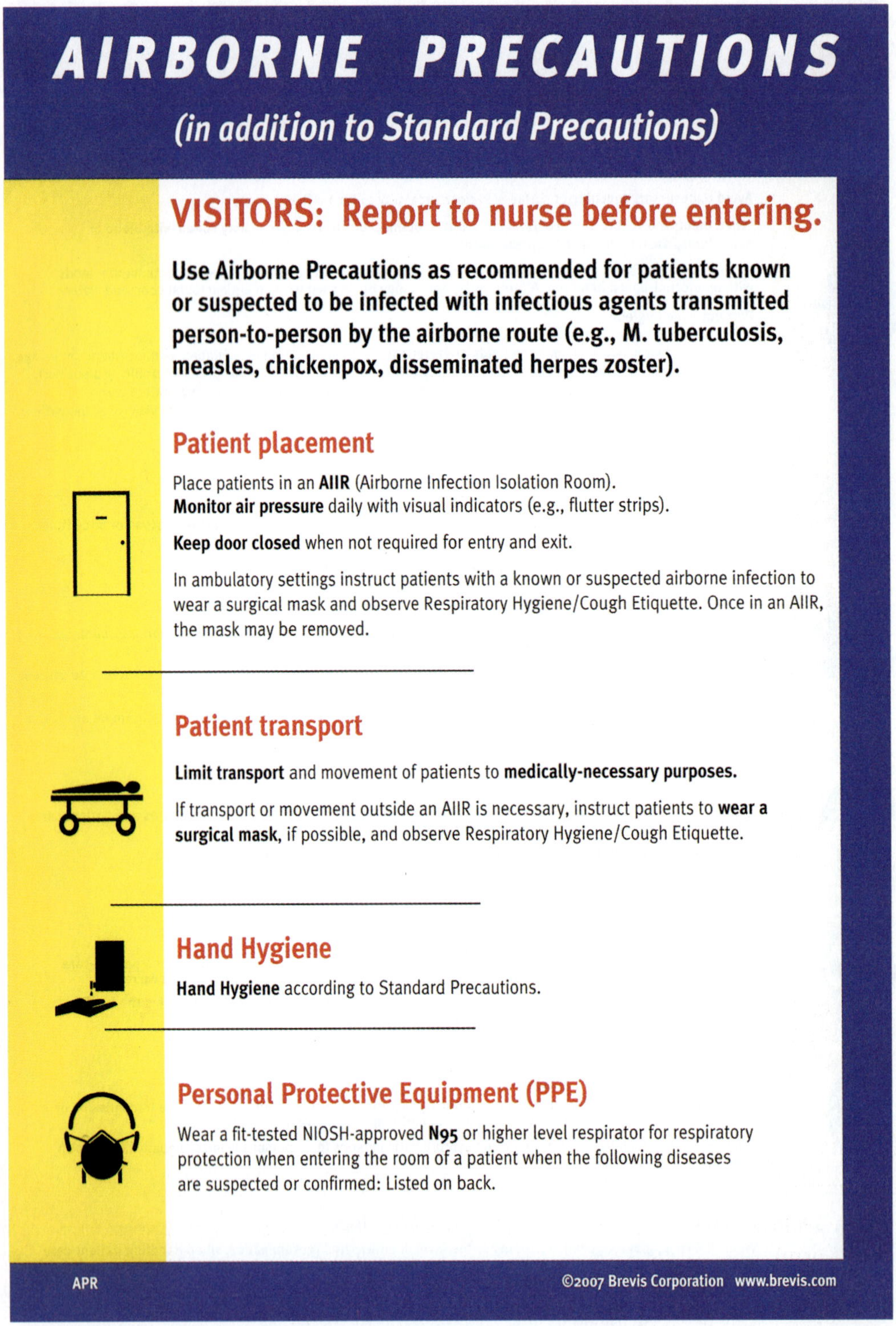
AIRBORNE PRECAUTIONS
(in addition to Standard Precautions)
VISITORS: Report to nurse before entering.
Use Airborne Precautions as recommended for patients known or suspected to be infected with infectious agents transmitted person-to-person by the airborne route (e.g., M. tuberculosis, measles, chickenpox, disseminated herpes zoster).
Patient placement
Place patients in an AIIR (Airborne Infection Isolation Room).
Monitor air pressure daily with visual indicators (e.g., flutter strips).
Keep door closed when not required for entry and exit.
In ambulatory settings instruct patients with a known or suspected airborne infection to wear a surgical mask and observe Respiratory Hygiene/Cough Etiquette. Once in an AIIR, the mask may be removed.
Patient transport
Limit transport and movement of patients to medically-necessary purposes.
If transport or movement outside an AIIR is necessary, instruct patients to wear a surgical mask, if possible, and observe Respiratory Hygiene/Cough Etiquette.
Hand Hygiene
Hand Hygiene according to Standard Precautions.
Personal Protective Equipment (PPE)
Wear a fit-tested NIOSH-approved N95 or higher level respirator for respiratory protection when entering the room of a patient when the following diseases are suspected or confirmed: Listed on back.
APR
©2007 Brevis Corporation www.brevis.com

Figure 10-10 Airborne Precautions, one category of Transmission-Based Precautions, for use in hospital settings. (Courtesy of Brevis Corp.)

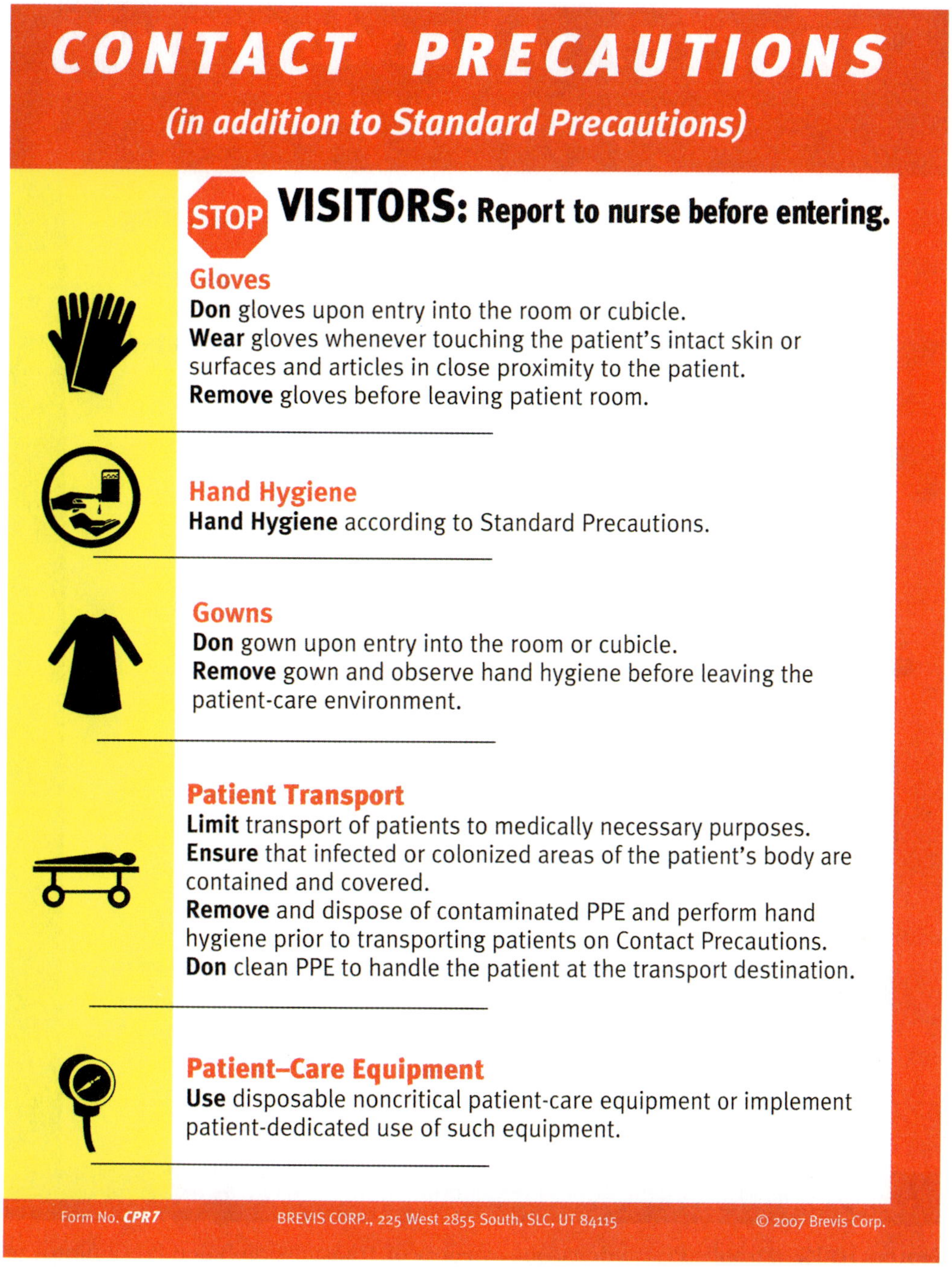

Figure 10-11 Contact Precautions, one category of Transmission-Based Precautions, for use in hospital settings. (Courtesy of Brevis Corp.)

Cerebrospinal fluid:

- Fluid aspirated, or withdrawn, during a lumbar puncture (spinal tap)
- Leakage of fluid due to trauma to the brain or spinal cord (through ear, nose)

Synovial fluid:

- Fluid aspirated during arthroscopic procedures

Pleural fluid:

- Fluid aspirated during thoracentesis, a surgical puncture of the thoracic cavity
- Fluid leakage caused by chest trauma

Pericardial fluid:

- Fluid around the heart exposed during cardiac surgery or caused by cardiac trauma

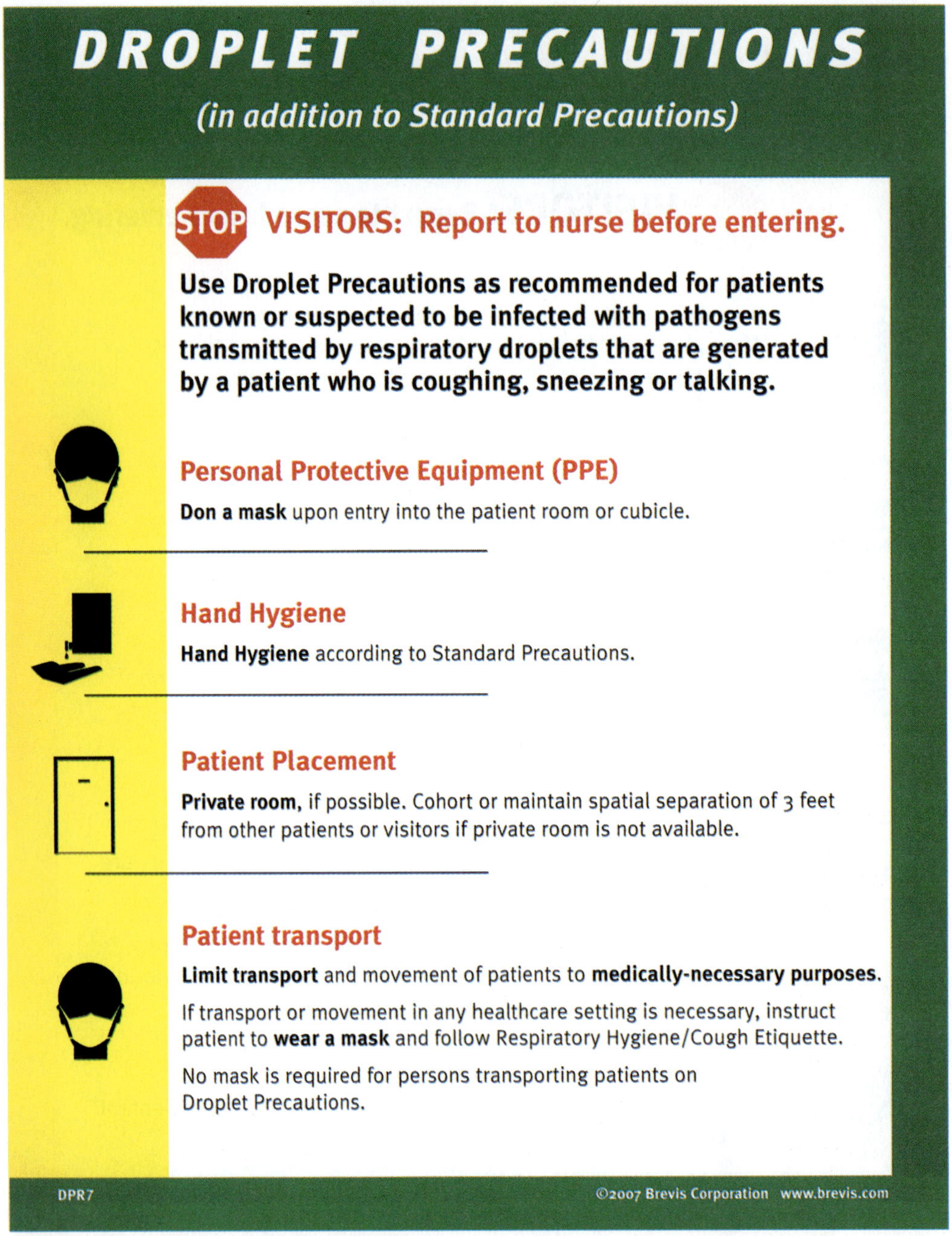

Figure 10-12 Droplet Precautions, one category of Transmission-Based Precautions, for use in hospital settings. (Courtesy of Brevis Corp.)

Peritoneal fluid:

- Fluid exposed during abdominal surgery (least likely fluid with which medical assistant will come into contact), but exposure can occur during a paracentesis

Semen:

- Seminal fluid as a laboratory specimen for sperm count in examination for fertility level

Amniotic fluid:

- Fluid aspirated during amniocentesis, a surgical puncture of the amniotic sac
- Vaginal leakage during pregnancy, labor, and delivery

Breast milk (possibility exists)

Sputum:

- Material coughed up and **expectorated** from the respiratory tract

Saliva:

- Oral mucous gland fluid in mouth during oral/dental procedures

Any other body fluid visibly contaminated with blood

Thus far, only blood and blood products, semen, vaginal secretions, and possibly breast milk have been directly linked to transmission of HIV; the virus is not spread casually or through close family contacts. There is not yet a vaccine to protect individuals from HIV.

HBV has been found in blood and blood products, vaginal secretions, semen, and saliva. Infection can spread through close family contacts, kissing, sexual contacts, intrauterinely, and during delivery. An infant may become a chronic **carrier,** one who has no symptoms but can transmit disease. If there has been an exposure to the virus, a prompt injection of immunoglobulin, an antibody, will help provide protection from the virus. HBV vaccine is available, and the series of three injections usually immunizes an individual from an attack of hepatitis B for approximately 18 years.

Some states require health care providers and allied health students to be immunized before employment and before admission into a health program in an educational institution. Also, many states require infants to be routinely immunized with HBV vaccine.

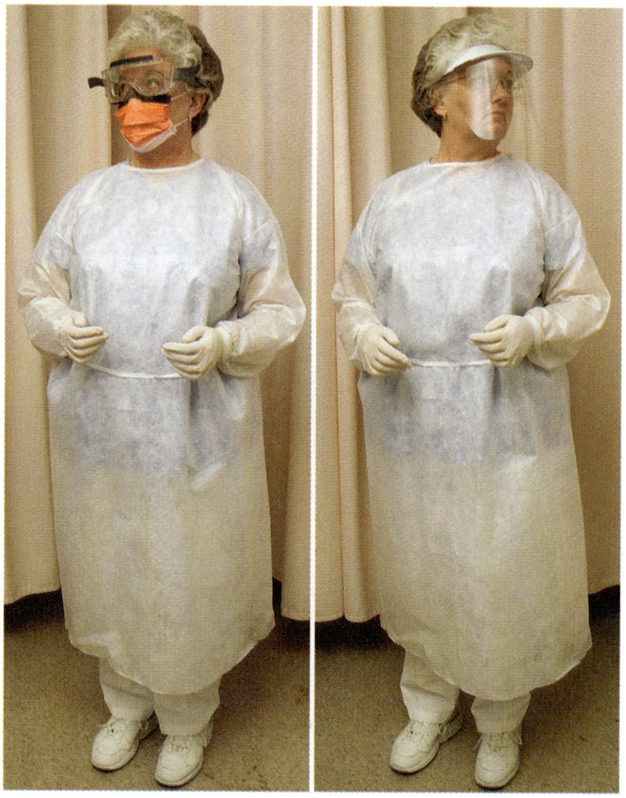

Figure 10-13 Medical assistant wearing personal protective equipment. (A) Goggles, mask, gown, latex gloves. (B) Full-face shield, gown, latex gloves.

Personal Protective Equipment

Standard and Transmission-Based Precautions all make use of barriers or personal protective equipment (PPE). The barriers consist of gloves, mask, gown, and goggles/face shield. Gloves reduce the risk for contamination to hands but do not prevent needles or other sharp instruments from penetrating the skin. Masks and protective eyewear reduce the contamination risk to mucous membranes of the eyes, nose, and mouth. Gowns protect clothing from contamination. Barriers or PPE are used in various combinations depending on the procedure or treatment being performed on patients. As a medical assistant, you may be exposed to infected blood and body fluids and must wear PPE (Figure 10-13).

Needlestick

One reason for exposure to blood is caused by accidentally sticking oneself with a dirty (used) needle after performing invasive procedures such as injections and venipuncture. In the past, needlesticks were common because of the practice of needle recapping. Contaminated (used) needles should never be recapped, broken off, removed from syringes, or manipulated by hand in any way. They are disposed of in the approved puncture-proof container designated for **sharps** (Figure 10-14). The disposal container for sharps must be in the closest proximity as practical to the area where sharps are used. If a needle is used and an appropriate disposal container is not nearby ("point-of-use disposal"), the **scoop technique** of recapping may be used, but only in this circumstance (no appropriate container nearby): the cap may be "scooped up" with the needle, using one hand, and then carried to the sharps container. The cap is not, under any circumstances, pushed into place over the needle (Figure 10-15). The risk to a health care provider of HIV infection caused by a needlestick is slight; however, the risk for HBV or HCV infection caused by a needlestick can be significantly greater.

OSHA mandates that (1) employers select the safest needle device available, (2) employers must involve employees in identifying these devices, and (3) employers maintain a log of injuries caused by contaminated sharps ([66FR5325]

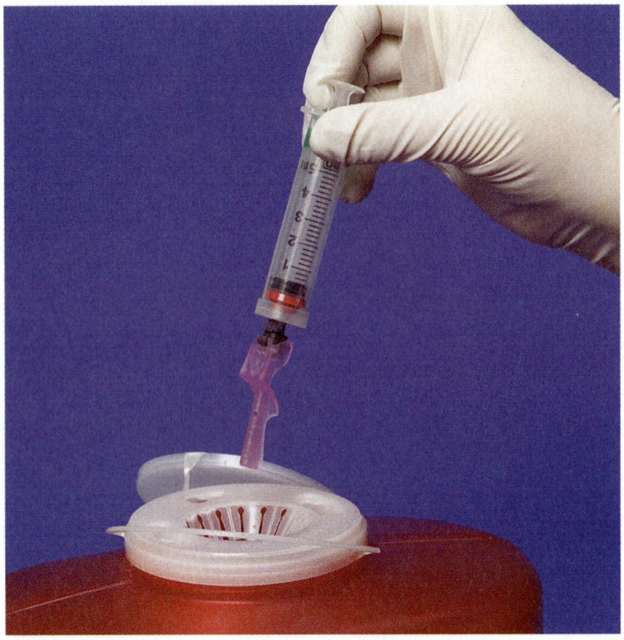

Figure 10-14 Discard the entire disposable safety syringe and needle into the biohazard puncture-proof sharps container.

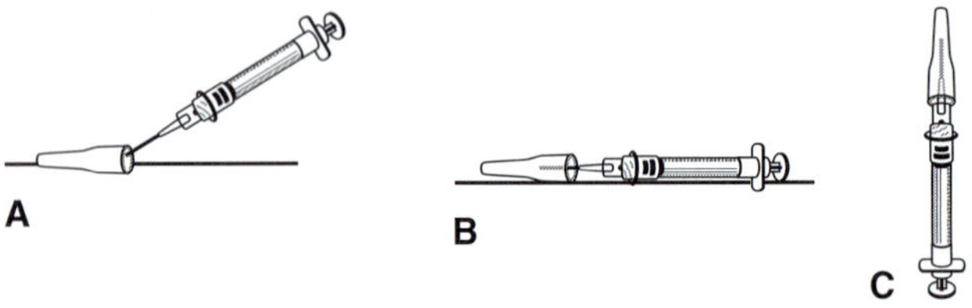

Figure 10-15 (A) Scoop into cap using one hand. Do not touch the cap with the other hand. (B) Slide needle into cap resting on table. (C) Holding the barrel of the syringe in one hand, carry to the sharps container. **Do not push the cap onto the syringe.**

OSHA 1910.1030). This is known as the "Needlestick Safety and Prevention Act." The act was added to the original act regarding engineering controls of the OSHA Bloodborne Pathogens Standard (Figure 10-16).

Desirable characteristics of safety devices include:

- The device is **jet injection.**
- The safety feature is built into the device.
- The device works passively (i.e., requires no activation by the user). If user activation is necessary, the safety feature can be engaged with a single-handed technique, allowing the worker's hands to remain behind the exposed sharp.
- The user can easily tell whether the safety feature has been activated. Some safety features have a sound, such as a click, indicating that the feature is engaged.
- The safety feature cannot be deactivated and remains protective through disposal.
- If the device uses needles, it performs reliably with all needle sizes.
- The device is easy to use and practical.
- The device is safe and effective in patient care.

Additional information regarding specific procedures to follow should an accidental needlestick occur, as well as other safety procedures included in the OSHA and CLIA rules and regulations, will be found later in this chapter and in Chapter 26.

Disposal of Infectious Waste

Infectious waste (contaminated items) is any item that has come in contact with patient blood or body fluids. These items must be handled with gloves and disposed of by placing them in the appropriate biohazard containers that are provided by an agency with which your employer has contracted (Figure 10-17). Infectious waste is either incinerated (burned) or subjected to sterilization by autoclave to render it harmless before it is disposed of in a sanitary landfill. For local rules and regulations of how to dispose of sharps and biohazard/infectious waste, contact your local Department of Health. Their staff can refer you to companies that specialize in the proper disposal of infectious waste and sharps. These companies follow strict state and federal regulations and can provide your clinic with containers, labels, and instructions. They will often work out a schedule for pickups, such as daily, weekly, monthly, or "on-call." Charges will usually be based on the amount of infectious waste that requires disposal.

Federal Organizations and Infection Control

The CDC is responsible for studying pathogens and diseases in an effort to prevent their spread. A division of the U.S. Public Health Department, the CDC has issued a number of guidelines over the last 25 years that have enabled health care professionals to practice responsible infection control. As diseases evolve and as new diseases are introduced into our society, the CDC revises and

EXAMPLES OF SAFETY DEVICES

Type of Device	Safety Features
Syringes and Injection Equipment	**Needleless or jet injection** – the medication/immunization is injected under the skin without a needle, using the force of the liquid under pressure to pierce the skin.
	Retractable needle – the needle (usually fused to the syringe) is spring-loaded and retracts into the barrel of the syringe when the plunger is completely depressed after the injection is given.
	Protective sheath – after giving an injection, the worker slides a plastic barrel over the needle and locks it in place.
	Hinged re-cap – after the injection, the worker, using the index finger, flips a hinged protective cap over the needle, which locks into place. This safety feature may be fused to the syringe or come separate and detachable from the syringe.
IV Access – Insertion Equipment	**Retractable** – the spring-loaded needle retracts into the needle holder upon pressing a button after use or the needle withdraws into the holder when withdrawn from the patient's arm.
	Passive – a metal safety clip unfolds over the needle as it is withdrawn.
	Shielded IV catheters (midline and peripheral) – a protective shield slides over the exposed needle.
	Hemodialysis safety fistula sets (butterfly) – a protective shield slides over the needle as it is withdrawn.
Blood-Collection and Phlebotomy	**Retractable needle** – the spring-loaded needle is pulled into the vacuum tube holder after use.
	Shielded butterfly needle – a protective shield slides over the needle after use.
	Self-blunting needle – after use, the needle is blunted while still in the patient.
	Plastic blood collection tubes – used to replace glass tubes.
Suture Needles	**Blunt suture needles** – used for sewing internal fascia.
Lancets	**Retracting lancet** – following skin puncture, the sharp automatically retracts back into the device.
Surgical Scalpels	**Retracting scalpel** – after use, the blade is withdrawn back into the body of the scalpel.
	Quick-release scalpel blade handles – a lever is activated that allows for a "touchless" attachment of the blade to the handle and releases it after use.

Figure 10-16 Examples of Safety Devices published by the U.S. Department of Labor. This publication includes information about various types of safety devises and their features. (Courtesy of the U.S. Department of Labor.)

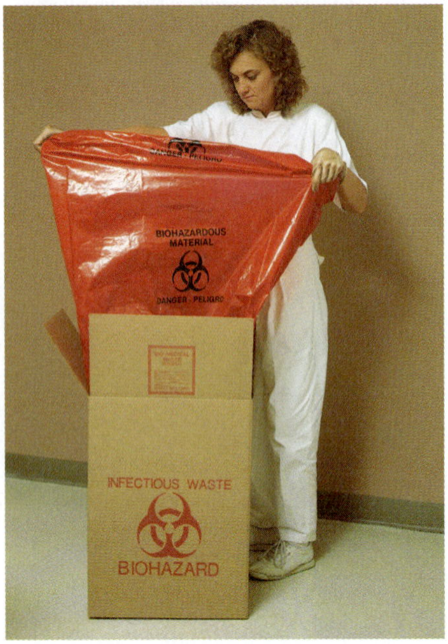

Figure 10-17 The medical assistant is placing a sturdy disposable plastic bag marked with the biohazard waste symbol into a durable cardboard box for collection of infectious waste material. When full, an authorized, licensed waste hauler will dispose of the box (usually by incineration) and provide documentation of its disposal.

updates existing guidelines or issues new control measures to contain the spread of infection.

In 1970, the CDC developed a system of seven **isolation categories** for patients with known infectious diseases. This category system included strict **isolation,** respiratory isolation, protective isolation, enteric precautions, wound and skin precautions, discharge precautions, and blood precautions.

In 1985, the agency released a set of guidelines known as Universal Blood and Body Fluid Precautions, or simply **Universal Precautions.** These infection control practices were written in response to the increase in AIDS and HBV, both bloodborne diseases, and other infectious diseases as well.

Beginning in 1991, the CDC infection control guidelines were reviewed and subsequently revised. In 1996, a new set of guidelines was released. Standard Precautions reflect improved recommendations intended to protect all health care providers, patients, and their visitors from a wide range of **communicable** diseases. At the same time that the CDC issued the new Standard Precautions, they also released a second tier of precautions called Transmission-Based Precautions. These are intended to be used in addition to Standard Precautions when caring for patients with known specific infectious diseases.

To understand the intent of these various CDC infection control guidelines, Standard Precautions and Transmission-Based Precautions are examined here in more detail.

OSHA REGULATIONS

OSHA regulations are intended to ensure that employers have a safe and healthful work environment for their employees. They represent requirements that employers must follow to ensure employee safety and health.

There are two standards that comprise the regulations: *The Occupational Exposure to Hazardous Chemicals in the Laboratory,* an amended version of the original standard *The Hazard Communication Standard,* and *The Bloodborne Pathogen Standard.*

The Bloodborne Pathogen Standard

The Bloodborne Pathogen Standard became effective in March 1992. It came about principally in the hope of reducing occupational-related cases of HIV and HBV infections among health care workers.

It covers all employees who can be "reasonably anticipated" to come into contact, as a result of performing their job duties, with blood and other potentially infectious materials. *The Bloodborne Pathogen Standard* seeks to limit exposure to bloodborne pathogens. The law covers:

- Exposure determination
- Methods of control of exposure, especially Standard Precautions
- HBV vaccine
- Postexposure follow-up
- Disposal of biohazardous waste
- Labeling
- Housekeeping and laundry functions
- Training for employee safety and documentation

See Figure 10-29 for an overview and summary of the OSHA *Bloodborne Pathogen Standard.*

Blood and Other Potentially Infectious Material.

Blood and other potentially infectious material are defined by the CDC and OSHA as the same human fluids listed previously as well as the following:

- Unfixed human tissue (alive or dead); e.g., breast tissue from a frozen section biopsy

- Any tissue culture, cells, or fluid known to be HIV-, HBV-, or HCV-infected

When the origin of a specimen is unknown, it must be handled as if it were infectious.

Bloodborne Pathogens. Disease-producing microorganisms are called pathogens; bloodborne refers to the manner in which the microorganisms can be transmitted—via blood or other potentially infectious material. Three pathogens of particular importance to health care professionals are HBV, HCV, and HIV.

Exposure Determination. Exposure determination requires an employer to list all the job classifications and employees in those job classifications who are exposed to blood and other potentially infectious material in the course of performing their jobs. Existing job descriptions can be used by the employer to identify the job categories that are considered high risk for exposure to blood and/or other potentially infectious material (Figure 10-18). It is important to note that exposure determination is made without regard to the use of PPE.

Plan to Control Exposure. Every employer who has an employee(s) who is identified and determined to be at risk for potential exposure must have a written exposure control plan (Figures 10-19 through 10-21). The plan must consist of methods of compliance for prevention of exposure, HBV vaccination and postexposure evaluation, communication of hazards to employee(s), documentation of the bloodborne standard, and a procedure for the determination of the events surrounding an exposure occurrence. The written plan must be employee accessible, updated regularly (at least annually), and modified when necessary and appropriate, especially to reflect changes in employee positions.

Methods of Compliance to Prevent Exposure. There are seven major strategies mandated by

Critical Thinking

Give eight examples of body fluids considered to be biohazardous substances. Explain under what circumstances medical assistants could become exposed to blood and body fluids.

SAMPLE

Exposure Classification Record of Employee

The following employee was classified according to work task exposure to certain body fluids as required by the current OSHA infection control standard on (Date) ____________ as follows:

Employee Name: ______________ SS# ___________

____ Category 1. "All procedures or other job related tasks that involve an inherent potential for mucous membrane or skin contact with blood, body fluids, or tissues, or a potential for spill or splashes of (blood or body fluids)."

____ Category 2. Tasks in which "The normal work routine involves no exposure to blood, body fluids, or tissues, but exposure or potential exposure may be required as a condition of employment." For example, receptionists, accounting, or insurance staff or others who may, as a part of their duties, be asked to help in clean up, instrument recirculation, laboratory, or other similar procedures where exposure may result.

____ Category 3. Tasks in which "The normal work routine involves no exposure to blood, body fluids, or tissues. Persons who perform these duties are not called upon as part of their employment to perform or assist in emergency medical care or first aid or to be potentially exposed in some other way."

Employer Signature __________________

Because of a change of job assignment, the above employee was reclassified according to tasks exposure on (Date) ________ as follows:

_______ Category 1

_______ Category 2

_______ Category 3

Employer's Signature ______________________

Because of a change of assignment, the above employee was reclassified according to task exposure on (Date) ______ ____ as follows:

_______ Category 1

_______ Category 2

_______ Category 3

Employer's Signature ______________________

NOTE: This record should be retained for length of employment plus thirty years.

Figure 10-18 Sample Exposure Classification Record of employee shows exposure categories into which employee's tasks fall. This record is kept for 30 years. (Courtesy of POL Consultants, 2 Russ Farm Way, Delanco, NJ 08075, 856-824-0800)

OFFICE WORK PRACTICE EXPOSURE CONTROL PLAN

Effective Date: ____________

Office of ________________________________

As of the above date the office will follow the rules below to reduce exposure and contamination:

- Observe Standard Precautions.
- Wear gloves when drawing blood and performing procedures/tests.
- Wash hands after removing gloves.
- Change gloves frequently during the day and between patients.
- Do not answer phone, handle papers, or word process while wearing gloves.
- Do not cap or break needles.
- Dispose of all needles in sharps containers.
- Do not allow sharps containers to fill beyond ⅔ full.
- Wear lab coats when performing tests.
- Leave lab coats in laboratory/work area.
- Dispose of all contaminated material in infectious waste (Biohazard) container.
- Disinfect the laboratory work surfaces frequently.
- Disinfect the examining room surfaces, daily and as needed.
- Sterilize nondisposable examination and testing equipment.
- Monitor sterilization procedure.
- Do not eat or drink in work area.
- Place gauze over tops of blood tubes when removing caps or use safety caps.
- Clean up all specimen and chemical spills properly and immediately.
- Label all chemicals according to OSHA regulations.
- Label refrigerator that blood is stored in.
- Centrifuges will have lids or specimens will be capped when spun.
- Centrifuges will be disinfected regularly.
- Hepatitis B vaccines will be offered to all employees.
- Employees will take a safety training program.

Figure 10-19 Office Work Practice Exposure Control Plan indicates a sample list of precautions to take to minimize employee risk exposure. (Courtesy of POL Consultants, 2 Russ Farm Way, Delanco, NJ 08075, 856-824-0800)

SAMPLE

Office Procedures Safety Form

PROCEDURE: ____________________

Type of hazard: ____________________

Person performing procedure: ____________________

Person assisting procedure: ____________________

Personal protective equipment used: ____________________

____

Proper techniques for safety:

____

____

____

What is done with used materials and soiled instruments?

____

____

____

What chemical products are involved?

____

____

____

What are the specific risks of procedure?

____

____

____

Additional comments:

____

____

____

____

Prepared By: ____________ Date: ____________

Figure 10-20 Sample Office Procedures Safety Form lists procedures, type of hazard, employee performing procedure, employee assisting with procedure, and personal protective equipment. (Courtesy of POL Consultants, 2 Russ Farm Way, Delanco, NJ 08075, 856-824-0800)

SAMPLE

Safety/Work Practice Controls for Office Procedures

Each office has special safety procedures that are unique to that particular practice. These are also known as work practice controls. The fundamental work practice control is using Standard Precautions. Work practice controls reduce the likelihood of exposure to hazards. Many times the risks can be eliminated by changing the way a procedure is performed. Make copies of the PROCEDURES SAFETY FORM. Fill in the information for any procedure that involves exposure to potentially infectious body fluids. File these procedures in the office operation section of your manual. Do not limit this section to only body fluid exposures. General safety for other hazards such as chemicals and X-ray should be listed as well. Common examples are listed below. Check the ones you do and add to this list.

____ Patient exams	____ Arthroscopies
____ Aspirations	____ Vaginal exams
____ **Inoculations**	____ PAP smears/IUDs
____ Taking blood samples	____ OB care
	____ Implanon
____ Lab testing	____ Vasectomies
____ Lesion excisions	____ Biopsies
____ Wound care	____ Sigmoidoscopies
____ Dressing changes	____ __________
____ Colposcopies	____ __________
____ Surgical procedures	____ __________
____ X-rays	

Figure 10-21 Sample Safety/Work Practice Controls for Office Procedures lists procedures that involve exposure to blood, body fluids, and other potentially infectious material. (Courtesy of POL Consultants, 2 Russ Farm Way, Delanco, NJ 08075, 865-824-0800)

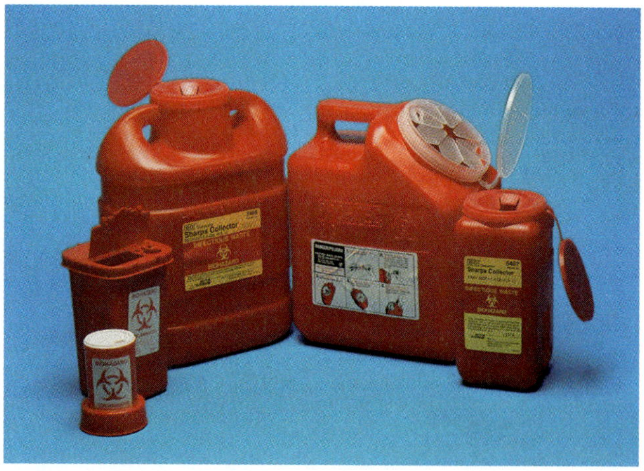

Figure 10-22 Various sizes of puncture-proof sharps containers. These and other biohazard waste containers are autoclaved when full and sent out to a biohazard agency for safe disposal.

OSHA for the prevention of exposure to bloodborne pathogens and other potentially infectious material.

1. *Standard Precautions.* Adherence to the CDC's Standard Precautions is required. Hand washing is stressed and employers must provide hand washing facilities and must ascertain that employees use them frequently and especially following exposure to blood or other potentially infectious material.
2. *Engineering Controls and Work Practice Controls.* Engineering controls and work practice controls consist of the physical equipment and mechanical devices an employer provides in an attempt to safeguard and minimize employee exposure. A common example of an engineering control is sharps disposal containers (Figure 10-22). Others are mechanical pipettes, fume hoods, splash guards, and eye wash stations (Figure 10-23). If and when occupational exposure continues after the engineering controls are in place, PPE must be used. Hand washing facilities or appropriate antiseptic hand cleanser (when hand washing facilities are unavailable) must be readily available.
3. *Personal Protective Equipment (PPE).* The employer must be certain that PPE is available and accessible and provide an alternative type of glove if an employee is allergic to those originally provided (see Latex Sensitivity box earlier in chapter.) Cleaning and laundering and disposal of PPE is the responsibility of the employer, and the employee does not incur any expense for them.

All PPE must be removed before the employee leaves the work site and placed in an appropriate

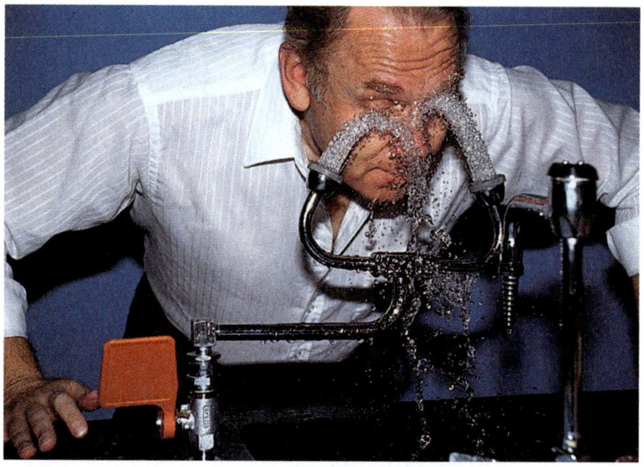

Figure 10-23 Emergency eyewash station: two streams of water or saline wash both eyes simultaneously and continuously.

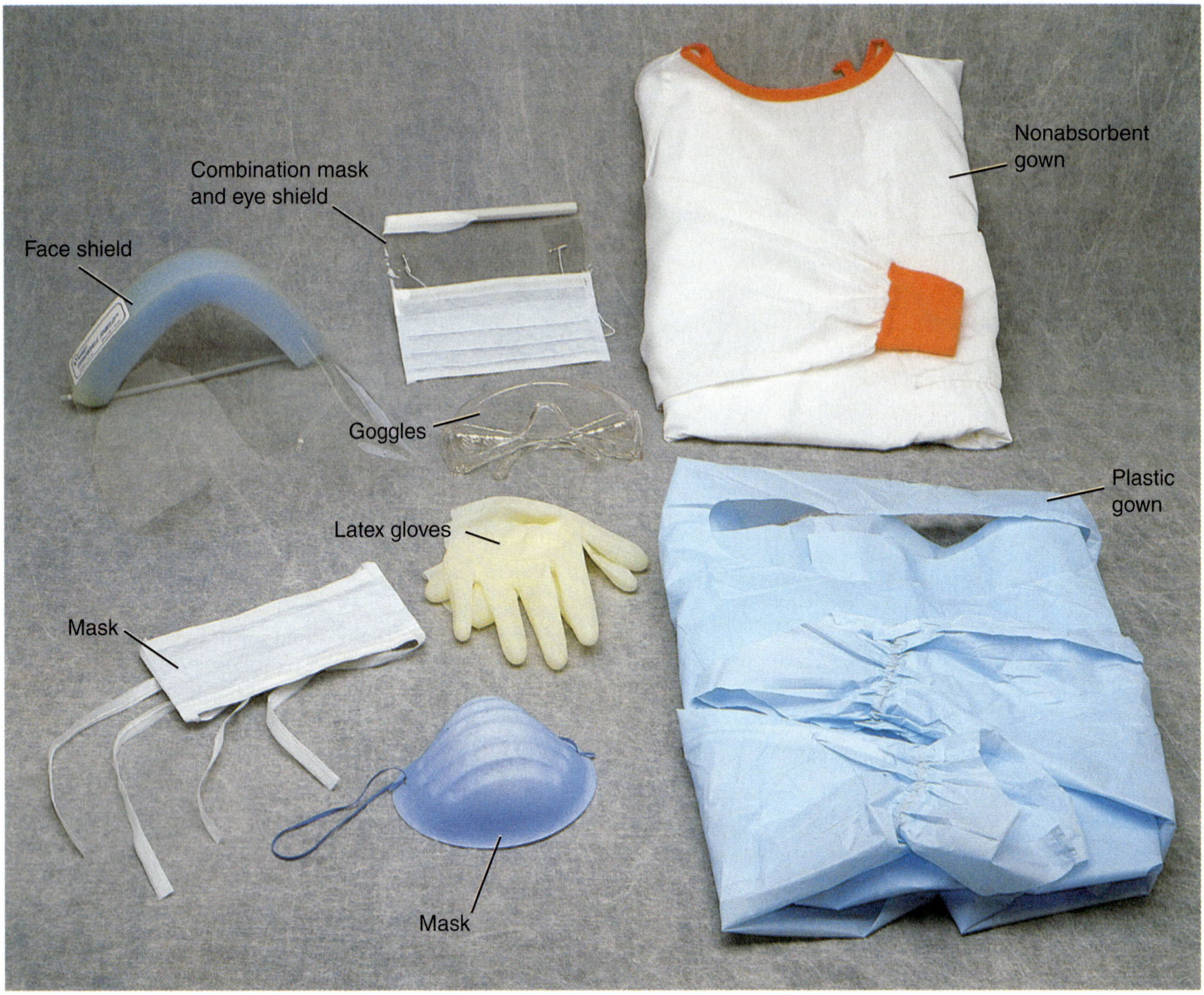

Figure 10-24 Personal protective equipment.

container that is supplied by the employer. Figure 10-24 shows PPE.

4. *Cleanliness of Work Areas.* The employer must maintain a work site that is clean and sanitary and have a written schedule for cleaning and decontaminating the work area after contact with blood and other potentially infectious material. **Spill kits** must be readily accessible (Figure 10-25).

Broken glass is placed in a sharps container after using cardboard or a dust pan and brush to remove it.

Laundry that is contaminated is handled with gloves and placed in a labeled container. If the laundry is damp or wet, gloves and other appropriate PPE must be worn, and the damp/wet laundry must be placed in a plastic bag(s) to prevent blood or other potentially infectious material from leaking through it. PPE cannot be laundered at home. All other Standard Precautions must be adhered to.

5. *Hepatitis B Vaccine.* HBV vaccine must be made available free of charge to every employee, full-time, part-time, or temporary, within 10 days of work assignment (Figure 10-26). This refers to employees who have the potential for occupational exposure, and who can "reasonably" be expected to have skin, eye, mucous membrane, or **parenteral** contact with blood or other potentially infectious material. The vaccine is given in three doses over a six-month period and is used to protect the employee from infection with HBV. It is an intramuscular injection with an approximate 96% rate of effectiveness.

An employee has the right to decline taking the vaccine but must sign a **declination form.** There is the option to reconsider receiving the vaccine at a later time.

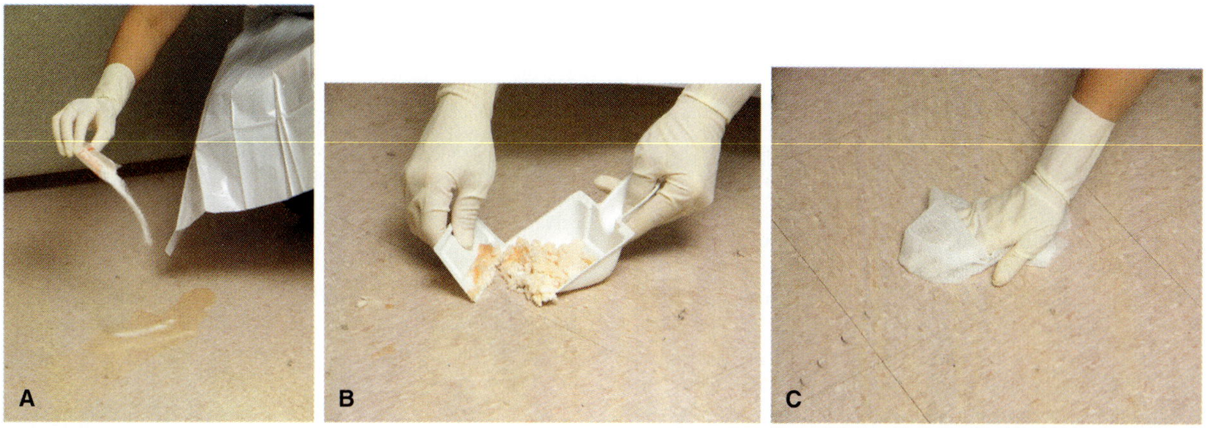

Figure 10-25 (A) Sprinkle coagulating powder over spill wearing protective clothing and gloves. (B) Scoop up spill with scoop from kit. (C) The spill area is then cleaned with a 10 percent bleach solution.

6. *Follow-Up After Exposure.* An accidental exposure is broadly defined as one in which blood, blood-contaminated body fluids, or body fluids or tissues to which Standard Precautions apply are introduced into a mucous surface, into nonintact skin, or into the conjunctiva via a needlestick, skin cut, or direct splash. If an incident exposes an employee to any of these, the employer must make available a confidential medical evaluation in which is documented:

   - The circumstances surrounding the event
   - The route or routes of exposure
   - The identification of the person who was the source of the exposure

   The following procedure describes the steps to take following an exposure incident:

   - Immediately wash exposed area with soap and warm water.
   - If mouth area is exposed, rinse with water or mouthwash.
   - If eyes are exposed, flush with large amounts of warm water.
   - Report incident to a supervisor immediately for documentation (Figure 10-27).

In addition, OSHA requires the following information:

   - The exposed employee must be tested for HBV, HCV, and HIV only if consent is given. An employee may refuse or may have blood drawn and stored for 90 days at which time the choice can be made whether to have the blood tested.
   - The source individual's blood, if permission is granted, is tested for HBV, HCV, and HIV and the employee shall know the results (unless protected by the law).
   - The employee is offered prophylaxis, gamma globulin, or HB vaccine after the exposure to HBV or HIV according to the current recommendation of the U.S. Public Health Service.
   - The employee is counseled regarding precautions to take to avoid possible transmission and is provided information on potential illnesses for which to be alert.
   - An OSHA 301 form must be filed.

7. *Medical Records.* Medical records of an employee who has suffered an occupational exposure must be kept for the length of employment plus 30 years, and confidentiality must be guaranteed.

   The following information is to be included in the employee's record: name and Social Security number, HB vaccination status with dates, results of any examinations or tests, a copy of the health care provider's written opinion, and a copy of the information that was provided to the health care provider.

   The records must be available to the employee, to OSHA, and anyone with the written consent of the employee, but *not* the employer.

Hazard Communication for Blood. The employer is required to label containers of **regulated waste,** refrigerators, freezers, and other containers that are used to keep or transport blood or other potentially infectious material with warning labels that are orange or orange-red and have the biohazard symbol affixed to them. Red bags can be used in place of labels. The labeling serves to

SAMPLE

Hepatitis B Employee Vaccination Form

MEMO: To all employees with occupational exposure to blood or other infectious materials on an average of one or more times per month.

OSHA and the CDC have identified the potential exposure of health care workers to hepatitis B virus (HBV) in the course of performing their duties in this office. For the protection of our employees, we are offering prescreening testing and the HBV vaccination with follow-up evaluation to all employees who are exposed to blood or other potentially infectious materials on an average of one or more times per month. *In accordance with recommended OSHA guidelines, this vaccine and testing will be offered at no cost to the employee.* You have the ability to decide whether or not you want the testing and/or vaccine. At the bottom of this memo, you may indicate your choice. Please return this memo with your signature and date to your immediate supervisor.

[ ] I want to receive the prescreening (optional)
[ ] I want to receive the vaccine and follow-up evaluation testing
[ ] I *do not* want the vaccine and testing and have read the following statement:

I understand that due to my occupational exposure to blood or other potentially infectious materials I may be at risk of acquiring hepatitis B virus (HBV) infection. I have been given the opportunity to be vaccinated with hepatitis B vaccine at no charge to myself. However, I decline hepatitis B vaccination at this time. I understand that by declining this vaccine I continue to be at risk of acquiring hepatitis B, a serious disease. If in the future I continue to have occupational exposure to blood or other potentially infectious materials and I want to be vaccinated with hepatitis B vaccine, I can receive the vaccination series at no charge to me.

________________ ________________
NAME DATE

________________ ________________
SIGNATURE SS#

PRESCREENING DATE ________ RESULTS __________
DATE OF VACCINATIONS ________________
DATE OF FOLLOW-UP EVALUATION __________
RESULTS ________________
NOTES:

Figure 10-26 Sample Hepatitis B Employee Vaccination Form provides employee information regarding hepatitis B vaccine and space to sign indicating whether employee declines vaccine. (Courtesy of POL Consultants, 2 Russ Farm Way, Delanco, NJ 08075, 856-824-0800)

SAMPLE

Post-Exposure Management Record

The following employee was the subject of an infectious exposure incident on (date) ______ and was examined and treated as follows:

Employee Name: ____________ SS# ____________
Type of Incident (describe) ________________

____

Route of Exposure: ________________

Source Patient Information:

____ Source patient could not be identified.
____ Source patient was identified but refused to contribute blood.
____ Source patient was identified and blood was secured from such patient. Results of blood testing of source patient's blood are attached to this form.

Employee hereby grants permission for tests for antibodies of human immunodeficiency virus (HIV-1) and/or hepatitis B virus and acknowledges that the employee has been counseled concerning such tests.

Employee Signature ____________ Date ________

The following test(s) were administered under supervision of a qualified provider:

____ Human Immunodeficiency Virus (HIV-1) Antibodies
____ Hepatitis B Virus Antibodies

Date(s) of Tests(s): ____________ Results of Test(s)—
See attached Provider's or Laboratory statement/report.

Employee hereby acknowledges that the employee was counseled and a written copy(ies) of the results of the above test(s) were furnished to such employee on (date):
____

Employee Signature ____________ Date ________

____ Additional follow-up was performed as indicated by attached reports.

NOTE: This record should be retained for length of employment PLUS thirty years.

Figure 10-27 Sample Post-Exposure Management Record can be used to document employee exposure to blood, body fluids, or other potentially infectious material; tests performed on the employee by a qualified provider; and test results. (Courtesy of POL Consultants, 2 Russ Farm Way, Delanco, NJ 08075, 856-824-0800) warn employees of the hazard possibility of container contents (Figure 10-28).

Information and Training for Employees. Employers must ascertain that employees take part in training sessions during working hours at no cost to employees. The initial session must be provided when occupational exposure may occur and annually thereafter. If employee tasks and job description change, training must take place at that time.

Training components are listed in Figure 10-29. Documentation of training sessions must be available and kept for 3 years.

OSHA REGULATIONS AND STUDENTS

With the passage of the OSHA law, all students with potential exposure to chemicals and bloodborne pathogens should follow all safety procedures as outlined by OSHA. Because students are not considered employees of a health care facility and are attending an educational institution, they do not fall under the OSHA guidelines. They should, however, take precautions to avoid contact with potentially infectious materials and toxic chemicals wherever learning is taking place (Figure 10-30).

BIOHAZARD LABELS

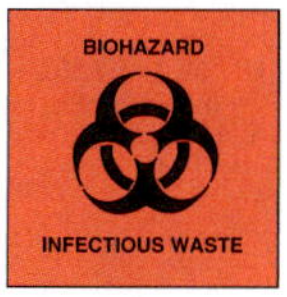

Containers that hold biohazardous materials must be properly labeled. Biohazardous materials include blood and body fluids as well as garments, gloves, masks, needles, gauze, wipes, aprons, and so on that may be contaminated with blood or other potentially contaminated body fluids. Labels shall be used to identify the presence of an actual or potential biological hazard.

CONSIDERATIONS:

- Labels shall be fluorescent orange or orange-red, with lettering or symbols in a contrasting color.
- Labels should be affixed onto or as close as feasible to the container by adhesive, string, wire, or other method.
- Red bags or red containers may be substituted for labels.
- If blood or control serum is stored in a refrigerator, the refrigerator shall be marked with a biohazard label.
- If blood is stored in a refrigerator for transport or same-day shipment, it does not need to be labeled but should be put in containment bags.

Figure 10-28 Biohazard labels alert employees to biohazardous materials, such as blood, body fluids, and other potentially infectious material.

Avoiding Exposure to Bloodborne Pathogens

Students can come into contact with blood and other potentially infectious material during laboratory practices and externships. The potential for exposure and contact increases whenever invasive procedures are being performed. Some examples of invasive procedures are:

- Phlebotomy, the process of withdrawing blood
- Administering an injection
- Performing or assisting with medical/surgical procedures such as suturing of wounds or removal of sutures; assisting with certain procedures such as Pap smears, arthroscopies, amniocentesis, thoracentesis, or lumbar puncture; dressing changes, colposcopies, vaginal exams, obstetrical care, vasectomies, biopsies, sigmoidoscopies, and colonoscopies are other examples in which students can contact blood and other potentially infectious material.

Students must be aware of and think about the procedures they are involved in and be certain that they use essential safety equipment (PPE) and procedures when necessary. Students should adhere to the same responsibilities that employees do.

PPE should be available in the student laboratory and used as necessary. Standard precautions must be strictly adhered to.

Students should always be on guard and make safety a priority by taking all precautions to avoid injuries. Some of the precautions are:

- Needles and other sharps (such as microscope slides and coverslips, sharp surgical instruments, and glass containers) should be handled with the same strict guidelines as outlined in the OSHA *Bloodborne Pathogen Standards* and the CDC's Standard Precautions.
- Obey all safety rules and know where the spill kits are located and how to clean up biohazard spills (see Figure 10-25).
- Know where the eyewash stations are and know how to operate them.

Be familiar with all the information about solutions and chemicals used in the laboratory as outlined in the Material Safety Data Sheet (MSDS) (see Chapter 26).

TRAINING COMPONENETS OF THE BLOODBORNE PATHOGEN STANDARD

Scope and Application

- The Standard applies to all occupational exposure to blood and other potentially infectious materials (OPIM), and includes part-time employees, designated first aiders, and mental health workers as well as exposed medical personnel.
- OPIM includes saliva in dental procedures, cerebrospinal fluid, unfixed tissue, semen, vaginal secretions, and body fluids visibly contaminated with blood.

Methods of Compliance

- General—standard precautions.
- Engineering and work practice controls.
- Personal protective equipment.
- Housekeeping.

Standard Precautions

- *All* human blood and OPIM are considered to be infectious.
- The *same* precautions must be taken with *all* blood and OPIM.

Engineering Controls

- Whenever feasible, engineering controls (devices that isolate or remove health hazards from the workplace) must be the primary method used to control exposure.
- Examples include needleless IVs, self-sheathing needles, sharps disposal containers, covered centrifuge buckets, aerosol-free tubes, and leak-proof containers.
- Engineering controls must be evaluated and documented on a regular basis.

Sharps Containers

- Readily accessible and as close as practical to work area.
- Puncture-resistant.
- Labeled or color-coded.
- Leak-proof.
- Closeable.
- *Routinely replaced* so there is no overflow.

Work Practice Controls

- Hand washing following glove removal.
- No recapping, breaking, or bending of needles.
- No eating, drinking, smoking, and so on in work area.
- No storage of food or drink where blood or OPIM are stored.
- Minimize splashing, splattering of blood, and OPIM.
- No mouth pipetting.
- Specimens must be transported in leak-proof, labeled containers. They must be placed in a secondary container if outside contamination of primary container occurs.
- Equipment must be decontaminated prior to servicing or shipping. Areas that cannot be decontaminated must be labeled.

Personal Protective Equipment (PPE)

- Includes eye protection, gloves, protective clothing, resuscitation equipment.
- Must be readily accessible and employers must require their use.
- Must be stored at work site.

Eye Protection

- Is required whenever there is potential for splashing, spraying, or splattering to the eyes or mucous membranes.
- If necessary, use eye protection in conjunction with a mask or use a chin-length face shield.
- Prescription glasses may be fitted with solid sideshields.
- Decontamination procedures must be developed.

Gloves

- Must be worn whenever hand contact with blood, OPIM, mucous membranes, nonintact skin, contaminated surfaces/items, or when performing vascular access procedures (phlebotomy).
- Type required —Vinyl or latex for general use.
  —Alternatives must be available if employee has allergic reactions (i.e., powderless).
  —Utility gloves for surface disinfection.
  —Puncture-resistant when handling sharps (i.e., Central Supply).

Protective Clothing

- Must be worn whenever splashing or splattering to skin or clothing may occur.
- Type required depends on exposure. Prevention of contamination of skin and clothes is the key.
- Examples —Low-level exposure lab coats.
  —Moderate-level exposure fluid-resistant gown.
  —High-level exposure fluid-proof apron, head and foot covering.
- *Note:* If PPE is considered protective clothing, then the *employer must* launder it.

Housekeeping

- There must be a written schedule for cleaning and disinfection.
- Contaminated equipment and surfaces must be cleaned as soon as feasible for obvious contamination or at end of work shift if no contamination has occurred.
- Protective coverings may be used over equipment.

Regulated Waste Containers (non-sharp)

- Closeable.
- Leak-proof.
- Labeled or color-coded.
- Placed in secondary container if outside of container is contaminated.

Figure 10-29 Overview of *The Bloodborne Pathogen Standard.* (Courtesy of the Occupational Safety and Health Administration, U.S. Department of Labor.)

TRAINING COMPONENETS OF THE BLOODBORNE PATHOGEN STANDARD

Laundry

- Handled as little as possible.
- Bagged at location of use.
- Labeled or color-coded.
- Transported in bags that prevent soak-through or leakage.

Laundry Facility

- Two options:
  1. Standard precautions for all laundry (alternative color coding allowed if recognized).
  2. Precautions only for contaminated laundry (must be red bags or biohazard labels).
- Laundry personnel must use PPE and have a sharps container accessible.

Hepatitis B Vaccination

- Made available within ten days to all employees with occupational exposure.
- At no cost to employees.
- May be required for student to be admitted to college health program as well as for externship.
- Given in accordance with United States Public Health Service guidelines.
- Employee must first be evaluated by health care professional.
- Health care professional gives a written opinion.
- If the vaccine is refused, the employee signs a declination form.
- Vaccine must be available at a future date if initially refused.

Post-Exposure Follow-Up

- Document exposure incident.
- Identify source individual (if possible).
- Attempt to test source if consent obtained.
- Provide results to exposed employee.

Labels

- Biohazard symbol and word *Biohazard* must be visible.
- Fluorescent orange/orange-red with contrasting letters may also be used.
- Red bags/containers may be substituted for labels.
- Labels required on —Regulated waste.
  —Refrigerators/freezers with blood of OPIM.
  —Transport/storage containers.
  —Contaminated equipment.

Information and Training

- Required for all employees with occupational exposure.
- Training required initially, annually, and if there are new procedures.
- Training material must be appropriate for literacy and education level of employee.
- Training must be interactive and allow for questions and answers.

Training Components

- Explanation of bloodborne standard.
- Epidemiology and symptoms of bloodborne disease.
- Modes of HIV/HBV transmission.
- Explanation of exposure control plan.
- Explanation of engineering, work practice controls.
- How to select the proper PPE.
- How to decontaminate equipment, surfaces, and so on.
- Information about hepatitis B vaccine.
- Post-exposure follow-up procedures.
- Label/color code system.

Medical Records

Records must be kept for each employee with occupational exposure and include:

- A copy of employee's vaccination status and date.
- A copy of post-exposure follow-up evaluation procedures.
- Health care professional's written opinions.
- Confidentiality must be maintained.
- Records must be maintained for thirty years plus the duration of employment.

Training Records

Records are kept for three years from date of training and include:

- Date of training.
- Summary of contents of training program.
- Name and qualifications of trainer.
- Name and job title of all persons attending.

Exposure Control Plan Components

- A written plan for each workplace with occupational exposure.
- Written policies/procedures for complying with the standard.
- A cohesive document or a guiding document referencing existing policies/procedures.

Exposure Control Plan

- A list of job classifications where occupational exposure control occurs (e.g., medical assistant, clinical laboratory scientist, dental hygienist).
- A list of tasks where exposure occurs (e.g., medical assistant who performs venipuncture).
- Methods/policies/procedures for compliance.
- Procedures for sharps disposal.
- Disinfection policies/procedures.

Figure 10-29 (continued)

(continues)

TRAINING COMPONENETS OF THE BLOODBORNE PATHOGEN STANDARD

- Procedures for selection of PPE.
- Regulated waste disposal procedures.
- Laundry procedures.
- Hepatitis B vaccination procedures.
- Post-exposure follow-up procedures.
- Training procedures.
- Plan must be accessible to employees and be updated annually.

Employee Responsibilities

- Go through training and cooperate.
- Obey policies.
- Use universal precaution techniques.
- Use PPE.
- Use safe work practices.
- Use engineering controls.
- Report unsafe work conditions to employer.
- Maintain clean work areas.

Cooperation between employer and employees regarding *The Bloodborne Pathogen Standard* will facilitate understanding of the law, thereby benefiting all persons who are exposed to HIV, HBV, HCV, and OPIM by minimizing the risk of exposure to the pathogens.

Meeting the OSHA standard is not optional and failure to comply can result in a fine that may total $10,000 for each employee.

To obtain copies of *The Bloodborne Pathogen Standard,* contact OSHA at 800-321-6742 or www.osha.gov.

Figure 10-29 (continued)

Student Safety Precautions

Gloves must be worn:
- During phlebotomy
- When giving injections
- When performing or assisting with invasive procedures
- When processing blood specimens

Eye protection with side projections must be worn:
- Whenever there is the potential for chemical exposure or the possibility of spray, splash, or splatter from blood or body fluids

Face shields or masks must be worn:
- When there is a chance of spray, splash, or splatter from blood or body fluids

Gowns or **aprons** must be worn:
- Where there exists any potential for exposure to contaminated materials

Lab coats must be worn and buttoned:
- When performing laboratory procedures

Figure 10-30 Student safety precautions.

An exposure to blood or other potentially infectious material experienced by a student must be immediately reported to the instructor if the accident occurs at the college or to the supervisor of the clinical agency and the externship coordinator if the student is exposed during externship. OSHA procedures as outlined earlier in this chapter should be followed with the exception of the filing of the OSHA 200 form.

Colleges require students studying the health professions to obtain the hepatitis B vaccine because it is approximately 96% effective against HBV. Because the vaccine is given in three doses over a period of 6 months, students should plan to have the injections in a timely fashion to be prepared for college laboratory courses and the externship period.

PRINCIPLES OF INFECTION CONTROL

By understanding the dependent nature of the chain of infection which holds that each link in the process must occur for infectious disease to occur, medical assistants can apply principles of infection control to eliminate or reduce the transmission of infectious microorganisms in the health care setting. Conscious and continual reliance on infection control is a professional standard and protects employees, patients, families, and the public from contracting infectious diseases. There are two general types of infection control: medical asepsis and surgical asepsis. Each is indicated in specific circumstances and each is achieved by the various techniques that are described in this chapter and in Chapter 19.

MEDICAL ASEPSIS

Medical asepsis is the use of practices such as hand washing, general cleaning and disinfecting of contaminated surfaces, and adherence to Standard and Transmission-Based Precautions. These measures are aimed at destroying pathologic organisms. These techniques are used to decrease the risk for transmission to others. Objects should be medically aseptic if they are to be used in procedures that are on the external body or if they will enter a usually contaminated body part, such as the mouth. Many things, such as our hands, cannot be sterilized or even disinfected, but they can be rendered clean of **gross contamination** and most pathogens by simple hand washing. Many items, such as stethoscopes or telephones, do not need to be sterile to be used on a variety of patients. These items do not enter into the body or into sterile areas of the body. These items should, however, be either cleaned or disinfected routinely. Sphygmomanometers and stethoscopes are used continuously throughout the day on different patients. Patients with hypertension, postsurgery patients, and patients having physical examinations routinely have blood pressure monitored. Both pieces of equipment contact patient's skin, clothing, or both, making the blood pressure equipment an indirect source of pathogens. Alcohol-based wipes or a simplified method of detergent cleaning should be used regularly to decontaminate blood pressure equipment. Medical asepsis also involves environmental hygiene measures such as equipment cleaning and disinfection procedures. Careful attention to methods of medical asepsis greatly reduces the presence of pathogens that could cause disease in others. Specific procedures to achieve medical asepsis include adherence to Standard and Transmission-Based Precautions. Standard Precautions and Transmission-Based Precautions are considered methods of medical asepsis. These precautions should be followed stringently to provide barriers between potentially infectious blood and body fluids and those people who may come into contact with the fluids. Use of PPE, disinfection, and waste control are crucial steps in practicing these precautions. Hand washing, sanitization, and disinfection of instruments or equipment are also essential.

Some specific examples of appropriate use of medical asepsis include:

- Wash hands before and after handling equipment and supplies, on arrival and before leaving, and before and after working with each patient even when gloves are worn.
- Handle all specimens as if they were contaminated.
- Use disposable equipment whenever possible and dispose of it properly in a biohazard waste container. All equipment is contaminated after patient use.
- Use PPE as outlined in Standard Precautions and wash hands after removal of any PPE, including gloves.
- Keep contaminated equipment and supplies away from clothing to prevent transmission of pathogens to self and others.
- Place dressing materials, gauze, cotton balls, and any other damp or wet contaminated absorbable material in a waterproof bag before disposal in the biohazard waste container.
- Any break in the medical assistant's skin should be covered with a sterile dressing.
- Items that fall to the floor are contaminated. Either discard or sanitize then disinfect them before using.
- If uncertain whether equipment or supplies are clean or sterile consider them contaminated. Clean or sterilize them before use.

Hand Washing

Hand washing is the most important aspect of all of the infectious control procedures. Proper hand washing removes gross contamination and reduces pathogens that could be transmitted by direct or indirect contact to others. Because hand washing is frequently required, the use of a good lotion is advised to reduce the possibility of skin breaks caused by dryness. Infectious diseases continue to present serious challenges. One of the biggest concerns is the spread of HIV, HBV, and HCV. In May 2007, the WHO issued nine patient safety solution recommendations. The Joint Commission has adopted the nine recommendations. Patient Safety Solutions No. 9 is entitled "Improved Hand Hygiene to Prevent Healthcare Associated Infection (HAI)." It can be applied to this chapter and to others because, according to the WHO, millions of people worldwide are suffering from hospital-acquired infections. "Effective hand hygiene is the primary measure for avoiding this problem," say the WHO and the Joint Commission.

Hand washing is the single, most effective way to lower the incidence of infectious disease transmission.

The CDC recommends that, as part of hand hygiene, when hands are visibly soiled with blood or other body fluids, they should be washed with either a nonantimicrobial soap or an antimicrobial soap and water. Procedure 10-1 describes medical asepsis hand wash. If hands are not visibly soiled, an alcohol-based hand rub or gel can be used routinely for decontaminating hands. When decontaminating hands with an alcohol-based hand rub, apply to palms of one hand and rub hands together covering all surfaces of hands and fingers, palms, back of hands, fingertips, and between fingers, wrists, and thumbs until hands are dry.

The CDC further recommends that hands be decontaminated in the following situations:

- Before and after patient contact
- After contact with blood or body fluids
- When caring for the patient if moving from a contaminated body site (mouth, rectum) to a clean body site (surgical wound, urinary meatus)
- After contact with inanimate objects such as medical equipment in close proximity to the patient
- Before inserting a urinary catheter
- After removing gloves and before donning gloves
- Before eating and after using restroom

Antimicrobial wipes *cannot* be used as a substitute for an alcohol-based hand rub. Wearing gloves is *not* a substitute for hand decontamination. Artificial fingernails or nail extenders cannot be worn when in direct contact with patients at high risk. Natural nails should be kept less than ¼ inch long.

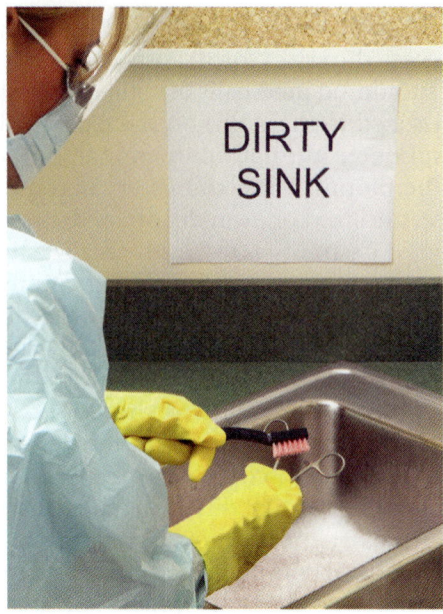

Figure 10-31 Medical assistant sanitizing an instrument.

Sanitization

Sanitization (washing) of instruments and equipment rids them of gross contamination and blood, body fluids, tissue, and other contaminated **debris.** Enzymatic detergent especially designed for medical instruments and a soft scrub brush are used to remove all contaminates from surfaces, crevices, hinges, and serrations. Use of enzymatic detergents will help break down the proteins found in body fluids and tissues. Water temperature should be warm but not hot. Heat coagulates protein, making it more difficult to remove. A critical component to promoting effective sanitization is to complete the procedure as soon as possible after contamination so that tissue or body fluids do not have the opportunity to dry on the instruments. Dried debris is more difficult to remove and may require much scrubbing. Instruments may be left to soak in disinfectant solution or water with a **solvent** if sanitization cannot be performed immediately after use (Figure 10-31).

To avoid the risk for punctures or cuts from sharp instruments during sanitization, heavy-duty gloves should be worn. Some facilities use an **ultrasonic cleaner** (Figure 10-32). It uses high-frequency sound waves and agitates the instruments (sanitizes them) before sterilizing them. Goggles are worn to protect eyes from splashing of contaminated debris during the scrubbing procedure. A plastic apron provides protection from splashing of clothing (see Chapter 19). Hot water may be used for rinsing to remove all residue and aid in the drying process. Check instruments for working condition. Drying thoroughly will prevent damage from rust or water spots.

Larger items such as instrument trays or Mayo stands, stools, chairs, examination tables, and lamps should also have a decontaminating sanitization process with thorough washing, rinsing, and drying.

See Procedure 10-4 for instrument sanitization. Gloves contaminated with blood and body

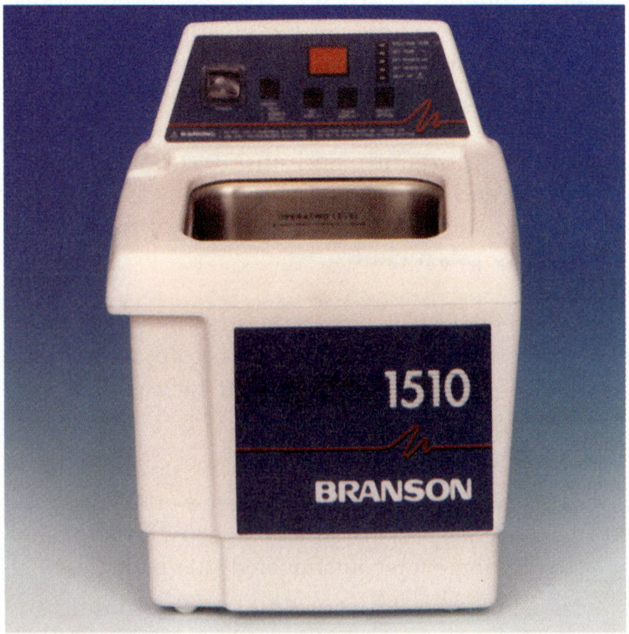

Figure 10-32 The Branson Ultrasonic Cleaner, model 1510. (Courtesy of Branson Ultrasonics Corp.)

fluids should be removed carefully to contain the contamination. Procedure 10-2 describes how to remove contaminated gloves, thereby preventing further exposure to biohazard substances.

Disinfection

Disinfection, a third procedure used in medical asepsis practices, consists of various chemicals that can be used to destroy many pathogenic microorganisms but not necessarily their spores. Disinfection chemicals are used on inanimate objects. Because of their **caustic** nature, these chemicals can irritate the skin and mucous membranes. Chemicals are used to disinfect items or equipment made from materials that could be damaged by heat or that are too large to fit into an autoclave such as stethoscopes, percussion hammers, examination tables, and Mayo trays and stands. These and other items that are chemically disinfected are used during *external* physical examination or procedures.

Boiling water (temperature 212°F) is considered a form of disinfection because it will kill some forms of microorganisms. It is important to note that this method *cannot* be considered a sterilization technique because the temperature is not high enough to kill the hepatitis virus, tuberculosis bacteria, or microbial spores. Articles such as nasal and ear specula can be sanitized and disinfected by vigorous boiling for at least 15 minutes, or soaked in a disinfectant according to manufacturer's instructions. The only reasonable use for boiling as a means of disinfection in today's medical setting is for items that:

1. Will *not* be used in invasive procedures
2. Will *not* be inserted into body orifices nor be used in a sterile procedure

Before either chemical disinfection or disinfection by boiling, articles must first be thoroughly sanitized and dried. Of special note are stainless steel gynecologic and proctologic examination instruments. These instruments are not sanitized with other instruments because of the risk for transmission of sexually transmitted diseases (STDs). They are sterilized in the autoclave after sanitization to eliminate transmission of microorganisms.

Chemical disinfectant solutions must be carefully prepared and used according to the manufacturer's instructions to ensure effective disinfectant properties. Medical offices should use the disinfectant solution that best meets the needs of the ambulatory care setting as to the quantity of instruments to be disinfected, cost, preparation requirements, storage needs, and handling procedures. When choosing a chemical disinfectant solution, pay close attention to the manufacturer's report of the chemical disinfectant properties of the product. Some solutions are effective against a wide spectrum of microorganisms, whereas other solutions may be selective for certain common microorganisms. When chemically disinfecting, items must be thoroughly sanitized and dried. Any debris or water left on the item being chemically treated will affect the chemical solution, thereby decreasing its effectiveness and compromising the disinfecting process.

For surfaces such as countertops, the least expensive and most readily available chemical is a 1:10 solution of ordinary household bleach (sodium hypochlorite). However, besides the obvious disadvantage of bleaching clothing, bleach is not easily rinsed, and it is only effective if the solution is mixed fresh daily. Nevertheless, its effectiveness is so highly respected that many medical laboratories depend almost entirely on bleach to chemically kill pathogens on countertops.

In summary, medical asepsis includes procedures for which all medical assistants must be responsible and qualified to incorporate into daily work practices. The responsibility for maintaining medical asepsis is the combined goal of the office staff and providers.

Maximum Process	Stethoscope	Chair	Ear Speculum	Vaginal Speculum	Fiberoptic Endoscope	Surgical Instrument	Skin
Sanitization	X	X	X	X	X	X	X
Chemical disinfection by wiping	X	X	X				
Chemical disinfection by soaking			X				
Boiling			X				

BIOTERRORISM

Bioterrorism is the use of biologic weapons (pathogenic microorganisms) to create fear in people. A bioterrorism attack is the deliberate release of biologic agents (weapons) such as bacteria, viruses, and toxins to cause death or illness in people, plants, or animals. The agents can spread through the air, food, and water. Terrorists can easily obtain and use biologic agents. The agents can be very difficult to detect and difficult to protect against. They have no odor, are invisible, have no taste, and can be spread quietly. Only small amounts are needed to kill or cause serious illness to hundreds of thousands of people. The agents can be put into food and/or water, absorbed through or injected into the skin, and dispensed as aerosols. Some diseases can be treated with pharmaceutical agents such as antibiotics and antitoxins.

The most dangerous disease threats are anthrax, botulism, pneumonic/bubonic plague, smallpox, and tularemia.

Anthrax, pneumonic/bubonic plague, and tularemia all can be treated with antibiotics. Smallpox is treated by early vaccination (within 4 days). The CDC has the vaccine (Table 10-7).

Table 10-7 Example of Six Agents that Could Be Used in a Bioterrorism Attack

Disease	Agent	Transmission	Vaccine Availability	Treatment
Anthrax	Bacterium	Inhalation Not spread person to person	Yes, but not readily available	Antibiotics
Botulism (severe food poisoning)	Toxin	Toxin in food Not spread person to person	Antitoxin (state, local health departments, and CDC have)	Antitoxin should be given as soon as disease is suspected
Plague (2 types: bubonic, pneumonic)	Bacterium found in rodents and their fleas	An infected flea bites someone Materials that are contaminated with bacteria can enter through nonintact skin Bubonic plague does not spread person to person Pneumonic plague occurs when bacteria are inhaled because it spreads through the air and from person to person	None	Antibiotics
Smallpox	Virus	Skin eruptions occur on arms, legs, feet, and face Virus settles in the nose and throat and spreads when infected person coughs, talks, or sneezes Can spread through ventilation systems Contact with contaminated clothes and bedding Highly contagious	After disease was eradicated, supplies of the virus were to be destroyed or locked away in two laboratories, one in the U.S. and the other in Russia Last immunization for smallpox was 1980 Immunity lasts for about 10 years	Symptomatic FDA has approved a new smallpox vaccine that will be used in the event of a bioterrorist attack
Tularemia	Bacterium (infected rabbits and ticks spread bacteria)	Human to human spread uncommon. Bacterium can enter nonintact skin, mucous membranes of eyes, respiratory tract, gastrointestinal tract	Yes	Antibiotics

Education plays a vital role in raising awareness and increasing the knowledge of health care professionals to aid them in being better prepared for threats to the public health. Protection against the agents should be started early. PPE and high-efficiency particulate air (HEPA) filters will filter most biologic agents from the air. Antibiotics given even before the agent is identified helps protect people, as do vaccines.

The Food and Drug Administration (FDA) has approved a new smallpox vaccine. The FDA said it is intended to inoculate people who are at high risk for exposure to smallpox, a highly contagious disease. The FDA-said the vaccine could be used to protect people during a bioterrorist attack. There is no FDA-approved treatment for smallpox.

According to the CDC, the threat that biologic agents will be used is more likely now than it has been throughout history. The WHO, the CDC, the Department of Homeland Security, and state and local public health departments are excellent resources for more information about bioterrorism (see Chapter 9).

Procedure 10-1

Medical Asepsis Hand Wash (Hand Hygiene)

STANDARD PRECAUTIONS:

PURPOSE:

To reduce pathogens on the hands and wrists, thereby decreasing direct and indirect transmission of infectious microorganisms. Average duration is 1 minute before beginning to work with patients, 15 seconds (CDC Hand Hygiene recommendation) following each patient contact.

EQUIPMENT/SUPPLIES:

Sink (preferably with foot-operated controls)
Soap (preferably liquid soap in foot-operated container; bar soap discouraged)
Water-based antibacterial lotion
Disposable paper towels
Nail stick or brush

PROCEDURE STEPS:

1. Remove all jewelry (plain wedding band is only acceptable jewelry). Push watch up on arm or remove. RATIONALE: Jewelry harbors microorganisms on the hands.
2. Prepare disposable paper towel (if using pull-down dispenser, prepare the amount of paper towel necessary for drying hands after wash; if using folded towels, have accessible). RATIONALE: After the hand washing, you may not touch any contaminated surface, such as the handle on a paper-towel dispenser or the water faucets.
3. Never allow your clothing to touch the sink; never touch the inside of the sink with your hands. RATIONALE: The sink is considered contaminated at all times (*NOTE:* Sinks must be sanitized and disinfected at the end of each day).
4. Turn on the faucet with a dry paper towel (Figure 10-33A). Discard paper towel after adjusting water temperature to lukewarm. RATIONALE: Lukewarm water is best for hand washing because excessively hot water may overdry the skin.
5. Wet hands and apply soap using a circular motion and friction; rub into a lather (Figure 10-33B). RATIONALE: This initial hand wash is to remove visible soil and some microorganisms. Interlace fingers to clean between them (Figure 10-33C).
6. Use an orange stick or brush at the first hand washing of each day (Figures 10-33D and E). RATIONALE: Nails harbor microorganisms. Even with trimmed nails, this step must be performed on a daily basis.
7. Rinse hands with hands pointed down and lower than elbows (Figure 10-33F). RATIONALE: When hands are held lower than elbows, pathogens and contaminated water run off the hands and not up on the forearms.
8. Repeat soap application and lather; interlace fingers well; wash with vigorous, circular motions all parts of hands including wrists; wash for at least one minute or longer depending on

continues

Procedure 10-1 (continued)

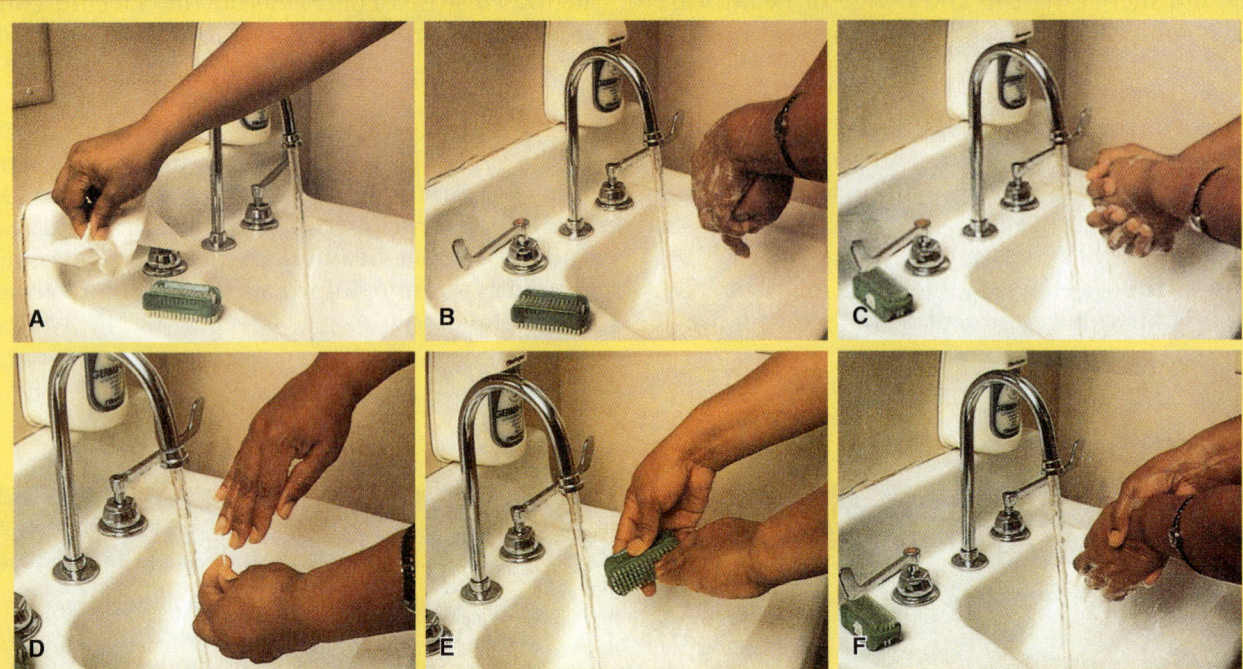

Figure 10-33 (A) Prepare towels for use. Turn on the faucet and adjust water to a lukewarm temperature. (B) Wet hands. Let water flow downward off hands and fingertips. (C) Use a circular motion to create friction and wash the palms and backs of hands. Interlace the fingers to clean between them. (D) Use an orange stick to clean under fingernails. (E) A hand brush may also be used to clean under fingernails. (F) Rinse hands thoroughly, letting the water flow downward off your hands and fingertips.

degree of contamination. RATIONALE: Appropriate length of hand washing is required to provide enough friction to remove soil and microorganisms.

9. Rinse well, keeping hands pointed downward. RATIONALE: Rinsing removes microorganisms, contaminated water, and soap from the hands.
10. Repeat hand washing for the first hand washing of the day or if necessary for contaminated or visibly soiled hands. Lather wrists using a circular motion and friction. Rinse arms and hands. RATIONALE: When the hands are excessively contaminated or soiled, two hand washings may be necessary to remove microorganisms from the hands.
11. Dry hands and wrists with disposable paper towel; do not touch towel dispenser after hand washing; blot instead of rubbing with towel; if sink is not foot operated, use a clean disposable towel to turn off water faucet. RATIONALE: Touching the towel dispenser contaminates the hands. Blotting the hands dry reduces drying of the skin. Turning faucet off with paper towel prevents recontamination from dirty faucet.
12. Discard paper towel in waste container. Do not leave contaminated towels for repeated use. *NOTE*: Repeat hand washing procedure before and after each patient contact, procedure, or meal. RATIONALE: Hand washing must be performed on a regular and frequent basis to ensure the reduction of microorganisms transmitted by hands.

Water-based antibacterial lotion can be applied to prevent chapped, **excoriated** skin. If skin is excoriated, the medical assistant may not be able to work because of breaks in the skin or may have to wear gloves during any patient contact.

Procedure 10-2

Removing Contaminated Gloves

STANDARD PRECAUTIONS:

PURPOSE:

To carefully remove and dispose of contaminated gloves to contain exposure.

EQUIPMENT/SUPPLIES:

Biohazard waste container

PROCEDURE STEPS:

1. Grasp the palm of the used left glove with the right hand to begin removing the first glove. Notice hands are held away from the body and pointed downward (Figure 10-34A and B). RATIONALE: Holding the hands away from the body will further prevent exposure to biological contaminants.
2. Turn the used left glove inside out and hold it in the right gloved hand. Be careful not to touch your bare left hand on the contaminated right glove (Figure 10-34C–E). RATIONALE: Turning the glove inside out helps isolate the biological contaminants.
3. Holding the glove that has been removed with the hand that still has the glove on, insert two fingers of the ungloved hand between your arm and the inside of the dirty glove (Figure 10-34F).

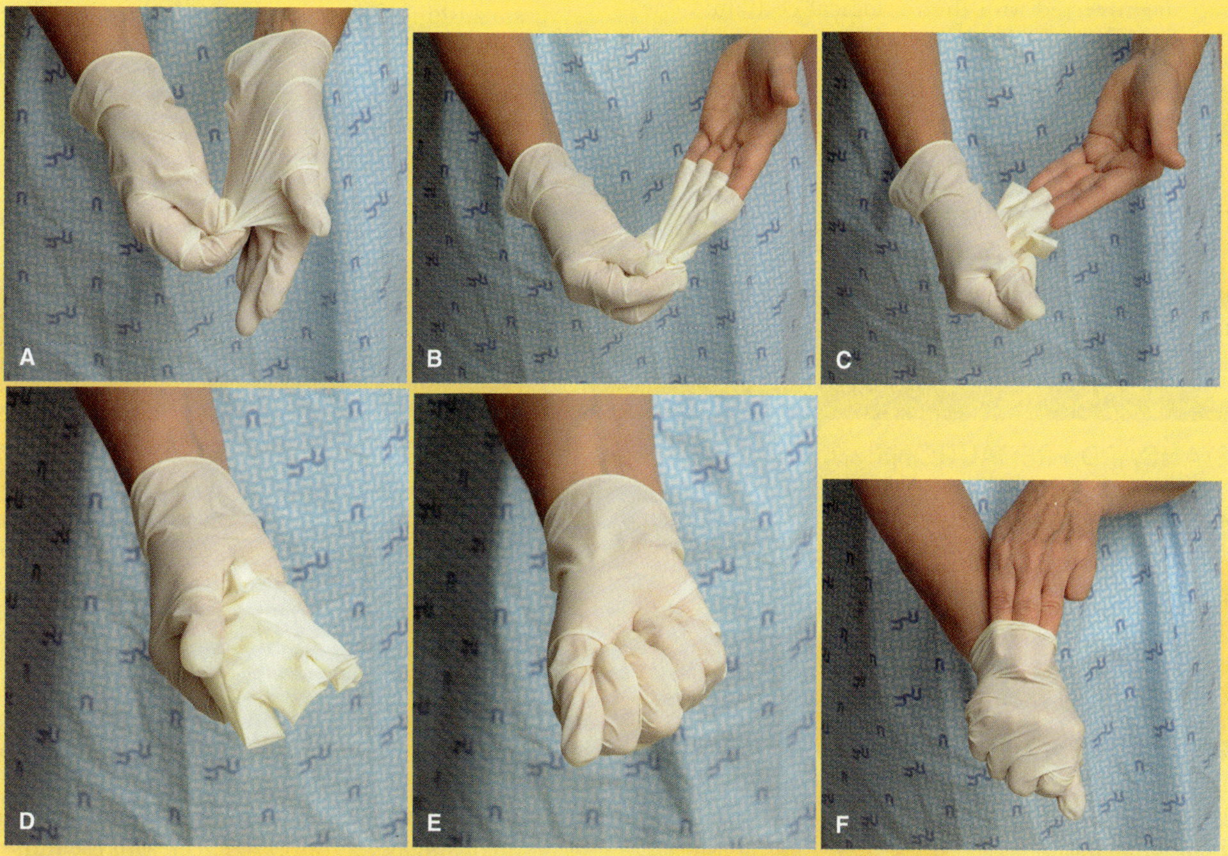

Figure 10-34 (A) Grasp the palm of the used glove with the right hand. (B) Begin removing the first glove. (C) Glove is turned inside out as it is being removed. Take care to not touch bare skin on the contaminated glove. (D) Inverted glove is completely removed into the contaminated glove. (E) Contain the inverted glove completely in the gloved hand. (F) Insert two fingers of the ungloved hand inside the back of the contaminated glove and turn it inside out over the other.

continues

Procedure 10-2 (continued)

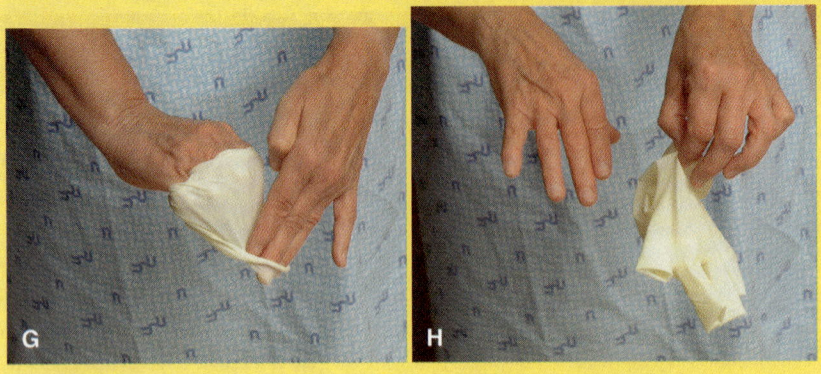

(G) Invert the second glove over the first. (H) One glove is now inside the other.

4. Turn the right dirty glove inside out over the other. One glove is inside the other and you can handle the gloves because the dirty, contaminated area is inside the gloves (Figure 10-34G and H). RATIONALE: Both gloves are inverted with the biological contaminates isolated.
5. Dispose of the inverted gloves into a biological waste receptacle. RATIONALE: All biological waste should be placed into a red biohazard bag.
6. Wash hands thoroughly. RATIONALE: Immediate washing of hands is an additional precaution.

Procedure 10-3

Transmission-Based Precautions: Donning a Gown, Mask, Gloves, and Cap (Isolation Technique)

STANDARD PRECAUTIONS:

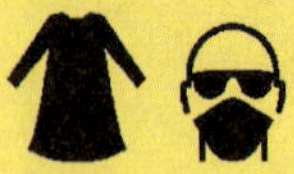

PURPOSE:
To provide barriers for medical assistant to be protected from airborne, contact, or droplet infectious diseases.

EQUIPMENT/SUPPLIES:
Disposable gowns
Disposable caps if needed
Disposable masks
Gloves (nonsterile and sterile)
Room with sink and running water
Paper towels
Other supplies relative to client's condition

PROCEDURE STEPS:
1. Review provider orders and agency protocols relative to the type of isolation precautions. RATIONALE: Provides for patient comfort and decreases the spread of microorganisms. Limits the number of personnel coming into the patient's room and the patient's exposure to microorganisms.
2. Place appropriate isolation supplies outside the patient's room and note type of isolation sign on the door (e.g., airborne, droplet, or contact). RATIONALE: Ensures staff follows isolation protocol and alerts visitors to check with the nurses' station before entering the room.
3. Remove jewelry, laboratory coat, and other items not necessary in providing patient care. RATIONALE: Decreases the spread of microorganisms.

continues

Procedure 10-3 (continued)

4. Wash hands and don disposable clothing:
   a. Apply cap to cover hair and ears completely.
   b. Apply gown to cover outer garments completely. Hold gown in front of body and place arms through sleeves (Figure 10-35A). Pull sleeves down to wrist. Tie gown securely at neck and waist (Figure 10-35B and C).
   c. Don nonsterile gloves and pull gloves over the cuff to cover completely.
   d. Apply mask by placing the top of the mask over the bridge of your nose (top part of mask has a metal strip) and pinch the metal strip to fit snugly against the skin of the nose.

   RATIONALE: Disposable garments act as a barrier in preventing the transmission of microorganisms from medical assistant to patient and protect the medical assistant from contact with pathogens.
5. Enter patient's room with all gathered supplies. RATIONALE: Prevents trips into and out of the patient's room and keeps supplies clean.
6. Assess vital signs and perform other functions (ECG, phlebotomy) of care to meet the needs of the patient. Record assessment data on a piece of paper, avoiding contact with any articles in the patient room. RATIONALE: Allows for data collection and the performance of patient care.
7. Dispose of soiled articles in the impermeable biohazard bags, which should be labeled correctly according to contents. If soiled, reusable equipment is removed from the room; label bag accordingly. RATIONALE: Impermeable biohazard bags prevent the leakage of contaminated materials, thereby preventing the transmission of infection. Labeling is a warning to other personnel that the contents are infectious.

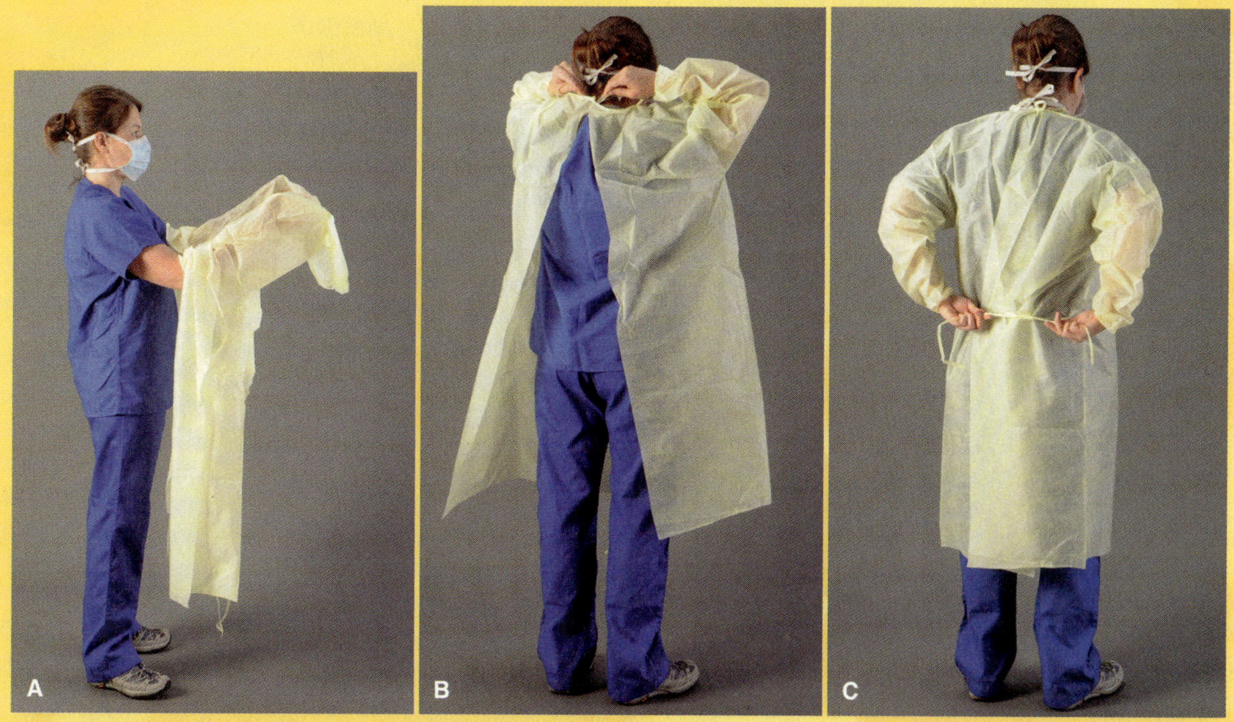

Figure 10-35 (A) Medical assistant has put on a mask and is donning the gown, pulling on the sleeves. (B) The neck of the gown is tied first and (C) the back of the gown, last.

continues

Procedure 10-3 (continued)

Exiting the Isolation Room: Removing Gown, Gloves, Mask, and Cap

1. Remove contaminated gloves (see Procedure 10-2). Wash hands and then untie waist tie of gown (Figure 10-36A).
2. Remove mask by untying bottom ties first, then top ties (Figure 10-36B). Holding mask by ties, place in contaminated waste.
3. Untie neckties of gown (Figure 10-36C). Wash hands. RATIONALE: Removes microorganisms from hands before proceeding.
4. Slip fingers of one hand inside cuff (Figure 10-36D) of the other hand. Pull the gown over the hand, being careful not to touch the outside of the gown.

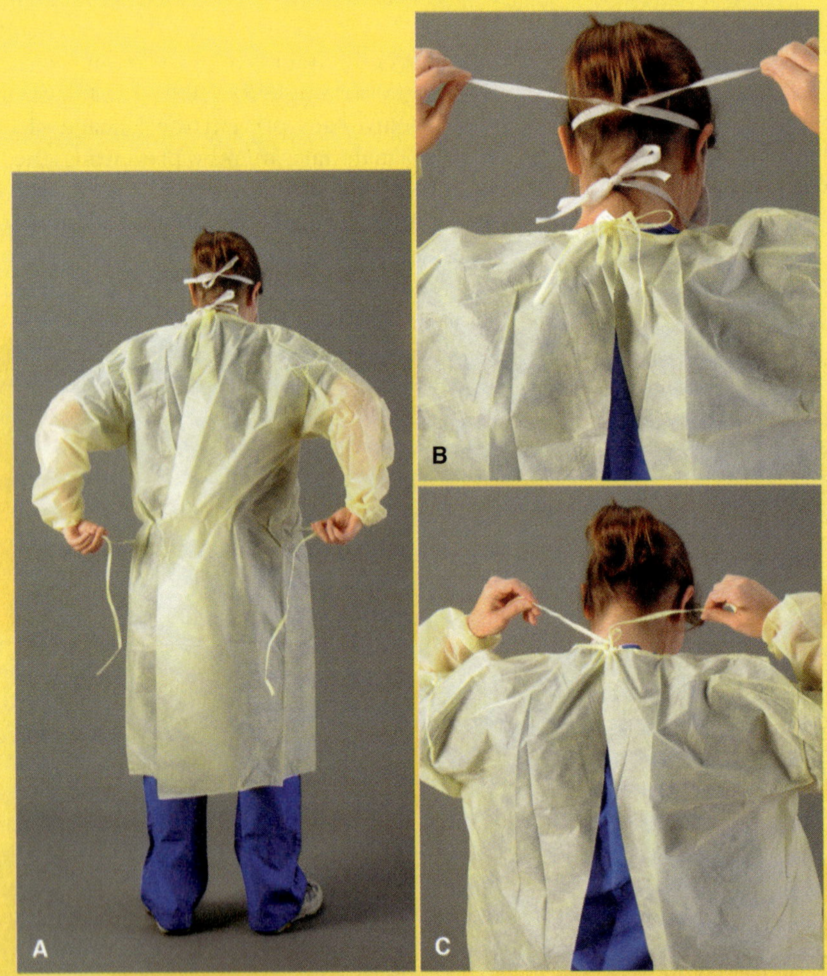

Figure 10-36 (A) When finished in the isolation room, the medical assistant removes the contaminated gloves (see Procedure 10-2), washes hands (see Procedure 10-1), and then unties waist tie of gown. Remove mask by untying bottom ties first, then top ties. (B) Holding mask by ties, place in biohazard container. (C) Untie neck ties of gown. Wash hands.

continues

Procedure 10-3 (continued)

5. Using the hand covered by the gown, pull down the gown over the other hand (Figure 10-36E).
6. Pull gown off your arms. Hold gown away from yourself and roll into a ball with the contaminated side inside (Figure 10-36F). RATIONALE: The gown is removed and folded, touching only the inside of the gown to prevent transmission of microorganisms to yourself.
7. Dispose of gown in biohazard container.
8. Wash hands thoroughly.
9. Document procedures performed on patient (vital signs, EKG, phlebotomy) in patient record or electronic medical record.

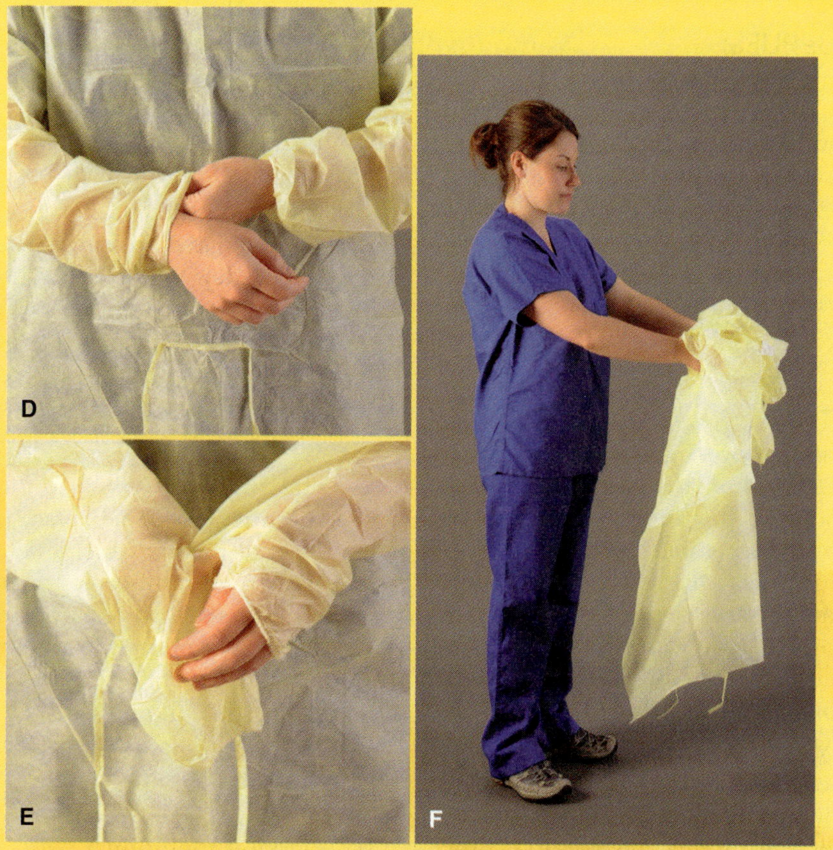

Figure 10-36 (continued) (D) Slip fingers of one hand inside cuff of the other hand. Pull gown over the hand, being careful not to touch the outside of the gown. (E) Using the hand covered by the gown, pull down the gown over the other hand. (F) Pull gown off arms and hold away from body and clothing. Roll into a ball with the contaminated side of gown on the inside. Wash hands thoroughly.

Procedure 10-4

Sanitization of Instruments

STANDARD PRECAUTIONS:

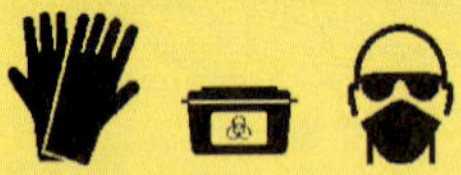

PURPOSE:

To properly clean contaminated instruments to remove tissue and debris.

EQUIPMENT/SUPPLIES:

Sink (or ultrasonic cleaner: follow manufacturer's instructions)
Sanitizing agent (low-sudsing detergent, approved chemical disinfectant, or blood solvent)
Brush
Disposable paper towels
Plastic apron
Disposable gloves, heavy-duty if cleaning sharps
Goggles
Biohazard waste container

PROCEDURE STEPS:

1. Wear heavy duty gloves, goggles, and apron. RATIONALE: Contaminated instruments pose a blood and body fluid precaution as indicated by OSHA standards. Disposable gloves must always be worn to sanitize instruments. Wear heavy-duty gloves if cleaning sharp instruments. Goggles are worn to protect eyes from splashing of contaminated debris during scrubbing procedure. A plastic apron provides protection from splashing of clothing.
2. As soon as possible after a procedure in which an instrument is contaminated, rinse the instrument in water and disinfectant solution; rinse again under running water. RATIONALE: Rinsing contaminated instruments as soon as possible after use removes debris and tissue that could quickly dry onto the instrument, making sanitization more difficult.
3. If contaminated instrument must be carried from one place to another for sanitization, place the instrument in a basin labeled "Biohazard." RATIONALE: Do not carry contaminated instruments in your hands. Biohazard basins must be sanitized and disinfected daily according to procedures for Standard Precautions.
4. Scrub each instrument well with detergent and water; scrub under running water, and be sure to scrub inside any edges, serrations, and all surfaces. RATIONALE: Thorough scrubbing removes tissue and debris from all areas of the contaminated instrument. If all tissue is not removed with scrubbing, the instrument may not be sterilized during sterilization procedures.
5. Rinse well with hot water. RATIONALE: Tissue and debris, as well as detergent, must be completely removed. Hot water will help remove all residue and aid in the drying process while rust and water spots will be eliminated.
6. After they are rinsed, place instruments on muslin or disposable paper towel until all instruments have been scrubbed and rinsed. RATIONALE: Often more than one instrument is sanitized; do not place sanitized instrument in the bottom of the sink or on a countertop without a disposable paper towel or muslin towel.
7. Dry instruments with muslin or disposable paper towels. RATIONALE: Wet instruments may rust or corrode. Check instruments for working condition.
8. Remove gloves and wash hands.

Case Study 10-1

Refer to the scenario at the beginning of the chapter.

CASE STUDY REVIEW

1. Explain the patient education Bruce can use to encourage adults to take advantage of available immunizations.
2. From where can Inner City Health Care Urgent Care Center, where Bruce is employed, order or obtain adult vaccines for immunizations?

Case Study 10-2

Your provider–employer asks you to help develop an exposure control plan. Include the measures the employer must take to eliminate or lessen an employee's risk for exposure to blood or other potentially infectious materials.

CASE STUDY REVIEW

1. How often will the plan be reviewed?

SUMMARY

Effective infection control measures are the first defense against the transmission of infectious diseases in the ambulatory care setting. Reliance on Standard and Transmission-Based Precautions, protective barriers, and basic principles of disinfection promotes professional and responsible clinical care for patients. When the processes of infection control are applied to all clinical procedures, the chain of infection may be broken by many varied means. Remember that an infectious disease will not spread to another person if the chain is sufficiently broken at any stage.

Infectious diseases spread and accidents occur through lack of education and carelessness. Medical assistants must understand the importance of the regulations and guidelines set forth by the federal government and follow through by helping employers and fellow employees implement them. In doing so, the health and safety of patients and health care workers can be protected, the spread of infectious diseases can be kept under control, and the risk for contracting a serious infectious disease such as HIV, HBV, or HCV will be greatly minimized.

Every medical office and ambulatory care setting must, by law, have clearly written and readily available manuals containing information about Standard Precautions and OSHA for the safe handling, storage, and disposal of blood, body fluids, and chemicals.

Through consistent use of Standard Precautions and adherence to OSHA laws, health care providers can acquire the behaviors and techniques needed to safeguard themselves and their patients.

Because of frequent changes in the laws, it is necessary for medical assistants and all other health care providers to keep abreast of the government mandates.

STUDY FOR SUCCESS

To reinforce your knowledge and skills of information presented in this chapter:

- Review the Key Terms
- Practice any Procedures
- Consider the Case Studies and discuss your conclusions
- Answer the Review Questions
  - Multiple Choice
  - Critical Thinking
- Navigate the Internet and complete the Web Activities
- Practice the StudyWARE activities on the textbook CD
- Apply your knowledge in the Student Workbook activities
- Complete the Web Tutor sections
- View and discuss the DVD situations

REVIEW QUESTIONS

Multiple Choice

1. Standard Precautions are issued by:
   a. Health and Human Services
   b. Centers for Disease Control and Prevention
   c. Food & Drug Administration
   d. Occupational Safety and Health Administration
2. *The Bloodborne Pathogen Standard* is primarily concerned with:
   a. reducing the transmission of HIV, HBV, and HCV infections
   b. protecting the employer from lawsuits
   c. regulating the use of personal protective equipment
   d. taking blood samples from patients
3. In the chain of infection, the location of the infectious agent is known as the:
   a. reservoir
   b. portal of exit
   c. portal of entry
   d. means of transmission
4. The stage in infectious disease in which symptoms are vague and undifferentiated is called the:
   a. incubation stage
   b. prodromal stage
   c. acute stage
   d. onset of disease stage

Critical Thinking

1. Analyze the importance of infection control and give five examples of how a medical assistant would practice responsible infection control in the ambulatory care setting.
2. Your patient has a draining wound. After you change the dressing, explain how to prevent the transmission of the microorganisms from the wound and dressing to you or another patient.
3. Give an example of how the proper disposal of contaminated objects can break a link in the chain of infection.
4. You notice a coworker sanitizing surgical instruments in preparation for sterilization. He or she did not scrub the serrations on the instruments well. What will be the result of his or her improper sanitization technique? Explain your answer.
5. Describe eight procedures/techniques that you could be performing on a patient that could expose you to bloodborne pathogens.
6. What becomes of the biohazard containers once they are full?
7. What alternative do you have if you do not have access to soap and water after performing a procedure on a patient?
8. Explain the differences between sanitization and disinfection.
9. Considering the growth requirements for pathogens, describe how to discourage bacterial growth in the patient examination room.

WEB ACTIVITIES

1. The U.S. Department of Labor Occupational Safety and Health Administration (OSHA) Web site (http://www.osha.gov) provides you with significant amounts of information about OSHA—the federal agency that seeks to protect health care workers from bloodborne pathogens. Visit the site to determine when the most recent changes have been made to *The Bloodborne Pathogen Standard.* What are they?
2. The HIV and Hepatitis.com Web site (http://hivandhepatitis.com/hep_b.html) gives information about simultaneous infections of HIV, HBV, and HBC. What are the statistics for persons who are infected with HIV and HBV, or HIV and HBC?
3. The Centers for Disease Control and Prevention National Center for Infectious Diseases Web site (http://www.cdc.gov) provides a tremendous amount of information regarding infectious diseases and hepatitis in particular. Information also is available about HIV and AIDS. Are there other hepatitis viruses in addition to A, B, and C? Look on this site for the treatment of choice for all hepatitis viruses you find, and describe what the most common side effects are of treatment.
4. Health information from WebMD Healthwise, Inc. P.O. Box 1989, Boise, ID 83701 (http://www.medscape.com) provides information on current recommendations for adult immunization in the United States. Check this site and determine if you, your adult relatives, and adult friends are current and up to date with the recommendations.
5. The Medical College of Wisconsin Web site (http://www.mcw.edu) provides an antibiotic guide and treatment recommendations for common infections. Visit this site to discover the likely antibiotic treatment for (1) pneumonia (community acquired), (2) pharyngitis (exudative), and (3) gonorrhea.
6. The National Coalition for Adult Immunization in Bethesda, Maryland, provides helpful information regarding adult immunizations on its Web site (http://www.medscape.com/NCAU/). Use this site to find facts about measles, mumps, and rubella such as: (1) Are these diseases preventable? (2) Who should get the vaccine? (3) How are measles, mumps, and rubella spread? (4) What risks are there for a woman and her fetus in her first trimester if she contracts rubella during that time?

REFERENCES/BIBLIOGRAPHY

Altman, G. B. (2004). *Delmar's fundamentals and advanced nursing skills* (2nd ed.). Clifton Park, NY: Delmar Cengage Learning.

Extensively drug-resistant tuberculosis. Retrieved June 22, 2007, from http://www.Medicine.Web.com.

Infectious Disease Epidemiology, Prevention and Control Division, STD and HIV Section, Minnesota Department of Health. (2007). *Hepatitis B and HIV/AIDS.* Retrieved June 9, 2007, from http://www.health.state.mn.us.

Josephson, D. L. (2004). *Intravenous infusion therapy for nurses principles and practices* (2nd ed.). Clifton Park, NY: Delmar Cengage Learning.

Keir, L., Wise, B. A., & Krebs, C. (2008). *Medical assisting administrative and clinical competencies* (6th ed.) Clifton Park, NY: Delmar Cengage Learning.

Occupational Safety and Health Administration Bloodborne Pathogens-1910.1030 (Regulations [Standards-29CFR]). Retrieved June 11, 2007, from http://osha.gov.

Pommerville, J. C. (2004). *Alcamo's fundamentals of microbiology* (7th ed.) Sudbury, MA: Jones and Bartlett Publishers.

Simmers, L. (2004). *Diversified health occupations* (6th ed.) Clifton Park, NY: Delmar Cengage Learning.

Taber's cyclopedic medical dictionary (21st ed.). (2002). Philadelphia: F. A. Davis.

Tamparao, C. D. & Lewis, M. A. (2005). *Diseases of the human body* (4th ed.) Philadelphia: F. A. Davis.

U. S. Department of Health and Human Services, Centers for Disease Control and Prevention. (2001). (Federal Register). Washington DC: U.S. Government Printing Office. Retrieved June 11, 2007, from http://cdc.gov/ncidod/hip/isolat/isoapp_a.html.

U. S. Department of Health and Human Services, Centers for Disease Control and Prevention. (2004). *Facts about pneumonic plague.* Retrieved June 14, 2007, from http:// www.emergency.cdc.gov/agent/plague/factsheet.asp.

THE DVD HOOK-UP

In this chapter, you learned about proper infection control guidelines.

During one of the scenes, Mr. Breech became very ill and vomited. The vomit sprayed on the medical assisting extern and on and around the sink area. The extern turned around and quietly told the medical assistant that there was blood in the vomit.

1. Do you think that the extern should have said something in front of the patient about the blood in the vomit? What might have been a more tactful way of letting the medical assistant know about the blood in the vomit?
2. During the aseptic hand cleansing scene, the extern did not clean under her nails because it was not the first hand wash of the day. Do you think that the medical assistant should have instituted a nail cleansing anyway, because of the particular circumstances? Why?

DVD Journal Summary

Write a paragraph that summarizes what you learned from watching today's DVD program. In one of the scenes, Sandy accidentally stuck herself on a used needle. She was quite frightened when she spoke with her supervisor. She wrestled with the idea of starting treatment. Do you think that Sandy was overreacting? What do you think you would do if you accidentally stuck yourself with a contaminated needle? Would you start treatment right away?

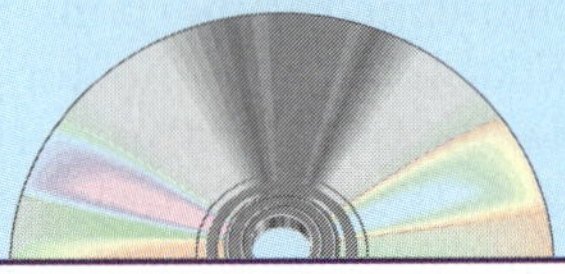

DVD Series	**Program Number**
Skills Based Series	4

Chapter/Scene Reference
- Watch entire program

The Patient History and Documentation

Chapter 11

KEY TERMS

Allergy
CHEDDAR
Chief Complaint
Clinical Diagnosis
Objective
Problem-Oriented Medical Record (POMR)
SOAP/SOAPER
Source-Oriented Medical Record (SOMR)
Subjective

OUTLINE

The Purpose of the Medical History
Preparing for the Patient
A Cross-Cultural Model
Patient Information Forms
- Demographic Data Form
- Financial Information Form
- Privacy Information Form
- Release of Information Form
- Medical History Form

Computerized Health History
The Patient Intake Interview
- Interacting with the Patient
- Displaying Cultural Awareness
- Being Sensitive to Patient Needs
- Approaching Sensitive Topics

Communication across the Life Span
The Medical Health History
- SOAP/SOAPER and CHEDDAR
- Chief Complaint
- Present Illness
- Medical History
- Family History
- Social History
- Review of Systems (ROS)

The Patient Record and Its Importance
- HIPAA Compliance
- Contents of Medical Records
- Continuity of Care Record

Methods of Charting/Documentation
- Source-Oriented Medical Records
- Problem-Oriented Medical Records

Electronic Medical Records (EMR)
Rules of Charting
- Abbreviations Used in Charting
- Chart Organization

OBJECTIVES

The student should strive to meet the following performance objectives and demonstrate an understanding of the facts and principles presented in this chapter through written and oral communication.

1. Define the terms as presented in the glossary.
2. Explain the purpose of the medical history.
3. Recall three functions to complete prior to a patient's appointment.
4. Compare/contrast the cross-cultural concerns between patients and providers.
5. Describe the four non-medical information forms to be signed by patients.
6. Discuss the medical assistant's general approach to the patient intake interview.

OBJECTIVES (continued)

7. Recall at least four circumstances to address in displaying cultural awareness.
8. Develop a strategy for communicating across the life span with patients.
9. Identify the components of the medical health history and their documentation.
10. Obtain a medical history from a patient.
11. Restate the function and meaning of SOAP/SOAPER and CHEDDAR charting.
12. List the characteristics of the patient's chief complaint and the present illness.
13. Compare/contrast the patient's medical, family, and social histories.
14. Discuss the rationale for including adult immunizations in health histories.
15. Explain how the review of systems is obtained and documented.
16. State five reasons why the medical record is important.
17. Identify three areas of concern regarding HIPAA compliance and the patient's chart.
18. Recall the rules for charting and documenting in the patient's chart.
19. Compare/contrast SOMR and POMR.
20. List the advantages of electronic medical records.
21. Review common charting abbreviations.
22. Describe the organization of a medical record.

Scenario

When clinical medical assistant Joe Guerrero, CMA (AAMA), of Drs. Lewis and King takes a patient history, he typically uses a form custom designed for the office. Joe uses the form as a guideline to be sure he gathers all pertinent information. However, he has learned that he must tailor his questions to the patient and sometimes will rearrange the order of the questions if necessary. Although Joe is adept at gathering specific and necessary patient information, he also is aware of patient concerns and sensitivities and adapts his approach to accomplish the task while making the patient feel at ease.

INTRODUCTION

A patient's medical record and all information in it, including the medical history, is key to competent medical care. Ideally, from the first encounter with the patient to any subsequent visits, all information regarding a patient's medical care is kept in one location—with the primary care provider.

A record created for all new patients will include a number of vital pieces of information. Established patients will have information updated upon each visit. Essential components of a complete medical record include present and past medical history, family and social history, chief complaints or problems, medications, allergies, laboratory results, summaries from other practitioners seen, and a host of other data related to the patient's health. A patient's record will also include demographic data, address, next of kin, and current insurance information.

Often, a family practice or internal medicine clinic will have a broad and rather extensive questionnaire for patients to complete which serves as the basis for the medical history. These questionnaires can be purchased or created on the computer, and they may be unique according to specialty. The questionnaire can be mailed to patients, even attached to an email to patients, so that questions can be answered in the quiet environment of their homes where they likely have access to the information requested. When patients are called the day before their appointment, they can be reminded to bring the completed questionnaire with them.

The role of the medical assistant in taking the patient history is to be as thorough as possible and still remain sensitive to the patient. Respect for the patient's privacy is to be balanced with the need for the kind of complete information that results in informed medical treatment and care.

The patient medical record is a collection of confidential patient information. Should a patient's medical record be introduced in court, it becomes a legal record of care given. It is essential that charting in the record be accurate, clear, concise, and complete.

Spotlight on Certification

RMA Content Outline

- Oral and written communications
- Charts
- Problem oriented records

CMA (AAMA) Content Outline

- Recognizing and responding to verbal and nonverbal communication
- Professional communication and behavior
- Evaluating and understanding communication
- Interviewing techniques
- Medical records
- Documentation/reporting
- Performing telephone and in-person screening
- Patient history interview
- Organization of patient's medical record

CMAS Exam Outline

- Basic health history interview
- Basic charting

THE PURPOSE OF THE MEDICAL HISTORY

The medical history is the basis for all treatment given by the primary care provider, on-call provider, any other provider, and any specialist consulted to treat the patient. During the history-taking process, information is revealed to help guide treatment for the patient. The medical history makes it easier to recall previous treatment and review notes and laboratory results.

In addition, medical histories give a base for statistical analysis for research, insurance data, and for any health department notices. The health history and chart notes are a legal record of patient treatment. This is especially important if the patient makes an injury claim against another party or if the patient makes a malpractice claim against the provider. If the records in the chart are precise and correct, the chart becomes a good defense; however, if the charting or documentation is sloppy or incomplete, the entire record may be questioned as insufficient. The best policy is to document everything concerning patient care.

PREPARING FOR THE PATIENT

Before the patient's visit and obtaining the medical history, perform the following:

1. Make certain the examination room is clean, tidy, and ready for the patient.
2. Check to see that all necessary supplies are available.
3. Review the patient's chart. Note the age, any possible need for assistance, and identified reason for appointment.

When everything is ready, go to the reception area for the patient. It is preferable to call the patient's full name (John Nichols or Mr. Nichols) unless the patient previously requested the use of the first name or a nickname. Speak clearly and plainly, making certain that your patient will be able to hear. When the patient stands, quickly determine if assistance is necessary. (The physical assessment has begun.) If assistance is warranted, make that offer and accompany the patient to the examination room, remembering later to note in the chart the assistance provided. A friendly greeting is appreciated and helpful; a greeting such as, "How are you today?" may not be appropriate.

Patients in the medical clinic generally are not feeling well and take that question seriously. Also, the reception area is not the appropriate place for the patient to begin sharing his or her medical issues. The following comments may be acceptable: "Did you have any trouble finding parking?" or "I really like the colors in the shirt you are wearing. They remind me of summer."

Once in the examination room and the door is closed, seat the patient comfortably and sit face-to-face with the patient to begin the interview. Build rapport with the patient. Use the patient's name often and make certain you pronounce it correctly. Finally, think globally. Ask about factors in the patient's life that might influence health. These topics might be sports, travel, pets, family, and hobbies. Not only does this provide information for the health history, it usually eases and relaxes the patient for the more difficult questions in the interview.

A CROSS-CULTURAL MODEL

It is important to understand that every patient interview is a cross-cultural one. Providers and patients view the gathering of the patient history and the personal visit differently. Health and illness are inseparable from social and cultural beliefs. Who patients are—their background, their belief system, their family orientation, and their cultural heritage—influences their choices in health care. Providers and patients have different concerns and anticipations, and the medical assistant conducting the interview who is aware of these perspectives will keep the following in mind:

- *Patient's chief concern:* The illness. The personal and social significance and the problems created by the illness are important to the patient.
- *Provider's chief concern:* Disease. The provider is concerned with the malfunctioning and maladaptation of biological and psychological processes.
- *Patient's idea of treatment success:* Being able to successfully manage an illness and its problems is often more important to the patient than curing the disease.
- *Providers's idea of treatment success:* Successfully managing treatments, medications, and procedures to control disease problems.

The medical assistant may find it helpful to ask certain questions of patients to help them move across cultures; for example:

Patient Education

Some patients may seem reluctant to answer your questions regarding birthplace or Social Security number. Noncitizens may fear deportation if they are identified in the health care system, especially if they are seriously ill. Remind these patients that you are there solely to assist them with their health care needs and encourage them to provide accurate information to assist you in appropriate diagnosis and treatment, because many diseases are specific to geographic locations.

1. What do you think caused your problem?
2. When do you think it started?
3. What effect does it have on you?
4. What are your concerns about this problem?
5. What kind of treatment do you expect?

These questions respect the patient's perception while providing helpful information to the provider.

PATIENT INFORMATION FORMS

A number of important forms are created in the medical setting at this time.

Demographic Data Form

The demographic data form (Figure 11-1) registers the patient's full name, address, mailing address if different, home and work telephone numbers, cell phone numbers, date of birth, Social Security number and all insurance information, person to be contacted in case of emergency, and a release of information signature.

Financial Information Form

Some facilities include the financial information form (Figure 11-2) to be signed. This form contains information on the financial policy of the practice, including billing, insurance billing, co-payment billing, and any finance charges added to monthly billings.

CODE

PATIENT INFORMATION

PLEASE PRINT

ACCOUNT

PATIENT	Mr. Mrs. Miss/Ms. Last	First	MI	HOME PHONE: ( )

Patient's Home Address	Street	City	State	Zip
Patient's Billing Address	Street	City	State	Zip
Social Security #	Date of Birth	Age	Sex	Driver's License #
Patient's Employer	Work Address		Work Phone:	
Spouse's Name	Spouse's Employer (Name & Address)		Work Phone:	
Emergency Contact: (Local Relative or Friend) Name	Address		Phone:	

REFERRED TO THIS OFFICE BY: ______

WHO IS YOUR PRIMARY PHYSICIAN? ______

INSURANCE PLEASE LIST ALL HEALTH CARE INSURANCE COMPANIES WHICH COVER THIS PATIENT:

PRIMARY: Name ______ Policy # ______ Subscriber ______

Insurance Address ______

SECONDARY: Name ______ Policy# ______ Subscriber ______

Insurance Address ______

MEDICARE # ______ (Please Include Letter)

MEDICAID # ______
(MEDI-CAL)

RESPONSIBLE PARTY	Mr. Mrs. Miss/Ms. Last	First	Middle
Address		Phone	
Occupation	Employers Name & Address	Bus. Phone:	

Please remember that insurance is considered a method of reimbursing the patient for fees paid to the doctor and is not a substitute for payment. Some companies pay fixed allowances for certain procedures, and others pay a percentage of the charge. It is your responsibility to pay any deductible amount, co-insurance, or any other balance not paid for by your insurance.

METHOD OF PAYMENT: CASH ______ CHECK ______ CREDIT CARD ______

PLEASE READ & SIGN THE FOLLOWING:
I directly assign all medical / surgical benefits to ______
and understand that I am financially responsible for all charges whether or not paid by insurance. I hereby authorize the doctor to release all information necessary to secure the payment of benefits. I further agree that a photocopy of this agreement shall be as valid as the original.

SIGN HERE ______ DATE: ______

FORM # 58-8421-01 • BIBBERO SYSTEMS, INC. • PETALUMA, CALIFORNIA © 10/85 (REV. 8/93) TO REORDER CALL TOLL FREE: 800-BIBBERO (800 242-2376) OR FAX: (800) 242-9330

Figure 11-1 Sample patient demographic form. (Courtesy of Bibbero Systems, Inc., Petaluma, CA.)

FINANCIAL POLICY

In order to reduce confusion and misunderstanding between our patients and the clinic, we have adopted the following financial policy. If you have any questions about this policy, please discuss them with our Billing Manager. We are dedicated to providing the best possible care and service to you and we regard your complete understanding of your financial responsibilities as an essential element of your care and treatment.

Unless other arrangements have been made in advance by yourself or your health coverage carrier, payment is due at time of service. For your convenience, we accept debit or credit cards or we can arrange a payment schedule.

YOUR INSURANCE:

We accept assignment of benefit from Medicare. We also have direct billing agreements with many insurance companies. We will bill those plans for whom we have an agreement and will only require that you pay the co-payment at the time of service.

If your medical plan determines a service is "not covered," you will be responsible for the entire charge. Payment is due upon receipt of statement from this office.

MINOR PATIENTS:

The adult accompanying the patient and the parent or guardian with custody will be billed for all services rendered to minor patients.

MISSED APPOINTMENTS:

In order to provide the best service and availability to our patients, we ask you to notify us 24 hours in advance if you know that you will be unable to keep the appointment. We reserve the right to charge for missed appointments.

I have read the financial policy and I understand it and agree to be bound by its terms.

_______________ Date __________

Figure 11-2 Sample financial information form.

Privacy Information Form

Since April 2004, the Health Insurance Portability and Accountability Act (HIPAA) privacy rule limited the circumstances in which individuals' protected health information (PHI) could be used or disclosed. It also required medical providers to give notice of its privacy practice to all patients. The notice must describe patients' rights, the facilities' practices related to PHI, and where and how to file a complaint if patients feel their rights have been violated. Health providers must make a good faith effort to obtain written acknowledgement from patients that the privacy notice was received.

The privacy notice has a number of components and can be lengthy. Many facilities have printed their notice in a brochure format. Details of the Privacy Rule can be found on the CMS Web site (http://cms.hhs.gov/HIPAAGenInfo/). Many varieties of privacy notices can be viewed online by searching for "HIPAA privacy notices."

There are civil penalties if a medical facility fails to comply with the Privacy Rule and criminal penalties if a person knowingly obtains or discloses PHI in violation of the HIPAA guidelines.

Release of Information Form

New patients may be asked to complete a Release of Information form (Figure 11-3) that is often created in the office. This form is sent to their former

AUTHORIZATION TO RELEASE HEALTH CARE INFORMATION

Patient __________ Date of Birth __________
SSN __________ Previous Name __________

I request and authorize __________________ to release the health care information of the patient named above to:

Name ______________________________
Address ______________________________

This request and authorization applies to:
(Please initial the appropriate box)

__ Health care information relating to the following treatment, condition, or dates of treatment:

____

__ All health care information **EXCLUDING** specific information relating to sexually transmitted diseases (including HIV/AIDS), alcohol or drug use, or visits related to psychiatric disorders or mental health.

__ All health care information **INCLUDING** specific information relating to sexually transmitted diseases (including HIV/AIDS), alcohol or drug use, or visits related to psychiatric disorders or mental health.

__ Other:______________________________

I understand that my express consent is required to release any health care information relating to testing, diagnosis, and/or treatment of HIV (AIDS virus), sexually transmitted disease, psychiatric disorders/mental health, or drug and/or alcohol use. If I have been tested, diagnosed, or treated for HIV (AIDS virus), sexually transmitted disease, psychiatric disorders/mental health, or drug and/or alcohol use, you are specifically authorized to release all health care information relating to such diagnosis, testing, or treatment.

______________________ / __________
Signature of patient or patient's authorized representative — Relationship to patient

____
Date

Figure 11-3 Sample release of information form.

providers to obtain past medical records and in some cases can be used to allow sharing of information with family members at the request of the patient.

If the patient has several providers, the examining provider will encourage the patient to choose one person to manage primary medical care so that all medical care and records are concentrated in one location. Under most managed care insurance policies, patients have one primary care provider (women may also have an obstetrician/gynecologist) who coordinates the patient's health care.

Medical History Form

The medical health history form can be as short as one page (8½″ × 11″) or as long and detailed as six to eight pages. This form includes information on:

1. Present health history, including why the patient is being seen
2. Health history, personal and family
3. Social history including marital status, sexual orientation, and occupation
4. Military service, including dates and assignment (alerts provider to screen for common veteran illnesses and inquire about Agent Orange exposure)
5. Body systems review/questionnaire
6. Medications currently being taken, including over-the-counter and prescription medications
7. Provider's review of systems (ROS) (completed by the provider)

The best form is neither too long nor too complicated. Patients may feel overwhelmed with a long form and may not finish it, stating they cannot remember all the information. The form that is simple and brief can provide adequate information in many instances. Some patients find a history form intimidating. It is often easier for these patients to talk directly with the medical assistant or the provider about the history, feeling a one-to-one exchange is more personal and private.

Many samples of health history forms can be viewed on the Internet. Facilities often ask patients who regularly use a computer and have Internet access to go online and print their health history form for completion prior to their appointment. Depending on the ambulatory care setting, this form can be tailored to include vaccines and immunizations, usage of recreational drugs, exercise and diet regimens, accident information (especially if patient was hurt on the job), and any other information suited to the provider's specialty. Health history forms can be printed in other languages, such as Spanish.

COMPUTERIZED HEALTH HISTORY

EHR Health care facilities may use totally computerized health histories. These can be of two types: patient-generated and provider-generated. In patient-generated health histories, the patient responds on the computer to various questions and then reviews information with the medical assistant for completeness. Patients who do not want to use a computer should be given the option of answering questions face to face. When using a provider-generated health history, the medical assistant completes the information on the screen during or after the patient interview. These programs are user-friendly and save time for both the patient and medical assistant. The medical assistant should remember to interact with the patient by looking up from the computer from time to time during the entry of information. It is easy to forget to look at patients as you ask them questions and enter the information. This habit can make the patient feel disconnected to the process.

THE PATIENT INTAKE INTERVIEW

Interacting with the Patient

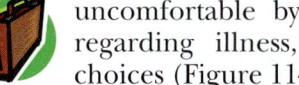

When the medical assistant takes the medical history, the first responsibility is to put the patient at ease (Table 11-1). A comfort level must be developed as the medical assistant guides the conversation, keeps it on track, and obtains the most information for the provider. Allowing conversation to wander, talking about other people, or letting the patient tell anecdotes does not help to complete the history. Explaining a term or concept that the patient does not understand is helpful. The medical assistant must remain professional and not be embarrassed or made uncomfortable by the patient's answers regarding illness, actions, or personal choices (Figure 11-4).

If the patient is already an established patient but has not seen the provider for several months or longer, update the medical history by asking if any illnesses have occurred in the time elapsed, if any new allergies to any medications or other substances have occurred, and the reaction to each. Document the chief complaint for

Table 11-1 General Approach to the History

1. Ensure an appropriate environment that is lit well, at a comfortable temperature, quiet, private, and free of distractions.
2. Sit facing the patient at eye level; the patient also should be seated. Ensure that the patient is as comfortable as possible, because obtaining the health history can be a lengthy process. Figure 11-4 illustrates an appropriate setting.
3. Avoid the use of medical jargon. Use terms the patient can understand.
4. Reserve asking intimate and personal questions until rapport is established.
5. Remain flexible in obtaining the health history. It does not need to be obtained in the exact order it is presented in this chapter or on the form.
6. Remind the patient that all information will be treated confidentially.
7. Ask the patient if he or she has any questions.

the current visit. The **chief complaint** is the problem that brings the patient to the provider. Sometimes patients bring several problems to discuss. Depending on the appointment schedule for the day, this may be difficult to accomplish. If there is time in the schedule, every effort should be made to accommodate patients. However, the medical assistant notes the chief complaint before the provider sees the patient to ensure the main problem is addressed.

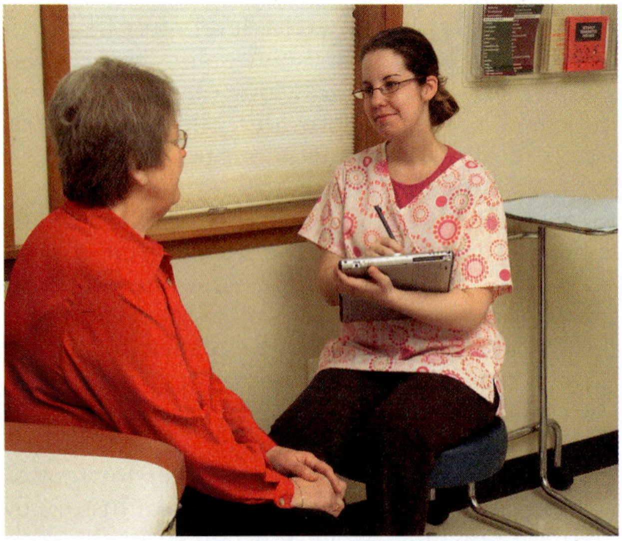

Figure 11-4 The medical assistant reviews the medical history from a computer tablet with a patient while still maintaining eye contact.

EHR Use of the electronic medical record (EMR) makes the patient intake process much easier. Little or no handwritten notes are necessary, and the data can be entered during the communication exchange between the medical assistant and the patient. Some settings allow the patient to see the data as they are entered. Figure 11-5 shows the importance of connecting all these data in a Total Practice Management System (TPMS).

Displaying Cultural Awareness

Remembering a cross-cultural model, the medical assistant begins the encounter with the patient aware of cultural differences and other problems that may inhibit communication. Any number of situations may arise that the medical assistant must be prepared to address. The medical assistant will overcome major obstacles if it is known that the patient does not speak English as a first language or needs an interpreter, if the patient is deaf and needs an interpreter, if the patient is from a culture in which the female patient does not disrobe for a male provider, or if the patient has a mental disorder making communication difficult.

If there is a language difficulty, the medical assistant may be required to arrange for an interpreter. There are language interpreters in most areas; especially in large urban areas, an interpreter might be found for nearly any language. If the patient is receiving medical care through Medicaid, special arrangements can be made for an interpreter through the state agency administering the program. Often the patient will bring a family member to interpret; however, if the matter is personal, the patient may not want to reveal personal matters with the family member present and may prefer an outside, objective interpreter. If the interpreter comes to the clinic as a contractor, a business associate contract should be completed to comply with HIPAA regulations. The contract is HIPAA not necessary for a family member, a volunteer, or a clinic employee serving as an interpreter.

The medical assistant will listen attentively to the patient. The patient may be uneasy talking to the provider and may be more comfortable telling the medical assistant about problems. Medical assistants can play an important part in

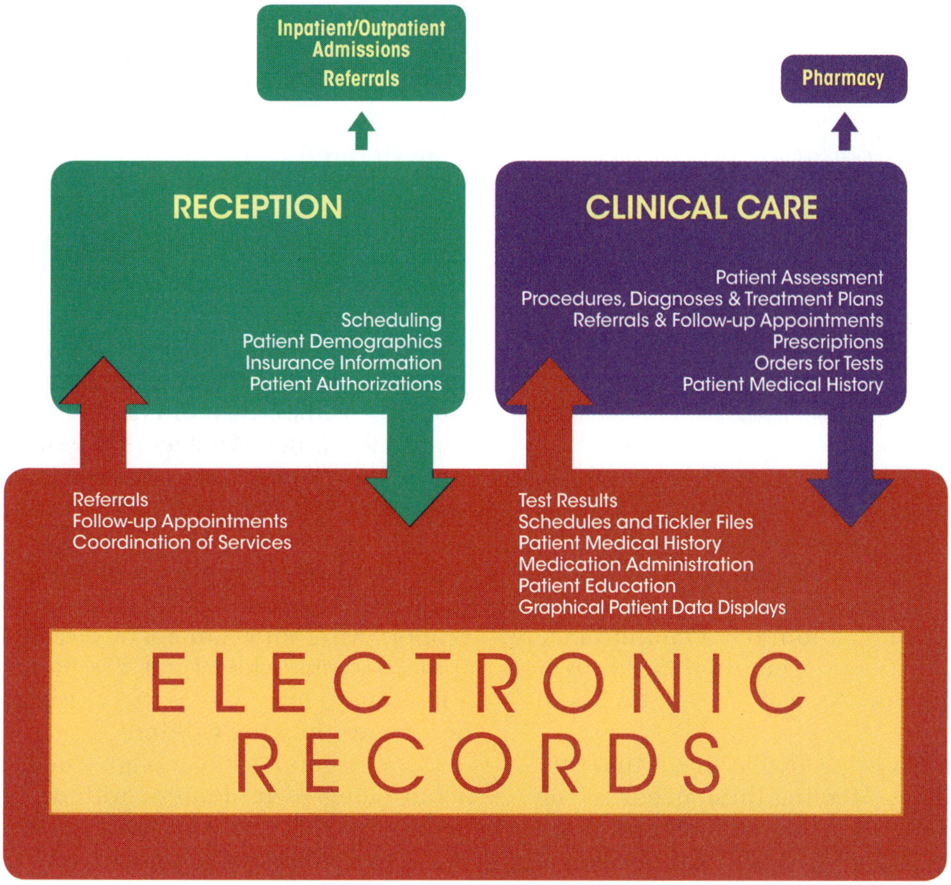

Figure 11-5 TPMS diagram illustrating the relationship between reception and clinical care activities to a patient's medical record.

the medical practice by listening and communicating with both the patient and the provider.

Being Sensitive to Patient Needs

Some patients are frightened, hostile, or depressed. It is important to be open to nonverbal and verbal communication in answer to questions. Some patients react positively to a hand placed gently on the forearm; it calms and reassures them. Others have a negative response, pulling away from any such contact. Maintaining a professional boundary with the patient is essential. Boundaries respect the patient's needs for privacy, nurturing, validation, and separation (see Chapter 4 for additional information).

The medical assistant will know when to touch the patient appropriately, always with permission either expressed or implied. (If the medical assistant tells the patient a blood pressure reading is next and reaches for the patient's arm and the patient extends an arm, permission to take the reading is implied. If, however, the patient pulls away and states no blood pressure is to be taken, permission is not given, and the reading must not be done at that time.) This is charted as "patient refused."

Trying to get information from a reluctant patient can be difficult and requires patience and understanding. If the patient is hesitant to discuss a problem, it is better not to press for information. Pressing for information may make the patient become defensive or angry and can impair communication altogether.

A patient may come to the clinic upset and crying. This patient must be made to feel more in control, that no one is going to rush care being given. Sometimes just taking a few moments to sit with such patients until they feel more settled is enough to calm them and enable the history-taking interview to proceed.

Uncommunicative patients require special questioning techniques. The medical assistant may have to supply a sample of problems to get these patients to acknowledge the health concerns they have. Or they may shrug their shoulders at every question and be unresponsive. Some patients may simply say, "I don't know. I just

Critical Thinking

With two others in your class, role-play a scenario where one person is the patient, another the medical assistant, and the third is an observer. A social history is being taken. Ask the patient about the use of any recreational drugs or chemicals. The patient responds, "Yes." What additional questions will you ask the patient? What will you include in the medical record?

don't feel well." If a relative has accompanied the patient to the appointment, it may be appropriate initially to have the relative present with the patient. In this way the patient has a familiar face in the unfamiliar, often frightening, clinic. It is always the patient's decision if anyone else is to be in the room.

Some patients have particular needs that they are willing to express. Meeting these needs is usually a minor matter and makes patients feel more comfortable. For example, "Can you help me undress and get into the gown?"

Approaching Sensitive Topics

Some of the most sensitive topics addressed in the health history include the use of alcohol, recreational drugs or chemicals, smoking, dietary habits, obesity, and sexual practices. An honest reporting on these topics can be important to the patient's well-being and treatment. Consider:

- Asking these questions in the later stages of the interview after rapport has been established.
- Using casual, direct eye contact without staring; this demonstrates the importance of the topic to the patient and your lack of embarrassment.
- Posing questions in a matter-of-fact tone.
- Adopting a nonjudgmental demeanor.
- Using the communication technique of "normalizing" when appropriate (e.g., "Some high school students drink alcohol/use drugs/engage in sexual relationships on a regular basis. Does this happen at your school? With you?").

If the medical assistant can enhance communication with the patient, communication between provider and patient will be more effective.

COMMUNICATION ACROSS THE LIFE SPAN

Keep in mind your patient's age when communicating and seeking information for the medical history. A parent or caregiver often accompanies a child. An infant will want to feel your physical support, your warmth, and a smile. As the child grows, time will be spent communicating with the child as well as the parent. During this time, you may be dealing with two patients, discussing with the parent the problem the child has and assisting the parent in understanding procedures, treatment, and so on. There can come a time, also, when a child may do much better without a parent present. This can be a sensitive issue for parents. Sometimes a couple of simple statements might help; for example, "Dr. Chalmers will want to establish some rapport with your son for a few minutes. Please come with me while I get the literature that she wants you to have. Often these visits can be harder on parents than the children."

Teenagers are old enough to make the decision about being seen alone or with a parent present. Some are comfortable; others are not. Teenagers who have had the same primary care provider since early childhood and have already established a relationship are more likely to feel comfortable without parents. Review a teenager's right to consent in Chapter 7.

Older adults may be accompanied by another adult and may request that individual be present during the interview. Others may prefer to be alone. Adults who have difficulty hearing, who are memory impaired, who are visually impaired, or whose language may not be understood are likely to be accompanied by another person. Some older adults find it difficult to answer questions in front of their children or even a spouse. Although it is not necessary for relatives, it is a

Patient Education

Some Asian cultures calculate age from conception, not from the actual birth date. For example, a newborn infant is considered to be 1 year old. The medical assistant needs to clarify the chronologic age with the patient or caregiver. This is particularly important for pediatric patients because of the link between age and developmental milestones.

good idea to have a HIPAA waiver signed by the patient, as long as they understand what is being signed. Remember that the intent of HIPAA is *not* to make communication more difficult or cumbersome; it is intended to protect a patient's privacy.

Chapters 15 and 17 have helpful suggestions for communications with children and with older adults.

THE MEDICAL HEALTH HISTORY

The patient's medical health history contains the following components:

- Personal data from the demographic form
- Chief complaint as noted at each visit by the medical assistant
- Present illness
  - Medications
  - Allergies
  - Other providers or alternative therapy practitioners being seen
- Medical history
- Family history
- Social and occupational history
- Review of systems by physician or provider

SOAP/SOAPER and CHEDDAR

SOAP charting is very common; SOAPER is increasing in popularity and is often used in clinics attached to teaching and research hospitals (Figure 11-6). **CHEDDAR** is another approach to charting that may be used. These charting methods encourage more comprehensive charting and make evaluating and managing the levels of service easier to document.

SOAP/SOAPER stands for the following:

S Subjective data; patient's complaint in his or her own words

O Objective, observable, measurable findings

A Assessment, probable diagnosis based on subjective and objective factors

P Plan for treatment, medications, instructions, return visit information

E Education for the patient

R Response of patient to education and care given

CHEDDAR charting encourages greater detail to SOAP/SOAPER. CHEDDAR stands for the following:

C Chief complaint, presenting problems, subjective information

H History—social and physical of presenting problem; contributing data

E Examination, body systems reviewed

Walter Pethokoukis
Date of Birth: 01/22/1949
Visit Date: 04/04/20XX

S: Patient returns after undergoing upper GI; not in as much discomfort as last visit. States he has been taking clear liquids and soft foods. Says he is hungry.
O: Lab results are back. Chem 7 shows slightly elevated glucose at 133. CBC and UA normal. Upper GI shows two small areas of ulceration.
A: Gastric ulcer.
P: Reduce omeprazole to 10 mg every day. Recheck glucose at return visit in 4 weeks.
E: Patient was advised not to smoke or chew tobacco, limit alcohol intake, and avoid aspirin, ibuprofen, and naproxen. Try acetaminophen instead. No diet restrictions indicated.
R: Patient was relieved; indicates there is no problem following the above plan and recommendation. MM/tim

Figure 11-6 Sample of a SOAP/SOAPER follow-up visit note.

D Details of problem(s) and complaint(s)

D Drugs and dosages; list of current medications, dosages, frequency

A Assessment; diagnostic evaluation, further testing, medications

R Return visit, if applicable

The medical assistant and the primary care provider in attendance to the patient both contribute to the completeness of the medical history using SOAP/SOAPER and CHEDDAR. A more detailed review of the information in these medical history components follows.

Chief Complaint

The **chief complaint** (usually abbreviated CC) is the specific reason that brought the patient to see the provider. It should be noted in as few words as possible but be very specific. It can be a direct quote from the patient.

A good example of a chief complaint notation might be: "I've had nausea and vomiting for three days." This is a **subjective** complaint in that it is known by the patient but cannot be seen or measured by the provider. It is specific, however, in relating the patient's condition. Another example is: "I hurt my ankle yesterday when I tripped over a curb." Again this is subjective but specific about cause, time of onset, and complaint. The ankle is visibly swollen and painful to touch. The swelling is an **objective** sign, a manifestation that can be seen, heard, or measured by any observer.

In contrast, a poor example of a chief complaint is "has not been feeling well." This notation tells nothing about what symptoms or problems the patient has been experiencing. It gives no specific clue as to the problem from the patient's perspective. The medical assistant should try to pinpoint a complaint to a body system, to a time frame, to discomfort in a specific area. The patient usually will respond to questions that offer several options.

Certain characteristics of each chief complaint should be ascertained for a complete history. These characteristics are:

- Location
- Radiation
- Quality
- Severity
- Associated symptoms
- Aggravating factors
- Alleviating factors
- Setting and timing

Present Illness

The present illness is usually reflected in the chief complaint. The chief complaint is expanded to give more information and detail. *Location* will describe the place where the symptom is located. Ask the patient to be as specific as possible. For instance, "I have pain on the inner thigh of my left leg" is more helpful than "my leg hurts." *Radiation* helps describe the symptom more by identifying how large an area the symptom covers. The patient might describe a "tingling sensation" all over my left leg, for instance. *Quality* addresses the characteristic of the symptom. The description might be "tingling and buzzing," or the pain described as "a dull ache" or "throbbing" or "stabbing." *Severity* of symptoms will include such descriptions as "keeps me awake at night," or "causes me to put little or no pressure on the leg." When the symptom is pain, patients may be asked to identify the pain on a scale of 1 to 10 with 10 being the most severe. *Associated symptoms* allows the patient to describe what other minor symptoms accompany the chief complaint. "Because I am limping and putting more weight on my right leg, my right hip aches much of the time." *Aggravating factors* and *alleviating factors* get at what makes the symptoms worse and what makes the symptoms decrease. "Walking fast or bending forward really hurts. Sitting down with my feet up on a stool makes it all feel better." You will also want to know what the patient has done to treat the problem and if any medications have been taken for the symptoms. The *setting* and *timing* have to do with when the symptoms started and what the patient was doing at symptom onset.

In the preceding example of nausea and vomiting, the patient may indicate inability to eat or take fluids. This would alert the provider to possible dehydration. Often the present illness is based on a prior health problem. For instance, a history of congestive heart failure gives a patient's symptoms of fluid retention, wheezing, and shortness of breath more importance because these are common complications. Without knowledge of the patient's medical history, these symptoms could be confused with bronchitis, asthma, or pneumonia.

Some practitioners will ask the medical assistant to address other topics in the present illness. These questions include the following:

- Are there any other problems you are experiencing at this time? This question allows patients to indicate if there is something other than the chief complaint about which they have concerns.

- What medications are you taking? Even though the patient's chart will indicate some of this information, this is not the case for a new patient. Most patients do not include any over-the-counter medications or alternative therapies they may be using. Some facilities will ask the patients to bring every medication they are currently taking with them to the first visit. Be certain to ask about over-the-counter items such as vitamins, pain medications, herbal remedies, and so on.
- Are you allergic to anything? Again, the medical chart may note any allergies, but this question alerts the staff to any potential problems and updates the chart. It is a safety measure important to both the patient and provider.

Medications and allergies should be reviewed each time the patient is seen in a medical facility. All medications are to be listed. Some patients will benefit from specific questions about over-the-counter medications. If there are no known allergies, it should be noted so the provider knows the topic has been discussed. When there are allergies, they usually are listed on every page of progress notes or on the summary page in an EMR. Some facilities have begun the practice of printing out the list of all medications and allergies to give to the patient who might want to provide it to any other practitioners.

Medical History

The medical history includes all the patient's health problems, major illnesses, and surgeries. If not included under present illness, all current medications are noted, including dosages and reasons for taking them, as well as all allergies to any medications and the specific allergic reaction to each. These are important to the medical history, because many health problems can overlap and affect the patient in several areas. A patient with a long history of diabetes mellitus may present with an ulcer on his foot. Whereas the same ulcer in an otherwise healthy patient will heal with little intervention, the diabetic patient may require major treatment and attention including debridement (removal of dead or damaged tissue or foreign debris), antibiotics, and close monitoring.

Medications have side effects and contraindications that can affect patients. **Allergies** to medications can be serious and need to be noted in a readily visible part of the chart. A red sticker is often placed in a conspicuous area on the inside cover of the paper chart noting allergies. In a similar fashion, notations will be made in the electronic chart usually on the summary page, to alert clinic providers and staff members of possible allergies. The information needs to be updated at least annually.

If possible, update immunizations for adults at this time. Childhood immunizations are regularly checked in pediatric examinations. Not all adults recall their records, but some questions can help providers determine if any immunizations are to be given. Refer to Chapter 10 for the immunization schedule for adults.

Family History

The family history can provide clues to the patient's present condition. By asking open-ended questions about medical problems of siblings, parents, and grandparents, the provider is alerted to hereditary and familial diseases and disorders such as coronary artery disease, hypertension, breast cancer, and so forth. Present ages of siblings, parents, and grandparents or causes of their death and age at time of death are noted. For instance, a family history of diabetes together with the patient's symptoms of frequent urination and thirst may make a diagnosis of diabetes mellitus a possibility. Be sensitive to cultural variances, however (see the Patient Education box).

Social History

The social history of patients includes their spouse/partner status; sexual habits; occupation; hobbies; and use of alcohol, tobacco, and recreational

Patient Education

In some cultures (e.g., Chinese, some Native Americans), it is disrespectful to speak of the dead. Thus, the patient may be reluctant to provide detailed information on the family health history of dead relatives. In these cases, you can ask the patient if there has been any history of specific diseases in the family and not focus on the specific individual if that person is deceased. The patient may be willing to share in which previous generation and which side of the family the condition existed. If these approaches are unsuccessful, explain to the patient the importance of this information, because it may provide clues to the patient's current health conditions.

drugs or other chemical substances. This part of the history includes those lifestyles and behaviors that may put the patient at greater risk for injury or disease than would normally be found from factors in the family history and medical history.

Patients may not want to answer questions pertaining to sexual history; attempt to return to these questions later. Ask if a medical assistant of a different sex would make the patient more comfortable in discussing sexual practice.

The adolescent patient may refuse to answer questions of a sexual matter or may provide false answers if the parent or caregiver is present. It may be best to ask the caregiver to leave the room at the completion of the health history so that you can ask the patient if there is anything else to note in the sexual history.

Be alert for cues that demonstrate the patient's desire for knowledge on sexual matters, such as questions or requests for written information. Answer the patient's questions, provide educational materials, and refer the patient to a specialist when indicated.

It may be necessary to inquire about the patient's home environment. Be attentive for clues that signal the necessity of performing an in-depth home environment assessment. Some clues include, but are not limited to, poor hygiene, frequent infections, smoke inhalation, burns, malnutrition, and falls (especially in older adults).

Review of Systems (ROS)

Once the medical history has been taken, it is time to prepare the patient for the examination. Note for the provider any questions for which you were unable to get a complete answer from the patient or any areas where you have concerns. Thank the patient for his or her time and information during the interview. In clear terms and not speaking too rapidly, explain to the patient the need to disrobe, put on a gown, and be seated on the examination table. (Chapter 21 describes how to transfer a patient in a wheelchair to the examination table.) *Always* ask if the patient needs assistance in disrobing. It is also wise to let the patient know that you can return in a few minutes to assist him or her onto the examination table if necessary. This allows you to see that the patient is comfortably settled and to give him or her an estimate of how long it will be before the provider is coming in for the examination.

The ROS is performed during the physical examination. When a patient is seen on a fairly regular basis, only the pertinent body system will be reviewed. In a complete physical examination, an orderly and systematic check of each part of the body is recorded. The provider asks questions concerning each organ and system of the body during the examination of the patient. The ROS, in conjunction with the physical examination, helps elicit information that is essential to the diagnosis of disease. The provider usually begins with an overall assessment and proceeds to check each body system in an organized manner. The order in which this is done may vary by providers, but all will check the cardiovascular, respiratory, gastrointestinal, genitourinary, and neurologic systems, as well as the extremities, the musculoskeletal system, and the skin.

Both positive and pertinent negative findings are documented in the ROS. When a response is positive, the patient is asked to describe it as completely as possible. Table 11-2 lists some symptoms and diseases that can be ascertained during the ROS. Many ambulatory care settings have preprinted ROS sheets. These are convenient, as positive findings can be circled and noted. Negative responses are not circled. In the EMR, the same is available as point and click.

By the completion of this portion of the history, the provider usually has an idea about the patient's condition.

To complete the examination, laboratory tests may be ordered depending on the findings and the probable diagnosis. These results, together with the history, examination, and patient symptoms, help to determine a **clinical diagnosis.**

Each piece of the patient's medical history documents integral parts of the patient's health. If any part is lacking, the current understanding of the patient's health is not complete.

Procedure 11-1 gives the steps for taking a paper medical history.

THE PATIENT RECORD AND ITS IMPORTANCE

The patient's record is a collection of confidential information that concerns the patient, care given to the patient, patient progress, and laboratory and other diagnostic test results that have been completed. This information is secured in a file folder or binder. The EMR is secured in appropriate computer storage, is viewed at the computer screen, and can be printed in part or whole for the provider as necessary. It is used for a variety of purposes, but primarily the record provides a foundation for planning patient care and making decisions about patient care. Other purposes for a medical record include using

Table 11-2 Review of Systems

General	Patient's perception of general state of health at the present time; difference from usual state; vitality and energy levels
Neurological	Headache, change in balance, in coordination, loss of movement, change in sensory perception/ feeling in an extremity, change in speech, change in smell, fainting, loss of memory, tremors, involuntary movement, loss of consciousness, seizures, weakness, head injury
Psychological	Irritability, nervousness, tension, increased stress, difficulty concentrating, mood changes, suicidal thoughts, depression
Skin	Rashes, itching, changes in skin pigmentation, black and blue marks, change in color or size of mole, sores, lumps, change in skin texture, odors, excessive sweating, acne, loss of hair, excessive growth of hair or growth of hair in unusual locations, change in nails, amount of time spent in the sun
Eyes	Blurry vision, visual acuity, glasses, contact lenses, sensitivity to light, excessive tearing, night blindness, double vision, drainage, bloodshot, pain, blind spots, flashing lights, halos around objects, glaucoma, cataracts
Ears	Hearing deficits, hearing aid, pain, discharge, lightheadedness, ringing in the ears, earaches, infection
Nose and Sinuses	Frequent colds, discharge, itching, hay fever, postnasal drip, stuffiness, sinus pain, polyps, obstruction, nosebleed, change in sense of smell
Mouth	Toothache, tooth abscess, dentures, bleeding/swollen gums, difficulty chewing, sore tongue, change in taste, lesions, change in salivation, bad breath
Throat/Neck	Hoarseness, change in voice, frequent sore throats, difficulty swallowing, pain/stiffness, enlarged thyroid
Respiratory	Shortness of breath, shortness of breath on exertion, phlegm, cough, sneezing, wheezing, coughing up blood, frequent upper respiratory tract infections, pneumonia, emphysema, asthma, tuberculosis
Cardiovascular	Shortness of breath that wakes patient up in the night, chest pain, heart murmur, palpitations, fainting, sleep on pillows to breathe better, swelling, cold hands/feet, leg cramps, myocardial infarction, hyper-tension, valvular disease, pain in calf with walking, varicose veins, inflammation of a vein, blood clot in leg, anemia
Breasts	Pain, tenderness, discharge, lumps, change in size, dimpling
Gastrointestinal	Change in appetite, nausea, vomiting, diarrhea, constipation, usual bowel habits, black and tarry stools, vomiting blood, change in stool color, excessive gas, belching, regurgitation or heartburn, difficulty swallowing, abdominal pain, jaundice, hemorrhoids, hepatitis, peptic ulcers, gallstones
Urinary	Change in urine color, voiding habits, painful urination, hesitancy, urgency, frequency, excessive urination at night, increased urine volume, dribbling, loss in force of stream, bed-wetting, change in urine volume, incontinence, pain in lower abdomen, kidney stones, urinary tract infections
Musculo-skeletal	Joint stiffness, muscle pain, back pain, limitation of movement, redness, swelling, weakness, bony deformity, broken bones, dislocations, sprains, gout, arthritis, osteoporosis, herniated disc
Female Reproductive	Vaginal discharge, change in libido, infertility, sterility, pain during intercourse, menses (last menstrual period, age period started, regularity, duration, amount of bleeding, premenstrual symptoms, intermen-strual bleeding, painful periods), menopause (age of onset, duration, symptoms, bleeding), obstetrical (number of pregnancies, number of miscarriages/abortions, number of children, type of delivery, complications), type of birth control, estrogen therapy

(continues)

Table 11-2 Review of Systems (continued)

Male Reproductive	Change in libido, infertility, sterility, impotence, pain during intercourse, age at onset of puberty, testicular pain, penile discharge, erections, emissions, hernias, enlarged prostate, type of birth control
Nutrition	Present weight, usual weight, food intolerances, food likes, food dislikes, where meals are eaten
Endocrine	Bulging eyes, fatigue, change in size of head, hands, or feet, weight change, heat/cold intolerances, excessive sweating, increased thirst, increased hunger, change in body hair distribution, swelling in the anterior neck, diabetes mellitus
Lymph Nodes	Enlarged, tenderness
Hematological	Easy bruising/bleeding, anemia, sickle cell anemia, blood type

it as a basis for communi-cation among caregivers, for statistical analysis in research, and for reporting infectious diseases to the health department. It is also a legal document and belongs to the provider or the agency in which the provider is employed. Chapter 7 discusses legal guidelines and medical records. Because it is a legal document, the medical record can be used to determine if patient care has been given according to the standards of care that the law recognizes; therefore, it must be complete, concise, accurate, and understandable. Many important items of information must be placed in the patient record and the medical assistant will be one of the professionals making chart entries.

HIPAA Compliance

HIPAA regulations focus on three vulnerable areas with respect to medical records and the patient's chart:

- Paper record storage and computer/server areas
- Fax machines
- Workstations

A patient's paper chart must be stored in secure and locked areas. It is important that only those persons with need for access to charts have a key to the stoage area. Locks should be changed periodically to ensure security. Sprinkler and fire detection systems should be installed and tested annually to protect paper records. Patients will respect and appreciate all procedures and policies to keep their history and medical records confidential and protected from harm.

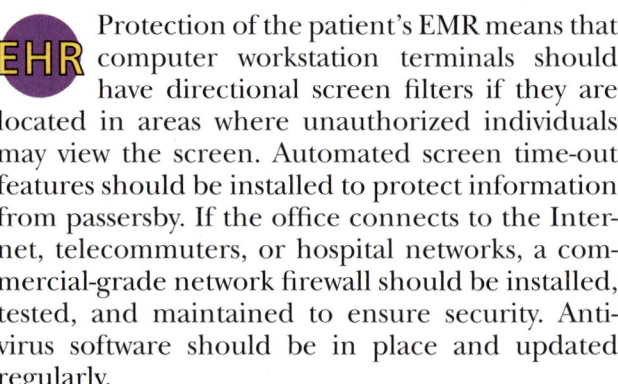

Protection of the patient's EMR means that computer workstation terminals should have directional screen filters if they are located in areas where unauthorized individuals may view the screen. Automated screen time-out features should be installed to protect information from passersby. If the office connects to the Internet, telecommuters, or hospital networks, a commercial-grade network firewall should be installed, tested, and maintained to ensure security. Antivirus software should be in place and updated regularly.

Faxing is a growing vulnerability to the threat of unintended disclosure of patient confidential information. Unintentional human, software, and telecommunication carrier code errors contribute to the security problem. Faxes are easily misdirected or intercepted by individuals for whom access was neither intended nor authorized. Only authorized personnel should have access to the fax machine area, and patient information should be faxed only with assurance that the same security is afforded where the fax is being sent.

Contents of Medical Records

Each patient has his or her own medical record. All patients' records hold standard information. In addition to the patient information forms previously mentioned, other important components of the record include:

- Informed consent forms
- Physical examination outcomes
- Laboratory and diagnostic test results
- The provider's diagnosis and plan of treatment

- Surgical reports
- Progress reports
- Follow-up care
- Telephone calls related to care
- Discharge summary
- Other communications (from other providers, laboratories, or agencies)
- Patient records from other providers
- Medication history

Continuity of Care Record

The Continuity of Care Record (CCR) was developed by a number of medical groups including the American Academy of Family Physicians and the American Academy of Pediatrics. The CCR makes it easier and more effective to transport patient medical information between providers. The CCR is intended to improve the continuity of patient care, reduce errors, and assure a minimum standard of information that is to be shared with another health care provider. The CCR includes patient and provider information, insurance data, patient's health status, recent care given, recommendations for future care, and the reason for referral or transfer. The patient's health status includes allergies, medications, immunizations, vital signs, pertinent laboratory results and recent procedures, and diagnoses. An expanded CCR likely includes any advanced directives the patient might have. During a time when much referral takes place, especially in managed care, or when patients are transferred from a hospital setting to an assisted living environment where care is likely provided by someone other than the current primary care provider, such a record is most beneficial.

The CCR is likely to be completed by providers, nurses, medical assistants, and ancillary personnel such as social workers and physical therapists, among others. It can include outpatient, community-based, and inpatient services. It should be machine readable, as well as human readable, and can be transferred through a number of electronic formats. At all times, however, the CCR is to be protected and designed to enhance patient confidentiality.

METHODS OF CHARTING/ DOCUMENTATION

There are two primary ways to maintain chart notes. These methods can be used in both paper and electronic records. They are:

- Source-oriented medical records
- Problem-oriented medical records

Source-Oriented Medical Records

The traditional or conventional method of charting, **source-oriented medical record (SOMR),** consists of a chronologic set of notes for each visit beginning with the patient's first visit (Figure 11-7). This form of charting makes it difficult to follow or track a specific patient problem. The caregiver must search through the record to locate information about a particular patient problem. Source-oriented notes may be typed by the medical transcriptionist from dictation after the provider has seen the patient.

The example of handwritten chart (Figure 11-8) notes shows the complete history taken at the time of examination including the present illness (if any), the medical history, allergies, family history, habits (social history), and ROS. The physical examination follows with each area noted. Impressions and changes in medications and plan finish the examination notes.

Problem-Oriented Medical Records

A more efficient way of keeping chart notes is the **problem-oriented medical record (POMR).** This method is used extensively today, especially by clinics or any medical practice where more than

Leo McKay
Date of Birth 01/22/1949
Office visit 04/01/20XX

This 57-year-old patient is seen after a several year absence because of abdominal pain which began approximately 2 weeks ago with progressively worsening abdominal pain. He has stopped eating to see if pain would improve, which it did not. Finally yesterday he stopped taking fluids as well. Until this episode, he was drinking several beers daily and smoking approximately 2 ppd.

Weight is 192. BP 152/88 rt. arm sitting P 78 R 18 T 97.6. He is a well-developed, moderately obese male in moderate distress. Abdomen is tense with some guarding at RUQ.

Abdominal pain - pt needs barium swallow, CBC, Chem 7 and UA. To restrict diet to clear liquids until seen in 2 days, omeprazole 20 mg every day.

JW/tlm

Figure 11-7 Sample of dictated and transcribed chart note.

Leo McKay 01/22/1949
04/01/XX 3:15 pm abdominal pain × 3 weeks
WT 192 BP 152/88 rt. arm sitting T 97.6 P78 R18
Pt complaining severe abdominal pain for 2 wks getting
progressively worse. Describes as burning, pressure.
Past Med. Hist. chronic Peptic Ulcer Disease
quit smoking 3 yr ago – now back to 2 ppd
Allergies–penicillin–hives 1950s
Family Hist noncontributory
Habits smokes 2 ppd
beer–several daily
ROS
HEENT noncontributory–PERRLA OU correct to 20/20
CR–clear, no rales, ronchi; murmurs
GI–some guarding. No masses, tenderness lower
abdomen. No nausea, vomiting, diarrhea
GU–clear
PE alert; oriented to time & place
HEENT–pupils nat teeth
fundi thyroid
carotids
} Ø
chest–clear
heart–no murmurs or enlargement
abdomen–Ø masses
rectal–soft brown stool in vault
extremities–neg.
neuro–reg.
skin–clear
Impression–Chronic Peptic Ulcer Disease
Hypertension, mild
Plan–Lab–CBC, Chem 7, UA, barium swallow
Rx–Omeprazole 20 mg every day
Return 3 days
M. Woo, MD 04/01/20XX

Figure 11-8 Sample of handwritten chart note.

one provider may see the patient. This method calls for a list of problems to be made, dated, and numbers assigned to them. When a patient is seen, the problems are identified by number throughout the record. This system makes it easier to follow the patient's progress.

The POMR has four major components:

- *The database:* The patient's medical history, results from laboratory and other diagnostic tests, and results of physical examination are the core of the record.
- *The problem list:* Each problem is listed individually and assigned a number and dated.
- *The diagnostic and treatment plan:* This component addresses the laboratory and other diagnostic tests completed and the provider's plan for treating the patient.
- *Progress notes:* These notes are entered on every problem initially recorded. Documentation is done chronologically and includes patient's complaints, problems, condition, treatment, and responses to treatment and care given.

The SOAP/SOAPER and CHEDDAR methods of charting can be used in either the source-oriented or the problem-oriented medical record.

Providers may dictate their notes to be typed by a medical transcriptionist and then filed in the chart (see Figure 11-7). These notes may follow the form seen in the handwritten chart note or as shown in Figure 11-8.

ELECTRONIC MEDICAL RECORDS (EMR)

The EMR can be viewed as simply a different mode of documenting and saving information related to a patient's care—computer storage versus paper storage. Most practitioners making the transition from paper to electronic records, however, seek a more efficient method for documenting patient care. Because EMRs are the mandate by 2010, paper medical records will be seen increasingly less in the future.

EMRs that are a part of a TPMS can be viewed at a computer terminal by a provider, updated, and saved very quickly. EMRs are available 24 hours per day and can be accessed by the provider from an outside location when necessary. More than one person can view the EMR at the same time. Storage of the EMR is not a serious problem; hundreds of medical records can be stored on one CD or disk. Errors are less likely in EMRs because of the lack of handwritten data. Medication errors are lessened when they are electronically transmitted to the patient's pharmacy, and there is no confusion over the provider's instructions of the medication or dosage. EMRs have the capability of "flagging" information or queries to providers to ensure accuracy and completeness.

Figures 11-9 and 11-10 show a sample EMR and follow-up note. The record grows in chronologic order, but problems are noted. Past health problems are shown at the top of each entry, and all current medications are shown on each sheet.

Remember, however, that an improperly implemented EMR is no more effective in quality patient care than is the well-kept paper record. In the EMR

Patient: Leo McKay
Date of Birth: 01/22/1949
Visit Date: 04/01/20XX

Chief Complaint: Abdominal pain
History: Has been ill over the last 2 weeks with progressively worsening abdominal pain.
Review of Symptoms: Patient denies the following:

- Chest pain, Chest pressure, Chest heaviness, Circulation problems, Palpitations, Rapid heartbeat, Irregular heartbeat, Ankle swelling
- Cough, Phlegm, Coughing up blood, Shortness of breath, Wheeze, Change in exercise tolerance
- Burning or pain on urination, Difficulty starting or stopping urination, Dribbling after urination, Incontinence of urine, Blood in urine, Cloudiness of urine
- Change in appetite, Unexpected weight loss, Nausea, Vomiting, Difficulty Swallowing, Belly pains, Gas pains, Change in bowel habit: change in frequency, shape, color, consistency, size of stool; Blood, Mucus, or Slime, Rectal pain or discomfort, Hemorrhoids
- Skin rash, New or changing moles, Excess bruising or bleeding
- Mouth sores, Denture problems, Sinus drainage or stuffiness, Facial pain
- Panic attacks, Anxiety, Depression, Sadness, Seizures, Problems with concentration or memory, Disturbance of sleep, Insomnia, Early wakefulness
- Dizziness, Fainting, Lightheadedness on standing, Headaches, Vision problems, Hearing problems, Numbness or tingling in arms or legs, Weakness in arms or legs

Medications, including Herbal, Vitamin, and Mineral Supplements

Drug	Dose	Freq.	Started
none			

Medical Problem List

Problem	When Dx'd	Active?
Peptic Ulcer	1985	no

List of Surgeries

Surgical Procedure	When
none	

Family History: Parents deceased, father died of heart attack, mother of breast cancer.
Social History: Divorced, no children
Habits: Smokes 2 ppd, Several beers daily
Allergies: Penicillin

Physical Examination

GENERAL: Well developed and well nourished gentleman in no distress. No jaundice, cyanosis, clubbing, or edema.
VITALS: Weight = 192, Temp = 97.6, Pulse = 78, R = 18, BP = 152/88
HEENT: Normocephalic and without evidence of trauma, tympanic membranes and external auditory canals are normal. Pharynx and mouth are normal.
NECK: supple, no masses or thyromegaly.
NODES: No cervical nodes palpable. No axillary or inguinal adenopathy.
CARDIOVASCULAR SYSTEM: Heart sounds: no murmurs, rubs or gallops, carotids with good upstrokes, no bruits heard. Peripheral pulses including radials, brachials, and femorals intact. Posterior tibial, and dorsalis pedis pulses intact.
RESPIRATORY SYSTEM: resps 18/min, trachea central, expansion, fremitus, resonance, and breath sounds normal.
ABDOMEN: soft, no masses, organomegaly, or tenderness. No loin or costo-vertebral angle tenderness. Inguinal canals are intact without herniae. Bowel sounds active.
GENITOURINARY: Penis without lesions or discharge, scrotum, testicles, epididymis and cords all normal
RECTAL: no masses, tenderness, or hemorrhoids. Soft brown stool in vault. Prostate normal in size, and shape without nodules or tenderness.
MUSCULOSKELETAL SYSTEM: Joints with full ROM, no joint tenderness or swelling. Muscle bulk symmetric and normal.
SKIN: without masses, skin tags, rash, blisters or ulcerations. Nails are normal without splinter hemorrhages.
NEUROLOGICAL SYSTEM: Alert and oriented to place, person, and time. Communicates with good word recognition and appropriate word usage. Cranial nerves and spinal nerves grossly intact.

Assessment and Plan

Problem	Plan/Status
Abdominal pain	Reports about two weeks of epigastric and retrosternal chest pain radiating up and to the left. Episodes of pain occur usually during the day and last for 3-4 hours. No associated dyspnea, palpitations, sweats, dizziness. No nausea, vomiting or diarrhea. No blood in the stool. To get barium swallow, CBC, Chem 7 and UA. Begin omeprazole 20 every day.

Follow-up appointment: 3 days
Mark Woo MD

Figure 11-9 Sample of electronic medical history and physical examination.

Leo McKay
Visit Date: 04/04/20XX

Symptoms: Feeling somewhat better.
Abdominal pain is less on the Omeprazole.
Exam: Weight = 185 BP = 150/84
Patient had barium swallow showing two areas of ulceration. Lab tests show normal findings for CBC and UA. Chem 7 shows slightly elevated glucose at 133.

Assessment	Plan
Gastric ulcer	Omeprazole 10 mg every day Recheck glucose at return visit.

Follow-up appointment: 4 weeks.

Mark Woo, MD

Figure 11-10 Sample of follow-up visit note in EMR.

there can be a tendency to rely too much on technology, causing providers to become careless in their entries. In any medical record, there is never room for inattention to detail and accuracy.

Keep in mind the standard accepted rules for charting in both the paper medical record and the EMR. Many of the rules are pertinent to both types of records.

Table 11-3 Charting Rules

Paper Records	Electronic Records
Always write in black or blue ink	Keyboarding must be accurate and appropriate.
After charting, sign with first initial, last name, and title.	Type personal or electronic signature after each chart activity.
Leave no space between chart entry and initial/ handwritten signature.	Leave no empty spaces between chart notes and electronic signature.
Do not erase or obliterate any entry.	Do not erase or obliterate any entry.
If an error is discovered, draw a single line through the mistake and write the correct information above it. "Corr" or "Correction" is written by the entry, which is dated and initialed. Red pen can be used for the correction and notation. Follow your clinic policy.	Errors made at the moment of entry are corrected as usual. Errors discovered later require a new document identifying the error, the correction, the date, and signature of the person making the correction. This document is added to the original document with a note. EMR software programs have variable time lockouts to prevent tampering with the chart.

RULES OF CHARTING

Charting is required for each medication, treatment/procedure, or provider and medical assistant action. Accounts of the patient's condition and activities must be charted in a clear and meaningful way. Information charted in the patient's record must be accurate, clear, complete, timely, and entered properly. There is a saying, "If it is not charted, it was not done." Some basic charting rules are given in Tables 11-3 and 11-4.

Abbreviations Used in Charting

Abbreviations are used extensively in charting to document information. Some are used as a short-hand to save time and space, whereas other abbreviations are used to give an exact meaning to a finding. For instance, the abbreviation N&V indicates "nausea and vomiting" without having to write out the entire expression. Table 11-5 lists commonly used abbreviations.

Although the use of abbreviations in medical charts is common, remember that there is an increasing expectation that the medical chart should be understandable to any person reading it, especially if it is required in any legal matter. The Joint Commission's *Journal on Quality and Patient Safety* reports that it is best not to use abbreviations when charting medications. Their findings report that the most common abbreviation resulting in medication error is the use of "qd" rather than "every day or once daily." Their report also noted that medication errors were more likely made during prescribing and were related to improper dose or quantity. Therefore, keep abbreviations to a minimum and use only standard abbreviations. Be prepared to provide any attorney a list of commonly used and accepted abbreviations in your medical practice. The Joint Commission posts a listing of prohibited abbreviations on their Web site (http://www.jointcommission.org) to further satisfy their goal of patient safety.

Table 11-4 Charting Rules That Apply to Both Paper and Electronic Charting

Leave no blank lines in the chart. Enter your data in the next available line.
Ditto marks may not be used.
Use only standard abbreviations that have been determined are not easily misinterpreted. See Abbreviations Common to Medical Charting (Table 11-5).
Avoid medical terminology unless absolutely certain of spelling and definition. Legal authorities advise keeping medical terminology to a minimum. The record must be understandable to the patient and to any authorized user.
Confirm the patient's name is on every page.
Use present tense. Never use future tense, such as "patient to be given a tetanus shot"; instead, wait until the injection is given, then chart the event.
Never chart for another person; chart only what you know, not what someone else has told you.
Describe events and behaviors; do not label them. "Patient was really angry" does not describe the event as well as "Patient yelled and threw the pencil on the counter."
Be as specific as you can. Charting "Patient complained of shoulder pain" is not as clear as "Patient complains of right shoulder pain when reaching overhead."

Table 11-5 Abbreviations Common to Medical Charting

BP or B/P	blood pressure
c̄	with
CBC	complete blood count
CC	chief complaint
CPE	complete physical examination
D&C	dilation and curettage
dx	diagnosis
ECG, EKG	electrocardiogram
EEG	electroencephalogram
ER	emergency room
GI	gastrointestinal
GU	genitourinary
GYN	gynecology
HEENT	head, eyes, ears, nose, and throat
I&D	incision and drainage
MI	myocardial infarction
N&V	nausea and vomiting
NVD	nausea, vomiting, and diarrhea
OPD	outpatient department
OR	operating room
P	pulse
PERRLA	pupils equal, round, reactive to light and accommodation
PT	physical therapy
R	respiration
ROM	range of motion
ROS	review of systems
s̄	without
SOAP	subjective, objective, assessment, plan
SOB	short of breath
T	temperature
T&A	tonsillectomy and adenoidectomy
UCHD	usual childhood diseases
URI	upper respiratory infection
UTI	urinary tract infection
WNL	within normal limits
XR	X-ray
>	greater than
<	less than
↑	increase
↓	decrease
Δ	change

Chart Organization

Chart notes in a paper medical record are kept in chronologic order for the primary provider. Laboratory tests results, hospital notes, consultations with other providers, and any correspondence should be kept in an orderly fashion.

The chart order presents current medications followed by laboratory reports and pathology reports, each in chronologic order. In the POMR system, often the list of medical problems is found above the current medications.

The provider's notes are in chronologic order with the most recent first. The radiographs and ECGs follow, including MRIs, mammograms, CT scans, exercise tolerance tests (ETTs), echocardiograms, and other similar tests. Following these are the hospital notes, including the history and physical, hospital consultations, and discharge summary. Consultations by other providers are grouped next, again in chronologic order.

The miscellaneous section may include anything from referrals for insurance companies to orders and updates from nursing homes or home health services. Finally, the correspondence section includes letters, insurance claim forms, and requests for prior medical records.

If a chart is kept in a specific order, information needed is easily gleaned by each member of the clinic staff.

Procedure 11-1

Taking a Medical History for a Paper Medical Record

PURPOSE:

To obtain a medical history from a patient new to the ambulatory care setting.

EQUIPMENT/SUPPLIES:

Patient history forms
Clipboard
Pen

PROCEDURE STEPS:

1. Introduce yourself to the new patient. Confirm identity of the patient and escort to the examination room or private area.
2. Make eye contact and use positive body language. RATIONALE: Puts patient at ease.
3. Explain the purpose and importance of obtaining the patient information. Ask the questions on the form, trying to get as much information as possible without letting the patient wander from the subject.
4. Ask each question clearly. Be sure patient understands all questions. Ask about allergies.
5. Repeat patient answers when needed to confirm. Be specific when documenting answers. Do not just write "yes" for tobacco use. List "2 packs per day." Be specific.
6. Write legibly using dark ink (blue or black).
7. Recheck the medical history form to be sure all parts are complete. Note any additional information provided by patient. Make sure numbers, dates, spelling, and other information are accurate and legible. RATIONALE: Ensures that all components of the medical history have been completed.
8. Prepare the patient for the review of systems and physical examination if this is indicated.
9. Document the procedure. RATIONALE: Identifies person responsible for taking the medical history.

Case Study 11-1

Review the scenario at the beginning of the chapter.

Maria Jover, a patient of Dr. Elizabeth King at Drs. Lewis and King, has finally convinced her teenage son to make an appointment for a physical. Adam Jover is 17 years old, outgoing, fun loving, and apparently healthy. But Maria is concerned that he may be engaging in harmful social activities and hopes that by seeing Dr. Winston Lewis, Adam may discover ways to protect himself and his health. Adam agreed to the appointment but is adamant that his mother not accompany him. At the ambulatory care setting, it is decided that Adam might be more forthcoming with a male medical assistant, so Joe Guerrero is scheduled to take Adam's medical history before Dr. Winston does an ROS.

CASE STUDY REVIEW

1. When Joe Guerrero first sits down with Adam to take the history, he notices that Adam is ill at ease and nervous. What can Joe do to reassure Adam that his privacy will be protected?
2. When Joe attempts to take the social history, Adam seems evasive about answering Joe's questions and finally admits that he doesn't want his mother, Maria, to know about his social activities. What is Joe's response?
3. By the end of the interview, it becomes apparent that Adam may be engaging in some behaviors that put him at high risk for contracting the human immunodeficiency virus. How can Joe provide Adam with guidance without alienating him?

Case Study 11-2

Harvey DiAntonio is a 52-year-old patient who lives at 45 W. Smith Avenue, Baltimore, Maryland, 21208. His date of birth is July 8, 1954. His phone number is 667-1870. He is a Baltimore City fire fighter and has been for 21 years. He has union medical insurance, and Blue Cross/Blue Shield (BC/BS) is his carrier. His number is 211-67-87-56. He also carries major medical and his policy is Diagnostic #4. He has been referred by the fire department practitioner, Dr. Alan Byers. Mr. DiAntonio's complaint is severe "gripping" pain in the anterior mid-chest sometimes radiating to the abdomen, neck, and both arms. Pain seems to occur with strenuous exercise and when walking uphill. Pain usually lasts 20 minutes with each episode. Pain does "ease up" when he ceases activity. Mr. DiAntonio states his episodes have occurred while he was shaving, climbing stairs at work, after a heavy meal, and during sexual intercourse. One episode last week was accompanied with dizziness, nausea, and fatigue. The episodes have been going on now once or twice a month for 5 months. Mr. DiAntonio's history is essentially noncontributory. It is questionable whether this is due to good health or the fact that the patient has not had a physical examination for 8 years. Surgeries include tonsillectomy and adenoidectomy, T&A, 1958, and appendectomy in 1964. Fractured rib, left side, in 1984 due to fire fighting incident. Usual childhood diseases. Hospitalized for observation, 1962, Sinai Hospital, for an unusually long episode of bronchitis. Social history shows that the patient is a pump operator on the job with much heavy exertion. Smokes 1½ to 2 packs of cigarettes per day and is a moderate drinker. He has a weight problem off and on and tends to eat too much while on duty. Lives in a one-story home. Hobbies include carpentry and music. Some family problems and tension exist as both of his children are in adolescence. Patient describes himself as "fun loving" with a "quick temper" and worries about meeting financial needs of the family. Is in a position to retire from active duty but states he could not tolerate the boredom.

Family history shows both parents deceased—mother of heart attack, age 59, and father of unknown cause at age 49. Has two siblings, one brother with history of hypertension and one sister living and in good health. Has two children both living and well. Family history otherwise negative.

Physical examination revealed a well-nourished, well-developed male in no acute distress at this time. Patient does seem a bit anxious about this examination. T. 98.6 - P. 94 - R. 24 - BP 175/104. Ht. 69", Wt. 198 pounds. HEAD, EYES, EARS, NOSE, THROAT—normal. NECK—supple. Trachea in midline. CHEST—normal in contour. Calcium deposit on left sixth rib probably due to history fracture. HEART—after careful examination with the patient recumbent and the scope placed lightly on the chest wall near the apex, a left atrial sound was heard (presystolic gallop). ABDOMEN—negative. EXTREMITIES—negative. GENITALIA—negative.

(continues)

Case Study 11-2 (continued)

SKIN—negative. NEUROLOGIC—negative. Laboratory tests performed show a hemoglobin of 11.0 gms. Awaiting results of serum cholesterol, calcium, phosphorus, and blood urea nitrogen. Chest radiograph essentially negative. EKG report showed atrial sounds occurring presystolically with long P-R intervals. DIAGNOSIS: (1) angina pectoris; (2) anemia; (3) hypertension. TREATMENT: Nitroglycerin tabs, sublingually as needed. To return to office in 2 weeks to follow medication effects. In consultation with patient, the patient was advised to control physical activity and quantity of food intake. Avoid extreme cold, 8 hours of sleep/night. Avoid emotional upsets. Attempt four meals/day. Low-fat 1,600-calorie diet. No smoking, moderate alcohol intake.

CASE STUDY REVIEW

1. Identify the following parts of the case study above and extract from the case study the portion that matches the appropriate medical history component.
   - Personal data
   - Chief complaint
   - Present illness
   - Medical history
   - Family history
   - Social history
   - Review of systems
2. Using appropriate terminology and abbreviations, make a charting entry for Mr. DiAntonio by using the SOAPER method of charting.

SUMMARY

The patient's medical history and the information that appears in the medical chart form the base for any and all treatment given to a patient. An efficient and effective medical chart tells the patient's story. It is critical that all information be accurate, documented appropriately, and complete in every way. Taking the medical history, maintaining the patient's chart, and documenting information is a major task for medical assistants. Increased use of the EMR makes charting easier and quicker for clinic staff personnel and providers. Errors are less likely in the EMR, and information is more readily available when needed. Changing from the paper medical chart to the electronic medical chart is time consuming and often seems overwhelming, but medical personnel using the EMR cannot imagine functioning without them.

STUDY FOR SUCCESS

To reinforce your knowledge and skills of information presented in this chapter:

- Review the Key Terms
- Practice any Procedures
- Consider the Case Studies and discuss your conclusions
- Answer the Review Questions
  - Multiple Choice
  - Critical Thinking
- Navigate the Internet and complete the Web Activities
- Practice the StudyWARE activities on the textbook CD
- Apply your knowledge in the Student Workbook activities
- Complete the Web Tutor sections
- View and discuss the DVD situations

REVIEW QUESTIONS

Multiple Choice

1. If the patient has difficulty with English, the medical assistant should:
   a. make the appointment for the patient and obtain the services of an interpreter to be present
   b. set the appointment after contact is made with the interpreter
   c. speak more loudly so the patient will understand
   d. suggest that the patient find a provider who speaks his or her first language
2. A helpful question to ask the returning patient is:
   a. Are you feeling bad today?
   b. Didn't you get better with the treatment prescribed last visit?
   c. Have you noticed any changes in your condition since your last visit?
   d. Do you realize you have gained six pounds since your visit last week?
3. When the patient reports not feeling well, the medical assistant should:
   a. mark the chief complaint as "patient not feeling well"
   b. ask helpful questions to help the patient express specific problems or symptoms
   c. pin down the symptoms by guessing what the problem could be
   d. let the provider work with the patient
4. Source-oriented medical records:
   a. are chronologic notes beginning with the patient's first visit
   b. have four major components
   c. are the best for finding information quickly
   d. are best when many providers see the patient
5. Name, address, telephone numbers, birth date, Social Security number, insurance information, and person to contact in an emergency is information referred to as:
   a. demographic data
   b. CCR of patient information
   c. social history
   d. none of the above
6. The chief complaint:
   a. often is referred to as the CC in the chart
   b. is a statement of objective findings made by the staff
   c. is subjective data as expressed by the patient
   d. a and c
7. Interviewing patients for their medical history requires:
   a. special credentials such as CMA or RMA
   b. cross-cultural interviewing and communication skills
   c. computer skills in medical note taking
   d. a major portion of the receptionist's time and energy
8. The CCR was developed:
   a. by medical groups including the American Academy of Family Physicians and the American Academy of Pediatrics
   b. to reduce errors and ensure certain information is shared among providers
   c. for input from all health care providers, nurses, and medical assistants
   d. all the above
9. Progress notes include:
   a. medical history and results of laboratory tests
   b. the provider's plan for treating the patient
   c. the CC, problems, conditions, treatment, and responses to care
   d. a and c
10. Subjective, objective, assessment, and plan charting is sometimes referred to as:
    a. SOAP
    b. POMR
    c. SOMR
    d. CCRP

Critical Thinking

1. Recall your last visit to your personal medical care provider. How well was the medical history taken? Was it done on paper or electronically? What was particularly helpful about the encounter? What was not helpful? Are there any ways in which you would like it to be changed? If so, describe the changes.
2. Compare and contrast the patient's chief concern with the provider's chief concern in the cross-cultural model. How can those concerns be brought together into one focus?
3. A male patient you are interviewing denies that he smokes, but his fingers are darkened with tobacco stain and he reeks of the tobacco odor. What questions might you ask to clarify his response?
4. The health and well-being of family members contributes what kind of information to a patient's medical history? When that information is essentially unknown for one reason or another, how is that information addressed in the chart?
5. There are two major "patient examples" of histories in this chapter: Mr. Leo McKay and Mr. Harvey DiAntonio. From the social and family history, identify how that information may or may not relate to the presenting problem.

WEB ACTIVITIES

1. With electronic medical records on the rise, there are many products coming on the market to make the transition from paper to electronic records easier and more efficient. Go to http://healthcare.scantron.com/patient-record/paros/htm for information about a system that allows health care providers and patients quick access to an EMR for patient histories. In this system, the patient fills out the history form using a digital pen which automatically captures the handwritten data by reading special paper on which the form is printed. When the patient completes the form, the pen is slid into a computer docking station and the captured information is instantly transferred to the EMR system. Discuss the advantages and disadvantages of such a system.
2. Search the Internet for information on the electronic POMR. Are you able to see samples? Discuss the advantages and disadvantages of the electronic record and the POMR.

REFERENCES/BIBLIOGRAPHY

U.S. Department of Health and Human Services, Centers for Disease Control and Prevention. *Recommended adult immunization schedule by age group and medical conditions, United States, 2006–2007.* Summary published by the Advisory Committee on Immunization Practices. Retrieved August 2007, from http://www.cdc.gov.

THE DVD HOOK-UP

In this chapter, you learned about the proper method for obtaining a patient's medical history and the proper technique for recording in a patient's chart.

In today's designated scenes, you observed Anita going over Mrs. O'Neil's patient history form. Anita first gathered information about the patient's personal history, and then the patient's familial history. Once Anita finished going over the history form, she asked Mrs. O'Neil what brought her into the office today.

1. Why did Anita need to ask the patient what brought her into the office today? After all, she just obtained the patient's entire medical history.
2. What do you think of Anita's personality? Do you think that she was a bit solemn?
3. Why must you also include over-the-counter medications when posting current medications being taken by the patient?

DVD Journal Summary

Write a paragraph that summarizes what you learned from watching today's DVD program. How do you feel about asking patients questions regarding sensitive subject matters such as sexual health and emotional stability?

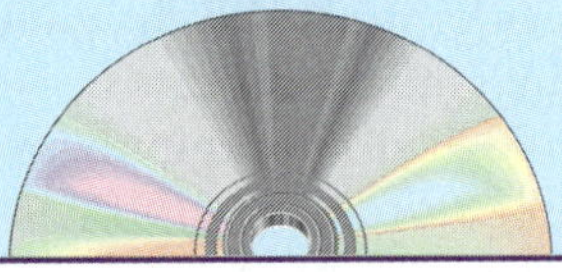

DVD Series
Skills Based Series

Program Number
6

Chapter/Scene Reference
- *Introduction to Taking a Patient History*
- *Preparing an Exam Room*
- *Patient Assessment and Measurement*

Vital Signs and Measurements

Chapter 12

KEY TERMS

Afebrile
Apical
Apnea
Arrhythmia
Atherosclerosis
Baseline
Bradycardia
Bradypnea
Cheyne–Stokes
Diastole
Dyspnea
Eupnea
Febrile
Frenulum
Hyperpnea
Hypertension
Hyperventilation
Hypotension
Hypoventilation
Increment
Lumen
Manometer
Meniscus
Orthopnea
Peripheral
Pulse Oximeter
Pyrexia
Rales
Stertorous
Stridor
Systole
Tachycardia
Tachypnea
Wheezes

OUTLINE

- The Importance of Accuracy
- Temperature
  - Terms Used to Describe Body Temperature
  - Phase Out of Mercury Thermometers and Other Mercury-Containing Equipment
  - Types of Thermometers
  - Measuring Temperature
  - Recording Temperature
  - Cleaning and Storage of Thermometers
- Pulse
  - Pulse Sites
  - Measuring and Evaluating a Pulse
  - Normal Pulse Rates
  - Pulse Abnormalities
  - Recording Pulse Rates
- Respiration
  - Respiration Rate
  - Abnormalities
- Blood Pressure
  - Equipment for Measuring Blood Pressure
  - Measuring Blood Pressure
  - Recording Blood Pressure Measurement
  - Normal Blood Pressure Readings
  - Blood Pressure Abnormalities
- Height and Weight
  - Height
  - Weight
  - Significance of Weight
- Measuring Chest Circumference

OBJECTIVES

The student should strive to meet the following performance objectives and demonstrate an understanding of the facts and principles presented in this chapter through written and oral communication.

1. Define the key terms as presented in the glossary.
2. Discuss normal and abnormal temperatures, including factors affecting temperature.
3. Identify and explain the procedures for using, caring for, and storing the various types of thermometers.
4. Discuss the Environmental Protection Agency's initiative to phase out mercury thermometers and other mercury-containing equipment.
5. Describe the locations and procedure for obtaining pulse rates.
6. Explain the procedure for obtaining respiration rates.
7. Identify and describe normal and abnormal pulse and respiratory rates and the factors affecting each.

OBJECTIVES (continued)

8. Describe the appropriate equipment and procedure for obtaining a blood pressure measurement.
9. Identify normal and abnormal blood pressure, including factors affecting blood pressure.
10. Describe the procedures for obtaining height, weight, and chest measurements of adults.
11. Accurately record measurements on the patient's chart or electronic medical record.
12. Explain two reasons why a professional individual shows responsibility by learning about the dangers of mercury.

Scenario

The medical office of Drs. Lewis and King, clinical medical assistant Joe Guerrero, CMA (AAMA), assists both providers in taking patients' vital signs. One of his favorite patients is Abigail Johnson, a friendly woman in her 70s who always has a kind disposition despite her financial and medical difficulties. Abigail is overweight and has hypertension, so her blood pressure is monitored on a regular basis to be certain that it is under control. In reviewing Abigail's chart, Joe notices that her blood pressure has been quite stable for the last few visits. He also checks her weight and notices that Abigail is slowly losing weight. Abigail's chart, with its history of blood pressure and other measurements, informs Joe's perspective and is a helpful record when evaluating the progress Abigail has made since she became a patient 3 years ago.

INTRODUCTION

One of the most important and commonly performed tasks of a medical assistant is obtaining and recording patient vital signs and body measurements. Vital signs, also sometimes referred to as cardinal signs, include temperature, pulse, respiration, and blood pressure, abbreviated TPR B/P. They are indicative of the general health and well-being of a patient and, with regular monitoring, may measure patient response to treatment. Vital signs, in total or in part, are an important component of each patient visit. Height and weight measurements, although not considered vital signs, are often a routine part of a patient visit.

Patients will exhibit vital sign readings that are uniquely their own. As a result, baseline assessments of vital signs are usually obtained during the patient's initial visit. These baseline results are used as a reference point for future readings, differentiating between what is normal and abnormal for the patient.

Two important habits must be developed by the medical assistant before taking a patient's vital signs: aseptic technique in the form of hand washing and recognition and correction of factors that may influence results of vital signs. Proper hand washing before taking vital signs will assist in preventing cross contamination of patients. Refer to the discussion on Standard Precautions and medical asepsis in Chapter 10. Also, emotional factors of patients must be recognized and addressed. Explaining procedures and allowing the patient the opportunity to relax will ease apprehension that may affect vital sign readings.

THE IMPORTANCE OF ACCURACY

Vital signs may be altered by many factors. Medical assistants must recognize and correct factors that may produce inaccurate results. For example, patients may exhibit anxiety over potential test results or findings of the provider. They may be angry or may have rushed into the office. A patient may have had something to eat or drink before the visit or may have had a long wait in the reception area. Patient apprehension and mood must always be considered by the medical assistant, because these factors can affect vital signs.

Spotlight on Certification

RMA Exam Outline

- Vital signs and measurements

CMA (AAMA) Content Outline

- Equipment preparation and operation
- Principles of operations
- Vital signs

CMAS Exam Outline

- Vital signs and measurements

The medical assistant may be required to take vital signs more than once during an office visit to ascertain a **baseline** and obtain an impression of overall well-being of the patient. Body measurements such as weight may be influenced by what the patient is wearing; height may be influenced by the patient's shoes and how his or her posture is while being measured.

Accuracy in taking vital signs is necessary because treatment plans are developed according to the measurement of the vital signs (Figure 12-1). Variations can indicate a new disease process or the patient's response to treatment. They may also indicate the patient's compliance with a treatment plan. Although taking vital signs is a task commonly performed by the medical assistant, it is never to be taken casually or lightly, and it should never be rushed or incompletely performed. Concentration and attention to proper procedure will help ensure accurate measurements and quality care of the patient. The following text discusses procedures used to measure the vital signs of children and adults. Procedures used for infant examinations are discussed in Chapter 15.

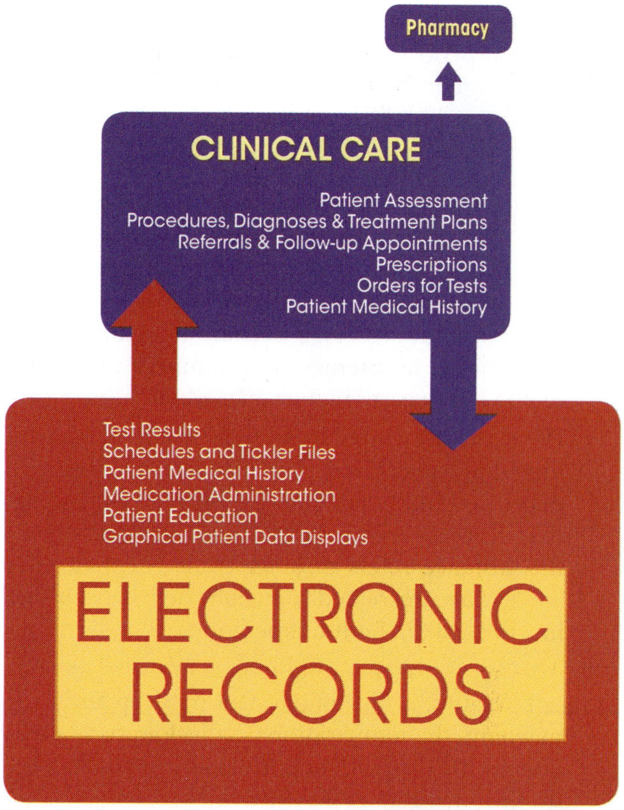

Figure 12-1 In a total practice management system, the patient's vital signs are often entered by the medical assistant during clinical care. Many programs have the ability to output vital signs data in a graph format, so a provider can easily note fluctuations in a patient's weight, blood pressure, normal temperature, etc.

TEMPERATURE

Body temperature is maintained and regulated by two processes functioning in conjunction with one another: heat production and heat loss.

Body heat is produced by the actions of voluntary and involuntary muscles. As the muscles move, they use energy, which produces heat. Cellular metabolic activities, such as the process of breaking down food sugars into simpler components (catabolism), are another source of heat.

The body loses heat by a combination of five processes:

1. *Convection.* The process by which heat is lost through the skin by being transferred from the skin by air currents flowing across it, such as a fan used on a hot day for cooling purposes.
2. *Conduction.* The transfer of heat from within the body to the surface of the skin and then to surrounding cooler objects touching the skin, such as clothing.
3. *Radiation.* Body heat lost from the surface of the skin to a cooler environment, much like a cool room becoming warm when occupied by many people.
4. *Evaporation.* A heat loss mechanism that uses heat absorption through vaporization of perspiration.
5. *Elimination.* Heat that is lost through the normal functioning of the intestinal, urinary, and respiratory tracts.

The delicate balance between heat production and heat loss is maintained by the hypothalamus in the brain. The hypothalamus monitors blood temperature and will trigger either the heat loss or heat production mechanism with as little as 0.04°F change in blood temperature.

Body temperature is measured in degrees and is influenced by several factors, including:

- An increase in temperature may result from a bacterial infection, increased physical activity or food intake, exposure to heat, pregnancy, drugs that increase metabolism, stress and severe emotional reactions, and age. Age becomes a factor in that infants have an average body temperature that is one to two degrees higher than adults.
- Decrease in temperature may result from viral infections, decreased muscular activity, fasting, a depressed emotional state, exposure to cold, drugs that decrease metabolic activities, and age. Age in this instance refers to older adults, in that older adults have decreased metabolic activity resulting in a decrease in body temperature.
- Another factor that can increase or decrease body temperature is time of day. During sleep and early morning, the temperature is at its lowest, whereas later in the day with muscular and metabolic activity, the temperature increases.

Because of the many factors influencing body temperature and the uniqueness of individuals, there is no "normal" temperature. The medical assistant must think of temperatures in terms of the "average," which for an adult is 98.6°F, or 37.0°C.

Terms Used to Describe Body Temperature

The following terms are used to describe body temperature:

- **Afebrile:** absence of fever
- **Febrile:** fever is present
- *Fever:* body temperature increased beyond normal range; **pyrexia** is another term for fever
- *Onset:* time when fever begins
- *Lysis:* body temperature gradually returns to normal after a period of fever
- *Crisis:* body temperature decreases suddenly to normal levels; the patient may perspire profusely (diaphoresis)
- *Intermittent:* a fluctuating fever that returns to or below baseline, then increases again
- *Remittent:* a fluctuating fever that does not return to the baseline temperature; it fluctuates but remains increased
- *Continuous:* a fever that remains above the baseline; it does not fluctuate but remains fairly constant

Figure 12-2 depicts types of fever.

Phase Out of Mercury Thermometers and Other Mercury-Containing Equipment

Glass mercury thermometers have been used for decades and have been common in health care agencies as well as the home. In recent years, concerns have arisen about mercury toxicity when mercury thermometers or other equipment containing mercury breaks and spills mercury into the environment.

This can create a mercury vapor in the indoor air, which is a serious problem. The mercury also can cause environmental damage if it enters lakes and rivers where it can contaminate fish, which are part of the food chain. Even small amounts of mercury can do great harm. The fetus is at risk because its developing nervous system is susceptible to mercury toxicity if a pregnant woman eats fish contaminated with mercury. When thermometers break or are disposed of improperly, the mercury can enter the atmosphere, especially if the mercury waste is burned in an incinerator.

If spilled mercury is not cleaned up (perhaps the individual using the thermometer is unaware that it is broken, and the mercury has seeped into a carpet or crevice), the mercury will evaporate and can reach dangerous levels in indoor air. There is medical literature that illustrates some cases of serious illnesses and even death from exposure to mercury from broken thermometers. Most cases involved young children. According to the Environmental Protection Agency (EPA), a 32-month-old child who was exposed to mercury became ill with hypertension, tachycardia, apathy, pulmonary edema, and coma. The mercury from a broken thermometer had not been cleaned up.

Even small mercury spills should be cleaned up as soon as possible. Becton-Dickinson, a thermometer manufacturer, makes the following recommendations for cleaning up a broken thermometer:

- Pick up the mercury with an eyedropper or scoop up the beads of mercury with a piece of heavy paper (cardboard, index card, or playing card).
- Place mercury, the dropper, heavy paper, and any broken glass in a plastic resealable bag. Place this bag into two more resealable bags, zipping each within the other, finishing up with the contents

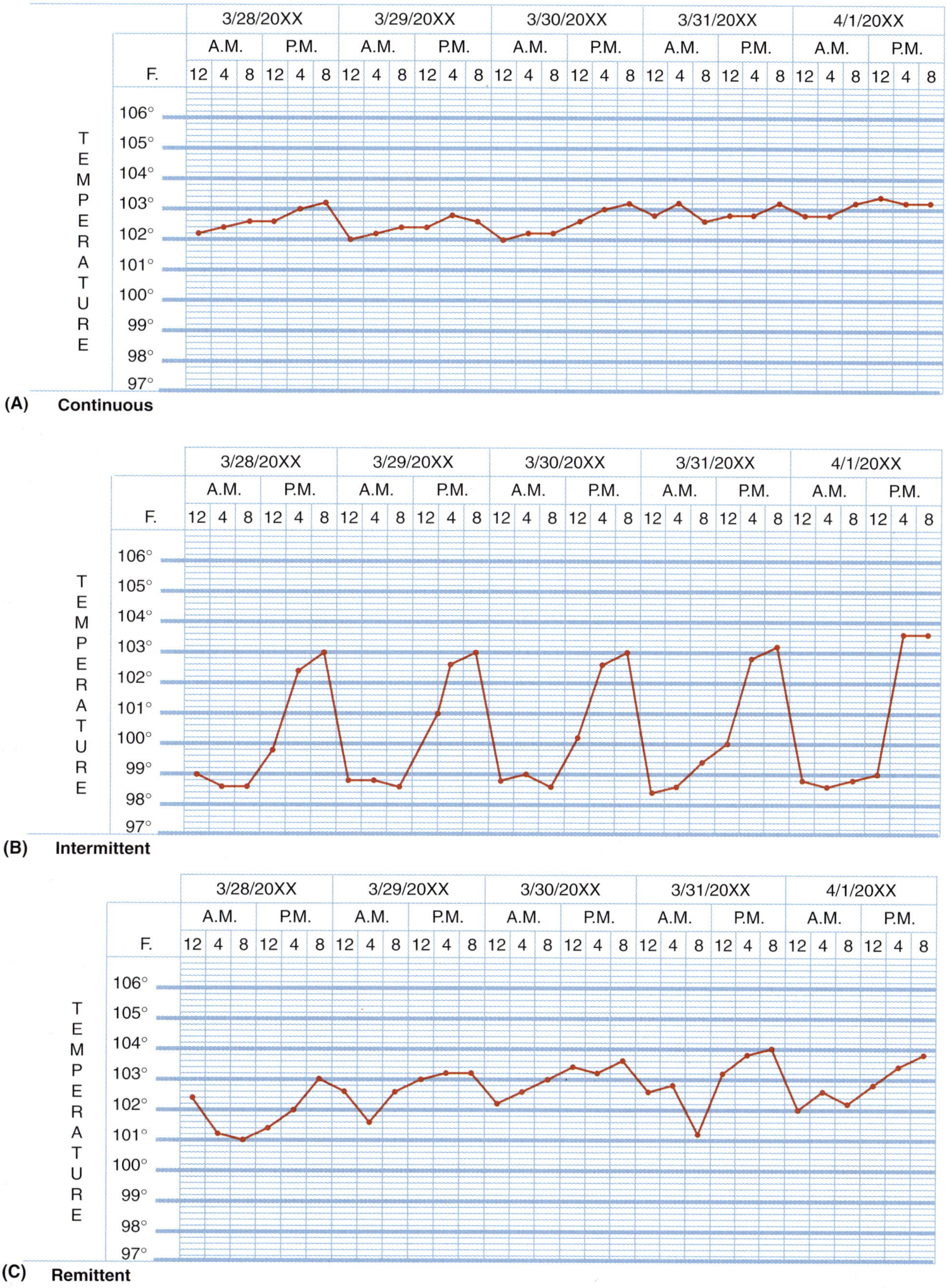

Figure 12-2 Types of fevers. (A) Continuous—remains above baseline. Does not fluctuate. (B) Intermittent—a fluctuating fever. Returns to or below baseline, then rises again. (C) Remittent—a fluctuating fever but does not return to baseline temperature. Remains elevated, but fluctuates.

bagged three times. Place this into a wide-mouth, sealable plastic container.

- Call the local health department for the nearest mercury disposal location. If no disposal location is available, dispose of the container according to local and state regulations. The health department can inform you regarding how to obtain the information.
- Leave windows open for about 2 days to ensure complete ventilation.

These recommendations can be applied to mercury spillage caused by other mercury-containing equipment. Do not do the following:

- Do not use household cleaning products. Combinations of some cleansers with mercury can release toxic gases.
- Do not use a broom or brush to clean up mercury; they only spread it around.
- Do not use a vacuum cleaner or shop vacuum. The mercury vapor escapes into the air and increases exposure to individuals in the area.

In 1998, the American Hospital Association signed an agreement with the EPA to eliminate mercury from their hospitals' waste systems. Hospitals and other health care agencies are phasing out the use of mercury thermometers and other medical equipment that contain mercury, such as sphygmomanometers, among others. Many states have recalled mercury thermometers and replaced them with digital ones.

The best alternative is use of nonmercury thermometers, such as digital and electronic. These can be used orally, rectally, or axillary. Also available are tympanic (ear canal) a temporal artery, and flexible, disposable, forehead, or oral thermometers (less accurate). There are no known risks with any of the above thermometers.

Types of Thermometers

The following are types of thermometers available for use in the ambulatory care setting:

- Disposable strips
- Electronic/digital
- Tympanic
- Temporal artery

Disposable Thermometers. Disposable thermometers are individually wrapped strips with heat-sensitive dots that change color to indicate temperature. They are used once and then discarded. There are strips for use on the forehead and others for oral use. Although strips are easy to use and prevent patient cross contamination, accuracy is questionable.

Electronic and Digital Thermometers. Electronic thermometers are widely used, handheld, battery-operated or plug-in units that have easy-to-read electronic display screens to indicate results (Figure 12-3). Electronic thermometers in Fahrenheit or Celsius scales are available. Probes are attached and are color-coded blue for oral and red for rectal. The probes have disposable plastic covers. The plastic cover acts as a barrier to prevent contamination of the probe and is replaced for each patient to prevent cross contamination. An accurate result can be obtained in approximately 10 seconds.

Inexpensive digital thermometers are widely available for home use (Figure 12-4). They are quick, easy to use, and accurate. Encourage your patients to switch to these from the mercury glass thermometers. These lightweight thermometers do not require recharging; their small imbedded batteries last for years but are not replaceable.

Suggest patients watch for "Turn in Your Mercury Thermometer Days." Some communities, in conjunction with local pharmacies, set aside a day or two each year for residents to take mercury thermometers to their local pharmacy. In exchange for the mercury thermometers, free digital thermometers are given as replacements.

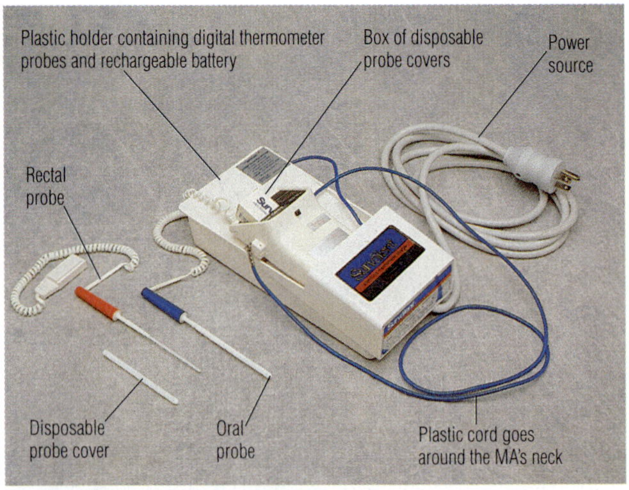

Figure 12-3 Electronic thermometers have interchangeable oral and rectal probes attached to a battery-operated portable unit.

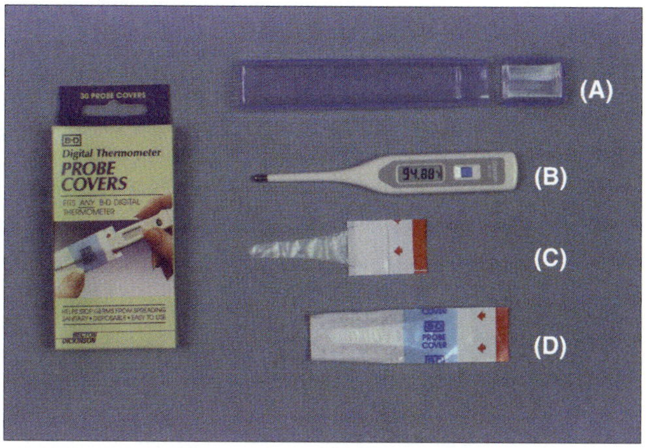

Figure 12-4 Digital thermometer. (A) Carrying case. (B) Digital thermometer. (C) Probe cover without backing. (D) Probe cover with backing.

Tympanic Thermometers. The use of tympanic thermometers is becoming more popular because they are fast, provide no discomfort to the patient, can be used on patients over 2 years of age as well as adults, and usually are accurate. They consist of a handheld unit with a probe tip that is inserted into the ear securely to make a seal. Disposable tips are used to prevent cross contamination. With the tympanic method of measuring body temperature, the procedure is complete in a few seconds. It is comfortable for the patient, nonthreatening to infants and children, and can be used when other methods are inappropriate. It is the thermometer of choice for pediatric patients older than 2 years. However, providers have found that inaccurate readings can result if patients have impacted cerumen in the ear of which they may be unaware. Also, if the patient has otitis media, a middle ear infection, the reading tends to be inaccurate and the procedure is painful.

The most commonly used thermometers are the digital/electronic, tympanic and temporal artery thermometer.

Temporal Artery Thermometers. A noninvasive thermometer known as a temporal artery thermometer, or TA thermometer, has been developed and is currently in use. Studies performed at Harvard Medical School and the Hospital for Sick Children found the TA thermometer to be more accurate than the aural (tympanic) and rectal thermometers. It is used on adults and children.

The temporal artery is a major blood vessel in the head. The thermometer measures the temperature of the skin surface over the temporal artery.

The thermometer has a probe that contains a sensor. When the TA thermometer is slid straight across the forehead (midline forehead), the infrared heat from the artery is picked up by the sensor (Figure 12-5). Software accurately determines and displays the temperature. The TA thermometer can also be used behind the ear lobe (if the forehead is wet with perspiration). See Procedure 12-3. There are many advantages to the TA thermometer: It can be used for patients of all ages; it is accurate, painless, fast, convenient, safe, comfortable, and noninvasive; and it can be cleaned with an alcohol wipe between patients.

Some considerations should be kept in mind when using a TA thermometer. If there is perspiration on the forehead, an inaccurate measurement could occur. Other sites that can be used are the femoral, axillary, and behind the ear. Scanning too rapidly can cause a false reading, as can a hat or hair covering the forehead. The TA thermometer must be the same temperature as the room in which it is used. It cannot be stored in the sun or

(A)
(B)

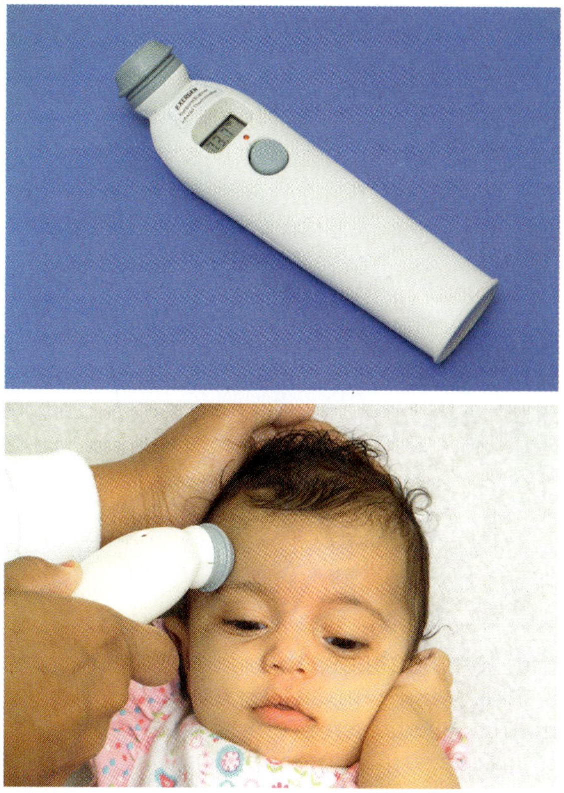

Figure 12-5 Using a temporal artery thermometer. (A) Temporal artery thermometer. (B) Slide thermometer across forehead.

Patient Education

Teach patients the importance of replacing mercury thermometers with an alternative such as digital, disposable, or aural (tympanic) thermometers. The risk for mercury poisoning is great if a mercury thermometer (or other mercury-containing item) is broken and the mercury escapes into the environment.

in a room where air-conditioned air has been blowing on the thermometer.

Measuring Temperature

To convert °F to °C:
Subtract 32 from F temperature, then multiply by 5/9.

Example:

$$5\overline{)324.9} = 64.9$$

64.9
5)324.9
30
24
20
49
45
4

To convert °C to °F:
Multiply C temperature by 9/5, then add 32.

Example:

$$\frac{36.1°C}{1} \times \frac{9}{5} + 32$$

36.1
× 9
324.9

64.9
5)324.9
30
24
20
49
45
4

or

65
+32
97° F

Oral Temperatures. To use an oral strip for taking a temperature, make certain that the package is not damaged, then peel it back to reveal the strip. Insert the strip into the patient's mouth. After the appropriate time interval has elapsed, remove the thermometer. The dots that have changed color are read using the scale located on the strip. Although convenient to use, accuracy is not always ensured with the strips, so these strips may not be the best choice for clinical use. Procedure 12-5 gives steps for taking an oral temperature using a disposable oral strip thermometer.

The procedure for obtaining an oral temperature with an electronic thermometer is quick, easy, and accurate (Procedure 12-1). Some electronic thermometers are stored on a recharging base. When removed from the base, they are turned on and ready for use. A disposable cover is placed over the probe, and the probe is placed in the patient's mouth. When temperature measurement is complete, the thermometer beeps and the temperature is displayed on the screen. The probe cover is ejected into a biohazard container without touching the container, and the unit is returned to the base. The temperature is then recorded in the patient's chart. Always read and follow the manufacturer's directions for use and care of a digital unit.

Aural Temperature. Taking a temperature with a tympanic thermometer is a fast, safe method for obtaining a patient's temperature (Figure 12-6). It is common in ambulatory care settings. Tympanic temperature can be obtained without discomfort for all patients except for children under 2 years of age.

The tympanic thermometer measures the patient's temperature by measuring the infrared waves produced by the tympanic membrane and records the temperature in less than 2 to 3 seconds on a digital screen. The tympanic membrane and the hypothalamus of the brain share the same blood supply, so an accurate measurement of the body temperature can be obtained.

The greatest benefits of the tympanic thermometer are that it gives nearly instant results; does not come into contact with mucous membranes, thereby minimizing cross contamination; uses a site that is readily accessible; is not affected by the patient smoking or drinking hot or cold liquids; does not require that the patient be conscious; and is an easy instrument to use. The unit is battery operated and uses a disposable probe cover or ear speculum.

Drawbacks to the tympanic thermometer have been demonstrated in pediatric patients with ear conditions such as otitis media. An inaccurate recording can result because fluid buildup in the inner ear limits infrared wave transmission.

The tympanic thermometer is a handheld unit that is inserted into the outer third of the ear canal. Procedure 12-2 gives steps for obtaining an aural temperature using a tympanic thermometer.

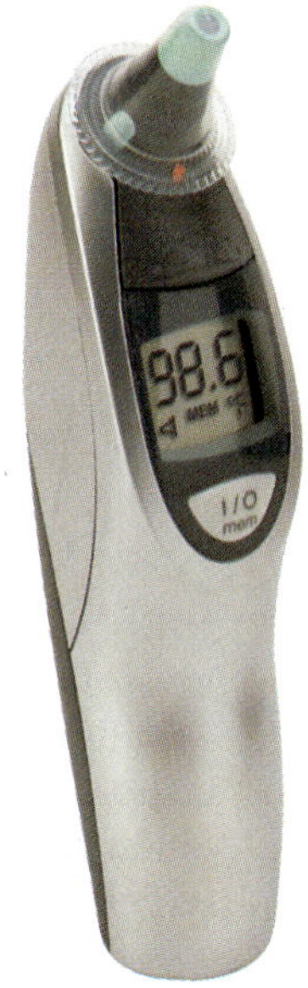

Figure 12-6 Thermo-scan tympanic thermometer. (Courtesy of Welch-Allyn.)

Rectal and Axillary Temperatures. The rectal and axillary methods for obtaining a temperature were widely used for infants, young children, and patients who were unable or uncooperative with oral temperature measurement. The new technology—tympanic, temporal artery, and electronic and digital thermometers—have simplified temperature measurement. These thermometers are safe, readily accepted by patients, greatly reduce microorganism transmission, are accurate, give a rapid reading, and are widely used in health care settings including ambulatory care. Although the newer eventually will replace the electronic digital method for measuring temperatures, including the rectal and axillary routes, the steps for obtaining rectal and axillary temperature measurements are included in Procedures 12-4 and 12-5.

Recording Temperature

Temperature may be taken on each visit to the provider's office to obtain a baseline for the patient. When recording the temperature in the patient's electronic medical record, the scale used for the results must be designated F for Fahrenheit and C for Celsius. The route used must be labeled as well; methods other than oral must be labeled according to the route used because there is a difference in the measurement. Use R for rectal, A for axillary, Tym for tympanic, and TA for temporal artery.

Temperatures is recorded as shown:

Oral	T 98.6°F
Rectal	T 99.6°(R) F
Axillary	T 97.6°(Ax) F
Tympanic	T 98.6°(Tym) F
Temporal artery	T 99.4°(TA) F

When a facility uses a tympanic thermometer exclusively, the route is known and therefore does not have to be labeled.

The medical assistant must read all manufacturer's instructions before using any digital, tympanic, or temporal artery thermometer. Each may have a slight difference in operating procedure.

Procedures 12-1 through 12-6 detail steps involved in taking temperature by various routes.

Cleaning and Storage of Thermometers

Oral and rectal thermometers should be separated. Storage depends on the policy of the facility.

Digital, electronic, tympanic, and temporal autery thermometers are cleaned according to the manufacturer's directions. The covers protect the probes from contamination. Each type of thermometer has a storage case or a wall-mounted base made especially for storing the unit. Disinfect these types of thermometers by wiping with a mild disinfectant as instructed by the manufacturer.

PULSE

The pulse rate consists of two phases of the heart action and can be felt when compressing an artery. As the heart contracts, it increases pressure on the arterial walls. The increased pressure passes through the arteries in a wave-like movement resulting in a slight expansion of the arterial wall (contraction). When the heart relaxes, (relaxation) the pressure is decreased in the arteries, resulting in the wall returning to its previous position. One contraction and one relaxation of the heart is equal to one heart cycle or heart beat. The pulse and heartbeat rate are usually identical in healthy individuals.

Pulse Sites

The pulse can be felt in areas of the body where an artery is close to the surface and to an underlying solid structure such as a bone. Common pulse sites include the radial, carotid, temporal, brachial, femoral, popliteal, and dorsalis pedis arteries (Figure 12-7). An apical pulse, located at the apex of the heart, may also be taken. Although the radial, brachial, and carotid arteries are the most frequently used sites for pulse rates, it is important to recognize pulse beats because circulation may be monitored by palpating the other sites. Pulse sites are also used when necessary as pressure points for controlling severe bleeding.

- The *radial* pulse is located at the thumb side of the wrist approximately 1 inch above the base of the thumb. This is the most commonly used site for obtaining a pulse rate.
- The *carotid* pulse, used during emergency situations and when performing cardiopulmonary resuscitation (CPR), is found between the larynx and sternocleidomastoid muscle in the front side of the neck on either side of the trachea. When measuring the pulse at the carotid site, compress only one side at a time.
- The *brachial* pulse is found in the inner aspect of the elbow called the antecubital space. This pulse site is the most commonly used site to obtain blood pressure measurements.
- The *temporal* pulse is located at the temple area of the head. It is rarely used to obtain a pulse rate but may be used to monitor circulation, control bleeding from the head and scalp, and to take a temporal artery temperature.
- The *femoral* pulse is located in the groin area. It is a deep artery and must be compressed firmly to be felt.
- The *popliteal* pulse is located at the back of the knee. The patient must be in a supine position with the knee flexed for it to be felt because the artery is deep within the knee. This artery is used for leg blood pressure measurements and to monitor circulation.
- The *dorsalis pedis* pulse is felt on the top of the foot slightly to the side of midline next to the extensor ligament of the great toe, between the first and second metatarsal bones. It is commonly used to monitor lower limb circulation.
- ***Apical*** *pulse* is found at the apex of the heart, located at the fifth intercostal space left side, midclavicular line, that is, between the fifth and sixth ribs perpendicular to the middle of the clavicle, left of the sternum. A stethoscope is required to obtain an apical pulse. Apical pulse is used for cardiac patients and patients with an arrhythmia, and to obtain infant pulse rates because they are difficult to obtain by the usual methods.

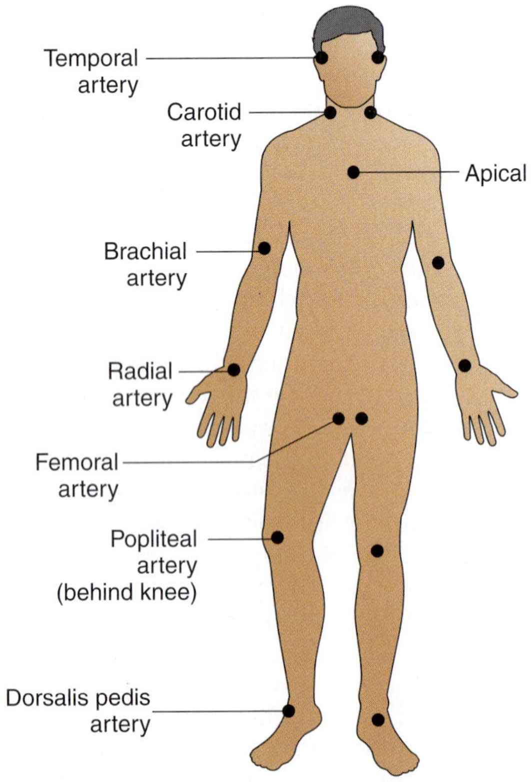

Figure 12-7 Pulse sites in the body.

Measuring and Evaluating a Pulse

When measuring a pulse rate, other characteristics besides the rate are noted, such as rhythm, volume of pulse, and condition of the arterial wall.

The rate is the number of pulsations or beats felt in 1 minute. The pulse is counted for 30 seconds, then the number is doubled. Pulse rates may vary according to age, activities, general health, sex, emotions, pain, and medications. The rate is lower when sleeping and higher when active or exercising. Rates for infants and children are greater than for adults. Well-conditioned athletes have a lower than average resting rate because their cardiovascular system has been developed to function more efficiently.

Rhythm of the pulse refers to the time between pulsations and regularity of the beat. Normal rhythm occurs when the beats are felt at regular intervals. In abnormal rhythms, **arrhythmias,** the interval between pulsations is altered by either an increased or decreased time span. Arrhythmias must be noted and reported because they may indicate heart disease.

The volume of the pulse refers to the strength of the beat that is felt. The pulsations may feel full, strong, hard, soft, thready, or weak. A pulse may have a regular rate and yet have a variation in intensity or volume. Volume should be noted and reported.

Condition of the arterial wall can be felt as the pulse is taken. The normal artery feels soft and elastic. The abnormal artery may feel hard, knotty, wiry, or a combination of these. These should be noted and reported because they may indicate cardiac disease.

Normal Pulse Rates

Average pulse rates vary from birth to adulthood. At birth, the pulse rate is much higher; as we age, it generally decreases.

NORMAL PULSE RATES

Birth		130–140 beats per minute
Infants		110–130 beats per minute
Children	1 year	110–130 beats per minute
	2 years	96–115 beats per minute
	3 years	86–105 beats per minute
	7–14 yerars	76–90 beats per minute
Adults		60–80 beats per minute

Pulse Abnormalities

Abnormalities may occur in the rate, rhythm, and feel of the arterial wall. Common pulse rate abnormalities include **bradycardia,** a pulse rate less than 60 beats per minute, and **tachycardia,** a pulse rate greater than 100 beats per minute. Common arrhythmias include a pulsation felt before expected, which is called a premature contraction, and sinus arrhythmia. An occasional premature contraction can occur in response to stress, caffeine, nicotine, alcohol, or lack of sleep. Sinus arrhythmia may occur during respiration and can be found in some children and young adults. The rate increases with inspiration and decreases with expiration. It usually does not require treatment.

When any pulse rate abnormalities or arrhythmias are felt, take the pulse for 1 full minute, note the frequency of the abnormality, record the abnormality, and alert the provider. The provider may want you to take an apical pulse (see Chapter 25).

Recording Pulse Rates

Pulse rates are normally recorded after the temperature; for example: T 98.6°F P 72 regular. Any unusual findings should be recorded and reported to the provider; for example: P 72 irregular × 2 minutes.

Procedure 12-7 describes measuring a radial pulse; Procedure 12-8 describes measuring an apical pulse.

RESPIRATION

The function of respiration (breathing) is the exchange of the gases oxygen and carbon dioxide. External respiration occurs when oxygen is drawn into the lungs when breathing in and carbon dioxide is expelled from the lungs when breathing out. Internal respiration occurs when oxygen is used by the cells for cellular function. Carbon dioxide is a by-product of cellular function and is expelled via exhalation as a waste product. Respiration is an involuntary act controlled by the medulla oblongata of the brain. The medulla oblongata measures blood levels of carbon dioxide and triggers a respiration when the level of carbon dioxide increases. Although it is an involuntary act, respiration may be altered by holding the breath or when hyperventilation occurs. One inspiration (inhalation) drawing in of air and one expiration (exhalation) expelling air together equals one respiration.

Abnormalities in the characteristics of respiration, such as rate, rhythm, and depth, are noted when measuring respiration.

Respiratory rate is the number of respirations per minute. The normal respiratory rate, **eupnea,** varies with age, activities, illness, emotions, and drugs. The average respiration rate to pulse rate is 1:4, one respiration to four pulse beats.

Respiratory rhythm refers to the pattern of breathing. It can vary with age, with adults having a regular pattern, but infants having an irregular pattern. Rhythm may be altered by laughing and sighing.

NORMAL RESPIRATORY RATES

Newborns	44 respirations per minute
Infants	20–40 respirations per minute
Children (1–7 years)	18–30 respirations per minute
Adults	12–20 respirations per minute

Depth of respiration is the amount of air that is inspired and expired with each respiration. In the resting state, the amount should be consistent. Depth is noted by watching the degree of rise and fall of the chest wall when measuring respiration rate.

Respiration Rate

Respiratory rate is measured by counting breaths for 30 seconds and doubling the amount. This will give the number of respirations per minute. It is important that patients not be aware you are measuring their respirations. The rate may change if the patient knows they are being counted. Procedure 12-9 gives steps for measuring respiration rate.

Abnormalities

Abnormalities of the respiration rate may be found in the rate, depth, rhythm, and sounds of respiration. Some rate abnormalities include apnea, tachypnea, bradypnea, and Cheyne–Stokes. Sleep apnea and narcolepsy are considered sleep disorders and involve the respiratory system.

Apnea is the temporary complete absence of breathing. It may result from a reduction in stimuli to the respiratory center of the brain. Apnea will occur when the breath is voluntarily held and in Cheyne-Stokes respiration. It can be a serious symptom of other conditions of the cardiovascular and renal systems. It also can result from a head injury such as a concussion.

Tachypnea is a respiratory rate greater than 40 respirations per minute. It may be caused by hysteria or be transient in the newborn. Excessive loss of carbon dioxide may occur if tachypnea is prolonged; there is a potential for this to lead to more serious problems.

Bradypnea is a decrease in the number of respirations and is commonly seen during sleep or because of certain diseases.

Cheyne–Stokes is a breathing pattern that starts with a period of apnea lasting 10 to 60 seconds followed by increasing depth and rate of respiration, which is then followed by a decrease in rate with apnea starting the cycle once again. This cycle may be normal for children but may indicate brain dysfunction in other age groups.

Orthopnea is a respiratory condition of severe **dyspnea** (labored breathing). Breathing is difficult in any position *other* than sitting erect or standing. This condition may be seen in patients with heart failure, angina pectoris, asthma, pulmonary edema, emphysema, pneumonia, and spasmodic coughing. Patients who experience orthopnea must be examined in a sitting position. Other positions will cause discomfort and may not be possible.

Abnormalities in the depth of respiration are divided into shallow abnormalities, such as hypoventilation, and deep abnormalities, such as hyperpnea and hyperventilation.

Hypoventilation occurs when respiration is decreased in rate and shallow in depth. It may result from a depression of nervous stimuli of the respiratory center in the brain.

Hyperpnea is respiration that is increased in both depth and rate. It is commonly seen with activities such as physical exercise. It can also be associated with pain, respiratory diseases, cardiac diseases, hysteria, and use of certain drugs.

Hyperventilation is a type of breathing in which the amount of oxygen drawn in during inspiration is greatly increased, resulting in a decrease in the amount of blood carbon dioxide. Hyperventilation may be associated with asthma, pulmonary embolism or edema, and acute anxiety. The patient can be treated by reducing the amount of oxygen inhaled during an inspiration. The patient may be instructed to hold one nostril closed while breathing or may be instructed to breathe into a paper bag. Either procedure will reduce the amount of inspired oxygen and bring the oxygen and carbon dioxide blood levels back to within normal range.

Sleep Apnea. Airflow during respiration that stops for more than 10 seconds is considered to be sleep apnea. The periods of apnea cause carbon dioxide to accumulate in the blood and oxygen to be depleted. For these reasons, sleep apnea can be dangerous. Oxygen depletion to the brain can cause memory impairment, cognitive changes, and daytime sleepiness. If the condition goes untreated, sleep apnea can result in cardiac arrhythmias, congestive heart failure, cerebral vascular accident (CVA), hypertension, and death.

Sleep apnea is associated with airway obstruction. The soft palate (especially in males who are overweight and who snore) can collapse while the patient is asleep. The result is apnea. The patient usually awakens from sleep enough to resume breathing.

Sleep apnea is diagnosed by sleep laboratory studies when apnea is observed while the patient is sleeping.

Treatment of sleep apnea consists of weight loss and continuous positive airway pressure (CPAP), a device that puts pressure on the airway while the patient sleeps. A mask is placed over the patient's face to keep the airway open. This prevents sleep apnea. A surgical procedure can be performed to remove parts of the soft palate and uvula.

Narcolepsy. Narcolepsy is another type of sleep disorder that causes patients to have daytime sleeping while driving, eating, or sitting in a movie theater. The patient can become paralyzed from the sleep, being unable to move, but can still breathe. The cause may be genetic.

The diagnosis is made by ruling out sleep apnea (through sleep studies) and by the history of repeated episodes of daytime sleeping for a few seconds to half an hour. The disorder is not under the patient's control.

Breath Sounds. The presence or absence of breath sounds can be indicative of respiratory problems. Sounds should be listened for and noted when taking the patient's respiratory rate.

Rales (pronounced "rawles") are rattling sounds heard during inspiration and expiration when the lung passageways contain secretions. The provider uses a stethoscope to auscultate or listen for rales, which are associated with some lung diseases. Rhonchi are sounds similar to snoring, usually produced by a rattle in the throat. These are also heard by auscultation.

Wheezes are high-pitched musical sounds heard on expiration. They can be the result of an obstruction in the bronchi and bronchioles of the lungs. Wheezes are commonly associated with asthma and emphysema, a chronic pulmonary disease characterized by dilated and damaged alveoli.

Stridor is a crowing sound heard on inspiration as a result of an obstruction of the upper airway. It is associated with laryngitis, a foreign body obstruction, and croup in children.

Stertorous respiration is described as a snoring sound with labored breathing. The sound usually is created by partial obstruction of the upper airway.

BLOOD PRESSURE

Blood pressure measures cardiovascular function by measuring the force of blood exerted on **peripheral** arteries during the cardiac cycle or heartbeat. The measurement consists of two components. The first is the force exerted on the arterial walls during cardiac contraction and is called **systole.** The second is the force exerted during cardiac relaxation and is called **diastole.** They represent the highest (systole) and lowest (diastole) amount of pressure exerted during the cardiac cycle. Blood pressure is recordedas a fraction, with the systolic measurement written, followed by a slash and then the diastolic measurement.

Example: systole/diastole or 120/80

Blood pressure may be affected by many factors, including blood volume, peripheral resistance, vessel elasticity, condition of the muscle of the heart, genetics, diet and weight, activity, and emotional state.

- Blood volume is the amount of blood within the arteries. Increased volume of blood increases blood pressure, whereas a decrease in blood volume decreases blood pressure, as in the case of a hemorrhage or severe dehydration.
- Peripheral resistance is the resistance to blood flow within the arteries. The resistance is in direct relation to the **lumen** of the arteries. The smaller the lumen, the more pressure needed to push blood through. The reverse is also true: the larger the lumen, the less resistance and less pressure needed to push the blood through. The size of the lumen can become smaller from deposits of fatty cholesterol (plaque), resulting in an increase in blood pressure.
- Vessel elasticity refers to the ability of arteries to expand and contract to provide a steady flow of blood. As a person ages, elasticity of the vessels is reduced. **Atherosclerosis** can cause an increase in arterial wall resistance, resulting in an increase in blood pressure.
- The condition of the heart muscle is extremely important to blood flow and blood pressure. A strong heart muscle provides a forceful pump resulting in efficient blood flow and normal blood pressure. A weak heart muscle results in an inefficient pumping action of the heart leading to a decrease in blood pressure and blood flow (see Chapter 25).

The viscosity of the blood also is a factor in blood pressure. Viscosity refers to how sticky a substance is, in this case, the blood. If the blood is sticky, it acts thicker. Imagine holding a bottle of thin syrup upside down over your pancakes. The thin syrup comes out of the bottle quite readily. Now imagine holding a bottle of thick molasses over the pancakes. Being very viscous, the molasses is thicker and much more difficult to pour. So it is with viscous blood; it is thicker and requires a lot more work for the heart muscle to move it through the vessels, thus increasing the pressure inside the walls of the arteries. In fact, it may be so viscous that it might not be able to reach the tiniest capillaries of the kidney, eyes, and other areas without substantial increase in blood pressure.

Equipment for Measuring Blood Pressure

Blood pressure is measured by the auscultatory (listening) method using a sphygmomanometer and a stethoscope (Figure 12-8). Three types of sphygmomanometers are commonly used in the ambulatory care setting: mercury, aneroid, and electronic (digital) manometers (Figures 12-9 to 12-12).

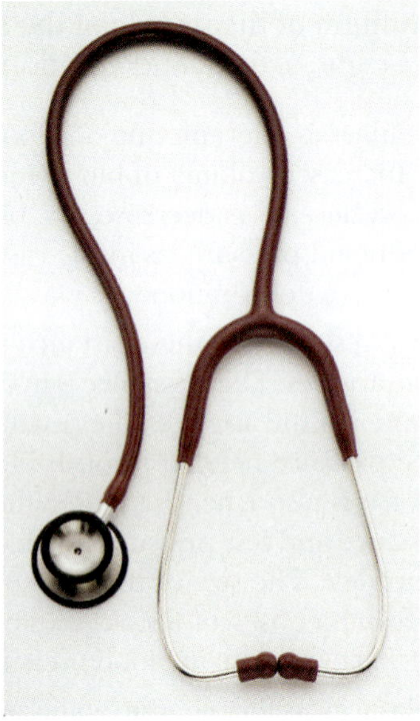

Figure 12-8 Adult stethoscope is used with a sphygmomanometer to measure blood pressure. (Courtesy of Welch-Allyn.)

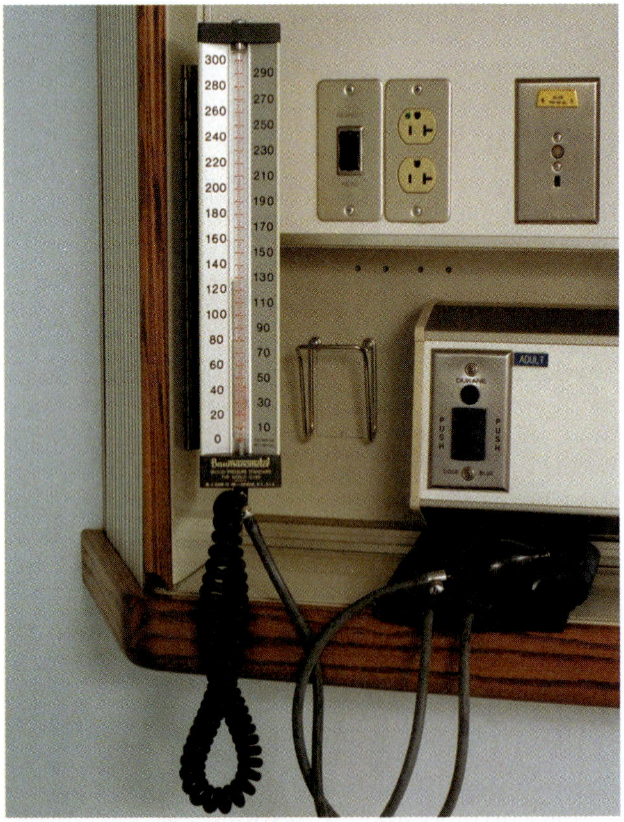

Figure 12-9 A mercury gravity sphygmomanometer.

Mercury sphygmomanometers are being phased out with other mercury-containing medical equipment, such as mercury thermometers. Aneroid and electronic blood pressure measuring devices are more commonly used. Many medical facilities continue to use mercury sphygmomanometers while phasing them out in agreement with the EPA, but the process has been slower than the phasing out

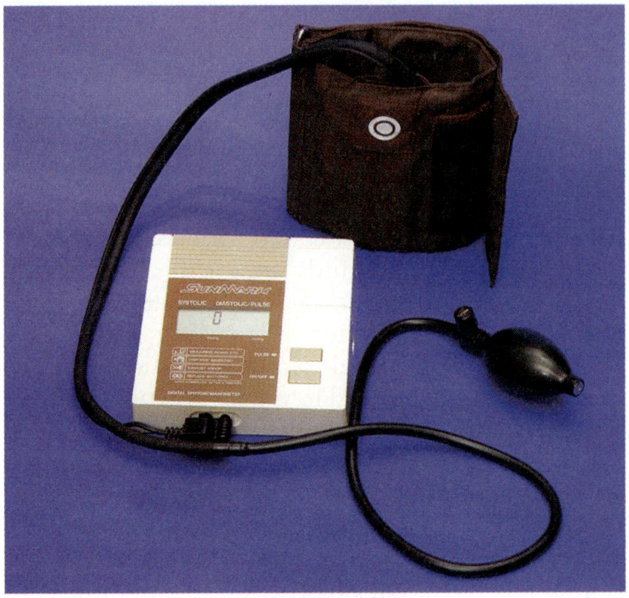

Figure 12-10 Digital sphygmomanometer.

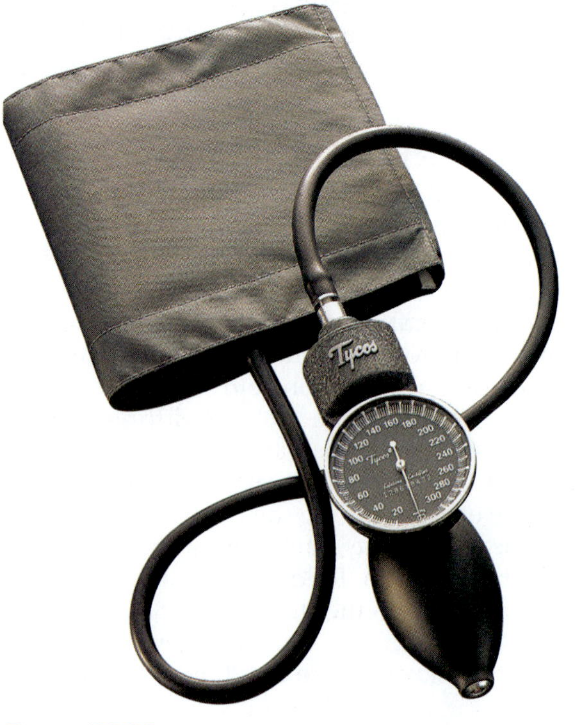

Figure 12-11 Aneroid sphygmomanometer. (Courtesy of Welch-Allyn.)

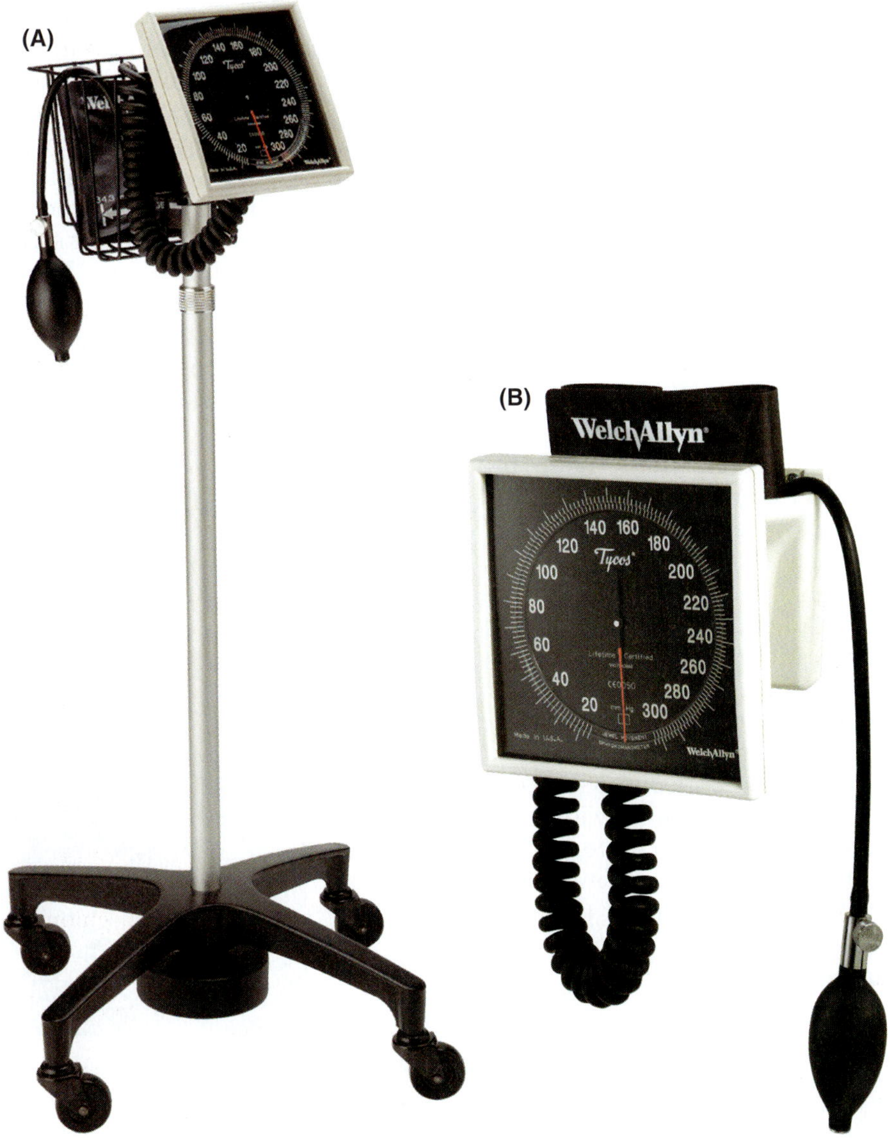

Figure 12-12 (A) Mobile aneroid sphygmomanometer. (B) Wall-mounted aneroid sphygmomanometer. (Courtesy of Welch-Allyn.)

of mercury thermometers; therefore, information about the mercury sphygmomanometers is provided in this chapter.

The mercury **manometer** consists of a cuff containing a rubber bladder attached by rubber tubing to a glass column of mercury. The blood pressure is read at the **meniscus** of the mercury as it descends the column. Mercury manometers are the most accurate method of blood pressure measurement and are considered the standard because blood pressure is measured in millimeters of mercury. Although the most accurate, mercury manometers do have disadvantages: they are not as portable as aneroid manometers, and there is always the danger of a mercury spill should the glass column break and cause health and environmental problems. Mercury manometers need to be cleaned and checked regularly for accuracy by a professional technician. Care in handling and storage is important to prevent air bubbles and dirt from forming in the column or breaking the glass containing the mercury.

The aneroid manometer is a cuff containing a rubber bladder attached to a dial. The blood pressure is read at the point of the needle descending the dial. Aneroid manometers need to be calibrated regularly because they do not maintain calibration easily. Care in handling and storage will decrease the loss of calibration. Although not as accurate as a mercury manometer, aneroid manometers are easily portable and there is no danger of a mercury spill.

An electronic syphmomanometer is automatic and registers blood pressure in digital form on a screen (Figure 12-13). No stethoscope is needed. Once the cuff is secured on the patient's upper arm, the medical assistant pushes a button and the cuff inflates; the medical assistant then releases the pressure slowly. A readout is visible on the screen (124/75). In addition to blood pressure reading, the unit can automatically measure pulse rate and other vital signs. A **pulse oximeter** (Figure 12-14) measures the amount of oxygen present in the patient's blood. The measurement automatically appears on the screen when the device is attached to the patient.

Cuff sizes for manometers range from the smallest pediatric cuff to the largest obese and thigh cuff (Figure 12-15). The appropriate cuff size is necessary to obtain an accurate blood pressure measurement. A cuff that is too small will give an artificially high blood pressure reading, whereas a cuff that is too large will give an artificially low reading. The selection of the cuff size depends on the size of the arm, not the age of the patient. Due to the size of the arm, it may be necessary to use an adult-size cuff on a child or a pediatric-size cuff on an adult. Adult cuffs should have a width that covers one third to one half the circumference of the arm. The length of the bladder should cover approximately 80% of the arm (about twice the size of the width). The cuff for a child should cover two thirds of the upper arm. The American Heart Association recommends if there has been a weight loss or gain of 10 pounds, then the cuff size should be reassessed for the appropriate size.

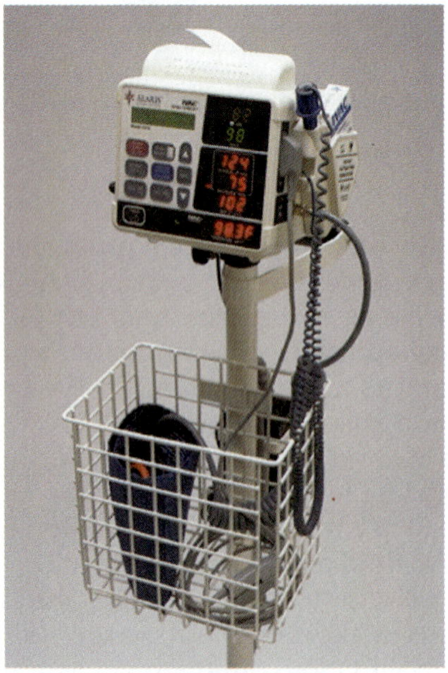

Figure 12-13 An electronic sphygmomanometer can measure pulse and other vital signs simultaneously.

Measuring Blood Pressure

The sounds heard during blood pressure measurement are named the Korotkoff sounds. The cause of the sounds is not known. They may be a result of distention of the vessels or the sound of the blood passing through the vessels. In either case, Korotkoff sounds have five distinct phases. Not all phases are heard easily, especially for beginners.

- *Phase I.* Begins with the first sound heard when deflating the cuff. It is a sharp tapping sound. Note this first sound as this will be the *systolic reading* of the blood pressure.

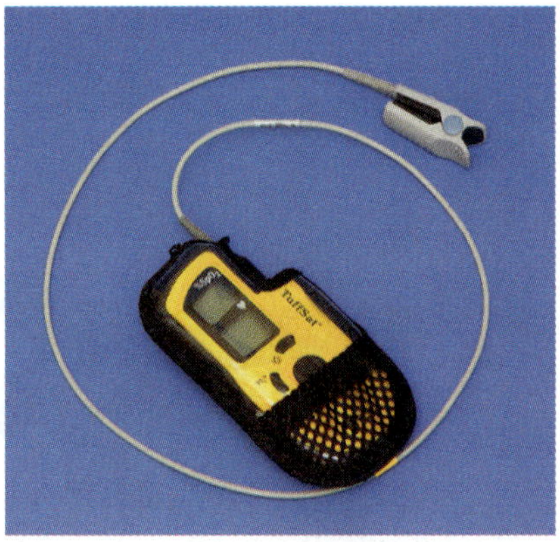

Figure 12-14 Pulse oximeter.

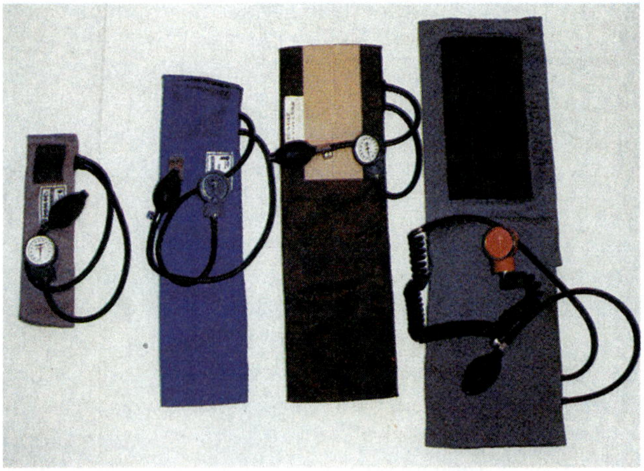

Figure 12-15 Blood pressure cuffs in sizes to fit the arm of a small child to the thigh of an adult. It is important to have the correct size to obtain an accurate reading.

- *Phase II.* This sound is the result of more blood passing through the vessels as the cuff is deflated. The sound is that of a soft swishing sound.
- *Phase III.* More blood continues to pass through the vessels as the cuff is deflated. The sound is a rhythmic tapping sound. If blood pressure measurements are not carefully followed and Phases I and II are missed, Phase III may erroneously be reported as the systolic pressure.
- *Phase IV.* Blood is now passing through the vessels fairly easily as the cuff is deflated. The sounds heard will be a muffling and fading of the tapping sounds. This phase may be used to record the diastolic pressure in children and in those patients where a tapping sound is heard to zero.
- *Phase V.* Blood is flowing freely at this time; a consequently all sounds disappear. The disappearance of sounds is noted and recorded as the *diastolic pressure.*

When measuring blood pressure, keep two things in mind: patient comfort and accuracy.

Auscultatory gap is heard in some patients. It is a time, usually between Phases I and II or III, when all sounds disappear. Within 20 to 30 mm Hg, or 20 to 30 **increments** on the aneroid, the sounds reappear. If the procedures are not followed carefully, the auscultatory gap is easily missed, and the blood pressure measurement is incorrect in that systolic and diastolic readings may be in error according to the length of the gap (Table 12-1).

Pulse pressure is the difference between the systolic and diastolic measurements. The normal range for pulse pressure is 30 to 50 mm Hg. The difference should be no more than one third of the systolic reading. For example, if the blood pressure is 120/80 a normal pulse pressure should be 120 minus 80 or 40. One third of the systolic reading of 120 is 40. Therefore, 40 mm Hg pulse pressure is within the normal range.

Table 12-1 Errors in Blood Pressure Measurement Procedures

Errors in measuring blood pressure must be avoided. Common errors include:
1. Improper cuff size.
2. The arm is not at heart level. Do not hold the arm up or let the patient hold up the arm. Pressure is increased when this is done.
3. Cuff is not completely deflated before use or after palpatory method, resulting in a higher pressure measurement.
4. Deflation of the cuff is faster than 2 to 4 mm Hg per heartbeat or 20–30 increments on the aneroid. Sounds are missed if this happens.
5. Reinflating the cuff during the procedure without allowing the arm to rest for 1 to 2 minutes.
6. Patient is not relaxed and comfortable. An anxious, apprehensive patient will have a reading that is higher than the actual blood pressure.
7. Improper cuff placement. Cuff is too loose, too tight, or not positioned correctly over the brachial artery.
8. Defective equipment in which there are air leaks in the bladder or valve, the mercury column is dirty, or air bubbles are present. Mercury and aneroid sphygmomanometers are not calibrated at zero.
9. Measuring blood pressure with thumb on the head of the stethoscope.
All of these errors are easily corrected by following careful procedure and by having the manometers calibrated and cleaned according to a regular maintenance schedule.

Recording Blood Pressure Measurement

The blood pressure is recorded on the patient chart or electronic medical recored in a fraction format. The position of the patient (sitting or lying down) may be noted. The arm used is also noted, particularly if the blood pressure was taken in both arms.

Example: 120/80, ® arm, supine or $\frac{120}{80}$ ® arm, supine

For children and those patients whose blood pressure can still be heard to zero, the beginning of Korotkoff Phase IV and zero both are recorded.

Example: 120/70/0 or $\begin{array}{c}120\\ \hline 70\\ \hline 0\end{array}$

Procedure 12-10 outlines the procedure for measuring blood pressure.

Normal Blood Pressure Readings

Normal blood pressure is low at birth and gradually increases with age until adulthood, at which point it should remain fairly constant. Blood pressure measurements are taken during yearly physical examinations beginning at age 3.

NORMAL BLOOD PRESSURE READINGS

In a healthy child, blood pressure is taken for the first time during the physical exam when the child is 3 years old. Blood pressure in children varies based on their gender and height percentile.

Child 10 years	100/65
Adolescent 16 years	118/75
Adult	Systolic less than 120 Diastolic less than 80
Prehypertension	120–139/80–89
High blood pressure	Above 140/90

Blood Pressure Abnormalities

There are only two possible blood pressure abnormalities: hypertension, blood pressure that is consistently above normal, and hypotension, blood pressure that is consistently below normal in which patients are unable to perform their normal activities without dizziness and extreme fatigue.

Hypertension. There are five types of **hypertension:** primary or essential, secondary, benign, and malignant.

- The most commonly seen form of hypertension is primary or essential. It is hypertension with no apparent cause or cure but is treatable. Treatment is designed to control hypertension and is a lifelong process. It will not be cured, just controlled. The American Heart Association (AHA) suggests that to diagnose hypertension, the diagnosis is based on the average of three readings at each of three visits to the provider's office after the initial baseline screening. According to the AHA, normal blood pressure for adults 18 years and older is less than 120/80, prehypertension is 120–139/80–89, hypertension stage 1 is 140–159/90–99, and hypertension stage 2 is ≥160/≥100.
- Secondary hypertension is the result of some underlying problem, such as renal disease, pregnancy, endocrine imbalances, obesity, arteriosclerosis, or atherosclerosis. Once the underlying problem is removed, the blood pressure returns to normal or near normal. Secondary hypertension can be successfully treated.
- Hypertension that has a slow progression but may progress to the same end point as malignant hypertension is referred to as benign hypertension.
- Malignant hypertension (no association with cancer) progresses rapidly with severe damage to the cardiovascular system, possibly to the point of death.
- White coat hypertension is hypertension that can occur in some individuals. It is caused by anxiety or fear when blood pressure measurements are taken by a provider.

Hypotension. **Hypotension** is blood pressure persistently less than normal, usually less than 90/60, although this may be normal for some healthy adults. Hypotension is defined as a blood pressure so low that the patient is unable to function normally. It is usually a result of various shocklike conditions such as hemorrhage, traumatic or emotional shock, central nervous system disorders, or chronic wasting diseases. With successful treatment of the underlying problems, the blood pressure usually will be in the range of normal readings.

Orthostatic hypotension, sometimes called postural hypotension, occurs when a person rapidly changes position from supine to standing, when

Patient Education

Hypertension is at epidemic proportions in the United States, and many patients are not treated because they do not know that they have the problem. It is known as the "silent epidemic" because most people do not experience any symptoms over a span of years. However, untreated or poorly treated hypertension over time can damage the heart, cause myocardial infarction, cause a stroke (cerebrol vascular accident), or lead to kidney failure.

There are several nondrug ways to reduce blood pressure, even for people who have inherited hypertensive tendencies. With the provider's advice, there are steps to take include: eating plenty of produce, grains, and low-fat dairy foods; cutting back on salt; stopping smoking; exercising regularly; maintaining a healthy weight; limiting alcohol intake; and reducing stress. It is easy to see that these recommendations all are lifestyle changes. They can significantly reduce blood pressure if practiced daily. Blood pressure must be monitored regularly by your provider.

standing in one position for too long, or as a side effect of certain medications. In this instance, the blood pressure has momentarily decreased, and the person experiences vertigo (dizziness) and may have blurred vision. These symptoms usually last only a few seconds, just long enough for the blood pressure to return to normal. Care should be taken when helping patients to an upright position from a supine position because orthostatic hypotension can lead to syncope (fainting) and injury from falling.

HEIGHT AND WEIGHT

Although not considered a vital sign, height and weight are routinely measured if warranted by the age and the physical condition of the patient. Many providers prefer that height and weight be measured as part of a yearly physical examination and otherwise may vary the frequency of patient height and weight measurements. Height and weight are normally measured simultaneously.

For children, height and weight are typically measured during each provider visit. The height of adults may be obtained on the initial visit only and weight taken on all visits. An adolescent or young adult may have height measured more frequently to plot body changes. Because older adult patients tend to lose the cushioning between vertebrae through osteoporosis as part of aging, they may need to have their height measured more frequently to check the stage of any degeneration.

Older adult patients require special attention by the medical assistant when measuring height and weight. It is especially important to assist older patients both on and off the scale, because the scale platform is movable, and older patients may lose their balance and fall if unassisted. A stand-alone walker can be placed over the scale platform to aid in stabilizing the patient.

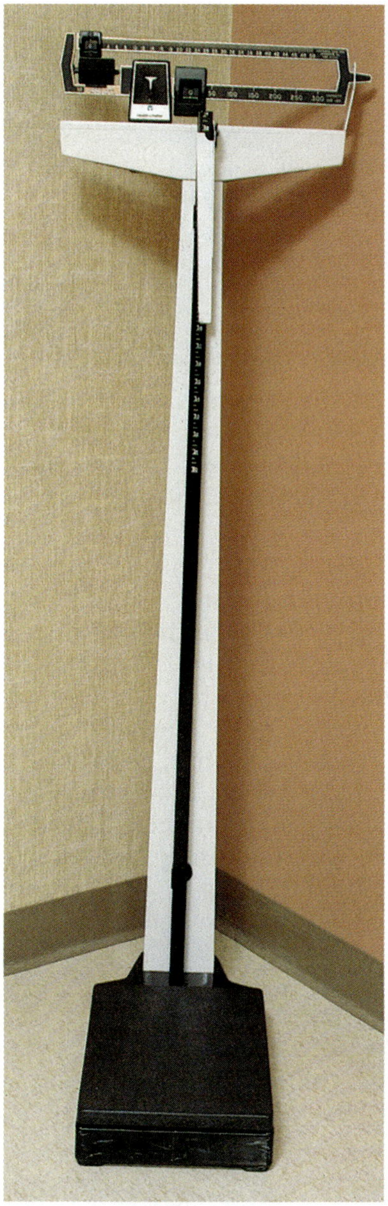

Figure 12-16A Traditional beam balance scale with measuring bar.

Height

To measure a patient's height, a scale with a measuring bar is necessary (Figure 12-16A). A paper towel is placed on the scale because the patient's shoes should be removed for accurate measuring.

> **Critical Thinking**
>
> Discuss the normal vital signs differences expected between an infant and an adult. Why do they occur?

The patient is asked to step on the scale and face away from the measuring bar. Assist patient onto the scale; the scale platform is movable and the patient could fall.

There are two reasons for having the patient's back to the scale. When the measuring bar is lifted, it could cause face or eye injuries if the patient were facing the bar. Lifting the measuring bar prior to the patient stepping on the scale can also lead to eye and face injuries in that the patient could inadvertently walk into the bar. Another reason to have the patient's back to the scale is if the patient does

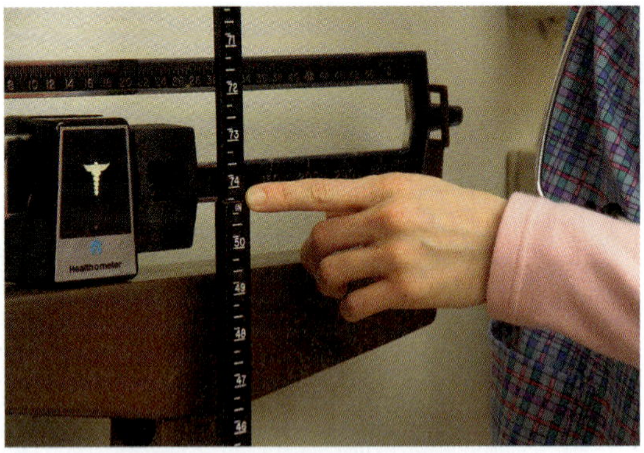

Figure 12-16B The height is read at the moveable point of the ruler. The bars are measured in one-quarter inches. Note the height measurement is 74.25 inches or 6 feet 2 ¼ inches.

not look straight ahead, the head is not level, which could result in a less than accurate measurement.

After the patient is on the platform, the measuring bar is placed firmly on the patient's head, and the line between where the solid bar and sliding bar meet is read. The bars are measured in quarter inches (Figure 12-16B). Children's heights are recorded in inches, whereas adults are recorded in feet and inches. Conversion from inches to feet is accomplished by taking the number of inches and dividing by 12. Procedure 12-11 gives steps for measuring height.

Weight

Provider preference and patient health dictate the frequency of measuring an adult's weight. Some providers require the patient's weight to be measured on each visit, whereas others do not if there are no health problems that require weight monitoring. Some health conditions that do require weight monitoring include obesity, eating disorders, hormone disorders such as diabetes and thyroid malfunction, hypertension, pregnancy, cancer, and some digestive disorders.

When measuring the weight of a patient, the medical assistant must maintain the patient's privacy. Most people are conscious of their weight and may become embarrassed if the measurement is taken where others may see and hear. Privacy is important and often overlooked. The medical assistant must also be careful of comments regarding a patient's weight, particularly with the obese patient and with those being treated for eating disorders (see Chapter 22). Encouragement for weight loss for the dieting patient is beneficial but must be done in privacy. Other comments are inappropriate.

Occasionally a patient will be instructed by the provider to monitor weight at home. It is important for the patient to understand the necessity of weighing at the same time each day because weight may vary significantly throughout the day. A normal routine is to measure weight before breakfast.

Before an accurate weight can be obtained, the scale must be calibrated. The point of the balance beam must be floating in the center when no weight is applied to the scale. Some scales are equipped with a screw at the end that can be turned slightly until the beam is in the correct floating position. Once it is centered, it is calibrated and ready for use (Figure 12-17).

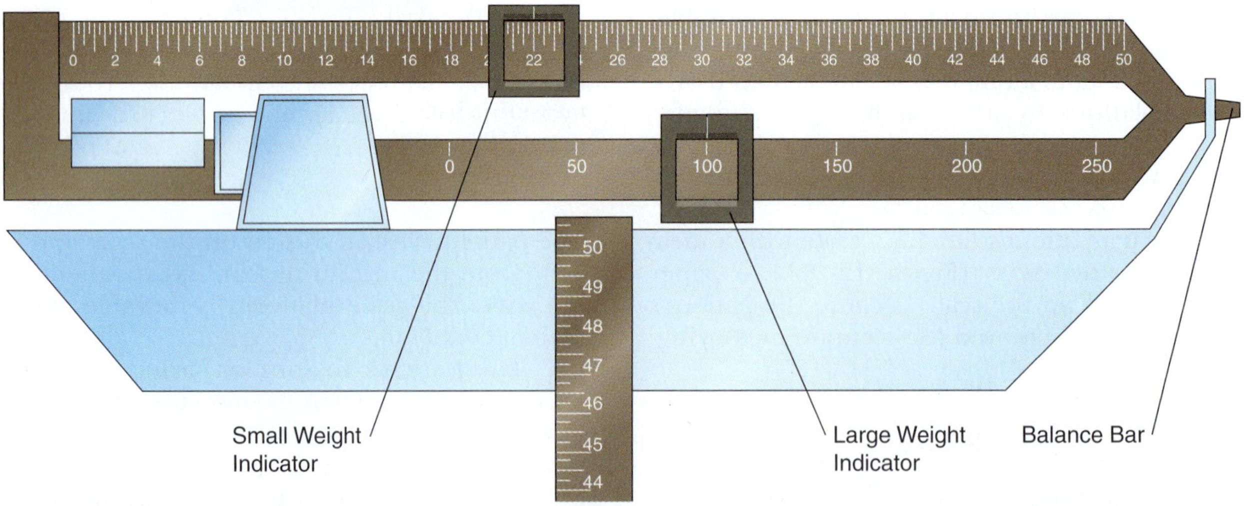

Figure 12-17 The upper bar indicates small pound weights (from 0–50 lb). The weight shown on the lower bar is measured in 50-lb increments. The lower measurement is added to the upper bar amount that is shown. The upper bar shows 22 lb; the lower bar measures 100 lb. Upper bar 22 lb plus lower bar 100 lb equal total weight 122 lb.

An eye-level digital scale with measuring bar measures height in the same way on the measuring bar of the digital scale as it is on the balance beam measuring bar. Weight measurement is quicker, easier, and usually safer taken on the digital scale. The scale platform is stationary, and the patient is assisted as needed onto the scale; the digital reading is ready in a few seconds (Figure 12-18).

The patient can wear normal indoor clothing, rather than disrobing, for weight measurement. Heavy coats or other outerwear should be removed. Heavy objects and purses should not be held during the procedure. A chair or counter should be provided to place these objects on while the procedure is being performed. Shoes should be removed. Procedure 12-12 gives steps for measuring adult weight.

Occasionally, as in the case of medication dosage, the medical assistant is required to convert pound weight into kilogram weight.

1 kilogram = 2.2 pounds

To convert pounds to kilograms:

Take the number of pounds and divide by 2.2

Example:

130 pounds divided by
2.2 = 59.09 kg

To convert from kilograms to pounds:

Take the number of kilograms and multiply by 2.2

Example:

50 kilograms multiplied by
2.2 = 110 lb.

Significance of Weight

The careful monitoring of a patient's weight may provide an insight into metabolic, nutritional, and emotional problems.

MEASURING CHEST CIRCUMFERENCE

Occasionally, the medical assistant is instructed to measure the chest of an adult. This procedure may be done on patients with emphysema and as a requirement for insurance and truck driver licenses. Two measurements are taken, one on the deepest inspiration and one on the deepest expiration. A comparison is then made to ascertain chest capacity. To perform the procedure, ask the patient to disrobe from the waist up. Place a tape measure around the chest at nipple level. Instruct the patient to inhale deeply while you measure, then ask the patient to exhale completely while you take the second measurement. Record the results as inspiration number and expiration number (see Chapter 18).

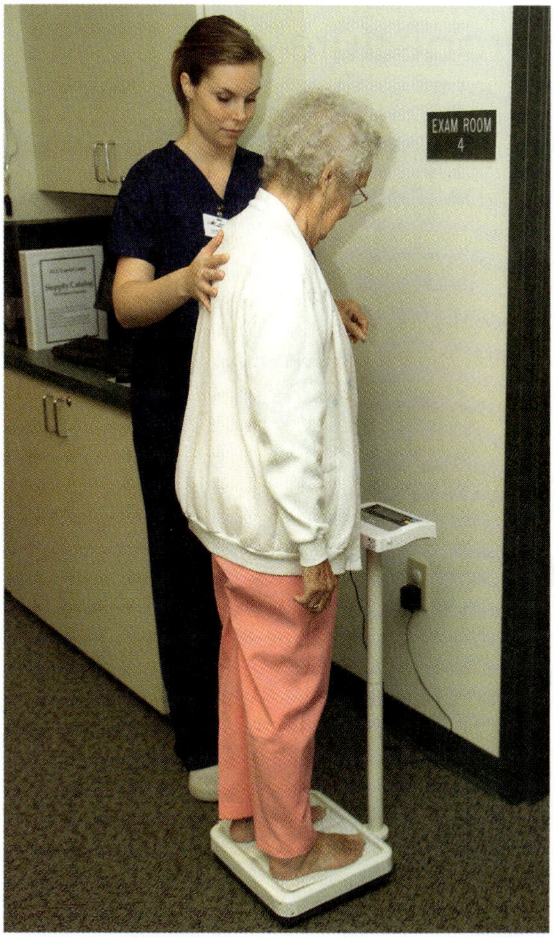

Figure 12-18 An electronic scale.

Critical Thinking

Discuss the methods the medical assistant may use to obtain patient cooperation when taking vital signs. Describe and demonstrate the appropriate charting procedure for normal vital sign results.

Procedure 12-1

Measuring an Oral Temperature Using an Electronic Thermometer

STANDARD PRECAUTIONS:

PURPOSE:

To obtain an oral temperature.

EQUIPMENT/SUPPLIES:

Electronic thermometer
Probe covers
Biohazard waste container

PROCEDURE STEPS:

1. Wash hands and follow Standard Precautions.
2. Assemble equipment.
3. Identify patient.
4. Position the patient in a comfortable position.
5. Determine if the patient has ingested hot or cold drinks or food or has been smoking within the previous half hour. RATIONALE: Ingesting hot or cold substances or smoking can result in an arbitrary increase or decrease in temperature results.
6. Explain the procedure. RATIONALE: To obtain patient cooperation and consent.
7. Select blue (oral) probe.
8. Cover with probe cover (Figure 12-19). RATIONALE: To prevent microorganism cross contamination.
9. Insert under the tongue to either side of the mouth (Figure 12-20). RATIONALE: Under the center of the tongue is the **frenulum,** which impedes placement in this area.
10. Instruct patient to close mouth without placing teeth on thermometer. RATIONALE: To prevent air leakage.
11. Leave in place until the beep is heard.
12. Remove thermometer after appropriate time has elapsed.
13. Read the results on the digital display window.
14. Discard probe cover in biohazard waste container.
15. Replace electronic thermometer in the base holder, if required for recharging.
16. Wash hands.
17. Record temperature in patient's chest or electronic medical record.

DOCUMENTATION

5/26/20XX 11:00 AM T 99.2°F, P 96, R 14. C. McInnis, RMA ———

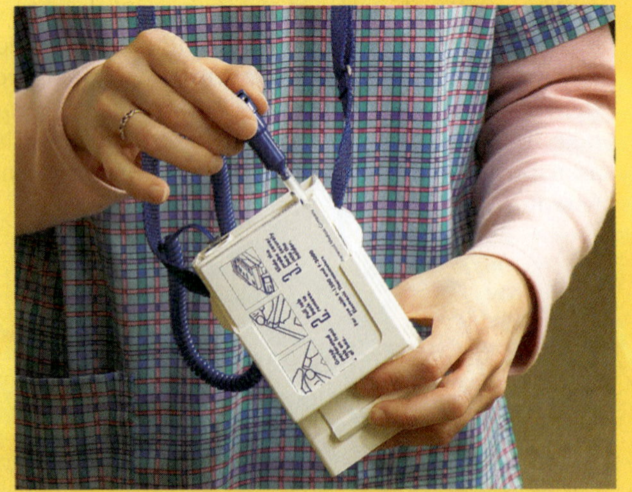

Figure 12-19 Slide the probe into the disposable cover, adjusting if necessary.

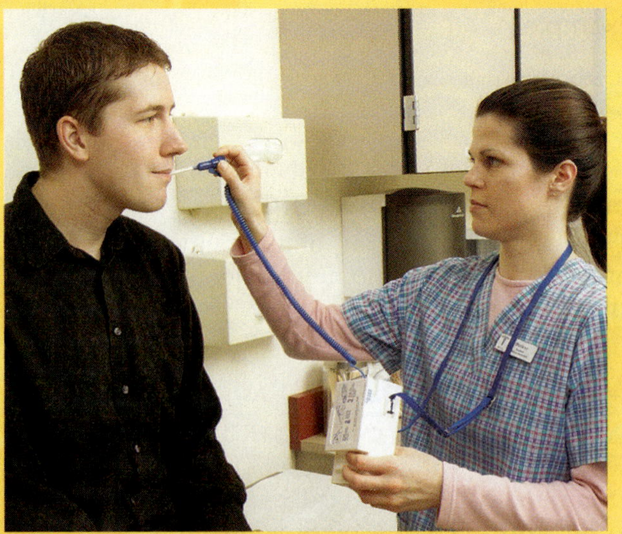

Figure 12-20 Insert the thermometer under tongue to either side of mouth.

Procedure 12-2

Measuring an Aural Temperature Using a Tympanic Thermometer

STANDARD PRECAUTIONS:

PURPOSE:
To obtain an aural temperature using a tympanic thermometer.

EQUIPMENT/SUPPLIES:
Tympanic thermometer (Figure 12-21)
Probe covers or ear speculum
Waste container

PROCEDURE STEPS:
1. Wash hands following Standard Precautions.
2. Assemble equipment.
3. Identify the patient.
4. Explain procedure. RATIONALE: This will help gain patient's cooperation and consent.
5. Place cover on thermometer (Figure 12-22).
6. Set thermometer to start.
7. Gently straighten ear canal up and back for adults and place probe into ear canal to seal the area and activate the system (Figure 12-23). RATIONALE: Air leaks will occur if the ear canal is not sealed.
8. Wait until the temperature is displayed on the screen.
9. Remove from the ear.
10. Discard cover into waste container by pressing the release button.
11. Wash hands.
12. Replace thermometer.

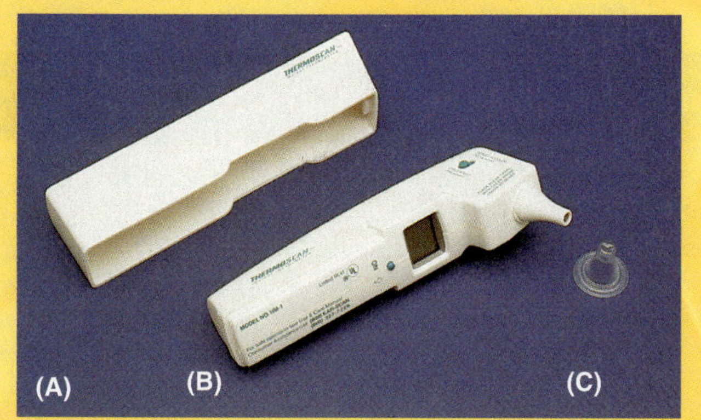

Figure 12-21 Tympanic thermometer: (A) Holder. (B) Tympanic thermometer. (C) Disposable speculum or cover.

13. Record temperature in patient's chart or electronic medical record, indicating tympanic measurement (Tym).

DOCUMENTATION
5/26/20XX 4:00 PM T 99.6° F (Tym), P 100, R 20. C. McInnis, RMA ———

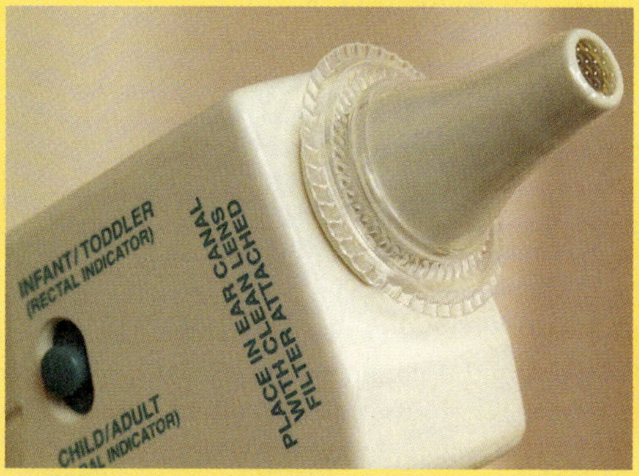

Figure 12-22 Attach the disposable speculum or cover to the tympanic thermometer to prevent spread of microorganisms between patients.

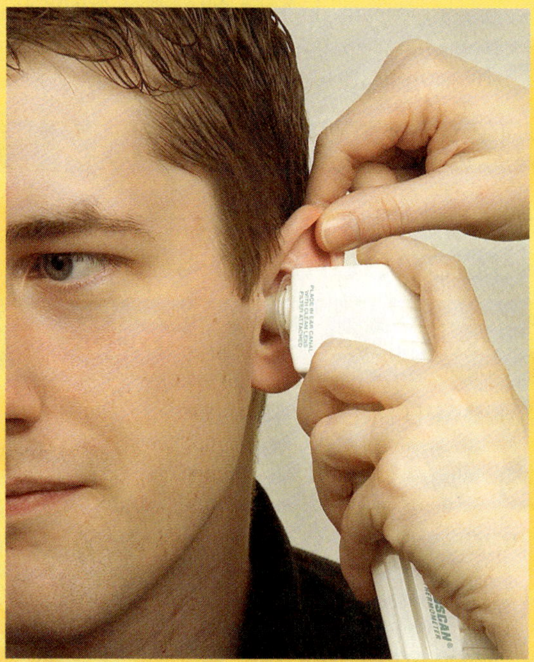

Figure 12-23 Pull up on the ear to straighten the auditory canal for an accurate reading.

Procedure 12-3

Measuring a Temperature Using a Temporal Artery (TA) Thermometer

STANDARD PRECAUTIONS:

PURPOSE:
To obtain a temporal artery temperature using a temporal artery (TA) thermometer.

EQUIPMENT/SUPPLIES:
Temporal artery thermometer
Alcohol wipes, probe cap or cover, or sheath

PROCEDURE STEPS:

1. Wash hands and follow Standard Precautions.
2. Assemble equipment. Clean probe with alcohol or attach a probe. RATIONALE: The lens of the thermometer must be clean to work properly.
3. Identify the patient. RATIONALE: To be certain you have the correct patient.
4. Explain the procedure. RATIONALE: Gain patient's cooperation and permission.
5. Remove perspiration from forehead, remove hat, push back hair from forehead. RATIONALE: False readings can occur from moisture (perspiration) on forehead cooling the skin or from a hat or hair covering forehead, raising the temperature.
6. Hold the probe in the center of patient's forehead flush against the skin. RATIONALE: Probe must be centered properly for accurate reading over area.
7. Press the scan button and hold while sliding the thermometer slowly across the forehead to the temple area hair line. There will be a tapping or clicking sound that will stop when the temperature has been reached.
8. Release the button and remove the thermometer from the forehead.
9. Read the display for temperature measurement.
10. Turn upside down and wipe probe with alcohol wipe. Let dry. Return to holder. RATIONALE: TA thermometer must be dry to work effectively.
11. Wash hands.
12. Record temperature in patient's chart or electronic medical record, indicating TA temperature.

PRECAUTIONS:
Check the manufacturer's manual. Some models cannot be used when oxygen is being used or when in close proximity to aerosols.

DOCUMENTATION:
8/31/20XX T. 99.8° F (TA) C. McInnis, RMA ———

Procedure 12-4

Measuring a Rectal Temperature Using a Digital Thermometer

STANDARD PRECAUTIONS:

PURPOSE:
To obtain a rectal temperature using a digital thermometer.

EQUIPMENT/SUPPLIES:
Digital thermometer with red probe (rectal)
Probe cover
Lubricating jelly on a 4 x 4 gauze or in packet
Gloves
Biohazard waste container

PROCEDURE STEPS:

1. Wash hands and don gloves following Standard Precautions.
2. Assemble equipment.
3. Identify patient.

continues

Procedure 12-4 (continued)

4. Explain procedure to patient. RATIONALE: Ensures understanding and gains patient cooperation and consent.
5. Remove patient's clothing from the waist down; drape as necessary. RATIONALE: Maintains patient's modesty, privacy, and warmth.
6. Position patient in Sims' position.
7. Place probe cover on red probe (rectal). RATIONALE: To prevent microorganism cross contamination. Red probe indicates rectal thermometer.
8. Lubricate with lubricating jelly. RATIONALE: Easier insertion of thermometer and safety for patient.
9. Spread buttocks and gently insert thermometer into the rectum past the sphincter (1½ inches) for adult.
10. Hold buttocks together while holding the thermometer. Do not let go of thermometer. RATIONALE: Holding buttocks together prevents air leaks and inaccurate recording. Holding onto thermometer ensures patient safety.
11. Hold in place until the beep is heard.
12. Read results on digital display window.
13. Remove from rectum.
14. Discard probe cover into biohazard waste container by pushing the release button.
15. Replace thermometer on holder base.
16. Remove gloves, discard in biohazard waste container, and wash hands.
17. Offer tissue to patient to wipe anus. Assist patient in dressing and position as necessary.
18. Record temperature in patient's chart or electronic medical record, indicating a rectal temperature (R).

DOCUMENTATION

5/28/20XX 8:00 AM T 99.6° F (R), P 104, R 20. C. McInnis, RMA ______________________

Procedure 12-5

Measuring an Axillary Temperature

STANDARD PRECAUTIONS:

PURPOSE:

To obtain an axillary temperature using a digital thermometer.

EQUIPMENT/SUPPLIES:

Digital thermometer
Sheath
Towelettes
Paper towels

PROCEDURE STEPS:

1. Wash hands following Standard Precautions.
2. Assemble equipment; place sheath on thermometer.
3. Identify patient.
4. Explain procedure. RATIONALE: This elicits patient cooperation and consent.
5. Ask patient to remove clothing to provide access to axilla.
6. Cover patient with gown as necessary to maintain patient modesty and warmth.
7. Wipe axillary area with dry towel or towelette to remove moisture. RATIONALE: Moisture in the axilla will cause inaccurate reading.
8. Place thermometer in axilla (Figure 12-24).
9. Ask patient to fold arm against chest or abdomen.
10. Leave in place for appropriate time according to manufacturer's instructions, usually 10 minutes.
11. Carefully remove.
12. Remove sheath and discard.
13. Read thermometer.

continues

Procedure 12-5 (continued)

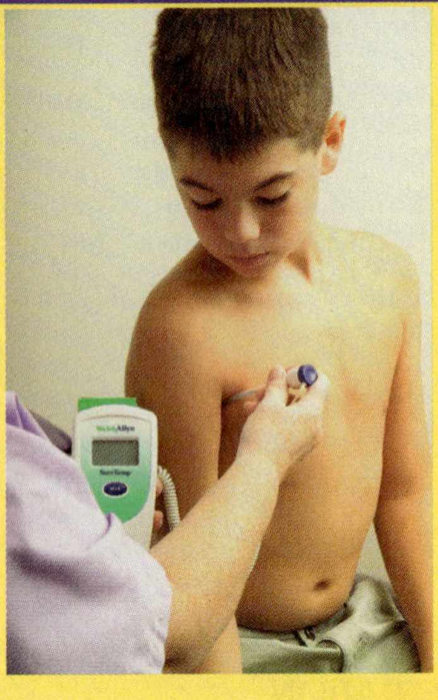

Figure 12-24 After placing thermometer in axilla, ask patient to fold arm against chest or abdomen.

14. Sanitize thermometer. Place on clean paper towel.
15. Wash hands.
16. Place clean thermometer in alcohol for 30 minutes.
17. Record temperature in patient's chart or electronic medical record, indicating axillary temperature (A).

DOCUMENTATION

4/30/20XX 2:00 pm T 97° F (A), P 64, R 12. J. Guerra, CMA (AAMA)

Procedure 12-6

Measuring an Oral Temperature Using a Disposable Oral Strip Thermometer

STANDARD PRECAUTIONS:

PURPOSE:
To obtain an oral temperature.

EQUIPMENT/SUPPLIES:
Oral strip thermometer (Figure 12-25)
Gloves
Biohazard waste container

PROCEDURE STEPS:
1. Wash hands following Standard Precautions.
2. Assemble equipment.
3. Identify patient.
4. Position the patient in a comfortable position.
5. Determine if the patient has ingested hot or cold drinks or food or has smoked within the previous half hour. RATIONALE: Ingesting hot or cold substance or smoking can result in an arbitrary increase or decrease in temperature results.
6. Explain the procedure. RATIONALE: To obtain patient cooperation and consent.
7. Apply gloves.
8. Insert disposable oral strip thermometer under the tongue to the side of the mouth. RATIONALE: Under the center of the tongue is the frenulum, the fold of mucus membrane that attaches the tongue to the floor of the mouth, which impedes placement in this area.
9. Instruct patient to close mouth tightly. RATIONALE: To prevent air leakage.
10. Leave in place for 60 seconds.
11. Remove thermometer after appropriate time has elapsed.

continues

Procedure 12-6 (continued)

12. Wait 10 seconds to read the dots.
13. Read temperature by locating the last dot that has changed color (Figure 12-26).
14. Discard strip in biohazard waste container.
15. Remove gloves and discard in biohazard waste container.
16. Wash hands.
17. Record temperature in patient's chart or electronic medical record.

DOCUMENTATION

4/16/20XX 3:15 PM T 101°F, P 100, R 22 (disposable oral thermometer reading) J. Guerra, CMA (AAMA) ———

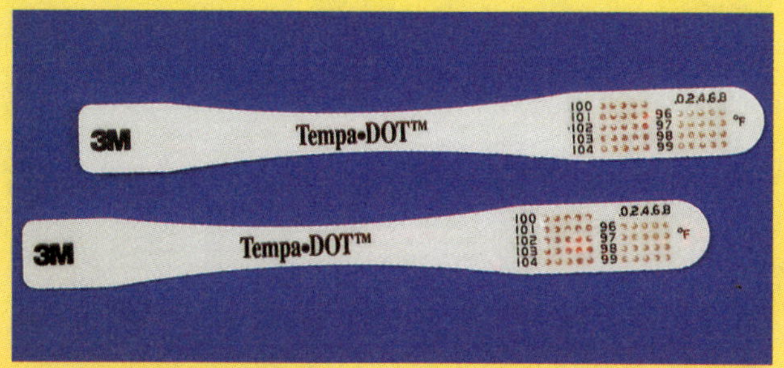

Figure 12-25 Disposable oral strip thermometer.

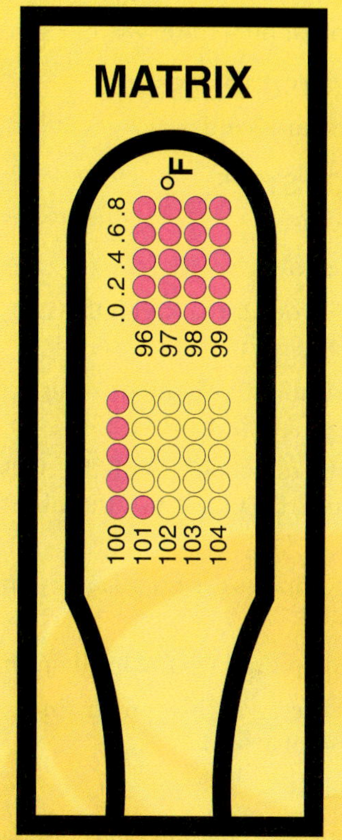

Figure 12-26 The reading on this disposable oral thermometer is 101°F.

Procedure 12-7

Measuring a Radial Pulse

STANDARD PRECAUTIONS:

PURPOSE:
To obtain a radial pulse rate.

EQUIPMENT/SUPPLIES:
Watch with second hand

PROCEDURE STEPS:
1. Wash hands.
2. Identify patient.
3. Explain procedure. RATIONALE: Ensures patient cooperation and consent.
4. Position patient with the wrist resting either on a table or on lap (Figure 12-27).
5. Locate the radial pulse with the pads of your first three fingers. Do not use thumb; it has its own pulse.
6. Gently compress the radial artery enough to feel the pulse.
7. Count the pulsations for 1 full minute.
8. Note any irregularities in rhythm, volume, and condition of artery.
9. Wash hands.
10. Record pulse in patient chart or electronic medical record after the temperature, noting any irregularities.

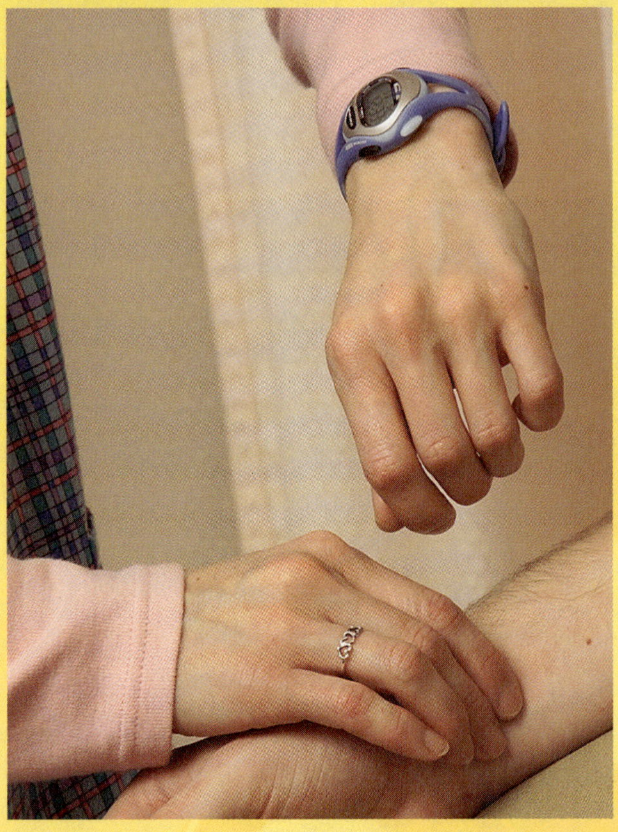

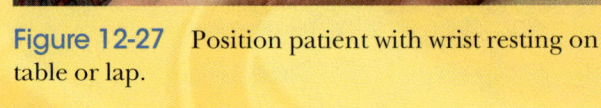

Figure 12-27 Position patient with wrist resting on table or lap.

DOCUMENTATION
2/10/20XX 3:00 pm T 98.2 °F P 80, regular and strong. D. Kolter, RMA ———

Procedure 12-8

Taking an Apical Pulse

STANDARD PRECAUTIONS:

PURPOSE:
To obtain an apical pulse rate.

EQUIPMENT/SUPPLIES:
Stethoscope
Watch with second hand
Alcohol wipes

PROCEDURE STEPS:
1. Wash hands.
2. Assemble equipment.
3. Wipe earpiece with alcohol wipes.
4. Identify patient.
5. Explain procedure. RATIONALE: Ensures patient cooperation and consent.
6. Assist patient in disrobing, removing clothing from the waist up.
7. Provide a gown or drape for patient modesty and warmth.
8. Position the patient in a supine position. RATIONALE: Easier access to apex of heart.
9. Locate the fifth intercostal space, midclavicular, left of sternum (Figure 12-28). RATIONALE: Location of apex of heart.
10. Place stethoscope on the site and listen for the lub-dub sound of the heart.
11. Count the pulse for 1 minute; each lub-dub equals one pulse.
12. Assist the patient to sit up and dress.
13. Wash hands.
14. Wipe earpieces, diaphragm, and tubing of stethoscope.
15. Record pulse in patient chart or electronic medical record with the designation of apical pulse (AP) to denote method of obtaining the pulse and note any arrythmias.

NOTE: Apical pulse and radial pulse are frequently taken simultaneously, with the radial pulse taken by another individual (Figure 12-29). Both pulse rates should be identical. A discrepancy may indicate a cardiac problem.

DOCUMENTATION
7/8/20XX 12 PM T 98.6°F, P (AP) 96 reg. (radial) 100 slightly irregular. Dr. King notified. D. Kolter, RMA ———

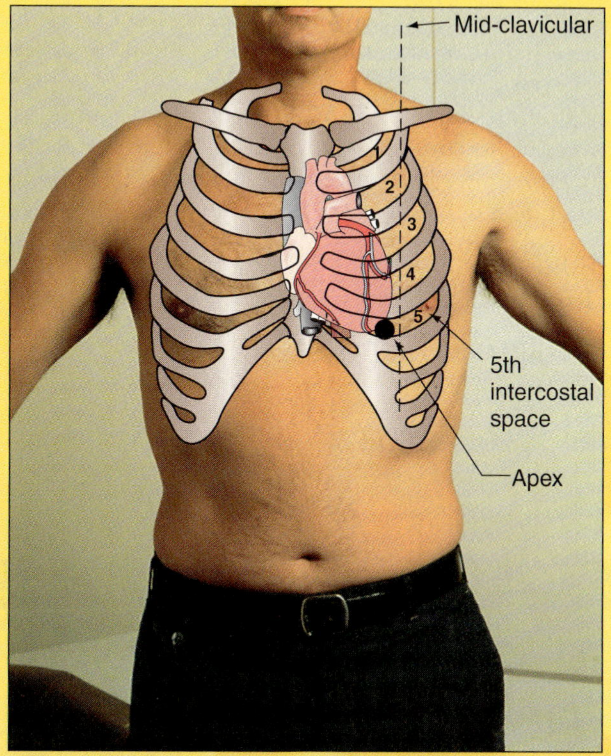

Figure 12-28 Locate the apical pulse by counting intercostal spaces. Locate the fifth intercostal space.

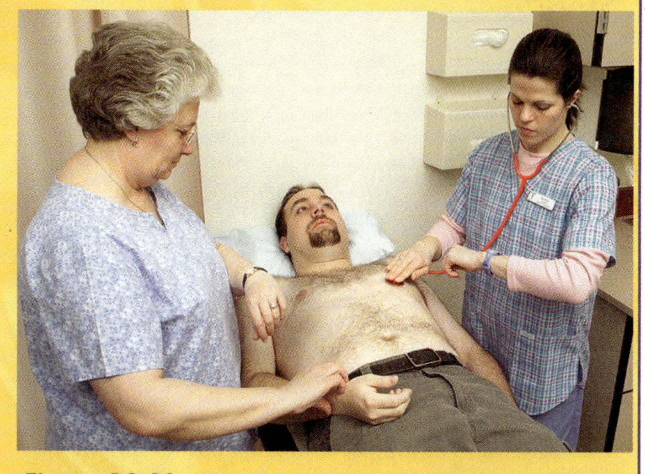

Figure 12-29 Sometimes apical and radial pulses are taken simultaneously.

Procedure 12-9

Measuring the Respiration Rate

STANDARD PRECAUTIONS:

NOTE: The respiration rate is normally taken immediately before or after the pulse rate. It should be taken without patient knowledge because respiration can voluntarily be altered. While counting respirations, it is best to continue grasping the wrist as if still taking the pulse. This procedure will assist in preventing alteration of breathing by the patient.

PURPOSE:

To obtain an accurate respiratory rate.

EQUIPMENT/SUPPLIES:

Watch with second hand

PROCEDURE STEPS:

1. Wash hands.
2. Identify the patient.
3. Position patient in a comfortable position.
4. Watch the rise and fall of the chest wall for 1 minute, or while holding the patient's arm, place it across the chest and feel for the rise and fall of chest wall. Alternatively, place a hand on the patient's shoulder and feel and watch for the rise and fall of the chest wall.
5. Note depth, rhythm, and breath sounds while counting.
6. Wash hands.
7. Record respiration rate in patient's chart or electronic medical record, noting any irregularities and sounds.

DOCUMENTATION

8/7/20XX 2:00 PM T 98.6°F, P 84. Rate and rhythm regular. J. Guerra, CMA (AAMA) ————————

Procedure 12-10

Measuring Blood Pressure

STANDARD PRECAUTIONS:

PURPOSE:

To measure blood pressure.

EQUIPMENT/SUPPLIES:

Stethoscope
Sphygmomanometer
Alcohol wipes

PROCEDURE STEPS:

1. Wash hands.
2. Assemble equipment, making sure that cuff size is correct. RATIONALE: Inappropriate cuff size will result in inaccurate measurement.
3. Clean earpieces of stethoscope with alcohol wipe.
4. Identify patient.
5. Explain procedure. RATIONALE: May be the first instance where blood pressure is measured; to allay anxiety and ensure cooperation and consent.
6. Position patient comfortably; feet flat on the floor, arm resting at heart level on the lap or a table. RATIONALE: Legs crossed may arbitrarily increase blood pressure; arm above heart level may result in inaccurate reading.
7. Bare the right upper arm. If clothing is restricting, have patient remove it. RATIONALE: Tight clothing on the arm can produce inaccurate results. Right arm is used for consistency, but if one arm measures a higher reading, then that arm is used consistently to measure the blood pressure.

continues

Procedure 12-10 (continued)

8. Palpate brachial artery.
9. Securely center the bladder of the cuff over the brachial artery above the bend of the elbow. RATIONALE: Cuff should be high enough so stethoscope does not touch it. Extraneous sounds may be heard. Be certain the gauge is on zero.
10. Palpate the radial pulse and smoothly inflate cuff until the pulse is no longer felt; note the number.
11. Quickly deflate the cuff and allow arm to rest for about one minute. Calculate peak inflation level. RATIONALE: This ensures that an auscultatory gap is not missed.
12. Make sure cuff is completely deflated.
13. Position stethoscope over the brachial artery and hold in position with the fingers only.
14. Inflate cuff smoothly and quickly to the peak inflation level plus 30 mm Hg (Figure 12-30).
15. Deflate the cuff at a rate of 2 to 4 mm Hg per heartbeat. RATIONALE: No matter how experienced you become, accurate blood pressure readings cannot be obtained if the cuff deflation is greater than 2 to 4 mm Hg per heartbeat.
16. Listen for Korotkoff Phase I; note when it appears.
17. Continue deflation, noting the Korotkoff phases.
18. Note when all sounds disappear, Korotkoff Phase V.
19. Continue deflating the cuff at the same rate for at least another 10 mm Hg after sounds have disappeared. RATIONALE: To hear an auscultatory gap should one be present.
20. Deflate the cuff quickly.
21. Remove the cuff.
22. Clean earpieces and diaphragm of stethoscope with alcohol wipes.
23. Wash hands.
24. Record blood pressure in patient's chart or electronic medical record.

NOTE: On a patient's initial visit and in patients with hypertension, the provider may want the blood pressure taken in both arms. There is normally a slight variation in pressure between the arms. If it is necessary to repeat the procedure, wait approximately 5 minutes before doing so.

DOCUMENTATION

2/16/20XX 3:00 PM BP 146/90 in right arm. BP 150/92 in left arm. D. Swingle, CMA (AAMA) ———

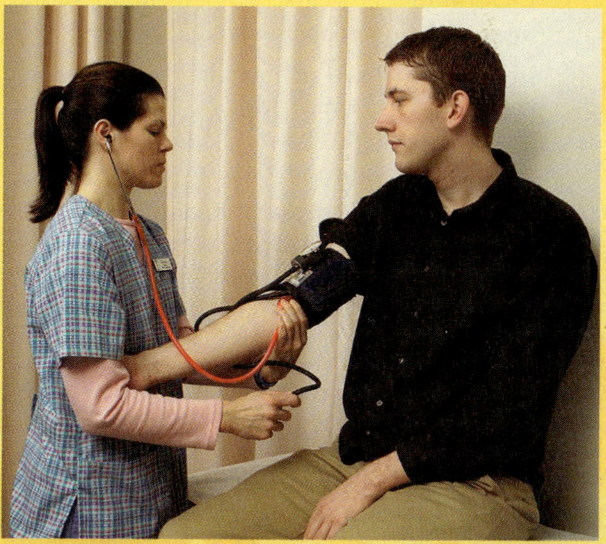

Figure 12-30 Inflate cuff smoothly and quickly.

Procedure 12-11

Measuring Height

STANDARD PRECAUTIONS:

PURPOSE:
To obtain the height of a patient.

EQUIPMENT/SUPPLIES:
Scale with measuring bar
Paper towel

PROCEDURE STEPS:
1. Wash hands.
2. Identify patient.
3. Explain the procedure to patient to ensure understanding, cooperation, and consent.
4. Instruct patient to remove shoes and stand on paper towel on scale with back against scale, looking straight ahead. RATIONALE: Back against scale aids patient safety.
5. Assist patient onto scale. RATIONALE: Scale platform is movable, and patient may become unsteady and lose balance and fall.
6. Lower measuring bar until firmly resting on top of head (Figure 12-31).
7. Assist patient's steping off the scale. Allow patient to sit and help with shoes if necessary.
8. Read line where measurement falls.
9. Lower measuring bar to its original position.
10. Wash hands.
11. Record height in patient's chart or electronic medical record.

DOCUMENTATION
3/4/20XX 2:00 PM Ht. 59 60. B. Abbott, RMA ———————

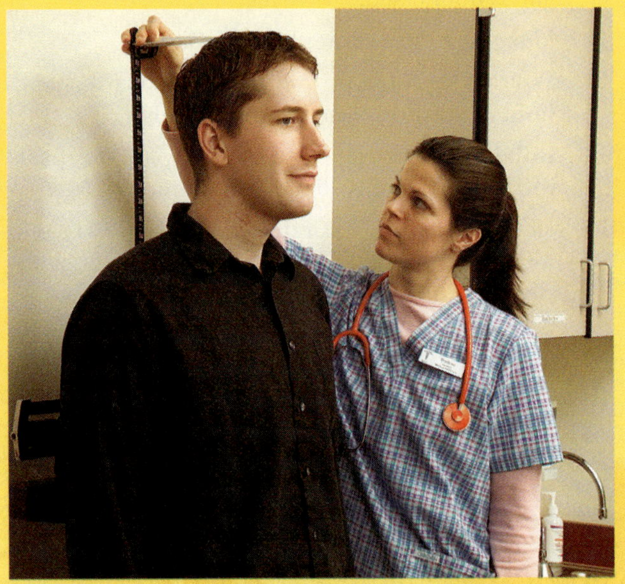

Figure 12-31 To measure height, have the patient stand with back against scale and keep head level.

Procedure 12-12

Measuring Adult Weight

STANDARD PRECAUTIONS:

PURPOSE:
To obtain the weight of the patient.

EQUIPMENT/SUPPLIES:
Balance beam or digital scale
Paper towels

PROCEDURE STEPS:

1. Wash hands.
2. Identify patient.
3. Explain the procedure to patient to ensure understanding and cooperation.
4. Place a paper towel on scale. RATIONALE: Paper towel protects patient's feet from microorganisms.
5. Instruct the patient to place heavy objects on the area provided, including heavy objects that may be in pockets.
6. Instruct the patient to remove shoes, jacket, and heavy sweater and step on the scale. Assist patient to the center of the scale. RATIONALE:The scale platform is movable, and the patient may become unsteady, lose balance, and fall. The platform on the digital scale is stationary, but assist the patient onto the scale platform and read the digital reading. If using a balance beam scale, continue with Steps 7 through14.
7. Move the lower weight bar (measured in 50-pound increments) to the estimated number (the patient may be asked for approximate weight).
8. Slowly slide the upper bar until the balance beam point is centered (Figure 12-32).
9. Read the weight by adding the upper bar measurement to the lower bar measurement (see Figure 12-17).
10. Assist the patient in stepping off the scale.
11. Provide a chair for the patient to sit and put on shoes. Return objects to the patient.
12. Return the weights to zero.
13. Wash hands.
14. EHR Record weight in patient's chart or electronic medical record.

DOCUMENTATION

5/2/20XX 3:00 P.M. Wt. 142 lbs. B. Abbott, RMA ————

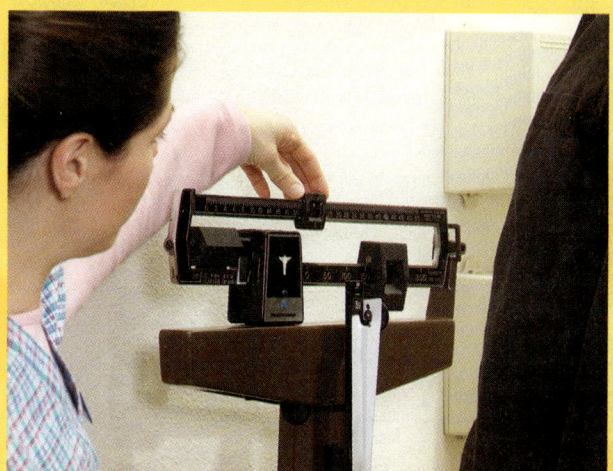

Figure 12-32 When weighing the patient, slide the upper bar until the balance beam point is centered.

Case Study 12-1

Refer to the scenario at the beginning of the chapter.

CASE STUDY REVIEW

1. There are three different kinds of sphygmomanometers. Give advantages and disadvantages of each.
2. When you weigh Mrs. Williams, you notice from her record that she has lost 10 pounds in 6 months. What questions will you ask her about her weight loss?
3. Height and weight measurements are important for many reasons. What do you consider the most important of the many reasons? What do you consider the least important reason? Why?

Case Study 12-2

Herb Fowler, a regular patient of Dr. Lewis at the medical facility of Drs. Lewis and King, is an African-American in his 50s. He has smoked for many years and only recently has thought about quitting smoking because of a chronic cough. Herb is significantly overweight but is having a hard time making the decision to give up smoking *and* change his diet. Although his blood pressure has been stable for the last few years, Audrey Jones, CMA (AAMA), is concerned when she takes Herb's vital signs during his most recent checkup. His weight is slightly up, and his blood pressure has jumped from 140/90 to 156/100.

CASE STUDY REVIEW

1. Is a blood pressure reading of 156/100 a cause for concern? Should Audrey take a second reading?
2. In addition to alerting the provider to the change in Mr. Fowler's blood pressure and weight, Audrey feels she may be able to provide advice to the patient (with provider permission). How can Audrey use her communication and medical assisting knowledge to counsel Herb Fowler on lifestyle changes?
3. To follow up, Audrey reviews her knowledge of hypertension and discusses the four types with the provider. What are the four kinds of hypertension and what are their characteristics?

SUMMARY

Throughout life, a patient will undergo various measurements to ascertain growth, development, and general health and well-being. The normal range for each of these measurements will vary according to the stage of life of the patient at the time of examination. The medical assistant must be aware of what to expect when measuring a patient in each life stage. Awareness of normal expectations for each stage of life will help the medical assistant to perform the procedures in a more effective and efficient manner and aid in observing any abnormal signs and measurements.

Together with differences seen with age, the medical assistant will see differences in patients because each patient has unique medical problems.

The medical assistant has a great responsibility when performing patient measurements and must ensure accuracy, patient safety, comfort, and confidentiality while obtaining accurate results.

STUDY FOR SUCCESS

- Review the Key Terms
- Practice the Procedures
- Consider the Case Studies and discuss your conclusions
- Answer the Review Questions
  - Multiple Choice
  - Critical Thinking
- Navigate the Internet by completing the Web Activities
- Practice the StudyWARE activities on your student CD
- Apply your knowledge in the Student Workbook activities
- Complete the Web Tutor section
- View and discuss the DVD situations

REVIEW QUESTIONS

Multiple Choice

1. This type of thermometer measures the temperature of the skin surface over the temporal artery:
   a. aural
   b. TA
   c. tympanic
   d. axillary
2. The artery commonly used for taking a patient's pulse is:
   a. carotid c. radial
   b. brachial d. popliteal
3. A blood pressure cuff that is too small for the patient's arm will:
   a. have no effect on the results
   b. give an arbitrarily low result
   c. give an arbitrarily high result
   d. have an effect on certain patients only
4. The term used to indicate a pulse rate significantly above the average is:
   a. bradycardia c. arrhythmia
   b. tachycardia d. sinus rhythm

Critical Thinking

1. Discuss the responsibilities of the medical assistant when measuring vital signs.
2. Describe the care and use for each of the various types of thermometers.
3. Discuss the reasons that a professional must be aware that mercury thermometers and other mercury-containing equipment are being phased out of use.
4. Demonstrate the procedure for converting temperatures from Fahrenheit to Celsius and vice versa and calculate the following conversions:
   a. 98.6°F = ________________ °C
   b. 39.1°C = ________________ °F
5. Discuss the rationale for not using the thumb for taking the pulse rate of a patient.
6. Discuss the reasons for taking the respiratory rate of a patient without the patient's knowledge.
7. Discuss the importance of using the appropriate blood pressure cuff size when measuring a patient's blood pressure.
8. Describe the following:
   a. hypertension c. apnea
   b. tachycardia d. remittent fever

WEB ACTIVITIES

1. Using a search engine, access information on the Internet from the American Heart Association regarding essential hypertension and answer the following:
   a. What population of people in the United States is at greatest risk for essential hypertension?

b. List four patient education tips for reducing blood pressure without the aid of medication.
c. Check the list of normal blood pressure readings in this chapter and compare it with what the American Heart Association says are normal blood pressure measurements at various ages.

2. Access information on the Internet from the National Research Council and list its recommendations for weight of the following women:

Height	Age	Weight in Pounds
5′ 2″	19–34 years	?
5′ 4″	19–34 years	?
5′ 6″	19–34 years	?

REFERENCES/BIBLIOGRAPHY

Environmental Protection Agency. (May 18, 2004, Federal Register, page 40517 [40CFR 273.81(a)]). *Mercury and the environment.* Retrieved from http://www.epa.gov.

Michigan State University. *Mercury containment initiative.* Retrieved March 22, 2004, from http://www.aware.msu.edu.

National Library of Medicine, National Institutes of Health. *Mercury facts.* Retrieved April 28, 2005, from http://cerhr.niehs.nih.gov/genpub/topics/mercury.html.

Taber's cyclopedic medical dictionary (22nd ed.). (2006). Philadelphia: F.A. Davis.

THE DVD HOOK-UP

This chapter discusses the proper techniques for obtaining the patient's vital signs and steps for measuring and weighing the patient.

This program illustrated many techniques for obtaining various vital signs. In the taking a radial pulse scene, the medical assistant noticed a problem with the patient's rhythm and decided to take an apical pulse as well. The chapter states that you should place the patient in a supine position and locate the apex of the heart when taking an apical pulse. The DVD program illustrated the medical assistant taking an apical pulse with the patient sitting in an upright position. It also had a more complicated technique for finding the apex of the heart.

1. How do you think you should manage a patient with an arrhythmia? How can you keep the patient from becoming concerned?
2. Which method do you think would work better for measuring an apical pulse: the method listed in the book or in the DVD program? Why?

DVD Journal Summary

Write a paragraph that summarizes what you learned from watching today's DVD program. At the end of the blood pressure scene, the medical assistant told the patient that her blood pressure was 158/100, which is quite elevated. Do you think it was wise of the medical assistant to tell the patient her reading? Do you think it is acceptable to tell patients their blood pressure when it is normal? Why or why not?

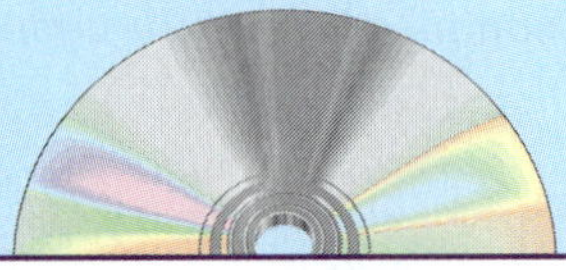

DVD Series: Skills Based Series
Program Number: 5
Chapter/Scene Reference
• *Watch entire program*

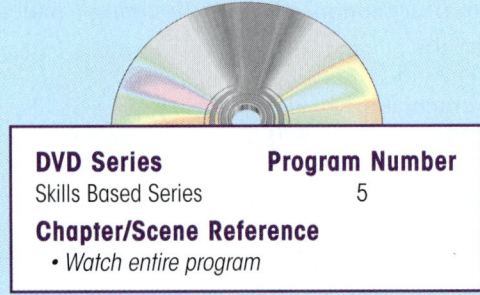

Chapter 13

The Physical Examination

KEY TERMS

Ataxia
Bruits
Catheterization
Cyanosis
Fenestrated Drape
Jaundice
Labyrinthitis
Pallor
Pyorrhea
Scleroderma
Symmetry
Tinnitus
Vertigo
Vitiligo

OUTLINE

- Methods of Examination
  - Observation or Inspection
  - Palpation
  - Percussion
  - Auscultation
  - Mensuration
  - Manipulation
- Positioning and Draping
  - Examination Positions
- Equipment and Supplies for the Physical Examination
- Basic Components of a Physical Examination
  - Patient Appearance
  - Gait
  - Stature
  - Posture
  - Body Movements
  - Speech
  - Breath Odors
  - Nutrition
  - Skin and Appendages
- The Physical Examination Sequence
  - Head
  - Eyes
  - Ears
  - Nose
  - Mouth and Throat
  - Neck
  - Chest
  - Breast
  - Abdomen
  - Genitals
  - Rectum
  - Reflexes
- After the Examination

OBJECTIVES

The student should strive to meet the following performance objectives and demonstrate an understanding of the facts and principles presented in this chapter through written and oral communication.

1. Define the key terms as presented in the glossary.
2. Describe the six methods used in physical examinations.
3. Name and describe seven positions used for physical examinations.
4. Discuss the purpose of draping and demonstrate appropriate draping for each position.
5. Identify at least 10 instruments and supplies used for examination of various parts of the body.
6. Identify eight basic components of a physical examination.
7. Describe the sequence followed during a physical examination.
8. Recall method of examination, instrument used, and position for examination of at least eight body parts.

Scenario

At the multiprovider Inner City Health Care facility, five providers are employed on a rotating basis, with two or three working at any one time. Clinical medical assistants Wanda Slawson, CMA (AAMA), and Bruce Goldman, CMA (AAMA), have developed a clear understanding of what each provider prefers in both room and patient preparation. Wanda and Bruce also coordinate with each other and with office managers Jane O'Hara and Walter Seals, both CMAs, to ensure patient comfort. Depending on the patient and the type of examination, Wanda will often assist with patient preparation when the patient is female and Walter will assist when the patient is male.

INTRODUCTION

Physical examinations are performed to obtain a picture of the health and well-being of the patient. An initial examination will provide a baseline reference for future examinations. The examination follows a standard routine, usually starting at the head and following through the entire body, including all major organs and body systems. Although the sequence of events for the physical examination is relatively standard, variations occur according to provider preference, type of practice, and patient's chief complaint. Diagnostic procedures such as laboratory tests and X-rays may be ordered or performed in the facility or sent to an outside laboratory. At the conclusion of the physical examination, the provider will have an impression of the patient's general health, a diagnosis if possible, and treatment plans. The provider uses information from three major sources to aid in making a diagnosis: the health history, the physical examination, and laboratory tests and diagnostic procedures.

The role of the medical assistant throughout the physical examination greatly depends on the provider. Some providers delegate many duties to the medical assistant, whereas others require little assistance. Commonly performed clinical medical assisting duties related to physical examinations can be divided into two categories: patient preparation and room preparation. Patient preparation includes patient explanation and preparation, positioning, draping, vital signs, specimen collection such as urine and blood, and electrocardiogram (ECG). Room preparation includes assembling the appropriate instruments and equipment for the provider and ensuring patient privacy and comfort.

Additional medical assisting duties include supporting the patient, handing the provider instruments and equipment as required, and taking notes to be entered into the electronic medical record (EMR). Throughout and after the examination, the medical assistant adheres to the principles of medical asepsis and Standard Precautions as required by Occupational Safety and Health Administration (OSHA). The effective medical assistant establishes an efficient but flexible routine providing for the needs of both the patient and the provider.

METHODS OF EXAMINATION

There are six methods used by the provider to examine the body. They include observation or inspection, palpation, percussion, auscultation,

Spotlight on Certification

RMA Content Outline

- Vital signs and measurements
- Medical history
- Patient positions
- Methods of examination
- Specialty examinations

CMA (AAMA) Content Outline

- Patient instruction
- Treatment area
- Equipment preparation and operation
- Principles of operation
- Patient preparation and assisting the provider

CMAS Content Outline

- Examination preparation

mensuration, and manipulation. The provider uses all in total or in part, depending on the type of examination being performed.

Observation or Inspection

Observation or inspection is the process of observing the patient. The general health, posture, body movements, skin, mannerisms, and care in grooming are noted. Closer observation focuses on body **symmetry** (correspondence in shape and size of body parts located on opposite sides of the body) and contour. Deformities and skin rashes are observed. Skin color is noted (Figure 13-1).

Palpation

Palpation is an examination of the body using touch and may be used to help verify observations. A body part or organ is felt for size and condition. Abdominal masses may be felt through the abdominal wall. Skin texture, moisture, and temperature can be felt. The contour of limbs and rigidity and position of bones and joints may be felt. Palpation may be performed with the use of fingertips, one or both hands, or the palm of the hand (Figure 13-2).

Percussion

Percussion is the process of eliciting sounds from the body by tapping with either a percussion hammer or fingers. The vibrations and sounds from underlying organs and cavities can be felt and heard. Using this method can determine the presence of air or solid material in the organ or cavity being checked. Healthy structures that are dense, such as the liver, produce a dull sound. Hollow structures such as the lungs should produce a more hollow sound. There are two methods used to perform percussion. The direct method is performed by tapping directly on the surface of the skin. The indirect method is performed by placing a finger or hand on the surface of the skin and tapping the hand (Figure 13-3).

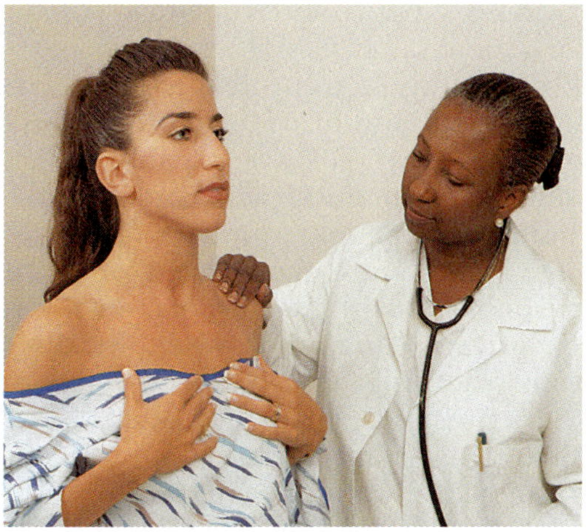

Figure 13-1 The provider uses observation to inspect the body for signs of disease.

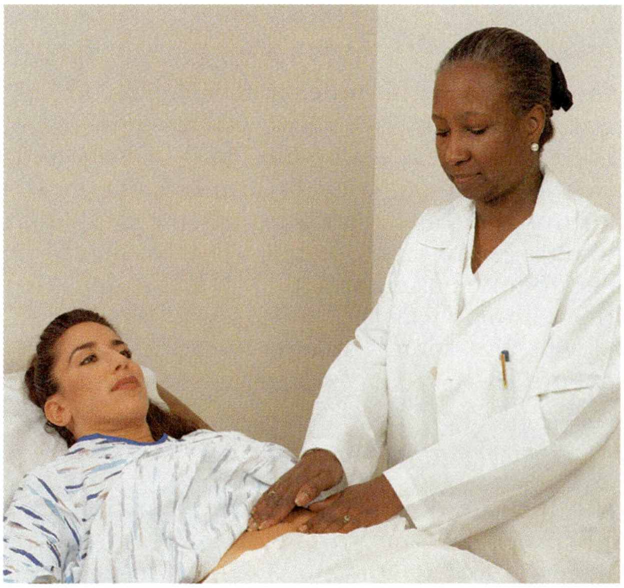

Figure 13-2 For palpation, the provider uses the hands and fingers to feel various body parts.

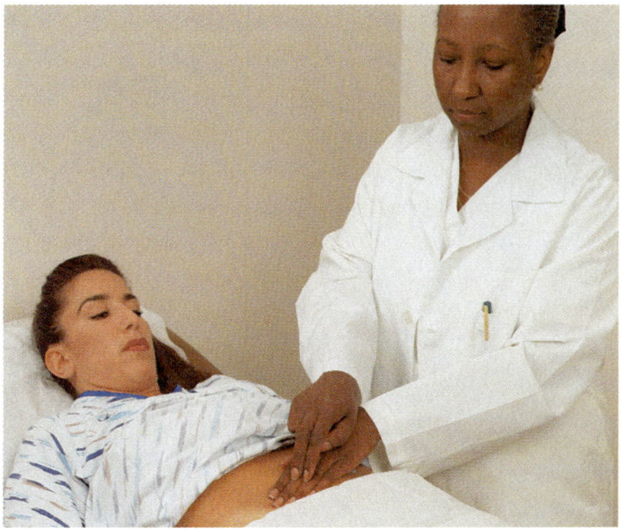

Figure 13-3 Percussion involves tapping on body parts and listening to sounds coming from body organs.

Auscultation

Auscultation is the process of listening directly to body sounds, normally with a stethoscope. The provider listens for lung and heart sounds such as murmurs, rales, or **bruits,** which generally are abnormal sounds heard on auscultation of an organ or vessel such as a vein or an artery. The abdomen is examined for bowel sounds that include the clicks and gurgles of normal bowel activity, the sounds that occur with peristalsis (Figure 13-4).

Mensuration

The mensuration method of examination uses the process of measuring. The measurements of height and weight, the length of a limb, and the amount of flexion and extension of an extremity are all forms of mensuration (Figure 13-5). Measurements of chest and infant head circumference are also forms of mensuration. In most instances, a tape measure is used to perform mensuration of an infant's head or circumference of a body part.

Manipulation

Manipulation checks the amount of flexion and extension of a joint by applying forceful passive movement on the joint. Range of motion of some joints may be checked using this method.

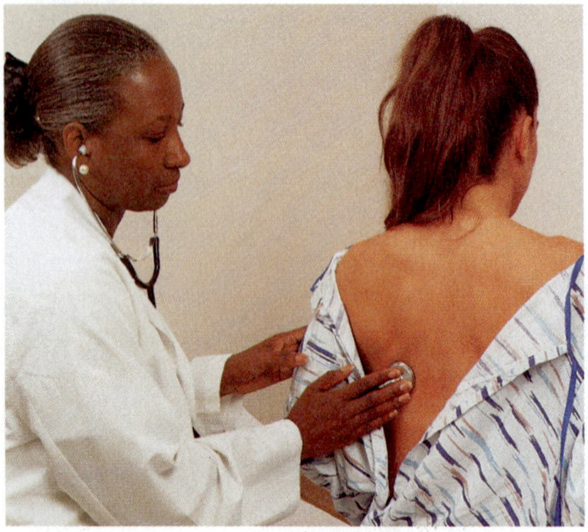

Figure 13-4 The provider is using a stethoscope to listen to heart and lung sounds. This is known as auscultation.

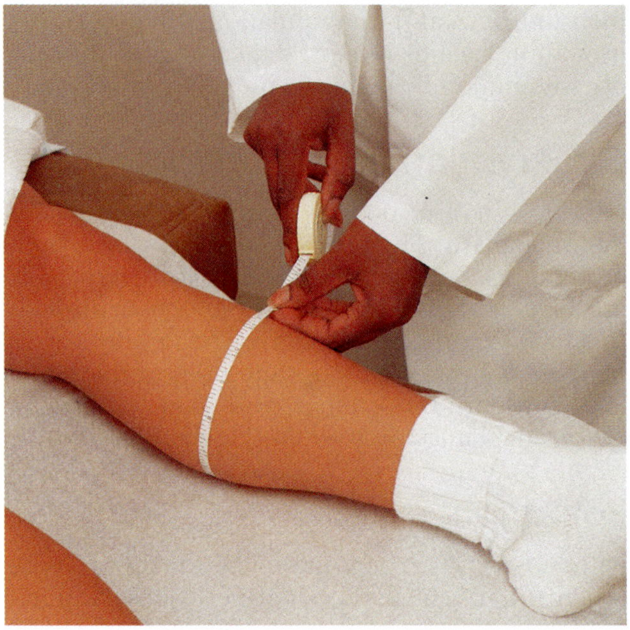

Figure 13-5 A tape measure may be used to measure the circumference of the calf of the patient's leg or other body part. This method of physical examination is known as mensuration.

POSITIONING AND DRAPING

Physical examinations require patients to be placed in various positions. Each position is designed to make examination of a particular area of the body easier and more efficient. The medical assistant may assist patients in undressing and will provide the appropriate drape and gown. The medical assistant also instructs patients about the appropriate position required for the examination and may assist patients into position by providing support and guidance. Always provide for patient safety.

Proper draping to protect modesty, prevent embarrassment, and provide comfort from chills is essential. If patients are capable of helping themselves, the medical assistant should leave the room while patients undress and put on a gown. If patients are disoriented or extremely ill, the medical assistant must stay in the room; patient privacy can be provided by discreetly removing clothing and covering patients as quickly as possible. When the patient is a child, the medical assistant should note the comfort level of the child while the child undresses. Children develop modesty at an early age and may be embarrassed by sitting on the examination table wearing only underwear. Respect a child's right to privacy by offering a gown or drape. Older adults will need assistance with undressing and draping. Care must be taken to provide as much modesty and privacy as possible as you assist patients of all ages.

Never turn your back on seriously ill or disoriented patients or young children. Ensure patient safety at all times.

Examination Positions

A number of positions may be required of patients during the physical examination. The position used depends on the type of examination. Seven positions can be used.

1. Supine (horizontal recumbent)
2. Dorsal recumbent
3. Lithotomy
4. Fowler's
5. Knee-chest
6. Prone
7. Sims'

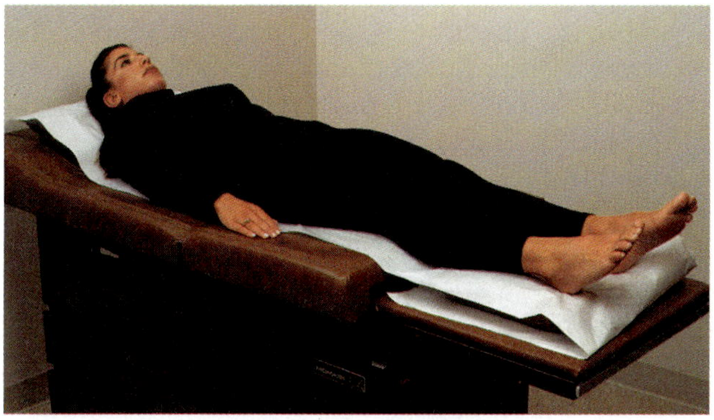

Figure 13-6 Supine or horizontal recumbent position.

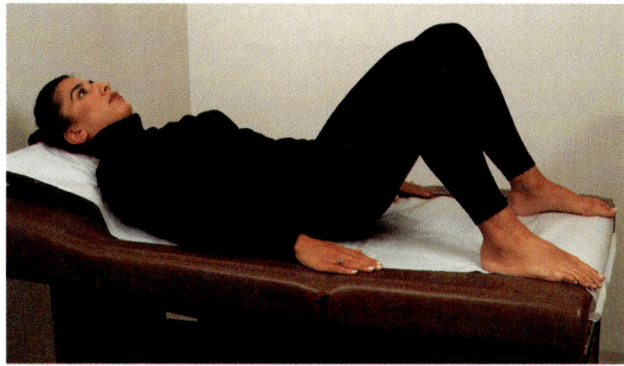

Figure 13-7 Dorsal recumbent position.

Supine (Horizontal Recumbent). The supine position is assumed when lying flat facing up (Figure 13-6). It is used for examination of the anterior surface of the body from head to toe. When the provider performs a physical examination on a female patient that includes a breast examination, the patient should be provided with a gown and instructed to wear it with the opening in the front. A drape is then placed over the lap or from the waist down.

Dorsal Recumbent. Patients lie on their back (dorsal) face up, legs separated, knees flexed with feet flat on the table (Figure 13-7). This is the most comfortable position for patients with back and abdominal problems. Examinations performed in this position include rectal, genital, head, neck, and chest, as well as abdominal palpation. It can also be used for urinary **catheterization.** Preteen and early teen girls requiring a pelvic examination may be placed in this position and will require careful instructions and procedure explanations. The patient is covered with a drape that is diamond shaped. One edge of the diamond can be lifted to examine the genitalia without exposing the rest of the body.

Lithotomy. Patients are assisted to lie on their back similar to the dorsal recumbent position except the buttocks should be as close to the bottom edge of the table as possible, and feet are placed in stirrups attached to the foot of the table (Figure 13-8). The lithotomy position is used for genital and pelvic examinations; it can also be used for urinary catheterization. At the conclusion of the examination, the patient should slide toward the head of the table before getting up from this position. Patients with special needs, such as older adults and those physically challenged as with severe arthritis, may not be able to assume this position. If this is the case, assist patient into Sims' position or modified dorsal position and

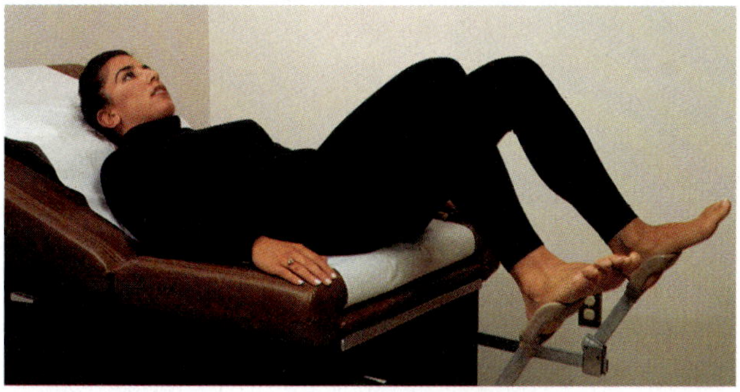

Figure 13-8 Lithotomy position.

the sigmoidoscopy, proctoscopy, or pelvic exam can be done in this position for these patients.

A modification of the dorsal recumbent position is often used for female external genitalia examinations, especially female urologic examinations, some gynecologic examinations, and examinations during pregnancy. This position consists of the patient lying on the examination table on her back, with her knees bent. The feet are together with the heels pulled up toward the buttocks. During the examination, the knees are relaxed apart. The provider may stand to the side of the patient during the examination. This position has many advantages over the lithotomy position if a full pelvic examination is not required.

Fowler's. Patients sit in a position with the back of the examination table raised to either 45 degrees (semi-Fowler's; Figure 13-9) or 90 degrees (high-fowler's; Figure 13-10). Legs rest flat on the table.

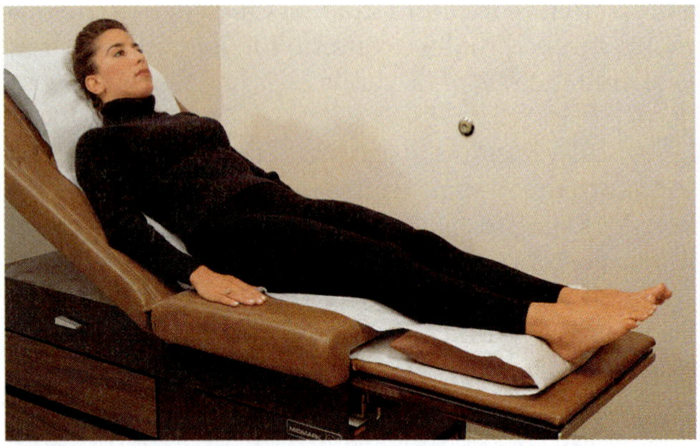

Figure 13-9 Semi-Fowler's position (45-degree angle).

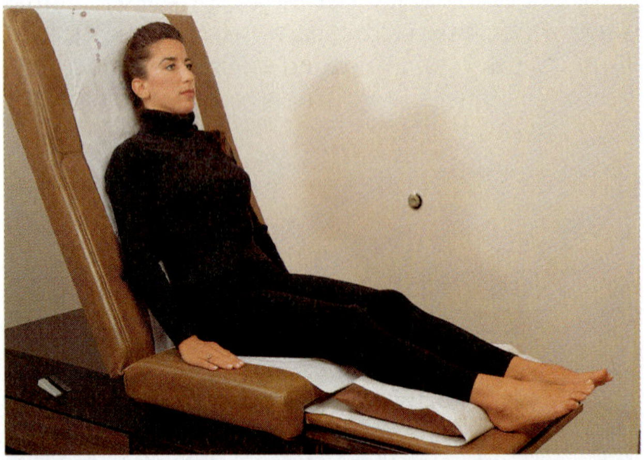

Figure 13-10 High Fowler's position (90-degree angle).

A pillow may be placed under the knees. This position is used for patients having cardiovascular or respiratory problems to facilitate their breathing, and for examination of the upper body and head.

Knee-Chest. The knee-chest position is rarely used. In this position, patients kneel on the examination table with buttocks elevated, back straight, and chest resting on the table. It is an uncomfortable position to get into, even with assistance, and it is difficult to maintain. Not only is it uncomfortable, but it is embarrassing and risky to place patients in the knee-chest position. The position has been used for proctologic examinations and sigmoidoscopy procedures; however, the proctologic table (Figure 13-11) has made the position unnecessary. The table is used in specialty offices, such as gastroenterology and proctology.

Proctologic. This position requires the use of a proctologic examination table (see Figure 13-11). The patient is instructed to undress from the waist down and to kneel on the knee board of the table. The patient then bends at the hips and rests the chest on the table. The head is supported by a head board. The table is then turned to elevate the buttocks. A triangular, diamond-shaped, or **fenestrated drape** covers the patient from the shoulders to the knees. This position is used for proctologic examinations.

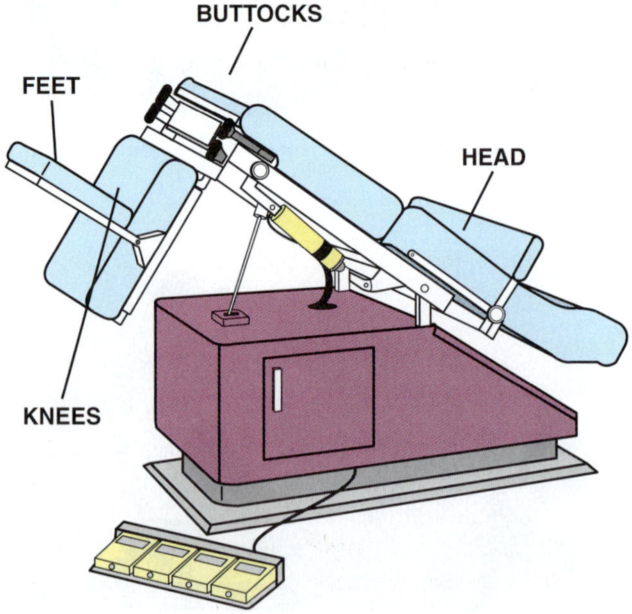

Figure 13-11 Proctologic table.

Prone. The patient is instructed to lie face down on the table with head turned to side; arms may be placed above the head or along the side of the body (Figure 13-12). The drape must cover from the mid-chest area to the legs. This position may be used for examining the posterior aspect of the body, including the back or spine and legs.

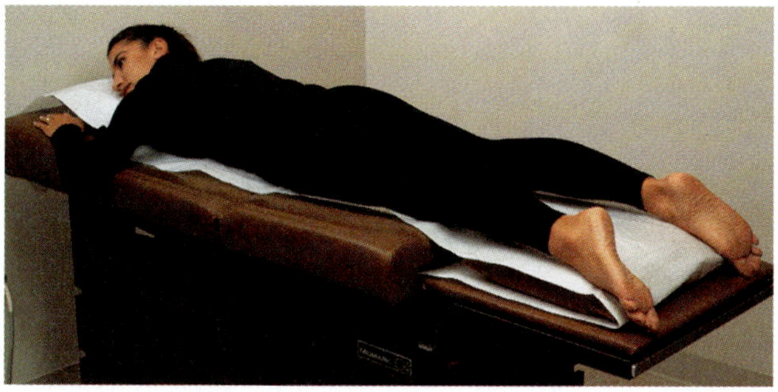

Figure 13-12 Prone position.

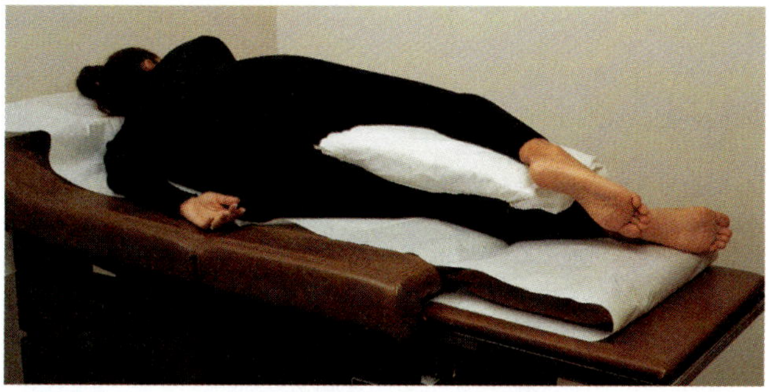

Figure 13-13 Sim's or lateral position.

Critical Thinking

Describe a type of examination that may be performed while the patient is placed in each of the following positions: (1) lithotomy, (2) Sims', (3) knee-chest, and (4) supine. Decide in what position you should place a patient and what manner of draping you would use for a Pap smear, examining a patient with shortness of breath, obtaining a rectal temperature, and an examination of the spine.

Sims' (lateral). The patient is instructed to lie on the left side; the left arm and shoulder may be drawn back behind the body (Figure 13-13). The left knee is slightly flexed to support the body, and the right knee is flexed sharply. A small pillow is provided for placement under the patient's head. A pillow may also be placed between the patient's legs if it will not interfere with the examination being performed. The drape should be large enough to cover the patient from the shoulders to the knees (triangle or diamond shape to expose rectum). This position may be used for vaginal or rectal examination, for obtaining a rectal temperature, for sigmoidoscopy, or for administering an enema.

Trendelenburg. Trendelenburg position can be used for two reasons. The first is to aid a person who is in shock. By lowering the head and elevating the legs, blood flow from the major vessels in the lower extremities will, by gravity, flow upward toward the brain and major organs. This may help to increase blood pressure enough to sustain the patient until taken to the emergency department (see Chapter 9). The other reason for Trendelenburg position is to elevate and incline the legs so that the abdomen and pelvic organs are pushed up toward the chest by gravity, making visibility and maneuverability easier for the provider doing either abdominal or pelvic surgery. In this case, the legs are elevated and inclined (see Chapter 19).

EQUIPMENT AND SUPPLIES FOR THE PHYSICAL EXAMINATION

Equipment and supplies used for physical examinations should be properly cleaned and ready for the provider's use (see Chapters 10 and 19 for proper cleaning and care of instruments). The list of instruments and supplies in Table 13-1 includes those that may be used in the physical examination. However, this is a limited list. Actual equipment and supplies needed vary with the provider and with the type of examination. Figure 13-14 shows some common instruments that may be used in the physical examination. (See Chapter 18, for instruments used in specialty examinations.) The medical assistant is responsible for room preparation prior to a physical examination. Equipment must be in working order (bulbs for scopes, good room lighting) and the room properly stocked with gowns, drapes, and other supplies, such as gloves, an antibacterial hand

Table 13-1 Some Common Instruments and Supplies Needed for a Physical Examination

Balance beam, digital, or electronic scale
Patient gown
Drape
Thermometer
Stethoscope
Sphygmomanometer
Alcohol wipes
Examination lights
Otoscope
Tuning fork
Ophthalmoscope
Penlight
Nasal speculum
Tongue depressors
Percussion hammer
Tape measure
Cotton balls
Safety pin
Gloves
Tissues
Lubricant
Emesis basin
Gauze sponges
Specimen bottles/slides—request forms
Biohazard and regular waste containers

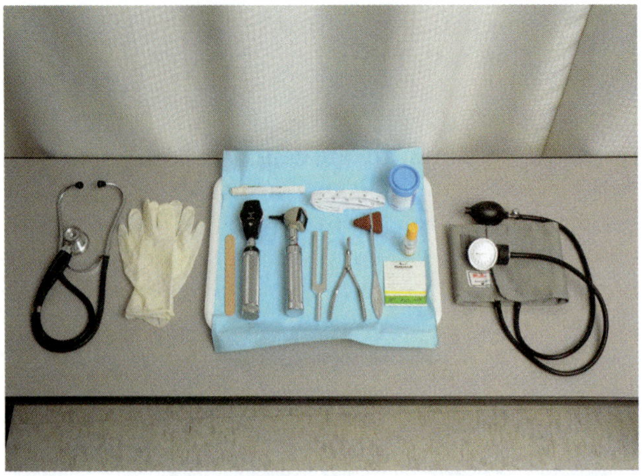

Figure 13-14 Instruments and supplies used in the physical examination: stethoscope, latex gloves, across top of tray: penlight, flexible tape measure, urine specimen container, tongue depressor, opthalmoscope, otoscope, tuning fork, metal nasal speculum, percussion hammer, Guaiac/occult blood slide, Guaiac/occult blood slide developer, and sphygmomanometer.

washing product, biohazard container, and any other materials needed to comply with Standard Precautions, such as a sharps container. In addition, the medical assistant is responsible for patient preparation. Urine, blood samples, and an ECG may be performed (if requested by the provider). Vital signs and height and weight will be measured. Signed consent forms, if needed, should be in the patient's record. If the patient needs help undressing and putting on a gown, the medical assistant provides assistance. Patient data can be documented

EHR

immediately using the computer to electronically record all of the information (vital signs, height and weight, known allergies, any medications the patient is taking) (Figure 13-15). Results of tests and the ECG usually are available within 24 hours and can be accessed in the patient EMR. Ensure patient confidentiality throughout the examination and documentation.

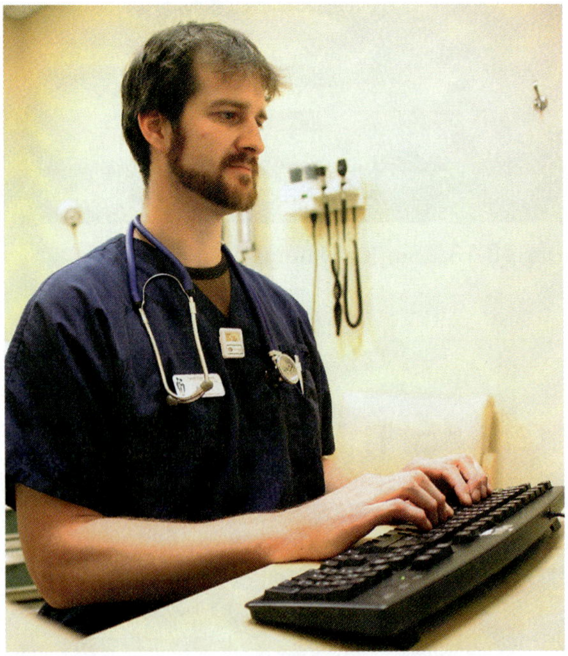

Figure 13-15 The medical assistant is able to document patient data immediately in the exam room computer.

BASIC COMPONENTS OF A PHYSICAL EXAMINATION

The physical examination of the patient begins as soon as the patient enters the office. The provider uses information from the health history, physical examination, and laboratory tests to aid in making a diagnosis. Figure 13-16 shows how these components are interrelated in a total practice management system. Although the physical examination is performed by the provider, it is important for the medical assistant to be aware of the various examination components and the significance of each as an indicator of patient well-being.

Patient Appearance

General appearance and actions are noted as the patient is received by the medical assistant and during the patient history (see Chapter 11). Skin color is checked, and general grooming, ease of conversation, and answers to questions are noted. Be aware of cultural differences while assisting with a physical examination. Some patients of other cultures may appear to you to be unclean in their appearance, have an unpleasant body order, have poor hygiene, or otherwise appear to be different from your culture. In some cultures, a daily bath is considered unnecessary, and body odor is not considered offensive. Regard your patient in a nonjudgmental way, taking into account the other's cultural beliefs. The medical assistant should be alert to a patient with abnormal skin color, confusion or disorientation, or difficulty in movement. Such a patient may have a serious problem and should be placed in an examination room and the provider contacted immediately.

The following aspects of the patient's health are evaluated by the provider through the method of physical examination known as observation.

Gait

Gait pertains to the manner or style of walking. The patient may have a limp, walk with feet wide apart, appear to be dragging one leg, or have difficulty maintaining balance. The provider observes the patient's gait by instructing the patient to walk on a designated straight line. Abnormal gait can include **ataxia,** uncoordinated wide-based walk; steppage, in which the leg stepping forward is raised high enough to raise the toes off the

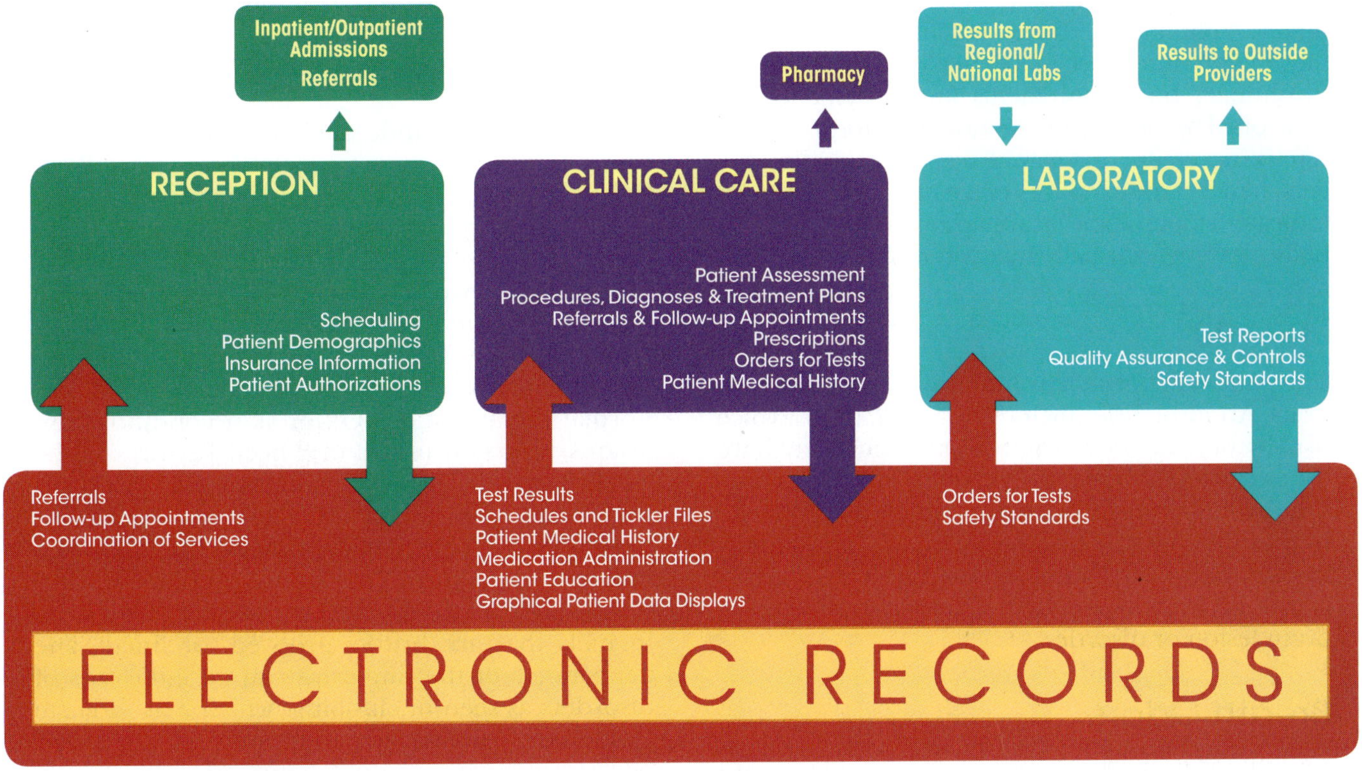

Figure 13-16 The provider uses the health history, physical examination, and lab tests to make a diagnosis. These components are integrated in a total practice management system.

ground; drag-to, in which the feet are dragged forward rather than lifted and moved; and spastic, in which the legs are held stiffly together and the feet are slightly dragged forward. Each of these gaits can indicate a disease process or health problem associated with poor neurologic functioning.

Stature

The height of the patient is measured. The provider looks for height, trunk, and limb proportion.

Posture

Because normal posture is erect with the head held up, a patient in pain may exhibit postural differences. The spine might be in a fixed position, or there may be limited motion in an extremity. The provider observes spine movement and alignment as the patient performs prescribed movements. Abnormalities can include kyphosis (humpback), which may be seen in older adult patients, particularly women with osteoporosis; lordosis, abnormal curvature of the lumbar area; and scoliosis, curvature of the upper spine.

Body Movements

Body movements may be either voluntary or involuntary. Voluntary body movements describe those movements intended to be made by the patient. Involuntary body movements are movements not controlled by the patient. Tremors are a form of involuntary movement that may be seen in the mouth, fingers, hands, arms, and legs of a patient. Tremors can indicate a neurologic health problem. Involuntary body movements usually are easily observed.

Speech

The patient's speech may indicate abnormal conditions. Abnormalities include aphonia, loss of voice usually because of laryngitis, but which may have other causes; aphasia, the inability to express oneself through speech or writing, which may indicate brain injury or disease; and dysphasia, an inability to use appropriate speech patterns, such as using words in the wrong order. This may indicate a brain lesion or disorder.

Breath Odors

Breath odors may be detected when speaking with the patient or when obtaining vital signs. A sweet fruity odor may indicate acidosis. This may result from diabetes mellitus, starvation, or renal disease. A musty odor may indicate liver disease, and an ammonia odor may indicate uremia.

Poor oral hygiene results in gingivitis (gum disease), caries (cavities), tooth loss, and foul breath odors. Gum disease and caries encourage the growth of microorganisms in the mouth and throat. Because of the vascularity of the oral cavity, microorganisms can enter into the circulatory system and travel to the heart, causing endocarditis. The importance of good oral health is necessary for general health and well-being. Regular dental checkups, cleaning, and daily flossing promote good health.

Nutrition

Various published charts contain guidelines for normal weight established by height and age. Overweight and underweight are defined as being above or below the published charts. Obesity and underweight are discussed in Chapters 12 and 22. Edema, which is excessive accumulation of fluids in the body tissues, causes weight gain. To test for edema, the provider presses a finger against the skin of the patient in an area over a bony prominence such as the ankle. If edema is present, pitting will be evident when the finger is removed. Fat tissue will not leave an indentation when pressed.

Skin and Appendages

Skin problems include abnormal skin color such as redness, pallor, cyanosis, jaundice, and vitiligo. **Pallor** is defined as lack of color or paleness often seen with anemia; **cyanosis** is a slightly blue or gray discoloration of the skin, often seen in patients with respiratory or cardiac problems; **jaundice** is a yellowing of the skin, often caused by obstructed bile ducts or liver disease; and **vitiligo** is characterized by white patches on the skin, observed against normal pigmentation. Other skin conditions are lesions, ulcers, bruises, and cancer. Texture may be smooth, rough, and scaly and have loss of elasticity. These findings may indicate health problems or excessive exposure to the sun. The nails can also indicate some forms of health problems. Infections, either local or systemic, may be observed in nails that are brittle, grooved, or lined. The appearance of the fingertips can be indicators of disorders as seen in clubbing, which may indicate congenital heart disease, and spooning, which may be seen in severe iron deficiency anemias. Abnormal hair distribution, as in facial hair on a female patient, may indicate hormonal changes.

HIPAA

When patients arrive for their appointments, the medical assistant will consider confidentiality to be of utmost importance. From the time the patient arrives until the patient leaves, there are multiple occasions to protect patient confidentiality. The medical history, personal finances, and insurance matters must be handled privately, out of the hearing range of others. Pertinent personal information that you may elicit from the patient that will be helpful to the provider during his or her examination also must be kept private. When the patient is undergoing testing such as electrocardiology that requires the patient to undress in preparation for the examination, care must be taken to avoid violating the patient's right to privacy. Respecting the dignity of all patients by protecting their privacy and confidentiality is a sign of a professional who is aware of patient rights.

THE PHYSICAL EXAMINATION SEQUENCE

A sequence is followed for a physical examination, although provider preference and the patient's chief complaint can produce a variation to the sequence.

The physical examination begins with the medical assistant taking and recording the patient's vital signs, height, and weight, and testing visual acuity as well as auditory ability when appropriate. Additional laboratory procedures, such as urinalysis and blood analysis or ECG may be performed as directed by the provider before the physical examination. Before the examination, a patient is instructed to empty the bladder, saving a urine specimen for analysis. The patient is then told what to expect during the examination. Any questions the patient has should be answered by the medical assistant or referred to the provider. The patient should be instructed about undressing (a private area should be provided for undressing). The medical assistant should be explicit as to what clothing is to be removed and what can be left on. If a complete physical examination is required, all clothing should be removed. A gown and drape are provided for the patient. The medical assistant may leave the room while the patient undresses unless the patient asks for help or is unable to manage alone. It is appropriate to knock before reentering the room.

It is customary for the medical assistant to remain in the room when the provider is examining a patient for the patient's comfort, to assist the provider, and as a deterrent to potential lawsuits.

The medical assistant places the instruments for the examination on the counter or Mayo stand, according to provider preference, but usually in order of use. When lamps are used for the examination, the medical assistant may turn them on and have them ready for the provider. Make sure that the light is not directed into the patient's eyes. When the patient is comfortably positioned on the examination table, inform the provider that the patient is ready. Normally the physical examination starts at the head and proceeds downward. Table 13-2 gives a detailed review of the components of the physical examination.

Head

The patient is in a sitting position for this examination. The face is checked for puffiness, especially around the eyes. Facial skin is checked for **scleroderma,** a tight and atrophied skin. The older adult patient may have fatty patches that appear raised and yellowish on the eyelids. The hair and scalp are checked. The head and neck are palpated for lumps and swelling.

Eyes

The appearance of the eyes is examined. The pupils of the eyes are checked for light and accommodation. When a penlight or flashlight is placed in front of the pupil, the pupil will constrict. The other pupil should constrict equally. The provider notes whether or not pupils are equal and react to light and accommodation (abbreviated as PERRLA). Pupils that do not constrict and return to normal equally may indicate a problem in the brain. A tonometer may be used to measure the intraocular eye pressure of patients older than 35 years. Normal eye pressure is 13 to 22 mm Hg. An increase above normal will be found in glaucoma. The provider uses an ophthalmoscope to view the blood vessels of the retina. This is done by turning out the lights in the room, allowing the patient's pupils to dilate. The patient is instructed to look straight ahead while the provider looks into the eye. Retinal changes may indicate disease such as hypertension. The sclera are checked for jaundice.

Table 13-2 Components of the Physical Examination

				Provider's Findings	
Body Part	**Position**	**Instrument Used**	**Method of Exam**	**Normal**	**Abnormal**
General appearance	Standing	—	Inspection	Patient is cooperative, good hygiene, good skin color, ease of gait	Uncooperative, behavior inappropriate, unkempt appearance
Skin	Supine Prone	Flashlight	Inspection Palpation	Good color, warm to touch; no lesion such as warts, moles, abscesses, rashes	Jaundice, cyanosis, pallor, redness, flakiness of skin, lesions, rashes
Head and neck	Supine or semi-Fowler's or sitting on edge of table	Light source	Inspection Palpation	Symmetry of head; hair not dry or oily and distributed evenly; scalp free of lesions and not dry; no lymph node enlargement	Asymmetry of head; alopecia, dry, flaky scalp; swelling, lumps or pain in head or neck
Eyes	Supine or semi-Fowler's or sitting on edge of table	Ophthalmoscope	Inspection Mensuration	Snellen test shows accurate visual acuity; able to identify color plates; no tearing; pupillary reaction to light equal; retina pink and blood vessels healthy; measurement of intraocular pressure within normal limits; no bulging of eyeballs	Poor visual and color ability; dull-appearing eyes; drainage; unequal pupils; clouded lens; unequal pupillary reaction; intraocular pressure increased; torturous, unhealthy retinal blood vessels; bulging eyeballs
Ears	Supine or semi-Fowler's or sitting on edge of table	Otoscope Tuning fork and audiometer	Inspection Percussion	Cerumen not impacted on tympanic membrane; tympanic membrane gray and intact; no discharge or pain; able to hear tuning fork or audiometer	Impacted cerumen; red, bulging tympanic membrane; discharge (pus or blood); inability to hear sound from tuning fork; poor auditory ability when checked with audiometer
Nose	Supine or semi-Fowler's or sitting on edge of table	Nasal speculum Flashlight Aromatic substance	Inspection	Mucous membranes moist and pink; able to detect specific odors; septum straight; nostrils equal in size; no abnormal discharge; no lesions	Dry, red, swollen mucous membranes; unable to detect odors; deviated septum; nostrils flaring; discharge, polyps noted
Mouth and throat	Supine or semi-Fowler's or sitting on edge of table	Flashlight Tongue depressors	Inspection	Gag reflex present; mucous membranes moist and pink; teeth intact, pink tongue; tonsils nonswollen, pink	No gag reflex; tongue rough; pallor of mucous membranes; dental caries; swollen tonsils

(continues)

Table 13-2 (continued)

				Provider's Findings	
Body Part	**Position**	**Instrument Used**	**Method of Exam**	**Normal**	**Abnormal**
Arms and hands	Supine or semi-Fowler's or sitting on edge of table	Percussion hammer	Inspection Palpation Percussion	Good muscle tone; normal range of motion; nails pink, smooth; ability to squeeze provider's hands with equal strength; normal reflexes	Poor muscle tone; poor range of motion; nails cyanotic; brittle, ridged nails; abnormal reflexes
Chest and lungs	Supine or semi-Fowler's or sitting on edge of table	Stethoscope Tape measure	Inspection Palpation Auscultation Mensuration Percussion	Axillary lymph nodes not palpable; lungs clear; no cough; ribs nontender; symmetrical chest wall; respirations and heart rate normal; normal chest sounds	Enlarged axillary lymph nodes; asymmetry of chest wall; respiration and heart rate abnormal; abnormal chest sounds
Heart	Supine or semi-Fowler's or sitting on edge of table	Stethoscope Sphygmomanometer Electrocardiogram (ECG)	Auscultation Palpation Mensuration	Normal heart function per ECG; regular rhythm, rate of heart sounds; no murmurs; blood pressure normal range; pulse points good quality	Abnormal heart function per ECG; irregularity of rhythm, rate; murmurs; blood pressure outside normal range; poor pulse quality
Breasts	Supine	—	Inspection Palpation	No lumps, tenderness, swelling, or thickening; no sores or lesions; no bleeding or discharge from nipples; no lymph node swelling in axilla; no dimpling or "orange peel" appearance	Lumps, tenderness, swelling, thickening; sores or lesions; bleeding or discharge from nipple; lymph node enlargement in axilla; "orange peel" appearance to breast tissue; dimpling of skin
Abdomen	Supine	Stethoscope Measuring tape	Inspection Palpation Auscultation Mensuration Percussion	Liver, spleen not palpable; symmetry to abdomen; no abnormal bowel sounds; no abnormal sounds from organs in abdomen; abdomen soft; no abdominal or inguinal hernias	Liver, spleen enlarged; asymmetric abdomen; increased or decreased bowel sounds; unusual sounds elicited from percussion of abdominal organs; abdominal distention; ascites; presence of abdominal, umbilical, or inguinal hernia

(continues)

Table 13-2 Components of the Physical Examination (continued)

				Provider's Findings	
Body Part	**Position**	**Instrument Used**	**Method of Exam**	**Normal**	**Abnormal**
Female genitalia and rectum	Lithotomy or dorsal recumbent or Sims'	Vaginal speculum Examination light Slides for occult blood (Hemoccult)	Inspection Palpation	External genitalia without lesions, sores, ulcerations; vaginal mucosa pink and without discharge; nontender ovaries; cervix smooth, noneroded, noninflamed; good muscle tone in perineal floor and rectum; negative stool for occult blood; nonpalpable lymph nodes in groin	Lesions, sores, ulcerations; discharge from vagina, cervix; painful ovaries; cervix ulcerated, inflamed; poor muscle tone in perineal and rectum floor; prolapse of uterus or bladder into vagina; hemorrhoids; positive hemoccult; enlarged inguinal lymph nodes
Male genitalia and rectum	Supine Standing	—	Inspection Palpation	Penis pink, no discharge; no lesions, sores, ulcers; testicles firm, nontender, and movable; rectal musculature intact; nonpalpable prostate; nonpalpable lymph nodes in groin	Discharge from penis; ulcers, sores, other types of lesions; testicles tender, swollen; relaxed anal sphincter; hemorrhoids; positive hemoccult slide; enlarged prostate; enlarged lymph nodes in groin
Legs and feet	Supine Prone	Tape measure	Inspection Mensuration Palpation	Normal muscle tone and range of motion; no edema; pulses normal; no varicosities; toenails smooth; no signs of fungus or other infection; calves equal in size	Muscle weakness; poor range of motion; edema; diminished pulse; varicose veins; toenails ridged, infected; unequal calf measurements
Neurologic examination	Supine	Percussion hammer Safety pin Cotton ball	Percussion Inspection	Normal reflexes; oriented to time and place; appropriate responses; normal responses to sensation; alert; steady gait; no vertigo or syncope	All reflexes disoriented; inappropriate responses; dulled response to pain and sensation; lethargic; unsteady gait; poor coordination; vertigo; syncope

Ears

An otoscope is used by the provider to examine the ears. The external ear is checked for redness in the ear canal and buildup of cerumen. A healthy tympanic membrane has a pearly gray appearance. A red appearance to the tympanic membrane may indicate infection in the middle ear, known as otitis media. **Vertigo** (dizziness) may indicate that the patient has an inner ear infection (**labyrinthitis**). **Tinnitus** (ringing in the ears) may indicate inner ear problems. Other symptoms of ear problems include pain, discharge, and deafness. The tuning fork is used in testing the sensations of hearing, including bone conduction and air conduction.

Nose

The nasal cavity is visualized by the provider with the use of a nasal speculum and flashlight. Discharge from the nose may indicate a postnasal drip in which the sinuses may be draining into the nose and throat. Other abnormalities may include obstruction because of a deviated septum. Polyps and ulcerations may be found in the nasal cavity. Epistaxis or nosebleed may be seen when the capillaries rupture on the surface of the nasal mucosa.

Mouth and Throat

The provider uses a tongue blade or depressor and a light source. The teeth and gums are checked for dental hygiene such as caries and the gums are checked for signs of **pyorrhea** (discharge of pus from the gums around the teeth). If the tonsils are present, they are checked for signs of infection, such as redness or white pockets of pus. The floor of the mouth is examined both visually and by palpation for indications of swollen glands and ulcerations.

Neck

The provider palpates the neck, looking for swollen lymph nodes. The thyroid gland is palpated anteriorly and posteriorly for size, symmetry, and texture. The patient is asked to swallow several times while the provider feels the thyroid gland. A small glass of water may be given to the patient to aid in swallowing. Range of motion is checked by having the patient turn the head in each direction. Care must be taken with older adult patients. The patient should be instructed to move the head slowly to avoid syncope.

Chest

The symmetry of the chest is observed, both anteriorly and posteriorly. Chest measurement may have been performed before the examination. The chest of a patient with emphysema will appear barrel-like in shape. While the patient is sitting, the provider listens to the lungs with a stethoscope. The patient may be instructed to take several deep breaths during this process.

Carefully monitor the patient, particularly the older adult patient, because deep breathing may cause dizziness. The provider is listening for abnormal lung sounds. The provider may examine the lungs by percussion. Heart sounds will be auscultated both anteriorly and posteriorly.

Breast

The patient is placed in a supine position and instructed to place the hand behind the head on the side on which the examination is taking place. The provider examines the breast for masses by using a circular motion, starting at the outer edge of the breast and working toward the center. The nipple is gently squeezed to see if there is any discharge. The patient is then instructed to change arm positions so that the other breast can be examined. With the patient in a sitting position, the provider observes the breasts for symmetry. Female patients should be instructed on the procedure for performing monthly breast self-examination. This may be an embarrassing procedure for the female patient. Maintain as much patient modesty as possible by carefully draping and giving emotional support (see Chapter 14 for more detailed information on breast examination and breast self-examination).

Abdomen

The patient is placed in a dorsal recumbent or supine position with the arms at the sides for examination of the abdomen. The drape is lowered to just above the pubic hair. The female patient wears a gown open in the front that can be pulled to the sides while still covering the breasts. The provider normally stands on the right side of the patient while performing this part of the examination. The abdomen is examined by palpation, percussion, and auscultation. Following the quadrants of the abdomen, the provider gently palpates the organs in each quadrant, working from side to side. The provider feels for organ size and location, as well as the presence of masses; percusses the abdomen listening for sounds from abdominal organs; uses the stethoscope to listen for abdominal sounds; and visually inspects the abdominal area for changes in skin color, scars, or other abnormalities. The contour of the abdomen may be flat or slightly convex. The presence of hernias is checked in both the supine and the standing positions. Patients with abdominal disorders may give a history of dyspepsia, dysphagia or excessive flatulence, nausea, vomiting, bloating, and pain.

Genitals

Refer to Chapters 14 and 16 for more detailed information about genitalia examinations.

Female Genitals. The patient is placed in the lithotomy position. The provider examines both the external genitalia and the reproductive organs. The rectum may be examined and a Hemoccult test done at the conclusion of the pelvic examination. (See Chapters 18 and 32 for information regarding the Hemoccult slide test.) After the examination, the patient is instructed to slide toward the head of the table and may be allowed to sit up slowly. Sitting up quickly may cause orthostatic hypotension and dizziness.

Male Genitals. Care must be taken to protect all patients' modesty and privacy. The provider begins the examination by inspecting and retracting the foreskin of the penis if the patient is uncircumcised. The glans penis is inspected for discharge and redness. The penis and scrotum are palpated for possible tenderness and masses. Because of the seriousness of testicular cancer, the patient will be instructed, usually by the provider, on the procedure for performing monthly testicular examinations (see Chapter 16).

Rectum

The provider may examine the rectum as a part of the male and female genitals examination. The patient may be placed in the Sims' position. The provider performs a manual examination. The prostate gland is examined by digital rectal palpation. The provider inserts the gloved index finger into the rectum and palpates the prostate gland for any masses or swelling (see Chapter 16). A lubricated rectal speculum may then be inserted for visual examination. Because this is uncomfortable for the patient, emotional support is important. The provider can visualize the rectum for bleeding, fissures, polyps, or other lesions.

Reflexes

The patient's reflexes in both the supine and sitting positions are observed by the provider. A percussion hammer is used. While sitting with the arm flexed, the elbow is lightly tapped to elicit movement from the biceps. The patellar or knee-jerk reflex is tested by tapping the area just below the patella at the knee. The Achilles reflex or ankle-jerk is tested by tapping the Achilles tendon. The Babinski reflex is tested on the sole of a relaxed foot (the great toe will flex) with the patient in a supine position. Reflexes determine the integrity of the neurologic system.

Procedure 13-1 outlines the steps in assisting with the physical examination.

AFTER THE EXAMINATION

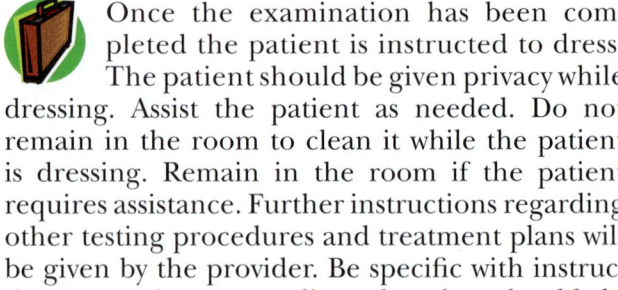

Once the examination has been completed the patient is instructed to dress. The patient should be given privacy while dressing. Assist the patient as needed. Do not remain in the room to clean it while the patient is dressing. Remain in the room if the patient requires assistance. Further instructions regarding other testing procedures and treatment plans will be given by the provider. Be specific with instructions to patients regarding what they should do after they are completely dressed.

Once the examination is finished and the patient has left the examination room, the equipment and supplies (including the examination table) should be sanitized, disinfected, and sterilized as appropriate.

Patient Education

Throughout the physical examination, from the time the patient arrives until the patient leaves, there are many opportunities for patient education. Written instructions should be given when necessary, and provider information should be clarified if needed (Figure 13-17).

Opportunities for teaching the patient how to adopt a healthy lifestyle are abundant. Regular exercise, no smoking, weight control, limiting alcohol consumption, and using stress reduction techniques, such as meditation, yoga, massage therapy, and so forth, all help to decrease blood pressure and reduce risk for heart attack, stroke, and other illnesses.

Critical Thinking

At the conclusion of the physical examination, the provider will have an impression of the patient's general health. What specific information can the provider obtain from the examination? From what sources other than the physical examination does the provider gain information to help in making a diagnosis?

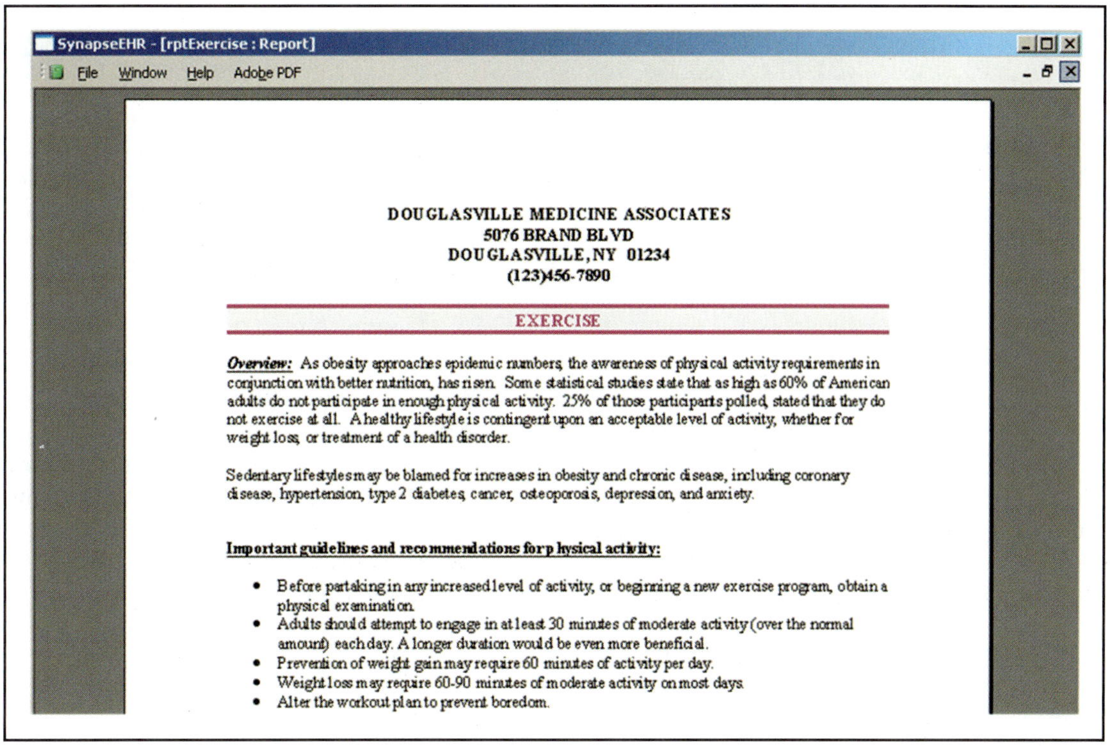

DOUGLASVILLE MEDICINE ASSOCIATES
5076 BRAND BLVD
DOUGLASVILLE, NY 01234
(123)456-7890

EXERCISE

Overview: As obesity approaches epidemic numbers, the awareness of physical activity requirements in conjunction with better nutrition, has risen. Some statistical studies state that as high as 60% of American adults do not participate in enough physical activity. 25% of those participants polled, stated that they do not exercise at all. A healthy lifestyle is contingent upon an acceptable level of activity, whether for weight loss, or treatment of a health disorder.

Sedentary lifestyles may be blamed for increases in obesity and chronic disease, including coronary disease, hypertension, type 2 diabetes, cancer, osteoporosis, depression, and anxiety.

Important guidelines and recommendations for physical activity:

- Before partaking in any increased level of activity, or beginning a new exercise program, obtain a physical examination.
- Adults should attempt to engage in at least 30 minutes of moderate activity (over the normal amount) each day. A longer duration would be even more beneficial.
- Prevention of weight gain may require 60 minutes of activity per day.
- Weight loss may require 60-90 minutes of moderate activity on most days.
- Alter the workout plan to prevent boredom.

Figure 13-17 Patient education forms can be printed from an electronic medical records software and given to the patient right in the exam room.

Procedure 13-1

Assisting with a Complete Physical Examination

STANDARD PRECAUTIONS:

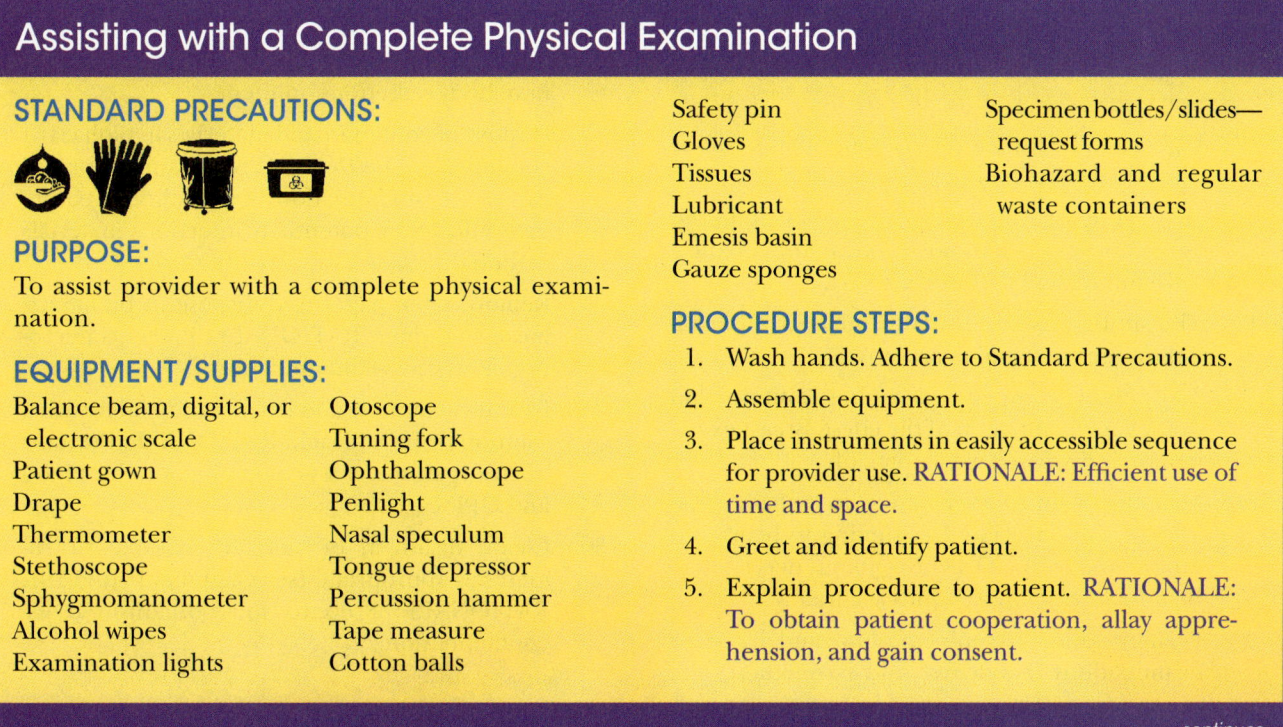

PURPOSE:

To assist provider with a complete physical examination.

EQUIPMENT/SUPPLIES:

Balance beam, digital, or electronic scale
Patient gown
Drape
Thermometer
Stethoscope
Sphygmomanometer
Alcohol wipes
Examination lights
Otoscope
Tuning fork
Ophthalmoscope
Penlight
Nasal speculum
Tongue depressor
Percussion hammer
Tape measure
Cotton balls
Safety pin
Gloves
Tissues
Lubricant
Emesis basin
Gauze sponges
Specimen bottles/slides—request forms
Biohazard and regular waste containers

PROCEDURE STEPS:

1. Wash hands. Adhere to Standard Precautions.
2. Assemble equipment.
3. Place instruments in easily accessible sequence for provider use. RATIONALE: Efficient use of time and space.
4. Greet and identify patient.
5. Explain procedure to patient. RATIONALE: To obtain patient cooperation, allay apprehension, and gain consent.

continues

Procedure 13-1 (continued)

6. Review medical history with patient (see Chapter 11 for obtaining patient history). RATIONALE: To ensure complete history has been obtained and is current.
7. Take patient vital signs, test visual acuity, and check hearing ability.
8. Obtain a urine specimen (see Chapter 30 for urine collection procedures).
9. Obtain all required blood samples (see Chapters 28 and 29 for blood specimen collection procedures).
10. Perform electrocardiogram (ECG) if directed by provider (see Chapter 25 for ECG procedure).
11. Provide patient with appropriate gown and drape.
12. Assist patient to disrobe completely; explain where the opening for the gown is to be placed. RATIONALE: To assist patient in maintaining modesty, privacy, and warmth.
13. Assist patient in sitting at the end of the table; drape patient across lap and legs. RATIONALE: Always drape patient to maintain modesty.
14. Inform provider when patient is ready.
15. When the provider arrives, remain by the patient ready to assist the patient and provider.
16. Position patient in a sitting or supine position for the head, throat, eye, ear, and neck examination.
17. Lights may be turned off to allow pupils to dilate for retinal examination.
18. Hand the provider instruments as required (some providers do not require the medical assistant to hand the instruments).
19. The sitting position is maintained for auscultation of the chest and heart.
20. Assist the patient into a supine position and drape for examination of the chest. Breast examination is discussed in Chapter 14.
21. Maintain a quiet atmosphere to enhance the ability of the provider in listening to heart and lung sounds. RATIONALE: Quiet is necessary to hear heart and chest sounds accurately.
22. Position patient in supine position and drape for examinations of abdomen and extremities.
23. Gynecologic examination may then be performed (see Chapter 14). Assist female patient into lithotomy position for gynecologic examination. Male genitals are examined.
24. If rectal examination is necessary, assist patient into Sims' position.
25. Place patient in prone position for examination of posterior aspect of body.
26. On completion of the examination, assist patient to sitting position and allow patient to sit at end of table for a few minutes. RATIONALE: Allows patient to recover from potential dizziness.
27. Ensure patient stability (check color of skin, pulse) before allowing patient to stand up. RATIONALE: Prevents the patient from fainting due to orthostatic hypotension.
28. Assist patient with dressing; provide privacy.

EHR

29. Enter any notes or patient instructions on computer in patient's EMR per provider orders.
30. Escort patient to provider's office for discussion of examination results.
31. Put on disposable gloves.
32. Dispose of gown and drape in biohazard waste container. RATIONALE: Prevents microorganism cross-contamination; gown and drape may have body secretions on them.
33. Dispose of contaminated materials in biohazard container. RATIONALE: Prevents microorganism cross-contamination of bloodborne pathogens and other potentially infectious materials (OPIM).
34. Remove table paper and dispose in biohazard waste container. RATIONALE: Prevents microorganism cross-contamination.
35. Disinfect counters and examination table with a solution of 10% bleach. RATIONALE: Prevents microorganism cross-contamination by blood and OPIM.
36. Clean, disinfect, or sterilize reusable instruments as appropriate (see Chapters 10 and 19). RATIONALE: Prevents microorganism cross-contamination.

continues

Procedure 13-1 (continued)

37. Remove gloves and discard in biohazard waste container. RATIONALE: Prevents microorganism cross-contamination by blood and OPIM.
38. Wash hands.
39. Replace table paper and equipment in preparation for the next patient.
40. Document the procedure on computer in patient's EMR.

EHR

DOCUMENTATION

11/8/20XX T 98.2, P 84, R 16 BP 124/76 Complete physical examination performed by Dr. Woo. Urinalysis negative, Hemoccult slide negative. Venipuncture performed and specimens sent to laboratory for complete blood count and electrolytes. Electrocardiogram completed. Patient given written instructions and appointment made for a colonoscopy. Says she understands the preparation for the colonoscopy. W. Slawson, CMA (AAMA) __________

Case Study 13-1

Refer to the scenario at the beginning of the chapter.

CASE STUDY REVIEW

1. Why do Wanda and Bruce prepare and assist for physical exams with patients of their own gender?

Case Study 13-2

At Inner City Health Care, clinical medical assistant Wanda Slawson is helping Liz Corbin, a part-time administrative/clinical medical assistant, learn to prepare the examination room and patients for the physical examination. In addition to alerting Liz to provider preferences, Wanda wants to be sure that Liz has a solid understanding of the methods of examination, positions and draping, and the components of the physical examination.

CASE STUDY REVIEW

1. In reviewing with Liz the methods of examination used by provider, what six primary methods would Wanda have Liz describe?
2. What patient positions would Liz need to know?
3. Wanda asks Liz to recall the various examination components and their significance. How should Liz respond?

Case Study 13-3

Mrs. Mason, a 72-year-old somewhat frail woman with arthritis and hypertensive heart disease, has an appointment today for a complete physical examination. It will include a basic physical examination and an examination of the pelvis because she has had bright red vaginal spotting.

CASE STUDY REVIEW

1. Discuss positions and draping for the physical examination, including pelvic examination for this patient.
2. Discuss any special safety needs for Mrs. Mason.
3. What additional supplies and equipment should be available for the provider?

SUMMARY

A complete physical examination will be performed during the patient's initial visit. Findings at this examination, both normal and abnormal, provide a baseline for future examinations.

The role of the medical assistant throughout the examination is twofold. The assistant assembles the necessary instruments and may hand them to the provider when requested. The medical assistant will also prepare the patient and obtain specimens as required by the examination and provider. Responsibilities to the patient include explanations and careful positioning, protecting modesty by careful draping, and, most important, providing comfort, emotional support, and safety. By performing these duties, the medical assistant can ensure patient compliance and provider efficiency.

STUDY FOR SUCCESS

To reinforce your knowledge and skills of information presented in this chapter:

- Review the Key Terms
- Practice the Procedures
- Consider the Case Studies and discuss your conclusions
- Answer the Review Questions
  - Multiple Choice
  - Critical Thinking
- Navigate the Internet by completing the Web Activities
- Practice the StudyWARE activities on your student CD
- Apply your knowledge in the Student Workbook activities
- Complete the Web Tutor sections
- View and discuss the DVD situations

REVIEW QUESTIONS

Multiple Choice

1. The method of examination that is the process of listening directly to body sounds is called:
   a. percussion
   b. auditory
   c. auscultation
   d. the direct method
2. The supine position is also known as:
   a. horizontal recumbent
   b. dorsal recumbent
   c. knee-chest
   d. Sims'
3. During the physical examination, ataxia might be observed, which relates to:
   a. stature
   b. posture
   c. body movement
   d. speech
4. When the patient asks a question of the medical assistant, the medical assistant should:
   a. refer all questions to the provider
   b. try to answer all questions, even if uncertain
   c. answer questions to the extent of knowledge; refer others to the provider
   d. ask the patient to please hold all questions until the examination is complete
5. When the abdomen is being examined, the patient is typically in a:
   a. supine position
   b. prone position
   c. Fowler's position
   d. Sims' position

Critical Thinking

1. Discuss the responsibilities of the medical assistant when preparing the patient for a physical examination.
2. Review the six methods used in the physical examination.
3. Evelyn Williams has a physical examination scheduled for today. She is recuperating from back surgery and still has pain when she moves to raise her legs. What position is most comfortable for her? Which body parts can be examined with her in this position?
4. Explain the sequence of a physical examination.
5. List the instruments and supplies needed for examining the following body areas:
   a. head
   b. reflexes
   c. chest
   d. abdomen
6. Describe the cleaning process that the following instruments will need after their use in an examination:
   a. nasal speculum
   b. tuning fork
   c. percussion hammer
   d. reusable otoscope speculum
7. List and describe the three sources of information the provider uses to aid in making a diagnosis.
8. List two procedures or tests the medical assistant might perform as part of the patient's physical examination.

WEB ACTIVITIES

1. Using one of the "gateways" for general health and medical information and its links to other sites, gather information about the U.S. government's guidelines for average adult height and weight measurements. According to the government tables, what is considered an appropriate weight for your height?
2. Explore the Web for information about the following conditions and their possible causes:
   - Changes in retinal blood vessels
   - Enlarged liver
   - Ascites
   - Varicose veins
   - Vertigo

REFERENCES/BIBLIOGRAPHY

Hegner, B. R., Acello, B., & Caldwell, E. (2008). *Nursing assistant: A nursing process approach* (10th ed.). Clifton Park, NY: Delmar Cengage Learning.

Keir, L., Wise, B., Krebs, C., & Kelley-Arney, C. (2008). *Medical assisting administration and clinical competencies* (6th ed.). Clifton Park, NY: Delmar Cengage Learning.

Simmers, L. (2004). *Diversified health occupations* (6th ed.). Clifton Park, NY: Delmar Cengage Learning.

Taber's cyclopedic medical dictionary (22nd ed.). (2003). Philadelphia: F. A. Davis.

Tamparo, C., & Lewis, M. (2005). *Diseases of the human body* (4th ed.). Philadelphia: F. A. Davis.

THE DVD HOOK-UP

This chapter discusses the proper techniques for positioning patients and various methods that providers use to examine the patient.

In the designated scene, the medical assistant is seen placing the patient in various positions. You probably noticed that many of the positions were awkward for the patient. It should be noted that the position that the DVD lists as the Trendelenburg position is not the true Trendelenburg position. The position illustrated in the DVD starts off by having the patient lying in a supine position. The medical assistant then carefully lifts the patient's legs and feet straight up in into the air. This is actually a maneuver that can be used in place of the Trendelenburg position when you do not have access to a tilt table.

1. What types of physical concerns do you need to be aware of when using this alternative maneuver to the Trendelenburg position?
2. What is the purpose of lifting the legs straight up into the air instead of just propping them up on some pillows?

DVD Journal Summary

Write a paragraph that summarizes what you learned from watching the scenes in today's DVD program. When positioning patients, you are going to see parts of the body that the patient may not be able to see. What would you do if you saw some fecal matter on the back part of the patient's upper leg?

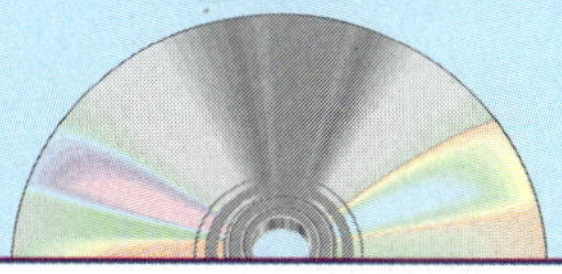

DVD Series — Skills Based Series

Program Number — 6

Chapter/Scene Reference
- *Positioning the Patient*

UNIT 5

Assisting with Specialty Examinations and Procedures

Obstetrics and Gynecology

Chapter 14

KEY TERMS

Abortion
Amniocentesis
Amniotomy
Bartholin Gland
Bimanual Examination
Braxton–Hicks
Candidiasis
Carcinoma in situ
Cervical Punch Biopsy
Cesarean Section
Chlamydia
Colposcopy
Condylomata
Congenital Anomalies
Coupling Agent
Cryosurgery
Diethylstilbestrol (DES)
Dilation
Dysmenorrhea
Dyspareunia
Dysplasia
Eclampsia
Ectopic
Effacement
Endometriosis
Erosion
Exfoliated
Formalin
Fulgarated
Genitalia
Gestation
Gestational Diabetes
Gravidity
Human Chorionic Gonadotropin

OUTLINE

Obstetrics
- Initial Prenatal Visit
- Subsequent or Return Prenatal Visits
- Disorders of Pregnancy
- Parturition
- Postpartum Period

Gynecology
- The Gynecologic Examination
- Gynecologic Diseases and Conditions
- Other Diagnostic Tests and Treatments for Reproductive System Diseases
- Complementary Therapy in Obstetrics and Gynecology

OBJECTIVES

The student should strive to meet the following performance objectives and demonstrate an understanding of the facts and principles presented in this chapter through written and oral communication.

1. Define the key terms as presented in the glossary.
2. Explain the importance of prenatal care, and discuss what examinations will be performed as part of the initial visit.
3. Explain why the initial prenatal visit is important.
4. List 12 conditions or diseases that can cause a pregnant woman and her fetus to be at greater risk for problems during the pregnancy.
5. List signs and symptoms and their possible corresponding conditions that the provider searches for during the prenatal history and physical examination.
6. Calculate an expected date of confinement (EDC) or expected date of birth (EDB) using Nägele's Rule.
7. Calculate an EDC (EDB) using a gestation wheel.
8. Explain the purpose of ultrasonography and amniocentesis.
9. List and describe six types of abortion.
10. Explain what occurs in each of the three stages of labor.
11. Describe what takes place during the postpartum examination.
12. List and describe the diseases and disorders that can affect the female patient.
13. Describe the laboratory tests and procedures that can help diagnose the diseases and disorders that can affect the female patient.

OBJECTIVES (continued)

14. Describe seven sexually transmitted diseases.
15. Explain the medical assistant's responsibilities with a gynecologic examination.
16. Describe breast self-examination and method of teaching patient breast self-examination.
17. Discuss menopause.
18. Describe the findings and concerns surrounding hormone replacement therapy.
19. Describe several methods of contraception.
20. Explain reasons for impaired fertility.
21. Describe three therapies that assist in reproduction.

KEY TERMS (continued)

Hyperemesis Gravidarum
Hypoxia
Hysterosalpingogram
Intraepithelium
Involution
Lamaze
Lochia
Meconium
Metrorrhagia
Multigravida
Nägele's Rule
Neonatal
Nullipara
Oxytocin
Parity
Parturition
Patent
Pelvic Inflammatory Disease
Placenta Abruptio
Placenta Previa
Polycystic
Postcoital
Preeclampsia
Prenatal
Primigravida
Prostaglandin
Puerperium
Sickle Cell Anemia
Stigma
Supine Hypotension
Tay–Sachs
Thalassemia
Titer
Trichomoniasis
Trimester
Ultrasonography
Vesicle
Viable
Wet Mount

Scenario

In the obstetrics department at Inner City Health Care, Wanda Slawson and Bruce Goldman, both certified medical assistants, are preparing for the day's appointments. Both take responsibility for being certain all rooms have appropriate equipment and supplies needed for today's patients. There are three ultrasonograms in addition to the pelvic examinations, Pap smear, and breast examinations scheduled for the afternoon. Wanda is responsible for assisting the provider with each of them. She is careful to follow all safety precautions before, during, and after assisting with examinations and procedures. She is careful to explain procedures to the patients and to direct any questions to the provider.

INTRODUCTION

Obstetrics is the medical specialty in which the provider treats the female patient from the prenatal period through labor, delivery, and during the 6-week postpartum period. Gynecology is the specialty that treats the medical and surgical disorders and diseases of the female reproductive tract. Both specialties are usually combined, and the provider who practices them is known as an obstetrician/gynecologist, or simply, an OB/GYN provider. Knowledge of the female anatomy, the laboratory tests and procedures for both specialties, the diseases and disorders that affect the female patient during her nonpregnant and pregnant states, and patient education are essential for the medical assistant who will care for these patients. The goal of the OB/GYN specialty is to promote the health and well-being of the woman and her baby.

Spotlight on Certification

RMA Content Outline

- Anatomy and physiology
- Patient education
- Obstetrics and gynecology

CMA (AAMA) Content Outline

- Medical terminology
- Anatomy and physiology
- Patient instruction
- Patient preparation and assisting the provider
- Collecting and processing specimens; diagnostic testing

CMAS Content Outline

- Medical terminology
- Anatomy and physiology
- Examination preparation

OBSTETRICS

Obstetrics is the branch of medicine that provides care to the mother and fetus during pregnancy, labor, delivery, and the postpartum period known as the **puerperium.** Pregnancy is a period of approximately 40 weeks from the day conception takes place (Figure 14-1). The puerperium is the period of 6 weeks after delivery when the mother's body is returning to its prepregnant state. Visits to the provider for prenatal and postnatal care are the initial **prenatal** visit, return visits, and the 6-week postpartum checkup.

Initial Prenatal Visit

The initial prenatal visit is of utmost importance and usually occurs after a woman has missed a second menstrual period or after an at-home pregnancy test result is positive. Some obstetricians recommend prepregnancy or preconception physical examinations. The information guide at this appointment can be used as a baseline on which to compare future tests and procedures. It is a risk assessment of maternal health for identification and prevention of complications. For example, blood pressure measurement performed prepregnancy and not during the first trimester can rule out pregnancy-induced hypertension. The prenatal visit is a time of health promotion for the expectant mother and her baby. It is also the time for diagnosis and treatment of maternal disorders that may have been present before the pregnancy or that may have developed during the course of the pregnancy. Growth and development of the fetus are followed and identification of problems that may impede a normal labor are sought. There is ongoing assessment of the expectant mother

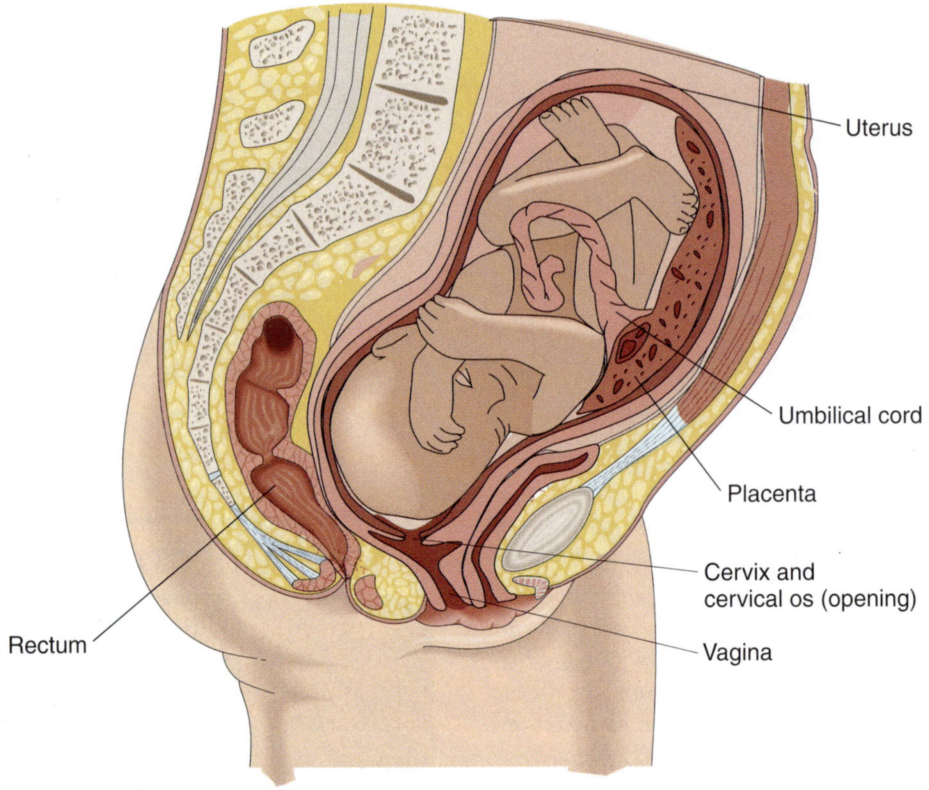

Figure 14-1 Normal uterine pregnancy.

and the fetus. Any abnormalities can indicate a problem or complication necessitating further testing and assessment. Early detection and management of conditions such as **gestational diabetes,** urinary tract infections, anemia, and **preeclampsia** can prevent serious complications.

The initial visit requires more time than subsequent visits because a thorough history and physical examination are done, including breast, abdominal, pelvic, and vaginal examinations. Pelvic measurements are taken to help ascertain if the pelvis is adequate for a fetus to be delivered vaginally.

The initial visit is followed by monthly visits and then weekly visits beginning at the 28th week, weeks 29–36 every 2 weeks, and at weeks 37–40 weekly. The routine visits consist of checking weight, measuring blood pressure, and testing blood and urine; education about nutrition, activity, and rest; and preparing for childbirth (see Procedure 14-1). Data are entered into the computer each time the patient has an appointment (Figure 14-2). They include findings from the provider's examination, vital signs, weight, blood and urine tests, and patient education for preparing for childbirth. Data are retrievable for comparison purposes and treatment options.

Many groups of women do not receive prenatal care. Lack of financial resources, insurance, or transportation and poor communication by health care providers are some of the reasons that some women do not participate in prenatal care. Modesty may deter some women from seeking prenatal care. Exposing the body to a man is viewed as a major violation of modesty in some cultures. This is why protecting the privacy of all patients is critical.

HIPAA

Cultural differences are another reason to keep the Health Insurance Portability and Accountability Act (HIPAA) regulation in mind. During pregnancy, some women's cultures demand modesty, and protecting their privacy is critical. Infertility is a **stigma** in some cultures. Maintaining confidentiality is a requirement of HIPAA for all patients.

The patient's partner may be unaware of the patient's obstetrical history such as previous pregnancies, abortion, or sexually transmitted diseases. Confidentiality is of utmost importance, and it is best to be alone with the patient when obtaining this type of medical information.

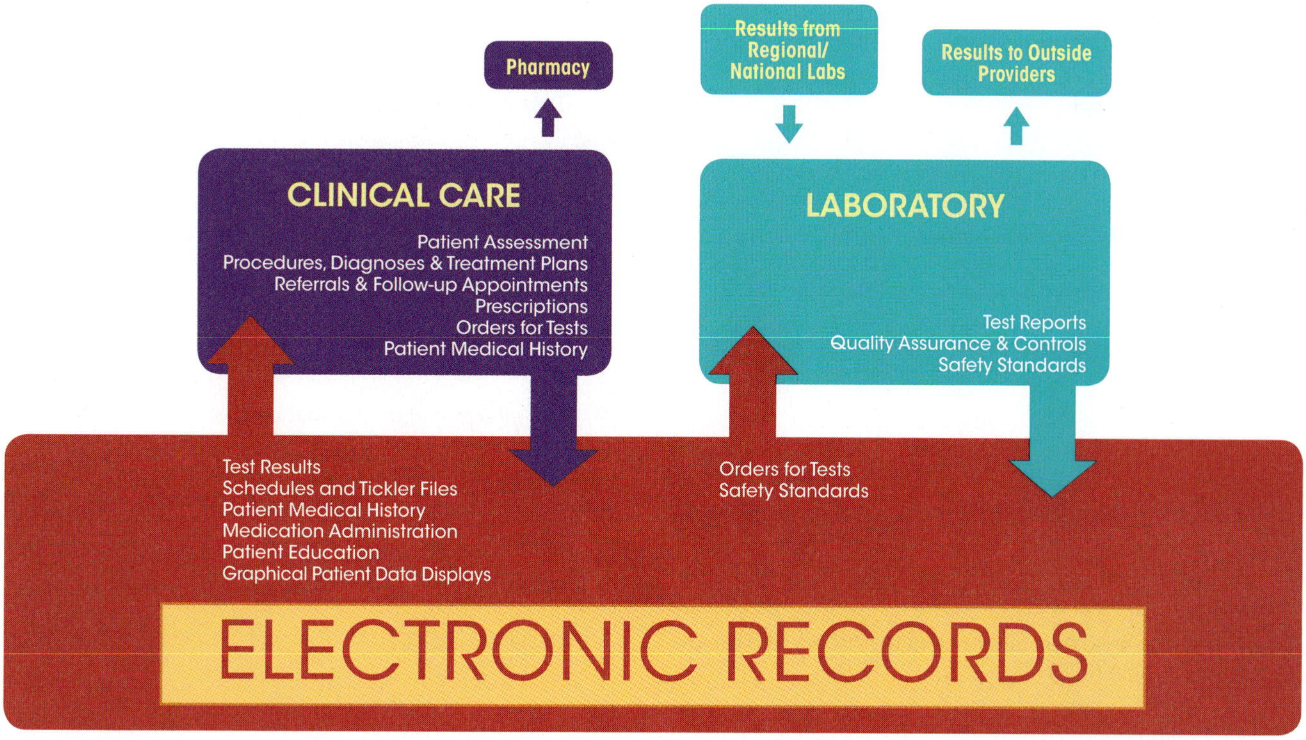

Figure 14-2 Clinical care and laboratory arms of the total practice management system data flow.

Certain cultures expect their women to observe practices believed to ensure a favorable pregnancy. Mexican women are advised not to watch an eclipse of the moon; the belief is that the baby will be born with congenital anomalies. Some Spanish women in the United States wear a braided cord around the midsection to ward off nausea and to ensure safe birth. Medals and beads, often worn by women, are believed to ward off evil spirits. Other cultures believe that inactivity during pregnancy will safeguard the mother and baby. There are also many dietary influences within different cultures. (Chapter 22 gives more information on culture, diet, and food choices.) Respect for all cultures is of great importance, and judgments should not be made that some women are ignorant or lazy. Incorporating customs and beliefs demonstrates that you value cultural diversity and women's self-esteem.

All women should be fully involved in their care. Women with physical or emotional disabilities must have their particular needs addressed. When necessary, make adaptations whenever possible for women who are mentally challenged, blind, deaf, or physically incapacitated.

Laboratory Tests. The laboratory tests and procedures that may be part of the initial prenatal visit are described in Table 14-1.

Patient Education

Whatever the pregnant woman ingests or inhales affects the fetus. Smoking during pregnancy poses serious risks to mother and fetus. Low birth weight, placenta abruptio, and deliveries before term are some of the possible effects to the fetus. Lung cancer, emphysema, and cardiovascular disease can affect the mother. Other kinds of substance abuse such as alcohol, cocaine, and other recreational drugs are commonly seen in pregnant women who are abused, such as in a domestic abuse situation; however, women do not have to be in an abusive situation to abuse drugs or alcohol. Ask the patient if she is in immediate danger. If so, a referral can be made to a community resource (e.g., women's shelter, hotline phone number, district attorney's office) or the provider can help devise a safety plan until the community resource steps in to help. (Chapters 7 and 23 provide more information about domestic violence and drug abuse.)

Patient Education. Patient education includes such topics as nutrition, dental care, rest, and exercise, as well as discussion about over-the-counter

Table 14-1 Laboratory Tests at the Initial Prenatal Visit

Laboratory Test	Disease or Condition
Complete blood count (CBC), hemoglobin, and hematocrit	To detect anemia or infection
Urinalysis with microscopic examination (pH, specific gravity, color, glucose, albumin, proteins, white and red blood cell counts, casts, acetone, **human chorionic gonadotropin** [HCG])	To screen for diabetes mellitus, renal disease, infection, hypertensive disease, pregnancy
Blood type, Rh factor	To detect Rh incompatibility
Rubella **titer**	To determine immunity to rubella
Renal function Alpha-fetoprotein (if initial visit is at 16-18 weeks gestation)	To evaluate renal impairment in women with history of diabetes mellitus, hypertension, or kidney disease
Tuberculin skin test	To screen for tuberculosis
Venereal Disease Research Laboratory (VDRL) and rapid plasma reagin (RPR)	To detect syphilis
Human Immunodeficiency Virus (HIV) with patient permission	To screen for HIV antibodies
Hepatitis B and C virus	To screen for hepatitis B and C viruses
Blood glucose	To screen for gestational diabetes
Cardiac evaluation electrocardiogram (ECG), chest radiograph, or echocardiogram	To evaluate cardiac function in women with history of heart disease or hypertension
Pap smear	To check for cervical dysplasia, herpes simplex virus 2
Vaginal, cervical, or rectal smear or culture for gonorrhea, chlamydia, and *Streptococcus* group B	To check for gonorrhea, chlamydia, human papilloma virus (HPV)

(OTC) remedies, prescription medications, and herbal products (Figure 14-3). Alcohol and tobacco and their dangers and potential harm to fetus and mother should also be discussed. Medications, alcohol, cigarettes, and mind-altering substances taken by the mother have harmful effects on the fetus and should not be used.

Before the birth, the expectant couple is encouraged to choose a method of feeding the infant. During the initial prenatal visit, benefits of breast-feeding the newborn are discussed. If the mother is HIV negative, breast-feeding is encouraged because it offers many nutritional, psychological, and immunologic benefits. Because the immune system of newborns is not fully developed, the high level of immunoglobulins in breast milk gives them protection against some

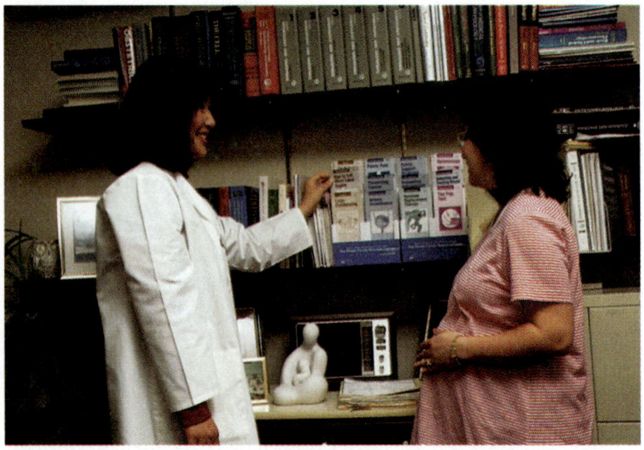

Figure 14-3 Supplying patients with information on a healthy pregnancy and potential risks and danger signs is an important responsibility of the medical assistant.

pathogenic diseases of the respiratory and gastrointestinal tracts. Close contact between mother and newborn is certain with breast-feeding, and bonding can readily take place. Breast-fed infants seem to have fewer allergic reactions. For the mother, one benefit of breast-feeding is that the uterus **involutes,** or returns more quickly to the nonpregnant state. Breast-feeding is the optimal way to feed a newborn. The services of a lactation consultant (available in most women's hospitals and some pediatric offices) can be helpful especially during the initial phase of breast-feeding. The consultant can provide hands-on instructions to the patient to optimize the experience for the mother and baby.

Formal childbirth education classes given in various languages teach the fundamentals of labor, delivery, and newborn care and feeding.

Prenatal History. The prenatal history will be comprehensive and include much of the same information that is obtained during the taking of a regular medical history. However, emphasis will be on identification of the high-risk patient. Particular attention is given to women who have a history of one or more of the following situations or conditions because they may place a woman and her fetus at greater risk during pregnancy:

- Use of legal drugs (OTC, prescription, tobacco, caffeine, alcohol), illegal drugs (marijuana, cocaine), and herbal products
- Age under 16 or over 35 years
- Rh-negative blood
- A history of repeated premature labors and deliveries, abortions, or stillbirths
- Genetic diseases in the family
- Previous **Cesarean section**
- Diabetes
- Hypothyroidism or hyperthyroidism
- Sexually transmitted disease
- Hypertension
- Nutritional deficiencies
- Cardiac problems
- Kidney conditions
- Epilepsy
- Headaches

Any of these conditions or diseases can place the woman and fetus at risk for serious complications.

During the initial prenatal visit, an obstetrical history is taken, which includes the **gravidity,** or total number of pregnancies, including the present pregnancy, regardless of duration. The history also includes the **parity,** the number of pregnancies carried to the point of viability regardless of whether the baby was born alive or dead. Multiple births, twins, and triplets count as one pregnancy (gravida) and one delivery (para). For example, a woman pregnant for the first time is referred to as Gravida 1, Para 0. After this woman delivers, regardless if the baby is born alive or dead, if it reached the age of **viability,** the history of the woman is Gravida 1, Para 1. Viability is the ability to grow and develop after birth. The term **multigravida** refers to a woman who has been pregnant more than once. **Nullipara** describes a woman who has not carried a pregnancy to viability.

Para sometimes has four letters that can be used to give more information about past deliveries. It does *not* include the present pregnancy. The four letters are FPAL:

F—number of full-term deliveries (37–40 weeks' gestation)

P—number of preterm or premature deliveries (20–36 weeks' gestation)

A—number of abortions (induced or spontaneous terminations before 20 weeks' gestation)

L—number of living children born to the patient who are still alive at the time of history data collection

For example, a woman has had four term pregnancies, delivered four live infants, but lost a child to leukemia at 7 years of age. This women is considered to be 4-0-0-3.

The present prenatal history includes information about the present pregnancy. The provider searches for problems indicative of high-risk factors. Identifying high-risk patients helps to limit maternal and newborn deaths and diseases. Some factors that indicate a patient is at high risk are inadequate nutrition; use of drugs such as alcohol, tobacco, or cocaine; existing medical conditions such as high blood pressure or diabetes; sexually transmitted disease; and poverty. The provider watches for signs and symptoms that indicate a potentially serious condition. Examples are listed in Table 14-2.

Subsequent or Return Prenatal Visits

Subsequent visits include weight, blood pressure, urinalysis, complete blood count with hemoglobin and hematocrit, measurement of the height of the uterine fundus (a tape measure is used by placing it on the anterior symphysis pubis and the crest of

Table 14-2 Signs and Symptoms of Potentially Serious Conditions

Signs and Symptoms	Possible Condition
Rapid weight gain	Preeclampsia
Headaches	Preeclampsia
Hypertension	Preeclampsia
Vision changes	Preeclampsia
Severe nausea and vomiting	Hyperemesis gravidarum/dehydration
Bleeding, discharge, abdominal pain/cramping	Threatened abortion, placenta previa, placenta abruptio
Edema	Preeclampsia
One-sided pelvic or abdominal pain	**Ectopic** pregnancy (Figure 14-4)
Chills, fever	Vaginal infection, sexually transmitted disease, other infections

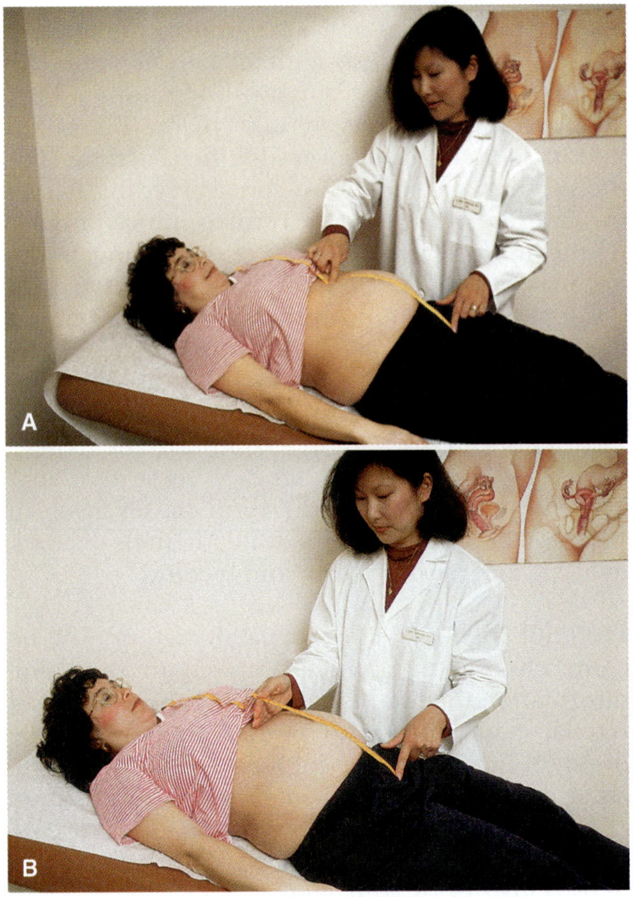

Figure 14-5 Fundal height is measured by placing the end of the tape at the symphysis pubis and extending it in either a (A) curved or (B) straight pattern to the fundus.

the uterus) (Figure 14-5), and fetal heart measurements (Figure 14-6). Generally, it is not possible to determine with accuracy the exact date of conception. Many formulas have been used for calculating the EDB (expected date of birth) or EDC (expected date of confinement). Although none is foolproof, **Nägele's rule** is the usual method used because it is reasonably accurate. Nägele's rule is to add 7 days to the first day of the last menstrual period (LMP), subtract 3 months, and add 1 year. An example is:

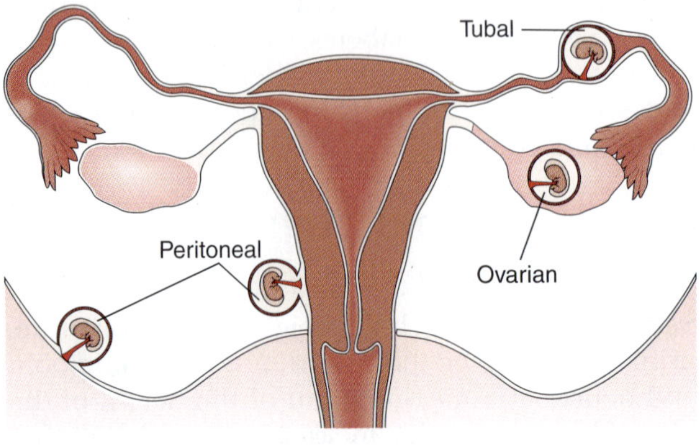

Figure 14-4 Sites of ectopic pregnancy.

The first day of LMP = July 10, 2007
Add 7 days = July 17
Subtract 3 months = April 17
Add 1 year = April 17, 2008

Another method to calculate EDB or EDC is to add 7 days to LMP and count forward 9 months. Most women give birth within 7 days before or after the EDB or EDC.

Pregnancy wheels help determine the EDC. Line up the arrow of the first day of the LMP, then read off the date that corresponds to the 40-week designation (Figure 14-7).

Vaginal examinations are only done periodically up to 2 to 3 weeks before the EDB or EDC. Patients are encouraged to attend classes in the **Lamaze** method of childbirth, as well as classes in the care of the newborn (Figures 14-8 through 14-10).

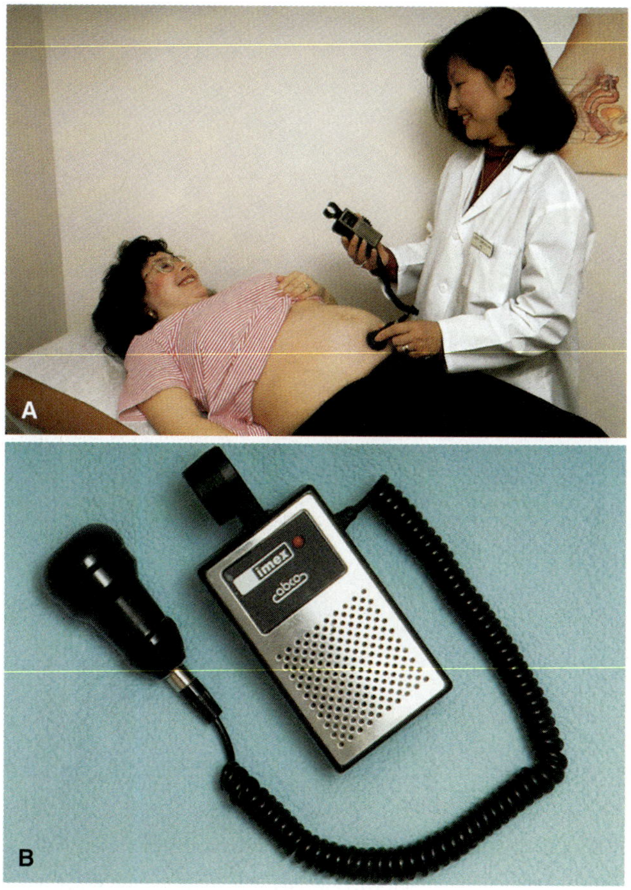

Figure 14-6 (A) Fetal heart tones are measured with a handheld Doppler. (B) Handheld Doppler.

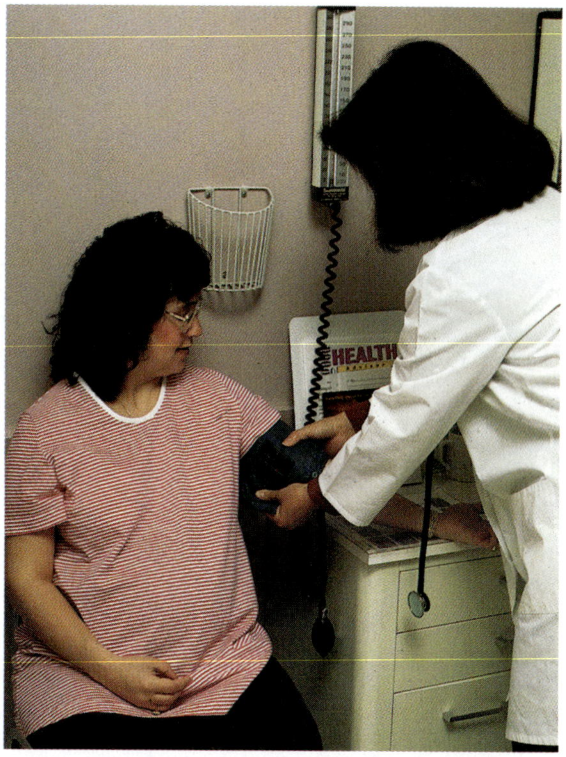

Figure 14-8 Blood pressure is measured at each prenatal visit.

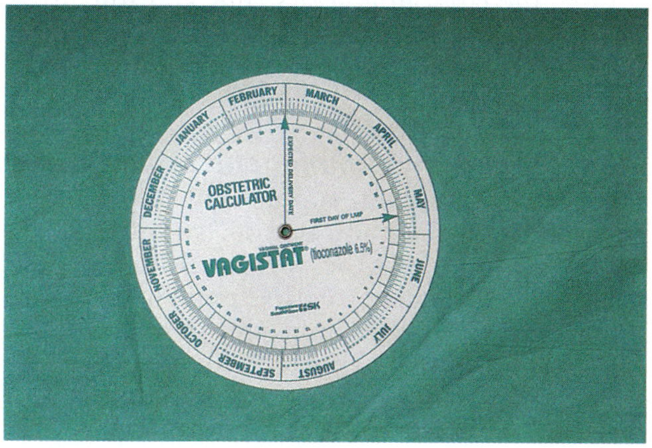

Figure 14-7 Gestation wheel. Place arrow labeled "first day of LMP" on date of last menstrual period (LMP). Read date at arrow labeled "expected delivery date."

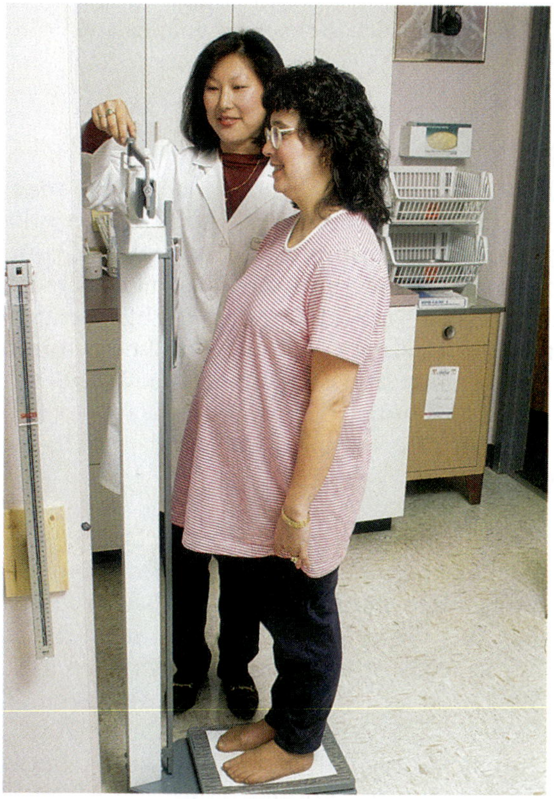

Figure 14-9 Weight gain is tracked throughout the pregnancy.

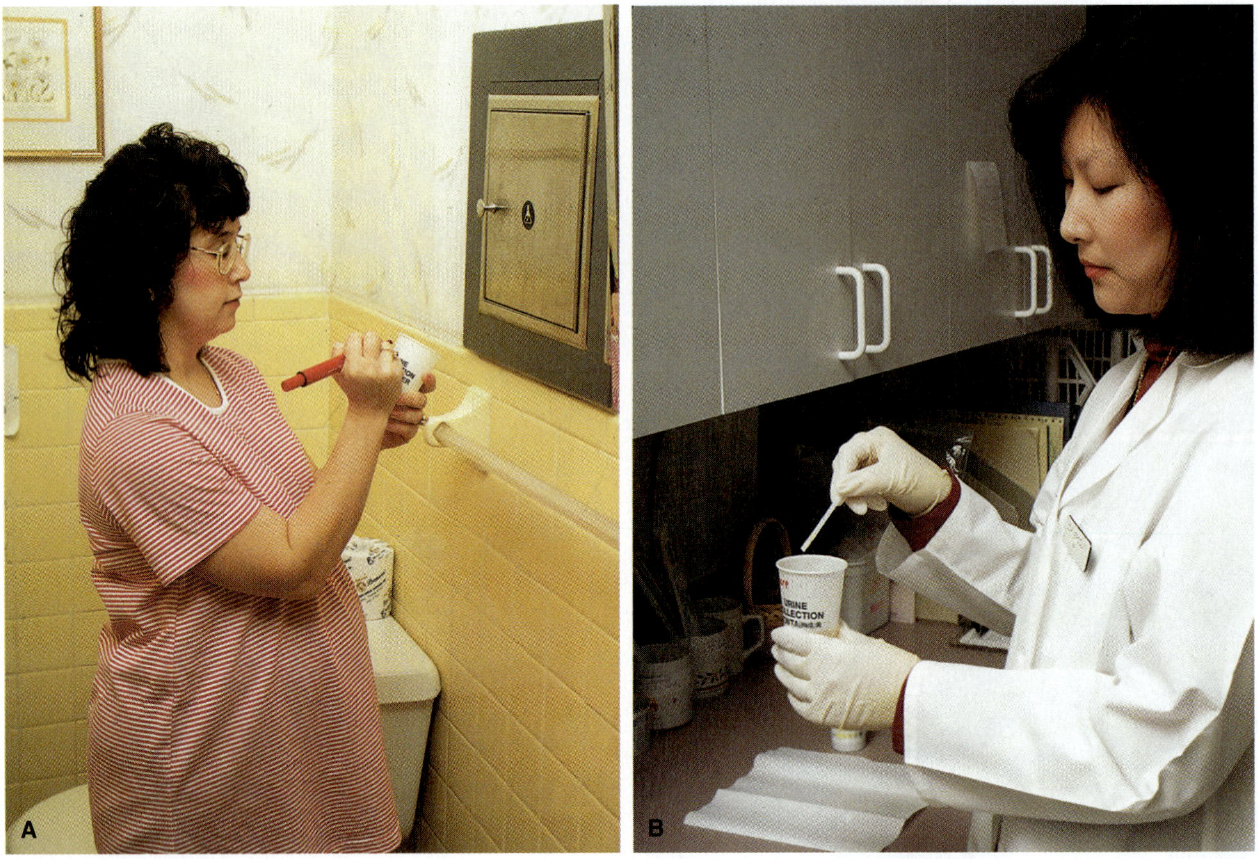

Figure 14-10 Urine is tested for glucose and protein at each visit. (A) Client provides a urine sample. (B) Medical assistant uses dipstick to check for glucose and protein.

Tests and Procedures

Alpha Fetoprotein. Another test that may be done during a subsequent visit is the mother's serum alpha fetoprotein (MSAFP) blood test. It is done about the 16th week of pregnancy. It is a screening test only, done to rule out neural tube defects, abdominal wall defects, and chromosomal problems such as Down syndrome. If the test is positive, additional testing such as an **amniocentesis** or an ultrasound will be used to help make a diagnosis.

Chorionic Villus Sampling (CVS). Chorionic villius sampling (CVS) is a test performed on women who are older than 35 years, have a history of chromosomal abnormalities, and are known carriers of a genetic disorder such as **thalassemia, sickle cell anemia,** or **Tay–Sachs.** The test is done at about 8 to 10 weeks' **gestation** and has an advantage over amniocentesis because the latter cannot be done before the 14th week. In one method of the CVS test, a sample of tissue that surrounds the fetus is taken through a catheter by means of suction. The sample is analyzed in the laboratory for genetic abnormalities. An ultrasonogram is done simultaneously with an amniocentesis to avoid possible injury to the fetus or placenta.

Ultrasonography/Amniocentesis. Two tests can be done that can supply vital information: **ultrasonography,** or ultrasound, and amniocentesis. Ultrasound can be performed in the first, second, or third **trimester.** It uses high-frequency sound waves to produce an image of the fetus. A **coupling agent** is spread onto the mother's abdomen to enhance penetration of sound waves through the tissue, and the scanning mechanism is moved over the abdomen. An image of the fetus can be viewed on a screen similar to a television screen. Photos are taken during the examination. The technique usually takes about a half hour. There are no known side effects to the fetus or mother, and ultrasound uses no X-rays. There is no pain involved, but slight discomfort can occur due to a full bladder. (A quart of fluid should be consumed 1 hour before the test and finished within 15 or 20 minutes.) A full bladder is essential to a good-quality ultrasound because it supports the uterus in position for good imaging. This procedure may be used to identify the number of fetuses, check the age of the fetus (number of weeks gestation), and detect some fetal abnormalities (e.g., Down syndrome; Figure 14-11).

A high-resolution three-dimensional ultrasonographic test is used more and more frequently to check for Down syndrome. The test is useful because it can detect chromosomal abnormalities. It can be done sooner in a pregnancy than blood testing and could minimize the need for CVS or amniocentesis, both of which create risks to the mother and fetus.

An amniocentesis is the surgical puncturing, with a long, thin needle, of the amniotic sac through the woman's abdomen. The purpose of this test is to obtain, by aspiration, a sample of amniotic fluid that contains fetal cells. The procedure can be done as early as 14 weeks and helps to diagnose genetic problems, **congenital anomalies** (present at birth), and chromosomal defects. It also can be used to determine the lung capacity of the fetus (Figure 14-12).

Ultrasonography is performed while the provider is doing the amniocentesis to identify the position of the fetus and placenta, thereby avoiding injury to either. There can be bleeding, leaking of amniotic fluid, and infection.

Percutaneous umbilical blood sampling (PUBS), also known as cordocentesis, is another procedure that can be done. It accesses fetal circulation by aspirating blood from the fetal umbilical cord vessels. Because the procedure is invasive, it is performed in conjunction with ultrasound. Many blood studies can be performed, and many conditions can be diagnosed using fetal cord blood, such as chromosomal abnormalities, infections within the uterus, and fetal hypoxia. Drug therapy and transfusions can be given through the umbilical vein in the fetal umbilical cord.

Fetal heart rate is another test. Monitoring can be done in one of two ways: a nonstress test monitors the fetus's heart rate while it is moving spontaneously, or a stress test monitors the fetal heart rate while the mother is stimulated with medication to have mild uterine contractions. Normally, the fetal heart rate will accelerate to a higher but safe limit while it is being stressed.

EHR Entering data electronically during each visit allows immediate access to the patient's medical record and comparisons of vital signs, laboratory values, ultrasounds, amniocentesis, and all other diagnostic tests and procedures to previous data entries. Baseline values are important, and timing of certain laboratory tests is crucial for accurate evaluation. Providers can refer back to it throughout the pregnancy. The electronic medical record (EMR) is a communication mechanism for organizing a patient's care. All data entry should be dated and include the time and your signature.

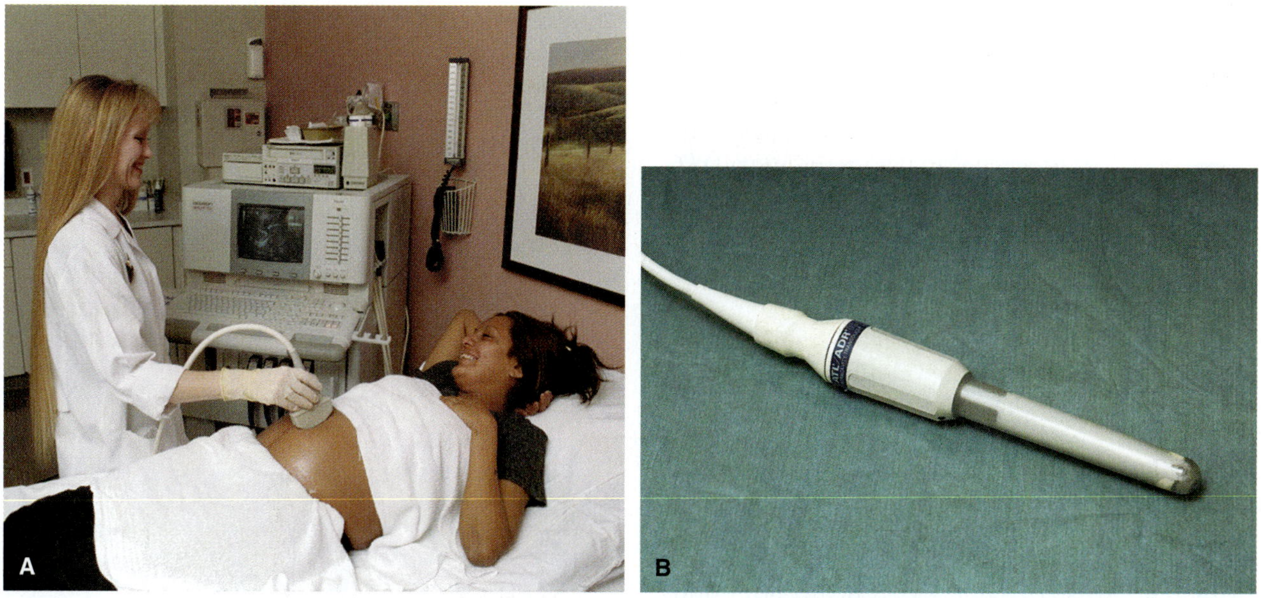

Figure 14-11 (A) Abdominal ultrasound. (B) Transducer for transvaginal ultrasound.

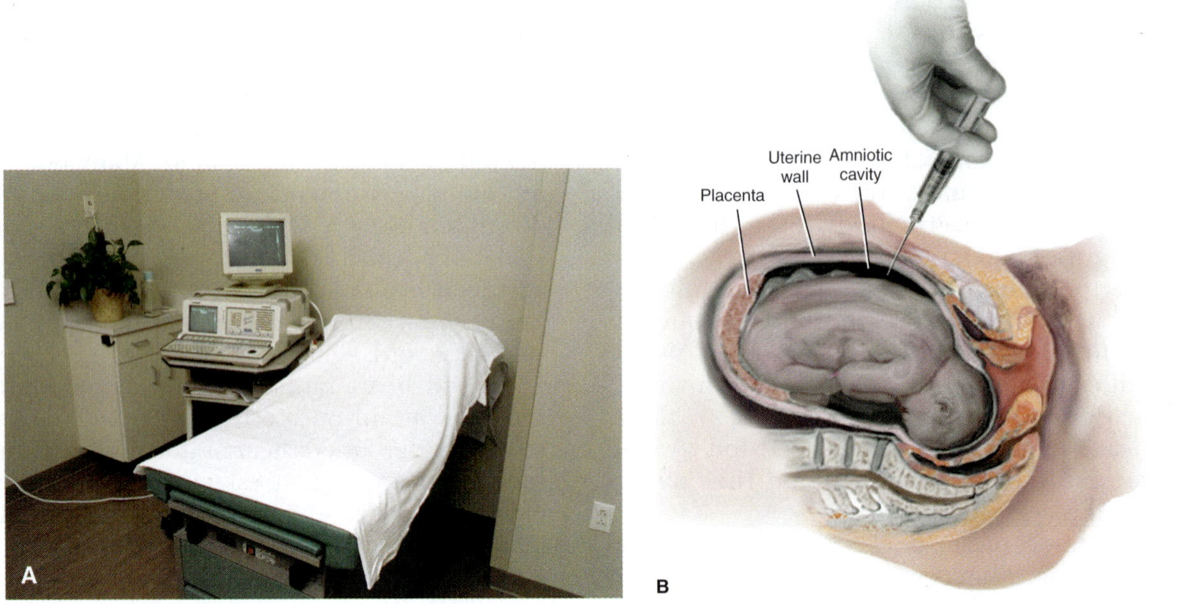

Figure 14-12 (A) An amniocentesis setup. (B) During amniocentesis, a sample of amniotic fluid is aspirated for evaluation. An ultrasonogram is done simultaneously with an amniocentesis to avoid possible injury to the fetus or placenta.

Disorders of Pregnancy

The following sections address some problems that may occur during pregnancy.

Abortion/Interruption of Pregnancy. The interruption of pregnancy before the fetus is viable is known as **abortion.** Six types of abortion are listed here:

1. *Spontaneous:* Unknown etiology (miscarriage)
2. *Complete:* Expulsion of all products of conception, fetus, and placenta with no surgical intervention
3. *Missed:* Fetus dies in the uterus and must be removed; usually a dilation and curettage (D&C) is the surgical procedure performed
4. *Incomplete:* Only parts of the fetus and placenta are expelled. Tissue remains in the uterus and a D&C usually must be performed.
5. *Threatened:* Bleeding from the uterus, but there are no contractions or dilation of cervix. Pregnancy continues.
6. *Induced:* Evacuation of the fetus and placenta from the uterus at the mother's request or because mother's health is in jeopardy.

Eclampsia. **Eclampsia** syndrome, also known as pregnancy-induced hypertension, can occur in pregnancy and result in convulsions unrelated to epilepsy or other brain conditions. It is a potentially life-threatening disorder characterized by hypertension, generalized edema, and proteinuria. It can put the woman and her fetus in grave danger and can be fatal if not treated. Preeclampsia is less severe. The symptoms are the same, except there are no convulsions. This is why weight is measured, blood pressure checked, and a urinalysis (including a check for protein) is routinely performed. Sudden significant weight gain, increase in blood pressure, and the presence of protein in the urine can indicate possible preeclampsia. The cause is unknown. Prophylaxis is of great importance. The problem is seen more often in women who have received inadequate prenatal care, especially poor nutrition, in **primigravida** (pregnant for the first time) younger than 18 years, in women with preexisting cardiovascular and renal conditions, as well as in women who are diabetic.

Gestational Diabetes. Gestational diabetes first appears during the second or third trimester of the pregnancy and usually disappears after the woman has delivered her baby or when the pregnancy terminates for any other reason. This type of diabetes is usually a milder form of the disease. Prompt detection (through blood and urine glucose testing) and

Critical Thinking

A 17-year-old girl has missed her period and has called the clinic describing sharp right quadrant pain. What tests/procedures will help the provider make a diagnosis?

therapy are essential to avoid fetal and **neonatal** (newborn) illness and death.

A blood glucose is drawn 1-hour after the patient is given a high-glucose drink. If the test result is elevated, than a 3-hour glucose tolerance test is done. Prenatal visits for the patient with gestational diabetes requires more frequent visits to the provider. The fetus is evaluated at each visit. Ultrasound evaluation of fetal growth is performed more often. The patient must control her diet and monitor blood glucose levels at home several times daily. A nutritionist will help by teaching the patient about a diabetic diet. The appropriate number of calories and percent of carbohydrates, proteins, and fats are calculated to keep the blood glucose as close to 100 mg/dL as possible. If the diabetic diet does not control blood glucose levels, insulin therapy is started. Usually the patient is admitted to the hospital if she has poorly controlled diabetes and has the additional factor of hypertension.

Pregnant women with gestational diabetes have a strong possibility of developing diabetes within their lifetime. The provider will order a blood glucose (1-hour glucose tolerance) when the woman is 6 to 8 weeks postpartum. The results will determine whether or not the patient's blood glucose level has dropped to the normal range.

Hyperemesis Gravidarum. **Hyperemesis gravidarum,** or excessive vomiting during pregnancy, can be harmful and is more than morning sickness, which is a common complaint during the first trimester. The cause of the condition is not known, but it is thought to be related to the cells that become the placenta and to the production of pregnancy hormones. The symptoms include uncontrollable nausea and vomiting, inability to eat, and exhaustion from inability to sleep. Severe dehydration can result and starvation may ensue. This complication is usually not fatal, but it is a severe problem that warrants immediate treatment. Treatment includes intravenous fluids to replace those lost through vomiting and mild sedation to aid rest and sleep.

Placenta Previa. **Placenta previa** occurs when the placenta implants low in the uterus and partially or completely covers the cervical os. It is an emergency. The cause is unknown. When labor ensues and the cervix begins to dilate, the placenta is pulled away from the wall of the uterus and causes bleeding. On occasion, the bleeding, which comes on suddenly and is painless, will stop spontaneously. If it continues, significant maternal blood is lost, and the fetus may suffer anoxia and die when the placenta separates from the blood supply (Figure 14-13B).

Ultrasonography can determine where the placenta is attached, at which time the diagnosis can be made and treatment begun. Treatment depends on the gestational age of the fetus and the percent of placenta that covers the cervical os. Cesarean section may be necessary to remove the placenta, control bleeding, and deliver the fetus safely.

Some of the factors associated with placenta previa are advanced maternal age, maternal smoking, and cocaine use. Maternal exposure to passive smoke and use of tobacco by the woman have been shown to be risky to the fetus, resulting in lower birth weight, premature birth, and infant death.

Placenta Abruptio. **Placenta abruptio** occurs when the placenta prematurely and abruptly separates from the uterine lining (Figure 14-13A). It

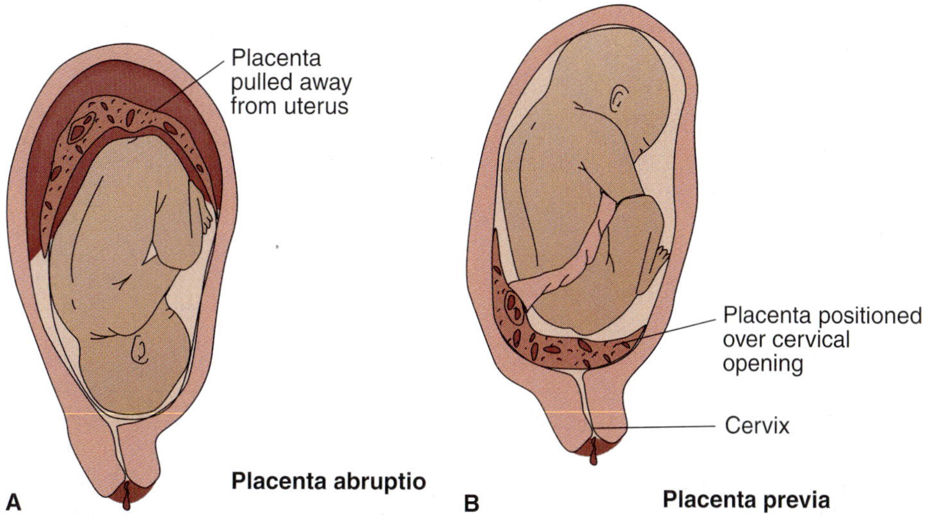

Figure 14-13 (A) Placenta abruptio. (B) Placenta previa.

can result in fetal distress and death and maternal shock and death. It usually occurs late in pregnancy but can occur during labor.

Factors that contribute to this complication are multiple pregnancies, chronic hypertension, trauma to the uterus, and sudden release of amniotic fluid. Delivery as soon as possible either vaginally or by Cesarean section is indicated. The prognosis of the newborn depends on the extent of **hypoxia** suffered during labor and delivery.

The infant should begin to cry and its color turn pink (hands and feet may remain blue for about a week). Abnormalities, if any, are documented. The Apgar score is an indication of the newborn's well-being. Assessments, in numbers from 1 to 10, are made at 1, 5, and 15 minutes. Five aspects of the newborn are evaluated: respiratory ease, heart rate, skin color, reflexes, and muscle tone. Each is assigned a number, which added together determines the newborn's Apgar score. The closer to 10 the score is, the closer the newborn is adapting to life outside the uterus. A lower score indicates a problem with the newborn's respirations, heart rate, color, and muscle tone. Oxygen and other measures may be necessary to stabilize a newborn with a low Apgar score.

Impaired Fertility. The inability to conceive and bear a child after a period of unprotected sex is known as impaired fertility. One reason for this problem is that couples delay pregnancy until later in life when fertility is naturally lower. The increase in the incidence of **pelvic inflammatory disease** (PID), endometriosis, substance abuse, and environmental factors such as pesticides and lead all can contribute to impaired fertility.

Diagnosis and treatment of impaired fertility requires a physical, emotional, and financial investment over a long period. To diagnose impaired fertility in the female patient, a complete history and physical examination are performed. Endocrine system and anatomic and physiologic abnormalities are sought. Laboratory tests on urine and blood are performed. Proof of ovulation can be determined by retrieving an ovum from the uterine tube, performing an endometrial biopsy, assessing mucus characteristics, and taking the basal body temperature. Levels of estrogen, progesterone, follicle-stimulating hormone, and lutenizing hormone are also measured. A **hysterosalpingogram,** a radiograph of the uterus and tubes after the injection of dye, reveals defects in either the uterus or tubes.

Laparoscopy can be performed to visualize the internal pelvic structures. Tubal patency, **endometriosis,** pelvic adhesions, or **polycystic** ovaries can be seen. Endometrial biopsy is done to examine the tissue and determine whether the endometrium is capable of accepting a fertilized ovum for implantation. Ultrasonography, either abdominal or transvaginal, can assess pelvic organs for abnormalities.

Tests that can be performed on a male to diagnose impaired fertility are semen analysis, hormone analysis, and biopsy of a testicle.

Once a diagnosis of impaired fertility has been made, a number of therapies are available to assist in reproduction. This is known as assisted reproductive technology (ART).

- In vitro fertilization (IVF), indicated for fallopian tube blockage and endometriosis: Eggs are retrieved from the woman's ovaries, fertilized with sperm from her partner in the laboratory, then transferred to her uterus.
- Gamete intrafallopian transfer (GIFT): Eggs are retrieved from the woman's ovaries. An egg and sperm from her partner are aspirated into a special catheter, then placed into the fallopian tube where fertilization may occur naturally.
- In vitro fertilization and gamete intrafallopian transfer (IVF + GIFT) with donor sperm: Eggs are retrieved from the woman's ovaries, fertilized with donor sperm in the laboratory, aspirated into a special catheter, then placed into the fallopian tube where fertilization may take place naturally.

Patient Education

Alcohol Exposure

Alcohol along with tobacco exposure during pregnancy is common. Drinking during pregnancy is the leading cause of childhood mental retardation. Two or more drinks a day while a woman is pregnant increases the risk of the newborn being born with fetal alcohol syndrome (FAS). Birth defects include small brain size, growth retardation, specific facial deformities (e.g., flat middle of the face, wide bridge of the nose, thin upper lip), and heart, kidney, and eye abnormalities. Behavioral problems (e.g., learning and attention difficulties, hyperactivity) occur. No safe amount of alcohol can be consumed during pregnancy, so abstention from all alcohol is necessary.

New technology allows retrieval sperm from the testicles if ejaculation is impossible. Sperm can be injected into the ovum, embryos can be frozen, and surrogate pregnancies are possible. With technology come the ethical and legal questions of donor eggs and embryos, pregnancies in older adult women, how to define who the parents are, what to do with frozen embryos after death or divorce, and other issues such as disposal of unused (extra) embryos.

In some cultures, a woman is deemed the responsible party for impaired fertility, and the impairment is thought to be caused by her sins, evil spirits, or her own deficiencies. The virility of a male is questioned unless he is able to manifest his sexual potency by having a child.

Incompatibility. The pregnant woman's blood type and Rh factor are determined at the first prenatal visit. If the woman has Rh-negative blood and the fetus has Rh-positive blood, problems can occur. When the fetus's blood (red blood cells) leak into the woman's body during birth, an Rh-negative woman may develop antibodies against the fetus's Rh-positive blood. The antibodies can pass through the placenta and kill the RBCs in the fetus. The fetus becomes anemic and jaundiced. Death of the fetus is possible if too much fetal blood is destroyed. When an injection of Rh-immune globulin (RhoGAM) is given at around the 28th week of pregnancy and 72 hours postpartum, and after percutaneous umbilical blood sampling (PUBS), CVS, abortion, or amniocentesis, then sensitization is prevented. Rh incompatibility should not occur with any subsequent pregnancy. RhoGAM must be given after every birth, abortion, miscarriage, amniocentesis, CVS, and PUBS to prevent sensitization.

Parturition

Parturition, or labor, is the process during which the uterus, through contractions, expels the fetus and placenta. There are three stages of labor:

- Stage I—Dilation: from onset of labor until complete **dilation** (expansion) and **effacement** (thinning and shortening) of cervix
- Stage II—Expulsion: from complete dilation and effacement through the birth of fetus (expulsion)
- Stage III—Placental: from birth of fetus through expulsion of the placenta

Labor is believed to be triggered by the release of **oxytocin** and **prostaglandins** after the level of other hormones decreases. When the oxytocin is released, it causes the muscles of the uterus to contract. **Braxton–Hicks** contractions, often referred to as false labor, can usually be differentiated from real labor because of their irregularity and tendency to disappear when the woman moves about and changes positions. When the woman is lying in supine position, the heavy, large uterus can press on the inferior vena cava and aorta, reducing blood flow back to the heart. The patient becomes pale, sweaty, and dizzy, and blood pressure drops. The condition is known as **supine hypotension**. When the patient is turned onto her side, the pressure on the vena cava is removed and the hypotension resolves.

If fetal membranes do not spontaneously rupture during labor, an **amniotomy** (artificial rupture of the membranes) can be done. The procedure uses a sterile amniohook, and it may shorten the length of labor (Figure 14-14).

Signs and symptoms to watch for during labor that indicate complications are heavy vaginal bleeding, sudden increase or decrease in blood pressure, increased activity by the fetus, headache, extreme restlessness, and visual changes. **Meconium,** the first stool of the newborn, in the vaginal discharge can indicate fetal distress.

Postpartum Period

The postpartum period is the time known as the puerperium during which the body returns to its nonpregnant state. It is usually 4 to 6 weeks after

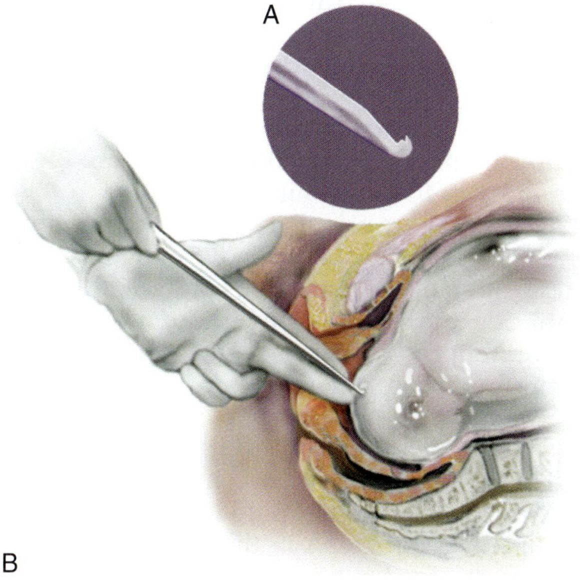

Figure 14-14 (A) Disposable amniohook used to rupture membranes. (B) Amniotomy technique.

delivery. The body undergoes changes during this time. The uterus involutes (returns to normal size) and healing of any injuries takes place.

A vaginal discharge, known as **lochia,** appears during the puerperium. It consists of tissue, blood, white blood cells, mucus, and bacteria. It can be described by its appearance. Lochia rubra is bright red and appears the first 3 days after delivery. Lochia serosa is pink or brown and is indicative of less blood. By about 10 days, the flow decreases, becomes whitish-yellow, and is known as lochia alba. Lochia usually disappears by the third week postpartum but may last for up to 6 weeks. Menstruation usually begins in a nursing mother 3 to 6 months after delivery, 2 months for nonnursing mothers. The mother is told to avoid heavy lifting, not to become fatigued, to eat a well-balanced diet, and to continue to take her prenatal tablets. Report any feelings of depression as soon as possible. An appointment in 6 weeks will evaluate the mother's general health, and the provider will discuss infant care, breast-feeding, the importance of exercise, good nutrition, and birth control. The medical assistant can stress the importance of yearly Pap smears and of monthly breast self-examinations because these are important aspects of patient education.

Contraception. Voluntary prevention of pregnancy is known as contraception. The opportune time to discuss contraception with the mother is soon after delivery and before discharge from the hospital. She should know what method of contraception she and her partner will use before resuming sexual activity. To discuss contraception at the 6-week postpartum checkup can be too late. Sexually transmitted disease (STD) protection should also be reviewed before discharge.

Written instructions about methods of contraception are important and help the patient understand options that are available.

Some nonprescription kinds of contraception are the various barrier methods: condoms; male (latex) and female (nonlatex); contraceptive foam; spermicide (nonoxynol-9) used with a condom to help prevent STDs; vaginal sponges that contain a spermicide; and abstinence.

Many types of prescription contraceptives are available (see Figures 14-15 to 14-19 and Table 14-3). They include hormonal contraception in the form of oral birth control pills; Implanon®, a surgical implant of progestin in the upper arm, which provides up to 3 years of contraception; a diaphragm used with a spermicide; a cervical cap to fit over the cervix; an intrauterine device (a small device made of copper or progesterone-medicated plastic; see Procedure 14-3); and vaginal rings.

Sterilization is a surgical procedure that renders the individual infertile. The woman's uterine tubes are **fulgarated** (destroyed by means of an electric current) or bands and clips are placed around the tubes to block them (ligation). Both fulgaration and ligation are considered to be permanent methods. Female sterilization can be performed immediately after giving birth or any time afterward during any phase of the menstrual cycle. Laparoscopic surgery is the usual approach. Tubal ligation and oral contraceptives are the top contraceptive choices in the United States (Figure 14-20).

The surgical procedure performed on a male to render him sterile is a vasectomy. It can be performed on an outpatient basis under localanesthesia. Small incisions are made into the scrotum above and to the side of each testicle. Each vas deferens is identified, ligated twice, and then severed (Figure 14-21). It is important for the patient to realize that sterility is not immediate because some sperm remain in the sperm ducts after vasectomy. One week to several months may elapse before the ducts are sperm free. Some form of contraception is necessary until two consecutive sperm counts are zero.

Another method of contraception approved by the Food and Drug Administration (FDA) is a medication known as RU-486, which is used to cause or induce an abortion. It's safety has been questioned by experts. Injectable contraceptives are available. Depo-Provera® is given intramuscularly every 3 months. Lunelle® is given intramuscularly monthly. These injectables are best given within the first 5 days of the menstrual cycle to be certain the woman is not pregnant. The majority of states mandate that health insurance cover the cost of contraception.

GYNECOLOGY

Gynecology is the specialty that studies diseases of the female reproductive tract and the breasts. The gynecologic examination is routinely performed in an office or clinic. It usually includes abdominal, pelvic, and breast examination and a Pap smear. It can be done as part of the female's complete physical examination, or it can be a separate examination performed in the gynecologist's office or gynecology clinic. Early diagnosis and treatment of problems associated with the female reproductive organs help the female to achieve optimum health of these organs and is the goal of the OB/GYN provider (Figure 14-22).

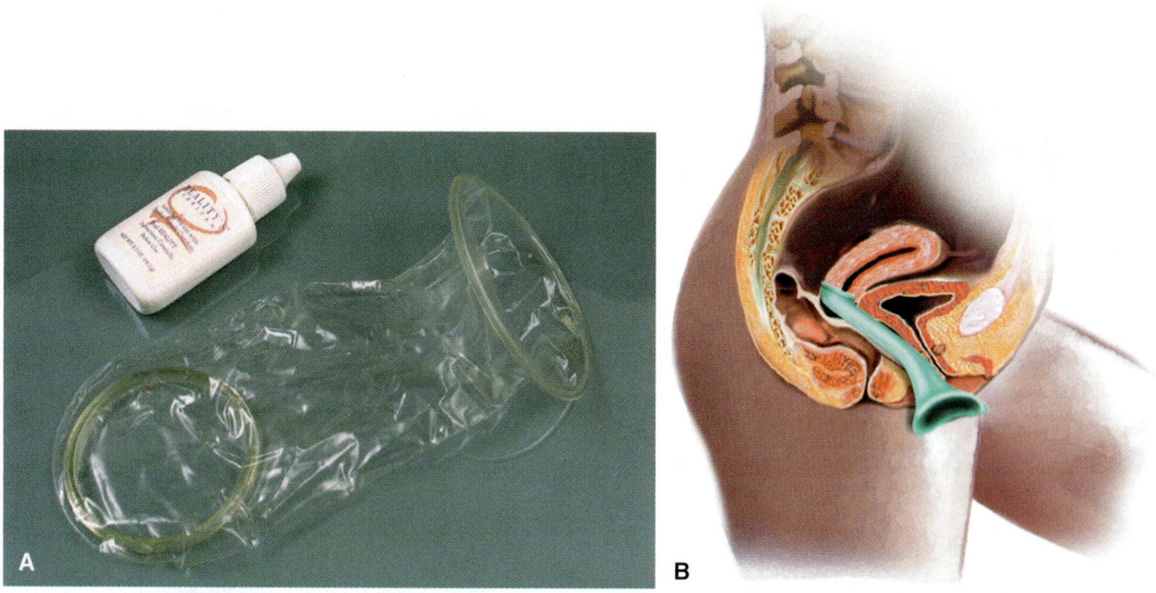

Figure 14-15 (A) Female condom. (B) Proper insertion of female condom.

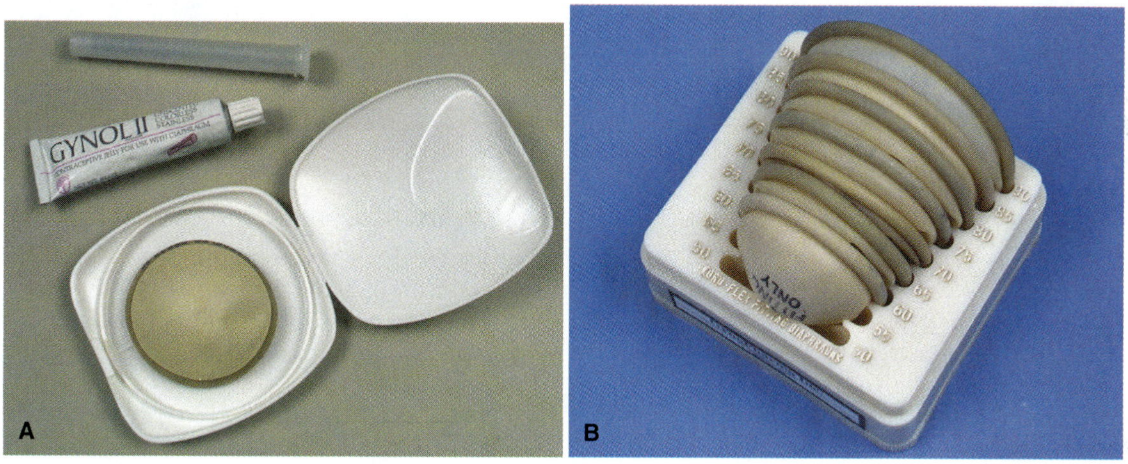

Figure 14-16 (A) Diaphragm with contraceptive jelly. (B) Various sizes of diaphragms. They must be fitted by the provider.

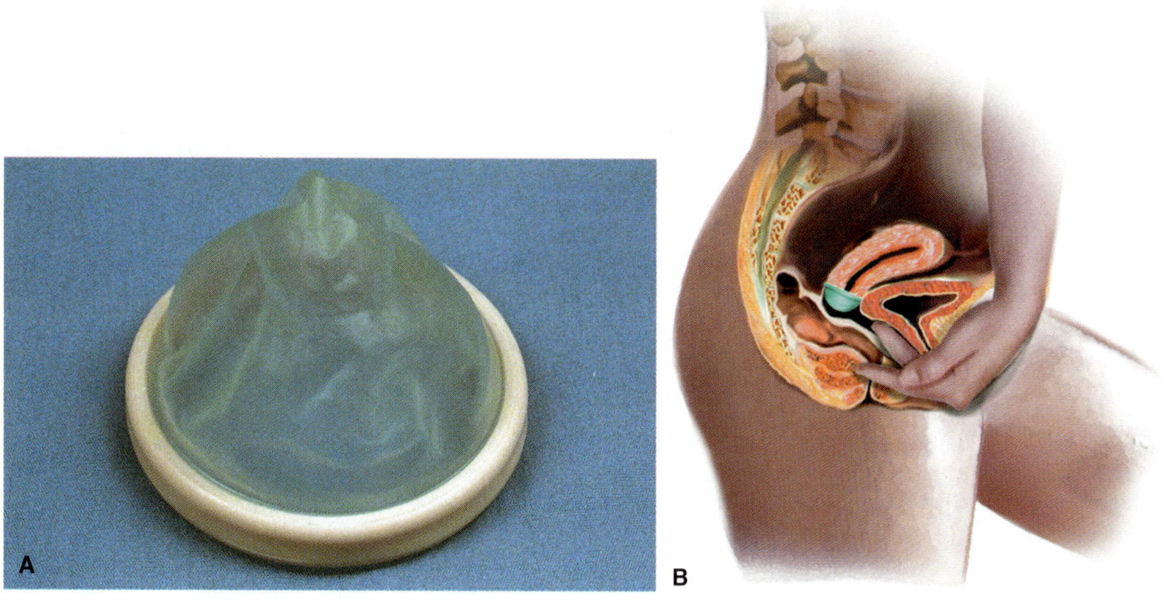

Figure 14-17 (A) Cervical cap. (B) Proper insertion of cervical cap.

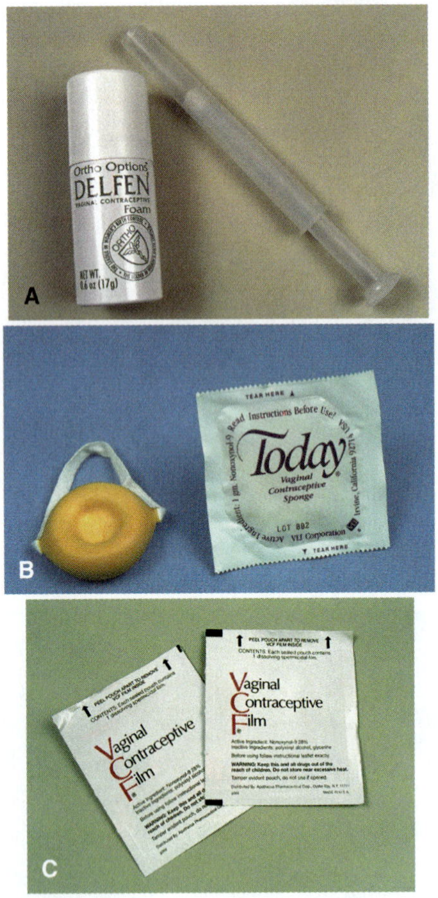

Figure 14-18 Spermicides. (A) Foam. (B) Sponge. (C) Film.

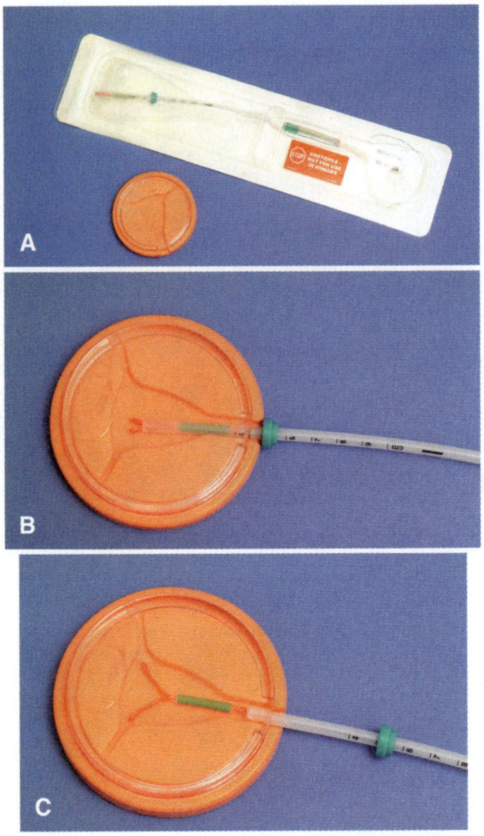

Figure 14-19 (A) Intrauterine device (IUD) and plastic uterus for patient education. (B, C) A plastic uterus can be used to demonstrate proper insertion and placement of IUD during a patient education session.

Table 14-3 Various Contraception (Birth Control) Methods

Method	Description	Effectiveness	Mechanism of Action
Barrier (over-the-counter condom) (see Figure 14-15)	Male and female condoms available. Male condoms are latex; female condoms are nonlatex.	Less effective than hormonal methods or IUD. Use with spermicide. Use to protect from STDs.	Inhibits sperm from entering the vagina. Used only once. To prevent STD and pregnancy, use a condom and another method of contraception.
Diaphragm (prescription needed) (see Figure 14-16)	Use with spermicide. Must be measured and fitted by provider. Fits up against the cervical opening so that cervix is within the cap.	Moderately effective if used correctly. Must fit perfectly. Spermicide is placed inside and around the diaphragm. Must remain in place for 6 hours after intercourse. Will last for years if cared for properly.	Provides barrier between sperm and opening to cervix.
Cervical cap (must be fitted by provider) (see Figure 14-17)	Made of rubber. Fitted to cover the cervix. Folded to insert into the vagina. Must be applied to cervix. Suction keeps the cap in place. Use with spermicide.	Moderately effective if used correctly, similar to diaphragm. Potential for infection because cap can be left in place up to 2 days. Must remain at least 6 hours after intercourse.	Provides rubber barrier between sperm and opening to cervix.

(continues)

Table 14-3 Various Contraception (Birth Control) Methods (continued)

Method	Description	Effectiveness	Mechanism of Action
Spermicide sponge foam cream/gel (over the counter) (see Figure 14-18)	Chemical known as nonoxynol-9.	When used alone, failure rate is high compared to other methods. Used with condom, diaphragm, or cervical cap, it is more effective. No bathing or douching for 6 hours after intercourse. Must allow 15 minutes before engaging in intercourse. Reapply spermicide with repeated intercourse.	Destroys sperm cells.
Hormonal pills (prescription needed for all hormonal contraceptives)	Various combinations of estrogen and progestin or progestin only.	Highest effectiveness rate when taken correctly. Can help reduce dysmenorrheal and heavy menses.	Prevents ovulation every month.
Injection	Intramuscular injection (Depo-Provera®) every 3 months. Lunelle®, injected once per month.	Highly effective. One of most effective contraceptives. Best given within first 5 days of menstrual period to be sure patient is not pregnant.	Prevents ovulation for 3 months. Stops ovulation for 1 month.
Patch	Applied to body and contraceptive is absorbed through the skin.	Highly effective. Worn for 1 week and then replaced same day of week for 3 consecutive weeks. Fourth week patch free.	Prevents ovulation for 1 month.
Vaginal ring	Small flexible ring inserted into the vagina. Releases steady flow of hormones. Left in for 3 weeks. Removed for 1 week.	Highly effective.	Prevents ovulation.
Lybrel* Seasonique*	Continuous contraception. No menstrual cycles for indefinite time period. Breakthrough bleeding possible. Continuous contraception for 3 months.	Effective. Highly effective.	Prevents ovulation. Reduces mood swings, migraines, and premenstrual syndrome (PMS). Prevents ovulation for 3 months.
Intrauterine device (IUD) (must be inserted by provider) (see Figure 14-19; Procedure 14-3).	T-shaped device made of copper. Good for 10 years. A second T-shaped device good for 1 year. Mirena® is an IUD that releases hormones. Remains in place for 5 years. To prevent STDs, IUDs should be used in conjunction with a condom.	Both highly effective. One of the most effective contraceptives.	Copper slowly released into uterus and kills sperm. Hormones in Mirena® cause thickening of the mucus in the cervix, so sperm cannot reach the ovum.

(continues)

Table 14-3 Various Contraception (Birth Control) Methods (continued)

Method	Description	Effectiveness	Mechanism of Action
Implantable (must be implanted by provider)	Device known as Implanon® is composed of one rod that is implanted. Lasts up to 3 years. Minor surgical procedure is required to implant and remove.	Highly effective. One of the most effective contraceptives.	Inhibits ovulation and changes the cervical and endometrial mucus.
	Essure® is a spring-like device implanted in fallopian tubes via the cervix.	Becomes more effective as scar tissue grows thicker. Use another form of contraceptive for at least 3 months.	Implanted device causes scar tissue to build up within the fallopian tubes, eventually blocking them. When blocked, neither sperm nor ovum can pass through.
Tubal ligation or hysterectomy (permanent method) (performed when the woman has a gynecologic problem that requires surgery and she wants permanent sterilization)	Sterilization procedure performed in which the fallopian tubes are tied or bands and/or clips are placed around the tubes to block them (ligation). The tubes can also be burned with electrocautery.	Considered permanent, but there is a small failure rate.	Fallopian tubes are severed and/or burned, banded, and/or clipped. Because fallopian tubes now are incapable of transporting either sperm or ovum, fertilization is not possible.
	Hysterectomy is the surgical removal of the uterus.	Permanent sterilization.	Uterus is surgically removed.
Family planning	Ovulation prediction (rhythm method). The woman charts her temperature and her changes in vaginal mucus and abstains from intercourse during the time she is ovulating (as predicted by temperature and mucus changes)	Can be effective if done correctly. However, method must be used consistently and the woman must realize that she may ovulate on a different day each month or at another time.	Prevents conception by avoiding intercourse during the period of ovulation.
Emergency contraception (**postcoital** contraception) also called Preven® or plan B (over the counter for age 18 and over, prescription if under 18)	Prevents unintended pregnancy when the woman has had unprotected sexual intercourse. Prevents unwanted pregnancy. Pills (known as "morning after pills") that contain birth control hormones can be taken as soon after unprotected sex as possible and up to 5 days after and still prevent pregnancy. Take a second dose 12 hours after the first dose. Will not interrupt an established pregnancy and will not harm the embryo. No prescription needed.	Very effective.	Not the same as RU-486, an abortion pill. Prevents ovulation or stops fertilization.
IUD made of copper, and the copper helps kill sperm. (Mirena® IUD cannot be used as an emergency contraceptive).		Very effective.	Kills sperm or prevents ovum fertilization.

*Newest oral contraceptives called extended hormonal contraceptives

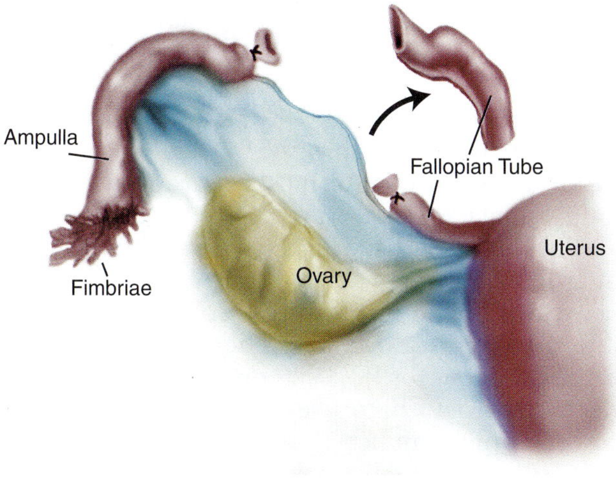

Figure 14-20 Tubal ligation.

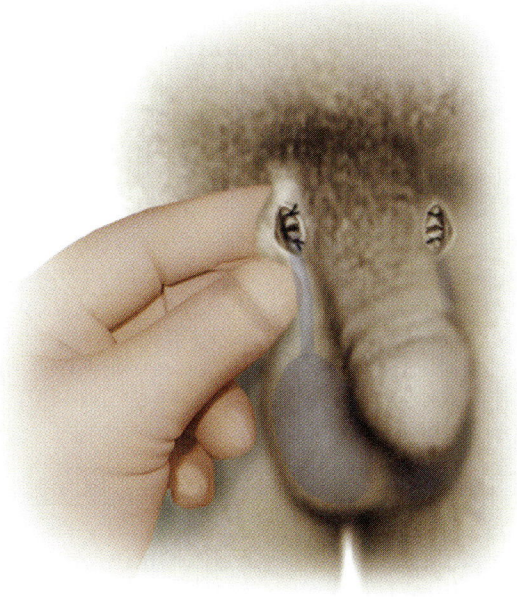

Figure 14-21 Vasectomy.

The Gynecologic Examination

It is recommended that a gynecologic examination be done annually on all women beginning when they become sexually active or by age 21 years. It is done to assess the female's health and to screen for cancer of the reproductive organs. It includes a breast examination by the provider and instructions for the patient about how to perform her own breast self-examination (BSE). It also includes a pelvic examination and Pap smear. Pap tests are done to detect cervical cancer. Women should be especially conscientioust in scheduling annual Pap tests and mammograms if they have a family history of breast, uterine, ovarian, or cervical cancer. Early detection of cervical and breast cancers and appropriate treatment may cure the disease. Women who have had a hysterectomy because of cancer should continue to be tested for pelvic cancer annually by having a Pap smear. Because the cervix has been removed, the specimen cells are taken from the inner vaginal vault instead. Even after hysterectomy, the woman still remains at risk for cancer cells to grow within the vagina and she should be encouraged to continue with her regular pelvic examinations and Pap tests. Others believe that in healthy women a Pap test done every 1 to 3 years is sufficient. The American Cancer Society (ACS) recommends that all women have a Pap test about every 3 years, after they become sexually active, or at age 21 years, whichever is sooner, then testing every year with the regular (conventional) Pap test or every 2 years with the newer liquid-based Pap test (e.g., ThinPrep®) should be done.

Further, the ACS recommends that at age 30 women who have had three sequential normal Pap tests be tested every 2 to 3 years with either

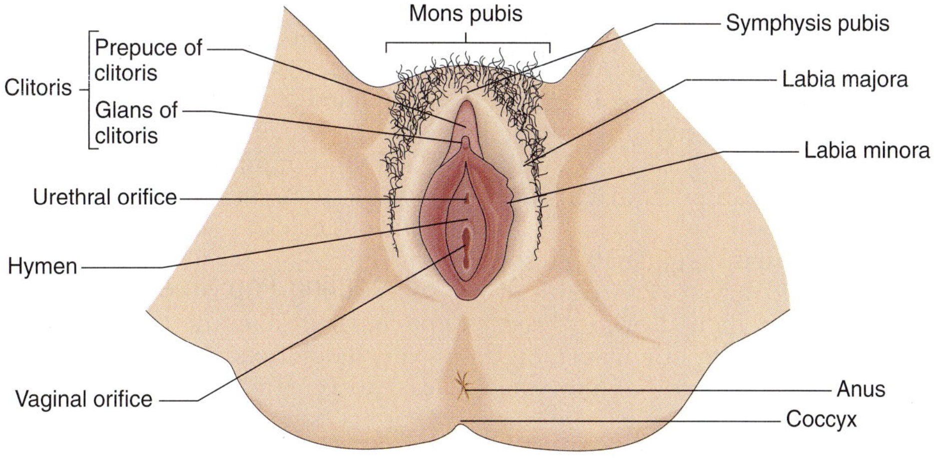

Figure 14-22 External genitalia of the female.

Patient Education

Post IUD Insertion

1. Report any bleeding other than spotting that occurs in the first 2 days.
2. Report fever, vaginal discharge, or pain at once.
3. A small percentage of IUDs are expelled from the uterus into the vagina during the first year. Another contraceptive should be used to prevent pregnancy.
4. There is a risk of perforation of the uterus, but this is most likely to occur during insertion.
5. There is no protection against STDs.
6. Some women experience headaches, breast tenderness, and mood swings. These symptoms usually subside in a few months.
7. It is possible (rare) to become pregnant with an IUD. It is recommended in this situation that the IUD be removed because it can cause miscarriage or premature birth.
8. The IUD can remain in place for as long as 10 years depending on the type.
9. An IUD must be removed by the provider.
10. An IUD is safe and highly effective.

the conventional Pap test or with the liquid-based Pap test and be tested for human papillomavirus (HPV) DNA.

Women 70 years or older who have had three sequential negative Pap tests in 10 years can stop cervical cancer testing.

Women with a history of cervical cancer, DES exposure before birth, HIV infection, or weak immune system should continue testing. Risk factors for cervical cancer are first sexual intercourse at an early age, multiple sex partners, sex with partners who have multiple partners, and a history of HPV.

Encourage patients to have regular Pap tests. Women at high risk should have a Pap test and a mammogram according to their provider's recommendations. If the patient is experiencing a vaginal discharge and there is a suspicion of a vaginal infection, smear(s) and cultures of discharge can be done to aid in diagnosis. (Chapter 31 provides more information.)

Human Papillomavirus (HPV) and Gardasil®. In June 2006, the FDA approved a vaccine that targets the virus responsible for most cervical cancers and condylomata (genital warts). The vaccine, called Gardasil, protects against four HPVs. According to an article on women's health on Web MD Medical News, two of the four viruses are responsible for 70% of all cervical cancers. The other two viruses are responsible for 90% of condylomata. Gardasil was approved to help prevent vaginal and vulvar cancers, which can be caused by HPV.

HPV is spread through sexual contact. According to the CDC, by age 50 years, at least 80% of women will have had an HPV infection. However, most women with HPV do not get cervical cancer. Gardasil is 100% effective in protecting against two of the HPV strains if the individual has not been exposed to the virus previously. The vaccine will not protect people already exposed to the virus. The vaccine does not contain a live virus. It lasts for at least 5 years.

The FDA approved Gardasil for girls and women aged 9 to 26 years. It is on the CDC's recommended vaccine schedule. Screening for cervical cancer (as with the Pap test) still is necessary because Gardasil does not protect against all HPV types. Pap tests also are essential for women who have not been vaccinated or who already are infected with HPV. The vaccine is not recommended during pregnancy.

The Advisory Committee on Immunization Practices (ACIP) recommends that girls 11 to 12 years of age be immunized with three doses of HPV vaccines, but the series can be started as early as age 9. The second and third doses should be given 2 and 6 months after the first dose.

HPV vaccines can be administered with other age-appropriate vaccines. Catch-up vaccinations are available for females 13 to 26 years of age who have not been vaccinated previously or who have not completed the full series. The vaccine is licensed only for females 9 to 26 years of age. Each dose is 0.5 mL given intramuscularly. Continuous research is being done to determine if HPV vaccine can be used on males.

Scheduling Pap Smear Tests. Encourage female patients to schedule their Pap smear and annual gynecologic examination on a date that will be easy to remember, such as April Fool's Day, Flag Day, tax day, or first day of summer. Keep a tickler file to remind patients who "forget." Women may believe that because they have had a hysterectomy, they no longer need their annual examination and Pap smear. Every woman should have an annual (or regular) examination even if the Pap test is not included. A woman who has had a hysterectomy because of cancer should continue to have Pap smears on a regular basis. Many women are not aware of this and need to be educated.

Other gynecologic problems may arise between annual gynecologic examinations and require an appointment. They include symptoms and problems such as severe **dysmenorrhea** (painful menses), lower abdominal pain, **metrorrhagia,** bleeding between menstrual periods, **dyspareunia** (painful intercourse), sexual dysfunction, infertility, and discomfort from menstrual symptoms. Women experiencing these problems should have a gynecologic examination, and the provider will determine a diagnosis based on the examination, the patient's history, symptoms, signs, and laboratory data. The data from previous appointments are available to the provider via the computer. Comparisons can be made quickly with previous entries, saving time and possibly preventing errors.

It is important to realize that patients' health practices related to culture, values, and belief systems are deeply ingrained and not easily changed. Being aware of some of these practices and beliefs will benefit both you and your patients. You will have a better understanding of their cultural heritage and beliefs that are different from yours, and this will help patients to be more comfortable. At times, it might be necessary to modify care according to the patient's cultural background and practice.

Female Circumcision.

Female circumcision is an ancient cultural custom that has been practiced worldwide for more than 2,000 years. Between 100 and 130 million women in 40 countries have had female circumcisions. Central Africa is one of the main areas where various forms of the procedure are performed.

There are four different types of female circumcision: (1) removal of the prepuce of the clitoris; (2) clitoridectomy, removal of prepuce and clitoris; (3) removal of prepuce, clitoris, upper labia minora, and some labia majora; and (4) infibulation, removal of all external genitalia (prepuce, clitoris, labia majora, labia minora). Some reasons given for this practice are that it is a right of passage, a sign of purity, marriage availability, sexual faithfulness, protection from rape and abortion, and for socialization into the role of a woman. Surgery is usually performed by a lay midwife, and a razor or broken glass is used; infections and hemorrhages are common. If an infibulation is performed, the two sides of the vulva are sewn together. Scar tissue forms over the vagina. A small opening for urination and menstruation is made by inserting a foreign object until the area heals. The most common reason given for this procedure is that it follows customs and tradition. During childbirth, the infibulation is cut to allow for delivery, then resutured after delivery.

Always view patients as individuals whose cultural beliefs and practices may differ greatly from your own. Treat them as you do all patients, with respect and empathy (see Chapters 15 and 16 for male circumcision).

Breast Examination.

The provider performs a breast examination on the patient as part of a gynecologic examination. Looking for redness, dimpling, and puckering, each breast is palpated and the axilla felt for lumps or thickening. Part of the medical assistant's responsibility is to teach patients how to perform the breast self-examination (BSE). Figure 14-23 provides illustrations for performing the BSE. The provider may supply several pamphlets and a breast model with lumps and thickening for enhancing patient education and awareness about the importance of the examination (Figure 14-24A and B).

Breast Self-Examination (BSE).

Provide the patient with these steps to follow:

1. Examine your breasts when they are not tender or swollen and at the same time each month, about 1 week after menses.
2. Women who are breast-feeding or pregnant or have breast implants can do a BSE.
3. Ask the medical assistant to review your technique when you have your yearly examination.
4. Lie on your back and put your right arm behind your head. This spreads out the breast tissue, making it easier to feel all of the tissue (Figure 14-23A).
5. Using your left hand and the finger pads of the three middle fingers (Figure 14-23B), feel for lumps or abnormalities in your right breast.
6. Use three degrees of pressure—light, medium, and strong (or firm)—to feel all of the tissue. Light pressure is used for skin and tissue just beneath the surface, and medium pressure is used for tissue in the middle of the breasts, strong pressure is used to feel the tissue closest to the ribs

Critical Thinking

A 27-year-old woman wants to schedule an appointment because she has some bright red bleeding after sexual intercourse. What conditions or diseases might this woman have? Discuss your reasons for choosing the conditions or diseases. What equipment and supplies might the provider require for her examination?

and chest. Use all three degrees of pressure on each spot on your breast before feeling another spot.

7. Use an up-and-down pattern as you move around the breast, starting at your imaginary seam line (straight down from the underarm) and moving up and down to the middle of the chest bone. Be certain you have examined your entire breast, from the collar bone to the ribs.
8. Do the same examination on your left breast, starting with step 4.
9. Looking in a mirror with hands pressing down on your hips, check your breasts for redness; dimpling; and change in shape, size, or contour (Figure 14-23C).
10. Examine each underarm while sitting or standing while your arm is raised slightly so that the area is easily felt.
11. The ACS recommends that women without symptoms of breast cancer aged 40 to 49 years have a mammogram every 1 to 2 years, and women aged 50 years and older, once a year (Figures 14-25 and 14-26).

The American College of Obstetricians and Gynecologists endorses the guidelines set forth by the ACS.

Breast cancer risk factors include:

- A family history of breast cancer
- Being female (males can get breast cancer, but there is much less chance)
- A biopsy of a breast lesion that showed atypical hyperplasia
- Early menarche (younger than 12 years)
- Late menopause (after 55 years)
- No children, or first child after 30 years of age
- More than 2 to 5 alcoholic drinks per week
- BRCA1 and BRCA2 gene mutations

According to the ACS, breast cancer is the second leading cause of death in women in the United States; the leading cause of death in women is lung cancer.

Diagnosis of breast cancer is made by the provider using some or all of the following diagnostic tools: mammography, tissue biopsy, MRI, ultrasound, and MRI-guided breast biopsies.

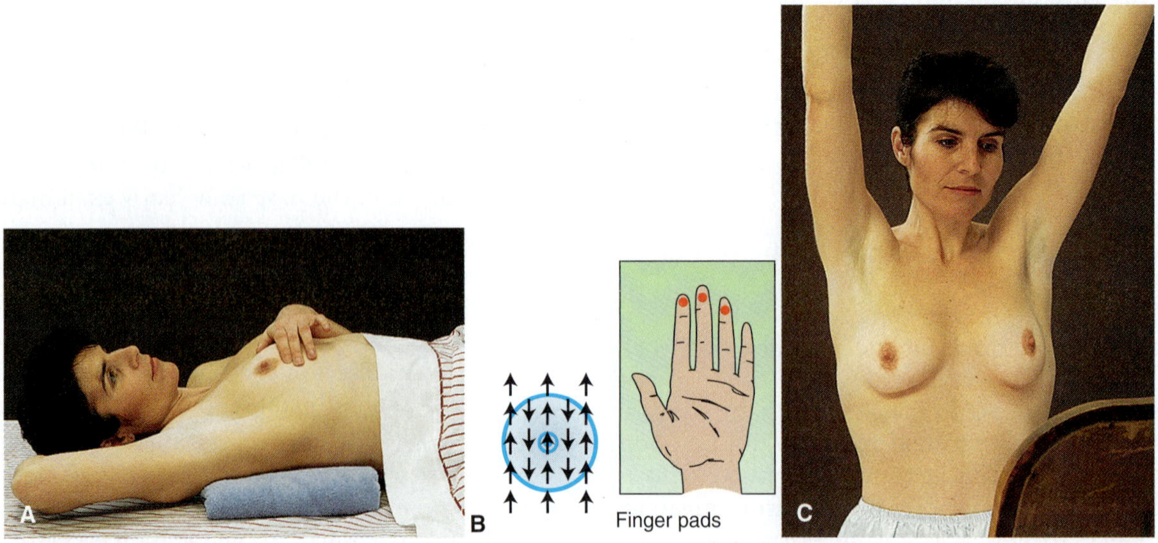

Figure 14-23 Breast self-examination. (A) Lie on your back and put your right arm behind your head. (B) Use the finger pads of your three middle fingers, making an up and down pattern to examine the breast. (C) Look in a mirror and observe the breasts for abnormalities.

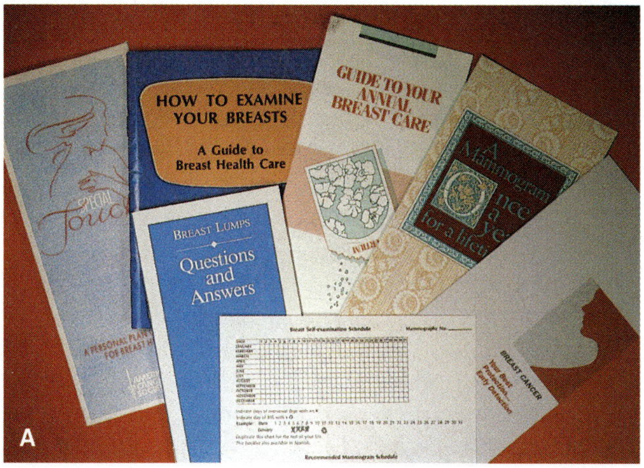

Figure 14-24A Informational pamphlets detailing the breast self-examination and its importance can be helpful to patients.

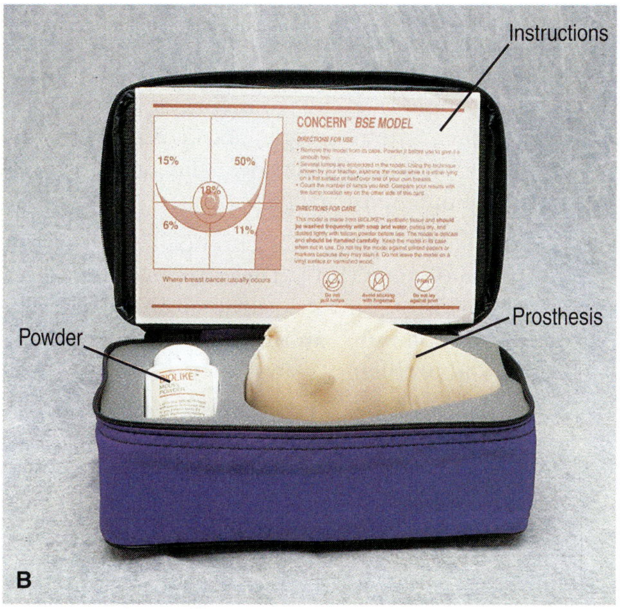

Figure 14-24B Breast self-examination model kit contains instructions for breast self-examination and powder to aid fingers in gliding over the breast prosthesis. The prosthesis contains lumps and thickened areas for identification and location.

The four standard treatment options for patients with breast cancer are surgery, radiation therapy, chemotherapy, and hormone therapy.

Hormonal therapy with tamoxifen acts against the effects of estrogen. In women who are at risk for breast cancer, tamoxifen reduces the chances of developing breast cancer. Tamoxifen for prevention of breast cancer continues to be studied.

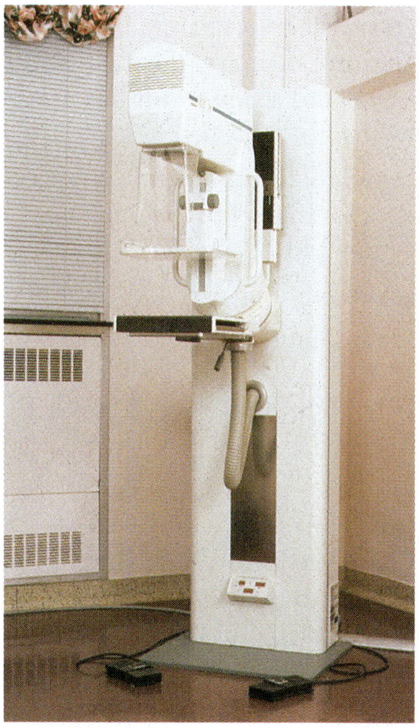

Figure 14-25 Breasts are compressed by the plates of mammographic X-ray unit.

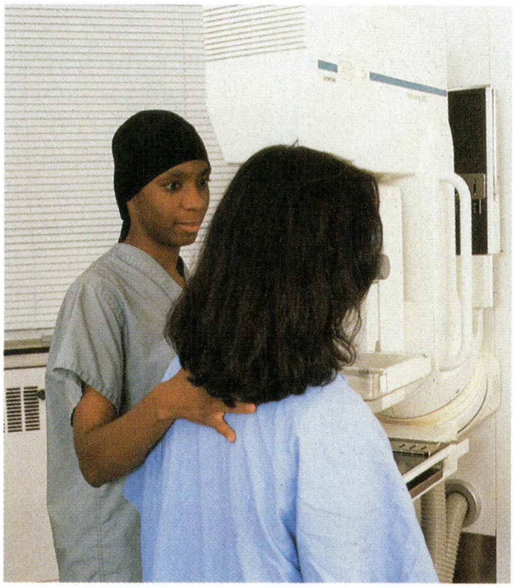

Figure 14-26 The technologist positions the patient for a mammography. The procedure requires the patient to move into various positions so that different angles of the breast tissue can be imaged.

Herceptin is a medication (nonhormonal) that can be administered to women with breast cancer if a sample of breast cancer cells shows a particular abnormal protein. Herceptin targets the abnormal protein.

Assisting with a Gynecologic Examination. The gynecologic examination consists of four parts:

1. Inspection of external **genitalia** (labia minora, labia majora, urinary meatus, clitoris, **Bartholin glands**, and vagina) for swelling, lesions, or ulcerations
2. Pelvic examination of cervix, uterus, tubes, and ovaries including a **bimanual examination;** may or may not include a Pap test
3. Rectal examination
4. Breast examination

The medical assistant should prepare the patient, equipment, and room before the examination.

Patient Education

Many women think that if they have had a hysterectomy because of cancer they no longer need to have Pap smears performed. This is not true, and it is up to health care professionals to educate them. If the hysterectomy was performed because of cancer, the cancer cells can reappear in the vaginal vault after the surgery. During the pelvic examination, because the cervix has been removed, the provider will scrape the inner walls of the vaginal vault for cells to include in the Pap smear.

Gynecologic Examination with Pap Equipment. On a Mayo tray near the end of the examination table, place the instruments and supplies the provider needs to perform the gynecologic or pelvic examination with Pap test. Figure 14-27 shows the equipment commonly needed for the examination. To aid in the inspection portion of the examination, you should place a gooseneck lamp at the foot of the table behind the stool on which the provider will sit (see Procedure 14-2).

In preparation for the annual examination, the patient is asked to avoid using tampons, foams, and gels; douching; and sexual intercourse for 2 days before a Pap test. Five days after menses is a good time to have a Pap test. Immediately before a pelvic examination, the patient is encouraged to empty her bladder. The urine may be collected for testing according to the clinic policy or the provider's preference and depending on any urinary tract complaints or symptoms the patient may have. If a Pap test is being performed, take a minute to interview the patient and gather the necessary medical and laboratory information. The data needed include:

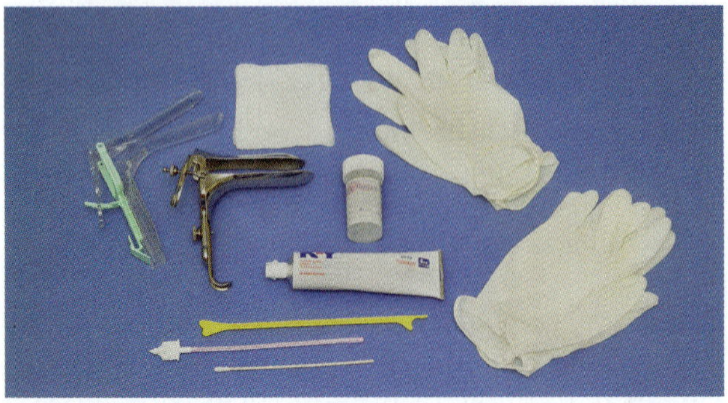

Figure 14-27 Setup for gynecologic examination including equipment for a Thin-Prep® Pap smear: transport medium container, spatula, cytology brush and broom, Specula (disposable and reusable), lubricant, gloves, tissues.

- Last normal menstrual period. This question will bring up information about breakthrough bleeding (if patient is taking oral contraceptives), dysmenorrhea, metrorrhagia, postcoital bleeding, perimenopausal irregularities, and other idiosyncrasies of the menstrual patterns.
- Hormonal therapies, either oral contraceptives or hormone therapy (HT). These are excellent questions for birth control history, successes/failures, problems/solutions, and menopausal issues, concerns, and problems.
- Surgical history, especially related to the genitourinary tract. These questions will initiate discussions about bladder problems and hysterectomies.
- Sexual history/habits. This will open discussions with the patient about disease prevention, birth control, hormonal problems, and menopausal conditions.
- Symptoms of diseases/disorders, such as pelvic or genital pain or discomfort; vaginal discharge, irritation, or itching; painful intercourse; dysuria; urinary frequency or incontinence; and breast pain or breast conditions/concerns.

EHR All the information gathered during the patient interview can be entered into the patient's medical record on the computer while sitting with the patient. There may be a health form on the computer for the medical assistant to fill out with the patient. The provider then will input the information and any other pertinent data gathered during the examination. The electronic medical record is stored and can be accessed at any time for laboratory and diagnostic tests and procedures, prescriptions, and previous data entry.

In preparation for the examination, have the patient undress and don a patient gown with the opening positioned in the front (for the breast examination) and a drape sheet. The patient is seated on the examination table. Provide the patient with privacy during the undressing. Ensure the patient's comfort by providing her with a blanket if she is cold and have her leave her socks on if her feet are cold.

During the breast and abdominal examinations, the patient is placed into the supine or dorsal recumbent position. Provide a pillow for comfort. For the pelvic examination, the patient is placed into the lithotomy position. Assist the patient into this position, providing leg and back support as needed.

During the pelvic examination and the Pap smear, the medical assistant assists the provider as needed (Figure 14-28). The tray of supplies should be at an appropriate height and position for access by the provider while seated. The vaginal speculum (metal or plastic) should be warmed to body temperature. Some examination tables are equipped with warming drawers for storing the specula so that they are warm and ready for use. The medical assistant may set up the pelvic exam/Pap smear supplies on a Mayo tray and position the gooseneck lamp so that the warmth from the light bulb can warm the speculum. The provider may hold the speculum under warm running water just before use. Whichever method is used, the provider will test the speculum to make sure it is not too hot before use. This is often done by touching the speculum on the patient's inner thigh to determine if the temperature is comfortable.

During the examination, the medical assistant will support the patient, hand the provider supplies as needed, and adjust the light source as needed. When the provider has obtained the appropriate cervical cells, the medical assistant will take the cytology broom or brush and uncap the ThinPrep container, swish the broom or brush vigorously in the ThinPrep solution until all the specimen has been deposited, dispose of the broom or brush in a biohazard container, reapply the cap, and complete the container label. If the patient is "status post hysterectomy," the provider will scrape cells (using the spatula) from the inner walls of the vaginal vault rather than from the cervix, which will no longer be present. Those cells are deposited into the ThinPrep solution in the same manner as a cervical specimen.

After the Pap test is performed, the provider will examine the internal organs. This is done using the bimanual (two-handed) examination (Figure 14-29). By inserting two fingers into the vagina and pressing on the outside abdominal wall, the shape,

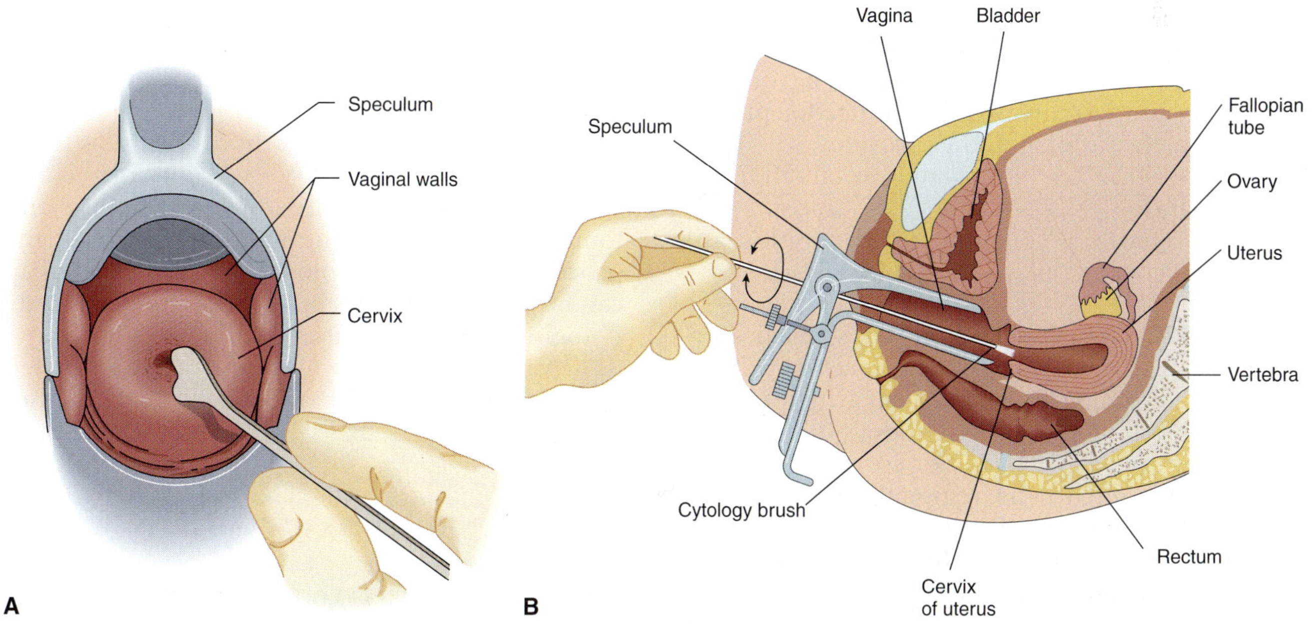

Figure 14-28 Use of speculum, cytology brush, and spatula to obtain material for a Pap smear. (A) The provider uses a spatula to obtain cells from the cervix. (B) The provider uses a cytology brush to obtain cells from the cervix.

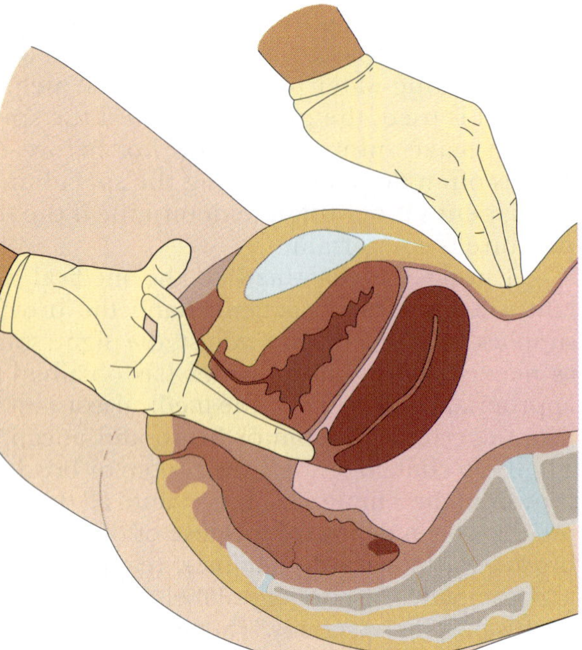

Figure 14-29 Bimanual pelvic examination.

consistency, movement, and positioning of the uterus and the ovaries can be felt. If any abnormalities are felt, further testing may be required. After the bimanual examination, a rectal examination is performed. This examination enables the provider to assess the back side of the uterus, which is not felt during the bimanual examination.

When the pelvic examination is completed, the medical assistant will help the patient off the table, offer tissue and the sink for her to clean up and wash her hands, and let her know you will be back in a few minutes. When you return, you may take the patient to the provider's office for private discussion. Occasionally, the provider will hold the discussion in the examination room after the patient has dressed.

The ThinPrep containe and cognisition are sent to the cytology laboratory (Figure 14-30).

Pap Smear. The conventional Pap smear is performed by scraping the patient's cervix with a spatula and cytology brush and smearing the cells onto a microscopic slide. The slide is then placed into a bottle of Pap fixative or sprayed with Pap fixative and sent to the regional laboratory for viewing. The ThinPrep Pap test differs in that the cells that are obtained on the collecting devices are swished vigorously into a vial of fluid transport medium rather than placed on a slide. The vial is sent to the regional laboratory for processing. Using the conventional method, approximately 80% of the specimen remains on the collecting device, with only about 20% being submitted on the slide. With the ThinPrep Pap test, virtually 100% of the collected cells are rinsed off the collecting device and submitted in the vial. The conventional Pap slide preparation results in an inconsistently distributed specimen containing blood cells, mucus, and other debris that can interfere with the viewing. The ThinPrep Pap test uses a ThinPrep processor to suspend the cervical cells; to eliminate the blood cells, mucus, and other debris; and to distribute a thin and even layer of cells onto a slide for analyzing. The ThinPrep Pap test slide is of better quality, is much clearer and easier to read, and increases accuracy for both the manual assessment and the computerized assessment. It greatly improves detection of precancerous cells.

Although the conventional Pap smear has undoubtedly saved countless lives by detecting cervical cancer, the ThinPrep Pap test is significantly more effective. Another advantage of the ThinPrep Pap test is that the same specimen may be used to determine the presence of HPV or chlamydia/gonorrhea if needed.

The federal government regulates laboratories that perform testing on Pap smears. Requirements are placed on the individuals who study the specimens for malignant cells, and they include specialized training. Limits are placed on the number of slides that can be read in one day. Proficiency testing, mandated by the Clinical Laboratory Improvement Act of 1988 (CLIA '88), ensures accuracy and precision of test results and is a requirement for Pap smear examination (Chapter 26 gives more information about CLIA '88).

A computerized method, known as AutoPap, is used to retest Pap smears that have been analyzed by technologists and found to be normal. The method duplicates the process that the technologists perform. AutoPap can be used for an initial Pap test as long as a technologists examines all abnormal smears.

Another test, known as ViraPap, can be used to screen for HPV in a Pap smear. There is higher

Critical Thinking

A 38-year-old woman has been diagnosed with HPV infection. What is the significance of this infection?

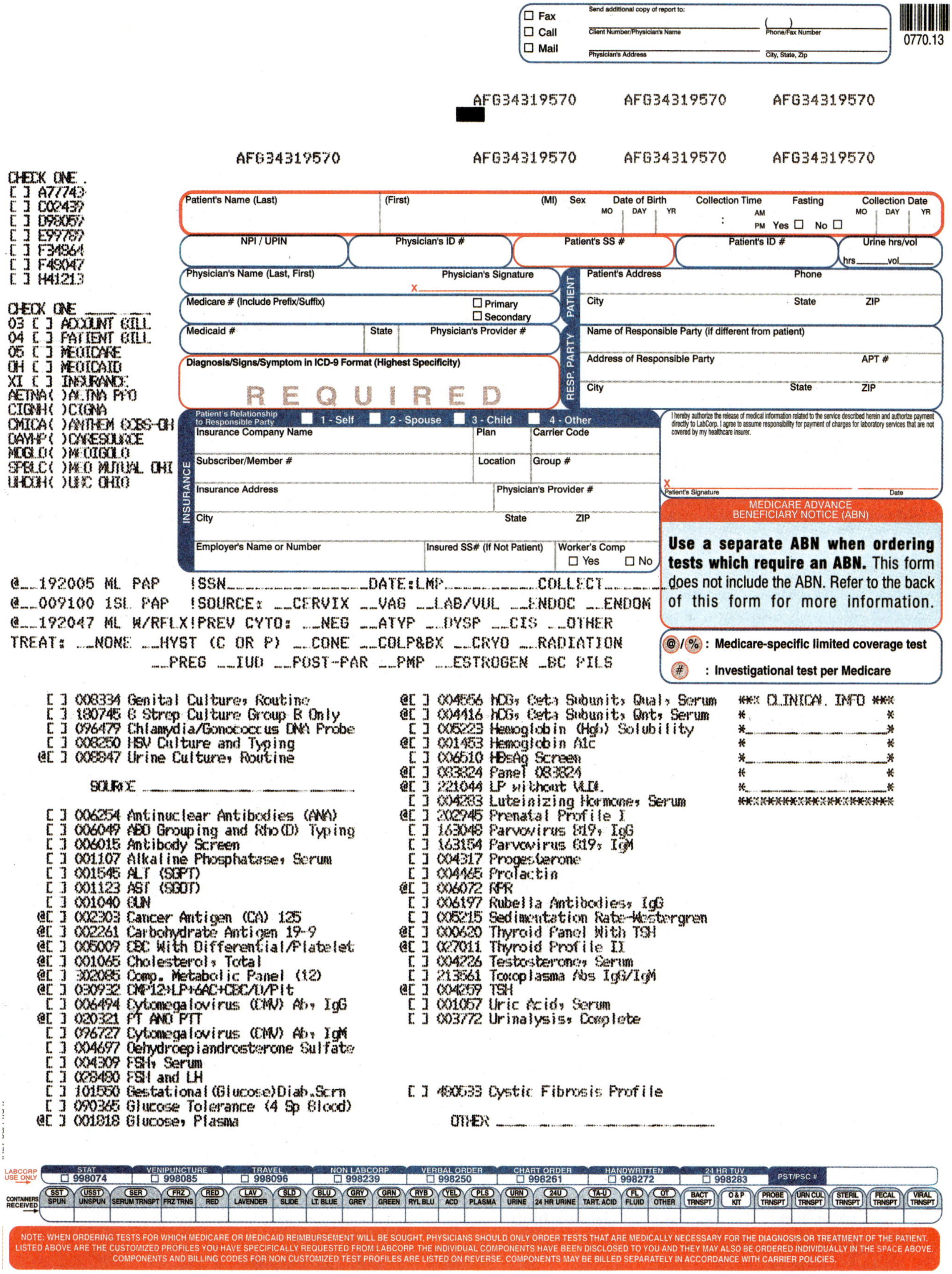

☐ Fax ☐ Call ☐ Mail
Send additional copy of report to:
Client Number/Physician's Name — Phone/Fax Number
Physician's Address — City, State, Zip
0770.13

AFG34319570 AFG34319570 AFG34319570
[redacted]
AFG34319570 AFG34319570 AFG34319570 AFG34319570

CHECK ONE .
[ ] A77743
[ ] C02439
[ ] D98057
[ ] E99787
[ ] F34864
[ ] F49047
[ ] H41213

CHECK ONE ________
03 [ ] ACCOUNT BILL
04 [ ] PATIENT BILL
05 [ ] MEDICARE
0H [ ] MEDICAID
XI [ ] INSURANCE
AETNA( )AETNA PPO
CIGNH( )CIGNA
CMICA( )ANTHEM BCBS-OH
DAYHP( )CARESOURCE
MDGLD( )MEDIGOLD
SPBLC( )MED MUTUAL OHI
UHDOH( )UHC OHIO

Patient's Name (Last) | (First) | (MI) | Sex | Date of Birth MO DAY YR | Collection Time AM PM | Fasting Yes ☐ No ☐ | Collection Date MO DAY YR

NPI / UPIN | Physician's ID # | Patient's SS # | Patient's ID # | Urine hrs/vol hrs_____vol_____

Physician's Name (Last, First) | Physician's Signature x
Medicare # (Include Prefix/Suffix) ☐ Primary ☐ Secondary
Medicaid # | State | Physician's Provider #
Diagnosis/Signs/Symptom in ICD-9 Format (Highest Specificity)
REQUIRED

PATIENT: Patient's Address | Phone; City | State | ZIP
RESP. PARTY: Name of Responsible Party (if different from patient); Address of Responsible Party | APT #; City | State | ZIP

INSURANCE: Patient's Relationship to Responsible Party ■ 1 - Self ■ 2 - Spouse ■ 3 - Child ■ 4 - Other
Insurance Company Name | Plan | Carrier Code
Subscriber/Member # | Location | Group #
Insurance Address | Physician's Provider #
City | State | ZIP
Employer's Name or Number | Insured SS# (If Not Patient) | Worker's Comp ☐ Yes ☐ No

I hereby authorize the release of medical information related to the service described herein and authorize payment directly to LabCorp. I agree to assume responsibility for payment of charges for laboratory services that are not covered by my healthcare insurer.
x Patient's Signature — Date

MEDICARE ADVANCE BENEFICIARY NOTICE (ABN)
Use a separate ABN when ordering tests which require an ABN. This form does not include the ABN. Refer to the back of this form for more information.

@ / % : Medicare-specific limited coverage test
# : Investigational test per Medicare

@__192005 ML PAP !SSN______________DATE:LMP__________COLLECT________
@__009100 1SL PAP !SOURCE: __CERVIX __VAG __LAB/VUL __ENDOC __ENDOM
@__192047 ML W/RFLX!PREV CYTO: __NEG __ATYP __DYSP __CIS __OTHER
TREAT: __NONE __HYST (C OR P) __CONE __COLP&BX __CRYO __RADIATION
__PREG __IUD __POST-PAR __PMP __ESTROGEN __BC PILS

[ ] 008334 Genital Culture, Routine
[ ] 180745 B Strep Culture Group B Only
[ ] 096479 Chlamydia/Gonococcus DNA Probe
[ ] 008250 HSV Culture and Typing
@[ ] 008847 Urine Culture, Routine

SOURCE ______________

[ ] 006254 Antinuclear Antibodies (ANA)
[ ] 006049 ABO Grouping and Rho(D) Typing
[ ] 006015 Antibody Screen
[ ] 001107 Alkaline Phosphatase, Serum
[ ] 001545 ALT (SGPT)
[ ] 001123 AST (SGOT)
[ ] 001040 BUN
@[ ] 002303 Cancer Antigen (CA) 125
@[ ] 002261 Carbohydrate Antigen 19-9
@[ ] 005009 CBC With Differential/Platelet
@[ ] 001065 Cholesterol, Total
@[ ] 322000 Comp. Metabolic Panel (14)
@[ ] 030932 CMP12+LP+6AC+CBC/D/Plt
[ ] 006494 Cytomegalovirus (CMV) Ab, IgG
@[ ] 020321 PT AND PTT
[ ] 096727 Cytomegalovirus (CMV) Ab, IgM
[ ] 004697 Dehydroepiandrosterone Sulfate
[ ] 004309 FSH, Serum
[ ] 028480 FSH and LH
[ ] 101550 Gestational(Glucose)Diab.Scrn
[ ] 090365 Glucose Tolerance (4 Sp Blood)
@[ ] 001818 Glucose, Plasma

@[ ] 004556 hCG, Beta Subunit, Qual, Serum
@[ ] 004416 hCG, Beta Subunit, Qnt, Serum
[ ] 005223 Hemoglobin (Hgb) Solubility
@[ ] 001453 Hemoglobin A1c
[ ] 006510 HBsAg Screen
@[ ] 083824 Panel 083824
@[ ] 221044 LP without VLDL
[ ] 004283 Luteinizing Hormone, Serum
@[ ] 202945 Prenatal Profile I
[ ] 163048 Parvovirus B19, IgG
[ ] 163154 Parvovirus B19, IgM
[ ] 004317 Progesterone
[ ] 004465 Prolactin
@[ ] 006072 RPR
[ ] 006197 Rubella Antibodies, IgG
[ ] 005215 Sedimentation Rate-Westergren
@[ ] 000620 Thyroid Panel With TSH
@[ ] 027011 Thyroid Profile II
[ ] 004226 Testosterone, Serum
[ ] 213561 Toxoplasma Abs IgG/IgM
@[ ] 004259 TSH
[ ] 001057 Uric Acid, Serum
[ ] 003772 Urinalysis, Complete

[ ] 480533 Cystic Fibrosis Profile

OTHER ______________

*** CLINICAL INFO ***
____
____
____
____
____
____
****

LABCORP USE ONLY: STAT ☐ 998074 | VENIPUNCTURE ☐ 998085 | TRAVEL ☐ 998096 | NON LABCORP ☐ 998239 | VERBAL ORDER ☐ 998250 | CHART ORDER ☐ 998261 | HANDWRITTEN ☐ 998272 | 24 HR TUV ☐ 998283 | PST/PSC #

CONTAINERS RECEIVED: SST SPUN | USST UNSPUN | SER SERUM TRNSPT | FRZ FRZ TRNS | RED RED | LAV LAVENDER | SLD SLIDE | BLU LT. BLUE | GRY GREY | GRN GREEN | RYB RYL BLU | YEL ACD | PLS PLASMA | URN URINE | 24U 24 HR URINE | TA-U TART. ACID | FL FLUID | OT OTHER | BACT TRNSPT | O & P KIT | PROBE TRNSPT | URN CUL TRNSPT | STERIL TRNSPT | FECAL TRNSPT | VIRAL TRNSPT

NOTE: WHEN ORDERING TESTS FOR WHICH MEDICARE OR MEDICAID REIMBURSEMENT WILL BE SOUGHT, PHYSICIANS SHOULD ONLY ORDER TESTS THAT ARE MEDICALLY NECESSARY FOR THE DIAGNOSIS OR TREATMENT OF THE PATIENT. LISTED ABOVE ARE THE CUSTOMIZED PROFILES YOU HAVE SPECIFICALLY REQUESTED FROM LABCORP. THE INDIVIDUAL COMPONENTS HAVE BEEN DISCLOSED TO YOU AND THEY MAY ALSO BE ORDERED INDIVIDUALLY IN THE SPACE ABOVE. COMPONENTS AND BILLING CODES FOR NON CUSTOMIZED TEST PROFILES ARE LISTED ON REVERSE. COMPONENTS MAY BE BILLED SEPARATELY IN ACCORDANCE WITH CARRIER POLICIES.

Figure 14-30 Laboratory requisition for OB/GYN practice.

incidence of cervical cancer in women who have HPV, and the test can help identify these women. Vaginal cancer can also be detected by a Pap smear. There is an increased risk for both cervical and vaginal cancer in daughters of women who used **diethylstilbestrol (DES)** during pregnancy.

Some advocate "at home" testing. The woman collects her cervical cells by inserting a small plastic applicator into the vagina up the cervix (as far as she can comfortably insert applicator) and moving it around to collect cells. The applicator is placed in a special container to preserve cells that will be tested by a laboratory. The ACS does not endorse "home" testing. Perhaps in the future "home" testing will become accurate for scientific use and accepted by the medical community.

One system for cytologic reporting of a Pap smear is a descriptive report that tells the provider exactly what cellular changes have taken place. The classification includes the grades of cervical **intraepithelial** neoplasia (CIN).

CIN 1 = mild **dysplasia** (abnormal tissue development)
CIN 2 = moderate dysplasia
CIN 3 = severe dysplasia or **carcinoma in situ**

Another system used to report Pap test results is the Bethesda System (TBS). The Bethesda System for reporting results of Pap tests has three main categories, some of which have subcategories:

Category 1 = negative for intraepithelial lesion or malignancy. These are known signs of cancer or precancerous cells or other abnormalities found.

Category 2 = epithelial cell abnormalities. The cells of the lining of the cervix show changes that might be cancer or precancerous. There are several subgroups within this group for squamous cells and glandular cells.

1. *Atypical Squamous Cells (ASCs).* The name given to what the cells look like under a microscope. It is difficult to determine whether the abnormal cells are caused by an infection, an irritation, or a precancerous condition. This group is divided again.

   a. *Atypical Squamous Cells of Uncertain Significance (ASC-US)* and *atypical squamous cells where high-grade squamous intraepithelial lesions (SILs) cannot be excluded.* A repeat Pap test is done; biopsy and/or colposcopy and HPV DNA testing may be recommended.

   b. *Squamous Interepithelial Lesions (SILs).* There are low- and high-grade SILs. All patients in this category require a colposcopy. High-grade SILs can develop into cancer if not treated. Treatment can cure both high- and low-grade SILs and prevent cancer from developing. The Pap test does not identify which SIL the patient has; rather, it shows that the results fit into one of the abnormal categories.

   c. *Squamous Cell Carcinoma.* This test result shows that the woman likely has an invasive squamous cell carcinoma. Further testing, colposcopy, and biopsy are needed to be certain of the diagnosis. If the biopsy proves positive, the provider will recommend surgery, radiation, and/or chemotherapy.

   d. *Adenocarcinomas.* These carcinomas are abnormalities of glandular cells. If a clear decision can not be made by the pathologist as to whether the cells are malignant, the term used is atypical glandular cells (AGS). Further testing is done to decide on a treatment plan.

Category 3 = other malignant neoplasms, including malignant melanoma, carcinoma, and lymphoma. These malignant neoplasms affect the cervix very rarely compared to squamous cell carcinoma and adenocarcinoma.

Pap Smear Results. The Pap smear usually is sent to a reference laboratory where a pathologist examines it and records the results on the cytology report form and in the computer. The form is returned to the provider, and the report can be accessed on the computer. Figure 14-31 lists some of the terms used on the cytology report form.

Gynecologic Diseases and Conditions

The female reproductive system is affected by many diseases and conditions caused by hormonal imbalance, cysts, infection, and tumors. Some of the more common disorders and diseases are covered here.

Infertility. Most women, with unprotected intercourse, will be able to conceive within a year. The inability to conceive can be caused by a problem with either the male or the female individual. Some common causes of infertility in a female patient are:

- Endometriosis
- Certain medications

atypical—not typical
CIN—cervical intraepithelial neoplasia
CIS—carcinoma in situ
condyloma—a lesion caused by human papillomavirus
dysplasia—precancerous lesion
epithelial—pertaining to epithelium
epithelium—cellular tissue that covers the surface of a body or that lines a body cavity
glandular—the cell making up the epithelium of a body cavity
HPV—human papillomavirus
lesion—a change in the tissue cells or a wound
malignant—a lesion that spreads out of the epithelium into underlying tissues
reactive changes—changes in cells caused by their reaction to infectious agents or a foreign body
reparative changes—changes in cells as they divide rapidly in an attempt to repair damaged tissue
SIL—squamous intraepithelial lesion (that lies within the squamous epithelium)
squamous—a type of cell that makes up the epithelium, the purpose of which is to protect underlying tissues

Figure 14-31 Terms and abbreviations used in cytology Pap test reports.

- Blocked fallopian tubes
- Problems ovulating
- Chronic stress
- Scar tissue from surgery, infection, or ectopic pregnancy
- Tumors

A woman who is having difficulty conceiving and has a history of any of the above will have a physical examination by a provider who specializes in infertility. The specialist will decide what tests and procedures are necessary. Hormone levels may be measured to look for hypothyroidism. Ovarian function can be determined through a surgical procedure, such as laparoscopy. A test for **patency** (openness) of the fallopian tubes can be performed by a hysterosalpingogram, a radiographic procedure done after injection of dye into the vagina, through the cervix, into the uterus, and out the fallopian tubes. The dye will pass through all of these organs if there is no blockage in any of them (see "Impaired Fertility" section earlier in this chapter).

Menopause. The period of time that marks permanent cessation of menstrual activity is known as menopause. It usually occurs between the ages of 35 and 58 years. There may be a gradual decline in monthly menstrual flow, or a woman may suddenly cease to menstruate. Natural menopause occurs when the ovaries produce less and less estrogen. This causes the ovaries to cease ovulation and, therefore, menstruation stops. Surgical menopause is caused by the surgical removal of both ovaries (bilateral oophorectomy). Symptoms occur soon after ovulation ceases with both natural and surgical menopause. Symptoms may last for a few months to several years and include mild to severe symptoms. Hot flashes, chills, nervousness, fatigue, apathy, mental depression, crying episodes, insomnia, palpitations, and headache are some common symptoms experienced by some women. A long-term effect of lower estrogen levels is osteoporosis. Hormone therapy (HT) was thought to prevent osteoporosis and heart disease. A federally funded HT study, the Women's Health Initiative (WHI), which was slated to run for 15 years, stopped testing in 2002 what had been the most widely prescribed estrogen and progestin combination. Safety concerns brought an early end (5.5 years) to the trial testing the long-term benefits and risks of combined estrogen and progestin therapy (HT). The testing was halted earlier than intended because it was determined that HT, specifically Prempro®, was more harmful than helpful. There were increased risks for breast cancer and cardiovascular incidents; therefore, researchers told the women in the study to stop taking the combination medication. This situation has left many women with few choices for treating menopausal symptoms such as night sweats, hot flashes, dyspareunia, mood swings, fatigue, and osteoporosis. Switching to something else is risky because no other hormones have been as well studied as estrogen and progestin in Prempro®. There are many safe options for prevention and treatment of osteoporosis.

Researchers continued to study the estrogen-only hormone after halting the estrogen–progesterone trial. Because progesterone was initially added to the estrogen to protect women from uterine cancer, the thinking was that healthy postmenopausal women who had a hysterectomy and were given the estrogen-only hormone would not be at risk. However, data showed an increase in stroke in postmenopausal women given estrogen only. As of February 2004, the estrogen-only arm of the WHI study was halted, and the recommendation is for only short-term use of the hormone for women with moderate-to-severe menopausal symptoms. The FDA has urged manufacturers to add warnings to their labels on the estrogen-only hormone about the increased risk for dementia, strokes, abnormal mammograms, and uterine cancer in women who have not had a hysterectomy.

Reanalysis of the data from the WHI found that the risk of heart disease was greatest in women who started HT 10 or more years after menopause began. Women with a history of heart disease or heart attack should not take menopause hormones. Older women also have an increased risk for clot formation around the plaque in their arteries. This plaque can rupture, causing a stroke or heart attack.

The American College of Obstetricians and Gynecologists and the National Institutes of Health recommended that HT is a reasonable choice and likely safe for women to use as short-term treatment of menopausal symptoms. Use of the lowest effective dose for the shortest period of time and yearly reevaluation of women taking HT should be done. However, HT increases the risk of breast cancer in women regardless of when they started HT.

Regardless of whether a woman chooses to use HT (a decision based on discussions with her provider) or decides against HT, the following behaviors are beneficial to all women:

- Do not smoke
- Keep blood pressure within normal limits
- Keep cholesterol level within normal limits
- Exercise regularly
- Maintain a healthy weight
- Get regular mammograms with ultrasound if necessary and Pap tests
- Practice good nutrition (go to the FDA Web site http://www.MyPyramid.gov for information)
- Avoid regular al]cohol use

Endometriosis. Endometriosis is a painful, common condition characterized by endometrial tissue adhering to tissue and organs outside of the uterus. It is primarily found in the pelvis, adhering to an ovary, fallopian tube, or pelvic peritoneum. It also can be found outside of the pelvis, even in the abdomen adhering to tissue and organs, such as the bowel. The cause is unknown. The abnormal and engorged endometrial tissue responds to hormonal stimulation (estrogen) and builds up along with the normal endometrium of the menstrual cycle. It sloughs off at time of menstruation and is painful. The blood has no way to leave the body and is discharged into the pelvic or abdominal cavities.

Endometriosis symptoms may respond to contraceptive medication because these pills suppress menstruation and no further treatment may be necessary (Figure 14-32). However, long-term hormonal treatment may help alleviate symptoms. Hysterectomy may be necessary if the woman does not respond to hormonal therapy.

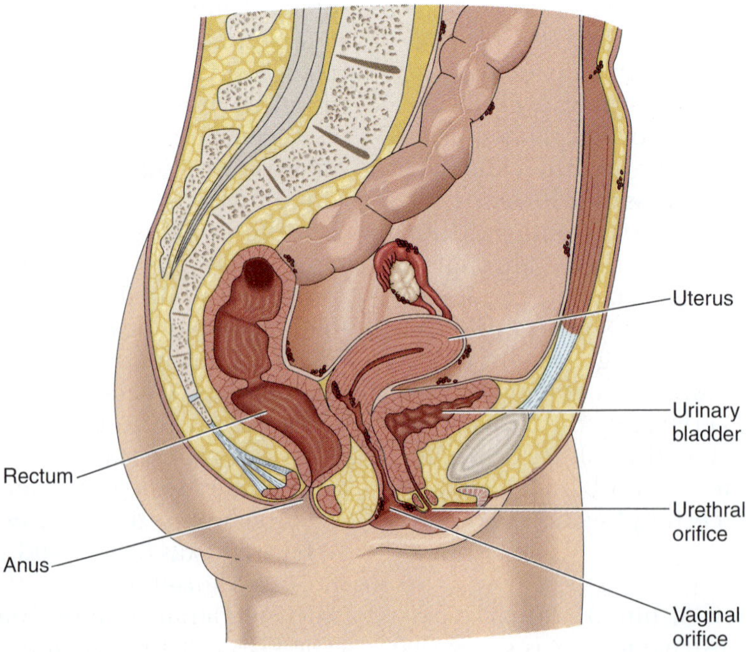

Figure 14-32 Endometriosis—common sites of endometrial implants.

Ovarian Cysts. Cysts that appear on the ovary are relatively common. As part of the menstrual cycle, the ovarian follicles enlarge and become graafian follicles. Only one graafian follicle ruptures at the time of ovulation. The follicles that do not rupture, but remain, are filled with fluid. They may enlarge and become cysts (Figure 14-33).

Ultrasonography will aid in viewing the ovaries. Most ovarian cysts resolve without treatment. Laparoscopy can be done to either drain or remove the cyst. Contraceptive therapy many times is helpful in resolving the cyst without surgery.

Direct viewing of the ovaries and surgery may be necessary because cancer of the ovary must be ruled out.

Ovarian Cancer. Because the symptoms of ovarian cancer do not appear until the disease has become established, it is difficult to make a diagnosis early in the disease process. Therefore, if a woman has any symptoms, the cancer usually has been present for some time. Symptoms may be pressure in the pelvis, lower abdominal discomfort, weight loss, bloating, and fluid in the abdomen. Diagnosis can be made by laparoscopic surgery and a biopsy. Hysterectomy and bilateral salpingo-oophorectomy are done, followed by radiation therapy or chemotherapy. The cause is not known.

Pelvic Inflammatory Disease (PID). PID involves some or all of the female reproductive tract and can be a serious infection. The causative microorganism is usually a sexually transmitted pathogen such as gonorrhea or chlamydia. The microorganism enters through the vagina and ascends through the cervix into the body of the uterus. It can spread out through the fallopian tubes into the pelvic cavity. Culture and sensitivity of the vaginal discharge are performed, and appropriate antibiotics are prescribed. Early treatment helps to lessen damage caused by scar tissue that forms in the pelvis and organs. Delayed treatment can cause septic shock, which can be life-threatening. Infertility and ectopic pregnancy are long-range problems that also can occur (Tables 14-4, 14-5, and 14-6).

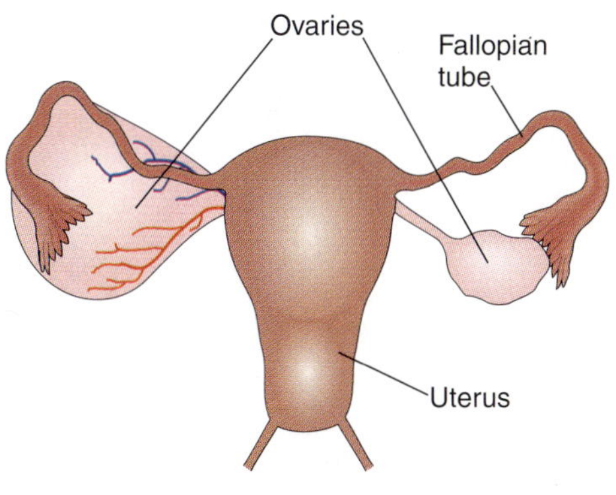

Figure 14-33 Ovarian cyst.

Other Diagnostic Tests and Treatments for Reproductive System Diseases

Colposcopy. **Colposcopy** is examination of the vagina and cervix by means of a lighted instrument that has a three-dimensional magnifying lens called a colposcope. The examination is done to determine if areas in the vagina or the cervix contain precancerous cells or tissue. The procedure is performed after an abnormal Pap test. It can also be performed to evaluate a lesion noted during a pelvic examination and to follow up after treatment of cervical cancer. Because the instrument has the ability to magnify tissue, the cervix can be more readily examined and a biopsy taken.

The patient is placed in lithotomy position and is prepared as she would be for a gynecologic examination. A nonlubricated speculum is inserted into the vagina. The vagina is swabbed with a long cotton-tipped applicator that has been moistened with saline. (This provides better visualization of the cervical tissue.) The cervix is then swabbed with acetic acid to dissolve mucus and provide a good contrast between normal and abnormal tissue. A staining medium can be used as another means of identifying abnormal cells. If the provider finds an area of abnormal tissue, a biopsy can be performed using cervical punch biopsy forceps (Figure 14-34). The specimen is examined by a pathologist to determine whether malignant cells are present.

Endometrial Biopsy/Sampling. An endometrial biopsy/sampling is often performed when patients are experiencing postmenopausal bleeding. It is a fairly simple procedure. The sampling device is housed in a long strawlike tube that slides through the cervical os quite easily. Once the end of the tube is inside the uterus, a plunger is pulled back. The action of pulling the plunger suctions a sampling of the endometrial tissue. This is a sterile procedure and requires an application of a cleansing solution (such as Betadine) to the cervix before performing the biopsy. Endometrial biopsy/sampling is quick and almost painless for the patient. The patient might experience slight cramping.

Table 14-4 Female Reproductive System Laboratory and Diagnostic Tests

Medical Tests or Procedures	Disease/ Disorder	Blood	Other	Radiography	Surgery
Pelvic examination	Bartholin gland infection		Exudate culture and sensitivity		Incision and drainage
Monthly breast self-examination	Breast cancer	Breast cancer gene detection BRCA1, BRCA2		Mammography Ultrasonography	Biopsy of breast lesion Lumpectomy
Pelvic examination Colposcopy	Cervical cancer		Pap smear		Cone biopsy Punch biopsy Dilation & curettage (D&C) Cryosurgery LEEP (loop electrosurgical excision procedure) Laser surgery Hysterectomy
Pelvic examination	Endometriosis		Urinalysis	Abdominal ultrasonography Chest radiograph	Laparoscopy Hysterectomy
Monthly breast self-examination	Fibrocystic breasts			Mammography Ultrasonography	Biopsy
Pelvic examination	Pelvic inflammatory disease	Complete blood count and differential (CBC)	Urinalysis Culture and sensitivity of vaginal discharge	Pelvic ultrasonography	Laparoscopy

Tests for Sexually Transmitted Diseases					
Pelvic examination	**Chlamydia**	Serology	Urinalysis Direct urethral or cervical smear using monoclonal antibodies ThinPrep Pap Test		
Pelvic examination Pap smear	**Condylomata**/ HPV (genital warts)		ThinPrep Pap Test	Excisional biopsy	
Pelvic examination	***Neisseria gonorrhoeae***	CBC	Urinalysis Direct smear of vaginal discharge, anal canal, and oropharynx Thayer-Martin culture ThinPrep® Pap Test	Pelvic ultrasonography	
	Hepatitis B and C and HIV	Virology	Liver function	Abdominal ultrasonography	Liver biopsy
Tests for Vaginitis					
Pelvic examination	**Candidiasis**	Blood glucose	Urinalysis **Wet mount:** direct vaginal smear with potassium hydroxide and/or saline (1 drop)		
Pelvic examination	**Trichomoniasis**		Urinalysis Wet mount: direct vaginal smear with isotonic saline (1 drop) and/or potassium hydroxide (KOH)		
Pelvic examination	**Bacterial vaginosis**	CBC	Culture and sensitivity of vaginal discharge		

Table 14-5 Female Reproductive System Disorders and Conditions

Bartholin Gland Infection. Infection of the mucous gland(s) that open near the vaginal opening.
Breast Cancer. Most common diagnosed cancer in females. A genetic cause has been identified for some breast cancers. Some symptoms are lump, thickening, swelling, dimpling, pain, and nipple discharge.
Cervical Cancer. A carcinoma of the cervix of the uterus caused by a progressive cervical dysplasia. Most common in women aged 30 to 40 years. A significant risk factor is seen in women who become sexually active early in their lives and who have multiple sex partners. Presence of HPV poses greater risk.
Cystocele. Herniation of the urinary bladder into the vagina. May cause urgency and frequency. Injury to the bladder during delivery of the fetus is one cause.
Endometriosis. Presence of endometrium in sites other than inside the uterus. May be found on the ovaries, fallopian tubes, large bowel, lungs, and pleura. Causes pelvic pain, dysmenorrhea, and infertility.
Fibrocystic Breasts. Benign cysts in breast tissue that increase or decrease in size during menses. Thought to be a normal variation in breast tissue due to monthly hormonal influence.
Pelvic Inflammatory Disease (PID). Pelvic reproductive organs become inflamed and infected by bacteria, viruses, or parasites. An ascending infection can ensue involving the vagina, cervix of uterus, body of uterus, fallopian tubes, and ovaries. Symptoms include vaginal discharge, pain, fever. May cause infertility. Majority caused by sexually transmitted disease (*Neisseria gonorrhea*, chlamydia).
Premenstrual Syndrome (PMS). Cluster of symptoms that occur monthly before the onset of menses thought to be caused by progesterone–estrogen imbalance. Symptoms include fluid retention, weight gain, irritability, and mood swings.
Rectocele. Herniation of the posterial wall of the vagina with the anterior wall of the rectum through the vagina.
Sexually Transmitted Diseases (STDs). Diseases caused by bacteria, viruses, and protozoa that are transmitted through sexual intercourse (vaginal, anal, oral). - *Chlamydia.* An invasion by an intracellular parasite causing urethritis, cervicitis, PID, proctitis, infant pneumonia, and conjunctivitis. - *Condylomata (HPV).* Genital warts caused by a virus. Grow around the external genitalia, rectum, and cervix. Associated with abnormal Pap smears. - *Neisseria gonorrhoeae.* An infection by a bacterium that can involve the cervix, urethra, fallopian tubes and ovaries, rectum, and mouth.
Vaginitis. Inflammation of the vagina that may be caused by bacteria, fungus, protozoa, chemical irritants, irritation from foreign bodies, vitamin deficiency, uncleanliness, and intestinal worms. - *Candidiasis.* A yeast (fungal) infection of the vagina caused by prolonged antibiotic therapy, pregnancy, or diabetes, which can change the normal vaginal flora leading to overgrowth of the fungus. - *Trichomoniasis.* An infection by a protozoan most commonly spread through sexual intercourse or may come from fecal contamination of the vagina.

Table 14-6 Common Sexually Transmitted Diseases

Pathology	Symptoms	Test	Treatment
AIDS	Flulike, lymphadenopathy, infections, malignancies, pneumonia	HIV CBC	Medication: antiretroviral medications such as zidovudine, didanosine, Ritonavir
Chlamydia	Usually asymptomatic	Vaginal culture ThinPrep® Pap test Urinalysis	Doxycyline, azithromycin
Condylomata	Warts on external and internal genitalia	Visual exam ThinPrep® Pap test HPV	Cryocautery or chemocautery preferred but electrocautery can be used Keratolytic agents such as Podofilox, CO_2 laser
Gonorrhea	Usually asymptomatic; yellowish-green discharge with dysuria in advanced stages	Gram stain or Thayer-Martin culture ThinPrep® Pap test	Ofloxacin, ceftriaxone, cefixine
Herpes simplex I and II	Itching and soreness followed by genital **vesicles,** which heal in 10 to 14 days	Visual exam Viral isolation by tissue culture	Acyclovir®, Valtrex, Famvir
Syphilis	Stage I: papule develops into ulcer, which develops into chancre on vulva Stage II: fever, general malaise, dermal and mucosal lesions Stage III: degeneration of central nervous system, lesions of internal structures	Venereal Disease Research Laboratory, fluorescent antibody test Dark-field exam Rapid Plasma Reagin (RPR) Culture and sensitivity of spinal fluid	Penicillin
Trichomonas	Milky white, frothy, malodorous discharge with genital burning and itching	Wet mount for microscopic examination	Oral Flagel®: partner(s) must also be treated

Cervical Punch Biopsy. The **cervical punch biopsy** is usually done in conjunction with a colposcopy to obtain a sample of cervical tissue for pathologic examination. The specimen is examined for malignant cells and the biopsy usually follows an abnormal Pap smear report.

The procedure is performed with the patient in lithotomy position and with a vaginal speculum in place. The provider may stain the cervix to aid in identifying abnormal tissue. If the colposcope is being used, it illuminates and magnifies the cervical tissue. The provider takes several tissue samples using the cervical punch biopsy forceps. If bleeding ensues, it can be controlled with a vaginal packing, or the area can be cauterized to stop the bleeding. The specimen is placed in a container with **formalin,** a completed requisition form is attached to the container, and it is sent to the pathology laboratory for examination. The patient may expect a small amount of

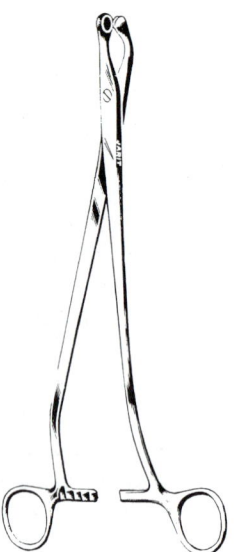

Figure 14-34 Toms-Gaylor uterine punch biopsy forceps. (Courtesy of Jarit Surgical Instruments.)

bleeding and should notify the provider if bleeding ensues that is greater than a menstrual period. A discharge that has a strong, foul odor is to be expected and can last for up to one month after the procedure.

Cervical Cone Biopsy. Another type of biopsy, known as a cone biopsy, can be performed. An inverted cone of tissue is excised by scalpel or laser under general anesthesia. In this procedure, a larger sample of tissue is excised to rule out invasive cancer and to remove the lesion. It is the most comprehensive specimen to diagnose a premalignant or malignant lesion. This is known as a cold knife biopsy.

Another type of cervical biopsy is the loop electrosurgical excision procedure (LEEP), also called large loop excision of the transformation zone (border between ectocervix and exocervix). This area is common for development of precancers and cancers. Either type of cervical cone biopsy can be used as a treatment to completely remove many precancers and very early cancers.

Cryosurgery. **Cryosurgery** is used to treat tissue by freezing temperatures. Chronic cervicitis and cervical **erosion** are two common problems treated in this manner (see Chapter 19 for information about cryosurgery). The freezing temperature causes cells to die; they are then cast off from the cervix and eventually replaced with healthy cells about a month after the procedure.

The procedure is performed with the patient in lithotomy position. The cervix is swabbed to remove mucus. The cryo probe is placed against the affected area of the cervix and the machine is turned on. The liquid nitrogen flows over the area for about 3 minutes and freezes the tissue. The tissue is allowed to thaw, and the treatment is repeated for another 3 minutes. The patient may have some pain similar to dysmenorrhea that may last for about a half hour. There should be no strong, foul odor, but there can be a discharge for up to 1 month. Patients should report any malodorous discharges because this may

Patient Education

Post Cervical Biopsy and Cervical Cone Biopsy

1. Rest for 24 hours after the procedure.
2. Do not lift heavy objects for two weeks.
3. Leave packing in place for 24 hours or as directed. Do not insert another tampon unless told to do so by the physician.
4. Report any bleeding greater than a normal menstrual period.

Patient Education

After Cryosurgery of Cervix

1. Expect a clear, watery, heavy discharge for several weeks, eventually tapering off.
2. Use only sanitary pads, not tampons. Change often, cleansing perineal area with each pad change.
3. Report signs of infection: fever, malodorous discharge, pain, nausea, or vomiting.
4. Do not engage in sexual intercourse, douche, or use tampons for 4 weeks (unless instructed otherwise by provider).
5. Expect a somewhat heavier than usual menstrual period the following month.
6. Report excessive bleeding.

indicate an infection. Healing usually takes 4 to 6 weeks.

Wet Prep/Wet Mount for Yeast, Bacteria, and Trichomonas. The wet prep or **wet mount** is an office procedure to determine the cause of vaginitis in women and urethritis in men. The provider takes a sample of the discharge on a cotton-tipped applicator, the medical assistant rinses it vigorously in a test tube containing a few drops (about 0.5 mL) of normal saline pressing the swab against the inside of the test tube to express all the specimen, places a drop of the solution onto a microscope slide, and covers it with a coverslip; then the provider views it microscopically for the following:

- If a yeast infection is present, budding yeast will be seen.
- If a bacterial infection is present, clue cells will be seen. Clue cells are vaginal epithelial cells that appear fuzzy with no clear cell edge. They appear this way because the outside edge is covered with bacteria.
- If trichomonas are present, they appear as motile single-cell protozoa. Movement will be noted. The trichomonas are sometimes identified in a microscopic portion of the urinalysis as well (see Procedure 14-4).

Potassium Hydroxide Prep for Fungus. After performing the previously mentioned test, a few drops of 10% potassium hydroxide (KOH) may be added to the remaining solution in the test tube and examined microscopically for fungi. The KOH destroys bacteria and vaginal epithelial cells, leaving only the cell walls of the fungus, which makes visualization easier. This slide is prepared in the same way as the wet prep: Place a drop of the solution onto a clean slide, cover with a coverslip. Dispose of all glass slides, coverslips, and test tubes into a sharps container (see Procedure 14-4).

Amplified DNA Probe Test for Chlamydia and Gonorrhea. The Amplified DNA Probe Test for Chlamydia and Gonorrhea is used as a screening tool for both men and women and on all pregnant women. It is not a culture. Two types of kits are available: the ProbeTec® blue kit for urethral specimens from the male patient (see Chapter 16) and the ProbeTec® pink kit for endocervical specimens from the female patient. The female kit contains preservative, swabs (one large swab and one small Mini-Tip Culturette Swab), and instructions. This test needs to be performed on the female patient before the digital/bimanual examination so that no lubricating jelly is present. Using the large swab, the provider will clean the cervix of any mucus, blood, and cellular debris and discard the swab. The Mini-Tip Culturette Swab is then inserted into the cervical canal and rotated for 15 to 30 seconds. Immediately it is placed into the transport tube. If the ProbeTec Wet Transport tube is used (Figure 14-35), the swab is broken off into the liquid before recapping. This test also may be used to test for chlamydia and gonorrhea in a urine specimen, following the manufacturer's instructions for collection and testing (see Procedure 14-5).

Laparoscopy. Laparoscopy is a procedure in which a lighted instrument is used to view the inside of the pelvic cavity. It can be helpful in diagnosing endometriosis and ovarian cysts or other abnormalities in the pelvic cavity. A tubal ligation, severing of the fallopian tubes, and an oophorectomy can be done laparoscopically. Laparoscopy can be done abdominally or vaginally (Figure 14-36).

Dilation and Curettage. Dilation and curettage (D&C) is a surgical procedure that involves dilating and scraping the cervix of endometrial tissue. It is commonly performed to remove any remaining tissue after an incomplete abortion or to

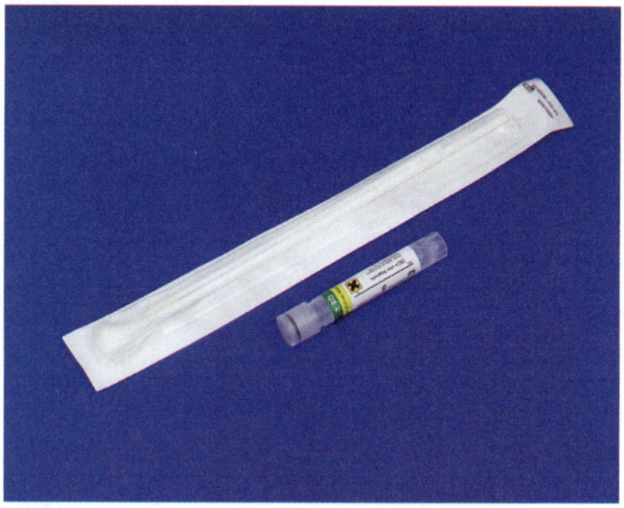

Figure 14-35 BD's ProbeTec Amplified DNA test kit for chlamydia and gonorrhea.

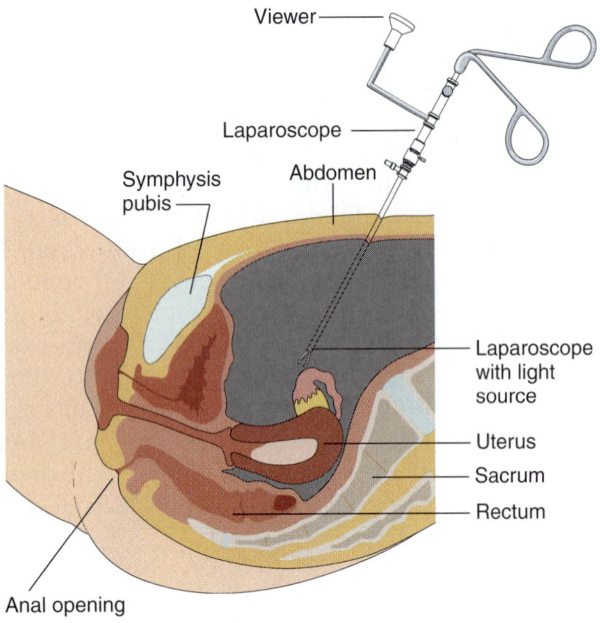

Figure 14-36 Laparoscopy.

examine the tissue if the patient has had abnormal uterine bleeding.

Diagnostic ultrasonography is used to help diagnose many gynecologic conditions, such as ovarian masses, fibroids, and endometriosis. The ultrasound can be performed transcervically or transvaginally (see Figure 14-11A and 14-11B.)

Complementary Therapy in Obstetrics and Gynecology

Most of the complementary therapy practiced today can be helpful to women in easing the discomforts of pregnancy and labor. In our stress-filled world, emotional calm can be provided through the use of some of these therapies.

Neonatal intensive care unit infants benefit from a calm, warm touch, rocking, hugging, and singing softly.

Information about any form of complementary therapy (stress reduction, imagery, acupuncture, biofeedback, massage therapy, music therapy, among others) should be obtained from the obstetrics patient at each visit. Consultation with the provider concerning their safety during pregnancy is advisable.

Caution is advised when the use of herbal medicine is considered during the pregnancy. Because herbal supplements are available over the counter and little is known about their effects on the fetus, women should be cautioned to avoid using any kind of herbal supplement during their first trimester. Women should ask their provider's advice about the use of the supplements after the first trimester.

Procedure 14-1

Assisting with Routine Prenatal Visits

STANDARD PRECAUTIONS:

PURPOSE:

To monitor the progress of the pregnancy.

EQUIPMENT/SUPPLIES:

Scale
Disposable gloves
Patient gown
Tape measure
Sphygmomanometer
Stethoscope
Doppler fetoscope and coupling agent
Urine specimen container
Urinalysis testing supplies
Biohazard waste container

PROCEDURE STEPS:

1. Wash hands.
2. Set up equipment.
3. Identify patient.
4. Obtain urine specimen. RATIONALE: A urine specimen for analysis is necessary for two reasons. An empty bladder facilitates the examination and is more comfortable for the patient. The urine sample will be tested.
5. Weigh patient. RATIONALE: Assesses gain or loss of weight to help determine fetal development and maternal nutrition.
6. Measure blood pressure.
7. Have patient disrobe from waist down and put on a gown open in the front. RATIONALE: An open gown facilitates access to the abdomen for examination and measurement of the fundal height.
8. Test the urine specimen while waiting for the provider. RATIONALE: Urinalysis is done for detection of glucose and protein, which may indicate disease.
9. Assist patient onto examination table and drape her. RATIONALE: The patient may be off balance and unsteady on her feet because of the enlargement of the abdomen. Provide for her safety.
10. Assist the provider as the examination is performed.
    - Hand the provider the tape measure to measure height of fundus
    - Hand the provider the Doppler fetal pulse detector for measurement of fetal heart rate. The medical assistant may spread the coupling agent onto the patient's abdomen.
11. After the examination, assist patient to sit for a few moments. Assess her color and pulse. RATIONALE: Orthostatic hypotension can occur when a patient rises from a recumbent position. Give the patient time for the blood pressure to go back to normal so she will not experience dizziness from decreased blood pressure.
12. Provide towel to patient to wipe off coupling agent.
13. Provide any instruction or clarification of provider's orders.
14. Apply gloves. Discard disposable supplies per OSHA guidelines. Disinfect equipment used.
15. Remove gloves.
16. Wash hands.
17. Set up for the next patient.
18. Record all information in patient's chart or electronic medical record.

DOCUMENTATION

4/14/20XX 2:30 PM Wt. 148 3/4 lbs., T 98.8°F, P 82, R 16, BP 118/72^{L} sitting. Urine dipstick negative for glucose and protein. Fundal height at 22 wks. FHR 120. Says she feels well and is sleeping and eating well. C. McInnis, CMA (AAMA) ___________________

Procedure 14-2

Assisting with Pelvic Examination and Pap Test (Conventional and ThinPrep® Methods)

STANDARD PRECAUTIONS:

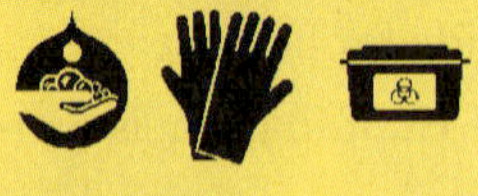

PURPOSE:

To assist the provider in collecting cervical cells for laboratory analysis for early detection of malignant cells of the cervix and to assess the health of the reproductive organs to detect diseases leading to early diagnosis and treatment.

EQUIPMENT/SUPPLIES:

Nonsterile gloves (2–3 pair)
Vaginal speculum, disposable or nondisposable
Warm water or warming light
Light source
Drape sheet
Patient gown
Tissues
Vaginal lubricant
Lab requisition (see Figure 14-30)
Urine specimen container
Urine testing supplies
Biohazard specimen bag
Biohazard waste container
Adjustable stool for provider

Supplies for the Pap test according to the method used for ThinPrep® Pap:

- Cervical spatula
- Brush and broom
- ThinPrep® container with solution

For conventional Pap test:

- Microscope slides
- Fixative and/or specimen bottle
- Cervical spatula
- Cytology brush

PROCEDURE STEPS:

1. Wash hands and assemble necessary supplies near patient.
2. Request that patient empty her bladder. (Instruct patient to save urine specimen and provide specimen container if ordered by provider.) RATIONALE: An empty bladder facilitates examination of the uterus and a urine specimen is frequently used for a urinalysis.
3. Provide patient with gown and request her to completely undress.
4. Explain procedure to patient.
5. Instruct patient to sit at end of table when ready for pelvic examination. Drape patient for privacy. If performing conventional Pap test, label the frosted end of the slide with a marking pencil. Include patient's name on slide. Indicate site from where specimen is collected: c = cervix, v = vagina, e = endocervical.
6. Assist patient into lithotomy position. Patient's knees should be relaxed and thighs rotated out as far as comfortable. Drape for privacy and warmth.
7. Encourage patient to breathe slowly and deeply through the mouth during examination. RATIONALE: Allows for relaxation of pelvic muscles and easier insertion of vaginal speculum.
8. Warm vaginal speculum with either warm water or under heat lamp or place on a heating pad. *NOTE:* Do not lubricate speculum. Lubricant obscures **exfoliated** cervical cells when Pap test is being performed.
9. Hand speculum and spatula, cytology brush, and broom to the provider as needed.
10. Apply gloves.
11. For conventional Pap test, hold slides for provider to apply smear of exfoliated cells, one for vaginal (v), one for cervical (c), and one for endocervical (e), in that order. If spraying Pap fixative, spray it over the slide within 10 seconds at a distance of about 6 inches. Allow to dry for at least 10 minutes. If using Pap fixative in a bottle, place slide directly into bottle. If using ThinPrep®, swish the cytology broom vigorously in the ThinPrep® solution until all the specimen has been deposited. Dispose of brush into

continues

Procedure 14-2 (continued)

biohazard container. RATIONALE: This maintains cell appearance and avoids contamination of cells. Avoid getting too close to slide with spray because this may destroy or damage cells. Slides must be fixed before they dry to protect the appearance of the cells.

12. For ThinPrep® Pap test, hand the speculum and cytology broom to the provider. Open the ThinPrep® solution container. When the cells have been obtained, take the broom and vigorously swish it into the container of solution until all the cells have been deposited. Replace the cap and label. Dispose of the broom into biohazard waste. RATIONALE: The ThinPrep® procedure requires that all cells obtained from the cervix be presented in the solution for complete testing.
13. Place lubricant on provider's gloved fingers without touching gloves, for bimanual and rectal examinations. The provider will insert the index and middle fingers into the vagina. The other hand is placed on the lower abdomen. The size, shape, and position of the uterus and ovaries are palpated.
14. The provider will insert one gloved finger into the rectum to check the ovaries and the tone of the rectal and pelvic muscles. Hemorrhoids, rectal fissures, or other lesions may be palpated.
15. Give the patient tissues to wipe genitalia and rectum.
16. Help patient to a sitting position, allowing her to rest a while. Check her pulse and skin color. RATIONALE: Some patients, especially older adult patients, can experience orthostatic hypotension.
17. Discard disposable supplies per OSHA guidelines. If stainless steel speculum was used, soak in cool water. Sanitize and sterilize as soon as convenient.
18. Remove gloves and wash hands.
19. Assist patient down and off the table if necessary.
20. Instruct patient to dress. Inform patient of how and when test results will be reported to her.
21. Prepare laboratory requisition (cytology request) form. Include provider name and address, date, source of specimen, patient's name and address, date of LMP, and hormone therapy if any. Place slides in slide container or ThinPrep® container into biohazard specimen bag. Place requisition into outer pocket of bag and send to laboratory.
22. Wash hands.
23. Document procedure in patient's chart or electronic medical record.

DOCUMENTATION

4/14/20XX 11:00 AM Wt. 138 lbs., T 98°F, P 68, R 20, BP 138/72^L sitting. Urine dipstick negative for protein and glucose. Pap smear performed by Dr. Woo. Slides of vaginal, cervical, endometrial cells sent to lab with requisition. Pelvic and rectal exams performed by Dr. Woo. Patient expressed no complaints of discomfort. BP 142/78 P 80. C. McInnis, RMA

Procedure 14-3

Assisting with Insertion of an Intrauterine Device (IUD)

STANDARD PRECAUTIONS:

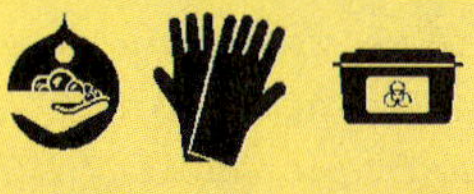

PURPOSE:

To assist the provider with the insertion of an intrauterine device (see Figure 14-19).

EQUIPMENT/SUPPLIES:

Nonsterile gloves (2–3 pair)
Sterile gloves
Vaginal speculum
Light source and stool for provider
Drape and gown
Tissue
Lubricant

continues

Procedure 14-3 (continued)

Prepackaged IUD
Biohazard waste container
Local anesthetic
Syringe and needle
Antiseptic such as Betadine® solution or swabs
Emesis basin for used items such as speculum

PROCEDURE STEPS:

1. Wash hands and assemble necessary supplies near patient.
2. Draw up local anesthetic into syringe as directed by provider.
3. Ask patient to empty her bladder. Save urine for pregnancy test. RATIONALE: If patient is pregnant, the IUD will not be inserted.
4. Ask patient to undress from the waist down and put on a gown.
5. Explain procedure to patient.
6. Give medication to patient for pain as prescribed by provider.
7. Help patient into lithotomy position. Drape for warmth and privacy.
8. Hand speculum to provider.
9. The provider does a pelvic examination after donning nonsterile gloves.
10. The provider checks for pelvic infection and position of the uterus. RATIONALE: An IUD cannot be inserted if the woman has a pelvic infection because the procedure can carry microorganisms into the uterus. The position of the uterus is important for the provider to know before insertion.
11. The provider swabs the cervix with an antiseptic and may inject a local anesthetic into the cervix.
12. The provider puts the IUD into the insertion device. The arms of the IUD flatten (the top of the "T")
13. The provider inserts the IUD with the insertion device through the cervix into the uterus.
14. The insertion tube is withdrawn completely.
15. Dispose of insertion device into biohazard waste container or emesis basin. The provider shortens the string on the IUD to 1–2 inches from the cervix and then removes speculum. Dispose of speculum into waste container or emesis basin. RATIONALE: The string is left long enough so the patient can feel for the string through her vagina after every period. The provider will have the patient check the string after the procedure. RATIONALE: Ensures that patient knows how to check for and find the string.
16. Place disposable speculum in biohazard waste container. Place nondisposable speculum into emesis basin.
17. Help patient into sitting position and allow her to remain seated while you check her pulse, skin color, and blood pressure if needed. RATIONALE: Some patients can experience orthostatic hypotension and become dizzy if they rise too quickly.
18. Discard disposable supplies according to OSHA guidelines. If stainless steel speculum was used, soak in cool water. Sanitize and sterilize later when convenient.
19. Remove gloves. Dispose in biohazard waster container. Wash hands.
20. Assist patient off table if she needs help.
21. Tell patient she can get dressed.
22. Explain to patient that she may experience light cramping and perhaps spotting for 1–2 days.
23. Make an appointment in 4–6 weeks for patient. Inform patient to make a yearly appointment thereafter for a check-up.
24. Document procedure in patient's chart or electronic medical record.

DOCUMENTATION

8/23/20XX 10:30 AM Pregnancy test negative. 1.0 mL of lidocaine injected into cervix by Dr. King. Pelvic examination done by Dr. King, and a copper IUD was inserted after anesthetic took effect. Small amount (approximately 15 mL) of bright red blood noted after insertion. Patient states she is "having slight cramping." BP 134/88, P 100 immediately after procedure. Patient able to feel string coming out of cervix into vagina. Explained to patient to call the office if she cannot feel the string, that sometimes the string tangles around the cervix and is hard to find. Told the patient that an ultrasound, if necessary, will show whether the IUD is still in place. Instructed patient to use another form of contraceptive until placement of IUD is confirmed. Blood pressure 10 minutes after procedure 124/82, P 92, color good. Patient left accompanied by her sister. C. McInnis, RMA ———

Procedure 14-4

Wet Prep/Wet Mount and Potassium Hydroxide (KOH) Prep

STANDARD PRECAUTIONS:

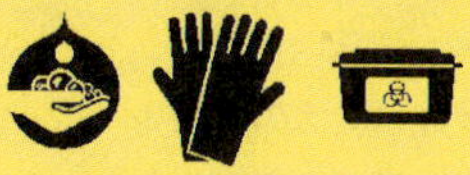

PURPOSE:

To test a vaginal specimen to determine the cause of vaginitis. The wet prep/wet mount tests for yeast, bacteria, and trichomonas; the KOH prep tests for yeast.

EQUIPMENT/SUPPLIES:

Cotton-tipped applicator
Small test tube
Normal saline (0.5 mL, or a few drops)
10% potassium hydroxide (KOH; 0.5 mL, or a few drops)
Two microscope slides and coverslips
Microscope
Vaginal speculum
Patient drape
Gloves
Other equipment as necessary for a vaginal examination

PROCEDURE STEPS:

1. Prepare the patient for a pelvic examination as outlined in Procedure 14-2 (Figure 14-37).
2. Place several drops of normal saline into a small test tube. RATIONALE: Preparing the test tube for the specimen.
3. Put on gloves.
4. Using the cotton-tipped applicator, the provider obtains a sampling of discharge from the vagina and hands it to the medical assistant. RATIONALE: The provider will complete the examination of the patient while the medical assistant prepares the sample for viewing.
5. Rinse the swab vigorously in the test tube containing saline, pressing the cotton tip against the inside of the test tube to express all the specimen. RATIONALE: It is important to get as much of the sample as possible for a more accurate diagnosis.
6. Dispose of the cotton-tipped applicator into a biohazard container. RATIONALE: All body fluid–contaminated supplies should be handled with care and disposed of according to Standard Precautions.
7. Apply a drop on a microscope slide and cover with a coverslip. Hand the slide to the provider for the microscopy examination. RATIONALE: Only a provider may perform the PPMP (Physician Performed Microscopy Procedure) for diagnosis, according to CLIA regulations.
8. Assist the patient back to a sitting position. Instruct her to dress and offer to assist if needed. RATIONALE: While the provider is viewing the slide, your responsibility is the safety and comfort of the patient.
9. In the laboratory, the provider will view the slide for yeast, bacteria, and trichomonas. RATIONALE: The provider will take the slide to the laboratory where the microscope is located.
10. After completion of the wet prep/wet mount, apply a few drops of KOH into the remaining solution in the test tube, place a drop on a fresh slide, and cover with a coverslip. RATIONALE: This is the second part of the microscopy test that can be performed on the vaginal secretion to diagnose the cause of vaginitis.
11. The provider will perform a microscopic examination for yeast. RATIONALE: This is a PPMP.
12. Dispose of all slides and the test tube into a sharps container. RATIONALE: As stated in Standard Precautions, all sharps must be disposed of in a sharps container.

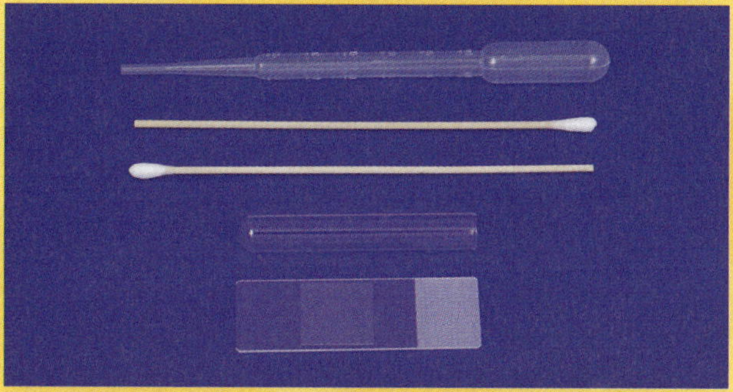

Figure 14-37 Supplies for wet mount and KOH prep: Pipette, cotton-tipped swabs, small test tube, and microscope slide with coverslip (not shown: saline and KOH solution).

continues

Procedure 14-4 (continued)

13. Disinfect the laboratory area and equipment. RATIONALE: As stated in Standard Precautions, all biohazard contaminated surfaces must be disinfected after contamination.
14. Return to the patient and assist as needed. RATIONALE: The patient may need assistance and direction.
15. Remove gloves. Wash hands.
16. Document procedure in patient's chart or electronic medical record. Input that a pelvic examination and wet prep were done, and that the provider examined the specimen. The provider will add his or her findings to the patient's electronic medical record. Be sure you sign the entry.

DOCUMENTATION

6/10/20XX 2:15 PM Wet mount and KOH prep done. Candidiasis identified. Patient given prescription for Gyne-Lotrimin 3 Vaginal suppositories (200 mg) at bedtime for three consecutive nights. J. Woo, MD.Patient will call on Monday to tell us how she feels. C. McInnis, RMA

Procedure 14-5

Amplified DNA ProbeTec Test for Chlamydia and Gonorrhea

STANDARD PRECAUTIONS:

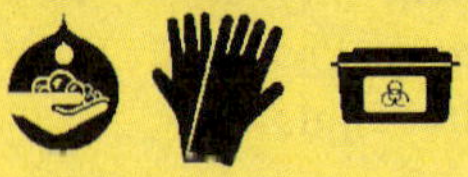

PURPOSE:

To test a vaginal specimen for diagnosis of chlamydia and gonorrhea and as a screening tool for the same for a pregnant woman.

EQUIPMENT/SUPPLIES:

Amplified DNA ProbeTec Kit (pink):

- Transport tube containing preservative
- Swabs (one large and one small Mini-Tip Culturette)

Vaginal speculum
Patient drape
Gloves
Other equipment as necessary for a vaginal examination

PROCEDURE STEPS:

1. Prepare the patient for a pelvic examination as outlined in Procedure 14-2.
2. Put on gloves.
3. Hand the large swab to the provider, who will use it to clean the cervix. RATIONALE: Mucus or blood on the cervix will interfere with the purity of the specimen.
4. Discard the large swab into the biohazard waste container. RATIONALE: According to Standard Precautions, all biohazard contaminated waste must be handled carefully and disposed of properly.
5. Hand the small Mini-tip Culturette Swab to the provider, who will insert the swab into the cervical os and rotate it for 15 to 20 seconds. RATIONALE: Accurate test results require obtaining adequate endocervical cells and secretions.
6. Immediately place the swab into the transport tube and recap. RATIONALE: The specimen must to be placed in the tube with preservative immediately to preserve it.
7. If using the ProbeTec Wet Transport tube, break the tip of the swab off into the the liquid before recapping. RATIONALE: The tip of the swab is scored and will snap off easily. This allows the entire specimen to be transported in a small amount of preservative.
8. Remove gloves. Wash hands.
9. Attach requisition to specimen.
10. Attend to your patient.
11. Document the procedure in the patient's chart or electronic medical record.

DOCUMENTATION

6/10/20XX 10:00 AM DNA ProbeTec test done by Dr. Woo. Entire specimen transported to laboratory. C. McInnis, RMA

Case Study 14-1

Refer to the scenario at the beginning of the chapter.
Mrs. Sanderson has an appointment today in the obstetric clinic at Inner City Health Care. Wanda is responsible for preparing Mrs. Sanderson for a repeat prenatal visit. Besides getting her patient ready, Wanda has other responsibilities to Mrs. Sanderson. Vital signs and certain laboratory tests must be done.

CASE STUDY REVIEW

1. What are some potential problems with Mrs. Sanderson's pregnancy that Wanda can discover and then can alert Dr. King?

Case Study 14-2

Maria Rodriguez has an appointment to see Dr. King today. It is her initial prenatal visit. She tells Liz Corbin, the medical assistant, as she is escorted from the reception area that she has been feeling "pretty good."

CASE STUDY REVIEW

1. Explain the importance of the initial prenatal visit. Discuss.
2. Name five specific diseases and conditions for which Dr. King will be on the alert during Maria's pregnancy, and what signs and symptoms to look for.
3. What laboratory and other procedural tests may be performed at the initial visit?
4. Discuss areas of patient education and health promotion that Liz will discuss with Maria at the initial visit.

Case Study 14-3

Annette Sanderson has made an appointment with Dr. King because she has had symptoms of vaginitis. When she arrives at the clinic, you take her chief complaint and history. She tells you that she has a milky-white, frothy vaginal discharge and that she itches in the genital area.

CASE STUDY REVIEW

1. What tests/procedures will you prepare for Dr. King in consideration of Annette's symptoms?
2. What is the most likely causative microorganism for these symptoms?
3. Describe the treatment that Dr. King may prescribe.

SUMMARY

Obstetrics and gynecology are two specialties that are usually practiced by the same provider. The OB/GYN provider will care for the health and well-being of the female patient in her pregnant and nonpregnant states. Knowledge of the numerous tests and procedures that are performed to diagnose and treat problems in the female patient are essential. Health promotion and patient education are of extreme importance whether the patient is an obstetric patient and scheduled for her initial prenatal visit or a gynecologic patient scheduled for yearly pelvic, Pap, and breast examinations.

STUDY FOR SUCCESS

To reinforce your knowledge and skills of information presented in this chapter:

- Review the Key Terms
- Practice any Procedures
- Consider the Case Studies and discuss your conclusions
- Answer the Review Questions
  - Multiple Choice
  - Critical Thinking
- Navigate the Internet and complete the Web Activities
- Practice the StudyWARE activities on the textbook CD
- Apply your knowledge in the Student Workbook activities
- Complete the Web Tutor sections
- View and discuss the DVD situations

REVIEW QUESTIONS

Multiple Choice

1. Which of the following conditions or diseases that an obstetrics patient experiences is considered to place her in the high-risk category?
   a. urinary tract infection
   b. 19 years of age
   c. both partners Rh negative
   d. poor nutritional habits
   e. poor hygiene
2. Using Nägele's Rule, calculate the expected date of birth of the baby of a patient whose last menstrual period was August 20, 2005.
   a. November 27, 2006
   b. December 13, 2006
   c. May 27, 2006
   d. April 20, 2006
3. The primary test performed at about the 16th week to check the fetus for neural tube defects is known as:
   a. alpha-fetoprotein test
   b. amniocentesis
   c. chorionic villus sampling (CVS)
   d. rubella titer
   e. Rh factor
4. The release of which of the following hormones is thought to cause labor to begin?
   a. progesterone
   b. estrogen
   c. oxytocin
   d. thyroxine
5. Ultrasonography is done to check for which of the following?
   a. gestational diabetes
   b. preeclampsia
   c. degree of effacement
   d. number of weeks of gestation
6. After a cervical punch biopsy, it is normal for the patient to experience which of the following?
   a. bleeding greater than a normal menstrual period
   b. no odor to vaginal discharge
   c. malodorous vaginal discharge
   d. severe abdominal cramps
7. To make the diagnosis of trichomoniasis, the medical assistant will need to prepare for which of the following?
   a. Pap smear
   b. ultrasonography
   c. wet mount
   d. culture and sensitivity
   e. blood glucose
8. To diagnose pelvic inflammatory disease (PID), the provider may order which of the following?
   a. culture and sensitivity
   b. Pap smear
   c. urinalysis
   d. rubella titer
   e. ultrasonography

9. Which of the following is/are primarily associated with abnormal Pap smears?
   a. endometriosis
   b. Bartholin cysts
   c. condylomata
   d. ovarian cysts
   e. PID
10. The primary purpose of colposcopy is to:
    a. treat advanced cancer of the vagina and cervix
    b. detect dysplastic cells of cervix after an abnormal Pap test
    c. treat PID in the fallopian tube
    d. treat endometriosis of the pelvic cavity

Critical Thinking Questions

1. A pregnant woman who has had no prenatal care has not had a period for 6 months. She has called the OB/GYN clinic to schedule an appointment because she has had vaginal bleeding. She continues to feel fetal movement.
   a. What laboratory tests or procedures will the provider order?
   b. What diagnosis is the provider most likely to make?
2. Lower abdominal and back pain that increases just before and during menses may be caused by what condition?
3. Emily Harris is scheduled to have a cervical punch biopsy. What is the primary reason for a cervical punch biopsy? Explain the post-biopsy instructions she will need.

WEB ACTIVITIES

Obstetrics

Access a Web site for expectant parents to locate information about the following:

1. Obtain fact sheets about each trimester.
2. Compile a list of tests, complications, and postpartum recovery.
3. Visit the National Library of Medicine Web site.
   a. What are the time frames for the various stages of labor?
   b. What are the various breech presentations?
4. Find a Web site that gives information about the Lamaze method of childbirth. Is this something you might consider for yourself or your partner?
5. Search the Internet for a Web site that gives information about postpartum exercise routines. Also visit http://www.medscape.com for information.

Gynecology

Locate a Web site specific to cancer of the female reproductive tract to complete the following:

1. What treatment options are available for cancer of the endometrium?
2. What tests are available to help diagnose the cancer?
3. Print a list of local support groups for women with endometrial cancer.
4. Visit the American College of Obstetricians and Gynecologists Web site for information about managing pregnant patients with the following disorders or conditions:
   a. hypertension
   b. cardiovascular disease
   c. Rh factor incompatibility
5. Visit the American Cancer Society's Web site. Find information about diethylstilbestrol (DES) and male offspring malignancies.

REFERENCES/BIBLIOGRAPHY

Centers for Disease Control and Prevention. (n.d.). *Genital HPV infection, CDC fact sheet.* Retrieved August 24, 2008, from http://www.cdc.gov/std/HPV/STDFact-HPV.htm.

Decision (pp. 165–192). Published by Rodale: Distributed to the trade by Holtzbrink Publishers, 2007.

Estrogen therapy: Not for prevention. (2004). *Consumer Report on Health,* 16(5), 3.

Littleton, L. Y., & Engebretson, J. C. (2002). *Maternal, neonatal, and women's health nursing.* Clifton Park, NY: Delmar Cengage Learning.

"The menopause–hormone discussion: how to weigh the risks," (June 11, 2007). Parker-Pope. Adapted from "The hormone decision." *The Wall Street Journal.* Published by Rodale: Distributed to the trade by Holtzbrink Publishers, 2007.

Morrison, R. W., & Lett, S. M. (2007). *Human papillomavirus (HPV) vaccine for VFC-eligible girls now available (memorandum).* Jamaica Plain, MA: The Commonwealth of Massachusetts, Executive Office of Health and Human Services, Department of Public Health, State Laboratory Institute. Retrieved August 24, 2008, from http://www.mass.gov/Eeohhs2/docs/dph/cdc/immunization/alerts_hpv_vaccine_availability.pdf.

National Cancer Institute. (2007). *Tamoxifen: Questions and answers.* Retrieved August 29, 2007, from http://www.cancer.gov/cancertopics/factsheet/therapy/tamoxifen.

National Cancer Institute Fact Sheet 4.21. *Human papillomavirus (HPV) vaccines: Questions and answers.* Retrieved October 5, 2008, from www.cancer.gov/cancertopics/factsheet/prevention/HPV-vaccine.

Spratto, G. R., & Woods, A. L. (2009). *2008/9 edition nurse's drug handbook.* Clifton Park, NY: Delmar Cengage Learning.

Taber's cyclopedic medical dictionary (21st ed.). (2002). Philadelphia: F. A. Davis.

Tamparo, C., & Lewis, M. (2005). *Diseases of the human body* (4th ed.). Philadelphia: F. A. Davis.

Web MD, Birth Control Health Center by Kelly Colihan, reviewed by Louise Change, MD, August 13, 2008. "More women ask for birth control." Retrieved October 5, 2008.

Web MD, Medical News Women's Health, Cervical Cancer Vaccine by Miranda Hitti, reviewed by Louise Chany, MD, September 12, 2008. "Gardisil approved to target more cancers." Retrieved October 5, 2008.

THE DVD HOOK-UP

In this chapter, you learned about the proper techniques for preparing a patient for a Pap and pelvic examination as well as a prenatal examination.

The selected scene from today's program illustrates Anita preparing a tray for a Pap procedure. Anita places the speculum into some warm water.

1. What are two reasons to place the speculum in water?
2. Why did Anita stay positioned above the drape?
3. What was the purpose of the Hemoccult Card?

DVD Journal Summary

Write a paragraph that summarizes what you learned from watching today's selected DVD scene. Think of how you feel when you have to have a pelvic examination. Do you like having the assistant in the room when you are examined? Why is it considered good practice for a female medical assistant to stay in the room with a male provider during a pelvic examination? What kinds of things will you do to make your patient feel more comfortable during a Pap/pelvic procedure?

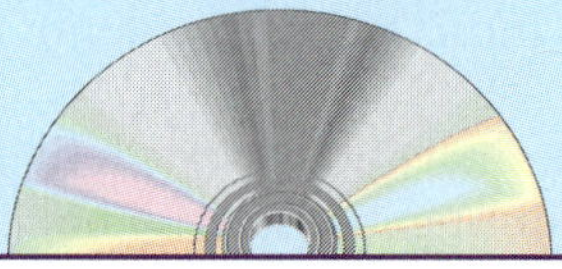

DVD Series	**Program Number**
Skills Based Series	6
Chapter/Scene Reference	
• *Pap Examination*	

Pediatrics

Chapter 15

KEY TERMS

Aerosolyzed
Cochlear Implantation
Exudate
Fontanel
Lyophilized
Myringotomy
Neonate
Organomercurial
Phenylketonuria (PKU)
Sensorineural
Suppurative
Tympanostomy

OUTLINE

OBJECTIVES

The student should strive to meet the following performance objectives and demonstrate an understanding of the facts and principles presented in this chapter through written and oral communication.

1. Define the key terms as presented in the glossary.
2. Describe the various theories of human development.
3. Describe pediatric care including measuring height, weight, head, chest circumference, and vital signs.

OBJECTIVES (continued)

4. Explain the process of collecting a urine specimen.
5. Explain the process of screening for hearing and visual impairments.
6. Describe common pediatric diseases and disorders.
7. Explain the importance of immunizations and scheduling of them.
8. Describe infant holds for injections and procedures.

Scenario

At Inner City Health Care, clinical assistant Bruce Goldman, CMA (AAMA), is responsible for encouraging parents to keep track of their children's immunization records. Bruce teaches parents the importance of immunizations for long-term health protection and the importance of following recommended vaccination schedules for maximum benefit.

INTRODUCTION

New techniques and developments occur frequently in medicine, and medical assistants must refine existing skills and learn new ones to be knowledgeable and proficient and to provide the most current, up-to-date quality care to patients. The medical assistant who works in a pediatrician's office or a pediatric ambulatory care setting that treats infants and children will need additional skills when providing pediatric care to patients.

Knowledge of the developmental stages, knowledge of diseases of infants and children, and the ability to gain the child's confidence and trust and the caregivers' cooperation are all skills required to provide for the physiological, emotional, and psychological needs of the pediatric patient. This chapter covers the specialty examination and the appropriate clinical procedures in pediatrics.

WHAT IS PEDIATRICS?

Pediatrics is the branch of medicine that cares for newborns, infants, children, and adolescents. Pediatricians are providers who diagnose and treat health problems and diseases specific to these age groups. This patient population has special needs, and medical assistants must be knowledgeable about the growth and development phases of life and diseases unique to pediatric patients. Children form judgments and have fears about health care providers. They need an atmosphere that is comfortable and one in which their physiological, emotional, and psychological needs are recognized and addressed.

Spotlight on Certification

RMA Content Outline

- Anatomy and physiology
- Patient education
- Vital signs and mensurations
- Pediatrics
- Parenteral medications
- Drugs
- Minor surgery
- Surgical supplies
- Surgical procedures

CMA (AAMA) Content Outline

- Psychology
- Adapting communication to an individual's ability to understand (e.g., patients with special needs)
- Equipment preparation and operation
- Patient preparation and assisting the provider

CMAS Content Outline

- Anatomy and physiology
- Vital signs and measurements
- Examination preparation

Medical assistants must gain the confidence and trust of the child and parent(s), allay fear, and help to promote positive relationships between the child and the provider and must themselves develop a positive relationship with the child. Children are likely to be cooperative when being examined or during a procedure if good rapport has been established. It is important to be honest with young patients and approach them at their level of understanding. Allow children to touch and hold a "safe" instrument, such as a stethoscope, and explain its purpose to them. Doing so can reduce anxiety and fear (Figure 15-1). It is important also for the medical assistant to recognize pediatric patients by their names no matter what their ages.

Taking a history of the child; assessing the child; measuring vital signs, height, weight, vision, and hearing; laboratory work; administration of injections; observing the parent–child interactions; and noting the child's development level are all responsibilities in which a medical assistant takes part.

The first physical examination of a newborn is performed immediately after delivery. The pediatrician assesses the **neonate's** ability to exist outside of the mother's uterus. A scoring system is used to determine the neonate's physical condition at 1, 5, and 15 minutes after birth. It is known as the APGAR (appearance, pulse, grimace, activity, and respiration) score. Muscle tone, skin color, respiration, heart rate, and response to stimuli are given a score 0, 1, 2, and so on, with the highest score 10. Infants with low APGAR scores need immediate attention, such as stimulation, oxygen, medication, and so on. Their condition is monitored closely (see Chapter 14).

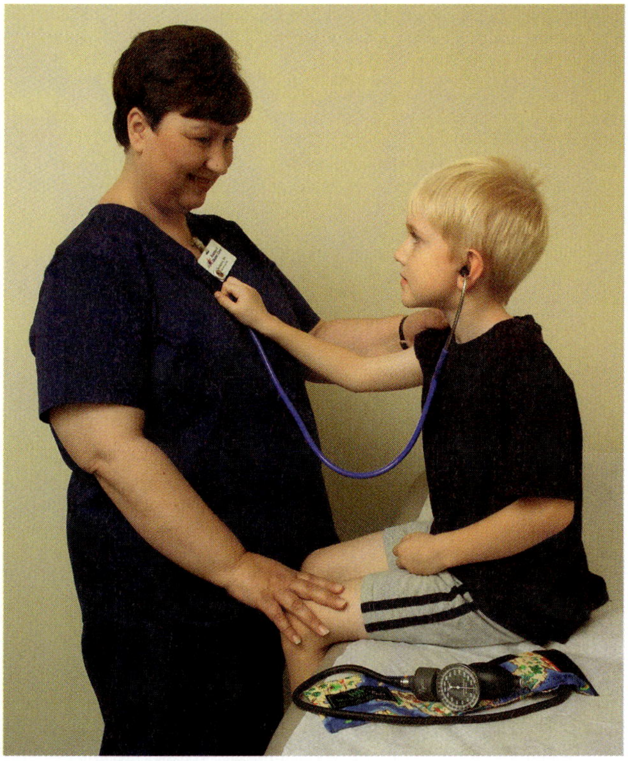

Figure 15-1 The medical assistant allows the child to touch the stethoscope and "listen" to her heartbeat to gain the child's cooperation.

Tests are done to detect problems the neonate may have. **Phenylketonuria (PKU),** iron deficiency anemia, lead poisoning, and hypothyroidism are problems for which neonates are screened shortly after the APGAR scoring is done.

Many patients seen in the pediatric setting are babies or children who are not ill. They are considered "well-baby" or "well-child" patients and are having routine checkups. Ill babies or children are often called "sick-child" or "sick-baby" patients. Well-baby appointments are regularly scheduled appointments during which time the provider examines the child and evaluates the growth and development of the child. Most offices schedule well-baby appointments after birth according to the following time frame: 1, 2, 4, 6, 9, 12, 15, 18, 24 months, and yearly thereafter.

The goal of well-baby visits or checkups is prevention of health problems and diseases. Typically, immunizations are given during these appointments. The charts shown in Figures 15-2, 15-3, and 15-4 include immunization schedules from the National Immunization Program. The program urges that all children be immunized because the vaccines provide the best defense against many dangerous childhood diseases. Immunizations protect children against hepatitis A and B, polio, measles, mumps, rubella, pertussis, diphtheria, tetanus, *Haemophilus influenza* type b, pneumonia, chicken pox, influenza, rotavirus, meningitis, and human papillomavirus (HPV) (see Chapter 14). Immunizations are given by mouth, injection, and intranasal spray. All of these need to be given before age 2 when children are most susceptible to infectious diseases. Vaccines protect children during these periods. HPV is the exception. It is given between ages 13 to 18 with the minimum age 9 years.

Preparation of Vaccines for Administration

Careful attention to both proper storage of vaccines and thorough patient preparation for immunization will promote effective vaccination results. Access to vaccination should be available to all patients, especially to families with young infants and children.

Recommended Immunization Schedule for Persons Aged 0 Through 6 Years—United States • 2009

For those who fall behind or start late, see the catch-up schedule

Vaccine ▼ Age ▶	Birth	1 month	2 months	4 months	6 months	12 months	15 months	18 months	19–23 months	2–3 years	4–6 years
Hepatitis B[1]	HepB	HepB		*see footnote 1*	HepB						
Rotavirus[2]			RV	RV	*RV*[2]						
Diphtheria, Tetanus, Pertussis[3]			DTaP	DTaP	DTaP	*see footnote 3*	DTaP				DTaP
Haemophilus influenzae type b[4]			Hib	Hib	*Hib*[4]	Hib					
Pneumococcal[5]			PCV	PCV	PCV	PCV				PPSV	
Inactivated Poliovirus			IPV	IPV	IPV						IPV
Influenza[6]					Influenza (Yearly)						
Measles, Mumps, Rubella[7]						MMR		*see footnote 7*			MMR
Varicella[8]						Varicella		*see footnote 8*			Varicella
Hepatitis A[9]						HepA (2 doses)				HepA Series	
Meningococcal[10]										MCV	

Range of recommended ages

Certain high-risk groups

This schedule indicates the recommended ages for routine administration of currently licensed vaccines, as of December 1, 2008, for children aged 0 through 6 years. Any dose not administered at the recommended age should be administered at a subsequent visit, when indicated and feasible. Licensed combination vaccines may be used whenever any component of the combination is indicated and other components are not contraindicated and if approved by the Food and Drug Administration for that dose of the series. Providers should consult the relevant Advisory Committee on Immunization Practices statement for detailed recommendations, including high-risk conditions: http://www.cdc.gov/vaccines/pubs/acip-list.htm. Clinically significant adverse events that follow immunization should be reported to the Vaccine Adverse Event Reporting System (VAERS). Guidance about how to obtain and complete a VAERS form is available at http://www.vaers.hhs.gov or by telephone, 800-822-7967.

1. **Hepatitis B vaccine (HepB).** ***(Minimum age: birth)***

   At birth:
   - Administer monovalent HepB to all newborns before hospital discharge.
   - If mother is hepatitis B surface antigen (HBsAg)-positive, administer HepB and 0.5 mL of hepatitis B immune globulin (HBIG) within 12 hours of birth.
   - If mother's HBsAg status is unknown, administer HepB within 12 hours of birth. Determine mother's HBsAg status as soon as possible and, if HBsAg-positive, administer HBIG (no later than age 1 week).

   After the birth dose:
   - The HepB series should be completed with either monovalent HepB or a combination vaccine containing HepB. The second dose should be administered at age 1 or 2 months. The final dose should be administered no earlier than age 24 weeks.
   - Infants born to HBsAg-positive mothers should be tested for HBsAg and antibody to HBsAg (anti-HBs) after completion of at least 3 doses of the HepB series, at age 9 through 18 months (generally at the next well-child visit).

   4-month dose:
   - Administration of 4 doses of HepB to infants is permissible when combination vaccines containing HepB are administered after the birth dose.

2. **Rotavirus vaccine (RV).** ***(Minimum age: 6 weeks)***
   - Administer the first dose at age 6 through 14 weeks (maximum age: 14 weeks 6 days). Vaccination should not be initiated for infants aged 15 weeks or older (i.e., 15 weeks 0 days or older).
   - Administer the final dose in the series by age 8 months 0 days.
   - If Rotarix® is administered at ages 2 and 4 months, a dose at 6 months is not indicated.

3. **Diphtheria and tetanus toxoids and acellular pertussis vaccine (DTaP).** ***(Minimum age: 6 weeks)***
   - The fourth dose may be administered as early as age 12 months, provided at least 6 months have elapsed since the third dose.
   - Administer the final dose in the series at age 4 through 6 years.

4. ***Haemophilus influenzae*** **type b conjugate vaccine (Hib).** ***(Minimum age: 6 weeks)***
   - If PRP-OMP (PedvaxHIB® or Comvax® [HepB-Hib]) is administered at ages 2 and 4 months, a dose at age 6 months is not indicated.
   - TriHiBit® (DTaP/Hib) should not be used for doses at ages 2, 4, or 6 months but can be used as the final dose in children aged 12 months or older.

5. **Pneumococcal vaccine.** ***(Minimum age: 6 weeks for pneumococcal conjugate vaccine [PCV]; 2 years for pneumococcal polysaccharide vaccine [PPSV])***
   - PCV is recommended for all children aged younger than 5 years. Administer 1 dose of PCV to all healthy children aged 24 through 59 months who are not completely vaccinated for their age.
   - Administer PPSV to children aged 2 years or older with certain underlying medical conditions (see *MMWR* 2000;49[No. RR-9]), including a cochlear implant.

6. **Influenza vaccine.** ***(Minimum age: 6 months for trivalent inactivated influenza vaccine [TIV]; 2 years for live, attenuated influenza vaccine [LAIV])***
   - Administer annually to children aged 6 months through 18 years.
   - For healthy nonpregnant persons (i.e., those who do not have underlying medical conditions that predispose them to influenza complications) aged 2 through 49 years, either LAIV or TIV may be used.
   - Children receiving TIV should receive 0.25 mL if aged 6 through 35 months or 0.5 mL if aged 3 years or older.
   - Administer 2 doses (separated by at least 4 weeks) to children aged younger than 9 years who are receiving influenza vaccine for the first time or who were vaccinated for the first time during the previous influenza season but only received 1 dose.

7. **Measles, mumps, and rubella vaccine (MMR).** ***(Minimum age: 12 months)***
   - Administer the second dose at age 4 through 6 years. However, the second dose may be administered before age 4, provided at least 28 days have elapsed since the first dose.

8. **Varicella vaccine.** ***(Minimum age: 12 months)***
   - Administer the second dose at age 4 through 6 years. However, the second dose may be administered before age 4, provided at least 3 months have elapsed since the first dose.
   - For children aged 12 months through 12 years the minimum interval between doses is 3 months. However, if the second dose was administered at least 28 days after the first dose, it can be accepted as valid.

9. **Hepatitis A vaccine (HepA).** ***(Minimum age: 12 months)***
   - Administer to all children aged 1 year (i.e., aged 12 through 23 months). Administer 2 doses at least 6 months apart.
   - Children not fully vaccinated by age 2 years can be vaccinated at subsequent visits.
   - HepA also is recommended for children older than 1 year who live in areas where vaccination programs target older children or who are at increased risk of infection. See *MMWR* 2006;55(No. RR-7).

10. **Meningococcal vaccine.** ***(Minimum age: 2 years for meningococcal conjugate vaccine [MCV] and for meningococcal polysaccharide vaccine [MPSV])***
    - Administer MCV to children aged 2 through 10 years with terminal complement component deficiency, anatomic or functional asplenia, and certain other high-risk groups. See *MMWR* 2005;54(No. RR-7).
    - Persons who received MPSV 3 or more years previously and who remain at increased risk for meningococcal disease should be revaccinated with MCV.

The Recommended Immunization Schedules for Persons Aged 0 Through 18 Years are approved by the Advisory Committee on Immunization Practices (www.cdc.gov/vaccines/recs/acip), the American Academy of Pediatrics (http://www.aap.org), and the American Academy of Family Physicians (http://www.aafp.org).

DEPARTMENT OF HEALTH AND HUMAN SERVICES • CENTERS FOR DISEASE CONTROL AND PREVENTION

Figure 15-2 The recommended immunization schedule for persons aged 0–6 years is approved by the Advisory Committee on Immunization Practices (http://www.cdc.gov/vaccines/recs/acip), the American Academy of Pediatrics (http://www.aap.org), and the American Academy of Family Physicians (http://www.aafp.org).

Recommended Immunization Schedule for Persons Aged 7 Through 18 Years—United States • 2009

For those who fall behind or start late, see the schedule below and the catch-up schedule

Vaccine ▼ Age ▶	7–10 years	11–12 years	13–18 years
Tetanus, Diphtheria, Pertussis[1]	*see footnote 1*	Tdap (Range of recommended ages)	Tdap (Catch-up immunization)
Human Papillomavirus[2]	*see footnote 2*	HPV (3 doses) (Range of recommended ages)	HPV Series (Catch-up immunization)
Meningococcal[3]	MCV (Certain high-risk groups)	MCV (Range of recommended ages)	MCV (Catch-up immunization)
Influenza[4]	Influenza (Yearly) (Range of recommended ages)		
Pneumococcal[5]	PPSV (Certain high-risk groups)		
Hepatitis A[6]	HepA Series (Certain high-risk groups)		
Hepatitis B[7]	HepB Series (Catch-up immunization)		
Inactivated Poliovirus[8]	IPV Series (Catch-up immunization)		
Measles, Mumps, Rubella[9]	MMR Series (Catch-up immunization)		
Varicella[10]	Varicella Series (Catch-up immunization)		

Range of recommended ages

Catch-up immunization

Certain high-risk groups

This schedule indicates the recommended ages for routine administration of currently licensed vaccines, as of December 1, 2008, for children aged 7 through 18 years. Any dose not administered at the recommended age should be administered at a subsequent visit, when indicated and feasible. Licensed combination vaccines may be used whenever any component of the combination is indicated and other components are not contraindicated and if approved by the Food and Drug Administration for that dose of the series. Providers should consult the relevant Advisory Committee on Immunization Practices statement for detailed recommendations, including high-risk conditions: http://www.cdc.gov/vaccines/pubs/acip-list.htm. Clinically significant adverse events that follow immunization should be reported to the Vaccine Adverse Event Reporting System (VAERS). Guidance about how to obtain and complete a VAERS form is available at http://www.vaers.hhs.gov or by telephone, 800-822-7967.

1. Tetanus and diphtheria toxoids and acellular pertussis vaccine (Tdap). ***(Minimum age: 10 years for BOOSTRIX® and 11 years for ADACEL®)***
- Administer at age 11 or 12 years for those who have completed the recommended childhood DTP/DTaP vaccination series and have not received a tetanus and diphtheria toxoid (Td) booster dose.
- Persons aged 13 through 18 years who have not received Tdap should receive a dose.
- A 5-year interval from the last Td dose is encouraged when Tdap is used as a booster dose; however, a shorter interval may be used if pertussis immunity is needed.

2. Human papillomavirus vaccine (HPV). ***(Minimum age: 9 years)***
- Administer the first dose to females at age 11 or 12 years.
- Administer the second dose 2 months after the first dose and the third dose 6 months after the first dose (at least 24 weeks after the first dose).
- Administer the series to females at age 13 through 18 years if not previously vaccinated.

3. Meningococcal conjugate vaccine (MCV).
- Administer at age 11 or 12 years, or at age 13 through 18 years if not previously vaccinated.
- Administer to previously unvaccinated college freshmen living in a dormitory.
- MCV is recommended for children aged 2 through 10 years with terminal complement component deficiency, anatomic or functional asplenia, and certain other groups at high risk. See *MMWR* 2005;54(No. RR-7).
- Persons who received MPSV 5 or more years previously and remain at increased risk for meningococcal disease should be revaccinated with MCV.

4. Influenza vaccine.
- Administer annually to children aged 6 months through 18 years.
- For healthy nonpregnant persons (i.e., those who do not have underlying medical conditions that predispose them to influenza complications) aged 2 through 49 years, either LAIV or TIV may be used.
- Administer 2 doses (separated by at least 4 weeks) to children aged younger than 9 years who are receiving influenza vaccine for the first time or who were vaccinated for the first time during the previous influenza season but only received 1 dose.

5. Pneumococcal polysaccharide vaccine (PPSV).
- Administer to children with certain underlying medical conditions (see *MMWR* 1997;46[No. RR-8]), including a cochlear implant. A single revaccination should be administered to children with functional or anatomic asplenia or other immunocompromising condition after 5 years.

6. Hepatitis A vaccine (HepA).
- Administer 2 doses at least 6 months apart.
- HepA is recommended for children older than 1 year who live in areas where vaccination programs target older children or who are at increased risk of infection. See *MMWR* 2006;55(No. RR-7).

7. Hepatitis B vaccine (HepB).
- Administer the 3-dose series to those not previously vaccinated.
- A 2-dose series (separated by at least 4 months) of adult formulation Recombivax HB® is licensed for children aged 11 through 15 years.

8. Inactivated poliovirus vaccine (IPV).
- For children who received an all-IPV or all-oral poliovirus (OPV) series, a fourth dose is not necessary if the third dose was administered at age 4 years or older.
- If both OPV and IPV were administered as part of a series, a total of 4 doses should be administered, regardless of the child's current age.

9. Measles, mumps, and rubella vaccine (MMR).
- If not previously vaccinated, administer 2 doses or the second dose for those who have received only 1 dose, with at least 28 days between doses.

10. Varicella vaccine.
- For persons aged 7 through 18 years without evidence of immunity (see *MMWR* 2007;56[No. RR-4]), administer 2 doses if not previously vaccinated or the second dose if they have received only 1 dose.
- For persons aged 7 through 12 years, the minimum interval between doses is 3 months. However, if the second dose was administered at least 28 days after the first dose, it can be accepted as valid.
- For persons aged 13 years and older, the minimum interval between doses is 28 days.

The Recommended Immunization Schedules for Persons Aged 0 Through 18 Years are approved by the Advisory Committee on Immunization Practices (www.cdc.gov/vaccines/recs/acip), the American Academy of Pediatrics (http://www.aap.org), and the American Academy of Family Physicians (http://www.aafp.org).

DEPARTMENT OF HEALTH AND HUMAN SERVICES • CENTERS FOR DISEASE CONTROL AND PREVENTION

Figure 15-3 The recommended immunization schedule for persons aged 7–18 years is approved by the Advisory Committee on Immunization Practices (http://www.cdc.gov/vaccines/recs/acip), the American Academy of Pediatrics (http://www.aap.org), and the American Academy of Family Physicians (http://www.aafp.org).

Catch-up Immunization Schedule for Persons Aged 4 Months Through 18 Years Who Start Late or Who Are More Than 1 Month Behind—United States • 2009

The table below provides catch-up schedules and minimum intervals between doses for children whose vaccinations have been delayed. A vaccine series does not need to be restarted, regardless of the time that has elapsed between doses. Use the section appropriate for the child's age.

Vaccine	Minimum Age for Dose 1	Minimum Interval Between Doses			
		Dose 1 to Dose 2	Dose 2 to Dose 3	Dose 3 to Dose 4	Dose 4 to Dose 5
CATCH-UP SCHEDULE FOR PERSONS AGED 4 MONTHS THROUGH 6 YEARS					
Hepatitis B[1]	Birth	4 weeks	8 weeks (and at least 16 weeks after first dose)		
Rotavirus[2]	6 wks	4 weeks	4 weeks[2]		
Diphtheria, Tetanus, Pertussis[3]	6 wks	4 weeks	4 weeks	6 months	6 months[3]
Haemophilus influenzae type b[4]	6 wks	4 weeks if first dose administered at younger than age 12 months 8 weeks (as final dose) if first dose administered at age 12-14 months No further doses needed if first dose administered at age 15 months or older	4 weeks[4] if current age is younger than 12 months 8 weeks (as final dose)[4] if current age is 12 months or older and second dose administered at younger than age 15 months No further doses needed if previous dose administered at age 15 months or older	8 weeks (as final dose) This dose only necessary for children aged 12 months through 59 months who received 3 doses before age 12 months	
Pneumococcal[5]	6 wks	4 weeks if first dose administered at younger than age 12 months 8 weeks (as final dose for healthy children) if first dose administered at age 12 months or older or current age 24 through 59 months No further doses needed for healthy children if first dose administered at age 24 months or older	4 weeks if current age is younger than 12 months 8 weeks (as final dose for healthy children) if current age is 12 months or older No further doses needed for healthy children if previous dose administered at age 24 months or older	8 weeks (as final dose) This dose only necessary for children aged 12 months through 59 months who received 3 doses before age 12 months or for high-risk children who received 3 doses at any age	
Inactivated Poliovirus[6]	6 wks	4 weeks	4 weeks	4 weeks[6]	
Measles, Mumps, Rubella[7]	12 mos	4 weeks			
Varicella[8]	12 mos	3 months			
Hepatitis A[9]	12 mos	6 months			
CATCH-UP SCHEDULE FOR PERSONS AGED 7 THROUGH 18 YEARS					
Tetanus, Diphtheria/ Tetanus, Diphtheria, Pertussis[10]	7 yrs[10]	4 weeks	4 weeks if first dose administered at younger than age 12 months 6 months if first dose administered at age 12 months or older	6 months if first dose administered at younger than age 12 months	
Human Papillomavirus[11]	9 yrs	Routine dosing intervals are recommended[11]			
Hepatitis A[9]	12 mos	6 months			
Hepatitis B[1]	Birth	4 weeks	8 weeks (and at least 16 weeks after first dose)		
Inactivated Poliovirus[6]	6 wks	4 weeks	4 weeks	4 weeks[6]	
Measles, Mumps, Rubella[7]	12 mos	4 weeks			
Varicella[8]	12 mos	3 months if the person is younger than age 13 years 4 weeks if the person is aged 13 years or older			

1. Hepatitis B vaccine (HepB).
- Administer the 3-dose series to those not previously vaccinated.
- A 2-dose series (separated by at least 4 months) of adult formulation Recombivax HB® is licensed for children aged 11 through 15 years.

2. Rotavirus vaccine (RV).
- The maximum age for the first dose is 14 weeks 6 days. Vaccination should not be initiated for infants aged 15 weeks or older (i.e., 15 weeks 0 days or older).
- Administer the final dose in the series by age 8 months 0 days.
- If Rotarix® was administered for the first and second doses, a third dose is not indicated.

3. Diphtheria and tetanus toxoids and acellular pertussis vaccine (DTaP).
- The fifth dose is not necessary if the fourth dose was administered at age 4 years or older.

4. *Haemophilus influenzae* type b conjugate vaccine (Hib).
- Hib vaccine is not generally recommended for persons aged 5 years or older. No efficacy data are available on which to base a recommendation concerning use of Hib vaccine for older children and adults. However, studies suggest good immunogenicity in persons who have sickle cell disease, leukemia, or HIV infection, or who have had a splenectomy; administering 1 dose of Hib vaccine to these persons is not contraindicated.
- If the first 2 doses were PRP-OMP (PedvaxHIB® or Comvax®), and administered at age 11 months or younger, the third (and final) dose should be administered at age 12 through 15 months and at least 8 weeks after the second dose.
- If the first dose was administered at age 7 through 11 months, administer 2 doses separated by 4 weeks and a final dose at age 12 through 15 months.

5. Pneumococcal vaccine.
- Administer 1 dose of pneumococcal conjugate vaccine (PCV) to all healthy children aged 24 through 59 months who have not received at least 1 dose of PCV on or after age 12 months.
- For children aged 24 through 59 months with underlying medical conditions, administer 1 dose of PCV if 3 doses were received previously or administer 2 doses of PCV at least 8 weeks apart if fewer than 3 doses were received previously.
- Administer pneumococcal polysaccharide vaccine (PPSV) to children aged 2 years or older with certain underlying medical conditions (see *MMWR* 2000;49[No. RR-9]), including a cochlear implant, at least 8 weeks after the last dose of PCV.

6. Inactivated poliovirus vaccine (IPV).
- For children who received an all-IPV or all-oral poliovirus (OPV) series, a fourth dose is not necessary if the third dose was administered at age 4 years or older.
- If both OPV and IPV were administered as part of a series, a total of 4 doses should be administered, regardless of the child's current age.

7. Measles, mumps, and rubella vaccine (MMR).
- Administer the second dose at age 4 through 6 years. However, the second dose may be administered before age 4, provided at least 28 days have elapsed since the first dose.
- If not previously vaccinated, administer 2 doses with at least 28 days between doses.

8. Varicella vaccine.
- Administer the second dose at age 4 through 6 years. However, the second dose may be administered before age 4, provided at least 3 months have elapsed since the first dose.
- For persons aged 12 months through 12 years, the minimum interval between doses is 3 months. However, if the second dose was administered at least 28 days after the first dose, it can be accepted as valid.
- For persons aged 13 years and older, the minimum interval between doses is 28 days.

9. Hepatitis A vaccine (HepA).
- HepA is recommended for children older than 1 year who live in areas where vaccination programs target older children or who are at increased risk of infection. See *MMWR* 2006;55(No. RR-7).

10. Tetanus and diphtheria toxoids vaccine (Td) and tetanus and diphtheria toxoids and acellular pertussis vaccine (Tdap).
- Doses of DTaP are counted as part of the Td/Tdap series
- Tdap should be substituted for a single dose of Td in the catch-up series or as a booster for children aged 10 through 18 years; use Td for other doses.

11. Human papillomavirus vaccine (HPV).
- Administer the series to females at age 13 through 18 years if not previously vaccinated.
- Use recommended routine dosing intervals for series catch-up (i.e., the second and third doses should be administered at 2 and 6 months after the first dose). However, the minimum interval between the first and second doses is 4 weeks. The minimum interval between the second and third doses is 12 weeks, and the third dose should be given at least 24 weeks after the first dose.

Information about reporting reactions after immunization is available online at http://www.vaers.hhs.gov or by telephone, 800-822-7967. Suspected cases of vaccine-preventable diseases should be reported to the state or local health department. Additional information, including precautions and contraindications for immunization, is available from the National Center for Immunization and Respiratory Diseases at http://www.cdc.gov/vaccines or telephone, 800-CDC-INFO (800-232-4636).

DEPARTMENT OF HEALTH AND HUMAN SERVICES • CENTERS FOR DISEASE CONTROL AND PREVENTION

Figure 15-4 Catch-up immunization schedule for persons aged 4 months–18 years who start late or who are more than one month behind. Information about reporting reactions after immunization is available at the VAERS Web site (http://www.vaers.hhs.gov) or by telephone via the VAERS national toll-free information line (800-822-7967). Suspected cases of vaccine-preventable diseases should be reported to the state or local health department. Additional information, including precautions and contraindications for immunization, is available from the National Center for Immunization and Respiratory Diseases Web site (http://www.cdc.gov/vaccines) or by telephone (800-CDC-INFO).

Table 15-1 Vaccine Administration Guidelines

Vaccine	Disease	About the Disease	Precautions and Contra-indications	Side Effects and Adverse Reactions	Vaccine Schedule
DTaP, DT, Td	Diphtheria, tetanus, pertussis	Diphtheria can cause breathing problems, paralysis, heart failure, and death; tetanus causes paralysis of the jaw—cannot open mouth or swallow; pertussis (whooping cough) causes severe coughing so infants have difficulty eating, drinking, or breathing or causes brain damage/death	Moderate to severe acute illness, neurologic disorder, allergic reaction to prior dose	Local reactions, fussiness, seizures, fever, allergic reaction	2 months, 4 months, 6 months, 15–18 months, 4–6 years; not given at 7 years or older
Inactive poliovirus (IPV)*	Poliomyelitis	Causes paralysis of skeletal muscles and diaphragm so that infants cannot breathe on their own	Allergic reaction to prior dose or to neomycin, streptomycin, or polymixin B; moderate to severe acute illness; pregnancy	Local reactions, allergic reaction	2 months, 4 months, 16–18 months, 4–6 years (booster)
Haemophilus influenzae type B (Hib)	Meningitis, pneumonia, epiglottitis, pericarditis	Causes bacterial meningitis, pneumonia, epiglottitis, septicemia, death	Moderate to severe acute illness, allergic reaction to prior dose	Fever, swelling, redness and/or pain; allergic reaction	2 months, 4 months, 6 months, 12–15 months (booster); children younger than 6 weeks old should not get vaccine
Combination vaccines containing Hib			Moderate to severe acute illness	Local reaction, allergic reaction	
• DTaP_Hib (TriHIBit)	Diphtheria, tetanus, pertussis, *Haemophilus influenzae*				Cannot be used at 2 months, 4 months, or 6 months; may be used as booster
• Hepatitis B-Hib (-Comvax)	Hepatitis B and *Haemophilus influenzae*				2 months, 4 months, 12–15 months; not given to infants younger than 6 weeks old
Hepatitis B (HBV)	Hepatitis B	Anorexia, fatigue, diarrhea, vomiting, liver damage, cancer, death	Pregnancy, moderate to severe acute illness, allergic reaction to baker's yeast	Mild systemic effects, soreness, fever, allergic reaction	Within 12 hrs of birth, 1–2 months, 6 months (3 doses needed)

(continues)

*Oral polio vaccine no longer recommended

Table 15-1 Vaccine Administration Guidelines (continued)

Vaccine	Disease	About the Disease	Precautions and Contra-indications	Side Effects and Adverse Reactions	Vaccine Schedule
Pediatrix, DTap, HepV, IPV	Diphtheria, tetanus, pertussis, *Haemophilus influenzae*, hepatitis B, inactive poliovirus		Moderate to severe acute illness	Mild systemic effects, local reaction, allergic reaction	2 months, 4 months, 6 months
Td	Tetanus, diphtheria		Moderate to severe acute illness, severe allergic reaction to prior dose	Soreness; swelling; severe allergic reaction; deep, aching pain in muscles of upper arm(s)	7 years or older then every 10 years for life
MMR	Measles, mumps, rubella	Measles can cause otitis media, pneumonia, seizures, brain damage, death; mumps can cause fever, swollen glands, deafness, meningitis, swelling of testicles or ovaries, death; rubella can cause pregnant women to have miscarriages or babies born with severe anomalies	Do not give if allergic to gelatin or the antibiotic neomycin, moderate to severe acute illness, breast-feeding, pregnancy, immunosuppressed individuals	Fever, mild rash, swelling of glands in cheeks and neck, seizures, temporary pain in joints, severe allergic reaction	Two doses: 12–15 months and 4–6 years (or any age if longer than 28 days from first dose)
Varicella	Chicken pox	Severe skin infection, pneumonia, brain damage, death; shingles (herpes zoster) may occur years later	Do not give if allergic to gelatin or the antibiotic neomycin, moderate to severe acute illness	Soreness and swelling at site, fever, mild rash, seizures, pneumonia	12–18 months or any age if never had chicken pox
HAV	Hepatitis A	Liver disease with flu-like symptoms, jaundice, nausea and vomiting, abdominal pain	Allergic reaction to prior dose, tell doctor if pregnant (safety of vaccine during pregnancy has not been determined)	Soreness at site, headache, severe allergic reaction	1 month before traveling or when at risk for infection (two doses needed 6 months apart); children 12–24 months with second dose 6 months later
Influenza Inactivated (I.M.) Live, intranasal (I.N.) Ages 5–49	Influenza (flu)	Fever, cough, chills, aches, death	Do not give to pregnant women, egg allergy, history of Guillain-Barré syndrome	Soreness, redness, fever, aches, allergic reaction	All children 6–23 months
Pneumococcal congugate	Pneumonia, bacterial meningitis	Meningitis, septicemia, otitis media, pneumonia, deafness, brain damage	Moderate to severe illness, allergic reaction to prior dose	Redness, swelling at site, fever, drowsiness	2 months, 4 months, 6 months, 12–15 months

(continues)

Table 15-1 (continued)

Vaccine	Disease	About the Disease	Precautions and Contra-indications	Side Effects and Adverse Reactions	Vaccine Schedule
Meningococ-cal	Meningitis	Infection of the brain and coverings of the spinal cord, septicemia, mental retardation, seizures, stroke, death	Severe allergic reaction to prior dose	Allergic reaction, redness or pain at site, fever	Not for children younger than 2 years (two doses needed 3 months apart)
Rotavirus (ROTA)	Kowasaki disease	Severe diarrhea, vomit-ing, fever, dehydration; cause unknown; serious in children; inflammation of small- and medium-sized arteries, including coronary arteries; no test to diagnose disease (signs and symptoms used to help diagnose)	Serious aller-gic reaction from previous vaccine dose, serious allergic reaction to vaccine com-ponent		2 months, 4 months, 6 months

Most of the recommended vaccines are administered in the child's first 15 to 18 months of life. Access involves cost of vaccines, appointment requirements, and time required to receive vaccines. Some offices permit walk-in vaccination administration with free or low co-payment fee only. Routine well-infant examinations should be scheduled according to the recommended vaccination schedule to promote and facilitate maintenance of the schedule.

Vaccine storage should follow specific manufacturer's guidelines. Some vaccine preparations require refrigeration or protection from light.

Vaccines have trade names, and manufacturers have been tested for safety. The package insert of each vaccine describes the vaccine including its route of administration, purpose, contraindications, and possible side effects (see Table 15-1). Because some vaccines are grown in bird eggs weakened by addition of chemicals or are made from animals, it is essential to know what allergies a child has. For example, a child who is allergic to eggs cannot receive an MMR, varicella, or influenza vaccine because of the possibility of the child being allergic to the egg protein that is used in the manufacturing of the vaccine (Figure 15-5). Symptoms of side effects, contraindications, and allergies must be known by the medical assistant, who will ensure that the parents are informed and have given written consent before the vaccines are given. After administration of vaccines (see Procedure 15-1), the medical assistant is responsible for documentation of the types of vaccines, site of administration, manufacturer's lot number, and side effects, if any have been reported by the parents (Figure 15-6). The provider will report any clinically significant adverse reactions to the Vaccine Adverse Event Reporting System (VAERS) and will file a VAERS Events Form for the National Immunization Program. Vaccine records can be kept electronically. All children must have a

Patient Education

Encourage parents to be aware of different vaccines and to keep track of vaccination schedules. By posting recommended schedules in visible locations in the ambulatory care setting, parents can be reminded.

Figures 15-2 and 15-3 illustrates the recommended vaccination schedule for children and adolescents, which is supported by the American Academy of Pediatrics, the Advisory Committee on Immunization Practices (ACIP), the Committee on Infectious Diseases (COID), the Commission of Public Health and Scientific Affairs (COPHSA), and the American Academy of Family Physicians (AAFP).

EMERGENCY TREATMENT

- If itching and swelling are confined to the injection site where the vaccination was given, observe patient closely for development of generalized symptoms.
- If symptoms are generalized, activate the emergency medical system (EMS; call 911) and notify the on-call provider. This should be done by a second person, while the vaccinator assesses the airway, breathing, circulation, and level of consciousness of the patient.
- The provider will administer aqueous epinephrine 1:1000 dilution subcutaneously. The standard dose is 0.01 mg/kg body weight, up to 0.3 mg maximum single dose in children and 0.5 mg maximum in a single dose for a pediatric patient.
- In addition, for anaphylaxis, the provider will administer diphenhydramine (Benadryl) either orally or by intramuscular injection. The standard dose is 1 mg/kg body weight, up to 30 mg maximum dose in children and 100 mg maximum dose in adolescents.
- Monitor the patient closely until EMS arrives. Perform cardiopulmonary resuscitation (CPR), if necessary, and maintain airway. Keep patient in supine position (flat on back) unless he or she is having breathing difficulty. If breathing is difficult, patient's head may be elevated, provided blood pressure is adequate to prevent loss of consciousness. If blood pressure is low, elevate legs. Monitor blood pressure and pulse every 5 minutes.
- If EMS has not arrived and symptoms are still present, the provider will repeat dose of epinephrine every 10–20 minutes for up to 3 doses, depending on patient's response.
- Record all vital signs; medications administered to the patient, including time, dosage, response; name of the provider who administered the medication, and other relevant clinical information.
- Notify the patient's primary care provider.

Figure 15-5 Emergency treatment for children and teens experiencing an allergic reaction to a vaccine

personal immunization record as part of their permanent medical record. It is mandated that the following information be included in the patient's electronic medical record with each immunization:

EHR

- Month, day, and year of administration
- Vaccine given
- Vaccine information sheet (VIS) given to a parent or guardian

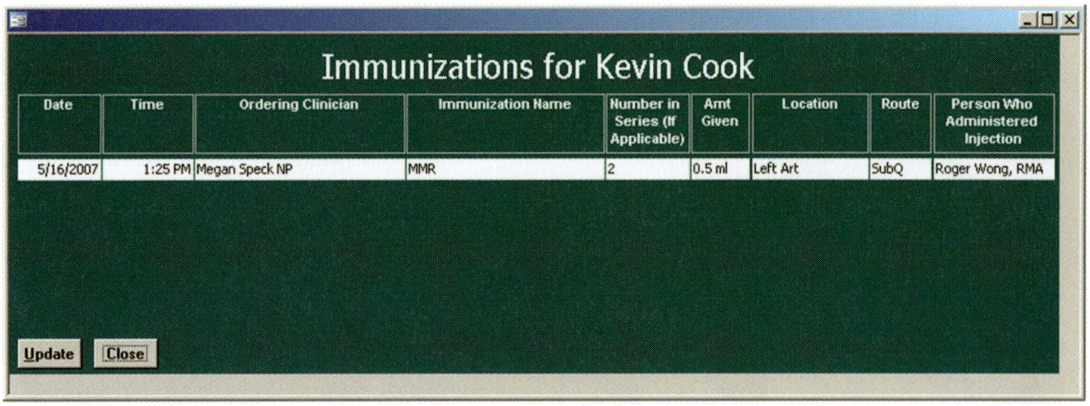

Date	Time	Ordering Clinician	Immunization Name	Number in Series (If Applicable)	Amt Given	Location	Route	Person Who Administered Injection
5/16/2007	1:25 PM	Megan Speck NP	MMR	2	0.5 ml	Left Art	SubQ	Roger Wong, RMA

A

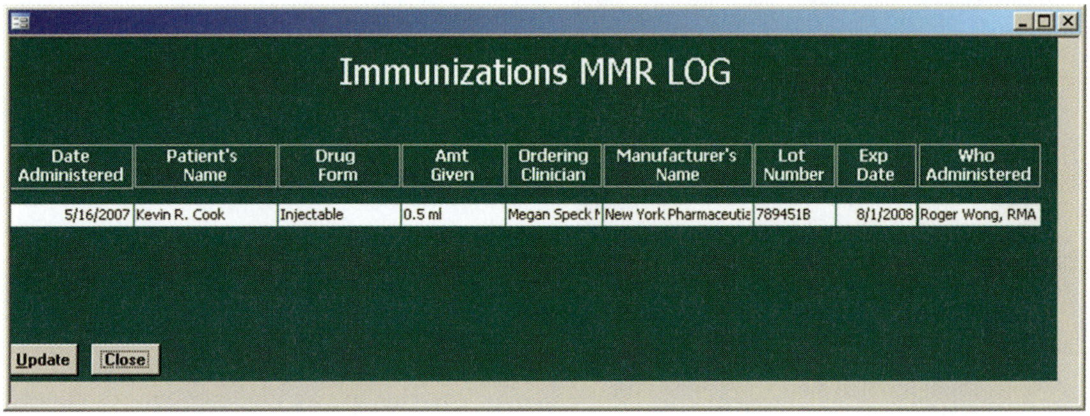

Date Administered	Patient's Name	Drug Form	Amt Given	Ordering Clinician	Manufacturer's Name	Lot Number	Exp Date	Who Administered
5/16/2007	Kevin R. Cook	Injectable	0.5 ml	Megan Speck N	New York Pharmaceutic	789451B	8/1/2008	Roger Wong, RMA

B

Figure 15-6 Immunizations recorded in (A) a patient's electronic medical record and (B) in the practice's global immunization log for that vaccine.

- Manufacturer name
- Lot number and expiration date
- Site and route of administration
- Name, address, and title of health care provider giving the vaccine
- Source of vaccine, (F) federal, (S) state, (P) private

Immunization recordkeeping is mandated by state and federal laws. Total practice management systems include immunization recordkeeping as part of clinical care (Figure 15-7). Procedure 15-2 gives more information about maintaining immunization records.

Vaccines stimulate the immune system to produce antibodies against pathogens (see Chapter 10). Some patients may have conditions or preexisting conditions that would contraindicate vaccine administration. Safe vaccine administration requires assessment and recognition of conditions that would contraindicate vaccine administration at any specific time. When any vaccine is not given because of an existing contraindication, careful documentation and notification of the provider are required.

Recommended Vaccination Schedule

The recommended vaccination schedule for infants and children is based on the premise that repeated doses of several vaccines are required and vaccine manufacturers recommend administering only compatible vaccines at any one visit to avoid drug interactions. If no contraindications are present at the various ages, vaccines should be administered according to the schedule to ensure complete vaccination by the age of 15 to 18 months, with booster vaccines on school entry and again every 10 years throughout adult life. Should any vaccine be missed for any reason, vaccine "catch-up" schedules are available to ensure adequate vaccine administration (see Figure 15-4).

Considerations for Vaccine Administration

- *Infection control.* Health care providers should follow Standard Precautions to minimize the risks of spreading disease during vaccine administration.

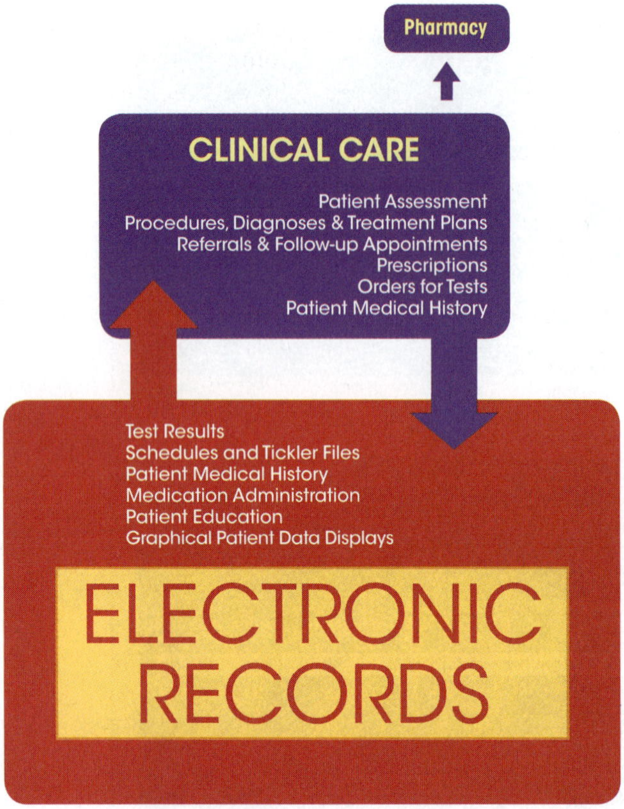

Figure 15-7 In a total practice management system, all the necessary data are documented at the time of clinical care, are electronically stored, and are accessible on demand.

- *Hand washing.* The single most effective disease prevention activity is good hand washing. Hands should be washed thoroughly with soap and water or cleansed with an alcohol-based waterless antiseptic between patients, before vaccine preparation, or any time hands become soiled (e.g., diapering, cleaning excreta).
- *Gloving.* Gloves are not required to be worn when administering vaccines unless the person administering the vaccine is likely to come into contact with potentially infectious body fluids or has open lesions on the hands. Office policy may require gloves be worn. It is important to remember that gloves cannot prevent needlestick injuries.
- *Syringe selection.* A separate needle and syringe should be used for each injection. A parenteral vaccine can be delivered in either a 1-mL or 3-mL syringe as long as the prescribed dosage is delivered. Syringe devices with engineered sharps injury protection are available, recommended by the Occupational Safety and Health Administration (OSHA), and required in many states to reduce the incidence of needlestick injuries and potential disease transmission. Personnel should be involved in evaluation and selection of these products. Staff should receive training with these devices before using them in the clinical area.
- *Needle selection.* Vaccine must reach the desired tissue site for optimal immune response. Therefore, needle selection should be based on the prescribed route, size of the individual, volume and viscosity of the vaccine, and injection technique. Typically, vaccines are not highly viscous; therefore, a fine-gauge needle (22–25 gauge) can be used.
- *Needle-free injection.* A new generation of needle-free vaccine delivery devices has been developed in an effort to decrease the risks of needlestick injuries to health care workers and to prevent improper reuse of syringes and needles. For more information on needle-free injection technology, see the Centers for Disease Control and Prevention (CDC) Web site: (http://www.cdc.gov/nip/dev/jetinject.htm).
- *Inspecting vaccine.* Each vaccine vial should be carefully inspected for damage or contamination prior to use. The expiration date printed on the vial or box should be checked. Vaccine can be used up to and including the last day of the month indicated by the expiration date unless otherwise stated on the package labeling. Expired vaccine should never be used.
- *Reconstitution.* Some vaccines are prepared in a **lyophilized** form that requires reconstitution, which should be done according to manufacturer guidelines. Diluent solutions vary; use only the specific diluent supplied for the vaccine. Once reconstituted, the vaccine must be either administered within the time guidelines provided by the manufacturer or discarded. Changing the needle after reconstitution of the vaccine is not necessary unless the needle has become contaminated or bent. Continue with standard medication preparation guidelines.
- *Prefilling syringes.* The CDC strongly discourages filling syringes in advance because of the increased risk of administration errors. Once the vaccine is in the syringe, it is difficult to identify the type or brand of vaccine. Other problems associated with this practice are vaccine wastage and possible bacterial growth in vaccines that do not contain a preservative. Furthermore, medication administration guidelines state that the individual who administers a medication should be the one to draw up and prepare it. An alternative to prefilling syringes is to use filled syringes supplied by the vaccine manufacturer. Syringes other than those filled by the manufacturer are designed for immediate

administration, not for vaccine storage. In certain circumstances, such as in large influenza clinics, more than one syringe can be filled. One person should prefill only a few syringes at a time, and the same person should administer them. Any syringes left at the end of the clinic day should be discarded. Under no circumstances should measles, mumps, and rubella (MMR), varicella, or zoster vaccines ever be reconstituted and drawn prior to the immediate need for them. These live virus vaccines are unstable and begin to deteriorate as soon as they are reconstituted with the diluent.

- *Labeling.* Once a vaccine is drawn into a syringe, the content should be indicated on the syringe. There are a variety of methods for identifying or labeling syringes (e.g., keep syringes with the appropriate vaccine vials, place the syringes in a labeled partitioned tray, use color coded labels or preprinted labels).
- *Multiple vaccinations.* When administering multiple vaccines, never mix vaccines in the same syringe unless approved for mixing by the Food and Drug Administration (FDA). If more than one vaccine must be administered in the same limb, the injection sites should be separated by 1 to 2 inches so that any local reactions can be differentiated. Vaccine doses range from 0.2 to 1 mL. The recommended maximum volume of medication for an intramuscular (IM) site varies among references and depends on the muscle mass of the individual. However, administering two IM vaccines into the same muscle would not exceed any suggested volume ranges for either the vastus lateralis or the deltoid muscle in any age group. The option to also administer a subcutaneous vaccine into the same limb, if necessary, is acceptable because a different tissue site is involved. If a vaccine and an immune globulin preparation are administered simultaneously (e.g., Td/Tdap and tetanus immune globulin [TIG] or hepatitis B vaccine and hepatitis B immune globulin [HBIG]), a separate anatomic site should be used for each injection. The location of each injection should be documented in the patient's chart or electronic medical record (Figure 15-8).
- *Nonstandard administration.* Deviation from the recommended route, site, and dosage of vaccine is strongly discouraged and can result in inadequate protection.
- *Needle gauge.* 22- to 25-gauge needle.
- *Needle length.* For all IM injections, the needle should be long enough to reach the muscle mass and prevent vaccine from seeping into subcutaneous tissue, but not so long as to involve underlying nerves, blood vessels, or bone. The vaccinator should be familiar with the anatomy of the area into which the vaccine will be injected. Decision on needle size and site of injections must be made for each patient based on the size of the muscle, the thickness of adipose tissue at the injection site, the volume of the material to be administered,

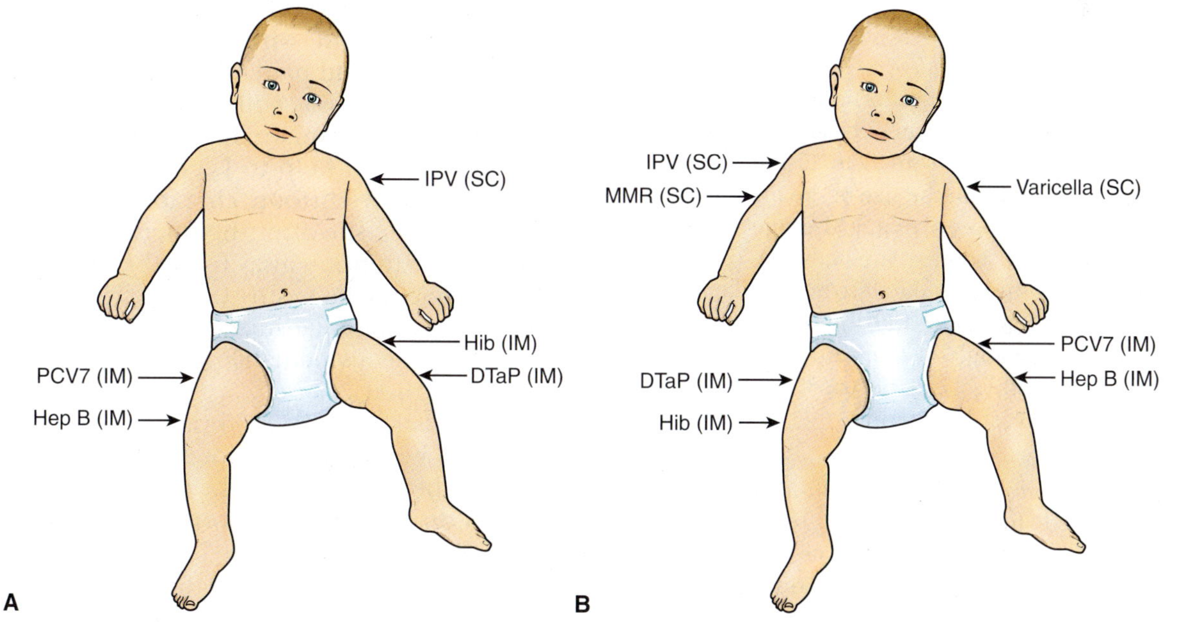

Figure 15-8 (A) An example of one way to give five doses at one visit. (B) An example of one way to give seven doses at one visit.

the injection technique, and the depth below the muscle surface into which the material is to be injected.

- *Infants (younger than 12 months).* For the majority of infants, the anterolateral aspect of the thigh is the recommended site for injection because it provides a large muscle mass. The muscles of the buttock have not been used for administration of vaccines in infants and children because of concern about potential injury to the sciatic nerve, which is well documented after injection of antimicrobial agents into the buttock. If the gluteal muscle must be used, care should be taken to define the anatomic landmarks. *If the gluteal muscle is chosen, injection should be administered lateral and superior to a line between the posterior superior iliac spine and the greater trochanter or in the ventrogluteal site, the center of a triangle bounded by the anterior superior iliac spine, the tubercle of the iliac crest, and the upper border of the greater trochanter.*
- *Injection technique.* This is the most important factor to ensure efficient intramuscular vaccine delivery. If the subcutaneous and muscle tissue are bunched to minimize the chance of striking bone, a 1-inch needle is required to ensure intramuscular administration in infants. For the majority of infants, a 1-inch, 22- to 25-gauge needle is sufficient to penetrate muscle in an infant's thigh. For newborn (first 28 days of life) and premature infants, a ⅝-inch needle usually is adequate if the skin is stretched flat between thumb and forefinger and the needle is inserted at a 90-degree angle to the skin.
- *Toddlers and older children (12 months to 10 years).* The deltoid muscle should be used if the muscle mass is adequate. The needle size for deltoid site injections can range from 22 to 25 gauge and from ⅝ to 1 inch based on the size of the muscle and the thickness of adipose tissue at the injection site. A ⅝-inch needle is adequate only for the deltoid muscle and only if the skin is stretched flat between thumb and forefinger and the needle is inserted at a 90-degree angle to the skin. For toddlers, the anterolateral thigh can be used, but the needle should be at least 1 inch long.
- *Adolescents and adults (11 years and older).* For adults and adolescents, the deltoid muscle is recommended for routine IM vaccinations. The anterolateral thigh can also be used. For men and women weighing less than 130 pounds (60 kg), a ⅝ to 1-inch needle is sufficient to ensure IM injection. For women weighing 130 to 200 pounds (60–90 kg) and men weighting 130 to 260 pounds (60–118 kg), a 1- to 1½-inch needle is needed. For women weighing more than 200 pounds (90 kg) or men weighing more than 260 pounds (118 kg), a 1½-inch needle is required.

Figure 15-9 gives information on administering vaccines.

Giving Injections to Pediatric Patients

Infants and toddlers who have injections must be held in such a way that they cannot move. This is done for two reasons: to protect the child from injury and to provide access to an injection site.

For a child from birth to about 2 years of age, the vastus lateralis muscle is the preferred site. It is readily accessible when the infant is lying supine on the examination table.

Children who are 2 to about 4 years old are not emotionally developed enough to understand the need for cooperation. You will need help from the parent or another staff member to hold the child securely, thus avoiding injury. The deltoid is the preferred site for this age group. One method used to restrict the child's movement is to seat the child on the parent's lap. The parent wraps his or her legs around the child's legs to limit movement. The parent or staff member holds down the noninjection arm. The injection can be given once the child is securely immobilized.

Keep the syringe and needle out of the child's sight, because pediatric patients learn quickly that doctor office visits many times mean an injection, and with the injection is some degree of fear and pain.

Do not tell the child that the injection will not hurt; rather, explain that it will sting for a short while, but it will help to keep him or her strong and healthy. A cartoon character adhesive strip applied to the site after the injection helps direct the child's attention away from the discomfort.

Although the vastus lateralis is the preferred site for intramuscular injections, the deltoid is used for subcutaneous pediatric injections (see Figures 15-10 and 15-11).

Sick-baby or sick-child visits are appointments that have been arranged for ill babies or children who will be examined by the pediatrician to determine a diagnosis and appropriate treatment for a particular problem.

Clinical responsibilities for medical assistants during either type of visit include the same or similar procedures as the adult examination. The instruments used for the pediatric physical examination

Administering Vaccines: Dose, Route, Site, and Needle Size

Vaccines	Dose	Route
Diphtheria, Tetanus, Pertussis (DTaP, DT, Tdap, Td)	0.5 mL	IM
***Haemophilus influenzae* type b (Hib)**	0.5 mL	IM
Hepatitis A (HepA)	≤18 yrs: 0.5 mL ≥19 yrs: 1.0 mL	IM
Hepatitis B (HepB) **Persons 11–15 yrs may be given Recombivax HB® (Merck) 1.0 mL adult formulation on a 2-dose schedule.*	≤19 yrs: 0.5 mL* ≥20 yrs: 1.0 mL	IM
Human papillomavirus (HPV)	0.5 mL	IM
Influenza, live attenuated (LAIV)	0.2 mL	Intranasal spray
Influenza, trivalent inactivated (TIV)	6-35 mos: 0.25 mL ≥3 yrs: 0.5 mL	IM
Measles, mumps, rubella (MMR)	0.5 mL	SC
Meningococcal, conjugated (MCV4)	0.5 mL	IM
Meningococcal, polysaccharide (MPSV4)	0.5 mL	SC
Pneumococcal conjugate (PCV)	0.5 mL	IM
Pneumococcal polysaccharide (PPV)	0.5 mL	IM or SC
Polio, inactivated (IPV)	0.5 mL	IM or SC
Rotavirus (Rv)	2.0 mL	Oral
Varicella (Var)	0.5 mL	SC
Zoster (Zos)	0.65 mL	SC
Combination Vaccines		
DTaP+HepB+IPV (Pediarix™) **DTaP+Hib (Trihibit™)** **Hib+HepB (Comvax™)**	0.5 mL	IM
MMR+Var (ProQuad®)	≤12 yrs: 0.5 mL	SC
HepA+HepB (Twinrix®)	≥18 yrs: 1.0 mL	IM

Injection Site and Needle Size

Subcutaneous (SC) injection

Use a 23–25 gauge needle. Choose the injection site that is appropriate to the person's age and body mass.

Age	Needle Length	Injection Site
Infants (1–12 mos)	⅝"	Fatty tissue over anterolateral thigh muscle
Children (≥12 mos), adolescents, and adults	⅝"	Fatty tissue over anterolateral thigh muscle or fatty tissue over triceps

Intramuscular (IM) injection

Use a 22–25 gauge needle. Choose the injection site and needle length appropriate to the person's age and body mass.

Age	Needle Length	Injection Site
Newborns (1st 28 days)	⅝"*	Anterolateral thigh muscle
Infants (1–12 mos)	1"	Anterolateral thigh muscle
Toddlers (1–2 yrs)	1"–1¼" ⅝"*–1"	Anterolateral thigh muscle or deltoid muscle of arm
Children & teens 3–18 yrs	⅝"*–1" 1"–1¼"	Deltoid muscle of arm or anterolateral thigh muscle
Adults ≥ age19 yrs		
Male or female less than 130 lbs	⅝"*–1"	Deltoid muscle of arm
Female 130–200 lbs Male 130–260 lbs	1"–1½"	Deltoid muscle of arm
Female 200+ lbs Male 260+ lbs	1½"	Deltoid muscle of arm

**If skin is stretched tight and subcutaneous tissue is not bunched.*

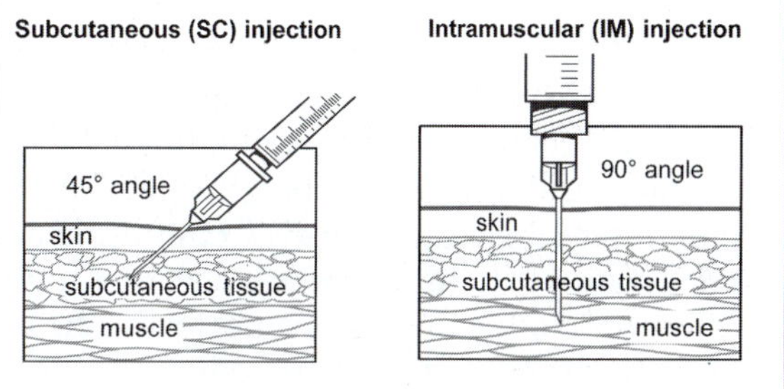

Please note: Always refer to the package insert included with each biologic for complete vaccine administration information. CDC's Advisory Committee on Immunization Practices (ACIP) recommendations for the particular vaccine should be reviewed as well.

Technical content reviewed by the Centers for Disease Control and Prevention, August 2007.
www.immunize.org/catg.d/p3085.pdf • Item #P3085 (8/07)

Immunization Action Coalition • 1573 Selby Ave. • St. Paul, MN 55104 • (651) 647-9009 • www.immunize.org • www.vaccineinformation.org

Figure 15-9 Administering vaccines: dose, route, site, and needle size. (From the Immunization Action Coalition, http://www.immunize.org.)

How to Administer Intramuscular (IM) Injections

Administer these vaccines via intramuscular (IM) route: Diphtheria-tetanus (DT, Td) with pertussis (DTaP, Tdap); Hib; hepatitis A; hepatitis B; human papillomavirus (HPV); inactivated influenza; meningococcal conjugate (MCV4); and pneumococcal conjugate (PCV). Administer inactivated polio (IPV) and pneumococcal polysaccharide (PPV) either IM or SC.

Patient age	Site	Needle size
Birth to 12 mos.	Anterolateral thigh muscle	5/8"* needle (newborns only), 1" (older infants), 22–25 gauge
12 mos. to 10 yrs.	Thickest portion of deltoid muscle—above level of axilla and below acromion (if adequate muscle mass). The anterolateral thigh may also be used.	5/8"*† to 1" needle, 22–25 gauge
Children and adults 11 yrs. and older	Thickest portion of deltoid muscle—above level of axilla and below acromion	1"–1½"*† needle, 22–25 gauge

*A 5/8" needle can be used if the skin is stretched tight and the subcutaneous tissue is not bunched.
†A 5/8" needle may be used in the deltoid muscle in children ages 12 mos. or older and in adults weighing less than 130 lbs.

Needle insertion

Use a needle long enough to reach deep into the muscle.

Insert needle at a 90° angle to the skin with a quick thrust.

(Before administering an injection, it is not necessary to aspirate, i.e., to pull back on the syringe plunger after needle insertion.¶)

Multiple injections given in the same extremity should be separated by a minimum of 1", if possible.

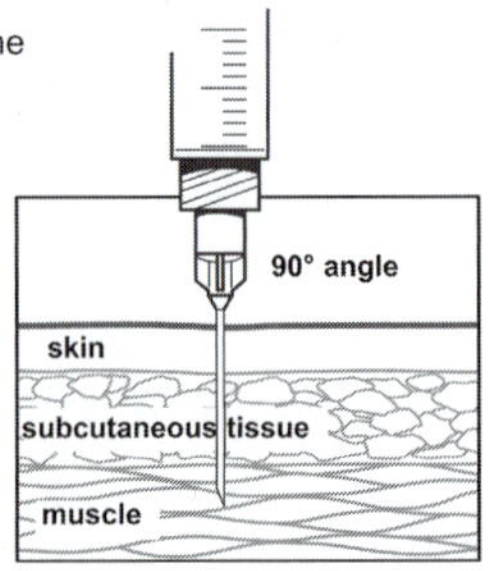

¶CDC. "ACIP General Recommendations on Immunization" at www.cdc.gov/nip/publications/ACIP-list.htm.

IM site for infants

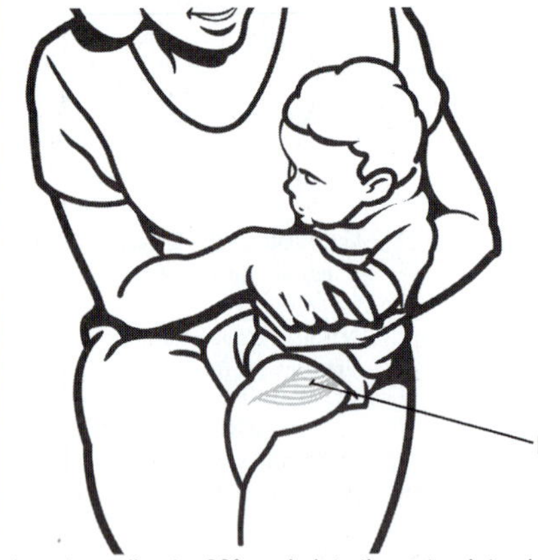

Insert needle at a 90° angle into the anterolateral thigh muscle.

IM site for children (after the 1st birthday) and adults

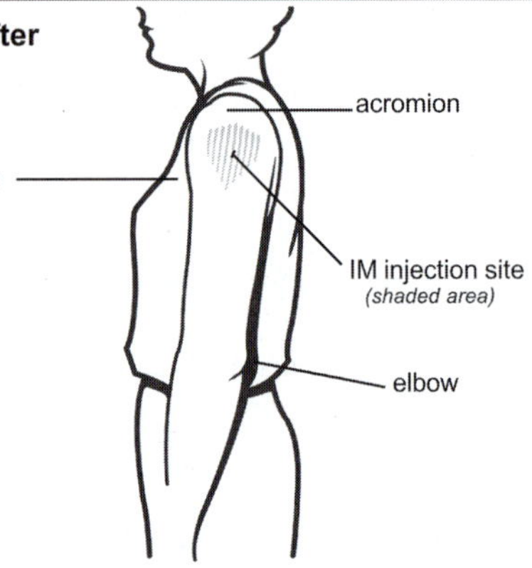

Insert needle at a 90° angle into thickest portion of deltoid muscle—above the level of the axilla and below the acromion.

Technical content reviewed by the Centers for Disease Control and Prevention, Jan. 2007.

www.immunize.org/catg.d/p2020.pdf • Item #P2020 (1/07)

Immunization Action Coalition • 1573 Selby Ave. • St. Paul, MN 55104 • (651) 647-9009 • www.immunize.org • www.vaccineinformation.org • admin@immunize.org

Figure 15-10 Administering intramuscular injections. The usual site for vaccine administration in infants is the vastus lateralis muscle of the upper thigh. (From the Immunization Action Coalition, http://www.immunize.org.)

are similar to those used for an adult physical examination. Vital signs are taken, visual acuity is measured, a urine specimen may be obtained, blood may be drawn and processed, height and weight measurements are taken, and head circumference is measured. To gain the child's confidence, begin the examination at the feet and work up to the head. These are some of the skills and procedures medical assistants will perform or with which they will assist during the pediatric office or clinic visit.

It is important for the medical assistant to know that parents may ask about vaccine safety and preservatives. The following information is helpful; however, the provider is the best individual to answer specific questions parents may have.

Preservatives have been used in vaccines for more than 70 years. According to the CDC, Thimerosol (an **organomercurial**, i.e., a mercury-containing compound) has been used as a preservative in multidose vials of vaccine. It was added in very small amounts to kill bacteria that could be or were introduced into the multidose vial through improper sterile technique when drawing the vaccines into a syringe. Fatalities from septicemia after vaccine administration using a multiple-dose vial have been reported.

There has been growing concern that the thimerosal in the vaccine is related to problems such as attention deficit hyperactivity disorder (ADHD), autism, and speech or language delays.

Many studies have been done over the last 30 years. The Institute of Medicine, the Immunization Safety Committee, the FDA, the CDC, and the National Institutes of Health (NIH) were involved throughout the studies. All have determined that there is no relationship between thimerosol and

How to Administer Subcutaneous (SC) Injections

Administer these vaccines via subcutaneous (SC) route: MMR, varicella, meningococcal polysaccharide (MPSV), and zoster (shingles). Administer inactivated polio (IPV) and pneumococcal polysaccharide (PPV) vaccines either SC or IM.

Patient age	Site	Needle size	Needle insertion
Birth to 12 mos.	Fatty tissue over the anterolateral thigh	5/8" needle, 23–25 gauge	Pinch up on SC tissue to prevent injection into muscle. Insert needle at 45° angle to the skin. (Before administering an injection, it is not necessary to aspirate, i.e., to pull back on the syringe plunger after needle insertion.*) Multiple injections given in the same extremity should be separated by a minimum of 1". *CDC. "ACIP General Recommendations on Immunization" at www.cdc.gov/nip/publications/ACIP-list.htm.
12 mos. and older	Fatty tissue over the triceps	5/8" needle, 23–25 gauge	

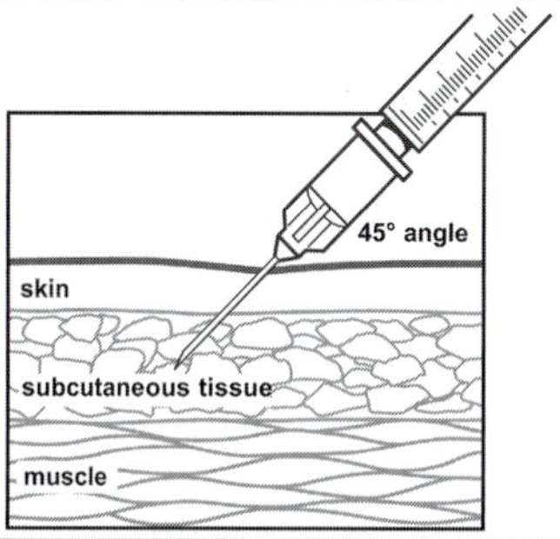

SC site for infants

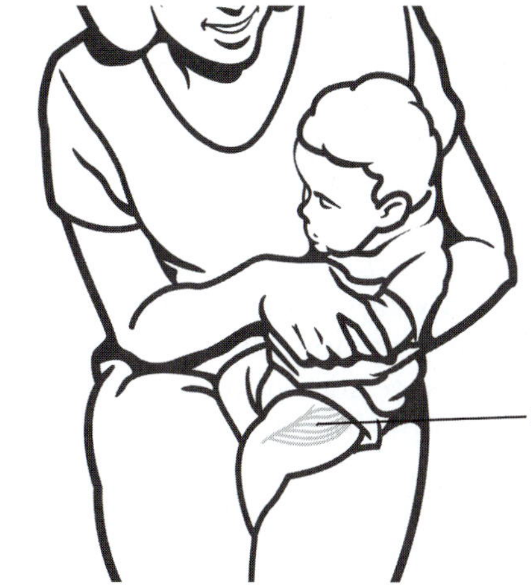

Insert needle at a 45° angle into fatty tissue of the anterolateral thigh. Make sure you pinch up on SC tissue to prevent injection into the muscle.

SC site for children (after the 1st birthday) and adults

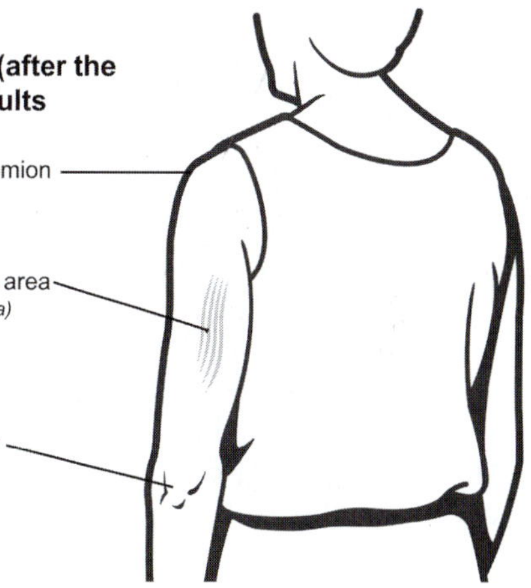

Insert needle at a 45° angle into the fatty tissue over the triceps muscle. Make sure you pinch up on the SC tissue to prevent injection into the muscle.

Technical content reviewed by the Centers for Disease Control and Prevention, Jan. 2007.

www.immunize.org/catg.d/p2020.pdf • Item #P2020 (1/07)

Immunization Action Coalition • 1573 Selby Ave. • St. Paul, MN 55104 • (651) 647-9009 • www.immunize.org • www.vaccineinformation.org • admin@immunize.org

Figure 15-11 Administering subcutaneous injections. Subcutaneous tissue can be found all over the body. The usual sites for vaccine administration are the thigh (for infants) and the upper outer triceps of the arm (for children older than 12 months). If necessary, the upper outer triceps area can be used to administer subcutaneous injections to infants. (From the Immunization Action Coalition, http://www.immunize.org.)

neurotoxicity from vaccine administration. The latest study in 2004 again investigated the situation and rejected the relationship between thimerosol and vaccines as a cause of neurotoxicity.

In 2000, the CDC, FDA, NIH, and the American Academy of Pediatrics (AAP) told the CDC to have thimerosol removed from all vaccines or to reduce it to trace amounts as soon as possible. There had been a movement by parents to remove all the preservatives. Parents still are involved in ongoing discussion about "reduced to trace amounts" in all routine vaccines for children 6 years and under. An exception, however, is inactivated flu vaccine. It contains thimerosol. A limited supply of preservative-free inactivated flu vaccine is available, but it is used for pregnant women, infants, and children. Perhaps over time all vaccines will be preservative-free.

THEORIES OF GROWTH AND DEVELOPMENT

Before providing more indepth information about the various stages of growth and development in children, it is important to review the major theorists who contributed to understanding human growth and development.

There are at least eight or nine theories of human development put forth by Freud (psychosexual), Erickson (psychosocial), Sullivan (interpersonal), Piaget (cognitive), Kohlberg (moral),

Bronfenbrenner (ecology), Pavlov, Skinner (behavioral), and Bandura (social learning). Each theory focuses on particular aspects of human development and its principles, strengths, and weaknesses.

No single theory can explain human development. The medical assistant can apply the theory or theories with relevance and understanding to each individual child or adult. This will allow for an inclusive approach to human development that is appropriate for children and families (Figure 15-12).

The following sections provide more information about growth and development at the various stages of a child's life (Figure 15-13).

Newborns

Even at a few days old, a newborn can imitate facial and manual gestures that adults make and can show a preference for certain colors (red, black, and white). The newborn can respond to auditory stimuli and is sensitive to being touched and handled. Respiratory rate is usually 30 to 60 breaths/min; breaths are somewhat irregular in depth and rhythm, shallow and abdominal. The heart rate ranges from 110 to 130 beats/min depending on whether the infant is awake or asleep. Urinary output is about 1 to 3 mL/hour or about 2 to 6 voidings a day.

Newborns can move and wiggle and can place themselves into dangerous or unsafe positions. One hand should always be kept on newborns whenever they are on top of any object because they can easily roll off. The safest place is in a crib with the sides raised.

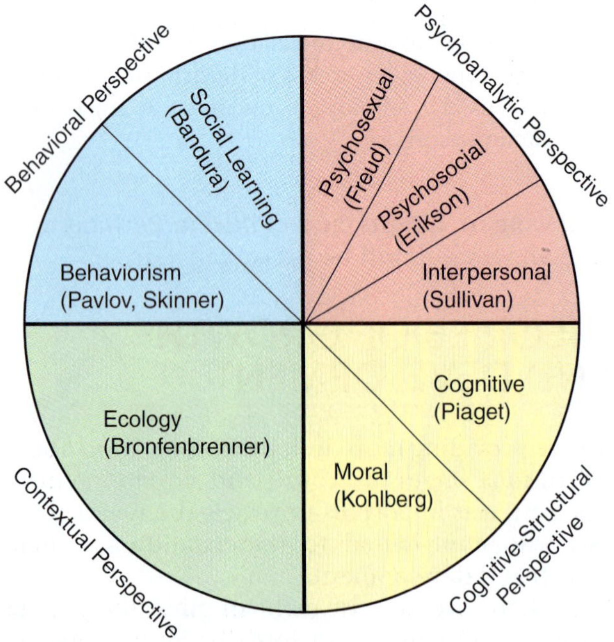

Figure 15-12 The eclectic nature of human development.

It is important to note the vital signs at different ages will vary according to size, age, and gender. Comparisons can be made by finding values within the electronic medical record.

Infants

The infant stage is from 1 month to 1 year. Gross and fine motor skills develop starting at the head and moving toward the feet.

The infant usually doubles his or her birth weight during the first 6 months; by 12 months, birth weight has tripled. Height increases about 1 inch per month. By 12 months, the infant's height has slowed, and there can be a 50% increase from the birth length.

Head size changes quickly to accommodate fast brain growth. By 1 year old, the infant's brain is about 66% of the size of an adult brain, but growth does slow during the second 6 months of the first year. The **fontanels** (anterior and posterior) close by 2 months old (anterior) and 12 to 18 months old (posterior). The infant cannot control head movement until about 4 months old. This is known as "head lag," and the amount of head lag can be determined by pulling the infant by the arms from a supine to a sitting position. Because the infant cannot control the head, it will fall back until about 4 months old, at which time the infant has no head lag and can control the head while sitting.

Gross and fine motor development occurs quickly during the infant stage, but once developed, the infant can begin to walk, first with help, then alone. By 1 year old, in addition to being able to walk alone, the infant can feed himself or herself finger foods, grasp with his or her index finger and thumb, place and remove small objects from a container, and hold a crayon and make a mark with it.

The medical assistant can be helpful in relaying information to the infant's parents or caregivers regarding growth and development, nutrition, hygiene, safety, and vaccines.

Toddlers

The toddler period covers 2 years in the child's life from about 1 to 3 years of age. During the toddler period, there is rapid change. The child is becoming more independent, is able to move about quickly, and is verbal and inquisitive. Environmental dangers are of utmost concern because of the

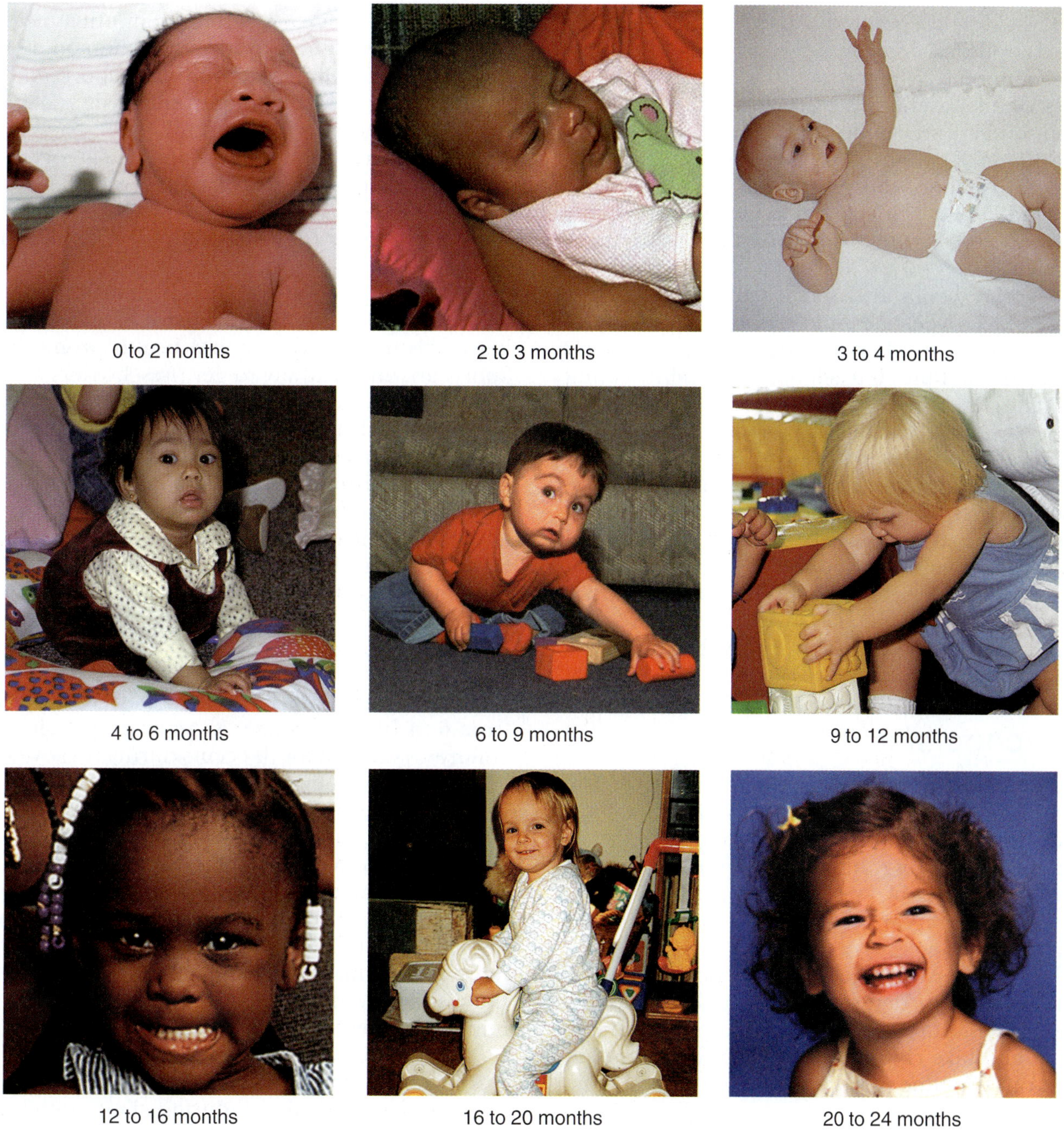

Figure 15-13 Growth and development stages of infants and toddlers.

toddler's rapid development of motor skills and lack of judgment. This is a time for discipline and guidelines but also for encouraging independence and natural curiosity. Most injuries and deaths occur as a result of airway obstruction, poisoning, drowning, falls, burns, and auto accidents.

During the 2 years that the toddler is developing, his or her physical growth slows. Height gain averages about 3 inches per year; weight gain is about 5 pounds per year. Most toddlers walk by 12 to 15 months old and climb stairs by 18 months old.

Bladder and bowel control usually occur during this period. Vital signs move closer to adult norms, respiration (25–30 breaths/min awake) and pulse rates (96–105 beats/min) slow, and blood pressure increases to greater than 90/50 mm Hg. Serum lead levels are checked during this time.

It is during the toddler period that rapid onset of respiratory distress can occur, and there is an increase in tendency for airways to collapse. Otitis media, tonsillitis, and upper respiratory infections are common.

Often parents or caregivers are concerned their toddlers are eating little or they focus only on one particular food. Most toddlers eat when they are hungry and caregivers worry unnecessarily. The toddler is less interested in food because of his or her slowdown in growth, thus fewer calories are needed.

Eating habits are established during the first 2 to 3 years of life, and good eating habits with children should start when they are toddlers. The early years are the time to teach lifelong healthy eating habits together with regular exercise. These two factors will significantly add years and quality of life because of disease prevention and maintenance of health. Many children in the United States are obese, perhaps because their parents are. A 2004 study reported in *Annals of Human Biology* found that almost half of children who were overweight at 1 year old were obese by 21 years old. The earlier that one can prevent obesity, the healthier one's children will be. Parents are their children's role models.

Preschoolers

The preschool years include ages 3 to 6 years. The child now has control over bowel and bladder, can dress and feed himself or herself, and can interact with others. During this period, preschoolers gain about 2 pounds of weight per year and 3 inches in height per year. Visual acuity rates decrease slightly.

The Denver Developmental Screening Test can be used to determine motor skills development levels. Running, jumping, skipping, jumping rope, and bike riding with training wheels usually occur in this time period. Preschoolers may begin to tie shoelaces.

Sexual curiosity is displayed, and questions about body parts, including genitalia, should be answered honestly. Children learn at this age that "private" body parts should not be touched by strangers.

Preschoolers learn through play and by imitating adult behaviors. It is now that children will play well with others and share. Preschoolers are creative and use their imaginations well.

During preschool years, a yearly physical examination should be done to note growth, vision, hearing, and blood pressure. Laboratory work includes a test for lead exposure, a tuberculosis test (once before beginning school), and a lipid profile. This age group suffers from otitis media, upper respiratory infections, and common stomach viruses. Teaching children the importance of good hand washing techniques and its significance in preventing illness is important.

Some preschoolers may refuse to eat for a few days or prefer one particular food everyday. Parents and caregivers should avoid issues over these matters. Instead, spend mealtimes in a pleasant way.

Regular physical activity is beneficial because it helps develop lifetime habits of exercise, leading to disease prevention and health promotion. Sports are an ideal way to get preschoolers active and to have fun. Noncompetitive activities such as dance, T-ball, karate, gymnastics, and bicycling also keep children active and healthy. Love of reading can be established now, especially when parents/caregivers read to their youngsters.

Playing near the road is an area of great concern for these children. They will listen to adults who set limits for their safety.

School-Aged Children

The school-aged group encompasses children from 6 to 12 years of age. A steady progression in children's rate of growth occurs during these years. Weight increases by about 5 pounds per year, and height increases about 2 inches per year. Muscle size increases, and the following motor skills continue to improve: climbing, running, jumping, throwing, catching, and balancing.

The circulatory and respiratory functions develop. The pulse and respiration rates slow. The pulse rate in this age group is about 90 beats/min; the average respiration rate is about 20 breaths/min. Both rates are while the children are at rest.

This period shows relatively few infectious diseases because of the immunity the children developed to microorganisms during their preschool years.

The last years of the school-aged period are known as prepuberty. Breast development, axillary and pubic hair, and body odor may appear as early as 9 or 10 years of age.

Peers begin to play a major role, and children seek support from their peers to begin gaining independence from their parents and family. Children have a sense of accomplishment when they focus their energy on sports, hobbies, and schoolwork and see themselves succeed in these activities.

Language is the way to communicate, and children use their language skills to socialize with their family and peers.

Usually school-aged children experience excellent health, and when they do become ill, it is usually a minor illness. The AAP recommends routine physical examinations about every 2 years, at ages 5, 6, 8, 10, 11, and 12 years old. Height, weight, vital signs, physical examination, vision and hearing tests, review of nutrition, scoliosis screening, and tuberculosis testing are checked. Use of recreational drugs, tobacco, and alcohol is addressed.

Booster immunizations of DPT (diphtheria, pertussis, tetanus) and MMR (measles, mumps, and rubella) are typically given between 4 and 6 years of age. Tetanus and diphtheria (Td) is usually repeated every 10 years.

Nutrition education is an ongoing process and children should be taught to eat breakfast daily and to make intelligent, healthy food choices. Good nutrition and physical activity are essential for their physical and emotional well-being and for long-range health maintenance and disease prevention.

Accidents in this age group are the leading cause of death. The increased independence, need for their peer's approval, and increased involvement in physically challenging activities are some of the reasons. Most injuries are related to auto accidents and firearms. Violent crimes against children in this age group have increased dramatically in the last 20 years.

School-aged children comprehend rules about safety with regard to automobiles, bikes, swimming, and firearms, but they frequently resist these rules.

This group of children suffers from not looking the "same" as their peers, bullying, stress (peer pressure, divorce, drugs), and both parents/caregivers working and not being home when the children go home after school (latchkey children).

Adolescents

The adolescent period of growth and development is noticeable for its wide range of physiological changes. It is the period between 11 and 21 years of age. During adolescence, there is a large growth spurt with gains in weight and height that occur rapidly. Boys can gain up to about 14 pounds and grow as much as 6 inches; girls gain up to about 10 pounds and grow up to 5 inches. Girls usually attain their adult height about 1 year before onset of menses; boys reach their adult height at about 13 years old, after axillary and pubic hair appear.

The average heart rate is about 60 to 70 beats/min; average blood pressure is 100/50 to 120/70 mm Hg. Girls have a slightly higher pulse and body temperature than boys; girls' systolic blood pressure is a bit less. Respiration rates in both sexes average about 16 to 20 breaths/min.

Adolescents direct their energy to nonfamily relationships and career goals. It is a time of conflict as adolescents try to become independent from their parents and establish their own identities.

The Department of Adolescent Health of the American Medical Association urges annual health screenings that focus not only on the physiological and psychological health of the adolescent, but also on such matters as physical activity, birth control, recreational drugs, alcohol, depression, suicide ideation, injury prevention, and school accomplishments.

Laboratory tests include human immunodeficiency virus (HIV) and other sexually transmitted diseases (gonorrhea, syphilis, chlamydia, and hepatitis B and C if sexually active). Tuberculosis testing is also recommended. The physical examination is comprehensive and includes vital signs, height and weight, vision and hearing testing, urinalysis, and complete blood count (CBC). At this time, the provider discusses issues of injury prevention (wearing seat belts, helmets for biking, no drinking and driving, contact sports, among others), violence prevention (gang memberships and anger management), nutrition (fast foods, high-sodium and fatty foods), how to avoid becoming overweight and obese, and regular physical activity. Motor vehicle accidents cause 50% of teenage deaths between ages 16 and 19 years, and they are common in drivers who use alcohol or other drugs.

To be effective at all stages of growth and development, the medical assistant must understand the age and maturity level of pediatric patients, the psychological changes that occur, and the psychosocial aspects of the child at various ages.

Communication with pediatric patients needs to be individualized, showing acceptance, empathy, honesty, and openness. Confidentiality must be maintained regardless of age. Parents and caregivers are involved with the care of their youngsters; therefore, they have the legal right to know the medical matters relating to their minor children. Adolescents may share information with the medical assistant that they do not want their parents or caregivers to know. It is important to stress that some matters may need to be shared with parents or caregivers, especially when adolescents are living at home (certain matters pertaining to birth control, abortion, pregnancy, and sexually transmitted diseases pose special problems). Some states allow minors to give their consent under these circumstances (see Chapter 7).

Medical assistants can teach parents and caregivers in various ways. Handouts, demonstrations, videos, and one-on-one instruction are helpful in keeping children safe and healthy.

The medical assistant must be caring, respectful, supportive, and nonjudgmental of all patients. The caregiver to pediatric patients must reflect these values. Family beliefs and values also must be taken into account. This will foster care for pediatric patients that is compliant and in the best interest of all.

GROWTH PATTERNS

Growth patterns provide valuable information to the pediatrician regarding the infant's physical progress. They are also used to calculate pediatric doses of medication. Height, weight, and head circumference are measured at each regularly scheduled appointment at the pediatric facility. The measurements are then plotted on a physical growth percentile chart that is part of the patient's permanent record (Figure 15-14).

MEASURING THE INFANT OR CHILD

Careful measuring of the infant or child and monitoring of growth patterns are essential and should be done in a consistent and accurate manner.

Length and Weight Measurements

To record or plot length and weight measurements, you must first locate one growth value, either length or weight, in the vertical columns of the physical growth percentile chart shown in Figure 15-15. Find the child's age in months in the horizontal rows. Locate the area where the growth value lines intersect on the graph and plot the length and weight by marking with a dot. Connect dots from previous values with a ruler to provide a neat and accurate graphic recording. The date, age, measurements, and comments should also be indicated at the bottom of the chart.

The curved lines printed across the growth charts show the normal range of growth of infants and children in the United States. The numbers on the right side of the chart, in the vertical boxes between age 34 and 35 months, show the percentiles of other children the same age. To determine into which percentile the infant falls in relation to other infants of the same age, follow the line (percentile) upward to the percentage values along the edge of the graph. The National Center for Health Statistics (NCHS) growth charts become a permanent record of the child's development. These give the provider a quick way to check the child's growth in relation to that of other children the same age. Growth charts aid in the diagnosis of growth abnormalities and nutritional disorders and disease. Hereditary factors also influence growth patterns; therefore, having the family's history is important.

Infant Holds and Positions

Lifting and carrying infants must be done safely. The medical assistant should be especially careful of the infant's neck. It should be supported whenever the infant is lifted or held. About the age of 4 months, an infant begins to be able to hold up its head without support. (Each infant's growth and development is unique; therefore, 4 months is an approximate age.)

There are two primary positions that the medical assistant uses when lifting or carrying an infant. The first is the upright position in which the anterior surface of the infant's body is held against the medical assistant's body with one hand, which supports the infant's buttocks. The other hand is placed behind the head and neck of the infant for support (Figure 15-16). This position can be used to carry the infant and to place him or her on the scale or examination table. The second position is called the cradle position; the medical assistant holds the infant under his back and neck with one arm, and the other arm supports the buttocks and legs (Figure 15-17). This position is commonly used by mothers when feeding their babies. It is comforting to infants when they are able to see the parent or the familiar person. A third position that is used less often is the "football" carry or position. The posterior of the infant lays across the medical assistant's dominant outstretched arm and hand, and the infant's legs straddle the medical assistant's arm. The medical assistant supports the head, neck, and back of the infant with the dominant hand and arm and keeps the infant close to the body (Figure 15-18). If transporting the infant in this position, the medical assistant uses the nondominant hand to protect the back and top of the infant's head. When the medical assistant is stationary, the nondominant hand can be used if needed. When done properly, this position keeps the infant safe and secure.

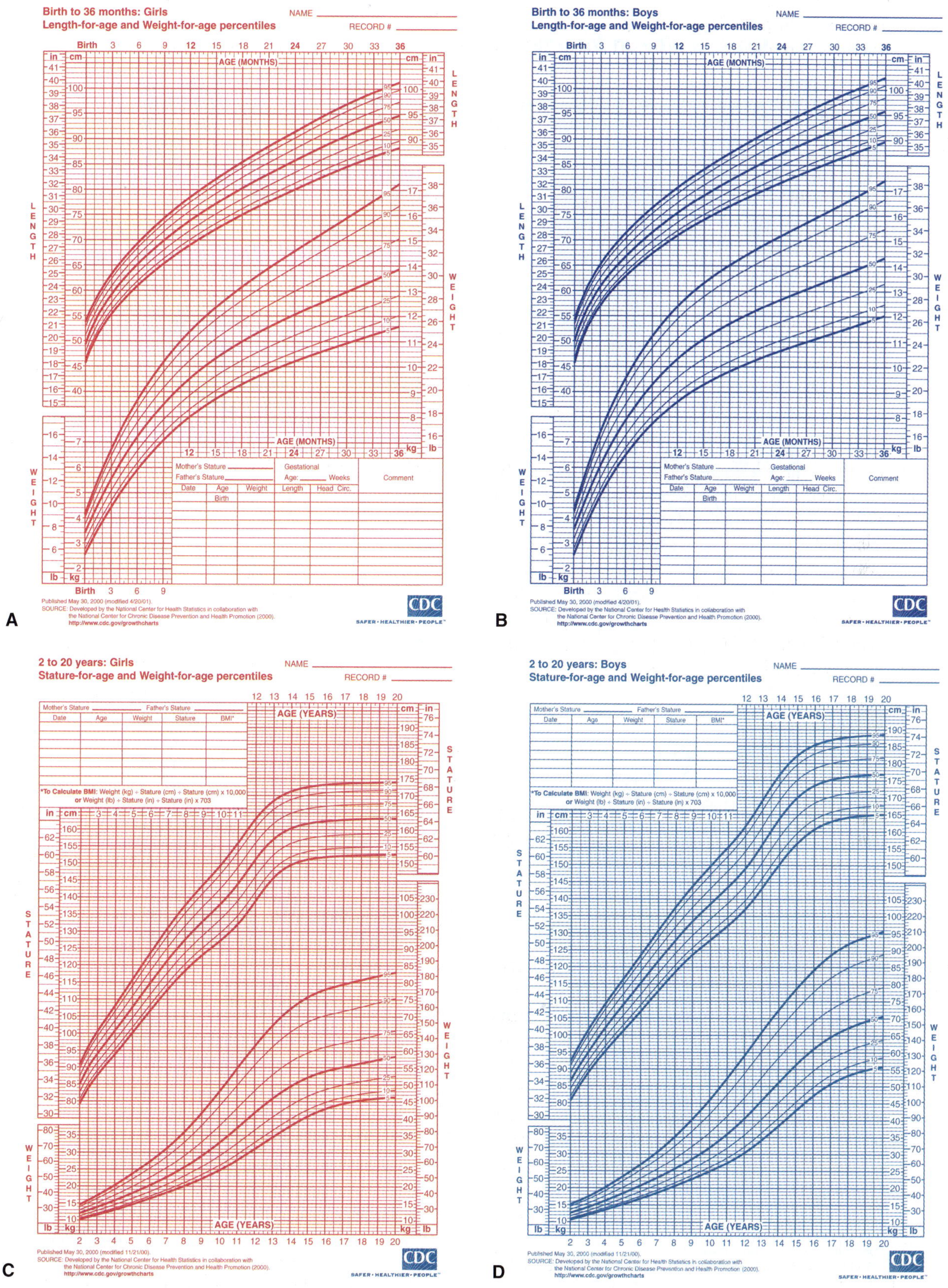

Figure 15-14 (A) Growth chart for girls' height and weight, age birth to 36 months. (B) Growth chart for boys' height and weight, age birth to 36 months. (C) Growth chart for girls' height and weight, age 2 to 20 years. (D) Growth chart for boys' height and weight, age 2 to 20 years. (Note that the growth charts shown in (A) and (B) provide space at bottom right of chart for date, age, weight, length and head circumference.) (Courtesy of the Centers for Disease Control and Prevention.)

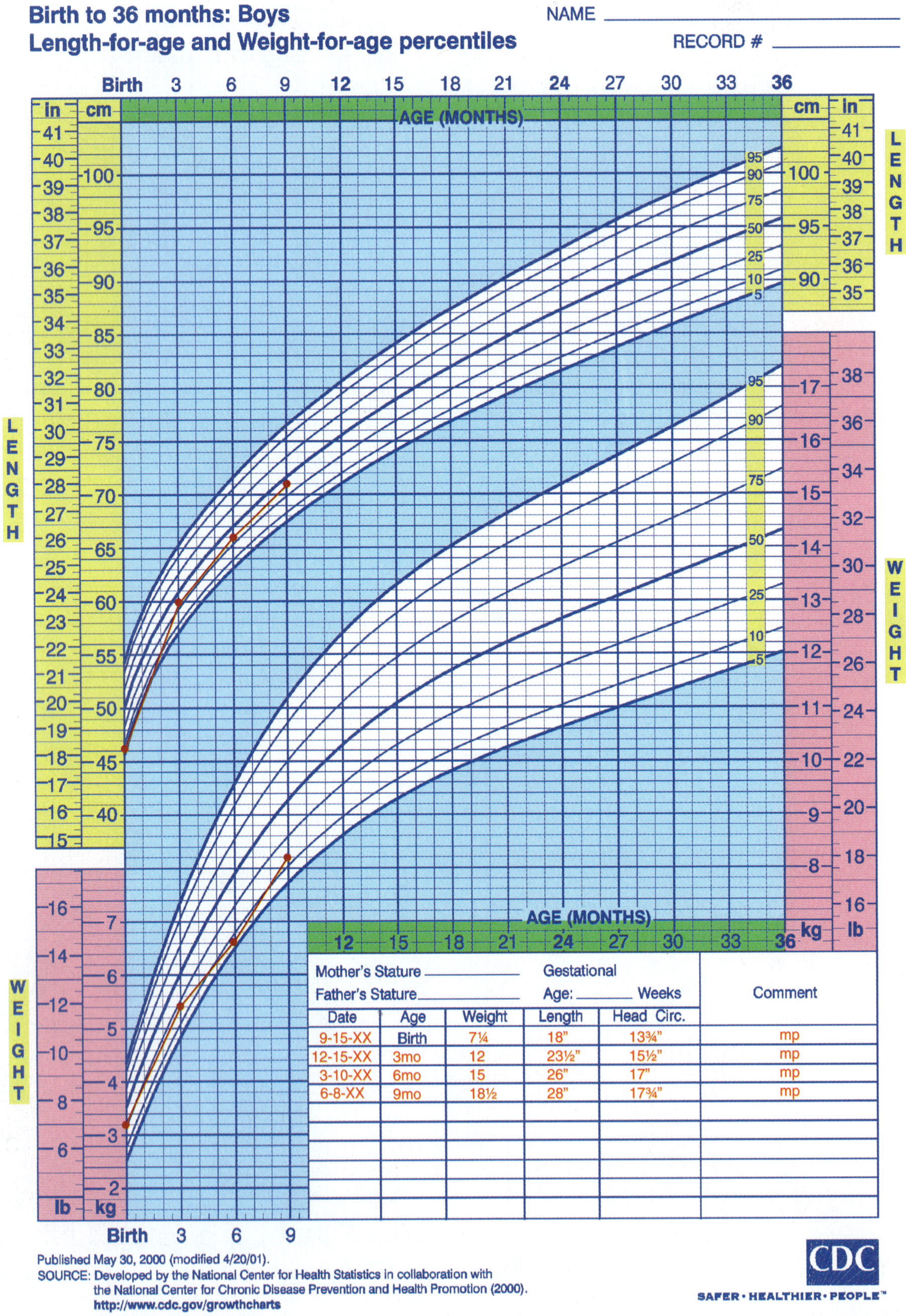

Date	Age	Weight	Length	Head Circ.	Comment
9-15-XX	Birth	7¼	18"	13¾"	mp
12-15-XX	3mo	12	23½"	15½"	mp
3-10-XX	6mo	15	26"	17"	mp
6-8-XX	9mo	18½	28"	17¾"	mp

Figure 15-15 Sample growth chart with information plotted at birth, 3, 6, and 9 months. Sections in this figure are highlighted to help you locate the values: length (yellow), weight (pink), age (green), and percentiles (white). (Courtesy of the Centers for Disease Control and Prevention.)

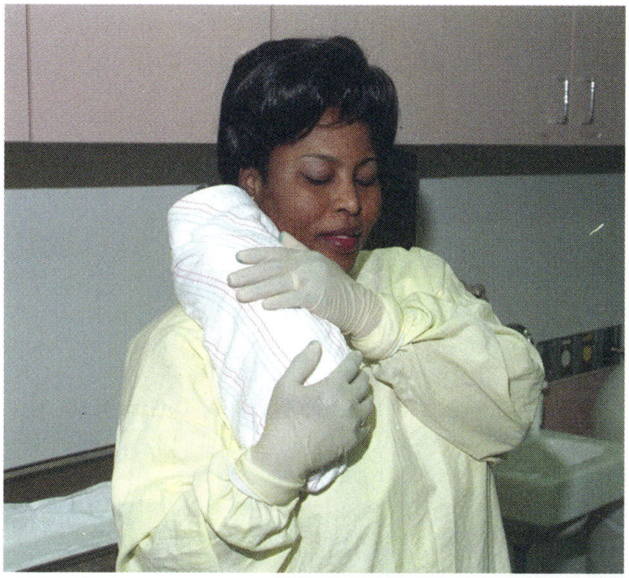

Figure 15-16 Infant carry—upright.

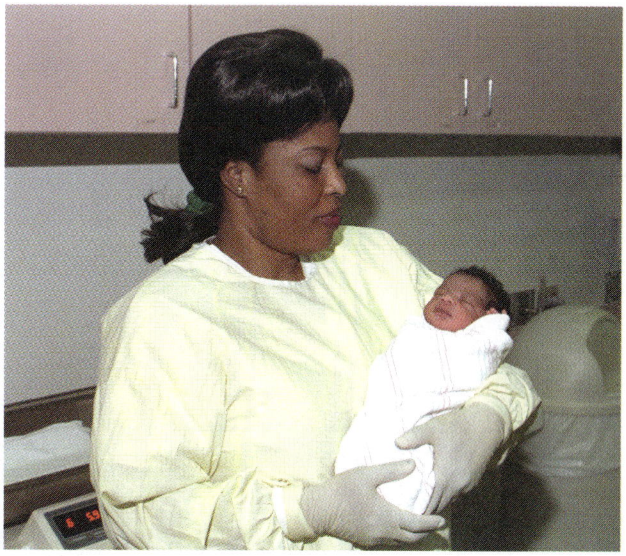

Figure 15-17 Infant carry—cradle.

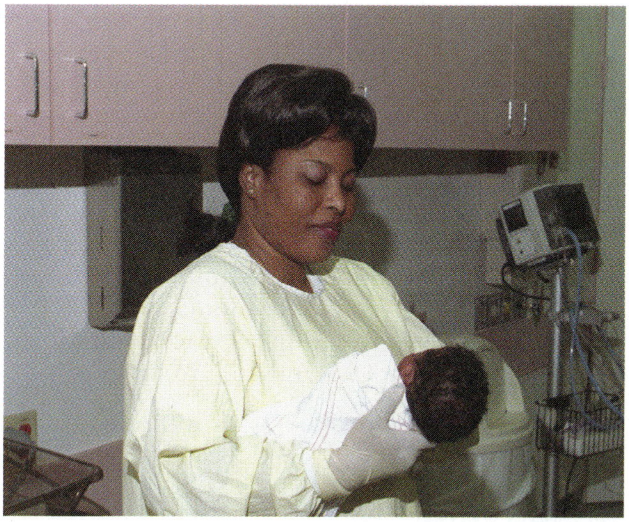

Figure 15-18 Infant carry—football.

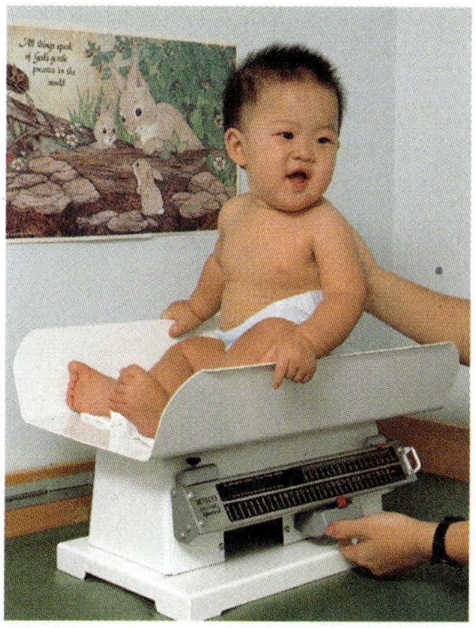

Figure 15-19 Infants who are able to sit and small children can be weighed on a platform scale.

Height and Weight Measuring Devices

Various devices are available for measuring height and weight in children. Infants and small children are weighed on an infant platform scale, which provides a measurement in pounds and ounces and kilograms and grams (Figure 15-19). The scale has a platform with curved sides in which the child may sit or lie. Weigh the infant or child in as few clothes as possible, removing the diaper and shoes or slippers. A small sheet, cloth diaper, or paper towel should be placed on the scale before weighing the infant or child, to avoid the transfer of microorganisms from bare skin. (The scale is sanitized and disinfected between patients.)

Infant length can be measured using an infant measuring board, which consists of a rigid headboard and movable footboard. Place the measuring board on a table and position the infant on his or her back on the board, with the head touching the headboard. Move the footboard up until it touches the bottom of the infant's feet (Figure 15-20).

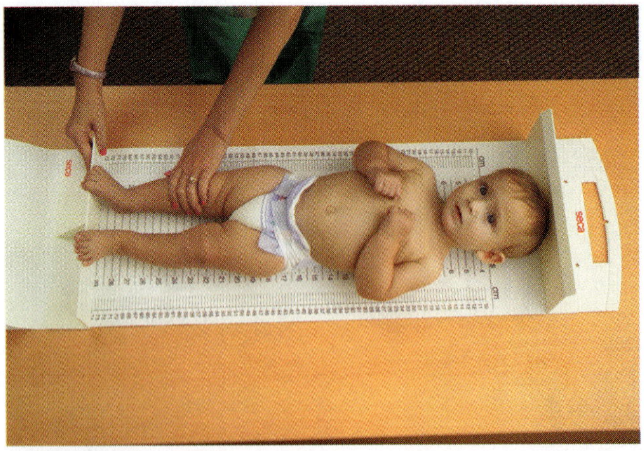

Figure 15-20 Measuring the recumbent length of an infant, from the vertex of the head to the heel.

An infant can also be measured on a pad by placing a pin into the pad or making a pencil mark at the top of the head and a second pin or mark at the heel of the extended leg. The length is the distance between the two pins. A tape measure can also be used. *NOTE:* 1 inch = 2.54 cm.

A stature-measuring device can be used to measure height once the child is able to stand erect without support. The device consists of a movable headpiece attached to a rigid measuring bar and platform (Figure 15-21). A paper towel should be placed on the platform before use to avoid the potential transmission of microorganisms from bare feet.

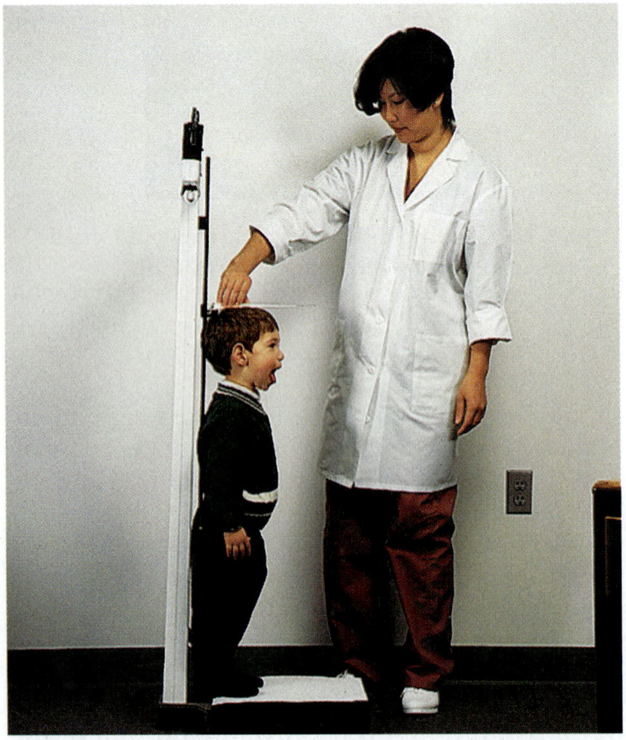

Figure 15-21 Measuring height in children.

Measuring Head Circumference

Head circumference measurement is routinely recorded on an infant's chart to alert the provider to any abnormal development. This procedure should be performed during routine visits until the child is 36 months old. Thereafter, it should be measured on a yearly basis until the age of 6 years. Head circumference measurement requires a flexible paper or metal measuring tape. A cloth tape may stretch and give a false measurement. Head circumference is plotted similarly to height and weight but on separate growth percentile charts for head measurements (Figure 15-22). Generally, head and chest circumference are equal at about 1 to 2 years of age. Rapid growth above the normal percentile may indicate hydrocephalus, a disorder in which excessive fluid accumulates around the brain causing an increase in intracranial pressure and possible brain damage. This could lead to mental and physical problems. Conversely, the growth of the head that falls below the normal percentile may indicate microencephaly caused by a premature closure of the fontanels. In this instance, there is not enough room for the development of the brain, and mental retardation can result. Head circumference for a newborn should be between 12.5 and 14.5 inches or 31.75 and 36.83 cm.

Measuring Chest Circumference

Measuring the chest circumference of an infant is not normally performed during routine examinations. It may be performed and monitored when there is a suspicion of overdevelopment or underdevelopment of the heart or lungs or calcification of rib cartilage. To measure the chest of an infant, snugly wrap the measuring tape around the chest at nipple level. It is preferable to read the measurement during the resting phase between respirations.

Occasionally it is necessary for the medical assistant to convert measurement results into inches or centimeters. To accomplish the task accurately, note that 1 inch equals 2.54 cm. (Procedure 15-3 gives steps for measuring infant chest and head circumference, weight, and height.)

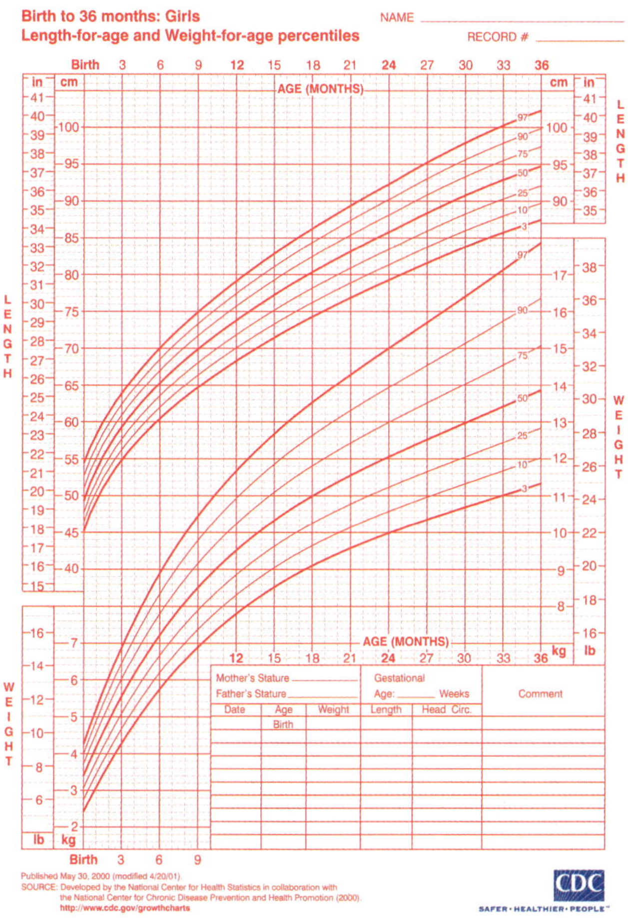

A

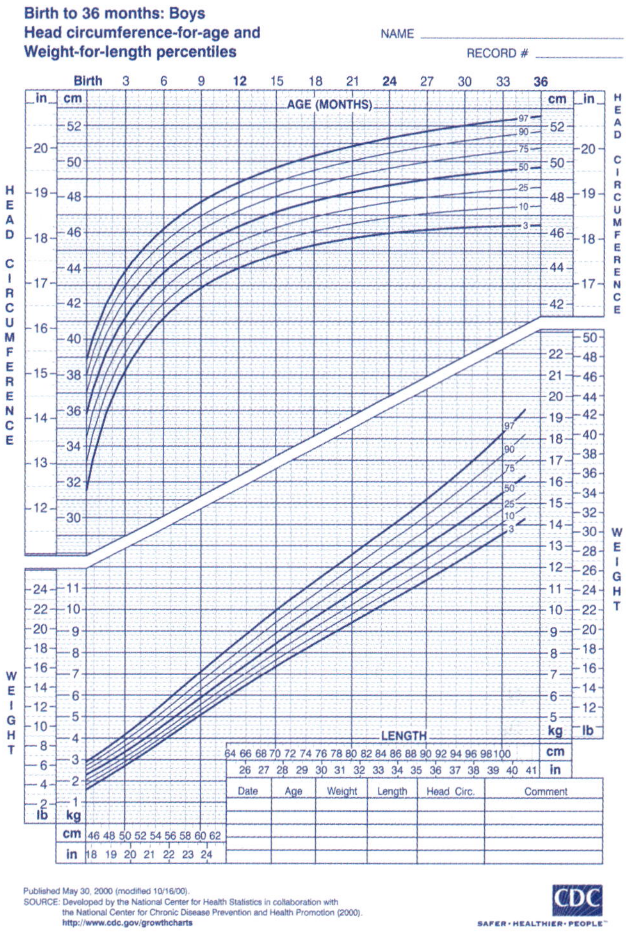

B

Figure 15-22 (A) Growth chart for girls' head circumference, birth to 36 months. (B) Growth chart for boys' head circumference, birth to 36 months. (Courtesy of the Centers for Disease Control and Prevention.)

Example:

To convert inches to centimeters, multiply the number of inches by 2.54:

Inches × 2.54 = Centimeters

Example:

To convert centimeters to inches, divide the number of centimeters by 2.54:

Centimeters ÷ 2.54 = Inches

Infant/Child Failure to Thrive

The failure of an infant or a child to grow and thrive may have many organic and inorganic causes. There may be social and emotional causes. Many causes an infant or a child failing to grow and thrive may be treated if found in time. The emotionally deprived infant needing affection will not grow, because of lack of growth hormone production. Once this child is given physical and emotional warmth, the growth hormone is produced and the child will grow. Other reasons for an infant failing to thrive may be because the infant has a chronic disease; has a diet that is inadequate especially in calories and proteins; has a disorder of the heart, brain, or kidneys; or has been improperly fed.

PEDIATRIC VITAL SIGNS

As with older children and adults, pediatric vital signs are commonly taken by the medical assistant. The vital signs are more fully covered in Chapter 12 for adult patients; however, specific procedures for taking an infant's temperature, pulse, respiration, and blood pressure are explained here. These procedures are done differently for infants than for older children and adults.

Temperature

Body temperature may be measured in Fahrenheit (F) or Celsius (C) degrees through oral, rectal, axillary, or tympanic routes. Many types of thermometers are used. Mercury (glass) thermometers have been replaced in ambulatory care areas and offices by digital thermometers, electronic thermometers, tympanic membrane sensors (aural), and temporal artery thermometers, which provide accurate temperature readings in less time. Broken mercury thermometers release vapors into the air that are toxic when inhaled and lead to mercury poisoning. They should not be used. Proper disposal of mercury is regulated by the health department and varies from state to state. Electronic and digital thermometers can display temperature within 15 to 60 seconds, depending on the model used. A reading can be obtained by infrared tympanic membrane and temporal artery sensor in a matter of seconds (see Procedure 15-3).

Oral Temperature. The oral route is used for children older than 5 years. Caution the child against biting down on the thermometer. Do not take an oral temperature if the child has a history of seizures.

Aural Temperature. The aural route uses the tympanic membrane thermometer. It is used on children older than 2 years because it is considered less accurate for children younger than 2 years. Otitis media and impacted cerumen are two other reasons why this route may not be selected. A reading can be obtained in a matter of seconds.

Rectal Temperature. Rectal temperatures may be taken with caution in infants and toddlers when other methods or routes are not advised. Place the child supine, with the knees flexed. An infant can also lie prone on a parent's lap. Do not force the thermometer. Rectal temperatures are not indicated for children who have had rectal surgery or for those who have diarrhea (see Procedure 15-4).

Axillary Temperature. Axillary temperatures are often preferable to rectal or oral temperatures for toddlers and preschoolers because they are safe and nonintrusive to take. Place the probe of the digital thermometer in the axillary space and have the child hold the arm close to the trunk. Leave in place until beep is heard. This route is not used if accuracy is critical.

Temporal Artery Temperature. Chapter 12 provides information and the procedure for taking a temperature using a temporal artery thermometer (TAT). Temporal artery thermometers are used almost exclusively.

Pulse

The apical pulse is heard at the apex of the heart, located at the fifth intercostal space left side, midclavicular line, that is, between the fifth and sixth ribs in the middle of the clavicle (usually below the nipple), left of the sternum. A stethoscope is required to obtain an apical pulse. The apical pulse is generally preferred over pulses from other locations for infants and small children (younger than 5 years). Each "lub-dub" sound is counted as one heartbeat. The pulse is counted for 1 full minute (see Procedure 15-4).

The normal pulse rate varies with age, decreasing as the child grows older (Table 15-2). The heart rate may also vary considerably among children of the same age and size. The heart rate increases in response to exercise, excitement, anxiety, and fever and decreases to a resting rate when the child is still.

Listen to the heart rate, noting whether the heart rhythm is regular or irregular. Children often have a normal cycle of irregular rhythm associated with respiration called sinus arrhythmia. In sinus arrhythmia, the child's heart rate is faster on inspiration and slower on expiration. Record whether the pulse is normal, bounding, or thready.

Table 15-2 Normal Heart Rate Ranges for Children

Age	Heart Rate Range (beats/min)
Newborns	130–140
Infants to 2 years	110–130
2 to 6 years	96–115
6 to 10 years	70–110
10 to 16 years	60–100

Respirations

In older children and adolescents, respiratory rate is counted in the same way as in an adult. In infants and children younger than 6 years, however, the respiratory rate is assessed by observing the rise and fall of the abdomen. Inspiration, when the chest or abdomen rises, and expiration, when the chest or abdomen falls, are counted as one respiration. Because these movements are often irregular, they should be counted for 1 full minute for accuracy. Normal respiratory rate varies with the child's age (Table 15-3; see Procedure 15-6).

Blood Pressure

The blood pressure of an infant is not normally taken unless requested by the provider. In children 3 years of age and older, blood pressure should be measured annually as part of a routine vital sign assessment.

Blood pressure can be measured using electronic or aneroid equipment and a pediatric cuff. The size of the blood pressure cuff is determined by the size of the child's arm or leg. A general rule of thumb is that the width of the inflatable bladder should be 40% of the circumference of the extremity used. If the cuff is too small, pressure will be falsely high; if too large, falsely low. Sometimes it is difficult to hear the blood pressure in an infant or small child. Use a pediatric stethoscope over pulse sites if possible.

If the pulse still cannot be auscultated, the blood pressure can be measured by touch. Palpate for the pulse. Keeping your fingers on the pulse, pump up the cuff until the pulse is no longer felt. Slowly open the air valve, watching the dial, and note the number where the pulse is again palpated. This is called the palpated systolic blood pressure (Table 15-4).

Table 15-3 Normal Respiratory Rate Ranges for Children

Age	Respiratory Rate (breaths/min)
Newborn	30–60
1 year	20–40
3 years	18–30
6 years	18–30
10 years	12–20
17 years	12–20

COLLECTING A URINE SPECIMEN FROM AN INFANT

Occasionally the medical assistant is required to obtain a urine specimen from an infant for laboratory testing. Special procedures and equipment are required for this procedure. The collection bag is clear plastic with adhesive tabs (clean catch bag) for application to the perineum of the infant (Figure 15-23; see Procedure 15-7).

The clean catch bag has been a popular way to obtain a clean catch specimen for urinalysis in pediatric patients. The urinalysis is essential to the provider's work-up of the patient. Not only is it time-consuming to wait for a child to void, but many times the bag is empty. There are risks of contamination of the specimen by the bag method. According to *The Internet Journal of Emergency Medicine,* a procedure known as direct urethral bladder catheterization is the preferred method for obtaining a sterile urine specimen. A very small catheter (5 French) is used. Using sterile technique, the catheter is inserted through the urethra into the bladder of the pediatric patient. The procedure used on an infant or child is the same as the procedures for performing a urinary catheterization on a male or female patient described in Chapter 18. Catheterization of a pediatric patient in order to obtain a sterile urine specimen is an invasive procedure performed by a licensed provider. A California study confirmed

Table 15-4 Normal Blood Pressure Ranges for Children

Age	Systolic (mm Hg)	Diastolic (mm Hg)
3 years	110	65
6 years	110	65
10 years	118	75
17 years	118	75

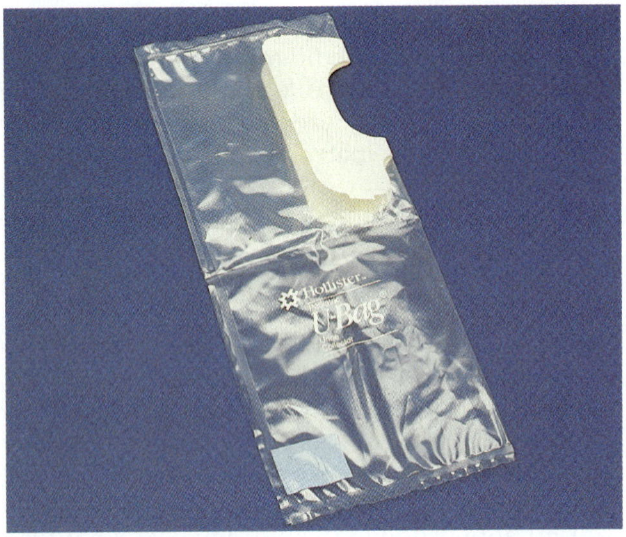

Figure 15-23 Pediatric urine collector. The collector is opened, and the paper backing is removed, exposing the adhesive surface. The collector is firmly attached over the child's cleansed genitalia to prevent leakage.

that catheterization is safe and effective particularly in the emergency department when a pediatric patient has a fever and symptoms of a urinary tract infection.

SCREENING INFANTS FOR HEARING IMPAIRMENT

In some hospitals, infants are screened for hearing impairment immediately after delivery. An automated system for checking hearing ability is used by some clinics. It is a more complex screening requiring the use of sensors. As the infant moves in response to sounds produced by the system, these responses are recorded by sensors attached to the infant. The procedure is a more definitive screening process. The medical assistant must maintain a quiet environment while these screening procedures are being performed because extraneous sounds may invalidate the results.

SCREENING INFANT AND CHILD VISUAL ACUITY

Measuring the visual acuity of an infant is difficult and is not usually performed unless visual impairment is suspected. Newborns will respond to light by tightly shutting their eyes and keeping them closed until the light is removed. Older infants will follow an object up and down when it is placed directly in front of the eyes. It is estimated that a newborn has the vision equivalent to 20/150, which will reach the adult level of 20/20 by the age of 6 months. The medical assistant will be required to maintain a nonstimulating environment while the provider is screening the infant, because any interference may invalidate results.

The kindergarten chart or Allen cards are used to test visual acuity in young children. It contains pictures in descending size, and the lines are labeled in the same manner as the Snellen Chart. The child is asked to identify the picture as the medical assistant points to it (Figure 15-24).

The E chart is a series of *E*s pointing in different directions in descending size. The size and labeling are the same as the Snellen chart. This chart is used for older children. The child will be asked to point in the direction of the *E* as the medical assistant points to it (Figure 15-25).

Make a game out of measuring young children's visual acuity because their attention span is very limited.

COMMON DISORDERS AND DISEASES

Young children grow and physically change very quickly. Their immune systems develop normally when they are healthy infants and children.

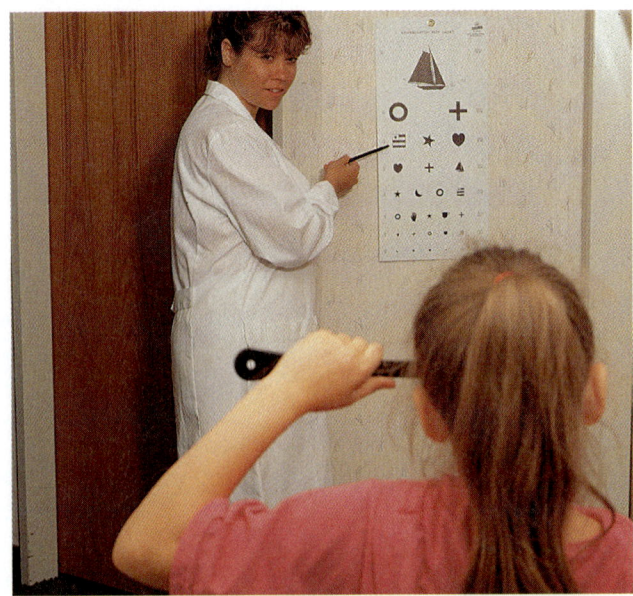

Figure 15-24 Measuring distance visual acuity of a child using a kindergarten vision screening chart.

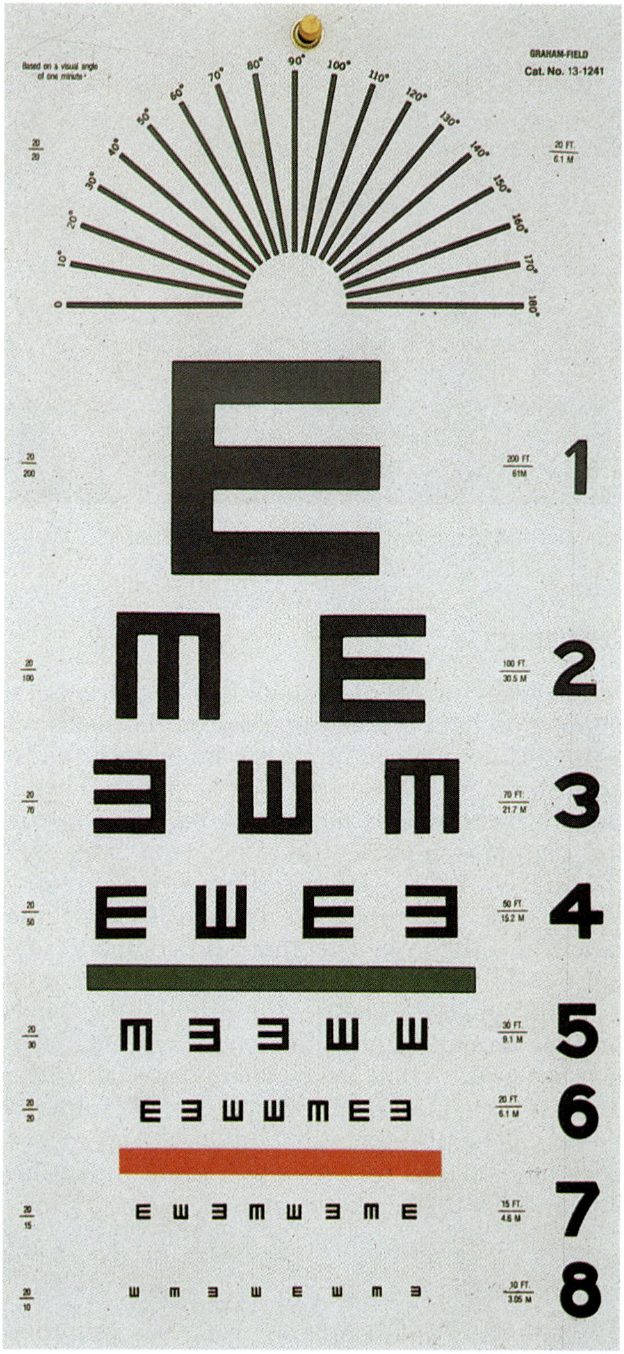

Figure 15-25 Snellen E or Big E chart for testing distance visual acuity of children.

Immunizations, together with their own developing immune system, give them protection from dangerous childhood diseases. Many life-threatening illnesses have been controlled because of scheduled immunization, the child's own developing immune system, and the wise use of antibiotics for infections.

Otitis Media

Otitis media is a commonly occurring disorder in infants and young children. It is characterized by inflammation of the middle ear. Fluid accumulates behind the tympanic membrane, resulting in a degree of temporary hearing loss. It is commonly known as a middle ear infection. Because of the infant and young child's eustachian tubes' connection to the nose and throat, bacteria that causes throat and respiratory infections can easily access the inner ear via the eustachian tube. The fluid in the middle ear can become infected by the bacteria present in the nose and throat. The fluid turns to pus and is known as **suppurative** otitis media. Pain and loss of hearing are common symptoms. Many young children have eustachian tubes that are horizontal and narrow, which predisposes them to otitis media. As children develop physically, they can outgrow otitis media.

The provider can diagnosis otitis media by visually examining the tympanic membrane with an otoscope. The membrane will be bulging and appear red and inflamed (Figure 15-26). If **exudate** or an oozing of pus is present, a culture and sensitivity can be done. The treatment for otitis media is antibiotics. To prevent antiobiotic overuse and pathogen resistance, providers attempt to prescribe antibiotic therapy only when necessary. Decongestants are helpful in some children. For chronic otitis media, a **myringotomy,** incision into the tympanic membrane, may be necessary to prevent rupture of the tympanic membrane and the scarring that results. Scarring can cause permanently impaired hearing ability.

Tympanostomy is a surgical procedure in which pediatric ear tubes are placed through the tympanic membrane to promote ongoing drainage. Chronic otitis media that is left untreated can result in permanent hearing loss.

Hearing loss causes serious major problems in a child's development. Treatment of hearing loss depends on its cause. Hearing aids may be helpful to amplify sounds if the loss is caused by sounds not being conducted to the inner ear. Sensorineural hearing loss does not improve with hearing aids. **Cochlear implantation,** approved by the FDA since 1990, is a procedure that can help children with bilateral **sensorineural** deafness.

The Common Cold

The common cold is aptly named because it is the most common and frequent disease that young children experience. Viruses are the usual

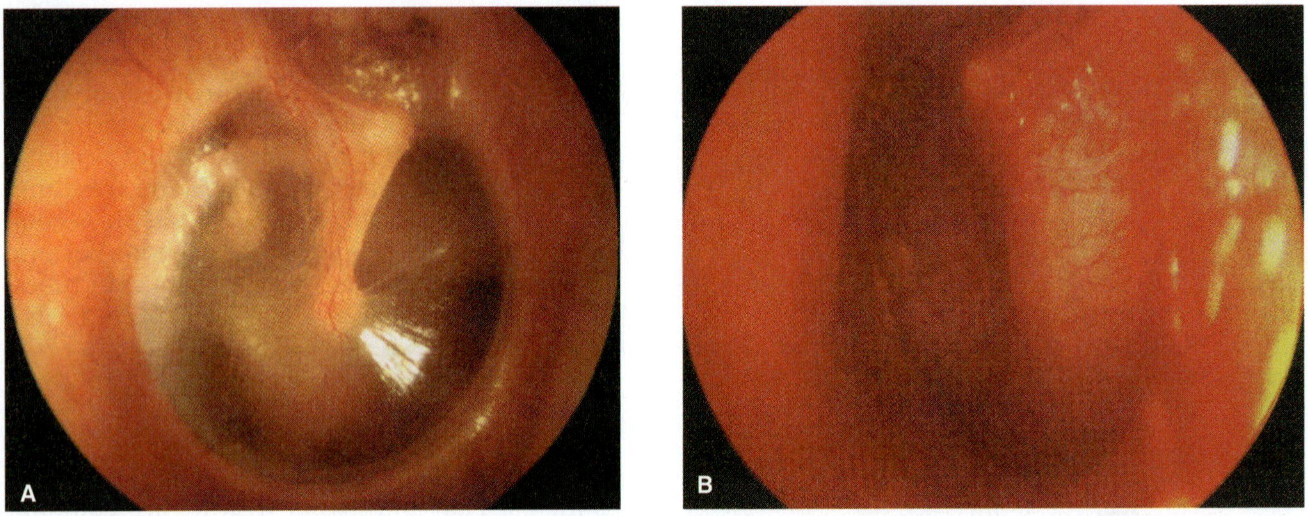

Figure 15-26 Comparison of (A) normal tympanic membrane and (B) acute otitis media.

microorganisms that cause a cold, and they are spread by direct contact and droplets through the air when children cough and sneeze. Some symptoms are inflammation of the nasopharynx, coughing, nasal discharge, sneezing, and fever. Treatment consists of getting sufficient rest, forcing fluids, and eating a well-balanced diet. Antibiotics are not helpful.

Tonsillitis

The tonsils are located in the back of the nose and throat. They aid in protecting the respiratory tract from infection but frequently become inflamed and infected while doing their job. The cause most often is group A beta-hemolytic streptococcus or a virus. Fever, cough, sore throat, and red, swollen tonsils are common symptoms. Diagnosis can be made by doing a culture and sensitivity of tonsillar exudate. Antibiotics will rid the child of infection if it is bacterial, and must be taken as prescribed. Tonsillectomy is considered for older children who have chronic tonsillitis.

Pediculosis

Infestation with the head louse is known as pediculosis capitus and is common among school-aged children. The parasites suck blood from humans and are highly contagious. Diagnosis can be made by visual examination of the hair and scalp and observing the eggs (known as nits) on the hair. Special medications applied to the hair is an effective treatment. Care should be taken to launder bed linens and clothing everyday. The louse is not a vector for disease.

Asthma

Asthma has increased dramatically in the general population but especially in children. The cause of asthma is not known, but it can be brought on by environmental substances, such as pollen, chemicals, cigarette smoke, mold, and dog and cat hair. Its symptoms include wheezing, coughing, and shortness of breath. It is a serious chronic respiratory disease. Spasms of the bronchi trap air and mucus in the lungs. The child will complain of a tight chest and will have shallow respirations and a nonproductive cough. The asthma attack may become an emergency situation. The pediatrician may refer the child to an allergy specialist who will test the child for various allergies. Respiratory therapy is helpful for some children. Airways can become damaged over time as a result of chronic inflammation.

Croup

The common viral condition croup has symptoms of a croupy or "barking"-type cough, a high-pitched sound on inspiration (stridor), and respiratory distress. The condition is often associated with an upper respiratory infection that leads to inflammation of the larynx, trachea, and bronchi. Respiratory obstruction can occur if severe, but children with croup generally are not seriously ill.

Pertussis (Whooping Cough)

Pertussis is a highly contagious respiratory tract infection caused by a bacterium. At the start, the disease appears to be a cold, but pertussis may become serious, especially in infants. Infected infants are at risk for pneumonia, seizures, brain diseases, and death. After about 2 weeks, the child has numerous rapid coughs that can last for months. Vaccines are available to prevent the disease. In recent years there have been outbreaks of pertussis in college-age individuals and adults. The thinking by providers is that these people have lost their immunity to pertussis and need to be revaccinated with a booster vaccine.

Respiratory Syncytial Virus

In most children, the virus causes mild cold-like symptoms. Death can occur in high-risk babies, such as premature infants, infants with a suppressed immune system, and infants with congestive heart failure. It is the most common cause of pneumonia in children under 1 year.

The virus spreads easily and rapidly through the air and can survive for 1 hour on hands and clothes and for several hours on toys, countertops, and other surfaces. There is no vaccine, but the infection can be treated with antiviral drugs such as ribavirin in **aerosolized** form. The drug inhibits the virus from replicating, so the sooner it is given, the better the results. This treatment is recommended only for severely ill and high-risk patients.

Attention Deficit Hyperactivity Disorder

Attention deficit hyperactivity disorder is a condition in which children have difficulties paying attention and focusing on the task at hand. Parents question whether the disorder is overdiagnosed. Many researches believe that the increase in diagnoses comes from improved techniques to detect the condition. There are three types of symptoms: hyperactivity, impulsivity, and inattention. Symptoms range from mild to severe.

The cause is uncertain, but researchers note that ADHD runs in families, with a possible genetic link. There also may be a link between ADHD and tobacco and alcohol use during pregnancy.

Diagnosis is made when a child is about 6 to 12 years old. Observation of the child's behavior is documented by parents, teachers, pediatrician, family care provider, psychologist, and psychiatrist. Tests are done to identify other medical problems that can help explain the child's symptoms such as hearing or vision impairment, lead exposure, anemia, and thyroid disease. Symptoms can be controlled, but there is no cure. Stimulant medications (e.g., Adderall, Ritalin, Concerta) and behaviorial therapy help control the symptoms.

Child Abuse

Child abuse has increased significantly in recent years. By law, health care professionals, including medical assistants, as well as others, must report suspected child abuse. The individual reporting the suspected abuse is protected against liability as a result of the reporting. If suspicion of abuse exists, the provider and health care professional should:

- Treat the child's injuries
- Send the child to the hospital if necessary
- Inform parents of the diagnosis
- Inform parents that the incident will be reported to the public and social service agency
- Notify child protective agency
- Document all information
- Provide court testimony if requested

Child abuse is any physical or mental injury, sexual abuse, negligence, or mistreatment of a child under 18 years of age. Some child abuse signs are:

- Bruises
- Broken bones
- Lacerations
- Burns (cigarette, rope, and burns from being immersed in scalding water)
- Poor hygiene
- Malnutrition
- Head injuries
- Neglected well-baby appointments

The AAP recommends parents be taught to monitor television, videos, DVDs, and other types of media to limit viewing time and exposure to violence. Children 2 years and younger should not be exposed to any of these media.

The cultural background of the family should be taken into consideration, as should some folk medicine practices. Latin American and Russian cultures treat headaches or abdominal pain by placing a cup on the skin, creating a vacuum, and placing a small amount of burning material on the skin. These children may present with burns. To treat minor ailments, Southeast Asians rub a coin or spoon in hot oil and rub it onto the child's neck, spine, and ribs, and a burn may occur.

MALE CIRCUMCISION

Circumcision of the male is the surgical removal of the foreskin (prepuce) of the penis. Female circumcision includes a variety of surgical procedures performed on a female's genitalia (see Chapter 18).

Male circumcision is a religious rite in the Jewish and Muslim religions. It is performed on a majority of males in the United States for hygienic reasons. The belief is that male circumcision is a prophylaxis against urinary tract infections and sexually transmitted diseases, especially HIV.

Most circumcisions usually are performed in the hospital shortly after birth. Some consider the procedure to be "cultural" surgery. It has become a tradition, and the majority of male babies are circumcised. According to the CDC, it is the most commonly performed neonatal surgical procedure in the United States.

The practice of circumcision arose during the nineteenth century when circumcision was deemed necessary for male infants. The belief was that not being circumcised resulted in males who habitually masturbated and/or suffered from insanity.

Proponents of circumcision say it is important for male babies to have penises that resemble their fathers', for improved hygiene, and for males to conform socially with peers.

Although circumcision is generally safe, it is not harmless surgery. The infant is restrained in a specially designed device on a table, and the surgery is performed using sterile technique with analgesia. (In the nineteenth century it was advocated that no analgesic be given so that the male would feel pain, thus accomplishing a means of averting masturbation.) Scientists have shown that during circumcision, without analgesia, the infant's heart rate and blood pressure rise. There is a risk of hemorrhage, sepsis, and laceration.

Advocates for not circumcising male infants claim there is no medical reason to perform the procedure. Research has shown that urinary tract infections and sexually transmitted diseases are no more common in noncircumcised infants than in circumcised infants. Some view the surgery as a profit-driven surgery. According to the AAP about 80% of American male babies are circumcised yearly. At one time the AAP had a pro-circumcision stance, but in 1975 it reversed its position stating there is "no absolute medical indication for routine circumcision of newborns." If it is performed, the AAP recommended that pain relief be provided.

Furthermore, those who are adverse to the surgery say that a child is normal when born and that circumcision results in loss of a body part, is unnecessary, leaves a scar, and removes a functioning body part in the name of custom or tradition. It is viewed as a nonessential, pathologic procedure and a violation of basic human rights because infants are too young and helpless to consent or refuse.

How can parents decide what to do? Circumcision or not? It is a choice they will make, and it will take courage. Deeply rooted cultural and traditional customs can be difficult to sort through. With courage, education, and research, parents can gain perspective about whether or not to circumcise their sons. The AAP has information available on its Web site (http://www.aap.org).

Some believe that elective circumcisions of males and females should not be accepted by conscientious health care providers.

Procedure 15-1

Administration of a Vaccine

STANDARD PRECAUTIONS:

PURPOSE:

To administer a vaccine.

EQUIPMENT/SUPPLIES:

Vaccines ordered by provider
Vaccine Information Statement (VIS)
Medication note
Appropriate syringe needles
Alcohol wipes
Gloves (if office/clinic policy)
Sharps container

PROCEDURE STEPS:

1. Check the provider's order. Write out a medication note. RATIONALE: Helps eliminate giving an incorrect medication or dose. Writing the vaccine order on the note prevents giving vaccine to the wrong patient.
2. Follow the six "rights" (see Chapter 24).
3. Perform medical asepsis hand washing following OSHA guidelines.
4. Work in a well-lighted, quiet, clean area.
5. Select the appropriate equipment (see Figure 15-9). RATIONALE: The appropriate size needle and syringe for the vaccine being given are important to prevent patient injury.
6. Give parents/guardians the Vaccine Information Statement (VIS) for the intended vaccine and give them time to read the VIS and ask questions.
7. Select the appropriate vial of vaccine. Check the label three times and check the medication note. RATIONALE: Safeguards patient from incorrect medication, dose, and route.
8. Check for expiration date on vial. RATIONALE: Expired medication is not safe to give.
9. Maintain sterile techniques throughout. RATIONALE: Compromising the vaccine or syringe and needle by poor technique can introduce microorganisms into the patient or vaccine with serious consequences.
10. Select the correct needle size (see Figure 15–9).
11. Shake the vial and/or reconstitute powder medication using all of the diluent. RATIONALE: Ensures medication is mixed properly.
12. Invert the vial and withdraw the correct dose of vaccine. Recheck the label on the vial and the medicine note. RATIONALE: Ensures you have the correct vaccine.
13. Wash hands and, if office/clinic policy, put on disposable gloves. RATIONALE: Gloves must be worn if the medical assistant has any openings in the skin or on the hands.
14. Restrain the child with parent's help. RATIONALE: Avoids injury to child.
15. Locate the appropriate site for administration. Cleanse the site with alcohol wipe and let dry. RATIONALE: The alcohol is an antiseptic and will lower the number of bacteria at the site. Letting the area dry lessens the sting when needle is inserted.
16. Inject the vaccine quickly and steadily at the appropriate angle.
17. Withdraw needle and syringe at angle of insertion. Immediately dispose of needle and syringe in sharps container.
18. Apply gentle pressure to injection site. Rub gently. RATIONALE: Vaccine will be distributed evenly.
19. Wash hands.
20. Fully document each immunization in the patient's chart or electronic record and on the vaccine administration record. Include lot number, manufacturer, site, VIS date, and your name and initials.
21. Update child's record of immunizations and remind parent or guardian to bring it to each visit.
22. Be aware of the location of the emergency drugs (epinephrine and others). RATIONALE: Medication must be readily available to counteract an allergic reaction.
23. Remove gloves (if worn) and wash hands.

Procedure 15-2

Maintaining Immunization Records

STANDARD PRECAUTIONS:

PURPOSE:

To establish and maintain a record of preventive immunizations against childhood diseases for the provider and parent or legal guardian.

EQUIPMENT/SUPPLIES:

Vaccine Administration Record
Vial of vaccine as ordered

PROCEDURE STEPS:

1. Give the parent or legal guardian the most recent copy of the Vaccine Information Statement (VIS). The statements explain risks and benefits of vaccines for each dose of vaccine given.
2. After the administration of a scheduled vaccine for the child, document in the patient's chart or electronic medical record and on the Vaccine Administration Record.
3. Using the medicine note and the vaccine vial, fill out the Vaccine Administration Record (Figure 15-27) according to which vaccine you administered. Note the headings, type of vaccine (use generic abbreviations, not the brand name), date given, month, day, year, dose, route, site, vaccine lot number and manufacturer, VIS; date on VIS, date given (VIS), and your initials as the individual who administered the vaccine.
4. The immunization record is kept by the provider and the parent or legal guardian. *NOTE:* Remind parent or legal guardian to keep immunization records safe and readily accessible for proof of immunization for daycare and school.
5. The data can be entered into the computer manually by the medical assistant and provider.

DOCUMENTATION

5/2/20XX DTaP 0.5 mL IM (R) vastus lateralis. Recorded on vaccine administration record. Parent given Vaccine Information Statement. W. Slawson CMA (AAMA) ———

continues

Procedure 15-2 (continued)

Vaccine Administration Record for Children and Teens

Patient name: ____________________

Birthdate: ____________________

Chart number: ____________________

Vaccine	Type of Vaccine[1] (generic abbreviation)	Date given (mo/day/yr)	Source (F,S,P)[2]	Site[3]	Vaccine		Vaccine Information Statement		Signature/ initials of vaccinator
					Lot #	Mfr.	Date on VIS[4]	Date given[4]	
Hepatitis B[5] (e.g., HepB, Hib-HepB, DTaP-HepB-IPV) Give IM.									
Diphtheria, Tetanus, Pertussis[5] (e.g., DTaP, DTaP-Hib, DTaP-HepB-IPV, DT, DTaP-Hib-IPV, Tdap, DTaP-IPV, Td) Give IM.									
***Haemophilus influenzae* type b[5]** (e.g., Hib, Hib-HepB, DTaP-Hib-IPV, DTaP-Hib) Give IM.									
Polio[5] (e.g., IPV, DTaP-HepB-IPV, DTaP-Hib-IPV, DTaP-IPV) Give IPV SC or IM. Give all others IM.									
Pneumococcal (e.g., PCV, conjugate; PPV, polysaccharide) Give PCV IM. Give PPV SC or IM.									
Rotavirus (Rota) Give oral (po).									
Measles, Mumps, Rubella[5] (e.g., MMR, MMRV) Give SC.									
Varicella[5] (e.g., Var, MMRV) Give SC.									
Hepatitis A (HepA) Give IM.									
Meningococcal (e.g., MCV4; MPSV4) Give MCV4 IM and MPSV4 SC.									
Human papillomavirus (e.g., HPV) Give IM.									
Influenza[5] (e.g., TIV, inactivated; LAIV, live attenuated) Give TIV IM. Give LAIV IN.									
Other									

1. Record the generic abbreviation for the type of vaccine given (e.g., DTaP-Hib, PCV), *not* the trade name.
2. Record the source of the vaccine given as either F (Federally-supported), S (State-supported), or P (supported by Private insurance or other Private funds).
3. Record the site where vaccine was administered as either RA (Right Arm), LA (Left Arm), RT (Right Thigh), LT (Left Thigh), IN (Intranasal), or po (by mouth).
4. Record the publication date of each VIS as well as the date it is given to the patient.
5. For combination vaccines, fill in a row for each separate antigen in the combination.

Technical content reviewed by the Centers for Disease Control and Prevention, February 2008.

www.immunize.org/catg.d/p2022.pdf • Item #P2022 (2/08)

Distributed by the Immunization Action Coalition • (651) 647-9009 • www.immunize.org • www.vaccineinformation.org

Figure 15-27 Vaccination Administration Record. (From the Immunization Action Coalition, http://www.immunize.org.)

Procedure 15-3

Measuring the Infant: Weight, Length, and Head and Chest Circumference

STANDARD PRECAUTIONS:

PURPOSE:

To obtain an accurate measurement of an infant's weight, length, and head and chest circumference for medical records and to screen for growth abnormalities.

EQUIPMENT/SUPPLIES:

Infant scale	Pen
Paper protector	Ruler
Flexible measuring tape without elasticity	Biohazard waste container
Growth chart	

PROCEDURE STEPS:

Measuring infant weight:

1. Wash hands. Explain procedure to parent(s).
2. Undress infant (including the diaper).
3. Place all weights to left of scale to check balance.
4. Place a clean utility towel on scale and check balance scale for accuracy, being sure to compensate for the weight of the towel. RATIONALE: The protection that the paper utility towel affords helps to reduce transmission of microorganisms and provides warmth because the scale is cool.
5. Gently place small infant on her back on the scale. Larger infants can sit on the scale. Place your hand slightly above the infant's body to ensure safety (Figure 15-28). RATIONALE: This will safeguard the infant from falling.
6. Place the bottom weight to its highest measurement that will not cause the balance to drop to the bottom edge.
7. Slowly move upper weight until the balance bar rests in the center of the indicator. A balanced scale will provide an accurate weight. Read the infant's weight while he or she is lying still.
8. Return both weights to their resting position to the extreme left.
9. Gently remove infant and apply diaper. (Parent can help with diapering and holding infant.)

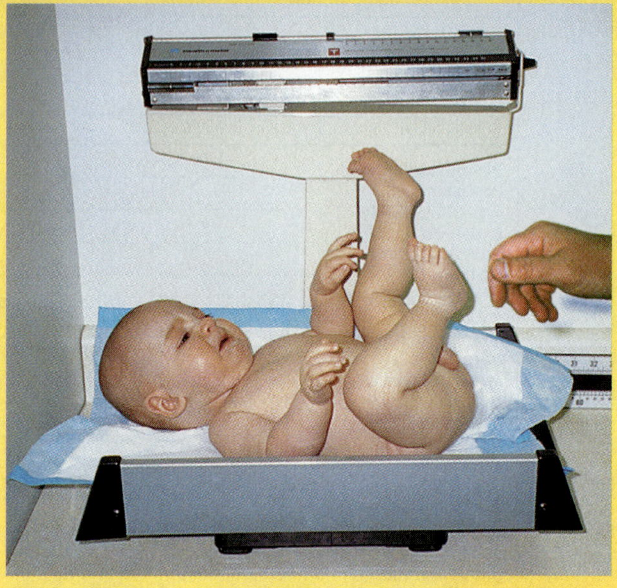

Figure 15-28 Infants who are unable to sit erect should be weighed on their back on the scale.

10. Discard used protective paper towel per Occupational Safety and Health Administration (OSHA) guidelines.
11. Sanitize scale.
12. Wash hands.
13. Document results according to office policy (pounds and ounces or kilograms) on growth chart, in patient's chart or electronic medical record, and parent's booklet if available. Connect dot from previous examination with a ruler to complete graph.

Measuring infant length:

1. Wash hands. Explain procedure to parent(s).
2. Remove infant's shoes.
3. Gently place infant on his or her back on the examination table. If the pediatric table has a headboard, ask parent to hold infant's head against headboard (end) of table at zero mark of ruler while you place infant's heels against footboard. Gently straighten infant's back and legs to line up along ruler. If there is no footboard (to place infant's feet against), use your right hand

continues

Procedure 15-3 (continued)

as a guide (Figure 15-29). If necessary, gently place your left hand over the child's legs at the knees to secure the child in place and straighten the legs so you can read the recumbent length from the head to the heel. RATIONALE: Sometimes it is difficult to straighten the legs.

4. Read length on the measuring device in inches or centimeters.
5. Give infant to parent to dress.
6. Wash hands.
7. Document measurement on growth chart, in patient's chart or electronic medical record, and parent's booklet if available. Connect dot from previous examination with a ruler to complete graph.

Measuring Head Circumference:

1. Wash hands and explain procedure to parent(s).
2. Talk to infant to gain cooperation. Infant may be held by parent or lie on examination table for procedure. Older children of 2 or 3 years may stand or sit if they will remain still.
3. Place the measuring tape snugly around the head from the occipital protuberance to the supraorbital prominence. This is the largest part of the head (Figure 15-30).
4. Read the measurement, which will be in either inches (to nearest ½ inch) or centimeters (to nearest 0.01 cm).

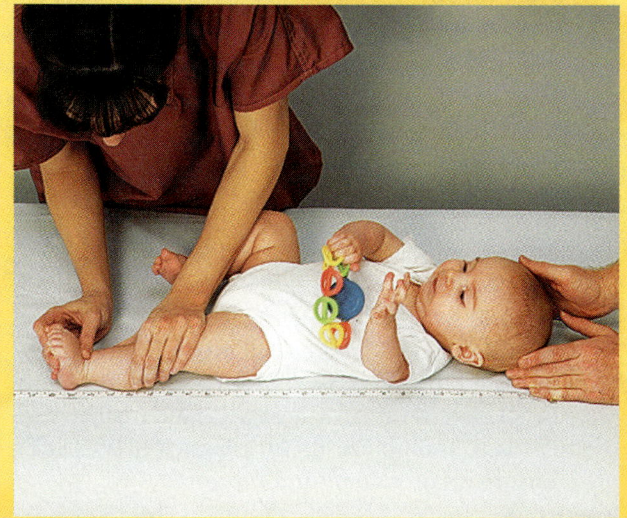

Figure 15-29 Measuring the recumbent length of an infant.

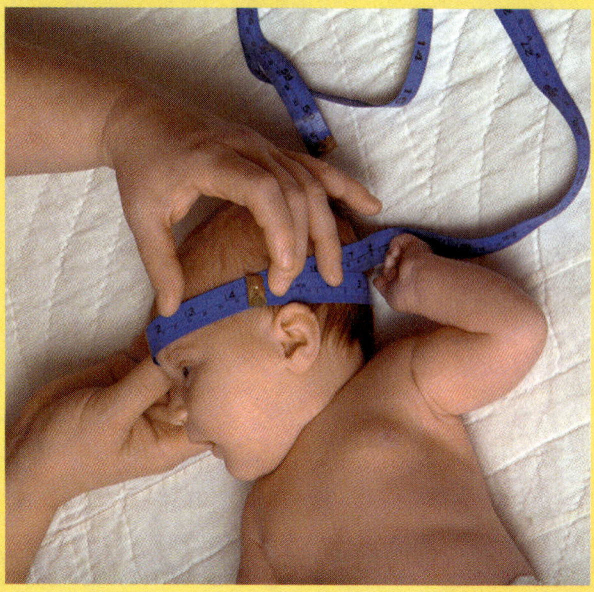

Figure 15-30 Measuring infant's head circumference.

5. Wash hands.
6. Document results according to office policy on growth chart, in patient's chart or electronic medical record, and parent's booklet if available. Connect dot from previous examination with a ruler to complete graph.

Measuring infant's chest circumference:

1. Wash hands and explain procedure to parent(s).
2. Use one thumb to hold tape measure with zero mark against the infant's chest at the midsternal area. With the other hand, bring the tape around/under the back to meet the zero mark of the tape in front. Take the measurement of the chest just above the nipples with the tape fitting around the child's chest under the axillary region. If you need assistance in holding the child still, ask the parent or another assistant. The measurement should be taken when the child is breathing normally and during the resting phase between respirations (Figure 15-31).
3. Read measurement to the nearest 0.01 cm or one-eighth inch.
4. Wash hands.
5. Document results in patient's chart or electronic medical record.

continues

Procedure 15-3 (continued)

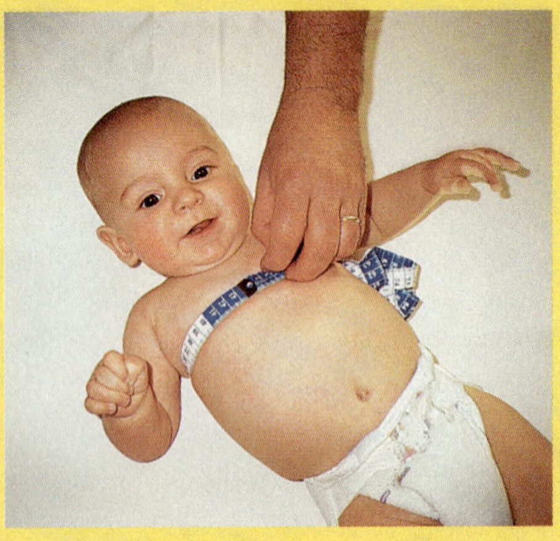

Figure 15-31 Measuring infant's chest circumference.

DOCUMENTATION

3/10/20XX 4:00 pm 6 months of age, wt. 15 lbs. Recorded on growth chart. C. McInnis, RMA

DOCUMENTATION

3/10/20XX 4:00 pm 6 months of age, length 26 inches long. Recorded on growth chart. C. McInnis, RMA

DOCUMENTATION

3/10/20XX 4:00 pm 6 months of age, head circumference 43 centimeters. Recorded on growth chart. C. McInnis, RMA

DOCUMENTATION

3/10/20XX 4:00 pm 6 months of age, chest circumference 30 centimeters. Recorded on growth chart. C. McInnis, RMA

Procedure 15-4

Taking an Infant's Rectal Temperature with a Digital Thermometer

STANDARD PRECAUTIONS:

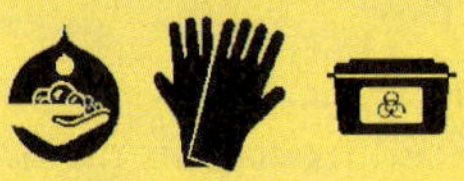

PURPOSE:

To obtain a rectal temperature using a digital thermometer.

EQUIPMENT/SUPPLIES:

Digital thermometer (red probe) and probe cover
Lubricating jelly
4 × 4 gauze sponges
Gloves
Biohazard waste container

PROCEDURE STEPS:

1. Wash hands.
2. Assemble equipment.
3. Identify patient.
4. Explain procedure to parent(s). RATIONALE: Gain cooperation and assistance in disrobing infant and positioning properly.
5. Remove infant's diaper.
6. Position infant in a prone (Figure 15-32A) or supine (Figure 15-32B) position having parent or another medical assistant safeguard infant.
7. Place sheath on thermometer. RATIONALE: Prevents microorganism cross contamination.
8. Lubricate with lubricating jelly. (Place lubricant on a 4 × 4 gauze sponge and place tip of thermometer in lubricant.) RATIONALE: Easier insertion of thermometer.
9. Apply gloves.
10. Spread buttocks, insert thermometer gently into the rectum past the sphincter; for an infant this is 0.5 inch (Figure 15-32B).
11. Hold buttocks together while holding the thermometer. If necessary, restrain infant movement by placing your arm across infant's back. Parent can immobilize infant's legs. RATIONALE: Ensure infant's safety and comfort.
12. Hold in place until beep is heard. Do not let go of the thermometer. RATIONALE: Movement by infant can cause thermometer to move and injure the infant.

continues

Procedure 15-4 (continued)

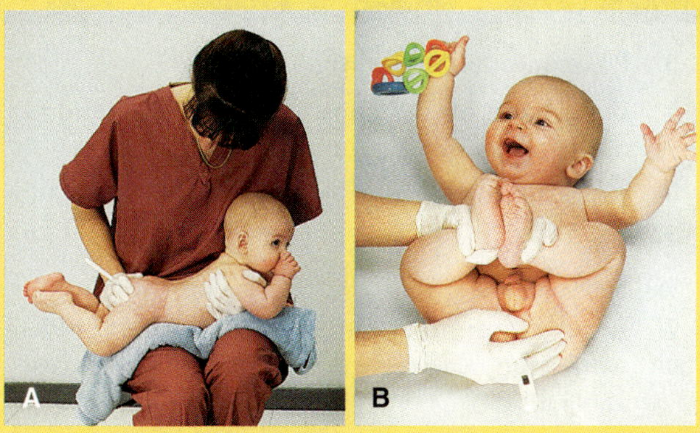

Figure 15-32 Taking the rectal temperature of an infant in (A) the prone position and (B) in the supine position.

13. Remove from rectum. Have parent attend to infant.
14. Note temperature reading.
15. Remove probe cover by ejecting it into a biohazard container.
16. Remove gloves, discard in biohazard waste container.
17. Wash hands.
18. Wipe probe with antiseptic wipe. Replace thermometer on holder.
19. Assist parent in dressing infant if necessary.
20. Record result in patient's chart or electronic medical record with designation of (R), indicating a rectal temperature.

DOCUMENTATION

5/3/20XX 4:00 P.M. T 99.8 (R). W. Slawson, CMA (AAMA) ———

Procedure 15-5

Taking an Apical Pulse on an Infant

STANDARD PRECAUTIONS:

PURPOSE:

To obtain an apical pulse rate.

EQUIPMENT/SUPPLIES:

Stethoscope
Watch with second hand
Alcohol wipes

PROCEDURE STEPS:

1. Wash hands.
2. Assemble equipment.
3. Identify patient.
4. Explain procedure to parent. RATIONALE: Gain co-operation an assistance.
5. Assist in disrobing infant if necessary.
6. Provide a drape for infant's warmth if necessary.
7. Position the infant in a supine position or sitting in the parent's lap. RATIONALE: The supine position may offer easier access to apex of heart if the child is calm.
8. Locate the fifth intercostal space, midclavicular line, left of sternum. RATIONALE: Location of apex of heart.
9. Place warmed stethoscope on the site and listen for the lub-dub sound of the heart.
10. Count the pulse for 1 minute; each lub-dub equals one heartbeat or pulse.
11. Wash hands.
12. Assist parent as needed.
13. Clean earpieces and diaphragm of stethoscope with alcohol wipes. RATIONALE: Prevents cross contamination of microbes between patients.
14. Record the pulse in the infant's or chart or electronic medical record with the designation of (AP) to denote method of obtaining the pulse. Note any arrhythmias.
15. Wash hands.

DOCUMENTATION

3/10/20XX 4:00 P.M. Pulse 140 (AP). Regular. W. Slawson, CMA (AAMA) ———

Procedure 15-6

Measuring Infant's Respiratory Rate

STANDARD PRECAUTIONS:

PURPOSE:

The respiratory rate is normally taken immediately before or after the pulse rate to obtain an accurate respiratory rate.

EQUIPMENT/SUPPLIES:

Watch with second hand

PROCEDURE STEPS:

1. Wash hands.
2. Identify the patient and explain the procedure to the parent. RATIONALE: To gain cooperation and assistance.
3. Position infant in a supine position.
4. Place hand on the chest to feel the rise and fall of the chest wall for 1 minute.
5. Note depth, rhythm, and breath sounds while counting.
6. Wash hands.
7. Record respiratory rate in patient's chart or electronic medical record. Note any irregularities and sounds.

DOCUMENTATION

3/10/20XX 4:00 PM Respirations 22. Regular. W. Slawson, CMA (AAMA)————————

Procedure 15-7

Obtaining a Urine Specimen from an Infant or Young Child

STANDARD PRECAUTIONS:

PURPOSE:

To obtain a specimen of urine from an infant or young child.

EQUIPMENT/SUPPLIES:

Urine collection bag
Urine cup
Laboratory request form
Biohazard transport bag
Gloves
Cleansing cloth
Towel
Biohazard waste container

PROCEDURE STEPS:

1. Wash and glove hands following Standard Precautions.
2. Assemble equipment.
3. Identify patient and explain procedure to parent(s). RATIONALE: To gain cooperation and assistance.
4. Instruct parent to remove diaper.
5. Wash and dry perineal area. RATIONALE: Cleaning area reduces microorganism level and provides better quality urine specimen.
6. Apply collection bag, secure with adhesive tabs (see Figure 15-22).
   a. Girls: spread perineum, place bag over labia.
   b. Boys: place bag over penis and scrotum.

continues

Procedure 15-7 (continued)

7. Replace diaper carefully.
8. Frequently check bag for urine.
9. Once specimen has been collected, remove bag carefully.
10. Prepare specimen as required. Send to laboratory in an appropriate container with a requisition or process the specimen in the office laboratory.
11. Remove gloves and discard in biohazard waste container.
12. Wash hands.
13. Record collection in patient's chart or electronic medical record.

DOCUMENTATION

3/10/20XX 4:00 PM Urine specimen collected via urine collection bag. Specimen sent to Bay Laboratory with requisition for routine urinalysis. J. Guerro, CMA (AAMA) ____________

Case Study 15-1

Refer to the scenario at the beginning of the chapter.

CASE STUDY REVIEW

1. In what ways can Bruce learn about new vaccines that are required for pediatric patients?
2. Other than the provider giving information, describe two ways in which Bruce can stay current with vaccines and immunizations.

Case Study 15-2

After examining Joey Little, Dr. King confirms the diagnosis of otitis media.

CASE STUDY REVIEW

1. Explain otitis media, the most common reason for its occurrence, and its treatment.
2. How can parents and caregivers be educated to help prevent otitis media?

SUMMARY

Caring for the health and well-being of infants and children throughout their various developmental stages and into adolescence is the responsibility of the pediatric practice.

Careful observation of the parent or caregiver and the child is helpful to the treatment and care given to the child. The medical assistant is responsible for reporting to the provider any suspicion of child abuse.

Opportunities abound for educating parents about topics that will keep their children healthy throughout life and include nutrition, sleep, immunizations, and exercise. Pamphlets, videos, and demonstrations are available to share with parents and caregivers.

Children need respect and should be treated with empathy, love, and honesty; in doing so, a positive relationship can be developed with the child.

STUDY FOR SUCCESS

To reinforce your knowledge and skills of information presented in this chapter:

- Review Key Terms
- Practice the Procedures
- Consider the Case Study and discuss your conclusions
- Answer the Review Questions
  - Multiple Choice
  - Critical Thinking
- Navigate the Internet by completing the Web Activities
- Practice the StudyWARE activities on your student CD
- Apply your knowledge in the Student Workbook activities
- Complete the Web Tutor sections
- View and discuss the DVD situations

REVIEW QUESTIONS

Multiple Choice

1. At what age should the first polio vaccine be given?
   a. birth
   b. 1 month
   c. 2 months
   d. 3 months
   e. 6 months
2. One procedure to treat otitis media is:
   a. suppuration
   b. tympanostomy
   c. ear irrigation
   d. otoscopy
   e. myringectomy
3. The pathogen usually responsible for causing tonsillitis is:
   a. *Staphylococcus aureus*
   b. meningococcus
   c. beta-hemolytic streptococcus group A
   d. beta-hemolytic streptococcus group B
4. Head circumference is measured on the child until what age?
   a. 12 months
   b. 24 months
   c. 36 months
   d. 72 months
5. An apical pulse is taken over which of the following sites?
   a. Third intercostal space on the left side
   b. Fourth intercostal space on the left side
   c. Fifth intercostal space on the left side
   d. Sixth intercostal space on the left side

Critical Thinking Questions

1. You notice when you undress a 2-year-old child to prepare for a physical examination that there are bruises on the buttocks and what appear to be burns on the feet. What course of action do you take?
2. Explain the importance of head circumference measurement.
3. Explain the importance of growth charts.
4. Describe the appropriate positions in which to place an infant for obtaining a rectal temperature.
5. Describe the appearance of the pediatric urine collector bag. What is the best way to make certain it will adhere to the child's body?
6. Explain the type of chart used to test visual acuity in young children.
7. When is it appropriate to use the tympanic thermometer when taking a child's temperature?
8. When taking an infant's rectal temperature, what precautions should be taken?
9. Chest circumference measurements on an infant are performed for what purpose?
10. What do the curved lines printed across growth charts indicate?

WEB ACTIVITIES

Search for the American Academy of Pediatrics Web site (http://www.aap.org) to answer the following:

1. What information is available about immunization for hepatitis A, B, and C?
2. What is the most recent recommendation that the American Academy of Pediatrics has made regarding varicella, influenza, and pneumonia immunizations?
3. Visit the Zero to Three Web site (http://www.zerotothree.org). Search for "healthy development for 24- to 36-month-old toddlers." Describe four to five ways parents can encourage their 2- to 3-year-old children to express themselves.
4. Visit the National Network for Child Care Web site (http://www.nncc.org). Search the site for information about fetal alcohol syndrome and birth defects. What specific problems can a newborn have if his or her mother consumed excessive alcohol during pregnancy?
5. Visit the American Academy of Family Physicians Web site (http://www.aafp.org). What information can you find about croup? List five symptoms that should alert parents to call their provider. What are pinworms? How do children get pinworms? How are pinworms detected? How are pinworms treated?

REFERENCES/BIBLIOGRAPHY

Ambroz, K. G., & Eilber, W. (2003). An enhanced method of pediatric urine collection. *The Internet Journal of Emergency Medicine 1*(1).

Clifton, J. C., 2nd. (2007). Mercury exposure and public health. In *Pediatric clinics of North America* (pp. 237–269). The National Library of Medicine and the National Institutes of Health. Retrieved July 2, 2008, from www.pubmed.gov.

Hegner, B. R., Acello, B., & Caldwell, E. (2008). *Nursing assistant: A nursing process approach.* Clifton Park, NY: Delmar Cengage Learning.

Keir, L., Wise, B., Krebs, C., & Kelley-Arney, C. (2008). *Medical assisting: Administrative and clinical competencies,* (6th ed). Clifton Park, NY: Delmar Cengage Learning.

Mandleco, B. L. (2004). *Growth and development handbook: Newborn through adolescent.* Clifton Park, NY: Delmar Cengage Learning.

Potts, N. L., Mandleco, B. L. (2002). *Pediatric nursing: Caring for children and their families.* Clifton Park, NY: Delmar Cengage Learning.

Taber's cyclopedic medical dictionary (20th ed.). (2006). Philadelphia: F. A. Davis.

Tamparo, C., & Lewis, M. (2005). *Diseases of the human body* (4th ed.). Philadelphia: F. A. Davis.

THE DVD HOOK-UP

In this chapter, you learned about the proper techniques for assisting with pediatric examinations.

The designated scene from today's program illustrates the medical assistant assisting with an infant examination. In the first scene, the medical assistant asks the patient's mother to remove everything but the diaper. The mother tells the medical assistant that the diaper is pretty wet; therefore, the medical assistant instructs the mother to change the diaper before she weighs the infant.

1. Why would removing the diaper altogether as suggested in this chapter be a better method for weighing the infant?

The medical assistant measures the infant by placing a mark above the head and below the foot after straightening out the foot and leg. Spencer is quite playful, making it difficult for the medical assistant to get an accurate reading. The marking for the foot actually had two lines.

1. How does the medical assistant know which mark to use?
2. Is this an accurate reading?

DVD Journal Summary

Write a paragraph that summarizes what you learned from watching today's DVD selected scene. How do you feel about working in pediatrics? Do you have children of your own? How does having children affect your ability to work in pediatrics?

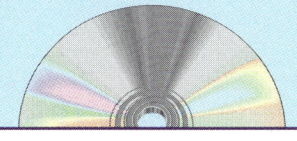

DVD Series **Program Number**
Skills Based Series 6

Chapter/Scene Reference
- *Infant Examination*

Chapter 16

Male Reproductive System

OUTLINE

OBJECTIVES

The student should strive to meet the following performance objectives and demonstrate an understanding of the facts and principles presented in this chapter through written and oral communication.

1. Describe the key terms as presented in the glossary.
2. Describe common disorders and diseases of the male reproductive system.
3. Explain benign hyperplasia of the prostate.
4. Identify signs and symptoms of the various disorders and diseases of the male reproductive system.
5. Explain erectile dysfunction, its causes, and its treatments.
6. Describe the common diagnostic tests and procedures used in the male reproductive system.
7. Explain testicular self-examination to a male patient.
8. Show compassion and empathy.

KEY TERMS

Cryptorchidism
Foley Catheter
Intravenous Pyelogram (IVP)
Libido
Metastasis
Nocturia
Orchidectomy
Residual Urine
Retention
Spermatogenesis
Transilluminator
Transurethral Resection of the Prostate (TURP)

Scenario

Joe Guerro, CMA (AAMA), finds many situations daily to educate patients because he knows how important it is. He keeps abreast of the latest techniques and procedures about diseases and problems of the male reproductive system. He attends lectures, workshops, and seminars when possible, and uses the Internet to obtain the latest information from the American Cancer Society about prostate cancer and as a resource for people with prostate cancer. With Dr. Woo's permission, Joe shares that information with patients.

INTRODUCTION

The male reproductive system consists of a pair of testes suspended in the scrotum, in which sperm and hormones are produced. The scrotum can contract and relax to help regulate temperature of the testes for optimum ***spermatogenesis.***

A system of tubes (the epididymis) transports the sperm to the outside of the body, and a penis transports the sperm into the female reproductive tract through the urethral opening. There are glands such as the prostate that secrete fluid that becomes part of the semen.

The male reproductive system is closely related to the male urinary system; thus, diseases and disorders of one system will naturally affect the other. Because the prostate gland encircles the male urinary urethra, any enlargement can cause urinary problems. The prostate gland is located directly next to the rectal wall. This location enables the provider to palpate the posterior of the prostate gland through the anterior rectal wall and, if necessary, perform an ultrasound and biopsy of the prostate using the rectal route. It is recommended that men have their prostate gland routinely evaluated at age 40 years, and then annually after age 50 years. During the annual examination of the prostate gland, the provider can assess the gland for enlargement, nodules, and other abnormalities. When the prostate becomes inflamed or irritated in any way, it can release a protein into the bloodstream. This protein is an antigen called prostate-specific antigen (PSA). Checking the PSA level can help the provider determine if there is some pathology of the prostate gland. It is important that blood be drawn for the PSA test before the digital rectal examination of the prostate, which can irritate the prostate gland, thus causing a slight increase of the PSA level.

Diseases, disorders, conditions, diagnostic tests, procedures, and treatments common to the male reproductive system are listed in Table 16-1.

Patient Education

1. Testicular cancer is one of the leading causes of death in men younger than 40 years.
2. Risk factors include an undescended testicle, **cryptorchidism,** and childhood mumps.
3. Prognosis is good when found in the early stages.

Spotlight on Certification

RMA Content Outline

- Anatomy and physiology
- Medical terminology
- Patient education
- Physical examinations
- Laboratory procedures
- Diseases and disorders

CMA (AAMA) Content Outline

- Medical terminology
- Anatomy and physiology
- Patient instruction
- Patient education
- Examinations
- Procedures
- Collecting and processing specimens; diagnostic testing

CMAS Content Outline

- Medical terminology
- Anatomy and physiology
- Examination preparation

Table 16-1 Male Reproductive System Diseases and Disorders

Disease/Disorder	Laboratory Diagnostics	Radiography and Technical Diagnostics	Medical/Surgical Diagnostics	Treatments
Prostatitis (inflammation of the prostate gland)	Complete blood count; urinalysis and culture; analysis of prostate secretion	Urodynamics (if not caused by a bacterium)	Digital rectal examination	Long-term treatment with antibiotics Increase fluid intake
Benign prostatic hypertrophy/enlargement of (BPH)	Prostatic-specific antigen (PSA); urinalysis	Intravenous pyelogram (IVP); pelvic ultrasound	Digital rectal examination; cystoscopy; ultrasound and biopsy	Medications; transurethral resection prostatectomy (TURP) is rare
Prostate cancer	PSA; urinalysis; acid phosphatase (blood)	IVP; pelvic ultrasound	Digital rectal examination; cystoscopy; ultrasound and biopsy	Prostatectomy; hormone manipulation; chemotherapy, radiation, or both
Epididymitis (inflammation of the tubes on the testis)	Complete blood count; Urinalysis and culture and sensitivity; culture and sensitivity of urethra	IVP; pelvic ultrasound	Physical examination	Antibiotics, scrotal support
Testicular cancer		Testicular ultrasound	Physical examination (palpation of testis); biopsy	Excision of the testis; radiation therapy; chemotherapy
Erectile dysfunction (ED) (inability of male to achieve erection)	Complete blood count; fasting blood sugar; lipid profile; testosterone level; urinalysis	Angiogram, rarely; magnetic resonance imaging of the brain, rarely	Physical examination; neurological examination; psychological evaluation	Oral medications; localized injected medication; penile implant; penile pump
Balanitis (inflammation of the glans of the penis)	Culture, rarely		Physical examination; skin culture	Localized soaks and frequent cleansing; antibiotics
Sexually transmitted diseases (STDs):				
Nonspecific urethritis (NSU)	Rule out other STDs; culture and sensitivity of urethral discharge			Increase fluid intake; antibiotics; possibly test/treat partner
Chlamydia	Urinalysis; urethral smear			Patient education; antibiotics; test/treat partner
Genital herpes (type II herpes simplex)	Culture of lesion			Patient education; antiviral medications; test/treat partner
Gonorrhea	Urethral smear			Patient education; antibiotics; test/treat partner
Syphilis	Urinalysis with culture; Venereal Disease Research Laboratory (VDRL) studies; culture of the lesion			Patient education; antibiotics; test/treat partner

TESTICULAR SELF-EXAMINATION

Early detection of testicular cancer relies heavily on the patient's willingness to perform self-examination of the testes on a regular basis. Patient teaching is valuable when used to educate the patient about self-examination for detection of abnormalities such as lumps or thickenings. Figure 16-1 illustrates a testicular self-examination, and Procedure 16-1 outlines steps for instructions usually given to the patient by the medical assistant. The testicular self-examination is best performed in the shower because the warmth will cause the scrotum to relax, making the examination easier and more effective.

DISORDERS OF THE MALE REPRODUCTIVE SYSTEM

Table 16-1 gives a summary of male reproductive disorders.

Testicular Cancer

Testicular cancer is the most common form of cancer in men between 20 and 35 years old; otherwise, it is rarely seen. Usually a painless lump is found in a testicle. An undescended testicle (cryptorchidism), and a history of mumps are predisposing factors. Diagnosis can be made by performing a biopsy after palpation of the testicle finds a mass. Surgery to excise the testicle, **orchidectomy,** followed by radiation and chemotherapy is the usual course of action. If caught early, there is a high cure rate. Monthly testicular examinations are recommended by the American Cancer Society for all men and are considered the best preventive measure for testicular cancer.

Testicular self-examinations (TSEs) are a common patient education topic. Many total practice management systems have an area for storing patient education information and forms. These forms (Figure 16-2) can be printed and given to the patient right in the exam room.

Epididymitis

Epididymitis is an inflammation of the epididymis, which is a small oblong body resting on and beside the posterior surfaces of the testes. It consists of a convoluted tube 13 to 20 feet in length. It constitutes the first part of the secretory duct of each testis. The patient's symptoms are chills, fever, pain in the inguinal region, and a swollen epididymis that

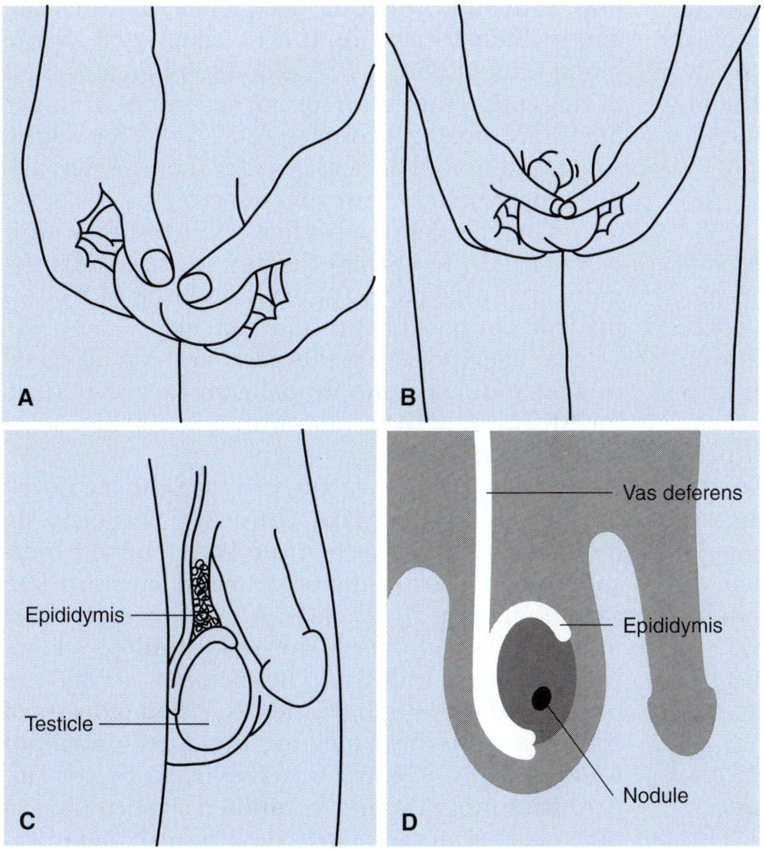

Figure 16-1 Testicular self-examination should be performed once a month after a warm bath or shower. The heat will relax the scrotum, making it easier to find abnormalities. (A) Stand in front of the mirror. Look for swelling on the skin of the scrotum. (B) Examine each testicle with both hands. Position your index and middle fingers under the testicle with the thumbs on top. Gently roll the testicle between your thumbs and fingers (having one testicle larger than the other is normal). (C) Find the epididymis (the soft tubelike structure at the back of the testicle). Do not mistake the epididymis for an abnormal lump. (D) If you find a lump, notify your provider immediately. Most lumps are found on the sides of the testicle, but some are located on the front. Testicular cancer is highly curable when detected early and treated promptly.

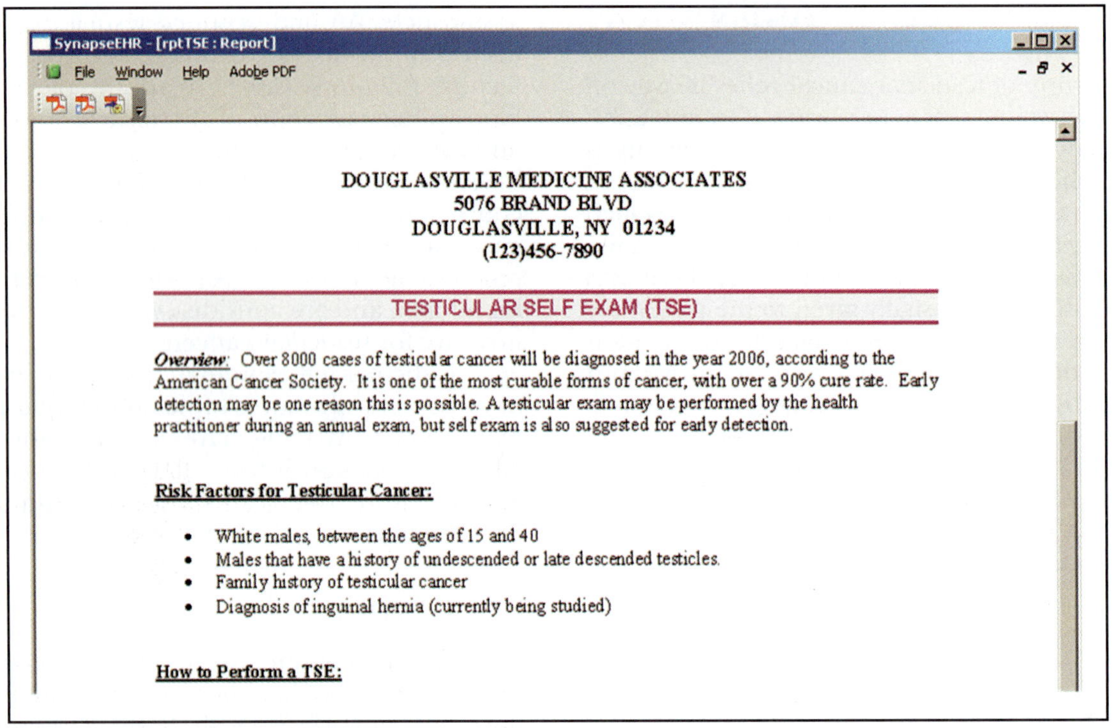

DOUGLASVILLE MEDICINE ASSOCIATES
5076 BRAND BLVD
DOUGLASVILLE, NY 01234
(123)456-7890

TESTICULAR SELF EXAM (TSE)

Overview: Over 8000 cases of testicular cancer will be diagnosed in the year 2006, according to the American Cancer Society. It is one of the most curable forms of cancer, with over a 90% cure rate. Early detection may be one reason this is possible. A testicular exam may be performed by the health practitioner during an annual exam, but self exam is also suggested for early detection.

Risk Factors for Testicular Cancer:

- White males, between the ages of 15 and 40
- Males that have a history of undescended or late descended testicles.
- Family history of testicular cancer
- Diagnosis of inguinal hernia (currently being studied)

How to Perform a TSE:

Figure 16-2 Testicular self-examination patient teaching forms can be printed in the exam room via the total practice management system and given to a patient.

can be seen on an ultrasonogram. It is primarily caused by a sexually transmitted disease (STD) such as chlamydia, gonorrhea, or syphillis. Other causes are urinary tract infections, trauma, prostatectomy, and prolonged indwelling **Foley catheter**. Treatment consists of antibiotics, scrotal support, and bed rest.

Prostatitis

Prostatitis, or inflammation of the prostate, occurs primarily in men older than 50 years. The prostate may enlarge and cause pain and discomfort, such as burning while urinating. There can be pain in the back, muscle aches, and urinary frequency. The cause may be bacterial, such as from gonorrhea, or it may be caused by another pathogen that produced a urinary tract infection. Urinalysis, urine culture, and digital rectal examination (to palpate the prostate) help in making a diagnosis. Treatment is usually medication, such as penicillin and pain medication, and the patient will be told to force fluids by increasing fluid intake significantly.

Prostate Cancer

Prostate cancer is the third leading cause of cancer death in men, after lung and colon cancer. **Metastasis** to the spine or pelvis is not unusual. The symptoms, if present, are similar to urinary obstruction, difficulty urinating, frequency of urination, and inability to urinate. It is of value to check the blood level of PSA. A PSA blood level greater than 2.5 mg/mL is the cutoff for normal values. Younger men have smaller prostates and lower PSA values. Any elevation of PSA level greater than 2.5 mg/mL in younger men is cause for concern.

The PSA is not a perfect test. Most men with elevated PSA levels have benign prostate enlargement, a normal part of aging. Low levels of PSA do not rule out possible prostate cancer.

At age 50 years, a PSA level and digital rectal exams should be done annually, and at age 40 years for African-American men with a family history of prostate cancer.

A new blood test for prostate cancer developed by Johns Hopkins University seems to be much more accurate than the PSA. The test measures blood levels of the protein and early prostate cancer antigen–2 (EPCA-2). According to a report in the periodical *Urology*, the new test shows a false-positive rate of only 3%. The majority of PSA tests performed show high PSA levels. When biopsies of prostates from these men are done, 80% turn out to be benign. A biopsy is necessary to be certain. An ultrasonogram and computed axial tomography (CAT) scan can help to determine if metastasis has occurred. Treatment may consist of prostatectomy, hormonal therapy, radiation, chemotherapy, and brachytherapy (internal radiation "seeds").

A prostatic ultrasound consists of a short probe inserted into the rectum. High-frequency sound waves are produced by the probe, and an image (either a photo or a video) of the prostate is recorded. A biopsy of the prostate can be done in conjunction with the ultrasound. The provider uses the ultrasound to guide a needle through the rectum into areas of the prostate that showed abnormalities on the ultrasound. The needle collects cells from the prostate through the rectum wall. The specimen is sent to the laboratory for analysis. Medical assistants are responsible for patient instruction and preparation and assisting with an ultrasound and biopsy of the patient.

A prostatectomy is major surgery done for prostate cancer and is performed through the abdomen or the perineum (the external region between the scrotum and the anus). Urinary incontinence, impotence, or both are possible complications.

If the cancer has metastasized, orchidectomy may be recommended because the surgery alters hormone production (loss of testosterone). Less testosterone can slow the metastasis but can lead to loss of muscle mass, osteoporosis, and sexual dysfunction.

An additional treatment consists of small pellets ("seeds") of a radioactive substance that are implanted in the prostate tissue through a small incision (brachytherapy). The seeds of radiation are concentrated in the prostate and destroy the prostate without harming surrounding tissue as external beam radiation does. Various medications such as those that reduce or suppress the production of testosterone may be helpful when combined with radiation or surgery, but they have the same possible side effects as orchidectomy.

Patients who have been tested for prostate cancer are monitored for progression of the cancer, which includes PSA every 3 months to 1 year, CAT and bone scans, and monitoring of the signs and symptoms that indicate cancer progression such as bowel and bladder function impairment, weight loss, pain, and fatigue.

Benign Prostatic Hypertrophy

Benign hypertrophy of the prostate gland or benign hypertrophic prostate gland, also known as benign prostatic hyperplasia (BPH), is common in men 50 years or older. Symptoms include **retention** (the inability to completely empty the bladder), a diminished flow of urine, and difficulty starting to urinate. Hesitancy and **nocturia** can occur. It is thought that the cause is aging and may be related to hormonal changes. The prostate enlarges and, because it surrounds the urethra, it causes constriction of the urethra and the associated symptoms. The provider can palpate the enlarged prostate gland when performing a rectal examination. This helps in making a diagnosis. Other tests may include the PSA, a urinalysis, and an **intravenous pyelogram (IVP)**; excretory urograph—(a radiograph of the kidneys, ureters, and bladder using a contrast medium). The enlarged prostate blocks urine flow and if **residual urine** stays in the bladder, infections can develop. The kidneys may cease functioning because they cannot drain urine properly into the bladder when it is full (Figure 16-3). Catheterization may be necessary (see Procedure 18-2).

The PSA blood test is used to detect abnormally high levels of a protein substance that may indicate prostate cancer. The American Cancer Society recommends that men aged 50 years and older have an annual PSA blood test.

Ultrasound can be used to view the prostate, bladder, or kidneys. A biopsy of the prostate, done in conjunction with an ultrasound, can help diagnose either BPH or cancer.

In some cases, treatment of BPH consists of medication that can relax prostate muscles, hormones that block prostate growth, or bladder relaxants. **Transurethral resection of the prostate (TURP),** removal of prostate tissue using a device inserted through the urethra, is the most common surgical treatment. Instruments are inserted through the penis and laser or radio waves can be used to remove the excess tissue (Figure 16-4). Possible risks of TURP include impotence and urinary incontinence. BPH does not cause or lead to cancer.

Critical Thinking

Describe brachytherapy. What is it used for?

Critical Thinking

List several sexually transmitted diseases that a male individual can contract.

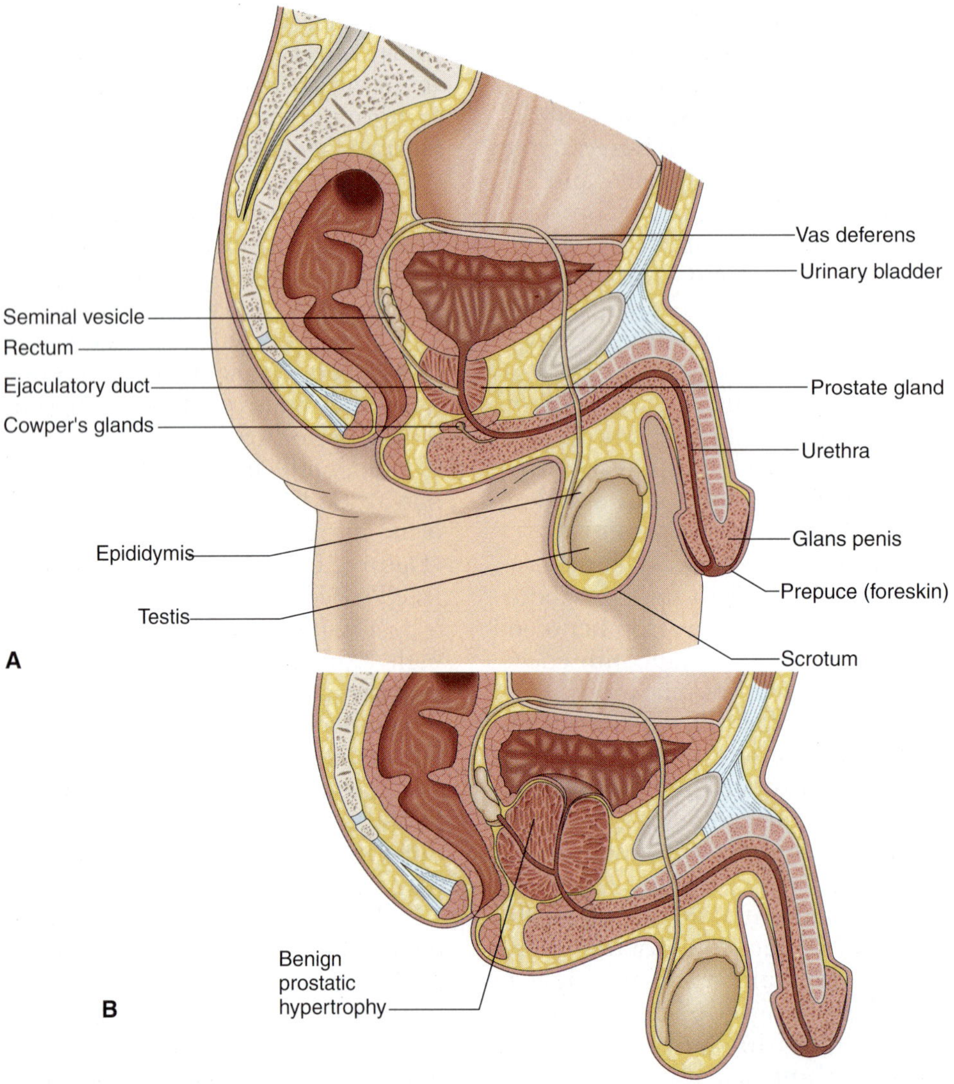

Figure 16-3 Normal and enlarged prostate. (A) Normal. (B) Enlarged.

Sexually Transmitted Diseases

STDs affect men and women; they can damage health and become life-threatening (Table 16-2). (See Chapter 14 for additional information regarding STDs.)

Balanitis

Balanitis is usually caused by poor hygiene in uncircumcised men. Bacteria, fungi, viruses, caustic soaps, and improper rinsing of soap while bathing also are causes. Symptoms and signs that occur include redness of the foreskin or of the penis, rashes on the head of the penis, malodorous discharge, and pain in the penis and foreskin. Diagnosis of balanitis may be made by the provider through examination of the penis and foreskin, skin culture for microorganisms, or both. If the cause is bacterial, then antibiotics can be used to treat balanitis. In severe cases, circumcision (surgical removal of prepuce of penis) may be necessary.

Infertility

When couples regularly have unprotected sexual intercourse, the majority of them usually conceive within 1 year. The inability or diminished ability to conceive is known as infertility.

An insufficient number or diminished motility of sperm can cause infertility. Other causes include an infection in the genitourinary tract or the presence of an STD, either of which can block the tract and prohibit sperm from being fully ejaculated. An injury to the blood or nerve supply in the area, radiation exposure, stress, and hormonal imbalances are other factors that can promote infertility.

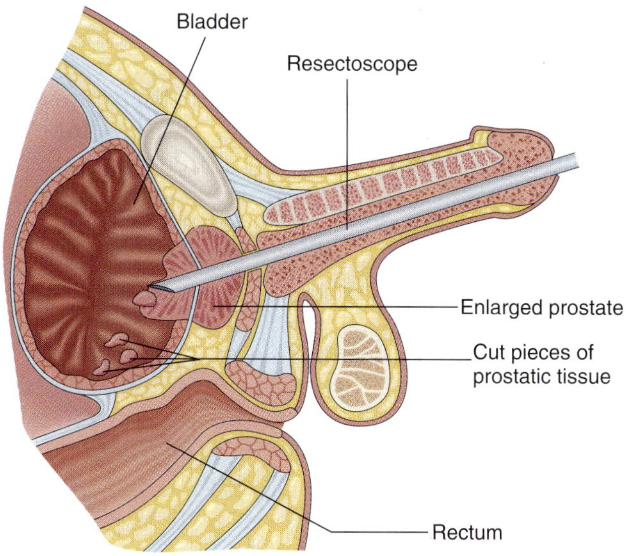

Figure 16-4 Transurethral resection of the prostate (TURP).

Table 16-2 Sexually Transmitted Diseases

Chlamydial infection	Common in male and female individuals. A prevalent sexually transmitted disease that often coexists with gonorrhea.
Genital herpes	Painful viral disease that is dormant and recurs periodically. There is no cure. Characterized by blisters similar to chicken pox. Common in male and female individuals.
Gonorrhea	Caused by a bacterium. Infection can spread, producing a stricture of the urethra or the vas deferens. Sterility can result if both vas deferens become involved.
Syphilis	Caused by a spirochete. Chancres develop. Can heal. If untreated, the disease progresses to stages two and three. Severe damage to the cardiovascular system and brain and vision and hearing loss occur. General paralysis and death can result. Highly contagious.
Hepatitis B and C virus and HIV	All caused by a virus. There is no care for any of the three.

A complete physical examination and medical history (including childhood illnesses such as parotitis [mumps]), semen analysis for count and motility, and tests for endocrine disorders can help determine the cause of infertility.

Treatment of a male patient with infertility depends on the cause. Treatments include surgery to remove a blockage, antibiotics to treat an infection, use of artificial insemination, or use of pharmaceuticals to treat the infertility.

Prevention of the factors that may cause infertility is preferable because the percentage of couples treated for infertility who successfully become pregnant is relatively low.

Erectile Dysfunction

Also called impotence, erectile dysfunction (ED) occurs when a man is unable to achieve or to sustain an erection of the penis during sexual intercourse. This condition or dysfunction is not normal at any age and is different from other issues that impede sexual intercourse, such as lack of **libido.**

Many men, at some point in their lives, can experience the inability to achieve an erection. This can happen on occasion from consuming too much alcohol or from extreme fatigue. This is not ED. The inability to achieve an erection more than 50% of the time is generally a reason for seeking treatment and is usually an indication of ED.

For an erection to occur, certain physiologic conditions must be present. There must be a stimulus from the brain and adequate circulation and nerve supply to the penis. If any of these conditions is impeded, an erection cannot be achieved. Some reasons why ED occurs include conditions or diseases that impair circulation (atherosclerosis) and nerve stimulation (nerve diseases) and psychological factors such as stress and depression. Medications such as those used to treat certain conditions such as hypertension can cause ED. Diabetes, multiple sclerosis, cerebral vascular accident (stroke), surgery on the prostate or bladder, and brain and spinal cord injuries are other causes of ED.

Treatment of the dysfunction is based on the cause. Referral to a urologist, psychologist, or both, is made if appropriate. Blood and urine tests will be done after the provider examines the individual for medical problems. Medications the patient may be taking will be addressed. Some of the ways ED can be treated include oral medications (Viagra, Levitra, Cialis), penile injections (medication injected into the penis), sex therapy, surgery such as penile implants (device surgically implanted to overcome

HIPAA

Because of the very nature of erectile dysfunction, many men are embarrassed if they have the disorder, feeling they are somehow less "manly" than other men. It is of extreme importance to be cautious and sensitive when caring for these patients. Confidentiality on the telephone and during conversations must be maintained. Protect your patient's privacy at all times. This is not only the law, but it is also an attribute of a professional medical assistant.

impotence), and vacuum pumps. A vacuum pump device is a pump put over the penis; air is pumped out of the cylinder, creating a vacuum. This vacuum causes blood to fill the penis, making it erect. Once the penis is erect, the pump can be removed.

Some experts say ED should be considered a possible risk factor for heart disease if arthero-sclerosis is present.

ASSISTING WITH THE MALE REPRODUCTIVE EXAMINATION

A female medical assistant usually is not required to assist the provider with the examination of the male reproductive system. The provider examines the penis and the foreskin of the penis in an uncircumcised patient. The penis and testes are examined for swelling, masses, or discomfort. A **transilluminator** may be used by the provider to check the prostate gland. A lighted instrument used to inspect a cavity or organ, the transilluminator is passed through the rectum to illuminate the prostate gland through the walls of the rectum. The provider perform a digital rectal examination to check the size of the prostate and also checks for an inguinal hernia.

When working in a total practice management system, the provider can complete the examination, orders tests and procedures, charts the findings, orders prescriptions as needed, and order a follow-up appointment for the patient—right in the exam room (Figure 16-5).

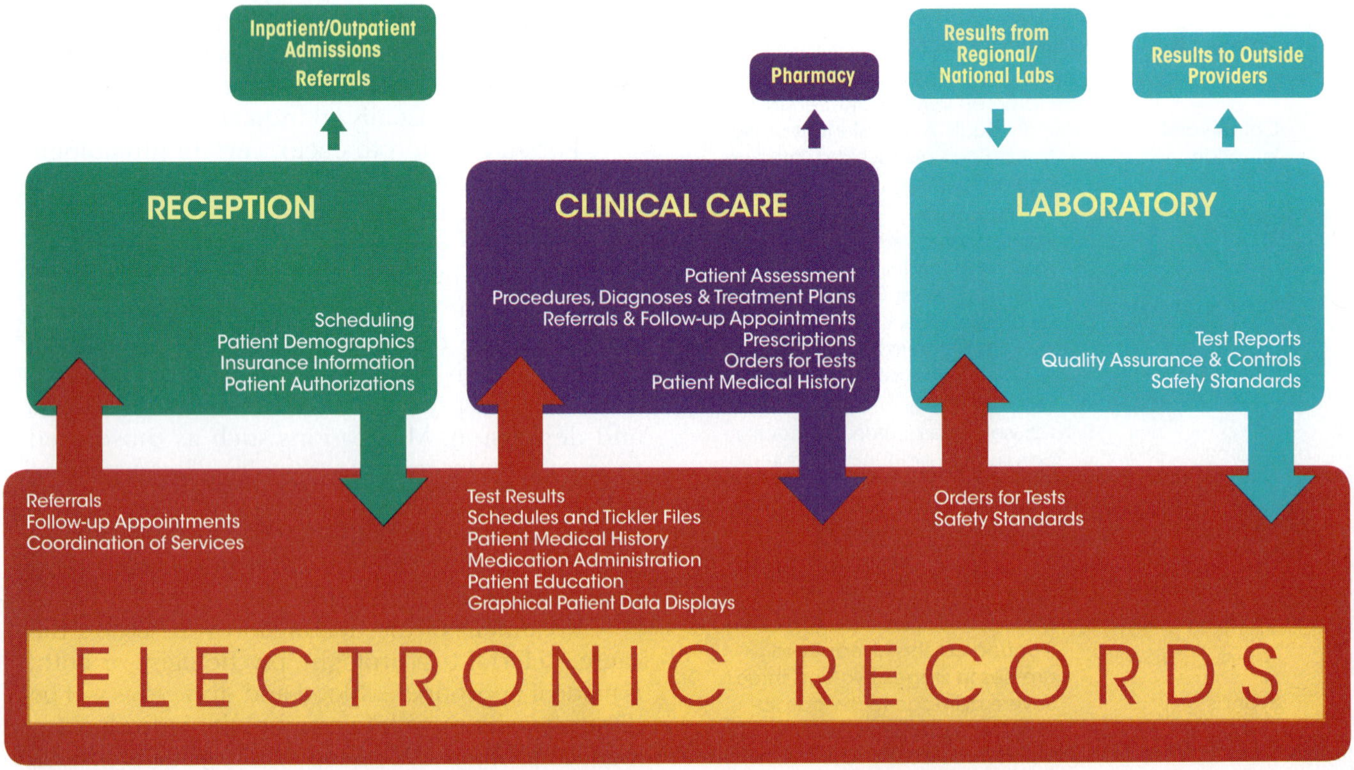

Figure 16-5 Clinical care, laboratory, and reception arms of a total practice management system.

DIAGNOSTIC TESTS AND PROCEDURES

Tests and procedures, in addition to those previously addressed, include vasectomy, semen analysis, and urodynamic studies.

Vasectomy

A vasectomy is performed to surgically sterilize the male individual. The vas deferens extends up into the abdomen where it connects to create the ejaculatory duct that opens into the urethra. By removing a portion of each vas deferens, sperm cannot travel to mix with semen, thereby causing the male to be sterile (Figure 16-6). See Chapter 19 for the vasectomy surgical procedure.

Semen Analysis

Semen testing is frequently performed in the provider's office or clinic to determine sperm cell counts before referring patients to a specialist who treats infertility. It is also done as part of a complete fertility workup and to evaluate the effectiveness of a vasectomy (see Chapter 32 for extensive information about semen analysis).

Urodynamic Studies

Urodynamic studies are a way of testing the lower urinary tract. A catheter is used to instill water into the bladder and the information is fed into a computer via electrodes. Bladder capacity, strength of contraction, and the ability to retain urine in the bladder can be measured.

Results from urodynamic studies can be stored electronically for readily accessible comparisons.

Critical Thinking

What test will be done at the first post-operative clinic visit following a vasectomy?

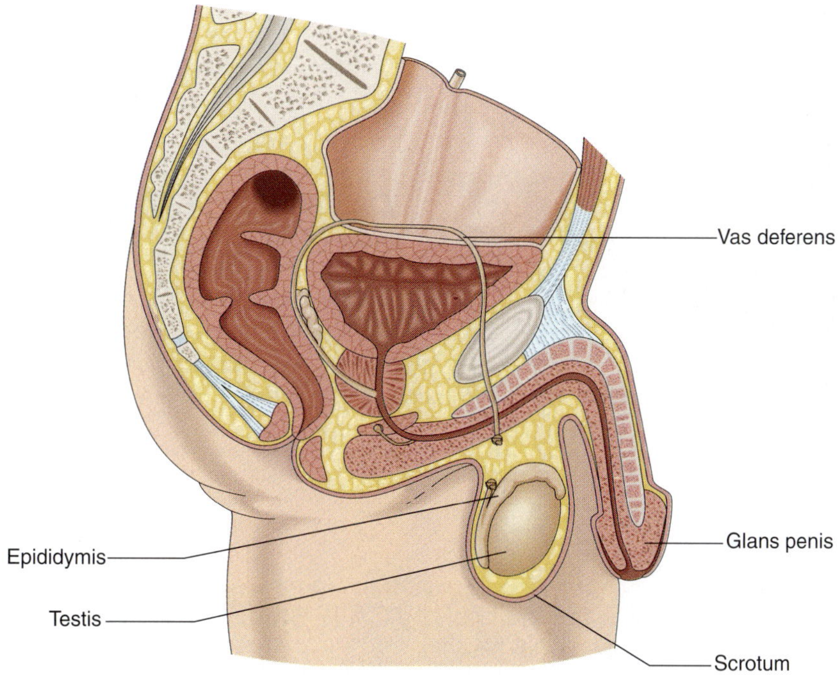

Figure 16-6 Vasectomy (one side).

Procedure 16-1

Instructing Patient in Testicular Self-Examination

PURPOSE:
To provide a patient with information concerning testicular screening for the presence of a painless mass in the scrotum.

EQUIPMENT/SUPPLIES:
Testicular self-examination card
Anatomy illustration

PROCEDURE STEPS:

1. Identify yourself and explain the procedure.
2. Instruct patient to examine his testicles in a warm shower. RATIONALE: The warmth causes the scrotal skin to relax.
3. Examine each testicle separately with both hands.
4. Place the index and middle fingers underneath the testicle and the thumbs on top. Roll the testicle gently between the fingers.
5. Locate the epididymis. Provide a chart to the patient that illustrates the testes and epididymis. RATIONALE: A lump can be similar in size to the epididymis and needs to be distinguished from the epididymis.
6. Look for swelling or changes in the scrotal area.
7. Encourage the patient to report anything unusual to the provider.
8. Document the education provided in the patient's chart or electronic medical record.

DOCUMENTATION

11/4/20XX Patient instructed on how to perform testicular self-exam. Patient returned the demonstration and had no questions. Joe Guerro, CMA (AAMA) ————————

Case Study 16-1

Refer to the scenario at the beginning of the chapter.
After Dr. Woo examines the patient, John Abbott, he asks you to schedule a pelvic ultrasound and a CT scan of the abdomen for the patient.

CASE STUDY REVIEW

1. What can be determined from these tests?
2. How will Dr. Woo know if Mr. Abbott's results show benign prostatic hypertrophy or prostate cancer? Will more tests be needed? If so, what are they?

Case Study 16-2

Adam Desmond has an appointment today in the clinic for a physical examination. His chief complaint is that he has been having trouble sitting through ball games or movies without having to go to the bathroom to urinate several times.

CASE STUDY REVIEW

1. How can the provider make a diagnosis of benign prostatic hyperplasia?
2 What preliminary tests might the provider order for Mr. Desmond today?

Case Study 16-3

John Toomey called Dr. King's office to say that he discovered "something hard in his right testicle, like a marble."

CASE STUDY REVIEW

1. What will Dr. King's examination consist of?

SUMMARY

A thorough knowledge of the diseases and disorders of the male reproductive system and the diagnostic tests and procedures that are performed for this specialty will enhance the quality of care given by the medical assistant.

STUDY FOR SUCCESS

To reinforce your knowledge and skills of information presented in this chapter:

- Review the Key Terms
- Practice the Procedures
- Consider the Case Studies and discuss your conclusions
- Answer the Review Questions
    - Multiple Choice
    - Critical Thinking
- Navigate the Internet by completing the Web Activities
- Practice the StudyWARE activities on your student CD
- Apply your knowledge in the Student Workbook activities
- Complete the Web Tutor sections

REVIEW QUESTIONS

Multiple Choice

1. Cancer of the prostate may be detected early by which of the following?
   a. prostate-specific antigen
   b. transurethral resection of the prostate
   c. semen analysis
   d. urine culture
2. The best preventive measure for testicular cancer is which of the following?
   a. yearly physical examination
   b. yearly intravenous pyelogram
   c. monthly self-examination
   d. monthly urinalysis with cultures
3. Benign prostatic hypertrophy (BPH) is thought to be caused by:
   a. excessive consumption of alcohol
   b. aging and hormonal changes
   c. recurrent epididymitis
   d. chronic chlamydia infections
4. Which of the following is a symptom of prostatitis?
   a. painful urination
   b. low sperm count
   c. eruptions on the scrotum
   d. high testosterone level

5. The most definitive way to diagnose cancer of the prostate is by which of the following?
   a. ultrasonography
   b. intravenous pyelogram
   c. biopsy of the prostate
   d. semen analysis

Critical Thinking

1. Describe how a testicular self-examination should be performed.
2. What is the purpose of severing the vas deferens?
3. List several symptoms of BPH and explain why the symptoms occur.
4. Describe the blood test that is helpful to diagnose prostate cancer.
5. At what PSA level does the provider consider the possiblity that the patient may have cancer of the prostate?
6. Explain why BPH is more common in men aged 50 years and older.
7. What age group is afflicted by testicular cancer, and how can the patient take action to detect it?
8. How is a rectal examination on a patient useful to the provider in determining a diagnosis for a patient who has nocturia?

WEB ACTIVITIES

Navigate the Internet to find a medical Web site, then answer the following questions:

1. Describe two treatment choices for BPH.
2. Search for information about internal radiation or "seeds" as a treatment choice for cancer of the prostate. What did you find?
3. Find two other disorders or diseases of the male reproductive tract (other than those in the text) and (a) describe what they are, (b) how they are diagnosed, and (c) how they are treated.
4. Discover what contraindications exist for some men whose provider is considering prescribing Viagra or one of the other medications for ED treatment.

REFERENCES/BIBLIOGRAPHY

Common male sexual problems—erectile dysfunction. Retrieved May 26, 2007 from http://www.webmd.com/sexual-conditions/guide/mens-sexual-problems.

Shuman, T. (ed.). (2006). *Sexual conditions guide.*

Taber's cyclopedic medical dictionary (20th ed.). (2005). Philadelphia: F. A. Davis.

Tamparo, C., & Lewis, M. (2005). *Diseases of the human body* (4th ed.). Philadelphia: F. A. Davis.

Warner, J. (Ed.). (2007). *Erectile dysfunction.* Retrieved May 29, 2007, from http://www.webmd.com/sexual-conditions/guide/mens-sexual-problems.

Chapter 17

Gerontology

KEY TERMS

Andropause
Arteriosclerosis
Cognitive Functioning
Cystitis
Dementia
Empathy
Geriatrics
Gerontology
Hyperthermia
Hypothermia
Incontinence
Macular Degeneration
Nevus
Pernicious Anemia
Presbycusis
Residual Urine
Senile
Transient Ischemic Attack (TIA)

OUTLINE

- Societal Bias
- Facts about Aging
- Physiologic Changes
  - Senses
  - Integumentary System
  - Nervous System
  - Musculoskeletal System
  - Respiratory System
  - Cardiovascular System
  - Gastrointestinal System
  - Urinary System
  - Reproductive System
- Prevention of Complications
- Psychological Changes
- The Medical Assistant and the Geriatric Patient
  - Memory-Impaired Older Adults
  - Visually Impaired Older Adults
  - Hearing-Impaired Older Adults
  - Elder Abuse
- Healthy and Successful Aging

OBJECTIVES

The student should strive to meet the following performance objectives and demonstrate an understanding of the facts and principles presented in this chapter through written and oral communication.

1. Define the key terms as presented in the glossary.
2. Identify expected physiologic changes that occur as part of the aging process.
3. List five common functional changes that can occur.
4. Describe prevention techniques for complications arising from age-related disorders.
5. Explain two myths about aging.
6. Explain the importance of communication with older adults.
7. Identify several techniques or strategies to communicate with visually and hearing-impaired older adults.
8. Describe strategies for healthy and successful aging.

Scenario

Mrs. Johnson is an 82-year-old patient of Dr. King, and she is scheduled for an appointment in the cardiac clinic. She is being evaluated for congestive heart disease and has had hypertension for many years. Her condition was difficult to control, but now she responds to medication. She has become a volunteer at the gift shop at St. Louis Hospital. She is an example of an older adult with chronic illnesses who has changed some long-time behaviors that were harmful to her health.

INTRODUCTION

Gerontology *is the scientific study of the problems associated with aging.* ***Geriatrics*** *is the branch of medicine that specializes in all aspects of aging: physiologic, pathologic, psychological, economic, and sociologic. The importance of studying gerontology is becoming more recognized because the expected life span is increasing. Thousands of people are living to be 100 years old or older. The aging population is growing rapidly, and according to the U.S. Census Bureau, by 2030, there will be 60 million people in the United States older than 65 years. The 80 and above age group is currently the fastest growing group. As a medical assistant, you will be experiencing the impact on the health care system of this growing population of people.*

Through knowledge of the physical and psychological changes that occur as an individual ages, as a medical assistant you will be better able to recognize the special needs of this group of people. You will draw on and use effective communication skills and provide quality health care to geriatric patients.

Spotlight on Certification

RMA Content Outline

- Conditions of states of health
- Health-related syndromes
- Patient education
  - Identify age-group specific responses and support
  - Understand and properly apply communication methods
- Employ active listening skills

CMA (AAMA) Content Outline

- Developmental stages of the life cycle
- Hereditary, cultural, and environmental influences or behaviors
- Adapting communication to an individual's ability to understand (e.g., patients with special needs: blind, deaf, elderly)
- Instructing individuals according to their needs
- Empathy
- Evaluating and understanding communication, observation, active listening, feedback
- Resource information and community services
- Patient advocate

CMAS Content Outline

- Use human relations skills appropriate to the health care setting
- Use effective written and oral communication

SOCIETAL BIAS

In our culture, there is a deeply ingrained bias about aging. Older adults are stereotyped, and there is much discrimination because of age. Myths and stereotypes are common, and the medical assistant can be an advocate for older adults and can be sensitive to these myths and stereotypes. Accurate information and useful concepts about aging must be communicated to the general public. Older adults oftentimes are viewed as sick, frail, powerless, sexless, and burdensome. As a society, we are obsessed with the negative, rather than the positive, aspects of aging. The most popular myth is, "To be old is to be sick." Recent studies indicate that older adults in the United States are generally healthier than their counterparts of nearly a decade ago. Even in advanced old age, a majority of the older

Critical Thinking

What do you consider common myths about older adults? What are your thoughts about these myths?

population has little functional disability. Years of research have debunked this myth. Because of better education about the practice of healthier lifestyles, to be old in the United States does not mean to be sick and frail. Thousands of people are living to be older than 100 years because of the recognition that healthy lifestyles are the most important factor in helping people to live long, healthy, productive lives. Such factors as good nutrition, regular exercise, stress reduction, yearly physical examinations, not smoking, and today's technology help forestall the aging process.

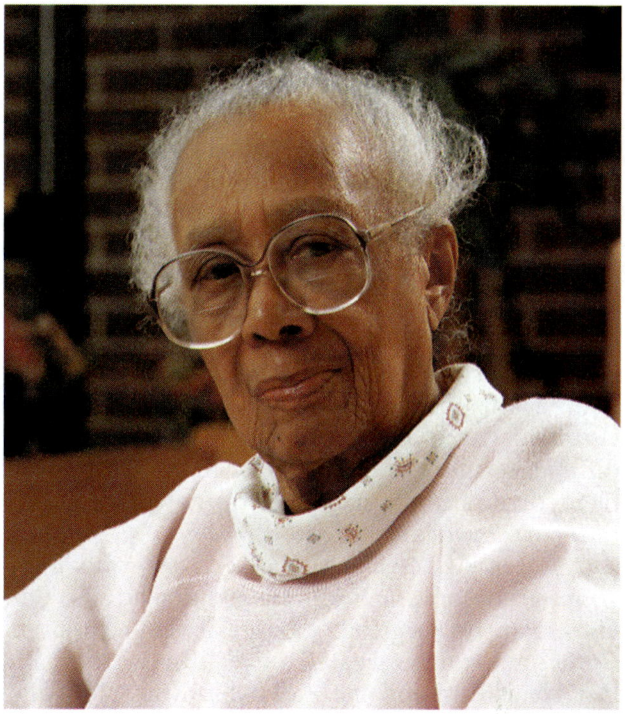

Figure 17-1 Note the many signs of aging.

FACTS ABOUT AGING

Following are general facts about aging:

- Aging is a progressive, universal, and slow process.
- There are no diseases specific to aging.
- As people age, not all functional changes are related to disease. Interest, personal and financial resources, family structure, genetics, and attitude all play a part. The individual's lifestyle is a major factor. For example, smoking, misuse of chemicals such as alcohol or drugs, type of diet, and lack of exercise all play a part in how people age.
- There is a wider range of what is considered "normal" function among older adults than among younger people. There is a greater variability among older people in their physical abilities, sizes, and characteristics than among younger groups (Figure 17-1).
- All older ages are not alike. People in their 60s, 70s, 80s, and 90s are all different.

PHYSIOLOGIC CHANGES

Although aging is a normal process, not all individuals age in the same way or at the same rate, because no two people have exactly the same genetic inheritance, personal lifestyle, or experiences in life. All of these factors strongly influence the ways in which we grow older. Some believe that the body endures wear and tear and stress during life and that because of this, eventually the body loses its ability to function as well as it had. Others believe that as people grow older, the body produces smaller and smaller amounts of various hormones and other chemicals that keep the body functioning. The fewer of these kinds of substances that are produced, the more susceptible an individual becomes to disease.

Every body system undergoes changes as we age. The changes are physiologic and psychological. As individuals move into their 60s and beyond, they will show physiologic changes that are part of the aging process. As people age, their body systems function less effectively, causing them to have difficulty performing their ordinary, everyday tasks of living. Also, as people grow older, they can become more susceptible to disorders and diseases. When taking the medical history of an older patient, it is evident that many have one or several chronic illnesses. Heart disease, diabetes, arthritis, hypertension, and vision and auditory impairments are common.

Although it is important to be knowledgeable about the physiologic changes that occur as part of aging, it is important to realize that the majority of older adults are free of serious, chronic health problems.

Senses

Vision. Many changes occur in the eye's ability to function. Pupil size diminishes, limiting the amount of light that can go through it to reach the retina. There is a diminished production of tears so the eye may be dry, red, and irritated. The lens may become cloudy, and the cornea thickens. There is increased sensitivity to glare. Several problems can occur as a result of these changes. There is less ability to see clearly at any distance and to discern various shades of colors. Older people will need eyeglasses to help correct their vision loss, but reading small print can remain difficult (Figure 17-2). Glare can be minimized by incorporating a process known as polarization into corrective lenses.

Cataracts, **macular degeneration,** and glaucoma are common findings in older adults. Cataracts can be surgically excised if they are large. Glaucoma can be treated medically or surgically but if left untreated can lead to blindness. Macular degeneration can lead to vision impairment. The macular of the retina is an important area in the visualization of fine details. Macular degeneration is the leading cause of visual impairment in adults older than 50 years, making it difficult to do fine work or such activities as threading a needle. Laser surgery may halt the progression of the degeneration.

Because of failing vision and impaired balance and coordination, older adults should be cautioned to use handrails whenever possible.

Hearing. Loss of hearing in the aging process is not uncommon. It usually occurs over a period of years, and the older person may not be aware of the loss. Loss of the ability to hear begins at about the third decade of life. Many times, individuals with hearing loss seem inattentive or confused and are thought to be mentally weak or **senile.** Presbyacusia or **presbycusis** is the progressive loss of hearing ability caused by the normal aging process.

Taste and Smell. Taste and smell diminish with age, making food less appealing because it no longer tastes as good as it once did (Figure 17-3). Taste buds decrease in size. Detecting odors becomes difficult and impaired, further lessening the desire for food. It is not unusual for older adults to lose weight and even to become malnourished because of the loss of the ability to taste and smell. Lacking the sense of smell can be dangerous because of the inability to smell smoke or gas and other dangerous fumes.

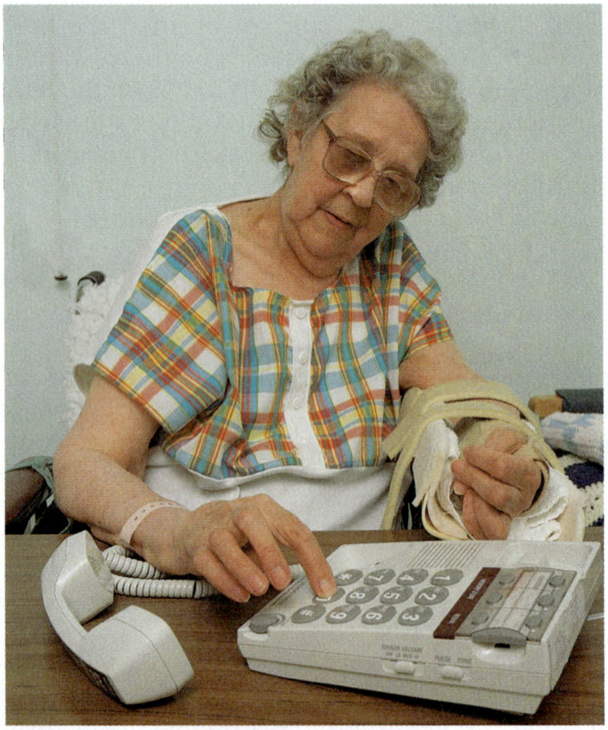

Figure 17-2 Good lighting and large numbers on a telephone can help improve vision.

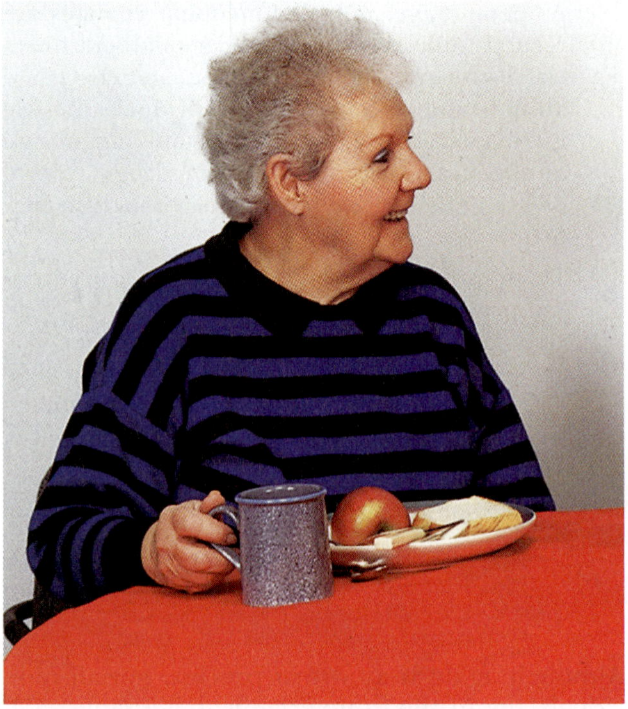

Figure 17-3 Older adults may add more salt and sugar to their food to compensate for their diminished sense of taste.

Integumentary System

Aging individuals' skin becomes more fragile with less subcutaneous and connective tissue. Exposure to sunlight is the major cause of wrinkled skin, liver spots, and leathery looking skin.

Sweat glands become smaller and the body becomes nonsensitive to heat and cold. **Hyperthermia,** an unusually high fever, and **hypothermia,** an unusually low body temperature, are serious problems, and exposure to excessive hot or cold temperatures should be avoided (see Chapter 21).

Hair loses color and becomes thinner. The skin dries and is less elastic. Fingernails and toenails thicken.

The development of skin cancer on the exposed skin surfaces is not uncommon in older adults. Basal and squamous cell carcinomas are the most common skin cancer types seen in this population. Both types of cancer can be serious if left untreated, but squamous cell cancer can metastasize. A complete skin assessment should be done on a yearly basis. Melanoma, a malignant tumor developing from a **nevus,** is the least common skin cancer, but it can be serious because it metastasizes readily. It is caused by exposure to the sun. Many older adults live in the Sunbelt areas of the United States and should be cautioned to wear sunscreen of at least SPF 15. People of all ages should protect their skin daily with a sunscreen of at least SPF 15, regardless of where they reside.

Nervous System

The brain shrinks in size as an individual ages because brain cells do not continue to divide throughout life as other cells do. Some loss of memory or delay in memory can be expected in many, but not all, aging people. Mental competence is the rule rather than the exception for older adults. Sudden loss of memory accompanied by confusion and inability to do tasks once able to be performed could be an indication of an organic problem, such as **transient ischemic attack (TIA),** a temporary interference of the blood supply to the brain, or a brain lesion.

Problems with balance, temperature regulation, diminished pain sensation, and insomnia can occur as part of the physical changes of aging that affect the nervous system.

Chronic illnesses from which many older people suffer often require several different medications to keep under control. Side effects of medication (over-the-counter, prescription, and herbals) can cause decreased mental capacity, as can malnutrition and substance abuse.

Loss of balance can be a problem for some older adults. Their coordination of muscles for movement may need more time for processing than it does with younger individuals. Older adults need to be reminded to be sure of their balance before starting to walk and to do so slowly. There is a general unsteadiness and lack of coordination not only because of the aging process, but also possibly because of medications the older adult takes (Figure 17-4). Older adults may need to use a cane to help steady their gait.

Musculoskeletal System

Musculoskeletal system changes are evident because older adults may have less muscle strength. This results in loss of mobility, and the activities of daily living become more difficult. There is less flexibility and joints can stiffen. Loss of height and a stooped appearance can result. Arthritis and osteoporosis are not unusual, and older adults can suffer fractured bones more easily. Poor nutrition, malnourishment, and lack of exercise all contribute to these conditions and prolong healing time as well (see Chapters 21 and 22).

Osteoporosis—a thinning of the long bones, pelvic bones, and vertebrae—is a fairly common problem in the aging population, with more women than men affected. This thinning of bone

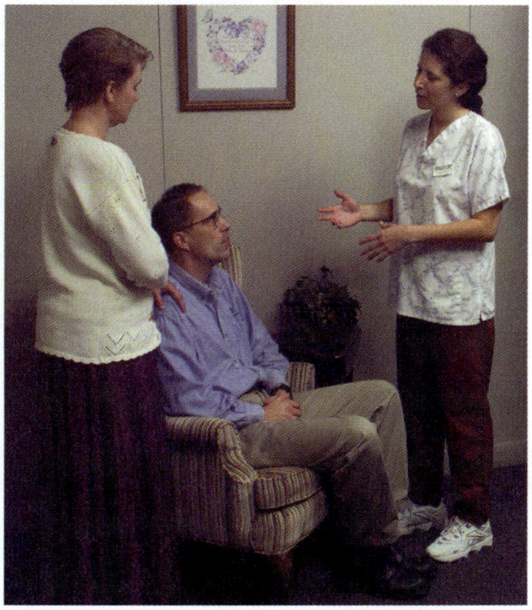

Figure 17-4 Older adults should be instructed to take their time when sitting, standing, and walking.

makes these individuals more susceptible to pain and fractures in these and other bones. New medications (Fosamax, Actonel, Evista) plus 1500 mg of calcium daily helps to slow the progress of osteoporosis. Vitamin D is essential for utilization of calcium. A deficiency of vitamin D in older adults occurs either because it is insufficient in their diets or because of insufficient exposure to sunlight. Vitamin D is added to milk.

Physical activity and a nutritional diet, including dairy products, can stall the development of bone and muscle loss; therefore, older adults should be encouraged to keep active by walking, gardening, swimming, bicycling, golfing, and so on. The pace of these activities should be suited to the individual's level of ability (Figure 17-5).

Respiratory System

Breathing capacity diminishes with age, and oxygen and carbon dioxide exchange is lessened. The rib and chest muscles become smaller and less efficient. Lungs lose their elasticity, and the older adult may be dyspneic, short of breath (SOB), and more prone to pneumonia.

As people age, there is a gradual decline in the muscle structure of the respiratory system, leading to a diminished ability to breathe deeply; thus, development of cough and pneumonia is not uncommon. Regular exercise can help to maintain the ability to breathe and cough effectively. In people who have been active throughout their lives, there is greater lung capacity.

Cardiovascular System

Heart disease and blood vessel disorders are the major cause of death in the United States. Lifestyle has been implicated as the most significant cause of cardiovascular disease. Blood vessels lose their elasticity, become narrower, and build up with plaque, and the arteries harden. This is known as **arteriosclerosis.** The myocardium loses some of its ability to pump effectively. This, together with narrowed and plaque-filled arteries, causes the heart to pump harder. Hypertension, or sustained high

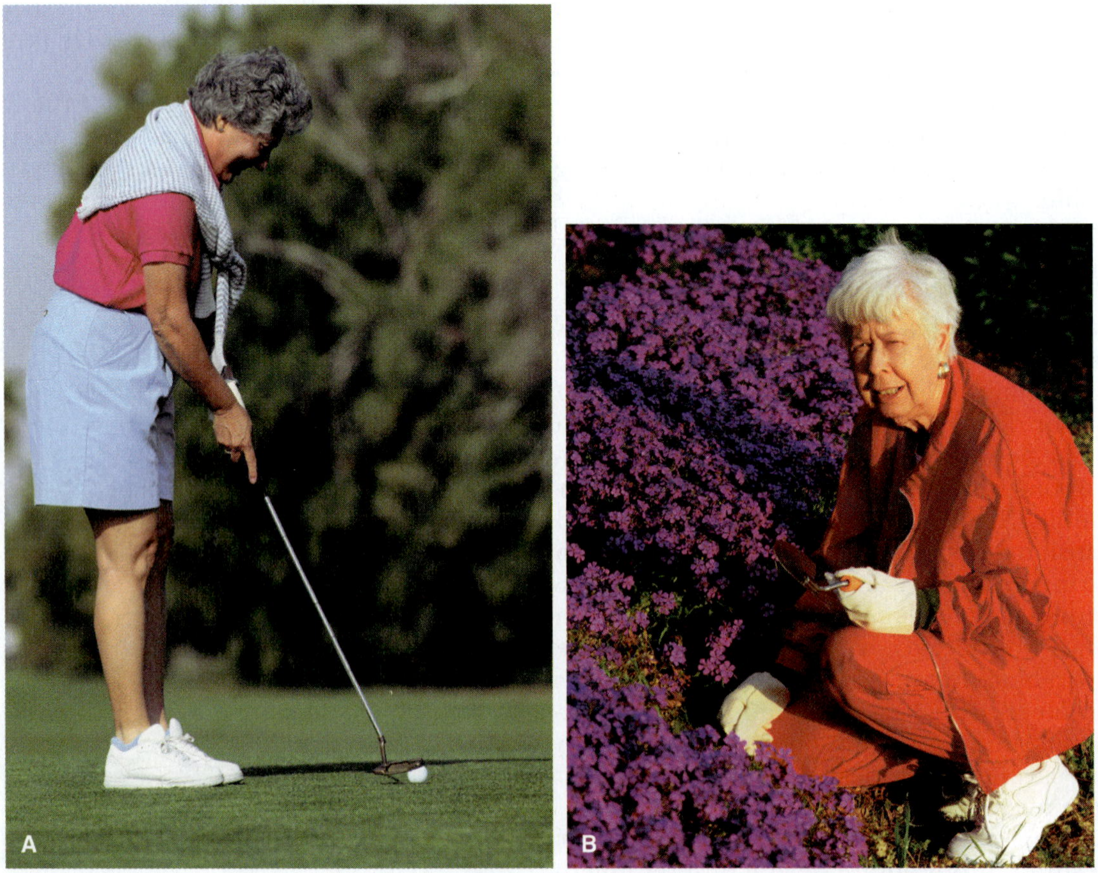

Figure 17-5 (A) A regular exercise program helps promote successful aging. (B) Gardening is a beneficial form of exercise.

blood pressure, is a direct result of these factors. Hypertension can contribute to the accumulation of plaque in artery walls. Congestive heart failure is the inability of the heart to pump effectively to meet the body's demand for blood. Myocardial infarction, or heart attack, is another result of arteriosclerotic heart disease. Regular exercise and a healthy diet are the most beneficial activities for older adults in order to maintain adequate cardiac output throughout their life spans.

Gastrointestinal System

Stomach secretions and motility slow as part of aging. Peristalsis slows, and food moves through the gastrointestinal tract more slowly. **Pernicious anemia** is a disorder that can occur when cells of the stomach lining fail to secrete the intrinsic factor. Associated with the absence of hydrochloric acid, pernicious anemia affects the nervous system and red blood cell formation.

Fewer calories are needed during this time because metabolism slows. Many overeat if they are lonely, gain weight, and may become obese. Eating is a social as well as a physiologic event, and if they have no one to eat with, many older adults will not prepare a meal or eat properly to have good nutrition. Loss of vigor and vitality occur. Malnourishment is not uncommon.

Poor eating habits, poor nutrition, overeating, or undereating can lead to dental problems. Poor dental hygiene leads to gum disease and loss of teeth, many times making the chewing of food difficult and discouraging. Sometimes cardiac problems, such as endocarditis and myocardial infarction, occur from gum disease due to the invasion of pathogens and inflammation.

Urinary System

With aging, the kidneys decrease in size, resulting in less urine production and output. With cardiovascular arteriosclerosis, blood flow to the kidney is less. Filtering of waste products from the blood is impaired. Medications are not excreted as quickly as they are in a young, healthy person. Levels of medication may increase to a dangerous level with impaired kidney filtration. The bladder walls become more inelastic, and the ability to empty the bladder completely becomes difficult. **Residual urine** remains in the bladder, and microorganisms can cause an infection. **Cystitis** is infection and inflammation of the bladder. Urinary **incontinence,** the uncontrollable loss of urine, can be the result of many factors, such as relaxed muscles in the female pelvic floor, cystitis, hypertrophy of prostate gland, and diabetes.

Reproductive System

Women experience menopause at about age 55 years. Estrogen produced by the ovaries ceases, and changes in the female are noticeable with shrinking of vulva and genitalia. Hot flashes are not uncommon because of blood vessel dilation and contraction. Vaginal secretions diminish, the vagina becomes smaller, and infections are more likely. Estrogen replacement therapy helps to lessen symptoms but is used only for short-term therapy in women who experience severe menopausal symptoms. Long-term use of estrogen and progesterone has been proved to increase the risk for heart disease and breast cancer (see Chapter 14 for information about hormone therapy).

Men continue to produce sperm well after 50 years of age; however, testosterone levels diminish and midlife changes occur in men. This is known as **andropause.** It is about this time that many men older than 50 years experience benign hypertrophy of the prostate (see Chapter 16). Medication may help in some cases; otherwise, surgery, a prostatectomy, may be performed.

Aging men and women maintain their sexual desires, and many enjoy sexual intercourse more when children are no longer in the home. They have more privacy and time to relax.

PREVENTION OF COMPLICATIONS

Older adults are at risk for complications as a result of changes in the structure and function of their body systems.

Accidents can happen because of impaired vision or the inability to hear a warning sound, such as a fire alarm.

Malnutrition and anemia can develop because of poor nutrition or poor absorption of food. This can be caused by lack of interest in food because of lack of sense of taste or smell.

Older adults may have diminished sensitivity and lack the ability to feel pain as well as a younger person does. Heat and cold applications can injure an aging person if not watched carefully. Simple fractured bones may go unnoticed for some time. Loss of balance, disorientation, and confusion may be signs of impaired nervous system function.

Because many older adults suffer from osteoporosis, bones are more easily fractured. Falls are more common because of a loss of vision and balance.

Respiratory tract infections are not unusual. Pneumonia is a serious complication in this group of people. Encourage fluid intake and activity to keep the lungs healthy.

Urinary infections are more common. Adequate fluid intake (eight 8-ounce glasses of liquid per day) help keep infections at bay. Incontinence occurs when pelvic floor muscles are relaxed after childbirth.

Circulatory problems because of cardiovascular disease can cause poor circulation to the extremities, especially the legs. Fluid retention with noticeable edema are a common complication, together with hypertension and congestive heart failure.

Vaginitis is more common because of vaginal dryness and irritation caused by lack of estrogen. The prostate gland enlarges, making urination difficult for men.

It is especially important for older adults to alert and consult with their providers when consuming an alternative substance or when considering engaging in an alternative therapy. Many older adults take prescription drugs for a variety of health problems, and there could be harmful effects because of the interactions of the prescribed medications with the alternative substance. Tai chi, massage therapy, yoga, art therapy, music therapy, and meditation are examples of some alternative or complementary therapies in which as older adult patients can participate. Balance, mobility, strength, creativity, and stress reduction are some of the benefits for older adults who choose to add these alternatives to enhance their health and well-being.

PSYCHOLOGICAL CHANGES

There is a great deal of variation in the psychological functioning of older adults. Among the factors that contribute are the person's health; psychosocial history; race; sex; and environmental aspects, such as education, support system, and social class.

The level of decline in an older adult's intelligence can be affected by social factors. People who maintain their intelligence tend to be in better health, have had more education, are in a higher socioeconomic group, and are involved with others and in their community.

Dementia affects memory, personality, and **cognitive functioning** (awareness, reasoning, judgment, intuition) and is permanent. Alzheimer's disease is a common form of dementia. Some research has shown that there may be a genetic, as well as environmental, link to the cause of Alzheimer's disease.

People who have had a stroke, which interferes with blood circulation to brain cells, may suffer from dementia, impairing brain functioning. Other forms of dementia include Parkinson's disease, caused by a deficiency of dopamine, a chemical in the brain; syphilis, caused by a bacterium that causes brain damage (which manifests about 20 years after initial infection); and Huntington's disease, a genetic disease. When caring for patients with dementia, protect them from injury, allow them to be independent if possible, and do not be critical or judgmental of their behaviors (it is unintentional) or what they say. Scientists have not determined what is in the minds of patients with dementia.

Depression in older adults can occur from loss of a spouse, chronic illness, or financial problems. When caring for older adults, look for signs and symptoms of depression such as poor hygiene, insomnia or excessive sleep, crying, depressed mood (sad every day, most of the day), inability to concentrate, and increased alcohol consumption. Personality seems to help determine how individuals adapt to changes that they experience as they grow older.

THE MEDICAL ASSISTANT AND THE GERIATRIC PATIENT

Many older adults experience dementia, mental illness, depression, stress, boredom, fear of the unknown, loss of independence, feelings of rejection and worthlessness, low self-esteem, loneliness, dependence, failed expectations, and disappointments. All of these factors coupled

HIPAA

Be cautious to limit access to patient health records only to those who need them to perform their jobs. Be sure to use passwords to safeguard databases and keep computer screens facing away from. patients Disclosure of suspected patient abuse is necessary to prevent serious threats or injuries to older adult patients and is required by law.

with the physiologic changes that can occur offer a special challenge to the medical assistant caring for the health and needs of this group of patients. Allow patients time to ventilate and express their concerns, allow for private and confidential discussion, and **empathize** with their situation by being aware of their feelings, emotions, and behavior. Good communication is essential for quality care of older adults. Do not talk to older adults as if they were children. Speak slowly and clearly. Face the individual while talking. Write instructions in addition to verbalizing them.

Memory-Impaired Older Adults

Geriatric care poses challenges when attempting to communicate with impaired older adults. The inability to communicate on a meaningful level can be frustrating and challenging, especially for the older person who is struggling to communicate but cannot find the right words. Following are some techniques that can be effective in improving verbal communication with older people experiencing memory impairment:

1. Talk to the person in a nondistracting place. It can be difficult for an older adult to concentrate or to sort things out when there are environmental distractions, such as other conversations, equipment noises, or people walking by.
2. Begin conversations with orientating information. Identify yourself, and call older adults by their preferred names. Explain the purpose of your visit.
3. Use short words and short, simple sentences with no pronouns.
4. Speak slowly and say individual words clearly.
5. Never "talk down" or be condescending. This is demeaning. Speak in an adult manner as you would to a coworker or friend. Provide the dignity and respect you wish to receive yourself.
6. Lower the tone (pitch) of your voice. A raised pitch is a signal that one is upset. A lower pitch is also easier for people with hearing impairments to understand.
7. Talk to the person in a warm and pleasant manner. Use nonverbal cues, such as facial expression, tone of voice, or touch, to show your feelings of affection and concern. Smiling, taking the older person's hand, or touching the person on the arm can vividly communicate that you are interested and really care.
8. When giving instructions, allow plenty of time for the information to be absorbed.
9. Give clear and simple instructions.
10. Ask the person to do one task at a time.
11. Listen actively. If you do not understand, apologize to the person by saying that you did not understand exactly what was said. It is extremely important to phrase responses in a way that does not damage the self-esteem of the older adult.
12. Avoid asking direct questions that require the person to remember a fact.
13. Focus on well behavior or things that you know the patient can still do.
14. Use humor when appropriate. If expressed naturally, humor brings much needed laughter, a dimension that is often lost in the health care setting.
15. Let the person know when you leave and if you are returning.
16. When discussing a case with another staff member, do so in private to protect patient confidentiality.

Visually Impaired Older Adults

Visually impaired people need to know you are present, but do not approach the individual until you make your presence known. Help by explaining his or her location, and identify others who may also be present (Figure 17-6).

Hearing-Impaired Older Adults

For the hearing-impaired older adult to communicate and understand instructions, there are some techniques the medical assistant should keep in mind. These strategies will be beneficial and will facilitate communication and understanding. These techniques include:

1. Face the hearing-impaired person directly and on the same level when possible. (If he or she is standing, the medical assistant should stand; if the patient is seated, the medical assistant should be seated).
2. Keep your hands away from your face while talking.
3. Reduce background noises when talking. Move to a quieter room away from extraneous sounds and activities.

Critical Thinking

Describe strategies for communicating with hearing-impaired patients.

Making Contact

Introduce yourself. Ask the visually impaired patient if he would like assistance. If he does, offer your arm by saying so and by touching your hand or forearm against his.

Grip

The patient grips your arm just above the elbow. The grip must be firm but not so tight that it becomes uncomfortable.

Stance

The patient stands next to you, slightly behind. His arm is bent and held close to his side. Relax your arm and let it hang naturally at your side.

Pace

The pace should be comfortable for both of you. If the patient tightens his grip or pulls on your arm, slow down; your pace may be too fast or he may be anxious. You should alert the patient to obstacles such as curbs, stairs, doors, and thresholds. Be specific, but do not confuse him with too much information.

Stairs

When approaching stairs, tell the patient. Let him know whether you are going to go up or down. Be sure you approach the stairs directly, not at an angle. Have the patient stand next to the handrail if there is one.

Pause at the top (or bottom) of the stairs and describe anything unusual about them. The patient will find the handrail and reach forward with his foot to locate the edge of the first step. Start down (or up) the stairs, keeping yourself one step ahead. Keep a steady pace.

When you reach a landing, stop immediately. (Do not take an extra step.) Doing so lets the patient know that there are no more steps, and he can then match his stride with yours.

The same procedure should be used when approaching curbs. Point out any changes in the terrain, even small ones.

Sitting

When guiding someone to a chair, walk up to it and place your hand on the back of the chair. Let the patient trail your arm down to its back. Tell him which way the chair is facing, and he can then seat himself.

If the chair lacks a back or is very large, bring the patient up to the chair so that his legs are against the front of it. He can then reach down to locate the arms and seat of it before he sits.

If the chair is at a table, describe the relationship of the chair, the table and the patient. Place one of his hands on the chair and the other hand on the table.

Doors

When approaching a closed door, tell the patient its position when open. For example, "The door opens away and to the left." Or say, "Take the door with your left hand." After you open the door and begin to walk through, the patient will have his hand ready to help hold it open as you walk through together. The patient will move his arm across the front of his body to find the door with the palm of his hand. He should close it behind you if it is not a self-closing door. Use the narrow passage technique in addition to this technique if the doorway is narrow.

Narrow Passage Technique

When coming to a narrow passage, tell the patient. Move your guiding arm to the center of your back. Slow your pace. He will move behind you and extend his arm, placing you in a single-file position. Once you pass through the narrow passage, bring your arm forward and return to the normal stance.

Figure 17-6 Sighted guide techniques.

4. Hearing-impaired individuals hear and understand less when they are tired or sick.
5. Get the person's attention before beginning to speak and do not talk from another room.
6. Speak in a normal tone; do not shout.
7. Be sure that light is not shining in the eyes of the hearing-impaired individual.
8. If the hearing-impaired patient has trouble understanding, reword what you have said. Do not repeat the same words again and again.
9. Written instructions are useful, but the medical assistant must be certain that what is written is understood.

Elder Abuse

What is elder abuse? Massachusetts law defines elder abuse as the committing or omitting of an act that results in serious physical or emotional injury to an older adult. All states have elder abuse laws. Abuse includes physical, emotional, and verbal abuse, and neglect. The law protects elders abused or neglected by caretakers.

All persons 60 years and older living in the community are protected under the law. Who must report elder abuse? Providers, medical interns, dentists, medical assistants, nurses, family counselors, police officers, psychologists, homemakers, licensed home health care aides, and many others may be required to report abuse. Agencies are also liable. Any person required to report abuse who fails to do so is subject to a fine. Anyone who has reasonable cause to believe an older adult has been abused may report it and has a moral obligation to protect older adults. In most states, the department responsible for elder affairs has established an elder abuse hotline to receive reports of abuse. Reports may also be made to the designated protective service agency in your community. Once reports are received by the elder protective services program, if appropriate, a caseworker will assess the situation to determine the nature and extent of the abuse. If abuse is confirmed, services will be provided to eliminate or alleviate abuse. Many social services are usually available. Mental health, legal, homemaker services, and alternative living arrangements may be provided (see Chapter 7).

Some signs and symptoms of mistreatment or abuse include:

Psychological Signs and Symptoms

- Increasing depression
- Anxiety
- Withdrawn/timid
- Hostile
- Unresponsive
- Confused
- New poverty
- Longing for death
- Vague health complaints
- Anxious to please

Physical Signs and Symptoms

- Lack of personal care
- Lack of supervision
- Bruises
- Welts
- Lack of food
- Beatings
- Neglect
- Unsatisfactory living conditions

There are other signs and symptoms, and not all of those listed by themselves indicate mistreatment, neglect, or abuse. If any seem to increase in number or severity, it may indicate a problem. By observing closely, you may be able to initiate corrective action or reduce or prevent the situation from deteriorating. Careful documentation in the patient's chart or electronic medical record over time can show continuous signs and symptoms of abuse.

Usually the victim is frail (weak), physically or emotionally, and dependent on the abuser for basic survival needs. The victim may be afraid to speak out for fear of retaliation. Many times the abuser is the caregiver or a member of the patient's family.

For information, contact elder protective services programs in the Yellow Pages of your phone book, or contact the Eldercare Locator toll free at (800) 677-1116 or via their Web site (http://www.eldercare.gov/public/resources/assessment.esp).

HEALTHY AND SUCCESSFUL AGING

Older adults are enjoying longer, healthier lives. Some reasons for healthy aging are the increase in the number of gerontologists (specialists who provide medical care only to older adult patients), greater awareness and involvement of older adults with their health care, improved nutrition, regular exercise, new medications, and advancing medical technology (Figure 17-7).

Some tips for healthy aging according to the National Institute on Aging of the National Institutes of Health are:

1. Eat a balanced diet.
2. Exercise regularly.
3. Get regular checkups.
4. Don't smoke.
5. Wear a seatbelt when in the car.
6. Practice safety to avoid falls and fractures.
7. Keep in contact with family and friends and stay active through work, community, and recreation.
8. Avoid overexposure to the sun and cold.

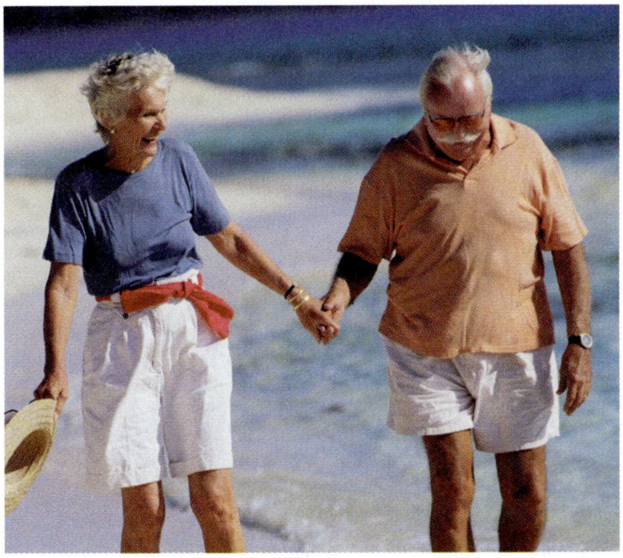

Figure 17-7 With improved geriatric care, older adults can look forward to longer, healthier lives.

9. Drink alcohol in moderation. Don't drink and drive.
10. Keep personal and financial records in order to simplify budgeting and investing. Plan for long-term financial needs and housing.
11. Keep a positive attitude toward life and engage in activities that make you happy.
12. Get vaccines: pneumonia, influenza, and herpes zoster (Zostavax). Zostavax is approved for people over age 60. It prevents herpes zoster (shingles).

Successful aging requires that healthy living and daily activities be combined. To age successfully, individuals need to be continually involved, must pursue what makes them happy, and make an effort to maintain a positive attitude. These actions of healthy habits should begin in childhood when they can be formed and encouraged. They become the responsibilities of each individual. Some activities that are important to successful aging are socialization with friends and family, intimacy, education, and employment (for income and social satisfaction). For successful aging to happen, the older person must make a commitment to work at it (Figures 17-8 through 17-10).

Critical Thinking

What are some strategies that older adults can do to keep mentally and physically stimulated?

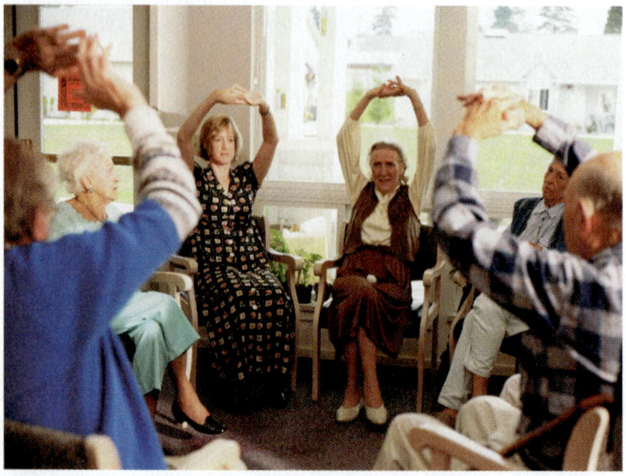

Figure 17-8 An exercise class in an assisted-living facility.

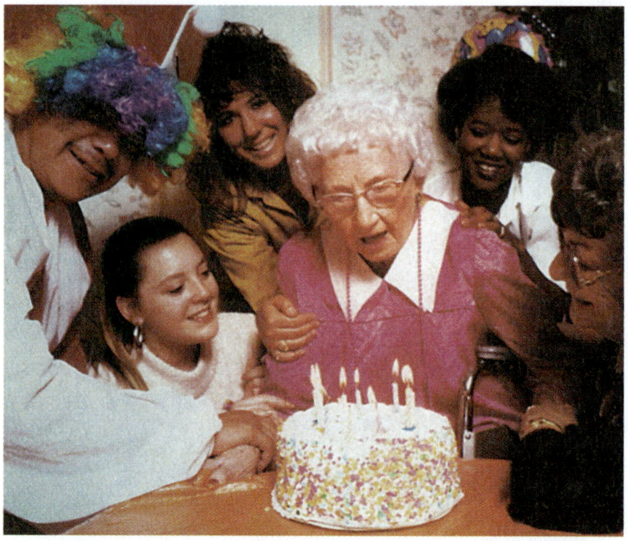

Figure 17-9 This woman is celebrating her 100th birthday and is surrounded by her family and friends.

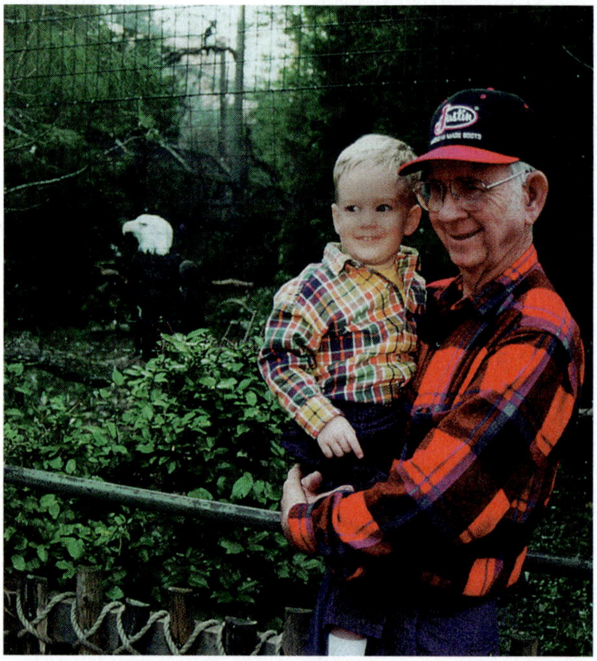

Figure 17-10 Caring for grandchildren is a very satisfying social relationship for many older adults.

Case Study 17-1

Refer to the scenario at the beginning of the chapter.

CASE STUDY REVIEW

1. Describe five strategies older adults such as Mrs. Johnson can use to help slow the aging process.

Case Study 17-2

Adelaide Robinson, 83 years old, has an appointment Thursday morning for a recheck of her most recent complaint. She tells you that she is moving slower than she did just 6 months ago, and she has noticed less flexibility as well.

CASE STUDY REVIEW

1. What are the possible causes of Mrs. Robinson's complaints?
2. What effect will these problems have on Mrs. Robinson's daily routine?
3. What might Dr. King suggest Mrs. Robinson do to help alleviate symptoms?

Case Study 17-3

Sally Donovan, 92 years old, is in the gerontology clinic today. Her main concern, problem, and reason for appointment is that she "cannot taste or smell much anymore and food doesn't taste good." She wants suggestions from the provider about how to improve her taste and smell so she can enjoy food more freely.

CASE STUDY REVIEW

1. What are some reasons that older adults lose their sense of taste and smell?
2. Describe any dangers that can be associated with loss of taste and smell.

SUMMARY

Many aging people live well into their 80s, 90s, and even to 100 years of age. They remain physically and mentally stimulated. They learn a foreign language, learn to play a musical instrument, love to read, garden, and volunteer. Older people are more aware today than ever before of the importance of a healthy lifestyle and of its significant contribution to their long and healthy life span.

Other older adults, because of genetic inheritance, wear and tear, and stress, and loss of chemicals and hormones, seem to age quickly and have little control over these factors.

Many others practice poor health habits, some by choice and others by circumstance. These habits contribute to chronic diseases, disability, and a shorter and unhealthy life span.

Above all, dispel myths about older adults. Be patient, kind, consistent, and thoughtful.

STUDY FOR SUCCESS

To reinforce your knowledge and skills of information presented in this chapter:

- Review Key Terms
- Consider the Case Studies and discuss your conclusions
- Answer the Review Questions
  - Multiple Choice
  - Critical Thinking
- Navigate the Internet by completing the Web Activities
- Practice the StudyWARE activities on your student CD
- Apply your knowledge in the Student Workbook activities
- Complete the Web Tutor sections

REVIEW QUESTIONS

Multiple Choice

1. The most chronic condition associated with older adults is:
   a. arteriosclerotic heart disease
   b. cystitis
   c. presbycusis
   d. pernicious anemia
2. An eye disease common to older adults that is characterized by fluid pressure buildup is:
   a. macular degeneration
   b. presbyopia
   c. cataract
   d. glaucoma
3. Joints in older adults become worn because:
   a. cartilage erodes in the joints
   b. osteoporosis makes bones brittle
   c. muscle fibers decrease
   d. vertebrae become thinner
4. Inability to cough deeply and raise mucus makes older adults more susceptible to which of the following?
   a. emphysema
   b. asthma
   c. pneumonia
   d. bronchitis
5. Residual urine refers to:
   a. catheterized urine for urinalysis
   b. first-voided specimen
   c. amount of urine left in bladder after voiding
   d. total amount of urine in the bladder when full

Critical Thinking

1. How can an older adult's food be made more appealing?
2. What are some ways that older adults can keep bones from becoming brittle?
3. Describe a vision problem that leaves older adults with difficulty seeing color intensity.
4. What are four causes of urinary incontinence?
5. Give three ways to enhance communication with older adults.
6. What is the best way to approach a visually impaired person?
7. Older adults in the United States are generally healthier today than older adults of 30 years ago. What are some of the reasons for this?
8. How can you encourage older adults to choose a healthy lifestyle?

WEB ACTIVITIES

1. Visit http://www.gov/aging/saha.htm. "The State of Aging and Health in America: 2007 Report" (pp. 5–6). "Healthy Brain Initiative." Discuss what strategies older adults can adopt to maintain brain function.
2. The American Psychological Association Web site (http://www.apa.org) gives information about psychology. Find information that pertains to older adults and their psychological health. What are some resources for mental health issues that can be helpful for older adults?
3. The U.S. government has a Web site (http://www.aoa.gov/) for concerns and information about aging. What government agencies can an older adult contact for help with health insurance questions?
4. The National Osteoporosis Foundation Web site (http://www.nof.org) provides information about osteoporosis. Retrieve information about osteoporosis that is useful for all older adults.
5. Locate a Web site for older adults who have arthritis. Find some techniques for these patients to make their activities of daily living less difficult.

REFERENCES/BIBLIOGRAPHY

Cox, H. (2001). *Later life: The realities of aging* (5th ed.). Upper Saddle River, NJ: Prentice Hall.

Hegner, B. R., Accello, B., & Caldwell, E. (2008). *Nursing assistant: A nursing process approach* (20th ed.). Clifton Park, NY: Delmar Cengage Learning.

Hogstel, M. O. (2001). *Gerontology: Nursing care of the older adult.* Clifton Park, NY: Delmar Cengage Learning.

Lodge, H. S. (2007). You can stop "normal" aging. *Parade Magazine,* March 6, 2007.

Markson, E., & Hollis-Sawyer, G. (2000). *Readings in social gerontology.* Los Angeles, CA: Roxbury Publishing Co.

Perls, T. (2007). Simple steps may slow aging. *Consumer Reports on Health, 19,* 1–4.

Simmers, L. (2008). *Diversified health occupations* (7th ed.). Clifton Park, NY: Delmar Cengage Learning.

Taber's cyclopedic medical dictionary (21st ed.). (2003). Philadelphia: F. A. Davis.

Examinations and Procedures of Body Systems

Chapter 18

KEY TERMS

Amblyopia
Amsler Grid
Appendicular Skeleton
Aseptic
Auricle
Axial Skeleton
Bariatrics
Biopsy
Bronchi
Bronchodilator
Carbuncle
Closed Fracture
Colonoscopy
Comedone
Demyelination
Dislocation
Dysuria
Electrocochleography
Emaciation
Erythema
External Respiration
Frequency
Furuncle
Hematuria
Hemoptysis
Immunoglobulin
Inhaler
Internal Respiration
Lesion
Lithotripsy
Malabsorption
Malaise
Morbid Obesity
Nephrolithotomy
Nitrogenous

OUTLINE

Urinary System
- Signs and Symptoms of Urinary Conditions and Disorders
- Diagnostic Tests
- Urinary Catheterization

Digestive System
- Signs and Symptoms of Digestive Conditions and Disorders
- Diagnostic Tests
- Bariatrics

Sensory System
- The Eye
- The Ear
- The Nose

Respiratory System
- Signs and Symptoms of Respiratory Conditions and Disorders
- Diagnostic Tests
- Spirometry
- Peak Expiratory Flow Rates
- Pulse Oximetry
- Inhalers

Musculoskeletal System
- Fractures, Casting, and Cast Removal

Neurologic System
- Components of a Neurologic Screening

Circulatory System

Blood and Lymph System

Integumentary System
- Allergy Skin Testing

OBJECTIVES

The student should strive to meet the following performance objectives and demonstrate an understanding of the facts and principles presented in this chapter through written and oral communication.

1. Define the key terms as presented in the glossary.
2. Describe how to perform a urinary catheterization.
3. Describe patient preparation for occult blood testing.
4. Differentiate between an instillation and an irrigation.
5. Discuss the different types of visual acuity charts and how to use them appropriately.
6. Explain the medical assistant's role when assisting with audiometry.
7. Describe the proper use of a metered dose inhaler.
8. Briefly discuss the role of the medical assistant during spirometry and pulse oximetry.

OBJECTIVES (continued)

9. Explain the medical assistant's role in cast application and cast removal and the guidelines for cast care.
10. List items required by a provider for a neurologic examination and explain the medical assistant's role in the examination.
11. Explain oxygen administration using a nasal cannula.
12. Describe how to perform a nasal irrigation.
13. Identify patient education information for sputum collections.

KEY TERMS (continued)

Nocturia
Nystagmus
Occluder
Oliguria
Opticokinetic Drum Test
Otoscope
Paresthesia
Phacoemulsification
Polyp
Proteinuria
Pyuria
Rosacea
Salicylates
Spirometry
Strabismus
Urgency

Scenario

At Inner City Health Care, a number of specialty examinations are scheduled for Tuesday the eighth. Administrative medical assistant Jane O'Hara, who is office manager, is careful to schedule patients requiring specialty procedures so that times do not overlap; before she schedules, Jane makes certain examination rooms are available with an extra margin of time between patients. Clinical medical assistants Wanda Slawson, CMA (AAMA), and Bruce Goldman, RMA, take responsibility to ensure that all supplies and equipment are assembled, that both provider and patient are comfortable with the physical environment, and that all safety precautions are followed before, during, and after the examination or procedure.

INTRODUCTION

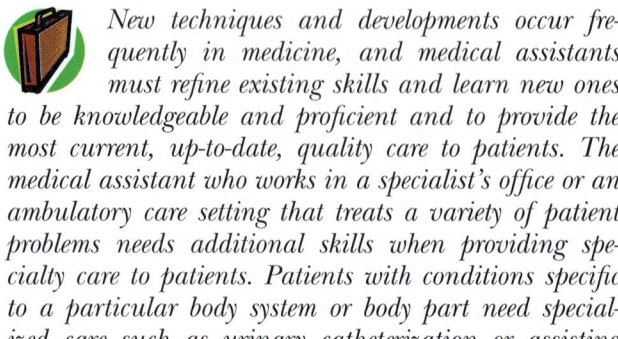

New techniques and developments occur frequently in medicine, and medical assistants must refine existing skills and learn new ones to be knowledgeable and proficient and to provide the most current, up-to-date, quality care to patients. The medical assistant who works in a specialist's office or an ambulatory care setting that treats a variety of patient problems needs additional skills when providing specialty care to patients. Patients with conditions specific to a particular body system or body part need specialized care such as urinary catheterization or assisting with a lumbar puncture. The medical assistant assists the provider with a multitude of clinical procedures that are an integral part of each specialty examination.

This chapter covers specialty and body system examinations and the appropriate clinical procedures in urology; endoscopy; and the sensory, respiratory, musculoskeletal, neurologic, circulatory, blood and lymph, and integumentary systems.

Each specialty description includes tables that contain information on diseases, disorders, and diagnostic tests and procedures used to confirm diagnoses. Other diseases and disorders and procedures related to each specialty are addressed in the body of the chapter.

Spotlight on Certification

RMA Content Outline

- Anatomy and physiology
- Disorders and diseases
- Patient instruction
- Asepsis
- Sterilization
- Instruments

CMA (AAMA) Content Outline

- Anatomy and physiology
- Communication
- Equipment
- Principles of infection control
- Treatment area
- Equipment preparation and operation
- Patient preparation and assisting the provider
- Collecting and processing specimen; diagnostic testing
- Methods of collection

CMAS Content Outline

- Anatomy and physiology
- Asepsis in the medical office
- Examination preparation

URINARY SYSTEM

The urinary system includes the kidneys, ureters, and bladder. The main function of the kidneys is to form and excrete urine, which contains waste products harmful to body tissues. The kidneys also regulate water balance in the body and help maintain the acid–base balance of body fluids.

Collecting and processing urine for laboratory analysis is covered in Chapter 30. Several other clinical and diagnostic procedures of the urinary system are covered in this section, including urinary catheterization and an overview of performing a urine drug screen and a diagnostic X-ray known as an intravenous pyelogram (IVP) or excretory urography used to diagnose disorders of the urinary tract.

Diagnostic tests, procedures, disorders, and conditions common to the urinary system are given in Tables 18-1 and 18-2.

Signs and Symptoms of Urinary Conditions and Disorders

Signs and symptoms of urinary tract diseases include any abnormality in urine or in the ability to urinate. Some common signs and symptoms are **dysuria** (painful urination), **proteinuria** (protein in the urine), **hematuria** (blood in the urine), **pyuria** (pus in the urine), **frequency, urgency, oliguria** (scanty urination), and **nocturia** (excessive urination at night). Patients may report flank or low back pain or experience fever, nausea, vomiting, general **malaise** (general discomfort), and fatigue.

Urinary tract infection (UTI) is the most common disorder of the urinary system, and it manifests itself with many of the above signs and symptoms. UTI is a broad diagnosis covering any infection of the urinary tract including the urethra, ureters, bladder, and kidneys. UTIs may be caused by virus or fungus, but by far the most common infection is caused by bacteria. The most common area is the bladder (cystitis).

Bacteria may reach the urinary tract through the blood (hematogenous infection) or enter the tract through the urethra (ascending infection). Hematogenous infection is less common and is usually the result of septicemia. In this case, the urinary tract is a site of secondary infection. Primary infection of septicemia may begin in the respiratory or gastrointestinal tract and is carried to the urinary tract through the blood.

Diagnostic Tests

The most commonly performed test to diagnose urinary system disorders is a urinalysis. Many different disorders of the urinary system can be identified, making this test extremely valuable. A specimen of urine can be analyzed for many components such as pH, specific gravity, protein, glucose, leukocytes, and blood. The specimen can be further analyzed by examination under the microscope to look for bacteria, white and red blood cells, crystals, and casts.

Urine culture and sensitivity can be performed and will indicate if a UTI is present so the appropriate antibiotic can be prescribed by the provider. To obtain a urine specimen for culture, there are two ways to collect the specimen: clean catch or by catheterization (insertion of sterile tube into urinary bladder; see Procedures 18-1 and 18-2 and Chapter 30).

Blood tests can be done to determine whether waste products are being adequately filtered out of the circulatory system. A test for kidney function confirms the status of glomeruli function.

Table 18-1 Urinary System Disorders

	Laboratory/Diagnostic Tests					
Disease/ Disorder	**Blood**	**Urine**	**Radiography**	**Surgery**	**Medical Tests or Procedures**	**Treatment**
Cancer of urinary bladder	Complete blood count	Urinalysis Culture and sensitivity of urine	Intravenous pyelogram Pelvic ultrasound Computed tomography scan	Biopsy of bladder with endoscopy	Cystoscopy	Resection of cancer (transurethral resection of a bladder tumor [TURBT]) Cystectomy Radium implants Chemotherapy
Cystitis	Complete blood count	Urinalysis including microscopic examination Culture and sensitivity of urine	Intravenous pyelogram		Cystoscopy	Appropriate antibiotic therapy
Glomerulonephritis	Blood urea nitrogen Creatinine Blood culture Sedimentation rate Electrolytes	Urinalysis Culture and sensitivity of urine	Intravenous pyelogram Ultrasound of kidneys X-ray of kidneys, ureters, and bladder		Biopsy of kidney(s)	Diuretics Antihypertensives Dialysis (if necessary) Kidney transplant
Polycystic kidneys	Blood urea nitrogen Creatinine Electrolytes	Urinalysis	Intravenous pyelogram Ultrasound of kidneys Computerized tomography scan			Dialysis Kidney transplant
Pyelonephritis	Blood urea nitrogen Creatinine Blood culture Electrolytes	Urinalysis	Intravenous pyelogram Ultrasound of kidneys			Appropriate antibiotics
Renal calculi	Complete blood count Uric acid	Urinalysis	X-ray of kidneys, ureters, and bladder (KUB) Ultrasound of kidneys, ureters, and bladder Intravenous pyelogram		Cystoscopy	**Lithotripsy** (crushing of a kidney stone) Surgery **(nephrolithotomy)**
Urinary tract infection	Complete blood count	Urinalysis Culture and sensitivity of urine			Cystoscopy	Appropriate antibiotics

Table 18-2 Description of Urinary Disorders and Conditions

Cancer of urinary bladder. Linked to cigarette smoking, industrial chemicals, and ingested toxins. Microscopic hematuria is one of the first Signs.
Cystitis. Inflammation of the urinary bladder. More common in female patients due to the short length of the urethra. *E.coli* may travel from the rectum to the bladder. Infectious organisms can invade the bladder during sexual intercourse. Frequency, burning, dysuria, and urgency are common symptoms.
Glomerulonephritis. Seen in children and young adults after streptococcal infection; strep throat, scarlet fever. Causes degenerative inflammation of glomeruli. Chills, fever, weakness are common symptoms. Edema and albumin in urine are common. Hypertension occurs.
Polycystic kidneys. A congenital anomaly. Kidneys contain multiple cysts and greatly dilated tubules do not open into renal pelvis. Hypertension, kidney failure, and death can result.
Pyelonephritis. Caused by pyogenic bacteria such as *E. coli*, streptococci, staphylococci, pregnancy, or calculi. May originate in the bladder and ascend to the kidneys. Pyuria, chills, fever, sudden back pain are symptoms. Dysuria is common. Tenderness in suprapubic area.
Renal calculi. May be present with or without symptoms. Cause intense pain when they lodge in the ureter(s). Formed by certain salts (perhaps calcium). Urinary urgency, nausea and vomiting, fever.

Two **nitrogenous** waste products normally filtered from the blood are urea and creatinine. A blood urea nitrogen (BUN) test checks the levels of these two wastes. High levels of waste products can result in uremia (waste products in the blood), a toxic condition of the blood that, if not reversed, leads to death (see Chapter 30).

An IVP, kidney-ureter-bladder (KUB) radiograph, and cystogram are radiologic examinations of the urinary tract.

Intravenous Pyelogram (Excretory Urography).

An IVP is used to examine the urinary tract (kidneys, ureters, and bladder) for blockage, narrowing, growths, and calculi. This urinary tract diagnostic radiograph is also used to diagnose disorders such as lesions, hydronephrosis (collection of urine in renal pelvis), and polycystic (many cysts) kidneys.

Patient Preparation for IVP. In studies of the urinary system, the IVP requires that the patient prepare with laxatives, enemas, and fasting (Table 18-3). The IVP consists of an intravenous injection of an iodine-based contrast medium that is used to define the structures of the urinary system. A retrograde pyelogram is a study of the urinary tract done by inserting a sterile catheter into the urinary meatus. Radiopaque contrast medium then flows upward into the kidneys. This diagnostic test is usually done in conjunction with cystoscopy. Patients should have iodine-sensitivity tests before the examination to determine the possibility of an allergic reaction. A voiding cystogram may be ordered in conjunction with an IVP. In this case, the contrast medium is instilled into the bladder by catheter and no special patient preparation is needed (see Chapter 20).

Table 18-3 Intravenous Pyelogram

Purpose	Patient Education	Precautions
To examine the urinary tract—kidneys ureters, bladder—for blockage, narrowing, growths, and calculi.	1. Light evening meal night before 2. Cathartic (laxative) 3. NPO after 9:00 PM 4. Cleansing enema(s) in AM	Contrast medium of iodine used for visualization (check with patient regarding seafood or iodine allergies) Warn patients of possible warm flushed sensation when dye is injected and that they may experience a metallic taste.

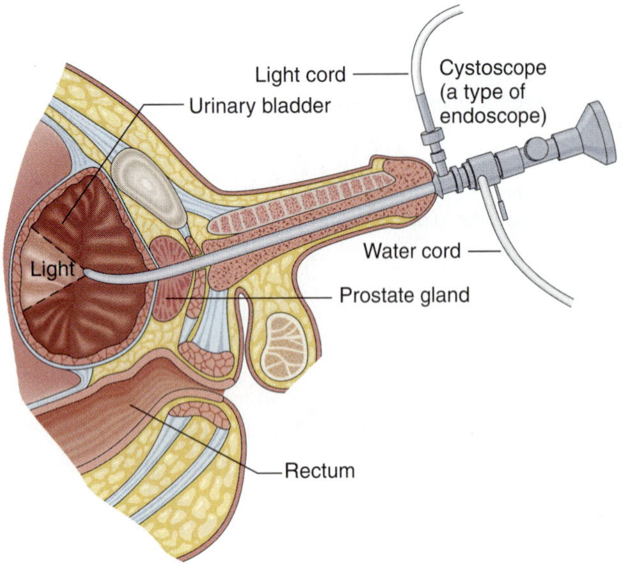

Figure 18-1 Cystoscopy.

Cystoscopy. Cystoscopy is a sterile procedure that uses a lighted scope (cytoscope) to view the urethra and bladder. Inflammation, bladder calculi (stones), **polyps,** and tumors can be seen using a cystoscope. A biopsy of the bladder can be done while performing a cystoscopy (Figure 18-1).

Biopsy of the Kidney. Biopsies of the kidney will help confirm a diagnosis. Using radiology and ultrasonography, a fine-gauge needle is inserted through the flank to remove a piece of kidney tissue for analysis and determination of possible malignancy.

Urinary Catheterization

In some states medical assistants can either perform or assist with urinary bladder catheterization, which is the introduction of a sterile catheter (tube) through the urethra into the bladder for withdrawal of urine. Figure 18-2 shows male and female anatomy for catheterization. There are basically four reasons to catheterize patients:

1. To obtain a sterile urine specimen for analysis
2. To relieve urinary retention
3. To instill medication into the bladder, after the bladder is emptied
4. To measure the amount of post-void residual urine

In some cases, this procedure is done by a urologist; however, some providers in obstetrics/gynecology and general and family practice

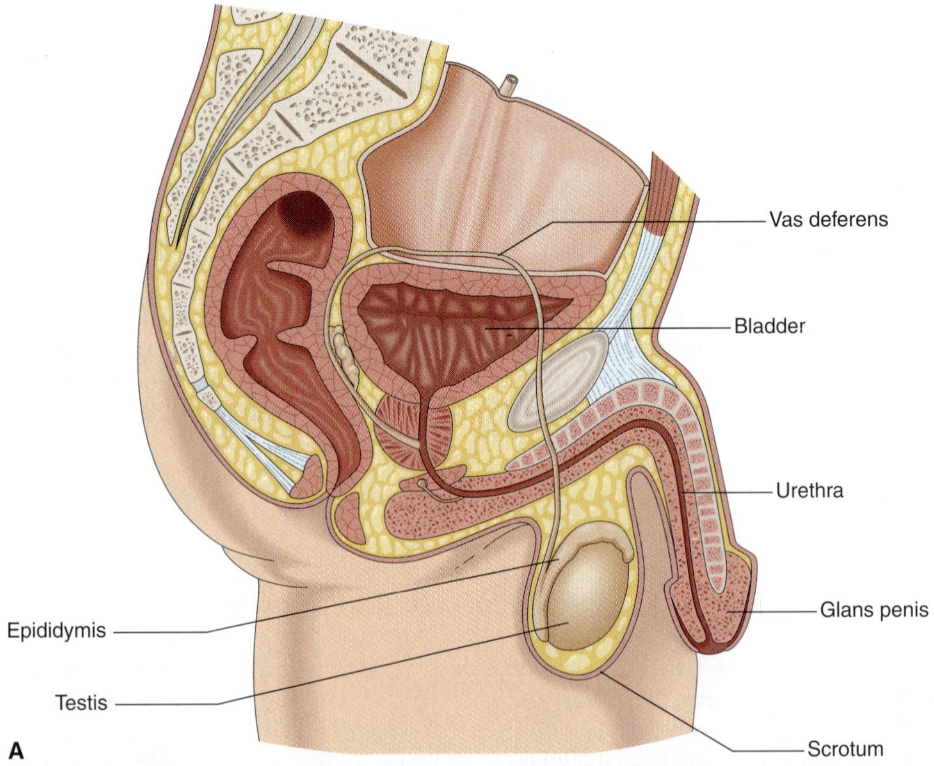

Figure 18-2 (A) Cross-sectional view of male anatomy showing urethra and bladder for catheterization. (continues)

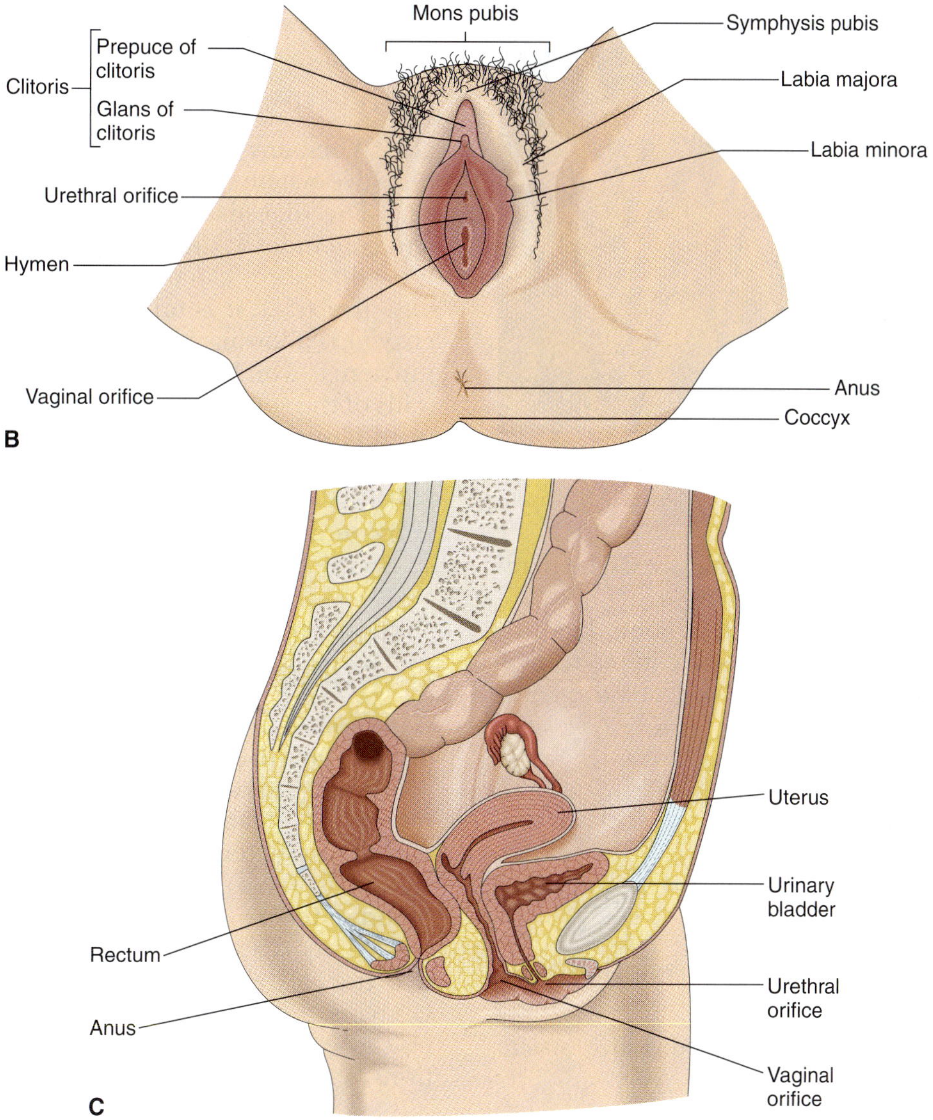

Figure 18-2 (continued) (B) External genitalia of the female. (C) Cross-sectional view of female anatomy showing urethra and bladder for catheterization.

perform or have the medical assistant perform the catheterization. Catheterizing male patients is generally performed by a male provider. The provider may order a culture and sensitivity of the urine obtained from catheterization if the patient is experiencing dysuria, frequency, hematura, and urgency. This is done to determine if microorganisms are present and, if so, what the causative microorganism is and which medication would irradicate it, in order to prescribe the appropriate antibiotics.

Sterile technique must be maintained throughout the catheterization. Contamination of any items during the procedure requires discarding the items and obtaining new sterile equipment before continuing the procedure (Figure 18-3).

Procedure 18-1 gives steps for performing a urinary catheterization of a female patient and Procedure 18-2 for a male patient.

Catheterization Equipment. Urinary catheters are sized according to a system of French sizes. A common size catheter is Fr 12. The higher the number the larger the diameter of the catheter. The provider orders the catheter size when ordering the catheterization procedure. Urethral catheters, sometimes called straight catheters, are used when the catheter is removed after the procedure. The Foley catheter is used when the catheter will remain in the urinary bladder (indwelling catheter). A suprapubic catheter (indwelling) is placed in the bladder during a surgical procedure. An

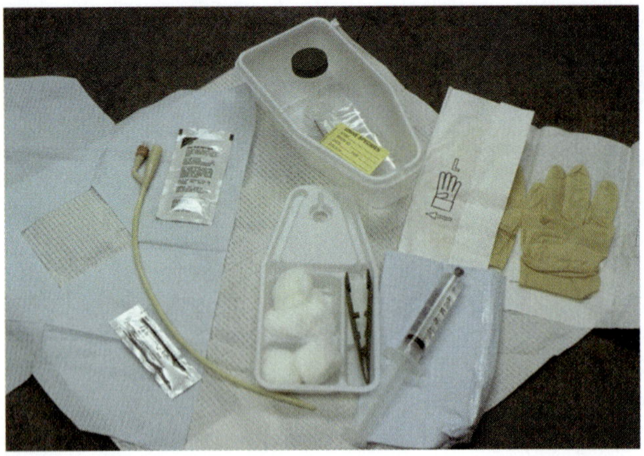

Figure 18-3 Catheterization kit.

incision is made in the suprapubic area. The bladder empties through the catheter.

Sterile, disposable catheterization kits are available that contain all necessary items to perform the procedure. Figure 18-4 shows the types of urinary catheterizations.

DIGESTIVE SYSTEM

The gastrointestinal system performs the following five functions:

1. Ingestion (taking in) of food and breaking it into smaller particles
2. Passage of food through the digestive system (peristalsis)
3. Digestion through secretions of digestive enzymes
4. Absorption of nutrients into the bloodstream
5. Defecation of the solid waste products of digestion

When any of these functions is hindered, the digestive system malfunctions.

The digestive process begins in the mouth and concludes at the anus. As food passes through the alimentary canal (gastrointestinal tract), or digestive tract, it is mixed with gastric juices and enzymes, allowing it to break down into smaller nutrients, which allows absorption through the walls of the small intestine. Contents that have not been absorbed travel through the large intestine and are excreted through the anus. Tables 18-4 and 18-5 list common tests, procedures, disorders, and conditions of the digestive system. Figure 18-5 shows the major organs of the digestive system.

Signs and Symptoms of Digestive Conditions and Disorders

Common signs and symptoms of disorders and diseases of the digestive tract include nausea, vomiting, stomach cramping, diarrhea, heartburn, loss of appetite, weight loss, indigestion, fatigue, hematemesis (vomiting blood), melena (blood in feces), and hematochezia (bright red blood in feces).

Many disorders and diseases of the digestive tract can cause these signs and symptoms. Gastritis, a common ailment of the stomach, can be caused by caffeine, aspirin and other medications, spicy foods, and alcohol. It is characterized

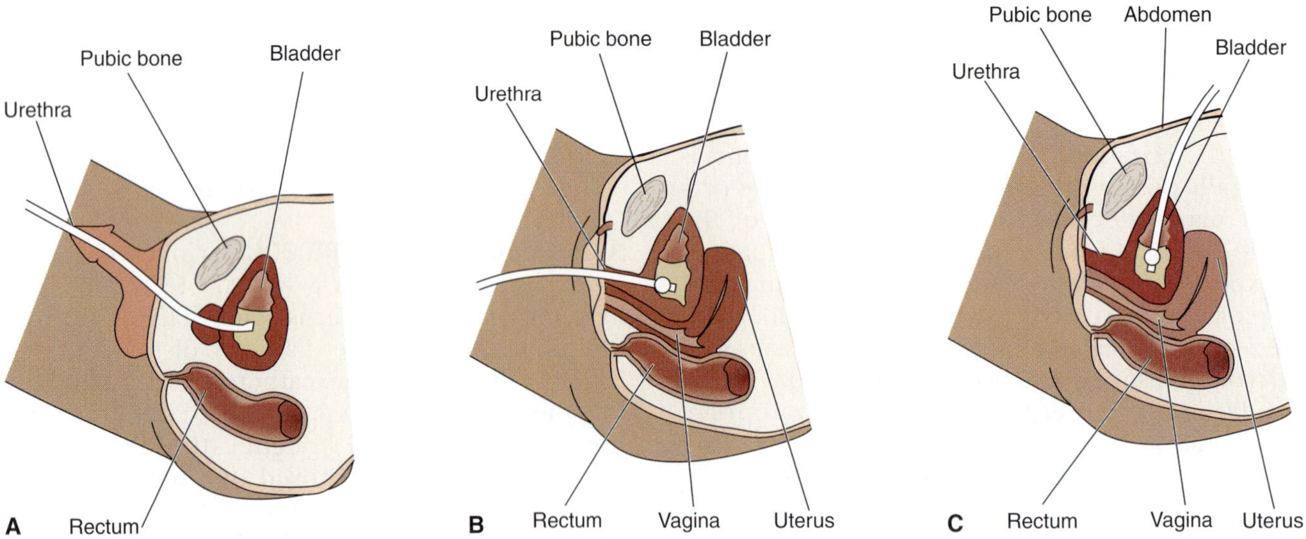

Figure 18-4 Types of urinary catheterizations: (A) Straight catheter. (B) Indwelling catheter. (C) Suprapubic catheter.

Table 18-4 Digestive System Disorders

	Laboratory/Diagnostic Tests						
Disease/ Disorder	**Blood**	**Urine**	**Other**	**Radiography**	**Surgery**	**Medical Tests or Procedures**	**Treatment**
Anorexia nervosa	Complete blood count Electrolytes Blood glucose	Urinalysis				Electrocardiography	Replacement of fluids and electrolytes if needed Psychiatric care
Appendicitis	Complete blood count	Urinalysis Pregnancy test		Abdominal ultra-sound		Rectal examination	Appendectomy
Bulimia	Complete blood count Electrolytes	Urinalysis				Electrocardiography	Replacement of fluids and electrolytes if needed Care of esophagus and teeth erosion Psychiatric care
Cholecystitis	Complete blood count Serum bilirubin	Urinalysis		Cholecystogram (oral or intravenous) Ultrasound of gall bladder			Cholecystectomy
Cholelithiasis	Complete blood count Serum bilirubin			Radioisotope scan Ultrasound of gall bladder Intravenous cholan-giogram			Cholecystectomy Asymptomatic—no treat-ment other than diet modifi-cation (low-fat diet)
Colon cancer	Complete blood count Electrolytes			Barium enema Abdominal ultrasound Computed tomog-raphy (CT) scan of abdomen	Biopsy of colon	Sigmoidoscopy Colonoscopy	Colectomy Resection of colon Radiation Chemotherapy
Crohn's disease	Complete blood count Electrolytes			Abdominal ultra-sound Barium enema Abdominal flat plate	Biopsy of colon	Sigmoidoscopy Colonoscopy Stool culture Pillcam	Nutritional support Medication (antibiotics, anti-inflammatories) Surgery of affected portion of colon (resection)
Diverticulitis	Complete blood count Erythrocyte sedi-mentation rate			Barium enema Abdominal flat plate		Sigmoidoscopy Colonoscopy	Antibiotics Surgery if bowel perforates (colectomy)

(continues)

Table 18-4 Digestive System Disorders (continued)

	Laboratory/Diagnostic Tests						
Disease/ Disorder	**Blood**	**Urine**	**Other**	**Radiography**	**Surgery**	**Medical Tests or Procedures**	**Treatment**
Drug-induced ulcer	Complete blood count Electrolytes		Guaiac test	Upper gastro-intestinal series	Biopsy of stomach	Gastroscopy	Cessation of: • Aspirin • Antiinflammatory drugs (Ibuprofen, Naproxen, etc.) • Corticosteroids • Iron • Methotrexate Treatments • Histamine H_2 blocking agents (Pepcid, Prilosec, Tagamet, Zantac)
Duodenal ulcer	Complete blood count		Breath test *H. pylori* Occult blood test	Upper gastro-intestinal series	Biopsy duo-denum	Upper endoscopy Esophagogastric duodenoscopy (EGD)	Medication: gastric secretion–blocking agent Antibiotics Lifestyle changes Small, frequent meals Gastrectomy if perforation
Enterobiasis	Complete blood count		Stool sample for ova and parasites			Perianal examination	Medication
Gastric ulcer	Complete blood count Serum albumin Transferrin		Guaiac test *H. pylori* Culture stomach secretions Breath test	Upper gastro-intestinal series Abdominal radio-graphs	Biopsy stom-ach lining	Upper endoscopy	Medication: gastric secretion–blocking agent Antibiotics Lifestyle changes Small, frequent meals Gastrectomy if perforation
Gastroenteritis	Complete blood count Electrolytes		Stool culture	Upper gastro-intestinal series		Upper endoscopy	Usually self-limiting Maintain electrolyte balance Antibiotics if indicated Infection control
Gastritis	Complete blood count		Samples of gastric content	Upper gastro-intestinal series	Biopsy of stomach	Gastroscopy	Antacid medications (Prilo-sec, Tagamet, Zantac) Antibiotics if needed

Gastro-esophageal reflux disease (GERD)				Esophageal ultrasonography Gastroscopy		Esophageal manometry	Medication Diet modification Weight loss
Hemorrhoids	Complete blood count				Hemorrhoid-ectomy	Physical examination Proctoscopy	Hemorrhoidectomy Ligation Cryosurgery
Hepatitis	Protein Bilirubin Liver functions Alkaline phosphatase Gammaglobulin	Urinalysis		Ultrasonography of liver	Liver biopsy	Liver scan	Hepatitis A • Immunoglobulin Hepatitis B • No specific treatment Hepatitis C • Medication (alpha-interferon; ribavirin)
Hiatal hernia (Figure 18-6)			pH studies of gastric secretions	Upper gastro-intestinal series Chest radiograph	Biopsy	Gastroscopy	Elevate head of bed for sleep Antacid medications (Prilosec, Tagamet, Zantac) Avoid foods that irritate stomach and esophagus Avoid overeating
Pancreatic cancer	Complete blood count			Ultrasonography Computerized axial tomography scan Endoscopic retrograde cholangiopancreatography (ERCP)		Percutaneous needle aspiration biopsy	Surgical resection (if possible) Radiation therapy Chemotherapy
Pancreatitis	Serum amylase Complete blood count Erythrocyte sedimentation rate			Ultrasonography Computerized axial tomography scan Endoscopic retrograde cholangiopancreatography (ERCP)			Analgesics Diet modification

Table 18-5 Description of Digestive Disorders and Conditions

Anorexia nervosa. An eating disorder of psychological origin. The individual does not eat and becomes **emaciated** (extremely thin) and malnourished because of the need to avoid weight gain.
Appendicitis. Acute inflammation of the appendix usually caused by infection or obstruction. Characterized by pain, nausea, vomiting, and fever.
Bulimia. A syndrome in which an individual binges on food and then purges by inducing vomiting. Laxative abuse is common. The reason individuals engage in this behavior is to avoid weight gain; it is of psychological origin.
Cholecystitis. Inflammation of the gallbladder. Usual cause is gall stones, but other causes may be bacteria or chemical irritants.
Colon cancer. Common malignancy characterized by change in bowel habits, diarrhea or constipation, and abdominal discomfort as tumor grows.
Crohn's disease. Chronic disease that exhibits inflammation of the ileum resulting in diarrhea, right lower quadrant pain, and attacks of diarrhea and frequent blood in the stools.
Diverticulitis. Inflammation of diverticula usually caused by impacted feces or bacteria in the sacs. Pain, cramplike, usually in left side of abdomen. Obstruction can develop.
Diverticulosis. Diverticula in colon without symptoms.
Drug-induced ulcers. Ulcers of the stomach or duodenum caused by taking salicylates (aspirin), corticosteroids, antiinflammatory medications (ibuprofen, naproxen), iron, and Methotrexate.
Duodenal ulcer. Lesion in the mucous membrane of the small intestine usually caused by hyperacidity or *Helicobacter pylori.*
Enterobiasis (pinworms). Intestinal parasites causing intestinal and rectal infection. Pruritus of the anus is a symptom.
Gastric ulcer. Caused by *Helicobacter pylori*, a bactrium, salicylates, smoking, and alcohol.
Gastritis. Inflammation of the stomach lining usually caused by an undefined irritant including alcohol, bacteria, or viruses. It can result in stomach discomfort, nausea, or vomiting.
Gastroenteritis. Inflammation of the stomach and intestinal tract. Causes nausea, vomiting, and diarrhea. May be caused by ingestion of pathogen.
Gastroesophageal reflux disease (GERD). A small valve in the lower esophagus (between the stomach and esophagus) leaks causing stomach acid to back up from the stomach to the esophagus. There is frequent heartburn and discomfort behind the sternum.
Hepatitis. Inflammation of the liver caused by infection from a virus resulting in hepatomegaly, anorexia, and jaundice. *Hepatitis A.* Spread by fecal contamination of food or water. *Hepatitis B.* Spread by blood and body fluids contamination through sexual contact, contaminated needles, perinatal fluids, semen. *Hepatitis C.* Spread by blood (i.e., transfusion), contaminated needles, and sexual contact. Refer to Chapter 10 for more information about hepatitis.
Hiatal hernia. Congenital or traumatic protrusion of stomach through the diaphragm into the chest cavity (Figure 18-6).
Pancreatic cancer. Cancer of the pancreas (usually the head). One of the leading causes of cancer deaths in the United States. Most commonly seen in the 60- to 70-year age group.
Pancreatitis (acute and chronic). Inflammation of the pancreas. Acute: can be a life-threatening event; pancreatic enzymes begin to digest the pancreas causing necrosis and hemorrhage. Chronic: a slow, progressive destruction of the pancreas thought to be from enzymes digesting the pancreas as seen in acute pancreatitis. May be idiopathic or related to alcoholism. Diabetes can be a complication of pancreatitis.

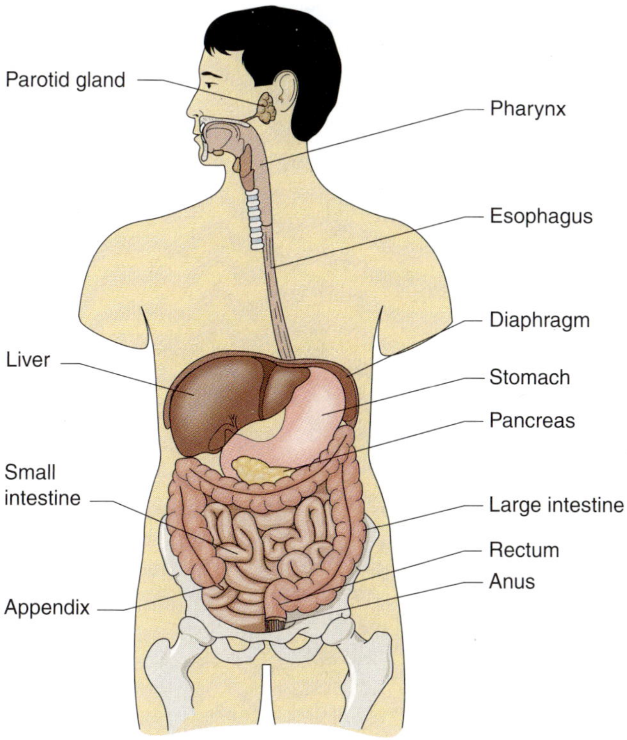

Figure 18-5 The digestive system.

by epigastric pain, nausea, and vomiting of blood (hematemesis). Gastroenteritis (inflammation of the stomach and small intestine), another common ailment, is also known as food poisoning, intestinal flu, and traveler's diarrhea. It can be caused by infections from contaminated food or water, drug reactions, and allergic reactions to particular foods. Peptic ulcers found in the stomach are called gastric ulcers and can be caused by the action of pepsin, an enzyme. It is an erosion (eating away of tissue) of the mucous lining of the stomach. **Salicylates** (such as aspirin), alcohol, smoking, oversecretion of hydrochloric acid, and stress seem to be implicated in this disease. Some gastric ulcers may be caused by the bacterium *Helicobacter pylori* and require antibiotic treatment. Ulcers found in the duodenum are called duodenal ulcers and are similar to gastric ulcers. A duodenal ulcer is an erosion of the mucous lining of the duodenum, a part of the small intestine. If the ulcer is determined to be caused by the bacteria, antibiotics will be prescribed. Both types of ulcers seem to run a chronic course. If they are not controlled, the ulcerated area can perforate (a hole caused by ulceration) and hemorrhage ensues. Contents of the stomach or intestine can spill out into the abdominal cavity and cause a serious complication called peritonitis (infectious organisms enter the membrane covering the internal organs). See Figures 18-7 and 18-8.

Diarrhea is characterized by frequent liquid bowel movements. Diarrhea and vomiting may have many causes such as allergic reactions, infections from food or water, or stress. Dehydration can become a problem if diarrhea continues for several days. Infants, children, and older adults are especially vulnerable to dehydration from vomiting and diarrhea.

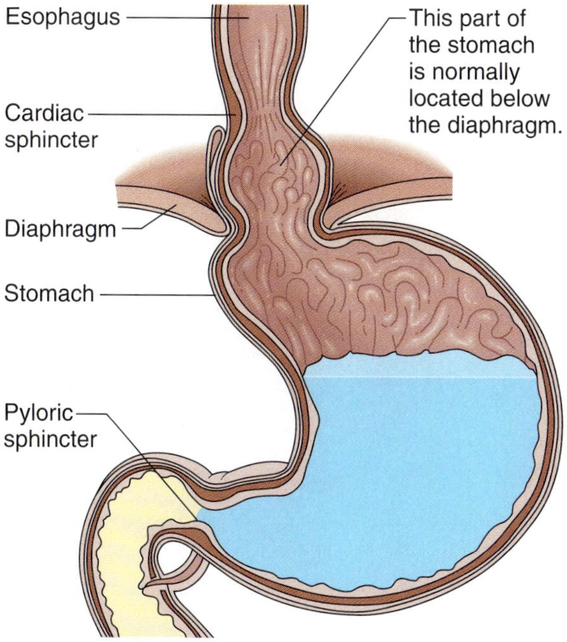

Figure 18-6 Hiatal hernia.

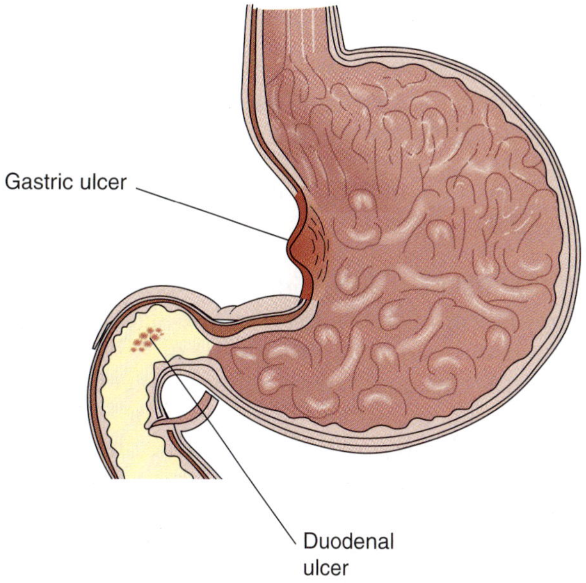

Figure 18-7 Peptic ulcers.

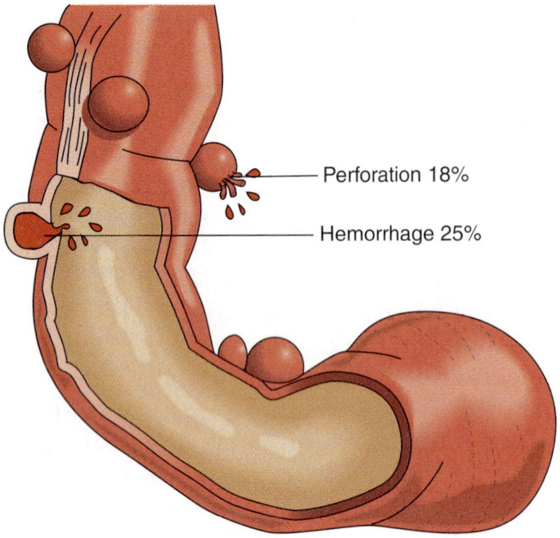

Figure 18-8 Diverticulosis.

Diagnostic Tests

Diagnostic tests for the digestive system commonly include radiography and endoscopy (viewing within the body with a lighted scope). An upper gastrointestinal (GI) series (barium swallow) is done to visualize the esophagus, stomach, and upper portion of the small intestine. A lower GI series (barium enema) visualizes the large intestine (see Figures 18-9 and 18-10 and Chapter 20).

Endoscopy allows the provider to look directly into the digestive organs with a lighted scope. Some examples of endoscopies used in the digestive tract are named by the organ being scoped:

Stomach: gastroscopy

Colon: colonoscopy

Sigmoid colon: sigmoidoscopy

Entire upper GI area: esophagogastroduodenoscopy (EGD); see Figure 18-11

Biopsies can be taken during an endoscopic procedure.

Sigmoidoscopy. Sigmoidoscopy is a diagnostic examination of the interior of the sigmoid colon. It is a useful aid in the diagnosis of cancer of the colon, ulcerations, polyps, tumors, bleeding, and other lower intestinal disorders. The sigmoidoscope is a flexible instrument with a light source and a magnifying lens, which permits visualization of the mucous membrane of the sigmoid colon.

Providers commonly use the flexible sigmoidoscope. Because it is flexible, it can be inserted farther into the colon, making it possible to view

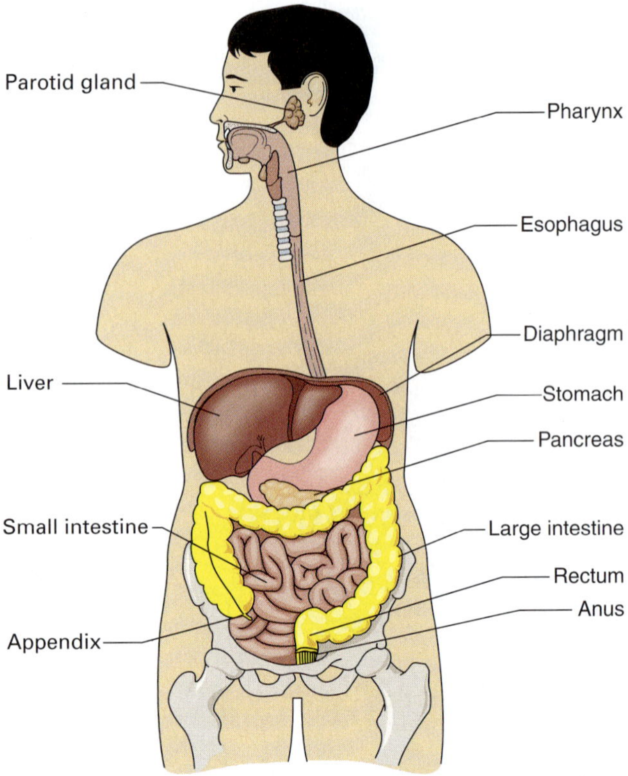

Figure 18-9 Lower gastrointestinal series; highlighted area is visualized.

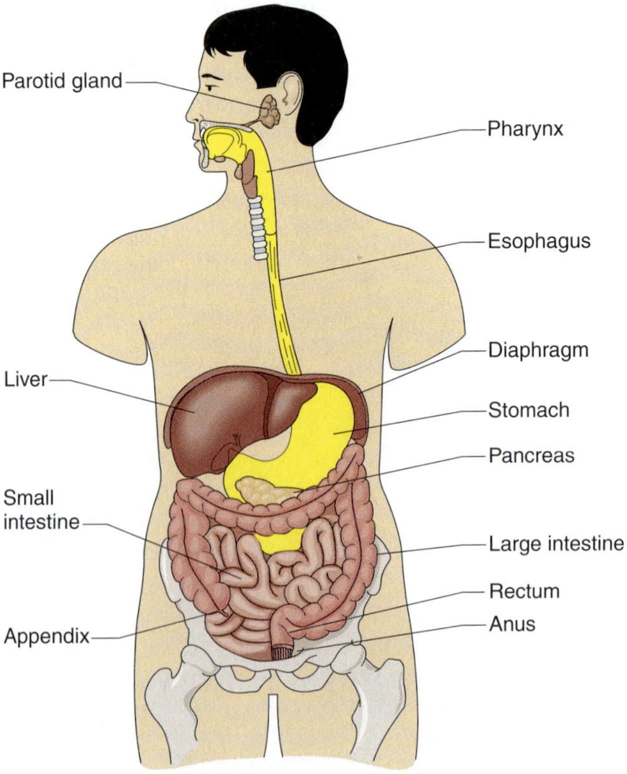

Figure 18-10 Upper gastrointestinal series; highlighted area is visualized.

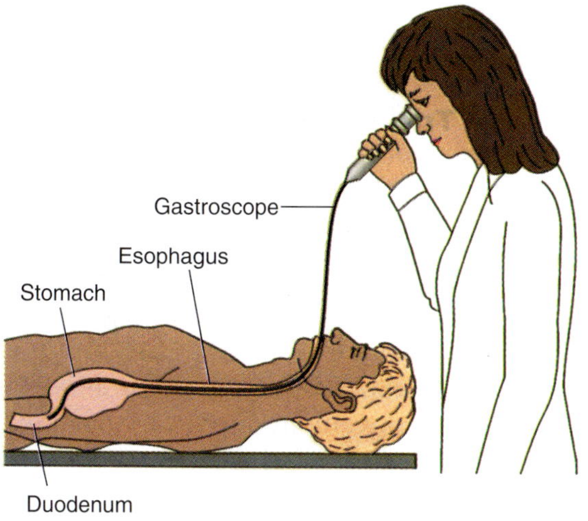

Figure 18-11 Esophagogastroduodenoscopy (EGD) procedure.

more of the mucous membranes of the intestines (Figure 18-12).

As with any examination of the pelvic or abdominal cavity, you should advise the patient to empty the bladder and evacuate the bowel before the procedure begins. This will make the examination easier for both patient and examiner. During the procedure the patient should be instructed to breathe through the mouth deeply and slowly to relax abdominal muscles. Patients may feel the urge to defecate during a colon examination because of the stretching of the intestinal wall from the instrument passing through and air being introduced with it. If patients use the breathing technique mentioned, this discomfort can be relieved. The procedure should last only a few minutes, especially if patients have followed preparation instructions.

Air is sometimes introduced into the sigmoid colon (by the examiner's use of the inflation bulb attached to the scope with tubing) to distend the wall of the colon for easier placement of the lumen of the endoscope. Patients find this to be uncomfortable and sometimes painful. The provider may need to use suction to remove mucus, blood, or fecal material that is obstructing the view of the sigmoid colon.

During these examinations, the medical assistant's roles are to hand necessary items to the provider and to give support to the patient.

Most often it is the medical assistant who teaches the patient how to prepare for the sigmoidoscopy and explains how the test is performed. For successful examination, proper preparation is essential. Have patients restrict dairy

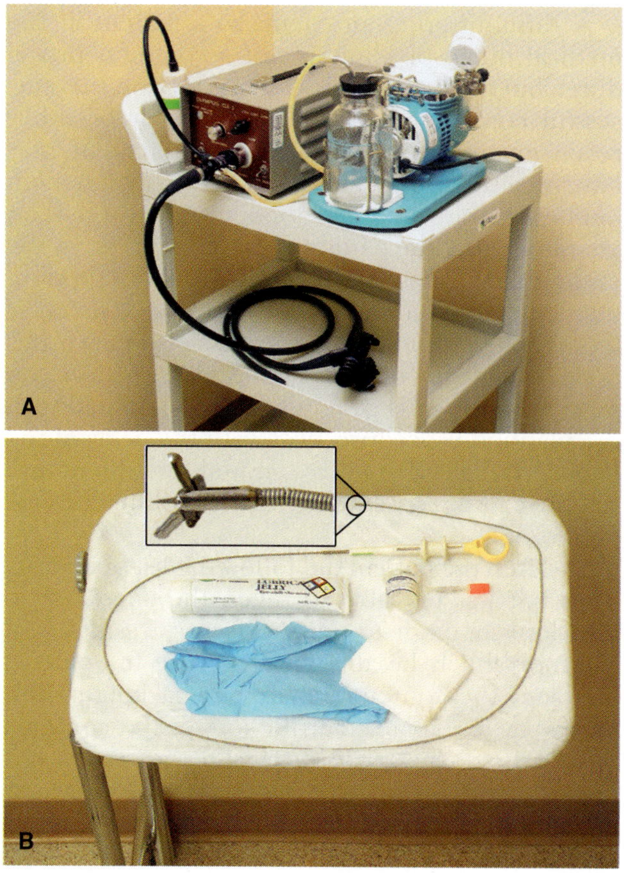

Figure 18-12 (A) Setup for a proctosigmoidoscopy with a flexible sigmoidoscope. (B) Control head of proctosigmoidoscopy.

products, raw fruits and vegetables, and grains and cereals from their diet, and encourage them to drink plenty of clear liquids and eat lightly the day before the scheduled appointment for the sigmoid colon examination. A plain commercial enema should be self-administered at home approximately 2 hours before the examinations. The provider may vary the instructions according to the patient's condition. If patients are not completely informed about preparations and the examination is attempted with unsatisfactory results, the examination will have to be repeated, which is both costly and inconvenient. Satisfactory results are obtained by giving patients both oral and written instructions.

There are occasions when, during an appointment for which the patient was "worked in" to the schedules, the provider believes that the patient's condition warrants examination of the sigmoid colon. In this case, the provider will order an enema to be given to the patient in the office.

Administering an enema to a patient in the medical office or clinic is not a common procedure, but it is sometimes necessary for the successful completion of a sigmoidoscopy or other rectal examination. Even though a patient may have received proper instructions and carried them out before the scheduled appointment, there is no guarantee that the patient achieved success. In the event that the patient comes in for the appointment and the colon is not sufficiently evacuated of feces for a sigmoidoscopy, the physician may order a cleansing enema so that the examination can be completed. It is generally best to proceed with the planned procedure, even with the delay of the enema. Usually this works out well for patient and staff, because rescheduling presents difficulties for everyone.

Often the patient did follow the list of instructions but was not able to retain the enema solution long enough to get satisfactory results. You will more likely be able to encourage the patient to retain the contents of the enema longer. You may want to explain that the longer the contents are retained, the more successful the results will be. Otherwise, it may have to be repeated, or the examination rescheduled. Be certain that you use an examination room that is close to the rest room for the patient's convenience when you administer an enema. Your patience and understanding are needed, because many patients are embarrassed to have an enema administered to them.

Some examinations, such as diagnostic sigmoidoscopy and X-rays, require the use of laxatives by the patient the day before or the morning of the examination. This may present a problem in the patient's personal or employment schedule if instructions are not made clear before the appointment is made. Most patients are fearful of what the diagnostic examination will disclose. Helping them choose a convenient appointment time and explaining the reasons for the preparations they must undergo is usually appreciated.

Proper positioning of the patient during the sigmoidoscopy is important for both the provider's viewing of the rectum and sigmoid colon and the patient's comfort. Proctology tables are designed especially for this procedure (refer back to Figure 13-11). They provide support of the patient's chest and head with the arm resting against the headboard as the table is tilted to the knee-chest position. Patients who cannot tolerate this position are assisted into Sims' position for the examination. Many providers find this acceptable and it is more comfortable for the patient. You should ask

Patient Education

With the provider's direction, you may discuss with your patients the following topics about their digestive health.

1. Remind them that laxatives and enemas should only be used by direction of the provider.
2. Constipation may be avoided/relieved by including fresh fruits and vegetables, cereals, and grains in the diet; drinking plenty of liquids (water); and getting regular exercise.
3. Instruct them that if they have any of the following symptoms persistently it could mean that a disease or an abnormal condition is present and consulting the provider is strongly advised: heartburn or indigestion, nausea or vomiting (especially if coffee grounds consistency), constipation or diarrhea, excessive gas or bloating, stool that is tarry (black), or other than a normal brown color.
4. Inform patients who are 40 years and older that they should routinely test their stool for occult blood every two years for screening of cancer of the colon, or more often if advised by the provider (if family history indicates). All patients older than 50 years should test annually for occult blood and have a colonoscopy.
5. Advise patients to include high-fiber foods in their diets, avoid fat (especially saturated fats) and cholesterol, and eat red meats sparingly.
6. Urge patients to eat a variety of foods (from the food pyramid) and to eat four to six small meals rather than one or two large meals daily to promote better utilization of nutrients and more energy.
7. Suggest to patients that they select snacks and beverages wisely such as fruits, vegetables, and juices over coffee/tea/soda and high-calorie sweets or chips.

about the provider's preference for patient position because there are many variations.

The provider may wish to view the intestinal mucosa after a normal bowel movement. More often, the patient is instructed to eat a light diet containing plenty of clear liquids and avoiding dairy products for 24 hours before the examination, and to have a plain cleansing enema the morning of, or 2 hours before, the examination. Still other provider's may wish patients to use laxatives the day before and an enema the night before and also the morning of the examination.

When making a diagnosis of hemorrhoids, fissures, and ulcerations, the provider usually begins investigative procedures by examining the anus and the interior of the rectum with a proctoscope. During the sigmoidoscopy, the provider may want to take a biopsy of questionable tissue from the sigmoid colon to aid in confirming the diagnosis. It is a good rule to have all possible necessary items available. When the patient has been prepared and the provider is ready to begin the examination, the medical assistant hands the necessary instruments and supplies to the provider as needed. Remember to advise patients to report any problems, such as bleeding, discharge, swelling, or any other unusual discomfort, after the procedure. A biopsy laboratory request form must be completed and accompany the tissue to the laboratory. Containers for biopsy specimens have a formaldehyde solution to preserve the tissue until the analysis is done.

Whereas the proctosigmoidoscope examines the rectum and sigmoid colon with a flexible scope, a procedure known as a **colonoscopy** (viewing the colon with a lighted scope) can be scheduled in the outpatient department of the hospital or endoscopy center or performed in the office or clinic. A flexible fiberoptic colonoscope is used, and the entire length of the large intestine (colon) can be examined for lesions such as tumors, polyps, fissures, and masses. Biopsies that consist of small tissue pieces can be removed with a snare-type instrument inserted through the colonoscope. The tissue is microscopically examined by a pathologist to determine whether a malignancy (cancer) is present in the colon (Figure 18-13). The patient may receive a muscle relaxant/tranquilizer to facilitate the examination. (See "Endoscopic Procedures" later in this chapter.)

Patient Education

After sigmoidoscopy, patients should drink plenty of clear fluids to help relieve the abdominal discomfort and flatulence. Patients may also find relief in lying in a prone position with a pillow across their midabdominal area to aid in the passage of gas.

Critical Thinking

Phyllis Lomeli, a new patient of Dr. Reynolds, has been experiencing gastrointestinal problems. Dr. Reynolds has ordered fecal occult blood tests for the patient. What diet instructions does the medical assistant give to the patient? What directions and supplies does the medical assistant give to the patient? When the guaiac slides are returned by the patient, how does the medical assistant develop and interpret them?

Fecal Occult Blood Test. Patients may be instructed to obtain three stool specimens at home for examination of a fecal sample for occult (hidden) blood. The patient will be given occult blood slides, applicators, and envelopes to take home (Figure 18-14). The patient will need to obtain two small stool samples from each of three separate bowel movements. Three separate samples are used to allow detection of blood from GI lesions that exhibit intermittent bleeding. The medical assistant's role is to instruct the patient about how to properly collect the stool specimens on the

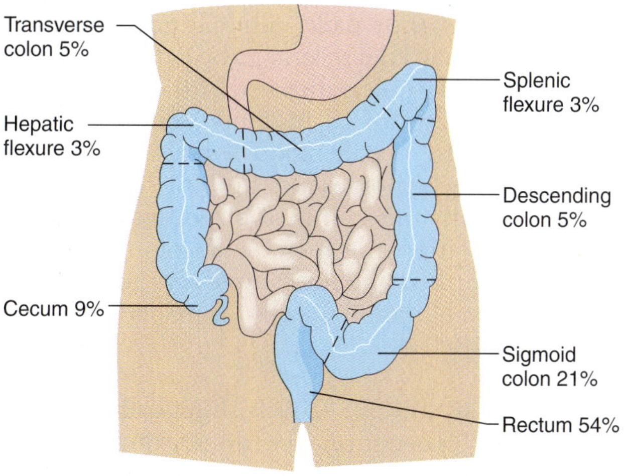

Figure 18-13 Incidence of colorectal cancer by site.

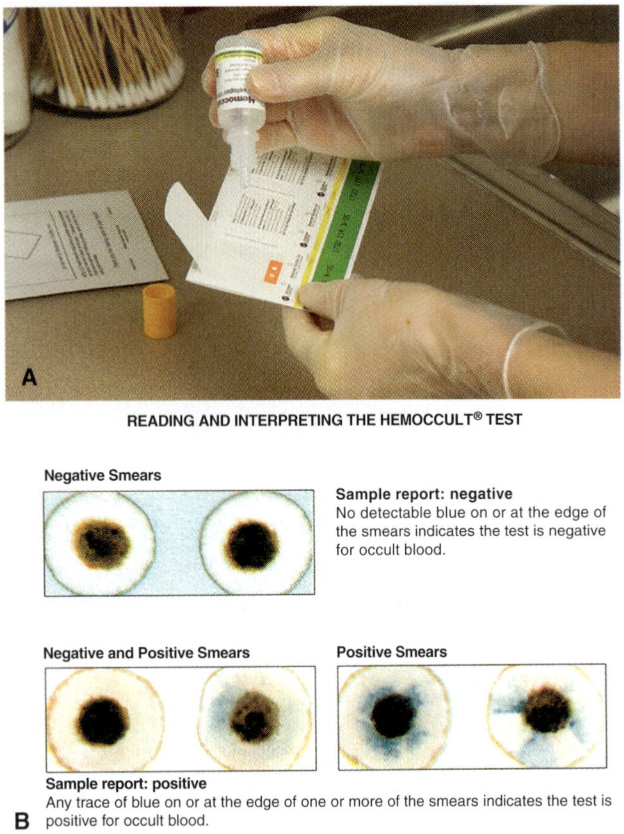

A
READING AND INTERPRETING THE HEMOCCULT® TEST
Negative Smears
Sample report: negative
No detectable blue on or at the edge of the smears indicates the test is negative for occult blood.
Negative and Positive Smears
Positive Smears
Sample report: positive
Any trace of blue on or at the edge of one or more of the smears indicates the test is positive for occult blood.
B

Figure 18-14 (A) Place the required number of drops of developing solution on the exposed guiac paper. (B) A change in color indicates that blood may be present in the stool.

test slides, and then how to care for and store the slides until they are returned to the office by the patient (see Procedure 18-3). Biohazardous material (feces) cannot be sent through the United States Postal Service.

For patients who have daily bowel movements, this will not be a problem. For patients who have difficulty with daily elimination, collecting the samples may take several days. Patients should not use laxatives unless directed by the provider.

Positive tests for occult blood require further testing, because occult blood testing is a screening tool only. Sigmoidoscopy and/or colonoscopy help to identify the source of bleeding. If a lesion is found in either the rectum or colon, a biopsy can be performed and the sample sent to the laboratory for examination of cells for malignancy (see Procedure 18-3).

Radiographic Studies of the Digestive System. Endoscopic procedures are done routinely but have not replaced the need for radiographic studies of the gastrointestinal tract. There are several diagnostic radiographic studies can be performed in order to study digestive structures and functions looking for disease. They include the upper GI series (barium swallow) (Figure 18-15), lower GI series (barium enema), and the cholecystogram. Table 18-6 lists the purpose, patient preparation, and procedures for each of these three studies.

Bariatrics

Millions of people in the United States are obese and are ill with or at serious risk for diabetes, heart disease, hypertension, certain cancers, stroke, sleep apnea, and many other conditions. Obesity affects every body system in a negative way. Emotional problems such as depression, rejection, low self-esteem, isolation, and chemical substance abuse are common. **Bariatrics** is the field of medicine that treats obesity and conditions associated with obesity.

Some obese patients decide, with their provider's recommendation, to undergo bariatric surgery because of the physical and emotional problems caused by their obesity. Prior to surgery, patients (with their provider's guidance) must bring their existing medical problems, such as uncontrolled diabetes, severe hypertension, hyperlipidemia, and gall bladder disease, under control. Stabilization is important to prevent serious complications before, during, and after surgery.

Bariatric surgery is performed to treat obesity and to help the patient lose weight. It can be

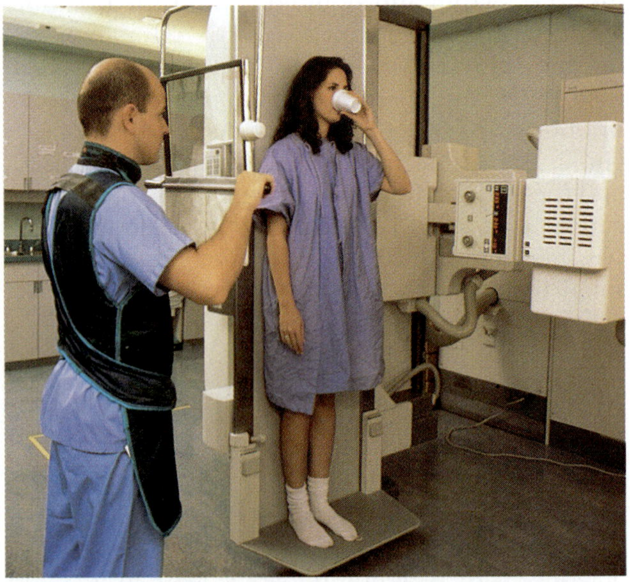

Figure 18-15 In a barium swallow test, barium sulfate is swallowed and radiographs are taken of the esophagus, stomach, and small intestine. This is also known as an upper gastrointestinal series.

Table 18-6 Patient Preparation and Procedure for Radiographic Studies of the Digestive System

Test	Purpose	Patient Prep	Procedure	Time
Barium swallow (upper gastrointestinal [GI] series)	To study the esophagus, stomach, duodenum of the small intestine for disease (ulcers, tumors, hiatal hernia, esophageal varices)	Day before radiograph: 1. Light evening meal 2. NPO after midnight Day of test: 1. NPO Postprocedural: 1. Increase fluid intake 2. Take laxative as prescribed	1. The patient is asked to drink a flavored barium mixture while standing in front of fluoroscope 2. The radiologist observes the passage down the digestive tract 3. The patient is turned to various positions to allow good visualization of the intestine 4. Radiographs are taken	1 hour
Barium enema (lower GI series)	To study the colon for disease (polyps, tumors, lesions)	Clear liquid 1 day prior (allowed: non-carbonated beverages, clear gelatin, clear broth, coffee and tea with sugar) No milk or milk products 8 oz water every hour until bedtime Prep kit: to include bottle of magnesium citrate, Dulcolax tab(s) Day before radiograph: 1. Late afternoon drink bottle of magnesium citrate 2. Early evening take Dulcolax tab(s) as prescribed 3. Light evening meal. NPO except water, after dinner Morning of procedure: 1. NPO 2. Cleansing enema Postprocedural instructions: 1. Increase fluid intake and dietary fiber 2. Report to provider if no bowel movement within 24 hours of test	1. The colon is filled with a barium sulfate mixture 2. The patient is turned in various positions to allow the barium to fill the colon. Air is injected to move the barium along the colon 3. When the colon is full, radiographs are taken	1–2 hours
Cholecystogram	To study the gall bladder for disease (stones, duct obstruction), inflammation	1. Evening before test fat-free dinner 2. Take dye tablets with 8 oz water 3. Cathartic or cleansing enemas may be prescribed 4. NPO after dinner and tablets	1. A series of radiographs is taken 2. A fatty meal may be given to stimulate the gall bladder to empty 3. Other radiographs can then be taken to check gall bladder function	1 hour

accomplished with a standard abdominal incision or laparoscope. Two procedures that can be performed are "banding" or "stapling" and gastric bypass surgery (Figure 18-16). With banding or stapling, the bottom of the esophagus (where it enters the stomach) is banded or stapled, thus shrinking the stomach. An adjustable port in the abdomen controls the tightness of the band or staples. In gastric bypass surgery, the surgeon creates a pouch out of a small portion of the stomach and attaches it directly to the small intestine, thereby passing the stomach and duodenum. As a result, absorption, which occurs in the small intestine, is reduced. Before surgery, patients are counseled

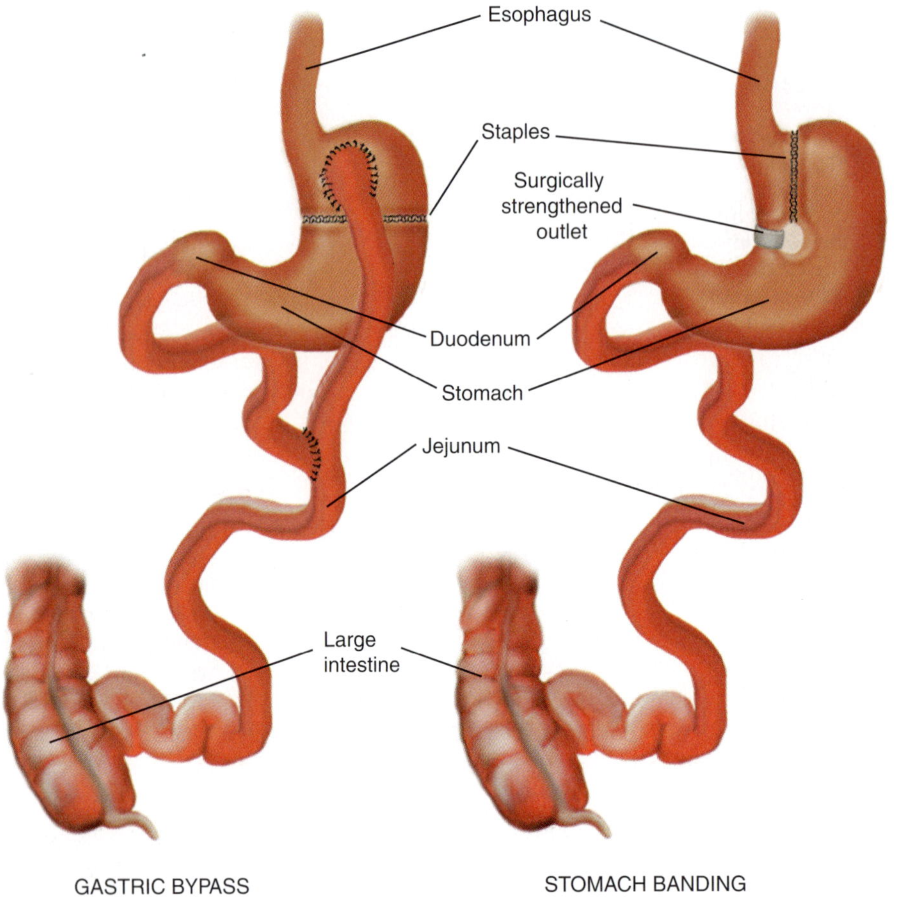

Figure 18-16 Gastric bypass and stomach banding are bariatric surgical procedures.

Patient Education

Follow specific package instructions.

The following steps should be followed 2 days before the fecal occult blood test and continued until three slides have been prepared:

1. Avoid red meats, processed meats, and liver. These release hemoglobin that can produce a false-positive result.
2. Avoid turnips, broccoli, cauliflower, and melons. These foods may contain a substance, peroxibase, that will cause a false-positive result.
3. Avoid aspirin, iron supplements, and large doses of vitamin C for 7 days before the test. These substances may cause gastric bleeding that can mask bleeding from a lesion.
4. Consume a high-fiber diet. Fiber provides roughage to promote bowel movement and encourage bleeding from any lesion that may be present.
5. Do not begin test during menses, for three days after menses, or if bleeding from hemorrhoids.
6. Drink plenty of fluids to help prevent constipation.
7. Store slides at room temperature and protect from heat, sun, and fluorescent lights.

about possible side effects, such as malabsorption, anemia, vomiting, diarrhea, hernias, and blood clots.

The surgery is considered for patients who are **morbidly obese** who have tried numerous weight loss and exercise regimens without results and are at serious risk for heart disease, stroke, cancer, and other conditions. Body mass index (BMI) is another factor considered when providers evaluate patients for surgery. A BMI around 30 to 40 (a general guideline) is one of the criteria used to determine which patients are candidates for the surgery (normal BMI is 18.5–24.9). The presence of other diseases is also a factor in the evaluation.

Caring for bariatric patients is challenging. Their emotional health is important. Being nonjudgmental and showing empathy for these patients is very important. They suffer from discrimination, prejudice, and isolation. Obesity is a chronic illness that requires patience and understanding.

SENSORY SYSTEM

The special senses of vision, hearing, equilibrium (balance), smell, touch, and taste permit the body to detect information about the environment. The eyes, ears, nose, taste buds, and skin are all sense organs that contain specialized receptor organs. Table 18-7 lists diseases and disorders and diagnostic tests and procedures for eyes and ears.

Patient Education

Several Web sites (e.g., CDC, Mayo Clinic, Weight Watchers) can automatically calculate BMI after inputting the patient's height and weight measurements. The following are formulas for determining BMI:

1. Multiply weight, in pounds, by 0.45 (130 pounds × 0.45 = 58.5).
2. Multiply height, in inches, by 0.025 (5 feet 6 inches or 66 inches × 0.025 =1.65).
3. Multiply the answer from step 2 by itself (1.65 × 1.65 = 2.72).
4. Divide the answer from step 1 by the answer from step 3 (58.5 ÷ 2.72 = 21.48).
5. If the BMI is less than 21, the individual is underweight.
6. If the BMI is equal to or greater than 25, the individual is overweight.
7. A BMI equal to or greater than 30 indicates obesity.

The Eye

The eye is the primary organ for sight and is one of the few organs of the body externally exposed. Its accessory structures—the eyelids, eyelashes, lacrimal ducts, and extrinsic muscles—provide protection for the eye. The anterior portion of the eyeball protrudes outward and the remainder is protected by the orbit.

The intraocular structures consist of some parts of the eye visible externally and parts visible only through an ophthalmoscope. The intraocular structures include the following:

- *Sclera:* white area covering the outside of the eye except over the pupil and iris
- *Cornea:* clear tissue covering the pupil and iris
- *Iris:* round disk of smooth and radial muscles giving the eye its color
- *Pupil:* round opening in the iris that changes size as the iris reacts to light and dark
- *Anterior chamber:* space between cornea and iris/pupil filled with clear fluid called aqueous humor
- *Posterior chamber:* space between the iris and lens that is filled with aqueous humor
- *Lens:* clear fibers enclosed in a membrane that refract and focus light to the retina
- *Posterior cavity:* space in the posterior part of the eyeball filled with thick, gelatinous material called vitreous humor
- *Posterior sclera:* white opaque layer covering the posterior part of the eyeball
- *Choroid layer:* layer between the sclera and retina containing blood vessels
- *Retina:* inside layer of the posterior part of the eye that receives the light rays (visual stimuli)

The mechanism of vision occurs after impulses leave the retina and travel through the optic nerves to the brain. At the optic chiasm, the nerve fibers cross and continue to the thalamus. These fibers synapse with other neurons that send the impulses to the right and left visual area of the occipital lobe of the brain. Because the tracts cross at the optic chasm, the stimuli coming from the right visual fields are translated in the visual area of the left occipital area, and the stimuli coming from the left visual fields are translated in the visual area of the right occipital lobe. Table 18-8 describes common

Table 18-7 Sensory System Disorders

	Laboratory/Diagnostic Tests					
Disease/ Disorder	**Blood**	**Other**	**Radio-graphy**	**Surgery**	**Medical Tests or Procedures**	**Treatment**
Amblyopia					Ophthalmologic examination	Cover the normal eye to force weaker eye to function
Cataract					Ophthalmologic examination Slit lamp	**Phacoemulsification** Surgical extraction
Chalazion				Excision		
Color blind-ness					Ishihara color plates	
Conjunctivitis		Culture and sensitivity of eye dis-charge		Stained smears of conjuncti-val scrap-ings		Antibiotic drops or antibiotics Ointment
Corneal abrasion					Fluorescein stain	Antibiotic ointment, dressing over affected eye
Diabetic retinopathy				Laser	Fluorescein agiography	Laser
Epistaxis	Complete blood count			Nasal	Blood pressure	Electrocautery
External otitis	Complete blood count	Culture and sensitivity of exudate			Otologic exami-nation	Antibiotic therapy Laser (if severe)
Glaucoma					Vision field testing Ophthalmologic examination includ-ing intraocular pressure Tonometry	Medicated eye drops Oral medication Laser surgery Conventional surgery or a combination
Impacted cearumen					Otologic exami-nation	Removal with curette Irrigation
Macular degeneration					Ophthalmologic examination Angiography **Amsler grid**	Laser Intraocular injections Intravenous medication Some untreatable

(continues)

Table 18-7 (continued)

	Laboratory/Diagnostic Tests					
Disease/ Disorder	**Blood**	**Other**	**Radio-graphy**	**Surgery**	**Medical Tests or Procedures**	**Treatment**
Ménière's disease					Audiometry, magnetic resonance imaging **Electrocochleography**	Medication, surgery only if severe
Motion sickness						Medication
Myopia					Ophthalmologic examination	Radial keratotomy
Nystagmus					**Opticokinetic drum test** Neurologic examination	Directed at cause (inner ear or central nervous system)
Hyperopia					Astigmatoscopy	Corrective lenses
Presbyopia					Snellen chart	Corrective lenses
Astigmatism					Ophthalmic exam	Corrective lenses
Nasal polyps				Biopsy of polyp (lesion)	Nasal examination	Electrosurgery
Otitis media	Complete blood count	Culture and sensitivity of exudate		Myringotomy Tympanostomy	Tympanography	Antibiotics Myringotomy
Otosclerosis					Audiometry Rinne test	Stapedectomy
Retinal detachment				Laser or surgery to reattach	Ophthalmologic examination	Laser
Sinusitis	Complete blood count	Culture and sensitivity of exudate	Sinus X-rays			Antibiotics for bacterial infection
Strabismus					Ophthalmologic examination Neurologic examination	Cover the normal eye to force weaker eye to function
Stye (hordeolum)		Culture and sensitivity if exudate present		Incision and drainage		Antibiotic ointment

Table 18-8 Description of Eye Disorders

Refraction and Other Disorders:
• *Astigmatism.* Irregular lens curvature or cornea shape causing improper focusing of objects.
• *Cataract.* Lens loses its transparent nature caused by changes in its proteins. Usually brought on by aging or sunlight.
• *Color blindness.* Inability to distinguish among colors. Caused by an absence of a cone photopigment, a genetic disorder.
• *Conjunctivitis.* Caused by a bacterial infection or irritant resulting in irritated and reddened conjunctiva. If caused by bacteria, conjunctivitis.
• *Corneal abrasion.* Caused by an injury to the cornea by a foreign body resulting in pain, tearing, redness, and possible infection.
• *Diabetic retinopathy.* Diabetes mellitus causes damage to the retina because the disease causes vascular changes. This is the leading cause of blindness in the United States.
• *Glaucoma.* Condition caused by increased intraocular pressure due to a buildup of aqueous humor. This results in mild visual disturbances with little or no pain but can lead to severe visual impairment if untreated.
• *Nearsightedness (myopia).* Caused by an elongated (shaped) eyeball and the image is focused in the front of the retina resulting in the inability to focus on objects at a distance.
• *Farsightedness (hyperopia).* Caused when the eyeball is irregularly shaped (shortened) and the image is focused behind the retina causing distance vision to be unclear.
• *Presbyopia.* Attributed to the aging process when the lens loses its elasticity and the ability to accommodate. Vision is hampered when items are close.
• *Retinal detachment.* Complete or partial separation of the retina from the choroid layer of the eye, leading to possible blindness.
• *Stye (hordeolum).* Inflamed sebaceous gland of the eyelid caused by bacterial infection. Erythema and tenderness at site are common symptoms.

eye disorders. Figures 18-17 and 18-18 illustrate the anatomy of the eye.

Signs and symptoms that are common to eye diseases and disorders are pain or burning in the eye (conjunctivitis) or around the eye (hordeolum), decreased visual acuity, and any visual changes such as seeing sudden flashes of light, which may indicate retinal detachment (see Figures 18-19 to 18-21).

Measuring Visual Acuity. A procedure commonly performed by the medical assistant is the measuring of a patient's visual acuity. This is only a screening process used when errors in refraction are suspected. The procedure must be performed in a well-lit, quiet area. While performing the procedure, the medical assistant must observe the patient for any action that may indicate difficulty with vision. These actions include squinting, wiping of the eyes, or leaning toward the chart. In near-vision acuity, these actions include holding the card nearer or farther than the stated position. The commonly used chart for distance visual acuity is the Snellen chart for the adult. Near-vision is commonly checked by using the Jaeger card.

The Jaeger chart used for checking clear vision is a small card that the patient holds between 14 and 16 inches from the eye. The medical assistant measures the distance for accuracy. This is the distance from which a person with normal vision is able to read printed material such as a newspaper. The Jaeger test consists of a series of reading material, the letters of which gradually become smaller. Record the last line number that the patient can easily read. The patient is checked with and without corrective lenses, and each eye is checked separately.

Errors in refraction is the term used to designate visual acuity abnormalities. The common visual abnormalities include myopia (nearsightedness), the ability to see only near objects clearly; hyperopia (farsightedness), the ability to see only distant objects clearly; and astigmatism, uneven curvature of the cornea resulting in a scattering of light rays producing blurry vision. Presbyopia (associated with the aging process) is an increase in farsightedness and a loss of lens elasticity that is necessary to accommodate for near vision (Figure 18-22).

The Snellen chart consists of the alphabet letters in various combinations starting at the top with a large E, and letters of descending size by line toward the bottom. Each line is labeled with the visual acuity measurement. The Snellen chart for children has pictures. Non–English-speaking patients may use a directional chart.

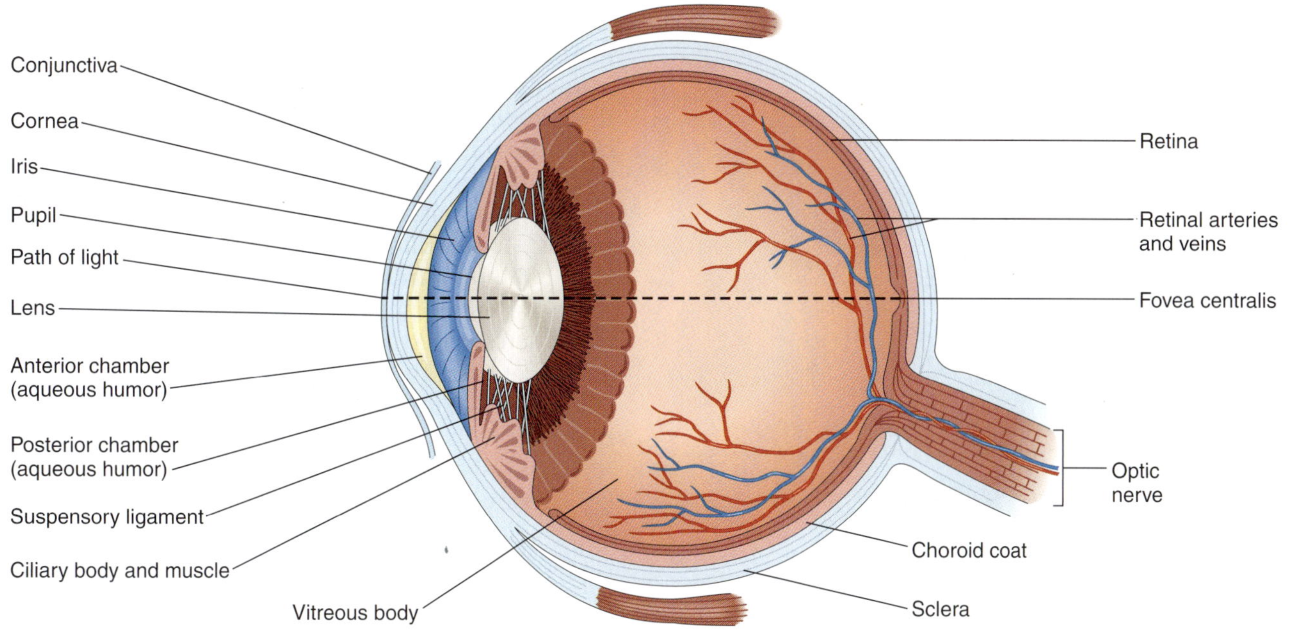

Figure 18-17 The eyeball—cross-sectional view.

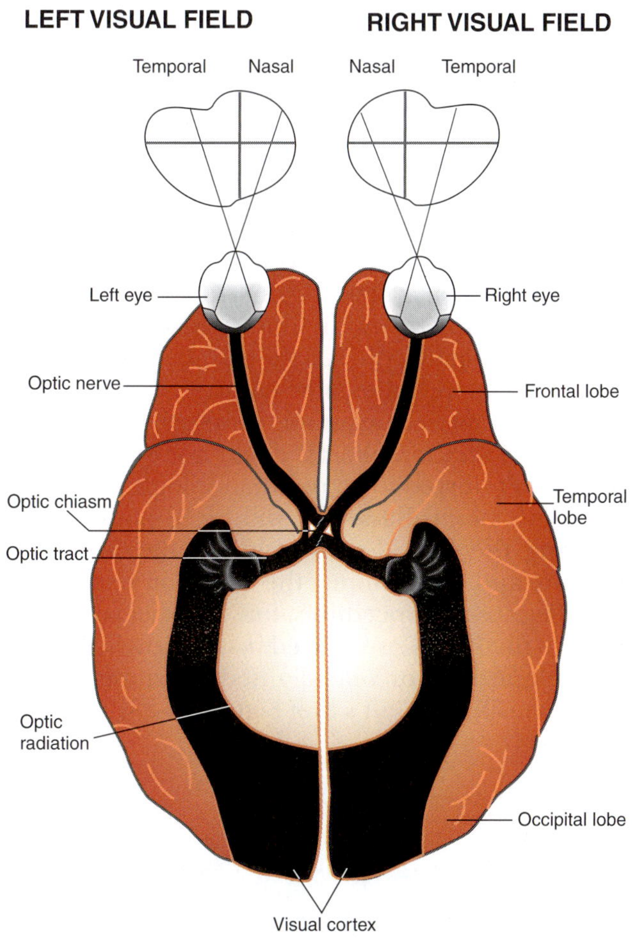

Figure 18-18 The visual pathways of the eye.

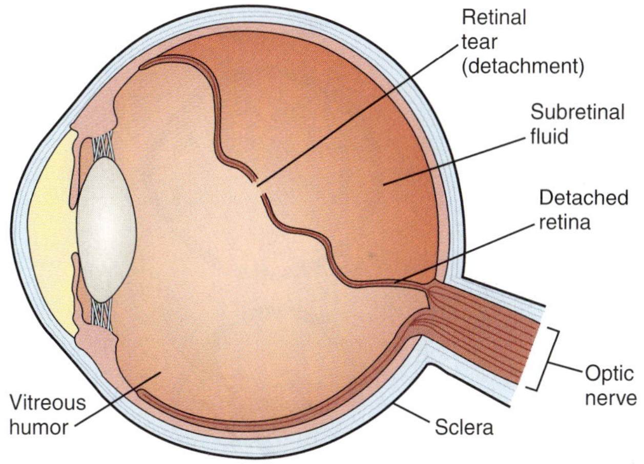

Figure 18-19 Detachment of the retina.

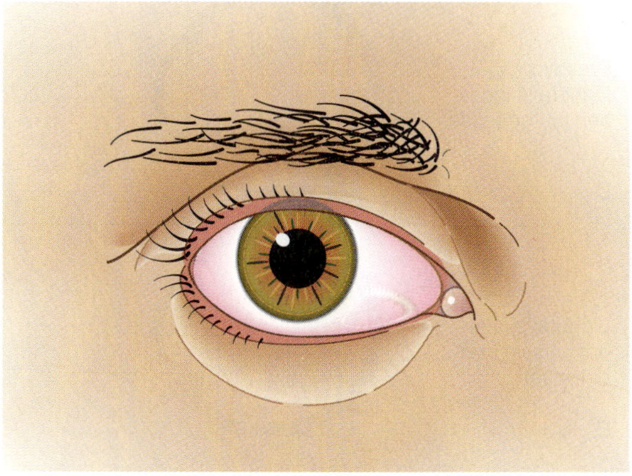

Figure 18-20 Conjunctivitis.

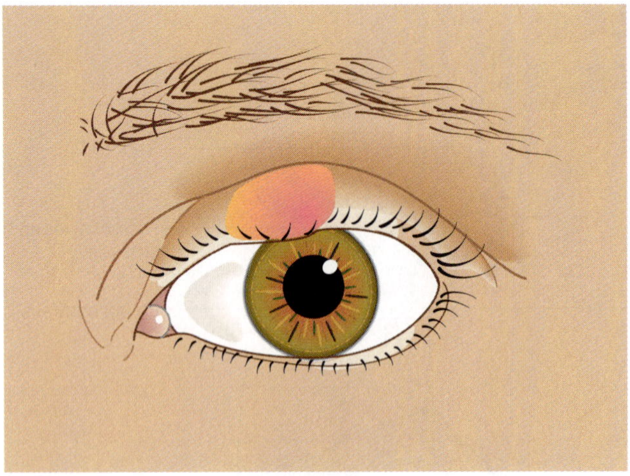

Figure 18-21 Stye (hordeolum).

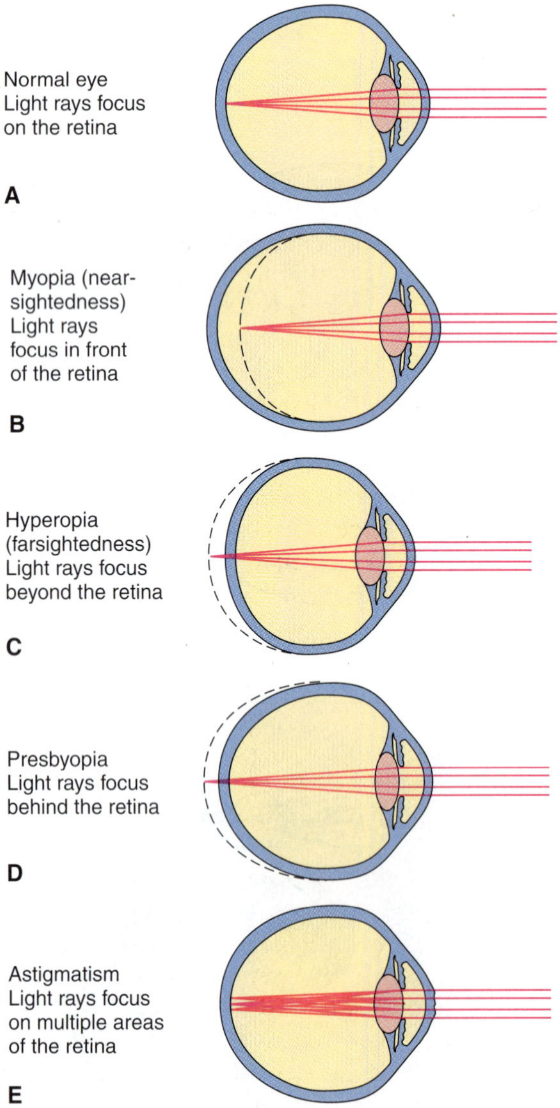
Normal eye
Light rays focus on the retina
A
Myopia (near-sightedness)
Light rays focus in front of the retina
B
Hyperopia (farsightedness)
Light rays focus beyond the retina
C
Presbyopia
Light rays focus behind the retina
D
Astigmatism
Light rays focus on multiple areas of the retina
E

Figure 18-22 (A) Normal eye vision. (B) Myopia. (C) Hyperopia. (D) Presbyopia. (E) Astigmatism.

Recording Visual Acuity. Visual acuity, both near and far, is recorded in a fraction format. The numerator indicates the 20-foot distance between the patient and the chart. The denominator indicates the visual acuity of the patient in relationship to the normal seeing eye. Normal vision is 20/20. This means that at 20 feet the eye is seeing what the normal eye would see at 20 feet. Should the vision be 20/30, this indicates that the eye is seeing at 20 feet what the normal eye would see at 30 feet away. A visual acuity of 20/15 indicates that the eye is seeing at 20 feet what the person with normal visual acuity would be able to see at 15 feet. Vision is recorded on the patient chart as right eye, left eye, and both eyes.

Example: Right 20/20 Left 20/20
Both 20/20

Patients should be screened with and without their corrective lenses and the results recorded in patients' charts or electronic medical records.

Color Vision. Checking color vision is not part of a routine examination. This procedure is usually performed on people who must distinguish color as part of their occupation (e.g., truck drivers, pilots, and salespeople). A commonly used color vision test is the Ishihara color graph. The Ishihara test chart book contains pages composed of varying sized and colored circles. Inside the circles are numbers or lines that can be traced. The patient is seated for the procedure with the book held 14 to 16 inches away and is instructed to identify the numbers as the page is turned or is instructed to trace the line from the indicated starting point to the end. Inability to see the number or to follow the line may indicate color blindness. Should this occur, the medical assistant must inform the provider as to what number(s) could not be seen. The patient is referred to an ophthalmologist.

The medical assistant will be responsible for assisting the provider in ophthalmologic examinations and performing the tests for visual acuity. Diagnostic procedures for the special senses involve the use of specialized instruments. The use of the ophthalmoscope (lighted instrument used to view inside patient's eye; Figure 18-23) assists in

Critical Thinking

List the steps the medical assistant must follow when performing a visual acuity test on a 9-year-old child and on a 3-year-old toddler.

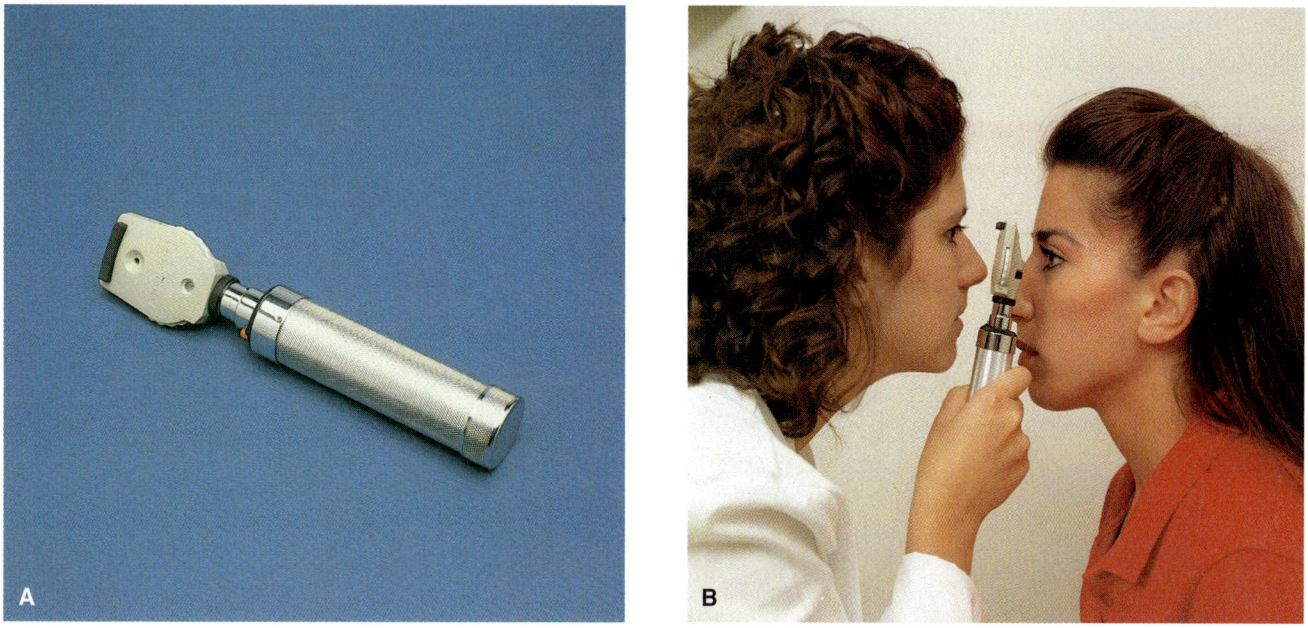

Figure 18-23 (A) The ophthalmoscope is used to identify eye disorders. (B) The provider uses the ophthalmoscope to view the interior of the patient's eye.

identifying disease-related problems. The interior of the eye can be examined.

Procedures 18-4 though 18-9 list the steps for specialty procedures for the eye.

The Ear

The structures of hearing and equilibrium are divided into the external ear, the middle ear, and the inner ear. The external ear includes the pinna **(auricle)** and the external auditory canal. The pinna is mostly cartilaginous tissue with a small amount of adipose tissue in the earlobe. The external auditory canal is about 1 inch in length and contains hair and wax (cerumen)-producing glands. The external ear and middle ear are separated by the tympanic membrane (eardrum).

The middle ear, also called the tympanic cavity, is a small space containing three bones, the malleus (hammer), incus (anvil), and stapes (stirrup). Next to the stapes is the oval window that leads to the inner ear. The eustachian tube connects the middle ear to the throat.

The inner ear is the most sophisticated part of the ear. It is responsible for both hearing and equilibrium (balance). The inner ear consists of a fluid-filled sterile space housing the vestibule, the semicircular canals, the round window, and the cochlea. The structures in the vestibule are responsible for maintaining equilibrium during movement of the head. The semicircular canals assist the body to adjust to changes in direction. The movement of fluid in this area can cause symptoms of dizziness. The cochlea is the organ of hearing.

The outer ear (auricle/pinna) picks up sound waves that are sent through the external auditory canal to the tympanic membrane. The membrane vibrates in reaction to the sound striking it. These vibrations pass through the three tiny middle ear bones through the oval window and into the fluid in the cochlea. Receptor cells respond and transfer the sounds into electrical impulses that travel to the brain via the acoustic nerve. The receiving area of the brain for auditory impulses is in the temporal lobe (Figure 18-24).

Diseases or conditions of the ear, if left untreated, can cause damage to nerves and tissues and can result in some degree of hearing impairment, from mild to deafness. Table 18-9 describes common diseases of the ear.

Measuring Auditory Ability. The simple methods of measuring hearing (gross hearing) are usually performed by the provider. The patient may be instructed to place a finger in one ear while the provider whispers one or two words in the other. The patient is then asked to repeat the words. A ticking watch may be placed by the patient's ear to ascertain hearing. A vibrating tuning fork may be placed on the mastoid process behind the ear and then on top of the head. The patient is asked

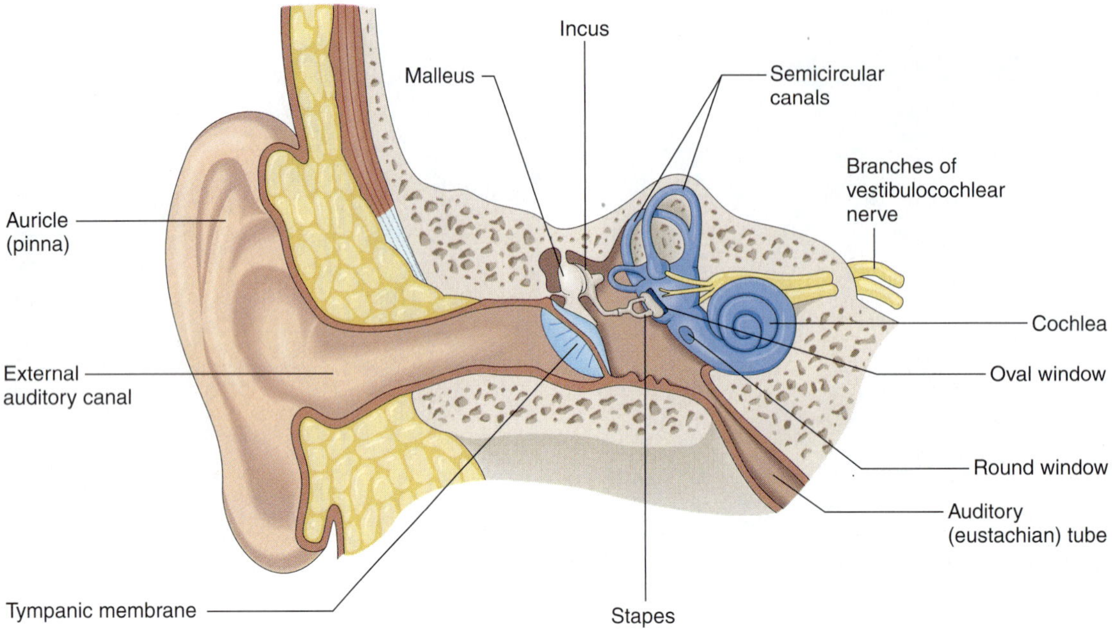

Figure 18-24 The ear.

if the sound vibrations could be heard or felt. This procedure will identify nerve or conduction deafness (Figure 18-25). Conduction deafness occurs when the sound wave is not transmitted to the middle ear. This type of deafness may be a result of the presence of impacted ear wax (cerumen) in the ear canal or a scarred tympanic membrane.

Cerumen, or ear wax, is a substance secreted by glands at the outer third of the ear canal. In some individuals it can accumulate and block the canal and become impacted (pressed firmly against the tympanic membrane). The sound waves cannot pass through the hardened cerumen to the middle ear, and hearing loss (conduction hearing loss) results.

To remove impacted cerumen, the provider may use a curette. The patient may have had ear drops prescribed before the physical removal of the impacted cerumen. The drops are instilled in an effort to soften the cerumen to facilitate its removal. An ear irrigation may be performed by flushing the ear canal with warm water or a solution ordered by the provider. Commercial solutions are available for patients to use at home (see Procedure 18-11).

A scarred tympanic membrane can occur from a ruptured or perforated tympanic membrane. This can occur from untreated acute otitis media or traumatic rupture. With acute otitis media, the tympanic membrane is red and bulges from accumulation of serous or purulent fluid behind it. The pressure of the fluid on the tympanic membrane may be so great that the membrane ruptures and drainage can be seen in the ear canal. The perforation or rupture will probably heal, but a small scar on the membrane will remain. Repeated ruptures from acute otitis media will cause repeated scarring and diminished hearing function (conduction hearing loss). A culture and sensitivity of the drainage (purulent or serous) will indicate the antibiotic to which the microorganism is sensitive.

Table 18-9 Ear Disorders

External otitis (swimmer's ear). Inflammation of ear canal. Symptoms are itchiness and crusting of ear canal.
Otitis media. Acute infection of the middle ear usually caused by bacteria. Symptoms are pain, fever, discharge, and decreased hearing acuity.
Otosclerosis. Conduction deafness caused by hardening of the stapes.
Ménière's disease. Characterized by deafness, vertigo, nausea, and tinnitus. Probable cause is edema of the labyrinth.
Impacted cerumen. Caused by accumulation of hardened cerumen that has built up against the tympanic membrane. Impaired hearing and tinnitus can result.

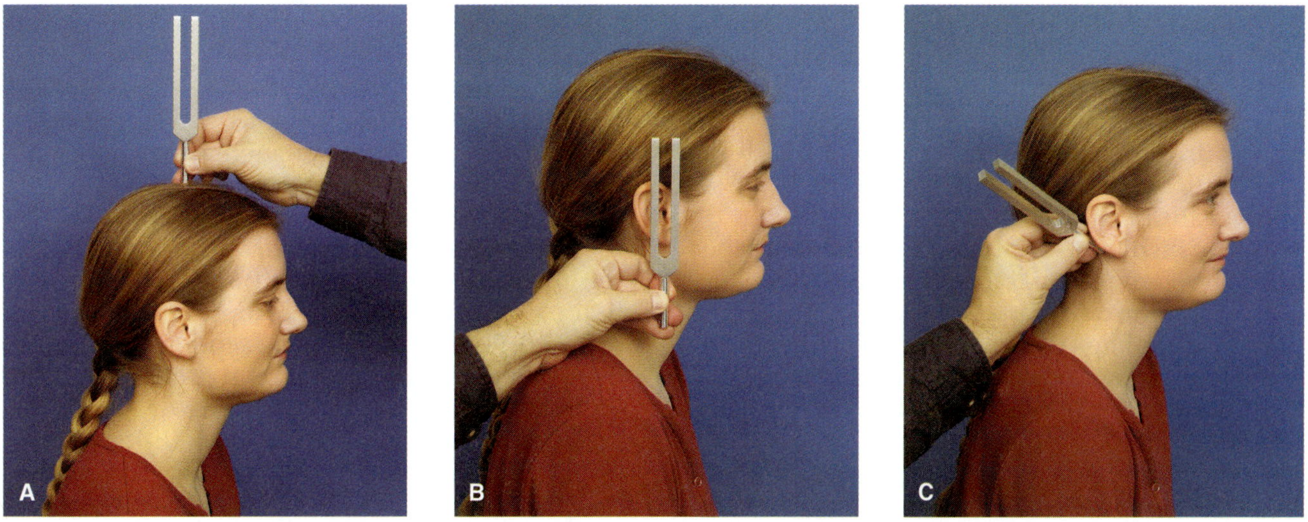

Figure 18-25 (A) The provider holds the tuning fork against the crown of the patient's head to determine which ear can hear the sound. (B) To check air conduction of sound, the provider holds the tuning fork 1 inch from the patient's auditory meatus. (C) The provider places the tuning fork on the bony prominence (mastoid bone) behind the patient's ear to check bone conduction of sound.

A myringotomy is a surgical incision into the tympanic membrane made to remove accumulated fluid caused by infection. Because the procedure is surgical in nature, the tympanic membrane can be incised to allow the fluid to drain. Scarring is minimized because the incision is made with a scalpel in a controlled location and will heal with less scarring. Tubes may be placed in the opening (tympanostomy) made by the myringotomy to equalize pressure and prevent fluid from accumulating (see Chapter 15).

Nerve deafness is a result of injury along the course of the nerves leading from the inner ear to the auditory centers of the brain.

A more complex procedure for measuring hearing may be performed by the medical assistant but more often by an audiologist, using an audiometer. A quiet room with no distractions is required for the procedure to be accurate. The patient is seated facing away from the medical assistant and the audiometer, then ear phones are placed over the ears. The patient is instructed to raise a hand when a sound is heard. The audiometer has two dials, one for the various wavelengths and the other for wave intensity. Starting at the lowest pitch, the intensity is increased until the patient responds to the sound. The next pitch is then tested in the same manner. This process continues until the highest pitched sound is tested. The results are obtained by noting the number of intensity at which the sound was heard. When performing the procedure, the medical assistant must not develop a pattern that can be detected by the patient. The ears should be tested in an alternating fashion to ensure accuracy (see Procedure 18-10 and Figure 18-26).

The medical assistant employed in an industrial medical facility may be required to monitor hearing of some employees. In this case, care must be taken to have the hearing test performed before the employee goes to work for the day. Hearing loss may result from the day's activities in some noisy facilities even when ear plugs are worn.

Tympanometry is a procedure used to ascertain the ability of the middle ear to transmit sound waves and is commonly performed on children to diagnose middle ear infections. A

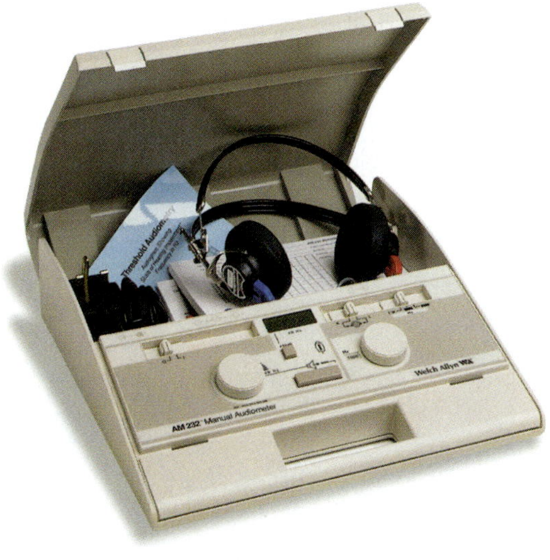

Figure 18-26 Manual audiometer. (Courtesy of Welch-Allyn.)

probe is inserted into the ear canal to measure the air pressure of the ear canal in relation to the air pressure found in the middle ear. Tympanogram is the recording produced by this procedure. The waves and peaks are measured providing an indication of possible middle ear abnormalities (Figure 18-27).

The medical assistant or the provider may perform the audiometry test. Diagnostic procedures for the ear involve the use of specialized instruments, including the **otoscope** (lighted instrument to examine the tympanic membrane), which assists in identifying disease-related ear problems (Figure 18-28).

Procedures 18-10, 18-11, and 18-12 describe steps for audiometry, ear irrigation, and ear instillation.

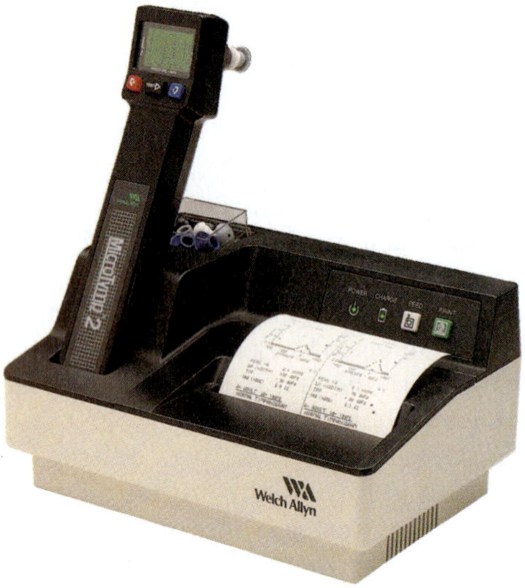

Figure 18-27 A portable tympanometric instrument with charger. A printout of the tympanogram can be seen. Testing is done in 1 second and is useful for diagnosing otitis media and other middle ear conditions, such as patency of tympanostomy tubes and otosclerosis. (Courtesy of Welch-Allyn.)

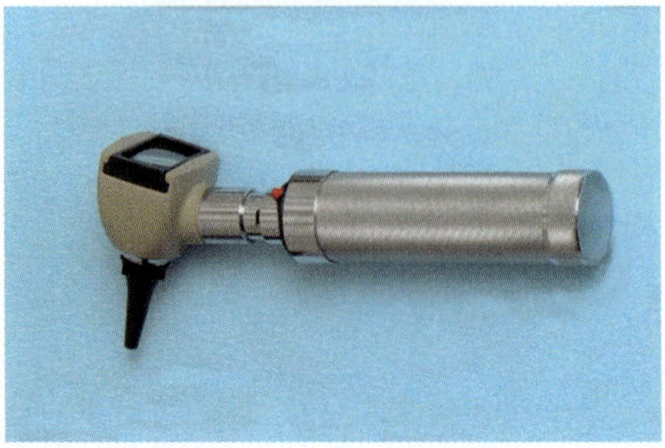

Figure 18-28 The otoscope is used to examine the patient's tympanic membrane.

The Nose

The provider inspects the exterior surface of the patient's nose for skin lesions such as **rosacea,** squamous or basal cell carcinoma, and other dermatologic problems. The provider examines and palpates to determine if the nose is patent and for the patient's ability to breathe in and out through the nose (through each nostril). The mucous membrane is checked for polyps, superficial blood vessels, and foreign bodies. The septum is noted for deviation. Epistaxis is a common problem and can be treated with electrocautery and/or nasal packing. Procedures 18-13, 18-14, and 18-15 describe steps for specialized procedures and examinations for the nose.

RESPIRATORY SYSTEM

The respiratory process is all important to the life process. **External respiration** allows for the exchange of carbon dioxide and oxygen across the cell walls into the airspaces of the lungs. **Internal respiration** is the exchange of these gases at the cellular levels of the organs.

The respiratory process begins with air entering the nose or mouth, where it passes through the pharynx, down into the trachea, into the **bronchi,** and then enters the lungs. Gas exchange takes place when the blood filters through the alveoli (smallest air sacs in the lungs) (Figure 18-29). Table 18-10 lists diagnostic procedures for respiratory diseases and disorders. Table 18-11 discribes respiratory disorders.

Signs and Symptoms of Respiratory Conditions and Disorders

If a patient's chief complaint indicates a respiratory condition or disorder, medical attention is essential. Some signs and symptoms include:

- Dyspnea
- Chest pain
- Fatigue
- **Hemoptysis**
- Chills and fever
- Hoarseness
- Wheezing
- Cough, productive or nonproductive

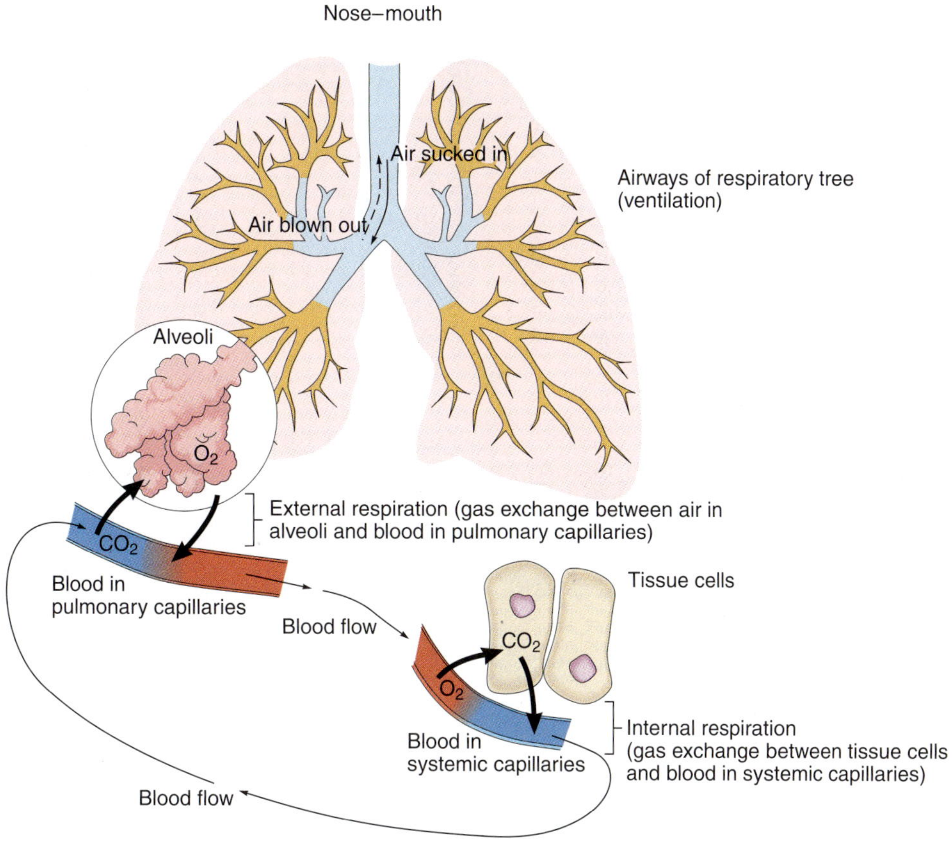

Figure 18-29 Gas exchange in the lungs and tissues.

Irrigations of the nose, collection of sputum specimens, and assisting with pulmonary tests are the roles of the medical assistant.

Diagnostic Tests

A fundamental test, auscultation of the chest, is used to check for abnormalities in breathing rate and quality. Lung function tests can be done. Chest X-rays are useful in helping to diagnose tuberculosis (Figure 18-30), lung lesions, pneumonia, and other respiratory conditions. Cultures of sputum can help diagnose infections in the respiratory tract. Bronchoscopy is used to take a sample of lung tissues (biopsy) for help in the determination of lung cancer and for culture of lung abcesses, washing, and irrigation. A spiral CT scan produces a sharper image of the lungs than a conventional CT scan.

Arterial blood gases measure the amount of oxygen and carbon dioxide in the arterial blood. Higher amounts of carbon dioxide and lower amounts than normal of oxygen indicate poor lung functions.

Pulmonary function tests such as spirometry are helpful. Procedures 18-16 through 18-19 describe specialized respiratory examinations and procedures.

Spirometry

The measurements of air flow, volume, and capacity are known as pulmonary function tests (PFTs). The patient's height, age, and sex are used in the PFT. Many times the provider requests the PFT be perfomed before the administration of a **bronchodilator** and again after the bronchodilator. This is useful in evaluating the effectiveness of the medication (see Procedure 18-18).

A commonly used tool in the medical office or clinic, **spirometry** (test to measure lung capacity) assists the provider in the evaluation of signs and symptoms of pulmonary disease by measuring the air capacity (air flow and volume) of the lungs (Figure 18-31). Many components of lung functions are measured including the following three components:

1. Forced virtual capacity (FVC), which represents the volume of air that can be exhaled from the lung after the lung is filled with air to meet its total capacity

Table 18-10 Respiratory System Disorders

	Laboratory/Diagnostic Tests					
Disease/ Disorder	**Blood**	**Other**	**Radiography**	**Surgery**	**Medical Tests or Procedures**	**Treatment**
Acute or adult respiratory distress syndrome (ARDS)	Complete blood count Blood chemistry Prothrombin time Partial thromboplastin time Arterial blood gases	Electrocardiography Urinalysis	Chest radiograph	Tracheotomy	Thoracentesis	Antibiotics Ventilator Oxygen
Asthma	Complete blood count Arterial blood gases	Sputum analysis Peak expiratory flow rate	Chest radiograph		Pulmonary function tests Skin testing for allergies	Medication (bronchodilators) Metered-dose inhaler Treatment of hypersensitivity
Bronchitis	Complete blood count	Sputum culture and analysis	Chest radiograph		Bronchoscopy	Antibiotics if secondary bacterial infection occurs
Emphysema (chronic obstructive pulmonary disease [COPD])	Complete blood count Arterial blood gases	Spirometry	Chest radiograph		Pulmonary function tests Pulse oximetry	Bronchodilators
Epistaxis	Complete blood count			Nasal cauterization	Blood pressure	Packing of nose, cautery
Influenza	Complete blood count		Chest radiograph			Symptomatic Antibiotics if secondary bacterial infection occurs
Laryngitis	Complete blood count	Throat culture Rapid strep test			Laryngoscopy	Throat lozenges Analgesics
Lung cancer	Complete blood count	Sputum cytology	Chest radiograph CT scan	Biopsy of lung tissue	Bronchoscopy	Surgery Chemotherapy Radiation

Nasal polyps				Biopsy of lesions	Nasal examination	Surgical excision
Pharyngitis	Complete blood count	Throat culture Rapid strep test				Lozenges Gargling
Pleurisy	Complete blood count		Chest radiograph			Taping of chest Antibiotics if bacterial Analgesics
Pneumonia	Complete blood count	Blood culture Sputum smear	Chest radiograph			Antibiotics if bacterial Symptomatic treatment if viral
Severe acute respiratory syndrome (SARS)	Complete blood count Blood chemistry Serum antibodies of SARS	Throat or nasopharyngeal swab Viral culture	Chest radiograph			Antiviral drugs Steroids Symptomatic treatment
Sinusitis	Complete blood count	Culture and sensitivity	Sinus radiographs		Nasal examination	Decongestants Antibiotics
Tonsillitis	Complete blood count Streptococcal antibody test	Throat culture		Tonsillectomy		Antibiotics
Tuberculosis	Complete blood count	Sputum culture Acid fast smear of sputum	Chest radiograph Bronchoscopy	Biopsy of lung tissue	Tuberculin skin test: Mantoux intradermal	Multiple anti-tuberculosis medications

Table 18-11 Description of Respiratory Disorders

Acute or adult respiratory distress syndrome (ARDS). A life-threatening condition that occurs when there is severe fluid buildup and hemorrhage in the lungs. ARDS is breathing failure that can occur in critically ill patients with underlying illnesses. There is a high mortality rate. Patients may be placed on isolation precautions (see Chapter 10).
Asthma. Inflammation and spasm of the smooth muscle of the bronchi brought on by an allergen or emotional upsets. Characterized by dyspnea and wheezing.
Bronchitis. Inflammation of the bronchi, caused by viral or bacterial infection with a dry, painful cough, progressing to a productive cough of greenish yellow sputum. Symptoms include cough, slight fever, chills, malaise, and soreness under the sternum.
Emphysema. Enlargement of the alveoli due to lost elasticity, usually brought on by a long-time irritant, such as cigarette smoking. Results in dyspnea, chronic cough, weight loss, and the appearance of a "barrel chest."
Epistaxis. A nosebleed. May be caused by trauma, chronic sinus irritation, drug abuse (esp. "snorting" drugs), hypertension, blood disorders, and high altitude.
Influenza. A viral infection of various strains of the upper respiratory tract. Sudden onset of chills, fever, cough, sore throat, gastrointestinal disorders are common. Can range from mild to life-threatening.
Laryngitis. Hoarseness, cough, aphonia caused by infections from nose or throat.
Lung cancer. Cancer that may appear in trachea, air sacs, bronchi, and other lung tissues and cells.
Nasal polyp. A tumor of the nose that can bleed easily. Should be removed surgically.
Pharyngitis. Inflammation of the pharynx caused by a bacteria, virus, or an irritant. Difficulty in swallowing, pain, redness, and inflammation of the pharynx are some of the symptoms. Streptococcus is the most common bacterial infection; influenza virus and the common cold virus are the most common viral agents involved. May be accompanied by fever, malaise, and headache.
Pleurisy. Inflammation of the pleura caused by bacteria or viruses. Symptoms include pain, fever, cough, chills, and dyspnea.
Pneumonia. Inflammation of the lungs caused by bacteria, fungi, viruses, and chemical irritants. Usually has sudden onset and is characterized by chills, fever, chest pain, cough, and purulent sputum. Symptoms include sore throat, fever, and lymphadenopathy.
Severe acute respiratory syndrome (SARS). An acute viral respiratory illness that begins with fever, headache, body aches, general malaise, and diarrhea. There may be mild respiratory symptoms at the onset. Most patients will develop pneumonia. The virus is spread by close person-to-person contact (i.e., kissing, hugging, sharing eating or drinking utensils, talking to someone within 3 feet [respiratory droplets], and touching someone directly). The patient will be placed on isolation precautions (see Chapter 10).
Sinusitis. Inflammation and infection of a sinus or sinuses. May be caused by allergies, bacteria, viruses, or polyps.
Tonsillitis. Inflammation of the tonsils usually caused by streptococcus. Tonsils become red and enlarged causing severe pharyngitis and fever.
Tuberculosis. Inflammatory infiltrations, formation of tubercles, abscesses, fibrosis, and calcification. Can lead to infection of other body systems. Is highly infectious. Airborne Precautions necessary to prevent transmission of the disease.

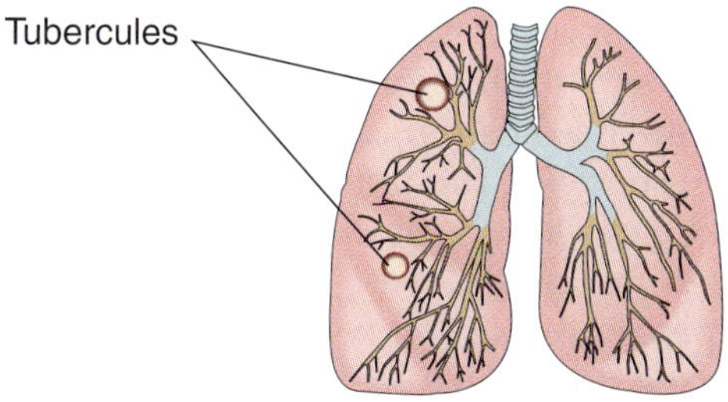

Figure 18-30 Tuberculosis.

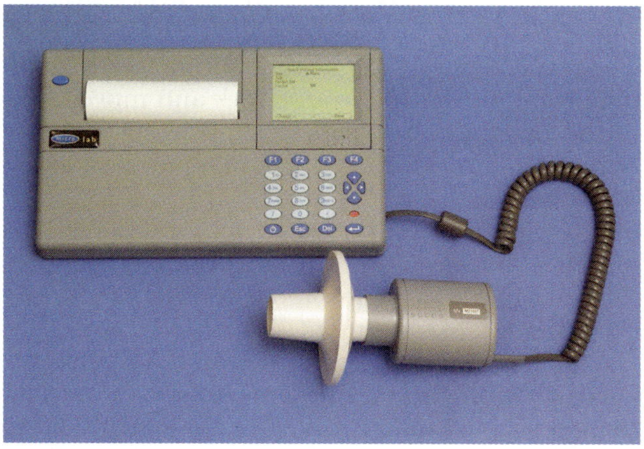

Figure 18-31 The spirometer is used to measure pulmonary function.

2. Forced expiration volume at 1 second (FEV), which is the volume of gas forcibly exhaled from the lungs after the first second and third second of expiration
3. Mean expiration flow (MEF) rate, which is a measure on a volume–time curve halfway through an exhalation

There are other measurements done after exhaling with force, after a normal exhalation, and how quickly the patient can exhale after a slow inhalation and others.

Most spirometers are computerized, and thus automatically calculate the lung functions. Results are stored in the electronic health record and readily accessible for comparison.

Peak Expiratory Flow Rates

Peak expiratory flow rates (PEFRs), as part of pulmonary function studies, help determine the extent of a patient's asthma or other pulmonary disorder. The PEFR is the measurement of the fastest rate of the flow of air that is exhaled from the lungs. It is measured with a peak flow meter. The PEFR is lower in an individual experiencing an asthma attack caused by impaired expiration and trapped air in the lungs.

Patient Education

Instruct Patient on Use of Peak Flow Meter

1. Slide the indicator to the bottom of the scale (may be done by the medical assistant).
2. Sit up straight or stand.
3. Hold the peak flow meter upright.
4. Inhale as deeply as you possibly can.
5. Form a tight seal around the mouthpiece with your lips.
6. Blow out as quickly and as hard as you can to exhale all of the air out of your lungs.
7. The force of your exhalation will cause the indicator to rise in the meter.
8. The medical assistant will have you use the peak flow meter twice more and will record the highest number.

NOTE: For accurate results, it is very important to inhale and exhale as completely as possible.

Pulse Oximetry

Pulse oximetry is test that uses a small probe with an infrared light. The probe is placed on the earlobe, toe, finger, or bridge of the nose. It evaluates the amount of oxygen saturation in the blood. This is helpful because cyanosis is not manifested until the saturation of oxygen is less than 85%. Pulse oximetry is useful in the diagnosis and evaluation of impaired respiratory and cardiac functions. A reading less than 95% indicates hypoxemia. It is not unusual for a patient being tested for sleep apnea to experience a pulse oximetry of under 75%.

The appropriate body part is selected, and a clip (sensor) is placed on it (typically the finger). One side of the sensor is an infrared light, and the other side is a photo detector. The infrared light passes through the tissues and blood vessels, and the detection measures the amount of light absorbed by hemoglobulin. This noninvasive procedure measures the amount of hemoglobin and can be performed on any patient, but especially those with impaired heart and lung function. Postoperative patients are attached to an oxygen pulse oximeter in the recovery room. The patient is likely to have shallow, less effective respirations because of the anesthesia or narcotics. The patient must not be wearing nail polish (see Procedure 18-19 and Figure 18-32).

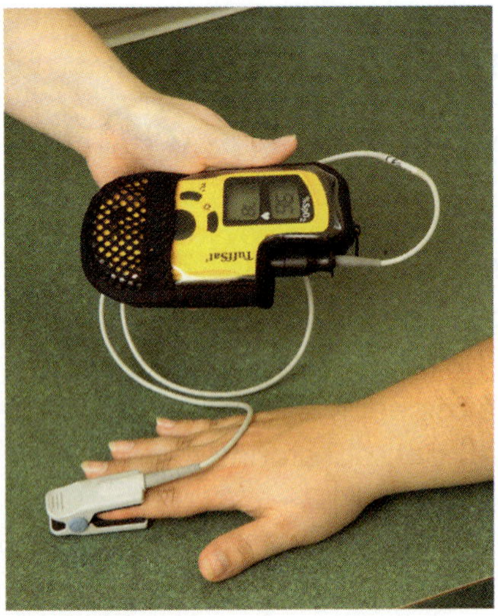

Figure 18-32 Apply the sensor to the selected site—in this case, the finger.

Inhalers

Inhalers are devices that are used to deliver medication into the lungs and are most often used to treat asthma. A number of different types of inhalers are available: metered dose inhaler (MDI), metered dose inhaler with spacer (MDIS), dry powder inhaler (DPI), and nebulizer.

The MDIS is the preferred method. A tube that attaches to the inhaler and holds the medication until the patient can breathe it in is called the *spacer.* It makes the MDI easier to use and helps get the medication into the lungs better. A mask can be attached to the spacer for children or for an individual who has difficulty inhaling correctly with a conventional spacer. However, an MDI can be used without a spacer.

Some medications for asthma are in the form of a powder and can be taken with a handheld device known as a DPI. This device delivers medication to the lungs when the patient inhales through the device. However, some patients cannot inhale through the device with sufficient force to breathe in the medication well.

A nebulizer is an apparatus that changes the medication for asthma from a liquid form into a mist for ease of inhaling the medication into the lungs. Nebulizers work well for infants and young children and for any person who is unable to use an MDIS. The different types of nebulizers all work in essentially the same way. The nebulizer hose is connected to an air compressor. The medicine cup is filled with the appropriate dose of liquid along with saline. If a single dose, the contents of the vial the are squeezed into the medicine cup. The hose and mouthpiece are attached to the medicine cup. The patient puts the mouthpiece into the mouth and exhales, and then breathes through the mouth until all the medication is used, about 10 to 15 minutes. Alternatively, the nebulizer can be used with a mask. The mask must fit well to prevent medication from getting in the eyes. The medicine cup and mouthpiece are washed with water and allowed to air dry (see Procedure 18-17).

MUSCULOSKELETAL SYSTEM

The muscular and skeletal systems interact to coordinate the supporting framework and movements of the body. The musculoskeletal system includes bones, joints, muscles, and surrounding tissue. The skeletal system provides support; protects vital organs; and allows for the attachment of ligaments, tendons, and muscles. The muscular system gives the body form and shape and is responsible for the coordination of movement.

Bones of the skeletal system store minerals for later use by the body. They are classified according to their shape. Bones provide for the attachment of muscles and joining of another bone, which allows for the passage of nerves and blood vessels. The skeletal system is divided into two parts: the **appendicular skeleton** (126 bones) and the **axial skeleton** (80 bones).

One of the top four reasons a patient visits a provider is for back pain. During the visit, the provider evaluates the patient for contributory factors for the pain by assessing the patient for deformities, asymmetry, and signs of restricted motion. The provider performs a functional assessment by observing the patient's gait (manner of walking) for indications of decreased mobility and postural changes associated with aging or injury. Flexion tests with a goniometer detect the degree of resistance applied to a given force, thus defining restricted motion and the amount of discomfort associated with movement. Supine straight leg raising (SLR) tests detect the amount of hamstring flexibility and can assess sciatic nerve damage.

There are more than 600 muscles in the body. Muscles are composed of bundles of muscle fibers, each with the ability to contract and relax. Any disease process that disrupts the balance between the muscular and skeletal systems severely hampers a person's ability to move effectively and painlessly (Tables 18-12, 18-13, and 18-14).

Diagnostic procedures involving the skeletal system involve the extensive use of various forms of radiographs and visual examination techniques. A bone biopsy may be ordered when additional diagnostic data are required.

Table 18-12 Musculoskeletal System Disorders

	Laboratory/Diagnostic Tests					
Disease/ Disorder	**Blood**	**Other**	**Radiography**	**Surgery**	**Medical Tests or Procedures**	**Treatment**
Carpal tunnel syndrome	Erythrocyte sedimentation rate Uric acid Complete blood count			Surgical repair	Electromyography	Cortisone injection Physical therapy Antiinflammatory drugs Splinting Surgery
Dislocation			X-ray of affected joint	Reduction		Reduction with anesthesia if necessary Surgical tightening of ligaments
Gout	Uric acid Complete blood count Erythrocyte sedimentation rate	Synovial fluid analysis Urinalysis	Skeletal x-rays			Bed rest when severe Ice to affected joint(s) Antiinflammatory agents Analgesics Corticosteroids Antigout drugs
Herniated disk			Myelogram Computerized tomography (CT) Magnetic resonance imaging (MRI)			Muscle relaxants Analgesics Brace for affected disk Epidural injection(s) of corticosteroids Surgical incision and release
Osteoarthritis	Complete blood count Sedimentation rate		Skeletal X-rays including vertebrae CT scan MRI			Physical therapy Antiinflammatory drugs Analgesics Muscle relaxants Corticosteroid injection into affected joint Surgery to replace knee, hip, or shoulder
Osteoporosis	Serum calcium Alkaline phosphatase Estrogen level Total protein Creatinine	Urine calcium Urine creatinine	Bone scan	Bone biopsy		Calcium supplements Vitamin D supplements and sunshine Drug therapy Weight-bearing exercises

(continues)

Table 18-12 Musculoskeletal System Disorders (continued)

	Laboratory/Diagnostic Tests					
Disease/ Disorder	**Blood**	**Other**	**Radiography**	**Surgery**	**Medical Tests or Procedures**	**Treatment**
Rheumatoid arthritis	Rheumatoid factor Antinuclear antibody test Lupus erythematosis test Erythrocyte sedimentation rate Complete blood count	Synovial fluid analysis	Skeletal X-rays	To correct deformity		Antiinflammatory drugs Corticosteroids Immunosuppression drugs Splinting of affected joints Exercises Replacement of joint with artificial joint
Rickets	Serum phosphorus Vitamin D Creatinine	Urine calcium Urine phosphorus Urine creatinine	Skeletal bone scan	Bone biopsy		Vitamin D and calcium supplements Sunlight exposure
Spinal curvatures • Scoliosis • Lordosis • Kyphosis			X-rays of spine			Exercise Brace Spinal fusion Body cast

Muscular system diseases and disorders can be treated by electromyostimulation (EMS). Electrical current directly stimulates motor nerves. A low frequency charge of electricity is given to muscle(s) through electrodes placed on the skin to elicit muscle contraction. The therapy improves muscle strength and is used to help strengthen atrophied muscles caused by surgery or injuries. EMS therapy can re-educate muscles that have become paralyzed. It can be used in sports training to improve muscle strength.

Therapeutic treatment of muscular system injuries caused by trauma is clinically handled by the use of cold and hot therapy and physical therapy including ultrasound therapy. These procedures are discussed in Chapter 21.

Fractures, Casting, and Cast Removal

Closed fractures of the wrist, forearm, fingers, lower legs, or upper arm are often treated in the ambulatory care setting. Table 18-15 lists types of fractures (see Chapter 9).

Types of casting materials used are the plaster (the mainstay for casting), synthetic or plastic cast, and the air cast. Plaster casts are formed by wetting bandage rolls impregnated with calcium sulfate and molding them to the injured body part. Synthetic casts are formed by using tape embedded with a polyester/cotton combination, fiberglass, or plastic resin. Air casts are a type of inflatable immobilizer and are used for sprains and postcast support. The type of casting material used is dependent on provider preference and the body part to which a cast is being applied. Synthetic casts are lighter, stronger, and more water resistant, but they have less room for swelling.

- *Short arm cast (SAC):* extends from the fingers to just below the elbow (fracture or dislocation of wrist and forearm)
- *Long arm cast (LAC):* extends from the fingers to the axilla, with a bend at the elbow (fracture of the upper arm)

Table 18-13 Muscular/Connective Tissue Disorders

	Laboratory/Diagnostic Tests					
Disease/ Disorder	**Blood**	**Other**	**Radiography**	**Surgery**	**Medical Tests or Procedures**	**Treatment**
Back pain		Urinalysis	X-ray of vertebrae	May be necessary	Computerized tomography (CT) Magnetic resonance imaging (MRI)	Treatment depends on diagnosis Analgesics Antiinflammatory medications Exercise Epidural corticosteroids Electronic stimulation device
Bursitis			MRI X-ray of affected joint for calcium deposits	Excision of bursa wall		Moist heat Immobilization Antiinflammatory medications Local injection of corticosteroids
Fibromyalgia	Rheumatoid arthritis antibody		Skeletal X-rays		Electromyography	Antiinflammatory medications may be useful Physical therapy Medication for sleep disturbances (antidepressants) Counseling Exercise
Strain, sprain			X-rays of affected body part to rule out fracture	May be necessary		Cold wet packs to area for 24 hours; follow with warm packs Antiinflammatory medications Elevate and rest affected part Immobilization or movement of affected part (per provider's recommendation) Physical therapy
Tendonitis			Arthrogram			Moist heat Antiinflammatory medications Local injection of corticosteroids Physical therapy

Note: Physical therapy should be encouraged from the onset. Patient can prevent further damage. Provide patient education.

Table 18-14 Description of Skeletal and Muscular Disorders

Bone
Carpal tunnel syndrome. Causes pain and weakness of hand and fingers. May cause **paresthesia** of hand and fingers. Caused by compression of the median nerve against the carpal bones. Usually results from repetitive tasks (such as using computer keyboard or mouse or rolling hair).
Cleft palate. Congenital disorder caused by nonunion of the maxillary bones. Surgical repair needed to close palate.
Fractures. Break in a bone classified according to angle, usually caused by trauma or pathology.
Herniated disk. A rupture of the cushioning mass between two intervertebral disks of the spine most often caused by injury or osteoarthritis. Causes back pain that may radiate into buttock(s) and down leg.
Osteoporosis. Diminished bone mass caused by lack of calcium deposits in the bone, predisposing patients to fracture.
Paget's disease. Chronic disease marked by a high rate of bone destruction and irregular bone repair. The new bone fractures easily. Cause unknown but may be hereditary.
Rickets. Abnormal bone softening caused by inadequate utilization of vitamin D, inadequate intake or loss of calcium. One symptom is night fever (known as osteomalacia in adults).
Spinal curvatures. Spinal defects with exaggerated curves caused by diseases of the spine, faulty posture, or congenital malformations. Scoliosis: right or left sideway curvature of the spine Lordosis: inward curvature of the lower spine (swayback) Kyphosis: outward curvature of the upper spine (hunchback)
Joints
Dislocation. A bone forcibly displaced from its joint usually caused by trauma.
Gout. Form of arthritis caused by metabolic disturbances in purine metabolism resulting in uric acid crystal deposits in the joints. Causes periodic attacks of arthritis pain and joint inflammation.
Osteoarthritis. Common, chronic inflammatory process of the joints, with overgrowth of bone and spur formation. Accompanies aging. Causes swollen joints and pain.
Rheumatoid arthritis. More serious and crippling form caused by inflammation of the synovial tissues of several joints, may be caused by antigen-antibody reaction. Systemic symptoms include fatigue, temperature elevation, sensory disturbances, pain, and joint deformities.
Muscle Disorders
Back pain. Localized discomfort usually in the lumbar area caused by stretching or straining of muscles.
Bursitis. Inflammation of the cavity found in connective tissue of a joint that is lined with synovial fluid usually caused by trauma.
Fibromyagia. Discomfort of muscles, tendons, ligaments, and soft tissues brought on by trauma, strain, and emotional stress.
Spasm. Sudden involuntary muscle contraction; can cause pain.
Sprains. Caused by trauma to a joint with torn ligament if severe.
Strain. Trauma to a muscle from violent contraction.
Tendonitis. Inflammation of tendons and attachments caused by trauma such as strain.

Table 18-15 Types of Fractures

Fractures can be simple, or closed, so called because the bone is broken with no penetration of the skin; or they can be compound, or open, so called because the broken bone has protruded through the skin and there is an open wound in addition to the fracture.
Two of the most common fractures are both simple fractures: Colles fracture and Potts fracture. Colles fracture is a fracture of the lower end of the radius. Potts fracture is a fracture of the lower part of the fibula and the malleolus of the tibia.
Fractures are described by their characteristics: *Greenstick.* The bone is bent on one side and fractured on the other. *Oblique.* The bone is fractured and runs obliquely to the axis of the bone. *Transverse.* The bone is fractured at a right angle to the axis of the bone. *Comminuted.* The bone is splintered into fragments. *Impacted.* The bone is fractured into fragments and the fragments have been driven into the interior of another bone. See Chapter 9.

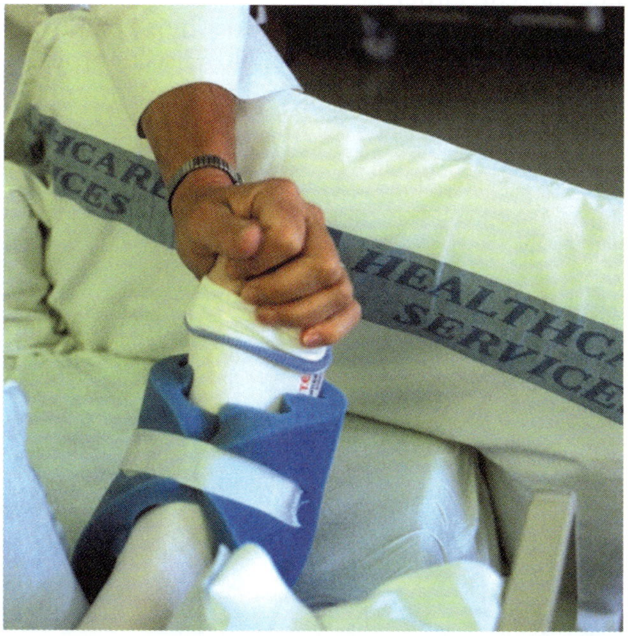

Figure 18-33 Ask the patient if she can feel you touching the extremities distal to the immobilized area.

- *Long and short leg casts:* extend from the thigh to the toes (LLC) or from below the knee to the toes (SLC) and usually include a walking heel

The medical assistant's role in cast application and removal consists of setting up supplies and assisting the provider. Patient teaching of cast care is also a primary function of the medical assistant. Procedures 18-20 and 18-21 outline steps in applying a plaster cast and assisting in cast removal (Figures 18-33, 18-34, and 18-35).

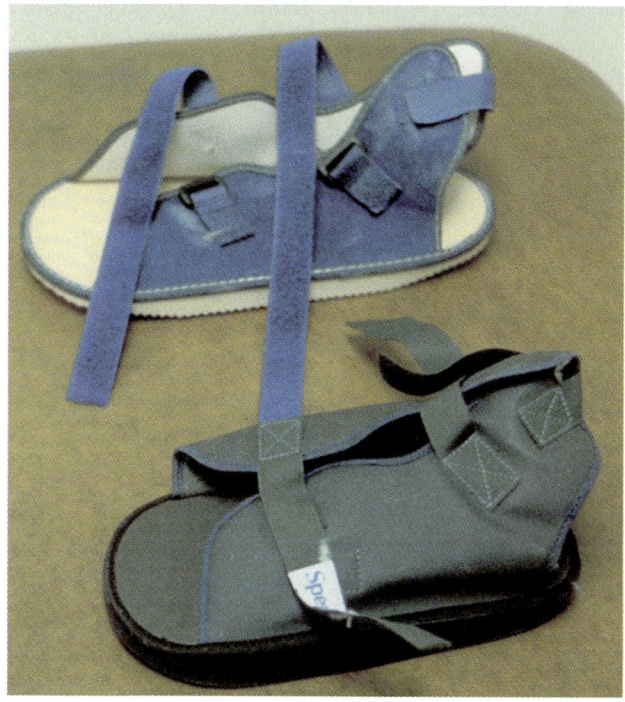

Figure 18-34 If the cast is on a lower extremity, and the patient will be ambulating, provide a cast boot for transfer.

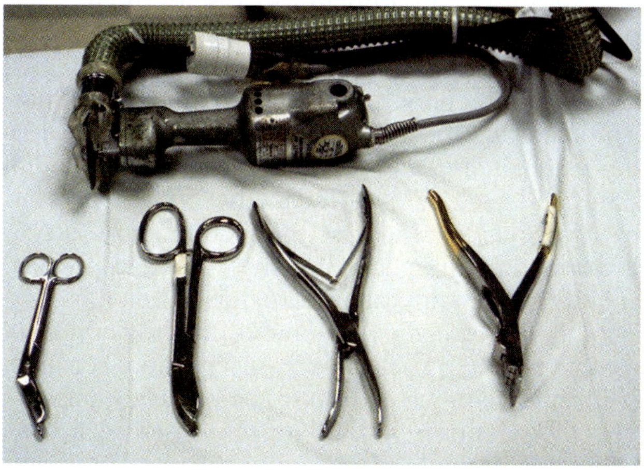

Figure 18-35 Cast cutter, cast splitter, and bandage scissors.

Patient Education

Cast Care Guidelines

The medical assistant should instruct the patient on managing and caring for a cast.

- Allow the casting material to dry by exposing it to the air and keeping it uncovered, even during the night. Applying pressure to the cast before drying can result in tissue damage under the pressure area.
- Elevate the casted extremity to aid in reducing swelling and pain. This allows for a better fitting cast, and thus less discomfort.
- Observe the fingers or toes for changes in color; temperature changes; and decreased sensation, pain, or tingling. This is called nerve and circulation assessment and could indicate the cast is too tight.
- Do not place objects into the cast to scratch irritated skin. A break in the skin will provide a breeding ground for bacteria. Do not use powder or creams.
- Do not get the cast wet. This could lead to malformation of the cast, resulting in misalignment of the extremity and breakdown of the skin. Cover with waterproof covering when bathing. If the cast gets wet, dry it with a hair dryer.
- Cleaning a cast can be accomplished by using a damp cloth.
- When decorating a cast, use only water-soluble paints or marking pens. This allows the cast to breathe, thus preventing tissue damage.
- Do not cut or trim the cast. Use masking tape if there is a sharp edge, or use a nail file to smooth a rough edge.
- Notify the provider if any of the following occurs:
  1. A bad odor coming from the cast. This may indicate an infection.
  2. Numbness, tingling, severe pain, difficulty moving, severe swelling, or cold fingers or toes. The cast may be too tight.
  3. A burning sensation over a bony area. The cast may be too tight.
  4. Bleeding or pink to red discoloration on the cast. There may be bleeding from a wound under the cast.

NEUROLOGIC SYSTEM

The nervous system functions to coordinate the activities of body systems and allows for the body to adapt to its internal and external environment. Diagnosis and treatment of the brain, spinal cord, and peripheral nerve (nerves away from spinal cord) disorders are often difficult because of the interdependence of one part of the system on another.

The provider screens the patient during a physical examination for neurologic signs and symptoms. The medical assistant's role in a neurologic screening is to observe and evaluate the patient's mental status and to assist or perform other tests as directed by the provider. Most of the examination is performed in conjunction with the complete physical examination, but it can also be done when a patient is exhibiting specific signs and symptoms of a neurologic problem such as lack of sensation, seizures, confusion, paralysis, or aphasia (inability to speak).

The equipment and supplies used in a neurologic screening test the patient's reflexes, touch, sense of smell, and degree of coordination to name a few (Figure 18-36). The provider pays particular attention to symmetric strength and notes unequal weakness on either side of the body. A patient's sex and body build are considered when examining muscle mass and tone. Table 18-16 lists neurologic diagnostic procedures. Table 18-17 describes neurologic disorders.

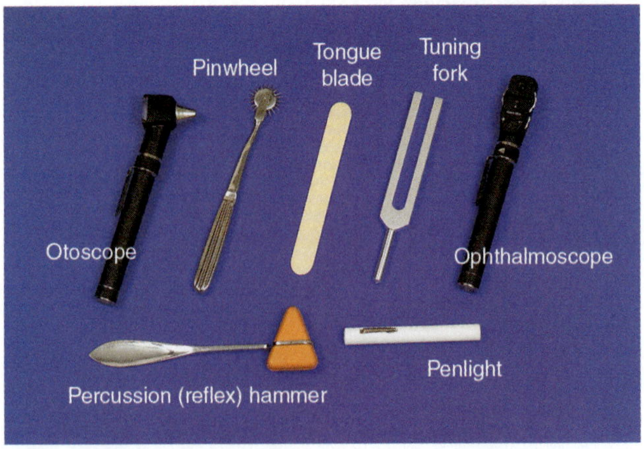

Figure 18-36 Supplies used in a neurologic examination.

Table 18-16 Neurologic System Disorders

	Laboratory/Diagnostic Tests					
Disease/ Disorder	**Blood**	**Other**	**Radiography**	**Surgery**	**Medical Tests or Procedures**	**Treatment**
Bell's palsy	Complete blood count		Magnetic resonance imaging (MRI) of brain			Warm moist heat Facial exercises Analgesics Eye patch if unable to close eye
Cerebral vascular accident (CVA) (stroke)			Cerebral angiography Computerized tomography (CT) MRI	To remove clots	Electroencephalography Lumbar puncture	Anticoagulant therapy Physical therapy Speech therapy Tissue-plasminogen activator (TPA)
Epilepsy			CT MRI		Electroencephalography	Antiepilepsy medication
Herpes zoster	Varicella-zoster antibody				Culture of cell scrapings from lesion	Analgesics Steroids Antiviral medication (Acyclovir, Famvir) Vaccine Zostavax
Multiple sclerosis			Bran scan CT MRI		Lumbar puncture	Steroids Medications: experimental Physical therapy Muscle relaxants Assistive devices
Rabies	Complete blood count Blood serum Reverse transcription polymerase chain reaction (RT-PCR)	Saliva Cerebral spinal fluid for antibodies to rabies virus				Wash wound immediately with soap and water Antirabies injections Medication for convulsions
Reye's syndrome	Complete blood count Serum ammonia	Liver function studies		Liver biopsy Brain biopsy	Lumbar puncture Examination of cerebrospinal fluid	Supportive Physical therapy Control of brain swelling
Sciatica	Blood serum		Myelogram CT MRI	Diskectomy (if caused by herniated disk)		Physical therapy Massage Exercise Analgesics Antiinflammatory drugs Surgery

(continues)

Table 18-16 Neurologic System Disorders (continued)

	Laboratory/Diagnostic Tests					
Disease/ Disorder	**Blood**	**Other**	**Radiography**	**Surgery**	**Medical Tests or Procedures**	**Treatment**
Tic douloureux				Biopsy of trigeminal nerve		Analgesics Surgery to dissect the trigeminal nerve
West Nile virus	Complete blood count	Cerebral spinal fluid	MRI		Neurologic work-up	No specific treatment Supportive

Table 18-17 Description of Neurologic Disorders

- *Bell's palsy.* Paralysis of seventh cranial nerve caused by an acute inflammation. Usually characterized by unilateral facial paralysis and pain, but it can be bilateral.
- *Cerebral vascular accident (CVA).* Loss of blood supply to the brain (anoxia). May be caused by a ruptured or clogged blood vessel or clot in the brain. Symptoms include sudden loss of consciousness and paralysis. Also referred to as a stroke.
- *Epilepsy.* Episodes of seizures caused by changes in electrical brain potentials that result in disturbed brain impulses or function.
- *Headache.* Diffuse pain in different parts of the head. May be acute or chronic with varying degree of pain and may be caused by a variety of reasons.
- *Herpes zoster.* An acute infectious viral disease caused by varicella-zoster virus. Painful vesicular eruptions. Known as "shingles."
- *Meningitis.* Inflammation of the membranes of the spinal cord or brain. Symptoms include a stiff neck, headache, anorexia, and irregular fever. Caused by either a bacterium or a virus.
- *Multiple sclerosis.* Chronic progressive disease characterized by **demyelination** (destruction of nerve covering) of nerve fibers. The cause is unknown. First symptoms are visual disturbances and muscle weakness.
- *Parkinson's disease.* A slowly progressive disease, usually occurring in later life, caused by a degeneration of brain cells due to lack of dopamine in the brain. Muscle rigidity and akinesia are common symptoms.
- *Rabies.* Caused by a virus and transmitted to humans by scratches or bites from animals infected with the virus. The disease infects the brain and spinal cord and causes acute encephalitis. It can be fatal.
- *Reye's syndrome.* A neurologic illness usually seen in young children after a viral infection such as influenza, varicella, Epstein-Barr. There may be a connection between the viral infection and aspirin. Cause is unknown, but characteristic symptoms include vomiting, rash, lethargy and neurologic involvement, seizures, and coma.
- *Sciatica.* Severe pain in the leg along the course of the sciatic nerve felt at the back of the thigh and running down the inside of the leg. Caused by compression of the nerve by a ruptured intervertebral disk or osteoarthritis. Characterized by sharp, shooting pain running down back of thigh. Leg movement aggravates the pain.
- *Tic douloureux.* Degeneration of or pressure on the trigeminal nerve (fifth cranial) causing severe stabs of pain that radiate from the angle of the jaw along one of the branches. Pain may be felt in the eye, lip, nose, tongue. Pain may come and go for hours.
- *West Nile virus.* A potentially serious illness that affects the central nervous system. Symptoms may include headache, stupor, disorientation, tremors, convulsions, and coma. Spread by bite of infected mosquitoes.

Patient Education

Post-Spinal Tap Instructions

1. Remain in a prone position for two to three hours to allow tissues to close over the puncture site and minimize cerebrospinal fluid (CSF) leakage and to allow CSF to be replenished.
2. Increase fluid intake because this helps to replace fluid loss.
3. Report any severe headaches or alterations in neurologic status (paralysis, numbness, and tingling).

Procedures performed to confirm a diagnosis of a neurologic problem or disease are limited to the use of various diagnostic imaging and electrical impulse studies. The medical assistant assists the providers during certain procedures. Patient teaching by the medical assistant before a procedure and active reinforcement during a procedure will promote patient cooperation. Procedure 18-22 outlines steps involved in removing cerebrospinal fluid from the lumbar area.

Components of a Neurologic Screening

During the neurologic screening examination, various functions are observed. Procedure 18-23 outlines the steps involved in a neurologic screening examination:

- Mental status
  - Level of consciousness (alert)
  - Memory (recall of past and present)
  - Cognition (ability to calculate and remember current events)
  - Mood (is it appropriate for the conversation)
  - Ideational content (hallucinations)
- Cranial nerve function
  - Cranial nerve I: aroma identification
  - Cranial nerve II: visual acuity, visual fields, optic disk
  - Cranial nerves III, IV, and VI: extraocular eye muscles
  - Cranial nerve V: sensations of the face, scalp, teeth
  - Cranial nerve VII: facial expressions, taste
  - Cranial nerve VIII: ear—hearing and equilibrium
  - Cranial nerves IX and X: gag reflex, saliva secretion, voice, slowing of heartbeat
  - Cranial nerve XI: neck and shoulder muscle
  - Cranial nerve XII: tongue

The provider continues with the neurologic examination by checking the patient for the following:

- Cerebral function
  - Memory
  - Muscle coordination
  - Sensory interpretation
  - Posture and gait
- Motor function
  - Muscle tone
  - Strength
  - Muscle mass
  - Twitching
- Sensory function
  - Touch (pain, light touch, vibration, position sense)
- Deep tendon reflexes

  Extremities:
  - Upper: biceps, triceps
  - Lower: quadriceps, achilles

  Additional tests:
  - Angiography provides visualization of the circulation of the blood throughout the brain.
  - Computerized tomography (CT) helps to diagnose hemorrhage and tumors (see Chapter 20).
  - Electroencephalography (EEG) records the electrical activity of the brain and helps to diagnose seizures and tumors.
  - Magnetic resonance imaging (MRI) helps to diagnose tumors and hemorrhage (see Chapter 20).
  - Electromyography (EMG) nerve conduction test, usually of the arms and legs.

CIRCULATORY SYSTEM

The circulatory system is composed of the heart and a complex network of blood vessels. Their function is to pump and transport the blood to all parts of the body, thus supplying oxygen and removing waste products from body tissues. Table 18-18 lists

Table 18-18 Circulatory System Disorders

	Laboratory/Diagnostic Tests					
Disease/ Disorder	**Blood**	**Other**	**Radiography**	**Surgery**	**Medical Tests or Procedures**	**Treatment**
Angina pectoris			Ultrasonography Angiography Cardiac catheterization	Coronary artery bypass Angioplasty	Electrocardiography Stress test	Nitrogycerin and other medications Coronary artery bypass surgery Angioplasty with stent Lifestyle changes
Congestive heart failure	Chemistry panel		Chest X-ray	Removal of part of myocardium	Electrocardiography Venous pressure	Medication Heart transplant Lifestyle changes
Coronary artery disease	Electrolytes Chemistry, low-density, lipoprotein, high-density lipoprotein, cholesterol, triglycerides	High sensitivity C-reactive protein (hsCRP)	Angiography Thallium stress test Cardiac catheterization	Coronary artery bypass Angioplasty	Electrocardiography	Medication Coronary artery bypass surgery Lifestyle changes
Essential hypertension	Electrolytes Chemistry panel	Urinalysis Kidney function	Chest X-ray		Electrocardiography Blood pressure	Medication Lifestyle changes
Mitral valve stenosis			Ultrasonography Echocardiography Cardiac catheterization	Valvotomy	Electrocardiography	Valve replacement Medication
Myocardial infarction	Cardiac enzymes Complete blood count		Thallium stress test Cardiac catheterization Ultrasonography	Coronary artery bypass Angioplasty	Electrocardiography	Oxygen Medication Lifestyle changes
Pericarditis	Complete blood count Erythrocyte sedimentation rate Cardiac enzymes Bacterial antibodies	Urinalysis Blood culture	Chest X-ray		Electrocardiography	Medication Antibiotics Pericardiocentesis

(continues)

Table 18-18 Circulatory System Disorders (continued)

	Laboratory/Diagnostic Tests					
Disease/ Disorder	**Blood**	**Other**	**Radiography**	**Surgery**	**Medical Tests or Procedures**	**Treatment**
Rheumatic fever	Complete blood count Streptococcal antibodies Erythrocyte sedimentation rate (ESR) Cardiac enzymes Kidney function Liver function	Throat culture	Echocardiography		Electrocardiography	Antibiotic therapy
Thrombophlebitis	Bleeding and clotting time Complete blood count	Urinalysis	Doppler ultrasonography Angiography Radioactive fibrinogen	Thrombectomy		Elevation of affected limb Medication (anticoagulant) Support hose
Varicose veins			Venography Doppler ultrasonography	Ligation and stripping Laser		Elastic stockings Sclerotherapy Ligation and stripping

circulatory system disorders and diagnostic procedures. Table 18-19 describes disorders of the circulatory sysem.

The variety of diagnostic procedures used to determine the patient's diagnosis are necessary because of the complexity of the cardiovascular system. The medical assistant assists with and performs some of the procedures used for clinical diagnosis. Electrocardiography (ECG) is explained in Chapter 25.

BLOOD AND LYMPH SYSTEM

The blood and lymph are excellent indicators of many underlying diseases. As blood circulates through body tissues and organs, it deposits nutrients and removes wastes. Failure to accomplish this leaves the body in a disease state. Blood cells include erythrocytes, leukocytes, and platelets, and each has its own function. Studying the results of laboratory findings assists the provider in making a diagnosis.

Lymph is important because of its filtering properties. The body's immune system relies heavily on the fact that the lymph passes through the lymph glands and bacteria and other substances are filtered out. Table 18-20 describes diseases and disorders diagnostic procedures for the blood and lymphatic system; Table 18-21 describes certain blood and lymph system disorders.

Common laboratory and diagnostic procedures requested by the provider include some of the following:

- *Complete blood count (CBC).* A routine test that includes a hemoglobin, hematocrit, and red and white blood cell count.
- *Differential.* Distinguishes among the various types of white blood cells.
- *Erythrocyte sedimentation rate (ESR)* (sedimentation rate). Done to time the speed of red blood cells settling to the bottom of a test tube.
- *Platelet count.* The number of platelets in a blood specimen.

Table 18-19 Description of Circulatory System Disorders

- *Angina pectoris.* Chest pain caused by lack of oxygen to the myocardium. Usual cause is coronary arteriosclerosis.
- *Congestive heart failure.* A syndrome characterized by the heart's inability to pump blood adequately to the body tissues. Characterized by congestion in the lungs, or edema of lower extremities, dyspnea on exertion, cough, and related edema.
- *Coronary artery disease.* Arteriosclerosis of the coronary arteries leading to impaired blood flow to the myocardium. Complete occlusion leads to myocardial infarction. May also be caused by thrombus in a coronary artery. Angina pectoris is the name of the chest pain that occurs due to lack of oxygen to the myocardium.
- *Essential hypertension.* Consistently high blood pressure of unknown cause.
- *Mitral valve stenosis.* Narrowing of mitral valve obstructing flow from atrium to ventricle. Usual cause is a rheumatic heart disease as a result of a streptococcal infection (throat or scarlet fever). Thrombi can form. Atrial fibrillation possible.
- *Myocardial infarction.* Death of myocardial tissue caused by anoxia to the myocardium. Symptoms include dyspnea, chest pain, nausea, vomiting, and diaphoresis.
- *Pericarditis.* Inflammation of the pericardium. Caused by tuberculosis, pyogenic organisms, uremia, and myocardial infarction. Characterized by fever, dry cough, dyspnea, and palpitations.
- *Rheumatic fever.* A systemic disease affecting the heart, joints, and central nervous system after a group A beta-hemolytic streptococcal infection. May occur without symptoms. Symptoms include fever, migratory joint pain, pericarditis, and heart murmur.
- *Thrombophlebitis.* An inflammation of a vein with thrombus formation, may be caused by trauma. Symptoms include pain and swelling in affected vein.
- *Varicose veins.* Enlarged, twisted, and engorged veins, commonly occurring in the saphenous veins but may occur in any vein in the body. Caused by conditions that hamper venous return, such as pregnancy, standing for long periods of time, and obesity. Symptoms include pain in feet and ankles, swelling, and leg ulcers.

- *Liver function studies.* Measure coagulation factors, prothrombin, and fibrinogen necessary for blood coagulation.
- *Schilling test.* Radioactive vitamins B_{12} and intrinsic factor measured in 24-hour urine specimen.

Procedures to collect blood specimens and venipuncture are explained in Chapter 28; hematology is discussed in Chapter 29.

INTEGUMENTARY SYSTEM

The integumentary system consists of the skin and its associated structures, such as hair, nails, nerve endings, and the sebaceous (oil) and sudoriferous (sweat) glands. This system provides protection for the body against invasion of microorganisms and trauma and helps regulate body temperature. Nerve endings sense pressure, touch, and pain. Structurally, the skin consists of two layers (Figure 18-37), which function differently from one another to perform specific activities.

- Epidermis is the outer layer of the skin that is composed of squamous epithelium and produces keratin and the pigment melanin.
- Dermis is the inner layer of the skin made up of connective tissue and contains blood vessels, nerve endings, and glands. Provides strength and elasticity.
- Subcutaneous connective tissue (hypodermis) is the layer on which the skin and muscles lie and consists of elastic and fibrous connective tissue and adipose tissue. Guards against heat loss and provides insulation.

Skin disorders frequently produce a **lesion** (injury or wound) unique to a specific skin disease, thus allowing for the diagnosis to be based on the appearance of the lesion, the patient's history, allergies, emotional well-being, and inherited diseases. If the lesion appears suspicious, the provider may perform a **biopsy** for tissue analysis. This procedure aids in the diagnosis and treatment of specific skin disorders. Table 18-22 lists integumentary system diseases and diagnostic procedures. Table 18-23 describes skin disorders of the integumentary system.

Table 18-20 Blood and Lymph System Disorders

	Laboratory/Diagnostic Tests					
Disease/ Disorder	**Blood**	**Other**	**Radiography**	**Surgery**	**Medical Tests or Procedures**	**Treatment**
Anemias	Ferritin Serum iron Complete blood count Red blood cell count Serum B_{12}	Gastric analysis	Ferrokinetic studies Radioactive B_{12}		Bone marrow	Depends on cause Increase dietary intake of iron or folic acid Vitamin B_{12} injections
Hodgkin's disease	Complete blood count Liver function		Chest radiograph Lymphangiography	Lymph node biopsy	Bone marrow	Radiation Chemotherapy
Infectious mononucleosis	Complete blood count Monoscreen Heterophile antibody Epstein–Barr virus Liver function					Analgesics Rest
Leukemia	Complete blood count Liver function Platelet count Bleeding time			Bone marrow transplant	Bone marrow	Chemotherapy Bone marrow transplant
Lymphedema			Lymphangiography			Antibiotics Surgery Lymphedema therapy

Table 18-21 Description of Blood and Lymph System Disorders

Anemias. All anemias are manifested by a reduction in circulating red blood cells and the amount of hemoglobin, which is the volume of packed red blood cells per 100 mL blood. Symptoms include pallor of the skin, nailbeds, and mucous membranes; weakness; vertigo; headache; drowsiness; and general malaise.

- *Iron deficiency.* Lack of reserve iron in the body and in red blood cells that lack hemoglobin resulting from inadequate dietary intake of iron, iron **malabsorption** (poor absorption of nutrients), blood loss, or pregnancy.
- *Pernicious anemia.* Lack of intrinsic factor in the stomach secretions (hydrochloric acid). Vitamin B_{12} cannot be absorbed. Red cells cannot develop properly.
- *Sickle cell anemia.* A hereditary chronic anemia characterized by abnormal red blood cells causing lysis of the cells and the formation of clumps in the blood vessels, impairing circulation. Not curable.

Hodgkin's disease. An idiopathic malignancy of the lymphatic system causing enlargement of lymphatic tissue, spleen, and liver. Symptoms include fever and night sweats. Often curable.

Leukemia. Overproduction of abnormal and immature white blood cells. Cause is unknown. Symptoms include anemia, fatigue, fever, and joint pain.

Lymphedema. Abnormal accumulation of lymph in the extremities caused by obstruction of the lymphatics. Symptoms include edema in arms or legs.

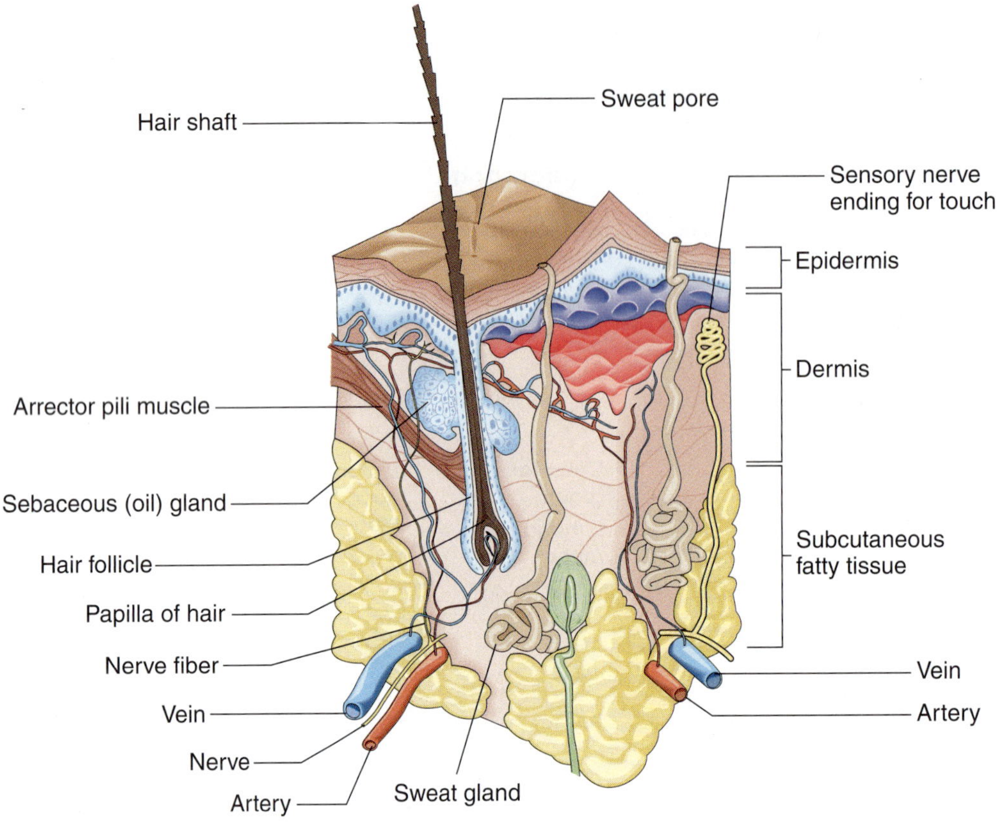

Figure 18-37 Cross-section of skin.

Diagnostic procedures involving the skin range from the simple to the complex. Simple observations such as skin color, texture, size and shape of a lesion, and patient history can lead to a quick diagnosis. Confirmatory procedures such as clinical studies of urine and blood, culture of a purulent lesion, radiographs, and biopsies of the affected tissues can further delineate the disease.

The clinical procedures for the skin most commonly performed by the medical assistant are obtaining wound cultures, applying a sterile dressings to the wound site, and allergy skin testing.

Allergy Skin Testing

Medical assistants often perform allergy skin testing. When performing allergy skin tests, severe allergic reaction is a distinct possibility. Emergency treatment must be available immediately and consists of the following: (1) notify provider immediately; (2) have patient lie down; (3) have epinephrine, benadryl, and corticosteroid injections ready to be administered; and (4) check patient's vital signs.

There can be a broad range of inflammatory responses to allergens. Some responses include urticaria (hives), swelling at the injection site, pruritus (itchiness), and redness. A response or reaction can be immediate, life-threatening, and systemic in nature. The allergen reaches the circulatory system triggering a massive release of substances (histamine) that can produce severe airway obstruction, vasodilation, hypotension, laryngeal edema, and shock (anaphylactic). See Chapter 9.

Three Kinds of Skin Tests. The scratch test, the patch test, and intradermal test are the three skin test procedures the provider can perform on patients to evaluate for allergies. Together with the patient's medical history, laboratory values, physical exam, and the skin test results, the provider compiles the data to determine the substances to which the patient is allergic (Figure 18-38).

Scratch Test. The back and arms are used for the scratch test. The skin surface is numbered in rows approximately two inches apart so that they can be identified. A small scratch is made on the surface of the skin and the allergen (a substance that causes allergy) is placed on the scratch. As

Table 18-22 Integumentary System Disorders

	Laboratory/Diagnostic Tests					
Disease/ Disorder	**Blood**	**Other**	**Radiography**	**Surgery**	**Medical Tests or Procedures**	**Treatment**
Abscess (furuncle, carbuncle)	Complete blood count Blood glucose	Culture and sensitivity of wound exudate		Incision and drainage		Antibiotics Incision and drainage
Acne		Culture of skin lesions				Antibiotics Steroids Retin-A
Corn, callus, wart (verucca), mole (nevus)				Excisional biopsy Electrocautery		Surgical excision
Dermatitis	Serum IgE			Biopsy of lesion		Depends of cause
Dermatophytosis		Culture			Wood's rays (ultraviolet rays)	Antifungal medication
Impetigo	Complete blood count	Gram stain of discharge from lesion				Antibiotics
Melanoma			Chest X-ray	Biopsy of lesion		Surgical excision Chemotherapy
Psoriasis				Skin biopsy		Medication Light therapy
Scleroderma	Sedimentation rate Rheumatoid arthritis factor Antinuclear antibodies	Urinalysis Kidney function tests	Gastrointestinal X-ray Chest X-ray	Tissue biopsy		Medication
Skin cancer				Biopsy of lesion		Surgical excision Laser therapy Radiation therapy

many as 50 allergens can be used at one time (Figure 18-39). A reaction to the allergen usually occurs within a half-hour. If the patient is allergic to a substance, a wheal (a hive) will develop at the scratch site. The site is compared with a scratch test with no allergens introduced into it, but just an allergy-free fluid. The provider reads the results, which are graded on a scale from 2 to 4. A number 2 reaction indicates a wheal larger than the control scratch reaction (which is minimal). A number 3 is given to a larger reaction, and a 4 is given to a reaction in which the wheal extends

Table 18-23 Description of Skin Disorders

Abscess. **Furuncle** "Boil." Acute circumscribed infection of the subcutaneous tissues and surrounding tissues caused by staphylococci. **Carbuncle.** A circumscribed inflammation and infection of the skin and deeper tissues accompanied by fever, leukocytosis, and sometimes prostration. Caused by staphylococcus and common in patients with diabetes.
Acne. Chronic inflammatory disease caused by blocked sebaceous glands, characterized by **comedones** (blackheads), papules, and pustules.
Corn and callus. Thickening and hyperplasia of the stratum corneum (outermost skin layer) caused by pressure or friction to the affected area.
Dermatitis. Caused by a specific irritant characterized by **erythema** or redness as in inflammation.
Dermatophytosis. A highly contagious infectious fungus infection of the skin. Common on hands and feet. When feet are infected, it is known as athlete's foot or tinea pedis.
Herpes zoster. An acute infectious disease caused by varicella-zoster virus. Characterized by inflammation of the ganglia of the spinal or cranial nerves. Painful, vesicular eruptions occur along the course of the nerves.
Impetigo. Contagious small pustules caused by a staphylococci or streptococci or a combination of both and spread by direct contact.
Melanoma. A malignant pigmented mole. Virulent and invasive. Can be caused by ultraviolet light exposure.
Nevus. A mole. Usually congenital.
Psoriasis. Chronic, genetically determined dermatitis, characterized by flat, reddened areas with silvery scales.
Scleroderma. Progressive thickening of the skin involving collagen tissue. Systemic involvement occurs. Cause is unknown.
Skin cancer. Malignant lesions on the skin surface caused by exposure to ultraviolet rays.
Verruca. A wart caused by a virus.

beyond the usual circumscribed area of the injection. The allergen extract should be wiped away from the scratch area that is exhibiting a number 4 reaction (see Chapter 10).

Patch Test. The suspected allergen is placed on the skin and is covered with a square of cellophane and held in place by tape. As many as 25 tests can be done at one time and results are read in 24 to 96 hours (Figure 18-40).

Intradermal Test. A small dose (0.1 mL) of an allergen is injected intradermally into the forearm. Ten to fifteen tests can be done simultaneously on each arm, and the patient can experience a severe reaction more quickly. This test is always done on the patient's forearm.

Patient Education

Teach patients that the following may be warnings of skin cancer (melanoma, basal cell, and squamous cell carcinoma):

1. Change in size, shape, or color of mole or wart
2. Scaliness
3. Oozing or bleeding
4. Pain

Teach patients to avoid exposure to the sun and to use a high number sunscreen even during winter months and overcast days. Early detection is necessary for successful treatment. Treatment is by surgical excision or electrosurgery (see Chapter 19).

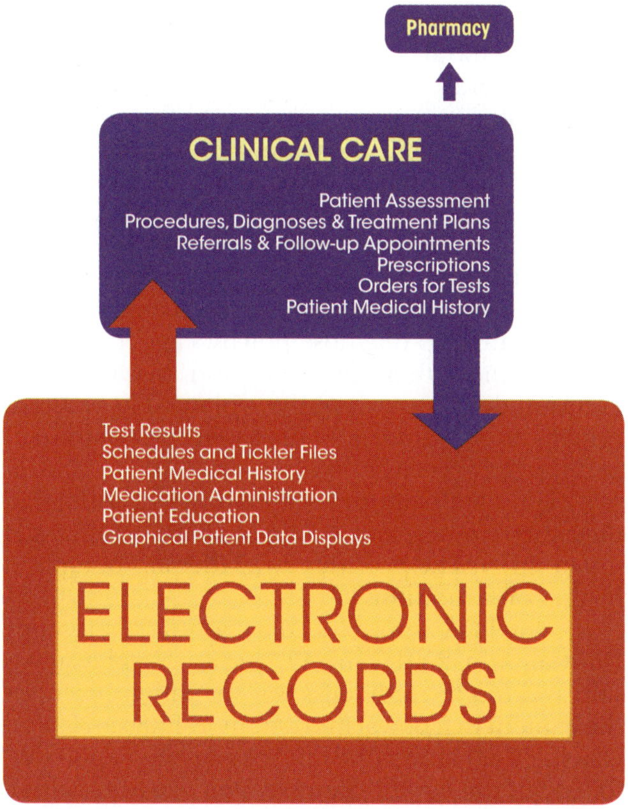

Figure 18-38 In a total practice management system, data entered during clinical care are available on demand and accessible for comparisons. It can help the provider develop a treatment plan.

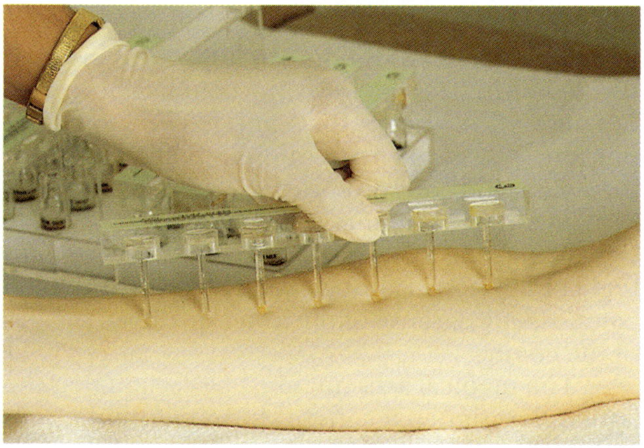

Figure 18-39 Allergy extracts are placed on the skin using a multiple applicator.

Radioallergosorbent Test (RAST). The RAST laboratory test is obtained by venipuncture and uses radioisotopes to measure minute, specific antibodies present in the circulating blood. Scratch, patch, and intradermal testing provide

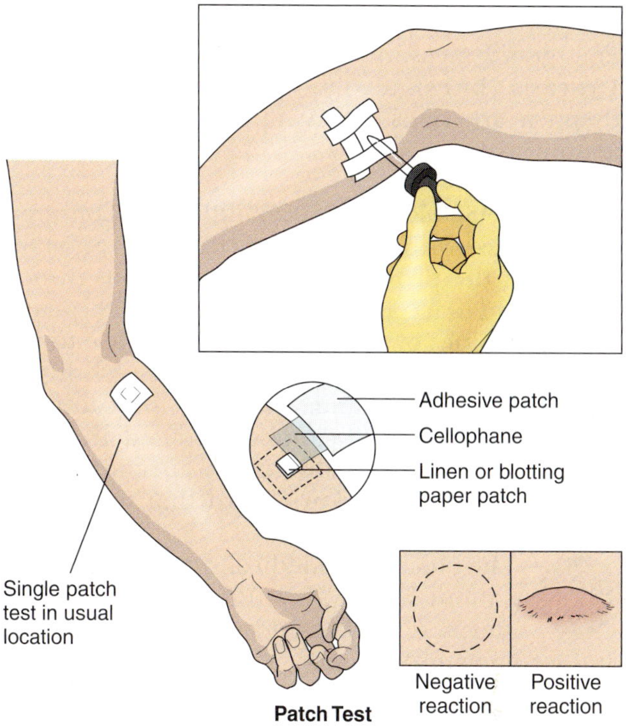

Figure 18-40 Patch test being applied. Tell the patient to keep the patch clean, dry, and covered until the provider reads the results.

immediate information about allergies and is less expensive.

After any type of allergy skin test or injection, the patient should remain in the office for 20 to 30 minutes to watch for an allergic reaction. If a reaction occurs, emergency medications and supplies (epinephrine, benadryl, and oxygen) must be readily available.

Once the allergies have been determined, the patient may choose to undergo immunotherapy. At regularly scheduled intervals (usually weekly), patients go to the office or ambulatory center and receive an injection of the substance (an extract) to which they are allergic. The dose of the extract given to patients is increased at each visit as long as the patient has had no reaction to the extract at the previous injection. This is done in order to provoke the production of large quantities of blocking antibody, primarily **immunoglobulin**.

Patients may bring their extracts (serum) from the allergist's office with them to the office or ambulatory center for you to administer to them. Extreme caution must be used because the substances being injected are the substances to which the patient is allergic, and anaphylaxis can occur.

Anaphylaxis is life-threatening and can be fatal if emergency measures are not taken immediately. Urticaria (hives), anxiety, weakness, pruritus, and dyspnea are signs and symptoms of impending anaphylaxis.

Medical Assistant Responsibilities. Common procedures with which the medical assistant can assist the provider are the cutaneous punch biopsy and wart and mole removal. The prime responsibilities of the medical assistant are to follow the principles of surgical **aseptic** technique, infection control, and standard precautions; provide the required supplies as needed; safely handle and transport the biopsy specimen; and document in the patient record that the biopsy was sent to the laboratory.

EHR The electronic medical record maintains patient history, including a list of allergies, test results, and the times, amount, and serum extract given.

Endoscopic Procedures. An endoscope is an instrument or device that is used to observe the inside of a hollow organ or cavity (to view within). Using an endoscope, procedures can be done on many internal organs without surgical intervention. These are known as fiberoptic endoscopic procedures or endoscopy, and they can be performed through a natural body opening or a small incision. A light source (fiberoptics) at the end of the endoscope permits the provider to observe within the body cavity for disorders such as polyps, tumors, cysts, stenoses, calculi, and malignancies. Biopsies and cultures can be taken during the procedure. Small lesions, such as polyps, can be totally removed during endoscopy. Photos can be taken for documentation also.

An endoscopic procedure known as capsule video endoscopy (CVE), wireless capsule endoscopy (WCE), or PillCam (all three are the same type of endoscopy) can be performed. The patient must fast for 10 hours before the procedure and needs a bowel preparation similar to a colonoscopy preparation. When the patient arrives at 7:30 AM at the gastroenterology clinic, sensor-like wires are attached to the abdominal wall (they look similar to electrocardiogram sensors) and an 8-hour battery-operated data recording device is attached to the patient's waist. The patient swallows a pill about 1 inch long and ½ inch wide that has a camera within it. The camera takes up to 57,000 color images (two photos per second) of the small intestine while the patient goes about normal activities. The camera "sees" areas overlooked by conventional endoscopy and small bowel X-rays. It photographs all 25 to 30 feet of the small intestines for evaluation of the patient's unexplained rectal bleeding, intermittent abdominal pain, and diarrhea. It can help diagnose polyps, cancer, Crohn's disease, and other disorders and diseases. The PillCam does not view the colon. The patient returns after 8 hours and drops off the equipment and the data receiver.

The data from the recorder are downloaded onto a computer, and the photos are compressed into a video. The provider views the photographed images on a monitor.

The FDA approved the capsule endoscopy (PillCam) in 2001. The FDA said the PillCam is safe and has few side effects. The patient excretes the camera in a bowel movement. A PillCam Colon is being used in Europe but has not been approved for use in the United States. A PillCam ESO, which was approved by the FDA in 2004, is used to look for abnormalities in the esophagus.

Another type of colonoscopy is known as virtual colonoscopy. It requires the same preparation as a conventional colonoscopy and can be used for patients who want a procedure they consider to be quicker and less painful.

The patient lies on the CT table, first on the back and then on the abdomen. A probe is inserted through the rectum into the colon. The probe inflates the colon with air. Computerized tomography and X-rays take three-dimensional pictures of the colon and software provides the radiographer with images on a monitor.

According to some gastroenterologists, virtual colonoscopy is not as good as a conventional colonoscopy because of the lower quality of images of the colon.

The medical assistant must be certain that the patient has signed a consent form before the procedure and that the patient has followed the preparatory instructions. Table 18-24 lists endoscopic procedures, their importance in diagnosis, and patient preparation.

Table 18-24 Endoscopic Procedures

Endoscopic Procedure	Importance in Diagnosis	Patient Preparation
Arthroscopy (examination and repair of joints)	Detects torn ligaments, examines for synovial problems. Surgery can be performed to repair joint.	NPO after 10:00 PM
Bronchoscopy (examines bronchial tree)	Detects lesions, obstructions, malignancies. Can take cultures and biopsies.	NPO for 12 hours before examination
Capsule video endoscopy	Helps diagnose Crohn's disease, polyps, and cancer of the small intestine.	Laxative NPO for 10 hours before procedure
Colonoscopy (views entire colon)	Detects polyps, tumors, bleeding, malignancies. Can take biopsies, remove polyps, take photos, take cultures.	Clear liquids for 2 days before NPO after 10:00 PM Night before bowel preparation: laxatives and enemas
Colposcopy (examines the cervix and vagina after an abnormal Pap test)	Biopsy lesions for abnormal cells.	No dietary restrictions Empty bladder
Cystoscopy (examines the urethra and bladder)	Identify lesions in the bladder, urethra; enlarged prostate gland. Biopsy	No dietary restrictions
Endoscopic retrograde cholangiopancreatography (ERCP) (examines the liver, gall bladder, bile ducts, and pancreas)	Helps diagnose problems in the liver, gall bladder, bile ducts, and pancreas, such as cholelithiasis, stenoses, and malignancies of these organs and structures.	NPO after 10:00 PM
Esophagogastroduodenoscopy (EGD) (examines esophagus, stomach, and duodenum)	Detects abnormalities in the esophagus, stomach, and duodenum, such as hiatal hernia, stenoses, tumors, ulcers, erosion. Biopsies, brushings, photos.	NPO after 10:00 PM
Gastroduodenoscopy	Examines stomach and duodenum for lesions, such as tumors, polyps, strictnress, and ulcers.	NPO after 10:00 PM
Gastroscopy	Examines stomach for ulcers, lesions, and malignancies.	NPO after 10:00 PM
Laparoscopy (examines the peritoneal cavity, abdomen, and pelvis)	Detects endometriosis, cysts, fibroids, ectopic pregnancies, and masses. Surgery can be performed, such as oophorectomy, biopsy, and tubal ligation.	NPO after 10:00 PM
PillCam	Evaluates unexplained rectal bleeding, intermittent abdominal pain, and diarrhea.	Laxative NPO for 10 hours before procedure
Proctosigmoidoscopy (views sigmoid colon and rectum)	Detects polyps, rectal abscesses, tumors, fissures, and fistulas.	Bowel preparation: 3-day special diet Laxative and enemas NPO after midnight the night prior
Wireless capsule endoscopy	Camera photographs entire small intestine with 57,000 colored images, two photos per second. Can photograph areas overlooked by conventional endoscopy and small bowel X-rays.	Laxative NPO for 10 hours before procedure

Procedure 18-1

Urinary Catheterization of a Female Patient

STANDARD PRECAUTIONS:

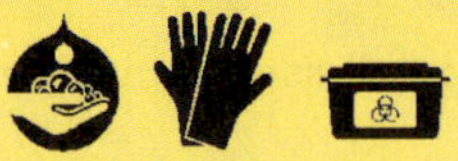

PURPOSE:

To obtain a sterile urine specimen for analysis or to relieve urinary retention.

EQUIPMENT/SUPPLIES:

Catheter kit (commercially available) containing:

- Sterile gloves
- Betadine® solution or swabs
- Lubricant
- Sterile fenestrated drape
- Sterile cotton balls
- Sterile urine container with label
- Sterile 2 × 2 gauze sponges
- Forceps (sterile)
- Sterile absorbent plastic pad

Additional items needed:

- Sterile catheter (size and type as ordered by provider)
- Biohazard waste container
- Laboratory requisition form
- Waxed paper bag

PROCEDURE STEPS:

1. Identify the patient and explain the procedure.
2. Wash hands and assemble supplies.
3. Place unopened catheter kit on Mayo stand near the patient.
4. Provide good lighting.
5. Have patient disrobe below the waist; provide a drape.
6. Position patient into a dorsal lithotomy position on an examination table. RATIONALE: This allows for access to the urinary meatus.
7. Drape patient with sheet exposing only external genitalia.
8. Open outer wrapping of sterile kit. This becomes a sterile field.
9. Place sterile absorbent plastic pad under patient's buttocks. Touching only the corners, empty contents of tray onto sterile field. Drape perineal area with fenestrated drape. Add sterile catheter to field.
10. Ask patient to keep knees apart. RATIONALE: This position provides good visualization of the urinary meatus.
11. Apply sterile gloves.
12. Pour Betadine over three cotton balls in appropriate compartment of the kit or open Betadine swabs.
13. Open urine specimen container.
14. Apply sterile lubricant to a gauze sponge and place tip of catheter in lubricant.
15. Instruct patient to breathe slowly and deeply during procedure. RATIONALE: This helps the patient relax the abdominal and pelvic muscles and facilitates easier insertion of the catheter.
16. Spread labia with nondominant hand. Dominant hand remains sterile. With dominant hand and sterile forceps, wipe genitalia with each of the three antiseptic soaked cotton balls, with a front to back motion. First, wipe the right labia using front to back motion. Discard cotton ball into waxed paper bag that is placed away from sterile area. Second, wipe the left labia repeating procedure, and last, wipe down the center, discarding cotton ball after each wipe. Discard forceps. Continue to hold labia apart until catheter is inserted. RATIONALE: Holding labia open will keep urinary meatus from becoming contaminated from labia while inserting catheter.
17. Place sterile catheter tray between the patient's legs, touching only the sterile surfaces of tray.
18. Using sterile gloved hand, pick up catheter and hold it about 3 to 4 inches from lubricated end. The other end of the catheter should go into the sterile catheter tray.
19. Gently insert lubricated tip of catheter into urinary meatus approximately 6 inches or until urine begins to flow.
20. Interrupt urine flow by clamping or pinching off. RATIONALE: Stop flow of urine while specimen container is positioned.
21. Position end of catheter into urine specimen container.
22. If analysis is needed, wait until catheterization is complete and pour urine into sterile container.

continues

Procedure 18-1 (continued)

23. Collect specimen by releasing clamp and collecting approximately 60 mL urine.
24. Allow remaining urine to flow into basin until flow ceases. Pinch catheter closed.
25. Remove catheter gently and slowly.
26. Dry area with remaining cotton balls.
27. Tighten lid on the urine specimen container.
28. Remove procedure items.
29. Position patient for comfort.
30. Assist patient in sitting up or relaxing in a horizontal recumbent position. Offer tissues and sink for hand cleansing.
31. Help patient to sit on edge of table. Check patient's color and pulse.
32. Discard disposable items per Occupational Safety and Health Administration (OSHA) guidelines.
33. If collecting specimen for analysis, label specimen container and attach to completed laboratory requisition form. Place in biohazard transportation bag.
34. Assist patient from examination table.
35. Remove gloves. Wash hands.
36. Don gloves.
37. Clean room and table. Remove gloves and discard in biohazard waste container.
38. Wash hands.
39. Document procedure in patient's chart or electronic medical record, noting the amount of urine collected. Document that specimen was sent to outside laboratory (if appropriate).

DOCUMENTATION

9/07/20XX 10:15 AM Catheterized with straight catheter to relieve urinary retention and to obtain specimen for urinalysis. 700 mL clear urine obtained. Urine specimen sent to laboratory with requisition for urinalysis. W. Slawson, CMA (AAMA)

Procedure 18-2

Urinary Catheterization of a Male Patient

STANDARD PRECAUTIONS:

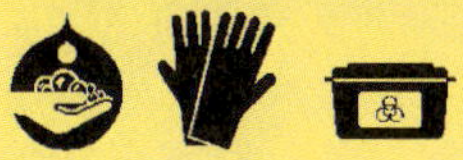

PURPOSE:

To obtain a sterile urine specimen for analysis or to relieve urinary retention.

EQUIPMENT/SUPPLIES:

Catheter kit (commercially available) containing:
- Sterile gloves
- Fenestrated drape (sterile)
- Betadine solution, or Betadine swabs
- Lubricant
- Sterile cotton balls
- Sterile urine container with label
- Sterile 2 × 2 gauze sponges
- Forceps
- Sterile absorbent plastic pad

Additional items needed:
- Sterile catheter (size and type as ordered by provider)
- Biohazard waste container
- Laboratory requisition form
- Waxed paper bag

PROCEDURE STEPS:

1. Identify the patient and explain the procedure.
2. Instruct patient to breathe slowly and deeply during procedure. RATIONALE: This helps the patient relax the abdominal and pelvic muscles and facilitates easier insertion of the catheter.
3. Wash hands and assemble supplies.
4. Place unopened catheter kit on Mayo stand near the patient.
5. Provide good lighting.
6. Have patient disrobe below the waist; provide a drape. Cover from umbilical area to pubic hairline.

continues

Procedure 18-2 (continued)

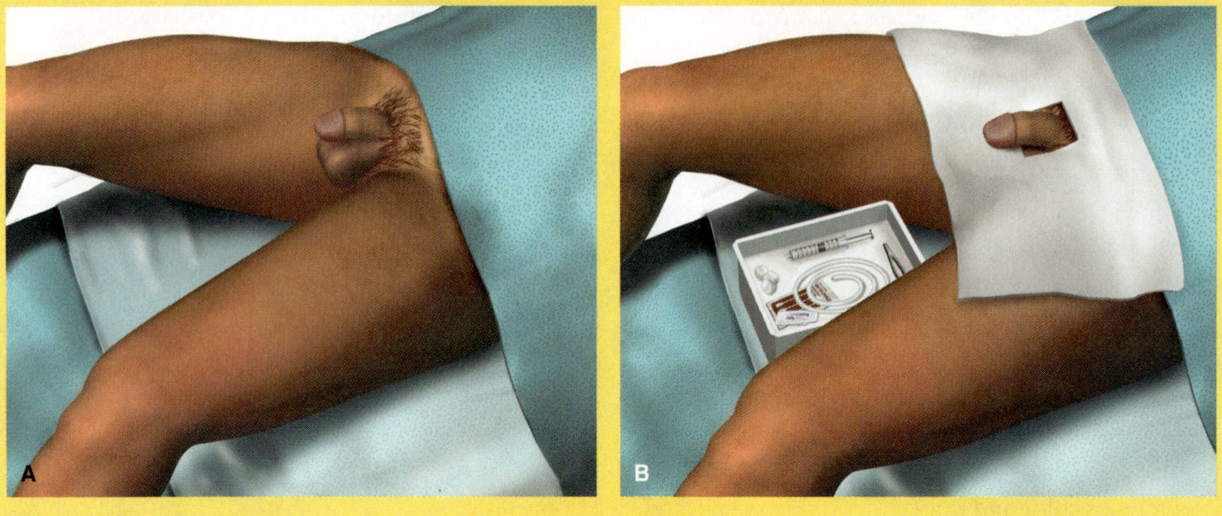

Figure 18-41 (A) First, have patient bend knees and separate legs. Then, place sterile underpad between patient's legs. (B) Open fenestrated drape. Be careful not to contaminate sterile underpad or drape. Place over penis.

7. Position patient lying on his back with knees bent and legs separated on an examination table. RATIONALE: This allows for access to the urinary meatus.
8. Open outer wrapping of sterile kit. This becomes a sterile field.
9. Place sterile underpad between patient's legs touching only corners. Empty contents of tray onto sterile field. Add sterile catheter to field (Figure 18-41A). RATIONALE: Provides sterile field.
10. Wash hands. Put on sterile gloves.
11. Open fenestrated drape and, being careful not to contaminate drape or gloves, position drape opening over penis (Figure 18-41B).
12. Apply sterile lubricant to a sterile gauze sponge and place tip of catheter in lubricant.
13. With nondominant hand, hold the penis just below the glans. In uncircumcised males, the glans must be pulled pack to expose the meatus. This is done entirely with the nondominant hand. RATIONALE: The dominant hand remains sterile so as not to contaminate remaining sterile equipment.
14. With the dominant hand, take the betadine swabs or sterile forceps and a cotton ball that has been dipped in Betadine, cleanse around the meatus in a circular motion from center toward outside. Use all three cotton balls or Betadine swabs (Figure 18-42). RATIONALE: Ensures that as many microorganisms as possible will be removed from the meatus and surrounding areas before insertion of sterile catheter.

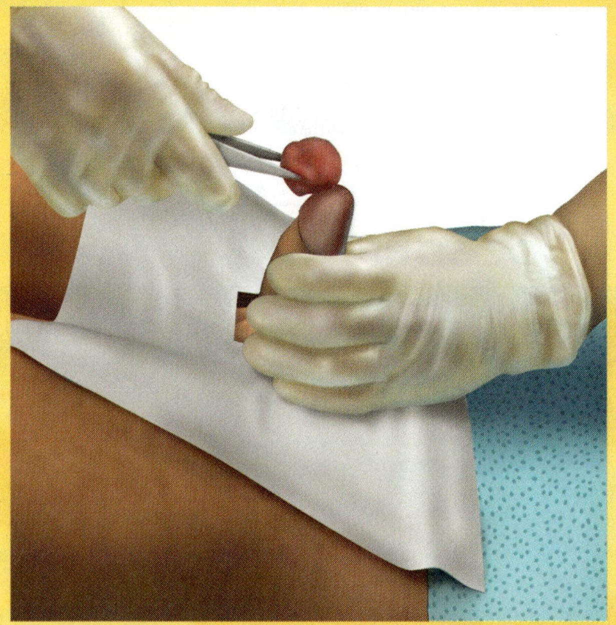

Figure 18-42 With dominant hand, take the sterile forceps and a cotton ball dipped in Betadine solution and cleanse around the urinary meatus moving from the center toward the outside. Use all three cotton balls and Betadine.

continues

Procedure 18-2 (continued)

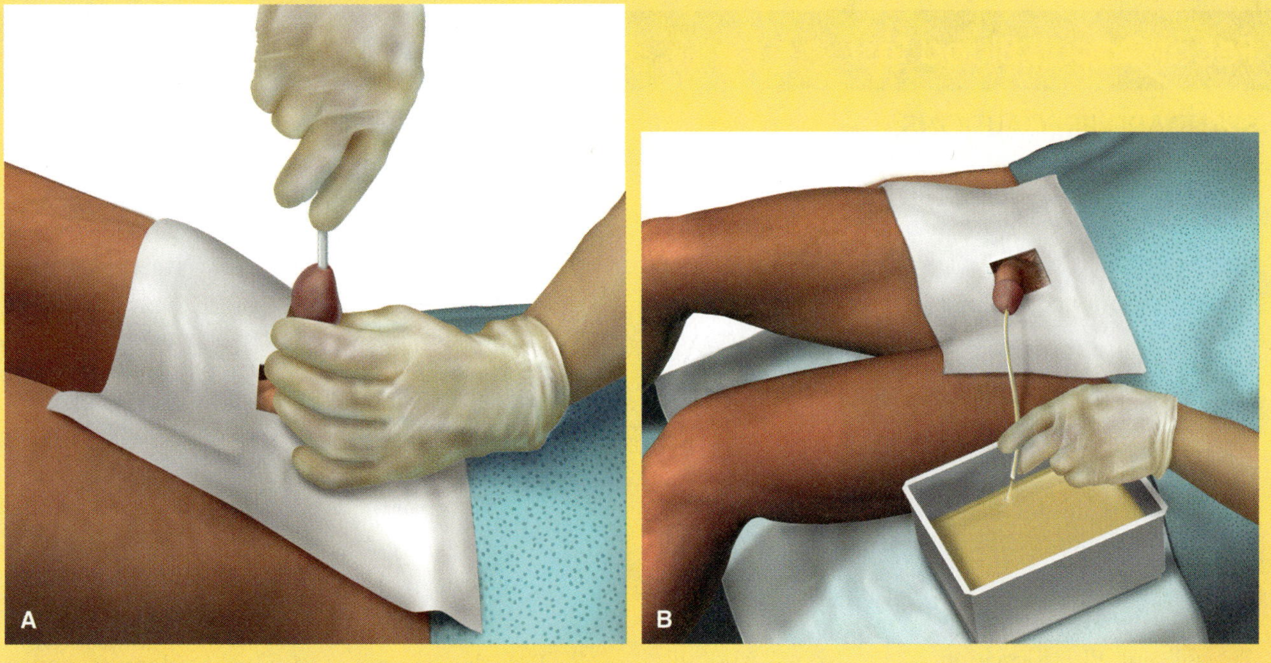

Figure 18-43 (A) With the dominant hand, take catheter out of lubricant. With the nondominant hand, hold the head of the penis so that the penis is in an upright, straight position. Insert the catheter about 6 inches until urine flows into the sterile kit. (B) Obtain a specimen if ordered.

15. With the dominant hand, take catheter out of lubricant; while holding the head of the penis upright and straight with the nondominant hand, insert the catheter approximately 6 inches until the urine flows into the sterile kit (Figure 18-43). RATIONALE: Holding the penis by the head so that the penis will be upright and straight facilitates insertion of the catheter. CAUTION: Do not force catheter. If problems arise attempting insertion, do not continue with procedure. Notify provider.
16. After urine flow ceases, remove catheter gently and slowly.
17. Dry penis with remaining cotton ball(s).
18. Position patient for comfort.
19. Discard disposable items per OSHA guidelines.
20. If collecting specimen for analysis, pour urine from sterile kit into sterile urine container.
21. Assist patient from examination table.
22. Remove gloves and wash hands.
23. Don gloves.
24. Clean room and table. Remove gloves and discard in biohazard waste container.
25. Wash hands.
26. Document procedure in patient's chart or electronic medical record, noting the amount of urine collected. Document that specimen was sent to outside laboratory (if appropriate) with a completed laboratory requistion.

DOCUMENTATION

9/07/20XX 10:15 AM Catheterized with straight catheter to relieve urinary retention. 700 mL clear urine obtained. W. Slawson, CMA (AAMA)

Procedure 18-3

Fecal Occult Blood Test

STANDARD PRECAUTIONS:

PURPOSE:

To test feces for occult blood.

EQUIPMENT/SUPPLIES:

Three occult slide test kits containing three slides, applicators, and envelope

PROCEDURE STEPS:

1. Check expiration dates on occult slides. RATIONALE: Outdated slides can give an inaccurate reading.
2. Identify the patient.
3. Fill out all information on the front flap of all three slides (Figure 18-44).
4. Explain the stool collection process; the patient will need to:
   a. Keep slides at room temperature, away from sunlight. RATIONALE: Sunlight destroys effectiveness of guaiac paper and could result in an inaccurate result.
   b. Place date on front flap, then open it.
   c. Use one end of the wooden applicator to apply a thin smear of the stool sample from the toilet to Box "A." *NOTE: Do not collect during menstrual cycle or if hemorrhoids are present.*
   d. Repeat the procedure using the other end of the applicator, taking a specimen from a different section of the same stool and applying a thin smear to Box "B." RATIONALE: Occult blood may be distributed differently throughout a bowel movement.
   e. Dispose of the applicator in a waste container.
   f. Close the cover after air drying overnight.
   g. Repeat the process with the next two bowel movements, on subsequent days.
5. Provide the patient with an envelope to return the slides to the provider's office. Review with patient instructions on diet and medication (Figure 18-45). Caution patient not to mail slides to the office. RATIONALE: Slides are considered biohazardous material.
6. Record that the test kit and instructions were given to patient.

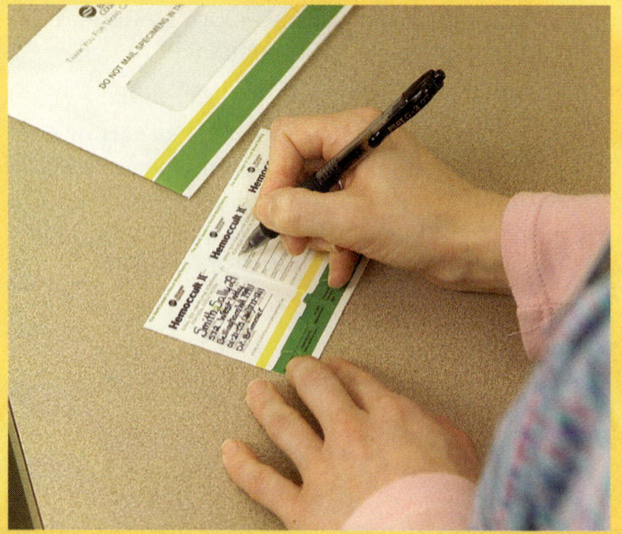

Figure 18-44 The medical assistant writes the patient's name, the date, and the specimen number on each occult slide.

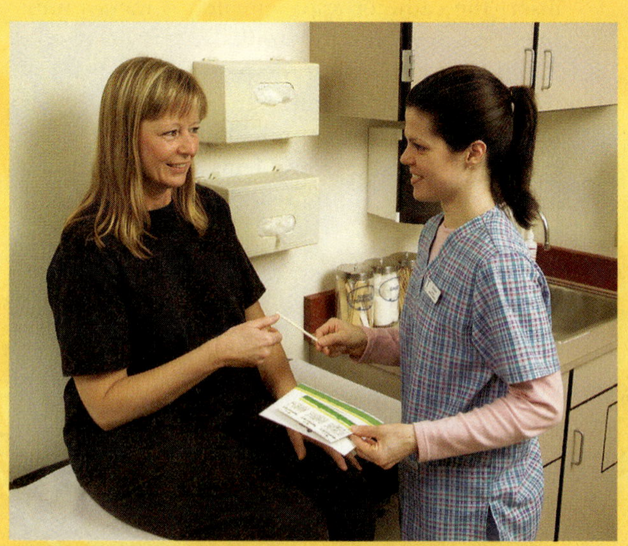

Figure 18-45 The medical assistant explains the process to the patient.

continues

Procedure 18-3 (continued)

Developing the Fecal Occult Slide

When the patient returns the fecal occult samples to the office, the medical assistant is responsible for developing the slides. Although most slides can be stored for up to 14 days before developing, the medical assistant should develop them as soon as possible because the patient may have already stored them for several days. Test results are important to ensure prompt treatment should a problem be discovered.

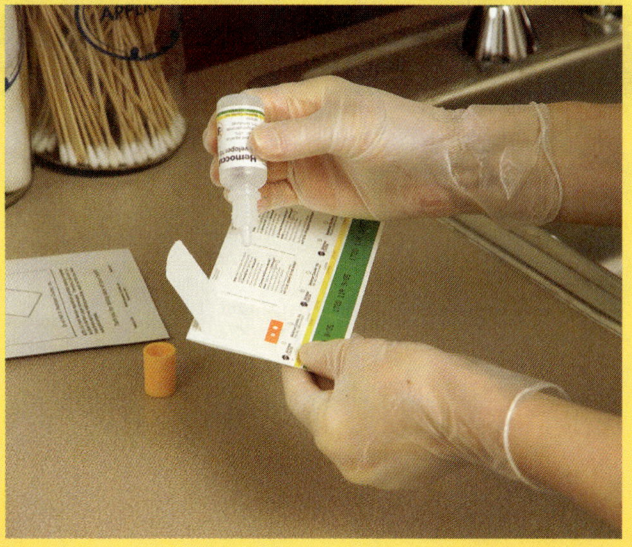

Figure 18-46 The medical assistant places developing solution on the slides.

EQUIPMENT/SUPPLIES:

Prepared fecal slides from patient
Good lighting
Occult blood developer
Reference card that accompanies kit
Gloves
Biohazard waste container

PROCEDURE STEPS:

1. Wash hands and check the expiration date on the developer.
2. Apply gloves and lay a surface protector (paper towels).
3. Open the window flap on the back of the slide.
4. Apply two drops of the developer to each Box "A" and "B," directly over each smear (Figure 18-46). RATIONALE: Paper contains the chemical guaiac, which will help identify occult blood.
5. Interpret the results within 30 to 60 seconds or per manufacturer's instructions. Record the results.
6. A positive reaction consists of a blue halo appearing around the perimeter of the specimen. Any blue color is positive.
7. Perform the quality-control procedure by processing the positive and negative monitor strip on each slide to confirm the test system is functional. RATIONALE: Failure of the positive strip to turn blue or of the negative strip to remain neutral indicates faulty supplies. Recheck expiration dates on slide and developer. Repeat test if necessary.
8. Dispose of all supplies according to OSHA guidelines.
9. Remove gloves and dispose in biohazard waste container.
10. Wash hands.
11. Document results in patient's chart or electronic medical record.

DOCUMENTATION

1/14/20XX 2:00 PM Given 3 occult slides, 3 wooden applicators, and an envelope with instructions. Instructed patient on dietary restrictions, collection of the stool specimens, and need to keep the slides at room temperature, away from sunlight. Patient instructed to bring specimens to office. J. Guerro, CMA (AAMA) ———————

5/12/20XX 3:00 PM Three hemoccult slides returned. Results: all three slides negative. Reported to Dr. Woo. Dr. Woo wants patient notified of results and to remind patient to make an appointment with her gastroenterologist for a colonoscopy. Spoke to patient. Understands slides were negative for hidden blood in the stool. She will make an appointment for a colonoscopy. W. Slawson, CMA (AAMA) ———————

Procedure 18-4

Performing Visual Acuity Testing Using a Snellen Chart

STANDARD PRECAUTIONS:

PURPOSE:

To perform a visual screening test to determine a patient's distance visual acuity.

EQUIPMENT/SUPPLIES:

Snellen eye chart placed at eye level (appropriate for age and reading ability of patient)
Pointer
Occluder
Alcohol wipes

PROCEDURE STEPS:

1. Wash hands and assemble equipment.
2. Prepare a well-lit room, free from distractions and with a distance mark 20 feet from the eye chart. Be certain there is no glare on the chart.
3. Explain the procedure to the patient. Patients should be tested with their glasses or contact lenses, unless otherwise indicated by the provider.
4. Instruct the patient to stand behind the mark and cover the right eye with the **occluder** (Figure 18-47). Instruct the patient to keep the left eye open under the occluder and not to apply pressure to the eyeball. RATIONALE: Closing of the eye not being tested may cause the person to squint when reading the chart.
5. Stand next to the chart, point to row 3, and instruct the patient to read each letter with the left eye, verbally identifying each letter read (Figure 18-48). If unable to read line 3, go to line 2 or 1. RATIONALE: Pointing to each row helps the patient to focus on one row of letters at a time. Beginning at row 3 saves time.
6. Record the results at the smallest line the patient can read with two or fewer errors. Vision is recorded as right eye, left eye, both eyes.

Examples: Right eye 20/25; Left eye 20/20; Both eyes 20/20

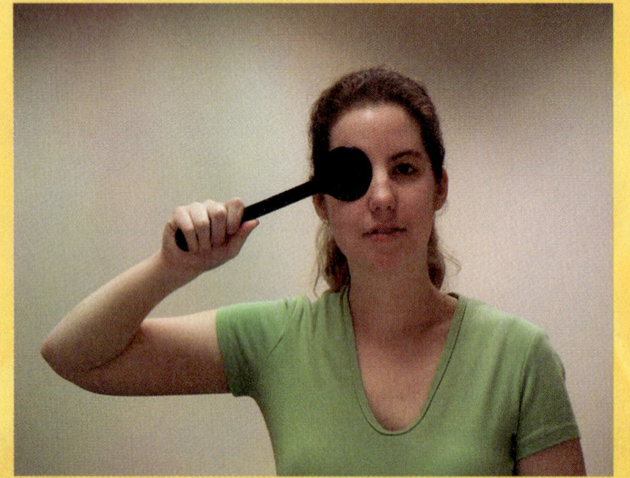

Figure 18-47 The patient covers the right eye with the occluder, keeping the eye open under the occluder.

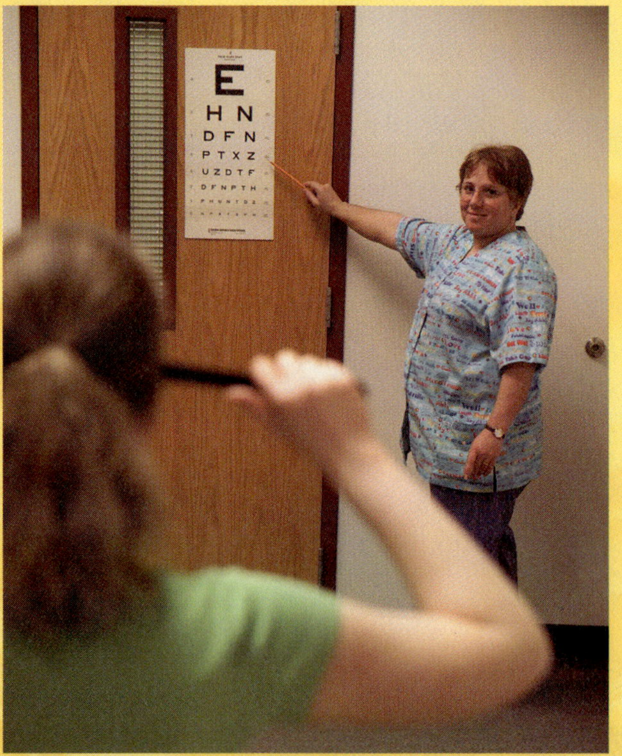

Figure 18-48 The patient uses the left eye to read the letters on the chart. The patient is instructed to start with row 3. Here she is reading row 4.

continues

Procedure 18-4 (continued)

RATIONALE: Visual acuity is recorded as a fraction. The number above the line on the chart is the distance the patient is standing from the chart. The number below the line on the chart is the distance from which a person with normal vision can read that row of letters.

7. Record the patient's reaction during the test. RATIONALE: Leaning forward, squinting or straining, or tearing from the eye may indicate eye problems.
8. When finished with the examination of the left eye, use the same procedure to test the right eye.
9. Disinfect occluder. Wash hands. Record the results in patient's chart or electronic medical record.

DOCUMENTATION

4/14/20XX 1:15 PM Visual acuity checked using Snellen chart. Results: right 20/30; left 20/20; both 20/20. B. Abbott, RMA ——————————

Procedure 18-5

Measuring Near Visual Acuity

STANDARD PRECAUTIONS:

PURPOSE:

To measure the near vision of the patient.

EQUIPMENT/SUPPLIES:

Appropriate near visual acuity chart (Jaegar)
3 × 5 cards or occluder

PROCEDURE STEPS:

1. Wash hands.
2. Identify patient.
3. Explain procedure to patient; provide occluder. RATIONALE: To obtain patient cooperation.
4. Position patient in a comfortable position.
5. Position the near visual acuity card 14 inches from the patient by measuring with a tape measure. RATIONALE: To obtain accurate results.
6. Have patient lightly (no pressure) cover the left eye with the occluder. RATIONALE: Pressure will cause blurring of the other eye.
7. Have patient read the paragraphs printed on the card.
8. Once patient has reached a line where more than two mistakes are made, note the visual acuity for that eye (allow the patient to repeat the line to verify acuity).
9. Repeat the process to measure the left eye.
10. Repeat the process to measure both eyes.
11. Record the result in the patient chart. Results are charted 14/14 for normal near visual acuity.
12. Discard the 3 × 5 card or disinfect the occluder. RATIONALE: To prevent microorganism cross-contamination.
13. Wash hands.
14. Record results in patient's chart or electronic medical record.

DOCUMENTATION

7/22/20XX 4:00 PM Near visual acuity checked. Results: 14/14. J. Guerro, CMA (AAMA) ——————————

Procedure 18-6

Testing Color Vision Using the Ishihara Plates

STANDARD PRECAUTIONS:

PURPOSE:
To assess a patient's ability to distinguish between the colors red and green.

Patient education:
1. Explain that the purpose of the test is to determine if the patient has a color vision deficiency.
2. Show patient plate number 12 as an example of the test process.

EQUIPMENT/SUPPLIES:
Ishihara plates (1–12) (Figure 18-49)

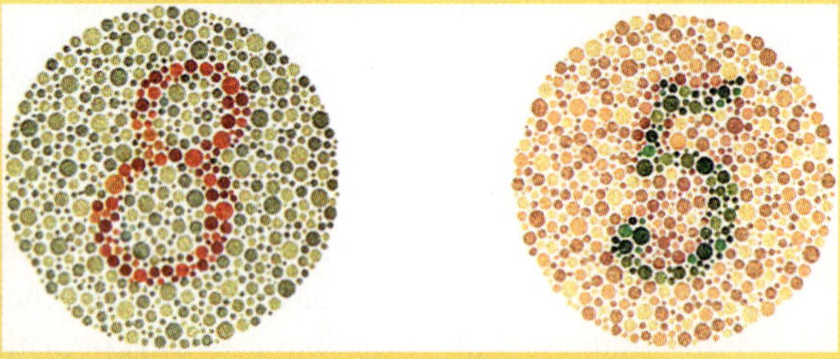

Figure 18-49 Ishihara plates are used to assess the patient's ability to distinguish between the colors red and green.

PROCEDURE STEPS:
1. Wash hands and assemble the equipment in a room lighted by daylight. RATIONALE: Direct sunlight or electric light may produce errors in the results because of an alteration in the appearance of shades of color.
2. Hold each plate 75 cm or 30 inches from the patient and tilted so that the plane of the plate is at a right angle to the line of the patient's vision.
3. Record the number given by the patient on each plate.
4. Assess the patient's readings and record. RATIONALE: If 10 or more plates are read correctly, the color vision is regarded as normal.

Source for error: Test plates should be kept covered when not in use. Undue exposure to sunlight causes a fading of the color plates, thus leading to inaccurate test interpretation

5. Document results in patient's chart or electronic medical record.

DOCUMENTATION
3/12/20XX 11:00 AM Color vision test performed using Ishihara plates. Twelve plates read correctly. L. Carlson, RMA ———

Procedure 18-7

Performing Eye Instillation

STANDARD PRECAUTIONS:

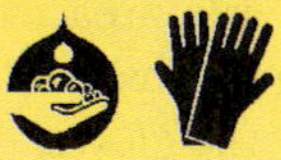

PURPOSE:

To treat eye infections, soothe irritation, anesthetize, and dilate pupils. Ophthalmic medication is supplied in liquid or ointment form. Use separate medication for each eye, if both are affected. Medication is sterile.

EQUIPMENT/SUPPLIES:

Sterile eye dropper for single use
Sterile ophthalmic medication, either drops or ointment, as ordered by the provider
Sterile cotton balls
Sterile gloves
Tissues

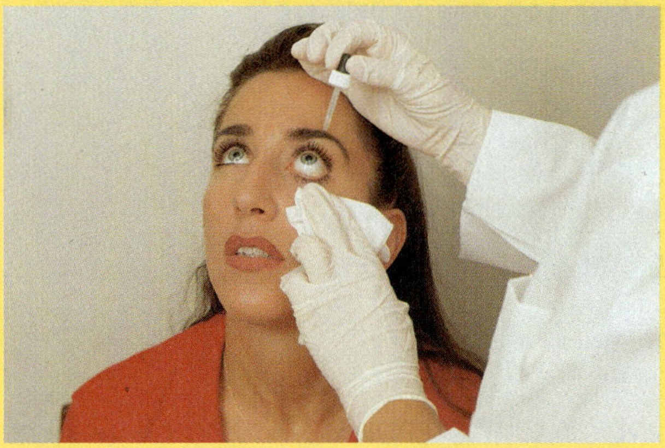

Figure 18-50 When medication is being instilled into the patient's eye, the patient should look up to the ceiling and the medical assistant should pull down on the lower lid. Contact with the eyeball should be avoided.

PROCEDURE STEPS:

1. Wash hands.
2. Assemble supplies using sterile technique.
3. Check medication carefully as ordered by the provider, including expiration date. Read label three times. RATIONALE: Verifies correct medication and ensures medication has not expired.
4. Identify patient.
5. Explain procedure to the patient and inform the patient that instillation may temporarily blur vision. RATIONALE: Blurring may occur due to medication.
6. Position the patient in a sitting or lying position.
7. Instruct the patient to stare at a fixed spot during instillation of the drops. RATIONALE: Allows for easier instillation.
8. Prepare medication using either drops or ointment.
9. Have the patient look up to the ceiling and expose the lower conjunctival sac of the affected eye by using fingers over a tissue to pull down (Figure 18-50).
10. Place the number of drops ordered in the center of the lower conjunctival sac or a thin line of ointment in the lower surface of the eyelid being careful not to touch the eyelid, eyeball, or eyelashes with the tip of the medication applicator. Carefully replace cover on bottle. Discard dropper. RATIONALE: A new dropper each time prevents contamination.
11. Have the patient close the eye and roll the eyeball. RATIONALE: Movement distributes the medication evenly.
12. If drops instilled, gently press on tear duct so medication will remain.
13. Blot excess medication from eyelids with cotton ball from inner to outer canthus. RATIONALE: Wipe from cleaner to dirtier.
14. Dispose of supplies.
15. Wash hands.
16. Record procedure in patient's chart or electronic medical record.

DOCUMENTATION

9/12/20XX 11:30 AM Ophthalmic drops (two) instilled in right eye. Eye red and swollen. No exudate noted. J. Bloom, RMA ———

Procedure 18-8

Performing Eye Patch Dressing Application

STANDARD PRECAUTIONS:

PURPOSE:
To apply a sterile eye patch.

EQUIPMENT/SUPPLIES:
Tape
Sterile eye patch
Sterile gloves

PROCEDURE STEPS:

1. Wash hands and assemble supplies.
2. Identify patient.
3. Explain the procedure. Ascertain if patient has a ride home. RATIONALE: Monovision is misleading, and the patient cannot see well enough to drive.
4. Position the patient in a sitting or supine position. RATIONALE: Easier to apply patch.
5. Instruct the patient to close both eyes during the application of the patch. Prepare sterile area by opening the sterile package and using the inside of the package as a sterile field. Apply sterile gloves.
6. Place the patch over the affected eye using sterile gloves.
7. Secure the patch with three to four strips of transparent tape diagonally from mid-forehead to below the ear.
8. Remove gloves.
9. Wash hands.
10. Document the procedure in patient's chart or electronic medical record and provide verbal and written care instructions to the patient.

DOCUMENTATION

8/1/20XX 2:30 PM Sterile eye patch applied to right eye. Eye appeared red. No exudate seen. Patient instructed not to drive with eye patch on. Wife to drive patient home. J. Bloom, RMA ______

Procedure 18-9

Performing Eye Irrigation

STANDARD PRECAUTIONS:

PURPOSE:
To irrigate the patient's affected eye.

a. To cleanse debris
b. To cleanse discharge
c. To remove chemicals
d. To apply antiseptic
e. To apply warmth for comfort

EQUIPMENT/SUPPLIES:
Sterile irrigation solution as ordered by the physician
Sterile bulb syringe (rubber)
Kidney-shaped basin to catch irrigation solution
Sterile cotton balls
Sterile gloves
Biohazard waste container
Towel
Pillow

continues

Procedure 18-9 (continued)

PROCEDURE STEPS:

1. Wash hands and assemble supplies. *NOTE:* If both eyes need to be irrigated, use separate equipment for each eye. RATIONALE: Prevents cross contamination.
2. Identify patient.
3. Explain the procedure to the patient.
4. Position the patient in a supine position.
5. Check expiration date on solution bottle.
6. Check label three times. Warm solution to body temperature (98.6°F). RATIONALE: More comfortable for patient.
7. Tilt head toward affected eye. Place towel on patient's shoulder. RATIONALE: Avoid cross contamination of unaffected eye by allowing the solution to flow from the affected eye into the kidney basin and away from unaffected eye.
8. Place the basin beside the affected eye. RATIONALE: Allows for the solution to drain into a catch receptacle.
9. Put on sterile gloves.
10. Moisten two to three cotton balls with irrigation solution and clean the eyelids and eyelashes of the affected eye from inner to outer canthus. Discard after each wipe. RATIONALE: Wipe from cleaner to dirtier.
11. Expose the lower conjunctiva by separating the eyelid with your index finger and thumb. RATIONALE: To facilitate flowing of solution.
12. Have the patient stare at a fixed spot. RATIONALE: More likely patient will blink less.
13. Irrigate the affected eye with sterile solution by resting the sterile bulb syringe on the bridge of the patient's nose, being careful not to touch the eye or conjunctival sac with the syringe tip. Allow the stream to flow from the inside canthus to the outer corner of the eye (Figure 18-51). RATIONALE: Prevents a flow of solution into the unaffected eye causing cross contamination.

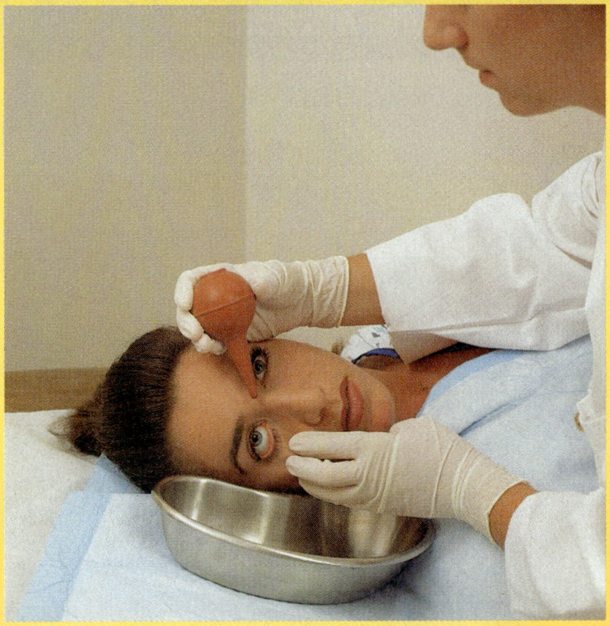

Figure 18-51 The medical assistant irrigates the patient's eye. Note that the solution will go from inner to outer canthus. The patient is turned toward the affected eye.

14. After irrigation, dry the eyelid and eyelashes with sterile cotton balls. The provider may add a staining solution to check for corneal abrasion.
15. Discard supplies in biohazard container.
16. Remove gloves.
17. Wash hands and document procedure in patient's chart or electronic medical record.

DOCUMENTATION

11/26/20XX 10:00 AM Right eye irrigated with 100 mL sterile normal saline (100°F). Eye appears slightly red. No exudate noted. Fluorescein stain (stain strip used for diagnosis and detecting foreign bodies or lesions on the cornea) instilled into right eye by Dr. Woo. Patient seemed to tolerate procedure well. Says she has "no discomfort." K. Bloom, RMA ———

Procedure 18-10

Assisting with Audiometry

STANDARD PRECAUTIONS:

PURPOSE:

To assist in testing patient for hearing loss.

Patient education:

1. Explain the use and purpose of the audiometer and that the test measures frequency of sound waves and ability of patient to hear various frequencies of sound waves (one frequency at a time).
2. When the patient hears a new frequency, signal the tester.

EQUIPMENT/SUPPLIES:

Audiometer with headphones
Quiet room

PROCEDURE STEPS:

1. Wash hands and assemble equipment and supplies.
2. Prepare room. Test must be held in a room without outside noises. RATIONALE: Outside interference may cause inaccurate test results, especially in the lower frequencies, which are more difficult to hear.
3. Identify and explain procedure to patient.
4. Position patient in a comfortable sitting position.
5. Have patient put on headphones. The procedure is done on each ear separately. RATIONALE: To test each ear for hearing loss.
6. If the medical assistant has been thoroughly trained to do the procedure, the provider will authorize the medical assistant to perform the audiometry. The audiometer is started at low frequency. The patient indicates when the sound is heard and the medical assistant plots it on the graph (the audiogram) (Figure 18-52).

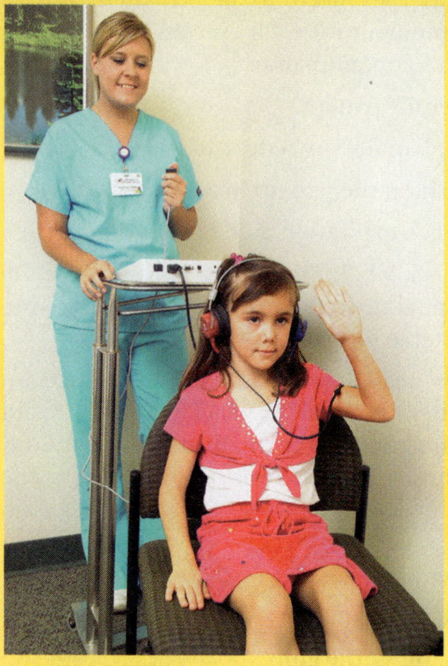

Figure 18-52 The patient raises her hand each time she hears a sound.

7. The frequencies gradually increase until completed.
8. The other ear is checked in the same manner.
9. The results are given to the provider for interpretation.
10. Equipment is cleaned following manufacturer's instructions.
11. Wash hands.
12. Document procedure in patient's chart or electronic medical record.

DOCUMENTATION

4/12/20XX 2:00 PM Audiometry performed. Results given to Dr. Woo. B. Abbott, RMA ——————

Procedure 18-11

Performing Ear Irrigation

STANDARD PRECAUTIONS:

PURPOSE:

To remove impacted cerumen, discharge, or foreign materials from the ear canal as directed by the provider.

EQUIPMENT/SUPPLIES:

Irrigation solution as ordered by the provider, warmed to 98.6–103°F
Ear irrigation syringe or bulb
Ear basin or emesis (catch) basin
Basin for warmed solution
Towel
Cotton balls
Otoscope

PROCEDURE STEPS:

1. Wash hands and assemble equipment.
2. Identify patient.
3. Explain the procedure and inform the patient that during the procedure a minimal amount of discomfort and dizziness may be experienced caused by solution coming into contact with the tympanic membrane. Be sure provider has examined the ear before irrigation. RATIONALE: Ensures irrigation needed.
4. Place the patient in a sitting position and use an otoscope to visualize the affected ear. Have patient tilt head toward affected ear.
5. Cleanse the outer ear with a wet cotton ball moistened with irrigation solution.
6. Gently pull the auricle upward and back to straighten the ear canal. RATIONALE: Allows better access to external ear canal.
7. Tilt the patient's head slightly forward and to the affected side (Figure 18-53). RATIONALE: This position allows the solution to flow into the basin by gravity.
8. Place towel on the patient's shoulder of the affected side.
9. Place the ear basin under the affected ear and have the patient hold the basin in place.

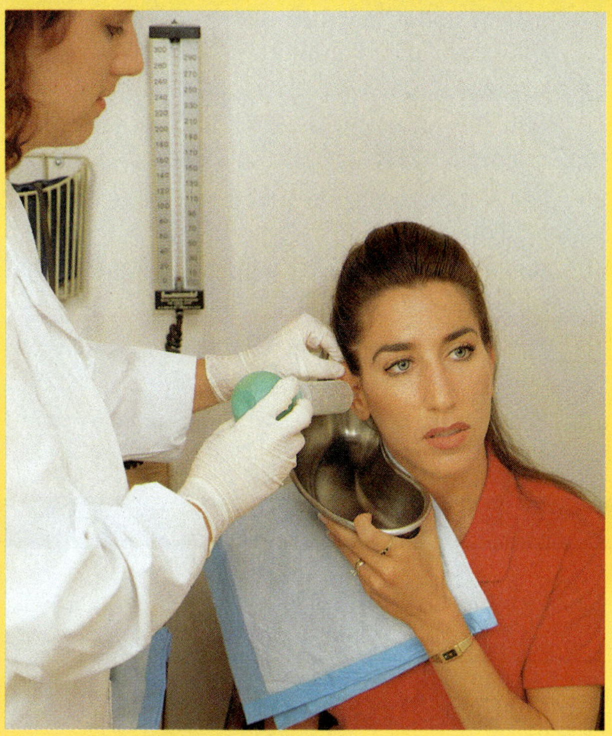

Figure 18-53 When irrigating the patient's ear, tip the affected ear to facilitate the flow of solution. The tip of the syringe does not occlude the opening to the external auditory canal.

10. Check label of solution three times for correctness and also check the expiration date of the solution.
11. Pour the solution into a basin and fill the syringe with the warmed irrigation solution as prescribed by the physician. Use about 30 to 50 cc solution at a time to warm the instrument. (Repeat Step 5.)
12. Straighten the external auditory canal by pulling back and upward on the auricle for adults.
13. Expel air from syringe and gently insert the syringe tip into the affected ear, being careful not to insert too deeply. Do not occlude external auditory canal. Direct the flow of the solution upward toward roof of canal. RATIONALE: Avoids injury to the tympanic membrane and prevents occlusion of external auditory canal, allowing solution to drain out.

continues

Procedure 18-11 (continued)

14. Repeat the irrigation, allowing the solution to drain from the ear, noting the return. Allow for free flow of return each time. Check with the patient about any discomfort or pain. Do not continue if pain is present.
15. Dry the outer ear and visualize the inner ear with the otoscope to verify the procedure has removed or dislodged the foreign body.
16. Notify the provider the procedure has been completed.
17. When the procedure is completed, remove the ear basin and towel.
18. Have patient lie on affected side on examination table for ear to continue draining.
19. Provide dry cotton balls to the patient to catch any further drainage if directed by the provider.
20. Provider will examine the tympanic membrane.
21. Dispose of supplies.
22. Wash hands.
23. Document the procedure in patient's chart or electronic medical record, noting return and amount. Provide postcare instructions:
    a. Report any pain or dizziness to the provider.
    b. Do not insert any foreign object (i.e., cotton applicator) into the ear canal.

DOCUMENTATION

6/4/20XX 3:30 PM Left ear irrigated with normal saline (100°F). Three pieces (size of pencil eraser) of cerumen in solution returns. No complaints of pain or dizziness. Inner ear and tympanic membrane appear clear. Dr. King notified of results. Examined by Dr. King. W. Slawson, CMA (AAMA) ————

Procedure 18-12

Performing Ear Instillation

STANDARD PRECAUTIONS:

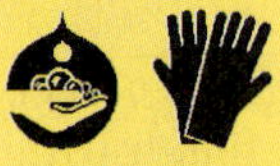

PURPOSE:

To soften impacted cerumen, fight infection with antibiotics, or relieve pain.

EQUIPMENT/SUPPLIES:

Otic medication as prescribed by the provider
Sterile ear dropper
Cotton balls
Gloves

PROCEDURE STEPS:

1. Wash hands and assemble supplies.
2. Identify patient.
3. Explain procedure to the patient.
4. Ask patient either to lie on unaffected side or to sit with head tilted toward unaffected ear. RATIONALE: Facilitates flow of medication.
5. Check otic medication three times against the provider's order and check expiration date of the medication. RATIONALE: Only otic medication can be used in the ear. Checking the medication three times minimizes medication error.
6. Draw up the prescribed amount of medication.
7. Gently pull the top of the ear upward and back (adult) or pull earlobe downward and backward (child) (Figure 18-54).
8. Instill prescribed dose of medication (number of drops) by squeezing rubber bulb on dropper into the affected ear.
9. Have the patient maintain the position for about 5 minutes to retain medication.
10. When instructed by the provider, insert moistened cotton ball into external ear canal for 15 minutes. RATIONALE: Moistened cotton

continues

Procedure 18-12 (continued)

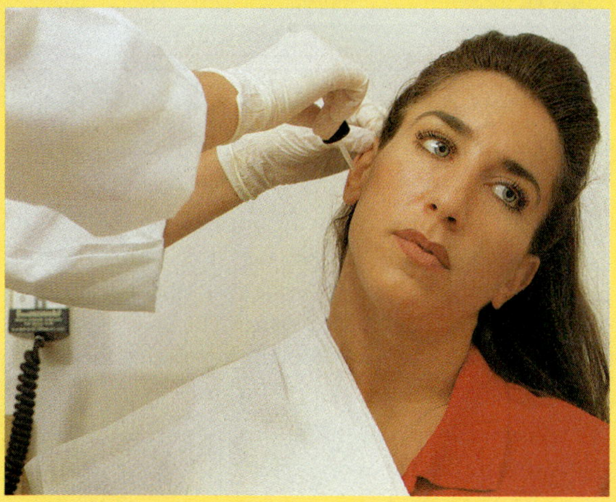

Figure 18-54 When instilling drops into patient's ear, have the patient tilt head so that the affected ear is uppermost.

ball will not absorb medication and will help retain medication in ear.

11. Dispose of supplies.
12. Wash hands.
13. Document procedure in patient's chart or electronic medical record.

DOCUMENTATION

12/10/20XX 4:00 P.M. Otic solution (four drops) instilled into patient's right ear. Moistened cotton ball inserted in ear. No exudate noted. W. Slawson, CMA (AAMA) ———

Procedure 18-13

Assisting with Nasal Examination

STANDARD PRECAUTIONS:

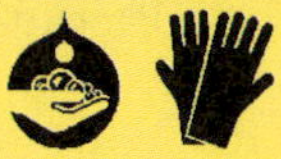

PURPOSE:

To assist the provider with the nasal examination when looking for polyps and engorged superficial blood vessels, and to assist in the possible removal of a foreign body.

Patient education:

When a foreign object is involved, instruct the patient not to blow the nose or to attempt to remove the object because this could cause tissue damage or push the object deeper into the nasal passage.

EQUIPMENT/SUPPLIES:

Nasal speculum
Light source
Gloves
Bayonet forceps
Kidney basin

PROCEDURE STEPS:

1. Wash hands and assemble supplies.
2. Identify patient.
3. Explain the procedure to the patient.
4. Place the patient in a sitting position.
5. Reassure the patient.
6. Hand the provider equipment and supplies as needed.
7. Clean equipment and dispose of supplies per OSHA guidelines.
8. Wash hands.
9. Document procedure in patients's chart or electronic medical record, noting foreign object if applicable.

DOCUMENTATION

2/4/20XX 4:30 P.M. Nasal examination done by Dr. Woo. Small polyp noted in left nostril. Arrangements made with Bayside Surgery for polyp removal on 2/10. B. Abbott, RMA ———

Procedure 18-14

Cautery Treatment of Epistaxis

STANDARD PRECAUTIONS:

PURPOSE:

Patient education:

Depending on the location and severity of the nosebleed, the provider will either pack the nasal canal or chemically cauterize the vessel. Generally, chemical cautery is attempted first; if that fails, nasal packing or a nasal balloon is inserted. If cauterization is performed, the patient should be instructed to not blow the nose or otherwise irritate/disturb the scab that will form. Cautery will sting, and the patient should be appropriately prepared.

EQUIPMENT/SUPPLIES:

Patient gown and drapes
Syringes and needles
Vienna nasal speculum
Light source (hands free)
Gloves, and other PPE if bleeding severe
Bayonet forceps
Epinephrine
Silver nitrate sticks
Cotton balls or gauze
Medicine cups
Local anesthetic (such as Xylocaine [lidocaine] with epinephrine or cocaine 4%)
Antibiotic/antiseptic ointment (such as triamcinolone)

PROCEDURE STEPS:

1. Wash hands, assemble equipment/supplies, and apply gloves.
2. Identify the patient and explain the procedure.
3. Give the patient a kidney basin and tissue and have the patient seated.
4. Assist the provider to visualize the area of treatment.
5. Assist the provider by handing the supplies and instruments as directed.
6. Assist the provider with applying the anesthetic (a syringe and needle may be used to remove Xylocaine from the vial and inject it into the medicine cup). The cotton balls or gauze are then soaked in the anesthetic and applied to the nasal membranes.
7. Assist the provider and the patient after the anesthetic has taken effect.
8. The provider will apply an epinephrine (vasoconstrictor)-soaked gauze to the site of bleeding and will use pressure on the outside of the nose to try to control the bleeding. This may be followed with electrocautery or silver nitrate. If not effective, a nasal packing may be needed if bleeding is not controlled well. The packing must be kept in place for 24 to 48 hours. The patient who has a nasal packing is instructed to make an appointment with an ear, nose, and throat specialist and to avoid aspirin and antiinflammatory medications. The provider will order an antibiotic for the patient.
9. Instruct the patient on postprocedure care.
10. Clean the equipment and dispose of contaminated supplies according to Standard Precautions and OSHA guidelines.
11. Wash hands.
12. Document the procedure in the patient's chart or electronic medical record.

DOCUMENTATION

8/6/20XX 2:45 PM Patient treated for epistaxis with epinephrine and pressure on the exterior of nose and silver nitrate cautery was also used. Bleeding finally controlled with a nasal packing. Instructions given to avoid blowing nose or otherwise irritate/disturb the scab and to call/return immediately if nose begins to bleed again. J. Guerro, CMA (AAMA)

Patient Education

Nasal Irrigation

Advise the patient that commercial nasal irrigation kits are available at the pharmacy or department store, or the patient can make her own solution of salt and warm water (1/2 teaspoon to a pint). Use a bulb-type syringe for irrigation. Instruct patient not to blow nose for 5 minutes after the irrigation. This could force the solution into the sinuses or ears and possibly cause an infection in either or both.

Procedure 18-15

Performing Nasal Instillation

STANDARD PRECAUTIONS:

PURPOSE:

To provide medication to the nasal membranes as ordered by the provider.

Patient education:

1. Instruct the patient to keep the head tilted back slightly during the procedure to allow the medication to cover the nasal tissues.
2. Do not blow nose immediately after treatment. Medication could be forced out of nose.

EQUIPMENT/SUPPLIES:

Medication, drops or spray, as ordered by provider
Medicine dropper (sterile)
Tissues

PROCEDURE STEPS:

1. Wash hands and assemble equipment.
2. Identify patient.
3. Explain procedure to the patient.
4. Position the patient with the head tilted back slightly.
5. Draw medication into dropper after checking medication three times and checking expiration date.
6. Place the dropper over the center of the outside of the affected nostril. Ask patients to inhale us you administer the drops. Care should be taken not to touch the inside of the nostril. RATIONALE: Touching the inside of the nostril will lead to contamination of the dropper.
7. Repeat the procedure for the other nostril if required. Dispose of dropper; recap medication container using sterile technique.
8. Instruct the patient to remain in position for 2 to 3 minutes. RATIONALE: Allow time for medication to be absorbed by the nasal membranes.
9. Provide cotton balls or gauze sponges to the patient when the patient returns to a sitting position. RATIONALE: Medication may drain from the nostrils.
10. Dispose of the supplies per OSHA guidelines.
11. Wash hands.
12. Document the procedure in patient's chart or electronic medical record.

DOCUMENTATION

4/13/20XX 6:00 PM Neosynephrine nasal drops (three drops) instilled into each nostril. W. Slawson, CMA (AAMA) ———

Procedure 18-16

Administer Oxygen by Nasal Cannula for Minor Respiratory Distress

STANDARD PRECAUTIONS:

PURPOSE:

To provide a low dose of concentrated oxygen to a patient during periods of respiratory distress (e.g., chronic obstructive pulmonary disease).

Patient education:

1. Demonstrate the position of the nasal prongs of the cannula into the nose. They face upward and the tab rests above the upper lip.
2. Describe how to clear the oxygen cylinder valve by turning it counterclockwise.
3. Oxygen supports combustion and a fire can start with oxygen in use. Friction, static electricity, a spark, or a lighted cigarette or cigar can cause ignition.

EQUIPMENT/SUPPLIES:

Portable oxygen tank with stand
Disposable nasal cannula with connecting tube
Flowmeter
Pressure regulator

PROCEDURE STEPS:

1. Wash hands.
2. Identify patient, and explain procedure to the patient.

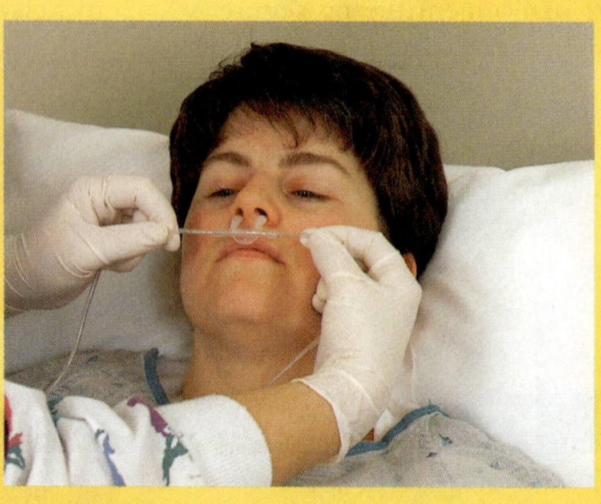

Figure 18-55 Insert cannula prong into nostrils.

3. Open the cylinder one full turn, counterclockwise.
4. Check the pressure gauge. RATIONALE: This will determine the amount of pressure in the cylinder.
5. Attach the nasal cannula to the tubing, and then to the flowmeter.

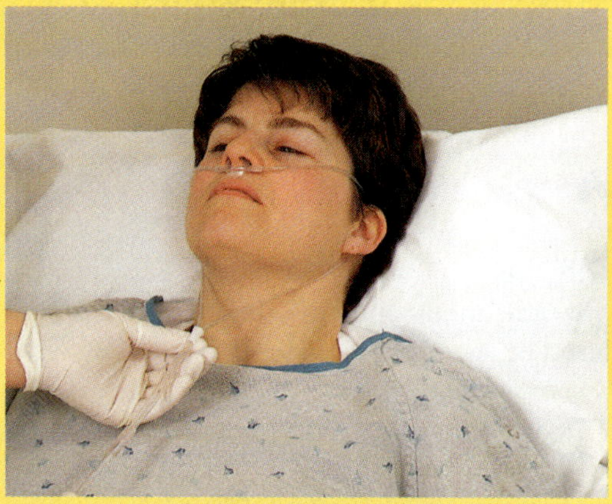

Figure 18-56 Adjust tubing.

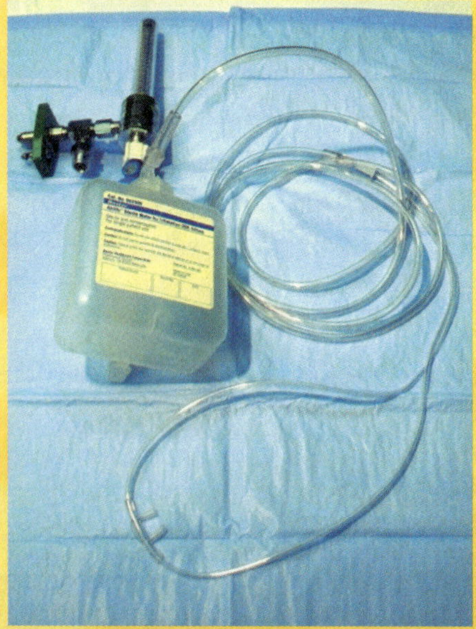

Figure 18-57 Nasal cannula and oxygen tubing attached to a humidifier.

continues

Procedure 18-16 (continued)

6. Adjust the flow rate according to the provider's order (oxygen is a medication).
7. Check for oxygen flow through the cannula.
8. Place the tips of cannula into the nares no more than 1 inch (Figure 18-55).
9. Adjust the tubing around the patient's ears (Figure 18-56) and secure it under the chin.
10. Answer patient's questions.
11. Wash hands.
12. Document the procedure in patient's chart or electronic medical record.

NOTE: Oxygen is usually humidified to prevent drying of respiratory mucosa (Figure 18-57).

DOCUMENTATION

4/19/20XX 2:45 PM Oxygen 3 L/minute by nasal cannula. Color slightly improved. Less cyanosis. J. Guerro, CMA (AAMA)

Procedure 18-17

Instructing Patient in Use of Metered Dose Inhaler

STANDARD PRECAUTIONS:

PURPOSE:

To instruct patient on the use of a handheld device known as a metered dose inhaler. The device delivers medication to the respiratory tract including the lungs. It is used to treat asthma, COPD, and other respiratory diseases and/or conditions.

Patient education:

1. Remind the patient to inhale slowly.
2. Close the mouth and lips around the mouthpiece.
3. Clean the inhaler by rinsing the mouthpiece in warm water.
4. Adhere to prescribed dose.

EQUIPMENT/SUPPLIES:

Handheld inhaler with mouth piece, and pressurized canister of medication as ordered by provider

PROCEDURE STEPS:

1. Wash hands and assemble equipment (Figure 18-58).
2. Identify patient.
3. Check medication order three times.
4. Demonstrate use of equipment to the patient and then have the patient repeat the demonstration.
5. Remove cap from metered dose inhaler (MDI) and shake well. RATIONALE: To mix medication thoroughly.
6. Instruct patient to sit upright, tilt head back slightly, and exhale fully. RATIONALE: Allows medication to reach all of the respiratory tract.

continues

Procedure 18-17 (continued)

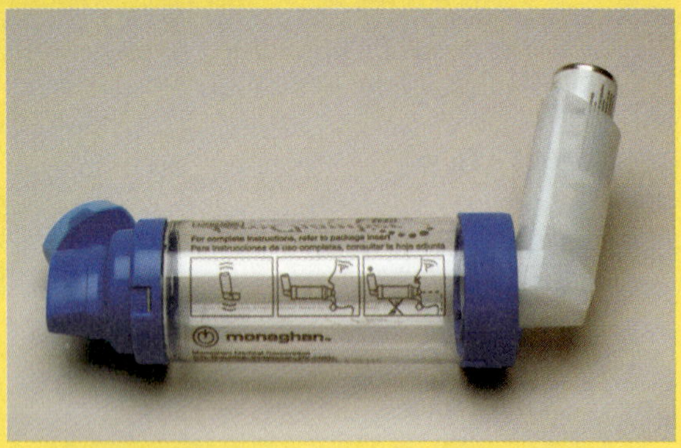

Figure 18-58 Metered dose inhaler and spacer.

7. While holding the inhaler, instruct the patient to open the mouth wide and place the MDI about ½ to 2 inches in front of mouth.
8. Inhale and exhale one more time.
9. On inhalation of the next breath, instruct patient to press down on the metal canister. RATIONALE: Releases medication.
10. The patient should inhale slowly and deeply (3–5 seconds).
11. Instruct patient to hold the breath for at least 10 seconds. RATIONALE: Medication can enter into lungs well.
12. Wait 1 minute, then repeat steps for each puff of medication ordered by the provider.
13. Check patient for any unusual effects.
14. Wash hands.
15. Put cap on the MDI when finished. If the patient's MDI contains a steroid, instruct the patient to rinse out mouth with water and mouthwash and to gargle after each treatment. RATIONALE: Prevents dry mouth, hoarseness, and microorganism growth.
16. Rinse mouthpiece and cap and let air-dry overnight.
17. Document in patient's chart or electronic medical record that patient was instructed in the use of an MDI. Encourage patient to cough. RATIONALE: Medication will loosen phlegm and mucus.

NOTE: The MDI can be used with or without a spacer (a tube that attaches to the inhaler and holds the medication until it can be breathed in) (see Figure 18-58). Spacers are made with masks for pediatric patients and for persons unable to breathe correctly through a standard spacer.

DOCUMENTATION

4/19/20XX 2:45 PM Instructed on use of handheld metered dose inhaler. Patient encouraged to cough following procedure. Performed procedure well. No adverse reactions noted. W. Slawson, CMA (AAMA) ———

Procedure 18-18

Spirometry

STANDARD PRECAUTIONS:

PURPOSE:

To prepare a patient for a spirometry to obtain optimum test results. To assist with diagnosis of asthma and chronic obstructive pulmonary disease (COPD).

Patient education:

1. Reinforce the importance of good posture during the process. RATIONALE: Good posture expands lungs more fully.
2. When blowing into the mouthpiece, the lips must seal tightly around it.
3. Explain the parameters needed for successful completion of the test.

Parameters:

1. Patient must refrain from the use of bronchodilators and tobacco for 24 hours before test.
2. Explain to the patient that maximum effort is required for accurate test results.
3. Patient must inhale deeply and quickly and exhale quickly and forcibly until no air can be expelled.

EQUIPMENT/SUPPLIES:

Spirometer
Disposable mouthpiece

PROCEDURE STEPS:

1. Wash hands and assemble equipment.
2. Identify the patient.
3. Explain the procedure and equipment to the patient. Allow the patient to breathe into the machine to become acquainted with the equipment (see Figure 18-31).
4. Measure patient's height and weight. Enter data into spirometer.
5. Place the patient in a comfortable position (sitting/standing). Loosen tie or collar. RATIONALE: Helps patient take as large an inhalation and exhalation as possible.
6. Instruct the patient not to bend at the waist when blowing into the mouthpiece.
7. Reinforce the inhalation process (deep breaths to fill the lungs to maximum capacity).
8. Instruct the patient to continue to blow into the mouthpiece until instructed to stop. RATIONALE: Provides more accurate result.
9. Be supportive and encouraging throughout the test.
10. Attend to patient's needs.
11. Discard disposable mouthpiece into biohazard container. Disinfect and sanitize equipment.
12. Wash hands.
13. Document the test results in the patient's chart or electronic medical record after they are reviewed by the provider.

DOCUMENTATION

12/22/20XX 4:00 PM Spirometry performed. Results given to Dr. Woo. J. Guerro, RMA

Procedure 18-19

Pulse Oximetry

STANDARD PRECAUTIONS:

PURPOSE:
To measure arterial oxyhemoglobin saturation within seconds by using an external sensor.

EQUIPMENT/SUPPLIES:
Pulse oximeter
Sensor
Soap and water or alcohol wipe
Nail polish remover, if needed

PROCEDURE STEPS:

1. Wash hands and assemble equipment.
2. Identify the patient.
3. Explain the procedure.
4. Select a site for the sensor (finger commonly used).
5. If patient has poor circulation, use another site (bridge of nose, earlobe, or forehead).
6. Clean site with alcohol wipe. Remove nail polish if necessary. Wash with soap and water. RATIONALE: Fingernail polish inhibits infrared light from passing through the oximeter.
7. Apply sensor (finger is placed within a clip) (see Figure 18-32).
8. Connect sensor to oximeter with a sensor cable.
9. Turn on oximeter. A tone and a pulse fluctuation can be heard. Adjust volume.
10. Alarms can be set to alert medical assistant to levels either too high or too low.
11. Check pulse manually and compare with oximeter. They should be the same.
12. Note results per manufacturer's instructions.
13. Notify supervisor of abnormal results (less than 95%).
14. Document procedure in patient's chart or electronic medical record, noting type of sensor used, site of application, and results.
15. Plug in oximeter for recharging when not in use so that the battery does not get low. *NOTE:* When measuring, cover the sensor with a towel to eliminate sensor's exposure to light. It could interfere with the sensor and give incorrect results.

DOCUMENTATION

3/16/20XX 4:00 P.M. Pulse oximetry 98%. G. Underwood, CMA (AAMA)

Procedure 18-20

Assisting with Plaster Cast Application

STANDARD PRECAUTIONS:

PURPOSE:

To assist provider in cast application.

EQUIPMENT/SUPPLIES:

Cast material:

Plaster bandage roll or synthetic tape
Container of warm water, which is lined with plastic or cloth to catch loose plaster
Water
Stockinette (3-inch width for arms, 4-inch width for leg casts)
Webril (sheet wadding) padding rolls
Bandage scissors
Rubber gloves
Sponge rubber for padding

PROCEDURE STEPS:

1. Identify the patient and explain of the procedure to patient.
2. Answer any questions about the injury or cast application.
3. Wash hands and assemble the equipment and supplies.
4. Position the patient in a sitting position or as required by the provider. Proper alignment must be maintained. RATIONALE: Proper alignment ensures fracture heals properly.
5. Put on gloves and drape patient.
6. Clean and dry the area to be casted, as directed by the provider. Chart any areas of bruising, redness, or open areas. RATIONALE: Appropriate documentation of skin condition is needed to assist in evaluation of the extremity at a later time.
7. Pad bony prominence with sponge rubber. RATIONALE: Protects from pressure.
8. Provide the correct width of stockinette for the area on which cast is being applied. RATIONALE: A stockinette that is too large will form creases, thus allowing for injury to tissues.
9. Provide provider with correct width of webril rolls. RATIONALE: Webril (soft cotton bandage) provider protection to the patient's skin, preventing pressure sores. Folds in the padding could lead to irritation of the skin.
10. Place the bandage in the container of warm water for 5 seconds. Remove from water and gently squeeze to remove excess water. Do not wring.
11. Assist with application of the cast material as requested by the provider.
12. Reassure patient as needed.
13. After cast application, clean any plaster off patient, review cast care instructions, and provide written instructions for cast care and isometric exercises (if prescribed by the provider). Reinforce any precautions given by the provider. RATIONALE: Reviewing possible complications with the patient enhances the immediate reporting of circulatory impairment and infection.
14. Discard water down the sink drain, being cautious to keep plaster from going down the drain. (Allow plaster to settle to bottom of basin first.) Discard plaster into trash receptacle.
15. Clean work area.
16. Remove gloves and wash hands.
17. Schedule patient for next appointment to have cast checked.
18. Document the procedure in patient's chart or electronic medical record.

DOCUMENTATION

12/14/20XX 2:00 PM Plaster cast applied to left arm by Dr. King. Fingers warm to touch. Patient says there is no tingling or numbness in her fingers. Instructed about cast care, exercises, and reporting of circulatory impairment and infection. Sling applied. Next appointment 12/28/20XX. S. Walsh, RMA ________________

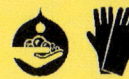

Procedure 18-21

Assisting with Cast Removal

STANDARD PRECAUTIONS:

PURPOSE:

To assist the provider with removal of a cast.

EQUIPMENT/SUPPLIES:

Cast cutter
Cast spreader
Bandage scissors
Bag for disposing of cast materials
Drape

PROCEDURE STEPS:

1. Wash hands.
2. Drape patient and area.
3. Explain the cast removal process to the patient. The cutter vibrates and does not spin. Some pressure and warmth may be experienced. RATIONALE: Explaining the procedure reduces apprehension and fears about being cut with the blade.
4. Reassure the patient that skin color and muscle tone will improve with therapy.
5. Hand the provider the equipment as requested.
6. After the procedure, provide written instructions for postcare.
7. Clean equipment.
8. Wash hands.
9. Document in patient's chart or electronic medical record cast removal and appearance of body part from which cast was removed. RATIONALE: Condition of the patient's arm size, skin appearance, and color are important factors to note for future evaluation.

DOCUMENTATION

6/12/20XX 2:45 P.M. Cast removed from left arm by Dr. King. Arm seems slightly atrophied. Skin color good, circulation seems good. Patient given skin care instructions. Appointment for physical therapy scheduled for 6/14/XX at 3:00 P.M. W. Slawson, CMA (AAMA) ——————

Procedure 18-22

Assisting the Physician during a Lumbar Puncture or Cerebrospinal Fluid Aspiration

STANDARD PRECAUTIONS:

PURPOSE:

To assemble supplies and position the patient for removal of cerebrospinal fluid from the lumbar area, which will be sent to the laboratory for analysis.

EQUIPMENT/SUPPLIES:

Drape
Xylocaine 1–2%
Syringe and needle for anesthetic
Sterile gloves
Disposable sterile lumbar puncture tray (to include):
- Skin antiseptic (povidone–iodine) with applicator
- Adhesive bandage
- Spinal puncture needle
- Three or four test tubes with corks or tops
- Drape
- Manometer
- Laboratory requisition
- Examination light
- Gauze sponges

PROCEDURE STEPS:

1. Reinforce provider's explanation of the procedure and answer questions.

continues

Procedure 18-22 (continued)

2. Verify the patient has signed a consent form.
3. Patient should be instructed to empty the bladder and bowel. RATIONALE: Patient cannot move during the procedure.
4. Wash hands and set up sterile field for the provider.
5. Cleanse the puncture site with antiseptic soap and water. Rinse.
6. Position the patient in a lateral recumbent position with the back at the edge of the examination table and a small pillow under the head. RATIONALE: Patient's alignment of the spine is best achieved in a horizontal position.
7. Drape patient for warmth and privacy.
8. Have the patient draw the knees up to the abdomen and grasp onto knees (Figure 18-59A) and flex chin on chest (fetal position). RATIONALE: Position allows for easier needle insertion into the subarachnoid space of the spinal cord because this position widens the spaces between the lumbar vertebrae. Procedure is performed at the fourth intervertebral space of the lumbar region (Figure 18-59B).
9. The provider swabs the puncture site with antiseptic such as Betadine®.
10. The provider drapes area with sterile fenestrated drape.
11. Assist provider to aspirate anesthetic.
12. Help the patient maintain this position until the needle has been inserted into spinal canal. RATIONALE: Movement by the patient could produce trauma to the spinal cord area.
13. Remind patient to breathe evenly and not to hold his breath or talk, because this may interfere with the pressure reading.
14. At the provider's direction, have the patient straighten his legs. RATIONALE: Muscle tension can give false pressure reading. The provider reads manometer to determine the pressure of the spinal fluid.
15. Provider collects spinal fluid into three test tubes.
16. After the procedure has been completed, the provider applies a sterile adhesive dressing to the puncture site. The patient is placed in a prone position for 2 to 3 hours, or as directed by the provider. RATIONALE: Helps prevent the possibility of cerebrospinal fluid from leaking through the puncture site.
17. Apply gloves. Cap specimens tightly.
18. Label samples with date, patient's name, and number CSF (#1, #2, #3).
19. Send the labeled specimens to the laboratory in a laboratory biotransfer bag with the appropriate laboratory requisition. Store in incubator. RATIONALE: An incubator preserves the specimens until they can be processed by a laboratory technologist.
20. Cleanse area using Standard Precautions.
21. Remove gloves.
22. Wash hands.
23. Document procedure in patient's chart or electronic medical record.

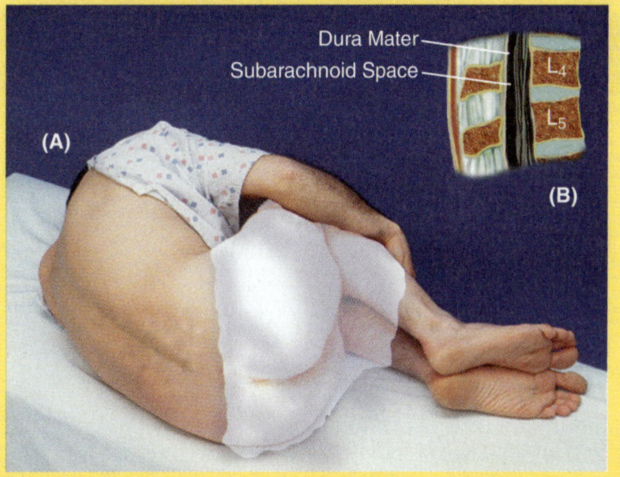

Figure 18-59 (A) Have the patient draw up the knees to the abdomen and grasp knees. Chin should flex on chest. (B) The site for the lumbar puncture.

DOCUMENTATION

6/12/20XX 3:10 PM Lumbar puncture performed by Dr. King. Three samples of cerebrospinal fluid obtained. Labeled #1, #2, #3. Taken to laboratory. Appeared to tolerate procedure. BP 142/82, P88. Instructed to remain flat for 3 hours and to drink increased amounts of fluids. J. Guerro, CMA (AAMA) ——————

Procedure 18-23

Assisting the Provider with a Neurologic Screening Examination

STANDARD PRECAUTIONS:

PURPOSE:

To determine a patient's neurologic status.

EQUIPMENT/SUPPLIES:

Percussion hammer
Safety pin or sensory wheel
Material for odor identification
Cotton ball
Tuning fork
Flashlight
Tongue blade
Ophthalmoscope

PROCEDURE STEPS:

1. Wash hands.
2. The mental status examination can be done by the medical assistant when taking the patient's medical history by observing the following: When taking patient's history, pay special attention to level of awareness, memory, cognition, and mood. When the patient answers questions during the history taking, note if behavior is appropriate for the circumstances.
3. The provider checks reflexes using the percussion hammer.
4. The provider checks the patient's sensory abilities; responses to skin sensations using a safety pin or sensory wheel and cotton ball; patient's ability to recognize the form of solid objects by touch (key, coin, paper clip); and patient's ability to identify specific odor. The provider also checks cranial nerves, performs finger to nose test, and checks patient's ability to touch heel to shin and ability to run the heel down opposite shin.
5. Assist the patient as needed during and after the examination.
6. Document procedure in patient's chart or electronic medical record.

DOCUMENTATION

8/22/20XX 3:20 PM Assisted Dr. Woo with neurologic screening examination. Made appointment for patient to see Dr. Sullivan, neurologist, on 9/4/XX at 3:00 PM. J. Backus, RMA ———

Case Study 18-1

Refer to the scenario at the beginning of the chapter.

Both medical assistants are responsible for ensuring that the supplies and equipment needed for the specialty examinations are available and that safety precautions are followed before, during, and after the examination.

CASE STUDY REVIEW

1. Determine what supplies and equipment should be assembled for the following specialty examinations: fecal occult blood testing, performing an eye instillation, performing an ear irrigation, and performing color vision testing.
2. Explain four safety precautions that must be in place when allergy skin testing is being performed.

Case Study 18-2

Corey Bayer is a 15-year-old patient at City Health Care. He sustained an injury to his right wrist today during soccer practice. Dr. Rice examined him and ordered a radiograph of the right forearm. The results show that Corey has sustained a Colles' fracture of the right wrist. Dr. Rice asks you to prepare the equipment to apply a cast.

CASE STUDY REVIEW

1. Describe cast application. What are the medical assistant's responsibilities?
2. After Corey's cast application, describe the cast care instructions that will be given to him and his mother.

Case Study 18-3

Dr. Rice has scheduled Anita Blanchette for a spirometry test and wants you to telephone her the day before the test to prepare her so that optimal results are obtained.

CASE STUDY REVIEW

1. What information do you give to Anita before her spirometry so that the best test results can be obtained?

SUMMARY

Medical assistants are a vital link in the health care team. A thorough knowledge and understanding of the various body system examinations and clinical procedures routinely performed as part of patient care will enhance the quality of care given.

Some of the specialty procedures are performed on a routine basis in the ambulatory care setting; others are performed occasionally and perhaps only in larger settings that offer specialized and primary care. Sometimes, to feel comfortable assisting with the less common procedures, medical assistants may need to broaden their base of knowledge by conducting independent research. Medical assistants who are willing to constantly expand their clinical understanding will not only fine-tune their professional skills but will derive greater satisfaction from their job performance.

STUDY FOR SUCCESS

To reinforce your knowledge and skills of information presented in this chapter:

- Review the Key Terms
- Practice the Procedures
- Consider the Case Studies and discuss your conclusions
- Answer the Review Questions
  - Multiple Choice
  - Critical Thinking
- Navigate the Internet by completing the Web Activities
- Practice the StudyWARE activities on your student CD
- Apply your knowledge in the Student Workbook activities
- Complete the Web Tutor sections
- View and discuss the DVD situations

REVIEW QUESTIONS

Multiple Choice

1. What is the name of the elevated skin lesions affecting the epidermis caused by the papillomaviruses?
   a. scleroderma
   b. moles
   c. calluses
   d. warts
2. What is the disorder that is characterized by discomfort of the muscles, tendons, ligaments, and soft tissues brought on by trauma, strain, and emotional stress?
   a. carpal tunnel syndrome
   b. bursitis
   c. gout
   d. fibromyalgia
3. What type of fracture has its bone fragments driven into each other?
   a. greenstick
   b. impacted
   c. oblique
   d. comminuted
4. What disease is caused by a degeneration of brain cells caused by lack of dopamine, bringing about muscle rigidity and akinesia?
   a. multiple sclerosis
   b. Bell's palsy
   c. Parkinson's disease
   d. tic douloureux
5. An acute circumscribed infection of the subcutaneous tissues caused by staphylococcus is a:
   a. comedone
   b. carbuncle
   c. verruca
   d. psoriasis

Critical Thinking

1. Is there an advantage to catheterizing a patient for urinalysis and culture and sensitivity? Why or why not?
2. What is the use and purpose of the audiometer? How is the test administered?
3. Explain the rationale when doing an eye irrigation that the flow of the irrigating solution is from the inside canthus to the outer canthus of the eye.
4. Differentiate among bronchitis, emphysema, and asthma.
5. What is the medical assistant's role when assisting in spirometry?
6. What are the cast care guidelines that the medical assistant gives to the patient?
7. When a mental status examination is given, what five areas are being reviewed?
8. Explain the medical assistant's role when assisting with a lumbar puncture.
9. Bariatrics is a relatively new specialty. Explain why obese patients might decide with their provider to undergo bariatric surgery. What are some medical problems that must be addressed before surgery? What are physical and emotional difficulties or problems bariatric surgical patients may have prior to surgery?

WEB ACTIVITIES

Use the Internet to search for information from a medical site to find answers to the following:

1. Using a search engine of your choice, go to Web MD and gather information about the following conditions:
   kidney stones
   polycystic kidneys
   Describe the etiology and treatment of each.
2. Search for possible treatments for sleep apnea.
   http://www.breathingdisorders.com
   http://www.sleepapnea.org
3. What are some long-term harmful effects of cigarette smoking?
   Check this Web site for information:
   http://www.tobaccofreekids.org
4. The National Digestive Diseases Clearinghouse is a useful source for learning about acute and chronic pancreatitis.
   What are the signs and symptoms of acute pancreatitis? How is a diagnosis made by the provider? What is the most common cause of chronic pancreatitis?
5. Adolescent cases of bacterial meningitis have increased since the 1990s.
   Is a particular group of adolescents at greater risk than other groups? How can meningitis be prevented?

REFERENCES/BIBLIOGRAPHY

Altman, G. B. (2004). *Delmar's fundamental and advanced nursing skills* (2nd ed.). Clifton Park, NY: Delmar Cengage Learning.

Asthma guide, overview and facts, treatment and self-care. Retrieved from http://www.webmd.com.

Chronic obstructive pulmonary disease overview and treatment overview. Retrieved October 4, 2008, from http://www.copdfoundation.org.

Delaune, S. C., & Ladner, P. K. (2002). *Fundamentals of nursing standards and practice* (2nd ed.). Clifton Park, NY: Delmar Cengage Learning.

Examinations and tests for COPD. Retrieved September 7, 2007, from http://www.webmd.com.

Metered dose inhalers and how to use them correctly. Retrieved October 11, 2008, from http://www.aafp.org/afp/20010815/603.html.

Miller-Keane. (1997). *Encyclopedia and dictionary of medicine, nursing and allied health.* (5th ed.). Philadelphia: W. B. Saunders.

Neighbors, M., & Tannehill-Jones, R. (2006). *Human diseases.* Clifton Park, NY: Delmar Cengage Learning.

Roe, S. (2003). *Delmar's clinical nursing skills and concepts.* Clifton Park, NY: Delmar Cengage Learning.

Section 4, Managing asthma long term overview. (2007). Retrieved October 11, 2008, from http://www.nhlbl.gov/idex.htm (pp. 277–280).

Spotlight on John McGuire, mobile spirometry unit. (2008). Retrieved October 11, 2008, from www.copdfoundation.org. 2(2).

Taber's cyclopedic medical dictionary. (2003). (22nd ed.). Philadelphia: F. A. Davis.

Tamparo, C., & Lewis, M. (2005). *Diseases of the human body* (3rd ed.). Philadelphia: F.A. Davis.

THE DVD HOOK-UP

This chapter discusses the proper techniques for assisting with specialty examinations.

The selected scenes from today's DVD program illustrated various procedures that are used to test the patient's vision and hearing.

When measuring distant vision, the program featured two separate charts that can be used to measure distant vision in children.

1. What were the names of the charts?
2. Which chart should be used for younger children? Which chart should be used for older children?
3. The procedure for measuring visual acuity in this chapter talks about using an occluder to cover the eye when testing vision. The scene for measuring visual acuity in the DVD program illustrates a patient using a small paper cup to cover the eye. Are there any advantages to using a cup versus an occluder?

DVD Journal Summary

Write a paragraph that summarizes what you learned from watching today's DVD selected scene. Imagine that you are testing the eyes of a pilot. To pass the flight physical, the pilot has to have perfect eyesight. You notice that the pilot is really straining to see the eye chart. His acuity test showed less than perfect vision. He tells you his eyes are just strained from flying all day and asks you to alter the results. What would you do in this situation?

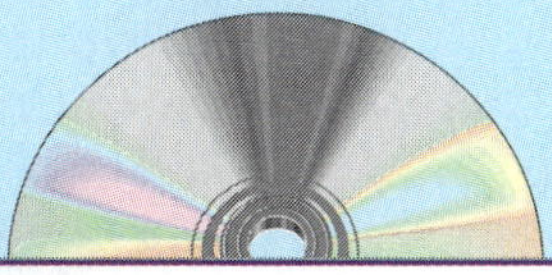

DVD Series	Program Number
Skills Based Series	6

Chapter/Scene Reference

- *Vision and Hearing Tests*

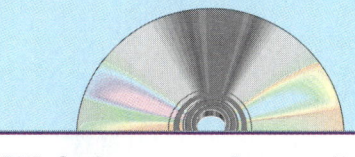

UNIT 6

Advanced Techniques and Procedures

Chapter 19

Assisting with Office/Ambulatory Surgery

KEY TERMS

- Allergy
- Anesthesia
- Antibacterial
- Approximate
- Avascularization
- Bandage
- Betadine®
- Caustic
- Cautery
- Contamination
- Dressing
- Epinephrine
- Exudate
- Fenestrated
- Friable
- Hibeclens®
- Hydrogen Peroxide
- Infection
- Inflammation
- Informed Consent
- Isopropyl Alcohol
- Ligature
- Liquid Nitrogen
- Mayo Stand/Instrument Tray
- Ratchets
- Silver Nitrate
- Sitz Bath
- Sodium Hydroxide
- Sterile Field
- Strictures
- Suppurant
- Surgery Cards
- Surgical Asepsis
- Suture

OUTLINE

- Surgical Asepsis and Sterilization
  - Hand Cleansing (Hand Hygiene) for Medical and Surgical Asepsis
- Sterile Principles
- Methods of Sterilization
  - Gas Sterilization
  - Dry Heat Sterilization
  - Chemical ("Cold") Sterilization
  - Steam Sterilization (Autoclave)
- Common Surgical Procedures Performed in Providers' Offices and Clinics
- Additional Surgical Methods
  - Electrosurgery
  - Cryosurgery
  - Laser Surgery
- Suture Materials and Supplies
  - Suture/Ligature
  - Suture Needles
  - Staples
  - Staple Removal
- Instruments
  - Structural Features
  - Categories and Uses
  - Care of Instruments
- Supplies and Equipment
  - Drapes
  - Sponges and Wicks
  - Solutions/Creams/Ointments
  - Dressings and Bandages
  - Anesthetics
- Patient Care and Preparation
  - Patient Preparation and Education
  - Informed Consent
  - Medical Assisting Considerations
  - Postoperative Instructions
  - Wounds, Wound Care, and the Healing Process
- Basic Surgery Setup
  - Basic Rules and Concepts for Setup of Surgical Trays
- Surgery Process
- Preparation for Surgery
  - Using Dry Sterile Transfer Forceps

OBJECTIVES

The student should strive to meet the following performance objectives and demonstrate an understanding of the facts and principles presented in this chapter through written and oral communication.

1. Define the key terms as presented in the glossary.
2. Define surgical asepsis and differentiate between surgical asepsis and medical asepsis.
3. List eight basic rules to follow to protect sterile areas.
4. State four methods of sterilization.
5. List supplies and equipment necessary to achieve surgical asepsis when using an autoclave.

OBJECTIVES (continued)

6. Explain competent wrapping and operation of the autoclave.
7. State storage measures and expiration periods for autoclaved materials.
8. Explain the sizing standards of suture material and the criteria used to select the most appropriate type and size.
9. Given a variety of surgical instruments, be able to identify each and describe its intended use.
10. Demonstrate the ability to select the most appropriate type of dressings for a given situation.
11. State advantages and disadvantages of Betadine®, Hibeclens®, isopropyl alcohol, and hydrogen peroxide when each is used as a skin antiseptic.
12. Define anesthesia, and explain the advantages and disadvantages of epinephrine as an additive to injectable anesthetics.
13. List five preoperative concerns to be addressed in patient preparation and education.
14. List five postoperative concerns to be addressed with the patient and the caregiver.
15. Demonstrate applying sterile gloves.
16. Demonstrate setting up a surgical tray, including laying the field, applying supplies and instruments, pouring a sterile solution, using transfer forceps, and covering the sterile tray.
17. Explain what is meant by alternative surgical methods.

KEY TERMS (continued)

Swaged
Thermolabile
Thermophile
Unsterile Field
Volatile

Scenario

It might be instructive to compare two different ambulatory care settings. At the multiprovider Inner City Health Care, minor surgery is performed on a routine basis. Certain days are dedicated to certain procedures. Because of the high volume of patients and different provider preferences, Inner City maintains two special rooms for minor surgery and has a large selection of instruments. At the smaller two-provider practice of Lewis and King, however, minor surgical procedures are less frequent and are conducted in the patient examination rooms.

INTRODUCTION

Office/ambulatory surgery differs from hospital surgery not only in complexity, but in the supplies, equipment, instruments, and personnel needed. Some office/ambulatory surgery is performed by the provider alone; some surgeries require the assistance of the medical assistant. Most ambulatory care settings do not need a large variety of surgical instruments but often need more than one of the more frequently used instruments. As a personal preference, special instruments may be purchased and maintained for a specific provider to use during a particular surgical procedure. These particular instruments are generally not used by the other providers.

*The equipment and supplies used in office/ambulatory surgery are usually portable and easily maintained. Larger practices that perform many office/ambulatory surgeries generally can afford the space and expense of maintaining a special room just for that purpose. Often patient examination rooms serve as small surgical suites with portable **Mayo stands/instrument trays**, supplies, and equipment brought into the room for the procedure.*

Whether assisting with office/ambulatory surgery is a routine or an infrequent event for the medical assistant, it is nonetheless important to be knowledgeable about sterile technique, the use and care of instruments and the room, as well as patient preparation for the surgery. Medical assistants should understand the preferences of each provider on staff to make the surgical procedure comfortable and effective for both patient and provider.

Spotlight on Certification

RMA Content Outline

- Asepsis
- Universal (Standard) Precautions
- Sterilization
- Instruments, care, and handling
- Minor surgery

CMA (AAMA) Content Outline

- Principles of infection control
- Surgical asepsis
- Equipment preparation and operation
- Autoclave/sterilizer
- Preparing/maintaining treatment areas
- Instruments, supplies, and equipment

CMAS Content Outline

- Asepsis in the medical office
- Exam preparation
- Basic pharmacology
- Understand concepts of asepsis, sanitization, disinfection, and sterilization
- Observe Standard Precautions

SURGICAL ASEPSIS AND STERILIZATION

Surgical asepsis means all microbial life (pathogens and nonpathogens) is destroyed before an invasive procedure is performed. Therefore, all equipment to be used is sterile. The terms *surgical asepsis* and *sterile technique* often are used interchangeably.

Regardless of the number and complexity of surgical procedures performed in the office or ambulatory care center, surgical asepsis must be strictly maintained. Surgical asepsis uses practices known as sterile techniques and the technique is always used during an invasive procedure. Some examples of invasive procedures include creating an opening in the skin such as a surgical incision, suturing a wound such as a laceration, giving an injection, or inserting a sterile catheter into a sterile body cavity such as the urinary bladder.

Because microorganisms are on virtually every surface such as skin, instruments, surgical instrument trays, clothing, and even in the air, it is necessary to destroy as many as possible before performing any surgical procedure. Surgical asepsis or sterile technique prevents microorganism entry into the body during an invasive procedure and, therefore, helps to protect the patient from infection. Once the items and areas are sterilized, every precaution must be taken to prevent **contamination** of the sterile items or areas either by a nonsterile item or surface or from airborne contamination. In this context, to contaminate means to make impure; for example, by introducing microorganisms or infectious material into or onto sterile goods or areas.

Living tissue surfaces such as skin cannot be sterilized but can be made as free of pathogens as possible before the use of a sterile covering. One example of this concept is the use of the surgical hand cleansing technique before applying sterile gloves (see Procedure 19-1). Another example of surgical asepsis is preparing the patient's skin with a surgical scrub solution before applying sterile drapes around the intended surgical site.

Refer to Chapter 10 for more complete information on the concepts of asepsis and aseptic techniques, including hand cleansing for medical asepsis.

The differences between hand cleansing for medical asepsis as discussed in Chapter 10 (see Procedure 10-1) and hand cleansing for surgical asepsis are addressed in the following section (Table 19-1).

Hand Cleansing (Hand Hygiene) for Medical and Surgical Asepsis

Hand cleansing (hygiene) for medical asepsis is defined as removing pathogenic microorganisms from the hands after they become contaminated. Medical hand cleansing is used many times throughout the day to cleanse the skin after removing contaminated gloves, assisting with patient care, and touching unclean surfaces.

Hand cleansing for surgical asepsis is defined as removal of as many microorganisms as possible before donning sterile gloves and performing surgery or a sterile procedure. Hand

Table 19-1 Differences between Medical and Surgical Hand Cleansing (Hygiene)

Medical Hand Cleansing (Hygiene)	Surgical Hand Cleansing (Hygiene)
Liquid soap and water sufficient for most routine clinical activities.	Performed before any surgical or invasive procedure.
One-minute duration.	Three to six-minute duration.
Wash hands and wrists.	Wash hands, wrists, and forearms to the elbows. Brush may be used.
Hands should be held down during rinsing.	Hands should be held up during washing and rinsing.
Scrub nails with brush; clean under nails with cuticle stick.	Scrub nails with brush and clean under each nail with cuticle stick.
Alcohol-based preparations are practical alternatives to soap and water on visibly clean hands.	Alcohol-based hand wash can be used after pre-washing hands to remove debris.
Apply lotion.*	Do not apply lotion.*
	Glove for sterility.
	Higher level of decontamination.

*The use of lotions is encouraged to help prevent chafing of the skin, especially with frequent hand cleansings. Nevertheless, studies have determined that lotions containing petroleum or mineral oil can break down latex and should be avoided if latex gloves are going to be worn within 1 hour after applying the lotion. If lotions are applied immediately before gloving, the use of water-based lotions is recommended. Of special interest to persons with latex sensitivities (see Chapter 10) is the fact that using lotions and creams containing petroleum products actually increases the amount of latex protein that is transferred from the gloves into the skin, thereby increasing the symptoms of latex sensitivity.

cleansing for surgical asepsis consists of meticulously scrubbing hands, wrists, and forearms before applying sterile gloves. Both medical and surgical aseptic hand cleansing techniques are designed to prevent exposing patients, health care workers, and the public to potentially harmful microorganisms. A brushless/waterless surgical hand cleanser can be used after prewashing hands to remove debris from hands and nails. The brushless cleansing agent has an antimicrobial additive that contains alcohol. The agent must be completely dry before donning gown and gloves.

Proper protocol when assisting with surgery requires the use of surgical hand cleansing at the beginning of each workday, as well as before every sterile technique, with the complementary use of medical hand cleansing before leaving the office and when returning and between patients and procedures. Any opening in the medical assistant's skin should be covered with a sterile adhesive dressing, and gloves are worn during any direct patient contact. See Chapter 10 for information on medical asepsis and Standard Precautions.

STERILE PRINCIPLES

Sterile principles are a set of guidelines designed to designate what items and areas are considered sterile and what actions cause contamination. Some areas are logical and clear, some are subtle and less clear. Some surfaces, such as skin, cannot be sterilized. Large items such as instrument stands and their trays cannot fit into an autoclave for sterilization. To create sterile areas and surfaces where sterility is not possible, sterile barriers should be used; sterile gloves can be worn over the hands. Sterile drapes can be applied to trays once they have been washed, rinsed, dried, and disinfected.

Guidelines to protect sterile items and areas include:

- A sterile object may not touch a nonsterile object.
- Sterile objects must not be wet. Moisture can draw microorganisms into or onto the sterile object.
- An acceptable border between a sterile area and a nonsterile area is 1 inch. The portion of a drape that hangs over the edge is considered nonsterile, no matter what its size. Sterile articles should be placed in the center of the **sterile field** and away from the edge as much as possible.
- Do not turn your back on a sterile field. If you cannot see the field, you cannot be aware of what touched it.
- Anything below the waist is considered contaminated. In support of this principle, all surgery trays should be positioned above the waist. All articles are to be held above the waist.
- All sterile objects (such as gloved hands) must be held in front and away from the body and above waist level.
- Do not cough, sneeze, or talk over a sterile field. Airborne particles may fall onto the sterile area and contaminate it.
- Do not reach over the sterile area. Contaminants may fall onto the area and clothing may touch, thereby contaminating the area. Spend as little time as possible reaching into the sterile area.
- Do not pass contaminated dressings or instruments over the sterile field.
- Arrange for the provider to place contaminated instruments into a separate container or area.
- Always be aware of actions to determine whether the sterile field has been contaminated. When in doubt, err on the side of safety.
- When opening sterile packages, the outer wrapper is contaminated. It should be opened without touching the inner contents, and the contents are then dropped onto the sterile field. Double wrapping can be used (see Procedure 19-3).
- Sterile solutions in bottles should be poured into sterile basins or cups on the sterile field without touching the rim of the bottle and without splashing solution onto the sterile field. If the sterile field is not polylined and becomes wet, it is considered contaminated because a field that is wet acts as a wick and draws microorganisms into the article. Using polylined drapes as sterile fields protects against contamination.

METHODS OF STERILIZATION

There are four methods of sterilization:

1. Gas sterilization
2. Dry heat sterilization
3. Chemical ("cold") sterilization
4. Steam sterilization (autoclave)

Gas Sterilization

Gas sterilization is accomplished in a gas oven large enough for wheelchairs and beds and takes hours for the extremely toxic gases to permeate and dissipate. These features make the gas oven useful in a large hospital setting but much too costly and impractical for the office.

Dry Heat Sterilization

Dry heat sterilization requires higher temperatures than steam sterilization and requires longer exposure times as well (at least 1 hour at 320°F). This method can be used for instruments that easily corrode, such as sharp cutting instruments. Powders, oils, ointments, rubber goods, and plastic tubing can be sterilized using the dry heat method. Procedures for wrapping are the same as when wrapping for steam sterilization (see Procedure 19-3). Dry heat is seldom used in today's medical office or clinic.

Chemical ("Cold") Sterilization

Chemical sterilization, or cold sterilization, may use the same chemical agents used to chemically disinfect instruments or fomites. However, the exposure time for chemical sterilization is achieved through prolonged immersion. Items must be sanitized first. The handling of instruments after chemical sterilization differs from handling procedures for instruments that are steam sterilized in that instruments must be handled with sterile gloves, rinsed with sterile water, and dried with sterile towels before placement on a sterile surface.

Chemical sterilization is an effective method used in many medical offices when the object being sterilized is too large or too heat sensitive for autoclaving (see following section for information on autoclaving). Fiber-optic endoscopes are one of the most common items sterilized with the use of chemicals. These items are delicate and unable to withstand the high heat of an autoclave. The necessary equipment for chemical sterilization is a container or basin of adequate size for the intended item (and should be maintained for that purpose only) with a well-fitting lid and the chemical of choice. A vent hood is required for safety. Two of the most popular brands of chemicals available through medical supply sources are Wavecide and Cidex. Both have advantages and disadvantages. Offices must make individual choices based on convenience, expense, and other personnel preferences.

The effectiveness of any of these products depends greatly on the strength of the solution. If the strength is a 1:1 ratio of water to chemical, effectiveness will be lost if the solution is not mixed according to that dilution. Any attempt to cut cost by mixing a weaker solution will greatly compromise the effectiveness. The item will not be sterile. Sometimes solutions are weakened unintentionally by placing wet items into them, thereby adding more water than is intended. For this reason, wet items must be carefully dried before chemical sterilization. A well-fitting tight lid is essential to prevent evaporation, which also interferes with the strength of the solution. The lid also lessens the chance of dust and airborne microbes from falling into the solution.

Another factor influencing the effectiveness of the sterilizing chemicals is exposure time. The manufacturer provides specific time charts for each purpose. Manufacturer's directions also include a time frame for replacing the solution. The ability of the solution to kill pathogens is directly related to its freshness or shelf life. Regardless of the chemical used for sterilization, ventilation is important.

When using commercial chemicals, make certain the lid is placed on the soak basin at all times except when placing or removing items. Care must be taken to avoid contact with skin, eyes, and mucous membranes. Wear protective gloves, goggles, and apron. The effects on skin can range from slight irritation to serious caustic burns.

Before any chemically sterilized items are used for patient contact, the chemicals must be thoroughly rinsed off using either sterile gloves or sterile transfer forceps to remove the item from the container. To maintain sterility, sterile water must be used for the rinsing process. Then dry with a sterile towel, and place onto a sterile field. This process is performed just before use of the item (see Procedure 19-2).

Steam Sterilization (Autoclave)

Steam sterilization is the most widely used method of sterilization used in the medical office. An autoclave, basically a pressure cooker, is used to achieve sterilization. The autoclave uses steam under pressure to obtain higher temperatures than can be achieved with boiling (Figure 19-1). Water reaches a maximum temperature of 212°F through boiling. When under pressure, water is converted to steam and is then able to reach a temperature of 270°F and higher. Exposing items to this extremely high heat and at least 15 pounds of pressure for a specific amount of time ensures that all microorganisms and their spores are killed. The autoclave is an inner sterilizing chamber surrounded by a metal jacket. This creates a middle steam chamber between the inner sterilizing chamber and the jacket. Inside the jacket is a reservoir for water. When water is poured into the reservoir, the autoclave door closed and secured, and the autoclave turned on, several processes occur. The water in the reservoir heats until vapor is produced. The vapor enters the middle steam chamber inside the jacket. The air in the steam chamber is pushed out and replaced with steam. Because the air has been pushed out, the pressure increases. The increase of pressure causes the steam to then enter the inner sterilizing chamber (where the items and instruments for sterilization are placed), which pushes out the air. With the air being displaced with steam, the pressure increases in the inner chamber. The steam under pressure is able to reach a much higher temperature than boiling water. When the steam is able to reach all surfaces of the items placed in the autoclave and exposure is maintained for adequate amounts of time, sterility of those items is ensured.

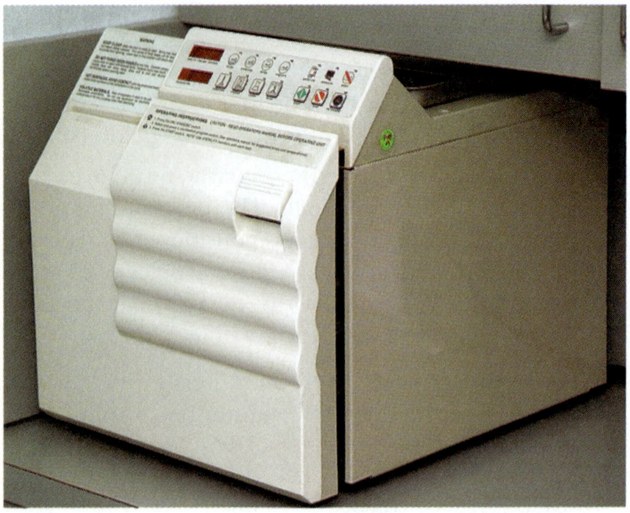

Figure 19-1 Commonly found in providers' offices, autoclaves are used for sterilization by steam pressure, usually at 270°F (118°C) for a specified length of time.

The recommended temperature for effective sterilization in an autoclave is 270°F. Unwrapped items should be sterilized for 20 minutes, loosely wrapped items for 30 minutes, and tightly packed items for at least 40 minutes. When uncertain about the proper amount of time necessary, the medical assistant should refer to the manufacturer's recommendations. The overall effectiveness of the autoclave in sterilizing contents is totally dependent on the medical assistant following proper operating procedure.

Only distilled water should be used to prevent mineral buildup in the machine. Before every use, check the water level and add to fill line if necessary. Distilled water is inexpensive and readily available.

How to Load Packages. It is of extreme importance that instruments and materials be positioned properly in the autoclave for the steam to circulate through and between packs and penetrate them. Do not overload the autoclave. Place items as loosely as possible inside the chamber. Leave a 1- to 3-inch space between packs and the walls of the autoclave. Correct positioning and spacing allows sterilization to take place provided the medical assistant adheres to proper temperature, pressure, and time requirements (Figure 19-2).

Autoclave Maintenance and Cleaning. The autoclave, like any piece of equipment in the medical office, needs regular cleaning and maintenance. Frequency of cleaning the autoclave depends somewhat on its usage. If the autoclave is used every day, the inner chamber should be washed with a mild detergent and cloth, rinsed, and dried on a daily basis. The outer jacket should be wiped clean of dust and soil. Follow the manufacturer's instructions and recommendations for cleansers. Omni® cleanser is a well-known brand of autoclave cleanser.

At least once a week or following the manufacturer's instructions, the autoclave should be drained of water and cleaned thoroughly. Cleaning the autoclave requires that it be drained, filled with cleaning solution, run through a 20-minute heated cycle, drained of solution, filled with distilled rinse water, run through another 20-minute heated cycle, drained of rinse solution, and filled with distilled water again. Then the inner shelves are removed and scrubbed, and the inner chamber is wiped clean. Because this process is fairly time-consuming and puts the autoclave out of use for a while, consideration should be given to scheduling the weekly cleaning at a time when personnel can devote the time and when the autoclave is not in demand for sterilization processes.

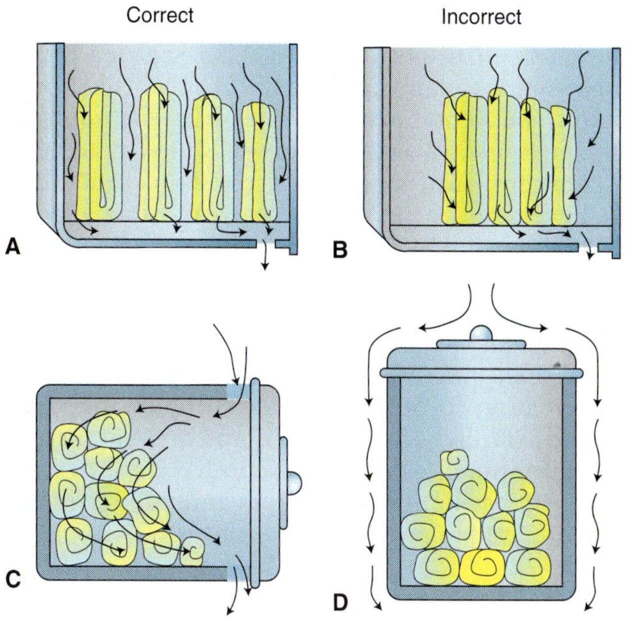

Figure 19-2 (A) Proper placement of packages in the autoclave allows steam to circulate and penetrate from all sides. (B) Packages incorrectly loaded in autoclave. (C) When placed correctly, the jar should lay on its side with the cover loosely in place to allow steam to freely circulate through the jar and properly sterilize the dressings. (D) Incorrect method. (Courtesy of Steris Corporation, Mentor, OH.)

General Rules to Ensure Proper Sterilization Using an Autoclave

- Articles placed into the autoclave must have been sanitized, rinsed, and dried.
- The articles are wrapped and placed to allow adequate exposure of all surfaces (see Figure 19-2). Instruments inside packages should have hinges open and serrations exposed.
- To prevent formation of trapped air pockets, containers should be placed on their sides with lids loosely in place.
- Any wrapping material used must be approved for autoclave use.
- Timing should not start until the gauges read 15 pounds of pressure and 270°F.
- When the cycle is complete, the door must be opened slightly to allow steam to escape. The sterile wrapped articles will be hot and damp and should be left in the autoclave to cool and dry. Microorganisms can contaminate the sterile articles through the damp wrapping if the door is opened too wide or if articles are handled while damp.

During the cleaning process, attention should be given to inspecting the rubber seal for cracks or wear. An extra replacement rubber seal should always be kept on hand. The seals are available through medical supply sources. Refer to the manufacturer's instructions for regularly scheduled replacement of the rubber seal and other recommended maintenance procedures.

Quality Control and Assurance for Autoclave. Quality control when using an autoclave consists of proper maintenance, proper operation, and observation of the temperature and pressure gauges. Equally important is the regular use of sterilization indicators and culture tests. Several types of sterilization indicators and culture methods are available:

- *Sterilization strips.* The strips contain a **thermolabile** dye that darkens when exposed to steam at the proper temperature and pressure for the proper amount of time. These indicators are placed in the center of the wrapped article (Figure 19-3).
- *Culture tests.* These are available as a culture strip containing heat-resistant spores. The strip is placed in the center of a wrapped article and placed in a fully loaded autoclave. After processing is complete, the article is unwrapped and the strip is placed into a culture medium. If the autoclave is functioning properly and the medical assistant has followed proper operating procedure, no growth should occur.

Also available through Becton-Dickinson Microbiology Systems is an ampule called the Kilit Ampule. These biological indicators are ampules that contain spores of the **thermophile** "*Bacillus stearothermophilus.*" After being processed through the autoclave, the Kilit Ampule is sent to a cooperating laboratory for week-long observation for survival of the bacilli spores. A written report of the results is generated by the laboratory and sent to the office for its records. The CDC recommends biological indicators.

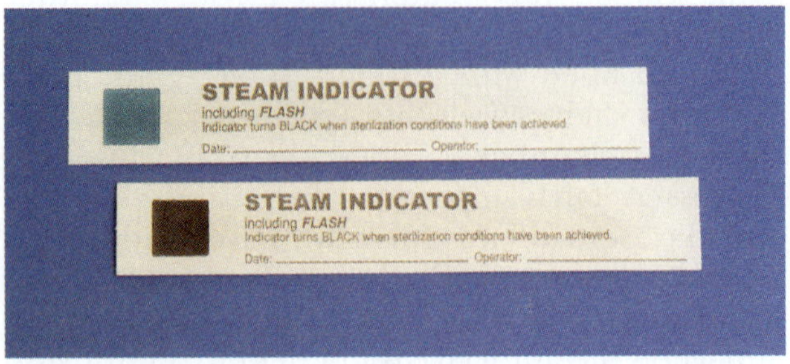

Figure 19-3 Types of sterilization indicators.

Autoclave Wrapping Material and Packaging Supplies. Wrapping or otherwise packaging surgical instruments and other surgical and medical articles before placing them in the autoclave will extend their shelf life. Before these articles are wrapped, they must first be sanitized, rinsed, and dried. Several materials are available for wrapping. Cost, convenience, visibility, time, space, and ease of use will help determine which to use. Many offices use a combination of materials.

- Muslin is a cloth wrap available in several sizes and colors. Even with the cost of the initial purchasing, occasional replacements, autoclave tape, and laundering, muslin is still an economical option. Besides these cost-effective advantages, many surgical instruments can be wrapped together in muslin, making up a convenient surgery/procedure set. One of the main disadvantages of muslin is the inability to view the contents. Another disadvantage is the need for constant examination for holes, tears, and wearing out of the cloth. Patching is not a reasonable option because iron-on patches impede penetration of steam and sewn-on patches create their own set of perforations. A defective muslin cloth should be discarded. Wrapping space and training of personnel are necessary when using cloth. Special autoclave tape is required to seal the package.
- Paper sterilization wrapping squares are available in many different sizes and types. This disposable type of material requires that a new paper be used each time items are sterilized, but it eliminates the need for laundering. Similar to cloth wrapping, paper wraps also lend themselves to larger sets of articles being wrapped together for surgery or procedural packs. As with muslin cloth, wrapping space and some personnel training are necessary. Paper wraps are opaque, making viewing of the contents impossible. Autoclave tape is required to seal the package.
- Sterilization pouches or bags may be plastic, paper, or a combination (Figure 19-4). They are fairly inexpensive and very easy to use. Because no wrapping is involved, additional work space is not required. Another advantage of bags is the visibility of the items inside. Some pouches are packaged on a continuous roll and are available in a variety of widths. This allows the medical assistant to cut the bag to fit the article. Because both ends must to be taped closed, it is difficult to remove the article while maintaining its sterility. Probably the best bag-type option is individual bags with the top end open for instrument placement and the bottom end factory closed with a peel-apart seal. The article is inserted into the

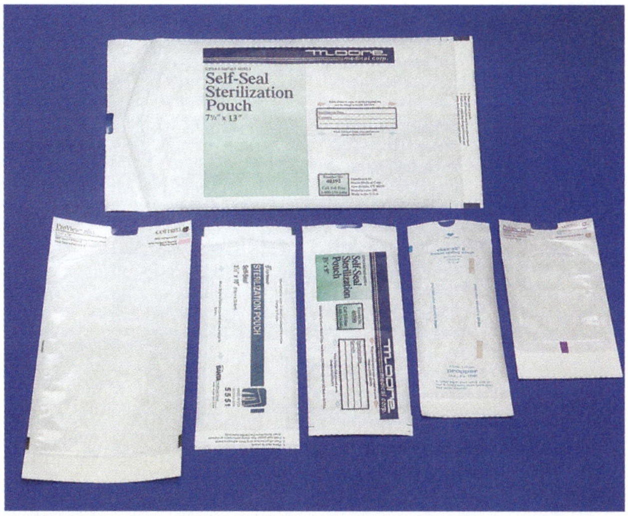

Figure 19-4 Various types and sizes of self-sealing bags for sterilization.

top opening, the bag is taped closed, and the package is sterilized (Figure 19-5). When needed, the sterile article is removed through the factory-sealed bottom end in a peel-apart sterile fashion. These individual bags need to be purchased in several sizes and are expensive but have the advantages of ease of use and item visibility and are probably the preferred method for most medical offices today.

Autoclave Tape. Autoclave tape is chemically treated to appear "striped" when exposed to heat. The striped pattern indicates exposure to high temperature but does not measure pounds of pressure or duration of exposure. Because of these limitations, autoclave tape does not assure that the wrapped package is sterile, only that it has been in a heated autoclave. The tape is placed on the outside of the package, so it does not assure that steam has penetrated to the inner article. It does help to determine if a package has been in the autoclave (Figure 19-6).

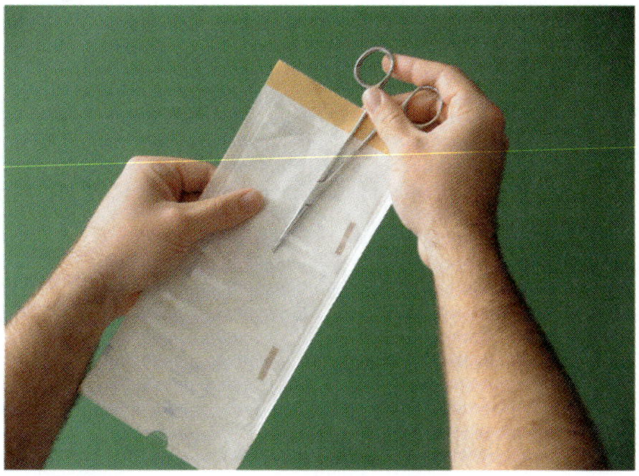

Figure 19-5 The medical assistant is placing a sanitized instrument into a sterilization bag for autoclaving by inserting the tips of the instrument in first.

Labeling Packages for Autoclave. Surgical packages should be labeled clearly. Clear bags usually have a designated place for labeling, and muslin- or paper-wrapped packages may be labeled across the autoclave tape. Proper labeling should include the name(s) of the articles in the pack, the date of sterilization, and the initials of the medical assistant responsible for the wrapping. The name of the instrument or article should be as specific as possible, especially when using the opaque cloth or paper wraps. If many instruments have been wrapped together for a specific surgery or for a specific provider, the label should clearly state which

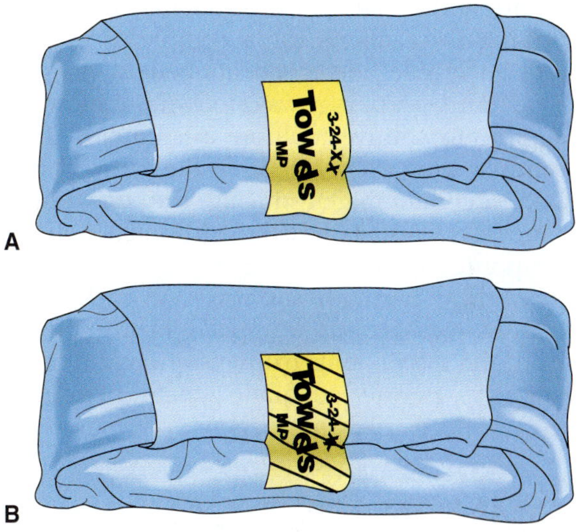

Figure 19-6 Package of towels (A) before and (B) after autoclaving. Note that the autoclave tape has a striped pattern indicating that the package was exposed to a high temperature. However, this does not assure sterility.

Critical Thinking

What is the purpose of OSHA's standards for bloodborne pathogens and whom does it cover?

surgery or surgeon. For example, a "laceration repair set" could contain all the necessary instruments for repairing a laceration. "Dr. Peterson's vasectomy set" would contain all the instruments Dr. Peterson needs to perform a vasectomy, including, perhaps, personal preference instruments. The date of sterilization helps determine the expiration of sterility and a "pull date" for resterilizing. Initialing the package allows for accountability if necessary. Labels should always be written with a permanent marker. Ballpoint pen should never be used because the ink will smear when wet. Caution should be taken to avoid puncturing through the package during labeling.

Wrapping Techniques. Articles must be wrapped in a specific way to ensure they remain sterile when opened. Wrapped surgical instruments need to be double wrapped. Some methods advocate placing both layers of wrapping material together and double wrapping the pack in one process. A much more useful method is the "wrapping twice" technique (see Procedure 19-3). The wrapping twice technique allows for additional options at the time of opening. Wrapping twice allows for a completely wrapped inner sterile package to be applied to the surgical tray. This wrapping twice technique eliminates struggling to control multiple instruments during the unwrapping process; and, if the inner package becomes contaminated during the unwrapping, the medical assistant has the additional option of unwrapping the inner package using the same technique without having to start over. All packs should be neatly and securely wrapped—firm enough to prevent the instruments from movement, but loose enough to permit adequate steam penetration (see Procedures 19-3 and 19-4).

COMMON SURGICAL PROCEDURES PERFORMED IN PROVIDERS' OFFICES AND CLINICS

All surgery has commonalities as well as specifics. The following on specific surgery or surgical procedures includes lists of needed instruments, supplies, and equipment, as well as basic patient preparation and postoperative instructions for some of the more frequently performed surgeries. The following procedures are suggested protocol only because providers will have preferences and techniques unique to them and their practices (Figure 19-7).

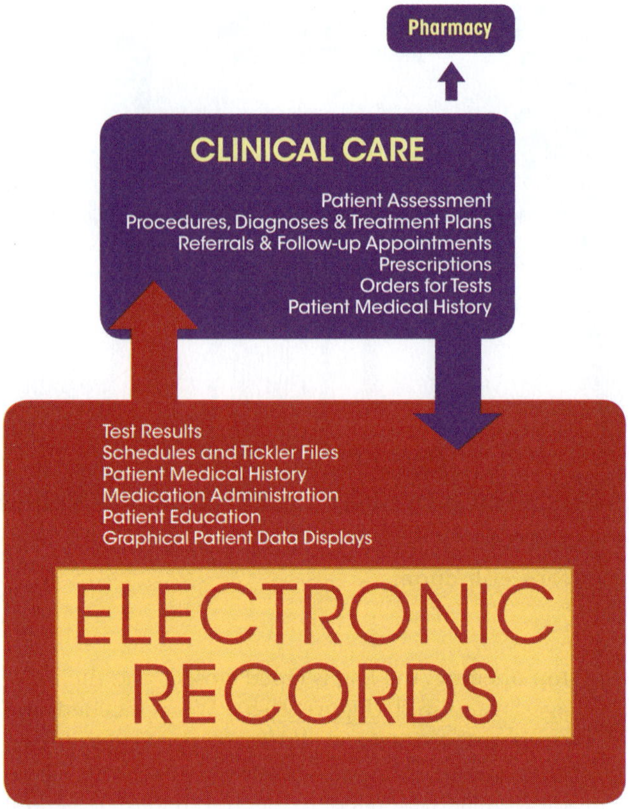

Figure 19-7 In a total practice management system, the provider's preferences for instruments, supplies, and equipment are electronically stored and immediately accessible to the medical assistant when setting up for various surgical procedures.

This section includes a general procedure for assisting with surgery and is followed by specific office/ambulatory surgical procedures, including:

- Assisting with Office/Ambulatory Surgery (Procedure 19-8)
- Dressing Change (Procedure 19-9)
- Wound Irrigation (Procedure 19-10)
- Preparation of Patient's Skin before Surgery (Procedure 19-11)
- Suturing of Laceration or Incision Repair (Procedure 19-12)
- Sebaceous Cyst Excision (Procedure 19-13)
- Incision and Drainage of Localized Infection (Procedure 19-14)
- Aspiration of Joint Fluid (Procedure 19-15)
- Hemorrhoid Thrombectomy (Procedure 19-16)
- Suture/Staple Removal (Procedure 19-17)
- Application of Sterile Adhesive Skin Closure Strips (Steri-Strips) (Procedure 19-18)

ADDITIONAL SURGICAL METHODS

Additional surgical methods are those methods not requiring the use of a surgical knife or scalpel but using other methods of cutting or destroying, such as electric current, heat, freezing, chemicals, or laser beam. The method used is determined by the provider's preference.

Electrosurgery

Electrosurgery uses an electric current in a concentrated area to either cut or destroy tissue whenever pathologic examination is not required. The equipment for electrosurgery consists of a power source, usually a small boxed unit, and a detachable handheld applicator with removable tips. The tips are available in various sizes and are removable for cleaning and sterilizing.

Electrosurgery is useful in removing benign skin tags and warts. The main advantage of electrosurgery is that the bleeding is controlled through the cauterization of the blood vessels as the electric current is applied. The terms *electrocoagulation, electrofulguration, electrodessication, electroscission, electrosection,* and *eletrocautery* all refer to various uses of electric current to either coagulate blood vessels, destroy tissue either with a spark or by drying, or cut tissue. Disposable battery-operated units designed for one-time use are available.

Cautery. The word **cautery** comes from the term *caustic* and means the application of a **caustic** chemical or destructive heat. Electrosurgery, cautery, and electrocautery are often used interchangeably. The burning of tissue, either chemically or electrically, is known as cauterization. Sometimes during surgical procedures unnecessary bleeding can be controlled by use of electrosurgical equipment (Figure 19-8). Tissues that do not need to be pathologically examined, such as benign skin tags, can be destroyed using cauterization. Some common chemicals used to destroy tissue and stop bleeding are **silver nitrate, liquid nitrogen,** and **sodium hydroxide.**

Chemical Tissue Destruction. Silver nitrate is available in a solid form, impregnated on the end of a wooden applicator stick. Silver nitrate is especially useful inside the nose to cauterize **friable,** easily broken, blood vessels in the treatment of epistaxis (nosebleed).

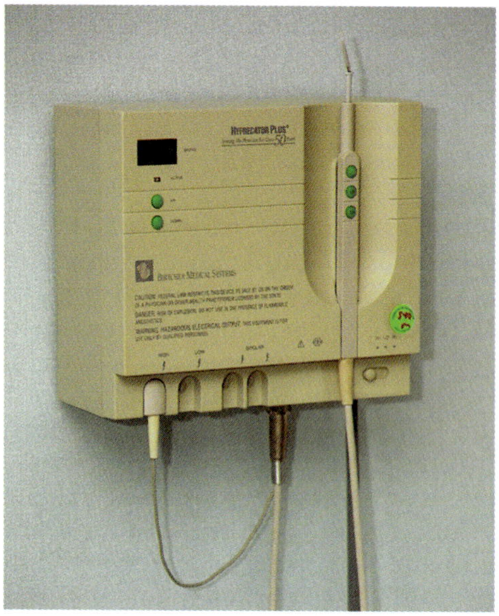

Figure 19-8 Electrosurgical equipment is used to destroy tissue, such as warts, or to coagulate blood vessels to decrease bleeding during surgery.

Liquid chemical caustic agents such as sodium hydroxide are used to permanently destroy the growth plates of toenails whenever total and permanent removal of the toenail is necessary.

Cryosurgery

Cryosurgery refers to the destruction of tissue by freezing. Some types of tissues react differently to heat than cold in the rate of healing and level of scarring. The cryogenic substance most often used to destructively freeze tissue is liquid nitrogen. Liquid nitrogen, often incorrectly referred to as dry ice, is extremely **volatile** (easily evaporated) and must be kept in a covered insulated canister. Liquid nitrogen is obtained when nitrogen gas is compressed under cold temperatures into a liquid. It is most often used to destructively "freeze" warts. Liquid nitrogen can be applied to cervical erosions to facilitate healing and growth of normal tissue, to remove lesions on the anus, and for cataract extraction, retinal detachment, prostate gland destruction, and removal of superficial lesions in the nose and throat. Some units are single purpose use. There is less trauma, more control of bleeding, and less pain with cryosurgery.

Many patients experience pain with liquid nitrogen because it is colder than other chemical cryosurgery options. Liquid nitrogen is usually kept in a large canister in a central location in the office and carefully transferred to a small thermos for transport into the treatment room. The medical assistant must take care to keep the canister and thermos covered because of the volatile properties (evaporation rate) of the liquid nitrogen.

The cryogenic properties of solid liquid nitrogen make it useful for freezing warts and nevi. Nitrous oxide is another chemical used in cryosurgery. Nitrous oxide requires a gas cylinder, a regulator, a pressure gauge, and a cryogun with assorted tips. Nitrous oxide is applied in a more direct and controlled pattern because of the precision of the probes, and nitrous oxide does not evaporate as readily as liquid nitrogen. The tank, probes, and other supplies can be expensive. Nitrous oxide is not as cold as liquid nitrogen; therefore, although it is not so uncomfortable for the patient, it is not as destructive. It is not appropriate for use with cancerous lesions, which must be completely destroyed. Because nitrous oxide is a carcinogen, the Occupational Safety and Health Administration (OSHA) requires that all nitrous oxide systems have outside venting. It is not practical for most ambulatory clinics.

All volatile gases are dangerous to inhale, and appropriate ventilation must be used. Refer to the Material Safety Data Sheet (MSDS) information (available in printed form or on the manufacturer's Web sites) for specific cautions.

Laser Surgery

Laser is an acronym for Light Amplification by Stimulated Emission of Radiation. The laser instrument converts light into an intense beam. By focusing the laser beam onto the target, the application can be extremely precise without damaging surrounding tissue. Over the past 2 decades, laser surgery has become less expensive, more readily available, and consequently much more widespread as a treatment of choice for surgery in dermatology, ophthalmology, nerve surgery, vascular surgery, plastic surgery, and others. Most specialty surgery uses laser in various ways. Because many providers use laser technology in the ambulatory care setting, medical assistants must be familiar with the dangers involved with laser surgery, and safety precautions must be implemented. Attending a laser education and safety workshop is recommended for all personnel intending to work with lasers.

The following precautions are designed to heighten awareness and serve as a safety guide:

- When the laser beam is focused on the target tissue, the cells explode and vaporize. Care should be taken not to inhale the vapors.
- Whenever high levels of electricity are used, care should be taken to avoid burns and to ensure that the equipment is always in good working order.
- Safety glasses should be worn by the provider, medical assistant, and, if possible, the patient.
- If the patient's skin has been prepared with flammable products such as alcohol-based antiseptics, the skin must be dry with no pooling of liquid. Read the product label for alcohol and other flammable substances.
- Sterile water should be readily available to extinguish any fire if the laser beam accidently ignites cloth or paper in the area.

SUTURE MATERIALS AND SUPPLIES

Suture/Ligature

The word **suture** can be used as a verb to describe the motion of sewing or as a noun to describe the material used to sew. Suturing, or sewing, a wound is a common procedure in provider's offices. The purpose is to **approximate,** or bring together, the edges of a wound. Suturing hastens healing and lessens scarring. Whether the wound is an accidental laceration or a surgical incision, the suturing process is basically the same. When suture material is used for tying off the ends of tubular structures during surgery, it is termed **ligature.** The terms *suture* and *ligature* both refer to suture material, but they are named according to their uses.

Most suture material used in office/ambulatory surgical procedures comes already fused, or **swaged,** to a needle and packaged in various lengths (Figure 19-9). These are also called atraumatic. Eighteen inches is a preferred length because it is short enough to be manageable yet long enough to complete most suturing procedures. Combinations of sizes and types of suture materials and sizes and shapes of needles are endless, but most providers use a select few. Selection from among the many different suture materials and needles is based on the needs of the tissue and tissue healing. Suture ranges in size on a scale from the smallest gauge below 0 (aught) to the largest gauge above 0. The scale from 6–0 to 4 includes all sizes from the smallest to the largest:

6–0, 5–0, 4–0, 3–0, 2–0, 0, 1, 2, 3, 4

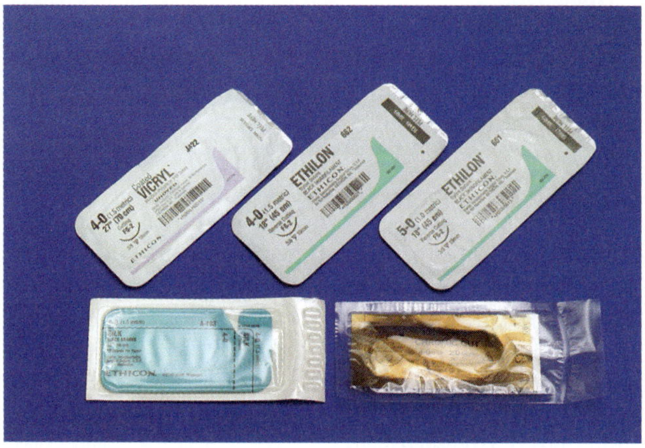

Figure 19-9 A variety of pre-packaged suture materials with needles of various sizes and shapes.

Sometimes 2–0 is labeled 00, 3–0 labeled 000, 4–0 labeled 0000, and so on. Ambulatory care settings use sizes 6–0 to 3–0.

If the tissue being sutured is delicate, as on the face or neck, smaller suture material such as 6–0 is used; the finer the stitch, the less scarring. Some sutures are made from materials that dissolve when they come in contact with the tissue enzymes. These are referred to as absorbable sutures. The original absorbable suture was called surgical gut or "cat gut." It was made from sheep intestinal tissue. Left "natural" or uncoated, it is called plain gut suture. It dissolves or is absorbed in about 1 to 2 weeks. If more time is needed to heal, surgical gut may be coated with chromion salts and is called chromion gut. It allows for a longer period of healing before dissolving. Absorbable gut suture is used for underlying tissues where removal is not reasonable and areas where suture removal is inconvenient. Individual body chemistries influence the exact absorption rate of both plain and treated gut suture. Surgical gut is rarely used now, having been replaced by man-made absorbable suture (such as Vicryl® and PDS® II). Suture is also made of nonabsorbable materials such as stainless steel, silk, cotton, nylon, and Dacron. Some are natural (cotton, silk) and some are synthetic/manmade (Dacron®, Ethilon®, Prolene®). Each type of suture material comes in a variety of options such as different colors for ease of visualization, braiding for additional elasticity and strength, and coatings for lubrications and to lessen irritability to tissues.

Suture Needles

The needles swaged (atraumatic) to the suture material are also varied (see Figure 19-9). For office/ambulatory surgery, the needles are usually curved. They are categorized according to size, shape, radius of curve, and type of point. Needles may be termed *cutting needles, round taper point needles,* or *blunt point needles.*

Staples

Many surgical incisions can be approximated using staples (made of stainless steel or titanium) and a stapler made for this purpose (Figure 19-10). The length, width, and number of staples depend on the tissue. They are safe to use, reduce blood loss, and reduce the length of time of the surgery. Wound healing is quicker, and there is less trauma. Staplers are made for specific types of tissues (e.g., blood vessels, skin, gastrointestinal tract, and so forth). It is more difficult to remedy incorrectly placed staples than it is for manually placed sutures.

Staple Removal

Staple removal (see Procedure 19-17) is done wearing sterile gloves and using sterile instruments. The staples are removed using a sterile prepackaged staple remover (Figure 19-11). The staple remover is carefully positioned under the staple and, when the handle is squeezed, the staple flattens out and it can be carefully lifted out. Cleanse with an antiseptic solution such as Betadine® and pat dry. Be certain all staples have been removed by verifying the number that were inserted with the number you have removed.

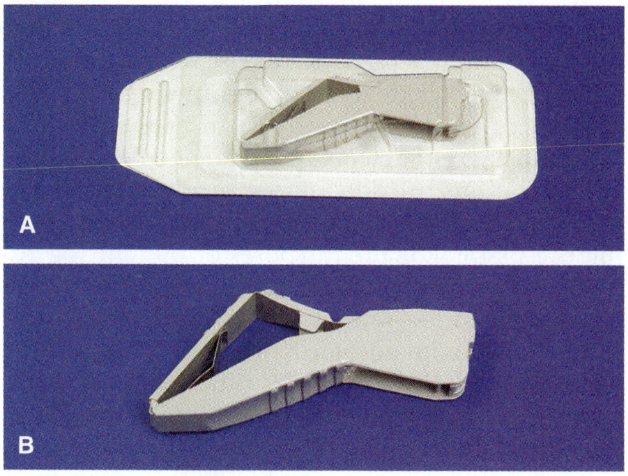

Figure 19-10 Disposable prepackaged skin stapler (A) in package and (B) out of package.

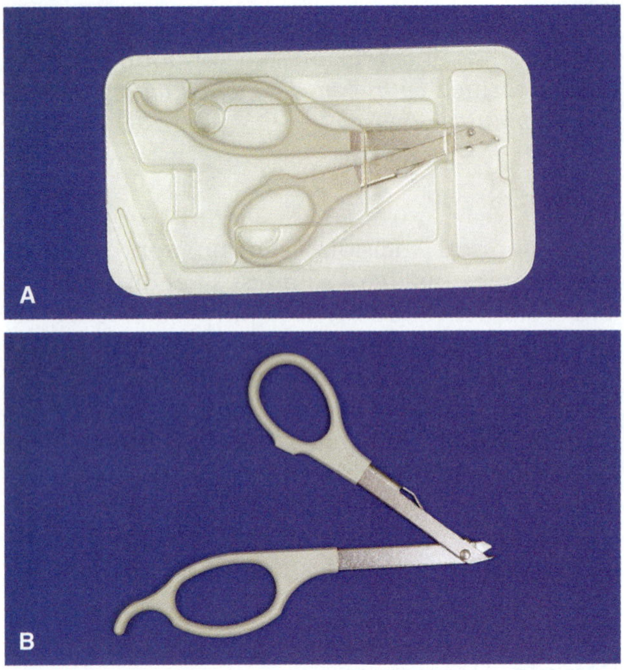

Figure 19-11 Disposable staple remover (A) in package and (B) out of package.

INSTRUMENTS

Structural Features

Rarely does the phrase "form determines function" have as much meaning as when discussing surgical instruments. One can almost always correctly imagine function simply by close examination of the instrument's design. Handles designed to be squeezed between the thumb and finger are called "thumb" handles. "Ring" handles are designed for the insertion of the thumb and finger into rings. **Ratchets** are locking mechanisms located between the rings of the handles and are used for locking the instrument closed. Ratchets are designed to close in varying degrees of tightness. Serrations are the crevices etched into the surfaces of the jaws of hemostats, some forceps, and needle holders. The serrations provide a more secure grip during use with slippery tissues without actually puncturing the tissue. For the purposes of puncturing tissue, forceps with teeth are an option. Teeth may be numerous or few but are always sharp and should approximate tightly when the instrument is closed. To help delicate tips match up properly, some thumb instruments have a guide pin built into the handle. The box-lock is a special type of hinge found on most ring-handled instruments, especially grasping instruments such as hemostats, forceps, and needle holders. Because the box-lock provides strength and aids in the prevention of warping, most instruments with ratchets also need the box-lock hinge. Other features include prongs, hooks, and loops (Figure 19-12).

Categories and Uses

Several companies publish and distribute large pictoral catalogs of well over 30,000 medical-surgical instruments. A glance through these references shows the many choices available. For ease of discussion, learning, and cataloging, most surgical instruments are placed according to their uses into three basic categories.

Instruments designed for specific purposes within medical specialties often do not readily fit into any one group and are called specialty instruments. This group includes long-handled gynecologic instruments, as well as other instruments designed to meet specific needs within specialty practices.

Scissors and Scalpels. Most of the cutting instruments are scissors. Scissors have ring handles and two blades and vary in size, shape, and function. Because scissors have two blades, the word *scissors* is always plural. Bandage scissors have one rounded tip to allow insertion under a bandage without causing injury to the patient. Bandage scissors do not have to be sterile to use. The two most common styles are the Lister bandage scissors and the finer finger bandage scissors (Figure 19-13).

Operating scissors are used to cut tissues and generally have very sharp blades. The blades may be curved or straight, and the tips may be sharp, blunt, or a combination of each. They are described as sharp/sharp (s/s), blunt/blunt (b/b), or sharp/blunt (s/b) (Figure 19-14). A special type of scissors, the Mayo dissecting scissors, may be straight or curved, with curved more often used, but are never described as sharp or blunt because the tips are specifically designed to be neither but have a beveled edge with slightly rounded points (Figure 19-15). Useful, delicately bladed scissors are iris scissors, originally named for usefulness in eye surgery but now widely used in many procedures. Iris scissors may be

Categories of Instruments

Cutting	Scissors and scalpels
Grasping/Clamping	Hemostats, forceps, clamps, and needle holders
Dilating/Probing	Specula, scopes, probes, retractors, and dilators

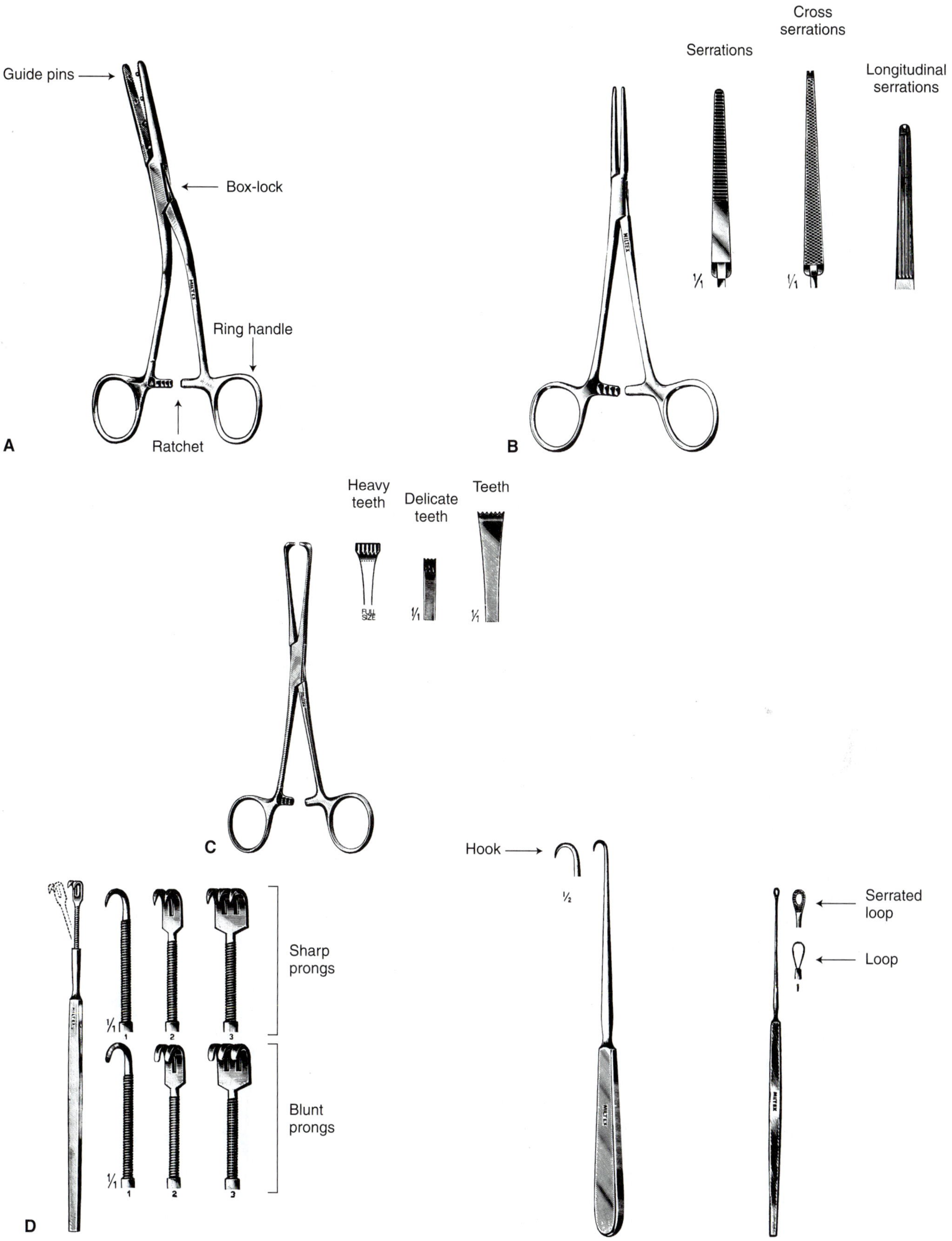

Figure 19-12 Structural features of instruments include (A) ratchets, box-locks, pins, and ring handle; (B) serrations; (C) teeth; and (D) prongs, hooks, and loops. (Courtesy of Miltex, Inc.)

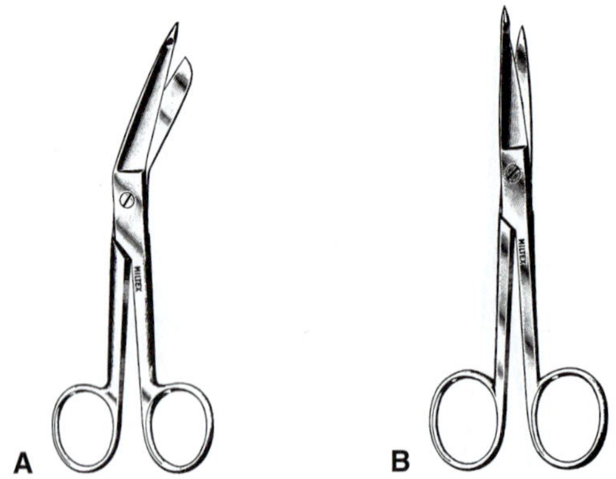

Figure 19-13 Bandage scissors (A) Lister bandage scissors, small; (B) Knowles finger bandage scissors, straight. (Courtesy of Miltex, Inc.)

either curved or straight (Figure 19-16). Suture scissors, also called stitch or stitch removal scissors, have a distinctively notched blade to facilitate the insertion of one tip under a suture (Figure 19-17). All of these scissors must be sterilized before use.

The scalpel is the knife used to cut the skin. The scalpel is actually a blade secured to a handle that, when combined, becomes a surgical knife or scalpel. Disposable one-piece units with a protective retractable blade are available (Figure 19-18). The most common blade sizes are #10, #11, and #15, with #11 often referred to as a "stab blade" because of its sharp point (Figure 19-19A). Handles vary in size, but the most popular are the sturdy #3 and #3L (long) and the more delicate #7 (Figure 19-19B).

Hemostats, Forceps, Clamps, and Needle Holders.

Grasping and clamping instruments are the largest of the instrument categories. They are used for many different tasks. Included in this category are the towel clamps or clips, needle holders, and forceps. Many forceps have locking mechanisms called ratchets. Forceps may have ring handles or use a squeeze concept like a tweezer. Forceps number in the hundreds, but most offices need only a select few. Like the word *scissors,* the word *forceps* is always plural. Hemostatic forceps, or hemostats, are used to grasp and clamp blood vessels. Their name means literally to "stop blood." Because blood vessels are slippery, hemostatic forceps have serrations for grasping and ratchets for locking tightly. Mosquito hemostatic forceps have fine tips, with serrations along the entire length of the tips. The Kelly hemostats have serrations only along partial length of the tips. The Kelly hemostatic forceps are sturdier, and some hemostatic forceps have teeth. All types may be straight or curved (Figure 19-20).

Allis tissue forceps are of a similar design to hemostatic forceps but have unique angular jaws with teeth. Another type of grasping instrument are thumb forceps, sometimes referred to as "pick-ups."

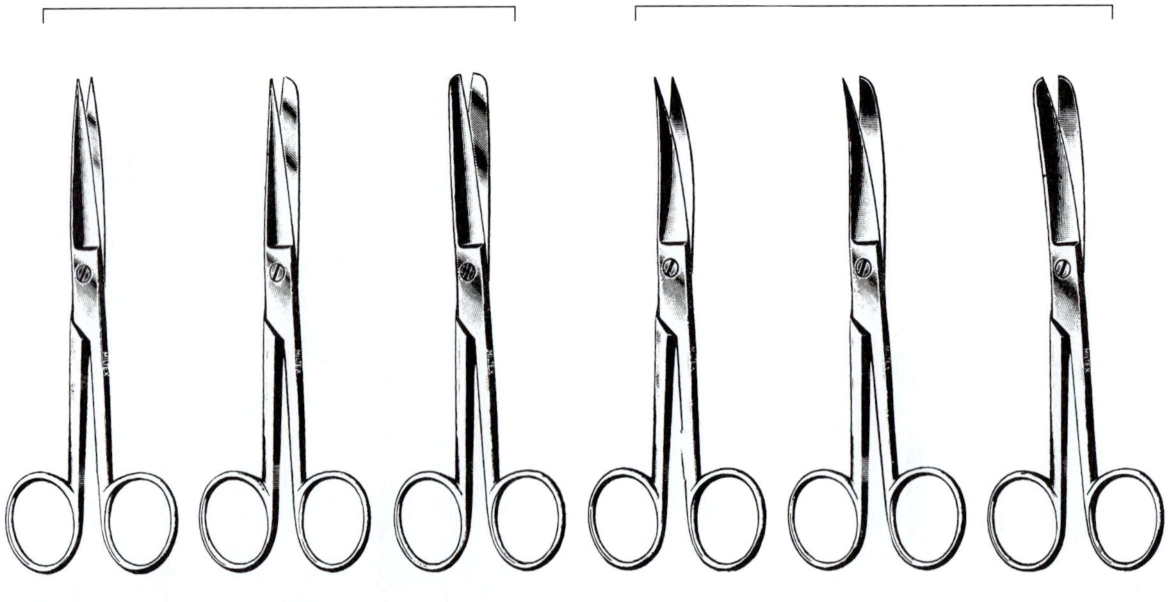

Figure 19-14 Standard operating scissors. (Courtesy of Miltex, Inc.)

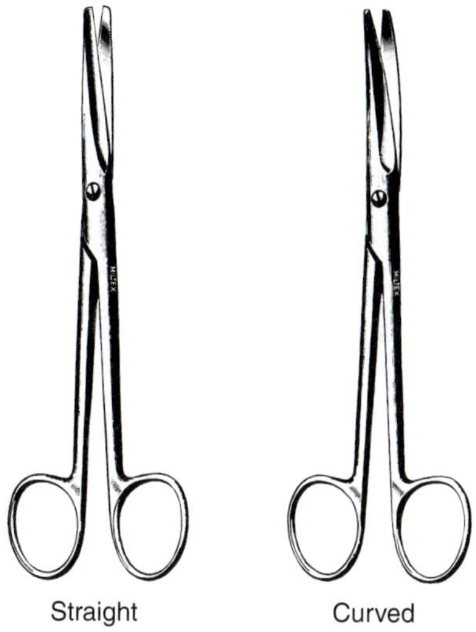

Figure 19-15 Mayo dissecting scissors. (Courtesy of Miltex, Inc.)

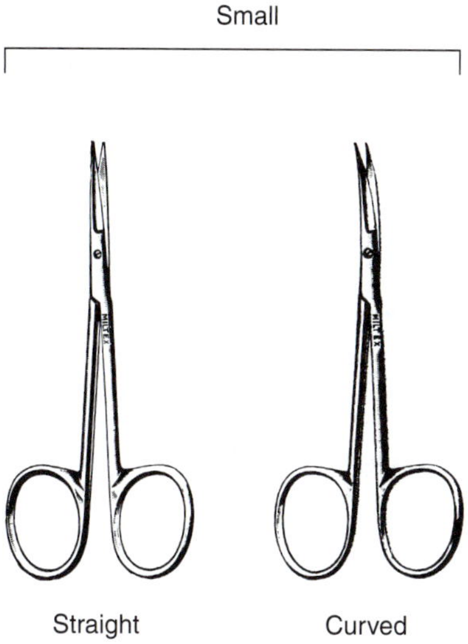

Figure 19-16 Iris scissors. (Courtesy of Miltex, Inc.)

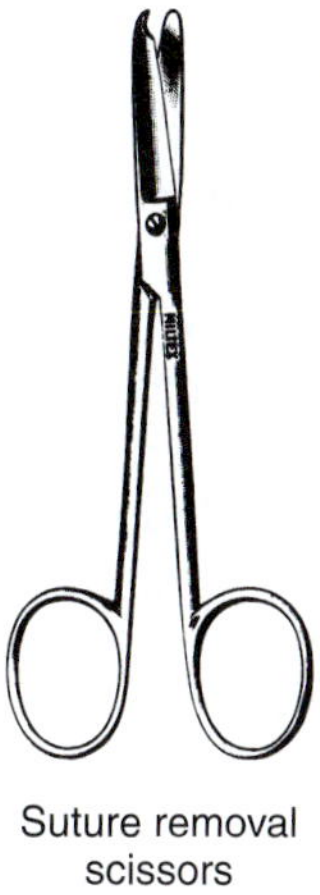

Figure 19-17 Suture or stitch removal scissors. (Courtesy of Miltex, Inc.)

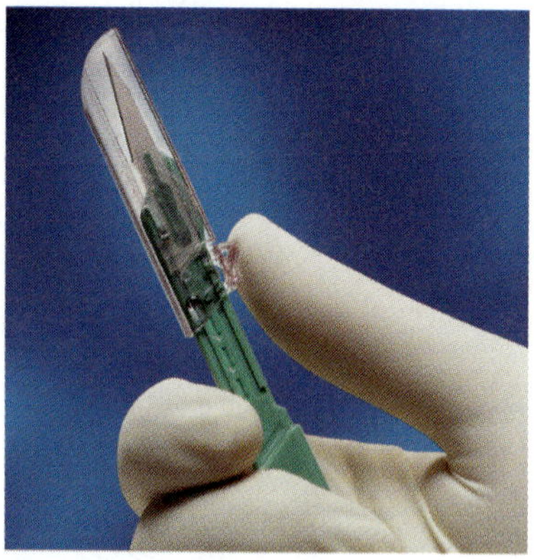

Figure 19-18 Disposable scalpels with a protective retractable blade help prevent sharps injuries. (Photo reprinted Courtesy of Becton Dickinson.)

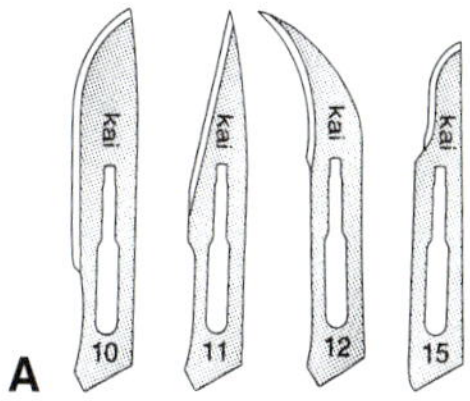

Figure 19-19A Surgical blades: #10, #11, #12, #15. (Courtesy of Miltex, Inc.)

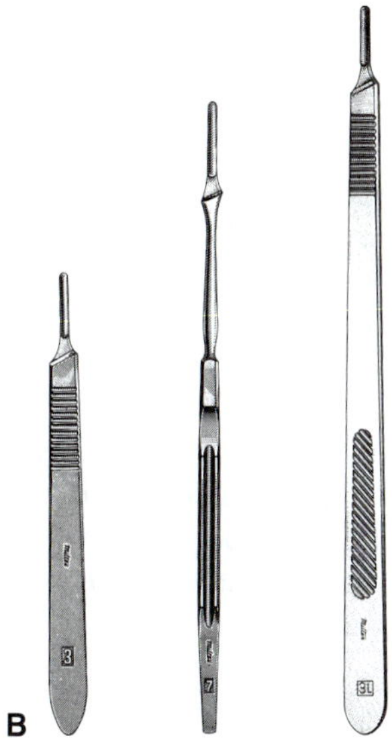

Figure 19-19B Scalpel handles: #3, #7, #3L. (Courtesy of Miltex, Inc.)

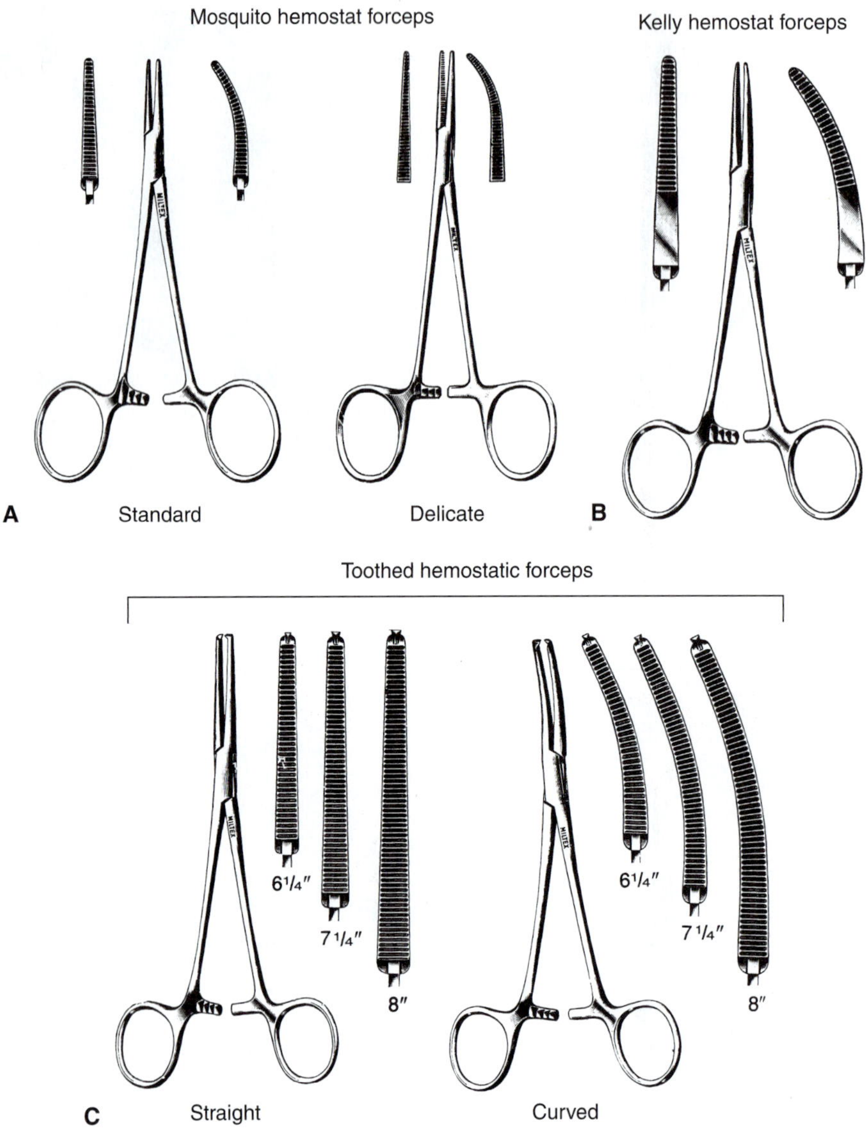

Figure 19-20 Hemostatic forceps include (A) mosquito hemostat forceps; (B) Kelly hemostat forceps; and (C) toothed hemostatic forceps. (Courtesy of Miltex, Inc.)

Thumb forceps do not have ring handles or ratchets but are more like the common tweezers. Thumb forceps with teeth are called tissue forceps because of their ability to grasp tissue. Dressing forceps (plain) do not have teeth and are useful for dressing wounds and applying sterile skin closure strips. Dressing forceps are also used to insert sterile gauze packing strips into wounds to facilitate drainage. The Adson, a special type of thumb forceps, is easily differentiated by the shape. Adsons may have teeth or be plain and have a finer tip.

The Lucae bayonet-type forceps, used in nose and ear procedures, have a thumb handle and are curved to allow the simultaneous use of other instruments and scopes and to facilitate viewing. In contrast, the Hartman ear forceps, duckbill ear alligator-type forceps, and the Hartman nasal dressing forceps have ring handles but also are bent for ease in ear and nose procedures. Figure 19-21 shows examples of each.

Splinter forceps do not have teeth and are used for pulling splinters. Many splinter forceps such as the plain splinter forceps and the Walter are of the thumb-handled style, but the physician's splinter forceps have ring handles and the Virtus have a spring-type handle (Figure 19-22).

Sponge forceps such as the Foerster may have rings on the tips and, as the name implies, are used to hold surgical gauze sponges. Sponge forceps may have long handles, making them useful for gynecologic procedures, and are called uterine sponge forceps. Many medical offices use uterine

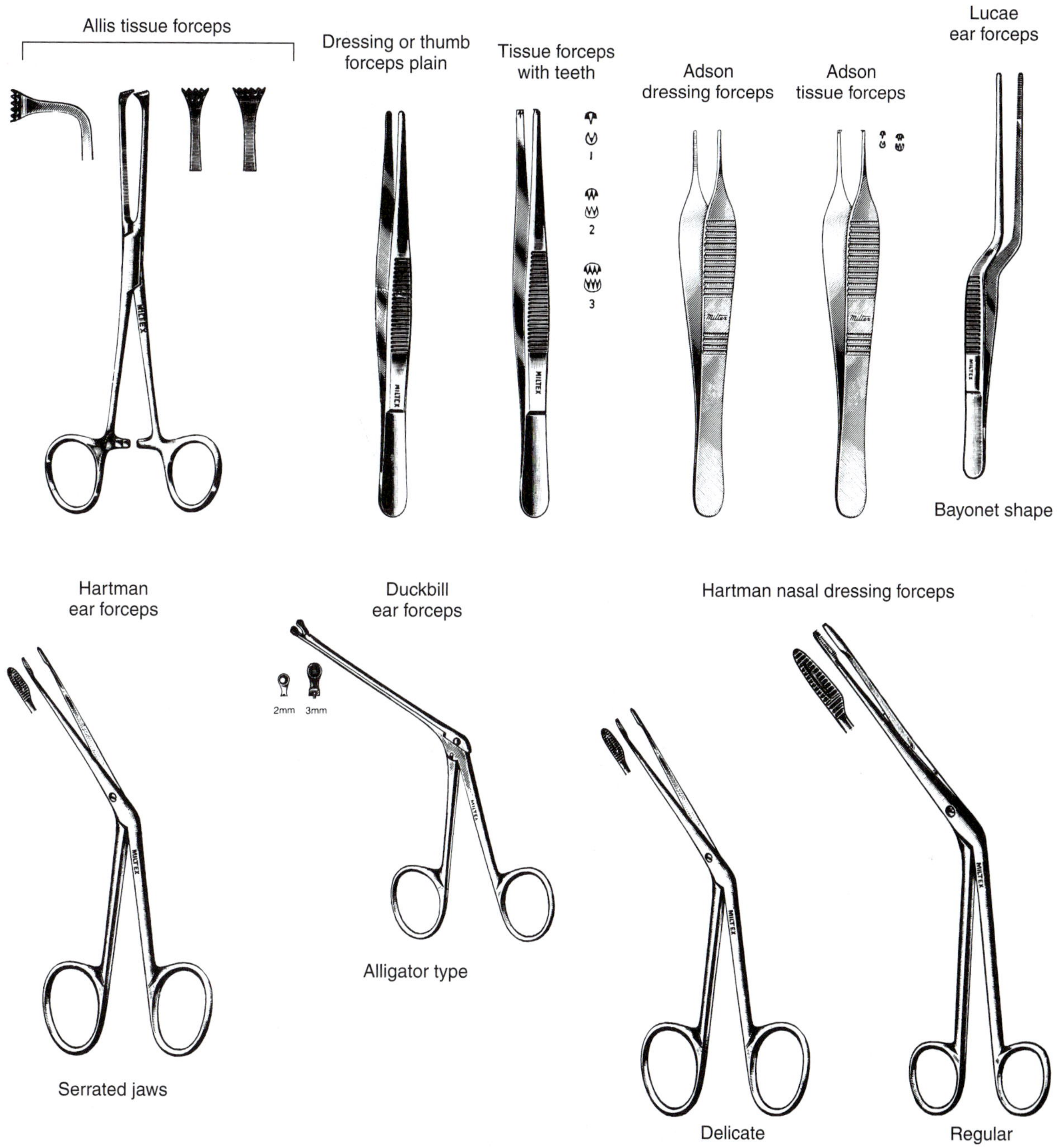

Figure 19-21 Tissue and dressing forceps. (Courtesy of Miltex, Inc.)

sponge forceps as transfer forceps (Figure 19-23). (see Basic Surgery Setup later in this chapter).

Towel clamps are used to attach surgical field drapes to each other and in some situations, such as when bisecting the vas deferens in a vasectomy, to clamp onto dissected tissue. In the case of a vasectomy, the Backhaus towel clamp is used to hold the dissected section of the vas deferens (Figure 19-24).

Needle holders are ratcheted instruments similar to hemostats but with a wider and more stout jaw. Often called needle drivers, they are designed to hold the needle firmly without crushing it while suturing. Most needle holders have a vertical ditch in the center of the jaw to disperse tension and help prevent slipping of the needle. Needle holders such as the Crile-Wood may have a special groove in which to place the needle during suturing. Some needle holders come in various sizes and some are equipped with a cutting edge that eliminates the need for a separate scissors to cut the suture material (Figure 19-25).

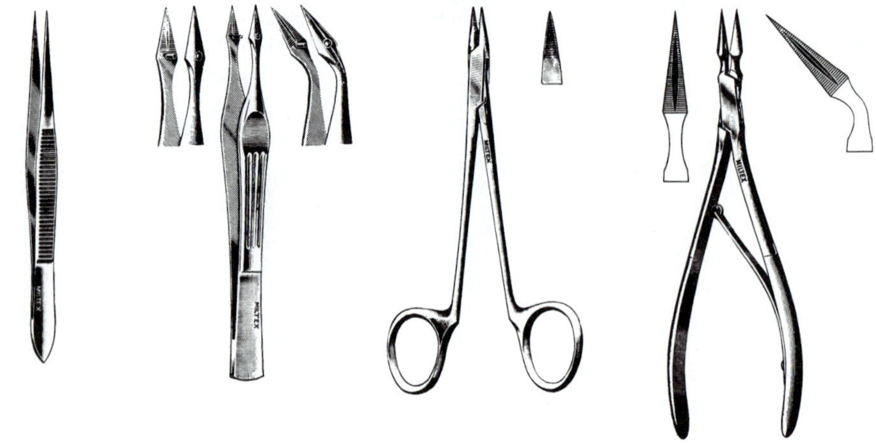

Figure 19-22 Splinter forceps. (Courtesy of Miltex, Inc.)

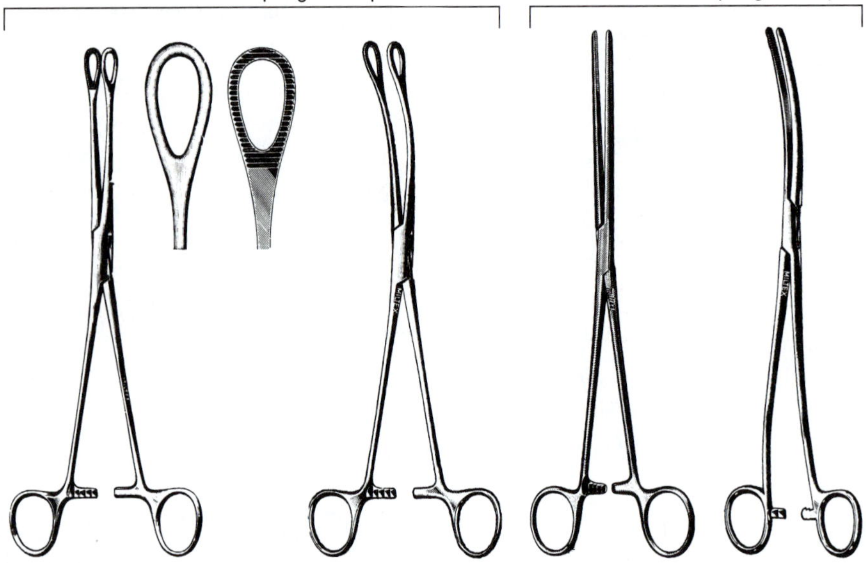

Figure 19-23 Sponge forceps. (Courtesy of Miltex, Inc.)

Specula, Scopes, Probes, Retractors, and Dilators.

The category of dilators and probes includes specula that are designed for enlarging and exploring body orifices (Figure 19-26). The vaginal speculum is available in various lengths and widths and may be made of metal or disposable plastic. The most common instrument for enlarging the nostril is the Vienna nasal speculum. This instrument is used with the Lucae bayonet forceps to perform procedures within the nose.

Scopes are lighted instruments used for viewing. The otoscope, used to visualize the ear canal and eardrum, has a small light aimed into an ear speculum. Ear specula may be disposable or reuseable. If reused, they are sanitized, chemically disinfected, rinsed, and dried between uses. Proctoscopes, anoscopes (Figure 19-27), and rigid sigmoidoscopes are used for viewing the rectum, anus, and the sigmoid portion on the large intestine and have guides called obturators to ease insertion. The light source for the proctoscopes and anoscopes is usually a separate lamp. Although the light sources cannot be sterilized, they can be meticulously disinfected. The speculum portion

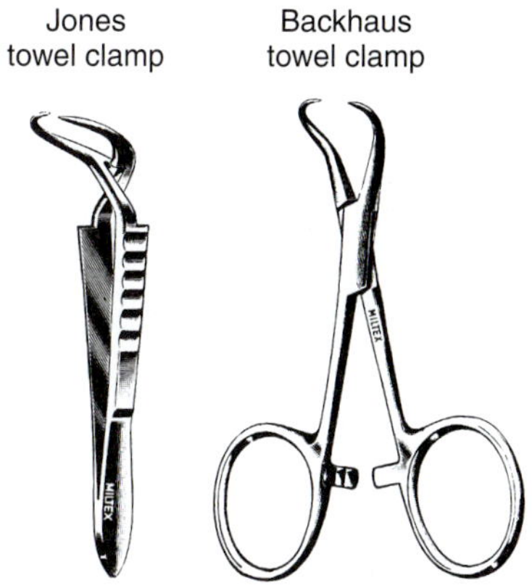

Figure 19-24 Towel clamps. (Courtesy of Miltex, Inc.)

that is inserted into the rectum may be made of disposable plastic or metal. Both the metal speculum and its obturator can sanitized and sterilized in the autoclave.

Another group of scopes are long, flexible, and much more complex and use fiber-optic light sources. Fiber-optic scopes are considered medical equipment rather than surgical instruments. Although considered to be medical equipment, these flexible scopes are inserted into body cavities and must be sanitized and sterilized between uses.

Probes are slender instruments used to probe into a hidden area, body cavity, or wound. Sounds are long, slender probing instruments used to determine the size and shape of the area being probed or to detect the presence of an unseen foreign body. Sounds may be calibrated in centimeters or inches (Figure 19-28).

Retractors used in office/ambulatory surgery are often called skin hooks and are used to hook onto and retract the edges of a wound to facilitate better viewing. Skin hooks are fine-tipped and delicate. As with all of the finer surgical instruments, special care should be taken to avoid damaging the delicate tips (Figure 19-29).

Dilators are double-ended metal rods with smooth, rounded tips, ranging in calibrated sizes from small to large. Dilators are inserted into narrowed or constricted ducts and tubes for the purpose of gradually dilating or enlarging the opening. Hegar uterine dilators are used to dilate the cervix to gain access to the inside of the uterus. Esophageal dilators are used to relieve **strictures,** or narrowing, of the esophagus. Urethral dilators are used to relieve strictures of the urethra (Figure 19-30).

Care of Instruments

Medical/surgical instruments require special care to prevent excessive wear and tear and unnecessary damage. Careful and frequent inspections will determine when instruments need to be replaced or repaired. Some basic rules and rationales include:

- Immediately after use, soiled instruments should be soaked. This prevents blood and other body fluids from drying onto the working surfaces of the instruments.

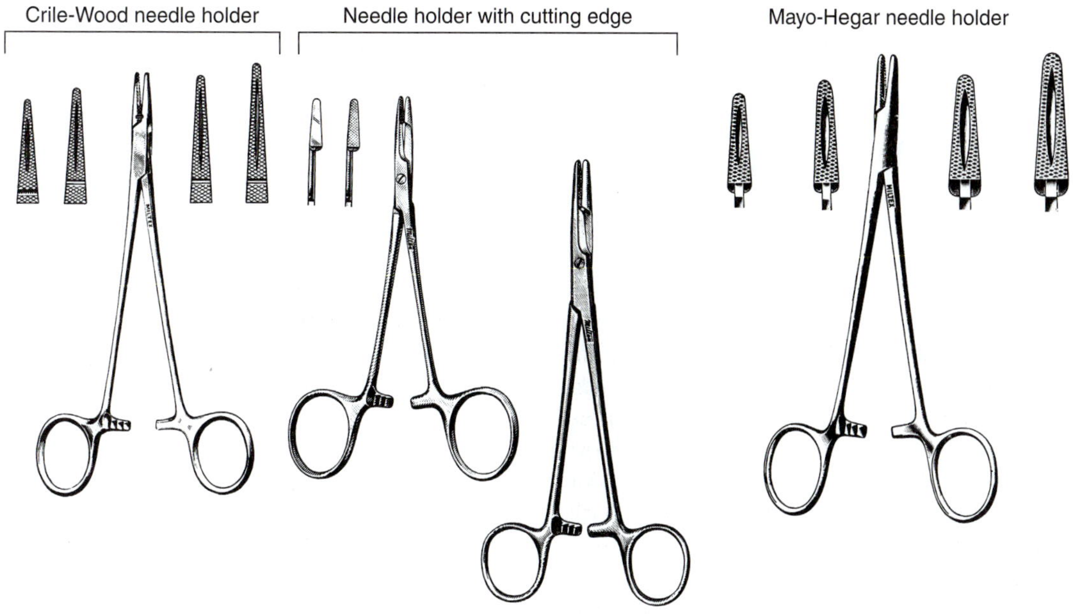

Figure 19-25 Towel clamps. (Courtesy of Miltex, Inc.)

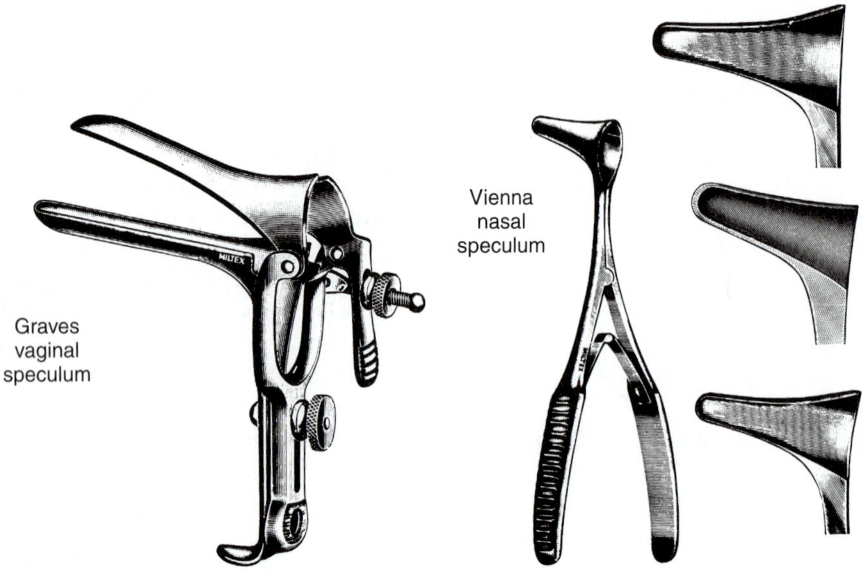

Figure 19-26 Specula and scopes are used to explore body openings by widening for better viewing. (Courtesy of Miltex, Inc.)

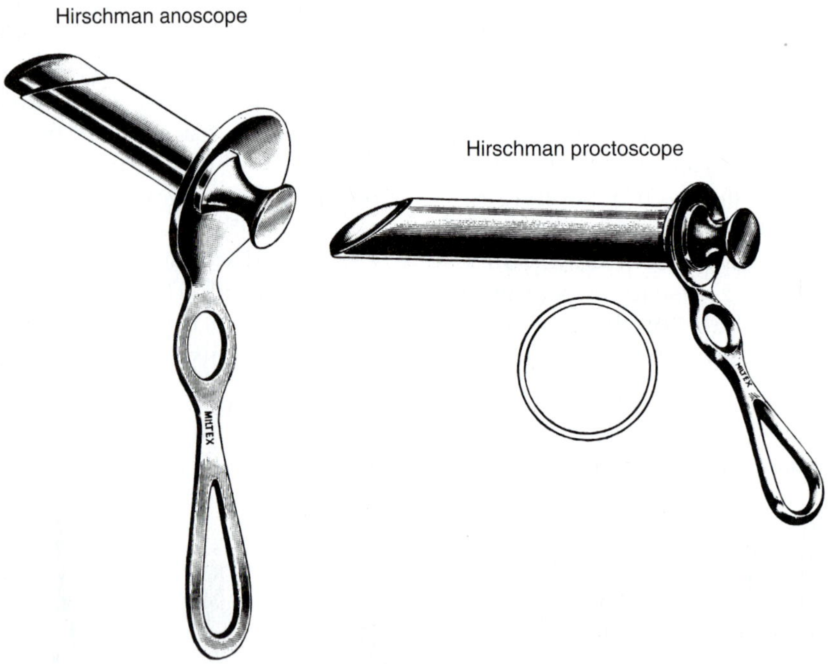

Figure 19-27 Scopes and specula are used to expose body orifices by opening for better viewing. (Courtesy of Miltex, Inc.)

- Soak solutions should be about room temperature and contain a neutral pH detergent with a protein/blood solvent. The proteins in the body fluids will not coagulate on the instruments in cool water and the neutral pH detergent will help prevent spotting and corrosion of the metals. Solvents will help break up the blood and proteins in the body fluids.
- Soak basins should be plastic to prevent damaging points and edges. If a metal soak basin is used, placing a towel on the bottom as padding will help prevent damage to the instruments.
- Heavy-duty rubber gloves should be worn when cleaning instruments to lessen the likelihood of being stuck or cut with the sharp points and edges.
- Goggles should be worn to protect eyes from splashes.
- Delicate instruments should be separated from heavier instruments to prevent the delicate instruments from being bent or otherwise damaged.
- Sharp instruments should be carefully separated from the other instruments and washed with extreme caution. The danger of being cut or

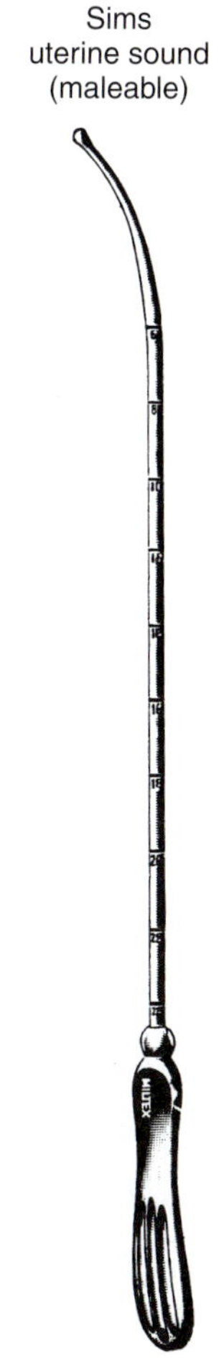

Figure 19-28 Uterine sound. (Courtesy of Miltex, Inc.)

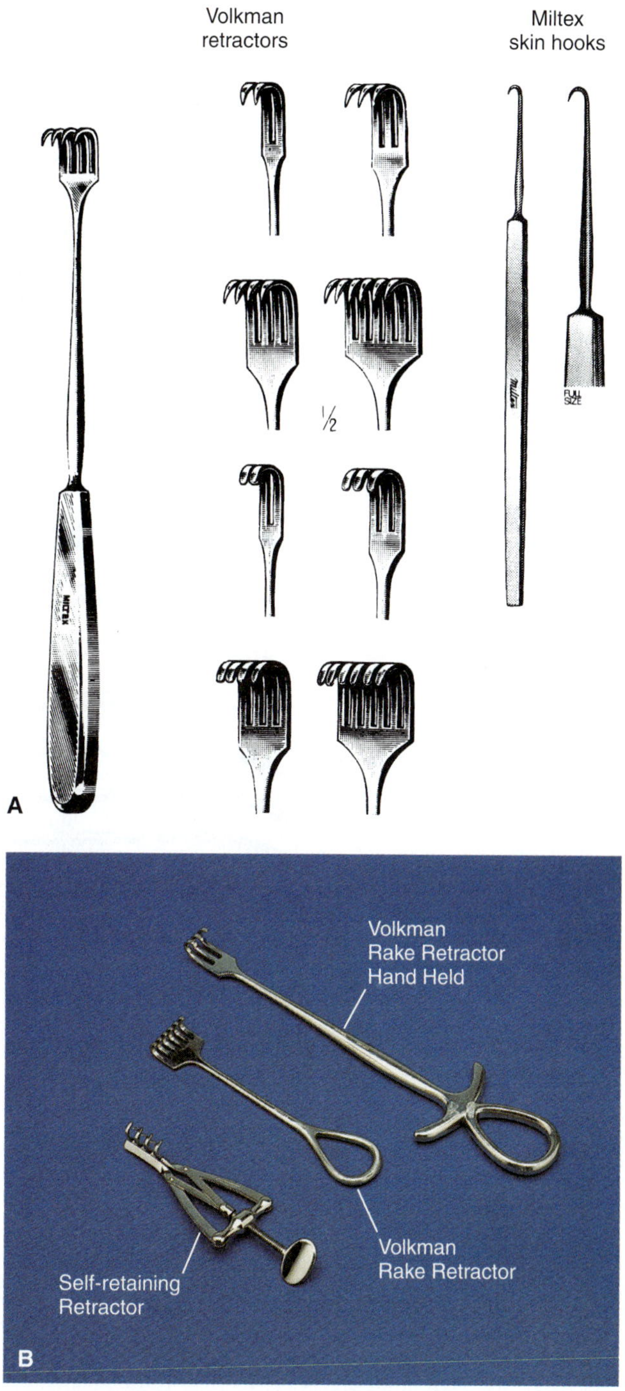

Figure 19-29 Various types of retractors (sharp and blunt). (Courtesy of Miltex, Inc.)

punctured is greater when cleaning sharp instruments than at most other times, and the sharp instruments are usually the most contaminated.

- A soft bristle brush should be used to scrub hinges, ratchets, and serrations. The brush should be firm enough to clean crevices thoroughly yet soft enough to prevent scratching instruments. Instruments with multiple parts must be taken completely apart.
- Immediately after sanitization, instruments should be thoroughly rinsed and dried to prevent spotting and water damage.
- Carefully inspect all surfaces, edges, and points. Check for nicks, dulling, and warping. Test blades for sharpness. Be sure the instrument is not bent or pitted. Handles should also be checked for nicks that may snag and tear surgical gloves, thus disrupting the protective barrier and causing contamination.
- Damaged or malfunctioning instruments should be repaired or replaced.

Ultrasonic Cleaning. Surgical instruments can be cleaned (sanitized) by using an ultrasonic cleaner. Instruments are placed into an ultrasonic container with special cleaning solution. Sound waves vibrate to loosen debris and contaminants. Place instruments with ratchets or hinges into the cleaner in an open position. The articles, when finished, are rinsed well, dried, and wrapped for sterilization. The process of sanitizing contaminated instruments by ultrasound is safe for all instruments including delicate instruments. It is preferred for endoscopes.

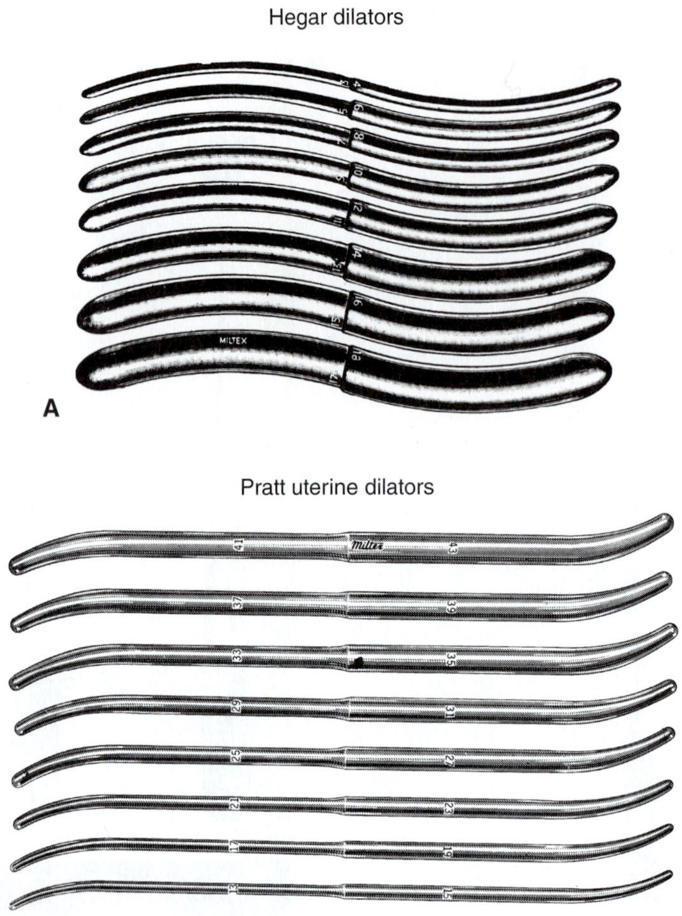

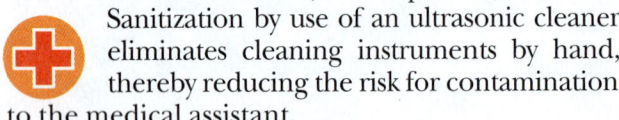

Figure 19-30 Two types of dilators. Hegar dilators arranged smallest to largest. Pratt dilators arranged largest to smallest. (Courtesy of Miltex, Inc.)

Follow manufacturer's directions for use and care of the ultrasonic cleaner (see Chapter 10).

Sanitization by use of an ultrasonic cleaner eliminates cleaning instruments by hand, thereby reducing the risk for contamination to the medical assistant.

- Instruments should be processed in the cleaner for the full recommended cycle time, usually 5 to 10 minutes.
- Place instruments in open position into the ultrasonic cleaner. Make sure that sharps blades and points do not touch other instruments.
- All instruments must be fully submerged.
- Do not place dissimilar metals (stainless, copper, chrome plated) in the same cleaning cycle.
- Change solution frequently—at least as often as the manufacturer recommends.
- Rinse instruments thoroughly with distilled water after ultrasonic cleaning to remove ultrasonic cleaning solution.

Chemical "Cold" Sterilization. This type of sterilization is sometimes referred to as "cold" sterilization, which indicates that heat-sensitive items such as fiberoptic endoscopes and delicate cutting instruments can be immersed in a chemical solution. The chemicals used are reliable and capable of destroying bacteria and their spores and, used in strict accordance with the manufacturer's instructions regarding length of immersion time, can ensure sterility.

Procedure 19-2 gives steps for chemical ("cold") sterilization.

SUPPLIES AND EQUIPMENT

The supplies necessary for office/ambulatory surgery are often disposable and should be replenished as needed. Most medical/surgical supply companies have catalogs and Web sites available for ordering, and many companies have sales representatives who make regular stops or are available by telephone or email to assist in the ordering process. Sales representatives are familiar with the products marked by their company and are extremely useful as a resource. Samples of new products are often available for trial, and optional choices are always offered. Medical/surgical supply companies frequently offer special prices for larger quantity purchases. If a medical/surgical supply item is being used frequently and storage space is available, buying in larger quantities might be more cost-effective. If a product currently being used is not meeting expectations, requesting optional trial products is usually the first step toward finding a better product. Following are some of the more commonly used supplies associated with office/ambulatory surgery.

Drapes

Drapes are used during surgery to create a sterile field over and around the surgical site. They are applied using sterile technique after the skin preparation.

Drapes are of different sizes and materials. A **fenestrated** drape is often used because it has an opening at the site of the surgery to be performed.

Sponges and Wicks

Surgical sponges are prepackaged squares of folded gauze used in surgery. In the provider's office, sponges are most often referred to by their size. A gauze square measuring 4 inches by 4 inches is called a 4 × 4 (Figure 19-31). The other most common sizes are 3 × 3 and 2 × 2. The gauge sponges are packaged in individual peel-apart packages of two or may be purchased in nonsterile bulk packages of two hundred. The individual packages are convenient, sterile, and useful for most purposes but cost more per sponge than the nonsterile bulk packages. For larger surgical needs, the medical assistant may wrap several bulk sponges together and autoclave them for later use. Most sponges are simply folded gauze, but some have cotton or rayon pads embedded in them to increase absorption ability and to create a softer texture. The medical assistant and the provider using the sponge probably have a preference among the different types and uses. Gauze sponges are used in wound cleansing, in skin preparation, as absorbable sponges during surgery, as dressings and coverings, and for padding. The ambulatory care setting may prefer to have different sizes and types in stock to meet different needs.

Sterile surgical wicks or wound packing strips are used when an infected wound must remain open for drainage. The sterile wicking material is made of narrow strips of gauze packaged in long lengths in opaque glass bottles (Figure 19-32). The most recognizable trade name is Iodoform®. The Iodoform® is sterile and packaged in multiple-use bottles. Extreme care should be taken to prevent contamination during removal of individual lengths. The bottle is opened using sterile technique, sterile dressing forceps are inserted into the bottle, the strip

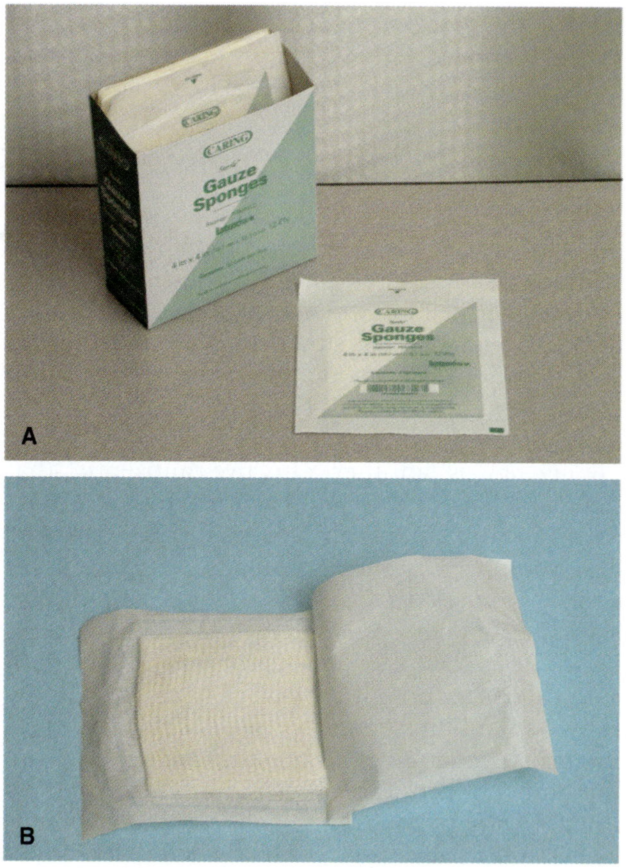

Figure 19-31 (A) Box of sterile gauze sponges. These are also referred to as 4 × 4s or, in surgery, as surgical sponges. (B) Peel-apart sterile open package of 4 × 4 gauze.

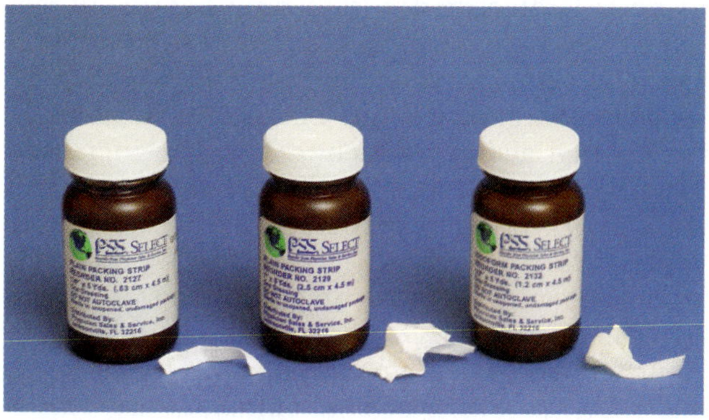

Figure 19-32 Various sizes of iodoform® gauze: ¼ inch, ½ inch, 1 inch, 2 inches.

is cut to the desired length using sterile scissors, and the lid is applied without compromising the sterility of the remaining wicking material in the bottle.

Solutions/Creams/Ointments

Many different soaps and solutions are available and effective as skin cleansers, preoperative scrubs, paints, soaks, and antiseptics. **Betadine®** (povidone-iodine) is a well-known antiseptic and is available as a surgical soap called a "scrub" and as a non-soap solution for preoperative skin preparation/paint. Betadine® comes in multiple-use bottles, in single use, and in individually packaged swabs. **Hibeclens®** is another effective antiseptic that does not have the staining tendencies of iodine. Medical/surgical supply companies have names and samples of other products. Consideration should be made to cost, effectiveness, ease of use, shelf life, and personal preferences. **Isopropyl alcohol,** a 70% alcohol solution, is of limited medical/surgical use, although because of its rapid volatility rate and its ability to dissolve oils, it is still preferred for skin preparation before injections and venipuncture. Isopropyl alcohol is available in bottles for use with cotton/rayon balls or in convenient individually packaged pledgets. Isopropyl alcohol can be irritating and is not effective as a preoperative skin preparation. **Hydrogen peroxide** is a noncaustic mildly effective skin antiseptic. It bubbles on contact with mucous membranes and other moist skin surfaces, dissolving blood and proteins, and has a mechanical cleansing action. Hydrogen peroxide is ineffective as a skin prep before surgery but is useful for cleaning after surgery. Many providers do not recommend using hydrogen peroxide on surgical wounds because of its abrasive "scrubbing action," which can cause increased scarring and irritations. Do not use or recommend the use of hydrogen peroxide without consulting your provider.

Antibacterial creams and ointments are sometimes applied topically on wounds to aid healing. Antibacterial creams are usually white, water-based, and nongreasy. Antibacterial ointments are usually clear and oil based. If a wound requires thorough cleaning between dressing changes, an antibacterial cream is preferred because of the ease of removal.

Some examples of sterile solutions are sterile saline, sterile distilled water, and Betadine® solution.

Silvadene® is the brand name of a sterile cream used on burns and other abrasion wounds. It is an excellent antibacterial cream but must be applied ⅛- to ¼-inch thick to help ensure that the dressing does not absorb all the cream, thus drying out the wound. Sterile tongue blades are handy to apply the Silvadene® cream to large area burns. Silvadene should be thoroughly removed and reapplied fresh with each dressing change. Silvadene is available by prescription only and comes in small tubes for individual use as well as larger jars for multiple use. Silvadene is fairly expensive. When using a multiple-use jar, as with any multiple-use container, extreme caution must be taken to avoid contamination of the product.

Dressings and Bandages

Dressings are the sterile material applied directly onto the surface of a wound or surgical site. **Bandages** are the supportive material applied over the top of dressings and are not sterile. A dressing, being sterile, should be handled with care to avoid contamination of the wound. Often a sterile nonstick pad or topical medication is applied to the wound to prevent the dressing from adhering to the wound.

Dressings are usually made of gauze and need to completely cover the wound. Dressings must be adequately absorbent for any wound drainage.

Bandages are used to keep dressings in place, to provide padding and protection, and to immobilize. Bandaging may consist of rolled gauze wrapped around the wound area with an additional sturdier wrap applied overall. An elastic bandage may provide additional support, and a triangular bandage, sling, brace, or splint provides even more. A unique type of bandage is the tubular gauze bandage. Tubular gauze bandages are used to cover appendages such as fingers, arms, toes, and legs and come in various sizes according to the size of the body part being covered. Chapter 9 provides information about wounds and bandages. Figure 19-33 illustrates various bandage-wrapping techniques.

Anesthetics

The word **anesthesia** means the loss of feeling or sensation. An anesthetic is any mechanism that causes this loss of feeling. The application of extreme cold can be an anesthetic because it causes numbness to nerve endings and thus the loss of feeling. Anesthetics may be inhaled, topically applied or sprayed, or injected directly into a vein (intravenously), the spinal column (intrathecally), or locally (subcutaneously) into the tissues at the site of the surgical procedure.

Injectable Anesthetics. Most anesthetics used in office/ambulatory surgery are administered locally through injection into the subcutaneous

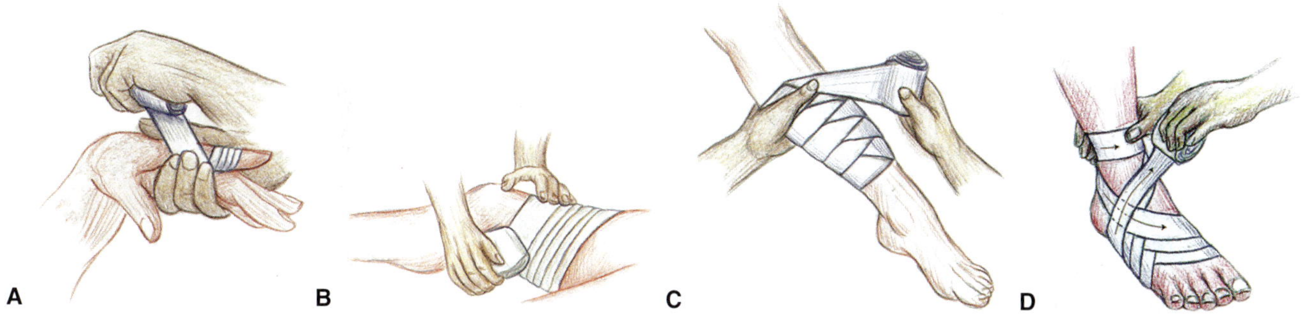

Figure 19-33 Bandage-wrapping techniques illustrating the circular, spiral, and figure-eight turns. (A) Circular turns are wrapped around a body part several times to anchor a bandage or to supply support. (B) Spiral turns begin with one or two circular turns, then proceed up the body part, with each turn covering two-thirds the width of the previous turn. (C) Reverse spiral turns begin with a circular turn. Then the bandage is reversed or twisted once each turn to accommodate a limb that gets larger as the bandaging progresses. (D) Figure-eight turns crisscross in the shape of a figure eight and are used on a joint that requires movement.

tissues. The nerves exposed to the anesthetic become temporarily unable to conduct sensations and feelings to the brain, thereby causing a lack of pain sensation in the area during the surgery. All synthetic local anesthetics have names that end in *-caine.* Some of the most common are Xylocaine (lidocaine), Novacaine (procaine), Marcaine, and Carbocaine. Local anesthetics are available in single-dose vials or ampules of 10 mL, but most medical offices prefer the cost-effectiveness of multiple-dose vials containing 30 to 50 mL. Local anesthetics are also available in varying strengths such as 0.5%, 1%, and 2%.

Injectable anesthetics may contain an additive called **epinephrine.** It has a red label. Epinephrine causes vasoconstriction and is used when reduced blood flow to the area is desired. The medical assistant is often delegated the responsibility of filling the syringe with the prescribed amount and strength of the ordered anesthesia or may assist the provider in drawing up the medication. Be sure to identify the drug and dose for the provider.

Anytime the medical assistant draws up a medication for the provider or pours a solution into a prep basin on the sterile tray, the original vial or bottle that the medication or solution comes from should be brought into the procedure room with the surgical/procedure tray and other supplies. The provider should check the vial and container before using the medication or solution to be sure it is exactly what has been ordered. A good practice is to set the vial or container on the counter within plain view for the provider to see. Often the provider verbally confirms what medication is in the syringe or what solution is in the prep basin before using them.

Anesthetics with epinephrine should not be used on fingers, toes, noses, or earlobes because of their vasoconstriction. Patients with circulatory complications may have even more restrictions/cautions on the use of epinephrine. This is one reason why it is important to bring the vial into the procedure room with the patient.

Drawing Techniques. If the provider plans to inject the anesthesia before applying sterile gloves, either the medical assistant or the provider may draw up the medication. The filled syringe is then placed on the side, rather than directly on the sterile field. This allows the provider to anesthetize the patient before beginning the sterile procedure. After the anesthesia has taken effect, the provider performs a surgical hand cleansing, applies sterile gloves, and begins the surgery.

When the provider applies sterile gloves before injecting the anesthesia, the sterile syringe may be placed directly on the sterile field either empty or filled. One person wearing sterile gloves may handle the syringe and draw up the medication while another person not wearing sterile gloves holds the vial. This method requires that the syringe and needle either be applied directly to the sterile tray or be handed directly to a "sterile" person. The medical assistant may draw up the anesthesia under sterile process when the sterile tray is set up. As stated previously, if the tray contains a filled syringe, the vial from which it was drawn should accompany the tray into the procedure room and be set on the counter for the provider to verify. Chapter 24 discusses the specific techniques for drawing up medications.

Topical Spray Anesthetics. Not all anesthesia is injectable. Topical (applied to the surface) anesthetics are available in liquid and spray form. The most common topical anesthetic used in the medical office is ethyl chloride spray. Ethyl chloride freezes the skin to allow for simple piercing or lancing. The anesthetic action usually only lasts for a few seconds; therefore, the procedure must be performed quickly. It is highly flammable. One example for the use of ethyl chloride spray is to briefly numb an area before an injection. A lesion that is infected is extremely painful to inject with a local anesthetic; however, by using ethyl chloride spray before the injection, the patient is able to remain still. Ethyl chloride spray may also be used before installing intravenous lines.

Table 19-2 summarizes supplies and equipment commonly used in minor surgery.

PATIENT CARE AND PREPARATION

Patient Preparation and Education

For the patient who will undergo a planned surgical procedure, there is time for patient preparation. Patients may need to modify their diet, adjust medication, acquire special supplies, adjust their personal home and work situations, obtain prior approval from their insurance, and prepare for the postoperative period. For the patient undergoing an unplanned procedure, such as a laceration repair, there is less time for preparation. In either case, the medical assistant needs to follow an established protocol about wound care, patient education, patient health consideration, and consent. In the case of an accidental wound, the medical assistant needs to

Table 19-2 Supplies and Equipment Commonly Used in Minor Surgery

Item	Use/Description
Anesthetics	A mechanism used to cause the loss of feeling. May be inhaled, topically applied, sprayed, or injected directly into a vein, the spinal column, or locally into the tissues at the site of the surgical procedure.
Bandages	Nonsterile supportive materials applied over dressings to keep the dressing in place. May be rolled gauze, elastic bandage, or tubular gauze bandage.
Creams and ointments	Antibacterial. May be used topically on wounds to promote healing. Creams are water-based; ointments are oil-based.
Drapes	Used to create a sterile field over and around the operation site. They are made in various sizes and different materials. A fenestrated drape is commonly used in surgery.
Dressings	Sterile material applied directly onto surface of a wound or surgical site. Usually made of gauze. Must be adequately absorbent and completely cover the wound.
Solutions	Used as skin cleansers, preoperative scrubs, paints, soaks, and antiseptics. Most common are Betadine®, an antiseptic often used in soap form as a scrub; Hibeclens®, an effective antiseptic without iodine's staining properties; isopropyl alcohol, a 70% alcohol solution favored for skin preparation before injections and venipuncture but not effective as a preoperative skin preparation; and hydrogen peroxide, a mildly effective abrasive skin antiseptic.
Sponges	Used in wound cleansing, skin preparation, as absorbable sponges during surgery, as dressings and coverings, and for padding. Also called 4 × 4s. Typically made of folded gauze, though some have cotton or rayon pads embedded in them to increase absorption.
Wicks	Used when an infected wound needs to remain open for drainage. Wicking material is made of narrow strips of gauze packaged in long lengths in opaque glass bottles, which should be opened using sterile technique (see Figure 19-32).

determine the cause of the wound and the date of the last tetanus injection. Chapters 10 and 23 provide specific information about tetanus and immunization schedules. The medical assistant must also check to determine whether the patient has allergies or sensitivities of any kind, particularly to medication and medically related substances.

Diet modifications include abstaining from eating and drinking for several hours before the surgical procedure, as well as restricting the types and amounts of certain foods or liquids consumed before and directly after the procedure. When patients are aware of special dietary needs after surgery, they can shop early and be prepared. An example of a medication treatment includes prescribing an antibiotic to be taken as a precaution against acquiring an infection after surgery or adjusting anticoagulant medications to prevent excessive bleeding during surgery. Each clinic, provider, procedure, and patient has individual requirements and preferences. The patient might be required to obtain special supplies for the convalescent period. For instance, immediately after a vasectomy a scrotal support is usually recommended. Crutches or special foot coverings might be necessary after foot or leg surgery. Specific wound dressing and bandages might need to be purchased before the surgery in anticipation of the postoperative need. Having another person accompany the patient to the clinic for the surgery is required for the safe return home. Knowing the planned period for recovery allows the patient to make the necessary arrangements for work, child care, and other personal situations.

Informed Consent

Before a surgical procedure, the patient's written consent must be obtained. For many medical and all surgical procedures, a written, **informed consent** form must be signed. An informed consent is a document that may be created specifically for a particular procedure or that may be an established document available for duplication. An informed consent document informs the patient of the medical or surgical procedure to be performed, describes the actual procedure in lay terms, cites alternative treatments, and lists the possible undesirable outcome and risks involved in the procedure. Chapter 7 provides additional information about informed consent and a model consent farm.

The cost of the procedure is important information. Some insurances companies and Medicare require patients to sign an Advanced Beneficiary Notice (ABN) if their out-of-pocket expenses will go above a certain amount. It is always a good idea to discuss financial arrangements with all patients before an elective procedure or surgery. In some offices, the bookkeeper or office manager comes into the examination room, sits down with the patient, and goes over the forms and financial arrangements. Any questions the patient has about the surgery should be answered completely by the provider, and an assessment should be made that the patient understands the answers. Even in the best of circumstances, results cannot be guaranteed. Most of the difficult situations between providers' practices and patients come from misunderstandings about unexpected outcomes. If patients are informed completely, even unplanned results are better tolerated.

Medical Assisting Considerations

The general health and condition of the patient before surgery is important when planning the recovery. A frail, weak man living alone may need home health care after even a simple surgical procedure. Some people may not be able to follow standard preoperative or postoperative instructions. The recovery may depend on the availability of supplies beyond what the patient can financially afford. If difficult circumstances can be identified before the surgery, arrangements can be made with home health care services, community assistance services, or friends and family. This can help avoid complications. Prior medical history should also be established and questions should be asked regarding **allergies** and sensitivities to medications and medical substances. A patient who has received a general anesthetic must be watched carefully for cardiopulmonary problems that can arise from the anesthesia. An elderly, weak patient who received a general anesthetic (inhalation or intravenous) may experience hypotension or hypoxia. A pulse oximeter is applied to the patient to monitor blood oxygen percentage (see Chapter 18). Vital signs are watched carefully.

Postoperative Instructions

Postoperative instructions should be written and clearly understood by the patient. If the patient has a caregiver at home, the postoperative instructions should be clearly understood by the caregiver as well. The telephone number of the clinic and an after-hours number should be written on the postoperative instructions and brought to the attention of the patient and caregiver. It is good practice to plan to call patients within the first postoperative day to check on their condition.

Wounds, Wound Care, and the Healing Process

There are many different types of wounds based on the type of injury incurred. Wounds may be classified as open or closed, accidental or intentional (surgical).

Lacerations, incisions, avulsions, and punctures are all examples of open wounds (Figure 19-34).

Ecchymosis, contusion, and hematoma are examples of closed wounds. They are caused by a blunt trauma that damages underlying tissues but leaves the skin intact (Figure 19-35).

Wounds are classified as superficial if the injury does not extend deeper than the subcutaneous tissues. Deep wounds extend beyond the subcutaneous layer. The size, location, and depth of the wound are important descriptors both for

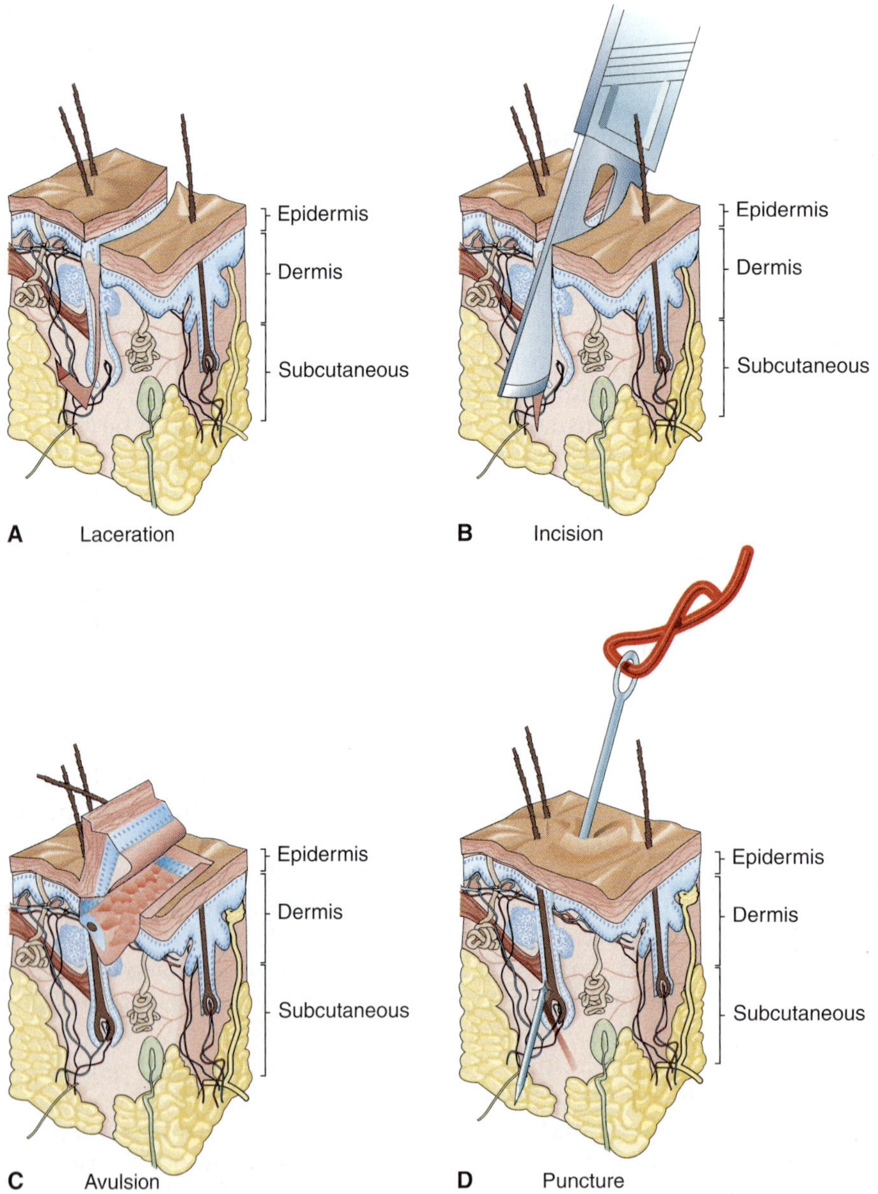

Figure 19-34 Open wounds. (A) Lacerations are accidental tearing of the body tissue usually made by sharp objects. The torn flesh may be smooth or jagged and often is difficult to clean and suture properly. There may be extensive bleeding. A cut from a sharp knife is an example of a laceration. (B) Incisions are intentional cuts typically made with a scalpel for surgical procedures. (C) Avulsions are accidental tearing away of a part or structures of the skin. (D) Punctures are holes or wounds made by a pointed object and can be either accidental or intentional. Puncture wounds have little bleeding because the point of entry is small. These wounds typically are not much larger than the instrument entering the skin. A puncture wound may also be the result of stepping on a nail.

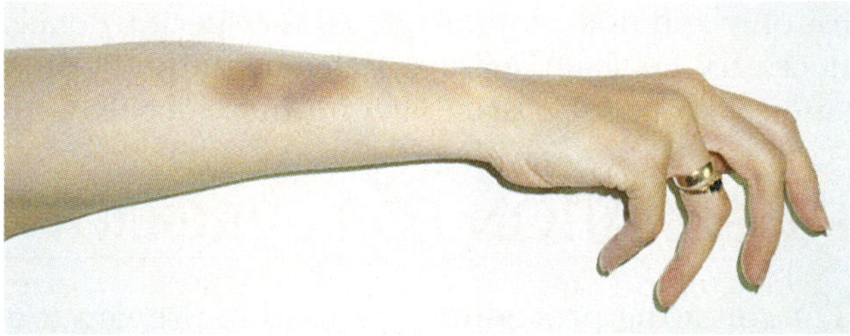

Figure 19-35 Closed wounds include contusions, ecchymoses, and hematomas. This photograph shows an ecchymosis.

Patient Education

The basic signs of inflammation are redness, heat, swelling, pain, and loss of function. Any one or more of these may be present in varying intensities during an inflammatory process. Most wounds will have a mild inflammation described as slightly red or pink, mild warmth, slightly tender to the touch, and mildly swollen. The symptoms are caused by increased blood supply to the traumatized area and the infiltration of white blood cells in reaction to the trauma. Patients should be taught to watch for an increase in the intensity of redness, pain, swelling, and heat or any drainage, fever, or lymph gland swelling, which can indicate an **infection** from invading pathogens. Patients should be given instructions as to what actions to take if these symptoms of infection are noticed. The instructions should include a name and telephone numbers to call during the day or night. The medical assistant should reassure the patient not to hesitate to contact the center or physician if infection is suspected.

the medical record and for proper insurance reimbursement. A typical description of a patient wound that is an intermediate laceration might be, "patient sustained a deep 3.5-cm laceration to the anterior surface of the right knee caused by a fall onto a rock." A puncture wound might be described as, "patient presents with a 2-cm deep puncture wound on the plantar surface of the left foot obtained from stepping on a rusty nail." Both statements describe not only the size, depth, location, and type of wound, but also the causative factor.

Inflammation is the body's natural reaction to trauma. Inflammation is also a normal process of wound healing. Occasionally, inflamed tissue will become infected if the trauma is caused by a pathogen. Although a certain degree of inflammation is expected, prevention of infection is a primary goal (see Chapter 10).

Chapter 9 describes wounds and emergency care of wounds.

The best treatment of infection is prevention. Instructing the patient about proper wound care is extremely important. Encourage the patient to keep the wound clean and dry. In certain circumstances, the provider may prescribe a warm soak solution or the application of a topical antibacterial medication. If the wound becomes infected and a **suppurant** is present, the provider may order a wound irrigation (see Procedure 19-10). Wound irrigation removes the accumulation of purulent **exudate** that impairs and delays healing. After the irrigation, a dry sterile dressing is applied (see Procedure 19-9). Protecting the wound from further trauma and contamination will also aid in the healing process. Opinions will differ on whether a wound is best left open to the air or covered with a dressing. Most health care providers will agree that covering a wound is preferred whenever contamination is likely (Procedure 19-9).

BASIC SURGERY SETUP

Preparing for surgery includes assembling supplies and equipment, setting up the surgery tray, getting the patient and room ready, and preparing to assist during surgery. The specific instruments, supplies, and equipment needed for each surgery should be listed on individual **surgery cards.** These cards may be 3 × 5 or 5 × 7 cards stored in a card file or full sheets of procedures compiled in a manual or notebook, or procedures can be found on the computer. Each provider will have individual instrument sets for each surgical procedure performed. Information on the surgery card or computer should include provider glove size, standing preoperative and postoperative instructions, type of skin preparation, and any additional information specific to the provider's needs or to the surgical procedure. The card file, whether manual or computerized, should be updated whenever chanages are made and may be the responsibility of the medical assistant.

Basic Rules and Concepts for Setup of Surgical Trays

In addition to basic sterile principles, the guidelines in Table 19-3 will help ensure the sterile field remains sterile.

SURGERY PROCESS

For ease in understanding the individual tasks involved in office surgery, Table 19-4 provides generic steps for setting up the surgical tray, preparing the room, preparing the patient, assisting with the surgery, and the terminal care process of the room and equipment. Table 19-4 is intended as a quick check-list only and does not include all the specific details necessary for each surgery. Refer to the individual surgical procedures that follow for more details.

PREPARATION FOR SURGERY

The following procedures are used in preparation for minor surgery:

- Applying Sterile Gloves (Procedure 19-1)
- Setting Up and Covering a Sterile Field (Procedure 19-5)
- Opening Sterile Packages of Instruments and Supplies and Applying Them to a Sterile Field (Procedure 19-6)

Table 19-3 Guidelines for Sterile Tray Setups

Set up the sterile surgery tray just before the surgery to minimize the chance of accidental contamination.
Immediately after the tray is set up, cover it with a sterile drape.
Once the tray is prepared and covered, move it directly into the surgery area rather than leaving it in a common area.
Inform the patient and others in the surgery room that the tray is sterile and should not be touched. Patients are often curious about instruments and may attempt to look under the cover if not cautioned against it.
If the medical assistant is interrupted while preparing the tray and it becomes necessary to leave the tray unattended, cover the tray and move it out of traffic paths to prevent it from being bumped.

Table 19-4 Preparations for Office/Ambulatory Surgery

Tray Setup

1. Wash hands.
2. Reference surgery card, manual, or computer.
3. Gather equipment and supplies.
4. Sanitize and disinfect Mayo instrument tray.
5. Wash hands.
6. Set up sterile field.
7. Place sterile instruments and supplies on the sterile field.
8. Apply sterile gloves or use sterile transfer forceps.
9. Arrange instruments and supplies in an organized and logical manner.
10. Medication may be drawn up with assistance (optional) (Figure 19-36).
11. Recheck tray for accuracy and completeness.
12. Remove gloves.
13. Cover and transport tray.
14. Add sterile solution (skin antiseptic) to tray if required.

Room Preparation

In preparing a room for a surgical procedure, all equipment should be clean and in good working order. Be certain to have spare parts such as light bulbs and filters readily available. Turn on equipment before the procedure to make sure all is working properly.

1. Check room equipment (light, stool, equipment, examination table, waste receptacle).
2. Check room supplies (tissue, extra gloves, and so on)
3. Arrange accessory supplies on the side counter in a logical order (pathology specimen bottle containing preservative, laboratory requisition, sterile glove package, dressings/bandages, postoperative medications, and instructions).

(continues)

Table 19-4 (continued)

Patient Preparation

1. Wash hands.
2. Greet patient and ensure identity.
3. Escort the patient to the procedure room and offer restroom facilities.
4. Discuss the patient's compliance to preoperative instructions.
5. Explain the procedure again and address any questions.
6. Review postoperative instructions.
7. Check for signed informed consent form and financial forms.
8. Have the patient remove appropriate clothing and position the patient on the examination table. Offer a drape, gown, pillow, and blanket for comfort.
9. Prepare the skin for the surgical procedure (see Procedure 19-11).

Assisting with the Surgery

1. Remove the sterile cover from the surgical tray while the provider applies sterile gloves.
2. Assist the provider with stool and lamp adjustment as needed.
3. If the medical assistant did not perform the skin preparation, assist the provider as needed during skin preparation and draping. The equipment and supplies for skin preparation are separate from the surgery tray and equipment (see Procedure 19-11).
4. Adjust the instrument tray and equipment around the provider.
5. Assist with drawing up local anesthetic or other medication as needed.
6. Apply clean gloves for protection or sterile gloves to assist.
7. Surgery begins.
8. The medical assistant either assists with sterile procedure or supports the patient as needed.
9. After surgery, assist with or perform dressing of wound.
10. Clean patient.
11. Dispose of biohazardous waste materials.
12. Remove contaminated gloves; wash hands.
13. Assist the patient after surgery.

Assisting the Patient after Surgery

1. Check patient vital signs.
2. Remain with patient to ensure patient safety. Allow patient to rest if necessary.
3. Assist patient off examination table and assist with clothing as necessary
4. Review written postoperative instructions with patient and caregiver. Dressing should be kept clean and dry. Patient should report any signs of infection.
5. Clarify any medication orders with patient and caregiver.
6. If not previously arranged, schedule follow-up appointment.
7. Document postoperative instructions in patient chart or electronic medical record.

Terminal Care of the Room and Equipment

1. Apply barrier gloves, gown, and goggles (if appropriate).
2. Dispose of drapes, table cover, pillowcase, and so on. Use biohazardous waste receptacle whenever appropriate.
3. Transfer contaminated surgical tray to cleanup area.
4. Using forceps, isolate sharps from surgical tray and dispose of them into designated sharps container.
5. Place instruments into a soak solution.
6. Sanitize Mayo instrument tray and all surfaces (examination table, stool, counter, lamp, machinery, and equipment).
7. Dispose of contaminated barrier gloves and apply protective gloves.
8. Disinfect all surfaces (examination table, stool, counter, lamp, machinery, and equipment).
9. Allow to air dry.
10. Sanitize, dry, wrap, and sterilize instruments.
11. It is the medical assistant's responsibility to make certain there are enough of each instrument and surgical set.

NOTE: During most surgical procedures, if tissue is excised, it is placed in a biopsy specimen jar containing formalin (a preservative) and sent to the pathology laboratory with an appropriately completed requisition (Figure 19-37).

- Pouring a Sterile Solution into a Cup on a Sterile Field (Procedure 19-7)
- Preparation of Patient Skin before Surgery (Procedure 19-11)

Setting up surgical trays for specific surgeries is addressed in the procedures of this chapter.

Critical Thinking

Dr. Woo asks you to assist him in repairing the laceration on Jaime Carrera's hand. Though you are unsure, you think you may have noticed a tiny hole in the palm of your left glove. What is your next step?

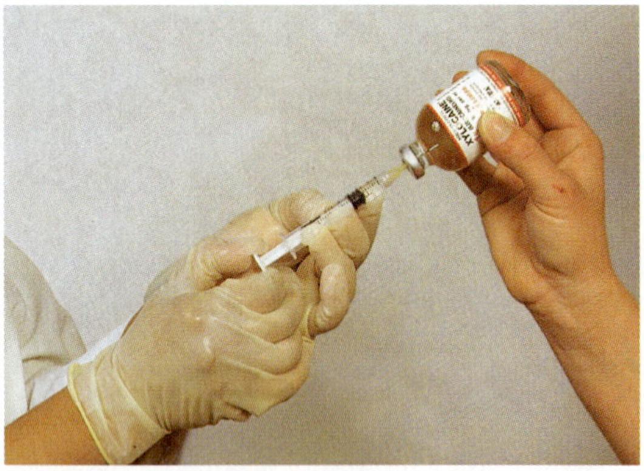

Figure 19-36 Hold the anesthetic solution in a convenient position so that the provider can fill the syringe without contaminating the needle.

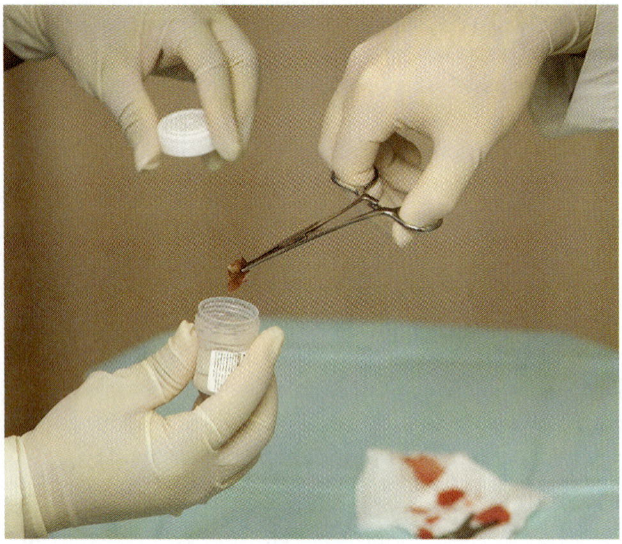

Figure 19-37 The provider places biopsy tissue into specimen jar. The specimen will be sent to the pathology laboratory for examination.

Critical Thinking

You are setting up a sterile surgical tray and have already applied your sterile gloves before you realize you forgot to place the suture package on the tray. You have several options. What are they, and what are the advantages and disadvantages of each?

Using Dry Sterile Transfer Forceps

Occasionally after a sterile tray has been set up and sterile gloves removed, an additional item needs to be applied to or removed from the tray. The use of dry sterile transfer forceps allows sterile items to be applied or sterile items on the tray to be rearranged without the application of another pair of sterile gloves (Figure 19-38). The practice of using wet sterile transfer forceps is no longer recommended. Instead, when the use of sterile transfer forceps is needed, dry sterile transfer forceps are unwrapped, used only once, and then reprocessed for sterilization and subsequent use.

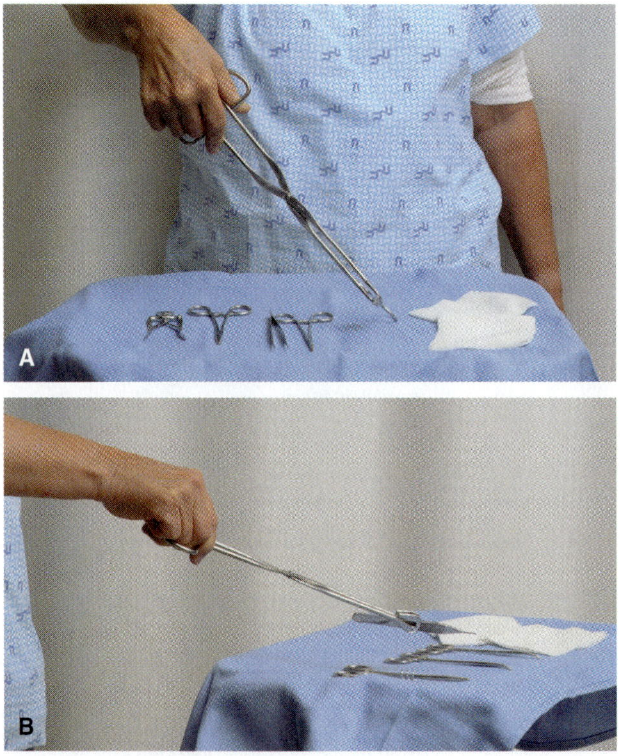

Figure 19-38 (A) If sterile gloves have been removed, use dry sterile transfer forceps to apply or rearrange sterile items on the Mayo stand. (B) Instruments and supplies can be moved around using dry sterile transfer forceps if necessary.

Procedure 19-1

Applying Sterile Gloves

STANDARD PRECAUTIONS:

PURPOSE:

Because hands cannot be sterilized, everyone performing sterile procedures must wear sterile gloves. This procedure provides direction on how to apply sterile gloves without compromising sterility.

EQUIPMENT/SUPPLIES:

Packaged pair of sterile gloves of appropriate size
Flat, clean, dry surface

PROCEDURE STEPS:

1. Remove rings and watch. Wash hands using surgical asepsis. RATIONALE: Rings and watches can snag and tear gloves, and therefore interfere with barrier protection.
2. Inspect glove package for tears or stains (Figure 19-39A). RATIONALE: Tears and stains indicate that the gloves are no longer considered sterile and must be disposed of or used for a nonsterile purpose.
3. Place the glove package on a clean, dry, flat surface above waist level. RATIONALE: Using a contaminated surface could compromise the sterility of the sterile package.
4. Peel open the package taking care not to touch the sterile inner surface of the package. Do not allow the gloves to slide beyond the sterile inner border (Figure 19-39B). RATIONALE: Care must be taken to maintain the sterility of the gloves.
5. The gloves should be opened with the cuffs toward you, the palms up, and the thumbs pointing outward. If the gloves are not positioned properly, turn the package around, being careful not to reach over the sterile area or touch the inner surface or the gloves. RATIONALE: Sterile gloves are packaged in this position for ease in application.
6. With the index finger and thumb of the nondominant hand, grasp the *inner* cuffed edge of the opposite glove. The glove should be picked straight up off the package surface without dragging or dangling the fingers over any nonsterile area. RATIONALE: Picking up the glove by grasping the inner cuff prevents the outer glove from becoming contaminated. Strict adherence must be made to the sterile principles listed in the beginning of this chapter.
7. With the palm up on the dominant hand, carefully slide the hand into the glove. Do not allow the outside of the glove to come in contact with anything and stand away from sterile package. Always hold the hands above the waist and away from the body with palms up (Figure 19-39C). RATIONALE: Keeping the palm up allows the glove to remain sterile in the palm area if it rolls slightly on the back of the hand.
8. With the gloved hand, pick up the glove for the remaining hand by slipping four fingers under the outside of the cuff. Lift the second glove up, keeping it held above the waist and away from the body. Do not allow the glove to drag across the package or touch nonsterile surfaces (Figure 19-39D). RATIONALE: The outside of the second glove is sterile and may only be touched by another sterile surface.
9. With the palm up, slip the second hand into the glove. Do not allow the outside of the gloves to touch nonsterile skin and be especially mindful of the thumb (Figure 19-39E).
10. Adjust the gloves on the hands as needed, but avoid touching the wrist area. Keep gloved hands above the waist and away from the body. Do not touch nonsterile surfaces with the gloved hands (Figure 19-39F and G).

continues

Procedure 19-1 (continued)

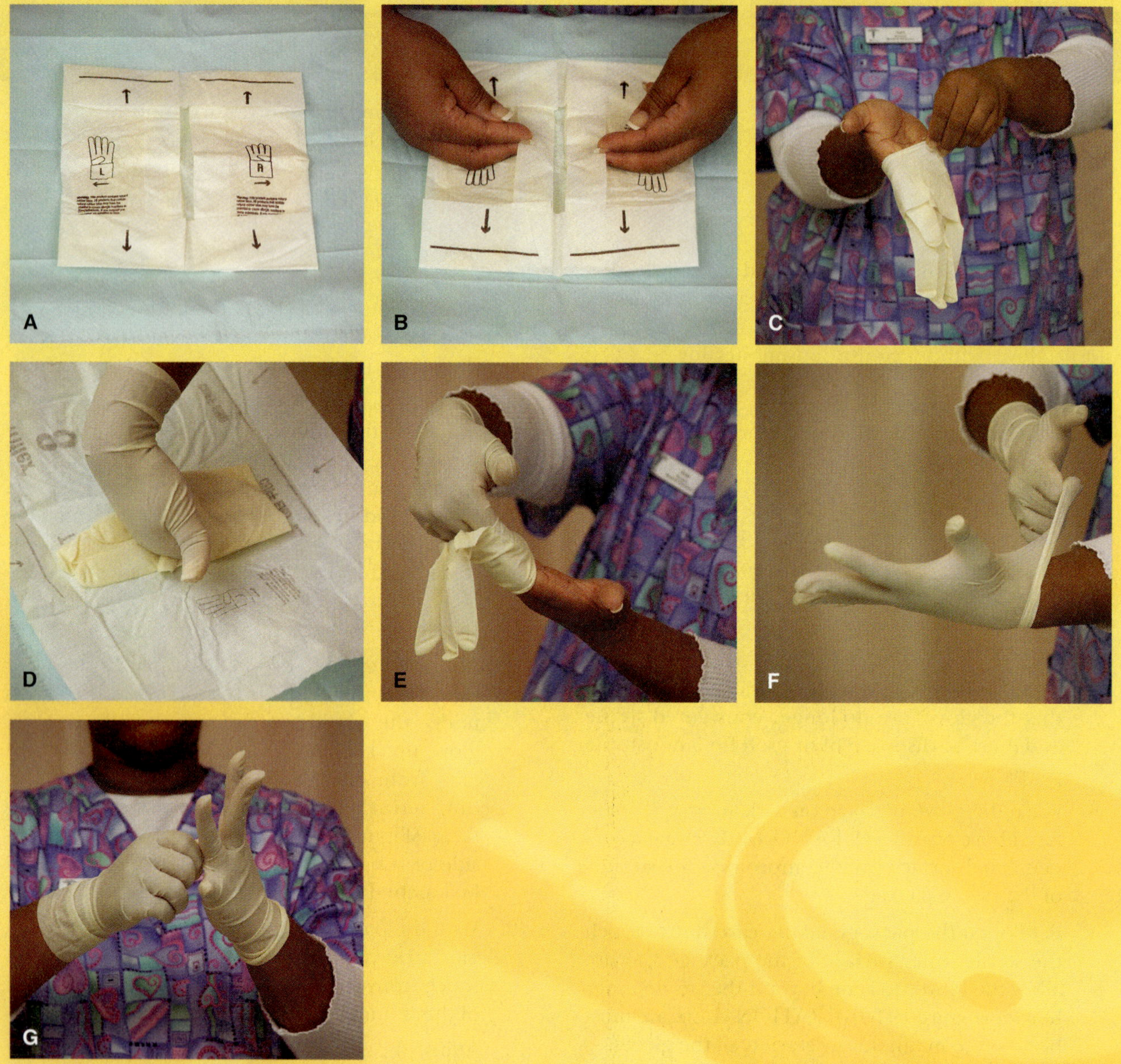

Figure 19-39 (A) Sterile gloves often are packaged with right and left clearly marked. (B) Using only the fingertips, reach in from each side and grasp the edges of the paper. Pull out and lay paper flat without touching any area except the very edges. (C) With the nondominant hand, grasp the *inner* cuffed edge of the opposite glove. Pick the glove up and step away from the sterile area, keeping your hands above your waist and away from your body. With palm up on the dominant hand, slide the hand into the glove. (D) Step back to the sterile area. With the gloved hand, pick up the glove for the remaining hand by slipping four fingers under the outside of the cuff. (E) With palm up, slip the second hand into the glove. Keep the gloved thumb in a "hitchhiking" position. (F) Keeping hands above the waist and away from the body, pull on the second glove. (G) Adjust gloves if desired, staying away from the wrist area. Keep gloved hands above the waist and away from the body.

Procedure 19-2

Chemical "Cold" Sterilization of Endoscopes

STANDARD PRECAUTIONS:

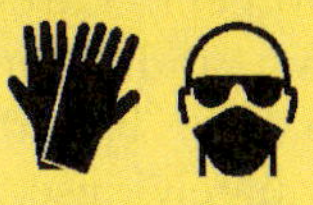

PURPOSE:

To sterilize heat-sensitive items such as fiber-optic endoscopes and delicate cutting instruments using appropriate chemical solution.

EQUIPMENT/SUPPLIES:

- Chemical solution such as Cidex Steris System® (percacetic acid)
- Airtight container
- Timer
- Sterile water
- Gloves (heavy-duty)
- Sterile towel
- Plastic-lined sterile drapes

PROCEDURE STEPS:

1. Sanitize items that require chemical sterilization. Rinse and dry. RATIONALE: Recall that debris and body proteins must be scrubbed from items before sterilization. Ultrasonic cleaning is best.
2. Read manufacturer's instructions on original container of chemical sterilization solution. RATIONALE: Each brand of chemical sterilization solution has specific preparation instructions and germicidal properties; choose the solution that best fits the needs of the ambulatory care setting. Keep the solution in its original container to reduce chances of accidental poisoning.
3. Put on gloves. RATIONALE: Heavy-duty gloves help protect from sharp items puncturing the skin. Chemicals are harsh on the skin.
4. Prepare solution as indicated by manufacturer; place the date of opening or preparation on the container and initial it. RATIONALE: Following manufacturer's instructions ensures sterility. Note the expiration date of solution.
5. Pour solution into a container with an airtight lid; avoid splashing (Figure 19-40A and B). RATIONALE: Chemicals should not be left exposed to open air to prevent evaporation and loss of potency, exposure to environmetal contaminants, accidental inhalation, or poisoning. Splashing may cause skin or mucous membrane contact and result in injury.
6. Place sanitized and dried items into the solution, completely submerging item(s). Avoid splashing when placing items into airtight container. RATIONALE: Total immersion is necessary for sterility to be achieved.

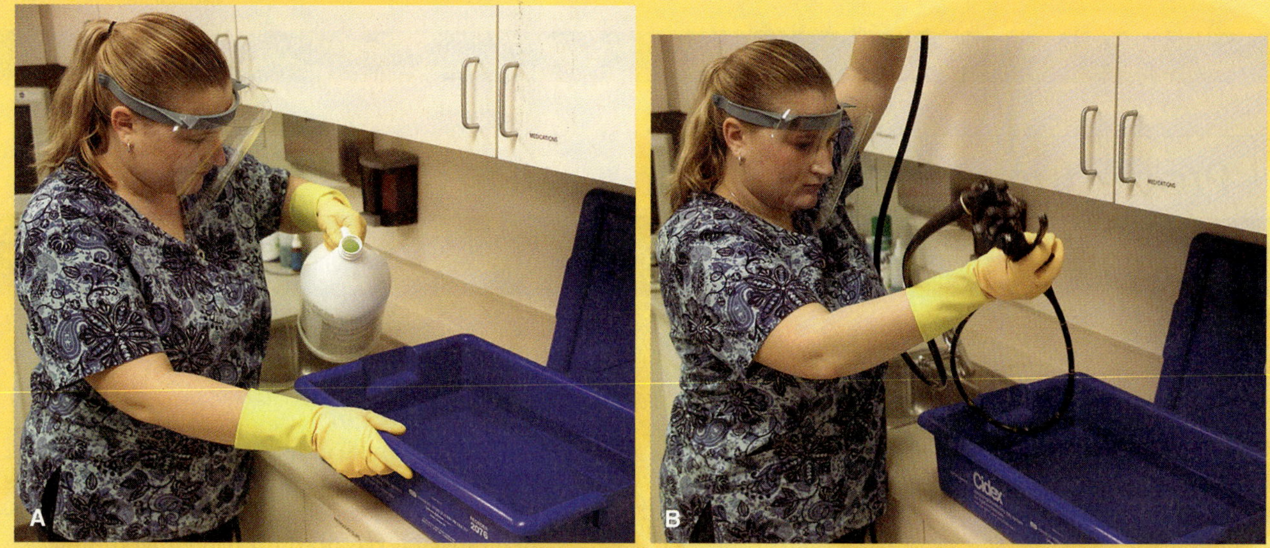

Figure 19-40 (A) Medical assistant pours chemical sterilization solution into a large soaking container. Note the use of heavy-duty gloves and face shield. (B) Medical assistant adds the endoscope to the chemical sterilization solution in the container.

continues

Procedure 19-2 (continued)

7. Close lid of container, label with name of solution, date, and time required per manufacturer, and initial (Figure 19-40C). RATIONALE: Exposure time is the required time indicated by the manufacturer to achieve sterility. Initialing work ensures accountability and responsibility.
8. Do not open lid or add additional items during the processing time. RATIONALE: Adding to the container interrupts the sterilization process and limits the effectiveness of the chemical.

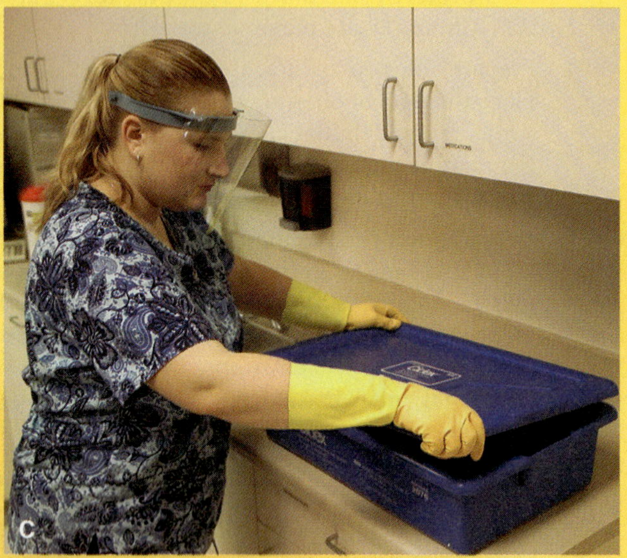

Figure 19-40 (continued) (C) Medical assistant secures lid tightly, then records the date, time of day, and her initials.

9. Following the recommended processing time, lift item(s) from the container using sterile gloved hands or sterile transfer forceps. Carefully hold item above sterile basin and pour copious amounts of sterile water over it and through it (endoscopes) until adequately rinsed of chemical solution. RATIONALE: Item(s) once processed are sterile and must be handled appropriately. Using sterile gloved hands or sterile transfer forceps ensures sterile-to-sterile contact and no contamination of the item(s). Sterile water is poured through the inner channels of endoscopes to rinse chemicals from the inside, as well as the outside.
10. Hold item(s) upright for a few seconds to allow excess sterile water to drip off.
11. Place the sterile item on a sterile towel (which has been placed on a sterile field) and dry it with another sterile towel. The towel used for drying is removed from sterile field. The use of sterile drapes that have a plastic polylined barrier layer between two layers of paper is recommended for the sterile field. RATIONALE: Plastic-lined sterile drapes create a barrier to prevent moisture from drawing contaminants from the metal surgical instrument tray or countertop up into the sterile area.

Procedure 19-3

Preparing Instruments for Sterilization in Autoclave

PURPOSE:

To properly wrap sanitized instruments for sterilization in an autoclave.

EQUIPMENT/SUPPLIES:

Sanitized instruments
Wrapping material (muslin or disposable wrapping paper)
Sterilization indicator
2 × 2 gauze or cotton balls (if instrument has hinges)
Autoclave wrapping tape
Permanent marker or felt-tip pen (Figure 19-41A)

PROCEDURE STEPS:

1. Prepare a clean, dry, flat surface of adequate size to lay the wrapping material. RATIONALE: A clean area reduces risk for contamination. Adequate space is required for proper wrapping.
2. Select two wraps of adequate size in which to wrap instruments.

continues

Procedure 19-3 (continued)

3. Place one square of wrapping material at an angle in front of you on the dry surface with one corner pointed directly toward you.
4. Place the sanitized instrument or articles to be placed in the autoclave just below the center of the wrap. Open instruments with hinges as wide as possible and place a 2 × 2 gauze or cotton ball in the opening (Figure 19-41B). RATIONALE: Instruments with hinged parts that are not spread open before autoclaving may not be properly sterilized.
5. Place one sterilization indicator with the instrument. RATIONALE: Sterilization indicators inside packages ascertain sterilization of each individual package. Indicators change colors when the required temperature has been reached, documenting the effectiveness of the sterilization. *NOTE:* Quality control for autoclave operation can be evaluated with sterilization indicators.
6. Bring the corner of the wrap closest to you up and over the article toward the center. Bring the tip of the same corner back toward you until it reaches the folded edge, creating a fan-fold effect. Smooth the edges of the fold. The article should remain completely covered (Figure 19-41C).
7. Fold one side edge toward the center line; fan-fold back to side, and crease (Figure 19-41D).
8. Repeat step 7 for the other side edge (Figure 19-41E).
9. Fold the package up from the bottom (Figure 19-41F).
10. Fold the top edge down and over the entire package (Figure 19-41G). RATIONALE: Final edge should wrap entire package for assurance of adequate coverage and protection once contents are sterilized. If wrap does not cover adequately, unwrap and start over with larger wrapping material.
11. To "wrap twice," place this package into the center of a second wrap (Figure 19-41H). Repeat Steps 7 through 10. RATIONALE: Double wrapping allows more control of multiple instruments when setting up a surgical tray.
12. Tape with autoclave tape across the point left exposed. RATIONALE: Autoclave tape indicates whether the package has been through the autoclave; it is not a form of sterilization indicator or quality control.
13. Label the tape with the name of the instrument or type of pack (i.e., laceration repair pack), date of sterilization, and your initials (Figure 19-41I).

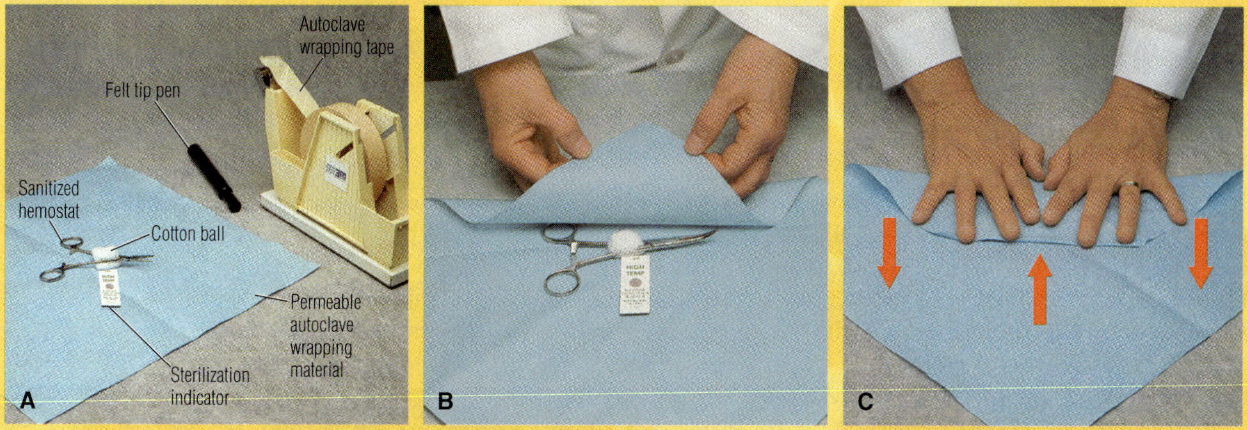

Figure 19-41 (A) Equipment needed to wrap surgical instruments or equipment for sterilization in an autoclave. (B) Place a cotton ball between the hinge joints of instruments to keep them open. Do not ratchet instruments closed. Pad the tips of sharp instruments. Put a sterilization indicator in with the instruments to be wrapped. (C) The wrapping paper is folded toward center. A small corner is turned back on itself.

continues

Procedure 19-3 (continued)

RATIONALE: Proper instrument labeling is required to identify wrapped sterilized instruments. Instruments wrapped and sterilized in paper or cloth wrappers are considered sterile for four weeks from the date of sterilization. Initialing packages ensures accountability and responsibility.

14. Place wrapped instruments in autoclave. RATIONALE: If wrapped instruments are not to be immediately autoclaved, do NOT date the package. Leave the package on a clean, dry surface and date the package just before autoclaving.

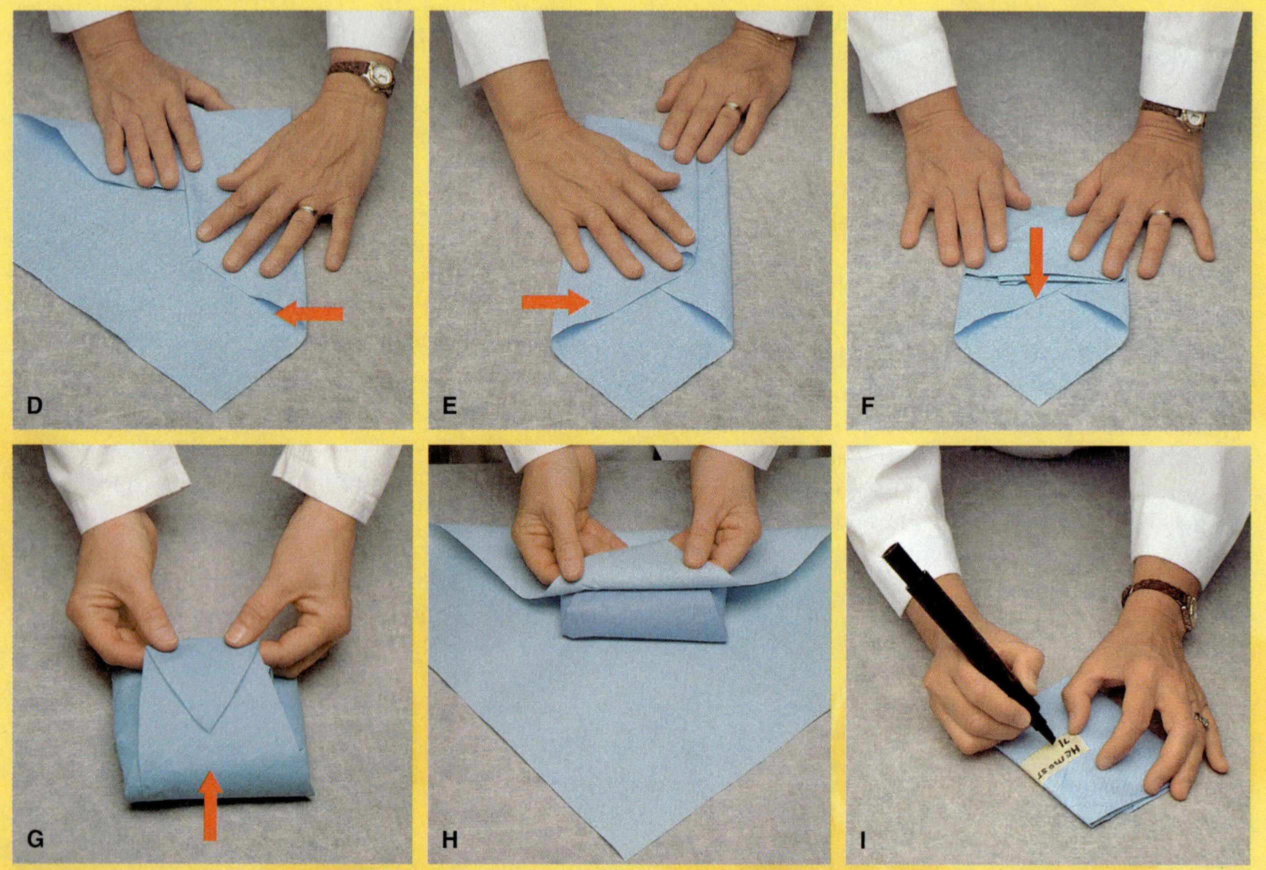

Figure 19-41 (continued) (D) Fold one side toward center, leaving small corner turned back on itself. (E) Fold other side toward center, leaving small corner turned back on itself. (F) The package is folded up from the bottom and secured. (G) Fold corner back on itself. (H) Wrap first package in another wrap. Double wrapping allows more control of multiple instruments when setting up a surgical tray. (I) Wrapped package is secured with heat-sensitive autoclave tape and labeled with the date, contents, and medical assistant's initials.

Procedure 19-4

Sterilization of Instruments (Autoclave)

PURPOSE:

To rid items of all forms of microbial (microorganisms) life for use in invasive procedures.

EQUIPMENT/SUPPLIES:

Steam sterilizer (autoclave)
Autoclave manufacturers instructions
Wrapped sanitized instrument package(s) with sterilization indicators placed inside package (or unwrapped item if removed with sterile transfer forceps)

PROCEDURE STEPS:

1. Check water level in the autoclave reservoir and add distilled water to fill line if necessary. RATIONALE: Not enough or too much water will impair the efficiency of the autoclave. Distilled water will not leave deposits (tap water leaves deposits) inside the autoclave. Deposits can impair the efficiency of the autoclave.
2. Depending on your autoclave, turn the knob to "fill" line and allow water into the chamber until it reaches the "fill" line. Turn the knob to the next position. This stops water from continuing to enter the chamber.

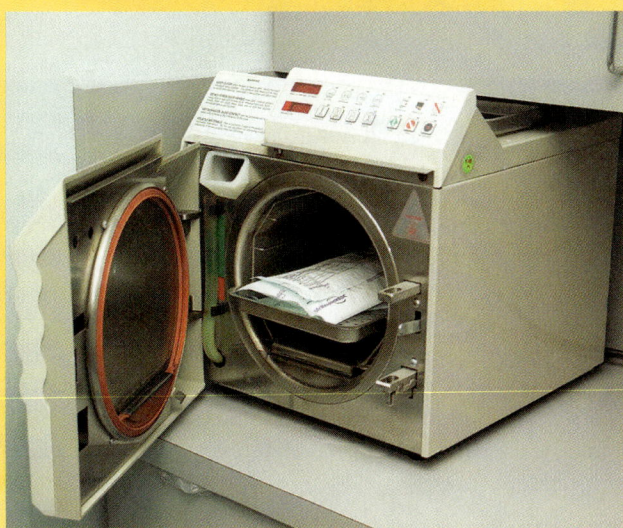

Figure 19-42 Load packages into the autoclave so that steam is able to reach all surfaces, allowing for proper sterilization.

3. Load packages into autoclave tray; allow room for steam to circulate (Figure 19-42). RATIONALE: Steam circulates in predictable patterns in an autoclave. When packages are loaded too closely or improperly, proper sterilization will not occur in individual packages.
   a. Load jars of dressings or cups on their sides, with tops ajar or loosely in place. RATIONALE: Steam is trapped within a jar when it is right side up; containers and goods will not be sterilized if loaded sitting up vertically.
   b. Load unwrapped instruments flat with handles opened, exposing all surfaces. RATIONALE: Steam must reach all surfaces.
4. Close autoclave door and seal. RATIONALE: Pressure cannot be achieved without a proper seal.
5. Turn on autoclave. When the temperature dial indicates 270°F (118°C) and 15 pounds of pressure has been achieved inside the autoclave, begin necessary exposure time by setting timer. RATIONALE: Proper heat, pressure levels, and exposure time must be achieved to kill all microorganisms within the autoclave. Careful note should be given to setting exposure time only after the proper temperature and pressure settings have been achieved.

Item	Required Exposure Time
Wrapped instrument packages or trays	30 minutes
Unwrapped items	15 minutes
Unwrapped items covered with cloth	20 minutes

6. After completion of the autoclave cycle, vent exhaust steam pressure from the autoclave by following the manufacturer's instructions. RATIONALE: Following the manufacturer's instructions carefully will ensure safe and proper use of the autoclave.
7. Open the door approximately 1 inch after the pressure gauge indicates zero (0) pressure and the temperature gauge indicates a decrease to at least 212°F. RATIONALE: You will not be able to open the door until the pressure is zero. Be

continues

Procedure 19-4 (continued)

aware that steam burns can occur when opening the door. Use caution.

8. Allow the contents to completely dry, approximately 30 to 45 minutes; do NOT touch contents until completely dry. RATIONALE: If packages are still wet or damp, microorganisms can enter a wrapped package, rendering it contaminated. Liquids travel along paper or cloth by capillary action and will be contaminated by microorganisms on countertops or from hands.
9. Remove wrapped contents with dry, clean hands and store in clean, dry closed cupboard or drawer. RATIONALE: Sterilized wrapped packages can be held with clean hands, because only the interior contents require maintenance of sterility. If the outer wrapper is required to remain sterile, remove with sterile transfer forceps and place on a sterile field or in sterile storage areas.
10. Remove unwrapped contents with sterile transfer forceps; resanitize and resterilize the transfer forceps following use. RATIONALE: Sterile transfer forceps must have been sterilized immediately prior to or along with the unwrapped item if they are to be used immediately in a sterile procedure. Place onto sterile surface.
11. Perform quality control on a regular basis, based on usage. RATIONALE: Quality control and maintenance of an autoclave is critical to assurance of proper operation. Accountability and responsibility to monitor quality control should be the responsibility of the medical assistant(s) most often responsible for sterilization.
    a. Monitor sterilization indicators with each use of sterilized instruments.
    b. Weekly perform quality control by documenting sterilization indicator outcome on a log; date and initial quality-control log entries.
12. Clean and service the autoclave regularly according to the manufacturer's guidelines. When sterilization is not being achieved, take equipment out of service and contact a service agency for repair. RATIONALE: It is the responsibility of the medical assistant to take out of service any equipment that is not operating properly as a component of risk management.
13. Keep a log of cleaning, services, and quality-control measures performed.

Procedure 19-5

Setting Up and Covering a Sterile Field

STANDARD PRECAUTIONS:

PURPOSE:

Disposable sterile field drapes or sterile towels are used to isolate a sterile area or field, as well as to cover the sterile field for use in surgery and sterile procedures. They are available in convenient peel-apart packages, fanfolded for ease of use, and often are two-tone in color to aid in differentiating one side from the other. Cloth drapes may be packaged separately and sterilized fanfolded.

NOTE: A variety of materials, both disposable and nondisposable, can be used to set up and cover a sterile field. All material has certain criteria to be safe for use and all have advantages and disadvantages. For example, woven textile fabrics are moisture retardant and are effective barriers to microbial penetration. Polylined paper disposable drapes are excellent barriers against microorganisms and moisture. Many times medical office preference is determined by financial consideration.

EQUIPMENT/SUPPLIES:

Disposable sterile polylined field drapes (two) or reuseable sterile towels (two) (muslin or linen with water-repellent finish)

continues

Procedure 19-5 (continued)

Mayo instrument tray/stand positioned above the waist with stem to the right

Sterile transfer forceps (if needed)

PROCEDURE STEPS:

1. Wash hands.
2. Sanitize and disinfect a Mayo instrument tray. Adjust tray to above waist level and have the stem to the right.
3. Select an appropriate disposable sterile field drape and place the drape package on a clean, dry, flat surface.
4. Open the package exposing the fanfolded drape. Ensure that the cut corners of the drape are toward you; turn the package if necessary (Figure 19-43A). RATIONALE: Sterile field drapes are fanfolded and positioned within the package to facilitate ease of use.
5. With thumb and forefinger of one hand, carefully grasp the top cut corner without touching the rest of the drape or towel and pick the drape or towel up high enough to ensure that as it unfolds it does not drag across a nonsterile area (Figure 19-43B). RATIONALE: The drape or towel will naturally unfold as it is lifted, so care must be taken to ensure that it is lifted quickly and allowed to unfold without touching a nonsterile surface.
6. Holding the drape or towel above waist level and away from the body, grasp the opposing corner so that both corners along the long edge of the drape are being held (Figure 19-43C).
7. Keeping the drape or towel above waist level and away from the body, reach over the Mayo tray with the drape or towel. Take care that the lower edge of the drape or towel does not drag across the tray (Figure 19-43D). RATIONALE: Sterile

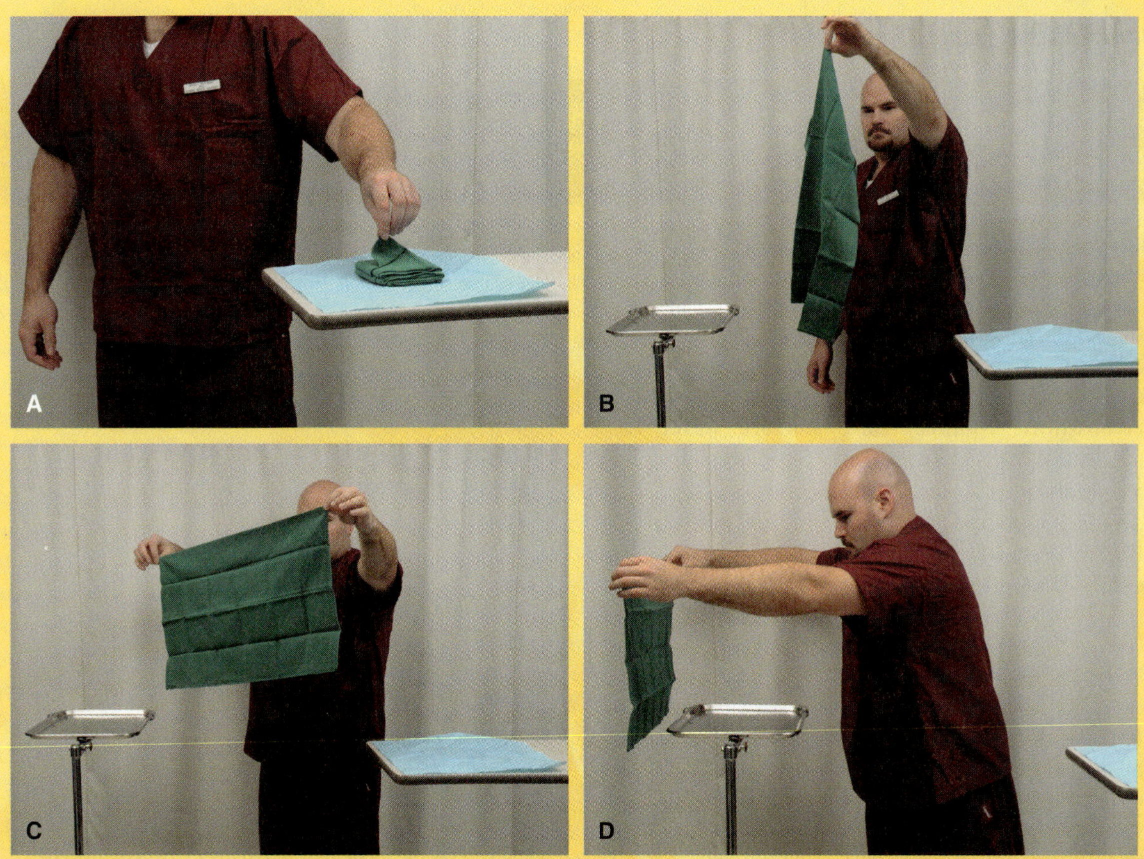

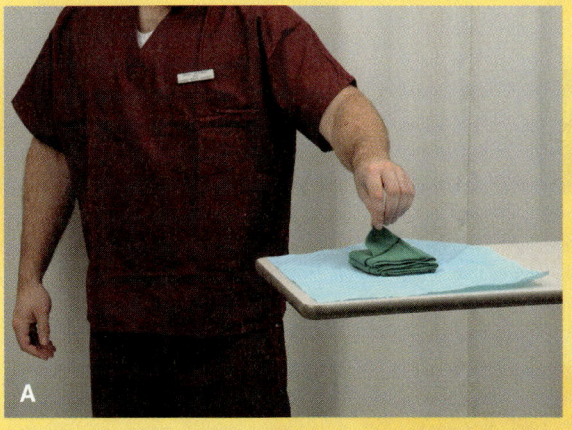

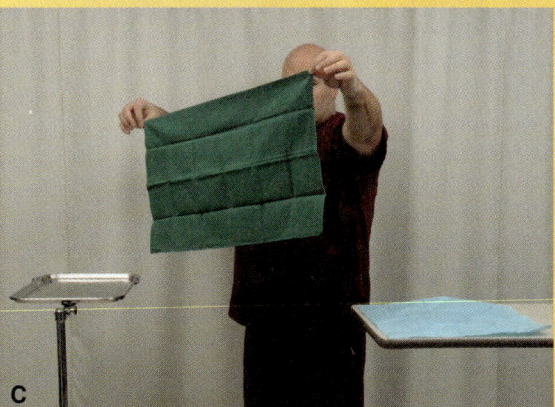

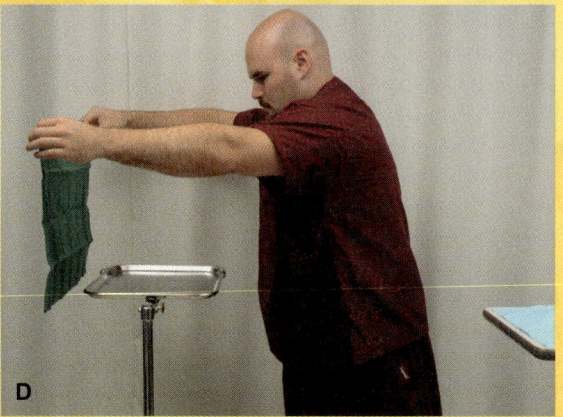

Figure 19-43 (A) Open the sterile drape package onto a flat, dry surface 90 degrees perpendicular to the Mayo tray. Grasp the corner of the sterile drape. (B) Pull the drape straight up, allowing it to unfold. Do not shake it out. (C) Carefully grasp another corner of the drape and apply the drape to the Mayo tray by pulling it toward you. Do not reach over the field; do not allow the "top" surface to touch anything. (D) Continue laying the drape as a sterile field.

continues

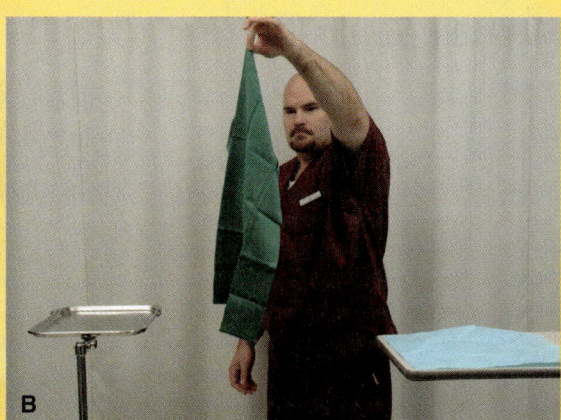

Procedure 19-5 (continued)

principles state that sterile items should be kept above the waist and not touch other objects.

8. Gently pull the drape or towel toward you as it is laid onto the tray. If adjustment is needed to center the drape or towel, do not touch the center of the drape or towel, or reach over the sterile field. Walk around or reach underneath the tray to move it or make adjustments. RATIONALE: The corners/edges that hang over the tray are no longer considered sterile.
9. After setting the instruments and supplies on the tray, it must be covered.
10. To cover the sterile field with a second sterile drape or towel, follow Steps 4 through 7; then instead of pulling the drape or towel toward you (as described in Step 8), which would necessitate reaching over the sterile field, apply the covering drape or towel by holding it up in front of the field. Adjust the lower edge so it is even with the lower edge of the field drape or towel (see Figure 19-44H). With a forward motion, carefully lay the cover over the sterile field (see Figure 19-44I). RATIONALE: Reaching over the sterile field would contaminate the tray.

Procedure 19-6

Opening Sterile Packages of Instruments and Supplies and Applying Them to a Sterile Field

STANDARD PRECAUTIONS:

NOTE: Sterile instruments and supplies are packaged in a manner that allows them to be opened and accessed without compromising sterility. Refer to other sections of this chapter for the specific steps of wrapping techniques, sterile gloving, and setting up sterile fields. The "wrapping twice" method of double wrapping was used in preparing the surgical packs for this procedure. Prepackaged items such as gauze squares should be in peel-apart packs.

PURPOSE:

To open sterile packages of surgical instruments and supplies and place them onto a sterile field using sterile technique.

EQUIPMENT/SUPPLIES:

Mayo instrument tray draped with sterile field
Sterile gloves
Wrapped-twice sterile surgical instruments
Prepackaged sterile surgical supplies

PROCEDURE STEPS:

1. Assemble supplies.
2. Wash hands and set up sterile field (see Procedure 19-5).
3. Position package of surgical instruments on palm of nondominant hand with outer envelope flap on top. (Figure 19-44A). RATIONALE: This will facilitate opening the pack while protecting its sterile contents.
4. Grasping the taped end of the top flap, open the first flap away from you. Do not touch the inside of the flap (Figure 19-44B).
5. Grasping just the folded back tips of the side flaps, pull the right-sided flap to the right. Then pull the left-sided flap to the left, taking care not to reach over the package (Figure 19-44C). RATIONALE: Pulling the tips of the flaps toward each side allows the inner portion of the package to be exposed without contamination.
6. Pull the last flap toward you by grasping the folded-back tip taking care not to touch the inner contents of the package (Figure 19-44D).

continues

Procedure 19-6 (continued)

RATIONALE: Pulling the last tip toward you allows you to avoid reaching over the inner contents of the package.

7. Gather all of the loose edges together to obtain a snug covering over your nondominant hand. Close your covered hand over the inner package and carefully apply the inner package to the sterile field (Figure 19-44E). RATIONALE: Gathering the loose edges prevents them from being dragged across the sterile field.

8. Open peel-apart packages using sterile technique by grasping both edges of the flaps and pulling them apart in a rolling down motion, keeping both hands together. The sterile item should be exposed gradually between the two peel-apart edges (Figure 19-44F). The sterile inner contents may then be offered to the sterile-gloved provider or applied to the sterile field using a flipping motion, or dropped as shown in Figure 19-44G, taking care not to contaminate either the package contents or the field.

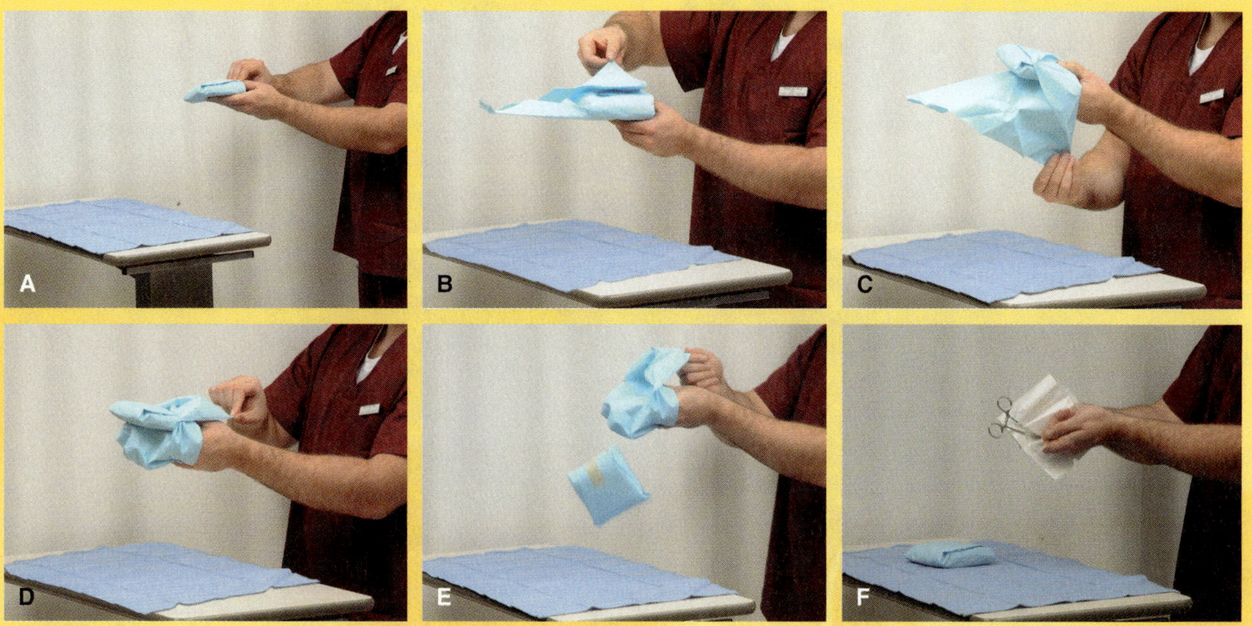

Figure 19-44 (A) To open a twice-wrapped pack, grasp the taped end of the top flap and open the first flap away from you. You should have the Mayo tray at or above waist height. Stand back from the sterile field. (B) Allow the pack to unroll on your hand. Do not touch the inside of the flap. Notice the medical assistant's thumb is under the flap, where she can securely grasp the inner pack. (C) Grasp just the folded back tips of the side flaps. First pull the right-sided tip to the right, then, reaching around or under, pull the left-sided tip to the left. Do not reach over the package. (D) Gather the loose edges together to form a snug covering over your nondominant hand. Securely grasping the wrapped inner pack, step toward your sterile field, and invert your hand. (E) Release (drop) the inner pack onto the center of the sterile field. Step back. (F) Open peel-apart packages using sterile technique, exposing sterile items slowly and gradually. Continue to peel back the sides of the package while securely holding onto the tip of the instrument.

continues

Procedure 19-6 (continued)

9. Apply sterile gloves. Arrange instruments and supplies in an organized and logical manner according to the provider's preference. RATIONALE: Instruments should be arranged in the order of use. All handles should be pointed toward the user. Instruments should be separated as much as possible within the space of the field so entanglement of instruments is not a problem.

10. Apply the sterile field cover (Figure 19-44H, I, and J) (see Procedure 19-5). RATIONALE: A sterile cover will need to be applied if the surgical tray will not be used immediately, needs to be moved, or if the medical assistant leaves the tray unattended.

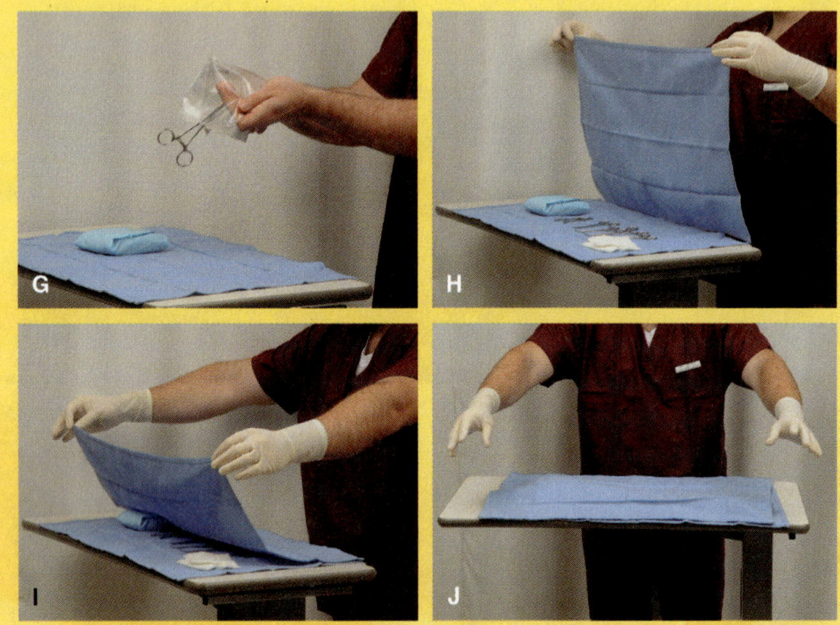

Figure 19-44 (continued) (G) Hold the sides of the package over your hand, step toward the Mayo tray, and apply the instrument, handle first, onto the sterile field. Apply other supplies as needed. Arrange instruments and supplies according to provider's preference using sterile gloves or sterile transfer forceps. (H) Apply the sterile drape cover to the surgical tray in a similar manner as the field was set up, except apply drape away from you. (I) Be sure the edges of the cover align with the edges of the field drape before letting go and applying the cover. (J) Do not adjust cover after it has been laid.

Critical Thinking

You have removed a double-wrapped instrument pack from the autoclave and notice a small tear in the outermost wrap. The innermost wrap appears to be intact. What would your action be? Why?

Procedure 19-7

Pouring a Sterile Solution into a Cup on a Sterile Field

STANDARD PRECAUTIONS:

NOTE: Occasionally, sterile solutions need to be poured into a sterile cup that has been placed onto the sterile tray. The solution is sterile, but the outside of the container is not; therefore, special precautions need to be taken to pour the solution into the cup without contaminating the sterile field. The solution is always poured after the tray has been moved into the surgical area to avoid spilling during transport.

PURPOSE:

To pour a sterile solution into a cup on a sterile tray in a sterile manner.

EQUIPMENT/SUPPLIES:

Covered sterile surgical tray with a sterile cup in upper right corner
Container of sterile solution (as ordered)

PROCEDURE STEPS:

1. Wash hands.
2. Transport the surgical tray into the surgical area before pouring the solution; or, the surgical tray can be set up for immediate use in the surgical area. RATIONALE: The solution may tip and spill during transport.
3. Read the label of the solution container three times and check the expiration date. RATIONALE: To eliminate the possibility of pouring the wrong solution or an outdated solution.
4. Remove the cap from the solution container, taking care not to touch the inner surface of the cap. Place the cap upside down on a nonsterile surface to avoid touching the inner surface of the cap with a nonsterile surface. When the cap is held in the hand, hold it right side up. RATIONALE: Touching the inside of the cap with either your hand or a nonsterile surface will contaminate the inside of an otherwise sterile container.
5. Read the label again to ensure accuracy. Place palm over the label to protect the label from stains. Pour a small amount of the solution into a bowl, cup, or sink that is outside the sterile field. RATIONALE: This action will cleanse the lip of the container.

NOTE: If the surgical tray is set up in a surgical area, the solution can be poured before covering the surgical tray with a sterile drape or towel.

6. Carefully pull back the upper right corner of the tray cover to expose the cup. Take care to only touch the corner tip of the cover and not reach over the exposed field. RATIONALE: Touching the underside of the cover or reaching over the exposed sterile field will contaminate the sterile surgical tray.
7. Approaching from the corner of the tray and using the cleansed side of the lip of the container, pour the needed amount of solution into the sterile cup (Figure 19-45). Precaution should be taken to avoid splashing, spilling, reaching over the field, or touching any of the sterile surfaces. RATIONALE: Splashing or spilling of the solution would cause the sterile field drape to become wet, which may cause contaminants to "wick" from the metal tray into the sterile field. Use of a polylined sterile field drape will create a barrier to avoid wicking.
8. Replace the corner of the drape cover using sterile technique or cover with a sterile drape or towel.
9. Replace the cap of the solution container using sterile technique.
10. Read the label again.

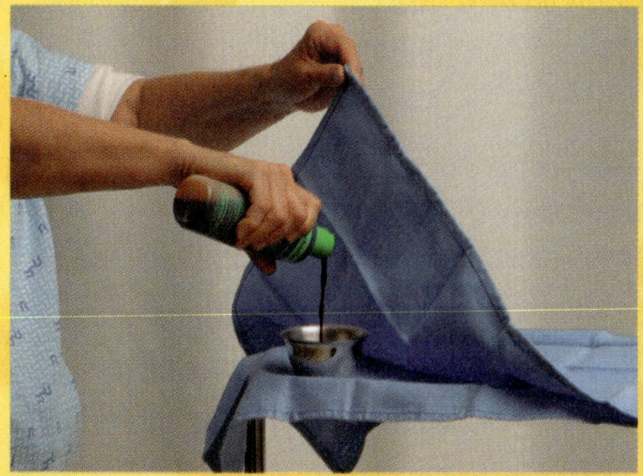

Figure 19-45 Approaching from the corner of the Mayo stand, pour the needed amount of solution into the sterile cup. Use the clean side of the container lip for pouring.

Procedure 19-8

Assisting with Office/Ambulatory Surgery

STANDARD PRECAUTIONS:

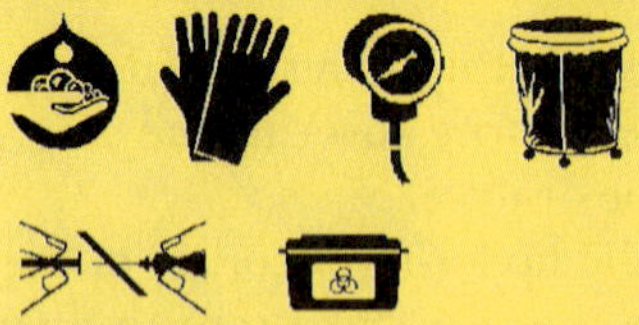

PURPOSE:

To maintain sterility during surgical procedures that require surgical excision.

EQUIPMENT/SUPPLIES:

Mayo stand:

- Needles and syringe for anesthesia
- Prep bowl/cup
- Gauze sponges
- Scalpel and blade
- Operating scissors
- Fenestrated drape
- Hemostats (curved and straight)
- Thumb dressing forceps
- Thumb tissue forceps
- Needle holder
- Suture pack
- Transfer forceps

Side table (unsterile field):

- Sterile gloves (in package)
- Labeled biopsy containers with formalin
- Appropriate laboratory requisition
- Anesthesia vial
- Alcohol wipes
- Dressing, tape, bandages
- Biohazard container
- Betadine ® solution

PROCEDURE STEPS:

1. Check room and equipment for readiness and cleanliness.
2. Wash hands.
3. Set up side table of nonsterile items. RATIONALE: Nonsterile items cannot be placed onto a sterile field because they will contaminate it.
4. Perform surgical asepsis hand cleansing.
5. Set up sterile field on a sanitized and disinfected Mayo stand or on a clean, dry, flat surface (see Procedure 19-5).
6. Add sterile items (see Procedure 19-6).
7. Apply sterile gloves or use sterile transfer forceps. Arrange instruments according to use. Remove gloves and forceps from area.
8. Wash hands.
9. Cover the sterile field with a sterile towel if not being used immediately.
10. Identify patient, explain the procedure, and prepare the patient. Refer to patient preparation in Table 19-4.
11. Prepare patient's skin (see Procedure 19-11).
12. Remove the sterile cover from the sterile setup as the provider applies sterile gloves. Lift the towel by grasping the tips of the corners farthest away from you and lifting toward you. Do not allow arms to pass over sterile field. RATIONALE: Avoids crossing over sterile field.
13. Assist the provider as necessary, being certain to follow the principles of surgical asepsis.
    - The medical assistant holds the vial of anesthesia while the provider withdraws the appropriate dose.
    - The provider injects the local anesthetic, applies Betadine® or other antiseptic to the surgical site, applies sterile drapes, and begins the surgery.
    - Adjust the instrument tray and equipment around the provider.
    - Ensure a good light source.
    - Comfort and support patient emotionally.
    - Assist with the surgery as directed by the provider (sterile gloves must be worn).
    - Hand instruments to the provider and receive used intruments from the provider and place in a basin or container out of patient's sight.
    - If necessary, hold biopsy container to receive specimen being excised. Do not contaminate the inside of the container. Hold the cover facing down. Tightly place cover on the container. Assist with or apply sterile dressing to the operative site.
14. Assist patient as necessary. Refer to Assisting the Patient after Surgery in Table 19-4.
15. The specimen container must be tightly covered; labeled with the patient's name, date, type, and source of specimen; and sent to the laboratory accompanied by the appropriate laboratory requisition.

continues

Procedure 19-8 (continued)

16. Wearing appropriate personal protective equipment (PPE), clean surgical or examination room.
    - Dispose of used gauze sponges in biohazard container and knife blades and other disposable sharps in puncture-proof sharps container.
    - Rinse used surgical intruments; soak, sanitize, and sterilize for reuse (see Chapter 10).
    - Remove gloves and other PPE and dispose of per Occupational Safety and Health Administration (OSHA) guidelines.
17. Wash hands.
18. Document in patient's chart or electronic medical record that the specimen was sent to the laboratory.

DOCUMENTATION

8/12/20XX 2:30 PM Skin tag from left axilla excised by Dr. King. Biopsy specimen in its entirety sent to laboratory. J. Guerro, CMA (AAMA) ———

Procedure 19-9

Dressing Change

STANDARD PRECAUTIONS:

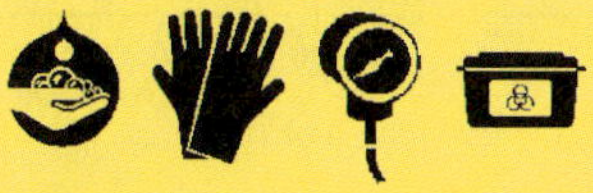

NOTE: After most surgical procedures have been completed, the wound is usually covered with a dry sterile dressing (DSD) that may need to be removed periodically so that the wound can be checked for healing or for suture removal. Another dry sterile dressing may then be applied. Burns require daily dressing changes.

PURPOSE:

To remove a wound dressing and apply a dry sterile dressing.

EQUIPMENT/SUPPLIES:

Sterile field:

Several sterile gauze sponges and other dressing material as needed or prepackaged sterile dressing kit
Sterile bowl with Betadine® solution or prepared sterile Betadine® swab sticks
Sterile dressing forceps
Sponge forceps

Side area (unsterile field):

Nonsterile gloves
Sterile gloves
Hydrogen peroxide
Container of sterile water
Cotton-tipped applicators
Adhesive strips
Antibacterial ointment/cream as ordered
Tape
Sponge forceps
Bandage scissors
Waterproof waste bag
Biohazard waste container

PROCEDURE STEPS:

1. Check provider's order.
2. Wash hands.
3. Prepare sterile field. Add gauze sponges, bowl with solution, and forceps.
4. Position a waterproof bag away from sterile area.
5. Pour Betadine® solution into sterile bowl or use Betadine swab sticks.
6. Identify the patient and explain the procedure.
7. Reassure and comfort the patient as needed.
8. Don nonsterile gloves or use forceps.
9. Loosen tape on dressing by pulling tape toward wound, or cut off bandage if necessary.
10. Carefully remove bandage; place in biohazard waste container. Do not pass over sterile field. RATIONALE: Passing dirty (used) bandage or dressing over sterile field contaminates it.

continues

Procedure 19-9 (continued)

11. Remove dressing, taking care not to cause stress on the wound (Figure 19-46A).
    a. If stuck to the wound, pour small amounts of sterile water over dressing; allow to soak for a short time. Remove dressing when loose enough to remove without resistance. Note type and amount of drainage if present.
12. Place used dressing in waterproof bag without touching inside or outside of bag. RATIONALE: Dirty (used) dressing can contaminate outside of bag.
13. Assess wound and note any drainage or signs of infection. Remove and discard gloves in waterproof bag.
14. Wash hands.
15. Apply sterile gloves.
16. Clean the wound with antiseptic solution as ordered (Figure 19-46B). Gauze may be held with forceps, or use swabs.
17. Dispose of used gauze in waterproof bag.
18. Using sterile cotton-tipped applicators, apply cream/ointment as ordered. Using sterile forceps or sterile gloves, apply sterile gauze sponge(s) to wound (Figure 19-46C).
19. Remove gloves, dispose of in waterproof bag. Wash hands.
20. Secure dressing with roller bandage and adhesive tape (Figure 19-46D and E) or elastic bandage.
21. Dispose of waterproof bag in biohazard container.
22. Wash hands.
23. Document procedure in patient's chart or electronic medical record, describing wound appearance (i.e., discharge, signs of infection, healing, and so on).

DOCUMENTATION

11/24/20XX 10:30 AM Dressing change to laceration left forearm. Small amount (dime-size) of serosanguinous discharge noted. No signs of redness or swelling in incisional area. DSD applied. Says she "feels fine and that my arm hurts very little." J. Guerro, CMA (AAMA) ———

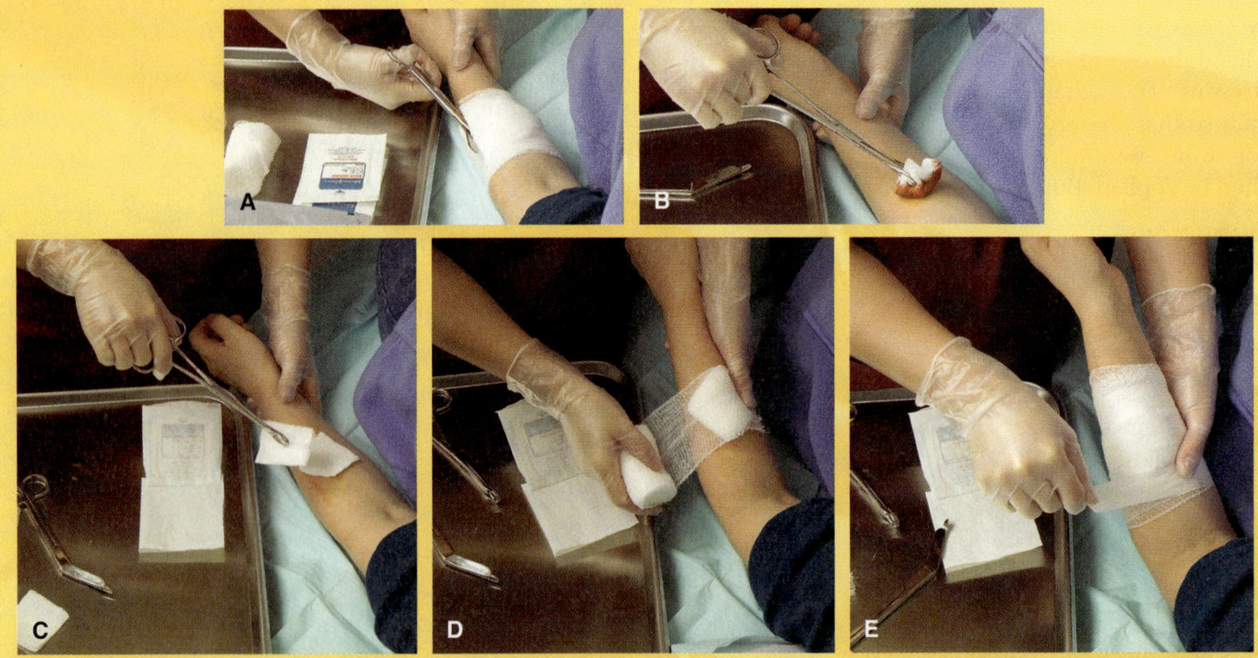

Figure 19-46 To change a dressing: (A) Gently remove dressing. Do not cause stress on wound. (B) Clean wound with Betadine® solution using sponge forceps. (C) Using dressing forceps, new sterile sponge forceps, a hemostat, or sterile gloves, apply sterile gauze sponge(s) to wound. (D, E) Secure dressing with elastic bandage and adhesive tape or roller bandage.

Procedure 19-10

Wound Irrigation

STANDARD PRECAUTIONS:

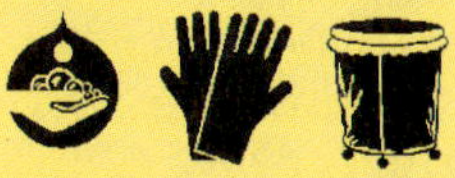

PURPOSE:

To irrigate a wound to remove the accumulation of exudate that impairs and delays healing.

EQUIPMENT/SUPPLIES:

On Mayo tray:

- Sterile gloves in package
- Sterile irrigation kit (irrigating syringe, basin, and container for solution)
- Sterile dressing material in package

Side area/unsterile field:

- Waterproof pad
- Sterile solution for irrigation (per provider's order)
- Nonsterile gloves
- Waterproof waste bag

PROCEDURE STEPS:

1. Check the provider's order. Select the correct solution and appropriate solution strength. It should be at least body temperature. (Solutions kept in warming closet.)
2. Identify the patient and explain the procedure.
3. Wash hands.
4. Place the waterproof pad under the body part that will be irrigated.
5. Position the patient in such a way that directs the flow of the solution into the wound. The basin catches the flow from the wound.
6. Don nonsterile gloves, remove the dressing, and dispose into waterproof waxed bag.
7. Note the wound's appearance, color, amount of discharge, and odor to the discharge. RATIONALE: Allows ongoing assessment of the wound.
8. Remove and discard gloves into biohazard container.
9. Wash hands.
10. Maintaining sterile technique, open the sterile irrigation tray and the dressings. Use the inner kit wrapping as a sterile field.
11. Pour the irrigation solution into the sterile solution bowl or container. (Should be at least room temperature.) RATIONALE: Room temperature solution is more comfortable for the patient.
12. Don sterile gloves.
13. Place the sterile basin against the edge of the wound. RATIONALE: The basin will collect the irrigation solution.
14. Fill the irrigating syringe (or bulb syringe) with the solution and carefully wash out the wound with the flow of solution (Figure 19-47A and B).
15. Continue to fill the syringe and continue to wash out the wound until the solution becomes clear and there is no drainage noted.

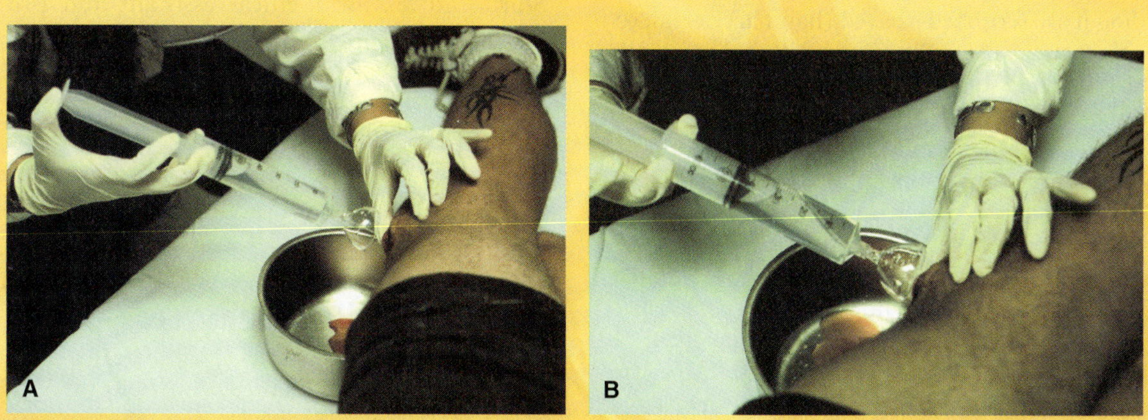

Figure 19-47 (A) Flush the wound gently. (B) Hold the syringe close to the wound, but do not touch the wound with the syringe.

continues

Procedure 19-10 (continued)

16. Dry the wound edge with sterile gauze.
17. Reassess the wound.
18. Apply a dry sterile dressing.
19. Remove gloves. Dispose in biohazard container.
20. Wash hands.
21. Document in patient's chart or electronic medical record.

DOCUMENTATION

8/6/20XX 2:30 PM Dressing removed from abdominal wound. Wound red and filled with serosanguinous exudate. Irrigated with 500 mL sterile normal saline (fluid returns were clear). Wound slightly red and clean-appearing after irrigation. Wound dried with sterile 4 3 4s. Dry sterile dressing applied. Patient states, "I feel much better now that my wound has been cleaned out. That only hurt a little." Patient says she does not want anything for pain. W. Slawson, CMA (AAMA) ——————————

Procedure 19-11

Preparation of Patient's Skin before Surgery

STANDARD PRECAUTIONS:

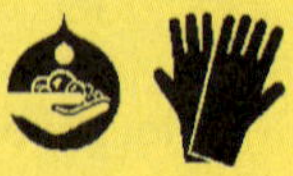

NOTE: The skin and hair contain many microorganisms, and the patient's skin must be prepared before surgery to remove as many of the microorganisms as possible. Wound infection results when microorganisms enter the body. The patient may be told to scrub the site of the surgery using antimicrobial soap on the night before surgery. Because it is impossible to sterilize the skin, the operative site and an area surrounding it are scrubbed, shaved (hair harbors microorganisms), washed, and painted with an antiseptic such as Betadine® solution. A skin prep self-contained unit is a sponge applicator with a cylinder of antiseptic solution inside. One brand is known as DuraPrep. It contains iodophor and isoprophyl alcohol. The medical assistant can use the unit with nonsterile gloves. The unit is compressed, the seal to the inner cylinder is broken, and the sponge end becomes the applicator. The mixture is thick and should be allowed to dry and not be blotted. Because it contains alcohol, which can be a fire hazard, the site must be dry before draping. The chemical action decontaminates the patient's skin.

PURPOSE:

To remove as many microorganisms as possible from patient's skin immediately before surgery.

EQUIPMENT/SUPPLIES:

Absorbent pads
Drape
Disposable prep kit (includes antiseptic solution, several sponges, razor, and a container for water, or self-contained skin prep unit)
Sterile water
Sterile bowl
Sterile gloves for medical assistant and provider (two pair)
If kit is unavailable, equipment needed is:
Sterile bowls (two)
Antiseptic solution
Sterile gauze sponges
Sterile razor
Basin for soiled sponges
Sterile transfer forceps

PROCEDURE STEPS:

1. Wash hands.
2. Assemble equipment.

continues

Procedure 19-11 (continued)

3. Identify patient.
4. Explain procedure, provide privacy, and drape patient if appropriate. Before the patient is prepped and draped for the procedure, ask the patient to state the location of the surgical site. Some facilities require that the appropriate site be marked with an indelible ink pen to be certain the correct site is identified.
5. Provide good light source.
6. Position patient for comfort and exposure of site.
7. Wash hands.
8. Protect area under preparation site with absorbent pads.
9. Open kit.
10. Put on sterile gloves or use sterile transfer forceps.
11. Apply antiseptic soap (Betadine®) with 4 × 4 sponges, beginning at operative site and moving outward in a circular motion from the center to away from center of prepared area. RATIONALE: Work from cleaner to least clean areas to prevent contamination.
12. Discard used sponges as necessary.
13. Using razor and holding skin taut, shave hair away from operative site, following hair growth pattern. RATIONALE: Prevents accidental nicks. Nicked skin can cause infection.
14. When hair has been removed, scrub again in a circular fashion as in Step 11 for about two to five minutes.
15. Rinse shaved area with sterile water and dry with a sterile 4 × 4 gauze sponge.
16. Remove and appropriately discard absorbent pad, 4 × 4 sponges, disposable prep kit, and gloves. RATIONALE: This removes used supplies and equipment from prepped skin area and prevents contamination.
17. Wash hands.
18. Using sterile transfer forceps, remove a sterile towel to place under operative site. RATIONALE: Placing a sterile towel under the operative area keeps site free from contamination.
19. Cover with a sterile towel. Instruct patient not to touch the area.
20. Pour antiseptic solution (Betadine®) into the sterile bowl. The provider puts on sterile gloves or uses sterile transfer forceps and, with a sterile 4 × 4 gauze sponge, paints the operative site with the antiseptic solution. Let dry. The provider covers the patient with fenestrated drape and begins the surgical procedure.

Procedure 19-12

Suturing of Laceration or Incision Repair

STANDARD PRECAUTIONS:

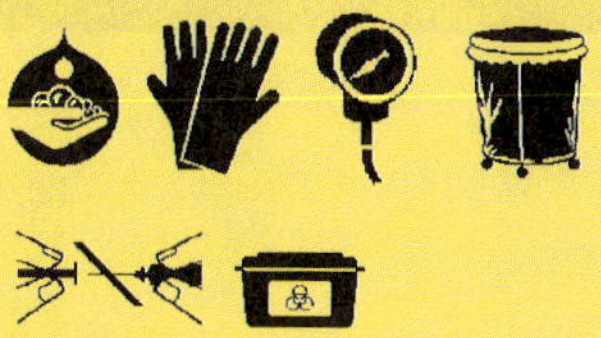

PURPOSE:

Suturing is recommended if a laceration or incision is gaping; is bleeding uncontrollably; is located on the face, neck, or a bend of a body part; or extends deep into underlying tissue. Suturing facilitates healing by approximating the edges of the wound. Suturing decreases scarring, helps decrease the likelihood of infection, and promotes healing. The wound and the surrounding area must be meticulously cleaned of any dirt and debris. Many providers have standard orders for wound cleaning before suture repair of either a laceration or incision-type wound such as a 10-minute soak in Hibiclens® solution and sterile water.

continues

Procedure 19-12 (continued)

EQUIPMENT/SUPPLIES:

Surgical tray:

- Syringe and needle for anesthetic
- Hemostats (curved)
- Adson tissue forceps
- Iris scissors (curved)
- Suture material and needle
- Needle holder
- Gauze sponges

Side table (unsterile field):

- Anesthetic as ordered by the provider
- Dressings, bandages, and tape
- Splint/brace/sling (optional)
- Sterile gloves in package

PROCEDURE STEPS:

1. Wash hands.
2. Identify the patient and explain the procedure. Check for signed consent forms.
3. Reassure and comfort the patient as needed.
4. Assess cause of wound and its severity.
   - Determine any known allergies and last tetanus booster.
   - Identify any health concerns to avoid possible complications.
   - Soak wound in an antiseptic solution as ordered by provider.
   - Clean and dry wound.
   - Position patient comfortably, lying down.
5. Assist the provider as needed.
6. Support the patient as needed.

Give postoperative care:

7. Apply sterile gloves.
8. Clean area around the wound and dry wound with sterile 4 × 4s or sterile towels.
9. Dress/bandage/splint wound following provider's preference.
10. Remove gloves.
11. Wash hands.
12. Check patient's vital signs.
13. Explain wound care to the patient (and caregiver) and provide written instructions including symptoms of infection and after-hours phone number.
14. Assist the patient with any concerns or questions.
15. Arrange for follow-up appointment and medication as ordered.
16. Don personal protective equipment.
17. Dispose of supplies per OSHA guidelines. Clean room, sanitize instruments, and sterilize for reuse.
18. Wash hands.
19. Document procedure in patient's chart or electronic medical record.

DOCUMENTATION

11/17/20XX 10:15 AM Patient sustained a 2 3 1.5-cm laceration on right elbow. Wound soaked in Hibeclens® solution and water for 10 minutes, and then dried. Dr. King sutured the laceration after injecting xylocaine (1%) into area around laceration site. Ten nonabsorbable Ethicon sutures used to close wound. Dry sterile dressing applied to wound. Given a prescription by Dr. King for Perodan, 1 tab PO q 4-6h prn for pain, and Amoxicillin 500 mg PO q 6 h. Postoperative instructions reviewed and she appears to understand. Last tetanus 12 years ago. Tetanus injection given I.M. right deltoid (0.5 cc). W. Slawson, CMA (AAMA)

Procedure 19-13

Sebaceous Cyst Excision

STANDARD PRECAUTIONS:

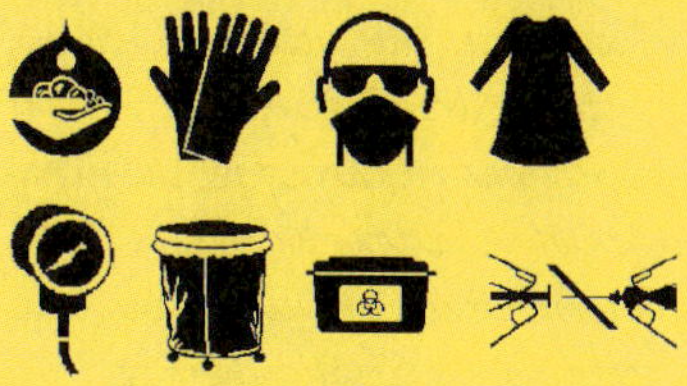

NOTE: A sebaceous cyst is a benign retention cyst, sometimes called a "wen." Sebaceous cysts are caused by an oil duct becoming "plugged," which causes the sebum (oil) to accumulate in the gland. Eventually the oil gland becomes distended. Sebaceous cysts that become inflamed or infected need to be removed. The patient may also elect to have a noninflamed sebaceous cyst removed if it is unsightly or located in a bothersome area. Incision and drainage of sebaceous cysts is usually not the treatment of choice because they tend to recur if the entire cyst is not completely excised. Ideally, the entire cyst sac is removed intact, but occasionally the sac ruptures during removal and large amounts of malodorous biohazardous sebum can be expelled. In preparation for this occurrence, extra gauze sponges, gloves, and goggles should be available.

PURPOSE:

To remove an inflamed or infected sebaceous cyst. To remove a sebaceous cyst that is not inflamed or infected but is located on an area of the body where the cyst is unsightly or where it may become irritated from rubbing.

EQUIPMENT/SUPPLIES:

Sterile field:

- Syringe/needle for anesthesia
- Iris scissors (curved)
- Mosquito hemostat (curved)
- Scalpel blade and handle
- Needle holder
- Suture material with needle
- Tissue forceps (two)
- Mayo scissors (curved)

Side area (unsterile field):

- Skin prep supplies
- Gauze sponges (many) (sterile, unopened)
- Fenestrated drape (a drape with an opening) in package
- Antiseptic solution as ordered
- Gloves (sterile and nonsterile)
- Personal protective equipment (PPE)
- Anesthesia as directed
- Dressing, bandages, tape
- Biohazard waste container
- Safety razor (optional)
- Alcohol pledgets
- Sterile culture tube (if needed)
- Biohazard specimen transport bag

PROCEDURE STEPS:

1. Wash hands.
2. Identify the patient and explain the procedure.
3. Reassure and comfort the patient as needed.
4. Determine any known allergies and last tetanus booster.
5. Check for signed consent form.
6. Identify any health concerns to avoid possible complications.
7. Position the patient comfortably, lying down.
8. Perform the skin preparation as directed (see Procedure 19-11).
9. Wear appropriate PPE including goggles if cyst is infected. RATIONALE: Purulent material may drain out of the wound and splash.
10. Assist provider to inject the anesthesia by holding the vial while the provider withdraws the appropriate amount of anesthesia. Continue to assist while the provider excises the cyst and sutures the surgical incision.
11. Support patient during surgery.

Give postoperative care:

12. Apply sterile gloves.
13. Clean area around the wound.
14. Dress and bandage as directed.
15. Dispose of items per OSHA guidelines. Remove gloves.
16. Wash hands.
17. Check the patient's vital signs.

continues

Procedure 19-13 (continued)

18. Explain wound care to the patient (and caregiver) and provide written instructions including symptoms of infection.
19. Assist the patient with any concerns or questions.
20. Arrange for follow-up appointment and medication as ordered.
21. Document procedure in patient's chart or electronic medical record, noting that the culture specimen was sent to laboratory if appropriate.

DOCUMENTATION

5/12/20XX 2:00 PM Sebaceous cyst (0.5 3 0.5 cm) excised by Dr. King. Moderate amount of purulent exudate noted as cyst ruptured during removal. Specimen of exudate obtained and sent to the laboratory for culture and sensitivity. Five nonabsorbable sutures used to close the incision. Wound cleansed with Betadine®; dry sterile dressing applied. Patient given verbal and written instructions on caring for the dressing and for watching for signs of infection. BP 118/74, P 88. Skin color good. Will call office for results of culture and sensitivity and to discuss the need for antibiotic therapy. Will return on 5/22/20XX or sooner if necessary. W. Slawson, CMA (AAMA) ———

Procedure 19-14

Incision and Drainage of Localized Infection

STANDARD PRECAUTIONS:

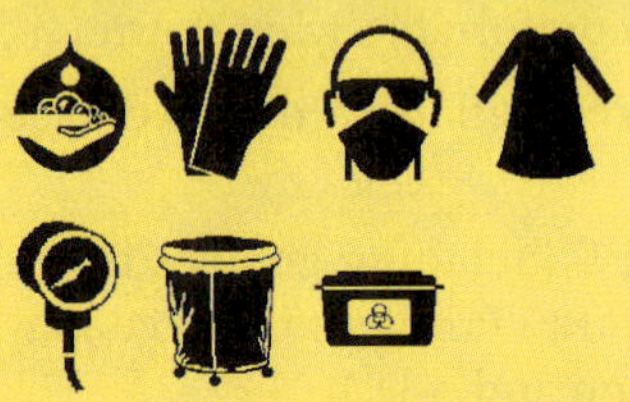

NOTE: An abscess is a localized accumulation of pus surrounded by inflamed tissue. The body attempts to isolate pus into a pocket or abscess as a means of protecting itself by walling off the pathogens and preventing them from spreading throughout the body. Incision and drainage is the procedure of cutting into an area (often an abscess) for the purposes of draining the fluid/material. A culture of the exudate can be done to identify microorganisms. Rather than suturing or otherwise closing the wound, the provider may place a gauze wick or a latex Penrose drain into the wound to facilitate continued drainage. The most commonly used type of wick is Iodoform. Iodoform is available in 5-yard lengths and widths of ¼, ½, 1, and 2 inches. Iodoform is packaged sterile in glass bottles under the Johnson & Johnson brand name of Nu Gauze (see Figure 19-32). Care must be taken when removing the desired length from the bottle to avoid contaminating the remaining gauze. To accomplish this, the medical assistant might hold the bottle and remove the lid to allow the provider to reach into the bottle with a sterile thumb dressing forceps and pull out the desired length. Sterile scissors are then used to cut the strip without contaminating the remaining wick. The Iodoform is packed into the wound with a short length exposed. After several hours or days of continued draining, the wick may be removed, and the wound allowed to heal without sutures. The patient may be prescribed an appropriate antibiotic.

The medical assistant should exercise caution by wearing appropriate PPE including goggles when assisting with this procedure because the exudate can be heavy and contains pathogenic microorganisms.

PURPOSE:

To incise and drain an abscess or other localized infection.

continues

Procedure 19-14 (continued)

EQUIPMENT/SUPPLIES:

Surgical tray:

Syringe/needle for anesthesia
Scalpel blades and handles
Thumb forceps
Mosquito hemostat (optional)
Gauze sponges (many) (sterile, unopened)
Fenestrated drape
Tissue forceps (two)
Mayo scissors
Iris scissors
Antiseptic solution such as Betadine® in sterile cup

Side area (unsterile field):

Skin prep supplies
Gloves (sterile and nonsterile)
Personal protective equipment (PPE)
Anesthesia as directed
Dressing, bandages, and tape
Specimen container with preservative and requisition (if culture is taken)
Biohazard specimen transport bag
Biohazard waste container
Extra sterile gauze sponges
Iodoform gauze wick or latex Penrose drain
Antiseptic solution
Sterile culture tube

PROCEDURE STEPS:

1. Wash hands.
2. Identify the patient and explain the procedure.
3. Reassure and comfort the patient as needed.
4. Determine any known allergies and last tetanus booster.
5. Check for signed consent form.
6. Identify any health concerns to avoid possible complications.
7. Position the patient comfortably, lying down.
8. Put on PPE, including goggles.
9. Perform the skin preparation as directed (see Procedure 19-11).
10. Assist the provider as needed to inject the anesthesia by holding the vial while the appropriate amount is aspirated for injection. The provider incises the abscess and inserts either Iodoform gauze or a latex Penrose drain into the wound to encourage drainage. No sutures are used. Specimen taken for culture and sensitivity.
11. Support the patient as needed.

Give postoperative care:

12. Apply sterile gloves.
13. Clean area around the wound with sterile 4 × 4s or sterile towels.
14. Dress and bandage as directed. Several thicknesses of dressing material will be needed to absorb exudate, or the accumulated fluid in the cavity.
15. Dispose of items per OSHA guidelines. Remove gloves.
16. Wash hands.
17. Check the patient's vital signs.
18. Explain wound care to the patient (and caregiver) and provide written instructions such as to apply warm moist compresses to wound. Explain to watch for symptoms of infection. Stress caution when handling contaminated items.
19. Assist the patient with any concerns or questions.
20. Arrange for follow-up appointment and medication as ordered.
21. Document procedure in patient's chart or electronic medical record.

DOCUMENTATION

6/20/20XX 10:00 am Incision and drainage of an abscess (2 × 1 cm) on the left buttock. Large amount purulent exudate noted. Wound packed with 1 inch iodoform gauze and DSD applied with large amount of 4 × 4s and abdominal dressings. Culture tube with specimen of exudate sent to laboratory with a requisition for C&S. BP 138/92, P 100. Postoperative wound care explained to patient and given written instructions as well. BP 142/72, P 88. J. Guerro, CMA (AAMA) ———

Procedure 19-15

Aspiration of Joint Fluid

STANDARD PRECAUTIONS:

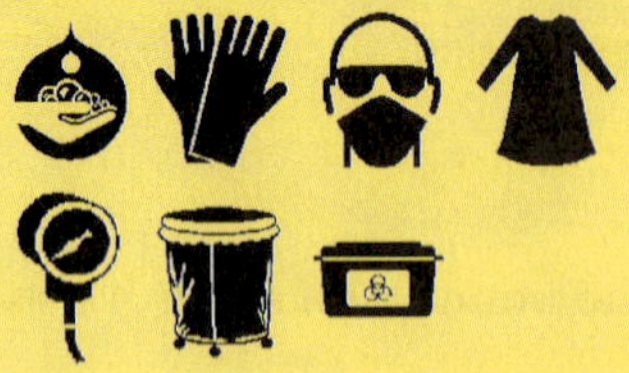

NOTE: The most common reason for aspirating fluid is to remove excess fluid from a joint, often the knee. A long, sterile, sturdy needle is inserted into the joint capsule and fluid is removed. Often a long-acting anesthetic and cortisone are injected at the same time. The fluid can be diagnostically examined for blood, pus, and fatty substances and also cultured for pathogens. After surgery the patient may be placed on antiinflammatory medications to treat the inflammation and antibiotics if the culture is positive for pathogens.

PURPOSE:

To remove excess synovial fluid from a joint after injury.

EQUIPMENT/SUPPLIES:

Surgical tray:

- Syringe/needle for anesthesia
- Gauze sponges
- Sterile basin for aspirated fluid
- Fenestrated drape (optional)
- Syringe/needle for drainage
- Sturdy hemostat or needle driver

Side area (unsterile field):

- Skin prep supplies
- Gloves (sterile and nonsterile)
- Personal protective equipment (PPE)
- Anesthesia as directed
- Cortisone medication as directed
- Culture tube
- Pathology requisition
- Specimen container
- Biohazard waste container
- Extra gauze sponges (sterile, unopened)
- Dressing, bandages, and tape
- Biohazard specimen transport bag

PROCEDURE STEPS:

1. Wash hands.
2. Identify the patient and explain the procedure.
3. Reassure and comfort the patient as needed.
4. Determine any known allergies, last tetanus booster, and which joint will be aspirated.
5. Check for signed consent form.
6. Identify any health concerns to avoid possible complications.
7. Position the patient comfortably, lying down.
8. Put on PPE if needed.
9. Perform the skin preparation as directed (see Procedure 19-11).
10. Assist the provider by holding the vial as anesthesia is aspirated. The provider injects anesthesia, inserts a long, sturdy needle into the synovial sac, and aspirates fluid with a large syringe. The aspirated fluid is put into a sterile bowl as the syringe fills with fluid. A hemostat is used to remove the syringe from the needle, leaving the needle in the joint. The syringe is reapplied to the needle, and the process continues until excess fluid is removed.
11. Support the patient as needed.

Give postoperative care:

12. Apply sterile gloves.
13. Clean area around the wound with sterile 4 × 4s or sterile towels.
14. Dress and bandage as directed.
15. Dispose of items per OSHA guidelines. Remove gloves.
16. Wash hands.
17. Check the patient's vital signs.
18. Explain wound care to the patient (and caregiver) and provide written instructions including symptoms of infection.
19. Assist the patient with any concerns or questions.
20. Arrange for follow-up appointment and medication as ordered.
21. Apply gloves and eye/mouth protection if sending specimen to laboratory. Place aspirated fluid into a sterile container and cover tightly.

continues

Procedure 19-15 (continued)

22. Send labeled specimen container and requisition to the pathology laboratory after placing specimen in biohazard transport bag.
23. Document the procedure in patient's chart or electronic medical record.

DOCUMENTATION

10/12/20XX 11:30 AM Left knee aspirated. 250 mL clear fluid withdrawn after injection of anesthetic. Sent to pathology department. Patient says she "feels better." Dressing applied to aspiration site. Postoperative verbal and written directions given. BP 118/64, P 72. Follow-up appointment made for discussion about results of analysis of fluid sent to laboratory. B. Abbott, RMA ———————————

Procedure 19-16

Hemorrhoid Thrombectomy

STANDARD PRECAUTIONS:

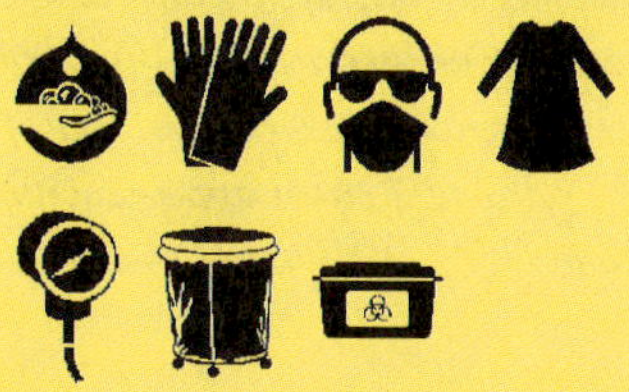

NOTE: Hemorrhoids are dilated or varicose veins in the rectum, either internal or external. Sometimes a blood clot can form in a protruding portion of the hemorrhoid and the vessel can become inflamed. The hemorrhoid is incised with a scalpel blade and the clot removed with a hemostat forceps. Suturing is not usually necessary. Soaking the area in a **sitz bath** can aid in healing. Hemorrhoidectomy can be performed in much the same manner as a hemorrhoid thrombectomy, and the supplies and equipment are similar. The anal sphincter is dilated, the hemorrhoid pedicle is tied, and then each hemorrhoid is removed with either laser, electrosurgery, or cryosurgery. Another alternative is to ligate the internal hemorrhoids after visualizing the area with an anoscope. Two rubber bands are placed around the pedicle of each hemorrhoid. They will slough off after a week to 10 days because of the loss of blood supply to them (**avascularized** hemorrhoid).

PURPOSE:

To incise inflamed hemorrhoids and remove thrombus. To remove hemorrhoids with laser, electrosurgery, cryosurgery, or banding.

EQUIPMENT/SUPPLIES:

Surgical tray:

- Syringe/needle for anesthesia
- Mosquito hemostat (curved)
- Sterile basin
- Gauze sponges
- Rubber bands
- Fenestrated drape

Side area (unsterile field):

- Skin prep supplies
- Gloves (sterile and nonsterile)
- Personal protective equipment (PPE)
- Anesthesia as directed
- Biohazard waste container
- Extra gauze sponges
- Soft absorbent pad, similar to sanitary napkin
- T-bandage (to hold pad in place)

PROCEDURE STEPS:

1. Wash hands.
2. Identify the patient and explain the procedure.
3. Reassure and comfort the patient as needed.

continues

Procedure 19-16 (continued)

4. Determine any known allergies and last tetanus booster.
5. Check for signed consent form.
6. Identify any health concerns to avoid possible complications.
7. Position the patient comfortably, according to provider's preference; usually on a proctologic table.
8. Assist with adequate draping for patient comfort.
9. Apply PPE if necessary.
10. Perform the skin preparation as directed (see Procedure 19-11).
11. Assist the provider to aspirate the appropriate amount of local anesthesia. After administering the anesthesia, the provider either bands or excises the hemorrhoids with a scalpel. Suturing is usually not necessary.
12. Support the patient as needed.

Give postoperative care:

13. Assist the provider in placing the soft absorbent pad against the wound. It may be held in place with a T-shaped bandage.
14. Dispose of used items per OSHA guidelines. Remove gloves and wash hands.
15. Assist the patient as needed.
16. Check the patient's vital signs.
17. Explain wound care to the patient (and caregiver) per provider. Sitting in a tub of warm water is soothing and aids healing. Provide written instructions including signs of complications such as excessive bleeding or pain.
18. Assist the patient with any concerns or questions.
19. Arrange for follow-up appointment and medication as ordered.
20. Document procedure in patient's chart or electronic medical record.

DOCUMENTATION

3/17/20XX 1:00 PM

A. Thrombus removed from hemorrhoid. Perineal pad applied and secured with a T-binder. Patient seemed to tolerate the procedure well. BP 110/70, P 88. Postoperative instructions, verbal and written, given to patient. Prescription for Percodan, 1 tab PO q 4-6 h prn given to patient. Return appointment made for 4/4/20XX. W. Slawson, CMA (AAMA) ——————

B. Internal hemorrhoids removed with electrosurgical equipment. Very little bleeding noted. Perineal pad and T-binder applied. Patient seemed to tolerate the procedure well. BP 110/68, P 72. Postoperative instructions given to patient (verbal and written). Prescription for Percodan 1 tab. PO q 4-6 h prn given to patient. Return appointment made for 4/4/20XX. W. Slawson, CMA (AAMA) ——————

Procedure 19-17

Suture/Staple Removal

STANDARD PRECAUTIONS:

NOTE: Many minor surgical procedures require that suturing be done to approximate the skin edges to promote healing. Because these sutures or staples are nonabsorbable, they must be removed when the wound has healed. The patient returns to the office or clinic to have the sutures or staples removed. The medical assistant removes the dressing and checks the wound. The provider also checks the wound for degree of healing and determines that the sutures/staples can be removed.

continues

Procedure 19-17 (continued)

PURPOSE:

To remove sutures from a healed surgical wound (as per provider).

EQUIPMENT/SUPPLIES:

(See Figure 19-48)
Gauze sponges
Bandage scissors
Biohazard waste container
Tape
Forceps
Suture removal kit (suture scissors or staple remover, thumb forceps, and 4 × 4s)
Sterile latex gloves
Antibiotic cream if ordered

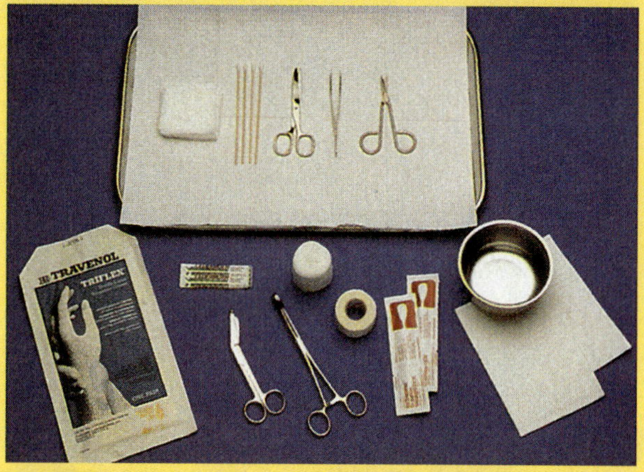

Figure 19-48 Equipment and supplies for suture removal.

PROCEDURE STEPS:

1. Identify patient.
2. Wash hands.
3. Glove and remove bandage. Dispose in biohazard container.
4. Wash hands.
5. Open suture or staple removal kit.
6. Apply sterile gloves.
7. If removing sutures: Using thumb forceps, gently pick up one knot of a suture. Gently pull upward toward suture line. RATIONALE: Less pressure is exerted on suture line.

   Using suture removal scissors, cut one side of the suture as close to skin as possible (Figure 19-49). RATIONALE: Holding knot with forceps and cutting suture as close to skin as possible, the suture will be pulled out from under the skin, avoiding contamination of the wound.
8. If removing staples: Gently apply instrument to staple. Gently squeeze handle of staple remover until staple is pinched outward and upward. Pull up.
9. Remove all sutures/staples in the same manner, noting number of sutures/staples removed. Dispose of the sutures/staples on a sterile gauze sponge.

   Examine the wound to be certain all sutures have been removed.
10. Apply antibiotic cream to area as ordered.

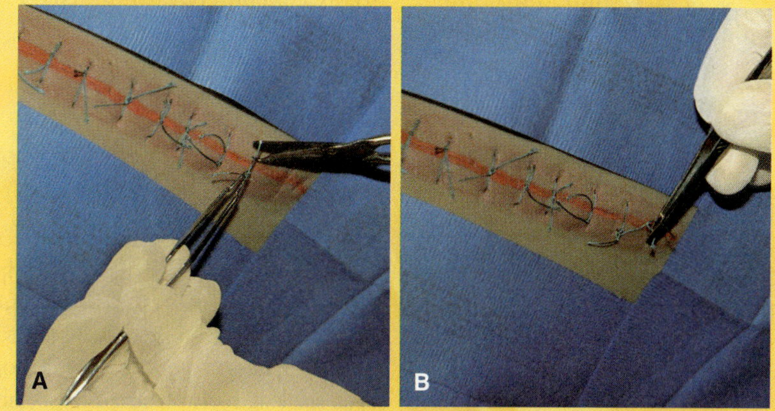

Figure 19-49 To remove sutures: (A) Grasp suture knot with thumb forceps. Place curved tip of suture removal scissors right next to the skin under the suture. Clip. (B) Gently pull the suture knot up and toward the incision with thumb forceps to remove.

continues

Procedure 19-17 (continued)

11. Apply dry sterile dressing if ordered by the provider (see Procedure 19-9).
12. Dispose of used items per OSHA guidelines.
13. Remove gloves.
14. Wash hands.
15. Check patient's vital signs if indicated.
16. Explain wound care and provide written instructions to patient.
17. Arrange follow-up appointment if necessary.
18. Document procedure in patient's chart or electronic medical record.

DOCUMENTATION

11/27/20XX 2:30 PM Ten sutures removed from right forearm. Wound appears clean, well healed. No discharge seen. Edges of wound well approximated. B. Abbott, RMA ———

OR

11/27/20XX 2:30 PM Six staples removed from right forearm. Wound appears clean, well healed. No discharge seen. Edges of wound well approximated. B. Abbott, RMA ———

Procedure 19-18

Application of Sterile Adhesive Skin Closure Strips

STANDARD PRECAUTIONS:

NOTE: On occasion, a superficial wound does not require sutures. However, the edges of the wound can be drawn together and sterile strips of adhesive used to hold the edges of the wound together to facilitate healing.

PURPOSE:

To approximate the edges of a wound after the removal of sutures. Sometimes used in lieu of sutures or to give additional support along with sutures.

EQUIPMENT/SUPPLIES:

Sterile field:

Suture removal instruments (as indicated)
Sterile adhesive skin closure strips
Iris scissors (straight)
Adson dressing forceps
Tincture of benzoin (optional)
Sterile cup
Sterile cotton-tipped applicators (for tincture of benzoin)

Side area (unsterile field):

Sterile gloves
Dressings, bandages, and tape
Waterproof bag

PROCEDURE STEPS:

1. Identify the patient and explain the procedure.
2. Position patient comfortably.
3. Wash hands and apply gloves.
4. Remove bandages and dressings (see Procedure 19-9).
5. Dispose in waterproof bag.
6. Remove gloves.
7. Wash hands.
8. Clean and dry wound (see Procedure 19-9).
9. Assess the need for skin closure strips and alert provider as indicated.
10. Wash hands.
11. Open container of tincture of benzoin.
12. Pour into sterile cup.
13. Apply tincture of benzoin to edges of wound if directed. Use sterile cotton-tipped applicator, taking care not to let it come into contact with the actual wound. RATIONALE: Tincture of benzoin is applied to the periphery of the wound to prepare it for application of the skin closure strips and to provide a better sticking surface and aid in easier removal with less skin irritation.
14. Open package of skin strips. Cut to size if needed. Remove strips from packaging one at a time using dressing forceps.

continues

Procedure 19-18 (continued)

15. Apply one end of a skin closure strip to one side of the wound. Place the first strip over the center of the wound (Figure 19-50A).
16. Secure the end to the skin by carefully pressing.
17. Stretch the strip across the edge of the wound and secure on the other side in the same manner. This motion should bring the edges together without puckering the skin.
18. Apply the next two closure strips at halfway points between the first strip and each end of the wound (Figure 19-50B).
19. Continue in this manner until the edges are approximated. Keep wound edges in alignment.

Give postoperative care:

20. Dress and bandage if necessary.
21. Dispose of used items per OSHA guidelines.
22. Remove gloves and wash hands.
23. Check the patient's vital signs, if indicated.
24. Explain wound care to the patient (and caregiver) and provide written instructions including symptoms of infection.
25. Assist the patient with any concerns or questions.
26. Arrange for follow-up appointment and medication as ordered.
27. Document procedure in patient's chart or electronic medical record.

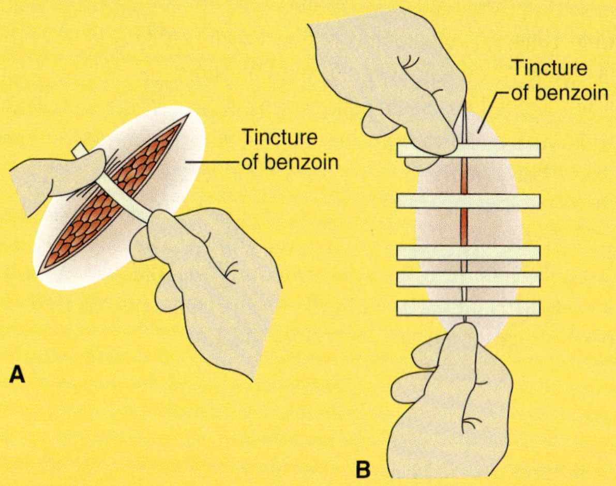

Figure 19-50 To apply skin closure strips: (A) Apply first strip in center of incision. (B) Apply closures to each side of center.

DOCUMENTATION

3/17/20XX 4:00 PM Nine skin closure strips applied to wound on shoulder after tincture of benzoin applied to skin around sutures. Suture line approximated well; no puckering of skin noted. Wound appears clean and to be healing. No redness or swelling. Patient says there is "very little discomfort." B. McQuestion, RMA

Case Study 19-1

Refer to the scenario at the beginning of the chapter. Distinguish between the types of surgery that would be performed in a high-volume patient practice and the surgery that would be performed in a smaller practice.

CASE STUDY REVIEW

1. List several types of surgery performed for the high-volume practice and the lower-volume practice.
2. Are there some surgeries common to both? If so, what are they?

Case Study 19-2

Cele Little, an 84-year-old patient at Inner City Health Care, is having office surgery performed on Thursday morning. Her sister, Dottie Tate, also a patient and also in her 80s, will come with Cele. A friend from the local senior citizen center has offered to drive them to the center and home again. Dottie is more nervous about the procedure, the removal of a bothersome cyst, than Cele. After talking with the sisters about the procedure, clinical assistant Wanda Slawson, CMA (AAMA), MLT, realizes this and wants to reassure Dottie but also wants her to be prepared to be caregiver to Cele.

CASE STUDY REVIEW

1. Where should Wanda begin in her communication with the two sisters?
2. What specific advice should Wanda give Cele and Dottie before the procedure?
3. What instructions should Wanda give the sisters to follow after the procedure?

Case Study 19-3

Letisha Brown has been scheduled to have a nevus excised from her upper back.

CASE STUDY REVIEW

1. Explain how you would prepare her for the surgery.
2. Explain how you would care for her after the surgery.
3. What will become of the excised nevus? Explain your actions.

SUMMARY

In assisting with surgery in the ambulatory care setting, the medical assistant needs to know sterile principles and understand the difference between medical and surgical asepsis. Knowledge of suture materials, instruments, and other supplies such as dressings and bandages is also critical. In preparing for surgical procedures, the medical assistant's communication skills will be needed, because patients can be apprehensive and will require both reassurance and education. In addition to understanding the basic process and preparations for assisting with minor surgery, the medical assistant should be aware of the steps involved in some of the more common surgical procedures.

STUDY FOR SUCCESS

To reinforce your knowledge and skills of information presented in this chapter:

- Review the Key Terms
- Practice the Procedures
- Consider the Case Studies and discuss your conclusions
- Answer the Review Questions
  - Multiple Choice
  - Critical Thinking
- Navigate the Internet by completing the Web Activities
- Practice the StudyWARE activities on your student CD
- Apply your knowledge in the Student Workbook activities
- Complete the Web Tutor sections
- View and discuss the DVD situations

REVIEW QUESTIONS

Multiple Choice

1. Which of the following describes the primary purpose of surgical asepsis?
   a. to prevent microorganisms from collecting on the Mayo stand
   b. to prevent microorganisms from causing inflammation
   c. to prevent microorganisms from entering the body during an invasive procedure
   d. to prevent microorganisms from multiplying
2. A basic rule to follow to protect sterile items is:
   a. a sterile object can touch a nonsterile object under certain circumstances
   b. it is safe to turn your back on the sterile field if you leave plenty of room between you and the field
   c. provide the provider a separate container for contaminated instruments
   d. gloved hands are held at the same height as the hip bone
3. Which of the following is the smallest size suture material?
   a. 0
   b. 2–0
   c. 4–0
   d. 1
4. Which of the following is an example of absorbable suture material?
   a. vicryl
   b. nylon
   c. silk
   d. cotton
5. What is the purpose of adding epinephrine to the local anesthetic?
   a. to prevent an allergic reaction
   b. to reduce blood flow in the operative site through vasoconstriction
   c. to reduce patient discomfort during the procedure
   d. to maintain patient vital signs
6. Which of the following actions might the physician take if a sebaceous cyst were infected?
   a. remove the cyst
   b. do a biopsy of the cyst
   c. perform cryosurgery on the cyst
   d. incise and drain the cyst

Critical Thinking

1. What would be the rationale behind leaving a wound open rather than suturing it? On what basis would the provider make the decision?
2. While you are preparing a patient for surgery, he confides in you that he doesn't have anyone to drive him home, but he only lives three miles away and plans to drive himself. How do you respond?
3. You have thoroughly explained the postoperative instructions to the patient and caregiver. Are written instructions also necessary? Why or why not?
4. While pouring a sterile solution into a bowl on the sterile field, you accidentally splash a very tiny amount of the solution onto the field. What is your next step? Explain your actions.
5. During an incision and drainage of a localized infection you notice a large amount of exudate from the site. What precautions should you take.

WEB ACTIVITIES

Search the Internet to explore the most current ambulatory surgical procedures for varicose veins, cataracts, and cholelithiasis.

1. Using a search engine of your choice, go to a Web site about ambulatory care.
   a. Look for the criteria that the patient must meet to be discharged after surgery.
   b. What are some common complications that can occur in the ambulatory center after any surgical procedure?
   c. Name two other surgeries other than those listed in your book that can be performed in an ambulatory center. Discuss them.
   d. List three to four advantages and disadvantages of ambulatory surgery.

REFERENCES/BIBLIOGRAPHY

Association of Surgical Technologists, Inc. (2008). *Surgical technology for the surgical technologists.* Clifton Park, NY: Delmar Cengage Learning.

Diversified health occupations. (6th ed.). (2004). Clifton Park, NY: Delmar Cengage Learning.

Phillips, N. (2004). *Barry and Kohn's operating room technique* (10th ed.). St. Louis, MO: Mosby.

Taber's cyclopedic medical dictionary (20th ed.). (2005). Philadelphia: F. A. Davis.

THE DVD HOOK-UP

This chapter discussed the proper technique for assisting with minor surgical procedures.

Today's DVD program illustrated how to assist with a sebaceous cyst removal. Eileen called the patient the day before the procedure to make certain that the patient was going to be there the day of the surgery. Eileen gave the patient some important information that he needed to know before having the surgery. The day of the surgery, Eileen escorted the patient back to the provider's office so that the provider could explain the procedure. Once the provider was finished explaining the procedure, Eileen took over and gave the patient his prescriptions and home-care instructions. Eileen had many duties during the procedure and had additional duties immediately after the procedure.

1. Why is it so important to contact the patient the day before the surgery?
2. What type of phone instructions did Eileen give the patient before the surgery date?
3. What type of instructions did Eileen give the patient the day of the surgery, before having the procedure? Why did Eileen give the patient instructions before the procedure?

DVD Journal Summary

Write a paragraph that summarizes what you learned from watching today's DVD program. What did you think about the testimony of the other medical assistant named Eileen regarding her first experience assisting the provider with a surgery? Would you have quit after the provider raised his voice and scolded you in front of the patient? What do you need to do now, while you are still in school, to ascertain that you do not break sterility when you get into the industry?

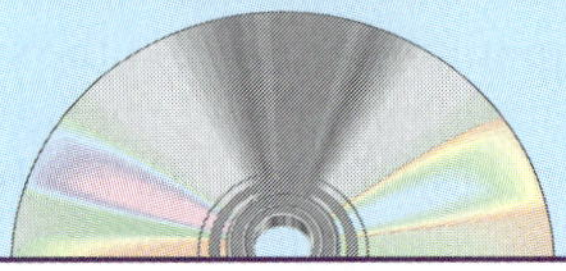

DVD Series	**Program Number**
Skills Based Series	14

Chapter/Scene Reference

- *Entire program*

Chapter 20

Diagnostic Imaging

KEY TERMS

Cathode
Claustrophobia
Doppler
Dosimeter
Echocardiogram
Esophageal Varices
Fluoroscope
Implantable Cardioverter-Defibrillator (ICD)
Ionizing Radiation
Isotope
Oscilloscope
Palliative
Radioactive
Radiograph
Radiolucent
Radionuclides
Radiopaque
Radiopharmaceuticals
Stomatitis
Transducer

OUTLINE

- Radiation Safety
- X-Ray Machine
- Contrast Media
- Patient Preparation
- Positioning the Patient
- Fluoroscopy
- Bone Densitometry
- Diagnostic Imaging
  - Positron Emission Tomography (PET)
  - Computerized Tomography (CT)
  - Magnetic Resonance Imaging (MRI)
  - X-Rays (Flat Plates)
  - Ultrasonography
  - Mammography
  - Filing Films and Reports
- Radiation Therapy
- Nuclear Medicine

OBJECTIVES

The student should strive to meet the following performance objectives and demonstrate an understanding of the facts and principles presented in this chapter through written and oral communication.

1. Define key terms as presented in the glossary.
2. Describe safety precautions for personnel and patients as they relate to ionizing radiation treatments.
3. Explain how fluoroscopy is used and explain its benefits.
4. Describe the various positions used during X-ray procedures.
5. Describe four X-ray procedures that require patient preparation.
6. Discuss the uses of ultrasonography, positron emission tomography, computerized tomography, magnetic resonance, and flat plates.
7. Discuss how radiographs are stored.
8. Explain the differences among radiology, radiation therapy, and nuclear medicine.
9. Recall four possible side effects of radiation.

Scenario

In the radiology department of Inner City Hospital, several patients are waiting to have their procedures performed. Wanda Slawson, CMA (AAMA), brings Don Waite to the department for an excretory urogram known as an intravenous pyelogram. She is careful to make certain that Mr. Waite has been properly prepared for the procedure. She does not want the procedure to have to be repeated because of the inconvenience and anxiety it may cause Mr. Waite, nor does she want there to be additional expense and time spent repeating the procedure.

INTRODUCTION

Radiology is a branch of medicine concerned with ***radioactive*** *substances, including* ***radiographs,*** *radioactive* ***isotopes,*** *and* ***ionizating radiation.*** *There are three specialties into which radiology can be classified: diagnostic radiology, radiation therapy, and nuclear medicine. All the specialties are extremely valuable tools that can be used to diagnose and treat diseases.*

X-rays were named when a German physicist, Wilhelm Roentgen, discovered them in 1895. He received the first Nobel Prize in physics for his discovery. Roentgen noticed while working with a ***cathode*** *ray tube that the rays of energy emitted could pass through skin, paper, wood, and other solid materials. Because he didn't know what the rays were, he called them X-rays.*

Radiologic procedures are not often performed in an office setting; rather, they are performed in the radiology department of a hospital, clinic, or a freestanding facility outside of the hospital or clinic.

Some radiographs, such as those looking for a fractured bone, require no preparation, whereas others, such as an excretory urography (intravenous pyelogram [IVP]) or a computerized axial tomography (CAT) scan, require special preparation.

Spotlight on Certification

RMA Content Outline

- Anatomy and physiology
- Patient education

CMA (AAMA) Content Outline

- Anatomy and physiology
- Medicolegal guidelines and legal requirements
- Scheduling and monitoring appointments
- Performing selected tests

CMAS Content Outline

- Anatomy and physiology
- Legal and ethical considerations
- Examination and preparation
- Appointment management and scheduling

RADIATION SAFETY

X-rays, though invisible to the human eye, are extremely powerful, and they can be beneficial or they can be dangerous and harmful. Exposure to radiation can destroy tissue and permanently damage the eyes, bone marrow, and skin. They are harmful to the developing embryo and fetus, causing severe anomalies and death.

The benefit of X-rays is the ability to use the information obtained from them to diagnose and manage a patient's disease. The diagnostic benefits outweigh the risks that may result from X-ray exposure. Radiographers are educated to be certain that patients receive as low a dose of radiation as possible but still obtain a useful radiograph, and that they and patients are protected from exposure to radiation that is not necessary. Radiation is rarely used during pregnancy because of the danger it poses to the fetus and embryo. The first trimester is the most critical because severe congenital anomalies can be the result of the fetus's or embryo's exposure to radiation. Women are routinely asked if there is a possibility of their being pregnant. X-rays of fertile women should be taken only when necessary and with a minimal exposure to the fetus or embryo. If a radiologic examination is necessary, a radiologic physicist calculates the dosage of radiation to estimate how little radiation to which the fetus or embryo should be exposed. The past guideline stated that X-rays of fertile women should not be taken until 10 days after the onset on their last menstrual period. The thinking was that women were unlikely to be pregnant during these 10 days. This guideline is now considered to be outdated because the ovum for the next

Critical Thinking

What are the effects of radiation on a fetus or an embryo?

Critical Thinking

What do some state laws require of personnel who take X-rays?

menstrual cycle is its most susceptible during this 10-day period.

In some states, medical assistants and other health care professionals who are not licensed to take radiographs are not allowed by law to take or assist with radiologic procedures. Licensure in those states (about 35 states) is mandated because of the possibility of severe injury to an unlicensed individual and to patients. In some states, a limited license is required. The medical assistant must undergo additional training and is limited to "skeletal films" (arms, legs, and so forth). Education and training in radiologic techniques is of utmost importance for the safety of the patient and health care worker. Medical assistants must have a basic understanding of radiology and radiology safety to instruct patients in the correct preparation for procedures and to keep patients and themselves safe. They must protect themselves from radiation exposure by not participating in procedures for which they have not been adequately educated and trained.

On March 30, 2007, a bill called the CARE bill (Consistency, Accuracy, Responsibility and Excellence in Medical Imaging and Radiation Therapy) was introduced before the U.S. Senate. If passed, it would require all persons who perform medical imaging (including X-rays) and radiation therapy (excluding ultrasound) procedures to meet specific federal education and credentialing standards in order to participate in Medicare and Medicaid. Presently, the law in some states requires only voluntary basic training standards. This situation allows individuals without formal education to perform imaging procedures.

The AAMA supports the legislation that would require specific educational and certification standards for individuals performing medical imaging.

Personnel in the X-ray department and others who are exposed to X-rays must wear a **dosimeter,** a small badge-like device worn above the waist. The dosimeter contains a strip of film that measures the amount of X-ray to which a person is exposed. The dosimeter film is read on a regular basis, and radiation exposure is reported to a supervisor. Exposure can come from the X-ray beam itself or from scattered rays that are produced when going through the patient's body.

Patients must wear lead aprons over the reproductive organs, and technicians must shield themselves with lead aprons and gloves when they are assisting. However, shields are not necessary when technicians are standing behind the lead wall and working the control panel. In addition, walls in rooms where X-rays are taken are lead-lined to absorb scattering rays.

X-RAY MACHINE

There are three main parts to an X-ray machine: the table, the X-ray tube, and the control panel. The tube is where the X-rays are produced and then come out as a beam of X-ray. Lead surrounds the tube except for the area where the beams of X-ray are sent out. The table on which the patient lies is movable in several directions, even upright or angled. The control panel is positioned behind a lead wall specially designed for shielding the radiographer from X-rays when an X-ray is being taken (Figure 20-1).

Photographic film is placed beneath or behind the patient's body and a radiograph, X-ray film, is produced by sending X-rays from the

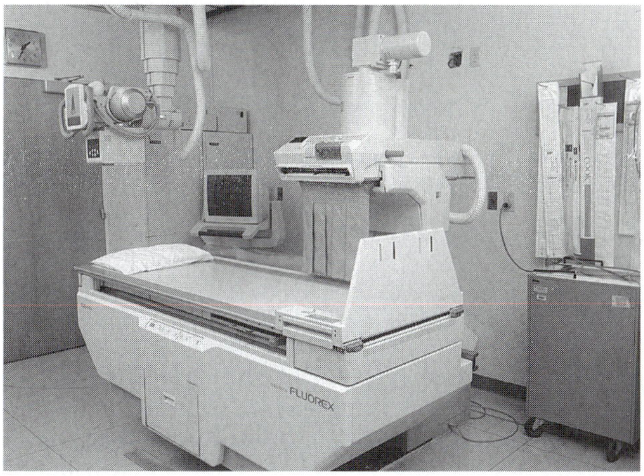

Figure 20-1 Radiography room prepared for procedure.

tube of the machine through the body and onto the film. After the film is processed, an image is created (see Figure 20-4A and B). Bone is denser than skin and other soft tissues, and therefore can absorb more X-rays. The image of the hand bones on the X-ray film is white due to absorption of the X-rays.

EHR Radiologic procedures can be done without using X-ray film (Figure 20-2). The technique, known as computed radiography (CR), uses similar equipment. Computers and laser technology are used to obtain and process digital images. CR images can be recorded on an imaging plate that is put through a computer scanner, which reads and digitalizes the images.

The technique provides clear images that assist the provider in making a diagnosis. The CR images can be sent to providers on the computer network for consultation or referral. Images are accessible in 3 minutes.

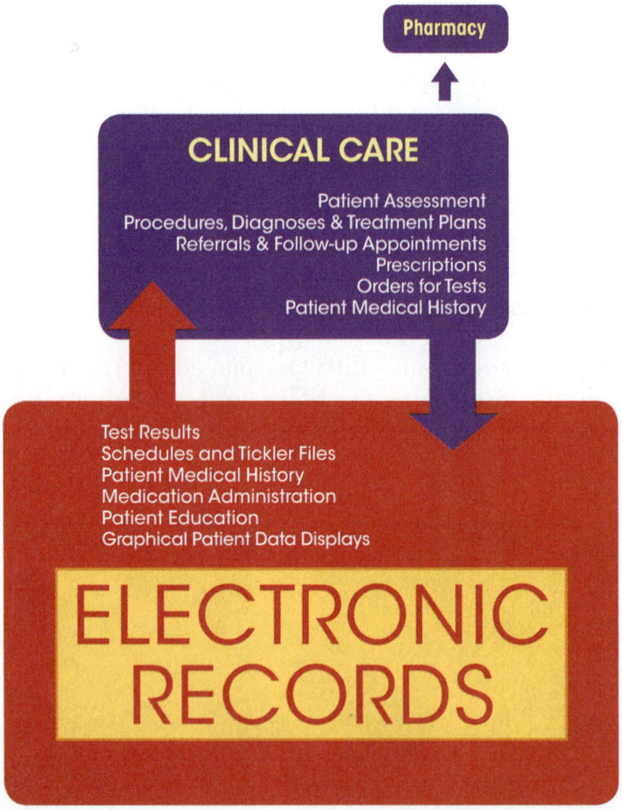

Figure 20-2 The clinical care arm of total practice management system data flow. Data about diagnostic imaging procedures are stored electronically. Examination reports and images are immediately available to providers on demand. Images can be sent to providers on the same network for consultation or referral.

The process produces excellent images without film. It makes film storage unnecessary, thereby reducing costs. Transmission of patient data is quicker.

CR equipment is costly, and technologists who use the equipment require training on its operation.

CONTRAST MEDIA

Various body structures are of different densities. Bone is denser than skin and, therefore, can absorb more X-rays, leaving fewer to be picked up by the X-ray film. Thus, an X-ray film of bone will appear white. A lung is less dense, and the X-rays can penetrate lung tissue. The lung appears black on the radiograph. If X-rays do not penetrate a structure easily, it is termed **radiopaque;** if they penetrate readily, it is termed **radiolucent.** Contrast media are radiopaque and help to obtain a radiographic image of an internal organ or structure that ordinarily would be difficult to see because the contrast media cause the organs or structures of the body to absorb more radiation (Figure 20-3A–C).

Some commonly used contrast media are barium sulfate, iodine compounds, air, and carbon dioxide. Barium is a chalky compound and, when mixed with water, can be swallowed by the patient or administered as an enema by a radiologic technician. It is not absorbed by the body. It is used for upper and lower gastrointestinal (GI) series of X-rays (Figure 20-4A and B). The patient is told to drink extra fluids to flush out barium after the procedure. Iodine salts are radiopaque and are used for kidney, gall bladder, and thyroid examinations. Some individuals are allergic to the iodine salts used as contrast media. Patients are asked whether they have any allergies, particularly allergies to foods that contain iodine, such as fish.

Air and carbon dioxide are used to visualize the spinal cord and joints but have been replaced by use of the magnetic resonance imaging (MRI) machine.

PATIENT PREPARATION

By law, without special education and training about X-rays, the medical assistant's role in X-ray procedures in most states is limited to giving patient preparation information and explanations about what the patient

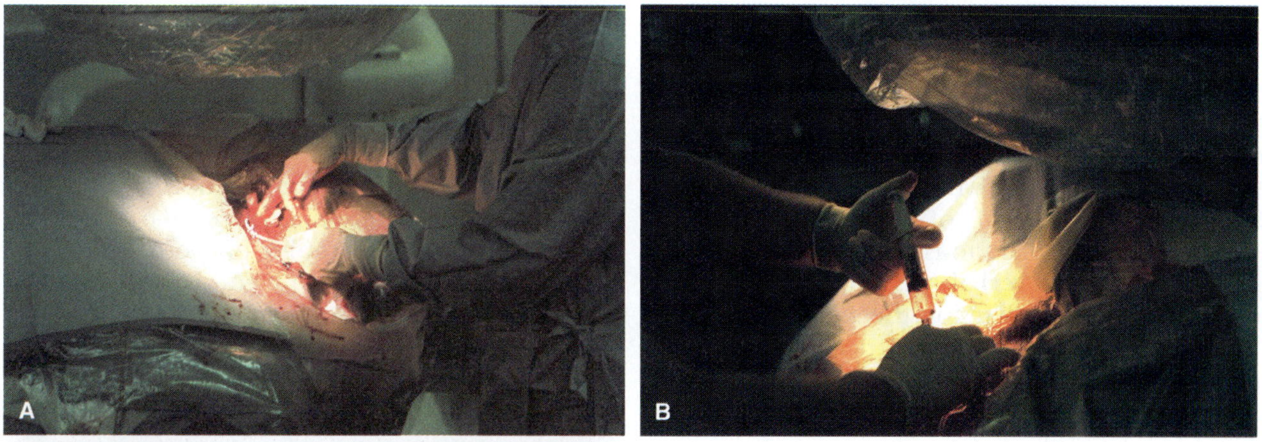

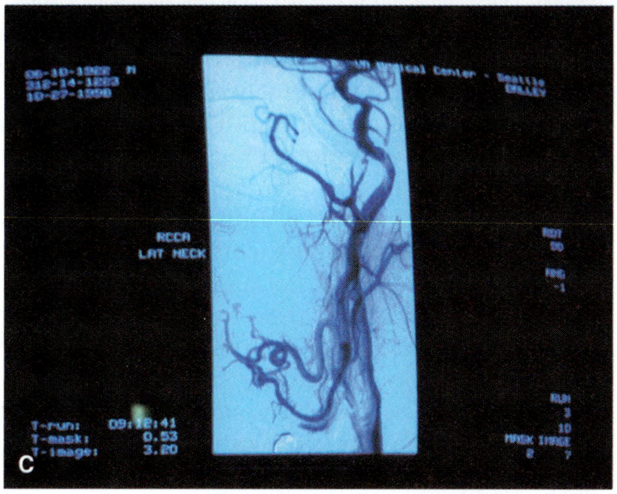

Figure 20-3 Angiography. (A) An intra-arterial catheter is inserted. (B) Radiopaque contrast material is injected. (C) The arteries are visualized.

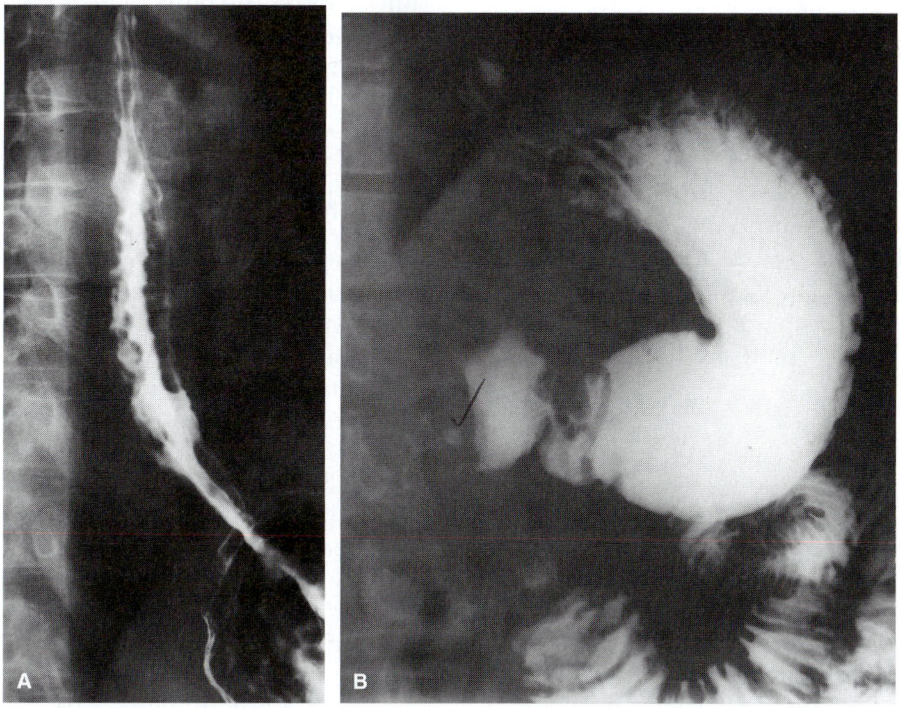

Figure 20-4 (A) Barium swallow showing esophageal varices. (B) Barium swallow showing duodenal ulcer.

can anticipate. A thorough knowledge of the procedure ordered by the provider is essential, and the medical assistant must be certain that patients understand the preparation they are about to undergo. Verbal explanations should be followed up with written instructions. Many patients, fearful of what the ordered X-ray will show, are anxious and frightened and can easily forget verbal instructions. Proper preparation is essential for the best results on the radiographs. Repeating a procedure because of inadequate preparation results in increased patient anxiety, time, expense, and inconvenience (Table 20-1).

POSITIONING THE PATIENT

The correct patient position is important for obtaining the best quality radiograph, and the type of examination that is necessary determines patient position. Some basic views are:

- *Anteroposterior view (AP):* the anterior surface of the body faces the X-ray tube and X-rays are directed from the front toward the back of the body.
- *Posteroanterior view (PA):* the posterior surface of the body faces the X-ray tube and X-rays are directed from back to front (Figure 20-5A and B).
- *Lateral view:* X-rays pass through the body from one side to the opposite side.
- *Right lateral view (RL):* X-rays are directed through the body from the left to the right side. The right side of the body is next to the film.
- *Left lateral view (LL):* X-rays are directed through the body from the right to the left side. The left side of the body is next to the film.
- *Oblique view:* the body is positioned at an angle.
- *Supine view:* the body is lying face up, on the back.
- *Prone view:* the body is lying face down, on the abdomen.

FLUOROSCOPY

Fluoroscopy is the process of using a **fluoroscope** to view internal organs and structures of the body so that they can be seen in motion immediately by the radiologist. The patient is usually given a contrast medium and placed between the X-ray tube and the fluoroscope. Fluoroscopy is used for procedures such as cardiac catheterization and for viewing the function of the stomach and intestinal structures to detect any abnormalities. A television screen and camera are available so that the radiographer can watch and take photos of the body system(s) in operation (Figure 20-6). Most fluoroscopes have radiographic properties and can be used for both fluoroscopy and X-rays. X-rays can be taken and recorded during fluoroscopy.

BONE DENSITOMETRY

An enhanced form of X-ray technology (low dose) is used during bone densitometry. X-rays check areas of the body (hip, hand, spine, foot) for signs of mineral loss and bone thinning. The test determines the density of bone and is used to diagnose osteoporosis, often found in women after menopause. It can occur in men as well. Bone densitometry can assess an individual's risk for fractures. It is a painless procedure.

The patient is told to refrain from taking calcium supplements for 24 hours prior to the examination, to wear loose clothing without metal zippers or buttons or a belt, and to remove jewelry and any metal objects. These items can interfere with the X-ray images.

Most machines have software that computes and displays the bone density on a computer monitor. The test takes from 10 to 30 minutes. The lower the density, the greater the risk for fractures.

DIAGNOSTIC IMAGING

Positron Emission Tomography (PET)

PET is a radiographic procedure that uses a computer and a radioactive substance. The radioactive substance is injected into the patient's body and gives off charged particles. They combine with particles in the patient's body to produce color images that reveal the amount of metabolic activity in an organ or structure.

PET is primarily a diagnostic medical imaging modality. It makes use of specialized, intravenously injected **radiopharmaceuticals** that emit positrons, which can be detected out of the body due to high-energy releases. Specialized detectors arranged around the patient sense the energy and map the location from which it originated inside the body. These radiopharmaceuticals can be chemically designed to localize in the heart, brain, or certain

Table 20-1 Examples of Diagnostic Procedures, their Purpose, Patient Preparation, and the Procedure

Test	Purpose	Patient Preparation	Procedure
Angiography	To visualize the inside of blood vessel walls. Helps to diagnose heart attacks, stroke, aneurysm (Figure 20-3).	NPO 6 to 8 hours before examination.	1. Contrast medium (iodine) injected into an artery or vein. 2. Catheter threaded to the appropriate site. 3. Digital angiography can be done and stored on computer disk.
Barium swallow (upper gastrointestinal [GI] series)	To study the esophagus, stomach, duodenum, and small intestine for disease (ulcers, tumors, hiatal hernia, **esophageal varices**) (see Figure 20-4).	Day prior: Light evening meal. NPO after midnight. Day of test: NPO. Postprocedural: Increase fluid intake. Take laxative as prescribed.	1. The patient is asked to drink a flavored barium mixture while standing in front of the fluoroscope. 2. The radiologist observes the passage down the digestive tract. 3. The patient is turned to various positions to allow good visualization of the intestines. 4. Radiographs are taken.
Barium enema (lower GI series)	To study the colon for disease (polyps, tumors, lesions).	Prep kit (usually supplied by provider's office), which includes bottle of magnesium citrate and Dulcolax tablet(s). Day prior: 1. Clear liquid allowed: carbonated beverages, clear gelatin, clear broth, coffee and tea with sugar. No milk or milk products. 2. 8 oz. of water every hour until bedtime. 3. Late afternoon, drink bottle of magnesium citrate. 4. Early evening, take Dulcolax tablet(s) as prescribed. 5. Light evening meal. NPO except water after dinner. Morning of procedure: NPO, cleansing enema Postprocedural: 1. Increase fluid intake and dietary fiber. 2. Report to provider if no bowel movement within 24 hours of test.	1. The colon is filled with a barium sulfate mixture. 2. The patient is turned in various positions to allow the barium to fill the colon. Air is injected to move the barium along the colon. 3. When the colon is full, radiographs are taken.
Cholangiography	To view the bile ducts for possible calculi or lesions.	May have cleansing enema 1 hour before examination. Meal preceding examination is withheld.	Contrast medium injected and radiograph of bile ducts is taken.
Cholecystography	To study the gall bladder for disease (stones, duct obstruction), inflammation.	1. Evening before test, fat-free dinner. 2. Patient takes dye tablets with 8 oz. of water. 3. Cathartic or cleansing enemas may be prescribed. 4. NPO after dinner and tablets.	1. A series of radiographs is taken. 2. A fatty meal may be given to stimulate the gall bladder to empty. 3. Other radiographs can then be taken to check gall bladder function.

(continues)

Table 20-1 Examples of Diagnostic Procedures, their Purpose, Patient Preparation, and the Procedure (continued)

Test	Purpose	Patient Preparation	Procedure
Cystography	To view the urinary bladder for lesions, calculi.	Day prior: Light evening meal. Laxative in evening. NPO after midnight.	Contrast medium injected and radiograph of the urinary bladder is taken.
Hysterosalpingography	To view the uterus and fallopian tubes for blockage and lesions. To check for pelvic masses.	Laxative evening before. Cleansing enema day of exam. Meal prior to examination is withheld.	Contrast medium injected and radiographs taken of uterus and fallopian tubes. Carbon dioxide may also be used.
Excretory urography (intravenous pyelogram) [IVP])	Visualization of kidneys, ureters, and bladder to detect kidney stones, lesions, strictures of urinary tract.	Eat a light evening meal and nothing after midnight. A laxative and enema are used to clean out the intestines to prevent a blocked view of the ureters behind the intestines.	A contrast medium of iodine salts is given intravenously after it has been determined that the patient is not allergic to iodine (see Chapter 18).
Mammography	To detect abnormalities in the breast, especially breast cancer.	Do not wear lotion, deodorant, or powders. Remove clothing from waist up. No contrast medium required.	Breast is positioned on the mammograph and compressed to flatten it. Two radiographs are taken of each breast, from the side and from above.
Retrograde pyelography	To view the kidneys and urinary tract for abnormalities.	Drink four to five glasses of water before examination unless sedated, then NPO.	Contrast medium injected and radiographs taken of the kidneys and urinary bladder.

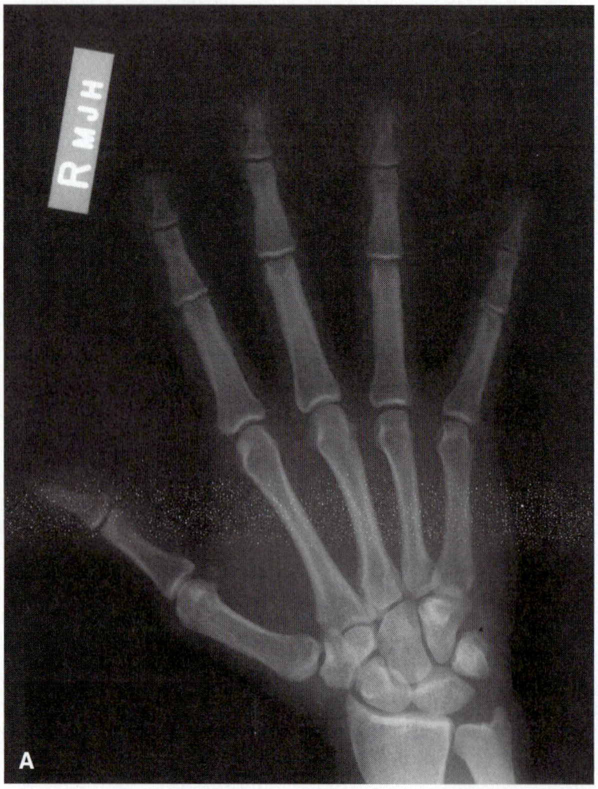

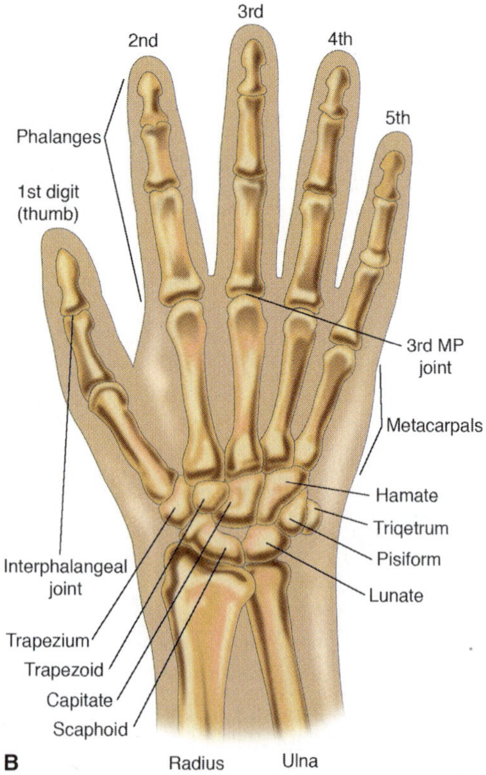

Figure 20-5 (A) Posteroanterior (PA) view of a hand. Note the dark spaces between the bones. This is because the bones (denser) pick up X-rays (absorb them) and appear white. The soft tissue (less dense) does not absorb X-rays and appears dark. (B) PA hand.

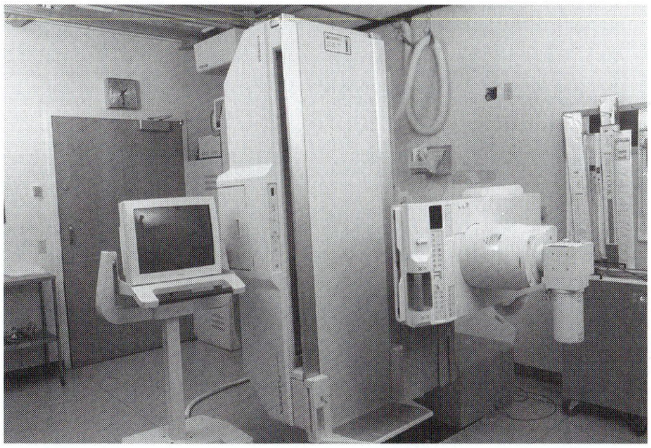

Figure 20-6 Fluoroscopy room ready for upper gastrointestinal study.

types of tumors (breast) throughout the body. A clinical image is formed by the accumulation of positron emissions in a target organ. The patient's emission pattern forms a clinical image. This image is compared with the normal distribution by the nuclear medicine provider.

Generally, low to moderate doses are used to diagnose disease in patients. The PET scan can detect cancer and the effects of chemotherapy. Certain nuclear medicine treatment studies use specialized radiopharmaceuticals that isolate in the area to be treated. These agents emit their energy locally, irradiate tissue, and usually do not leave the body, unlike diagnostic radiopharmaceuticals. The properties and intent of diagnostic radiopharmaceuticals are different from therapeutic radiopharmaceuticals (Figure 20-7A–C).

Computerized Tomography (CT)

CT uses a small amount of radiation. The beams penetrate body tissues to produce a series of cross-sectional images of the body part being examined. It allows images of structures that cannot be seen with regular X-rays. It is a noninvasive test that usually requires no preparation.

EHR The CT machine has software and hardware for storing and managing information. The images can be examined on a

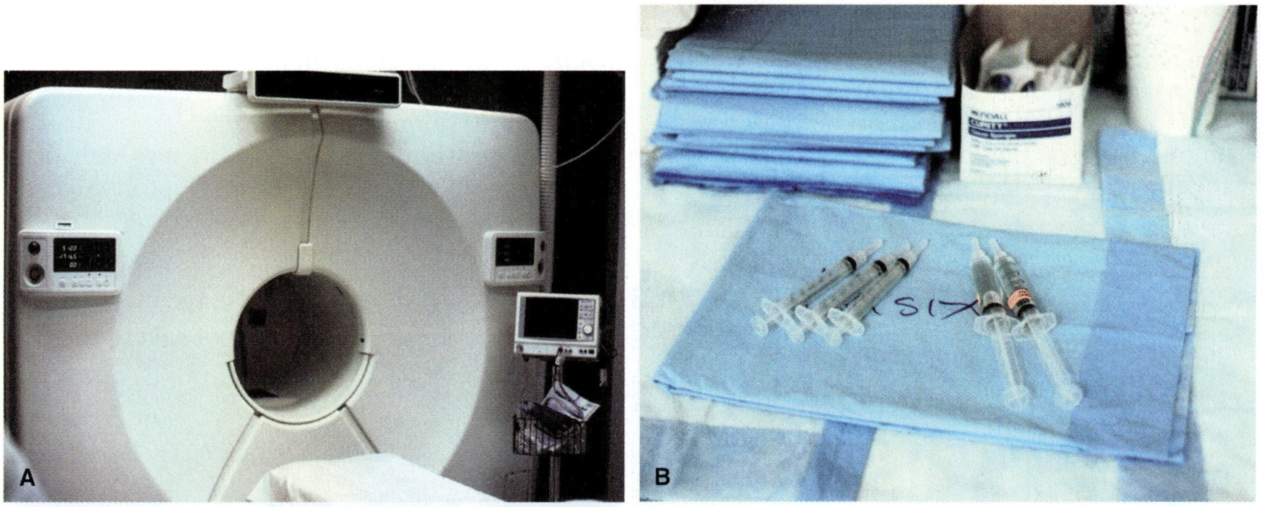

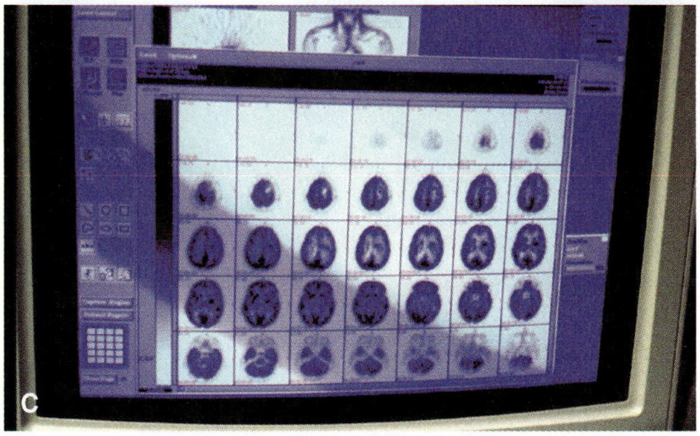

Figure 20-7 (A) Position emission tomography (PET) scanner. (B) Medications ready for injection. (C) PET scan output images.

computer monitor, and hard copies of the images can be made. It rotates 360 degrees around the patient to obtain cross-sectional images that are processed by a computer and can be viewed on a monitor and on film. It can also be used to guide biopsies, plan surgery, and identify internal organ injury due to trauma. It is ideal for early detection of tissue tumors such as childhood cancers and abdominal tumors, and it helps in directing radiation therapy for tumor masses. The cardiac CT is more useful for diagnosing coronary artery disease than cardiac stress testing. On occasion, a contrast medium is injected for a better view of internal structures. If contrast medium is used, the patient must be NPO (have nothing by mouth) for 4 hours before being placed onto a motorized table that moves the body part to be examined into a scanner that surrounds that part of the patient. An entire body can be scanned in 15 to 20 minutes (Figures 20-8A and B). Newer multislice CT scanners produce thinner slices in a shorter time with greater detail.

Magnetic Resonance Imaging (MRI)

EHR

Images produced by MRI are of exceptionally high quality. No ionizing radiation is used, and it is a noninvasive, safe, and painless procedure that can produce computer-processed images. All body areas can be viewed by MRI, but it is especially helpful for soft tissues. It is good for the spine, pelvis, and joints and is superior for visualizing the brain. It shows more detail than CT. The examiner can see through fluid-filled tissue with exceptional detail using an MRI machine. The computer forms the visual image.

A noninvasive test, magnetic resonance angiography (MRA), evaluates arteries and veins throughout the body and is very useful for showing neck and brain blood flow. The computer converts the data into digital images of slices. No catheterization is needed, but a contrast medium may be given intravenously. The procedure helps diagnose blood vessel and heart disorders as well as strokes. Another imaging technique, functional MRI, measures split-second nerve cell activity of the brain.

Another application of the technology is breast imaging using an MRI that is linked to the computer. Hundreds of detailed pictures of the breast are taken from several angles. The patient lies on the table on her abdomen, and the breasts drop into a hollow in the table. Breast MRI is not used for routine breast cancer screening. It is primarily used to evaluate breast implants for leaks and to assess abnormalities seen on a conventional mammogram. Breast MRI does not take the place of conventional mammography and ultrasonography and is not routinely used to diagnose breast cancer.

For MRI, the patient lies on a table. The machine has an electromagnet. Three types of MRI machines are available: closed MRI, open-air MRI, and open MRI (Figure 20-9).

The conventional closed MRI has high magnetic strength. According to Lexington Medical

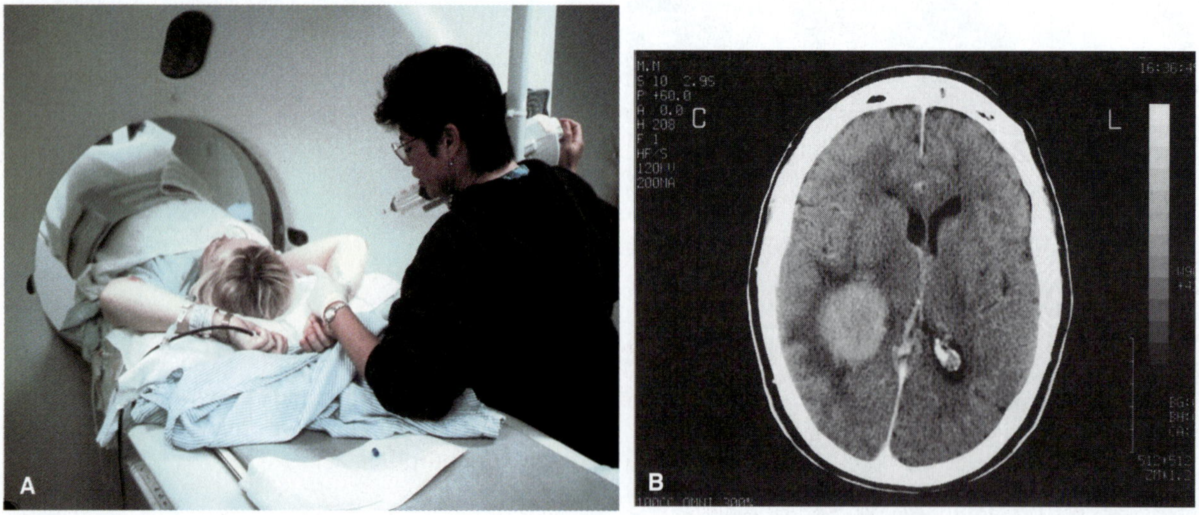

Figure 20-8 (A) Computed tomography (CT) scanning. Instruct patient to lie still. (B) This axial CT scan demonstrates a meningioma surrounded by edema.

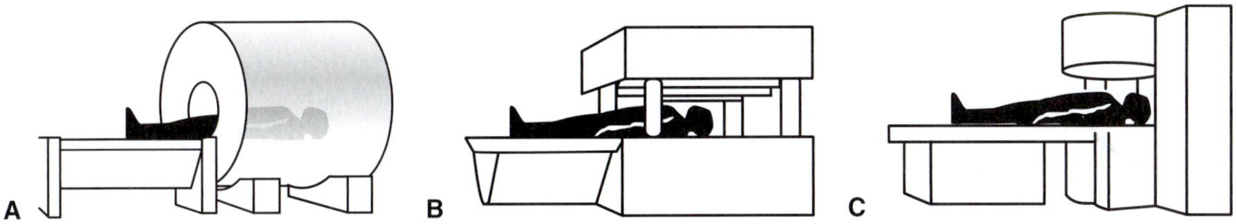

Figure 20-9 Three types of MRI machines: (A) closed MRI, (B) open-air MRI, and (C) open MRI.

Center, nine of ten MRI machines used in hospitals and clinics are the closed MRI. It produces high-quality images.

The open-air type MRI has open sides and ends. Most open machines have low-strength magnets and are not as powerful as the closed MRI. Images are of lesser quality.

The open type MRI is an advanced MRI machine that is completely open on all sides. It eliminates patient **claustrophobia** and can accommodate obese patients. It has a powerful magnet that is much stronger than the magnet used in open-air type MRIs. Greater image detail results in information providers need to make a diagnosis (Figure 20-10).

A drawback to MRI and CT is that they cannot be used in patients with a pacemaker; an **implantable cardioverter-defibrillator (ICD)**; or metal clips, pins, or other permanent hardware left in place on an internal organ or structure as part of a surgical procedure. The metal may become damaged during testing. Controlled studies investigating whether patients with implantable devices such as a pacemaker and/or an ICD can undergo CT and/or MRI are inconclusive. The FDA has not approved either procedure for these patients. Some researchers found that newer CTs and MRIs did not cause difficulties for patients with implantable-devices compared with earlier models, which did cause minor difficulties in some patients. An MRI is not as useful as conventional radiographs or a CT scan for diagnosing fractured bones.

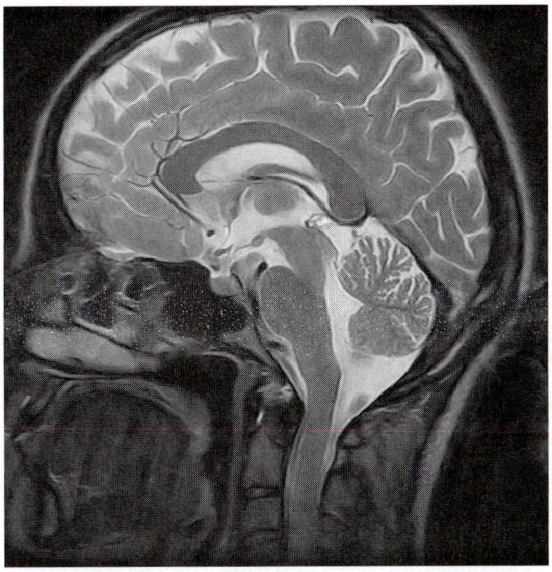

Figure 20-10 A sagittal MRI of the head. (Courtesy of GE Healthcare.)

Patients are asked to remove all objects that have metal (watches, belts, hairpins, rings, other metal jewelry) and credit cards because of the strong magnet in the MRI machine. Loose, comfortable clothing without zippers or snaps should be worn. The procedure takes about 45 minutes to an hour, during which time the patient must remain still. The technician, although not in the room with the patient, has a camera and microphone with which to communicate with the patient. An intermittent tapping sound can be heard throughout the procedure, and earphones are available if the patient wants them.

X-Rays (Flat Plates)

Flat plates are also known as "plain" films because they require no special technique or use of contrast medium. This type of X-ray is used on various parts of the body and is helpful in diagnosing problems in the skull, abdomen, chest, sinuses, and bone.

Ultrasonography

Ultrasonography, CT, and MRI allow for greater imaging detail than conventional radiographs. Ultrasonography, or ultrasound, has been available longer than the other technologies. High-frequency sound waves (inaudible to the human ear) are used to image internal soft tissues. It can be used to help diagnose problems in the abdominal organs, liver, gall bladder, uterus, ovaries, and spleen (Figure 20-11). It cannot be used for skeletal structures or the lungs.

Doppler ultrasonography is a noninvasive technique used to evaluate blood flow through the major arteries and veins of the neck, arms, and legs. It can reveal blockages such as plaque or thrombi (blood clots). An **echocardiogram,** an ultrasound of the heart, can view the heart and determine its size, shape, and position and the motion made by the valves opening and closing (Figure 20-12). Ultrasound has advantages over other methods of viewing internal organs and structures in that it uses no X-rays and allows for continuous viewing while organs and structures are in motion.

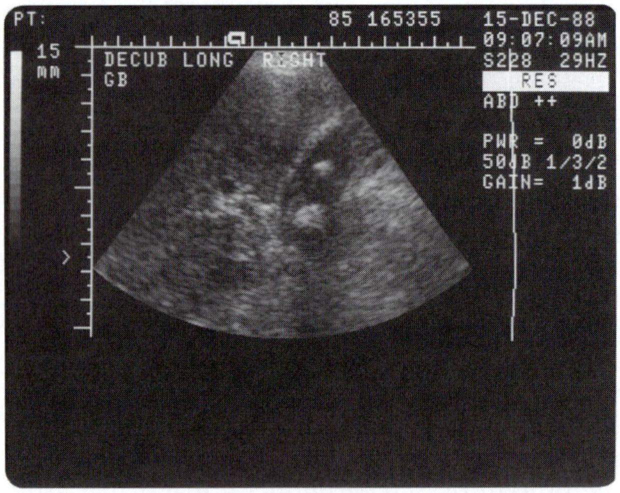

Figure 20-11 Sonogram of gall bladder with gallstones.

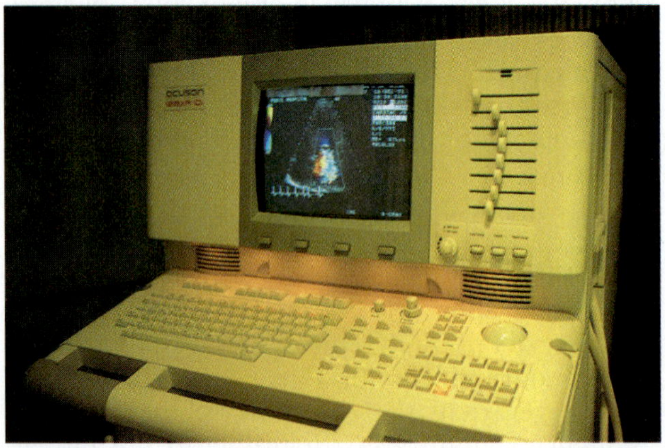

Figure 20-12 Echocardiograph machine. (Photo by Marcia Butterfield. Courtesy of W.A. Foote Memorial Hospital, Jackson, Michigan.)

During ultrasound, a **transducer** is used with a coupling agent, and sound waves are emitted from the head of the transducer. The transducer is placed firmly on the patient's body over the organ to be examined. The sound waves pass through the skin and bounce off the body's tissues and are reflected back to the transducer. These echoes are displayed on an **oscilloscope,** showing a visual pattern or picture. The image or record produced is known as a sonogram or echogram. A permanent film for the patient's record and videotape can also be made.

Integration of ultrasonography with a computer stores data and then produces three-dimensional images. Ultrasonography can be used to guide the provider while performing a biopsy.

Ultrasonography, because it is noninvasive (procedure does not puncture skin or enter the body), is widely accepted for obstetrical use. Gestational age can be determined, congenital anomalies detected, multiple fetuses noted, ectopic pregnancy

Patient Education

Magnetic Resonance Imaging (MRI)

1. Determine if the patient has followed the preparation instructions, if there were any.
2. Explain the procedure and what the patient can expect.
3. Have patient remove all metal objects (jewelry, watch, and so on). The magnet in the MRI machine is strong, and metal can disrupt images.
4. Have patient empty bladder before the procedure because it takes about 45 minutes and patient cannot move during that time.
5. Explain to patient that machine makes humming and tapping noises.
6. Tell patient that the intravenous contrast medium may be slightly uncomfortable when injected into vein.
7. Remind patient to lie still and not to move.
8. Tell patient that there is a microphone for communication between the patient and technician.

diagnosed, and fetal size and position determined (see Chapter 14).

Ultrasound takes 15 to 45 minutes, and the preparation depends on the body part being examined. An obstetrical ultrasound may require the patient to have a full bladder to push aside the intestines. An ultrasound of the gallbladder and liver requires the patient to have had nothing to eat or drink for 8 to 12 hours before the examination. The patient must remain still unless requested to change positions. Therapeutic ultrasonography is discussed in Chapter 21.

Mammography

More than any other X-ray, the mammogram must be of the highest resolution and contrast. High resolution and contrast call for an increase in exposure to radiation, but mammography currently is safer than ever because of strong regulations (the only fully regulated radiography examination by the federal government) and improved technology. The machines used for mammography must meet stringent requirements. They are used with special screens, film, and cassettes. Currently, the equipment can produce high-resolution and extremely high-contrast images with exposures that are lower than ever. Digitalization helps improve images. Although some newer mammography equipment is digitalized, according to some experts, it produces images that are only slightly better than those produced by nondigitalized equipment. Imaging techniques help providers perform biopsies of the breast, especially of abnormal areas that cannot be felt but are seen by conventional mammography or with ultrasound. A type of needle biopsy, stereotactic-guided biopsy, involves the exact location of the abnormal area in three dimensions using conventional mammography. (Stereotatic refers to use of a computer and scanning devices to create three-dimensional images.) A sterile needle is inserted into the precise location, and tissue or cell samples can be obtained. The samples are examined by a pathologist who looks for cancer cells.

Computer-Aided Detection (CAD). Computer-aided detection uses the computer to bring suspicious areas on a mammogram to the radiologist's attention. The CAD scans the mammogram with a laser beam and converts it into a digital signal that is processed by the computer. The image is displayed on a video monitor, with the suspicious area highlighted. The radiologist can compare the digital image with the conventional mammogram to see if any of the highlighted areas were missed on the initial review and require further investigation. CAD technology may improve the accuracy of a screening mammogram. Researchers continue to seek ways to reduce the exposure of X-rays to the patient even further. Chapter 14 provides more information on mammography.

Filing Films and Reports

Because radiographs are part of the patient's permanent record, they must be safeguarded from the environment. Conditions such as heat, moisture, light, and radiation can damage them. Processed films are stored in special envelopes with the patient's name, date, and identification number marked on the outside. They are stored in a cool, dry place. The films are the property of the hospital or other facility where the films were taken and usually remain where they were taken. Storage on-site makes them accessible for future use for comparison purposes and eliminates the possibility of their being lost if they were allowed to be taken away from the facility where they were processed. Written reports of the findings are prepared by the radiologist and sent to the patient's provider(s) (Figure 20-13). Computed radiography eliminates the need for film storage (hard copy).

RADIATION THERAPY

Radiation therapy is generally used to treat tumors that cannot be surgically removed or are inaccessible for surgical removal, and for treatment of a malignant tumor that was surgically excised but a portion of the tumor remains. It is a specialty within cadiology. When used to treat inaccessible or inoperable tumors, the treatment is considered **palliative** treatment. The treatments shrink the tumor, thereby lessening the symptoms. The treatments can be either external, with direct radiation aimed through the surface of the skin to an area within the body, or internal, using various

Critical Thinking

Describe how radiation therapy helps to destroy malignant neoplasms.

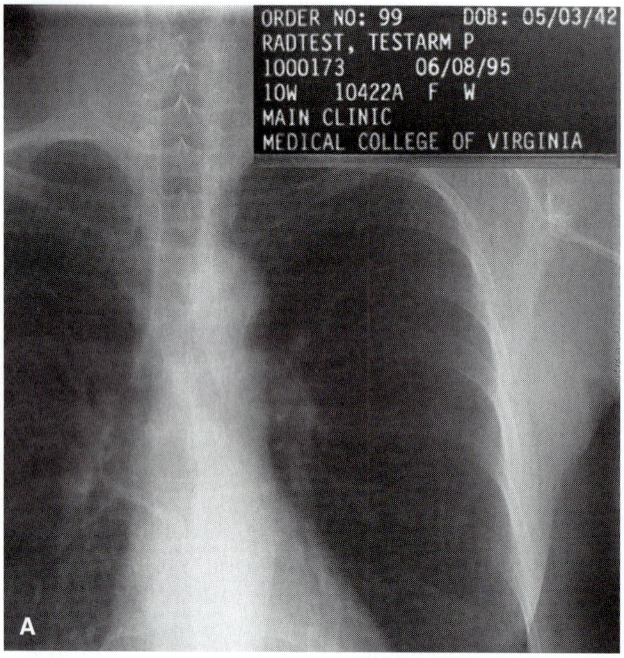

Figure 20-13A Radiograph showing patient identification information.

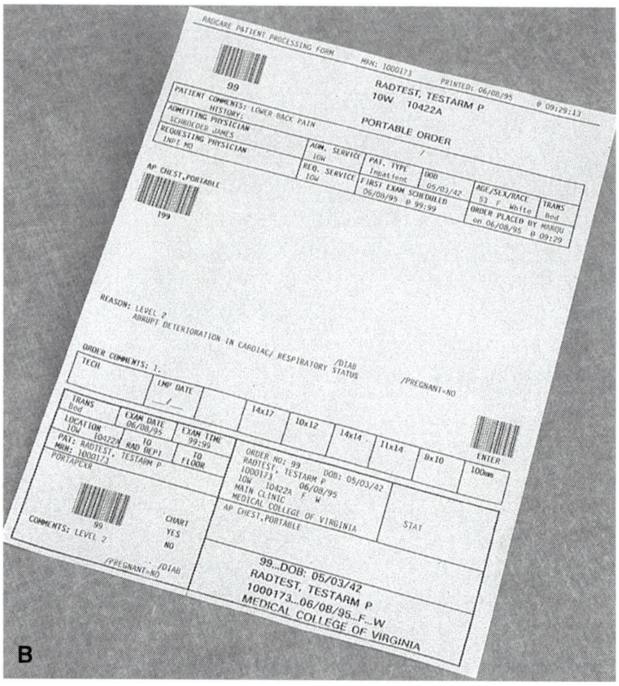

Figure 20-13B Sample requisition form.

applications of radioactivity such as seeds or beads that are planted inside the body and left there for a certain amount of time. The radiation is the same as X-rays, with doses carefully calculated. The aim of radiation therapy is to interfere with cell growth and to disrupt the DNA. The object is to destroy as many of the malignant cells as possible without harming healthy cells surrounding the tumor. Possible side effects are nausea, vomiting, hair loss, anorexia, bone marrow suppression, and **stomatitis.**

NUCLEAR MEDICINE

Nuclear medicine is the branch of medicine involved with the use of radioactive (emits rays or particles from nucleus) substances for diagnosis, therapy, and research. Specific training is necessary for this speciality.

Radioactive substances are administered to the patient either by mouth or by injection. The radioactive compounds, known as **radionuclides,** travel to an organ or area in the body that attracts them and creates an image of that area. The gamma rays omitted are detected by camera.

If the radionuclide is in an area that is abnormal, such as a tumor, the area is referred to as "hot." If the radionuclide does not concentrate in the abnormality, but surrounds it instead, the area is refered to as "cold". Both hot and cold areas are suggestive of abnormalities.

EHR The provider may order a nuclear medicine scan for the following reasons: to analyze kidney function, image blood flow through the heart, scan lungs, measure thyroid function, identify bleeding into the colon, determine the spread of cancer, bone scan, brain scan, and others. Nuclear imaging techniques use a camera and a nearby computer to detect emissions of the rays, measure the amount of radioactivity, and provide a digitalized image of the organ (e.g., the thyroid gland).

Data gathered from all of these diagnostic imaging devices are stored electronically in a hospital information system (HIS). Picture archiving and communication systems (PACS) store all radiologic exam results and are available online to providers on demand. The level of access to the data can be defined by each system. The benefits of these systems are that the examination reports and images will not become lost and no time is spent waiting for a report.

Case Study 20-1

Refer to the scenario at the beginning of the chapter.

CASE STUDY REVIEW

1. What is the patient preparation for excretory urography (IVP)?
2. What should Wanda tell Mr. Waite about what to expect as he begins to have his procedure?

Case Study 20-2

Gloria McDermott is scheduled to have a GI series of X-rays next week because of persistent episodes of stomach pain that is unrelieved by the medication Dr. King has prescribed for her.

CASE STUDY REVIEW

1. How will you explain to her the purpose of the test?
2. What will you tell her about how to prepare for the examination?

Case Study 20-3

Raymond Brunnelle has had a series of X-rays, a GI series, a cholecystogram, and an MRI of his abdomen. He has scheduled an appointment with a gastroenterologist and asks you to get all of the films for him.

CASE STUDY REVIEW

1. What is your response to his request?
2. Explain why they should be kept on-site.

SUMMARY

Radiology and diagnostic imaging are helpful in the diagnosis and treatment of diseases and conditions because procedures can be done to visualize internal structures and their functions. Radiation is not without its risks to personnel and patients, but by following specific safety precautions, the health and safety of all involved can be safeguarded.

The three specialty areas are radiology, radiation therapy, and nuclear medicine.

STUDY FOR SUCCESS

To reinforce your knowledge and skills of information presented in this chapter:

- Review the Key Terms
- Consider the Case Studies and discuss your conclusions
- Answer the Review Questions
  - Multiple Choice
  - Critical Thinking
- Navigate the Internet by completing the Web Activities
- Practice the StudyWARE activities on your student CD
- Apply your knowledge in the Student Workbook activities
- Complete the Web Tutor sections

REVIEW QUESTIONS

Multiple Choice

1. Which of the following radiologic procedures does *not* require a contrast medium?
   a. hysterosalpingogram
   b. mammogram
   c. cholecystogram
   d. angiogram
2. A cholecystogram requires which type of contrast medium?
   a. air
   b. tablets
   c. carbon dioxide
   d. barium
3. A cholangiogram will examine:
   a. upper GI tract
   b. lower GI tract
   c. bile ducts
   d. kidneys and ureters
4. In which of the following positions does the posterior aspect of the body face the X-ray tube and the anterior face the film?
   a. oblique
   b. anteroposterior
   c. posteroanterior
   d. prone
   e. supine
5. The radiologic procedure of choice for brain imaging is:
   a. computerized tomography
   b. positron emission tomography
   c. magnetic resonance imaging
   d. ultrasonography
   e. thermography

Critical Thinking

1. Describe the purpose of a lead apron and lead-lined walls in the radiology department.
2. For what is thermography used?
3. How are X-rays used to diagnose?
4. How are X-rays used to treat patient diseases or conditions?
5. What is contrast media? How is it used and why?
6. To whom do X-ray films belong once they are taken and processed?
7. What special precautions should be taken when a patient is having excretory urography (IVP), especially the initial time?

WEB ACTIVITIES

1. Visit the American Society of Radiologic Technicians at http://www.asrt.org. What is available at this Web site?
2. Use Google to find a Web site for "The history of MRI." Describe how long it took for the first MRI to produce one image.
3. Using a search engine of your choice, locate information about how CT scans work. What is the fundamental concept of how a CT scan operates?
4. Using a search engine of your choice, find information about how nuclear medicine works. Name three types of techniques that use nuclear medicine. How is an image obtained?
5. Locate a Web site about medical radiation safety. Find a guide about radiation protection for the patient. What are the benefits and risks of a mammogram? Excretory urogram (IVP)?

REFERENCES/BIBLIOGRAPHY

Bone mineral density test. MedlinePlus Medical Encyclopedia. Retrieved February 18, 2008, from http://www.nlm.nih.gov/medlineplus/ency/article/007197.htm.

Carlton, R. R., & Adler, A. M. (2001). *Principles of radiographic imaging: An art and a science* (3rd ed.). Clifton Park, NY: Delmar Cengage Learning.

Cornuelle, A., & Gronefeld, D. (1998). *Radiographic anatomy positioning: An integrated approach.* Stanford, CT: Appleton and Lange.

Cowling, C. (1998). *Radiographic positioning procedures, Volume II: Advanced imaging procedures.* Clifton Park, NY: Delmar Cengage Learning.

Metler, F. A., Jr., & Guiberteau, M. J. (2005). *Essentials of nuclear medicine imaging* (5th ed.). Philadelphia: W. B. Saunders.

Orenstein, B. W. (2006). Hot issues—MRI and implantable devices. *Radiology Today,* 7(4), 8.

Taber's cylopedic medical dictionary. (22nd ed.). (2005). Philadelphia: F. A. Davis.

Rehabilitation and Therapeutic Modalities

Chapter 21

KEY TERMS

Abduction
Activities of Daily Living (ADL)
Adduction
Ambulation
Body Mechanics
Circumduction
Diathermy
Dorsiflexion
Effleurage
Eversion
Extension
Flexion
Gait
Gait Belt
Goniometer
Goniometry
Hemiplegia
Hydrocollator Pack
Hypertension
Inversion
Modalities
Petrissage
Plantar Flexion
Pronation
Range of Motion (ROM)
Rehabilitation Medicine
Rotation
Supination
Thermotherapy
Ultrasound
Vasoconstriction

OUTLINE

OBJECTIVES

The student should strive to meet the following performance objectives and demonstrate an understanding of the facts and principles presented in this chapter through written and oral communication.

1. Define the key terms as presented in the glossary.
2. Define rehabilitation medicine and explain its importance in patient care.
3. Discuss the importance of correct posture and body mechanics, and demonstrate how to safely transfer patients and lift or move heavy objects using proper body mechanics.
4. Describe safety precautions and techniques used when helping a patient to ambulate and demonstrate how to assist the patient to safely stand and walk.
5. Demonstrate how to safely care for the falling patient.
6. Describe assistive devices and the importance of each in helping patients to ambulate.
7. Demonstrate how to measure patients for a walker, crutches, and a cane and help them ambulate safely with each device.
8. Describe the ambulation gaits used with crutches.
9. Discuss the safety precautions and techniques used when pushing a wheelchair.

OBJECTIVES (continued)

10. Explain the importance of joint range of motion and the method used to measure joint movement.
11. Explain the importance of therapeutic exercise and the types of therapeutic exercises used in patient rehabilitation.
12. Describe electromyography and its purpose.
13. Explain the purpose of the electrostimulation of muscle.
14. Explain the body's physiologic reactions to heat and cold therapeutic modalities.
15. Be able to identify and describe the various types of hot and cold modalities, and describe how ultrasound works.
16. Describe various conditions for which massage therapy is used.

Scenario

In a large urgent care center such as Inner City Health Care, a team of therapists is responsible for providing patients with a high level of rehabilitative care. However, the clinical medical assistants at Inner City also are involved on a daily basis in the care of patients who have experienced injuries such as fractures or severe back pain. Clinical medical assistant Wanda Slawson, CMA (AAMA), MLT, and clinical medical assistant Bruce Goldman, CMA (AAMA), are often responsible for transferring patients and getting them safely from the reception area to the examination room and from wheelchair to examination table. Although acutely aware of the needs and safety of the patient, Wanda and Bruce also make sure they protect themselves by using proper body mechanics, by observing good posture, by using their arm and leg muscles and not their back muscles, and by always bending from the hips and knees, not the waist. Wanda's and Bruce's observation of these important principles protects their health and ensures the safety of their patients.

INTRODUCTION

Physical disability affects millions of people in the United States, regardless of age, race, or socioeconomic status. Every year thousands of people survive strokes, head or spinal cord injury, or other debilitating illness or injury that leaves them unable to perform complete independent function. Some of these individuals recover completely. Others recover to their fullest ability, living the rest of their lives with some type of disability. Still other patients experience chronic conditions such as arthritis or severe back pain that incapacitates them to the extent they cannot work or completely care for themselves.

Rehabilitation medicine *is a field of medical disciplines that uses physical and mechanical agents to aid in the diagnosis, treatment, and prevention of diseases or bodily injuries. Its goal is to aid in the restoration of those functions that have been affected by the patient's condition. For those who have experienced permanent loss of ability, it seeks to find practical substitutions for that loss, thereby assisting patients to make the most of their remaining abilities.*

Most rehabilitation services are prescribed by the provider in charge of a patient's care and, depending on the patient's condition, can include a recommendation to one or several rehabilitation specialists. Most likely, that specialist will be a physical therapist, occupational therapist, speech therapist, or sports medicine specialist, although the field of rehabilitation medicine is certainly not limited to these four areas of specialty.

Professional rehabilitation therapists, in whichever field they practice, are specifically trained and licensed in their field of expertise to assess, plan, and execute the patient's treatment in an overall effort to restore that patient to the highest level of physical and social independence possible. The medical assistant, as a member of an

Spotlight on Certification

RMA Content Outline

- Personal and physical safety
- Body mechanics
- Treatment and medication
- Patient education
- Therapeutic modalities

CMA (AAMA) Content Outline

- Treatment area
- Equipment preparation and operation
- Principles of operations
- Physical therapy modalities
- Wheelchair/stretcher

CMAS Content Outline

- Employ effective written and oral communication
- Prepare patients for clinical examination
- Patient information and community resources
- Process Workers' Compensation/disability reports and forms

interdisciplinary health team, can use medical assisting skills to enable patients to regain normal or near-normal function after an illness or injury. Chapter 7 provides information on legal considerations and the Americans with Disabilities Act (ADA).

THE ROLE OF THE MEDICAL ASSISTANT IN REHABILITATION

As a medical assistant, you may find yourself working in one of the rehabilitation fields. Such opportunities might include an ambulatory care setting with a specialty in physical therapy or sports medicine, an orthopedic surgeon's practice, the occupational or speech therapy department of a large suburban hospital, or other outpatient clinic or medical office. For the more chronically ill, nursing homes and rehabilitation hospitals also focus on restoring patients to as much independence as possible.

Even if you do not work in the field of rehabilitation and therapeutic modalities, you may be referring patients for treatments and perhaps even performing insurance coding or rehabilitative and therapeutic modalities. Either way, a good working knowledge of the field is important for a well-rounded understanding of today's medical treatments.

Whatever the rehabilitation setting, you will most likely find that you are a member of an interdisciplinary team of health care professionals who bring a broad knowledge base to patient care (Table 21-1). However, the provider is responsible for prescribing any type of rehabilitative medicine.

It is important to remember that patients seeking rehabilitation treatment may have substained a tremendous loss of physical ability, leaving them vulnerable to feelings of helplessness. They may be able to perform only limited **activities of daily living (ADL)** or normal daily self-care such as brushing their teeth, getting dressed, and eating. Perhaps they cannot even do the simple tasks we take for granted every day, leaving them completely dependent on another person for help.

Understanding and encouragement are vital to the recovery process of these patients. While working with disabled persons, remember that certain tasks may be challenging to them. More than likely they are acutely aware of their impairment and feel frustrated at their loss of function and discouraged about the future. Some patients may suffer some speech impairment, making communication difficult or impossible. Respect for their dignity will build their self-esteem and have a positive effect on their treatment.

Patients' safety is essential. Many have a loss of ability to move and are vulnerable to falls.

Table 21-1 Some of the Specialized Fields of Rehabilitation Medicine

Physical Therapy/ Physiotherapy	The treatment of disorders with physical and mechanical agents and methods to restore normal function after injury or illness.
Occupational Therapy	The use of activities to help restore independent functioning after an injury or illness.
Speech Therapy	The diagnosis and treatment of speech disorders.
Sports Medicine	A branch of medicine that specializes in the treatment and prevention of injuries caused by athletic participation.

PRINCIPLES OF BODY MECHANICS

The medical assistant's work with disabled persons may require great physical effort, particularly if patients are incapable of lifting or moving themselves. Moving patients or heavy, awkward objects can be hazardous for the patient as well as the caregiver if not performed correctly.

Body mechanics is the practice of using certain key muscle groups together with good body alignment and proper body positioning to reduce the risk for injury to both patient and caregiver. Always be conscious of using proper body mechanics, not just on the job, but in everything that requires moving, lifting, pushing, or pulling heavy or awkward objects.

Posture

Practicing good body mechanics starts with good posture. Good posture protects the entire body, particularly the back, whether standing, sitting, or lying down.

Glance at yourself sideways in a full-length mirror. When standing, does your posture most resemble that in Figure 21-1A or 21-1B? When the body's muscle groups and body parts are in proper alignment, as shown in Figure 21-1B, the body is said to be in balance. Good balance is important for your body to function at its best. It enables you to lift, push, and pull easily and safely.

Frequently check your posture by reminding yourself to keep your chin and chest up, shoulders back, pelvis tilted slightly inward, feet straight and shoulder-width apart, and weight evenly distributed to both legs with a slight bend in your knees.

Using the Body Safely and Effectively

The spine is a flexible rod, designed to bend in many directions and hold the back steady. However, the muscles of the back are small and not meant for lifting heavy loads. They can be easily damaged if called on to work beyond their natural ability. The muscles in the arms and legs, however, are large and were designed for heavy work. Rely on these muscles when lifting and

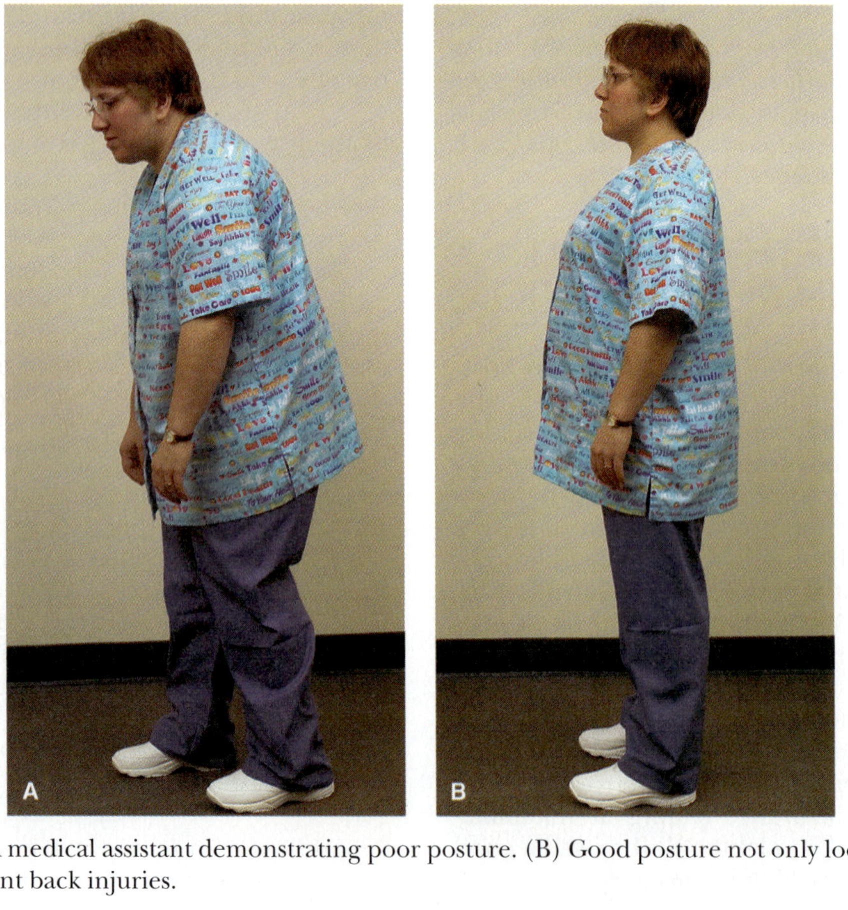

Figure 21-1 (A) A medical assistant demonstrating poor posture. (B) Good posture not only looks more professional but can prevent back injuries.

carrying heavy objects, bending over or bending down, or moving patients.

It is important to keep several basic rules in mind whenever performing any task:

- Keep the back as straight as possible and feet shoulder-width apart to provide a good base of support (Figure 21-2).
- Always bend from the hips and knees, which enables the largest muscles of the legs to do the hard work, but *never* bend from the waist (Figure 21-3).

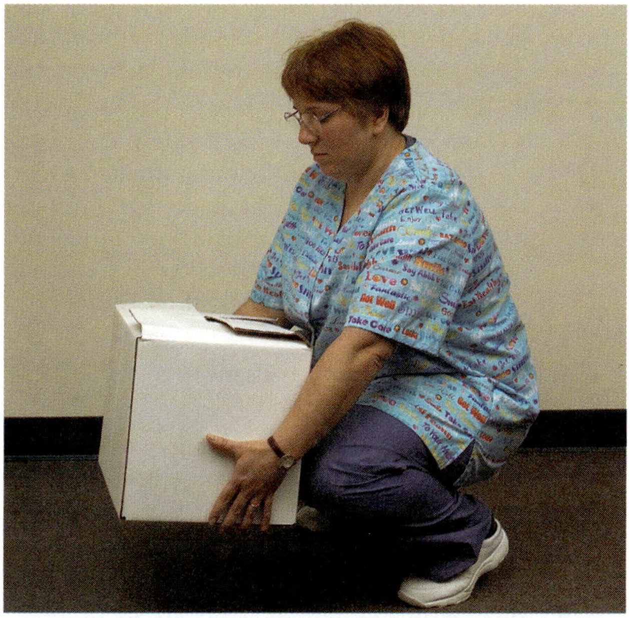

Figure 21-2 Provide a good base of support by keeping the back straight and feet apart.

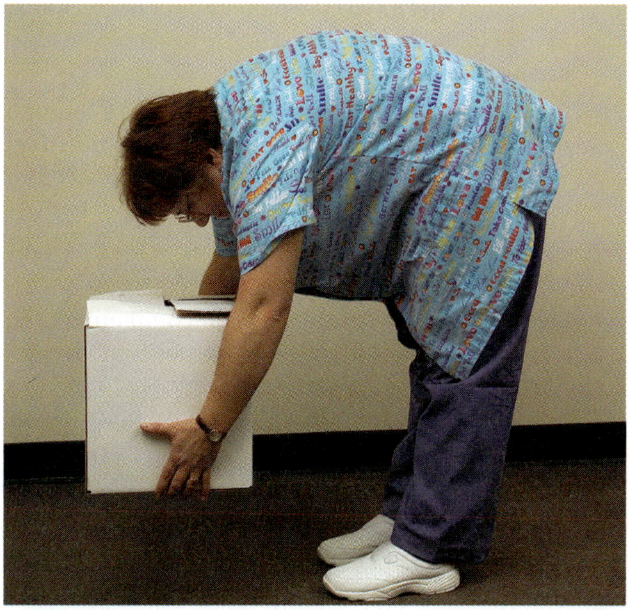

Figure 21-3 Never bend from the waist.

- Pivot the entire body instead of twisting it.
- Use the body's weight to push or pull any heavy object.
- Obtain help if unable to move a patient or object that is too heavy.
- Hold heavy objects close to the body (Figure 21-4).
- Make sure the path is clear and the area to receive the object is ready before lifting or moving it.
- Get into the habit of wearing a body support if a job includes much lifting.

Lifting Techniques

When lifting patients or moving or lifting heavy objects, certain techniques should be used to prevent back injury:

- Get as close as possible to the object or person being lifted, because this allows the center of gravity to be maintained over the base of support.
- Keep the feet apart, one slightly in front of the other, and knees slightly bent.
- Use the large muscles of the legs and arms to lift, not back muscles.
- Keep the back straight to transfer the workload to larger arm and leg muscles.
- Bend from the hips and knees, squat down, and push up with leg muscles.

TRANSFERRING PATIENTS

It may be necessary to transfer patients if they cannot walk or lift themselves. Such patients may have a wide variety of disabilities, from severe back pain to **hemiplegia,** or paralysis of one side of the body resulting from a stroke, accident, or other condition. Frail older adults also require particular care when being transferred, because they are more prone to bruising and broken bones, and they may be unsteady on their feet.

As a safety precaution, it is important to remember good body mechanics when transferring patients. The act of lifting and moving someone can throw off one's center of gravity and therefore the base of support. Provide a wider base of support by moving the feet farther apart and bending slightly, using strong arm and leg muscles to lift.

Before beginning any transfer, observe certain precautions:

- Make sure the equipment is stable and firm. Lock the brakes of the wheelchair and make sure the

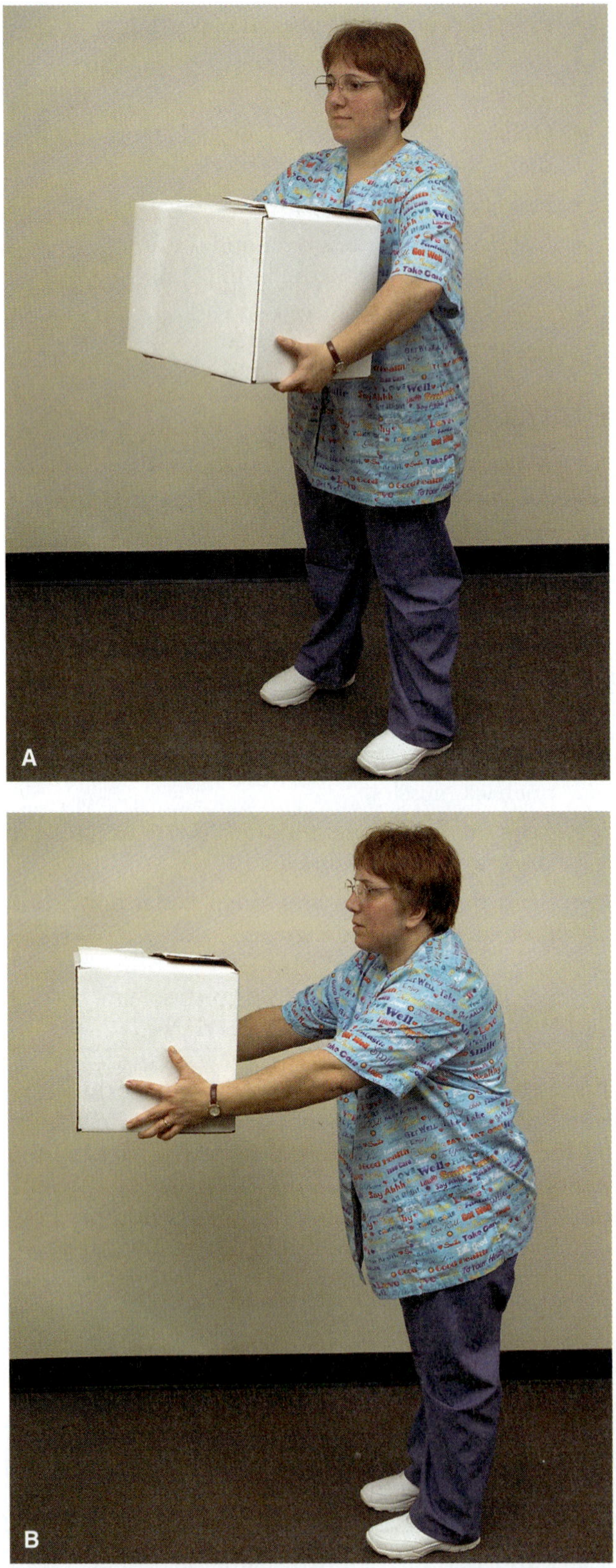

Figure 21-4 (A) When carrying heavy objects, hold them close to the body. (B) Never carry heavy objects out in front.

examination table or other surface will not move during the transfer.

- Check that there are no obstructions to trip over when making the transfer.
- Take small shuffling steps, and avoid crossing the feet.
- It is best if the transfer surfaces being used are close to the same height. If possible, lower the examination table or bed to the height of the wheelchair.
- Position the equipment according to the patient's physical limitations or disability. If the patient is stronger on one side, make sure that is the side on which the transfer will take place. It not only makes the transfer easier, it gives the patient more confidence.
- Always use a **gait belt,** a safety belt worn around the patient's waist, when transferring a patient. Lift the patient by grasping the belt from underneath and lifting up. Never lift a patient by the arms, or under the armpits, because this could cause injury to you and the patient.
- Take advantage of any assistance the patient can provide in lifting and moving.
- Never have patients put their arms around your neck or on your shoulders, because it could cause you to be injured.
- Make sure both you and the patient are wearing footwear that will not slip or hinder the transfer process in any way. If a prosthesis or brace is involved, make sure it is secure and will not present a problem.
- Thoroughly explain to the patient what you intend to do, and make sure the patient understands what to expect during the transfer. Instructions need to be simple and repeated when necessary.
- Practice good body mechanics. Get close enough to the patient so you can lift with your legs (Figure 21-5). Always bend at the hips instead of the waist.
- Ascertain beforehand whether assistance will be needed with the transfer.
- Finally, take sufficient time when completing each step. Many patients will want to help themselves. Respect their courage and determination, but remember that safety is of the utmost importance.

Procedure 21-1 gives the proper steps for transferring patients from a wheelchair to an examination table. Procedure 21-2 outlines steps for transfer from examination table to wheelchair.

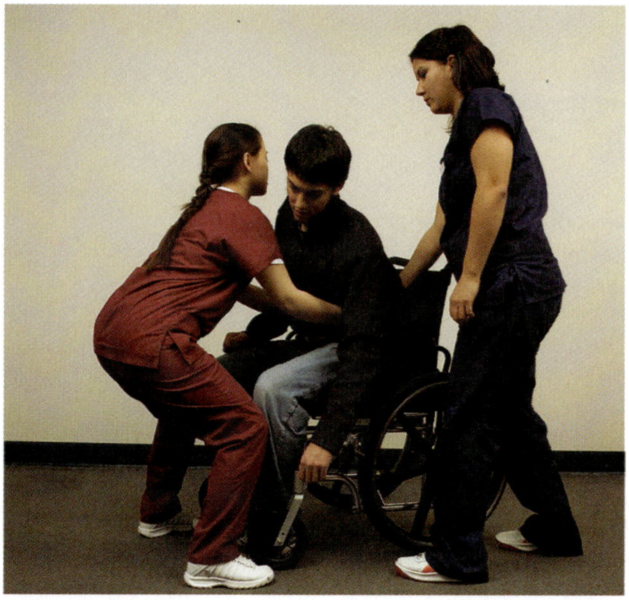

Figure 21-5 When a patient or object is too heavy, get help if necessary. Consider wearing a body support to protect the back if a job requires frequent lifting.

ASSISTING PATIENTS TO AMBULATE

Despite great strides that have been made in providing access for disabled persons, **ambulation,** or walking, is a functional activity that still provides the ultimate level of independence and freedom. For many patients, being able to ambulate again gives them tremendous satisfaction, because the act of walking more than anything else signifies their return to wellness. Some patients take months to walk again by undergoing exercises and treatment designed to strengthen specific muscles. They may still need help while in your office or a clinic specializing in orthopedics or sports medicine.

Before assisting with any type of ambulation, there are several safety issues to remember:

- Make sure the patient is ready to walk. If a patient has trouble sitting well or cannot balance once standing up, walking should not be attempted.
- The patient should be wearing good shoes that are flat, supportive, and have a rubber sole.
- Check to be certain there are plenty of handholds or railings within easy reach should the patient become unstable during walking.
- A gait belt provides a firm hold on the patient should the patient require assistance with stability at any time. For the patient just starting to walk, this device should be used and held by the caregiver throughout the session.
- Monitor the patient when standing and throughout the ambulation session for signs of fatigue and vertigo.
- Ambulate only as long as the patient has strength. Never push the patient beyond endurance.
- Never hurry a patient.
- Be ready should a patient start to fall. Generally, patients will fall toward their weaker side, but sometimes their legs lose stability and they go straight down.

Procedures 21-3 and 21-4 detail the steps involved in assisting patients to stand and walk and in caring for a falling patient.

ASSISTIVE DEVICES

For some patients, the extent of their physical disability may determine that ambulation is only possible with the help of an **assistive device,** or walking aid such as a walker, crutches, or cane. For others, their physical disability is such that mobility is not possible at all without the use of a wheelchair.

Some assistive devices provide stability and support, whereas others require more coordination. Depending on the patient's condition, one assistive device may be used until the patient has gained enough strength and coordination to move on to another type of assistive device, with the ultimate goal of walking unaided. The device a patient needs depends both on the disability and the patient's recuperation curve and is prescribed after careful evaluation by the attending provider or other health professional (Table 21-2).

Whatever device a patient will be using, medical assistants may be called on to measure the patient for the correct size and provide instruction in its proper use and care. Once the patient has become proficient on level surfaces, provide instruction on sitting; standing; turning around; and negotiating stairs, curbs, ramps, doors, and other obstacles. In addition, patients should be taught how to protect themselves should they fall while alone and how to get back up.

Walkers

Walkers are best used for patients who require maximum assistance with balance and coordination, because walkers provide stability and support

Table 21-2 Types of Assistive Devices

Assistive Device	Features	Patient Requirements
Walkers		
Standard	• Adjustable • Rubber tips	• Requires upper body strength • Provides maximum stability and support • Excellent for older adults
Rolling	• Legs have wheels • Otherwise same as regular walker	• Good for patients who need walker only for balance and not support
Crutches		
Axillary	• Wooden or steel • Worn under axillae	• Requires good upper body strength and balance • Not recommended for older adults • Best for younger persons with lower extremity or hip fractures that will heal in a short time • Provides greatest range of ambulation
Forearm (Lofstrand or Canadian)	• Shorter than axillary crutches • Has metal cuff worn around forearm	• Less stable than axillary crutches • Best for long-term crutch use • Reduces stress on axillary vessels and nerves • Requires upper body strength and more stability and coordination • Provides most maneuverability of all crutches
Platform	• Platform affixed to a crutch • Patient bears weight on forearm	• Best for patients with severe arthritis or poor use of hands • Does not require as much upper body strength • Requires good balance
Canes		
Standard	• Single leg • Curved handle • Rubber tip	• Good for patients with only one good arm, lateral instability, or balance conditions
Quad (four-point)	• Single cane resting on a platform with four legs • Rubber tips on legs	• Better for patients with more severe conditions • Does not require as much coordination, but still requires balance and upper body strength in one arm
Walkcane or Hemiwalker	• Has four legs that come all the way up to a handlebar • Rubber tips on all legs	• Provides most stability of all canes • Best for hemiplegic patients who require extra support on one side

when patients are standing or walking. They provide patients with the ability to ambulate independently with confidence. To use one, patients must be strong enough to be able to hold themselves upright while leaning on the walker.

Various styles of walkers are available. The two most widely used walkers are those that have rubber tips on the legs (stationary walkers), and those with wheels on the bottom of the legs (rolling walkers). Walkers that have wheels can be easily pushed ahead by the patient while walking and are best for patients who primarily need a walker for balance.

Most walkers are made of aluminum and are lightweight; most can be easily folded for storage

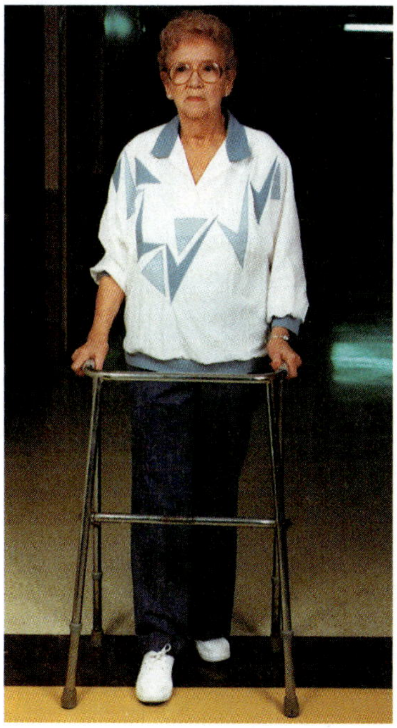

Figure 21-6 Proper fit for a walker. Note the patient's elbows are flexed at a 30-degree angle.

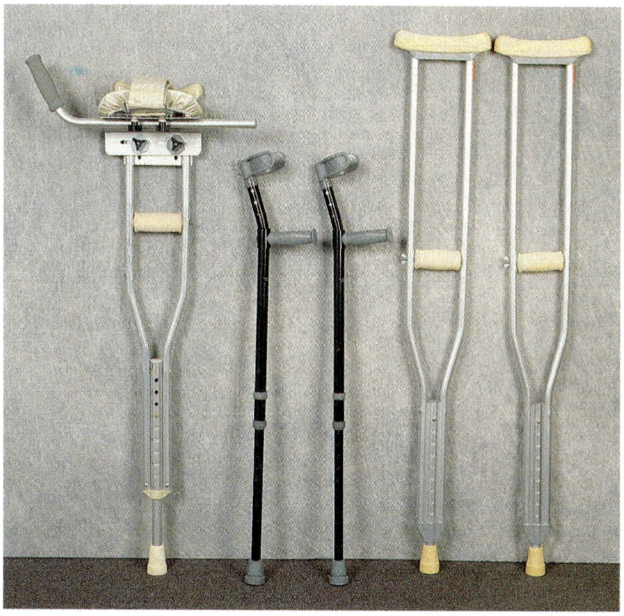

Figure 21-7 Types of crutches, from left to right: platform, forearm (or Lofstrand), and axillary.

or transport. The major disadvantage is that they must be used on level ground and cannot be used on stairs. Walkers are also difficult to use when attempting to go through doorways and in small areas around the house.

Fitting a Walker. Most walkers can be adjusted for a proper fit. The height of the handgrip should be adjusted to the individual patient just below the patient's waist, or at the top of the femur so the elbow can be bent at a 30-degree angle when the patient is standing with hands on the handgrip (Figure 21-6).

Procedure 21-5 provides steps for assisting a patient to ambulate with a walker.

Crutches

Crutches provide the ambulating patient with a great deal more mobility and flexibility. They provide good stability and support, therefore allowing for a broad range of gait patterns and ambulating speeds.

Three basic types of crutches are prescribed, depending on the patient's physical limitations and abilities: axillary crutches, forearm crutches (also called Lofstrand or Canadian crutches), and platform crutches (Figure 21-7).

Axillary crutches are made of wood or aluminum and are used primarily for individuals who need crutches temporarily while a lower extremity heals. Axillary crutches are ideal for stronger patients and pediatric patients who have minor injuries; they are not recommended for frail older adults because upper body strength and balance are required to use them (Figure 21-8). These crutches are easily transported and can be used to maneuver on stairs or in tight places.

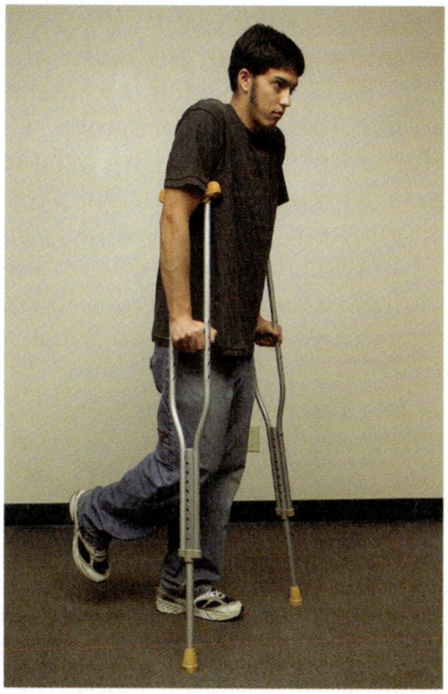

Figure 21-8 Patient using axillary crutches.

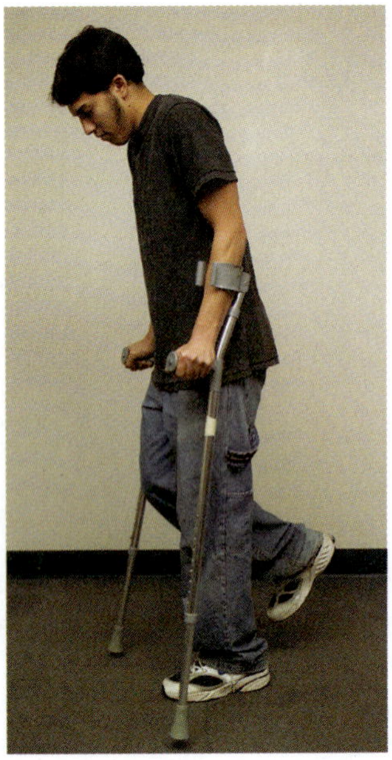

Figure 21-9 Patient using Lofstrand or forearm crutches.

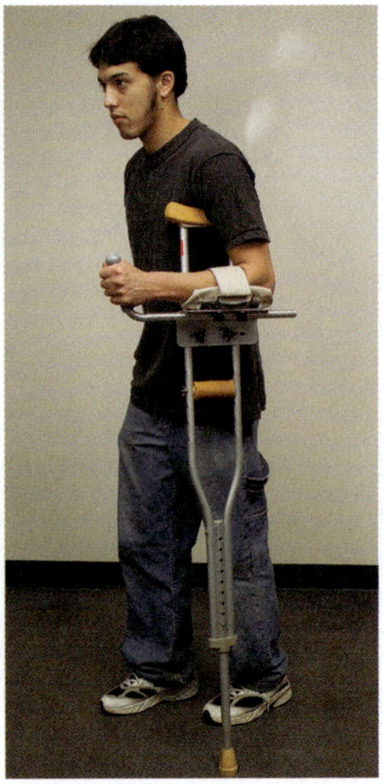

Figure 21-10 Patient using a platform crutch. This crutch is an ideal substitute for a cane if the patient cannot bear weight in his upper arm or on his hand.

Forearm crutches, or Lofstrand or Canadian crutches as they are also known, are shorter and provide less stability than axillary crutches. Forearm crutches are fixed with a metal or hard plastic cuff that fits around the patient's forearm. The weight is borne almost exclusively on the hand grip, requiring a great deal of upper body strength and coordination to use. This type of crutch is generally recommended for patients who will need crutches permanently or for a long period because they do not put any pressure on the axillary vessels and nerves (Figure 21-9).

The *platform crutch* is a third type of crutch that is recommended for patients who cannot grip the handles of other types of crutches or bear weight through their wrists or hands. The crutch has a platform attached to the top that includes a hand grip. It is high enough for the patient to use with the elbow bent at a right angle. The patient bears his or her weight completely on the forearm, which requires stability, strength, and coordination. The platform crutch is an ideal substitute for a cane when a patient only requires minimal weight transfer but cannot bear weight on or grip with the hands (Figure 21-10).

Measuring a Patient for Axillary Crutches. To determine the right height of the crutches, the patient should stand tall. Be sure the patient is wearing good walking shoes. Adjust the height of the crutch so it is about two to three fingers, or 2 inches, below the patient's axillae, or armpits (Figure 21-11). Adjust the hand grips so the patient's elbows are bent at about a 20- to 30-degree angle. Position the crutch tips about 2 inches lateral and 6 inches anterior to the foot. When the patient is standing correctly, the crutch tips and patient's feet should form a triangle (Figure 21-12).

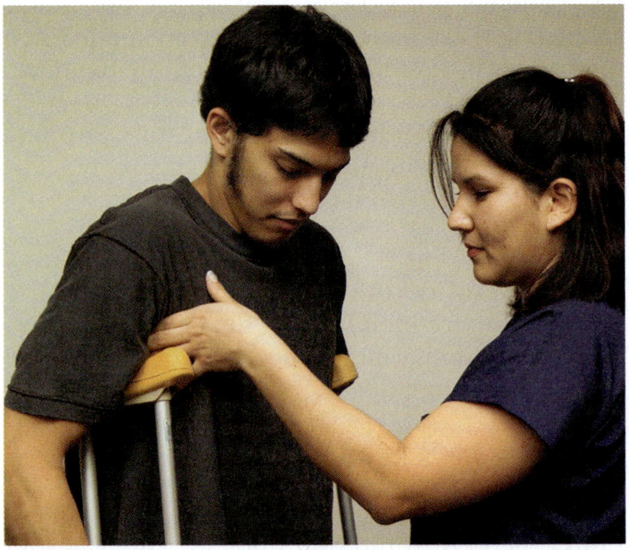

Figure 21-11 Measuring for axillary crutches. Note the height is about two to three fingers below the patient's axillae.

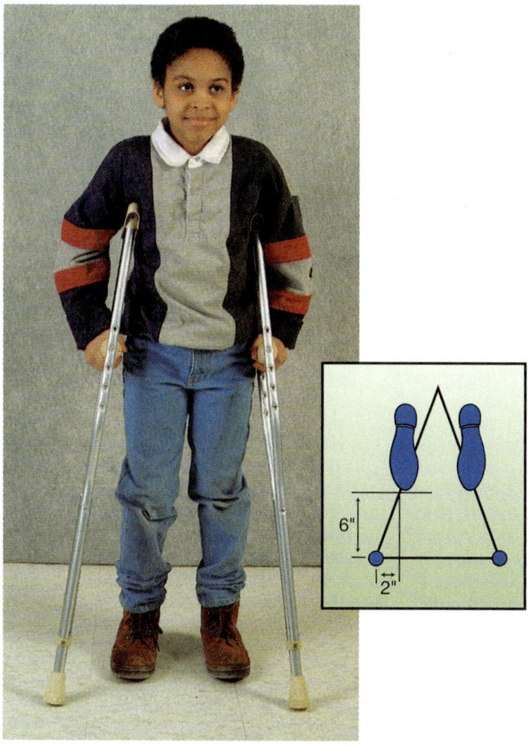

Figure 21-12 The distal end of the crutch should be 2 inches lateral and 6 inches anterior to the foot to form a triangle.

Procedure 21-6 gives steps for teaching patients to ambulate with axillary crutches.

Crutch-Walking Gaits. The type of **gait,** or walk, a patient uses depends on the patient's injury and condition and is determined by the provider or licensed therapist. In crutch-walking gaits, each time the patient's foot or crutch touches the ground it is called a *point.* There are five gaits that are commonly used in crutch ambulation. The number of points in the gait relates to the number of feet and crutch tips that are on the ground at the same time.

Common crutch-walking gaits include two-point, three-point, four-point, swing-to, and swing-through gaits.

Two-Point Gait. There are two types of two-point gaits:

1. The first type is a nonweight-bearing gait. Patients place the crutch tips about 18 inches in front of them. They push off, taking the weight off their body and transferring it to their hands, then bring their strong leg forward past the crutches.
2. The second gait, called the two-point alternating gait, is used when the patient can bear weight on both legs. The opposite foot and crutch are advanced forward at the same time (Figure 21-13). This gait is a more advanced gait and is used after the four-point gait has been mastered.

Three-Point Gait. This gait is used when the patient can only bear partial weight on one leg, or just touch that foot to the floor. Both the crutches and the weak leg are advanced at the same time. The body weight is then transferred forward to the crutches, and the stronger leg is advanced and placed slightly in front of the crutches (Figure 21-14).

Four-Point Alternating Gait. This is a slower gait that is used for patients who can bear weight on both legs and move each leg separately. The patient moves one crutch forward, then the opposite foot. The patient then moves the other crutch forward, then the opposite foot (Figure 21-15).

Swing-To Gait. Patients start with the crutches at their side. They move both crutches forward, transfer their weight forward, and swing both feet together up to the crutches.

Swing-Through Gait. Start with the crutches at the side. Move both crutches forward. Transfer the weight and swing both feet through the crutches, stopping slightly in front of the crutches.

Sitting. The patient backs into a straight chair with armrests until the seat of the chair touches the back of the legs. Crutches are held in the hand on the strong side and opposite the weak leg. With the other hand the patient can grasp the armrest of the chair and lower slowly into the chair.

Standing. The patient holds both crutches in the hand on the strong side, moves forward in

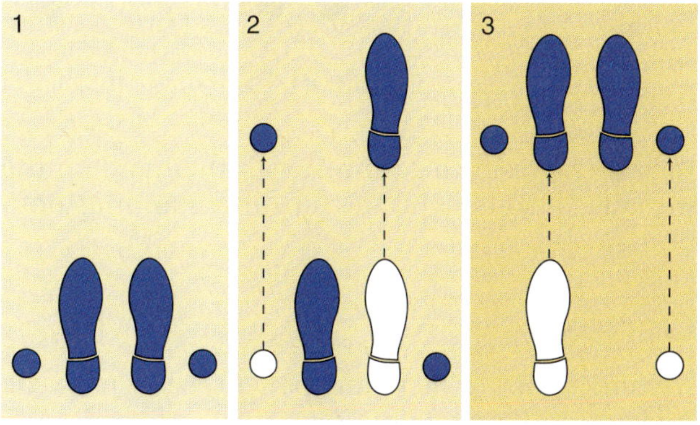

Figure 21-13 Two-point gait. The patient is bearing weight on both legs.

Patient Education

When instructing patients in the use of axillary crutches, impress on them the importance of putting all their weight on their hands, not on the axillae. Many patients using crutches for the first time mistakenly put the pressure on their axillae, which can damage the axillary nerve. Also reinforce the need for wearing flat, nonskid shoes when using crutches.

Throw rugs and other obstacles in the home or work area are a danger to patients on crutches. Remind them to have such hazards removed. Teach patients to examine crutches daily for the following:

- Check that the wing nuts that adjust the crutches are tight.
- Check the crutch tips for wear and tear.
- Check the foam pads of the hand grips and axilla rests for tears.

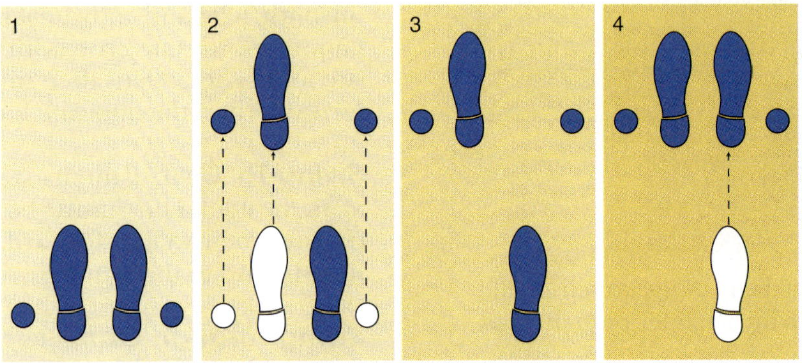

Figure 21-14 Three-point gait. The left leg is the weaker leg and bears no weight.

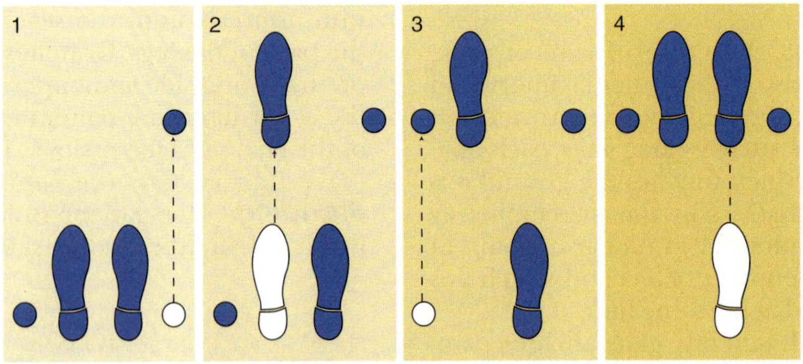

Figure 21-15 Four-point gait. The patient is bearing weight on both legs.

the chair, grasps the armrest with the hand on the weaker side, then pushes up to a standing position.

Canes

A cane is used when the patient has one weak side and will need this assistive device for a longer period than crutches. It is also useful for patients who have a general but minor weakness on one side or those who have poor balance.

Canes come in three basic types, are made of either aluminum or wood, and have rubber tips. Some are adjustable and some are not (Figure 21-16). The first type of cane is called a *standard,* or single-tipped, cane (Figure 21-17). It has a curved handle for gripping, and the newer canes have a hand grip attached. The standard cane is used for patients with less severe walking conditions who need a small amount of support.

The second type of cane is a four-legged, or *quad,* cane. It is a single cane that rests on a

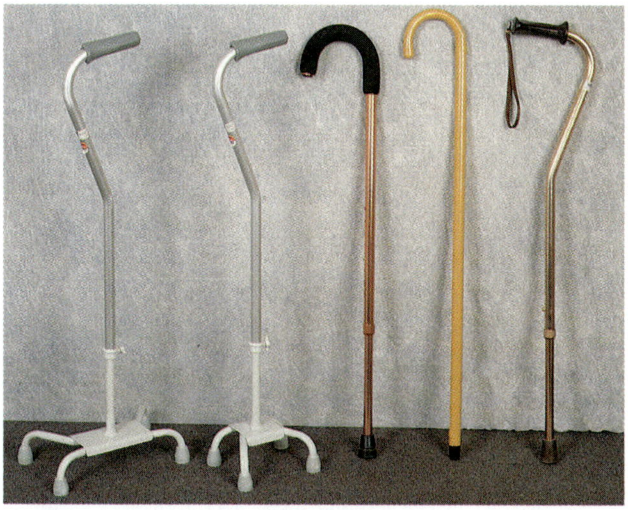

Figure 21-16 Types of standard canes: quad canes and single-tip canes.

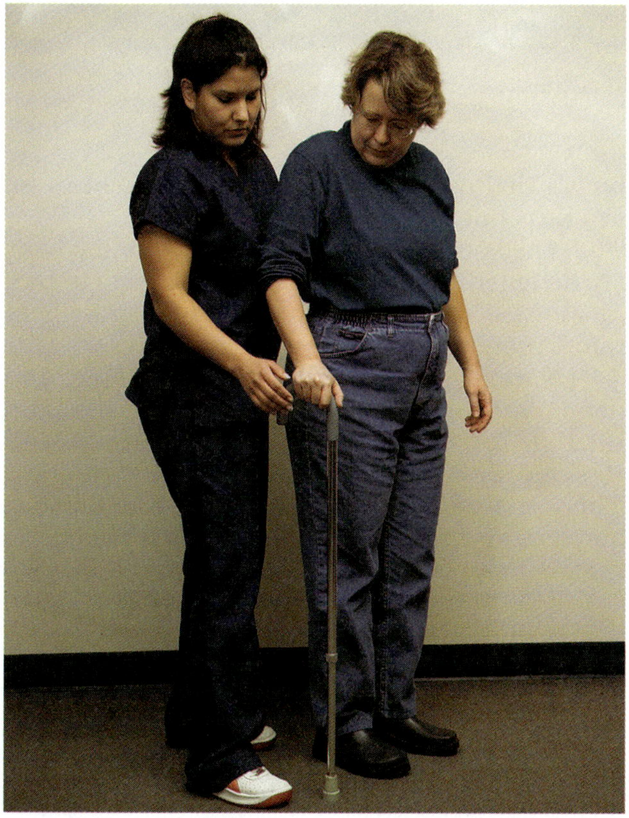

Figure 21-17 A standard cane being used by a hemiplegic patient.

four-legged platform, provides stability and a wide base of support, and is for patients with more severe walking difficulties.

The third type of cane is a *walkcane.* It has four legs and a handlebar for gripping and provides the best support of all canes. This type of cane is also referred to as a Hemiwalker because it is ideal for hemiplegic patients who need the extra stability of this wide base. When the cane is the correct height, the elbow is flexed at a 20- to 30-degree angle.

Procedure 21-7 outlines the steps for teaching a patient how to walk safely with a cane.

Wheelchairs

Wheelchairs are mobile chairs that enable patients with severe ambulation conditions, or no ability to ambulate at all, to otherwise get around. Some must be moved manually, either by the patient or by someone else. Others are motorized and can be controlled completely by the patient (Figure 21-18).

With the many advancements in wheelchair design, patients with chronic conditions no longer are restricted to a home or hospital environment. Today, all public buildings and many private ones have handicapped access ramps as an alternative to stairs, remote-controlled doors, elevators that can accommodate a wheelchair, and other amenities that enable wheelchair patients to get around almost as well as if they were ambulating.

Many types of wheelchairs can be modified to suit a patient's particular disability and lifestyle. There are even wheelchairs that enable patients to participate in sports activities. Many car manufacturers can modify a van to accommodate a wheelchair, and some are equipped to allow wheelchair patients to drive.

Patients who will be using a wheelchair for a long time are taught how to maintain it. Depending on their abilities, they check it regularly to make sure all the parts are working correctly, and, if they are able, to make any necessary repairs. Patients are taught to use the wheelchair safely and how to maneuver into and out of difficult spaces.

If a patient is being pushed by someone else, that individual must learn basic safety rules for transporting a patient:

- Make sure that the brakes are locked when transferring a patient into and out of a wheelchair, and if a patient must be left alone in the wheelchair for any length of time, lock the brakes (Figure 21-19).
- Make sure the patient's feet are placed on the footrests when the wheelchair is in use.
- Be certain the patient feels safe.
- Always back into and out of elevators.
- Stay to the right in corridors.
- Back down slanted ramps.

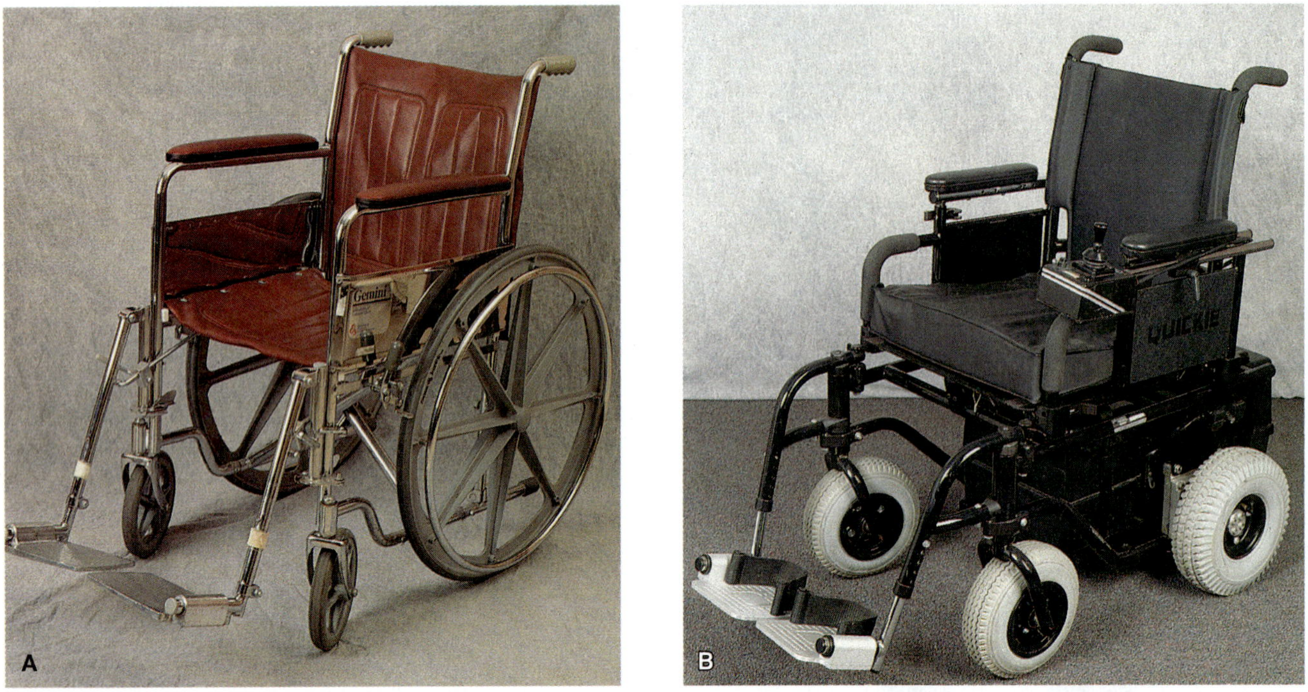

Figure 21-18 (A) A manual wheelchair. (B) A motorized wheelchair.

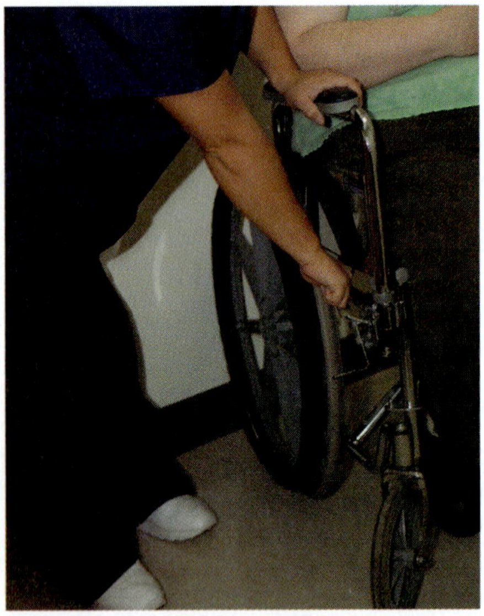

Figure 21-19 The patient's wheelchair should be locked when transferring a patient in and out of it, or when the patient is left alone in the wheelchair for any length of time.

THERAPEUTIC EXERCISES

Range of Motion

The musculoskeletal system is a complex joining of bones, joints, ligaments, and tendons. Not only does it give structure to the body and protect the body's vital organs, it allows for movement so we can carry out a multitude of activities.

The bones of almost all the joints of the body are designed to move as well. Each joint has its own **range of motion (ROM),** the amount of movement that is present in a joint.

Normal ROM varies among people and depends on several factors, such as age, sex, and whether the motion being performed is passive (assisted motion) or active (voluntary motion). There is a standard ROM for all movable joints, and it is this standard that is used when evaluating the joint movement of a particular patient.

The measurement of joint motion is called **goniometry.** Joint movement is measured with an instrument called a **goniometer** and is always expressed in degrees. For example, the average person lying flat with arms to the sides can move the elbows from a 20-degree hyperextension (extending the arm beyond its normal limits) to 0-degree extension, through to 150 degrees of flexion, or bending (Figure 21-20).

ROM evaluation is one of several tools used when developing a therapeutic program for a patient (Figure 21-21).

As a medical assistant, you need to be familiar with ROM exercises (Figure 21-22). ROM exercises are designed to maintain joint mobility and are performed either passively (someone else does the movement) or actively (the patient does the movement).

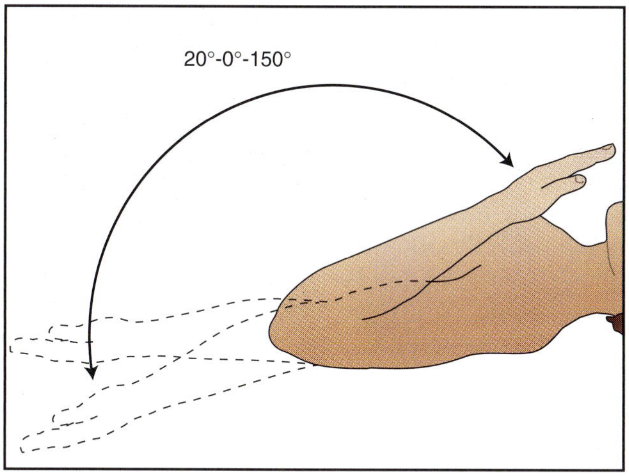

Figure 21-20 Joint mobility is measured against standard ranges of motion and is always expressed in degrees.

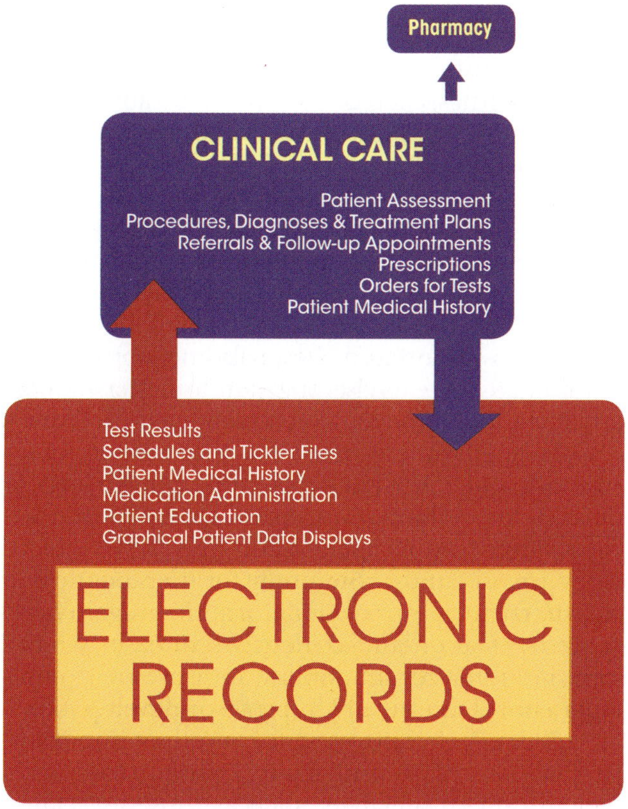

Figure 21-21 Clinical care arm of the total practice management system (TPMS). Patient rehabilitative procedures and therapeutic modalities treatment plans ordered by the provider are part of the TPMS data flow. Treatment plans, progress notes, and follow-up appointments are recorded in the patient's medical record and readily accessible to the provider for continuity of patient care.

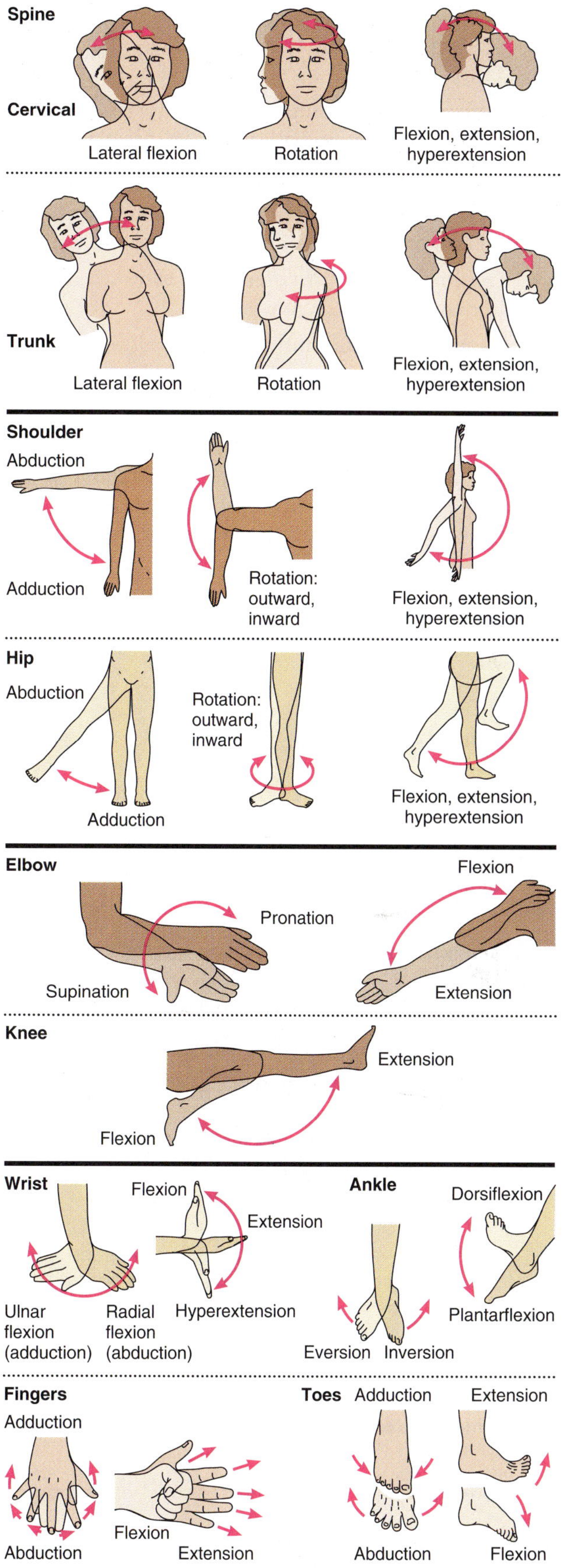

Figure 21-22 Range of motion (ROM) exercises for specific joints.

Joint movement has a special vocabulary, and it is helpful to learn the terms and their definitions (Table 21-3).

Before performing ROM exercises on a patient, the caregiver will need to observe some general precautions:

- Always move the patient's limbs gently, within pain tolerance and the flexibility of the limb.
- Use slow, careful movements that allow the muscles time to adjust to the movement.
- Always support the limb above and below the joint.
- It is best to perform passive ROM with the patient in the supine position.
- ROM should never cause pain. If the patient reports pain at any time, the ROM exercises should be discontinued until the provider or other health care professional can determine the source of pain.
- Repeat each movement several times or as prescribed by the provider.
- Provide for patient privacy.

Table 21-3 Terminology of Joint Movement

Abduction	Motion away from the midline of the body
Adduction	Motion toward the midline of the body
Circumduction	Circular motion of a body part
Dorsiflexion	Moving the foot upward at the ankle joint
Eversion	Moving a body part outward
Extension	Straightening of a body part
Flexion	Bending of a body part
Hyperextension	A position of maximum extension, or extending a body part beyond its normal limits
Inversion	Moving a body part inward
Plantar Flexion	Moving the foot downward at the ankle
Pronation	Moving the arm so the palm is down
Rotation	Turning a body part around its axis
Supination	Moving the arm so the palm is up

Muscle Testing

The other tool used for evaluating the movement abilities of a patient is muscle testing. Whereas goniometry focuses on joint movement, muscle testing evaluates the motion, strength, and task potential of a given muscle. *ROM* testing for muscles determines how flexible and resilient a muscle may be. *Strength testing* shows how hard a muscle can work. *Task potential* of a muscle means how well a muscle can aid in accomplishing a given activity. As a medical assistant, you may assist with testing the patient for joint mobility, posture, and strength of muscles.

Types of Therapeutic Exercise

Without constant exercise, the musculoskeletal system would deteriorate. Joints would become stiff and contractures, or deformities, could develop. Muscles would atrophy, or shrink and lose strength. Bones would lose vital minerals such as calcium and phosphorus. The body's overall circulation would decrease, which in turn would create a separate set of unhealthy conditions.

Like drugs, exercise has a powerful and systemic effect on the body. It involves the function of joints, bones, muscles, nerves, tendons, ligaments, as well as the circulatory and respiratory systems. Therapeutic exercises are prescribed after careful evaluation by a trained specialist and are tailored to each patient depending on that patient's individual condition and rehabilitation goals. It is the role of the medical assistant to understand the goals and objectives of the therapeutic exercise program to better support and encourage patients to complete their program.

Whereas an athlete uses exercise to build strength and endurance to attain a certain level of performance, therapeutic exercises are prescribed for a variety of therapeutic and preventive effects. They are used most commonly for therapeutic reasons to correct or prevent deformities, regain body movement after an accident or disease, restore joint motion after immobility, improve neuromuscular coordination, and improve or develop ADLs.

Exercise is also used for another important reason: It can prevent many common problems brought on by inactivity, such as those associated with respiration and circulation.

A variety of exercise programs are used for therapeutic or preventive purposes:

1. *Active exercises,* which are self-directed and performed by the patient without assistance
2. *Passive exercises,* which are performed by another person with no voluntary participation from the patient

3. *Assisted exercises,* which help the patient voluntarily move weakened muscles with the use of an assistive device, such as a therapy pool
4. *Active resistance exercises,* which provide voluntary movement against various types of manual or mechanical pressure to increase muscle strength

Electromyography

Electrical activity of muscles can be recorded on a graph or film to help determine how well muscles contract. An electromyograph is the instrument used to test the electrical activity of a muscle. An electrode (using a small gauge needle) is inserted through skin into the muscle, and measurements of muscle strength are made.

Electrostimulation of Muscle

An electric current of low voltage can help stimulate muscles to exercise by innervating the sensory and motor nerves for that muscle. It is helpful for a patient who has nerve damage to the muscle and cannot voluntarily move the muscle. The purpose is to prevent atrophy of the muscle and help restore muscle function.

The low current of electricity passing through the patient's muscle acts similarly to the patient's own nerves causing the muscle to contract and relax. The stimulation is helpful to retrain a patient after experiencing an injury to a muscle or muscle group. Disposable gel electrodes are applied, and low-voltage current stimulates muscles to prevent atrophy of muscle.

A method of using electric current to stimulate nerves is known as *transcutaneous electric nerve stimulation* (TENS). It is used for patients who have severe pain, for example, chronic lower back pain from an injury. In this method, electrodes are attached to the patient's skin over a painful area. It causes interference with the transmission of painful stimuli, thus reducing the patient's pain sensation. Many patients with chronic severe pain need narcotics to ease the pain. However, TENS can control the pain and lesson the need for addictive drugs. TENS can be used by patients at home.

THERAPEUTIC MODALITIES

Sometimes, therapeutic exercise is not the best or only way to restore injured or painful joints and tissues. A patient's condition may respond equally well to certain physical agents, called **modalities,** which take advantage of the properties of heat, cold, electricity, light, and water to improve circulation, minimize pain, and correct or alleviate muscular and joint malfunction.

Many modalities have been around for centuries, and some can easily be performed by the patient or caregiver at home. Modalities can be used locally to treat a small area at a time or systemically to alter a patient's temperature or soothe many groups of painful muscles or joints. The patient's condition and rehabilitation program both influence the modality or combination of modalities used.

A provider order is required for any therapeutic modality.

Heat and Cold

Heat, or **thermotherapy,** acts on the body by causing vasodilation (dilation of the blood vessels). The effect of heat increases circulation to an area and acts to speed up the repair process. Heat can be used to:

- Relax muscle spasms
- Relieve pain in a strained muscle or sprained joint
- Relieve localized congestion and swelling
- Increase drainage from an infected area
- Increase tissue metabolism and repair
- Combat local infection
- Increase circulation
- Improve mobility before exercise

However, because heat dilates the blood vessels and increases circulation, it also acts to speed up the inflammatory process, which can lead to more serious problems, such as increased bleeding and swelling. Heat should not be used longer than its prescribed length of time.

Cold applications, or cryotherapy, are used to constrict blood vessels and slow or stop the flow of blood to an area. This process, also called **vasoconstriction,** slows down the inflammatory process, which can reduce or prevent swelling of inflamed tissues, reduce bleeding, numb the pain sensation by acting as a topical anesthetic, and reduce drainage to an area.

By understanding how heat and cold affect the body, it is easier to observe whether they are having the desired therapeutic effect. Because heat and cold modalities can be extremely effective, they are widely used for treating certain physical conditions. However, the effects of heat and cold modalities depend on several conditions: the type of modality used, the length of time it is applied, the patient's condition, and the area or areas being treated.

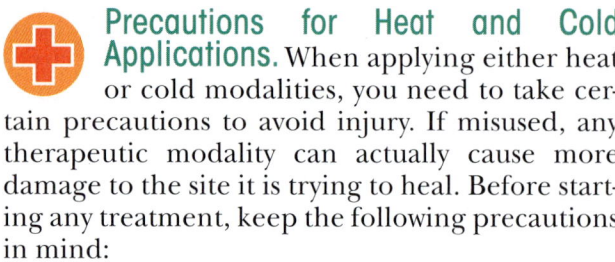

Precautions for Heat and Cold Applications. When applying either heat or cold modalities, you need to take certain precautions to avoid injury. If misused, any therapeutic modality can actually cause more damage to the site it is trying to heal. Before starting any treatment, keep the following precautions in mind:

- Infants and patients who cannot report a burning sensation should be watched carefully. Infants and older adults are particularly susceptible to burns.
- Heat and cold sensitivity varies with patients; check patients frequently and never leave them alone.
- Never have a patient lie on a heating pad because severe burning can result. Place a rubber cover over the heating pad if using with moist dressings.
- Always wrap appliances, whether warm or cold, with cloth before applying them to the skin.
- Only soak or immerse patients in water between 104°F and 113°F (40–45°C). Temperatures of 116°F (47°C) or greater can cause burning.
- Never use heat within the first 48 hours of an acute inflammatory process and never apply heat to newly burned skin.
- Watch carefully persons with impaired circulation; cardiovascular, renal, sensorineural, or respiratory conditions; or osteoporosis. Tell patient to report pain or numbness.
- Excessive cold can damage tissues.
- Lack of sensation to a therapy may mean impaired circulation to an area, and the patient may be unable to report a burning sensation.
- Heat concentrates in metal materials, so have patients remove all jewelry and other metal objects, and administer the treatment on nonmetal tables and chairs.

EHR

- Document in the patient's chart or electronic medical record the type of modality, length of time applied, color of patient's skin, and any discomfort.

Moist and Dry Heat

Moist Heat Therapies. Moist heat refers to heat modalities that feel moist against the skin. Moist heat penetrates better than dry heat and aids in improving circulation, relaxation, and mobility.

Warm Soaks. Warm soaks are generally used for soaking the extremities and can be administered easily at home by the patient or caregiver. The patient's body part is gradually immersed in plain or medicated water no hotter than 110°F (44°C) for a short time, usually no more than about 15 minutes. The patient should be positioned to be comfortable. Observe the patient's skin for excessive redness and, if noticed, remove the limb at once. Always dry the skin carefully by patting, not rubbing, it.

Total body immersion in water 104–113°F can be administered in a whirlpool bath or special Hubbard tank. This treatment is often prescribed to promote relaxation, circulation, and movement of limbs in preparation for exercise. The mechanical action of agitating water moving over the body in a whirlpool is called hydromassage and can both relax muscles and stimulate circulation. The Hubbard tank is a bit larger and provides room for limited body exercise without the effects of gravity.

Sitz Bath. A sitz bath is a bath of warm water in which only the hips and buttocks (perineum) are immersed for relief of pain and discomfort from conditions such as rectal surgery and episiotomy. It is therapeutic and cleansing and will help relieve discomfort by reducing swelling and improve healing by stimulating blood flow.

Warm Wet Compresses and Packs. A warm wet compress is usually applied to a small area. It is prepared by soaking and wringing out either a square of gauze or other absorbent material (such as a clean washcloth) and applying it for a limited time to the affected area (Figure 21-23). Warm compresses can be administered easily at home. A warm pack is used for a larger area and generally involves the use of a professional warm pack (**hydrocollator**) administered in the clinical setting. This type of warm pack is soaked in water 150–170°F, removed with tongs and drained, and placed over larger areas such as the back or shoulders. Check color of patient's skin frequently.

Paraffin Wax Bath. This type of treatment is most often used for chronic joint disease, such as rheumatoid arthritis. The bath mixture of seven parts paraffin to one part mineral oil is heated to melting (about 127°F) and the body part is dipped in the mixture several times until a thick coat of wax builds up. The body part is then wrapped in foil, cloth, or plastic wrap to help insulate the heat, then left on for 30 minutes or less. Once peeled off, the circulatory effects of this treatment can last up to several hours. It is an excellent modality for warming up joints before ROM or other exercises. This modality, ordered by the provider, will be carried out in the physical therapy department by a professional therapist (Figure 21-24).

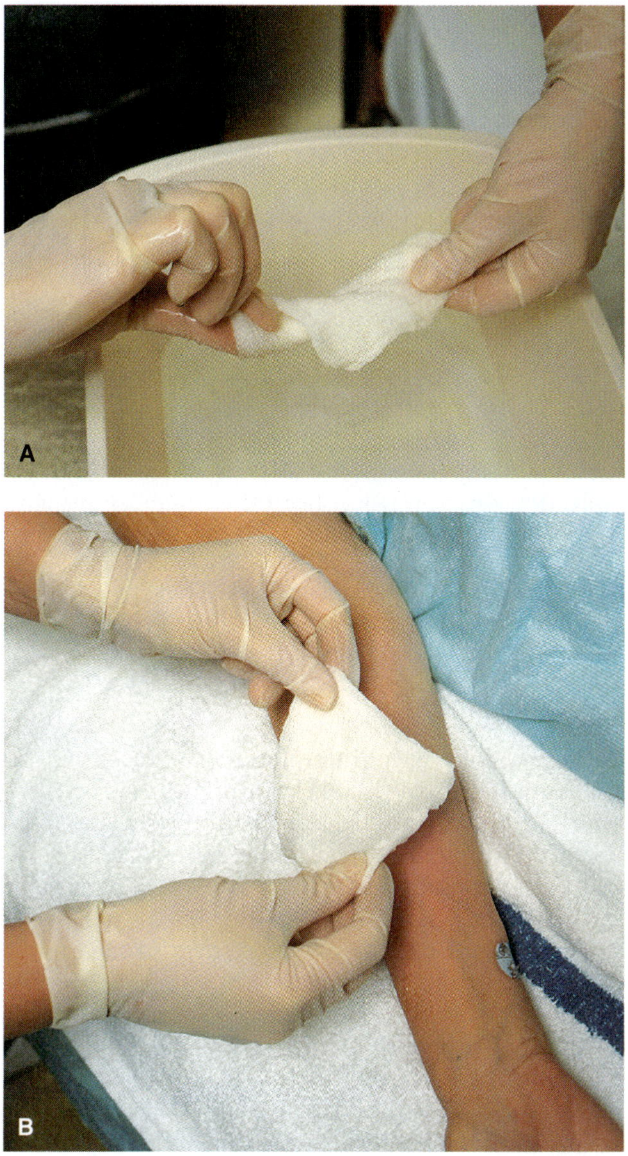

Figure 21-23 (A) Dip warm compresses frequently into a basin of warm water to keep them warm. (B) Apply compresses directly to the skin. *NOTE:* Limb will be wrapped in a towel that will then be covered with a blue plastic wrap. This helps keep the compresses warm.

Dry Heat Therapies. Dry heat applications feel dry against the skin and do not penetrate like moist heat. They are used more to improve circulation for the purposes of relieving swelling and healing wounds, as well as to relax muscles and reduce muscle spasms. Most dry heat modalities can be performed easily by the patient or caregiver at home.

Heating Pads and Packs. Heating pads and commercially prepared packs are used for smaller areas and should always be covered with a cloth before applying against the skin. Never let a patient lie directly on a heating pad because burns can result. Set the switch on the heating pad to a low or medium setting and observe the proper time of exposure.

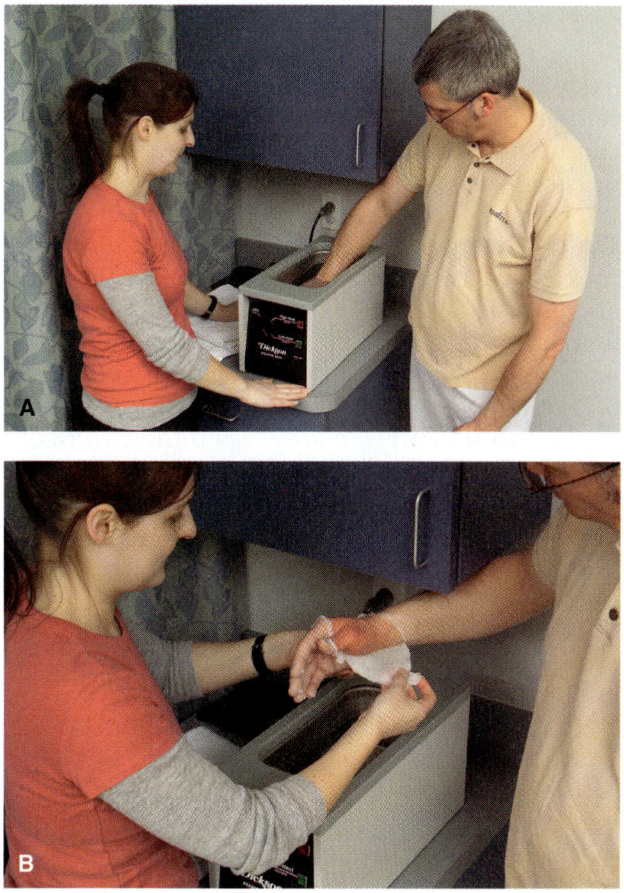

Figure 21-24 (A) A body part is dipped into the paraffin bath three or four times to create a layer of warm wax on the skin. (B) After the wax has been in place for 20 to 30 minutes, it is peeled off and discarded.

An Aquamatic K-Pad® is a commercial pad that is safer to use than a heating pad or commercially prepared pack because you can maintain a constant temperature and regulate that temperature more carefully. It is a pad with tubes that are filled with distilled water and heated by a control unit. The pad must be covered and left on the patient for no more than about 30 minutes. The temperature usually is set between 95 and 100°F.

Moist and Dry Cold

Moist Cold Therapies. Moist cold therapies refer to cold modalities that feel moist against the skin. Moist cold, as with moist heat, penetrates better than dry cold and is used to prevent swelling or edema, relieve pain or tenderness, and reduce body temperature. Most cold therapies can be performed easily at home by the patient or caregiver.

Cold Compresses and Packs. Cold compresses are used for smaller areas, and cold packs are used for larger areas. For a cold compress, immerse the cold cloth, gauze, or other clean material in a basin filled with ice and cold water or solution prescribed. Wring out the cloth and apply it to the affected area. Keep the cloth cold by immersing it several times throughout the treatment or use a syringe to add cold water to the compress. Cold or ice packs are administered in the same manner. Check patient's skin frequently.

Dry Cold Therapies. Dry cold treatments are used for the same reasons as moist cold treatments but are better for bleeding and acute injuries. Dry cold is also an excellent therapy for sprains, strains, burns, or bruises.

The temperature used depends on the area being treated and the method used, as well as the patient's tolerance for cold temperatures. In general, the colder the temperature, the shorter the duration of exposure.

Ice Packs. Dry cold treatments include ice packs and commercially prepared chemical ice packs or cold packs. Always cover the pack with cloth before applying it to the skin (Figure 21-25). Generally, ice packs can be kept on the body longer than heat packs, about 30 minutes. Check color of patient's skin frequently (see Chapter 9). A commercial ice pack can be used for smaller areas and can usually be chilled in the freezer. Because they do not freeze and become solid, these ice packs are pliable, making them ideal for contouring to the body part being treated. The cold packs are usually single-use. They must be activated by a blow to the pack before applying or by squeezing the pack.

Critical Thinking

How do heat and cold affect the body's physiology and for what conditions should each be used?

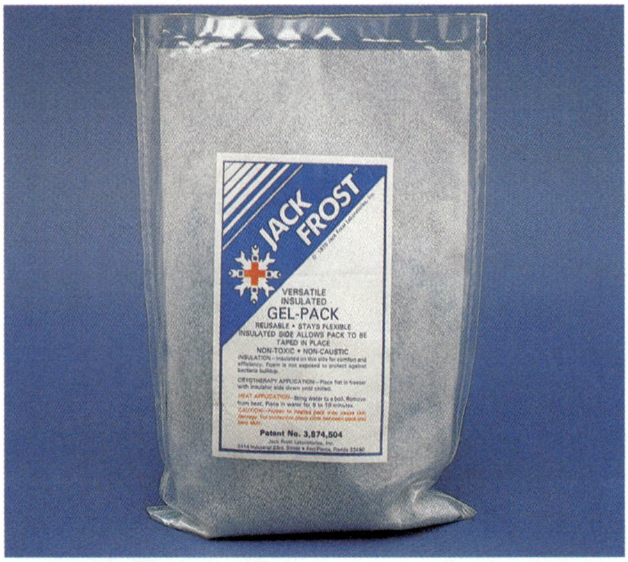

Figure 21-25 A chemical ice pack. These should be covered with a cloth before applying to the skin.

Ultrasound

Ultrasound is a high-frequency acoustic vibration that is part of the electromagnetic spectrum, and its frequencies are beyond the perception of the human ear. This type of treatment uses high-frequency sound waves that are converted to heat in the deeper tissues.

Ultrasound is an effective form of treatment for chronic pain or acute injuries such as sprains or strains. It relaxes muscle spasms, increases the elasticity of tissue such as tendons and ligaments, and stimulates circulation, which, in turn, speeds up the healing process.

Ultrasound waves travel best in tissue that has a high concentration of water, such as muscles. They cannot penetrate and move through tissue such as bone that has a low water content. In fact, ultrasound treatment must be used carefully near bones, particularly those

Patient Education

Neither heat nor cold applications should be left on the skin for prolonged periods, because both can have counterproductive effects if not monitored carefully. When applying heat or cold, periodically check the skin for signs of paleness or redness. If the patient experiences any numbness or tingling reaction, discontinue the application. Report the observations, and document.

near the surface, because their waves are capable of concentrating in one area and causing damage.

Because ultrasound waves cannot be conducted through air, a special gel is applied to the skin surface that acts as a conduit. The sound waves are generated through an applicator that is rubbed over the gel. This applicator must be kept moving to prevent any internal damage caused by too high a concentration of sound waves. The duration of treatment lasts anywhere from 5 to 15 minutes, depending on the condition being treated and the recommendation of the physician or other health care provider. It is important to note that, because of its potential dangers, ultrasound treatment should only be administered if the medical assistant or other caregiver is specially trained in its safe and effective use.

Massage Therapy

Massage therapy has become recognized as a modality that is basic to physical therapy. The majority of states require a massage therapist to be licensed in order to practice the profession.

History shows massage therapy is one of the earliest practices for helping the body restore healthy functioning. It is used to relieve minor aches and pains, thus helping patients feel relaxed and refreshed. Massage therapy is safe and advantageous for most individuals, from infants to older adults.

Some physiologic benefits include increased metabolism, promotion of healing, soothing of muscles, relief of discomfort and pain, and improved circulation. Massage therapy can be used to manage the pain associated with conditions such as whiplash injury, muscle spasm, sciatic nerve pain, arthritis, and many other health problems.

Therapists use their hands to handle or touch the soft tissues of the patients' body. The movements stimulate the patients' circulation, help relieve discomfort, improve range of motion, and relax muscles. Some of the movements include percussion (tapping), rubbing, pressing, **petrissage** (kneading), and **effleurage** (stroking) of the soft tissue (Figure 21-26).

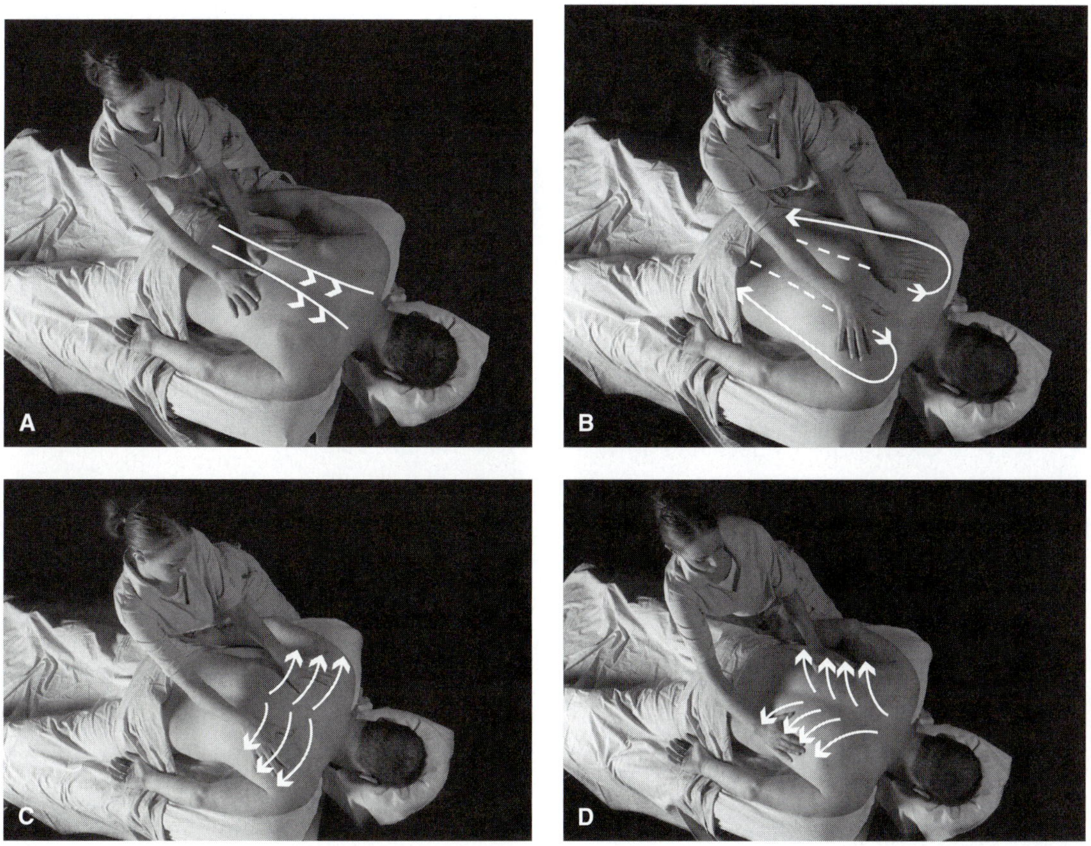

Figure 21-26 (A) The therapist applies long strokes up along the muscles on each side of the spine. (B) Effleurage strokes are used up the back and over the shoulders. Effleurage or gliding strokes are applied in the direction of venous blood and lymph flow. (C) The muscles of the back are stroked outward. (D) Fan stroking is applied to the back.

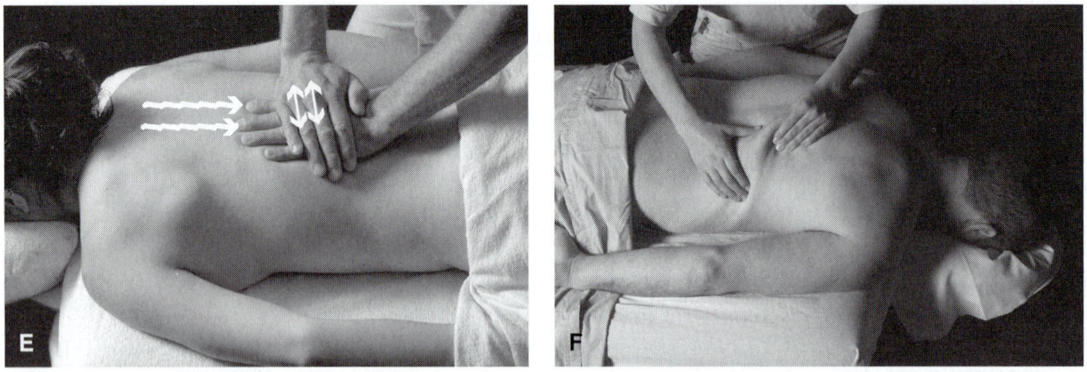

Figure 21-26 (continued) (E) Vibration movements are applied to the vertebrae, and vibrations go back and forth as the therapist moves down along the spine. (F) Petrissage is applied to the entire side opposite the therapist.

Massage therapy is inappropriate for patients with open wounds, neuropathies, shock, severe upper respiratory illnesses, varicose veins, phlebitis, high blood pressure, and often patients with osteoporosis (bones can easily break).

There are psychological benefits as well. Massage therapy relieves stress and tension; refreshes the patient thereby lessening fatigue; and regenerates energy.

Massage therapy has been accepted and recognized by the medical community and the community-at-large as a complementary or alternative form of medicine.

Procedure 21-1

Transferring Patient from Wheelchair to Examination Table

STANDARD PRECAUTIONS:

PURPOSE:

To move a patient safely from a wheelchair to the examination table.

EQUIPMENT/SUPPLIES:

Stool with rubber tips and a handle for gripping
Gait belt

PROCEDURE STEPS:

1. Wash hands.
2. Identify the patient and introduce yourself. Explain to the patient what you are going to do.
3. Place the wheelchair next to the examination table and lock the brakes. **CAUTION:** The side nearest the examination table should be the patient's stronger side to allow the patient to balance on that leg during the transfer.
4. Place the gait belt snugly around the patient's waist and tuck the excess end under the belt (Figure 21-27A).
5. Move the footrests up and out of the way. Have the patient place feet on the floor. Newer wheelchairs have removable footrests. Taking them off enables you to put the wheelchair closer to the examination table. There is also less chance of being bumped or bruised by the wheelchair.
6. Position the stool in front of the examination table as close to the wheelchair as possible (Figure 21-27B).
7. Have the patient move to the edge of the wheelchair.

continues

Procedure 21-1 (continued)

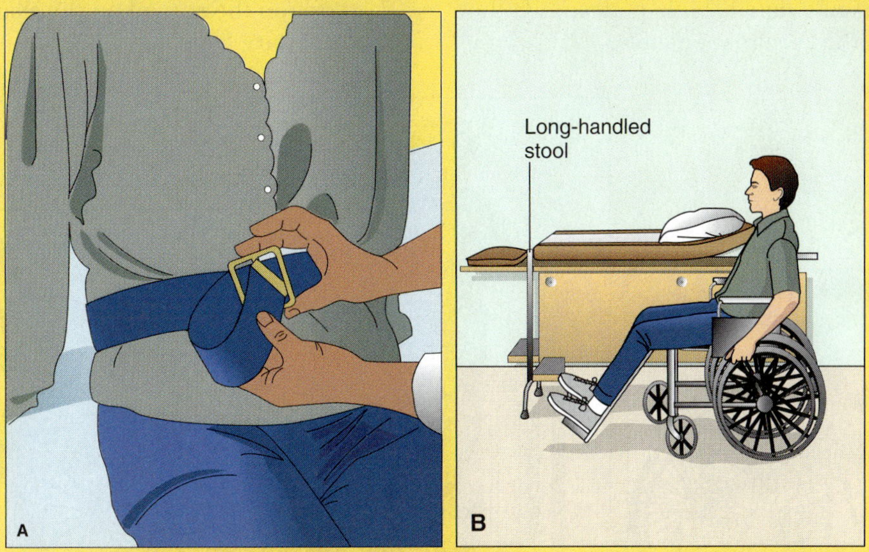

Figure 21-27 (A) The gait belt is always applied snugly around the patient's waist before attempting to move or ambulate with the patient. (B) Position the long-handled stool in front of the examination table and as close to the wheelchair as possible.

8. Stand directly in front of the patient with your feet slightly apart. Bending at the hips and knees, grasp the gait belt and have the patient place his or her hands on the armrests of the wheelchair so he or she can push up when you give the signal (Figure 21-27C). If the patient does not have the upper body strength to push off, simply let the arms rest in front of him or her.
9. Give a signal and lift the gait belt upward, pushing with your knees. If the patient has the strength in the legs, he or she should push with the legs in addition to pushing up with the arms.
10. Still grasping the gait belt, have the patient step onto the stool with the foot closest to the examination table, and pivot so the back is to the examination table (Figure 21-27D). Make sure the buttocks are lifted slightly higher than the bed. Support the patient's weaker, outer leg with your leg furthest from the examination table.
11. Have the patient grasp the stool handle and place the other hand on the examination table.
12. Gently ease the patient to a sitting position on the examination table.
13. Position the patient on the examination table as necessary.
14. Move the wheelchair and stool out of the way.

Modification: Two-Person Transfer

1. Place the gait belt snugly around the patient's waist and tuck the excess end under the belt.
2. Have one person stand in front of the patient and the other to the side.
3. Both persons should grasp the gait belt from underneath. Have the patient place the hands on the armrests of the wheelchair.
4. On one person's signal, both persons pull the patient straight up. The patient should also push up with the hands, but if there is little upper body strength to push off, simply let the arms rest in front (Figure 21-28).
5. The person nearest the examination table moves the wheelchair out of the way, whereas the other pivots the patient and has the patient place his or her stronger leg on the stool. If the patient has the upper body strength, he or she should also grasp the handle of the stool.

continues

Procedure 21-1 (continued)

6. On one person's signal, both persons lift the patient onto the examination table.
7. Position the patient on the examination table as necessary.

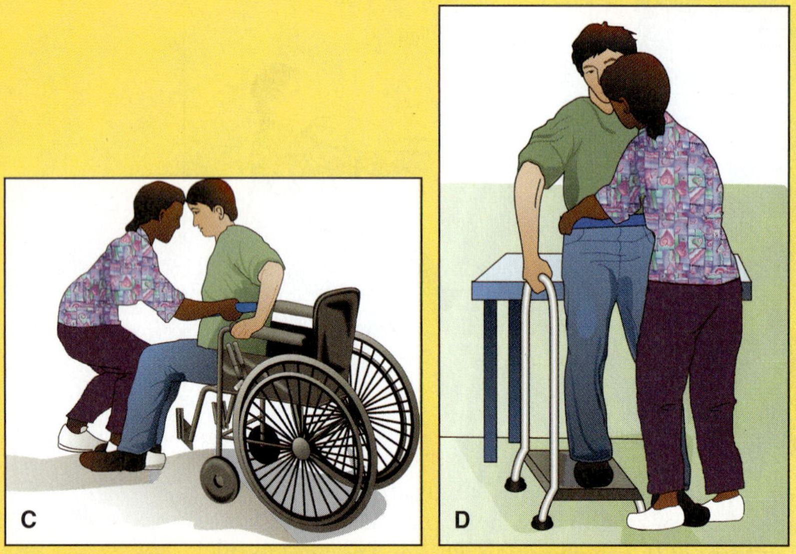

Figure 21-27 (continued) (C) Before lifting, observe proper body mechanics to avoid injuring yourself or the patient. (D) Check that the patient's foot is firmly placed on the stool before completing the transfer.

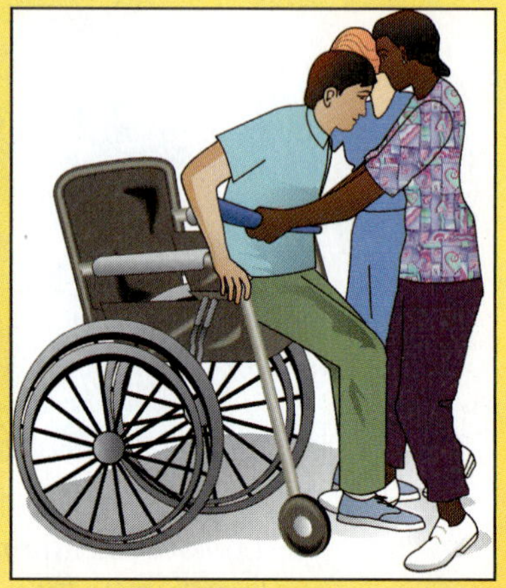

Figure 21-28 A two-person transfer is used when the patient does not have the upper body strength to help move himself or herself.

Procedure 21-2

Transferring Patient from Examination Table to Wheelchair

STANDARD PRECAUTIONS:

PURPOSE:

To move a patient safely from the examination table to a wheelchair.

EQUIPMENT/SUPPLIES:

Stool with rubber tips and a handle for gripping
Gait belt

PROCEDURE STEPS:

1. Wash hands.
2. Identify the patient and introduce yourself. Explain to the patient what you are going to do.
3. Position the wheelchair next to the examination table and lock the brakes. *NOTE:* Place the wheelchair so it is closest to the patient's stronger side so the patient can transfer weight onto the stronger foot as he or she gets down.
4. Position the stool next to the wheelchair.

continues

Procedure 21-2 (continued)

5. Assist the patient to rise to a sitting position. Place the gait belt snugly around the patient's waist and tuck the excess end under the belt.
6. Place your arm under the patient's arm and around the shoulders, and your other arm under the knees. Pivot the patient so the legs are dangling over the side of the examination table.
7. Keeping a hand on the patient, move so you are directly in front.
8. Grasp the patient by placing your hands under the gait belt. Plant your feet shoulder's width apart and bend your knees so you will have a strong base of support.
9. On your signal, pull the patient slightly toward you so the feet come down onto the stool. The patient should push off the examination table and grasp the stool handle for support.
10. Still grasping the gait belt, have the patient step onto the floor with the strong leg, and pivot at the same time so the back is to the wheelchair.
11. Have the patient grasp the armrests of the wheelchair.
12. Bending from your knees and hips, gently lower the patient into the wheelchair and make sure the patient is comfortably seated.
13. Lower the footrests and place the feet on them.

Procedure 21-3

Assisting the Patient to Stand and Walk

STANDARD PRECAUTIONS:

PURPOSE:

To help a patient ambulate safely.

EQUIPMENT/SUPPLIES:

Gait belt

PROCEDURE STEPS:

1. Wash hands.
2. Identify the patient and introduce yourself. Explain to the patient what you are going to do.
3. Lock the brakes on the wheelchair, if the patient is using one. Place the patient's feet on the floor and move the foot plates out of the way.
4. Instruct the patient to slide forward in the chair.
5. Place the gait belt around the patient's waist and tuck the excess end under the belt.
6. Standing directly in front of the patient, grasp the gait belt from underneath and assist to stand on your signal. At the same time, have the patient push up on the armrests of the wheelchair.
7. Steady the patient momentarily and watch for balance, strength, and skin color. If necessary have patient sit back in wheelchair and take his or her pulse and/or blood pressure.
8. If the patient appears steady and has balance, strength, and good skin color, proceed by standing slightly behind and to the side of the patient's weaker side.
9. Grasp the gait belt with one hand and place the other hand on the patient's bent arm for support. Note the gait belt is grasped with your fingers under the belt, palm up and elbow bent (Figure 21-29).
10. Start with the same foot as the patient and keep in step with him or her.
11. Document the procedure in the patient's chart or electronic medical record, including date, time, duration of ambulation, response of patient, and instructions given.

continues

Procedure 21-3 (continued)

Modification: Two-Person Assist with Ambulation

1. Perform the preceding steps 1 through 5.
2. Have a person stand on either side of the patient. Grasp the gait belt from underneath with one hand, and place the other hand on the patient's back for support.
3. During ambulation, there should be a person on either side of the patient and slightly behind (Figure 21-30). Both persons should be grasping the gait belt throughout the ambulation session.
4. Document the procedure in the patient's chart or electronic medical record, including date, time, duration of ambulation, response of patient, and instructions given.

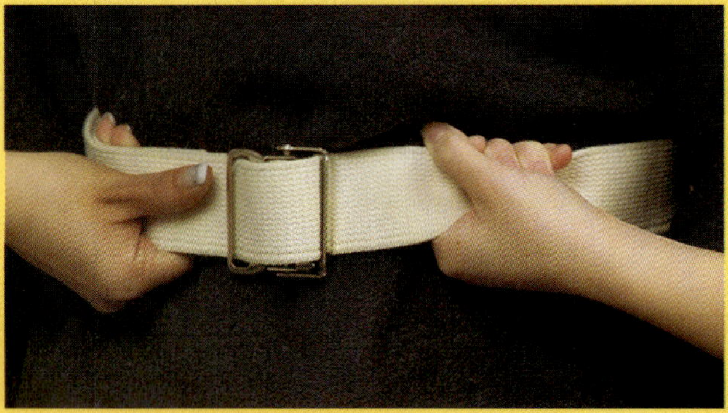

Figure 21-29 Firmly grasp the gait belt from underneath, with the palm up and elbow bent.

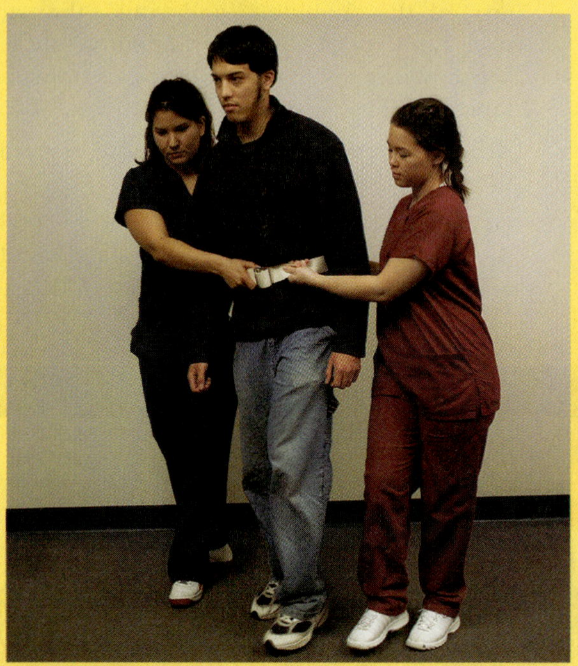

Figure 21-30 When two persons are assisting with ambulation, they should stand on either side of the patient.

DOCUMENTATION

7/14/20XX 2:30 PM Patient states she has been doing "fairly well" in physical therapy. She says she walks short distances, about 10 feet. Assisted with ambulation. Seems steady on her feet. Says she feels "very good." W. Slawson, CMA (AAMA) ———

DOCUMENTATION

7/14/20XX 2:30 PM Patient has been to physical therapy a total of 15 times. Dr. Woo wants patient to ambulate to see her progress. Assisted patient to ambulate with another person assisting. Did very well. Walked about 100 feet. Color remained good. P 100. B. Beckus, RMA ———

Procedure 21-4

Care of the Falling Patient

PURPOSE:
To help the patient fall safely to prevent injury.

EQUIPMENT/SUPPLIES:
Gait belt (should already be on patient)

PROCEDURE STEPS:

1. Keep a firm hand on the gait belt. **CAUTION:** Never grab clothing, because it can shift and become unstable.
2. If the patient falls backward, widen your stance to become a more stable base of support to fall against (Figure 21-31). Gently guide the patient to the floor, call for assistance, and take pulse and blood pressure.
3. If the patient falls to either side, steady back onto the feet. To do this, you will need to move your foot in the direction of the fall. Inquire whether the patient would like to terminate the ambulation session and check for signs of fatigue. If necessary, call for assistance. Check blood pressure and pulse.

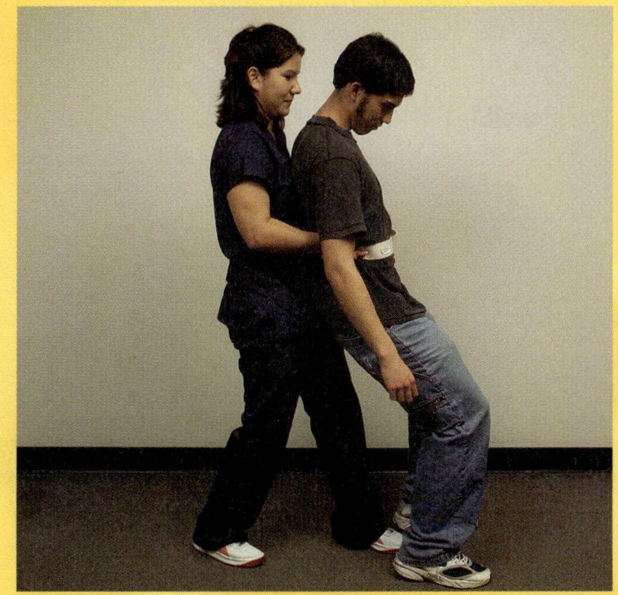

Figure 21-31 Support a falling patient with a wide base of support.

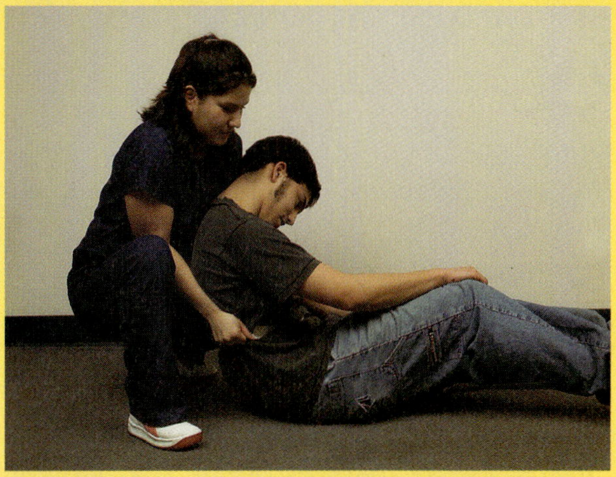

Figure 21-32 Ease the falling patient to the floor and try to protect the head.

4. Should the patient fall forward, support him or her around the waist. Step forward with your outer leg and gently lower to the floor, making sure to protect from injury (Figure 21-32). Call for assistance and take blood pressure and pulse.
5. Have the patient examined by the provider before moving patient again.
6. Document the fall in an incident report and in the patient's chart or electronic medical record.

DOCUMENTATION

1/21/20XX 11:30 AM While walking to exam room with assistance the patient suddenly began to fall forward with knees buckling. Says she feels "faint." Eased to the floor gently. Did not strike any body parts during fall. BP 110/60, P 108 (lying on floor). BP and pulse rechecked when patient placed in wheelchair. BP 120/78, P 92. Dr. King notified. B. Abbott, RMA ———

Procedure 21-5

Assisting a Patient to Ambulate with a Walker

STANDARD PRECAUTIONS:

PURPOSE:

To allow a patient to ambulate independently and safely with a walker.

EQUIPMENT/SUPPLIES:

Walker
Gait belt

PROCEDURE STEPS:

1. Wash hands.
2. Identify the patient and introduce yourself. Explain to the patient what you are going to do.
3. Apply the gait belt snugly around the patient's waist and tuck the excess end under the belt.
4. Check the walker to be sure the rubber suction tips are secure on all the legs. Check the handrests for rough or damaged edges that could cut or pinch the patient. The adjustments should be tightened so they will not slip.
5. Be sure the patient is wearing good walking shoes with a rubber sole.
6. Check the height of the walker. The handrests should be level with the tip of the patient's femur, and the elbows should be flexed at a 30-degree angle.
7. Position the patient inside the walker, and instruct the patient to hold onto the handles while keeping the walker in front.
8. Position yourself behind and slightly to the side of the patient.
9. Have the patient lift the walker and place all four legs of the walker in front so the back legs are even with the patient's toes.
10. Instruct the patient to lean forward and transfer the weight and step into the walker, first with the stronger leg, then the weaker leg. Make sure the stronger leg is brought past the weaker leg.
11. Monitor the patient carefully. Be alert for signs of fatigue and be ready to assist the patient to fall without injury.
12. If the walker has rollers, the patient simply rolls the walker ahead a comfortable distance, then walks into it. The patient can also walk normally with a rolling walker by simply rolling it in front and leaning into the gait, using the walker for support.
13. Document the date, time, duration of ambulation, response of patient, and instructions given in the patient's chart or electronic medical record.

DOCUMENTATION

2/12/20XX 1:35 PM Patient assisted with ambulation using a walker for the first time. Walked approximately 50 feet. Did well. Walked to reception desk and back. No change in color. P 100. J. Guerro, CMA (AAMA) ————

Procedure 21-6

Teaching the Patient to Ambulate with Crutches

STANDARD PRECAUTIONS:

PURPOSE:
To teach the patient how to ambulate safely using crutches.

EQUIPMENT/SUPPLIES:
Crutches
Gait belt

PROCEDURE STEPS:

1. Wash hands.
2. Identify the patient and introduce yourself. Explain to the patient what you are going to do.
3. Assemble the crutches and be sure they are in good working order. Make sure there are rubber suction tips on the bottom ends, and that they are not worn or torn. Check the bar and handrest to be sure they are covered with padding, and that the padding is not cracked or worn. Be sure the wing nuts are tight.
4. Check the measurement of the crutches. Pediatric crutches must be used for pediatric patients.
5. Apply the gait belt and assist the patient to stand and place the crutches under the axillae.
6. Instruct the patient to carry the weight completely on the hands and not on the axillae.
7. Have the patient put all the weight on the good leg, and bend the weak leg slightly so it will not drag on the floor.
8. Assist the patient with the required gait.
9. Wash hands.
10. Document the date, time, duration of ambulation, and instructions given in patient's chart or electronic medical record.

DOCUMENTATION

3/24/20XX 4:45 P.M. Crutches adjusted to patient's height. Three-point gait used. Tolerated well. J. Guerro, CMA (AAMA) ———

Procedure 21-7

Assisting a Patient to Ambulate with a Cane

STANDARD PRECAUTIONS:

PURPOSE:
To teach patients how to walk safely with a cane.

EQUIPMENT/SUPPLIES:
Appropriate cane for patient
Gait belt

PROCEDURE STEPS:

1. Wash hands.
2. Ascertain what type of cane the provider or therapist indicates your patient is to use and assemble the equipment.
3. Identify the patient and introduce yourself. Explain to the patient what you are going to do.
4. Check the cane to be sure the bottom has a rubber suction tip that is not worn. If a quad

continues

Procedure 21-7 (continued)

or walkcane is to be used, make sure all the legs have rubber suction tips.

5. Apply the gait belt snugly around the patient's waist if needed and tuck the excess end under the belt. Assist the patient to a standing position.
6. Place the cane relatively close to the body to the side of the foot of the strong leg. Adjust the cane so the handle is at the level of the patient's hip joint (Figure 21-33).
7. During weightbearing, the patient's elbow should be flexed 20 to 30 degrees.
8. The cane and the involved leg are advanced simultaneously.
9. Have the patient move the weak leg forward while transferring the weight to the cane.
10. Have the patient move the strong leg forward past the cane.
11. Follow along behind and to the side of the patient's weak side.
12. Wash your hands.
13. Document the date, time, duration of ambulation, response of patient, and instructions given in patient's chart or electronic medical record.

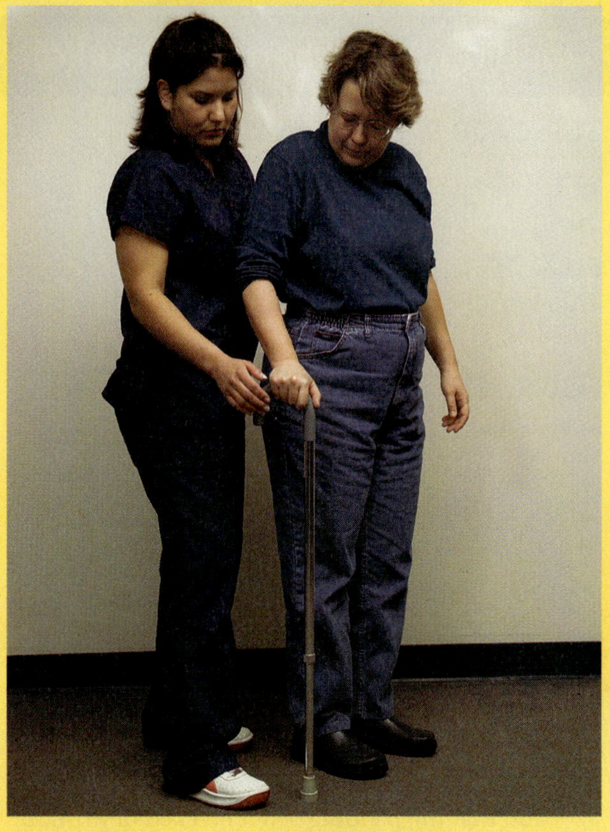

Figure 21-33 When placing the cane, be sure the handle comes to the top of the patient's hip and elbow is flexed 20 to 30 degrees.

DOCUMENTATION

4/17/20XX 10:30 AM Standard cane adjusted to patient's hip joint. Ambulated about 100 yards and seemed to tolerate it well. W. Slawson, CMA (AAMA)

Case Study 21-1

Refer to the scenario at the beginning of the chapter.

Mrs. Williams comes to Inner City Urgent Care because she fell when she tripped on a scatter rug at home. Her son helped her to the clinic. Her left ankle is swollen and painful.

CASE STUDY REVIEW

1. What action(s) should you take immediately to help Mrs. Williams?
2. After X-rays, Dr. King determined that Mrs. Williams has an ankle fracture, and he applied a cast to it. He wants you to fit Mrs. Williams to crutches and teach her how to use them. What gait will Dr. King have you teach the patient? Why?

Case Study 21-2

It is a mild summer afternoon in the city of Carlton, the home of Inner City Health Care. The softball season is in full swing, and Inner City has treated its share of players and spectators who have had minor injuries. On this particular Tuesday, Bill Schwarz, a regular patient, comes in late in the day in obvious pain. Bruce Goldman, the clinical medical assistant on duty, quickly gets the patient into a wheelchair. From the patient's description of the situation and the pain, Bruce suspects a sprained ankle. Dr. Woo is on call and is available to examine the patient immediately. Dr. Woo asks Bruce to transfer Bill from the wheelchair to the examination table.

CASE STUDY REVIEW

1. What are some of the general principles the medical assistant should observe during any transfer?
2. Summarize the steps involved in transferring the patient from the wheelchair to the examination table.
3. What are possible treatment choices Dr. Woo may use?

Case Study 21-3

After diagnosing Mr. Schwarz with a sprained left ankle, Dr. Woo has prescribed an Ace bandage to the ankle, crutches, and an ice pack to be applied to the ankle. He has also given Mr. Schwarz a prescription for pain relievers and has recommended that Mr. Schwarz stay off his feet as much as possible. He is to keep the leg elevated with an ice pack on it.

CASE STUDY REVIEW

1. Explain what you would tell Mr. Schwarz about applying the ice pack to his ankle at home.
2. What patient education can be used in this situation?

SUMMARY

Rehabilitation medicine is a field of medical disciplines that specializes in both preventing disease or injury and restoring physical function. It uses a combination of physical and mechanical agents to aid in the diagnosis, treatment, and prevention of diseases or bodily injury, including exercise and a variety of treatment modalities.

Much of what a medical assistant might do on the job in this field involves some form of lifting or moving of heavy objects. It is important to remember to use good body mechanics to prevent back or other injury. When transferring patients, good body mechanics ensures the safety of both caregiver and patient. If necessary, get someone to help with the transfer.

Helping patients to ambulate safely after a period of sedentary recuperation is an important part of a rehabilitation program. If they are not able to ambulate on their own, patients can be fitted for a variety of assistive walking devices, including walkers, crutches, and canes. Crutch walking, by far the most common use of an assistive device, can be done using one of several walking patterns, or gaits, depending on the patient's condition, strength, and stability. Whatever assistive device is used, it is important that the patient be measured correctly for that device and taught how to periodically check it for safety.

In addition to ambulation, there are a number of other types of therapeutic exercises. Depending on the patient's condition, an exercise program can be prescribed after evaluating the patient's joint ROM and muscle strength. Joints and muscles must be exercised regularly to prevent muscle atrophy or joint contractures, as well as improve circulation and maintain or improve overall health. ROM and other exercises can be performed by the caregiver, the patient, or a combination of the two.

In addition to exercise, a variety of therapeutic modalities might be used as part of the patient's rehabilitation program. The various properties of heat, cold, light, electricity, and water act on the body to improve circulation, minimize pain, or correct or alleviate joint and muscle malfunction. Heat dilates the blood vessels, thereby increasing circulation to an area and speeding up the repair process. Cold constricts the blood vessels, slowing circulation and therefore the inflammatory process. Ultrasound and other electrical **diathermies** use an electrical current to create heat in the deeper tissues of the body. It is important to understand how each modality affects the physiologic functioning of the body and observe certain safety precautions to avoid injuring the patient.

STUDY FOR SUCCESS

To reinforce your knowledge and skills of information presented in this chapter:

- Review the Key Terms
- Practice the Procedures
- Consider the Case Studies and discuss your conclusions
- Answer the Review Questions
  - Multiple Choice
  - Critical Thinking
- Navigate the Internet by completing the Web Activities
- Practice the StudyWARE activities on your student CD
- Apply your knowledge in the Student Workbook activities
- Complete the Web Tutor sections
- View and discuss the DVD situations

REVIEW QUESTIONS

Multiple Choice

1. Brushing teeth, getting dressed, and eating are referred to as:
   a. rehabilitation medicine
   b. activities of daily living
   c. assistive behaviors
   d. occupational therapy
2. Hemiplegia is defined as:
   a. inability of the patient to ambulate properly
   b. severe back pain
   c. paralysis of one side of the body
   d. confinement to a wheelchair
3. Ambulatory assistive devices include:
   a. gait belts
   b. walkers, canes, and crutches
   c. wheelchairs
   d. stools with handholds
4. Motion away from the midline of the body is called:
   a. adduction
   b. pronation
   c. extension
   d. abduction
5. Supination involves:
   a. placing the patient in the supine position
   b. moving the arm so the palm is up
   c. bending a body part
   d. straightening a body part

Critical Thinking

1. Define rehabilitation and explain its importance in patient care.
2. If a patient should fall to the side, what action would you take to ensure safety?
3. Describe the procedure for measuring for axillary crutches.
4. What kind of patient would need a forearm crutch?
5. In crutch-walking gaits, what is a *point*?
6. Describe the five different types of crutch gaits.
7. List the six safety rules for transporting a patient in a wheelchair.
8. What is joint range of motion, how is it measured, and how is the measurement expressed?
9. Describe how ultrasound works and identify the patient conditions for which it is an effective treatment.
10. Explain how to avoid internal damage to the patient when an ultrasound treatment is being performed.

WEB ACTIVITIES

1. Search the Internet for information online about the Americans with Disabilities Act of 1990.
   a. To what group of people does the act apply?
   b. What does the act provide for these individuals?
   c. Does the act have any influence over access to physicians' offices and clinics? Explain.
2. Visit the American Physical Therapy Association (APTA) Web site to find information about (1) repetitive stress injuries, (2) spinal cord injuries, and (3) sports injuries. What therapies can be prescribed for each of these?

REFERENCES/BIBLIOGRAPHY

Beck, F. (2006). *Theory and practice of therapeutic massage* (4th ed.). Clifton Park, NY: Delmar Cengage Learning.

Hegner, B., & Caldwell, E. (2008). *Nursing assistant: A nursing process approach* (10th ed.). Clifton Park, NY: Delmar Cengage Learning.

O'Sullivan, S. B., & Schmitz, T. (2000). *Physical rehabilitation: Assessment and treatment* (4th ed.). Philadelphia: F. A. Davis.

Taber's cyclopedic medical dictionary. (22nd ed.). (2003). Philadelphia: F. A. Davis.

Weiss, R. C. (1999). *The physical therapy aide: A work text.* Clifton Park, NY: Delmar Cengage Learning.

THE DVD HOOK-UP

This chapter discusses the medical assistant's role in assisting with various types of modalities and rehabilitation therapy.

In the first scene of this program, Carla, the medical assistant, helped Jerry through the door. She noticed that Jerry was having a difficult time maneuvering the crutches and the door at the same time, so she took that opportunity to conduct some patient education.

1. Do you think that Carla should have waited until the patient was in the examination room to instruct the patient? Why or why not?
2. In general, what is the public's attitude about rehabilitative therapy?
3. Why does the patient start with the weak leg first, when using a cane or walker?

DVD Journal Summary

Write a paragraph that summarizes what you learned from watching today's DVD program. Many times when a patient has an injury to an extremity, it prohibits him or her from being able to shower properly. What will you do if another coworker starts talking to you about the way a patient looks or smells?

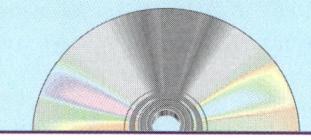

DVD Series
Skills Based Series

Program Number
7

Chapter/Scene Reference
- *Entire program*

Chapter 22 Nutrition in Health and Disease

OUTLINE

OBJECTIVES

The student should strive to meet the following performance objectives and demonstrate an understanding of the facts and principles presented in this chapter through written and oral communication.

1. Define the key terms as presented in the glossary.
2. Describe the relation of nutrition to the functioning of the digestive system.
3. Identify the seven basic nutrient types.
4. Explain the relationship and balance among the three energy nutrients.
5. Distinguish between water-soluble and fat-soluble vitamins.
6. Discuss herbal supplements.
7. Explain the reason for nutrition labels on food packaging.
8. Read and interpret nutrition facts and ingredients on three food packages.
9. Discuss various therapeutic diets, and explain how each can help to control a particular disease state or accommodate a change in the life cycle.

KEY TERMS

Amino Acid
Antioxidant
Ascorbic Acid
Basal Metabolic Rate (BMR)
Beriberi
Cachectic
Calorie
Carotene
Catalyst
Cellulose
Cheilosis
Cholecalciferol
Cobalamin
Coenzyme
Digestion
Diuretic
Electrolytes
Extracellular
Fat-Soluble
Folic Acid
Glycogen
Homeostasis
Major Mineral
Metabolism
Niacin
Nutrient
Nutrition
Oxidation
Pellagra
Preservative
Processed Food
Pyridoxine
Riboflavin
Saturated Fat
Scurvy

KEY TERMS (continued)

Thiamin
Tocopherol
Trace Mineral
Water-Soluble
Xerophthalmia

Scenario

This morning at Inner City Health Care, clinical medical assistant Wanda Slawson, CMA (AAMA), was conferring with Dr. Rice on three of the center's patients whose diets needed modification. With the help of Dr. Rice, Wanda was putting together dietary plans for patients Edith Leonard, who is in her early 70s and is losing weight because she is not eating well enough or often enough; Corey Boyer, who is in the prime of adolescence and capable of eating large quantities of food with little nutritional value; and Annette Samuels, who recently discovered she was pregnant. All these patients have different nutritional requirements, and Wanda wants to encourage all to review and modify their diets.

INTRODUCTION

The human body is in a constant state of fluctuation. The outside environment is constantly changing, and the body requires ***homeostasis,*** *or a continual internal environment, which, in turn, gives us a requirement for nutrients. The nutrients we take into our bodies replenish the materials we have used. In this way, homeostasis is maintained, and our bodies have a relatively balanced internal environment.* ***Nutrition*** *is the study of the taking of nutrients into the body and how the body uses them.*

The normal healthy individual will consume and use close to what the body needs to stay healthy. However, some individuals either do not consume enough nutrients or consume too much of a particular type of nutrient. These are poor diets that can cause particular disease states, and the diet must be modified to return the patient to good health. In addition, specific disease states, such as diabetes mellitus, warrant a change from a normal diet to control the progress of the disease. The human body also goes through many changes in a lifetime and with these changes come new nutritional needs. Protecting health requires paying attention to strategies to prevent disease. The choices made regarding foods consumed and the quality of nutritional intake have a significant impact on the quality and longevity of life. Healthy food choices contribute to living longer and preventing major health issues.

This chapter explores the balance of nutrients required for good health and examines therapeutic modifications to the diet that should take place at various life stages or in the presence of disease. The astute medical assistant will recognize the role of nutrition in maintaining health and will use a knowledge of nutritional principles to encourage patients to adopt a healthy lifestyle.

NUTRITION AND DIGESTION

Nutrition includes ingestion, digestion, absorption, and metabolism of food. Good nutrition results in longer life spans and healthier individuals through the control of preventable diseases.

Spotlight on Certification

RMA Content Outline

- Disorders and diseases
- Health and wellness
- Nutrition

CMA (AAMA) Content Outline

- Developmental stages of the life cycle
- Patient instruction
- Basic principles (food pyramid)
- Special needs (diets)

CMAS Content Outline

- Know various disorders and diseases

The food eaten by an individual is used to build and repair cells and tissues of the body. Therefore, it is important to have knowledge and information about nutrition and to make appropriate food choices for optimum health. A well-nourished individual is less susceptible to infection and disease.

Patient education is important especially when the normal diet must be modified to treat the patient's illness. The medical assistant can answer patient questions only through a knowledge of good nutrition and what constitutes the therapeutic diets prescribed by the provider.

Digestion involves the physical and chemical changes to food that the body makes to make it absorbable. Absorption is the transfer of the nutrients from the gastrointestinal tract into the bloodstream. Without absorption, the body would not receive the nutrients. Figure 22-1 shows the digestive system and its basic functions.

TYPES OF NUTRIENTS

Nutrients serve many purposes in the body. Some nutrients provide energy for the body to perform activities such as the pumping of the heart, the division of cells, or the contraction of muscles. Nutrients also provide building blocks so that proteins or phospholipids can be made within the body, or they can act as catalysts to help processes such as the clotting mechanism proceed at a faster rate. Essentially, ingested substances that help the body stay in its homeostatic state can be called **nutrients.**

Nutrients can be divided into two groups: those that provide energy and those that do not. Both groups are necessary for good health. Table 22-1 lists examples of each of these two groups. Those that provide energy are composed of three types: carbohydrates, fats (lipids), and proteins. Each of these three substances is used in ways other than making energy, but it is important to remember that these are the only substances from which the body can derive energy. Nutrients that do not provide energy are also important and perform other vital functions as described previously. These nutrients include vitamins, minerals, water, and fiber.

Energy Nutrients (Organic)

The three energy nutrients—carbohydrates, fats, and proteins—have one thing in common: all can be converted into energy.

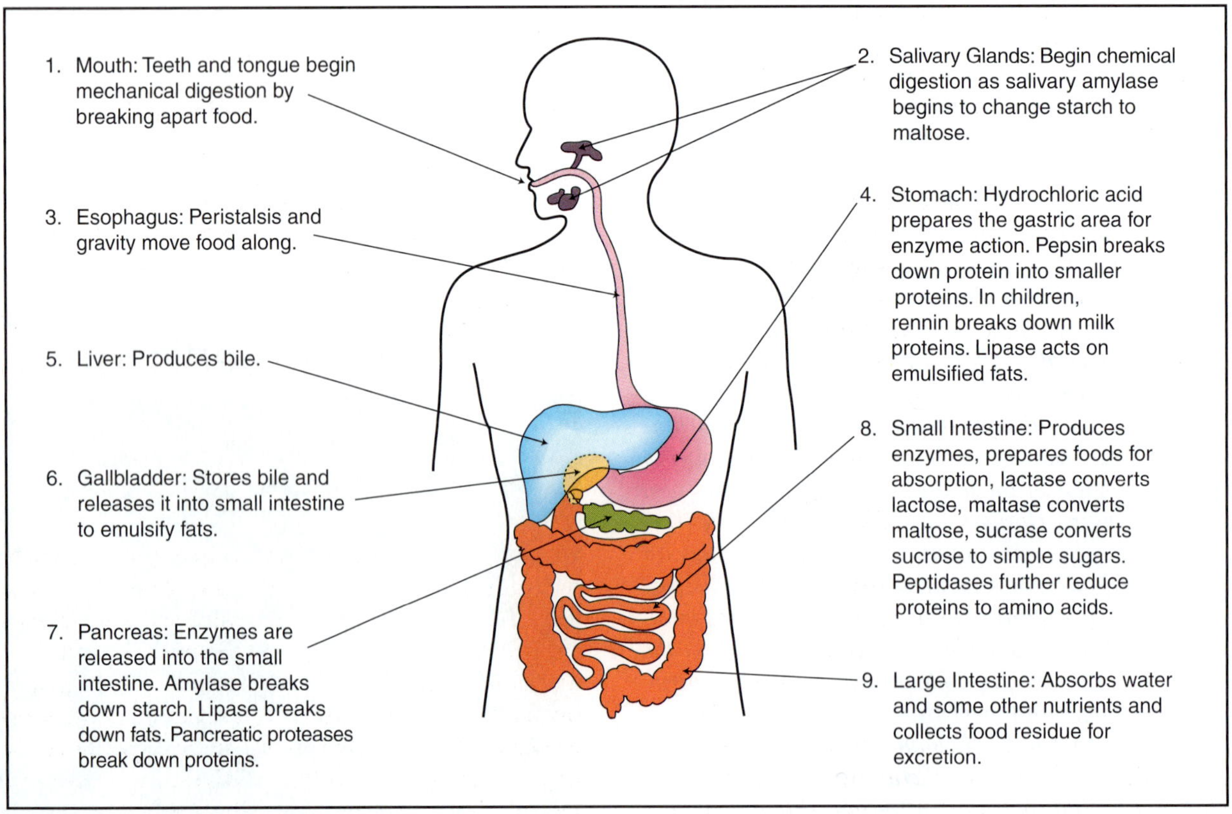

1. Mouth: Teeth and tongue begin mechanical digestion by breaking apart food.
2. Salivary Glands: Begin chemical digestion as salivary amylase begins to change starch to maltose.
3. Esophagus: Peristalsis and gravity move food along.
4. Stomach: Hydrochloric acid prepares the gastric area for enzyme action. Pepsin breaks down protein into smaller proteins. In children, rennin breaks down milk proteins. Lipase acts on emulsified fats.
5. Liver: Produces bile.
6. Gallbladder: Stores bile and releases it into small intestine to emulsify fats.
7. Pancreas: Enzymes are released into the small intestine. Amylase breaks down starch. Lipase breaks down fats. Pancreatic proteases break down proteins.
8. Small Intestine: Produces enzymes, prepares foods for absorption, lactase converts lactose, maltase converts maltose, sucrase converts sucrose to simple sugars. Peptidases further reduce proteins to amino acids.
9. Large Intestine: Absorbs water and some other nutrients and collects food residue for excretion.

Figure 22-1 The digestive system.

Table 22-1 Types of Nutrients

Energy Nutrients (Organic)	**Function**
Carbohydrates (CHO)	Provide energy
Fats (lipids)	Provide energy
Proteins	Build and repair tissues
Other Nutrients	**Function**
Vitamins	Regulate body processes
Minerals	Regulate body processes
Water	Regulate body processes
Fiber	Regulate body processes

Carbohydrates. Carbohydrates provide the major source of energy and are made up of carbon, hydrogen, and oxygen. Although many compounds are made up of these three elements, it is the ratio of these elements that is important. Carbohydrates are made up of units called sugars. The scientific term for sugar is *saccharide,* and carbohydrates can exist as monosaccharides, disaccharides, or polysaccharides.

A monosaccharide is composed of a single unit of sugar, whereas disaccharides have two units of sugar. Together, monosaccharides and disaccharides are known as simple sugars. Examples of monosaccharides are glucose, fructose, and galactose. Glucose is the sugar that the body uses most efficiently, thus most ingested sugar is broken down in the intestines and converted to glucose in the liver. Fructose is found largely in fruits, whereas galactose is a product of lactose digestion. Examples of disaccharides are lactose, maltose, and sucrose. Lactose is found primarily in milk or milk products. Maltose is a product of starch breakdown. Sucrose is one of the sweetest sugars and is what we commonly refer to as table sugar. It occurs naturally in many fruits and vegetables, as well as sugar cane and the sugar beet, which are commercial sources of refined sugar.

Polysaccharides are also known as complex carbohydrates. They are made up of many units of sugar connected together. The most common polysaccharides are starches, glycogen, and fiber. Starches are the most important dietary complex carbohydrate. **Glycogen** is only ingested in small quantities, but is an important carbohydrate form for storage of glucose in the body. Fiber is a special polysaccharide because it cannot be digested.

Because the simple sugars are composed of only one or two units of sugar, their digestion takes little time, and absorption occurs soon after ingestion. The body initially experiences a large increase in sugar concentration in the blood, which is brought down to within a normal range by the release of insulin. The complex carbohydrates require more time to digest, and as a result there is a slow absorption of the single-carbohydrate units as the larger starch molecule is broken down. This is demonstrated in Figure 22-2. In this case, there would be a moderate increase in the sugar levels in the blood, and this would continue for a longer period. A continuous level of sugar in the bloodstream is necessary for a constant energy supply (Figure 22-3). The principle sources of carbohydrates are fruits, vegetables, cereal grains, and sugar.

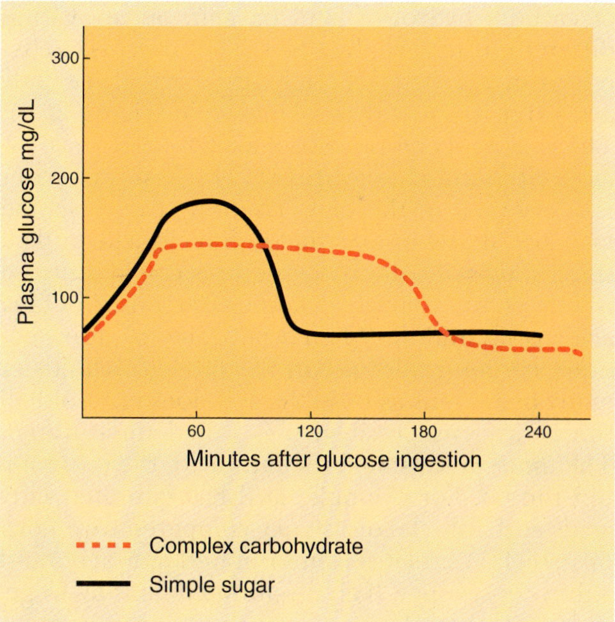

Figure 22-2 This graph shows how complex carbohydrates (red broken line) and simple sugar (black line) are used by the body (in minutes) after glucose ingestion. Simple sugar peaks to approximately 120 to 160 mg/dL in 60 minutes and returns to a normal level within 120 minutes. Complex carbohydrates (red broken line) never increase to more than approximately 130 to 140 mg/dL during a 60-minute period; that level is maintained for the next 180 minutes and then returns to normal.

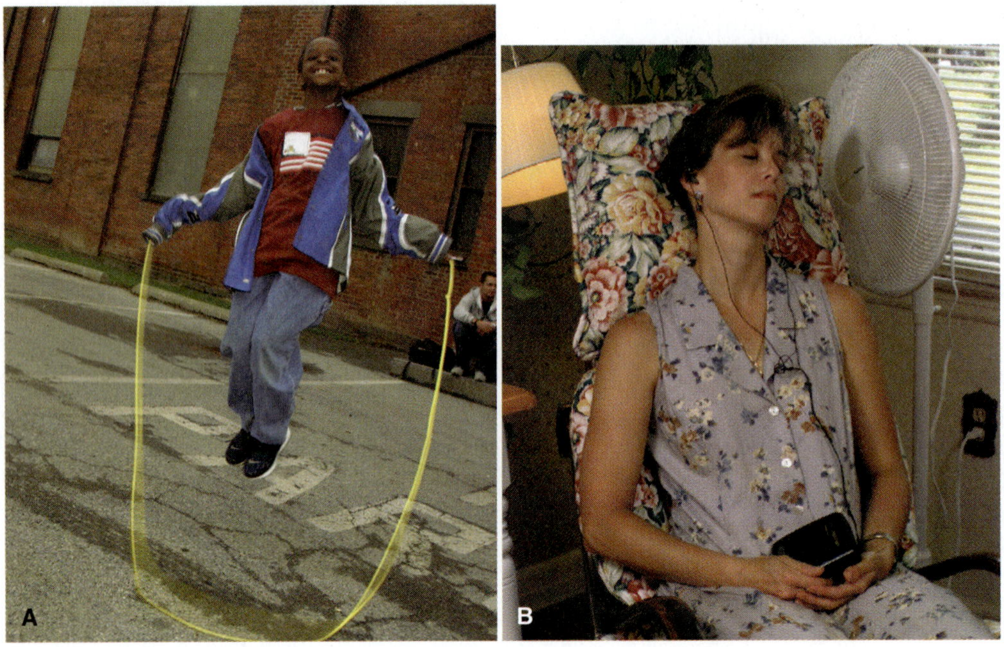

Figure 22-3 The need for carbohydrates is constant whether you are (A) active or (B) at rest.

Fats. Fats, also called lipids, are also composed of carbon, hydrogen, and oxygen, but in a ratio different from carbohydrates. They exist as triglycerides in the body. A triglyceride has three fatty acids attached to a glycerol molecule (Figure 22-4). The fatty acid component of a triglyceride has several important characteristics. The first is whether it is essential to the diet. The only true essential fatty acid in the human diet is linoleic acid, and all other fatty acids the body requires can be derived from this. Another important characteristic of fatty acids is saturation. When a fatty acid is saturated, every carbon molecule on the fatty acid holds as many hydrogens as possible. If it does not hold all the hydrogens possible, it is called unsaturated. The more unsaturated the fatty acid, the more liquid the fat. For example, lard has saturated fatty acids and a thick consistency compared with corn oil, which has relatively unsaturated fatty acids and a thin consistency. If an unsaturated fat is hydrogenated, combined with hydrogen, it becomes more saturated. **Saturated fats** are more common in foods from animal sources than from plant sources. Generally, saturated fatty acids tend to increase the level of fats and cholesterol in the blood.

Trans unsaturated fatty acids (trans fats) are unhealthy fats because they increase low-density lipoproteins (LDL), bad cholesterol, and decrease high-density lipoproteins (HDL), good cholesterol.

Trans fats are produced by a process known as hydrogenation. Vegetable oil (liquid) is heated and hydrogen is added to it. This makes the product solid at room temperature. It gives certain foods a longer shelf life (stays fresh longer) and a better taste. The process, however, turns healthy fat (vegetable oil) into unhealthy fat, trans fats.

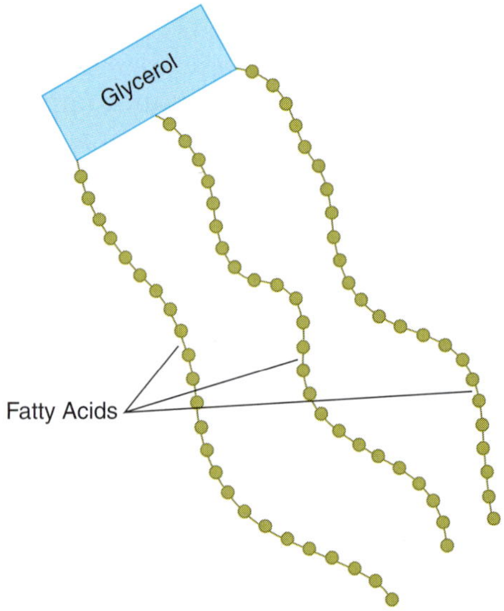

Figure 22-4 A triglyceride has three fatty acids attached to a glycerol molecule.

Trans fats are found in meat and dairy products, as well as stick margarine, solid shortening, and many commercially prepared foods. Foods that are considered convenience foods such as snacks, potato chips, cookies, crackers, and cakes are high in trans fats. Margarine, fast foods, cereal, doughnuts, and french fries are also examples. Experts recommend that the daily amount of trans fats be as close to zero as possible. The FDA requires that all food packaging labels show the amount of trans fats per serving in the product. Table 22-2 lists some common foods and their grams of total fat and trans fat per serving.

Proteins. Although protein is also composed of carbon, hydrogen, and oxygen, it contains one more important element: nitrogen. The basic structural unit of protein is the **amino acid.** There are 22 amino acids in proteins. Eight of these are needed in the diet for the body to function normally. One more, histidine, is essential only during childhood. The rest of the amino acids can be synthesized from the eight, provided that they are present in adequate quantities. A complete protein is so named because it has all eight of the essential amino acids. An incomplete protein does not contain all of these. The best sources for complete proteins are meats and animal products such as milk and eggs. Most plants provide only incomplete proteins and must be combined with complementary incomplete proteins to obtain all eight amino acids (Figure 22-5).

Although protein is described as an energy nutrient, its main function is not to provide energy but to provide amino acids to be used as building components of body proteins, which can be used as enzymes, hormones, and as the basic structural unit in all body tissues and cells. The body uses carbohydrates and fats as its primary energy sources; however, when these are in short supply, the body diverts its use of protein for structural purposes to use it as an energy source. This has detrimental effects on the body.

Table 22-2 Grams of Fat per Serving of Some Common Foods

Product	Serving Size	Total Fat	Saturated Fat	Trans Fat
Butter	1 tbsp	10.8	7.2	0.3
Cake (pound)	1 slice	16.4	3.4	4.3
Cookies (filled with cream)	3	6.1	1.2	1.9
Doughnut	1	18.2	4.7	5.0
French fries (fast food)	Medium	26.9	6.7	7.8
Granola bar	1 bar	7.1	4.4	0.4
Margarine (stick)	1 tbsp	11.0	2.1	2.8
Margarine (tub container)	1 tbsp	6.7	1.2	0.6
Mayonnaise	1 tbsp	10.8	1.6	0.0
Milk (whole)	1 cup	6.6	4.3	0.2
Potato chips	Small bag	11.2	1.9	3.2
Ramen noodle soup	42 g	7.2	3.2	0.9
Shortening (solid)	1 tbsp	13.0	3.4	4.2
Wheat crackers	50 g	10.0	2.0	4.0

Source: Food and Drug Administration Center for Food Safety and Applied Nutrition; U.S. Department of Agriculture National Nutritional Database.

Patient Education

Trans Unsaturated Fatty Acids

- Use a margarine that is soft at room temperature; it is lower in trans fat. Some margarines are available that are entirely trans fat free.
- Olive oil is a wise choice for salads and for dipping bread, and butter is a better option than margarine.
- Olive oil and canola oil are best for sautéing and frying.
- Make foods from scratch to avoid trans fats. Foods such as breads, dips, salad dressings, cereals, and soups can be made without hydrogenated fats.

If a food label lists hydrogenated oil or shortening as one of its main ingredients (usually one of the first listed ingredients), it has a large amount of trans fats in it. Avoid the product altogether, or eat only small amounts.

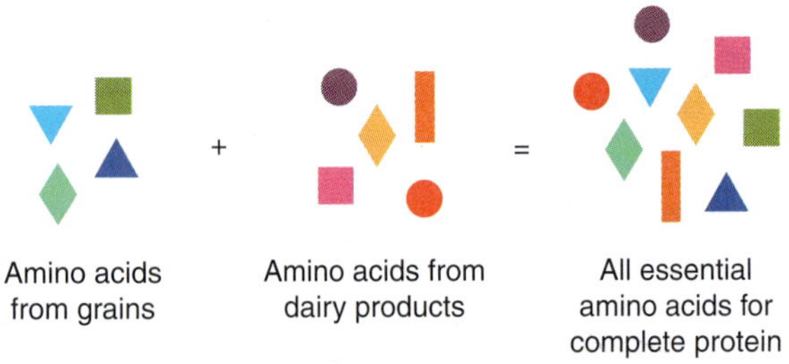

Figure 22-5 Some foods, such as grains and dairy products, may not have all the essential amino acids when considered separately. Combined, however, these form a complete protein and therefore are considered complementary.

Deficiencies in protein usually occur together with deficiencies in total Calories. Failure to thrive is caused by a lack of protein in infants and young children.

Energy Balance. Although all of the energy nutrients are capable of supplying energy to the body, they do so in different ways and in varying amounts. The amount of energy that a substance is able to supply can be measured in large **Calories.** Nutrition is discussed in terms of the large Calorie, which is always capitalized to distinguish it from the small calorie. The large Calorie (abbreviation: C or Cal) is also expressed as a kilocalorie (abbreviation: kcal). One thousand small calories equal one large Calorie or one kilocalorie.

Carbohydrates and proteins both give four Calories for each respective gram. So, if 10 g pure carbohydrate were ingested, it would yield 40 Calories.

$$\frac{10\text{ g}}{\text{carbohydrate}} \times \frac{4\text{ Calories}}{1\text{ gram of carbohydrate}} = 40\text{ Calories}$$

Similarly, if 10 g protein were used for energy, it would yield 40 Calories.

$$\frac{10\text{ g}}{\text{protein}} \times \frac{4\text{ Calories}}{1\text{ gram of protein}} = 40\text{ Calories}$$

Fats, in comparison, yield nine Calories for every gram of fat. Fats, therefore, are a more energy-rich food source than carbohydrates or proteins because they give more Calories for every gram used. If 10 g fat were used, it would yield 90 Calories.

$$\frac{10\text{ g}}{\text{fat}} \times \frac{9\text{ Calories}}{1\text{ gram of fat}} = 90\text{ Calories}$$

The total of all changes, chemical and physical, that take place in the body is called **metabolism.** The metabolic rate concerns itself with the changes in the body with respect to energy. It is the balance between the energy that is brought into the body and the energy used by the body. Energy is used during every action of the body, including voluntary activities such as walking or riding a bicycle and involuntary activities such as breathing and cellular repair.

The level of energy required for activities that occur when the body is at rest is called basal metabolism. The **basal metabolic rate (BMR)** varies according to several factors. For example, the BMR is higher in individuals with leaner body mass (muscle) because more energy is needed to fuel the muscles than to store fat. BMR also is higher in individuals during periods of high growth rate, such as in children and pregnant women.

Ideally, an individual will take in as many Calories as the body will use each day. When a person takes in more Calories than will be used, the body will store the excess energy in the form of fat. When a person uses more energy than is brought into the body, the body breaks down these stores. When the stores of fat are depleted, the body will start to break down its protein structures.

For an optimal energy balance in the body, the largest percentage of Calories in the diet should come from carbohydrates. Ideally, the percentage should be 50% to 60% of total calories consumed. The percentage of Calories attributable to fat should not be greater than 30%, with a percentage closer to 20% being preferred. Proteins should make up 10% to 20% of Calories in the diet.

Take note that these values are the percentage of the total Calories derived from each energy nutrient—not the percentage of grams. This distinction is important because of the difference in Calories derived from each energy nutrient. Figure 22-6 gives an example of these calculations. Note the percentages of fat, carbohydrate, and protein found in the "mystery" food. All fall outside of the recommended percentages for each.

In many cultures outside of the United States, rice, bread, and noodles are the basis of the diet. In the United States, we have available great amounts of food from the dairy and meat groups. Unfortunately, dairy products and meats, although containing many good nutrients, also contain a great deal of fat. Studies have shown that many Americans are obese (as defined as weight being at least 20% greater than what their ideal weight should be). The U.S. diet is too high in fat, has too many calories, has too much salt and cholesterol; and has insufficient amounts of complex carbohydrates and fiber. As a result, many illnesses and diseases occur, such as heart disease, high blood pressure, diabetes, and cancer.

Label for Mystery Food:	*Amount Per Serving*
Calories	149
Total Fat	9g
Total Carbohydrate	14g
Total Protein	3g

The first calculation to make is one that converts grams to Calories.

$$9 \text{ grams of fat} \times \frac{9 \text{ Calories}}{\text{gram}} = 81 \text{ Calories due to fat}$$

$$14 \text{ grams of carbohydrate} \times \frac{4 \text{ Calories}}{\text{gram}} = 56 \text{ Calories due to carbohydrate}$$

$$3 \text{ grams of protein} \times \frac{4 \text{ Calories}}{\text{gram}} = 12 \text{ Calories due to protein}$$

The next calculation is to find the percentage of total Calories due to each of the energy nutrients.

$$\frac{81 \text{ Calories due to fat}}{149 \text{ total Calories}} = 54\%$$

$$\frac{56 \text{ Calories due to carbohydrate}}{149 \text{ total Calories}} = 38\%$$

$$\frac{12 \text{ Calories due to protein}}{149 \text{ total Calories}} = 8\%$$

Figure 22-6 Calculations of percentages of total calories from fat, carbohydrate, and protein.

Because obesity in the United States has become such a serious problem, there has been much interest in modifying the U.S. Department of Agriculture's pyramid for ideal weight. Health experts believe that the emphasis on 6 to 11 servings from the bread, cereal, rice, and pasta groups (carbohydrates) is a contributing factor to obesity. Ongoing studies and research has led to redesign of the pyramid with less emphasis on the carbohydrate group and more emphasis placed on the fruits, vegetables, whole grains, legumes, and nuts (Figure 22-7).

The new food pyramid has specific information about portions and calories. It can help individuals get individualized nutrition and exercise advice.

Each color on the pyramid represents a food group:

- *Orange* represents grains. The recommendation is to eat 5–8 ounces of grain per day, 3 of which should be from whole grain breads, pasta, rice, cereal, or crackers.
- *Green* represents vegetables. For a low calorie per day intake, 2½ cups of vegetables should come from all five vegetable groups several times a week.
- *Red* represents fruits. Two cups daily is the recommended intake.
- *Yellow* represents oils. Most oil should come from nuts, fish, and vegetable oil, while limiting butter, lard, stick margarine, and shortening.
- *Blue* represents milk. Three cups per day of fat-free or low fat milk or milk products is recommended.
- *Purple* represents beans and meat. Choose lean meat and poultry and use fish, beans, nuts, seeds, and peas.
- The *action figure* represents physical activity (Table 22-3).

The new government Web site (http://www.mypyramid.gov) allows individuals to input their age, gender, and activity level. By doing so, they get a recommendation about their personal daily calorie intake and physical activity level.

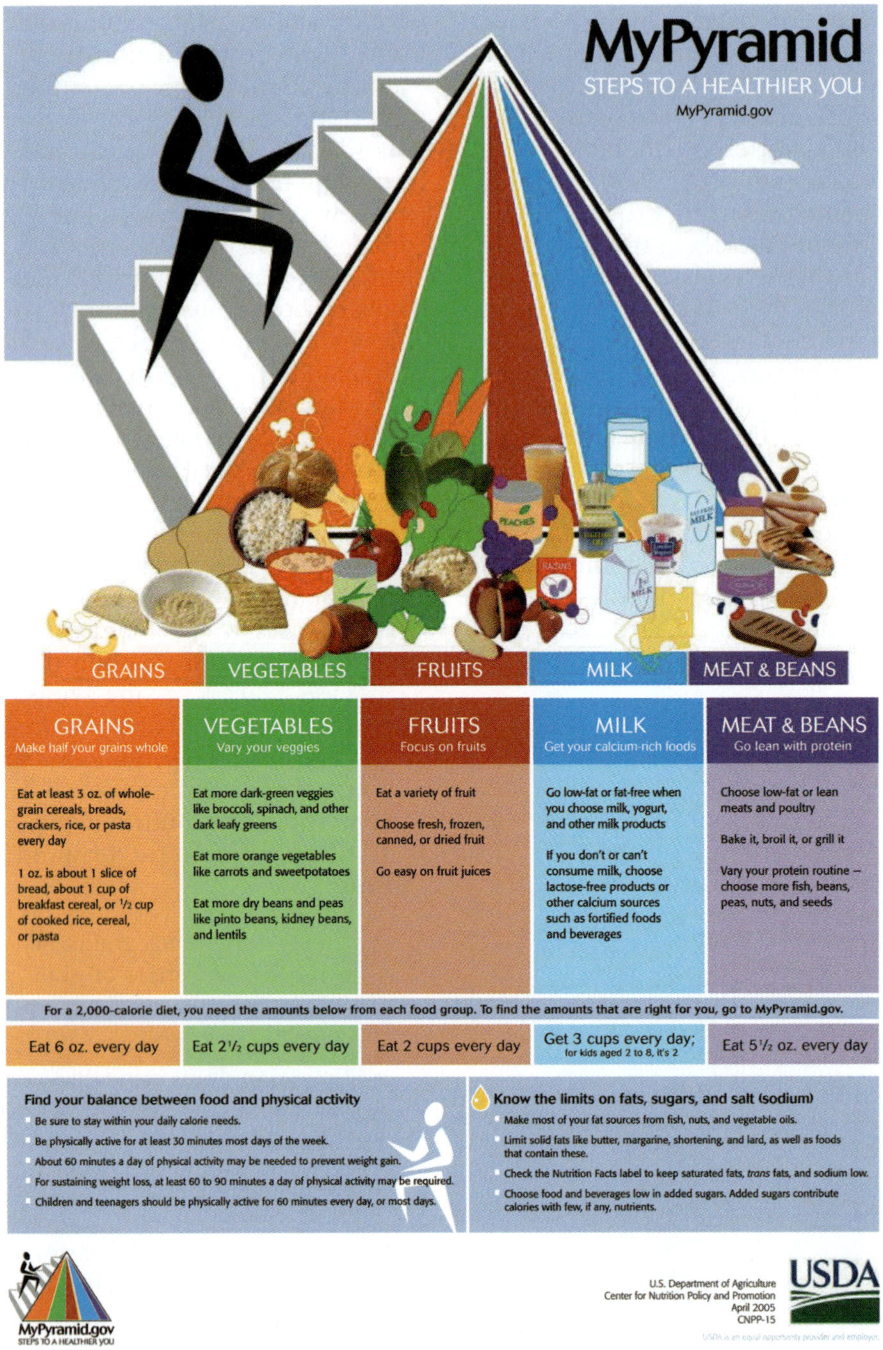

Figure 22-7 The U.S. Department of Agriculture's guide to a balanced diet takes the shape of a pyramid. The foundation of a good diet is made up of a balance between food and physical activity. (Courtesy of U.S. Department of Agriculture.)

Other Nutrients (Inorganic)

Many other nutrients are essential to maintaining good health. Although they do not provide the body with energy, they perform a variety of necessary functions. They include vitamins, antioxidants, herbal supplements, minerals, water, and fiber.

Vitamins. Vitamins are a class of nutrient in which each specific vitamin has a function entirely its own. They are complex molecules and are required by the body in minute quantities. Vitamins were first named as letters of the alphabet. These names have been supplemented with chemical names and both should be learned. Vitamins generally have one of

Table 22-3 Health Benefits of Regular Physical Activity

Increase physical fitness
Helps build and maintain healthy bones, muscles, and joints
Builds endurance and muscular strength
Helps manage weight
Lowers risk factors for cardiovascular diseases, colon cancer, and type 2 diabetes
Helps control blood pressure
Promotes psychological well-being and self-esteem
Reduces feelings of depression and anxiety

Source: *Nutrition and Your Health: Dietary Guidelines for Americans* (6th ed.), 2005

two functions: to facilitate cellular metabolism by acting as a coenzyme with a catalyst, and to act as a component of tissue structure. A **catalyst** allows a chemical reaction to proceed at a much quicker rate and without as much energy input, and the **coenzyme** is the nonprotein part that acts with it. Neither a catalyst nor its coenzyme is used in the reaction, thus each can be used again and again. Vitamins that work with catalysts are only needed in minute quantities.

Vitamins are divided into two classes based on solubility. The vitamins that are not soluble in water are said to be fat soluble. This is important because the **fat-soluble** vitamins are not carried into the bloodstream easily and are stored in fatty tissue, especially the liver. The **water-soluble** vitamins are not so easily stored, and blood levels must be maintained by constant dietary intake. Toxicity can occur with high doses of either type of vitamin but is more likely to occur with the fat-soluble vitamins because they are stored in the body. The vitamins are listed in Table 22-4.

Table 22-4 Vitamin Sources and Functions

Name	Food Sources	Functions	Deficiency/Toxicity
Fat-Soluble Vitamins			
Vitamin A (carotene or retinol)	Animal Liver Whole milk Butter Cream Cod liver oil Plants Dark green leafy vegetables Deep yellow or orange fruit Fortified margarine	Antioxidant Dim light vision Maintenance of mucous membranes Growth and development of bones	Deficiency Night blindness **Xerophthalmia** Respiratory infections Bone growth ceases Toxicity Cessation of menstruation Joint pain Stunted growth Enlargement of liver
Vitamin D (cholecalciferol)	Animal Eggs Liver Fortified milk Plants None	Bone growth	Deficiency Rickets Osteomalacia Osteoporosis Poorly developed teeth Muscle spasms Toxicity Kidney stones Calcification of soft tissues

(continues)

Vitamins are divided into two classes based on water solubility: fat soluble and water-soluble vitamins.

Table 22-4 Vitamin Sources and Functions (continued)

Name	Food Sources	Functions	Deficiency/Toxicity
Vitamin E (alphatocopherol, betatocopherol, deltatocopherol, gammatocopherol)	Animal None Plant Wheat germ Margarines Salad dressing Nuts	Antioxidant	Deficiency Neurologic defects Destruction of red blood cells (RBCs) Toxicity Hypertension
Vitamin K (phytonadione)	Animal Egg yolk Liver Milk Plant Green leafy vegetables Cabbage	Blood clotting	Deficiency Prolonged blood clotting Toxicity Hemolytic anemia Jaundice
Water-Soluble Vitamins			
Thiamin (vitamin B_1)	Animal Liver Eggs Fish Pork Beef Plants Whole and enriched grains Legumes	Coenzyme in oxidation of glucose	Deficiency Beriberi Gastrointestinal tract, nervous and cardiovascular system problems Toxicity None
Thiamin	Animal Pork Beef Liver Eggs Fish Plants Whole and enriched grains Legumes Brewer's yeast	Metabolism of carbohydrates Maintains normal appetite and nervous system function	Deficiency Cardiovascular system, nervous system and gastrointestinal system disorders Toxicity None
Riboflavin (vitamin B_2)	Animal Poultry Milk Fish Plants Green vegetables Cereals Enriched bread	Aids release of energy from food	Deficiency **Cheilosis** Glossitis Photophobia Toxicity None

(continues)

Table 22-4 (continued)

Name	Food Sources	Functions	Deficiency/Toxicity
Pyridoxine (vitamin B_6)	Animal Pork Milk Eggs Plants Whole grain cereals Legumes	Synthesis of nonessential amino acids Conversion of tryptophan to niacin Antibody production	Deficiency Irritability Depression Dermatitis Toxicity Liver disease Rare
Vitamin B_{12} (cobalamin)	Animal Seafood Meat Eggs Milk Plants None	Synthesis of RBCs Maintenance of myelin sheaths	Deficiency Degeneration of myelin sheaths Pernicious anemia Toxicity None
Niacin (vitamin B_3, nicotinic acid)	Animal Milk Eggs Fish Poultry	Transfers hydrogen atoms for synthesis of adenosine triphosphate	Deficiency **Pellagra** Toxicity Vasodilation of blood vessels
Folate (folic acid)	Animal Liver Plants Spinach Asparagus Broccoli Kidney beans	DNA synthesis Synthesis of RBCs Protein metabolism	Deficiency Anemia Glossitis Macrocytic anemia Neural tube defects Toxicity None
Biotin	Animal Milk Liver Plants Legumes Mushrooms	Coenzyme in carbohydrate and amino acid metabolism Niacin synthesis from tryptophan	Deficiency None Toxicity None
Pantothenic acid (vitamin B_5)	Animal Eggs Liver Salmon Plants Mushrooms Cauliflower Peanuts Yeast	Metabolism of carbohydrates, lipids, and proteins Synthesis of acetylcholine	Deficiency None Toxicity None

(continues)

Table 22-4 Vitamin Sources and Functions (continued)

Name	Food Sources	Functions	Deficiency/Toxicity
Vitamin C (ascorbic acid)	Fruits All citrus Plants Broccoli Tomatoes Brussel sprouts Potatoes	Prevention of scurvy Formation of collagen Healing of wounds Release of stress hormones Absorption of iron Antioxidant	Deficiency Scurvy Muscle cramps Ulcerated gums Toxicity Increase uric acid level Hemolytic anemia Kidney stones

There are four fat-soluble vitamins, which include vitamins A, D, E, and K. The first one, vitamin A, has two forms. The form that is used by the body is retinol, which is found in animal foods. The form found in plants is carotene. **Carotene** is converted into retinol in the body. Vitamin A is part of the pigment rhodopsin found in the eye and is responsible in part for vision, especially night vision. Vitamin A also gives strength to epithelial tissue and is required for healthy skin and mucous membranes. It is also an antioxidant. Sources of vitamin A include animal fats, butter, and cheese.

Vitamin D, also called **cholecalciferol,** is the fat-soluble vitamin involved in the metabolism of calcium in the body. It not only helps with absorption of this important mineral, but also with formation and maintenance of bone tissue. Vitamin D can be made in the body with exposure to sunlight. Rickets, osteomalacia, and osteoporosis are diseases caused by a deficiency in vitamin D. When deficiencies occur, especially during childhood, malformation of the skeleton is seen. Sources of vitamin D include milk, cod liver oil, and egg yolk.

Another fat-soluble vitamin is vitamin E, or **tocopherol.** It too is an **antioxidant,** possibly reducing the likelihood of **oxidation** of substances. This ability to reduce oxidation has recently led to suggestions that vitamin E may slow the aging process, but its true effectiveness is yet to be demonstrated. Vitamin E is found in lettuce and other green leafy vegetables, wheat germ, and rice.

Vitamin K is a fat-soluble vitamin required for the production of prothrombin. Prothrombin is one agent responsible for the clotting of blood. Deficiencies can result in prolonged blood clotting time and hemorrhage. Vitamin K is synthesized by intestinal bacteria, and bile is required for its absorption. About half of the body's requirement for vitamin K is fulfilled in this way. Sources of vitamin K include fats, fishmeal, oats, alfalfa, wheat, and rye.

Antioxidants.

Antioxidants are an important topic in nutrition. Some think they are as important as the discussion about fats. Antioxidants are powerful and beneficial to us. The four primary antioxidants are betacarotene (vitamin A), vitamin C, vitamin E, and selenium.

When our bodies use oxygen to burn (oxidize) food for energy, the process results in the formation of free radicals. Most times our bodies take care of the free radicals by producing enzymes to fight them.

If free radicals are excessive, health can be seriously impaired. Evidence has shown that excess free radicals cannot be fought successfully and the body cannot get rid of them.

The radicals attack the cells' DNA and blood vessel cells, contributing to cardiovascular disease, strokes, arthritis, cataracts, and other diseases that may be degenerative in nature. These are seen in older adults.

Free radicals are not only a by-product of oxidation, they form with exposure to environmental influences such as water and air pollution, cigarette smoke, and certain foods, like fried foods.

Antioxidants fight free radicals through those enzymes in our bodies, those we ingest in food, and those we take as supplements. Vitamins A (as betacarotene), C, E, and selenium provide powerful benefits because they fight against oxidation that produces free radicals.

Vitamin C, or **ascorbic acid,** is a water-soluble vitamin. Vitamin C is a constituent of connective tissue and acts to hold cells together. A deficiency of vitamin C causes **scurvy,** in which the walls of the capillaries become so weakened that they burst. Vitamin C also helps with wound healing and with the absorption of iron. Sources include most fresh fruits (especially citrus fruits) and vegetables (especially tomatoes).

The last group of water-soluble vitamins is the B-complex vitamin. It is important to remember that each vitamin in the B-complex is a separate vitamin with distinct functions. Vitamin B_1, or **thiamin,** helps in the conversion of glucose to energy. The disease **beriberi** is caused by thiamin deficiency and is characterized by neuritis, edema, and cardiovascular changes. Sources include whole grain cereals, peas, beans, vegetables, and brewer's yeast. Vitamin B_2, or **riboflavin,** is also involved in energy production. It is important in the production of proteins and is necessary for normal growth. Sources include eggs, liver, milk, brewer's yeast, and green vegetables. A third B-complex vitamin, **niacin,** works with both thiamin and riboflavin in the production of energy. Lack of niacin results in gastrointestinal and central nervous system disturbances. All three of these vitamins are important throughout the body.

Vitamin B_6, or **pyridoxine,** has an important role in protein metabolism, especially the synthesis of proteins. It is also important in the metabolism of fats and carbohydrates. Vitamin B_6 is found in rice, beans, and yeast. Another B-complex vitamin, **folic acid,** is involved in the formation of DNA and the formation of red blood cells. Folic acid is found in liver, yeast, and green leafy vegetables. Vitamin B_{12}, or **cobalamin,** is another vitamin important to the functioning of red blood cells. This vitamin is responsible for the synthesis of the heme portion of hemoglobin, and deficiencies in vitamin B_{12} result in the disease pernicious anemia. Because vitamin B_{12} is only found in animal foods such as liver, kidney, and dairy products, pernicious anemia may be a problem for some vegetarians. Pernicious anemia may also occur when there is decreased production of a factor within the stomach that is required for vitamin B_{12} absorption. Other B-complex vitamins, pantothenic acid, vitamin B_5, and biotin, are generally responsible for energy metabolism.

Multivitamin supplements may help reduce the risk for certain diseases, especially in individuals who do not eat nutritionally sound diets. Individuals who may be more likely to suffer vitamin deficiencies because of poor nutrition include the elderly, mentally challenged individuals, young children without proper care, alcoholics, and patients with chronic diseases such as Crohn's disease, cystic fibrosis, and celiac disease. Some studies show a reduced risk for coronary artery disease in patients who take a multivitamin coupled with antioxidants. Researchers believe that B vitamins and antioxidants may help keep plaque from forming in arteries.

Most patients who are healthy and eat a nutritious diet do not need a supplement in the form of a multivitamin. A balanced diet is the best overall source of nutrients. Some people may need a supplement because they are at risk for disease such as cancer and heart disease. Examples of people at high risk are patients who have a chronic illness such as AIDS or cancer; who have gastrointestinal problems that impair digestion or absorption; who are dieting; who are vegans or vegetarians; pregnant and breast-feeding women; and patients older than 50 years (many older than 50 years have difficulty absorbing B vitamins from food, and their level of vitamin D may be low because of lack of sunshine and eating poorly).

Patients should check with their provider before beginning to take multivitamin supplements.

Herbal Supplements. Herbs are medicinal plants and are also known as botanicals or phytomedicines. Many have been used as far back as Roman times and used as traditional herbal medicine.

Many patients use herbs for the treatment of illnesses and diseases and to maintain health. It is part of a movement toward alternative or complementary therapy. The herbal supplements can be found in health food stores, pharmacies, supermarkets, large outlet stores, through the mail, and on the Internet.

Herbs are made from dried plants and plant juices. Herbal teas are made by placing the herb into boiling water. Natural hormones can be found in soy products.

Some supplements are helpful; other supplements are harmful and are banned in several countries but may be available in the United States. The Food and Drug Administration (FDA) is exempt from having authority over dietary supplements, although under the Dietary Supplement Health and Education Act of 1994, the FDA must prove a product is unsafe before it can order its removal from store shelves. An example of a potentially unsafe herbal supplement that the FDA removed from the shelves in 2004 is ephedra. It was used as an anorectic and a bronchodilator, acts as a stimulant, and can increase blood pressure and pulse to dangerous levels. In 2005, a federal judge struck down the FDA's year-long ban on ephedra and supplements containing ephedra. A Utah supplement company challenged the ban that prompted the judge's ruling. In 2006, the ruling was appealed to the U.S. Court of Appeals for the Tenth Circuit in Denver, Colorado, and the Appeals Court upheld the FDA's ban on ephedra. Sale of ephedra or supplements containing ephedra are illegal in the United States. Although ephedra is an illegal and banned substance, it is widely used by athletes.

Be sure to ask patients about all substances or remedies they may be using, including herbs, vitamins, teas, or others. Most patients do not consider supplements to be medicines and may not think to mention them when asked what medications they are taking. Herbs can interact unfavorably with certain prescription and over-the-counter medications.

Minerals. Minerals differ from vitamins in two distinct ways. Whereas vitamins are complex molecules, minerals are singular elements. Another way that minerals differ from vitamins is that although vitamins are only required in minute quantities, some minerals are required in larger amounts. The foundation of the classification of minerals falls into two groups: major and trace minerals. No matter how small the quantity required of either a mineral or vitamin, all are vital to a healthy body. Some minerals are considered **electrolytes,** in that they become ionized and carry a positive or negative charge. The levels of these minerals in the bloodstream must be carefully balanced for the body to function in a healthy state.

There are seven **major minerals** (Table 22-5). They are calcium, phosphorus, sodium, potassium, magnesium, chloride, and sulfur.

Calcium (Ca) is the mineral present in the largest quantity in the body because of its involvement in the structure of bone and teeth. It is also important in blood clotting, muscle contraction, and nerve conduction. Its levels in the blood must be kept at narrow limits to ensure that the nervous and muscular tissues can function. This is especially important for the beating heart tissue. When there is a deficiency of calcium in the diet, calcium is taken from the bones to keep the blood calcium levels constant. The resulting deficient peak bone mass may put a person at risk for osteoporosis. This condition develops when there is not enough calcium in the bones and the bones become porous and easily broken.

Women older than 60 years are at greater risk for osteoporosis than are men. There are no symptoms of the disease, and the first indication for the patient is when he or she sustains a fracture caused by weakened bones.

Most adults in the United States older than 60 years do not consume enough calcium in their diets and risk development of osteoporosis. Dairy products contain high amounts of calcium, as do sardines, figs, oranges, almonds, greens, and beans.

Supplemental estrogen for menopausal women was once a common preventative for bone loss. Since 2002, estrogen has not been given as a preventive measure because a large study by the Women's Health Initiative showed an increased risk for heart disease, stroke, cancer, and breast cancer in postmenopausal women who took estrogen.

Phosphorus (P) is another mineral important in bone formation. Phosphorus also is involved in numerous activities associated with energy metabolism, as well as maintaining a proper pH balance in the blood.

Sodium (Na) and potassium (K) are two minerals that act as electrolytes. Together they work to maintain proper water balance. They also help in maintenance of proper pH balance and are involved in nerve and muscular conduction and excitability. In addition, potassium is involved in protein synthesis and release of insulin from the pancreas.

Magnesium (Mg) is another mineral that is involved with energy metabolism. It also functions in nerve and muscle excitability and is stored in bone.

Chloride (Cl) is important in pH balance and is the major **extracellular** (outside the cell) anion. It is also a major component of gastric secretions in the form of hydrochloric acid.

The last major mineral is sulfur (S). It is a component of one of the amino acids, and therefore is found in protein. It is also involved in energy metabolism.

The **trace minerals** are required in smaller quantities but are as important as the major minerals. Some of the more important trace minerals include iron, copper, chromium, molybdenum, selenium, manganese, iodine, zinc, cobalt, and fluorine.

Iron is vital to life because of its role in the heme molecule, which carries oxygen to every cell in the body. Iron-deficiency anemia results when the diet is low in iron and is characterized by small, pale red blood cells. Iron is also part of the molecule myoglobin, found in muscle cells, and is involved in a number of metabolic reactions.

Copper, chromium, molybdenum, selenium, and manganese are trace minerals important as factors in a number of metabolic reactions. Selenium acts as an antioxidant and has been receiving much of the recent publicity that vitamin E has. Iodine is also involved in metabolism but is unique in that the only place that iodine is found is in the thyroid hormone produced by the thyroid gland. Without it, the thyroid gland would be unable to regulate the overall metabolism of the body.

Zinc is an important constituent of many parts of the body but most notable is its involvement with the immune system and growth of tissues. Deficiencies lead to decreased ability to heal and reduced

Table 22-5 The Seven Major Minerals and Their Food Sources

Name	Food Sources	Functions	Deficiency/Toxicity
Calcium (Ca)	Milk exchanges Milk, cheese Meat exchanges Sardines Salmon Vegetable exchanges Green vegetables	Development of bones and teeth Permeability of cell membranes Transmission of nerve impulses Blood clotting Normal heart action	Deficiency Osteoporosis Osteomalacia Rickets Poor bone and teeth formation
Phosphorus (P)	Milk exchanges Milk, cheese Meat exchanges Lean meat	Development of bones and teeth Transfer of energy Component of phospholipids Buffer system	Deficiency (Same as calcium) Anorexia Weakness
Potassium (K)	Fruit exchanges Oranges, bananas Dried fruits Legumes	Contraction of muscles Maintaining water balance Transmission of nerve impulses Carbohydrate and protein metabolism	Deficiency Hypokalemia Toxicity Hyperkalemia
Sodium (Na)	Table salt Meat exchanges Beef, eggs Milk exchanges Milk, cheese	Maintaining fluid balance in blood Transmission of nerve impulses	Toxicity Increase in blood pressure
Chloride (Cl)	Table salt Meat exchanges Eggs	Gastric acidity Regulation of osmotic pressure Activation of salivary amylase	Deficiency Imbalance in gastric acidity Imbalance in blood pH
Magnesium (Mg)	Vegetable exchanges Green vegetables Bread exchanges Whole grains	Synthesis of adenosine triphosphate Transmission of nerve impulses Activator of metabolic enzymes Relaxation of skeletal muscles	Unknown, perhaps mental and emotional disorders
Sulfur (S)	Meat exchanges Eggs, poultry, fish	Maintaining protein structure Formation of high-energy compounds	Unknown

immune resistance. Cobalt is part of vitamin B_{12} and is therefore important for the functioning of red blood cells. Fluorine is involved in calcified tissues. Its involvement in strengthening teeth has led to the fluoridation of most public water supplies. Its role in the prevention of osteoporosis has been suggested but is still under investigation.

Water. Water is an important nutrient. The human body can go far longer without food than it can without water. Water has a multitude of functions in the body. It is the major solvent of the body and is the medium in which most biochemical reactions of the body take place. As a solvent, water is essential for the removal of toxic waste from the body. In addition, it is an important component of many structures; the body is composed of 50% to 60% water. Being the major component of blood, water serves as a transporter. Another function of water is its lubricating role, especially in joints and in the digestive system. In addition, water helps control temperature within the body by eliminating excess heat through the evaporation of water secreted in the form of perspiration.

Because the body cannot efficiently store water, water that is lost daily must continually be replenished. Water is lost through perspiration, feces, urine, and respiration. Water can be replenished in part from foods that are ingested, but additional water should also be consumed. It is suggested that six to eight glasses of water be taken in per day. Although other beverages are important sources of water, it should be considered that caffeine and alcohol are **diuretics** and may cause the body to lose water through increased urinary output.

Fiber. Although most fiber is carbohydrate in composition, it is included in its own section because of its special characteristics. Fiber comes only from plant sources. An adequate supply of fruits, vegetables, and grains is necessary to ensure enough fiber in the diet. Fiber cannot be digested and therefore is not absorbed into the body. Although fiber is not digested, it is important for the proper functioning of the gastrointestinal tract because it adds bulk to feces as it is passed through the intestines; therefore, it gives the muscles of the tract something against which to work. Lack of fiber in the diet has been implicated in such gastrointestinal disorders as diverticulitis, constipation, and colorectal cancer.

There are several types of fiber. Most are carbohydrates and include **cellulose,** gums, mucilages, algal polysaccharides, pectins, and hemicellulose. Another important fiber, lignin, is not a carbohydrate. It is recommended that the diet contain 20 to 35 g of fiber per day. The U.S. diet tends to be far below this recommendation (approximately 11 g), in part because of the consumption of processed foods. During processing, fiber is often removed. Fiber levels should be increased gradually to prevent gastrointestinal distress, which can include diarrhea or flatulence.

READING FOOD LABELS

When assisting patients to change or modify their diets, the medical assistant must be knowledgeable not only about types of nutrients, but about how these nutrients are expressed in the foods we eat. The nutritional analysis presented on a package's food label is a helpful guide to understanding levels of fat, cholesterol, sodium, carbohydrate, protein, and vitamins contained in a particular food.

Many of the foods we eat are **processed foods,** which are cooked or packaged with parts removed or ingredients added. We rely on the labels on the cans, bottles, and boxes to tell us what nutrients are inside. The government wants to make it easier for people to understand the labels.

The government also wants to prevent food companies from fooling people into thinking something has good nutrition when it really does not. Food companies often put words on their labels to make people believe a product is healthy. Words like "healthy" and "light" or "lite" are not adequately descriptive. To discover what is in the package and if it is healthy, it is important to read the nutrition label (Figure 22-8).

Items on the Nutrition Label

Serving Size. The nutrition information given is for one serving of the food. In this case, one serving is one-half cup of the food. The package contains four servings.

Calories. The label lists the number of calories per serving, as well as the number of calories from fat per serving. This number should be less than 30% of the total calories. For example, if the total calories is 100, the calories from fat should be 30 or less.

The Percentage (%) Daily Value. The percentage (%) daily value is the amount of a nutrient obtained by eating one serving of the product. The amount is given in a percentage based on a diet of 2,000 calories a day. For example, if the packaged food has 3 g fat, the total fat from eating one serving is 5% of the total fat that should be ingested in an entire day.

Fat and Cholesterol. Because it is important to eat a low-fat diet, nutrition labels list both the total amount of fat and the amount of saturated

Nutrition Facts	
Serving Size ½ cup (130g)	
Servings Per Container About 4	
Amount Per Serving	
Calories	110
Calories from Fat	0
	% Daily Value*
Total Fat 0g	**0%**
Sodium 340mg	**14%**
Total Carbohydrate 20g	**7%**
Dietary Fiber 6g	**25%**
Sugars 2g	
Protein 8g	
Calcium 6% • Iron 10%	
Not a significant source of saturated fat, trans fat, cholesterol, vitamin A and vitamin C.	
*Percent Daily Values are based on a 2,000 calorie diet.	

Figure 22-8 Labels on food packages give facts about the ingredients and nutrition of the food in the package.

fat and trans fat per serving. Saturated fat comes from an animal source and contains more cholesterol than unsaturated fats, which come from vegetable sources. The cholesterol content is also listed.

Sodium. The amount of sodium per serving is listed. This category is especially important for patients on a sodium-restricted diet, such as those with cardiac disease and hypertension.

Carbohydrates. The total amounts of carbohydrates per serving is listed together with the amount of carbohydrates that come from simple sugar. These two types of carbohydrates are separated for individuals who are trying to eat more complex carbohydrates and less simple sugar.

Other Information. The amounts of fiber, protein, and some vitamins and minerals are listed.

Ingredients. The ingredients contained in a packaged food are listed on the label. The item that is in the largest quantity is listed first. For example, if a product lists flour first and water second, there is more flour than water in the product. **Preservatives,** or chemicals added to food to keep it fresh longer, and artificial flavors and colors are often added to processed foods.

Comparing Labels

Look at some labels from snack foods that people eat when they want something crunchy and salty. Figure 22-9 shows labels from potato chips, pretzels, and snack crackers. When comparing products, compare equal amounts. These products list the serving as 30 or 28 g. That is close enough to compare the labels.

In reviewing these labels, note the amount of fat and saturated fat in each item. It might be assumed that potato chips, which are fried, would be high in fat. It may be surprising that the snack crackers have high fat content. Pretzels are the clear winner for a low-fat snack.

Although the labels show total fat and saturated fat, the amount of trans fatty acids (TFA) is not listed. Previously, food labels included trans fats within the total fat amount. The FDA now requires the amount of TFAs be listed in the label. All three snack items contain TFAs. These snacks should be avoided or used sparingly.

In terms of sodium, calories, and sugar, pretzels have the most sodium, but all three are high in sodium.

All three are low in sugar. Their calories are nearly the same as are the amounts of fiber and protein. The pretzels have the most carbohydrates, and the crackers have the most artificial flavors, colors, and preservatives.

Critical Thinking

Following is information from a label for peanut butter. Calculate the percentage of calories from fat, protein, and carbohydrate.

Serving size	2 tbsp
Calories	204
Protein	9 g
Carbohydrates	6 g
Fat	16 g

NUTRITION AT VARIOUS STAGES OF LIFE

For the nutrients discussed in the preceding sections, ranges of suggested normal requirements were given. These ranges should be used as a guide, remembering that each individual is unique, and requirements will vary.

Patient Education

Encourage patients to read and evaluate food labels. Typically, they should look for:

- The lowest amount of fat, saturated fat, and trans fat. Calories from fat should not be more than 30% of total calories.
- No cholesterol or low cholesterol. Total cholesterol should be less than 300 milligrams (mg) per day.
- Low sodium content. Total sodium should be less than 2,400 mg per day.
- High fiber. Fiber intake should be as high as possible.
- Vitamins and minerals. Some vitamins and minerals occur naturally and sometimes they are added to food during processing.

A

Nutrition Facts
Serving Size 1 oz. (28g/About 15 chips)
Servings Per Container About 12

Amount Per Serving	
Calories 140	Calories from Fat 60
	% Daily Value*
Total Fat 6g	**10%**
Saturated Fat 1g	**5%**
Polyunsaturated Fat 2g	
Monounsaturated Fat 3.5g	
Trans Fat 0g	
Cholesterol 0mg	**0%**
Sodium 130mg	**5%**
Potassium 75mg	**2%**
Total Carbohydrate 18g	**6%**
Dietary Fiber 2g	**9%**
Sugars 3g	
Protein 2g	

Vitamin A 0%	Vitamin C 0%
Calcium 0%	Iron 2%
Vitamin E 8%	Thiamin 2%
Niacin 2%	Vitamin B_6 4%
Phosphorus 6%	Magnesium 4%
Zinc 2%	

*Percent Daily Values are based on a 2,000 calorie diet. Your Daily Values may be higher or lower depending on your calorie needs:

	Calories:	2,000	2,500
Total Fat	Less than	65g	80g
Sat Fat	Less than	20g	25g
Cholesterol	Less than	300mg	300mg
Sodium	Less than	2,400mg	2,400mg
Potassium		3,500mg	3,500mg
Total Carbohydrate		300g	375g
Dietary Fiber		25g	30g

Calories per gram:
Fat 9 • Carbohydrate 4 • Protein 4

Ingredients: Whole Corn, Sunflower Oil, Whole Wheat, Rice Flour, Whole Oat Flour, Sugar, Salt, Whey Protein Concentrate, Dry Buttermilk, Whey, Sour Cream (Cultured Cream, Nonfat Dry Milk), Onion Powder, Natural Flavors, Hydrolyzed Soy Protein, Cultured Whey, Corn Starch, Autolyzed Yeast Extract, Mozzarella Cheese (Pasteurized Part Skim Milk, Cheese Cultures, Salt, Enzymes), Citric Acid, Garlic Powder, Gum Arabic, Glycerol, Disodium Phosphate, Spice, and Artificial Color (Including Red 40, Blue 1).
CONTAINS WHEAT, MILK, AND SOY INGREDIENTS.

B

Nutrition Facts
Serving Size 6 Crackers (15g)
Servings Per Container About 24

Amount Per Serving	
Calories 60	Calories from Fat 15
	% Daily Value*
Total Fat 1.5g	**2%**
Saturated Fat 0.5g	**3%**
Trans Fat 0g	
Polyunsaturated Fat 0.5g	
Monounsaturated Fat 0.5g	
Cholesterol 0mg	**0%**
Sodium 160mg	**7%**
Total Carbohydrate 11g	**4%**
Dietary Fiber less than 1g	**1%**
Sugars 1g	
Protein 1g	

Vitamin A 0%	Vitamin C 0%
Calcium 0%	Iron 2%

*Percent Daily Values are based on a 2,000 calorie diet. Your Daily Values may be higher or lower depending on your calorie needs:

	Calories:	2,000	2,500
Total Fat	Less than	65g	80g
Sat. Fat	Less than	20g	25g
Cholesterol	Less than	300mg	300mg
Sodium	Less than	2,400mg	2,400mg
Total Carbohydrate		300g	375g
Dietary Fiber		25g	30g

Ingredients: Enriched flour (wheat flour, niacin, reduced iron, thiamin mononitrate [vitamin B_1], riboflavin [vitamin B_2], folic acid), partially hydrogenated soybean and/or cottonseed oil† with TBHQ for freshness, sugar, contains two percent or less of salt, leavening (baking soda, sodium acid pyrophosphate, monocalcium phosphate), corn syrup, high fructose corn syrup, sodium stearoyl lactylate, sodium sulfite, soy lecithin.
†Less than 0.5g *trans* fat per serving
CONTAINS WHEAT, AND SOY INGREDIENTS.

C

Nutrition Facts
Serving Size 18 Pretzels (30g)
Servings Per Container about 8

Amount Per Serving	
Calories 120	Calories from Fat 0
	% Daily Value*
Total Fat 0g	**0%**
Saturated Fat 0g	**0%**
Trans Fat 0g	
Cholesterol 0mg	**0%**
Sodium 320mg	**13%**
Total Carbohydrate 25g	**8%**
Dietary Fiber 2g	**8%**
Sugars 3g	
Protein 3g	

Vitamin A 0%	Vitamin C 0%
Calcium 0%	Iron 2%

*Percent Daily Values are based on a 2,000 calorie diet. Your Daily Values may be higher or lower depending on your calorie needs:

	Calories:	2,000	2,500
Total Fat	Less than	65g	80g
Sat Fat	Less than	20g	25g
Cholesterol	Less than	300mg	300mg
Sodium	Less than	2,400mg	2,400mg
Total Carbohydrate		300g	375g
Dietary Fiber		25g	30g

Calories per gram:
Fat 9 • Carbohydrate 4 • Protein 4

Ingredients: Organic wheat flour, water, organic oat flour and oat bran, organic evaporated cane juice, salt, yeast, sodium bicarbonate.
Allergy information: Produced in a facility that handles peanut butter.

Figure 22-9 Examples of food label from (A) potato chips, (B) wheat crackers, and (C) pretzels.

Critical Thinking

Evaluate your own diet. Write down every item you eat in a day and find the values of the nutrients contained in the foods. A medical dictionary is a good source for listing the nutrient value of selected foods. If you are eating prepared foods, read the package food label. Remember, you are trying to get an idea of your average daily diet, so do not change your diet for your analysis unless you plan to maintain it. What is the balance of your energy nutrients? Are you getting enough vitamins and minerals? Are you getting adequate fiber? What modifications could you make?

Pregnancy and Lactation

Pregnancy and lactation both cause marked changes in a woman's body and both require an increase in various nutrients. During pregnancy, not only does the growth of the fetus require additional nutrients, but the growth of the placenta, the increase in adipose tissue in the mother, the increased volume of blood, and the growth of breast tissue also require additional nutrients.

The increased demand for nutrients is not just a demand for Calories, but also for other specific nutrients to be increased, most notably protein. Protein requirements are nearly double during pregnancy. Because of the role vitamins play in metabolism and structure, they are needed in greater quantities than usual. In addition, calcium, phosphorus, and iron are needed in such high amounts that usually a vitamin supplement is prescribed. It is important that diet modifications are not simply an increase in Calories but include quality foods high in minerals, vitamins, and protein.

Pregnancy is an important time for both fetus and mother. It is normal and healthy for the mother to gain weight. Her provider will determine the appropriate amount of weight gain based on the individual. During lactation, the requirement for higher levels of nutrients continues; however, overall, it is not as high as during pregnancy. A baby is more likely to be healthy and develop normally if the mother has good nutritional habits during pregnancy and breast-feeding. A baby born to a mother who is malnourished may suffer from mental retardation and be of lower birth weight. Lower birth weight babies (less than 5.5 pounds) have a greater mortality rate than do babies of normal weight.

Breast-Feeding

There are several reasons why breast-feeding is encouraged. The nutrition the infant receives from breast milk is a perfect combination of water, lactose (sugar), fat, and protein. There are more than 100 ingredients in breast milk that are not found in formula milk. There are no allergic reactions to mother's milk. (On occasion, if the mother eats a particular food, the infant may react by being fussy.) Breast-feeding is nutritionally sound, economical, and sterile. Breast milk is easily digested and does not easily cause gastrointestinal upsets. Breast-fed babies receive temporary antibodies to many diseases from their mothers. Mother and infant bond during breast-feeding. Breast-feeding helps contract the uterus and bring it back to its nonpregnant state, thus helping to control postpartum bleeding.

While breast-feeding, the mother will continue to require nutritious foods taken from the food pyramid and will need to increase her intake of Calories. If she consumes inadequate Calories, the amount of milk produced will be decreased. When the mother terminates the period of breast-feeding (6 months is recommended for the greatest benefit to the infant), caloric intake should be reduced to avoid gaining weight.

Infancy

Infancy is a time of continuous growth, and many of the mother's nutritional requirements during pregnancy are still required by the baby after birth. In the first year of life, the baby will triple birth weight. The infant will need two to three times more Calories per kilogram (kg) of body weight than the normal adult. This is true for protein as well, and most of the vitamins and minerals are required at greater levels per kilogram. Most of these can be furnished with breast milk or formula; however, once iron stores have been used up, usually in 3 to 6 months, the infant will require an iron supplement, which is why pediatricians prescribe infant liquid iron supplement. Because of the high rate of growth, especially of the nervous system, infancy is an important time to be sure nutritional requirements are met. However, according to some pedintricians, overfeeding in infancy might lead to childhood doesity.

Critical Thinking

Write a response to a teenage girl who refuses to gain weight during her pregnancy.

Childhood

Good eating habits develop during childhood. One way parents who have good eating habits can teach their children how to eat healthfully is by example. Family eating habits, physical activity, and lifestyle help children to adopt healthy habits. Poor habits are established during childhood and are often difficult to alter. This can lead to lifelong health problems, such as obesity, diabetes, and cardiovascular diseases. The affects of poor nutrition not only are physical but can be emotional as well. When an obese child is "picked on" in school, anxiety, low self-esteem, depression, and irritability can result.

Childhood obesity is a serious problem, leading to type 2 diabetes because the disease is related to being overweight and having a poor diet. Obese children have a greatly increased chance of becoming obese as adults if they are obese before becoming a preteen (around age 11 years). Osteoporosis and cardiovascular diseases are other problems obesity can cause.

The availability of electronic devices, such as computers, video games, and television, contribute greatly to a child's reluctance to be active. Bike riding, jumping rope, swimming, and running are activities that most children enjoy if encouraged to engage in them.

Fast foods and carbonated sodas contribute to obesity because of their high fat and Calorie content. They are even banned from some schools because they are consumed readily and are poor choices at any age.

Clearly, parental education (and therefore of their children) about exercise and good nutrition is an excellent way to stop childhood obesity and type 2 diabetes. By following *MyPyramid for Kids and MyPyramid for Adults,* parents and children can learn to be active every day and to make healthy food choices. The government Web site (http://www.MyPyramid.gov) gives ideas on how everyone in the family can eat better and exercise more (Figures 22-10 and 22-11).

Adolescence

During adolescence, individuals experience the greatest levels of growth. The period of growth varies from person to person but generally begins

A Close Look at MyPyramid For Kids

MyPyramid for Kids reminds you to be physically active every day, or most days, and to make healthy food choices. Every part of the new symbol has a message for you. Can you figure it out?

Be Physically Active Every Day
The person climbing the stairs reminds you to do something active every day, like running, walking the dog, playing, swimming, biking, or climbing lots of stairs.

Eat More From Some Food Groups Than Others
Did you notice that some of the color stripes are wider than others? The different sizes remind you to choose more foods from the food groups with the widest stripes.

Choose Healthier Foods From Each Group
Why are the colored stripes wider at the bottom of the pyramid? Every food group has foods that you should eat more often than others; these foods are at the bottom of the pyramid.

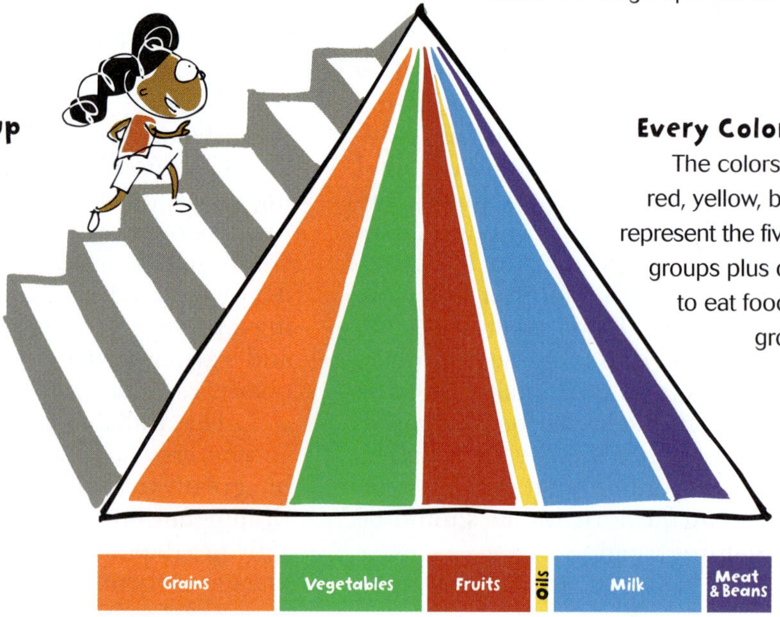

Every Color Every Day
The colors orange, green, red, yellow, blue, and purple represent the five different food groups plus oils. Remember to eat foods from all food groups every day.

Make Choices That Are Right for You
MyPyramid.gov is a Web site that will give everyone in the family personal ideas on how to eat better and exercise more.

Take One Step at a Time
You do not need to change overnight what you eat and how you exercise. Just start with one new, good thing, and add a new one every day.

MyPyramid.gov
STEPS TO A HEALTHIER YOU

U.S. Department of Agriculture
Food and Nutrition Service
September 2005
FNS-388

USDA is an equal opportunity provider and employer.

teamnutrition.usda.gov

Figure 22-10 The U.S. Department of Agriculture's MyPyramid for Kids reminds children to be physically active every day, or most days, and to make healthy food choices. (Courtesy of the U.S. Department of Agriculture.)

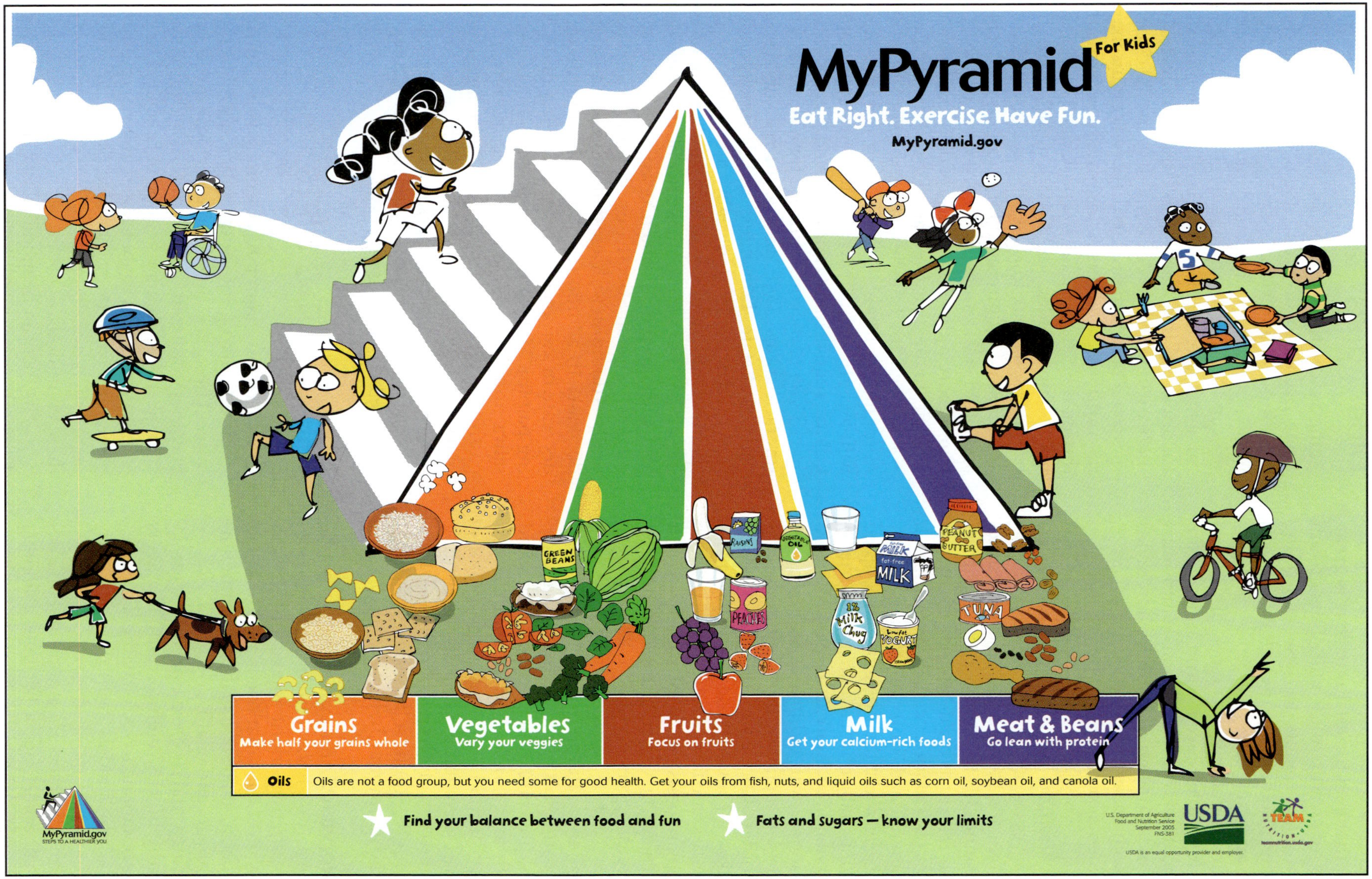

Figure 22-11 The U.S. Department of Agriculture's Guide to a balanced diet for children. It takes the shape of a pyramid. A good diet is made up of a balance between food and physical activity. (Courtesy of the U.S. Department of Agriculture.)

sooner with girls. Except for times of pregnancy and lactation, the need for total nutrients is greatest at this stage of growth. At the end of the growth spurt, nutrient requirements decrease, and young adults must then also decrease the amount of food they consume and exercise regularly.

Two particular nutrients that especially need to be altered during adolescence are iron and calcium. Iron requirements increase for the female individual as she begins menstruation. Calcium requirements increase for both male and female individuals as bone development is occurring at a rapid rate.

Bulimia and Anorexia Nervosa. Two eating disorders that may occur at any age are bulimia and anorexia nervosa, and they are serious in all individuals. Girls are more likely than boys to suffer from these problems. The diets of adolescent girls in general are deficient in Calories, vitamins, protein, and, as previously mentioned, iron and calcium. Many girls have concerns about their weight and, coupled with poor eating habits; when taken to extreme, can result in bulimia or anorexia nervosa. When a patient is diagnosed with bulimia or anorexia nervosa, the provider monitors the patient's weight gain or loss, orders laboratory tests at each office visit, and makes an appropriate treatment plan. EHR These tasks are facilitated in a total practice management system, as the patient's weight pattern can be viewed graphically and test results can be easily accessed (Figure 22-12).

Bulimia. Bulimia, although not usually life threatening, can result in electrolyte imbalance, dental caries, malnutrition, dehydration, and eroded mouth and esophagus. Individuals with bulimia binge on food and then purge (vomit). Use of laxatives is common. Girls fear becoming overweight and usually binge on high-Calorie dessert-type foods, then self-induce vomiting. Psychological therapy may help.

Anorexia Nervosa. Anorexia nervosa can be life threatening. It is characterized by the individual severely restricting caloric intake and exercising excessively. Problems that occur are low blood pressure, alopecia, altered metabolism, amenorrhea, brain damage, and death.

Both bulimia and anorexia nervosa seem to have some basis in U.S. culture, with teenagers (mostly women) wanting to look like the slim super models and fashion models (with distorted body images) seen in movies and in magazines.

These eating disorders are serious, and relapses are not unusual. Sometimes it becomes a lifelong struggle, and repeated therapy sessions are needed.

Older Adults

Aging is a natural process of the body. Although aging occurs in different stages and at different rates for each individual, some generalities can be made. As we age, our cellular metabolism tends to slow and, coupled with a general decline in physical activity, results in a decreased requirement for Calories. At the same time, there may be an increase in nutrient requirement in special circumstances. There is always an increased requirement for nutrients, vitamins, and protein in particular during illness, especially the prolonged illness that may occur in older adults. With aging, there may be increased breakdown of cells; as a result, there is an increased requirement for nutrients that repair and build cells and tissues. There is also a need to ingest more nutrients because of decreased absorption within the digestive tract. Thus, although there is less need for Calories, there is more need for nutrient-rich foods. Less need for Calories along with less physical activity may lead to weight gain if Calorie requirement is not reduced.

This may become difficult for older adults for several reasons. One may be an individual's psychological state. Loneliness and depression affect many older adults, especially after the loss of a spouse. Older adults may not like the idea of eating alone. The economic status of the individual also may present problems, as after retirement income generally decreases. Physiologically, taste tends to diminish with age and interest in food may decrease. In addition, problems with teeth and a decrease in salivary gland secretions may make eating painful. Many medications cause a decrease in saliva production. Also, decreased motility in the gastrointestinal tract may lead to constipation, making eating uncomfortable. All these factors, as well as a general unwillingness to break old habits, may make it difficult to change the diet to keep up with the body's aging process.

THERAPEUTIC DIETS

Thus far this chapter has examined the nutrient requirements of the body under normal conditions. There are times, however, when the body becomes diseased and nutrient requirements change. These changes may be necessitated by disease states such as diabetes mellitus or conditions resulting from a poor diet such as obesity. Therapeutic diets are designed to overcome or control these conditions.

The diet can be modified in a number of ways. The number of overall Calories can be adjusted, or

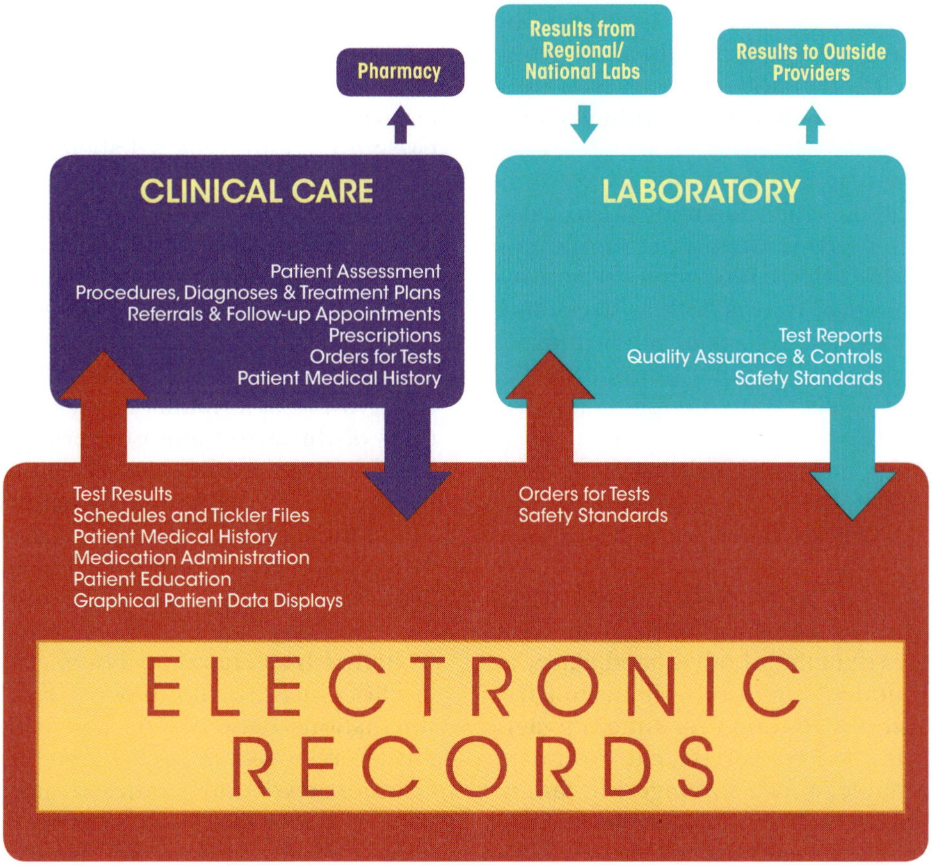

Figure 22-12 The clinical care and laboratory arms of the total practice management system (TPMS). Laboratory test results and mensurations are tracked in the patient's electronic medical record and are accessible to providers when determining an appropriate treatment plan.

one type of nutrient can be restricted or encouraged. The consistency, texture, and spiciness of food can be varied. The frequency of eating can be increased or decreased. When counseling patients, remember that habits are hard to change. The medical assistant should be supportive and encouraging.

Weight Control

Overweight and underweight are both weight disorders. The problem in defining overweight or underweight stems from the fact that there is no ideal weight for an entire population. There is only an ideal weight for the individual. Ideal weight can depend on many factors including age, sex, lean muscle mass, bone structure, and physical activity. Obesity is generally considered more than 20% overweight. Underweight is weight 10% to 15% below average. Height–weight tables now generally give ranges that vary more than 20 pounds. The ratio of fat tissue to lean muscle mass is a better indicator of whether individuals are at their ideal weight than a specific weight.

Individuals will gain weight if they consume more Calories than they need. Conversely, individuals will lose weight if they use more Calories than they ingest. In either case, the individual must bring the amount of Calories ingested into balance with the amount used. For the overweight individual, this means either decreasing Calorie consumption or increasing Calorie usage, or both. For the underweight individual, it usually entirely involves increasing Calorie consumption.

Weight loss has become a big business. However, individuals do not need to spend tremendous amounts of money to lose weight; patient education about low-Calorie, low-salt foods and a moderate exercise program are basic starting points for weight loss. Because losing more than 1 to 2 pounds a week can put an individual into nutritional deficiency, goals should not be set higher than this. Modifications made to the diet should then be maintained even after the weight is lost and should be continued throughout life. Losing weight takes much effort, and the patient needs constant encouragement and support from medical personnel and family.

Obesity has become a serious health problem. It is defined as severely overweight and having a body mass index (BMI) of 30 or above. BMI uses height and weight to calculate an individual's total amount of body fat.

Genetics may play a role in obesity. Several genes affect the rate at which the body burns calories. Playing a major role in obesity are family eating habits, other lifestyle habits, physical activity levels, and psychological factors such as stress and depression. Major causes are lack of physical exercise, oversized portions of high-fat foods, and the accessibility of fast foods. Many people eat more food than their bodies need.

Obesity causes increased risk for hypertension, heart and lung disease, hip and knee problems, certain cancers, and diabetes, and it shortens the life span.

Parents can be role models and teach their children to eat nutritious foods and not to consume more calories than their bodies need. Parents should provide nourishing foods, limit inactivity such as television and computer time, engage the entire family in regular exercise, eat at regular mealtimes at the table, and encourage the family to drink plenty (six to eight glasses) of water daily. By parents setting good examples when their children are young, the children will learn that healthy eating habits and regular exercise will improve the quality of life (fewer illnesses) and prolong the length of life.

The American Heart Association and the American Cancer Society are community resources available with information about reducing the risk for heart disease and cancer. Keeping weight under control and regular exercise helps prevent heart attacks, hypertension, and certain cancers.

Because there has been a great deal of media attention given to the problem of obesity and the diseases it can cause, many people are looking for a quick fix to lose weight. There are many claims that people can lose weight without exercising or eating healthy foods. Most claims about weight loss products are deceptive or false.

Individuals who want to lose weight must strive to eat a healthful diet over time. A healthful diet together with regular exercise can reduce their risk for hypertension, coronary artery disease, and certain cancers (colon and breast).

Diabetes Mellitus

Diabetes mellitus is a disease in which there is either reduced or no production of insulin, or in which there is reduced or no response to insulin. Approximately 5% of the population has diabetes mellitus (type 1 or type 2) in some form. Most patients with this disease are not dependent on insulin and can control their condition by monitoring diet, exercise, and weight (type 2 diabetes).

Normally, after a meal, the body secretes the hormone insulin, which makes its way to all cells of the body. Insulin signals the cells that the glucose is available and should be brought in so that it can be converted to energy. If the cells do not receive this signal, or do not respond to it, their ability to use glucose is markedly reduced. Because the body uses glucose as its main energy source, the ramifications of this affect almost every tissue of the body. In addition, the high levels of glucose that remain in the bloodstream put a tremendous strain on the kidneys and other major body organs, causing problems such as myocardial infarction, vascular diseases, neuropathy, and infections.

The effects of diabetes mellitus can be controlled with a general goal of maintaining a regular level of glucose in the bloodstream, avoiding large fluctuations between high and low levels. There are several ways suggested to accomplish this. Total Calories need not be altered, unless the diabetic patient is overweight. However, the ratio of carbohydrate, fat, and protein must be closely monitored. Total carbohydrates should be increased, but simple sugars should be avoided. Because of the longer rate of digestion and absorption of complex carbohydrates, these will be released over a longer period and prevent a sudden high level of glucose in the bloodstream, and these are the type of carbohydrates diabetics need. Increasing fiber content also increases the time of absorption and decreases the likelihood of sudden increases in glucose levels in the bloodstream. Regular snacks may be added between meals to maintain levels of glucose. The trend is for patients to take charge of their own care. The role of educator for the medical assistant will be an important one to facilitate patient self-management.

Type 2 Diabetes and Obesity. Obesity has become epidemic in the last 10 years and is the most significant factor in the increase in diabetes. Children and young people who are obese are being diagnosed with type 2 diabetes at an extremely high rate. The longer individuals have diabetes, the greater their risk for development of the complications of the disease, heart disease, stroke, kidney disease, blindness, and infections. Diabetes is a major cause of death.

Prevention of type 2 diabetes is of utmost importance. Changes in lifestyle such as weight loss, regular exercise, and a nutritious diet can prevent type 2 diabetes. If a patient has type 2 diabetes, it can be controlled by diet and exercise and by medication (see Chapter 24 for more information about diabetes and insulin).

Cardiovascular Disease

Cardiovascular disease is currently the leading cause of death in the United States. The unfortunate aspect is that much of it is preventable. Cardiovascular disease encompasses a variety of problems. Two of these problems, hypertension and atherosclerosis, often work hand in hand to perpetuate one another until a myocardial infarction occurs. It is important to remember that the conditions leading up to a myocardial infarction do not occur overnight. They have been developing slowly over many years, often asymptomatically. These conditions can be reduced or prevented with lifestyle modifications such as a healthy diet, moderate exercise, cessation of smoking, and weight management. This section focuses on a healthy diet to prevent cardiovascular disease.

Hypertension, or increased blood pressure, is often of unknown cause. Sometimes it has a familial connection. When the blood pressure is only moderately increased, certain diet modifications can be used to reduce it. If it is severe, drug therapy may be used in conjunction with diet therapy. One of the largest diet factors in controlling increased blood pressure is restricting sodium, because it can play such an important role in maintenance of water levels in the body. Some individuals are salt sensitive. An increased volume of blood and water will increase the pressure on the blood vessel walls. Eliminating sodium includes more than simply eliminating use of table salt. Foods that are particularly high in sodium include smoked meats, luncheon meats, olives, pickles, chips, crackers, catsup, and cheese. In some cases, eliminating foods with only moderate salt levels may be indicated. These may include certain meats, breads containing baking powder or baking soda, shellfish, and some vegetables.

Atherosclerosis is another condition that can lead to a myocardial infarction. Atherosclerosis is hardening of the arteries because of deposits of fatty substance. It should not be confused with arteriosclerosis, which is a hardening of the arteries because of loss of the elasticity of the arterial wall. Atherosclerosis leads to arteriosclerosis, which generally occurs because of a lack of exercise and increased blood cholesterol levels. The elasticity can be regained by increasing activity, although it should be started slowly and under a physician's guidance. Atherosclerosis and arteriosclerosis often occur together. Smoking and hypertension will increase the likelihood of development of both of these conditions.

The conditions of atherosclerosis and arteriosclerosis facilitate each other. The fatty deposits associated with atherosclerosis tend to occur at points of damage to the inner walls of the artery. One of the causes of this damage is high pressure at points where there may be narrowing because of deposits that are already there, or because of the constriction of blood vessels due to nicotine. Carbon monoxide brought into the bloodstream during smoking also causes damage to the arterial walls. The deposits and hardening increase the blood pressure, which, in turn, causes more damage and more deposits. It is a cycle that is difficult to stop. The best solution is prevention.

Fats and cholesterol in the diet have been strongly implicated in atherosclerosis. It is not only total fat that is important, but also types of fat ingested. The effect of high levels of fats and cholesterol in the diet will vary among individuals, and the factor in atherosclerosis is the levels of these substances in the bloodstream. Some individuals are able to ingest high amounts of fat and cholesterol without the body maintaining high levels of it in the blood. Unfortunately, this is not the case for everyone, and fat and cholesterol levels in the bloodstream must be closely monitored. Fat levels are measured by looking at triglycerides and lipoproteins. Lipoproteins are a complex made of fatty acids and proteins and are used to carry fat and cholesterol in the bloodstream. LDLs are used by the body to transport fats and cholesterol to the body tissues. These are the lipoproteins more likely to deposit cholesterol and fat into the arterial wall. HDLs carry fats and cholesterol to the liver to be broken down and used. These lipoproteins are more likely to remove fats and cholesterol from the deposits in the arterial walls. HDL levels can be increased by exercise.

The Nurses' Health Study, done by Harvard University, showed an association between the intake of hydrogenated fats (trans fats) and heart disease. The women who consumed high levels of foods that contained hydrogenated fats experienced a much greater risk for having a heart attack than did the women who consumed few hydrogenated fats. Harvard School of Public Health researchers have found that hydrogenated fats are responsible for the thousands of premature heart disease deaths in the United States every year.

Trans fats have also been implicated in increasing the risk for type 2 diabetes.

If total serum cholesterol and LDL levels are found to be increased, the individual must modify the diet, and, if severe enough, drug therapy may be indicated. The percentage of Calories from fat should be kept to less than 20% to 30% of total daily dietary intake, with less than a third of these coming from saturated fats. Cholesterol consumption should be less than 200 mg per day.

If a person experiences a myocardial infarction, it is important that the heart muscle be allowed to rest to facilitate proper healing. This includes bed rest, initially with a gradual progression to limited activity over about a 2-week period. Then the patient is allowed to resume full activity. Rehabilitation consists of cessation of smoking; control of hypertension; weight reduction through a low-fat, low-calorie diet; and a program of exercise. All help to improve myocardial function.

Cancer

Some substances ingested or inhaled are thought to be carcinogenic. For example, nitrites that are found in foods such as smoked ham or bacon are thought to cause cancer of the stomach and esophagus. Smoking tobacco, although not a food, has been implicated in cancers of the mouth, larynx, esophagus, and lungs. High fat in the diet has been shown to be associated with cancer of the breast, uterus, and colon.

High fiber in the diet may protect from colon cancer. Foods with vitamins A and C protect from cancer of the stomach, lung, and bladder. Fruits and vegetables, legumes, and foods with soy may protect from certain cancers.

Wise choices of foods from the food pyramid, avoiding foods with known carcinogens, keeping weight under control, and practicing a healthy lifestyle will improve the quality and length of life.

Cancer is a disease that comes in a variety of forms. It generally means that normal regulatory mechanisms within a cell have broken down. The result is that cells continue to grow in an unrestrained manner, diverting energy and nutrients from the patient's body to the cells' uncontrolled growth. There are many stages through which these cells may go, and they will go through them at varying rates. The ramifications of this new growth will vary depending on what types of cells are affected.

For these reasons, each cancer patient will have varying nutritional requirements. However, there are some generalities that can be made. First, there is definitely a need for increased Calories. Because the new growth has the ability to divert nutrients to itself, the result is the body receives fewer nutrients. It will then break down its own tissue. In addition, there is an increased need for nutrients to supply the immune system with energy and nutrients in its attempt to destroy the cancerous cells.

The patient who is receiving chemotherapy or radiation treatment has an even greater need for increased nutrients. These therapies are directed at killing cells that are rapidly dividing. This includes not only the cancerous cell but also healthy cells such as those of the lining of the gastrointestinal tract and hair follicles. Increased nutrients are needed for repair and replacement of the lost cells, and protein levels in particular should be increased. Because of the disturbance of the gastrointestinal lining, digestion and absorption may also be decreased. It is important that the patient maintain as healthy a nutritional status as is possible rather than having to make up for nutritional deficiencies.

The patient may experience loss of appetite, as well as nausea and vomiting. There are several ways to cope with this. First, food should be made as appealing as possible. If the patient has difficulty swallowing, food can be liquefied in a food processor. Generally, food will be better tolerated if it is slightly chilled; extremes of temperature should be avoided. Several smaller meals may be easier to eat than three large meals.

If patients lose large amounts of weight because of worry or concern or as a result of chemotherapy and/or radiation, they may become **cachectic.** In such cases, a tube is passed into the patient's stomach or duodenum through the nose, and liquid feedings are given through the tube. Another method for providing nutrition to a patient who is unable to take in necessary amounts of food is through a catheter (sterile tube) inserted into the subclavian vein to the superior vena cava, known as total parenteral nutrition (TPN). Feedings via the catheter provide very good nutrition and can be given for prolonged periods.

DIET AND CULTURE

Medical assistants are likely to come into contact with patients from many different ethnic groups. Many of these patients will have diets based on traditional cultures, and some of the foods they eat, or the way they combine foods, may be unfamiliar to the medical assistant. Often, diets in other cultures are sensible, with foods chosen or combined to make up a complete protein. The medical assistant who has some knowledge of ethnic food choices can help reassure patients that the dietary changes they need to make are within the parameters of their own cultures. Table 22-6 presents some highlights of the food choices of different ethnic groups.

Vegetarian diets are fairly common around the globe, including in the United States. With a good variety of grains, vegetables, fruits, and dairy products, a vegetarian diet can supply an individual with all the required nutrients. Pernicious anemia, a disease caused by lack of cobalamin (vitamin B_{12}), is sometimes associated with vegetarian diets that do not contain enough animal product (see the section on vitamins in this chapter). One type of vegetarian, vegan, does not eat any product associated with animals, including milk or eggs. This type of diet is particularly susceptible to nutritional deficiencies.

In speaking with patients about diet and dietary changes, it is important to remember that patients choose their diets for a variety of reasons, including cultural, religious, or ethical beliefs. The medical assistant should respect the patient's reasons for following a certain diet while encouraging any modifications.

Table 22-6 Sample Food Choices of Various Cultural, Religious, and Ethnic Groups

Culture/Region/ Group	Diet and Food Choices
Native American	It is thought that approximately half of the edible plants commonly eaten in the United States today originated with the Native Americans. Examples are corn, potatoes, squash, cranberries, pumpkins, peppers, beans, wild rice, and cocoa beans. In addition, they used wild fruits, game, and fish. Foods were commonly prepared as soups and stews, and dried. The original Native American diets were probably more nutritionally adequate than their current diets, which frequently consist of too high a proportion of sweet and salty, snack-type, empty calorie foods. Native American diets today may be deficient in calcium, vitamins A and C, and riboflavin.
U.S. Southern	Hot breads such as corn bread and baking powder biscuits are common in the U.S. South because the wheat grown in the area does not make good quality yeast breads. Grits and rice are also popular carbohydrate foods. Favorite vegetables include sweet potatoes, squash, green beans, and lima beans. Green beans cooked with pork are commonly served. Watermelon, oranges, and peaches are popular fruits. Fried fish is served often, as are barbecued and stewed meats and poultry. There is a great deal of carbohydrate and fat in these diets and limited amounts of protein in some cases. Iron, calcium, and vitamins A and C may sometimes be deficient.
Mexican	Mexican food is a combination of Spanish and Native American foods. Beans, rice, chili peppers, tomatoes, and corn meal are favorites. Meat is often cooked with the vegetable as in chili con carne. Corn meal is used in a variety of ways to make tortillas and tamales, which serve as bread. The combination of beans and corn makes a complete protein. Although tortillas filled with cheese (called enchiladas) provide some calcium, the use of milk should be encouraged. Additional green and yellow vegetables and vitamin C–rich foods would also improve these diets.
Puerto Rican	Rice is the basic carbohydrate food in Puerto Rican diets. Vegetables commonly used include beans, plantains, tomatoes, and peppers. Bananas, pineapple, mangoes, and papayas are popular fruits. Favorite meats are chicken, beef, and pork. Milk is not used as much as would be desirable from the nutritional point of view.
Italian	Pastas with various tomato or fish sauces and cheese are popular Italian foods. Fish and highly seasoned foods are common to Southern Italian cuisine, whereas meat and root vegetables are common to northern Italy. The eggs, cheese, tomatoes, green vegetables, and fruits common to Italian diets provide excellent sources of many nutrients, but additional milk and meat would improve the diet.
Northern and Western European	Northern and Western European diets are similar to those of the U.S. Midwest, but with a greater use of dark breads, potatoes, and fish, and fewer green vegetable salads. Beef and pork are popular, as are various cooked vegetables, breads, cakes, and dairy products.

(continues)

Table 22-6 Sample Food Choices of Various Cultural, Religious, and Ethnic Groups (continued)

Culture/Region/ Group	Diet and Food Choices
Central European	Citizens of Central Europe obtain the greatest portion of their calories from potatoes and grain, especially rye and buckwheat. Pork is a popular meat. Cabbage cooked in many ways is a popular vegetable, as are carrots, onions, and turnips. Eggs and dairy products are used abundantly.
Middle Eastern	Grains, wheat, and rice provide energy in these diets. Chickpeas in the form of hummus are popular. Lamb and yogurt are commonly used, as are cabbage, grape leaves, eggplant, tomatoes, dates, olives, and figs. Black, very sweet (Turkish) coffee is a popular beverage.
Chinese	The Chinese diet is varied. Rice is the primary energy food and is used in place of bread. Foods are generally cut into small pieces. Vegetables are lightly cooked, and the cooking water is saved for future use. Soybeans are used in many ways, and eggs and pork are commonly served. Soy sauce is extensively used, but it is salty and could present a problem with patients on low-salt diets. Tea is a common beverage, but milk is not. This diet may be low in fat.
Japanese	Japanese diets include rice, soybean paste and curd, vegetables, fruits, and fish. Food is frequently served tempura style, which means fried. Soy sauce (shoyu) and tea are commonly used. Current Japanese diets have been greatly influenced by Western culture.
Southeast Asian	Many Indians are vegetarians who use eggs and dairy products. Rice, peas, and beans are frequently served. Spices, especially curry, are popular. Indian meals are not typically served in courses as Western meals are. They generally consist of one course with many dishes.
Thailandese, Vietnamese, Laos, and Cambodian	Rice, curries, vegetables, and fruit are popular in Thailand, Vietnam, Laos, and Cambodia. Meat, chicken, and fish are used in small amounts. The wok (a deep, round fry pan) is used for sautéing many foods. A salty sauce made from fermented fish is commonly used.
Jewish	Interpretations of the Jewish dietary laws vary. Those who adhere to the Orthodox view consider tradition important and always observe the dietary laws. Foods prepared according to these laws are called kosher. Conservative Jews are inclined to observe the rules only at home. Reform Jews consider their dietary laws to be essentially ceremonial and thus minimize their significance. Essentially the laws require the following: • Slaughtering must be done by a qualified person, in a prescribed manner. The meat or poultry must be drained of blood, first by severing the jugular vein and carotid artery, then by soaking in brine before cooking. • Meat or meat products may not be prepared with milk or milk products. • The dishes used in the preparation and serving of meat dishes must be kept separate from those used for dairy foods. • A specified time, 6 hours, must elapse between consumption of meat and milk. • The mouth must be rinsed after eating fish and before eating meat. • There are prescribed fast days—Passover Week, Yom Kippur, and Feast of Purim. • No cooking is done on the Sabbath—from sundown Friday to sundown Saturday. These laws forbid the eating of: • The flesh of animals without cloven (split) hooves or that do not chew their cud • Hind quarters of any animal • Shellfish or fish without scales or fins • Fowl that are birds of prey • Creeping things and insects • Leavened (contains ingredients that cause it to rise) bread during the Passover Generally, the food served is rich. Fresh smoked and salted fish and chicken are popular, as are noodles, egg, and flour dishes. These diets can be deficient in fresh vegetables and milk.

(continues)

Table 22-6 (continued)

Culture/Region/Group	Diet and Food Choices
Roman Catholic	Although the dietary restrictions of the Roman Catholic religion have been liberalized, meat is not allowed its adherents on Ash Wednesday and Fridays during Lent.
Eastern Orthodox	Followers of this religion include Christians from the Middle East, Russia, and Greece. Although interpretations of the dietary laws vary, meat, poultry, fish, and dairy products are restricted on Wednesdays and Fridays and during Lent and Advent.
Seventh Day Adventist	Generally, Seventh Day Adventists are ovolacto-vegetarians, which means they use milk products and eggs, but no meat, fish, or poultry. They may also use nuts, legumes, and meat analogues (substitutes) made from soybeans. They consider coffee, tea, and alcohol to be harmful.
Mormon (Latter Day Saints)	The only dietary restriction observed by Mormons is the prohibition of coffee, tea, and alcoholic beverages.
Islamic	Adherents of Islam are called Muslims. Their dietary laws prohibit the use of pork and alcohol, and other meats must be slaughtered according to specific laws. During the month of Ramadan, Muslims do not eat or drink during daylight hours.
Hindu	To the Hindus, all life is sacred, and small animals contain the souls of ancestors. Consequently, Hindus are usually vegetarians. They do not use eggs because they represent life.
Vegetarians	There are several vegetarian diets. The common factor among them is that they do not include red meat. Some include eggs, some fish, some milk, and some even poultry. When carefully planned, these diets can be nutritious. They can contribute to a reduction of obesity, high blood pressure, heart disease, some cancers, and possibly diabetes. They must be carefully planned so they include all needed nutrients. Lacto-ovo vegetarians use dairy products and eggs but no meat, poultry, or fish. Lacto-vegetarians use dairy products but no meat, poultry, or eggs.
Vegans	Vegans avoid all animal foods. They use soybeans, chickpeas, and meat analogues made from soybeans. It is important that their meals be carefully planned to include appropriate combinations of the nonessential amino acids to provide the needed amino acids. For example, beans served with corn or rice, or peanuts eaten with wheat, are better in such combinations than any of them would be if eaten alone. Vegans can show deficiencies of calcium; zinc; vitamins A, D, and B_{12}; and, of course, proteins.
Zen macrobiotic diets	The macrobiotic diet is a system of 10 diet plans developed from Zen Buddhism. Adherents progress from the lower number diet to the higher, gradually giving up foods in the following order: desserts, salads, fruits, animal foods, soups, and ultimately vegetables, until only cereals—usually brown rice—are consumed. Beverages are kept to a minimum, and only organic foods are used. Foods are grouped as Yang (male) or Yin (female). A ratio of 5:1 Yang to Yin is considered important. Most macrobiotic diets are nutritionally inadequate. As the adherents give up foods according to plans, their diets become increasingly inadequate. These diets can be especially dangerous because avid adherents promise medical cures from the diets that cannot be attained, and thus medical treatment may be delayed when needed.

Procedure 22-1

Provide Instruction for Health Maintenance and Disease Prevention

PURPOSE:

To instruct patients about how to exercise more responsibly and take control of their health in order to extend their lives and enjoy healthy years.

With the provider's permission, medical assistants have many opportunities on a daily basis to educate patients about ways to stay healthy and r educe the risk of disease. Patient education boxes throughout the textbook relate specific behaviors patients can adopt to prevent diseases and measures they can take to preserve health.

EQUIPMENT/SUPPLIES

Discussion
DVDs
Videos
Print material
Authentic Web-based interactive information
Community resources directories
Seminars
Classes (self-directed and self-paced)

PROCEDURE STEPS:

1. Gather materials being used for guidelines for health and disease prevention.
2. Arrange a quiet area for patient and medical assistant.
3. Assess patient's learning style and preference. RATIONALE: The patient's age, physical limitations, and learning preferences need to be taken into consideration by the medical assistant. It is important to communicate clearly and at the level of the patient's understanding and knowledge.
4. Include the patient's family if appropriate. RATIONALE: The patient's family will learn along with the patient and provide instruction and encouragement to the patient at home.
5. Teach patients to take an active role in their health. Tell them that prevention is an important aspect in maintaining health. Instruct them to:
   - Get regular screenings for cancer when age appropriate, such as yearly physical examination, Pap smear, mammogram, occult blood testing, colonoscopy, urinalysis, electrocardiogram, chest X-ray, blood tests for anemia, chemistry profiles, hearing and vision tests.
   - Avoid tobacco.
   - Get regular exercise at least 30 minutes most days (walk dog, bicycle, rake leaves, do housework, swim).
   - Eat a balanced diet (see myPyramid worksheet at http://www.mypyramidtrackerworksheet.gov)
   - Practice safety to prevent injuries (make sure smoke detectors work, wear seat belts, don't drink and drive).
   - Control weight, blood pressure, and cholesterol.
   - Watch sun exposure and use a sun block factor of at least SPF 30 all year.
   - Keep vaccine immunizations current.
   - Practice food safety by preparing food with clean hands and on clean surfaces.
6. Instruct patients who do not have a computer that they may be able to gain online access at a public library. Some Web sites they can visit to learn more about strategies to prevent disease are:
   - General health: http://www.healthfinder. gov
   - Cancer: http://www.cancer.gov
   - Osteoporosis: http://www.osteo.org
   - Nutrition: http://www.usda.gov
   - Nutrition: http://www.fda.gov
   - Alcohol and drug abuse: http://www.niaa.nih.gov
   - Depression:http://www.nimh.nih.gov/health/topics/depression/index.html
   - Heart and lung: http://www.nhlbi.nih.gov
   - Product safety: http://www.cpsc.gov
7. Document the education session in the patient's chart or electronic medical record.

Case Study 22-1

Review the scenario at the beginning of the chapter.

CASE STUDY REVIEW

1. List and explain four possible reasons for Mrs. Leonard's not eating enough.
2. What strategies might you use to educate the teenager Corey Boyer about his consuming "fast" food?
3. Annette Samuels is pregnant and has particular needs. Search online for dietary/nutritional requirements for pregnant women. Name five of the most important nutrients that Annette needs during pregnancy.

Case Study 22-2

Anita Ferguson is a new patient at Inner City Health Care. She is a 16-year-old girl who is 4 months pregnant and came to the urgent care center only a couple of weeks ago. After Wanda Slawson, CMA (AAMA), took Anita's medical history, and after Anita was examined by the provider, Wanda set aside time to answer any questions Anita might have about her pregnancy. Anita is obviously scared; she wants the baby, but she does not want her life to change. According to the history, Anita has lost a few pounds in the last 2 weeks.

CASE STUDY REVIEW

1. What patient education can Wanda provide to alert Anita to the importance of diet and weight gain during pregnancy?
2. What foods should Wanda encourage Anita to eat?
3. If Anita resists Wanda's suggestions and has not gained any weight by the next visit, how should Wanda proceed?

Case Study 22-3

Dr. Lewis prescribed a diabetic diet for Mrs. Johnson.

CASE STUDY REVIEW

1. Describe what is included in a diabetic diet.
2. Describe the patient education you would use to help Mrs. Lewis understand the diet and to help her reach her goal of improved health.

SUMMARY

Seven types of nutrients are required by the body for maintenance of good health. Carbohydrates, fats, and proteins provide energy for the body. Vitamins, minerals, fiber, and water cannot provide energy but are responsible for many vital processes within the body.

Some individuals take herbal supplements. Making the provider aware of which supplements is an important responsibility of the medical assistant.

Nutritional needs change at various points in the life cycle. During pregnancy, lack of nutrients can be detrimental to the development of the fetus and the health of the expectant mother. The need for nutrients is great during infancy and childhood, with the greatest need for total nutrients occurring during adolescence. During adulthood, the requirement for Calories decreases. With the decrease in basal metabolism that occurs with aging, the requirement for Calories decreases even more.

At times of disease, the diet of the individual must be modified to help relieve stress put on the body by the disease, to give energy to fight the disease, and, in cases where the disease is diet related, to decrease the severity of the disease.

It is important to have adequate nutritional intake during every stage of life. The healthier one is, the better one feels and enjoys a good quality of lfe. Nutritional status should be examined and adjustments made if necessary with the goal of helping patients maintain a healthy body.

STUDY FOR SUCCESS

To reinforce your knowledge and skills of information presented in this chapter:

- Review the Key Terms
- Consider the Case Studies and discuss your conclusions
- Answer the Review Questions
  - Multiple Choice
  - Critical Thinking
- Navigate the Internet by completing the Web Activities
- Practice the StudyWARE activities on your student CD
- Apply your knowledge in the Student Workbook activities
- Complete the Web Tutor sections

REVIEW QUESTIONS

Multiple Choice

1. The transfer of nutrients from the gastrointestinal tract into the bloodstream is:
   a. ingestion
   b. digestion
   c. absorption
   d. elimination
2. Fats are considered a(n):
   a. mineral
   b. vitamin
   c. energy nutrient
   d. fiber
3. The total of all chemical and physical changes that take place in the body is called:
   a. homeostatis
   b. metabolism
   c. a catalyst
   d. an antioxidant
4. What is the significance for the provider in determining the patient's use of herbal supplements?
   a. The FDA has authority over these dietary supplements, therefore they are safe.
   b. They are unsafe if bought in a supermarket.
   c. They may interact with over-the-counter and prescription medications.
   d. They are not considered medicines. It is not significant to inform the provider.
5. Another name for vitamin C is:
   a. tocopherol
   b. carotene
   c. biotin
   d. ascorbic acid

Critical Thinking

1. For each of the following vitamins and minerals, suggest some symptoms that might appear if there were a deficiency:
   vitamin A
   vitamin K
   vitamin C
   thiamin
   riboflavin
   cobalamin (vitamin B_{12})
   calcium
2. Consider the functions of the various regions of the digestive system, and look up in a medical dictionary each of the following procedures. Describe the problems that might exist with the following procedures if diet modifications do not take place:
   colostomy
   gastrectomy
3. Explain why a breakfast high in complex carbohydrates is an important goal.
4. Figure 22-6 shows calculations of percentages of total calories from fat, carbohydrate, or protein. Are the percentages healthy or unhealthy? What are the recommended percentages of total calories from fat, carbohydrate, and protein?
5. What are some things to consider when assessing the diet of an older adult?
6. Find five things a person can do to decrease the risk for heart disease. Compile a list from the class. How many of the items are associated with diet? How many of the items involve you?
7. Describe how the diet can be used to control diabetes mellitus. When a person becomes dependent on insulin, should the diet continue to be used?

WEB ACTIVITIES

1. Search community agencies on the Web for information about the following diseases and the role nutrition plays in prevention of the disease:
   a. diabetes mellitus
   b. arteriosclerotic heart disease
   c. hypertension
2. Explore the FDA's site and find the amount of trans fats in one serving of:
   a. apple pie
   b. a jelly doughnut
   c. shredded wheat
   d. ice cream
3. Explore the National Center for Chronic Disease Prevention and Health Promotion and Physical Activity at Web site (http://www.cdc.gov/nccdphp/dnpa/index.htm) and discuss with your classmates four diseases that can be prevented through nutrition and exercise. Explain how and why.
4. Using a search engine, find a site for discussion about anorexia nervosa and bulimia. Describe these eating disorders. Is there any treatment for them?
5. Visit http://www.healthmonitor.com to calculate your body mass index (BMI) and decide if it is within a healthy range.
6. Use the government Web site (http://www.mypyramid.gov) to help you determine how your dietary habits rate according to the food pyramid.
7. Use www.cfscan.fda.gov/~dms/Foodlabel/html to access information on how to use food labels of pasta. How much cholesterol and saturated fat is there? Look at nutrition facts on a box.

REFERENCES/BIBLIOGRAPHY

Centers for Disease Control and Prevention. (2007). *Overweight and obesity.* Retrived May 24, 2007, from http://www.cdc.gov.

Ephedra. (2007). Retrieved May 25, 2007, from http://www.wikipedia.org/wiki/ephedra.

Richardson, M. (2004). Calcium absorption in postmenopausal women. *Harvard Women's Health Watch,* 5, 1–3.

Roth, R. A. (2007). *Nutrition and diet therapy.* (9th ed.). Clifton Park, NY: Delmar Cengage Learning.

Spratto, G. R., & Woods, A. L. (2004). *PDR nurses drug handbook.* Clifton Park, NY: Delmar Cengage Learning.

Taber's cyclopedic medical dictionary. (20th ed.). (2006). Philadelphia: F. A. Davis.

Chapter

23 Basic Pharmacology

OUTLINE

OBJECTIVES

The student should strive to meet the following performance objectives and demonstrate an understanding of the facts and principles presented in this chapter through written and oral communication.

1. Define the key terms as presented in the glossary.
2. Recall five medical uses for drugs.
3. Describe three types of drug names and give an example, for one drug, of all three names.
4. List five sources of drugs.
5. Describe the Federal Foods, Drug, and Cosmetic Act and the Controlled Substance Act of 1970.
6. Name the five controlled substances schedules and describe appropriate storage of the substances.
7. Define the law in terms of administering, prescribing, and dispensing drugs.
8. Describe how to use the four most commonly used sections of the *Physician's Desk Reference* (PDR).

KEY TERMS

Abuse
Administer
Anaphylaxis
Contraindication
Dispense
Pharmacology
Prescribe
Pruritus
Urticaria

OBJECTIVES (continued)

9. Describe the principal actions of drugs and three undesirable reactions.
10. Describe routes of drug administration and drug forms.
11. Describe handling and storing of drugs.
12. List emergency drugs and supplies.
13. Recall commonly abused drugs and describe their physical and emotional effects.
14. Critique the legal role and responsibilities of the medical assistant.

Scenario

Policy at Drs. Lewis and King dictates that a patient medication history is taken on the first appointment, routinely updated, and reviewed whenever medication is prescribed, dispensed, or administered. Both administrative and clinical medical assistants work together to ensure that this policy is carried out. When making a patient appointment, administrative medical assistants ask patients to bring with them any medications (keeping them in the labeled container) that they are currently using. When taking or updating a patient history, clinical medical assistants Audrey Jones, CMA (AAMA), and Joe Guerrero, CMA (AAMA), ask a number of questions of patients regarding medications, prescription, over-the-counter, and herbal supplements, and gently probe to ensure that patients include all medications in the history and describe any allergy or hypersensitivity they may have to certain drugs.

INTRODUCTION

__Pharmacology__ is the study of drugs, the science that is concerned with the history, origin, sources, physical and chemical properties, uses, and effects of drugs on living organisms. Medical assistants in the ambulatory care setting need to understand basic pharmacology including the uses, sources, forms, and delivery routes of drugs; must know and be able to implement the intent of the law regarding controlled substances and other medications; and must have a knowledge of drug classifications and actions to be able to caution patients when taking prescription or nonprescription drugs. In addition, the medical assistant must be able to educate patients about a drug's intended purpose and the correct way to take the drug for maximum effectiveness.

This chapter provides an overview of pharmacology; it is considered a review for medical assistants who have had a formal course in the subject. Information on dosage, calculation, and medication administration can be found in Chapter 24.

MEDICAL USES OF DRUGS

A drug is defined as a medicinal substance that may alter or modify the functions of a living organism. There are five medical uses for drugs:

Spotlight on Certification

RMA Content Outline

- Anatomy and physiology
- Medical law
- Medical ethics
- Patient education
- Asepsis
- Clinical pharmacology

CMA (AAMA) Content Outline

- Anatomy and physiology
- Medicolegal guidelines and requirements
- Principles of infection control
- Pharmacology
- Emergencies

CMAS Content Outline

- Anatomy and physiology
- Apply principles of medical law and ethics to the health care setting
- Asepsis in the medical office
- Recognize and respond to emergencies
- Understand basic pharmacological concepts and terminology

- *Therapeutic.* Used in the treatment of a condition to relieve symptoms. An example is an antihistamine that may be used in the treatment of an allergy.
- *Diagnostic.* Used in conjunction with radiology and other diagnostic imaging procedures to allow the physician to pinpoint the location of a disease process. An example is dye tablets used in the X-ray study of the gallbladder.
- *Curative.* Used to kill or remove the causative agent of a disease. An example is an antibiotic.
- *Replacement.* Used to replace substances normally found in the body. Hormones and vitamins are examples of replacement drugs.
- *Preventive or Prophylactic.* Used to ward off or lessen the severity of a disease. Examples are immunizing agents such as vaccines.

DRUG NAMES

Most drugs have three types of names: chemical, generic, and trade or brand name.

- The *chemical name* describes the drug's molecular structure and identifies its chemical structure.
- The *generic name* is the drug's official name and is assigned to the drug by the U.S. Adopted Names Council. A generic drug can be manufactured by more than one pharmaceutical company. When this is the case, each company markets the drug under its own unique trade or brand name. Generic names begin with a lowercase letter.
- A *trade* or *brand name* is registered by the U.S. Patent and Trademark Office and is approved by the U.S. Food and Drug Administration (FDA). The ® symbol following a drug's trade or brand name indicates that the name is registered and protected for 17 years. No other manufacturer can make or sell the drug during that time. Once the patent expires, any manufacturer can sell the drug under its generic name or a new trade name. The original trade name cannot be reused. The brand name begins with a capital letter.

Example:

Chemical name: 1, 4, 3, 6-dian hydrosorbitol-2, 5 dinitrate
Generic name: isosorbide dinitrate
Trade/Brand name: Sorbitrate®

When providers prescribe a drug, they may use either the generic or trade name. It is not uncommon for providers to prescribe the generic form of a drug because it is usually less costly for the patient. To reduce costs, some insurance companies pay for only generic brands. Sometimes, providers specify drugs by their trade names. Some states allow patients to request that their pharmacist dispense the generic drug equivalent unless the provider has specified that the drug be dispensed by its trade name. Also, in some states, a pharmacist may select a generic form of a drug if not specifically directed otherwise by the provider. Generic and trade name drugs have the same chemical composition and must adhere to identical FDA standards; therefore, according to most state laws, they can be used interchangeably. The drug label reflects the drug products dispensed.

HISTORY AND SOURCES OF DRUGS

Drugs prepared from roots, herbs, bark, and other forms of plant life are among the earliest known pharmaceuticals. Their origin can be traced back to primitive cultures where they were first used to evoke magical powers and to drive out evil spirits. Having discovered that certain plants were pharmacologically useful, a search was begun for sources of drugs.

Today this search continues. In addition to plants, drugs are derived from animals and minerals and are produced in laboratories using chemical, biochemical, and biotechnologic processes.

Plant Sources

The leaves, roots, stems, or fruit of certain plants may contain medicinal properties. For example, the dried leaf of the foxglove plant *(Digitalis purpurea)* is a source of digitalis, a cardiac glycoside used in the treatment of certain heart conditions.

Herbals fit into this plant source category. The disadvantage of many natural herbals on the market today is that some drugs derived from plants may not be standardized. In any given crop, there may be plants that are more or less potent than their neighboring plants. This lack of consistency is related to the amount of sunshine and water a particular plant receives, as well as the nutrients in the soil. Another disadvantage of natural plant drugs is the pesticides that may be present. These may be man-made pesticides applied to the plants or taken up by the plant through the environment (soil, water, and air); they may also be natural pesticides originating from the plant itself to defend itself from molds, insects, and other threats. These pesticides all pose biologic threats to our chemical and biologic functions. These foreign chemicals can be interpreted by our bodies as irritants, free radicals, antigens, and antagonists. Patients should be cautioned to purchase only reputable, standardized, natural herbal products for these reasons.

Animal Sources

A few drugs are obtained from tissues such as the adrenal glands of animals. Examples of drugs obtained from animals are adrenaline and cortisone, extracted from the adrenal glands of animals. Adrenaline is used for allergic reactions and cortisone is an antiinflammatory. Premarin® is another example. It is derived from urine produced by pregnant mares. It is used for treating menopausal symptoms in some women.

Mineral Sources

Some naturally occurring mineral substances are used in medicine in a highly purified form. One such mineral is sulfur, which has been used as a key ingredient in certain bacteriostatic drugs. It is now prepared synthetically and used in the treatment of urinary and intestinal tract infections.

Herbal Supplements

With the increased interest in alternative or complementary medicine, many patients and some practitioners use herbal products for treatment, prophylaxis, and maintenance of health and care of disease. *Phytomedicine* is the term used to describe the use of plants to promote optimum health.

Native cultures since ancient times had great respect for their medicine men and women because they knew about plants and herbs for medicinal purposes. Such diseases and conditions as cardiac arrhythmia, pain, blood thinning, digestive upsets, and increased urinary output (diuresis) have been treated with success with herbal medicine.

European providers use herbal medicines routinely in their practices and have had classes on the topic throughout medical school.

In the United States, it was not until 1974 that the FDA passed an act known as the Dietary Supplement Health and Education Act (DSHEA). The act examines any dietary supplement such as herbal products and may remove it from the market if it presents a significant or unreasonable risk for illness or injury when used according to its labeling or under ordinary conditions of use.

The DSHEA gathers and thoroughly reviews evidence about the pharmacology of a product, uses peer-review scientific literature on safety and effectiveness, examines adverse event reports, and includes public comments for information about associated health risks.

Self-medication with herbal products is less in the United States than worldwide, but sales in the United States have been increasing yearly. There has been an abundance of interest by the public in herbal products because of the media attention given to them and their benefits.

Many providers combine herbal products (together with nutrition) in their practice(s), and certain herbal treatments have become part of the practitioner's treatment regimen.

Some examples of herbs and their uses are as follows: cascara—laxative; feverfew—headaches; garlic—antibacterial; licorice—gastritis, cough, menopause; St. John's wort—depression and anxiety; and saw palmetto—prostate health.

There are risks associated with self-medication with herbal products. Patients need to be informed that taking certain medications together with herbal products can produce dangerous interactions. It is important for you as the medical assistant to gather information about all medications, prescriptions, over-the-counter medications, and herbals. Pregnant patients should inform their provider about what they are taking and should be cautioned about possible harm to the fetus (see Chapter 14). It is important to remember that any medication and any herb can cause an allergic reaction and have side effects.

The dietary supplement ephedra, also known as Ma huang, had been prohibited from being sold since April 2004 because, according to DSHEA of 1994, ephedra presented an unreasonable risk for illness and injury. The herbal supplement had been promoted for use in weight loss and control and for enhancing performance in sports activities. Evidence showed modest effectiveness for weight loss with no clear health benefit. It was confirmed that, in many instances, the substance increased blood pressure and caused tachycardia, chest pain, myocardial infarction (MI), cerebral vascular accidents (CVA), seizures, psychosis, and death.

In 2005, the ban on ephedra was lifted because it had been challenged in court, and the judge ruled for the company that manufactures ephedra. During 2005 and 2006, ephedra was sold again. In August 2006, the FDA's ban on all ephedra and ephedra-like drugs was upheld. It now is illegal in the United States. In October 2006, the manufacturing company filed a petition for a

Patient Education

If you want to use herbal therapy, you should find a qualified herbalist and work with him or her and your practitioner. Herbal products are not regulated or standardized by an agency or organization (see earlier for information about DSHEA). Report at once symptoms that seem unusual. Herbal products should be used for the shortest amount of time needed to obtain results. Keeping track of herbs taken, for what purpose they are being taken, and the effect on symptom control is important and provides information about which products are helpful and those that are not. Journals, newsletters, and the Internet can provide information about herbal medicine. These publications can be explored for information and are a valuable resource. Relevent publications include *Herbalgram*, *Phytomedicine*, *Alternative Medicine Alert*, and *Alternative and Complementary Medicine*.

rehearing on the issue. Ephedra remains illegal and is likely to remain so. Congress is rewriting laws so it will be easier for the FDA to take action and ban substances they believe are harmful.

Synthetic Drugs

Synthetic drugs are artificially prepared in pharmaceutical laboratories. By combining various chemicals, scientists can produce compounds that are identical to a natural drug or create entirely new substances. An advantage of synthetic drugs over natural is the ability to standardize doses. Thousands of drugs are now produced synthetically. Examples are Motrin® (ibuprofen), Feldene® (piroxician), and Prilosec® (omeprazole).

Genetically Engineered Pharmaceuticals

Scientists are now capable of creating new strains of bacteria using a technique known as gene splicing. Through this process, hybrid forms of life have been created that benefit human beings by providing an alternative source of drugs, such as Humulin® (insulin) for the diabetic patient and interferon for use in treatment of cancer. These drugs can be manufactured in large quantities; thus, they are less expensive than natural substances.

DRUG REGULATIONS AND LEGAL CLASSIFICATIONS OF DRUGS

Qualified medical practitioners who prescribe, dispense, or administer drugs must comply with federal and state laws. The laws govern the manufacture, sale, possession, administration, dispensing, and prescribing of drugs. All drugs available for legal use are controlled by the Federal Food, Drug, and Cosmetic Act. The law protects the public by ensuring the purity, strength, and composition of foods, drugs, and cosmetics. It also prohibits the movement in interstate commerce of altered and misbranded food, drugs, devices, and cosmetics. Enforcement of the act is the responsibility of the FDA, which is part of the Department of Health and Human Services (DHHS).

Controlled Substance Act of 1970

One category of drugs—those with potential for abuse or addiction—is regulated by the Controlled Substance Act of 1970. It controls the manufacture, importation, compounding, selling, dealing in, and giving away of drugs that have the potential for abuse and addiction. The drugs are known as controlled substances and include heroin and cocaine and their derivatives, other narcotics, stimulants, and depressants. The Drug Enforcement Agency (DEA) of the U.S. Justice Department monitors and enforces the act, which is also known as the Comprehensive Drug Abuse Prevention and Control Act. Under federal law, providers who prescribe, administer, or dispense controlled substances must register with the DEA and renew their registration as required by state law (Form DEA 224).

Applications for registration are available online (http://www.deadiversion.usdoj.gov). A licensed provider is issued a registration that must be renewed at regular intervals (Figure 23-1). The renewal form is sent approximately 2 months before the expiration date.

Controlled Substances Schedules. Controlled substances are classified according to five schedules:

- *Schedule I* specifies drugs that have a high potential for abuse and are not accepted for medical use within the United States. Examples are heroin, lysergic acid diethylamide (LSD), and marijuana.
- *Schedule II* drugs include those that also have a high abuse potential but have an accepted medical use

Form-224

APPLICATION FOR REGISTRATION
Under the Controlled Substances Act

APPROVED OMB NO 1117-0014
FORM DEA-224 (10-06)
Previous editions are obsolete

INSTRUCTIONS

Save time - apply on-line at *www.deadiversion.usdoj.gov*

1. To apply by mail complete this application. Keep a copy for your records.
2. Print clearly, using black or blue ink, or use a typewriter.
3. Mail this form to the address provided in Section 7 or use enclosed envelope.
4. Include the correct payment amount. FEE IS NON-REFUNDABLE.
5. If you have any questions call 800-882-9539 prior to submitting your application.

IMPORTANT: DO NOT SEND THIS APPLICATION **AND** APPLY ON-LINE.

DEA OFFICIAL USE :

Do you have other DEA registration numbers?

☐ NO ☐ YES

MAIL-TO ADDRESS Please print mailing address changes to the right of the address in this box.

FEE FOR THREE (3) YEARS IS $551
FEE IS NON-REFUNDABLE

SECTION 1 APPLICANT IDENTIFICATIION ☐ **Individual Registration** ☐ **Business Registration**

Name 1 (Last Name of individual -OR- Business or Facility Name)

Name 2 (First Name and Middle Name of individual - OR- Continuation of business name)

Street Address Line 1 (if applying for fee exemption, this must be address of the fee exempt institution)

Address Line 2

City State Zip Code

Business Phone Number Point of Contact

Business Fax Number Email Address

DEBT COLLECTION INFORMATION

Mandatory pursuant to Debt Collection Improvements Act

Social Security Number (***if registration is for individual***)

Provide SSN or TIN.
See additional information note #3 on page 4.

Tax Identification Number (***if registration is for business***)

FOR Practitioner or MLP ONLY:

Professional Degree : *select from list only*

Professional School :

Year of Graduation :

National Provider Identification:

Date of Birth (*MM-DD-YYYY*): M M - D D - Y Y Y Y

SECTION 2 BUSINESS ACTIVITY

Check one business activity box only

☐ Central Fill Pharmacy
☐ Retail Pharmacy
☐ Nursing Home
☐ Automated Dispensing System
☐ Practitioner (DDS, DMD, DO, DPM, DVM, MD or PHD)
☐ Practitioner Military (DDS, DMD, DO, DPM, DVM, MD or PHD)
☐ Mid-level Practitioner (MLP) (DOM, HMD, MP, ND, NP, OD, PA, or RPH)
☐ Euthanasia Technician
☐ Ambulance Service
☐ Animal Shelter
☐ Hospital/Clinic
☐ Teaching Institution

FOR Automated Dispensing System (ADS) ONLY:

DEA Registration # of Retail Pharmacy for this ADS

An ADS is automatically fee-exempt. Skip Section 6 and Section 7 on page 2. You must attach a notorized affidavit.

SECTION 3 DRUG SCHEDULES

Check all that apply

☐ Schedule II Narcotic
☐ Schedule II Non-Narcotic
☐ Schedule III Narcotic
☐ Schedule III Non-Narcotic
☐ Schedule IV
☐ Schedule V

☐ Check this box if you require official order forms - for purchase or transfer of schedule 2 narcotic and/or schedule 2 non-narcotic controlled substances.

NEW - Page 1

Figure 23-1 Licensed providers who prescribe, administer, or dispense controlled substances must register with the Drug Enforcement Agency (DEA) of the U.S. Justice Department. The registration must be renewed at regular intervals. Shown here is Form 224 for a new application for registration with the DEA. Form 224(A) is for registration renewal.

SECTION 4

STATE LICENSE(S)

Be sure to include both state license numbers if applicable

You MUST be currently authorized to prescribe, distribute, dispense, conduct research, or otherwise handle the controlled substances in the schedules for which you are applying under the laws of the **state** or jurisdiction in which you are operating or propose to operate.

State License Number (required) ☐☐☐☐☐☐☐☐☐☐☐☐☐☐☐☐ Expiration Date (required) / / MM - DD - YYYY

What state was this license issued in? ______

State Controlled Substance License Number (if required) ☐☐☐☐☐☐☐☐☐☐☐☐☐☐☐☐ Expiration Date / / MM - DD - YYYY

What state was this license issued in? ______

SECTION 5

LIABILITY

IMPORTANT

All questions in this section must be answered.

1. Has the applicant ever been **convicted of a crime** in connection with controlled substance(s) under state or federal law, or is any such action pending? YES ☐ NO ☐

   Date(s) of incident MM-DD-YYYY: ☐☐-☐☐-☐☐☐☐

2. Has the applicant ever surrendered (for cause) or had a **federal** controlled substance registration revoked, suspended, restricted, or denied, or is any such action pending? YES ☐ NO ☐

   Date(s) of incident MM-DD-YYYY: ☐☐-☐☐-☐☐☐☐

3. Has the applicant ever surrendered (for cause) or had a **state** professional license or controlled substance registration revoked, suspended, denied, restricted, or placed on probation, or is any such action pending? YES ☐ NO ☐

   Date(s) of incident MM-DD-YYYY: ☐☐-☐☐-☐☐☐☐

4. If the applicant is a **corporation** (other than a corporation whose stock is owned and traded by the public), association, partnership, or pharmacy, has any officer, partner, stockholder, or proprietor been **convicted of a crime** in connection with controlled substance(s) under state or federal law, or ever surrendered, for cause, or had a **federal** controlled substance registration revoked, suspended, restricted, denied, or ever had a **state** professional license or controlled substance registration revoked, suspended, denied, restricted or placed on probation, or is any such action pending? YES ☐ NO ☐

   Date(s) of incident MM-DD-YYYY: ☐☐-☐☐-☐☐☐☐ *Note: If question 4 does not apply to you, be sure to mark 'NO'. It will slow down processing of your application if you leave it blank.*

EXPLANATION OF "YES" ANSWERS

Applicants who have answered "YES" to any of the four questions above **must provide a statement to explain each "YES" answer.**

Use this space or attach a separate sheet and return with application

Liability question # ______ Location(s) of incident: ______

Nature of incident:

Disposition of incident:

SECTION 6 EXEMPTION FROM APPLICATION FEE

☐ Check this box if the applicant is a federal, state, or local government official or institution. Does not apply to contractor-operated institutions.

Business or Facility Name of Fee Exempt Institution. **Be sure to enter the address of this exempt institution in Section 1.**

☐☐

FEE EXEMPT CERTIFIER

Provide the name and phone number of the certifying official

The undersigned hereby certifies that the applicant named hereon is a federal, state or local government official or institution, and is exempt from payment of the application fee.

______ Signature of certifying official (**other than applicant**) ______ Date

______ Print or type name and title of certifying official ______ Telephone No. (required for verification)

SECTION 7

METHOD OF PAYMENT

Check one form of payment only

☐ Check — Make check payable to: **Drug Enforcement Administration**. See page 4 of instructions for important information.

☐ American Express ☐ Discover ☐ Master Card ☐ Visa

Credit Card Number ☐☐☐☐☐☐☐☐☐☐☐☐☐☐☐☐ Expiration Date ☐☐ - ☐☐

Sign if paying by credit card

______ Signature of Card Holder

______ Printed Name of Card Holder

Mail this form with payment to:

U.S. Department of Justice
Drug Enforcement Administration
P.O. Box 28083
Washington, DC 20038-8083

FEE IS NON-REFUNDABLE

SECTION 8

APPLICANT'S SIGNATURE

Sign in ink

I certify that the foregoing information furnished on this application is true and correct.

______ **Signature of applicant (sign in ink)** ______ Date

______ Print or type name and title of applicant

WARNING: Section 843(a)(4)(A) of Title 21, United States Code states that any person who knowingly or intentionally furnishes false or fraudulent information in the application is subject to imprisonment for not more than four years, a fine of not more than $30,000, or both.

NEW - Page 2

Figure 23-1 (continued)

within the United States. Examples are amphetamines and cocaine. Because of their high potential for abuse, a special DEA form must be used to order these drugs. The form is not necessary for Schedule III and IV drugs. A written prescription is required for Schedule II drugs and the prescription cannot be renewed. Examples of Schedule II drugs are morphine, codeine, Ritalin, and Percocet.

- *Schedule III* drugs have a low-to-moderate potential for physical dependence, yet have a high potential for psychological dependency. Some examples are barbiturates and various drug combinations containing codeine and paregoric. Prescriptions for Schedule III drugs can be either written or oral. They can be refilled, but only five times within 6 months. Schedule III drugs are accepted for medical use in the United States.
- *Schedule IV* drugs have a lower potential for abuse and have an accepted use in the United States. Examples of these drugs include chloral hydrate and diazepam. Prescriptions for Schedule IV drugs may include refills, but refills are limited to five times within 6 months.
- *Schedule V* drugs have the lowest abuse potential of controlled substances. Some examples from this schedule are Lomotil® and Donnagel®. Some drugs from Schedule V may include refills, but refills are limited to five times within 6 months.

On occasion, the DEA will reclassify drugs and move them from one schedule to another.

So that they can be readily identified, controlled substances are labeled with a large C with a Roman numeral inside it to indicate from which schedule the drug has come; for example, CII represents a Schedule II drug.

The provider's DEA number must appear on each prescription for controlled substances.

A copy of the federal law and a complete list of controlled substances and their schedules are available from any DEA office or online.

Storage of Controlled Substances. Federal law requires that all controlled substances be kept separate from other drugs. They must be stored in a well-constructed metal box or compartment that has a double lock. Controlled substances must be protected from possible misuse and abuse, and persons who administer controlled substances must record them in a separate record book. The record must be maintained on a daily basis and kept for a minimum of 2 to 3 years, depending on state laws. Patient name, address, date of administration of the controlled substance, drug name, dose, and route and method of administration must be included in the record.

Record keeping applies only to persons who administer or dispense controlled substances. Record-keeping data can be stored electronically.

Controlled substances (Schedule II) stored and used on the premises must be counted at the end of each workday, verified by two individuals for accuracy of count, and recorded on an audit sheet. An inventory record of Schedule II drugs must be submitted to the DEA every 2 years.

Because of the increase in office and clinic drug theft and substance abuse, as well as the stringent federal laws that apply to storing, dispensing, and administration of controlled substances, many offices and clinics do not keep controlled substances on the premises. However, agencies that do have controlled substances on the premises must comply with the DEA disposal policy.

Controlled Substance Disposal Policy (per DEA). The DEA Disposal Policy for Controlled Substances requires that controlled substances be accounted for when they are disposed of. One option is the company Universal Solutions, which is contracted with the DEA and will dispose of expired or unused controlled substances. Certain forms (DEA Form 41) must be completed, and the provider must have current certificate of registration (DEA Form 222) with the DEA. Records of disposed controlled substances must be kept for 2 years. Application forms are completed and signed by the provider. A copy of the provider's DEA certificate of registration is included and sent to Universal Solutions (controlled substances are not sent at this time). Shipping instructions from Universal Solutions will be sent along with a label. Follow the instructions provided and ship to Universal Solutions. The company will confirm receipt of the material and its eventual destruction. Copies of application and confirmation of destruction must be sent to the DEA. Applications for forms for disposal of controlled substances are available from the nearest DEA office or online (http://www.usdoj.gov/dea).

Medical Assistant Role and Responsibilities. Medical assistants are required to know the legalities that surround controlled substances. Medical assistant responsibilities may include:

1. Monitor the provider's DEA registration renewal date.
2. Maintain legally designated records and inventories of all drugs (Figure 23-2), including samples. This can be done electronically.

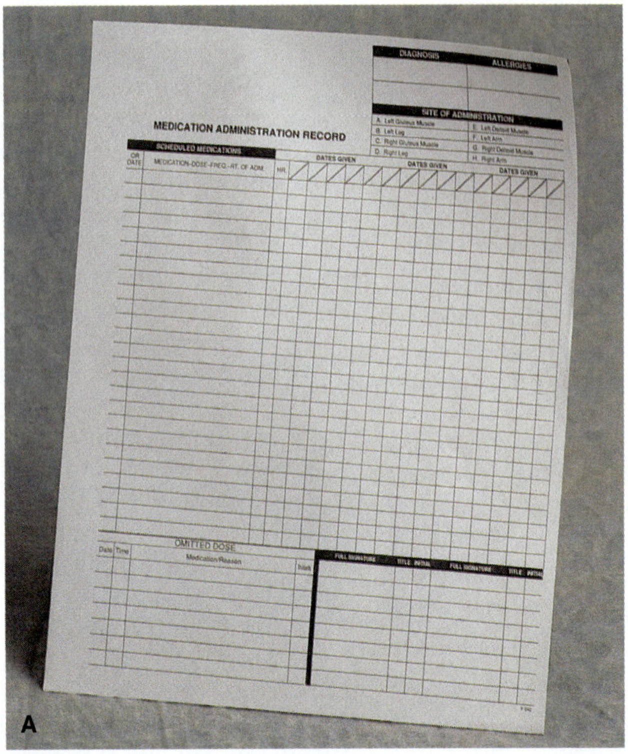

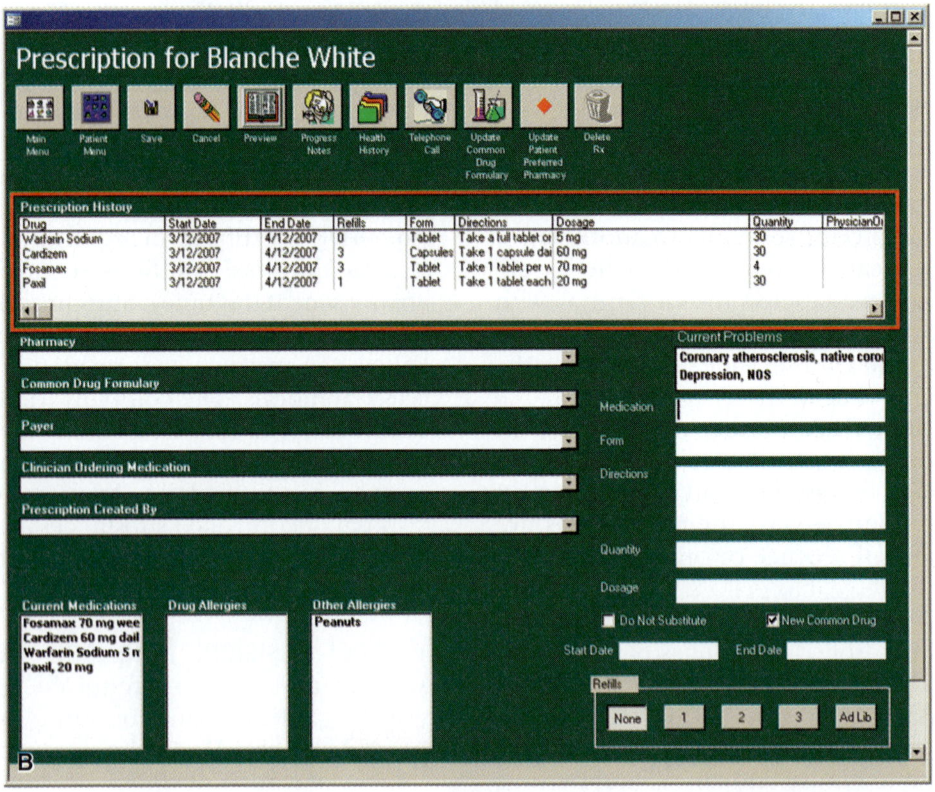

Figure 23-2 It is important to maintain patient medication records both for the safety of the patient and to protect the practice. (A) A paper-based patient medication record. (B) The patient medication record as part of the patient's electronic medical record.

3. Provide security for all drugs, in particular controlled substances (Schedule II).
4. Provide security for prescription pads.
5. Properly destroy expired drugs and document.
6. Know and understand federal and state laws that regulate drugs, including all controlled substances and samples.

EHR The computer and its software have the capability of storing information regarding the due date for the provider's DEA registration renewal, maintaining legal records and inventories on all drugs including samples, keeping track of expiration dates of drugs and when they are destroyed, accessing the latest information regarding new DEA laws, and e-prescribing.

Since 2006, the DEA has been reluctant to approve regulations covering e-prescribing of controlled substances. The reluctance and lack of DEA policies have been a hurdle to widespread adoption of e-prescribing. Presently, some providers can e-prescribe medications other than controlled substances (which require handwritten and signed prescriptions). This requires two separate systems, e-prescribing and handwritten prescriptions, and providers object, viewing this as time-consuming.

A proposal known as the Medicare Electronic Medication and Safety Protection Act, if approved, would penalize providers who write prescriptions by hand after 2011. The government is offering a one-time grant to help offset the costs to providers who implement e-prescribing technology.

The DEA is preparing to allow e-prescribing of controlled substances as of 2008. It has sent a proposed rule to the Department of Justice (DOJ). The rule requires review from the DOJ and the Office of Management and Budget (OMB) before the rule can be enacted.

E-prescribing of medications is safe, efficient, and effective. It can improve patient safety. The next section on Prescription Drugs discusses how e-prescribing is beneficial to providers and patients.

Prescription Drugs

State laws require that licensed practitioners who prescribe drugs must write and sign an order for the dispensing of drugs. This process is known as writing a prescription. Some examples of drugs that require a prescription are all of the controlled substances, except for Schedule I, which is not accepted for medical use in the United States, and other categories such as digoxin, a cardiac drug, and epinephrine, a vasoconstrictor.

Medical assistants need to advise patients after the provider prescribes a drug. Patients should also read warning labels on medication containers (Figure 23-3). Prescription drugs are also called legend drugs.

EHR The July 20, 2007, issue of *Medical Economics,* a periodical for providers and other medical professionals, reported the results of a survey they conducted, which showed physicians ranked computer systems high on timely access to records, better quality of care, and better documentation. E-prescribing is a feature many providers appreciated (Figure 23-4). Providers have instantaneous and remote access to records, in addition to many other capabilities. Some are:

- Automatically alerts to allergies and drug interactions
- Automatically calculates doses of medication according to the patient's age and weight
- Recommends brand and/or generic drug substitutions
- Prints prescriptions and faxes them to the patient's pharmacy

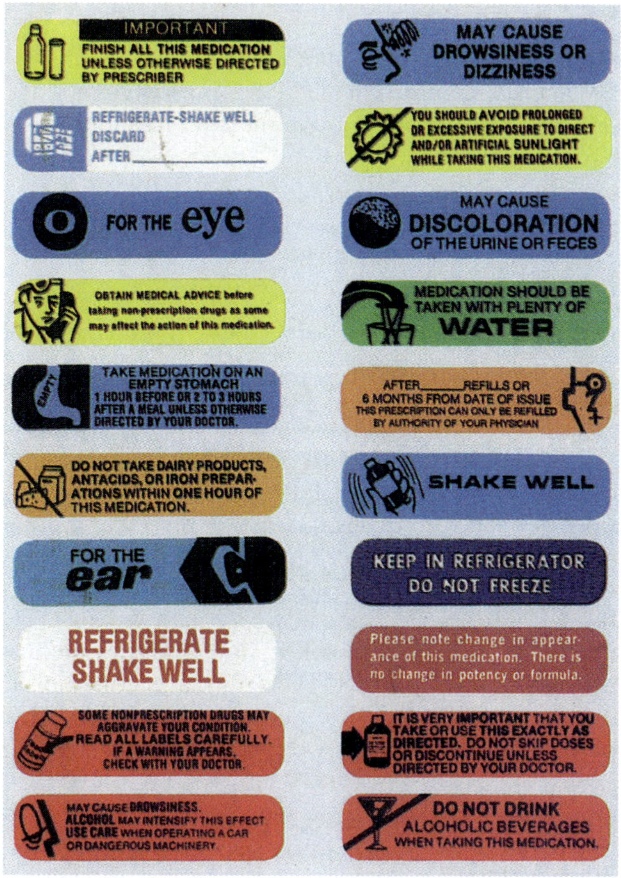

Figure 23-3 Warning labels are placed on prescription medication containers, and patients should be advised to read and adhere to the precautions or instructions.

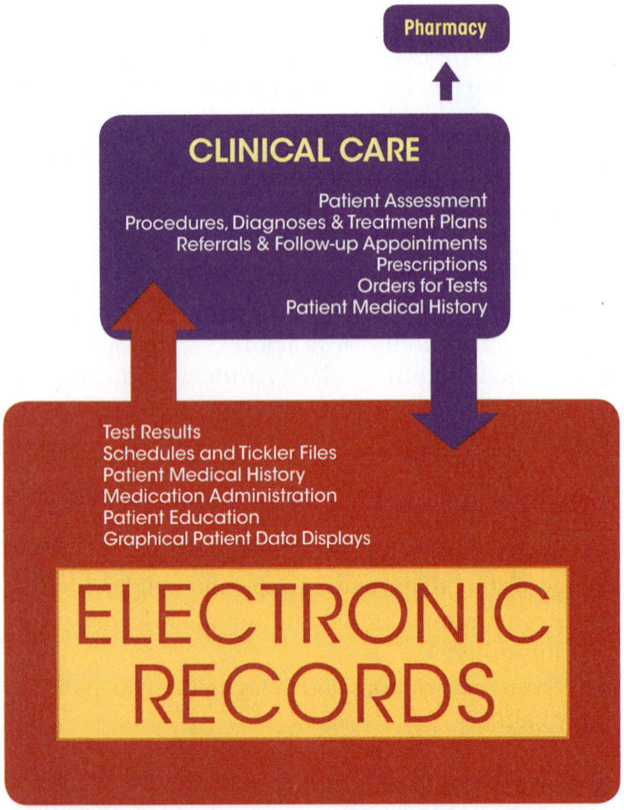

Figure 23-4 The clinical care arm of the total practice management system (TPMS). E-prescribing sends prescriptions and prescription refills directly to the patient's pharmacy.

- Integrates with a drug reference such as the *Physician's Desk Reference* (PDR)
- Contains and upgrades patient's demographics
- Automatically processes renewals or refills

Nonprescription Drugs

Drugs that are frequently referred to as over-the-counter (OTC) drugs fall into the category of nonprescription drugs. These drugs are readily accessible to the public. They do not require a prescription because the FDA considers them safe to use without a provider's advice. Examples of OTC drugs are aspirin, ibuprofen, and vitamins such as vitamin C. Although OTC drugs are considered safe, it is useful for the medical assistant to offer patients some guidelines (Figure 23-5).

Proper Disposal of Drugs

All drug labels contain an expiration date (Figure 23-6). When that date has been reached, the drug must be removed from the shelf and destroyed (see Procedure 23-1).

Patient Education

Guidelines for patients who take prescription medications include:

1. Take exactly as directed.
2. Inform the provider or the medical assistant of unusual or adverse reactions.
3. Continue to take the medication for the duration of the prescribed number of days, weeks, and so on.
4. If you want to discontinue the medication, inform your provider or the medical assistant.
5. Do not take other medications or herbs concurrently without checking with your provider or medical assistant.
6. Do not take someone else's prescribed medication.
7. Store all medications away from children.
8. Discard unused medication properly. Many states require that unused medications be turned into a community's biohazard waste collection. Medication substances have been found in some water supplies.
9. Heed warning labels on medication containers.

An expired drug cannot be dispensed or administered because it could be harmful.

When disposing of expired drugs, it is no longer recommended that expired and unused medications, prescriptions or over-the-counter, be released into the sewage system. Various antibiotics and hormones have been discovered in the water supplies. Pharmacists have been asked to allow patients to take their expired and unused medications to their pharmacies. Pharmacists can arrange to have the medications incinerated. Some communities have 1 day a year set aside for disposal of biohazard substances, including these medications.

If a medication is removed from its original container, it should not be used (for example, the patient refused the medication); do not replace it in the container. Dispose of it as outlined earlier.

Outdated and expired controlled substances (Schedule II) are handled differently. They must be returned to the pharmacy (as required by law). If a

Because patients are more aware and better informed about their health care needs, they are becoming more involved in making choices and decisions about their health care. When they choose to take over-the-counter (OTC) drugs, they need information and guidance. Over the past few years, some previous prescription drugs have been changed to OTC drugs. The safety of these drugs can only be ensured if patients take them as directed.

Patients need to realize that OTC medications:

1. Can interact with other drugs (either prescribed, herbal, or other OTCs) and cause undesirable or adverse reactions or complications
2. May be used in lieu of seeking professional help and thereby interfere with the need for medical care
3. Can mask symptoms and exacerbate an existing condition
4. May have several active ingredients, which may be found to be undesirable
5. Have a safe minimum dose, which may not have the desired therapeutic effect

Figure 23-5 Guidelines for patients when taking nonprescription (over-the-counter) medications.

controlled substance (Schedule II) has been either dropped onto the floor (and is thus unfit to be given to a patient) or has spilled (if in liquid form), a witness should verify the action and proper documentation must take place.

The local DEA office and local police must be notified and the appropriate paperwork completed if there has been a loss or theft of a controlled substance (Schedule II).

Administer, Prescribe, Dispense

There are three ways to handle drugs in the provider's office or clinic: by prescribing, dispensing, or administering them. To **prescribe** a drug means that the licensed practitioner with prescriptive authority (provider, physician assistant, or nurse practitioner) gives a written order to be taken to the pharmacist to be filled. To **dispense** a drug means to give (hand over) the medication as ordered by the provider to the patient to be taken at another time. To **administer** a drug means to give it to the patient by mouth or injection or any other method of administration as ordered by the provider.

Patient Education

Many patients keep unused medications past their expiration date. This presents a potential health hazard, because some medications lose their potency after a period, whereas others become toxic. It is best to inform patients to discard any unused portion of medication by the stated date. Encourage patients to check their medicine cabinets at the same time every year so it becomes a routine practice.

Although state laws vary, some states allow certain professionals, including medical assistants, to prepare and administer medications under the licensed practitioner's supervision. Usually, it is the provider and pharmacist who dispense medications. However, medical assistants can also dispense samples of drugs under the provider's direction. Although medical assistants act as the provider's agent when they prepare and administer medication, they are ethically and legally responsible for their own actions and can be subject to legal action should harm come to a patient. The law requires that individuals who prepare and administer medications know the medications and their side effects.

DRUG REFERENCES AND STANDARDS

The strength, purity, and quality of drugs differ depending on how they are manufactured. To control the differences, standards have been set. By law, the various drug products must meet standards that are set forth by the FDA. A special reference book, *United States Pharmacopeia/National Formulary*, and Web site list the drugs for which standards have been established. These resources are recognized by the U.S. government as the official list of drug standards, which are enforced by the FDA. Every 5 years the information is updated in an attempt to include all drug products in the United States. Naturals and herbals are not regulated.

Other useful books used as references include the *Compendium of Drug Therapy*, the *Desk Reference for Nonprescription Drugs*, and the *Physician's Desk Reference* (PDR), which is published annually by Thomson Healthcare in cooperation with pharmaceutical companies. The PDR is published annually and supplements to the PDR are available two times a year. The supplements contain the newest drugs that were not yet available when the PDR was printed; thus, the supplements contain the most current information. The supplements are organized in the the same way as the PDR. The PDR is available in print, on the

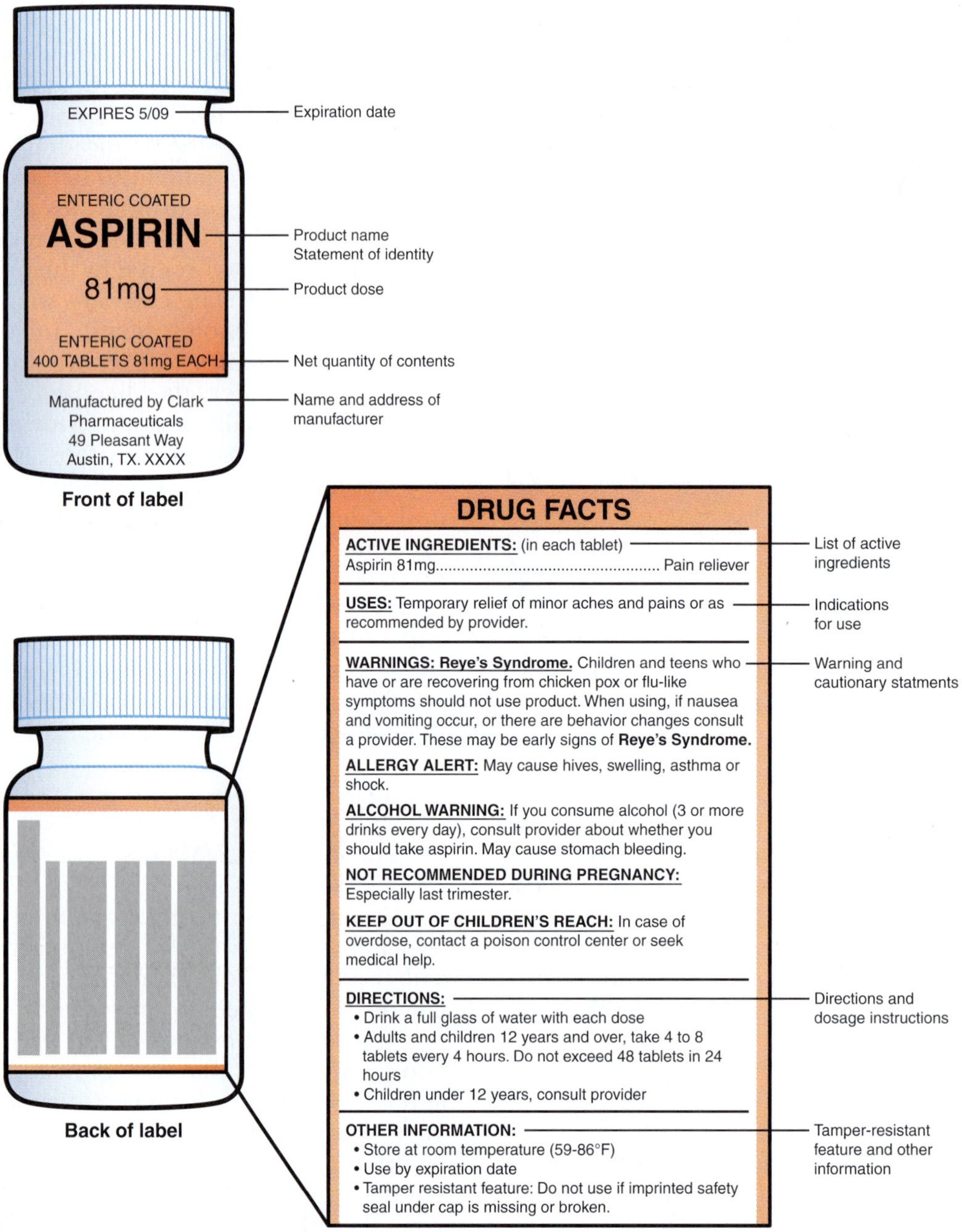
EXPIRES 5/09
Expiration date
ENTERIC COATED
ASPIRIN
Product name
Statement of identity
81mg
Product dose
ENTERIC COATED
400 TABLETS 81mg EACH
Net quantity of contents
Manufactured by Clark Pharmaceuticals 49 Pleasant Way Austin, TX. XXXX
Name and address of manufacturer
Front of label
Back of label
DRUG FACTS
ACTIVE INGREDIENTS: (in each tablet)
Aspirin 81mg.. Pain reliever
List of active ingredients
USES: Temporary relief of minor aches and pains or as recommended by provider.
Indications for use
WARNINGS: Reye's Syndrome. Children and teens who have or are recovering from chicken pox or flu-like symptoms should not use product. When using, if nausea and vomiting occur, or there are behavior changes consult a provider. These may be early signs of Reye's Syndrome.
Warning and cautionary statments
ALLERGY ALERT: May cause hives, swelling, asthma or shock.
ALCOHOL WARNING: If you consume alcohol (3 or more drinks every day), consult provider about whether you should take aspirin. May cause stomach bleeding.
NOT RECOMMENDED DURING PREGNANCY: Especially last trimester.
KEEP OUT OF CHILDREN'S REACH: In case of overdose, contact a poison control center or seek medical help.
DIRECTIONS:
• Drink a full glass of water with each dose
• Adults and children 12 years and over, take 4 to 8 tablets every 4 hours. Do not exceed 48 tablets in 24 hours
• Children under 12 years, consult provider
Directions and dosage instructions
OTHER INFORMATION:
• Store at room temperature (59-86°F)
• Use by expiration date
• Tamper resistant feature: Do not use if imprinted safety seal under cap is missing or broken.
Tamper-resistant feature and other information

Figure 23-6 Medication labels contain valuable information essential to the safe and effective use of the drug.

Web, and for PDAs. The PDR is one of the most widely used reference books and is found in most offices and clinics. It is divided into sections of drug information, which are followed by other useful drug information such as a list of products, poison control 800 telephone numbers, conversion tables, and a guide to management of drug overdose (Figure 23-7).

Providers use electronic technology to assist them when they need references to drugs, their interactions, brand and generic names, and doses according to patient's needs. Some providers use personal digital assistants (PDAs), hand-held electronic devices that give them the information they need. The PDR comes with a CD-ROM, and an individual can register online to access medications information (http://www.PDR.net).

How to Use the PDR

The five most commonly used sections of the PDR list drugs according to:

- Brand name and generic name index, section 2
- Classification or category, section 3

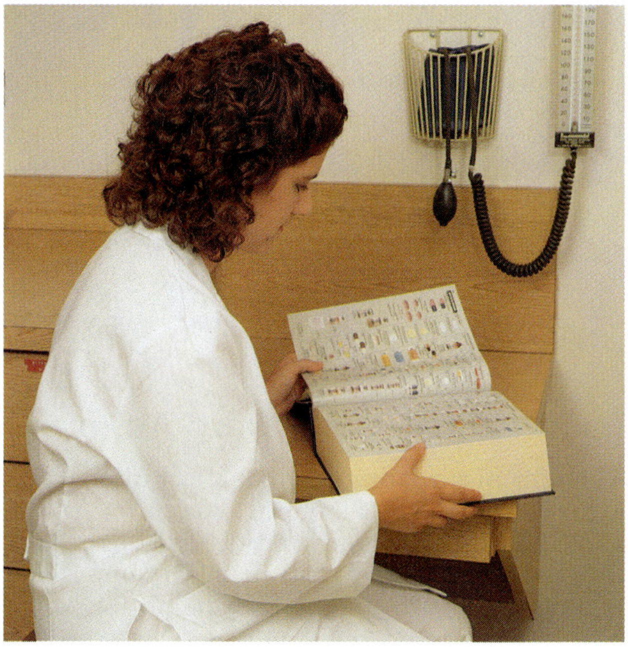

Figure 23-7 *The Physician's Desk Reference* (PDR) is a valuable resource for the medical assistant who wishes to obtain information about a specific medication.

- Product identification guide, section 4
- Product information and alphabetical arrangement by manufacturers, section 5

Section 2 of the PDR is the alphabetized section used for finding the page numbers for generic and brand name drugs. Each drug, whether generic or brand, has a page number listed to enable you to locate a specific drug. Each time a brand name appears, it is followed by the manufacturer's name and page number to check for more information. When more than one page number appears, the first number refers to the photo section (Product Identification Guide), section 4; the last number refers to the prescribing category, section 3 (Product Category Index). Generic named drugs are underlined; brand names are not.

The PDR has many other sections within it, such as the Key to Controlled Substances category, the U.S. Food and Drug Administration telephone directory, telephone numbers for poison control centers, and herb and drug interactions.

The following guidelines will assist you as you learn to use the PDR.

1. If you know the brand or generic name of the drug, turn to section 2 and locate the drug in the alphabetical listing. The manufacturer's name will be in parentheses, followed by a page number or two page numbers. The first number is the product identification page number, section 4. The second number is the product information, section 5.

Example:

Look up Zithromax® capsules in a current PDR.

Zithromax (Pfizer)
Note all the information provided for a drug.

- *Description.* Gives the origin and chemical composition of the drug.
- *Clinical Pharmacology.* Indicates the effect of the drug on the body and the process by which the drug exerts this effect.
- *Indications and Uses.* States the various conditions, diseases, types of microorganisms, and so on, for which the drug is used.
- *Contraindications.* States when the drug should not be given to a specified person.
- *Warnings.* Gives the potential dangers of the drug.
- *Precautions.* States the possible unfavorable effects that the drug may have on a patient.
- *Adverse Reactions.* Lists the undesired side effects or toxicity of the drug.
- *Dosage and Administration.* States the amount (usual daily dose for adults and children) and time sequence of administration.
- *How Supplied.* Lists the various forms of the drug and their dosages.

2. If you know the classification of the drug, turn to section 3 and locate the category of the drug.

Example:

Antibiotics
Macrolide
Zithromax® capsules (Pfizer)

NOTE: All controlled substances listed in the PDR are indicated with the symbol C with the Roman numeral II, III, IV, or V printed inside the C to designate the schedule in which the substance is classified.

Example:

Duramorph® C-II, morphine sulfate USP

Other Reference Sources

On occasion, you may not find the drug that you are looking for listed in the PDR. When this happens:

- Refer to another drug reference book, or go online
- Ask a pharmacist about the drug
- Refer to the packet insert that comes in the drug package

The package insert that most manufacturers provide with their products is an important source of information about a particular drug. This is a brief description of the drug, including its clinical pharmacology, indications and usage, **contraindications** (any symptom or circumstance that indicates that the use of a particular drug is inappropriate when it would otherwise be advisable), warnings, precautions, drug interactions, adverse reactions, overdose, dosage, and administration. The package insert can be a valuable source of information about drugs that might not be listed elsewhere, or if a PDR is unavailable.

Information about some older medications, such as digoxin, can be found in the package insert because they may have been deleted from the current PDR. You or your employer can become registered to use the PDR. A version of the PDR is available.

CLASSIFICATION OF DRUGS

Drugs can be classified (arranged in groups) in a number of ways. Some examples are:

- Drugs used to treat or prevent disease (examples are hormones and vaccines) (see Chapter 10)
- Drugs that have a principal action on the body (examples are analgesics and antiinflammatory drugs)
- Drugs that act on specific body systems or organs (examples are respiratory and cardiovascular drugs)
- Drug preparation (examples are suppository, liquid)

Table 23-1 lists common drug classifications. See Appendix B for the 50 top prescribed brand name medications, or visit the following Web site: http://www.drugtopics.modernmedicine.com. Look under facts and figures for the top 200 brand name drugs for 2007.

PRINCIPAL ACTIONS OF DRUGS

In general, drugs can be grouped as follows: those that act directly on one or more tissues of the body; those that act on microorganisms; and those that replace body chemicals.

Certain drugs have selective action, such as stimulants, which increase cell activity, and depressants, which decrease cell activity.

Other drugs may have what is known as:

- *Local action.* The drug acts on the area to which it is administered.
- *Remote action.* A drug affects a part of the body that is distant from the site of administration.
- *Systemic action.* The drug is carried via the bloodstream throughout the body.
- *Synergistic action.* One drug increases or counteracts the action of another.

Factors That Affect Drug Action

The four principal factors that affect drug action are: absorption, distribution, biotransformation, and elimination. These factors depend on the individual patient, the form and chemical composition of the drug, and the method of administration.

1. *Absorption* is the process whereby the drug passes into the body fluids and tissues.
2. *Distribution* is the process whereby the drug is transported from the blood to the intended site of action, site of biotransformation, site of storage, and site of elimination.
3. *Biotransformation* is the chemical alteration that a drug undergoes in the body, usually in the liver.
4. *Elimination* is the process whereby the drug is excreted from the body. Elimination occurs via the gastrointestinal tract, respiratory tract, skin, mucous membranes, and mammary glands.

Undesirable Actions of Drugs

Most drugs have the potential for causing an action other than their intended action. For example:

1. *Side effect.* An undesirable action of the drug that may limit the usefulness of the drug.
2. *Drug interaction.* Occurs when one drug potentiates—increases or diminishes the action of another drug. These actions may be desirable or undesirable. Drugs may also interact with various foods, alcohol, tobacco, and other substances.
3. *Adverse reaction.* An unfavorable or harmful unintended action of a drug, such as an allergic reaction.

A patient may experience an allergic reaction to a drug after administration. It is often mild and may exhibit itself in the form of a rash, **urticaria,** or **pruritus.** On occasion, a severe reaction or **anaphylaxis** can occur, which is hypersensitivity to a drug or other foreign protein. It is the least common

Table 23-1 Common Classifications of Drugs and Their Actions

Classification (with Phonetic Spelling)	Action	Examples of Drugs Commonly Used in Ambulatory Care Setting
Analgesic (an"al-je'sik)	An agent that relieves pain without causing loss of consciousness	Acetaminophen (Tylenol), acetylsalicylic acid (aspirin), ibuprofen (Advil, Motrin)
Anesthetic (an"es-thet'ik)	An agent that produces numbness May be local or general depending on the type and how administered	lidocaine HCl (Xylocaine), procaine HCl (Novacaine) } Both are local anesthetics
Antacid (ant-as'id)	An agent that neutralizes acid	Amphojel, Gelusil, Mylanta, Milk of Magnesia
Antianemic (an"ti-an-em'ic)	An agent that replaces iron	Iron, ferrous sulfate
Antianxiety (an"ti-ang-zi'e-te)	An agent that relieves anxiety and muscle tension	Benzodiazepines: diazepam (Valium), chlordiazepoxide HCl (Librium), alprazolam (Xanax)
Antiarrhythmic (an"te-a-rith'mik)	An agent that controls cardiac arrhythmias	Lidocaine HCl (Xylocaine), propranolol HCl (Inderal)
Antibiotic (an"ti-bi-ot'ik)	An agent that is destructive to or inhibits growth of microorganisms	Penicillins (Pentids, Duracillin, Polycillin, Pipracil, Augmentin) and others
Anticholesterol or antihyperlipidemic (an"ti-ko"less;ter-ol)	An agent that reduces cholesterol	Zocor, Lipitor, Crestor, Mevacor
Anticholinergic (an"ti-ko"lin-er'jik)	An agent that blocks parasympathetic nerve impulses	Atropine, scopolamine, trihexyphenidyl HCl (Artane)
Anticoagulant (an"ti-ko-ag'u-lant)	An agent that prevents or delays blood clotting	Heparin sodium, Dicumarol, warfarin sodium (Coumadin)
Anticonvulsant (an"ti-kon-vul'sant)	An agent that prevents or relieves convulsions	Carbamazepine (Tegretol), Phenytoin (Dilantin), Ethosuximide (Zarontin)
Antidepressant (an"ti-dep-res'ant)	An agent that prevents or relieves the symptoms of depression	Monoamine oxidase (MAO) inhibitors: isocarboxazid (Marplan), phenelzine sulfate (Nardil), tricyclic: amitriptyline HCl (Elavil), imipramine HCl (Tofranil), sertraline HCl (Zoloft), paroxetine HCl (Paxil), trazodone (Desyrel), fluoxentine (Prozac)
Antidiarrheal (an"ti-di-a-re'al)	An agent that prevents or relieves diarrhea	Pepto-Bismol, Kaopectate, Diphenoxylate HCl (Lomotil)
Antidote (an-ti'dot)	An agent that counteracts poisons and their effects	Naloxone (Narcan)
Antiemetic (an"ti-e-met'ik)	An agent that prevents or relieves nausea and vomiting	Tigan, Dramamine, Phenergan, Reglan, Marinol, Compazine

(continues)

Table 23-1 Common Classifications of Drugs and Their Actions (continued)

Classification (with Phonetic Spelling)	Action	Examples of Drugs Commonly Used in Ambulatory Care Setting
Antihistamine (an"ti-his'ta-min)	An agent that counteracts histamine	Dimetane, Benadryl, Seldane, Allegra
Antihypertensive (an"ti-hi"per-ten'siv)	An agent that prevents or controls high blood pressure	Methyldopa (Aldomet), clonidine HCl (Catapres), metoprolol tartrate (Lopressor)
Antiinflammatory (an"ti-in-flam'a-to-re)	An agent that counteracts inflammation	Naproxen (Naprosyn), aspirin, ibuprofen (Advil, Motrin)
Antimanic (an"ti-man'ik)	An agent used for the treatment of the manic episode of manic-depressive disorder	Lithium
Antineoplastic (an"ti-ne"o-plas'tik)	An agent that kills or destroys malignant cells	Busuflan (Myleran), cyclophosphamide (Cytoxan)
Antipsychotic	An agent that helps in schizophrenia and chronic brain syndrome	Haloperdol (Haldol), chlorpromazine (Thorazine)
Antipyretic (an"ti-pi-ret'ik)	An agent that reduces fever	Aspirin, acetaminophen (Tylenol)
Antitussive (an"ti-tus'iv)	An agent that prevents or relieves cough	Codeine, dextromethorphan (Pertussin, Romilar)
Antiulcer (an"ti-ul'ser) (H_2 blockers)	An agent that relieves and heals ulcers by blocking hydrochloric acid	Cimetidine (Tagamet), anitidine (Zantac), omeprazole (Prilosec)
Antiviral (an"ti-viral)	An agent that fights a specific virus	Zovirax, Retrovir, Denavir
Bronchodilator (brong"ko-dil-a'tor)	An agent that dilates the bronchi	Isoproterenol HCl (Isuprel), albuterol (Proventil)
Contraceptive (kon"tra-sep'tiv)	Any device, method, or agent that prevents conception	Envid-E 21, Ortho-Novum 10/11-21; 10/11-28 Triphasil-21, Ovral 28, Alesse, Levlen
COX-2 Inhibitor (kox-2 in-hib-it-or)	An agent that inhibits COX-2 (an enzyme) found in joints or other body parts that are inflamed	Celebrex
Decongestant (de"con-gest'ant)	An agent that reduces nasal congestion or swelling	Oxymetazoline (Afrin), phenylephrine HCl (Neo-Synephrine), pseudoephedrine HCl (Sudafed)
Diuretic (di"u-ret'ik)	An agent that increases the excretion of urine	Chlorothiazide (Diuril), furosemide (Lasix), mannitol (Osmitrol)

(continues)

Table 23-1 (continued)

Classification (with Phonetic Spelling)	Action	Examples of Drugs Commonly Used in Ambulatory Care Setting
Expectorant (ek-spek'to-rant)	An agent that facilitates removal of secretion from bronchopulmonary mucous membrane	Guaifenesin (Robitussin)
Hemostatic (he"mo-stat'ik)	An agent that controls or stops bleeding	Humafac, Amicar, vitamin K
Hypnotic (hip-not'ik)	An agent that produces sleep or hypnosis	Secobarbital (Seconal), chloral hydrate, ethchlorvynol (Placidyl)
Hypoglycemic (hi"po-gli-se'mik)	An agent that reduces blood glucose level	Insulin, chlorpropamide (Diabinese), tolbutamide (Orinsase)
Laxative (lak'sa-tiv)	An agent that loosens and promotes normal bowel elimination	Metamucil powder, Dulcolax, Docusate sodium (Colace)
Muscle relaxant (mus'el re-lak'sant)	An agent that produces relaxation of skeletal muscle	Robaxin, Norflex, Paraflex, Skelaxin, Valium
Nonsteroidal antiinflammatory drug (NSAID)	An agent that relieves mild to moderate pain due to headache, toothache, dysmenorrhea, backache	Aspirin (Bufferin, Ecotrin), ibruprofen (Advil, Excedrin, Motrin), naproxen (Aleve, Anaprox, Naprosyn), ketorofex (Orudis)
Proton-pump inhibitor (prōtōn pump in-hib-it-or)	An agent that suppresses gastric acid (GERD) ulcers	Acifex, Nexium, Protonix
Sedative (sed'a-tiv)	An agent that produces a calming effect without causing sleep	Amobarbital (Amytal), butabarbital sodium (Buticaps), phenobarbital
Tranquilizer (tran"kwi-liz'er)	An agent that reduces mental tension and anxiety	Diazapem (Valium), Alprazolam (Xanax), chlordiazepoxide (Librium)
Vasodilator (vas"o-di-la'tor)	An agent that produces relaxation of blood vessels; reduces blood pressure	Isorbide dinitrate (Isordil), atenolol (Tenormin), nitroglycerin, diltiazem (Cardizem)
Vasopressor (vas"o-pres'or)	An agent that produces contraction of muscles of capillaries and arteries; increases blood pressure	Metaraminol (Aramine), norepinephrine (Levophed)

allergic reaction but can become severe quickly and result in dyspnea and shock. Loss of consciousness and death can result. To help prevent an allergic reaction or minimize its risk, the medical assistant should attempt to ascertain before administration of every drug whether the patient has any known allergies. The medical assistant should be aware of signs and symptoms of allergic reaction and notify the provider immediately so that appropriate emergency treatment can be given. One or two injections of epinephrine usually reverses the life-threatening symptoms of anaphylaxis and is followed by administration of an antihistamine such as Benadryl®. In severe cases that do not respond to this treatment, oxygen and immediate transfer to the emergency department is necessary.

DRUG ROUTES

Drugs are manufactured in a variety of forms and for various purposes. The route of a drug refers to how it is administered to the patient, and thereby transported into the patient's body. Certain medications can be administered by more than one route, whereas others must be administered via a specific route.

The route of administration is determined by a number of factors. One factor is the action of the medication on the body, either local or systemic. Intravenous medication reaches the systemic circulation rapidly via the bloodstream and quickly becomes effective. Injections of medication and medications absorbed through mucous membranes such as suppositories and sublingual nitroglycerine are absorbed quickly. Oral medications take longer to act because they must be digested by the stomach and then be absorbed into the bloodstream.

Another factor in route selection is the physical and emotional state of the patient. The patient's consciousness level, emotional status, and physical restrictions are considered when selecting a route to administer medication.

A third factor to consider is the characteristics of the drug. An example is insulin. Insulin is destroyed by digestive enzymes; therefore, the route of administration must be by injection.

The most frequently used routes of administering medication to the patient are oral and parenteral routes: oral medications are taken by mouth, parenteral generally by injection. Other routes of administration include:

- Direct application to the skin—topical (lotions, creams, liniments, ointments, transdermal [patch] systems)
- Sublingual (tablets, liquid, drops)
- Buccal (tablets)
- Rectal (suppositories, ointments)
- Vaginal (suppositories, creams, applications)
- Inhalation (sprays, aerosols)
- Instillation (liquid, drops)

FORMS OF DRUGS

Drugs are compounded in three basic types of preparations: liquids, solids, and semisolids. The ease with which a drug's ingredients can be dissolved largely determines the variety of forms manufactured. Some drug agents are soluble in water, others in alcohol, and others in a mixture of several solvents.

The method for administering a drug depends on its form, its properties, and the effects desired. When given orally, a drug may be in the form of a liquid, powder, tablet, capsule, or caplet. If it is to be injected, it must be in the form of a liquid. For topical use, the drug may be in the form of a liquid, powder, or semisolid. Oral and injectable medications are examples of preparations designed for internal use.

Liquid Preparations

Liquid preparations contain a drug that has been dissolved or suspended. Depending on the solvent used, the drug may be further classified as an aqueous (water) or alcohol preparation or as an aerosol or mist. When prescribed for internal use, liquid preparations other than emulsions are rapidly absorbed through the stomach, intestinal walls, or lungs.

Solid and Semisolid Preparations

Tablets, capsules, caplets, troches or lozenges, suppositories, and ointments are examples of solid and semisolid preparations. These products offer great flexibility as a means of dispensing different dosages of drugs. Figure 23-8 shows types of tablets and capsules.

Other Drug Delivery Systems

Technologic advances have introduced new ways by which drugs can be introduced into the patient. In addition to the conventional preparations, the following therapeutic systems offer special delivery of medication to targeted areas.

Transdermal System. The transdermal system of medication delivery consists of a small adhesive patch that may be applied to intact skin near the treatment site. For example, Transderm Scop®, used for preventing motion sickness, may be applied behind the ear; Nitro-Dur® (Figure 23-9), used for preventing angina pectoris, may be applied to the chest; Estraderm®, used to treat menopausal symptoms, may be applied to the trunk; and Nicoderm®, used to relieve the body's craving for nicotine, may be applied to any area above the waist. A transdermal system generally consists of four layers (Figure 23-10):

1. An impermeable backing that keeps the drug from leaking out of the system
2. A reservoir containing the drug
3. A membrane with tiny holes that controls the rate of drug release

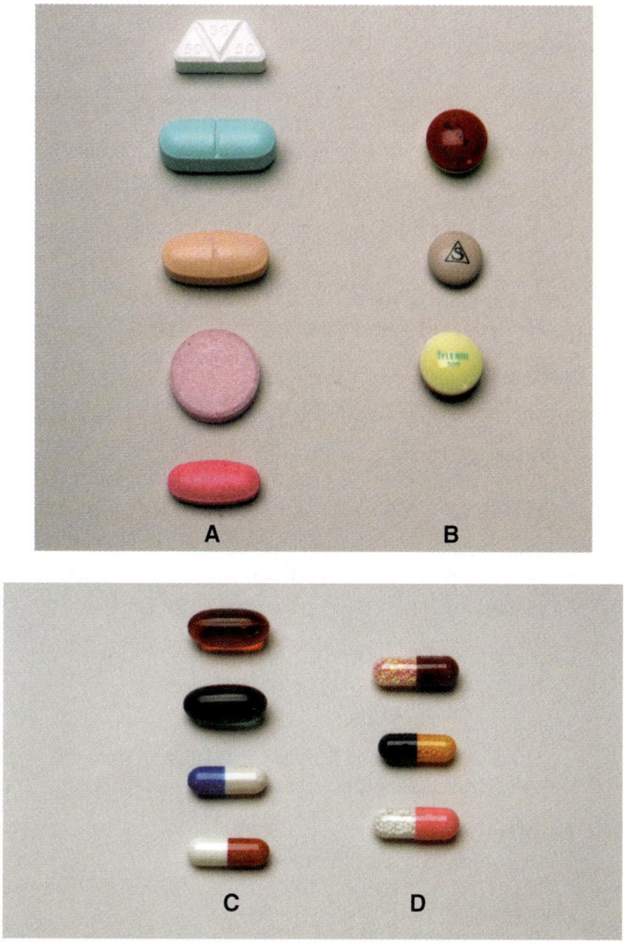

Figure 23-8 Drugs are manufactured in various forms, including solid preparations such as tablets and capsules. (A) Tablets, scored and unscored. (B) Enteric-coated tablets. (C) Capsules and gelatin-coated capsules. (D) Timed-release capsules.

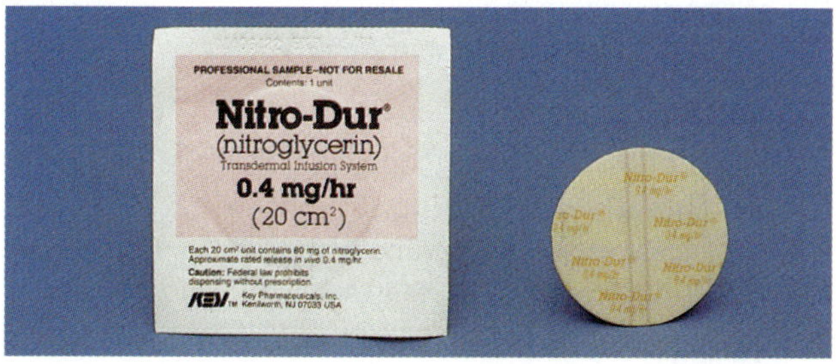

Figure 23-9 Nitro-Dur® is a transdermal system of delivering medication used for prevention and for long-term management of angina pectoris. It can be applied to the chest.

4. An adhesive layer or gel that keeps the device in place

Inhalation Medications. Medication for respiratory diseases and conditions such as asthma, bronchiectasis (permanent dilation of one or more bronchi), bronchitis, and others may require treatment with inhalation medication from an aerosolized inhaler or a nebulizer. Some of the commonly prescribed medications are bronchodilators such as aminophylline, albuterol, isuprel, epinephrine, and cortisone-type medications. Oxygen may be prescribed for hypoxia caused by respiratory diseases. Oxygen may be prescribed for cardiovascular collapse, congestive heart failure, and pneumonia among other examples. (See Chapter 18 for information about nebulizers, inhalers, and oxygen administration.)

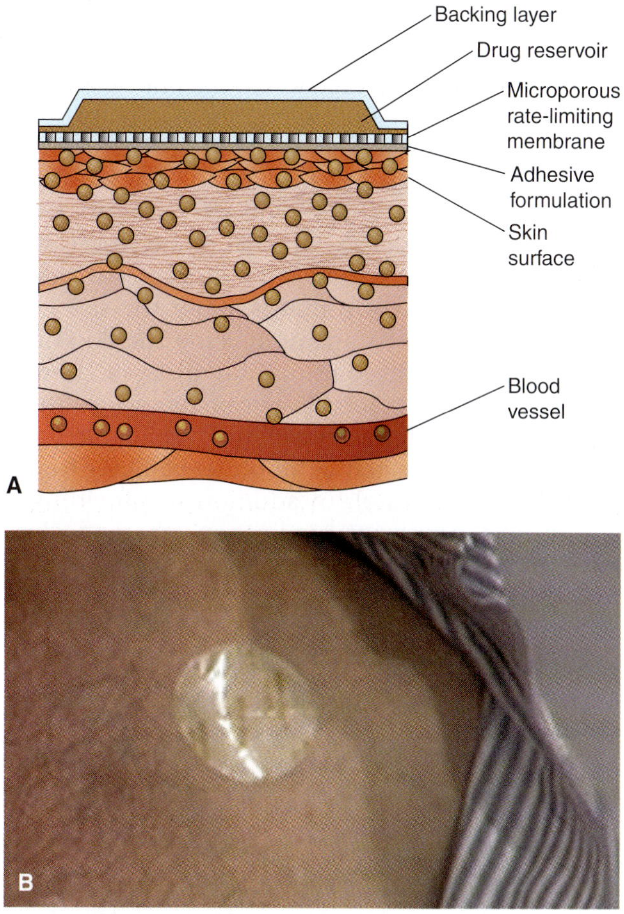

Figure 23-10 (A) The multilayer unit comprising TransdermNitro® delivers nitroglycerin into the bloodstream in a consistent, controlled manner for 24 hours. The thin unit contains a backing layer, a reservoir of nitroglycerin, a unique rate-limiting membrane, and an adhesive layer that has a priming dose of nitroglycerin. (B) The patch is applied to the skin. *(Courtesy of Novartis.)*

Eye-Curing Lens. Another innovative drug delivery system is one in which a drug, contained between two ultrathin plastic membranes, is placed inside the lower eyelid. It appears to cause little or no discomfort and provides a controlled release of the medication for an extended period. Pilocarpine, a miotic that causes contraction of the pupils, is being used in this method for the treatment of glaucoma.

Implantable Devices. Implantable devices are available in several shapes and sizes and are positioned just beneath the skin near blood vessels that lead directly to the area to be medicated. For example, an infusion pump that is about the size of a hockey puck can be implanted below the skin near the waist to provide continuous delivery of chemotherapy to patients with liver cancer or insulin to a diabetic. This device, which has a refillable drug reservoir, is connected by an outlet catheter to the patient's blood vessel. In addition to providing a continuous supply of medication, these devices have the advantage of delivering greater doses with fewer side effects than can be realized through the systemic route.

STORAGE AND HANDLING OF MEDICATIONS

Certain precautions should be followed if the ambulatory care setting keeps medications on the premises. The goal should be to store all medications in their original containers in a separate room in a locked cabinet. Many medications require storage in a certain manner, such as a dark area or in a dark container (to keep light away from them) or in the refrigerator. Some must be kept in glass containers only because plastic may react with the medication's chemical composition. The drug label indicates proper storage and handling for each medication.

Keep medications that are for internal use separated from those intended for external use.

Access to medications is simplified if they are organized in the storage area either according to their classification (diuretic, hormones) or according to the alphabet. Always check expiration dates.

EMERGENCY DRUGS AND SUPPLIES

The ambulatory care setting should maintain a tray, box, cabinet, or crash cart (see Chapter 9 for contents of crash cart) especially and solely for drugs and supplies needed in an emergency such as anaphylaxis or other form of shock. The drugs listed in Table 23-2 are a sample of

Table 23-2 Examples of Common Emergency Drugs

Adrenaline (a-dren'a-lin) or **epinephrine** (ep-i-nef-rin)	A vasoconstrictor. Relieves anaphylactic shock.
Albuterol (al-bú-ter-ol)	A bronchodilator. Relaxes smooth muscle of the respiratory tract.
Atropine (a-trō-peen)	Helps restore heart rate.
Benadryl (ben'a-dril)	An antihistamine that relieves allergic symptoms.
Compazine (com-pa'zeen)	An antiemetic. Relieves symptoms of nausea and vomiting.
Dextrose (deks'trose) 50%	Used for hypoglycemia to counteract hyperinsulinism.
Diazepam (dī-az′-e-pam)	Helps control seizures. Antianxiety.
Digoxin (di-jox'in)	Cardiac drug. Used for congestive heart failure, arryhthmias. Slows and strengthens heartbeat.
Diuril (di'ur-il)	Promotes excretion of urine.
Hydrocortisone (hi"dro-cort'i-zon)	An antiinflammatory. Used to suppress swelling and shock.
Insulin (in'sah-lin)	Diabetic coma.
Isuprel (īcé-ū-prel)	Heart block.
Lidocaine (lī′-dō-kāne)	Controls ventricular arrhythmia.
Narcan (nar'can)	Antidote. Used in narcotic overdose.
Nitroglycerin (ni"tro-glis'er-in)	Vasodilator. Dilates coronary arteries. Used in treatment of angina pectoris.
Valium (val'e-um)	Antianxiety, muscle relaxant. Used to calm anxious patients and to relax muscles. Valium is a Schedule IV drug, and therefore must be kept in a locked cabinet.
Verapamil (ver-ap'a-mil)	For cardiac arrhythmia, stable and unstable angina.

NOTE: Ipecac syrup, no longer used to induce vomiting, has proven to be cardiotoxic, and several cases of aspiration have occurred.

some general drugs to keep readily available for emergencies.

Other supplies and equipment to keep together with the drugs on the emergency cart are:

- Intravenous (IV) materials such as IV fluids, needles, tubing, syringes, alcohol, swabs, constriction band, and tape
- Sphygmomanometer
- Stethoscope
- Oxygen and mask
- Airways
- Defibrillator
- Suction equipment (nasopharyngeal)
- Personal protective equipment

Check the tray on a regular basis (weekly, monthly, depending on use) according to need. Check the oxygen tank and gauge. Replace items that have been used as soon as possible, and discard drugs and supplies that have reached their expiration dates. Document that the tray has been checked and updated. (See Chapter 9 for more information about emergencies and emergency drugs used in the office and other ambulatory areas.)

Bioterrorism

Bioterrorism is the name given to the use of biologic weapons (pathogenic microorganisms) to create fear in people. There are many biologic agents that can be used in an attempt to cause serious diseases. Most diseases can be treated with pharmaceutical agents such as antibiotics and antitoxoids.

The most dangerous disease threats are anthrax, botulism, pneumonic/bubonic plague, smallpox, and tularemia.

Anthrax, pneumonic/bubonic plague, and tularemia can all be treated with antibiotics. Botulism is treated with botulism antioxides supplied by public health authorities. Smallpox is treated by early vaccination (within four days). The Centers for Disease Control and Prevention has the vaccine.

Education plays a vital role in raising awareness and increasing the knowledge of health care professionals to aid them in being better prepared for threats to the public health. The World Health Organization, the Centers for Disease Control and Prevention, and state and local public health departments are excellent resources for more information about bioterrorism. (See Chapter 9 for information about emergencies, Chapter 10 for infectious diseases, and Chapter 24 for information on antibiotics.)

DRUG ABUSE

There has been an enormous increase in the **abuse,** or misuse, of legal and illegal drugs. Any drug can be abused, whether it is penicillin, alcohol, or a controlled substance such as cocaine. Medical assistants, while caring for patients, may unexpectedly come in contact with patients who abuse or misuse drugs.

Medical assistants must be able to recognize the symptoms of drug abuse in a patient or coworker and report it to the provider. Health professionals, including providers, are among individuals who can have a problem with drug or alcohol abuse, and it must be reported to the proper professional association (see Chapter 7 for more information on drug abuse).

There are many programs available for treatment of drug abuse. Detoxification and rehabilitation are examples of treatment programs. The National Institute on Drug Abuse, which is part of the National Institutes of Health of the U.S. Department of Health and Human Services, provides information, treatment options, and specific programs for drug abuse on their Web site (http://www.nida.nih.gov/podat/podatindex.html).

Table 23-3 gives examples of drug types most commonly abused.

In addition to the drugs of abuse listed in Table 23-3, another drug of abuse is dextromethorphan. It is an antitussive (cough suppressant) that has been an over-the-counter medication for more than 30 years and is a component of several cough medications. One of the drugs is coricidin HBP (cough and cold tablets), also known as "ccc," "robo," or "red devils." Primarily it is used by youths as a recreational drug for its euphoric effects, but an overdose can result in coma and death. The cough and cold medications are easily available and often are shoplifted by persons who abuse them.

The same social pressures that influence young people to try alcohol are responsible for introducing people of all ages to the previously mentioned drugs and other chemical substances. Because it is easier to prevent drug abuse than it is to break an established habit, most efforts to combat drug abuse are directed at the young. However, people of all ages, including older people, may be or become abusers.

Table 23-3 Drugs of Abuse—Uses and Effects

				Dependence	
Drugs	**Controlled Substance Schedule**	**Trade or Other Names**	**Medical Uses**	**Physical**	**Psychological**
Narcotics					
Heroin	Substance I	Diamorphine, Horse, Smack, Black tar, *Chiva, Negra (black tar)*	None in United States, analgesic, antitussive	High	High
Morphine	Substance II	MS-Contin, Roxanol, Oramorph SR, MSIR	Analgesic	High	High
Hydrocodone	Substance II, Product III, V	Hydrocodone with acetaminophen, Vicodin, Vicoprofen, Tussionex, Lortab	Analgesic, antitussive	High	High
Hydromorphone	Substance II	Dilaudid	Analgesic	High	High
Oxycodone	Substance II	Roxicet, Oxycodone with acetaminophen, OxyContin, Endocet, Percocet, Percodan	Analgesic	High	High
Codeine	Substance II, Product III, V	Acetaminophen, Guaifenesin or Promethazine with Codeine, Fiorinal, Fioricet or Tylenol with Codeine	Analgesic, antitussive	Moderate	Moderate
Other Narcotics	Substance II, III, IV	Fentanyl, Demerol, Methadone, Darvon, Stadol, Talwin, Paregoric, Buprenex	Analgesic, antidiarrheal, antitussive	High-Low	High-Low
Depressants					
Gamma Hydroxybutyric Acid	Substance I, Product III	GHB, Liquid Ecstasy, Liquid X, Sodium Oxybate, Xyrem®	None in United States, anesthetic	Moderate	Moderate
Benzodiazepines	Substance IV	Valium, Xanax, Halcion, Ativan, Restoril, Rohypnol (Roofies, R-2), Klonopin	Antianxiety, sedative, anticonvulsant, hypnotic, muscle relaxant	Moderate	Moderate

Tolerance	Duration (hours)	Usual Method	Possible Effects	Effects of Overdose	Withdrawal Syndrome
Yes	3–4	Injected, snorted, smoked	Euphoria, drowsiness, respiratory depression, constricted pupils, nausea	Slow and shallow breathing, clammy skin, convulsions, coma, possible death	Watery eyes, runny nose, yawning, loss of appetite, irritability, tremors, panic, cramps, nausea, chills, sweating
Yes	3–12	Oral, injected	Same as above	Same as above	Same as above
Yes	3–6	Oral	Same as above	Same as above	Same as above
Yes	3–4	Oral, injected	Same as above	Same as above	Same as above
Yes	3–12	Oral	Same as above	Same as above	Same as above
Yes	3–4	Oral, injected	Same as above	Same as above	Same as above
Yes	Variable	Oral, injected, snorted, smoked	Same as above	Same as above	Same as above
Yes	3–6	Oral	Slurred speech, disorientation, drunken behavior without odor of alcohol, impaired memory of events, interacts with alcohol	Shallow respiration, clammy skin, dilated pupils, weak and rapid pulse, coma, possible death	Anxiety, insomnia, tremors, delirium, convulsions, possible death
Yes	1–8	Oral, injected	Same as above	Same as above	Same as above

(continues)

Table 23-3 Drugs of Abuse—Uses and Effects (continued)

Drugs	Controlled Substance Schedule	Trade or Other Names	Medical Uses	Dependence: Physical	Dependence: Psychological
Other Depressants	Substance I, II, III, IV	Ambien, Sonata, Meprobamate, Chloral Hydrate, Barbiturates, Methaqualone (Quaalude)	Antianxiety, sedative, hypnotic	Moderate	Moderate
Stimulants					
Cocaine	Substance II	Coke, Flake, Snow, Crack, *Coca*, *Blanca*, *Perico*, *Nieve*, Soda	Local anesthetic	Possible	High
Amphetamine/ Methamphetamine	Substance II	Crank, Ice, Cristal, Krystal Meth, Speed, Adderall, Dexedrine, Desoxyn	Attention deficit/ hyperactivity disorder, narcolepsy, weight control	Possible	High
Methylphenidate	Substance II	Ritalin, Concerta, Focalin, Metadate	Attention deficit/ hyperactivity disorder	Possible	High
Other Stimulants	Substance III, IV	Adipex P, Ionamin, Prelu-2, Didrex, Provigil	Vasoconstriction	Possible	Moderate
Hallucinogens					
MDMA and Analogs	Substance I	(Ecstasy, XTC, Adam), MDA (Love Drug), MDEA (Eve), MBDB	None	None	Moderate
LSD	Substance I	Acid, Microdot, Sunshine, Boomers	None	None	Unknown
Phencyclidine and Analogs	Substance I, II, III	PCP, Angel Dust, Hog, Loveboat, Ketamine (Special K), PCE, PCPy, TCP	Anesthetic (ketamine)	Possible	High
Other Hallucinogens	Substance I	Psilocybe mushrooms, Mescaline, Peyote cactus, Ayahausca, DMT, Dextromethorphan (DXM)	None	None	None
Cannibis					
Marijuana	Substance I	Pot, Grass, Sinsemilla, Blunts, *Mota*, *Yerba*, *Grifa*	None	Unknown	Moderate

*Not regulated

Tolerance	Duration (hours)	Usual Method	Possible Effects	Effects of Overdose	Withdrawal Syndrome
Yes	2–6	Oral	Slurred speech, disorientation, drunken behavior without odor of alcohol, impaired memory of events, interacts with alcohol	Shallow respiration, clammy skin, dilated pupils, weak and rapid pulse, coma, possible death	Anxiety, insomnia, tremors, delirium, convulsions, possible death
Yes	1–2	Snorted, smoked, injected	Increased alertness, excitation, euphoria, increased pulse rate and blood pressure, insomnia, loss of appetite	Agitation, increased body temperature, hallucinations, convulsions, possible death	Apathy, long periods of sleep, irritability, depression, disorientation
Yes	2–4	Oral, injected, smoked	Same as above	Same as above	Same as above
Yes	2–4	Oral, injected, snorted, smoked	Same as above	Same as above	Same as above
Yes	2–4	Oral	Same as above	Same as above	Same as above
Yes	4–6	Oral, snorted, smoked	Heightened senses, teeth grinding, dehydration	Increased body temperature, electrolyte imbalance, cardiac arrest	Muscle aches, drowsiness, depression, acne
Yes	8–12	Oral	Illusions and hallucinations, altered perception of time and distance	Longer, more intense "trip" episodes	None
Yes	1–12	Smoked, oral, injected, snorted	Illusions and hallucinations, altered perception of time and distance	Unable to direct movement, feel pain, remember	Drug-seeking behavior*
Possible	4–8	Oral	Illusions and hallucinations, altered perception of time and distance	Unable to direct movement, feel pain, remember	Drug-seeking behavior*
Yes	2–4	Smoked, oral	Euphoria, relaxed inhibitions, increased appetite, disorientation	Fatigue, paranoia, possible psychosis	Occasional reports of insomnia, hyperactivity, decreased appetite

(continues)

Table 23-3 Drugs of Abuse—Uses and Effects (continued)

				Dependence	
Drugs	**Controlled Substance Schedule**	**Trade or Other Names**	**Medical Uses**	**Physical**	**Psychological**
Tetrahydrocannabinol	Substance I, Product III	THC, Marinol	Antinauseant, appetite stimulant	Yes	Moderate
Hashish and Hashish Oil	Substance I	Hash, Hash oil	None	Unknown	Moderate
Anabolic Steroids					
Testosterone	Substance III	Depo Testosterone, Sustanon, Sten, Cypt	Hypogonadism	Unknown	Unknown
Other Anabolic Steroids	Substance III	Parabolan, Winstrol, Equipose, Anadrol, Dianabol, Primabolin-Depo, D-Ball	Anemia, breast cancer	Unknown	Yes
Inhalants					
Amyl and Butyl Nitrite		Pearls, Poppers, Rush, Locker Room	Angina (amyl)	Unknown	Unknown
Nitrous Oxide		Laughing gas, balloons, Whippets	Anesthetic	Unknown	Low
Other Inhalants		Adhesives, spray paint, hair spray, dry cleaning fluid, spot remover, lighter fluid	None	Unknown	High
Alcohol					
Alcohol		Beer, wine, liquor	None	High	High

Tolerance	Duration (hours)	Usual Method	Possible Effects	Effects of Overdose	Withdrawal Syndrome
Yes	2–4	Smoked, oral	Euphoria, relaxed inhibitions, increased appetite, disorientation	Fatigue, paranoia, possible psychosis	Occasional reports of insomnia, hyperactivity, decreased appetite
Yes	2–4	Smoked, oral	Same as above	Same as above	Same as above
Unknown	14–28 days	Injected	Virilization, edema, testicular atrophy, gynecomastia, acne, aggressive behavior	Unknown	Possible depression
Unknown	Variable	Oral, injected	Same as above	Same as above	Same as above
No	1	Inhaled	Flushing, hypotension, headache	Methemoglobinemia	Agitation
No	0.5	Inhaled	Impaired memory, slurred speech, drunken behavior, slow-onset vitamin deficiency, organ damage	Vomiting, respiratory depression, loss of consciousness, possible death	Trembling, anxiety, insomnia, vitamin deficiency, confusion, hallucinations, convulsions
No	0.5–2	Inhaled	Impaired memory, slurred speech, drunken behavior, slow-onset vitamin deficiency, organ damage	Vomiting, respiratory depression, loss of consciousness, possible death	Trembling, anxiety, insomnia, vitamin deficiency, confusion, hallucinations, convulsions
Yes	1–3	Oral	Impaired judgments, uncoordinated movements, slurred speech, blurred vision	Motor vehicle accidents, gastritis, liver damage, brain damage, domestic violence	Anxiety, shakiness, depression, hallucinations, sweats, increased blood pressure, seizures

Procedure 23-1

Proper Disposal of Drugs

STANDARD PRECAUTIONS:

PURPOSE:

To properly dispose of drugs that have reached their expiration dates.

EQUIPMENT/SUPPLIES:

Drugs (oral and parenteral) that have reached their expiration dates

PROCEDURE STEPS:

1. Gather expired drugs, either prescription or over-the-counter. RATIONALE: Expired drugs cannot be dispensed nor administered because they can be harmful to patients.
2. According to agency policy and state law, the drugs can be taken to the pharmacy or drug supply company from which they were ordered, and the pharmacist can make arrangements to have expired drugs incinerated. Another option is for the provider to contract with an outside company to incinerate the expired drugs. RATIONALE: Disposal of drugs into the sewage system, either by flushing down the toilet or down the sink, is discouraged and is prohibited in some states (medication substances have been found in some municipal water supplies).
3. Only if the label or accompanying patient information specifically instructs flushing drugs down the toilet or sink can you do so. RATIONALE: The FDA advises that only a certain few drugs can be flushed or thrown into the trash. The label or accompanying information will give instructions.
4. Wash hands.
5. Document instructions in the computer that the drugs with expired use by dates were disposed of either by returning them to the pharmacy or by having the contracted agency incinerate them. Be sure to save receipts.

   NOTE: Patients can be instructed to determine if their communities have pharmaceutical take-back programs or hazardous waste disposal programs that allow them to bring unused drugs to a central location for proper disposal.

DOCUMENTATION

2/17/XX Drugs from the crash cart, drugs in the medication closet, and drug samples all checked for expiration dates. Expired medications were removed and returned to the pharmacy for incineration. Drugs inventoried and restocked with new replacements. C. McInnis, RMA ———

Case Study 23-1

Refer to the scenario at the beginning of the chapter.

Mrs. Anderson has an appointment to see Dr. Lewis. While Audrey Jones is updating data in the patient's electronic medical records, Mrs. Anderson, tells Audrey that she has brought in with her a bag of medications. She tells Audrey that she cleaned out her medicine cabinet and found some expired prescription medications. Audrey recognizes an opportunity to educate Mrs. Anderson about unfinished prescribed medication.

CASE STUDY REVIEW

1. What should Audrey tell her, and what can Audrey do with the expired medications?

Case Study 23-2

Maria Jover reports vaginal discharge and discomfort. Dr. King confirms the diagnosis of a yeast infection by performing a smear and identifying the microorganism. Dr. King prescribes over-the-counter vaginal suppositories. After asking Maria if she has any questions, clinical medical assistant Audrey Jones proceeds to help Maria understand the self-administration of this particular medication.

CASE STUDY REVIEW

1. The patient, Maria, asks Audrey Jones whether she can use some vaginal suppositories she bought last year. How should Audrey respond?
2. Maria tells Audrey that the last time she had a vaginal yeast infection she only used part of the recommended number of suppositories because the infection cleared up. How should Audrey respond?
3. Maria does not really like using suppositories. Should Audrey ask Dr. King to prescribe another form of medication for the yeast infection? What other forms might be available?

Case Study 23-3

Dr. Lewis keeps a small quantity of various controlled substances on the premises for use in an emergency situation.

CASE STUDY REVIEW

1. What are the legalities that surround controlled substances as Joe Guerrero, the clinical medical assistant, is concerned?
2. What are his responsibilities?

SUMMARY

Medical assistants must know state and federal laws that govern the distribution and administration of medications and understand their role and responsibilities in light of these laws. Knowledge of drug regulations; the legal classifications of drugs, including controlled substances; and prescribing, administering, and dispensing of drugs is essential to ensure compliance with the law.

Available resources and reference books will provide valuable information about pharmaceutical products, their classifications, routes, forms, storage and handling, and side effects.

Emergency drugs and supplies should be available on a crash cart or a tray or cabinet for the sole use in an office emergency.

With the increase of drug abuse and misuse, it is important for medical assistants to recognize the signs of drug abuse in patients and coworkers and to report abuse to the provider or supervisor.

STUDY FOR SUCCESS

To reinforce your knowledge and skills of information presented in this chapter:

- Review the Key Terms
- Practice the Procedure
- Consider the Case Studies and discuss your conclusions
- Answer the Review Questions
  - Multiple Choice
  - Critical Thinking
- Navigate the Internet by completing the Web Activities
- Practice the StudyWARE activities on your student CD
- Apply your knowledge in the Student Workbook activities
- Complete the Web Tutor sections

REVIEW QUESTIONS

Multiple Choice

1. Which of the following drugs is commonly used in an emergency such as anaphylactic shock?
   a. lomotil
   b. interferon
   c. cytoxan
   d. epinephrine
2. Which of the following types of drugs do providers prescribe most frequently?
   a. generic
   b. official
   c. chemical
   d. brand
3. An example of a drug that can be obtained from an animal is:
   a. digitalis
   b. cortisone
   c. imferon
   d. sulfur
4. Which of the following is an example of a controlled substance?
   a. Nembutal
   b. Keflin
   c. Inderal
   d. Aldomet
5. After you have poured a medication and taken it to the patient, he refuses to take it. You should:
   a. give it to another patient who has the same medication prescribed
   b. return the refused medication to its original container
   c. save it for the next time the patient is due for another dose
   d. dispose of it by returning it to the pharmacist to dispose of. Document.

Critical Thinking

1. Drugs are derived from various sources. List five sources of drugs.
2. How does the Federal Food, Drug, and Cosmetic Act protect the public?
3. The _________ is recognized by the U.S. government as the official list of standardized drugs.
4. Describe the principal factors that affect drug action.
5. While preparing an injection of Demerol® (meperidine), you accidentally drop and break the ampule, spilling its contents. Describe what actions you would take.
6. Name five emergency drugs that may be found on a crash cart or emergency tray. Describe the use and actions of each.
7. Under what circumstances can a medical assistant dispense stock medication?
8. Audrey Jones is considering taking a new position with a provider who is opening an office in another state. Audrey will be responsible for the clinical aspect of the practice. Where can Audrey find information about laws that apply to her in regard to administering medications? Where can she get information about the storage and handling on the premises of narcotics?
9. List several drug references and briefly describe the contents of the PDR.
10. After lunch, a newly hired medical assistant is helping you get Lenore McDonell back into her wheelchair after her physical examination. You strongly suspect that the medical assistant has been drinking alcohol, because she is uncoordinated in her movements and there is a strong odor of what seems to be alcohol on her breath. Describe your next action.

WEB ACTIVITIES

Explore on the Internet for information regarding the Drug Enforcement Agency.

1. Print a copy of Schedules I–V of the controlled substances.
2. Find to which schedule the following controlled substances belong: phencyclidine (PCP), amphetamines, cocaine, and heroin.
3. Using a search engine of your choice, gather information about over-the-counter (OTC) analgesics such as aspirin and nonsteroidal antiinflammatory drugs (NSAIDs).
   a. What risks can be associated with taking these drugs?
   b. Look for surveys that have been done by the National Consumers League on adults who used an OTC pain reliever in the past year.
   c. What percentage exceeded the recommended dose?
   d. What percentage had not spoken to a health care professional about possible risks associated with these products?

REFERENCES/BIBLIOGRAPHY

Broderick, M. (2003, September). Spotting drug abuse. *RN Magazine, 66*(9), pp. 48–53.

Centers for Disease Control and Prevention. (2007). *Public emergency preparedness and response.* Retrieved September 11, 2007, from http://www.bt.cdc.gov.

Facts & figures. (2007). Retrieved October 15, 2008, from http://www.drugtopics.modernmedicine.com.

Rice, J. (2006). *Principles of pharmacology for medical assisting* (4th ed.). Clifton Park, NY: Delmar Cengage Learning.

Spratto, G. R., & Woods, A. L. (2007). *Physician's desk reference—nurses drug handbook.* Clifton Park, NY: Cengage Delmar Learning.

Taber's cyclopedic medical dictionary (22nd ed.). (2003). Philadelphia: F. A. Davis.

United States Drug Enforcement Agency (DEA). (2007). *Drugs of abuse publication chart.* Retrieved February 16, 2008, from http://www.usdoj.gov/dea/pubs/abuse/chart.htm.

U.S. Food and Drug Administration, Department of Health and Human Services. (2004, February 6). *FDA issues regulations prohibiting sale of dietary supplements containing ephedrine alkaloids and reiterates—it advises that consumers stop using these products.* Retrieved September 11, 2007, from http://www.cfisan.fda.gov/~lrd/fpephed6.html.

WebMD Health. (2006). *Crash carts and their typical contents and indications.* Retrieved October 15, 2008, from http://vcdmc.vcdavis.edu/cne/resources/clinical_skills_refreshed/crash_cart.

Wooten, J. M. (2003, April). Medicine cabinet staples are not without risks. *RN Magazine, 66*(4), 96.

World Health Organization. (n.d.). *Health aspects of biological and chemical weapons.* Retrieved September 10, 2007, from http://www.who.int.

Chapter 24

Calculation of Medication Dosage and Medication Administration

OUTLINE

KEY TERMS

Administering
Apnea
Body Surface Area (BSA)
Compounding
Dispensing
Hypoxemia
Meniscus
Nomogram
Parenteral
Phytomedicines
Port
Precipitate
Retrolental Fibroplasia
Status Asthmaticus
Taut
Unit Dose

OBJECTIVES

The student should strive to meet the following performance objectives and demonstrate an understanding of the facts and principles presented in this chapter through written and oral communication.

1. Define the key terms as presented in the glossary.
2. Discuss the legal and ethical implications of medication administration.

OBJECTIVES (continued)

3. Describe the medication order.
4. Describe the parts of a prescription.
5. Define drug dosage.
6. State what information is found on a medication label.
7. Understand ratio and proportion.
8. Use the metric, household, and apothecary systems of measurement and convert between metric and apothecary systems.
9. Understand units of medication dosage.
10. Correctly calculate dosages for adults and children.
11. List the guidelines to follow when preparing and administering medications.
12. Describe safe disposal of syringes, needles, and biohazard materials.
13. Understand intravenous therapy.
14. Describe site selection for administration of injections.
15. Understand allergenic extracts.
16. Describe inhalation medication and its administration.

Scenario

At Drs. Lewis and King's practice, office policy dictates that a medicine card must be written out before the administration of any medication to a patient. Clinical medical assistant Joe Guerrero, CMA (AAMA), is careful to check the provider's order, then prepare the medicine card before preparing and administering medication. He notes that the card contains the patient's name, the provider's order, and the date, time, and route the medication is to be administered. After giving the medication to the patient, Joe documents the fact in the patient file, and then, according to procedure, tears and discards the medicine card.

INTRODUCTION

Despite the fact that many ambulatory care centers use what is known as the unit dose type of medication preparation, there remains a responsibility for medical assistants to know and understand how to calculate dosages of medication and to safely administer them to patients.

This chapter addresses calculation of adult and pediatric dosages of medication using the metric and household systems. It also emphasizes the legal aspects of medication administration and discusses oral and parenteral medication administration.

LEGAL AND ETHICAL IMPLICATIONS OF MEDICATION ADMINISTRATION

Members of the health care profession who prepare and administer medications are ethically and legally responsible for their own actions. Under law, these individuals are required to be licensed, registered, or otherwise authorized by a physician.

Each state has enacted laws governing the practice of medicine, nursing, and pharmacy. These laws vary from state to state; therefore, it is essential that

Spotlight on Certification

RMA Content Outline

- Medical law
- Patient education
- Asepsis
- Sterilization
- Specialty examinations
- Allergy
- Clinical pharmacology
- First aid and emergency response

CMA (AAMA) Content Outline

- Legislation
- State compliance
- Documentation/reporting
- Drug Enforcement Administration (DEA)
- Principles of infection control
- Principles of asepsis
- Preparing and administering medications
- Pharmacology
- Emergencies
- First aid

CMAS Content Outline

- Medical office emergencies
- Asepsis in the medical office
- Pharmacology
- Understand basic pharmacological concepts and terminology
- Risk management and quality assurance

medical assistants become familiar with the laws of the state in which they are employed before administering any medication. In some states, the only health professional authorized to give injections, other than a physician, is a registered nurse. In other states, legislation gives physicians broad authority to delegate responsibility for administering medication to other health care workers such as medical assistants. Laws have been passed in some states specifying which qualified and properly educated and trained persons may perform certain medical acts.

Regardless of the differences in state authorization laws, the courts will not permit the careless action of health care workers to go unpunished, especially when such actions result in harm or death to the patient. Under the law, those administering medications are expected to be knowledgeable about the drugs that they administer and the effects the drug(s) may or will have on the patient. Many states have uniform disciplinary acts. Never administer a medication without thorough knowledge of the drug. It is the medical assistant's responsibility to know the information about a medication listed in Figure 24-1 before administering it to a patient. You are an agent of the provider and accountable for your actions.

Ethical Considerations

Anyone who has access to medications may be tempted to use them for personal benefit. To do so not only is unethical, it is considered to be illegal. The conversion to personal use of medications intended for another is unethical and may cause harm to the patient. It is also unethical and illegal to take any medication that belongs to your employer, even aspirin or drug samples, without proper authorization.

The Medication Order

The medication order is given by the provider. It is for a specific patient and denotes the drug to be given, the dosage, the form of the drug, the time for or frequency of administration, and the route by which the drug is to be given.

The Prescription

The prescription is a written legal document that gives directions for **compounding**, **dispensing**, and **administering** a medication to a patient. There are nine parts to a prescription (Figure 24-2).

1. Drug name (generic and brand)
2. Action
3. Uses
4. Contraindications
5. Warnings when indicated
6. Adverse reactions
7. Dosage and route
8. Implications for patient care
9. Patient teaching
10. Special considerations

Figure 24-1 Medical assistants should have a thorough knowledge of any medication they administer to a patient and should consult references such as the *Physician's Desk Reference* (PDR).

Parts of a Prescription

1. The physician's name, address, telephone and fax numbers, and DEA registration number.
2. The patient's name, date of birth, address, and the date on which the prescription is written.
3. The *superscription* that includes the symbol Rx ("take thou").
4. The *inscription* that states the names and quantities of ingredients to be included in the medication.
5. The *subscription* that gives directions to the pharmacist for filling the prescription.
6. The *signature* (Sig) that gives the directions for the patient.
7. The physician's signature blanks. Where signed, indicates if a generic substitute is allowed or if the medication is to be dispensed as written.
8. REFILL 0 1 2 3 p.r.n. This is where the physician indicates whether or not the prescription can be refilled.

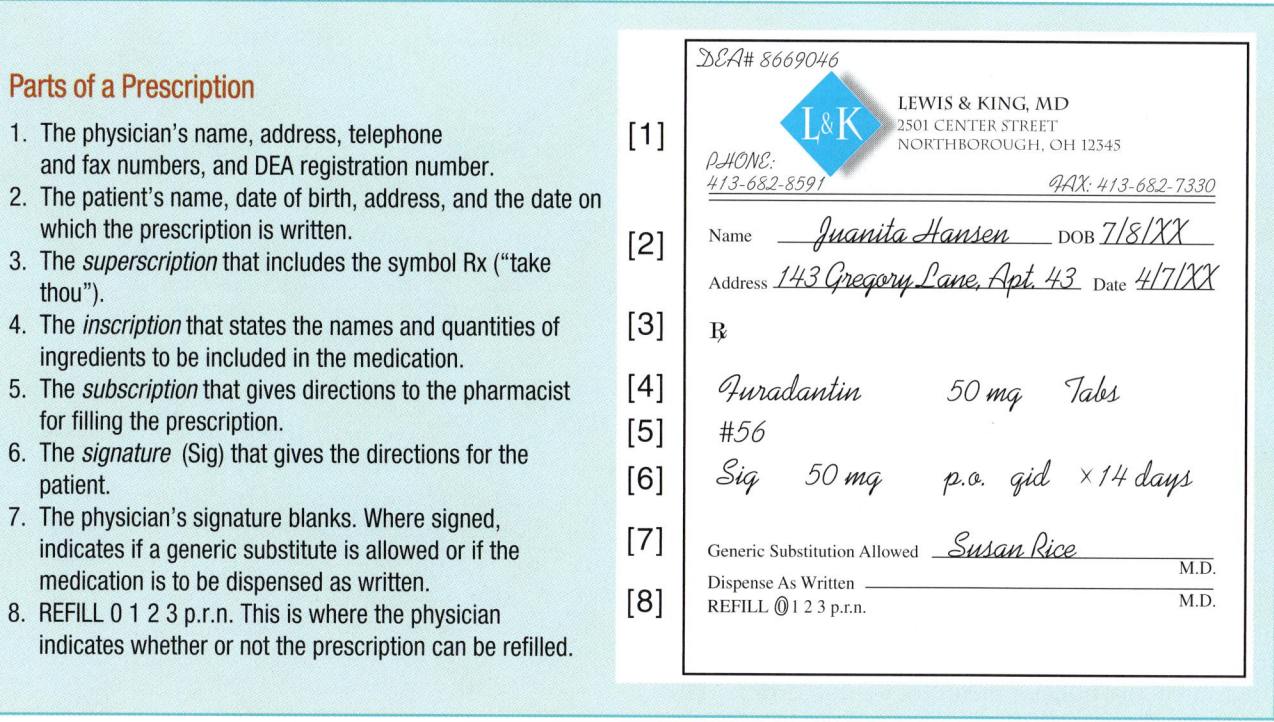

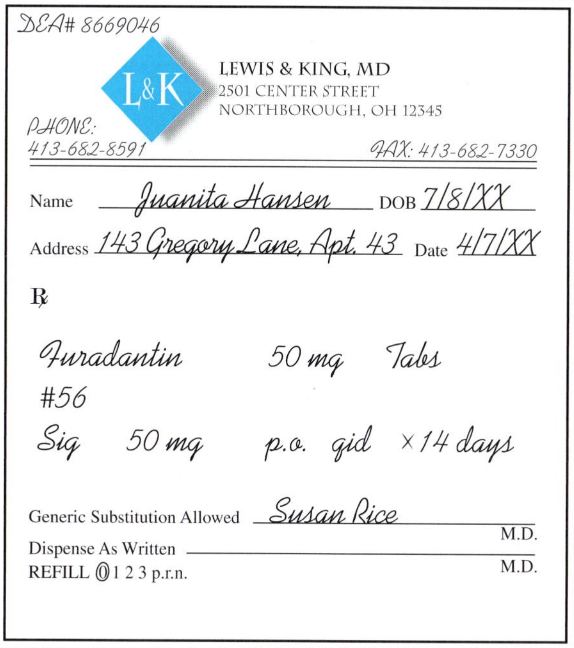
DEA# 8669046
L&K
LEWIS & KING, MD
2501 CENTER STREET
NORTHBOROUGH, OH 12345
PHONE:
413-682-8591
FAX: 413-682-7330
[1]
Name Juanita Hansen DOB 7/8/XX
Address 143 Gregory Lane, Apt. 43 Date 4/7/XX
[2]
℞
[3]
Furadantin 50 mg Tabs
[4]
#56
[5]
Sig 50 mg p.o. qid × 14 days
[6]
Generic Substitution Allowed Susan Rice M.D.
Dispense As Written M.D.
[7]
REFILL ⓪ 1 2 3 p.r.n.
[8]

Figure 24-2 Prescriptions are written legal documents that give directions for compounding, dispensing, and administering a medication. Prescriptions have eight distinct elements.

The purpose of a prescription is to control the sale and use of drugs that can be safely and effectively used only under the supervision of a licensed provider. Federal law divides medicines into two main classes: prescription or legend medicines and over-the-counter (OTC) medicines. The prescription is written by the provider and signed with an ink pen or e-prescribed. The pharmacist fills the prescription according to the provider's order. Once the prescription has been filled, the assigned prescription number and all other information can be entered into a computer. The hard copy of the prescription is filed and kept for a minimum of 7 years. Schedule II controlled substances prescriptions (see Chapter 23 for a description of schedule II medications) are kept separate from other prescriptions and are stamped with a red C (C for controlled) and filed separately. Schedule III through V prescriptions are stamped with a red C and filed.

HIPAA

HIPAA E-prescribing is the process of electronically accessing the patient's medical history, prescribing a medication, and selecting a pharmacy.

EHR The Medicare Prescription Drug, Improvement and Modernization Act (MMA) of 2003 and the Health Insurance Portability and Accountability Act (HIPAA) of 1996 have recommended e-prescribing standards. Medications handled electronically have reduced the problems of medication errors. Patients enjoy the ease of e-prescriptions because they do not have to drop off the prescription and then return to pick it up. Some states already have e-prescriptions in patients' electronic medical records. However, the possibility of a breach in confidentiality exists whenever electronic medical records are used.

Prescriptions for Controlled Substances. Federal laws require that the provider follows specific procedures when prescribing controlled substances (Table 24-1).

All prescriptions for controlled substances must be dated and signed on the date issued, bearing the full name and address of the patient and the name, address, and Drug Enforcement Administration (DEA) number (see Chapter 23) of the provider. The prescription must be written in ink or typewritten and signed by the provider's own hand.

Prescription Abbreviations and Symbols. It is important to be knowledgeable of the most common

Table 24-1 Requirements for Prescriptions for Controlled Substances

	Verbal Order or Prescription	Written Prescription	Refills
Schedule I	NOT FOR MEDICINAL USE		
Schedule II	No	Yes	No
Schedule III	Yes	Yes	5 × within 6 months
Schedule IV	Yes	Yes	5 × within 6 months
Schedule V	Yes	Yes	Yes

abbreviations used by the provider when an order for a prescription drug is given. The abbreviations are a clear and concise means of writing orders. This medical shorthand is an international language used by professional and nonprofessional people involved with patient care. Medical assistants should memorize all abbreviations in Table 24-2 so that they can prepare medications safely and accurately for administration.

The Joint Commission requires that facilities comply with the Joint Commission's minimum requirement for the banning of certain abbreviations, acronyms, symbols, and their *do not use* list. This ban, as part of the Joint Commission's 2004 patient safety goals, has been applied to protect patients from errors during documentation. The ban was reaffirmed in 2005 by the Joint Commission.

Table 24-3 lists abbreviations no longer allowed by the Joint Commission. Table 24-4 lists abbreviations and symbols that can be misinterpreted and are under consideration for possible inclusion on the "Do Not Use" list in the future.

Patients should be inquisitive when at the provider's office, clinic, pharmacy, or hospital and should ask questions about the medications they are prescribed or being given (see Patient Education box).

Many medications sound alike and look alike, which can cause confusion and errors. The Joint Commission recommends that pharmaceutical manufacturers examine their practices in naming their medications and make changes to alleviate confusion and errors. Table 24-5 lists a few sound-alike, look-alike medications. The United States Pharmacopeia regularly updates a complete list of

Table 24-2 Common Prescription Abbreviations and Symbols

Abbreviation or Symbol	Meaning
aa	of each
ac	before meals
ad lib	as desired
aq	water
bid	twice a day
c̄	with
cap	capsule
dil	dilute
elix	elixir
g	gram
gr	grain
gt or gtt	drop (drops)
h	hour
IM	intramuscular
IV	intravenous
kg	kilogram
L	liter
liq	liquid
m or min	minim
mg	milligram
mL	milliliter
mm	millimeter
NPO	nothing by mouth
non rep	do not repeat
p̄	after
pc	after meals
per	by or with
po	by mouth
prn	as needed

(continues)

Table 24-2 (continued)

Abbreviation or Symbol	Meaning
pt	patient
q	every
qh	every hour
q (2, 3, 4) h	every (2, 3, 4) hours
qid	four times a day
qs	of sufficient quantity
Rx	take
$\bar{s}$	without
sol	solution
ss	one-half
stat	at once
tab	tablet
Tbs	tablespoon
tsp	teaspoon
tid	three times a day
tr	tincture
ung	ointment

sound-alike, look-alike medications on their Web site (http:// www.USP.org).

DRUG DOSAGE

The dosage or dose is the amount of medicine that is prescribed for administration. It is determined by the provider or qualified practitioner who considers the following important factors: age, weight, sex, and other factors as well.

Age

The usual adult dose is generally suitable for the 20- to 60-year age group. Infants, young children, adolescents, and older adults require an individualized dosage regimen.

Weight

The average adult dosage is based on 150 pounds (about 68 kilograms). Individuals who weigh less or more than this should have the dosage based on **body surface area (BSA)** or kilogram of body weight.

Sex

Many medications are contraindicated during pregnancy and breast-feeding. It is important that these two factors be known before any dose of medication is prescribed.

Table 24-3 Dangerous Abbreviations No Longer Allowed

Do Not Use	Possible Misinterpretation	How to Avoid Problem
U (for unit)	Mistaken for a four (4), zero (0), or cc	Write out the word "unit"
IU (for international unit)	Mistaken for IV or ten (10)	Write out "international unit"
Q.D., every day; Q.O.D, (every other day)	Mistaken for one another	Write "daily" Write "every other day"
Trailing zero (X.0 mg) Lack of preceding zero (.X mg)	Decimal point is missed and dose is either too much or not enough	Do not write a zero by itself after the decimal point (X mg) Always use zero before a decimal point (0.X mg)
mS mSO_4 $MgSO_4$	Can be interpreted to mean morphine sulfate or magnesium sulfate	Write out "morphine sulfate" Write out "magnesium sulfate"

Table 24-4 Additional Abbreviations, Acronyms and Symbols that May Be Misinterpreted (for Possible Future Inclusion in the Official "Do Not Use" List)

Do Not Use	Possible Misinterpretation	How to Avoid Problem
> (greater than) < (less than)	Can be misinterpreted as number seven (7) or the letter "L" Confused for one another	Write out "greater than" and "less than"
Apothecary units	Unfamiliar to many practitioners Confused with metric units	Use metric units
@	Mistaken for number two (2)	Write "at"
cc	Mistaken for U (units) when written poorly	Write out "mL" or "milliliters"
µg	Mistaken for mg (milligrams) causing 1,000× overdose	Write out "mcg" or micrograms

Table 24-5 Sound-alike, Look-alike Medications

Accupril (hypertension)	Aciphex (heartburn, ulcers)
Rimantidine (flu)	Ranitidine (heartburn)
Oxycontin (pain)	Oxybutynin (urinary incontinence)
Paxil (depression)	Plavix (prevent heart attack and stroke)
Pravachol (high cholesterol)	Propranolol (hypertension)
Singulair (asthma)	Sinequan (depression, anxiety)
Clonazepam (anticonvulsant)	Chlorazepate (anti-anxiety)
Darvon (analgesic)	Diovan (hypertension)
Clonazepam (anticonvulsant)	Lorazepam (anti-anxiety)

Other Factors

Other factors that determine the dosage of a medication include the following:

1. Physical and emotional condition of patient
2. Disease process, especially kidney disease because of impaired excretion
3. Presence of more than one disease process
4. Causative microorganism(s) and the severity of the infection
5. Patient's medical history, allergies, and idiosyncrasies
6. Safest method, route, time, and amount to effect the desired maximum result

THE MEDICATION LABEL

The medication label can be a source of valuable information to the medical assistant and the patient. Regardless of whether administering a prescription drug or taking a nonprescription product, an understanding of the information provided on the label is essential to the safe and effective use of any medicine. In addition to the name and address of the manufacturer, other important items of information on a medication label include:

- The trade or brand name for the medication
- The generic name (or listing of active and inactive ingredients)
- The National Drug Code (NDC) numbers that can be used to identify the manufacturer, the product, and the size of the container
- The dosage strength in a given amount of the medication
- The usual dosage and frequency of administration
- The route of administration
- Precautions and warnings
- The expiration date for the medication

Other information that may be on a medication label includes directions for storage and directions for mixing or reconstituting a powdered form of the drug (see Figure 23-6).

CALCULATION OF DRUG DOSAGES

The preparation and administration of medications is one of the most important and critical tasks that medical assistants perform. Today, drugs are more potent and more likely to cause physiologic changes in the body; therefore, anyone who administers medications must do so with extreme care.

Incorrectly calculated or measured dosages are the leading cause of error in the administration of medications. A drug error is a violation of a patient's rights. It is important that medical assistants develop a working knowledge of mathematics to calculate or measure accurately a medication that is to be administered to a patient.

According to the Institute of Medicine (IOM), each year medications kill several thousands of hospital patients and injure another 1.5 million. About half of these deaths and injuries result from side effects; the other half result from errors. Because the majority of prescriptions are written in the provider's offices, the figures are likely to be proportionately higher. E-prescribing will reduce the number of errors. Hospital prescriptions and all OTC medications, vaccines, and blood will require standardized and universal bar codes to help prevent medication errors. Reading the bar code with a scanner can correlate the medication bar code with a patient identification bar code.

The IOM states that only a small percent of health care agencies use a bar code medication system. Studies have shown that use of bar codes (bar code on medication matches bar code on patient's wrist) results in far fewer errors.

The IOM wants health care agencies, especially hospitals, to computerize their prescription systems by 2008 and to begin using them by 2010. According to the IOM, fewer than 10% of hospitals have computerized prescriptions systems. The system works when a provider inputs data on the computer. For example, the patient's height and weight and medication are entered and the computer calculates the dose. There is no paper, illegible handwriting, or miscalculation of the dose. The computer fills in the correct dose as part of the prescription (Figure 24-3).

Additionally, the IOM recommended to the FDA that they lessen the confusion about sound-alike medications and simplify look-alike labels and packaging.

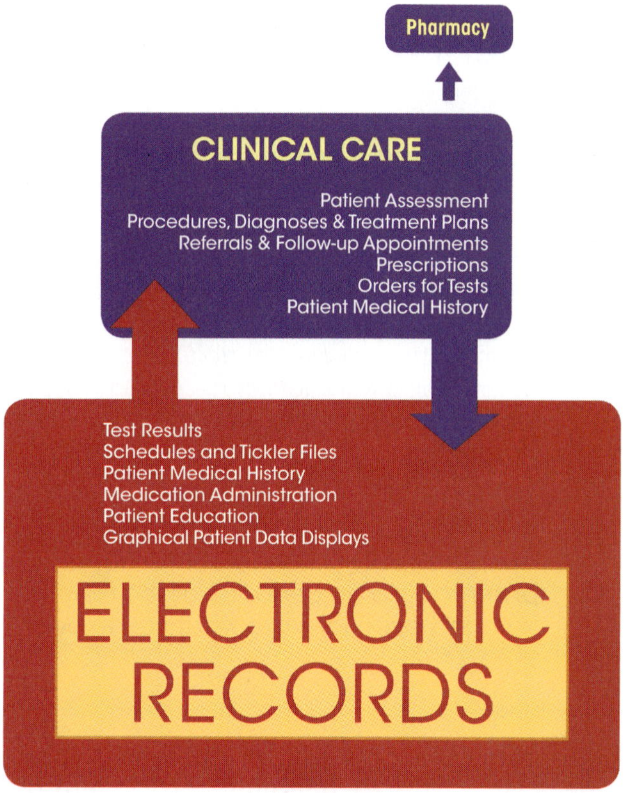

Figure 24-3 The clinical care arm of the total practice management system (TPMS). Medication errors can be minimized when prescriptions are written electronically. The computer calculates the dose according to the patient's height and weight and can send the prescription to the pharmacy.

Understanding Ratio

Ratio is a method of expressing the relationship of a number, quantity, substance, or degree between two similar components. For example, the relationship of one to five is written 1:5. Note that numbers are side by side and separated by a colon.

In mathematics, a ratio may be expressed as a quotient, a fraction, or a decimal.

Ratio Expressed as a Quotient. A quotient is the number found when one number is divided by another number. The ratio one to five written as a quotient is $1 \div 5$.

Ratio Expressed as a Fraction. A fraction is the process of dividing or breaking a whole number into parts. The ratio one to five written as a fraction is $1/5$ or $\frac{1}{5}$.

Ratio Expressed as a Decimal. A decimal is a linear array of numbers based on 10 or any

Patient Education

Patients should:

1. Question the provider, pharmacist, and staff administering the drug about the drug and its possible side effects.
2. Be sure the prescription has been written legibly. Many drugs sound alike (e.g., Ambien® for insomnia and Amen® for menstrual cycle control; Xanax® for anxiety and Xantac® for heartburn and ulcers; Fosamax® for osteoporosis and Flomax® for enlarged prostate).
3. Always check the label at the pharmacy to make sure it is clearly written.
4. Always check your medication at the pharmacy to be certain that the medication and directions are what you expect.
5. Have the provider or pharmacist explain the name and purpose of each new medication that is being prescribed. Be sure you understand.
6. Keep an updated list of all medications, prescriptions, OTC vitamins, minerals, and **phytomedicines.**
7. Take medications as directed, and do not discontinue use until the appropriate date as indicated by the provider.
8. Store medicines away from heat and humidity in their original containers.
9. Ask the provider or pharmacist what you should do if you miss a dose.

multiple of 10. To express the ratio one to five as a decimal, divide the denominator (5) into the numerator (1).

$$\text{(denominator)}\ 5\overline{)1.0}^{\ 0.2}\ \text{(numerator)}$$

The ratio may be expressed as:

A quotient	*A fraction*	*A decimal*
1 ÷ 5	⅕ ($\frac{1}{5}$)	0.2

Understanding Proportion

Proportion is a process of expressing the comparative relationship between a part, share, or portion with regard to size, amount, or number. In mathematics, a proportion expresses the relationship between two ratios. In setting up a proportion, the ratios are separated by : or an = sign. In this text, the equal sign (=) is used to separate ratios.

Example:

6 : 4 = 3 : 2

Read:

Six is to four equals three is to two.

The four terms of a proportion are given special names. The *means* are the inner numbers or the second and third terms of the proportion.

Example:

6 : 4 = 3 : 2 (4) (3)

means

4 × 3 = 12 (*means*)

6 × 2 = 12 (*extremes*)

The *extremes* are the outer numbers or the first and fourth terms of the proportion.

Example:

6 : 4 = 3 : 2 (6) (2)

extremes

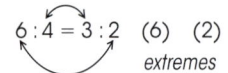

In a true proportion, the product of the means equals the product of the extremes.

Example:

means (16) (1)

8 : 16 = 1 : 2

extremes (8) (2)

16 × 1 = 16 (*means*)

8 × 2 = 16 (*extremes*)

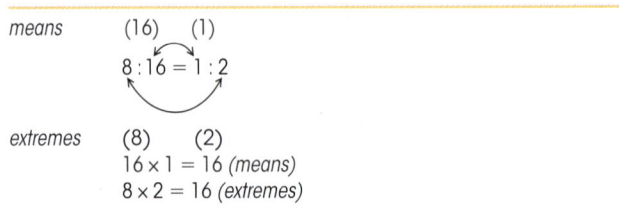

Solving for *x*. The proportion is a useful mathematical tool. When a part, share, or portion of the problem is unknown, then *x* represents the unknown factor. You can determine the unknown by solving for *x*. The unknown factor *x* may appear any place in the proportion.

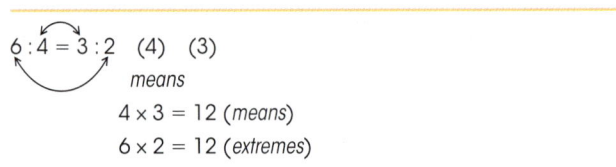

Now solve for x in the problem: $3:4 = x:12$.

1. Multiply the term that contains the x and place the product to the left of the equal sign ($4x$).
2. Multiply the other terms and place the product to the right of the equal sign (36).
3. To find x, divide the product of x into the product of the other terms.

$$4x = 36$$
$$x = \frac{36}{4} \text{ or } 36 \div 4$$
$$x = 9$$

After finding the unknown factor, check your mathematical skills by determining if you have a true proportion. This technique is called proof or proving your answer. To prove your answer:

1. Place the answer you found for x back into the formula where x was.

$$3:4 = 9:12$$

2. Now multiply the means by the means, and the extremes by the extremes.
3. The results will equal each other.

Formula: $3:4 = x:12$

Proof: $3:4 = 9:12$

$$4 \times 9 = 36$$
$$3 \times 12 = 36$$

Weights and Measures

Two systems of measurement are used in pharmacology to calculate dosages: metric and household. The metric system is used throughout the world as the official language of communication in scientific and technical fields. It is based on the decimal system: the number 10 or multiples of 10.

Metric System Guidelines. The following guidelines are helpful when learning basic facts about the metric system:

1. Arabic numbers are used to designate whole numbers, e.g., 1, 250, 500, 1,000.
2. Decimal fractions are used for quantities less than one, e.g., 0.1, 0.01, 0.001, 0.0001.
3. To ensure accuracy, place a zero before the decimal point, e.g., 0.1, 0.001, 0.0001.
4. The Arabic number precedes the metric unit of measurement, e.g., 10 grams, 2 millimeters, 5 liters.
5. The abbreviation for gram should be capitalized (Gm) or written as (g) to distinguish it from grain (gr).
6. The abbreviation for liter is capitalized (L).
7. Prefixes are written in lowercase letters, e.g., milli, centi, deci, deka.
8. Capitalize the measurement and symbol when it is named after a person, e.g., Celsius (C).
9. Periods are no longer used with most abbreviations or symbols.
10. Abbreviations for units are the same for singular and plural. An *s* is not added to an abbreviation to indicate a plural.

The Seven Common Metric Prefixes. It is important to know common metric prefixes to have a solid foundation for determining metric equivalents. When a metric prefix is combined with a root of physical quantity, you arrive at multiples or submultiples of the metric system.

Example:

- **milli** (prefix): one-thousandth of a unit
  meter (root): a measure of length
  millimeter: one-thousandth of a meter
- **kilo** (prefix): one thousand units
  liter (root): a measure of volume
  kiloliter: one thousand liters
- **micro** (prefix): one-millionth of a unit
  gram (root): a measure of mass and/or weight
  microgram: one-millionth of a gram

Prefixes:

micro (mi'kro)	= one millionth of a unit written as 0.000001
milli (mil'i)	= one-thousandth of a unit written as 0.001
centi (sen'ti)	= one-hundredth of a unit written as 0.01
deci (des'i)	= one-tenth of a unit written as 0.1
deka (dek'a)	= ten units written as 10
hecto (hek'to)	= one hundred units written as 100
kilo (kil'o)	= one thousand units written as 1000

Fundamental Units:
Following are the fundamental units of the metric system:

meter (m)	length
liter (L)	volume
gram (Gm, g)	mass and/or weight

The meter is the fundamental unit of length in the metric system and originally formed the foundation for the entire system. A meter is equal to 39.37 inches, which is slightly more than a yard, or 3.28 feet.

A millimeter is about the width of the head of a pin. It takes approximately 2½ centimeters to make an inch; a decimeter is approximately 4 inches.

Meter (m)	=	**Length**
1 millimeter (mm)	=	0.001 meter
1 centimeter (cm)	=	0.01 meter
1 decimeter (dm)	=	0.1 meter
1 meter (m)	=	1 meter
1 dekameter (dam)	=	10 meters
1 hectometer (hm)	=	100 meters
1 kilometer (km)	=	1,000 meters

The liter is the metric unit of volume. A liter is equal to 1.056 quarts, which is 0.26 gallon or 2.1 pints.

A milliliter is equivalent to one cubic centimeter (cc), because the amount of space occupied by a milliliter is equal to one cubic centimeter. The weight of one milliliter of water equals approximately one gram. It takes approximately 15 milliliters to make 1 tablespoon. It takes 15 or 16 minims to make one milliliter.

Liter (L)		**Volume**
1 milliliter (mL)	=	0.001 liter
1 centiliter (cL)	=	0.01 liter
1 deciliter (dL)	=	0.1 liter
1 liter (L)	=	1 liter
1 dekaliter (daL)	=	10 liters
1 hectoliter (hL)	=	100 liters
1 kiloliter (kL)	=	1,000 liters

The gram is the metric unit of mass and weight. It equals approximately the weight of 1 cubic centimeter or 1 milliliter of water. A gram is equal to approximately 15 grains or 0.035 ounce.

Gram (Gm, g)		**Mass and Weight**
1 microgram (mcg)	=	0.000001 gram
1 milligram (mg)	=	0.001 gram
1 centigram (cg)	=	0.01 gram
1 decigram (dg)	=	0.1 gram
1 gram (Gm, g)	=	1 gram
1 dekagram (dag)	=	10 grams
1 hectogram (hg)	=	100 grams
1 kilogram (kg)	=	1,000 grams

The metric equivalents most frequently used in the medical field are:

Length
2½ centimeters (cm) = 1 inch

Volume
1,000 milliliters (mL)= 1 liter (L)

Weight

1,000 micrograms (mcg)	= 1 milligram (mg)
1000 milligrams (mg)	= 1 gram (Gm, g)
1000 grams (g)	= 1 kilogram (kg)
1 kilogram	= 2.2 pounds (lb)

Household Measurements. Household measurements are approximate measurements. They are more frequently used in the home than in the medical field, but the medical assistant should be familiar with the common household measurements listed in Table 24-6.

Because medications can be prescribed in either metric or household measurements, it is important to know equivalents between both to calculate the dose of prescribed medication (Table 24-7).

Metric System Conversion. The process of changing into another form, state, substance, or product is known as *conversion*. In the metric system, changing from one unit to another involves multiplying or dividing by 10, 100, 1,000, and so forth. This can be done by the proportional method or by moving the decimal in the correct direction.

Proportional Method for Converting Metric Equivalents. There are six basic steps in the proportional method, plus an additional step to prove the answer. The following example will serve as a model for future applications of the proportional method of converting metric equivalents.

Table 24-6 Common Household Measures

60 drops (gtt)	is equal to:	1 teaspoon (t or tsp)
3 teaspoons (tsp)	is equal to:	1 tablespoon (T or tbsp)
2 tablespoons (tbsp)	is equal to:	1 ounce (oz)
8 ounces (oz)	is equal to:	1 measuring cup (c)
16 tablespoons or 8 ounces	is equal to:	1 measuring cup (c)
2 cups (c)	is equal to:	1 pint (pt)
2 pints (pt)	is equal to:	1 quart (qt)
4 quarts (qt)	is equal to:	1 gallon (gal)

Drop (gt) = approximate liquid measure depending on kind of liquid measured and the size of the opening from which it is dropped.

Table 24-7 Approximate Equivalents Among Metric and Household Systems

Metric	Household
DRY	
60 mg	
1 Gm	¼ tsp
15 Gm	1 tbsp (3 tsp)
30 Gm	1 oz (2 tbsp) 1 lb (16 oz)
1 kg	2.2 lb
LIQUID	
	1 gt
1 mL	15 gtt
5 mL	1 tsp
15 mL	1 tbsp (3 tsp)
30 mL	1 fl oz (2 tbs)
500 mL	(1 pt or 2 cups)
1,000 mL	4 cups (1 qt)
LENGTH	
2.5 cm	1 in
1 m	39.37 in

Example:

Convert 1,500 milligrams to grams.

1,500 mg = _____ g

Step 1.

Because the unknown factor in the given formula is the number of grams contained in 1,500 milligrams, substitute the symbol *x* for grams in the equation.

Step 2.

Setting up the proportion requires that you know metric equivalents. For example, in this problem you have to know that 1,000 milligrams (mg) = 1 gram (g).

Step 3.

Since you know that 1,000 mg is equal to 1 g, you can create one-half of the equation. Write the equivalent and place it on the left of the equal sign.

1,000 mg : 1 g =

Step 4.

Now that you have the left side of the equation, set up the right side by using the designated metric value 1,500 mg : *x* g. Always write the smallest equivalent as to the largest equivalent, for example, mg : g. By being consistent, it is less likely errors will occur.

1,000 mg : 1 g = 1,500 mg : *x* g

Step 5.

Note that you have an equal equation:

mg : g = mg : g

The first values on either side of the equal sign are milligrams, and the second values on either side are grams.

Step 6.

Now solve for the unknown (*x*) by multiplication and division. Multiply the means by the means and the extremes by the extremes. *NOTE:* Once the proportion is correctly set up, simply use the numbers as you multiply and divide.

1,000 : 1 = 1,500 : *x*

1,000*x* 5 1,500
x 5 1,500 4 1,000
x 5 1.5

```
         1.5
1,000)1,500.0
      1,000
        500.0
        500
```

Step 7.

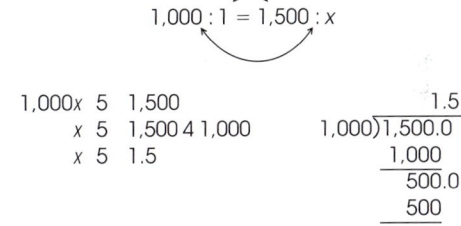

To make sure the answer is correct, prove the work: Place the answer 1.5 g into the formula where *x* once was. Now multiply the means by the means and the extremes by the extremes.

1,000 mg : 1 g 5 1,500 mg : 1.5 g
1,500 5 1,500

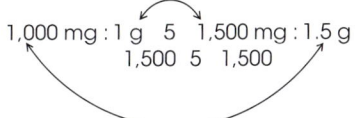

MEDICATIONS MEASURED IN UNITS

Medications such as insulin, heparin, some antibiotics, hormones, vitamins, and vaccines are measured in units. These medications are standardized in units based on their strengths. The strength varies from one medicine to another, depending on the source, condition, and method by which it is obtained.

How to Calculate Unit Dosages

When calculating medications that are ordered in units, use either the proportional method or the formula method.

The Proportional Method

Example:

The provider orders 4,000 USP units of heparin given deep subcutaneously. On hand is heparin 5,000 USP units per milliliter.

Step 1.

Use the following proportion to calculate the dose:

Known unit on hand	:	Known dosage form	=	Dose ordered	:	Unknown amount to be given
5,000 Units:		1 mL	=	4,000 Units:		x mL
		5,000x	=	4,000		
		x	=	$\frac{4}{5} = \frac{4}{5}$ mL or 0.8 mL		

Use a tuberculin syringe to draw up 0.8 mL, or convert $\frac{4}{5}$ mL to minims.

Step 2.

Convert $\frac{4}{5}$ mL to minims. *NOTE:* There are 15 or 16 minims per milliliter.
Multiply:

$$\frac{4}{\cancel{5}_1} \times \frac{\cancel{15}^3}{1} = \frac{4}{1} \times \frac{3}{1} = 12 \text{ minims}$$

Administer 12 minims (of 5,000 Units/mL for correct dose of 4,000 Units) to the patient.

The Formula Method

Example:

The provider orders 450,000 Units of Bicillin 1M. On hand is Bicillin 600,000 Units per milliliter.

Step 1.

Use the following formula to calculate the dose:

$$\frac{\text{Dose ordered (desired)}}{\text{Dose on hand}} \times \text{Quantity (per mL)} = \text{Amount to give}$$

$$\frac{450{,}000 \text{ units}}{600{,}000 \text{ units}} \times 1 \text{ mL} = \frac{450{,}\cancel{000} \text{ units}}{600{,}\cancel{000} \text{ units}} = \frac{45}{60} = \frac{3}{4}$$

$$\frac{3}{4} \times 1 \text{ mL} = \frac{3}{4} \text{ mL}$$

Step 2.

You may convert to minims. If you do, multiply $\frac{3}{4}$ by 16.

$$\frac{3}{\cancel{4}_1} \times \frac{\cancel{16}^4}{1} = 12 \text{ minims}$$

The patient will receive 12 minims of Bicillin 600,000 Units for the ordered dose of 450,000 Units.

Insulin

Insulin is a chemical substance (hormone) secreted by the beta cells of the islets of Langerhans in the pancreas. Insulin is necessary for the proper metabolism of blood glucose and maintenance of the correct blood sugar level. Inadequate secretion or no secretion of insulin, as in the disease diabetes mellitus, results in hyperglycemia and subsequent excessive production of ketone bodies. Eventual coma can occur.

Patients' needs are individualized according to the severity of their disease; treatment includes taking insulin, controlling diet, and exercise. The diet is well-balanced and consists of the correct number of calories distributed among carbohydrates, fats, and proteins. Patients are taught to monitor blood and urine glucose levels at home throughout the day, because the dosage of insulin taken depends on the amounts of glucose detected. Uncontrolled diabetes mellitus can result in serious complications such as circulatory problems, especially in the feet and legs; kidney disease; loss of vision; bedsores; infection; and gangrene. Special care of the feet is essential. The mouth and teeth require excellent oral hygiene.

Diabetes

The National Diabetes Data Group of the National Institutes of Health organized the various forms of diabetes into the following categories:

Type 1	Insulin-dependent diabetes mellitus (IDDM)
Type 2	Noninsulin-dependent diabetes mellitus (NIDDM)
Type 3	Women who developed glucose intolerance in association with pregnancy (gestational)
Type 4	Other types of diabetes associated with pancreatic disease, hormonal changes, adverse effects of drugs, or genetic or other anomalies

Individuals with type 1 diabetes (IDDM) must take insulin on a regular basis to maintain life. Other insulin delivery devices besides the syringe and the needle can be used for injection. With an insulin pen, the patient can turn a dial on the top until the correct dose of insulin is displayed through a small window. Once the correct dose is chosen, the dial "locks" itself to prevent the pen from losing insulin or from the dial moving forward to give an unintended larger dose. The pen has a needle similar to the insulin syringe, and the patient presses the plunger and the dose of insulin is delivered under the skin.

Another delivery device is a jet injector. High-pressure air sends a fine mist of insulin through the skin. No needles are required. This device may be suitable for patients who dislike needles.

Patient Education

Encourage patients with diabetes to enroll in diabetic education classes, which are offered at most local hospitals. Patients also need to realize that treatment of diabetes is a lifelong commitment and that they must abide by everything that the hospital teaches.

The insulin pump is a small device outside of the body that pumps insulin through a flexible tubing that is connected to a catheter that is under the skin of the abdomen, thigh, or buttocks. The pump is programmed to deliver a steady flow of the correct dose of insulin 24 hours a day. The pump can allow the patient to add insulin in a short time if needed. Although it is convenient and helps keep the patient's blood glucose under control, the pump can be damaged if the patient engages in certain physical activities. Patients still must regularly monitor their blood glucose levels.

Other devices not yet approved but being worked on for approval are an insulin patch and a dry powder that is inhaled into the lungs through the mouth, then from the lungs into the bloodstream. The dosage of insulin is expressed in units and is individualized by the provider for each patient. The amount of insulin that a person must take is based on blood and urine glucose levels, diet, exercise, and the individual's needs (Table 24-8).

It is *extremely important* that the *exact dosage of insulin be given to the patient.* Too little or too much insulin can cause serious problems ranging from a blood sugar level too low or too high, to coma, and even death. It may be the medical assistant's responsibility to administer insulin and to teach patients or their families how to administer insulin.

When administering insulin, the U-100 syringe (1 mL) is preferred. U-100 means there are 100 units of insulin per milliliter. Insulin dosage should always be expressed in units rather than in milliliters. For example, if the provider orders 30 units of U-100 NPH insulin, use a U-100 syringe and draw up 30 units of U-100 NPH insulin.

Table 24-8 Insulin Preparation Units 100

Type of Insulin	Onset	Appearance
Rapid-Acting Humalog Lispro	5 minutes after injection Peaks in 1 hour Works for 2–4 hours	Clear, colorless
Regular or short-acting Humulin R Novolin Actrapid	30 minutes after injection Peaks in 2–3 hours Works for 3–6 hours	Clear, colorless
Intermediate Lente L Humulin NPH	2–4 hours after injection Peaks in 4–12 hours Effective 12–18 hours	Cloudy
Long-lasting Ultralente Lantus	6–10 hours after injection Effective 20–24 hours	Clear, colorless
Premixed Humalog Mix 75/25	5 minutes after injection Duration 1–24 hours	Clear, colorless
Humulin 70/30	1–2.5 hours after injection Peak 7–15 hours Duration 24 hours	Clear, colorless
Humulin 50/50	15–20 minutes after injection Peak 1–4 hours Duration 1–24 hours	Clear, colorless

Precautions to Observe When Administering Insulin. The following precautions must be observed when administering insulin:

- Be sure to use the proper insulin, the one ordered by the provider. Refer to Table 24-8 for various insulin preparations.
- Do not substitute one insulin for another.
- Use the correct syringe, U-100.
- Dosage of insulin is always measured in units and is individualized for each patient.
- Check the label for the name and type of insulin, strength, and expiration date.
- Make sure the insulin has the proper appearance. Refer to Table 24-8 for proper appearance of various insulins.
- When insulin is not in use, store it in a cool place and avoid freezing.
- When mixing insulins in one syringe, be certain they are compatible. NPH and Regular are compatible. Regular and lente are not compatible.
- Avoid shaking the insulin bottle. Roll gently in palms of hand to mix. This method prevents bubbles in the medication.

- Use a subcutaneous needle, but inject at a 90-degree angle.
- Insulin pens are available prefilled with 300 units of insulin.
- Use a site rotation system and select an appropriate site. Insulin injection sites must be rotated to prevent tissue damage. Record site used (Figure 24-4).
- Do not massage after injection.
- Always follow the provider's order and office policy when mixing insulins.

Oral Hypoglycemic Medication. Persons with type 2 diabetes mellitus are known to have noninsulin-dependent diabetes mellitus (NIDDM). Type 2 diabetes has a gradual onset, usually seen in adults over 40 years of age. With the obesity epidemic in the United States, individuals are contracting type 2 diabetes at earlier ages (obesity contributes to and can cause type 2 diabetes). The pancreas in patients with type 1 diabetes secretes no insulin; in type 2, the pancreas has some ability to secrete insulin. Most individuals with type 2 diabetes do not have to inject insulin, although a few do. Exercise and diet management may be sufficient for type 2 diabetics to lose enough weight and not require oral hypoglycemic medication. For the majority, however, exercise and diet are not enough to bring the blood sugar to an acceptable level. Medication works by stimulating the pancreas to secrete more insulin, by making cells more receptive to insulin, and by slowing the body's carbohydrate absorption. Some oral hypoglycemics are Orinase, Tolinase, Micronase, Glucotrol, Glucophage, and Starlix.

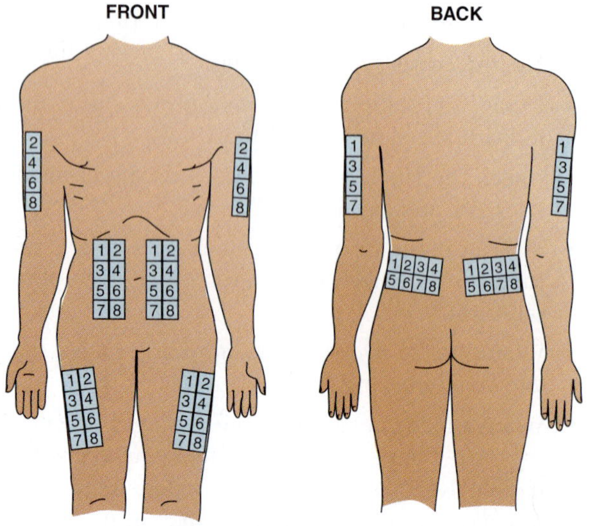

Figure 24-4 Sites and rotation for insulin administration.

CALCULATING ADULT DOSAGES

Two measures, weight and volume, are used to determine the amount of medication that is to be administered. The weight of a medication may be expressed as any of the following:

- milliequivalent (mEq)
- microgram (mcg)
- milligram (mg)
- gram (Gm, g)
- unit

The volume of a medication may be expressed as a:

- milliliter (mL)
- minim (m)
- dram (dr)
- ounce (oz)
- by a variety of household measures, such as the teaspoon (tsp)

Many different methods can be used when calculating the dosage to be administered. Two of the most useful methods—the proportional method and the formula method—are described next.

The Proportional Method

Example:

The provider orders 0.2 g of Equanil tabs. The dose on hand is 400 mg tabs.

Step 1.

Determine whether the medication ordered and the medication on hand are available in the same unit of measure.

Step 2.

If the medication ordered and the medication on hand are not in the same unit of measure, convert so that both measures are expressed using the same unit of measure.

Conversion: To change 0.2 g to mg

$$1{,}000 \text{ mg} : 1 \text{ g} = x \text{ mg} : 0.2 \text{ g}$$
$$x = 200 \text{ mg}$$
or
$$\text{multiply } 0.2 \times 1{,}000 = 200$$

Step 3.

Now use the following proportion to calculate the dosage. Remember that 0.2 g was converted to 200 mg.

Known unit on hand	:	*Known dosage form*	=	*Dose ordered*	:	*Unknown amount to be given*
400 mg	:	1 tab	=	200 mg	:	*x* tab

$$400 : 1 = 200 : x$$

$$400x = 200$$

$x = \frac{\overset{1}{\cancel{200}}}{\underset{2}{\cancel{400}}}$ (Reduce fraction to lowest terms)

x = ½ tab of 400 mg

Step 4

Prove your answer. Place your answer in the original formula in the *x* position.

400 mg : 1 tab = 200 mg : ½ tab

200 = ½ of 400

200 = 200

The Formula Method

Example:

The provider orders 0.2 g of Equanil tabs. The dose on hand is 400-mg tabs.

Step 1.

Determine whether the medication ordered and the medication on hand are available in the same unit of measure.

Step 2.

If the medication ordered and the medication on hand are not in the same unit of measure, convert so that both measures are expressed using the same unit of measure.

Conversion: To change 0.2 g to mg

1,000 mg : 1 g = *x* mg : 0.2 g

x = 200 mg

or

multiply 0.2 × 1,000 = 200

Step 3.

Now use the following formula to calculate the dosage.

$$\frac{\text{Dose ordered (desired)}}{\text{Dose on hand}} \times \frac{\text{Quantity}}{1} = \text{(Amount to give form of drug)}$$

$\frac{D}{H}$ 3 Q 5 Amount to give

The provider ordered 0.2 g of Equanil tabs (0.2 g converts to 200 mg). The dose on hand is 400 mg tabs.

$\frac{200 \text{ mg}}{400 \text{ mg}}$ 3 1 tab 5 $\frac{200}{400}$ or ½ tab

Give ½ tab of 400 mg.

CALCULATING CHILDREN'S DOSAGES

Each child is an individual with differences in age, size, and weight. In the past, formulas such as Young's, Clark's, and Fried's rules were used to calculate pediatric dosages. These formulas determined what fraction of an adult dose was appropriate for a child. Because each child does not develop in the same way during a given time span, these formulas have been replaced by more exact methods of determining the correct dosage of medication for a child.

Today, there are two basic methods used to calculate children's dosages:

- According to kilogram of body weight
- According to BSA

The body weight method is generally the method of choice, because most medications are ordered in this way and it is easier to calculate. The BSA is an exact method, but one must use a formula and a **nomogram** (a device-graph that shows relation among numeric values) to determine a correct dosage (Figure 24-5).

Body Surface Area

The BSA is considered to be one of the most accurate methods of calculating medication dosages for infants and children up to 12 years of age. This method requires the use of a nomogram that estimates the BSA of the patient according to height and weight.

The body surface area is determined by drawing a straight line from the patient's height to the patient's weight. Intersection of the line with the surface area column is the estimated BSA. This figure is then placed in the following formula:

$$\frac{\text{BSA of child (m}^2\text{)}}{1.7 \text{ (m}^2\text{)}} \times \text{adult dose} = \text{child dose}$$

This formula is based on the average adult who weighs 140 pounds and has a body surface area of 1.7 square meters (1.7 m^2).

Example:

Marion Carrera is a 4-year-old child who is 40 inches tall and weighs 38 pounds (BSA 0.7). The provider has ordered Demerol for pain. The average adult dose of Demerol is 50 mg per mL. What dosage will be given to Marion according to the BSA method?

$$\frac{0.7 \text{ (m}^2\text{)}}{1.7 \text{ (m}^2\text{)}} \times \frac{50 \text{ mg}}{1} = \text{child's dose}$$

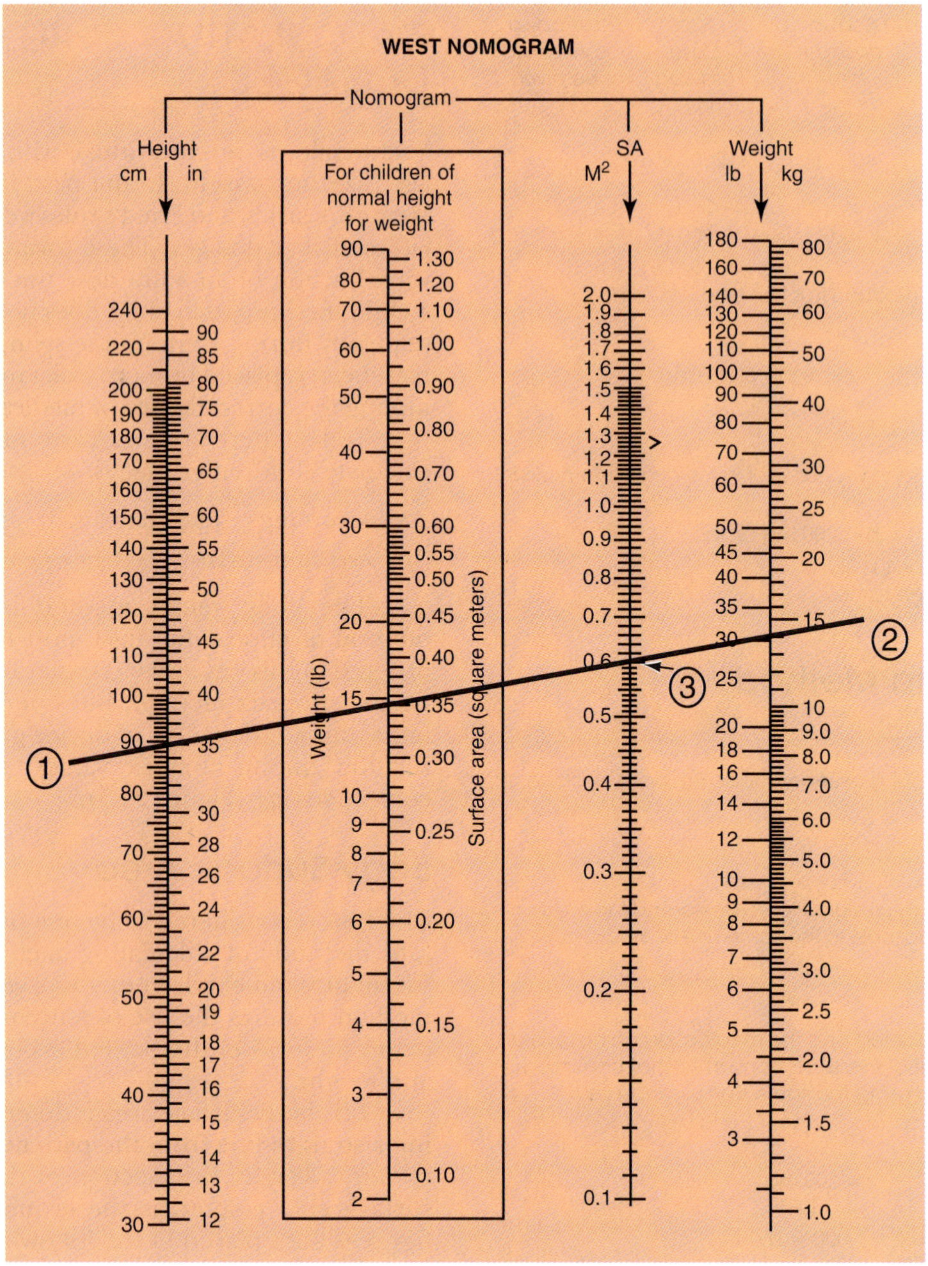

Figure 24-5 Body surface area (BSA) is determined by drawing a straight line from the patient's height (1) in the far left column to his or her weight (2) in the far right column. Intersection of the line with BSA column (3) is the estimated BSA (m^2). For infants and children of normal height and weight, BSA may be estimated from weight alone by referring to the enclosed area. (From Behrman, R. E., Kleigman, R. M., & Arvin, A. M. (1996). Nelson textbook of pediatrics (15th ed.). Philadelphia: W. B Saunders, Reprinted with permission from Elsevier.)

$$\frac{0.7\ (m^2)}{1.7\ (m^2)} \times \frac{50}{1} = \frac{35}{1.7} = 20.5\text{ mg} = 20.5\text{ or }21\text{ mg}$$

Now use the formula $\frac{\text{Desired}}{\text{Have}} \times$ Quantity to convert mg to mL.

$$\frac{21\text{ mg}}{50\text{ mg}} \times 1 = x\text{ mL}$$

$\frac{21}{50}$ =0.42 mL administered in a tuberculin syringe

Kilogram of Body Weight

It may be the responsibility of the medical assistant to calculate the amount of dosage ordered by the provider according to the patient's body weight. Today, many medications are ordered in this manner; therefore, it is essential that you learn how to calculate dosage according to this method. The following example will guide you step by step through the mathematical process of calculating dosage according to kilogram of body weight.

There are 2.2 pounds in 1 kg.

Example:

The provider ordered the antiepileptic agent Depakene (valproic acid) 15 mg/kg/day capsules for Clark Kipperley, who weighs 110 pounds. The medication is to be given in three divided doses.

Step 1.

To express pounds in kilograms, divide the weight in pounds by 2.2. Convert the patient's weight to kilograms:

$$110 \div 2.2 = 50 \text{ kilograms}$$

Step 2.

Now, calculate the prescribed dosage by placing 50 in the appropriate place:

$$15 \text{ mg}/50/\text{day}$$
$$15 \times 50 = 750 \text{ mg/day}$$

Step 3.

To determine the amount of each dose, divide 750 by 3 (divided doses).

$$750 \text{ mg} \div 3 = 250 \text{ mg}$$

Depakene is available in 250-mg capsules and 250-mg/5 mL syrup. The provider ordered the medication in capsules, so Clark will receive a 250-mg capsule every 8 hours for a total of 3 doses a day.

In the same example, use the proportional method to calculate kilogram of body weight.

Step 1.

To convert 110 pounds to kilograms, set up the proportion as follows:

$$2.2 \text{ lb} : 1 \text{ kg} = 110 \text{ lb} : x \text{ kg}$$

Step 2.

Now, solve for x.

$$2.2 : 1 = 110 : x$$
$$2.2x = 110$$
$$x = 50$$

Step 3.

Now, calculate the prescribed dosage by placing 50 in the appropriate place: mg/50 kg/day

$$15 \times 50 = 750 \text{ mg/day}$$

Step 4.

To determine the amount of each dose, divide 750 by 3 (divided doses).

$$750 \div 3 = 250 \text{ mg per dose}$$

ADMINISTRATION OF MEDICATIONS

Regardless of a medication's form or the route by which it is administered, certain basic guidelines must be followed. These guidelines are:

1. Practice medical asepsis (see Chapter 10 for specific medical asepsis rules.) Wash your hands before and after administering a medication. Remember Occupational Safety and Health Administration (OSHA) guidelines and Standard Precautions (see Chapter 10 for Standard Precautions.)
2. Work in a well-lighted area that is free from distractions.
3. Follow the "Six Rights" of proper drug administration (see following section).
4. Always check for allergies before administering any medication.
5. Give only drugs ordered by a licensed practitioner who is authorized to prescribe medications.
6. Never give a medication if there is any question about the order.
7. Be completely familiar with the drug that you are administering before giving it to the patient. Look it up in the PDR or online.
8. Always check the expiration date on the medication label.
9. Never give a drug if its normal appearance has been altered in any way (color, structure, consistency, or odor); it may be outdated, contaminated, or stored incorrectly.
10. Make out a medication note (Figure 24-6) for medications, dose, route, and time exactly as ordered by the provider using the provider's order from the patient's record as a guide. Do not rely on memory.
11. Give only those medications that you have actually prepared for administration. Trust only your own actions.
12. Do not allow someone else to give a medication that you have prepared. Depend on yourself to give the correct medication.
13. Once you have prepared a medication for administration, do not leave it unattended; it could be misplaced or spilled.
14. Be careful in transporting the medication to the patient. Do not spill or drop.
15. When administering oral medications, stay with the patient until you are certain that the medication has been taken, to be sure patient swallowed medication.

A medication note is written out prior to administration of any medication to the patient in the ambulatory care setting. The information is taken directly from the provider's order sheet of the patient's record. An example follows.

Information needed:

Patient name: Abigail Johnson

Provider's order: Cardizem (diltiazem hydrochloride) 180 mg po stat. Winston Lewis, MD.

The medicine note is then used to be certain you have the correct patient, and to document the information on Mrs. Johnson's record. Following documentation, tear up the medication note and discard.

Room 3
Johnson, Abigail
Cardizem
180 mg
po
stat
10/24/XX – 10 A.M.

Figure 24-6 A medication note is used to prepare, administer, and record medications, dose, route, and time as ordered by the provider.

16. Shake (to mix) all liquid medications that contain a **precipitate** before pouring. A precipitate is a substance that separates from a solution if allowed to stand. This mixes the liquid for the proper medication.
17. When pouring a liquid medication, hold the measuring device at eye level or place it on a flat surface and squat down so you can observe it at eye level. Read the correct amount at the lowest level of the **meniscus**, which is the top surface of the column of liquid.
18. Do not contaminate the cap of a bottle while pouring a medication. Place the cap with the rim pointed upward to prevent contamination of that portion that comes into contact with the medication.
19. Keep all drugs not being administered in a safe storage place.
20. Carefully follow the procedural steps for the type of medication that you are giving or the type of procedure you are performing.
21. Always keep safety precautions in mind. The United States Department of Health and Human Services, Public Health Service, and Centers for Disease Control and Prevention recommend following Standard Precautions for prevention of hepatitis B and C viruses and human immunodeficiency virus and other bloodborne diseases (see Chapter 10 for specifics about Standard Precautions).

The "Six Rights" of Proper Drug Administration

The "Six Rights" have been developed as a checklist of activities to be followed by those who give medications. This easy-to-remember list should always be followed to ensure the proper administration of any drug:

1. *Right drug.* To be sure that the correct drug has been selected, compare the medication order with the label on the medication bottle. A frequent check of the medication label is a good way to avoid a medication error. One should make a practice of reading the label on each of the following three occasions:

First:	When the medication is taken from the storage area.
Second:	Just before removing it from its container.
Third:	On returning the medication container to storage or before discarding the empty container.

2. *Right dose.* It is essential that the patient receive the right dose. If the dose ordered and the dose on hand are *not the same,* carefully determine the correct dose through mathematical calculation. When calculating dosage, it is advisable to have another qualified person verify the accuracy of your calculations before the medication is administered.
3. *Right route.* Check the medication order to be sure that you have the right route of administration (Figure 24-7A).

4. *Right time.* You are responsible for medicating the patient at the proper time. Check the medication order to ensure that a drug is administered according to the time interval prescribed. For a drug to be maintained at the proper blood level, care must be taken to administer it at the right time (Figure 24-7B).
5. *Right patient.* Before administering any medication, always be sure that you have the right patient. A good safety practice is to correctly identify the patient on each occasion when you administer a medication. In a hospital, the patient's identification bracelet is always checked. In the ambulatory care facility, call the patient by name or ask the patient to state his or her name (Figure 24-7C).
6. *Right documentation:* The recording process is the vital link between provider, patient, and medical assistant. It is an account of the essential data that are collected and preserved. The patient's chart is a legal document; therefore, all data should be recorded in ink or entered into the computer. The data should be accurate and clearly stated. It is important that certain data about drug administration be entered into the patient's chart (Figure 24-7D):

- Patient's name
- Date and time of administration
- Name of the medication and the amount (dosage) administered
- Route by which the medication was administered
- Any unusual reactions experienced by the patient
- Any complications in administering the drug (patient refusing to take the medication, difficulty in swallowing)
- If the medication was *not* given, state why and dispose of the medication according to agency policy and federal and state laws
- Patient data, such as blood pressure, pulse, respirations, when appropriate
- Your name or initials and title

Medication Errors

Medication errors should not happen when personnel follow the "Six Rights" of proper drug administration and the essential medication guidelines; however, honest mistakes will be made periodically. A medication error occurs when any of the following happen:

1. A drug is given to the wrong patient
2. The incorrect drug is given
3. The drug is given via an incorrect route
4. The drug is given at the incorrect time
5. The incorrect dose is administered
6. Incorrect data are entered on the patient's chart or electronic medical record

When a medication error occurs, follow standard procedure:

a. Recognize that an error has been made.
b. Stay calm. Assess the patient's condition and reactions to the medication.
c. Report the error immediately to the provider. Give the details of the mistake and the patient's reactions.
d. Follow the provider's order for correcting the error.
e. Document the error in the patient's chart or electronic medical record or the facility's record form:
   - Describe the type of error.
   - Describe the patient's reactions.
   - Describe the steps taken to correct the error.
   - State date, time, and your name.

Patient Assessment

Before administering any medication, carefully assess the patient's condition. An assessment should include, but is not limited to, the following conditions:

1. *Age.* Is the medication and route suitable for the patient at a particular stage in life? The stages of life include infancy, childhood, adolescence, adulthood, and old age. During infancy, early childhood, and old age, a smaller dose of medication may be required than would be appropriate for the other stages in life.
2. *Physical conditions.* Potential problems associated with the patient's physical condition must be considered. Female patients during pregnancy or while breast-feeding should not be given certain medications because they may be contraindicated.
3. *Body size.* The amount of medication given and size of the needle used are directly related to the size of the patient. Pediatric and geriatric patients usually have less subcutaneous and muscular tissue per BSA than the average adult (see Figure 24-5). Small, thin patients usually require less medication, and a shorter needle may be used to reach

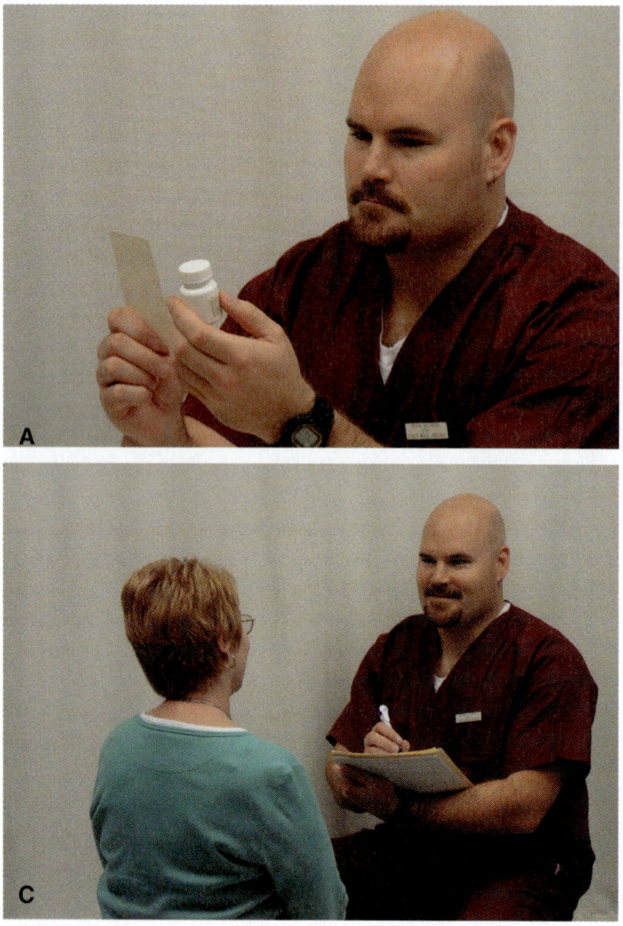

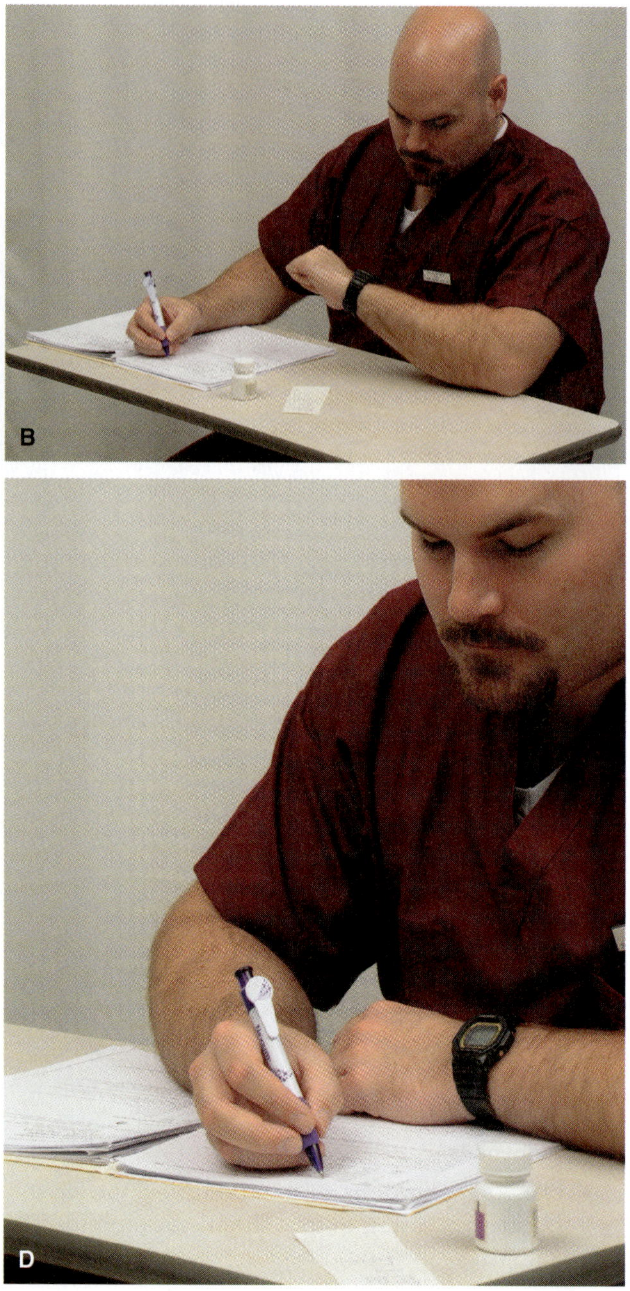

Figure 24-7 (A) Medical assistant checks the right drug, the right route, and the right dose of medication to administer. (B) Medical assistant checks for the right time to administer medication to the patient. (C) Medical assistant assesses patient before administering the medication. The medical assistant ascertains he has the right patient and asks the patient if she has any allergies. (D) Medical assistant documents administration of medication in patient's chart.

the appropriate tissue level. On the other hand, the large or obese patient may or may not require more medication than the average adult and a longer needle to reach the appropriate tissue level.

4. *Sex.* Consider differences that are related to the sex of the patient.
   - *Build.* Muscular patients generally have more muscular tissue. Obese patients have more adipose tissue. Always inspect and palpate muscle tissue with this in mind when determining the appropriate needle length to reach muscle tissue.
   - *Skin texture.* Some patients have tougher skin than others. A young person's skin might have more tone than that of an older adult. Slightly more force is required to penetrate skin that is tough or lacking in tone.
5. *Injection site.* Always inspect and palpate the skin before administering an injection. The following body areas should be avoided when choosing the site for an injection:
   - Any type of skin lesion
   - Burned areas
   - Inflamed areas
   - Previous injection sites

- Any traumatized area
- Scar tissue (vaccination, keloid)
- Moles, warts, birthmarks, tumors, lumps, hard nodules
- Nerves, large blood vessels, bones
- Cyanotic areas
- Edematous areas
- Paralyzed areas
- Arm on same side as mastectomy, or other lymphatic compromise

Correct injection sites are illustrated later in this chapter.

ADMINISTRATION OF ORAL MEDICATIONS

Oral medications are easily and economically administered. There are, however, several disadvantages associated with the oral route. For instance, the drug may:

- Have an objectionable odor/taste
- Cause discoloration of the teeth, mouth, and tongue
- Irritate the gastric mucosa
- Be altered by digestive enzymes
- Be poorly absorbed from the digestive system because of illness or nature of the medication
- Not be taken by the patient
- Have less predictable effects on the body when given orally than when given by the parenteral route (by injection)
- Not be able to be swallowed if in tablet, capsule, or caplet form

Equipment and Supplies for Oral Medications

Three measuring devices commonly used in the administration of oral medications are the medicine cup, the water cup, and the medicine dropper. The medicine cup (Figure 24-8) comes in various sizes and shapes, depending on its manufacturer and its intended use. Cups may be calibrated in fluid ounces, fluidrams, milliliters (mL), and tablespoons.

The water cup is a small plastic or paper cup that is disposable. The average water cup holds three ounces of liquid.

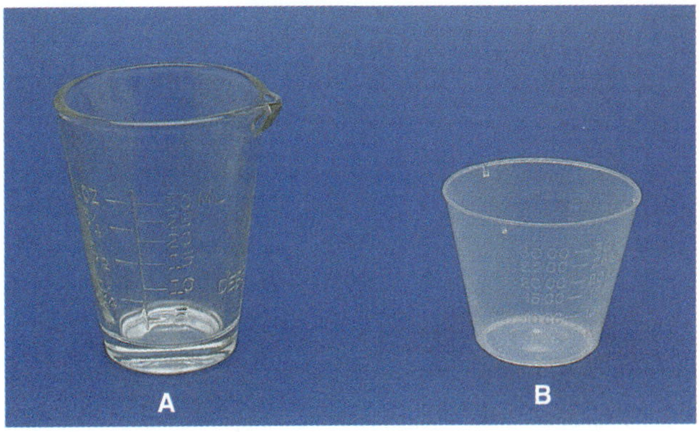

Figure 24-8 Medicine cups: (A) glass; (B) plastic.

The medicine dropper (Figure 24-9) may be calibrated in milliliters, minims, or drops. Medicine droppers are often included with the bottle of medication. Uncalibrated droppers may be provided when the medicine is administered only in drops. The size of the drop varies with the size of the dropper opening, the angle at which it is held, the force exerted on the rubber bulb, and the viscosity of the medication.

It is important that the appropriate measuring device be selected for a medication and the prescribed dosage accurately measured. The selection of the measuring device depends on the physical structure of the medication (solid or liquid), the amount of medication prescribed, the size of the measuring device, and the calibrations on the container.

Procedure 24-1 give steps for administration of oral medications.

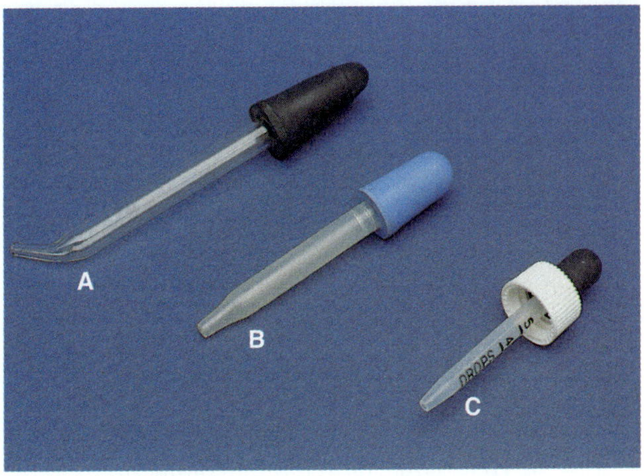

Figure 24-9 Various types of medicine droppers: (A) glass; (B) plastic; (C) plastic calibrated.

ADMINISTRATION OF PARENTERAL MEDICATIONS

The term **parenteral** is used to describe the injection of a substance into the body via a route other than the alimentary canal/digestive system. The most frequently used parenteral routes are:

- *Subcutaneous.* Just below the surface of the skin. A subcutaneous injection is usually given at a 45-degree angle.
- *Intramuscular.* Within the muscle. An intramuscular injection is given at a 90-degree angle, passing through the skin and subcutaneous tissue, and penetrating deep into muscle tissue.
- *Intradermal.* Within the dermal layer of the skin. An intradermal injection is given at an angle between 10 and 15 degrees.
- *Intravenous.* Within or into a vein.

Medications that have been prepared for use by injection are available in multiple-dose form (vials) and in unit dose form (ampules and cartridge-needle units) (Figure 24-10.) **Unit dose** forms are premeasured amounts, packaged on a per-dose basis.

- *Ampule.* A small, sterile, prefilled glass container that usually holds a single dose of a hypodermic solution.
- *Cartridge-needle unit.* A disposable sterile cartridge containing a premeasured amount of medication. This unit is designed for use in a nondisposable cartridge-holder syringe such as the Tubex® or Carpuject®.
- *Vial.* A small, sterile, prefilled glass bottle with rubber stopper containing a hypodermic solution.

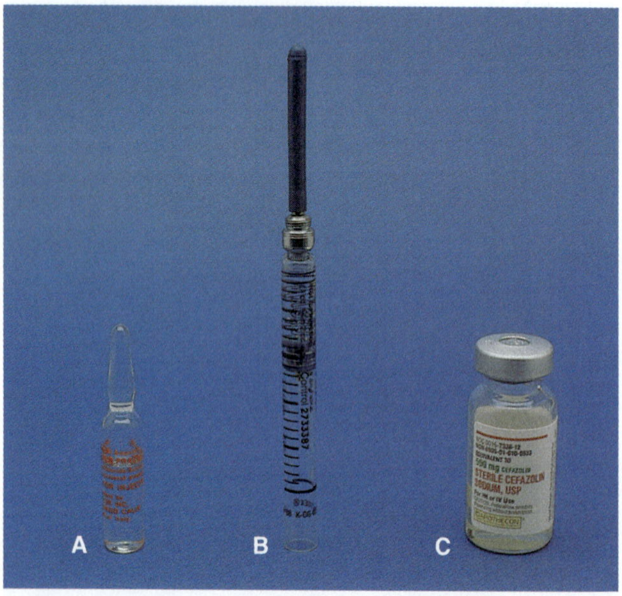

Figure 24-10 Medications given parenterally. (A) Ampule. (B) Sterile cartridge with premeasured medication. (C) Vial of powder for reconstitution.

Hazards Associated with Parenteral Medications

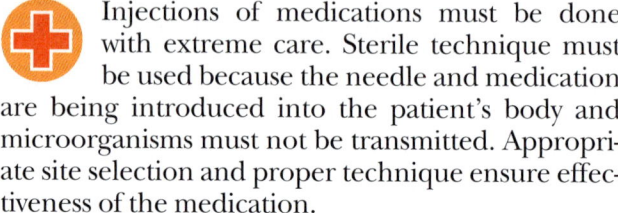

Injections of medications must be done with extreme care. Sterile technique must be used because the needle and medication are being introduced into the patient's body and microorganisms must not be transmitted. Appropriate site selection and proper technique ensure effectiveness of the medication.

Additional dangers to be aware of when administering medications parenterally (by injection) include:

- Allergic reaction (if present) will be swift
- Injury to bone, nerve, or blood vessel
- Breaking of needle in tissue (rare)
- Injecting into a blood vessel instead of tissue (this is avoided by checking for blood return, on aspiration).

Reasons for Parenteral Route Selection

The parenteral route is selected because of:

- Rapid response time to medication
- Accuracy of dosage
- Need to concentrate medication in a specific body part or area (into a joint or local anesthetic)
- Inability to administer orally because the medication is destroyed by gastric juices, or the patient is incapable of taking medication orally

Because parenteral medications are intended for use by injection, they must be injected as liquids. Some medications are supplied in powder form and must be reconstituted to a liquid form for injection (see Procedure 24-8).

Because they must be in liquid form, the amount of parenteral medications is expressed in terms of volume (milliliters, minims, or ounces). The strength of the drug contained in the liquid is usually expressed in terms of its weight (milliequivalents, micrograms, milligrams, grams, or units).

Therefore, medications ordered for parenteral use are often ordered by both weight and volume.

The parenteral route of drug administration offers an effective mode of delivering medication to a patient when a rapid and direct result is desired. The effect of a parenteral medication is faster than one given by the oral route; however, the accuracy of dosage calculation for both is important.

Parenteral Equipment and Supplies

Syringes. Syringes are classified as disposable, nondisposable, or a combination of these two types. Most syringes used are plastic. They also may be classified according to their intended use. In addition to the standard hypodermic syringes that are in general use, there are special-purpose syringes for irrigations or oral feedings, tuberculin syringes, and insulin syringes.

Disposable Syringes. Disposable syringes are those that are sterilized, prepackaged, nontoxic, nonpyrogenic, and ready for use. They are available as a syringe-needle unit and are generally enclosed in individual peel-apart packages of durable paper or clear plastic. They are available in sizes from 1 to 60 milliters. The 1-, 3-, and 5-mL syringes are the ones most often used when parenteral medications are administered.

A disposable syringe-needle unit consists of a syringe with an attached needle. The needle is covered by a hard plastic sheath to prevent it from accidentally penetrating the package or sticking the user. The unit may be sealed within a peel-apart package or encased in a rigid plastic container that has been heat sealed to ensure sterility. Labeling usually includes the manufacturer's name, type and size of the syringe, gauge and length of the needle, and a reorder number. Packages are usually color coded for ease of identification. Always read the label. Disposable syringes are generally preferred for the administration of parenteral medications because they ensure sterility and sharp needles. Also, disposable syringes eliminate the need for resterilizaton, which is costly, time-consuming, and possibly unsafe if not done properly.

Nondisposable Syringes. Nondisposable syringes are usually made of specially strengthened glass resistant to thermal shock. These units, consisting of round glass barrels with individually fitted plungers, are manufactured to exacting specifications.

Nondisposable glass and plastic syringes are available in sizes from 1 to 50 milliters. They may be used by providers to perform special procedures such as paracentesis, thoracentesis, thoracotomy, and tracheotomy.

Combination Disposable/Nondisposable Cartridge-Injection Syringes. A cartridge-injection system, such as the plastic Carpuject® (Figure 24-11) or the metal Tubex®, consists of a disposable cartridge-needle unit and a nondisposable cartridge-holder syringe. The cartridge-needle unit is factory sealed and sterile and contains a precisely measured unit dose of medicine. The cartridge-holder syringe may be made of durable chrome-plated brass or of plastic. These reusable syringes are designed for quick and safe loading and unloading of cartridge-needle units, which are manufactured in various sizes and dosage capacities and contain a wide range of medications (Figure 24-12).

The combination of disposable/nondisposable syringe system is easy to use and convenient. When using this system, be careful to read the label and compare the medication order with the label. For example, the provider may order Demerol® 25 mg and the cartridge is 50 mg/mL. Give ½ mL and properly discard the other ½ mL according to office policy. Another person must witness the disposal of the Demerol®, which is a controlled substance.

Parts of a Syringe. The component parts of a syringe consist of a barrel, plunger, flange, tip (Figure 24-13), and a safety shield on a safety syringe.

- The *barrel* is the part that holds the medication and has graduated markings (calibrations) on its surface for use in measuring medications.

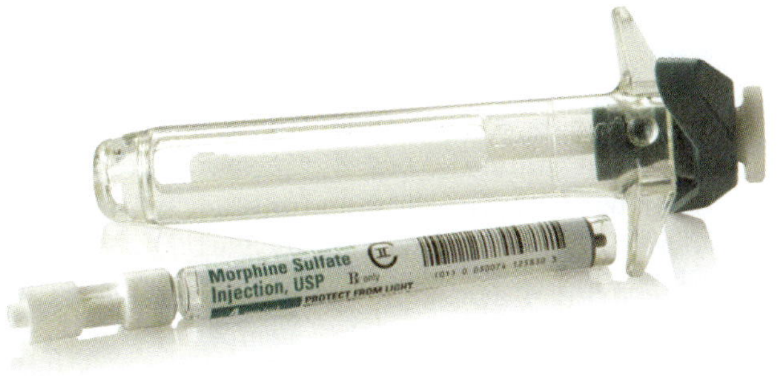

Figure 24-11 The Carpuject® is a type of cartridge-injection system with a click-lock mechanism for safety. (Courtesy of Hospira, Inc.)

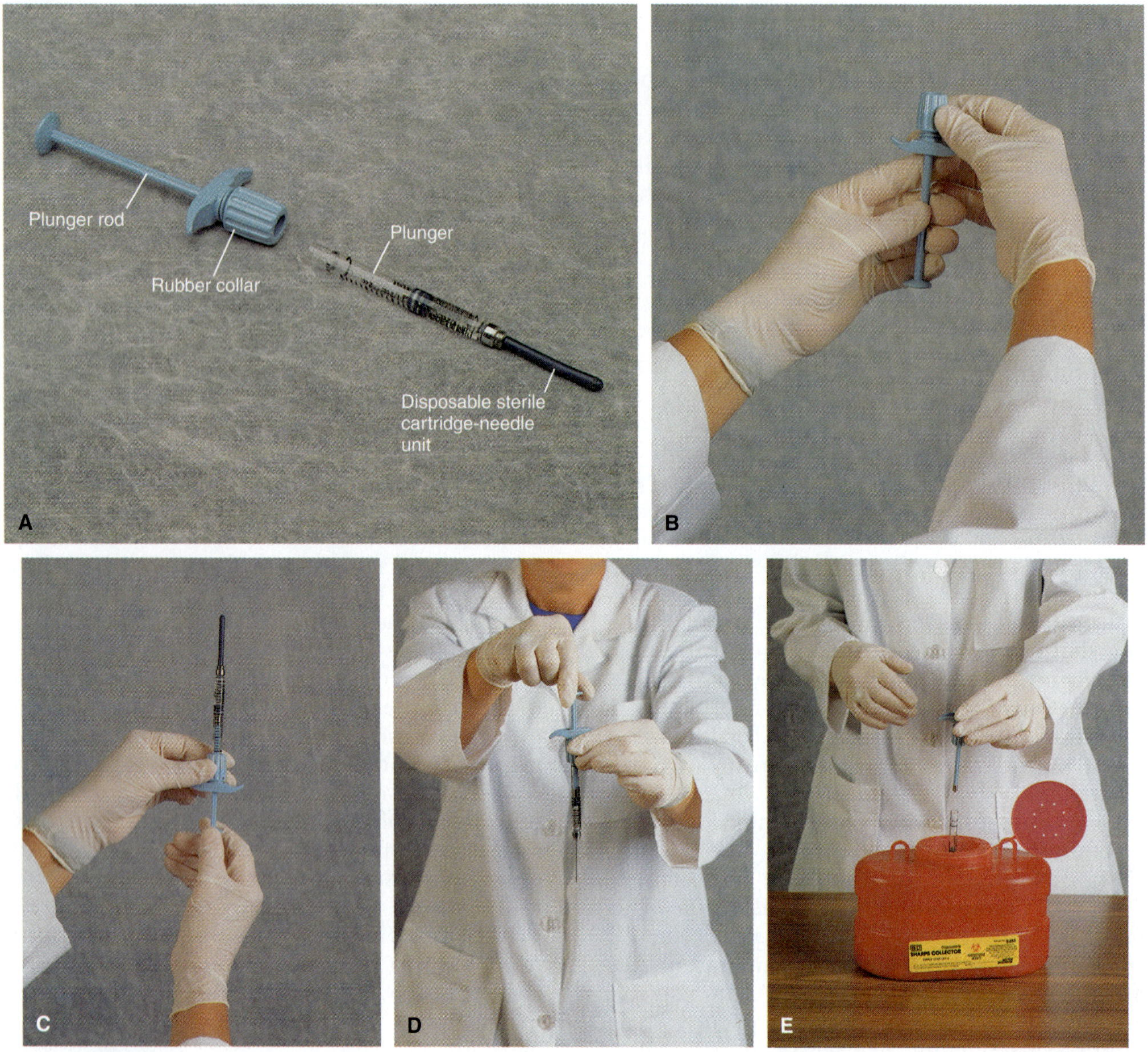

Figure 24-12 (A) Reusable cartridge holder with disposable sterile cartridge needle unit. (B) Turn ribbed collar to open position. (C) Insert the sterile cartridge-needle unit into the open end of the injector. The ribbed collar is firmly tightened. The plunger of the injector and the plunger of the cartridge-needle unit are tightened and ready for use. (D) The medical assistant prepares to dispose of the cartridge-needle unit. The needle is not recapped. The plunger rod is disengaged by unscrewing. The ribbed collar is loosened. (E) The medical assistant holds the cartridge-needle unit over a sharps container, and the unit drops into the container.

- The *plunger* is a movable cylinder designed for insertion within the barrel; it provides the mechanism by which a medication (or other substance) is drawn into or pushed out of the barrel.
- The *flange* is at the end of the barrel where the plunger is inserted. It forms a rim around the end of the barrel where the plunger is inserted and has appendages against which one places the index and middle fingers when drawing up solution for injection. The flange also prevents the syringe from rolling when laid on a flat surface.
- The *tip* is at the end of the barrel where the needle is attached.
- The safety shield is pulled over the needle while withdrawing it. Safety needles have a mechanism to either sheath the needle, retract it, or blunt it. (Figure 24-14).

The parts of a syringe that must remain sterile during the preparation and administration of a parenteral medication are the inside of the barrel, the section of the plunger that fits inside the

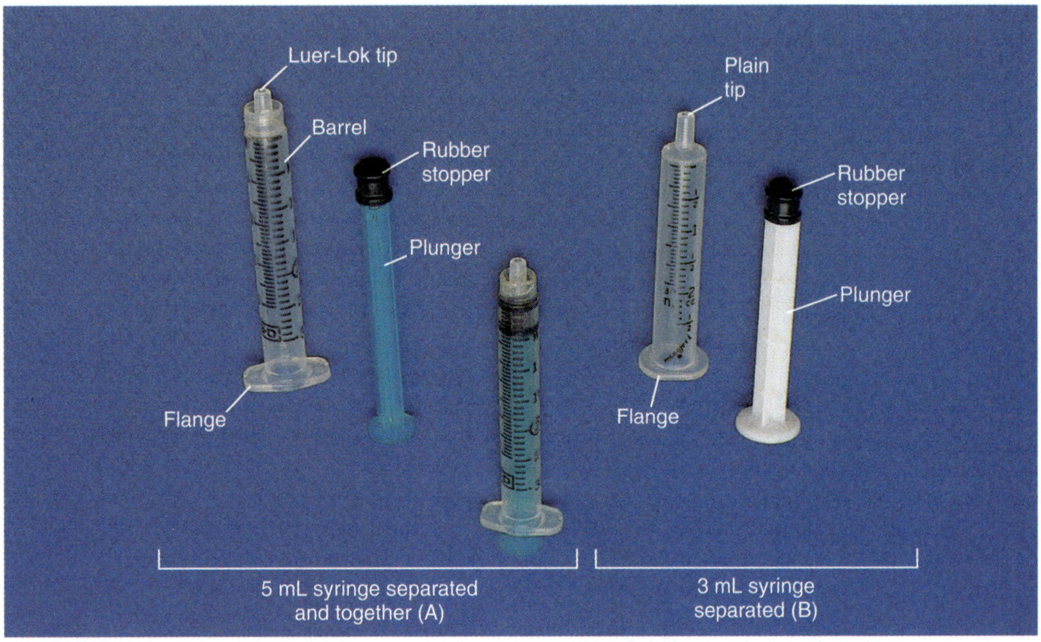

Figure 24-13 Parts of a syringe. (A) A 5-mL syringe separated and unseparated with Luer-Lok® tip. (B) A 3-mL syringe separated with plain tip.

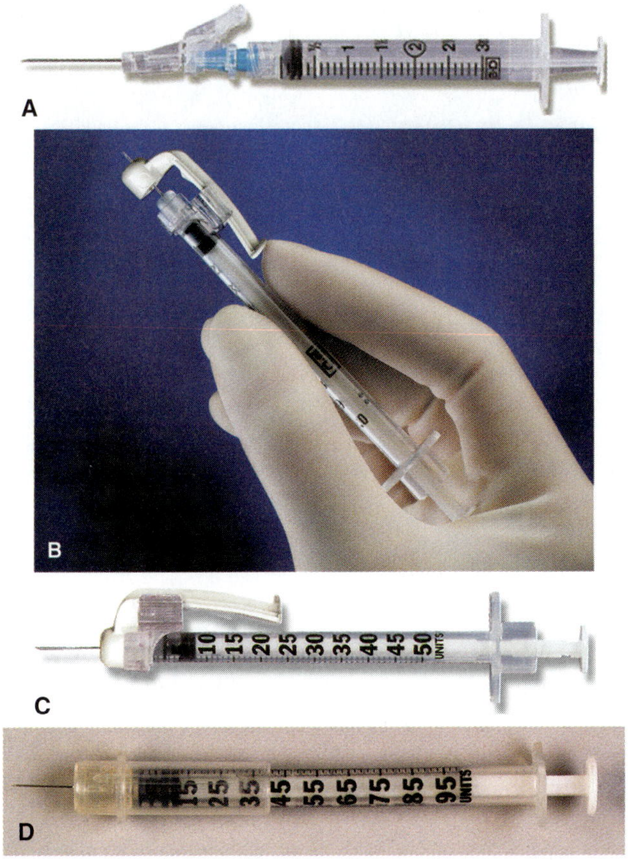

Figure 24-14 Types of safety syringes. (A) Hypodermic safety syringe, 3 mL with protective needle guard. (B) Tuberculin syringe 1 mL. (C) Lo-dose unit 100 insulin syringe. (D) Standard units 100 insulin syringe. (Courtesy of BD.)

barrel, and the syringe tip to which the needle is to be attached.

Types of Syringes and Uses. Syringes are named according to their sizes and uses. Table 24-9 lists the types, sizes, calibrations, and uses of syringes used in the administration of parenteral medications. Figure 24-14 shows various sizes of safety syringes.

One should always choose a needle with sufficient length to reach the desired tissue level (Table 24-10). A large person may require a longer needle to reach the correct body tissue than would be required for a smaller person. The delivery of medication to the proper tissue level is important. A concentrated or irritating medication that is intended for deep intramuscular injection could be delivered instead into the subcutaneous tissue of an obese patient if one selects a needle that is too short. Such an inappropriate injection may cause a sterile abscess and necrosis. This unnecessary complication can be avoided by considering the size of the patient when choosing the length of the needle.

Needles. Both disposable and nondisposable needles are available for use with syringes. Of these, the most frequently used are disposable needles, which are individually packaged in sterile paper or plastic containers. Disposable needles and syringe-needle units are available with a color-coded sheath. The

Table 24-9 The Most Frequently Used Syringes for Parenteral Medications

Type of Syringes	Size and Calibration	Typical Uses
Hypodermic	3 milliliter Calibrated 0.1 15/16 minims/milliliters	Intramuscular and subcutaneous injections
Hypodermic	5 milliliter Calibrated 0.2	Venipuncture and intramuscular injections
Hypodermic	Larger sizes (10, 30, and 60 milliliter)	Medical/surgical treatments, aspirations, irrigations, venipunctures, gavage (tube-to-stomach) feedings
Tuberculin	1 milliliter Calibrated 0.1 and 0.01 16 minims/milliliters	To inject minute amounts for intradermal injections, allergy testing, allergy injections
Insulin	U-100 (0.5 milliliter) U-100 (1 milliliter)	Lo-Dose® administration of insulin Insulin administration

Table 24-10 Syringe-Needle Combinations for Various Parenteral Routes

Subcutaneous Injection	Intramuscular Injection	Intradermal Injection
3-mL syringe/25G, ⅝ inch needle	3-mL syringe/23G, 1 inch needle	1-mL syringe/25G, ⅝ inch needle
3-mL syringe/26G, ⅜ inch needle	3-mL syringe/22G, 1½ inch needle	1-mL syringe/26G, ⅜ inch needle
3-mL syringe/27G, ½ inch needle	3-mL syringe/21G, 1½ to 2 inch needle	1-mL syringe/27G, ½ inch needle
U-100 (1 mL)/26G, ½ inch needle for insulin		

sheath protects the needle and identifies its gauge and length. Common needle gauges (G) range from 16 to 32, and their lengths vary from ⅜ to 2 inches. The needle's gauge is determined by the diameter of the lumen or opening at its beveled tip. The larger the gauge, the smaller the diameter of its lumen. For example, a 32-gauge needle is much smaller than a 16-gauge needle.

Nondisposable needles are made of high-quality stainless steel. They are equipped with a mounting hub that has a cylindrical opening designed to slip over the lock onto the tip of a syringe, such as a Luer-Lok®. See Figure 24-15 for various sizes and types of needles.

Parts of a Needle. Figure 24-16 shows the parts of a needle used to administer parenteral medications.

- The *point* is the sharpened end of the needle. The point is formed when the end of the shaft is ground away to form a flat, slanted surface called the *bevel*.

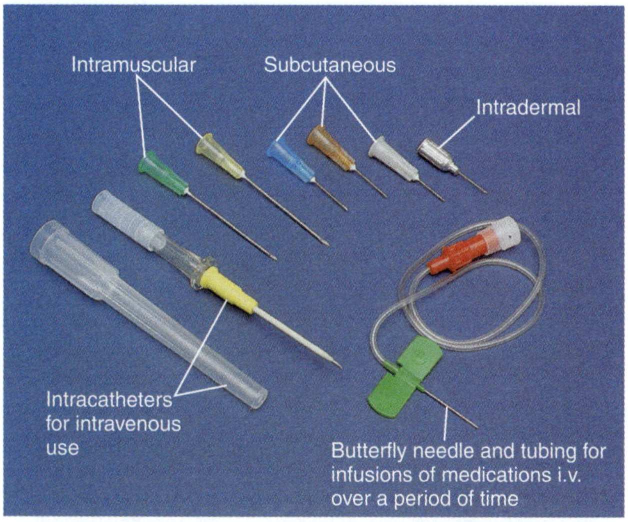

Figure 24-15 Various sizes and types of needles. Different colored hubs denote needle gauges.

- The *lumen*, the hollow core of the needle, forms an oval-shaped opening when exposed at the beveled point.
- The hollow steel tube through which the medication passes is the *shaft*.
- The other end of the shaft attaches to the *hub*, which is part of the needle unit that is designed to mount onto the syringe.
- The point at which the shaft attaches to the hub is called the *hilt*.

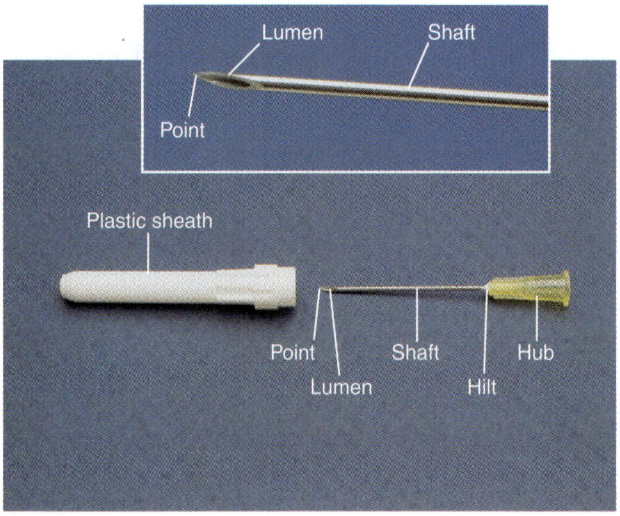

Figure 24-16 Parts of a needle and needle sheath. Inset shows point, lumen, and shaft.

The Safe Disposal of Needles and Syringes. The careless disposal of used needles and syringes may present a health risk to any person coming into contact with the used equipment. An accidental stick by a contaminated needle could transmit diseases such as hepatitis B, hepatitis C, syphilis, Rocky Mountain spotted fever, tuberculosis, malaria, varicella zoster, and human immunodeficiency virus (HIV). Used needles and syringes should be discarded in a rigid, puncture-proof container (Figure 24-17). Never recap a needle after giving an injection. Do engage safety feature. Most needlesticks occur while recapping. Refer to Chapter 10 for OSHA regulations.

Most sharps-related injuries (needlesticks) occur in the hospital with inpatients. However, any health care worker who administers parenteral medications is at risk for an injury. Other types of sharps-related injuries besides disposable needles include suture needles, butterfly needles, scalpel blades, phlebotomy needles, and IV catheter stylets.

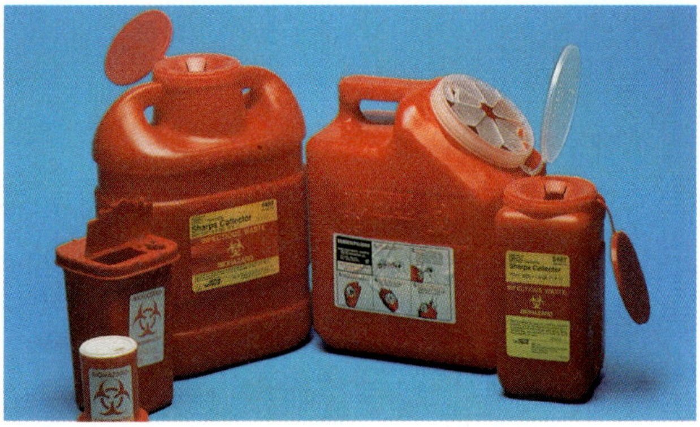

Figure 24-17 Place used needles, point down, in puncture-proof sharps containers.

A number of pathogens can enter the body during a sharps-related injury, but of greatest concern are hepatitis B and C viruses and HIV (see Chapter 10 for details about these and other bloodborne pathogens).

The National Alliance for the Primary Prevention of Sharps Injuries (NAPPSI) consists of medical device makers, health organizations, and health care providers whose goal is the prevention of sharps-related injuries. Besides safety needles (see information on retractable needles in Chapter 10), laser scalpels, and needleless drug delivery systems such as patches and inhaled medications, a needleless injection system is available (fluid under pressure). There are glues and adhesives available to approximate surgical incisions. These alternative methods are helpful in reducing sharps-related injuries; however, phlebotomy and IV therapy still require a needle. Legal regulations (CDC and OSHA) require use of the safest needle available.

Proper use and disposal of sharps is the utmost importance to health care workers and others. Avoid needles if there are other methods available, and never recap used needles. Engage the safety mechanism and dispose of needles and syringes immediately after use.

Sharps Collectors. Sharps collector systems eliminate the need to reshield the needle, thereby reducing the risk for an accidental needlestick.

Needles are placed into the container as a whole unit after safety mechanisms are engaged. Sharps containers need to be within reach any time injections are given.

PRINCIPLES OF INTRAVENOUS THERAPY

Patients who are unconscious, uncooperative, experiencing severe nausea and vomiting, have had severe burns, or have a significant amount of blood loss may need an intravenous infusion. All of these situations result in the patient losing body fluids, resulting in loss of homeostasis. The provider will order the fluids to be replaced by intravenous infusion according to the patient's condition or disease. The fluids will be specific for the needs of a particular patient. Some infusions maintain the patient's water (fluids) and electrolyte needs. For example, some elderly people who live alone and do not feel well, perhaps have pneumonia, may not eat well or drink enough liquid to maintain the body's balance of fluids and electrolytes. If the situation goes on for a few days, during which time the patient becomes dehydrated, the patient will need IV fluids. Symptoms of dehydration are dry mouth, dark urine, and lightheadedness. It can lead to changes in the body's chemistry and become life-threatening.

Severe nausea and vomiting can quickly dehydrate an individual and eventually can lead to kidney failure. The patient needs replacement of fluids and electrolytes through an intravenous infusion. (If a patient is vomiting, any attempt at taking in fluids orally is not likely to be successful.)

When a patient is prescribed intravenous fluids, the provider takes into consideration the patient's age, weight, height, and clinical laboratory results.

When patients are receiving an intravenous infusion, they must be watched carefully. The flow rate is ordered by the provider. Blood pressure should be monitored. Breathing and chest tightness should be reported. Excessive volume (too much fluid too quickly) can result in overhydration and possible serious adverse cardiac and pulmonary consequences.

Inserting a needle or cannula into a vein for purposes of an infusion is an invasive procedure, and the possibility exists for microorganisms to enter the patient's body. Everything must be sterile because microorganisms can enter the bloodstream and cause serious problems. Infection at the site of needle entry is possible. Phlebitis (inflammation of the vein) can occur from the patient moving about and causing the needle to irritate the vein. The IV fluid can infiltrate the tissues around the needle site, causing pain, swelling, and possibly tissue damage. The IV must be terminated and a new site used to restart it. Monitor the skin around the injection site for swelling and redness. Standard Precautions must be used to avoid exposure to the patient's blood and/or body fluids. The fluid is infused into the patient drop by drop. The flow of the solution is carefully monitored. The rate of the IV flow is crucial, and the number of drops per minute must be accurate. Other essential factors for IV infusion are that the prescribed fluid amount and the amount of time required for the infusion to finish are correct, and that the drop factor is calculated using a mathematical formula.

Electronic devices for IV infusion are battery operated, electronically operated, or a combination of both. The devices are safe and accurate and can be programmed to a specific drop per minute rate. The device has an alarm that signals if there is a problem and signals when the infusion is finished.

Equipment for an IV comes in a sterile kit. Within the kit are the needle and cannula for entering the vein, the tubing to attach to the needle and cannula (shielded), and a plastic (usually) or glass container of the prescribed fluid. The equipment institutes a "basic" administrating set and is what is generally seen in ambulatory care (Figure 24-18). The tubing has a roller-type clamp for adjusting the drop rate. Some tubing is made with a **port** that gives ready access for addition of other fluids by using another infusion set simultaneously. The tubing can become kinked and slow down the flow of fluid. If the needle is not securely attached to the tubing, the fluid may leak out at the attachment site.

IV therapy or infusion is ordered by the provider for a variety of patient conditions. It provides for medication to be given for a rapid response, replaces fluids and electrolytes, helps to raise blood pressure when the patient suffers from shock due to blood or fluid loss, and can be used for nutritional supplements. Access to a vein when needed will have

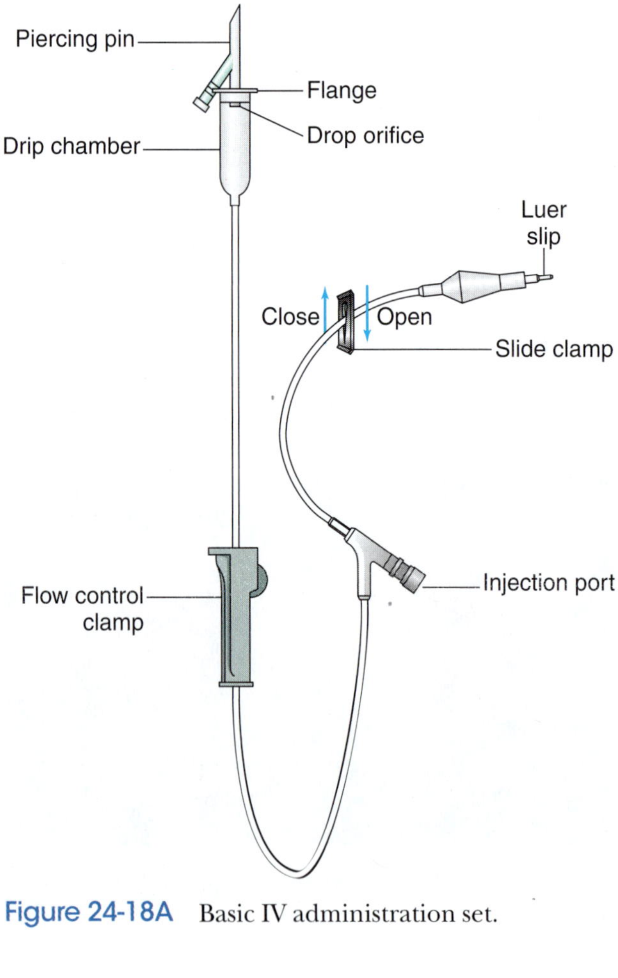

Figure 24-18A Basic IV administration set.

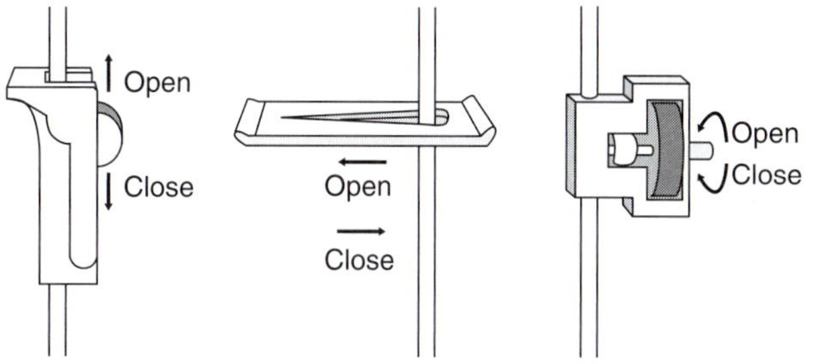

Figure 24-18B Administration set tubing clamps.

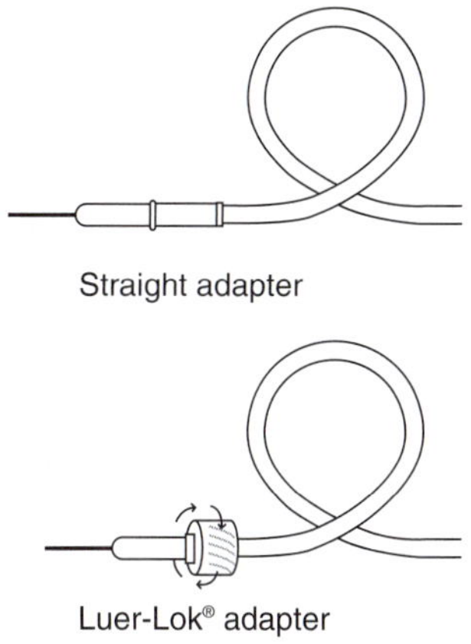

Figure 24-18C Straight and Luer-Lok® cannula hub adapters.

a systemic effect in a short period of time. The vein is accessible for emergencies. The route is useful for unconscious patients and provides a rapid route for countering poisonous substances or inappropriate medication response.

Veins may "collapse" (very difficult to find) as a result of the patient's condition (dehydration, hypotension, blood loss), and locating an accessible vein may be difficult. The provider may order that the vein be kept opened (by continuous IV infusion). This is abbreviated KVO (keep vein open) or TKO (to be kept open) for immediate accessibility.

Some IV solutions commonly used for infusions in ambulatory settings are:

- 5% dextrose in water
- Saline solutions
- Dextrose in normal saline
- Lactated Ringer's solution

Although IV therapy is not a procedure medical assistants perform, they must be knowledgeable about the procedure, understand the purpose for IV infusions, recognize the precautions concerning this invasive procedure, and realize that state laws vary regarding IV infusion.

All persons providing health care to patients are legally responsible for their own actions. See Chapter 28 for information regarding phlebotomy.

It is important to realize that IV infusion is an invasive procedure much like the phlebotomy procedure. The veins for IV infusion are similar to those used for venipuncture in the hands and arms.

SITE SELECTION AND INJECTION ANGLE

The selection of a proper site for a subcutaneous, intramuscular, or intradermal injection and the correct angle of insertion for each will ensure that the medication is delivered to the correct tissue type (Figure 24-19).

A subcutaneous injection is given at an angle of 45 degrees just below the surface of the skin wherever there is subcutaneous tissue. The shaded areas shown in Figure 24-20A are the usual sites for subcutaneous injections because they are located away from bones, joints, nerves, and large blood vessels.

An intramuscular injection is given at a 90-degree angle, passing through the skin and subcutaneous tissue and penetrating deep into muscle tissue. Body areas normally used for intramuscular injections are the dorsogluteal area, ventrogluteal area, deltoid muscle, and vastus lateralis.

After locating an appropriate vein, an IV injection is given at a 25-degree angle penetrating the skin and introducing the needle into the vein. The antecubital, median cephalic, median basilic, and median cubital veins are common sites appropriate for IV injections (see Chapter 28 for more information about vein selection).

Intradermal injections are given at an angle between 10 and 15 degrees into the dermal layer of the skin. The body areas used for intradermal injections are the inner forearm and the middle of the back (Figure 24-20B). These two sites are used because the skin in these areas is thin and contain little hair.

Marking the Correct Site for Intramuscular Injection

To give a safe injection, it is necessary to become familiar with the anatomic structures associated with the injection site. With knowledge of where such structures are located, it is easier to mark injection sites that avoid bones, nerves, and large blood vessels.

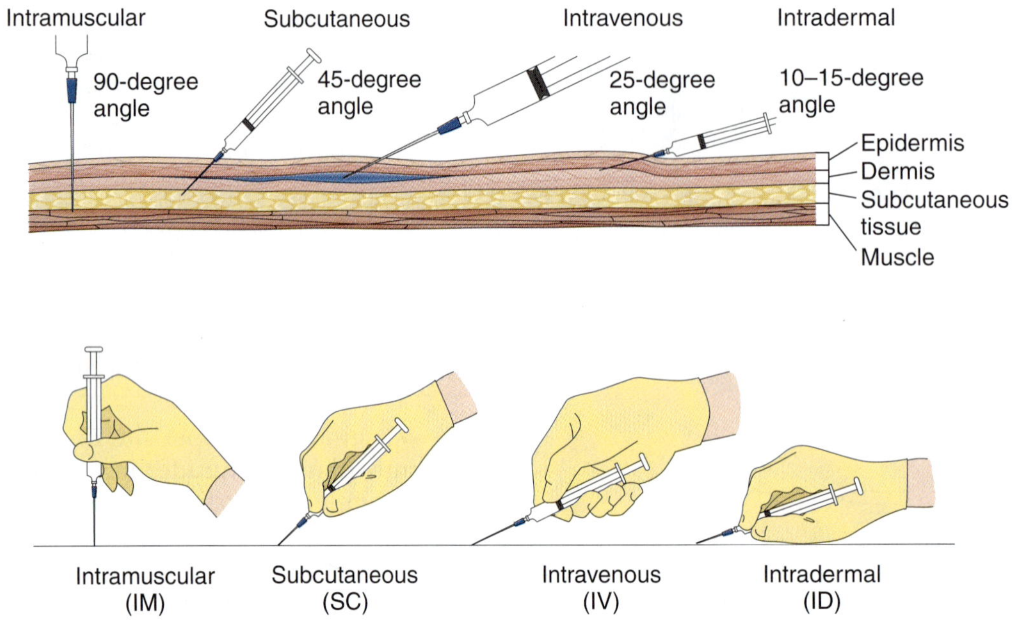

Figure 24-19 Angles of injection for intramuscular, subcutaneous, intravenous, and intradermal injections.

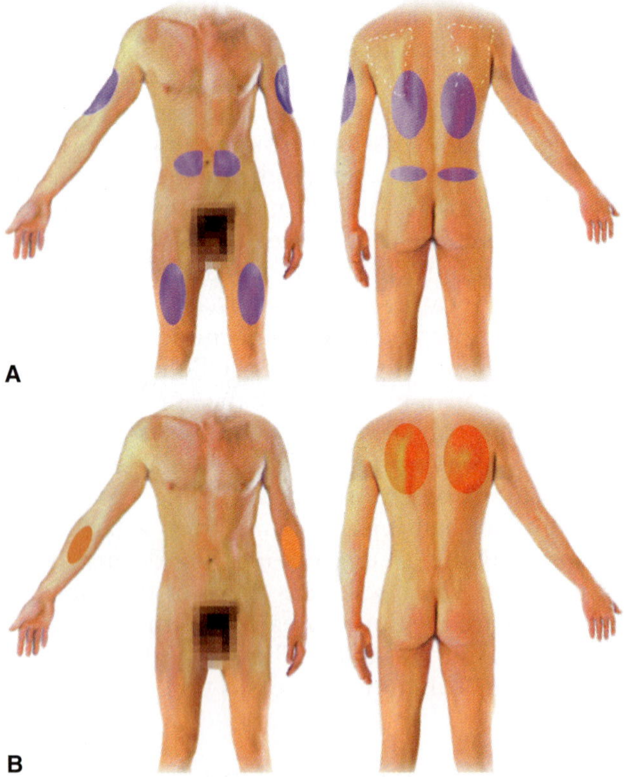

Figure 24-20 Injection sites: (A) subcutaneous; (B) intradermal.

Dorsogluteal Site. The dorsogluteal site is the traditional location for giving most (adult) deep intramuscular injections (Figure 24-21A). Commonly referred to as the "upper outer quadrant of the buttocks," this description can be easily misinterpreted and result in an injection into the inappropriate area. To locate the correct site for a dorsogluteal injection, locate the superior posterior iliac spine and place a small *x* on this spot. Then locate the greater trochanter of the femur and mark this spot. Draw (or imagine) a diagonal line between the two locations. The area above and outside this line and about 3 inches below the iliac crest is the correct location of the dorsogluteal site.

Extreme caution should be used when giving intramuscular injections in the dorsogluteal area. Improper site selection can result in damage to the sciatic nerve or injection into the superior gluteal artery or vein. This site is contraindicated for infants and is used only as a site of last resort in children because of less muscle development. This muscle mass may be degenerated in older adults, the nonwalking, or the emaciated patient.

Ventrogluteal Site. The ventrogluteal site (gluteus medius muscle) can generally accommodate the majority of medications ordered for intramuscular injection. It may be used for individuals from infancy to adulthood. The ventrogluteal site is relatively free of major nerves and vessels, thereby making it a choice site for intramuscular injections. To locate the ventrogluteal injection site, palpate to find the greater trochanter, the anterior superior iliac spine, and the bony ridge of the iliac crest (Figure 24-21B). With these three locations identified, place the palm of your hand against the greater trochanter with the tip of your index finger on the anterior superior

- Volume of drug administered:
  Usual 1.0 mL to 2.0 mL
- Needle sizes frequently used:
  20G to 23G. 1inch to 1½ inches
  (greater length needed for very obese individuals)
- Acceptable patient position:
  Prone
- Angle of injection:
  90° angle to flat surface upon which prone patient is lying
- Advantages of site:
  Large muscle mass accommodates deep IM/Z-track injections.
  Injection not visible to patient.
- Disadvantages of site:
  Boundaries of the upper, outer quadrant are often arbitrarily selected and may exceed margin of safety.
  Danger of injury to major nerves and vascular structures if incorrect site or technique is used.
  Subcutaneous fat in area is often very thick; an injection intended for muscle may in fact be subcutaneous.

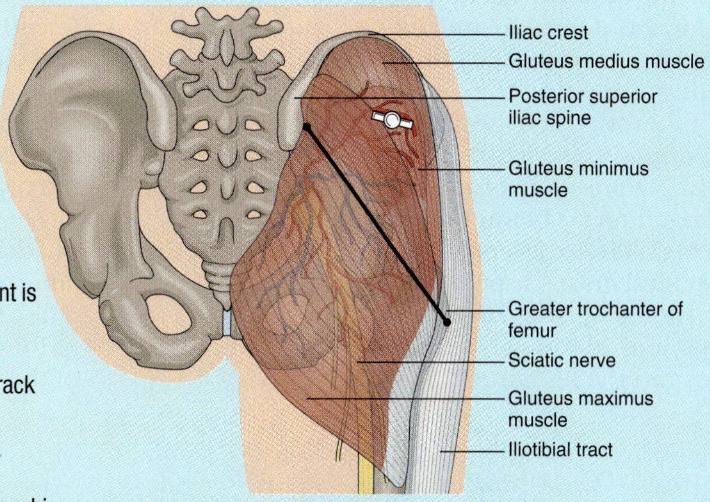

- Additional considerations:
  IM injection using the dorsogluteal site requires strict adherence to proper anatomical site location and injection technique.

Figure 24-21A Injection technique for dorsogluteal site, adult and pediatric (2 years and older).

- Volume of drug administered:
  Usual 1.0 mL to 2.0 mL
  Adult 1.0 mL (2 years and older)
- Needle sizes frequently used:
  20G to 23G. 1 inch to 1½ inches
- Acceptable patient positions:
  Supine, lateral
- Angle of injection:
  Angle the needle slightly toward the iliac crest
- Advantages of site:
  Relatively free of major nerves and vascular branches.
  Well localized by bony anatomic landmarks.
  Thinner layer of subcutaneous fat than dorsogluteal site.
  Sufficient muscle mass for deep IM/Z-track injections.
  Readily accessible from several patient positions.
- Disadvantages of site:
  Health professional's unfamiliarity with site.
- Additional considerations:
  Serves as alternative to dorsogluteal and vastus lateralis for deep IM/Z-track injections.

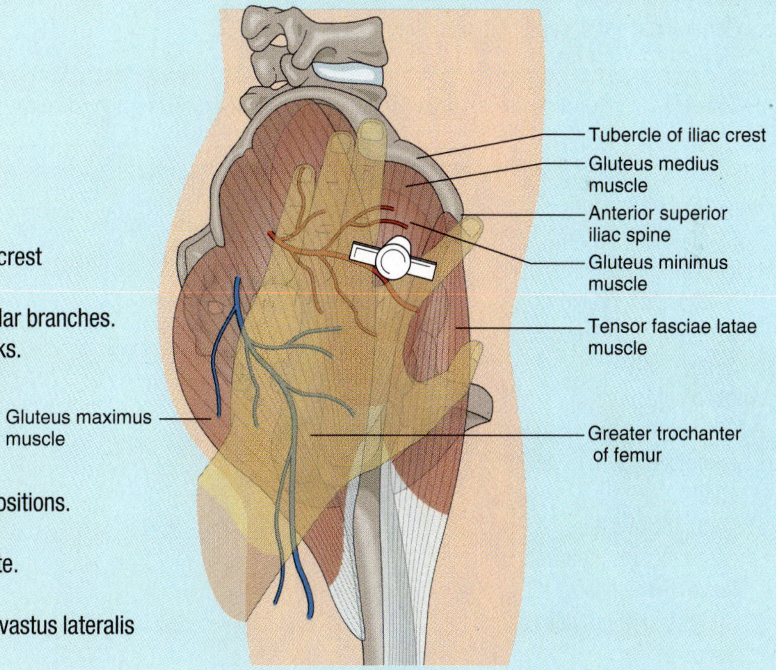

Figure 24-21B Injection technique for ventrogluteal site, adult and pediatric (2 years and older).

iliac spine. Then spread your middle finger as far from the index finger as possible. Place an *x* in the center of the triangle formed by the middle and index fingers to mark the correct injection site.

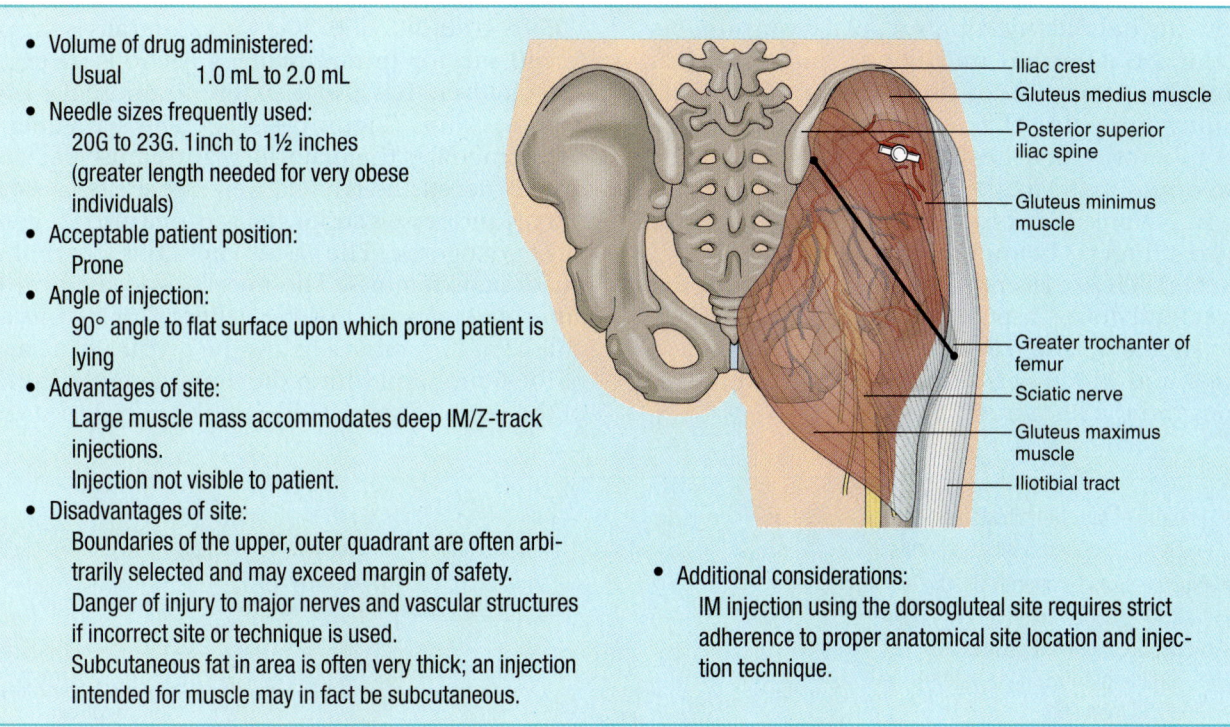

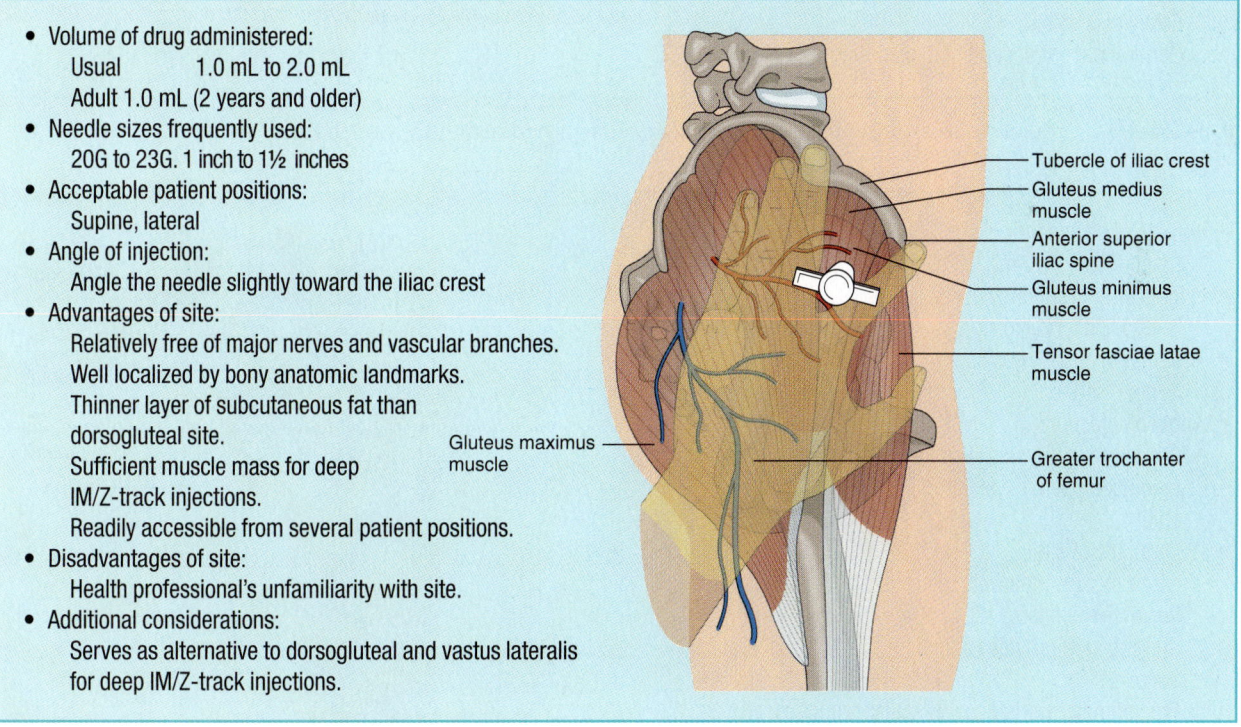

Deltoid Muscle. The deltoid muscle is a small but adequate site for certain intramuscular injections. These intramuscular preparations include vaccines, narcotics, sedatives, and vitamin preparations. The site should not be used for an infant. To locate the deltoid injection site, place your fingers on the shoulder and find the acromion (lateral triangular projection of the spine of the scapula forming the point of the shoulder) and the deltoid tuberosity that lies lateral to the side of the arm, opposite the axilla (Figure 24-21C). The correct injection site is 1 to 2 inches (about the width of three fingers) below the acromion.

CAUTION: Do not inject medicine into the upper and lower aspects of the deltoid muscle. Care should be taken to avoid brachial and axillary nerves and blood vessels, the radial nerve, acromion, and the humerus.

Vastus Lateralis Site. The vastus lateralis is the preferred site for intramuscular injections in infants and children. It is also used for intramuscular injections in adults (Figure 24-21D). This site generally accommodates the majority of intramuscular injections ordered and is a relatively safe site because the nerves and vessels supplying the area are not generally endangered. The vastus lateralis is a part of the quadriceps femoris. The muscle is located on the anterolateral aspect of the patient. For infants and children, the site lies below the greater trochanter of the femur and within the upper lateral quadrant of the thigh (Figure 24-21E).

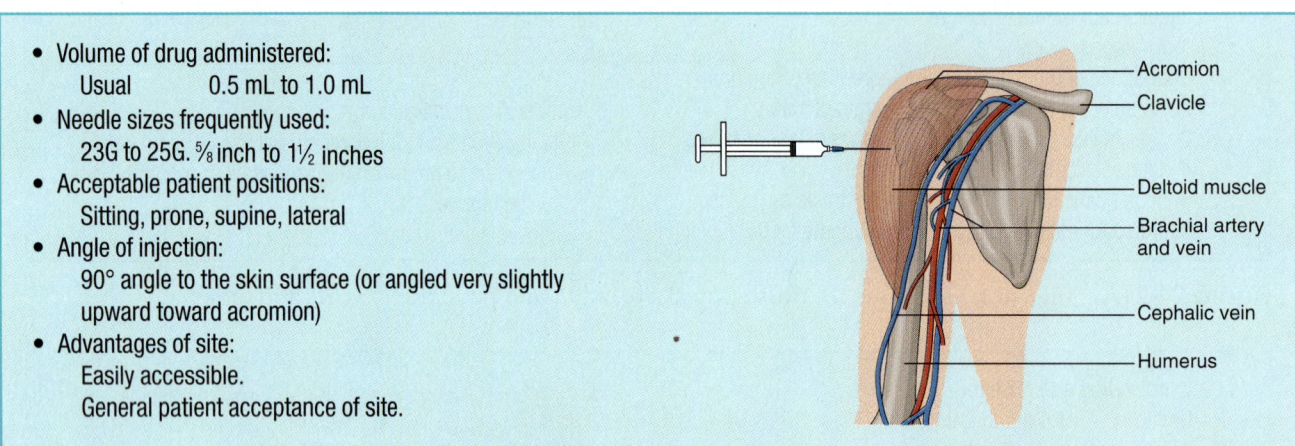

- Volume of drug administered:
  Usual 0.5 mL to 1.0 mL
- Needle sizes frequently used:
  23G to 25G. ⅝ inch to 1½ inches
- Acceptable patient positions:
  Sitting, prone, supine, lateral
- Angle of injection:
  90° angle to the skin surface (or angled very slightly upward toward acromion)
- Advantages of site:
  Easily accessible.
  General patient acceptance of site.

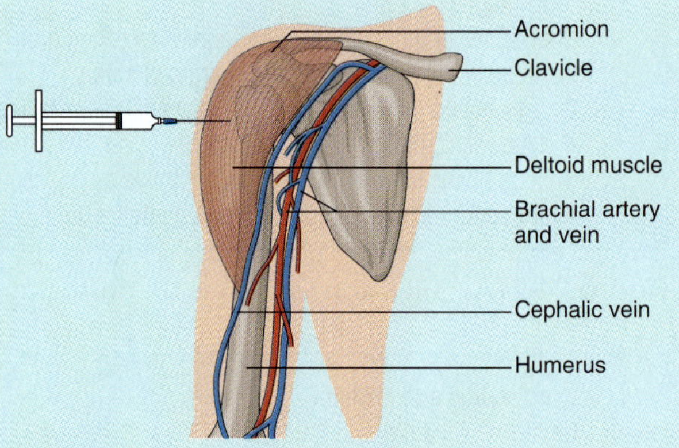

Figure 24-21C Injection technique for deltoid site, adult and pediatric (15 months and older).

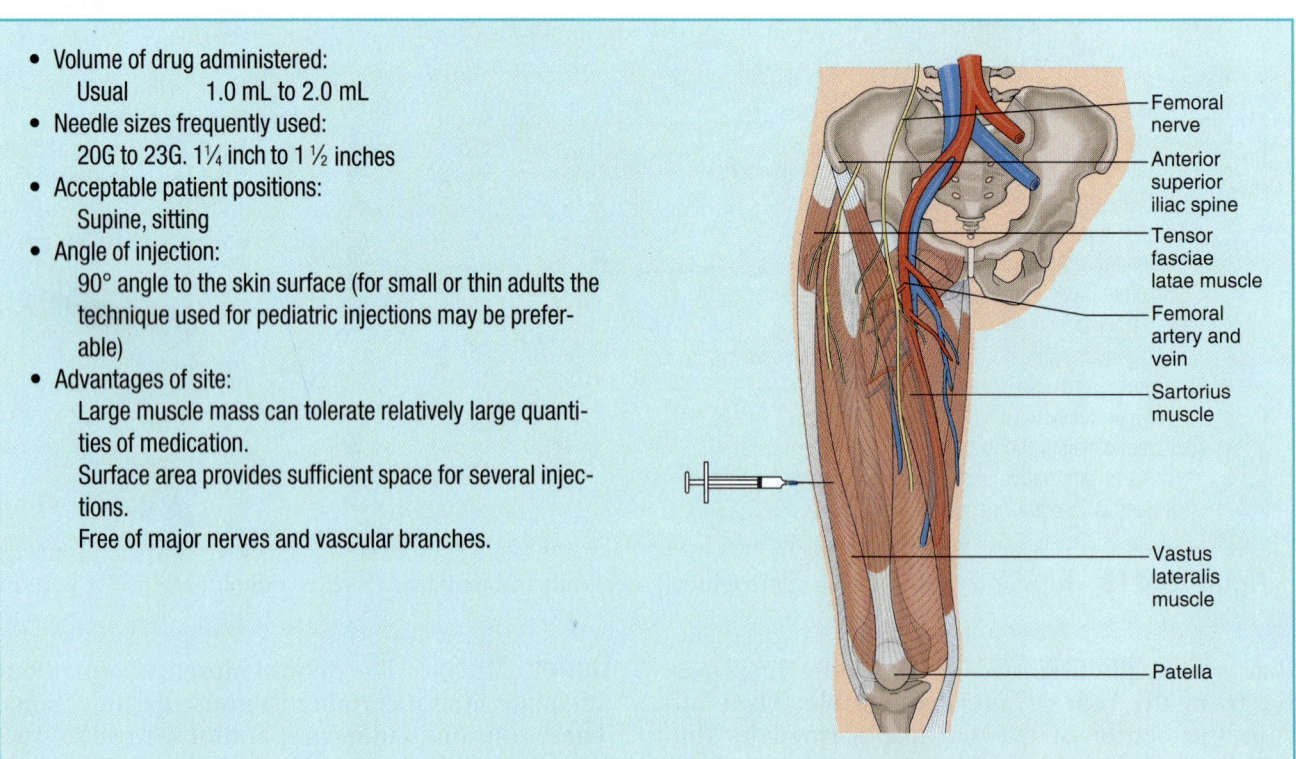

- Volume of drug administered:
  Usual 1.0 mL to 2.0 mL
- Needle sizes frequently used:
  20G to 23G. 1¼ inch to 1 ½ inches
- Acceptable patient positions:
  Supine, sitting
- Angle of injection:
  90° angle to the skin surface (for small or thin adults the technique used for pediatric injections may be preferable)
- Advantages of site:
  Large muscle mass can tolerate relatively large quantities of medication.
  Surface area provides sufficient space for several injections.
  Free of major nerves and vascular branches.

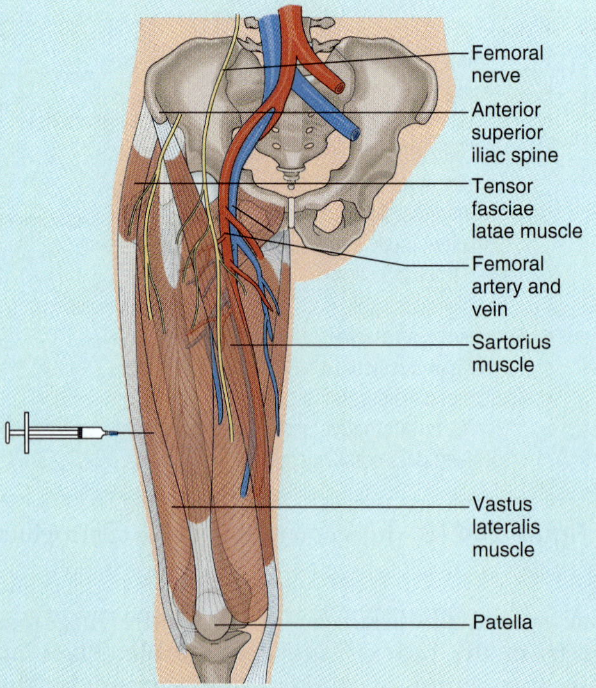

Figure 24-21D Injection technique for vastus lateralis site, adult and pediatric (2 years and older).

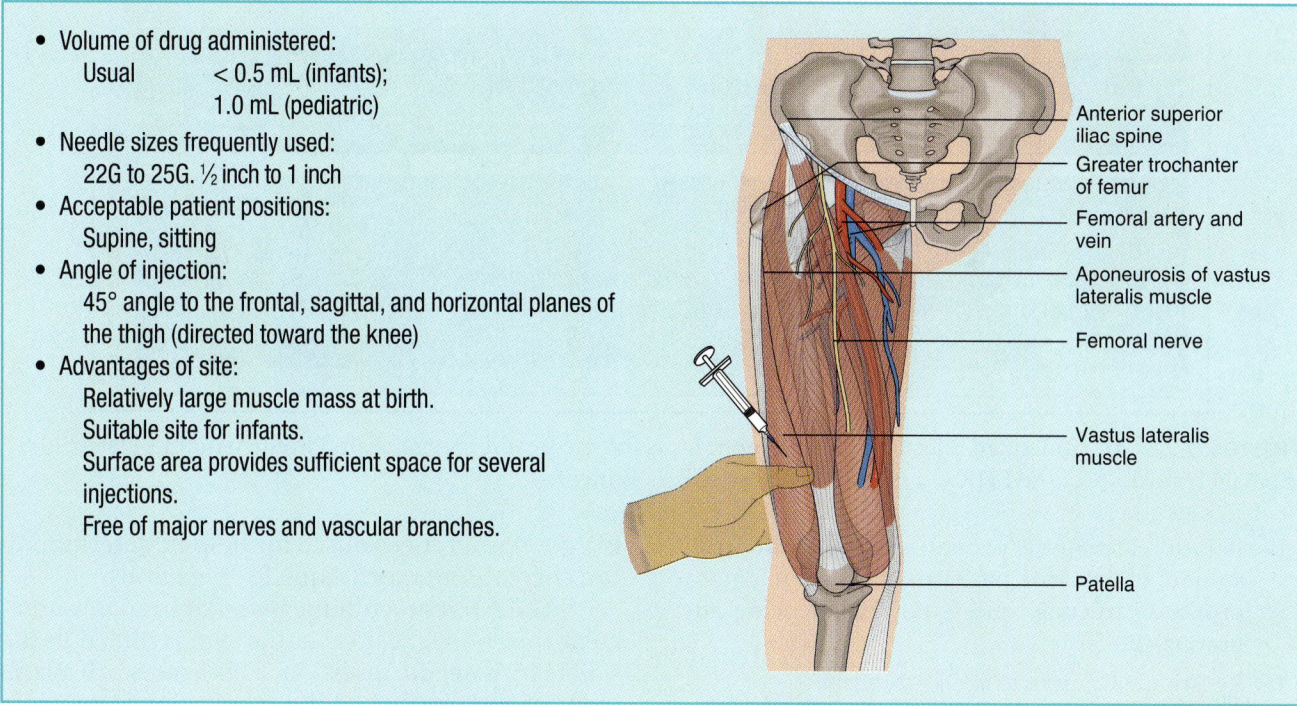

- Volume of drug administered:
  Usual < 0.5 mL (infants);
  1.0 mL (pediatric)
- Needle sizes frequently used:
  22G to 25G. ½ inch to 1 inch
- Acceptable patient positions:
  Supine, sitting
- Angle of injection:
  45° angle to the frontal, sagittal, and horizontal planes of the thigh (directed toward the knee)
- Advantages of site:
  Relatively large muscle mass at birth.
  Suitable site for infants.
  Surface area provides sufficient space for several injections.
  Free of major nerves and vascular branches.

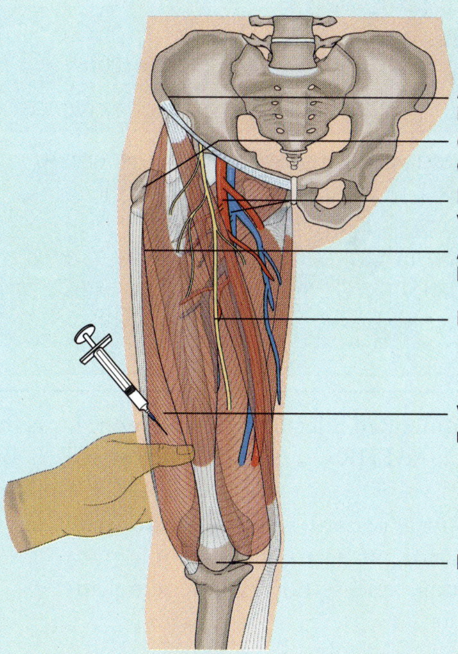

Figure 24-21E Injection technique for vastus lateralis site, pediatric (newborn to 2 years of age).

For the adult patient, the correct injection site is within the middle third of the muscle.

BASIC GUIDELINES FOR ADMINISTRATION OF INJECTIONS

Regardless of the type of injection, basic guidelines must be followed to safeguard the patient. These guidelines are presented according to the sequence of the events to which they relate:

1. Adhere to the "Six Rights" of proper drug administration.
2. Always evaluate each patient as an individual.
3. Select a needle–syringe unit that is the appropriate size for the proper administration of a parenteral medication.
4. Correctly prepare the appropriate parenteral equipment and supplies for use. Wash hands and put on gloves. Always use OSHA guidelines and follow standard precautions.
5. Select the correct site for the intended injection.
6. Prepare the patient properly for the injection.
7. For subcutaneous and intramuscular injections, use a smooth, quick, dartlike motion to insert the needle into the patient's skin. Use the correct angle of insertion (45 or 90 degrees) for the injection.
8. Once the needle is inserted, gently pull back on the plunger (aspirate) to ensure that the needle is not in a blood vessel.

   CAUTION: If blood appears in the syringe on aspiration, smoothly withdraw the needle, properly discard the used unit, and prepare another injection for administration. Repeat the preceding steps.
9. Slowly inject the medication into the patient.
10. With a quick, smooth motion, remove the needle from the injection site. Immediately activate the safety mechanism and discard the syringe–needle unit in a puncture-proof container. Cover the injection site with a dry, sterile cotton swab and gently massage the site.

    CAUTION: Do not massage the site when administering insulin, Imferon, or heparin.
11. Remove the cotton swab and check for bleeding. If bleeding occurs after applying pressure for 30 seconds, apply a sterile adhesive strip to the injection site.
12. Remove gloves.
13. Observe the patient for any signs of hypersensitivity. Take precautions to ensure the patient's safety.
14. Properly and immediately discard the used equipment and supplies.
15. Wash hands.
16. Follow documentation procedures in patient's chart or electronic medical record, noting administration of the medication (Figure 24-22).

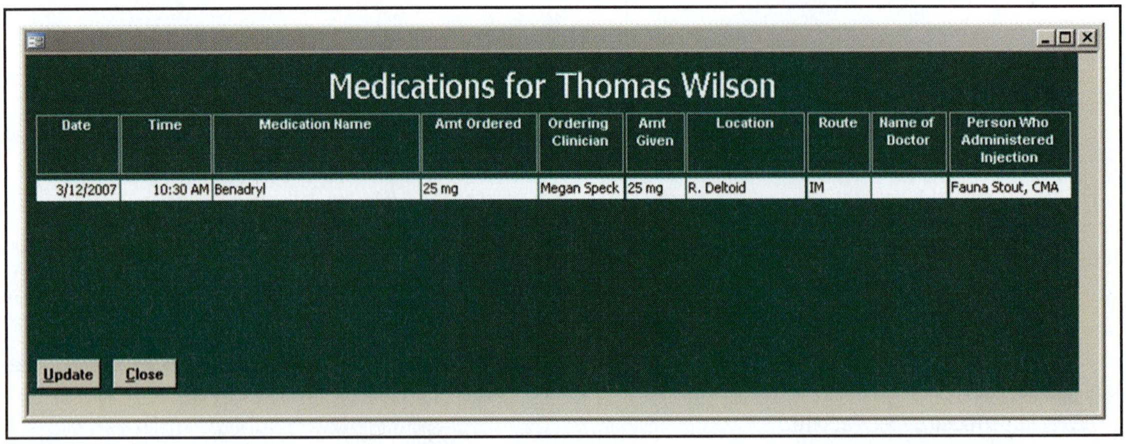

Medications for Thomas Wilson

Date	Time	Medication Name	Amt Ordered	Ordering Clinician	Amt Given	Location	Route	Name of Doctor	Person Who Administered Injection
3/12/2007	10:30 AM	Benadryl	25 mg	Megan Speck	25 mg	R. Deltoid	IM		Fauna Stout, CMA

Update Close

Figure 24-22 Document all injections. This screen shows the medication documented in the patient's electronic medical record. (Synapse EHR screen shot courtesy of E. S. Butler).

17. Before releasing the patient, wait the appropriate amount of time and make sure the patient is given proper instructions and is not experiencing any unusual effects.
18. Return medications to shelf/storage.

Procedures 24-1 through 24-9 provide steps as follows:

- Procedure 24-1: Administration of Oral Medications
- Procedure 24-2: Withdrawing Medication from a Vial
- Procedure 24-3: Withdrawing Medication from an Ampule
- Procedure 24-4: Administration of Subcutaneous, Intramuscular, and Intradermal Injections
- Procedure 24-5: Administering a Subcutaneous Injection
- Procedure 24-6: Administering an Intramuscular Injection
- Procedure 24-7: Administering an Intradermal Injection of Purified Protein Derivative (PPD).
- Procedure 24-8: Reconstituting a Powder Medication for Administration
- Procedure 24-9: Z-Track Intramuscular Injection Technique

Z-TRACK METHOD OF INTRAMUSCULAR INJECTION

Imferon is an example of a medication that is administered using the Z-track method. This medication and others that are irritating to the subcutaneous tissues and may discolor the skin are given in this manner. (The *Physician's Desk Reference* [PDR] is a good reference source for help in determining the correct route technique for injections.)

The Z-track technique is similar to an intramuscular injection, except that the skin is pulled to the side before needle insertion. This causes a displacement of the tissues and the medication enters in a manner that will not allow it to seep back into the subcutaneous tissues and up to the skin's surface. Because the medications are irritating, for the comfort of the patient, change the needle on the syringe after aspirating the medication from the ampule or vial before injecting the patient with the medication (see Procedure 24-9).

ADMINISTRATION OF ALLERGENIC EXTRACTS

It may be the responsibility of the medical assistant to administer allergenic extracts. It is important to observe the following:

- Allergic extracts are *always* given in subcutaneous tissue, *never* in the muscle.
- Use a tuberculin syringe with a 25G, ⅝-inch needle, 26G, ⅜-inch needle, or 27G, ½-inch needle or 1-mL allergist syringe (Figure 24-23).
- Use a site rotation system for each injected extract.
- Correctly document the procedure and dosage.
- Allergenic extracts should be refrigerated; they should retain potency for 10 to 12 weeks.
- Adverse reactions such as itching, swelling, and redness should be reported immediately to the provider.
- Severe reactions such as anaphylactic shock have occurred; therefore, emergency equipment and supplies must be available for use. Epinephrine and Benadryl must be readily accessible. (See Chapters 9 and 23 for emergency supplies.)

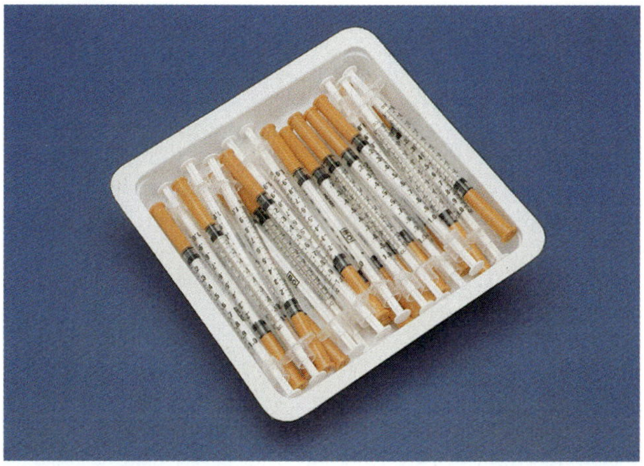

Figure 24-23 Allergist syringes.

- Allergy testing is done when the provider is present.
- Patient must wait 20 to 30 minutes after injection to be certain there has been no reaction.

Example:

Patient's Name:

Date	Dose	Site
6/24/XX	1st 0.01 mL SC	Lt. arm
6/27/XX	2nd 0.02 mL SC	Rt. arm
6/30/XX	3rd 0.03 mL SC	Lt. arm

The patient should be observed for 20 to 30 minutes after the injection of an allergenic extract.

Susceptible individuals can experience development of allergic reactions to many foreign substances. It is wise for the patient with allergies to be aware of those substances and others that are known allergens.

ADMINISTRATION OF INHALED MEDICATIONS

The act of drawing breath, vapor, or gas into the lungs is known as *inhalation*. Inhalation therapy may involve the administration of medicines; water vapor; and such gases as oxygen, carbon dioxide, and helium.

An inhaler may be used to deliver medications to the lungs. Medications that use an inhaler include bronchodilators, mucolytic agents, and steroids. Inhalers are useful in the delivery of treatment for chronic obstructive pulmonary disease (COPD) and reversible obstructive airway disease. An inhaler is a small, handheld apparatus, usually an aerosol unit, that contains a microcrystalline suspension of medication. When activated, it produces a fine mist or spray containing the medication. This suspension is then drawn into the respiratory tract, settling deep into the lungs and alveoli. See Chapter 18 for information about pulmonary diseases and procedures.

Implications for Patient Care

Patients should be instructed to follow the prescribed medication regimen. The prescribed medicine and the type of inhaler to be used will determine the method of administration. A handheld inhaler may be used for oral or nasal inhalation, depending on the type ordered by the provider.

Inhalation therapy may be contraindicated in patients with delicate fluid balance, cardiac arrhythmias, **status asthmaticus**, and hypersensitivity to the medication. As with any medication, the provider will determine the treatment regimen for each patient. See Chapter 18 for information about pulmonary diseases and procedures.

Administration of Oxygen

Oxygen is a colorless, odorless, tasteless gas that is essential for life. When the body does not have an adequate supply of oxygen, a state of **hypoxemia** (lack of oxygen in the blood) develops, and irreversible damage to vital organs is possible. When

Patient Education

- Patients should be advised to avoid overuse of the inhaler. Tolerance, rebound bronchospasm, and adverse cardiac effects can occur from overuse. Instruct the patient to notify the provider should the prescribed dose of medication fail to produce the desired effect.
- Instruct the patient to perform good oral hygiene, including rinsing of the mouth and mouthpiece of equipment, after the inhalation treatment (to prevent the possible growth of fungi).
- Caution the patient against the continued use of a metered-dose canister after the stated number of actuations. If the medication contains adrenaline, fatalities can occur if heart rate and blood pressure increase significantly.

a lack of oxygen threatens a person's survival, supplemental oxygen must be prescribed and administered immediately, and arterial blood gas analysis will be necessary after oxygen administration has been started. If the situation is not an emergency or life threatening, arterial blood gas analysis can be performed before the provider prescribes the dosage and method of administration. The normal range for oxygen in the arterial blood is 80 to 100 mm Hg (millimeters mercury). Oxygen is supplied in tanks (Figure 24-24) for use in the ambulatory care setting, but in a hospital setting, oxygen is piped in through a wall pipe system.

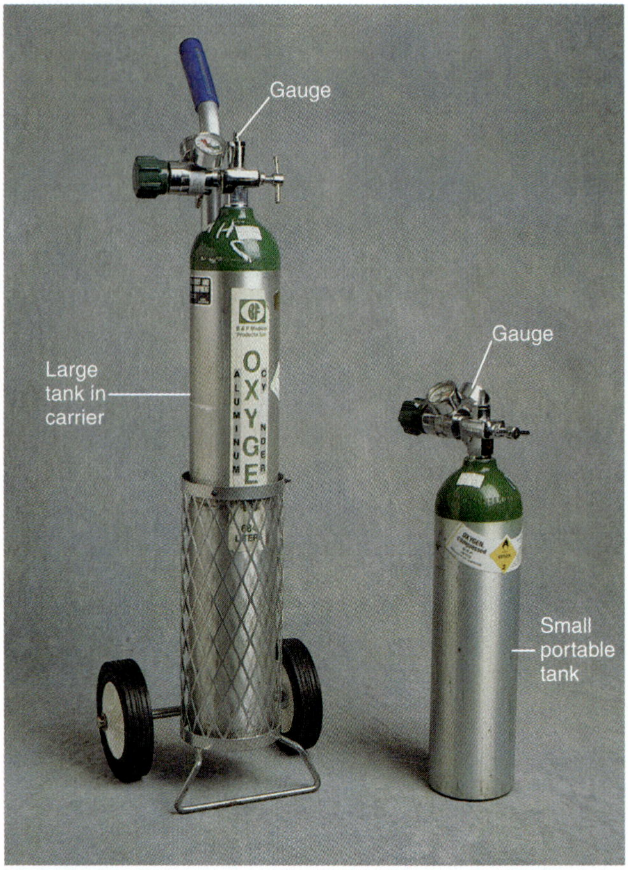

Figure 24-24 Oxygen tanks. Note gauge at top of tanks.

Dosage. When oxygen is to be administered, dosage is based on individual needs. Because oxygen is a drug, the provider will prescribe the flow rate, concentration, method of delivery, and length of time for administration. Oxygen is ordered as liters per minute (LPM) or L/min and as percentage of oxygen concentration (%).

It is the medical assistant's responsibility to follow provider orders and adhere to the guidelines for proper drug administration. Always assess the patient as an individual, explain the procedure, and carefully observe the patient for signs of improvement or symptoms of oxygen toxicity.

CAUTION: Oxygen toxicity may develop when 100% oxygen is breathed for a prolonged period. As with any other drug, toxicity depends on dose, time, and the patient's response. The higher the dose, the shorter the time required to develop toxicity. Symptoms of oxygen toxicity are substernal pain, nausea, vomiting, malaise, fatigue, numbness, and a tingling of the extremities.

High concentrations of inhaled oxygen cause alveolar collapse, intraalveolar hemorrhage, hyaline membrane formation, disturbance of the central nervous system, and **retrolental fibroplasia** in newborns.

NOTE: **Apnea** (absence of breathing) can result when giving oxygen at a flow rate greater than 2 liters per minute to patients with COPD, especially those with emphysema.

Methods of Oxygen Delivery. Many methods are available today for the delivery of oxygen. The more commonly prescribed methods include the use of nasal cannulas, nasal catheters, and masks. Other methods of delivery involve the use of isolettes, hoods, and tents.

Nasal Cannula. When a low concentration of oxygen is desired, the nasal cannula (Figure 24-25) is the simplest and most convenient method for the administration of oxygen. Made of plastic, the nasal cannula consists of two hollow prongs through which oxygen passes, and a strap or other device to secure it to the patient's head (Figure 24-26). Do not place the direct flow of oxygen against the patient's nasal mucosa, because this causes tissue dehydration. Flow rates greater than 2 to 4 L/min require humidification.

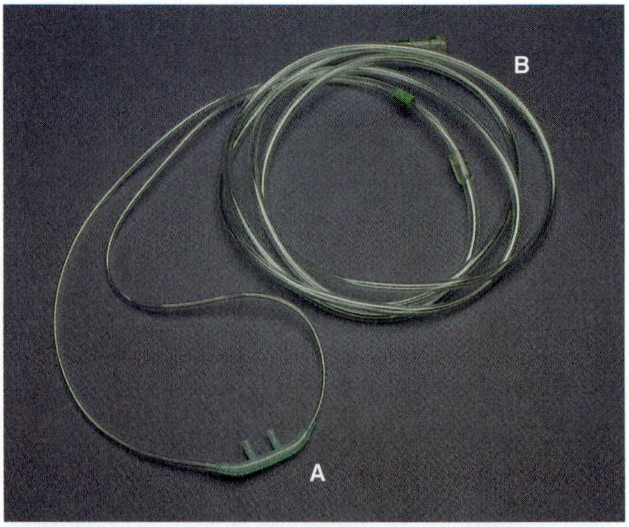

Figure 24-25 (A) Oxygen cannula. (B) Tubing.

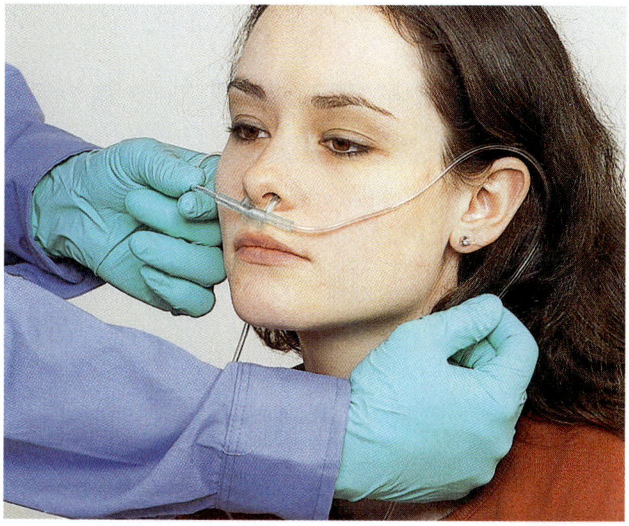

Figure 24-26 Medical assistant adjusts nasal cannula around patient's ears for oxygen administration.

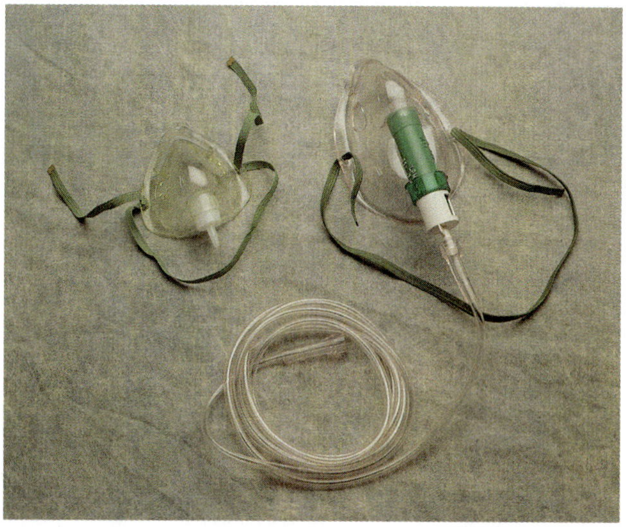

Figure 24-27 Oxygen masks: (A) without tubing; (B) with tubing.

Nasal Catheter. The nasal catheter is a disposable plastic tube that has small holes at the inserted end. These holes diffuse the flow of oxygen for better distribution to lung tissue with minimum dehydration. The nasal catheter is seldom used today because it causes mucous membrane irritation and has to be changed every 8 hours. Because of the discomfort caused to the patient by the catheter, the nasal cannula is the preferred method for the delivery of oxygen.

Mask. The common types of masks used for inhalation therapy include plastic disposable, partial rebreather, nonrebreather, and Venturi (Figure 24-27). These devices are used when the patient requires high humidity and a precise amount of oxygen. To be effective, the mask must be fitted snugly to the patient (Figure 24-28).

CAUTION: Oxygen must be humidified before delivery to the patient to prevent drying of the respiratory mucosa.

Oxygen Safety Precautions. Oxygen supports combustion; thus, there is the danger of a fire being started when oxygen is in use. Extreme caution should be exercised when oxygen is being administered because ignition can be caused by friction, static electricity, or a lighted cigar or cigarette. In the provider's office, oxygen is generally stored in tanks. These tanks must be checked on a regular basis and replaced as necessary. See Chapter 18 for information about pulmonary diseases and procedures.

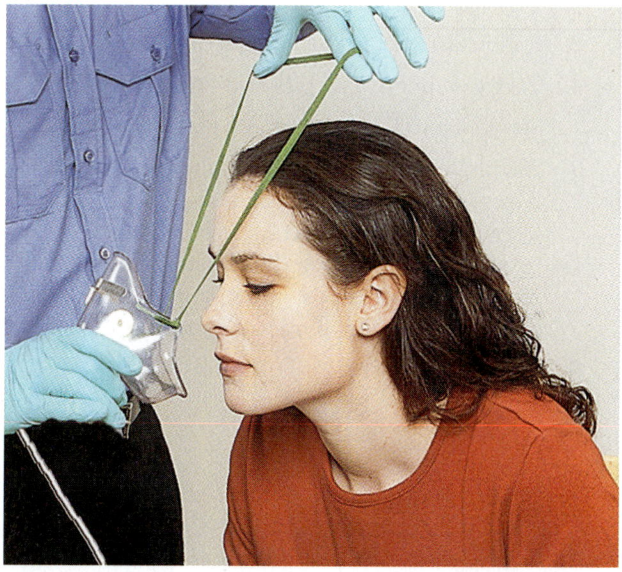

Figure 24-28 Medical assistant adjusts oxygen mask around patient's head.

Patient Education

Explain safety measures to the patient who uses oxygen at home. Cigarettes, lighters, candles, and other smoking materials should not be used in the room where oxygen is used. Instruct the patient to wear nonstatic-producing clothing, such as cotton.

Procedure 24-1

Administration of Oral Medications

STANDARD PRECAUTIONS:

PURPOSE:

Correctly administer an oral medication after receiving the provider's order and assembling the necessary equipment and supplies.

EQUIPMENT/SUPPLIES:

Proper medication
Medication note
Medicine cup
Water, milk, or juice for patient

PROCEDURE STEPS:

1. Verify the provider's order.
2. Follow the "Six Rights" (Figure 24-29A).
3. Perform medical asepsis handwash.
4. Work in a well-lighted, quiet, clean area.
5. Assemble equipment and supplies. RATIONALE: A well-lighted area for preparing medications is important because you must be able to see well to accurately pour medications. A quiet area is free from distractions, and medical asepsis helps fight transmission of microorganisms.
6. Obtain the correct medication using the medicine note.
7. Compare the medication label with the medication note (first time). RATIONALE: Reading from a medicine note helps prevent errors while pouring the medication.
8. Check the expiration date. RATIONALE: Outdated medication may be deteriorated or altered in some way and be harmful to the patient.
9. Calculate dosage if necessary.
10. Correctly prepare (a, b, or c) (Figure 24-29B and C).
    a. Multiple-dose solid medication
    b. Unit dose medication
    c. Liquid medication
11. Compare medicine label with medication note (second time).
12. Properly transport the medicine.
13. Identify the patient. Explain the procedure.
14. Assess patient. Take vital signs if indicated. RATIONALE: Always assess the patient for body size, physical condition, age, and gender to be certain the dose and route are appropriate prior to administration of certain medications. BP or pulse may need to be taken to ascertain if the vital signs are within normal limits.
15. Assist patient to a comfortable position.
16. Check medication label a third time.

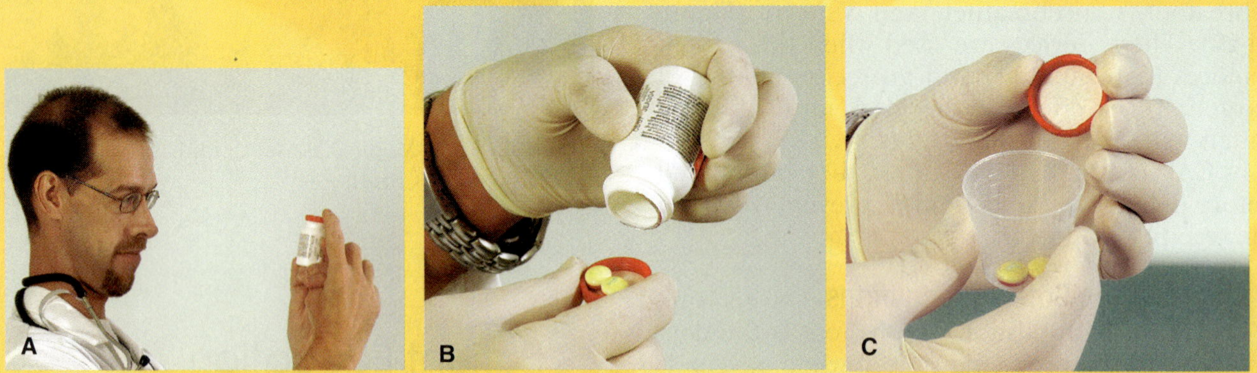

Figure 24-29 (A) Medical assistant checks for right drug, right dose, right route, and expiration date before pouring medication. (B) Medical assistant pours capsules from the cover of the medicine container into a medicine cup before administering medicine to patient. The medication is poured into cover to avoid contamination of medicine. (C) Medical assistant administers the medication, being certain that patient takes the medicine.

continues

Procedure 24-1 (continued)

17. Administer the medication. Provide water. Be certain that the patient takes the medicine. RATIONALE: Some patients, for various reasons, may deliberately not swallow their medication.
18. Provide for the patient's safety: Observe the patient for any adverse reactions.
19. Care for equipment and supplies according to OSHA guidelines.
20. Document administration of the medication in patient's chart or electronic medical record. (Figure 24-29D and 24-29E).
21. Return the medication to the shelf/storage area.

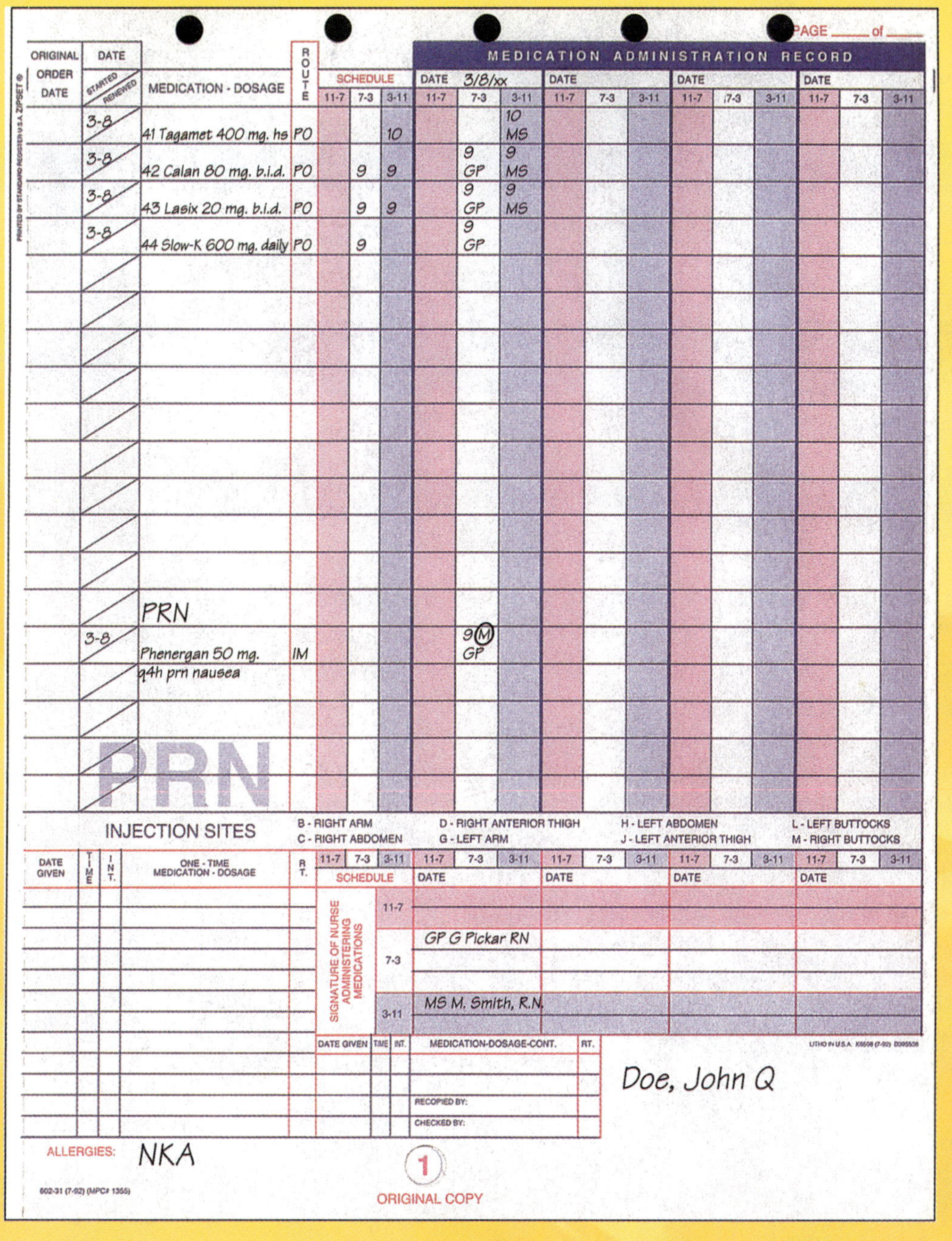

Figure 24-29 (continued) (D) Example of medication administration record for patient's chart.

continues

Procedure 24-1 (continued)

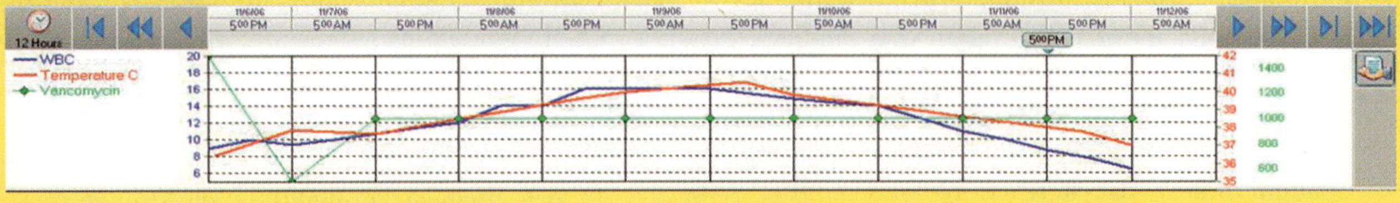

Figure 24-29 (continued) (E) The computer makes a graph when the appropriate patient data is input. The patient's white blood cell count (WBC), temperature (in Celsius), and antibiotic (Vancomycin) are shown. The patient has an infection, and the computer-generated graphic shows the patient's response to the antibiotic. The WBC and temperature climb over a period of 4 days, then began to drop in response to the antibiotic. The provider has access to the information on demand.

Procedure 24-2

Withdrawing Medication from a Vial

STANDARD PRECAUTIONS:

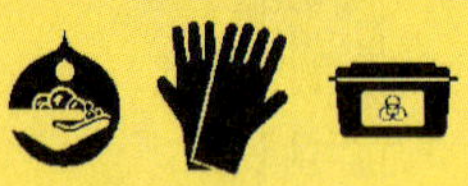

PURPOSE:

Medication is supplied in a variety of packaging. Medication from a vial must be drawn into a syringe for parenteral injection.

EQUIPMENT/SUPPLIES:

Medication order	Vial of medication
Medication note	Alcohol wipes
Appropriate syringe and needle with cover	Disposable gloves
	Sharps container

PROCEDURE STEPS:

1. Read the medication order and assemble equipment. Check for the "Six Rights." Read the vial label by holding it next to the medicine card (first time).
2. Wash hands. Apply gloves.
3. Select the proper size needle and syringe for the medication and the route (e.g., for subcutaneous injection of insulin, 100-U insulin syringe and 25G, ⅝-inch needle). If necessary, attach the needle to the syringe.
4. Check the vial label against the medication note (second time).
5. Remove the metal or plastic cap from the vial. If the vial has been opened previously, clean the rubber stopper by applying an alcohol wipe in a circular motion (Figure 24-30A).
6. Remove the needle cover by pulling it straight off.
7. Inject air into the vial as follows:
   a. Hold the syringe pointed upward at eye level. Pull back the plunger to take in a quantity of air that is equal to the ordered dose of medication.
   b. Leave vial on tabletop/countertop.
   c. Insert the needle through center of the rubber stopper of the vial. Inject the air by pushing in the plunger (Figure 24-30B).
8. Invert the vial. Hold the vial and the syringe steady. Pull back on the plunger to withdraw the measured dose of medication. Measure accurately. Keep the tip of the needle below the surface of the liquid; otherwise, air will enter the syringe. Keep syringe at eye level (Figure 24-30C).
9. Check the syringe for air bubbles. Remove them by tapping sharply on the syringe. Push the air bubbles back into the vial (Figure 24-30D). Check measurement for accuracy, and draw more medication if needed.
10. Remove the needle from the vial. Replace the sterile needle cover (Figure 24-30E) using "scoop"

continues

Procedure 24-2 (continued)

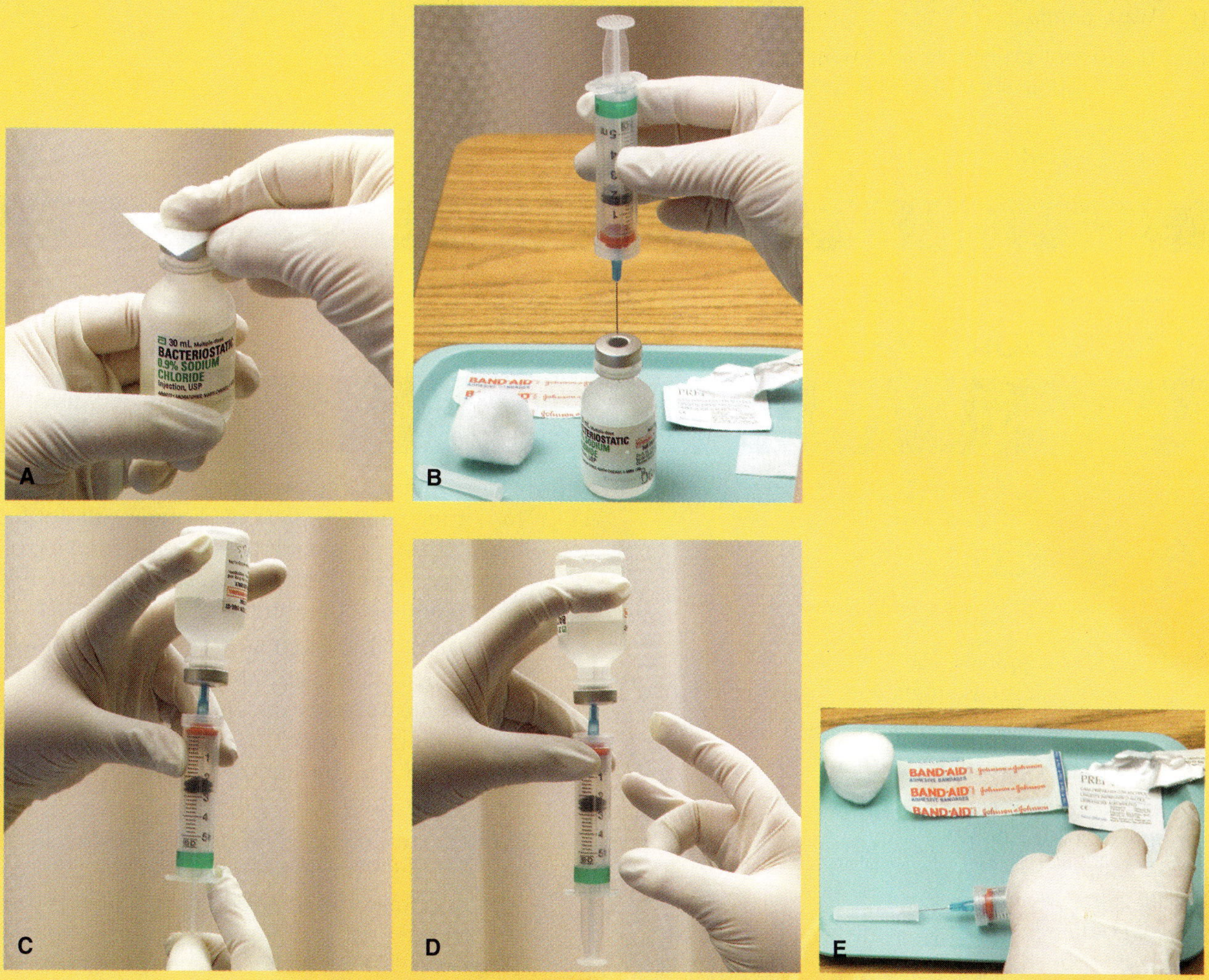

Figure 24-30 (A) Disinfect the rubber stopper on the medication vial with an alcohol wipe. (B) Keeping the bevel of the needle above the fluid level, inject an amount of air equal to medication quantity to be withdrawn. (C) Hold syringe pointed upward at eye level and with the bevel of the needle in the medication. Pull back plunger and aspirate the quantity to be withdrawn. (C) Hold syringe pointed upward at eye level and with the bevel of the needle in the medication. Pull back plunger and aspirate the quantity of medication ordered. (D) Tap syringe to eliminate air bubbles. Hand should hold syringe while tapping it. (E) After the correct dose has been withdrawn, recover the sterile needle using "scoop" method. Place medicine on a tray with medication note, the medication vial, and an alcohol wipe and safely transport to the patient.

method. RATIONALE: The needle cover can be replaced because it is sterile and has not been used on a patient.

11. Check the vial label against the medication note (third time).
12. Place the filled syringe and medication vial on a medicine tray with an alcohol wipe and the medication note. The dose is now ready for injection.
13. If medication is a tissue irritant, change to another sterile needle. RATIONALE: Tissue irritants can cause tissue necrosis. Activate safety mechanism.
14. Immediately after the injection, activate the safety mechanism. Discard the syringe-needle unit into a sharps container.
15. Remove gloves and dispose in biohazard waste container.

continues

Procedure 24-2 (continued)

16. Wash hands.
17. Document procedure in patient's chart or electronic medical record.
18. Return the vial to the proper storage area. Destroy medication note.

DOCUMENTATION

8/9/20XX 2:30 PM Vitamin B_{12} (Cyanocobalamin) 100 mcg IM (R) deltoid area. W. Slawson, CMA (AAMA) ———

Procedure 24-3

Withdrawing Medication from an Ampule

STANDARD PRECAUTIONS:

PURPOSE:

Medication is supplied in a variety of packaging. An ampule is a sterile, glass, single-dose container of liquid medication. It is aspirated into a syringe for injection.

EQUIPMENT/SUPPLIES:

Medicine tray and medication note
Ampule of medication
Alcohol wipes
Sterile gauze sponges
Sharps container
Sterile filter needle and syringe
Gloves

PROCEDURE STEPS:

1. Check the provider's order. Write out medication note.
2. Wash hands and gather equipment. Put on gloves.
3. Select ampule of medication. Read label and check medication note for correct medication, dose, route, and time (first time). Check medication expiration date.
4. Flick ampule of medication (medication will often get "trapped" above the neck of the ampule). A sharp flick of the wrist will help force all of the medication down below the neck of the ampule into the body of the ampule (Figure 24-31A). RATIONALE: This is important to ensure all medication is available in the body of the ampule to calculate the correct dose. If some of the medication remains trapped above the neck in the top of the ampule, some medication will not be available for use and it is possible to give an incorrect dose, especially if the patient is to receive the entire contents of the ampule.
5. Thoroughly disinfect the neck with an alcohol swab. Check label (second time). RATIONALE: The needle will enter the opening of the ampule and wiping the neck of the ampule before removal of the top ensures disinfection of the neck or opening of the ampule.
6. With a sterile gauze, wipe dry the neck of the ampule. Completely surround the ampule with the gauze and forcefully snap off the top of the ampule by pulling the top toward you (Figure 24-31B). RATIONALE: Ensure medical assistant safety from possible injury from broken glass. Discard top in sharps container.
7. Place opened ampule down on medicine tray. Check label (third time).
8. With a prepared sterile syringe-needle unit that has a filter on the needle, aspirate the required dose into the syringe (Figure 24-31C). Cover needle with sheath using scoop method and transport it with medication ampule to patient on the medicine tray. RATIONALE: Filtered needles prevent glass particles from being aspirated with medication.
   a. There is another method used to aspirate the contents of an ampule. The needle and syringe unit can be inserted into the open ampule and then inverted. The medication can be drawn into the syringe because surface tension prevents the medication from leaking out of the ampule.

continues

Procedure 24-3 (continued)

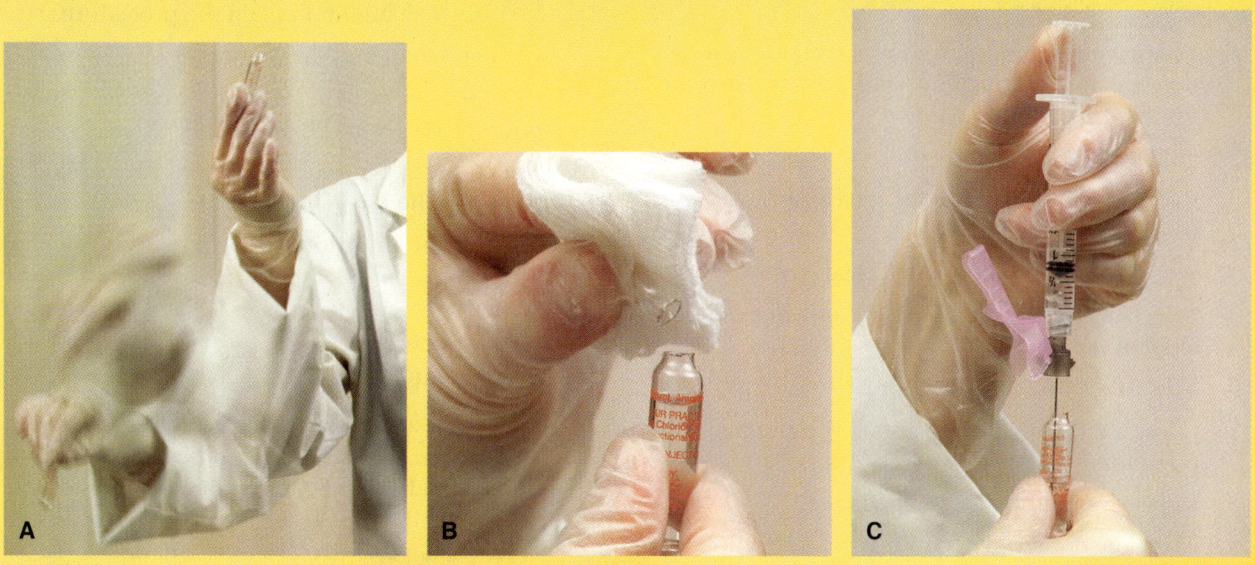

Figure 24-31 (A) Hold ampule by the top and force all the medication into the bottom of the ampule by a snap of the arm and wrist. (B) Remove top from ampule. Snap away from you by pulling top toward you. (C) Draw the required dose into syringe.

9. Change needles. **RATIONALE: The filter needle may contain glass particles.**
10. Identify the patient.
11. Administer medication.
12. Discard syringe–needle unit into sharps container. Alcohol wipes and gauze are discarded in biohazard waste container if there is any blood on them.
13. Remove gloves and dispose in biohazard waste container. Dispose of ampule into sharps container.
14. Wash hands.
15. Document procedure in patient's chart or electronic medical record. Destroy medication note.

DOCUMENTATION

5/12/20XX 11:20 AM Phenergan 25 mg IM (R) dorsogluteal area. B. Abbott, RMA ———

Procedure 24-4

Administration of Subcutaneous, Intramuscular, and Intradermal Injections

STANDARD PRECAUTIONS:

PURPOSE:

To properly administer subcutaneous, intramuscular, and intradermal injections.

EQUIPMENT/SUPPLIES:

Medicine tray
Medication as ordered by the provider and medication note
Appropriately sized needle and syringe
Alcohol wipes
Disposable gloves
Sharps container
Cotton ball

continues

Procedure 24-4 (continued)

PROCEDURE STEPS:

1. Verify the provider's order. Write out medication note taking information from provider's order sheet from patient record.
2. Follow the "Six Rights."
3. Perform medical asepsis hand cleansing. Adhere to OSHA guidelines.
4. Work in a well-lighted, quiet, clean area.
5. Select the appropriate syringe and needle and alcohol wipe.
6. Select the correct medication.
7. Compare the medication label with the medication note (first time).
8. Check expiration date on medicine.
9. Calculate dosage, if necessary.
10. Prepare syringe and needle for use (Figure 24-32A–D).
11. Withdraw medication from vial.
12. Compare medicine label with the medication note (second time).
13. Place filled syringe and needle on the medicine tray with medication note and vial. Check the medication label with the medicine note (third time).
14. Transport the medicine to the patient with medication note.
15. Identify the patient. Explain the procedure.
16. Assess the patient. Put on gloves.
17. Prepare the patient for the injection (drape, position, allay apprehension).
18. Select an appropriate injection site. Follow a rotating schedule if appropriate.
19. Cleanse the injection site with a sterile alcohol wipe. Use a circular motion, working from the center out to about 2 inches beyond the planned injection site.
20. Allow the skin to dry.
21. Inject medication after first aspirating to be certain needle is not in a blood vessel (except for intradermal injection). Immediately activate safety mechanism and dispose of syringe and needle in a puncture-proof container.
22. Massage injection site with an alcohol wipe unless contraindicated (such as insulin, Imferon, heparin).
23. Observe the patient for signs of difficulty.
24. Inspect the injection site for bleeding, apply adhesive strip if necessary.
25. Properly dispose of used equipment and supplies. Remove gloves.
26. Perform medical asepsis handwash.

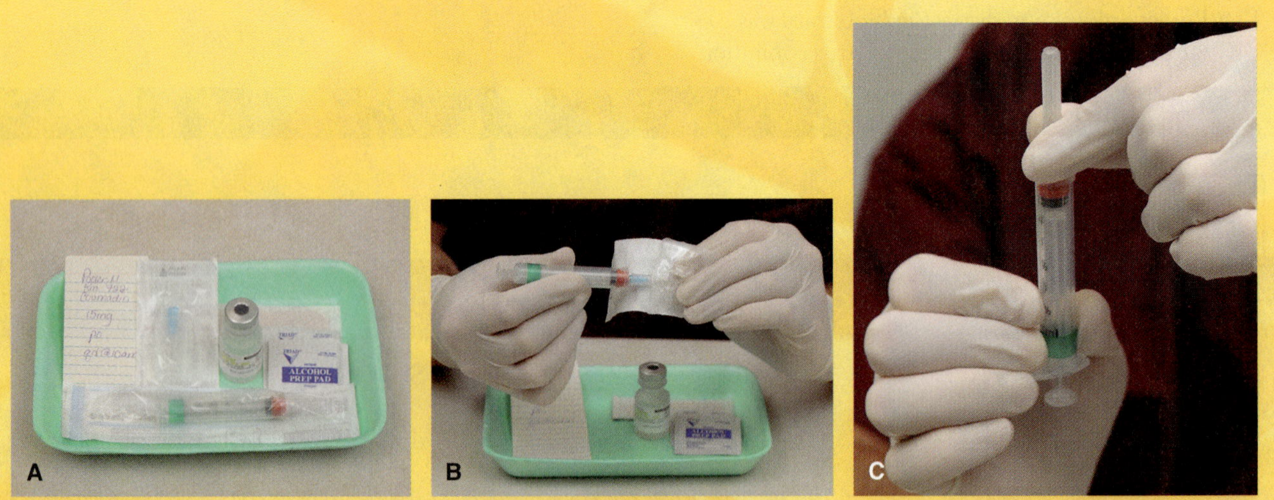

Figure 24-32 Preparing syringe–needle unit for use. (A) Assemble the equipment and supplies needed to draw up medication from a vial. (B) Open the sterile syringe and needle from packages. (C) Secure the needle by twisting it clockwise.

continues

Procedure 24-4 (continued)

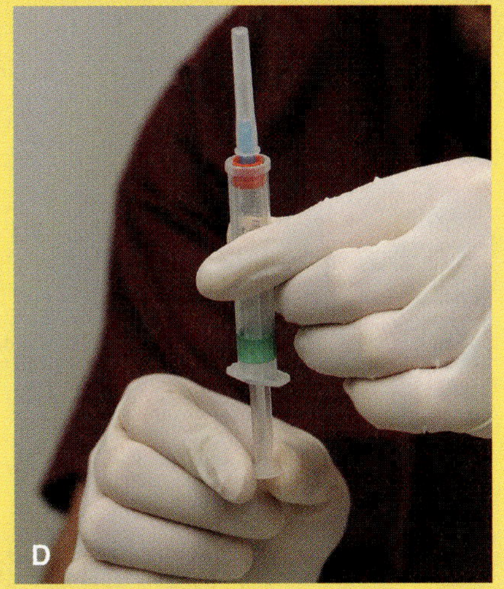

Figure 24-32 (Continued) (D) Pull the plunger to check for ease of gliding operation.

27. Correctly document procedure in patient's chart or electronic medical record. Return the vial to storage. Destroy medication note.

Procedure to follow should the medical assistant sustain an accidental needle-stick after the injection:

- Thoroughly wash the site where the stick occurred.
- Cleanse the skin with an antiseptic.
- Report the incident to your supervisor and manager.
- Document the incident and retain a copy for yourself.
- Obtain medical attention. Be tested for hepatitis B and C viruses and HIV.
- Fill out appropriate OSHA paperwork (200 form).

Procedure 24-5

Administering a Subcutaneous Injection

STANDARD PRECAUTIONS:

PURPOSE:

Correctly administer a subcutaneous injection after checking the provider's order and assembling the necessary equipment and supplies.

EQUIPMENT/SUPPLIES:

Medication ordered by provider	Alcohol wipes
Medication note	Gloves
Appropriately sized needle and syringe	Sharps container
	Adhesive strip
	Medicine tray

PROCEDURE STEPS:

1. Verify the provider's order. Write out a medication note.
2. Follow the "Six Rights."
3. Perform medical asepsis handwash. Adhere to OSHA guidelines.
4. Work in a well-lighted, quiet, clean area.
5. Select the appropriate equipment and supplies.
6. Select the correct medication.
7. Compare the medication label with the medication note (first time).
8. Check expiration date on medicine.
9. Calculate dosage, if necessary.
10. Correctly prepare the parenteral medication.
11. Compare medication label with the medication note (second time).
12. Correctly transport the medicine to the patient on the tray, with the vial and medication note.
13. Identify the patient. Explain the procedure.
14. Assess the patient. Put on gloves.
15. Prepare the patient for the injection (drape, position, allay apprehension).
16. Check syringe with the medication note (third time).

continues

Procedure 24-5 (continued)

17. Select an appropriate injection site.
18. Correctly cleanse the site with an alcohol wipe using a circular motion starting with the injection site and moving outward to a 2-inch diameter. Allow skin to dry.
19. Remove needle guard.
20. Grasp skin to form a 1-inch fold.
21. Insert needle quickly at a 45-degree angle (Figure 24-33).
22. Aspirate to be certain needle is not in a blood vessel.
23. Slowly inject the medicine.
24. Quickly remove the needle and syringe and activate the safety mechanism. Release the skin.
25. Immediately dispose of needle and syringe in a sharps container.
26. Cover site. Massage (unless contraindicated as with insulin, Imferon, and heparin).
27. Provide for patient's safety.
28. Properly dispose of used supplies. Remove gloves and wash hands. Return medication vial to storage.
29. Document procedure in patient's chart or electronic medical record. Destroy the medication note.

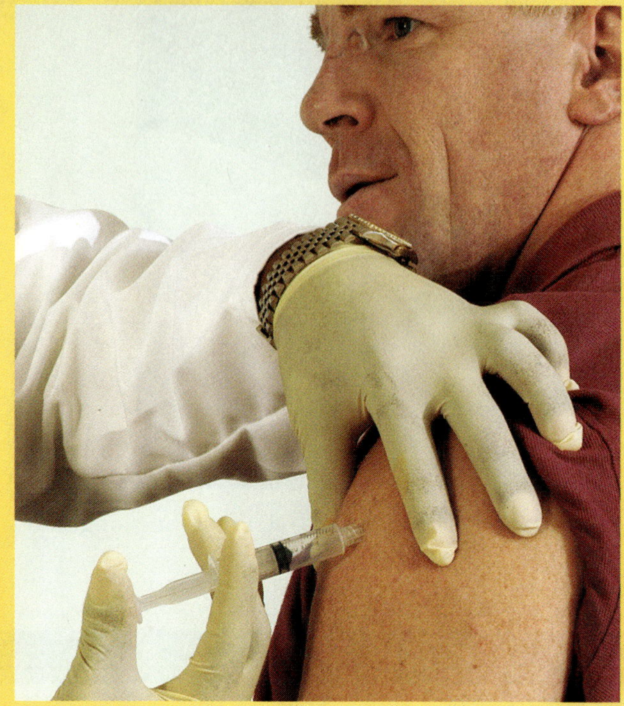

Figure 24-33 Insert needle at 45-degree angle into upper arm.

DOCUMENTATION

12/16/20XX 10:00 AM Sandostatin 100 mcg subcutaneously (L) deltoid. S. Jones, CMA (AAMA) ——————

Procedure 24-6

Administering an Intramuscular Injection

STANDARD PRECAUTIONS:

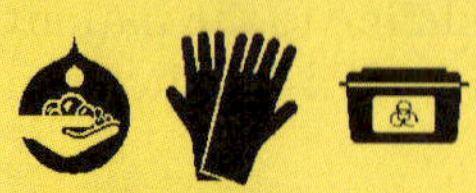

PURPOSE:

Correctly administer an intramuscular injection after receiving a provider's order and assembling the necessary equipment and supplies.

EQUIPMENT/SUPPLIES:

Medication ordered by provider with medication note
Appropriately sized needle and syringe
Alcohol wipes
Gloves
Sharps container
Medicine tray
Adhesive strip

continues

Procedure 24-6 (continued)

PROCEDURE STEPS:

1. Verify the provider's order. Write out a medication note.
2. Follow the "Six Rights."
3. Perform medical asepsis handwash. Adhere to OSHA guidelines.
4. Work in a well-lighted, quiet, clean area.
5. Obtain the appropriate equipment and supplies.
6. Obtain the correct medication.
7. Compare the medication label with the medication note (first time).
8. Check expiration date.
9. Calculate dosage, if necessary.
10. Correctly prepare the parenteral medication.
11. Compare medicine label with the medication note (second time).
12. Transport the medicine to the patient on tray, with the vial.
13. Identify the patient. Explain the procedure.
14. Assess the patient. Put on gloves.
15. Prepare the patient for the injection (drape, position, allay apprehension).
16. Compare the medication note with the medication (third time).
17. Select an appropriate injection site.
18. Correctly cleanse the site with an alcohol wipe using a circular motion and covering a 2-inch diameter. Allow the skin to dry.
19. Remove needle guard.
20. Stretch the skin **taut,** pulling it tight.
21. Using a dartlike motion, insert needle to the hub at a 90-degree angle (Figure 24-34).
22. Release the skin.
23. Aspirate to check for blood.
24. Slowly inject the medication.

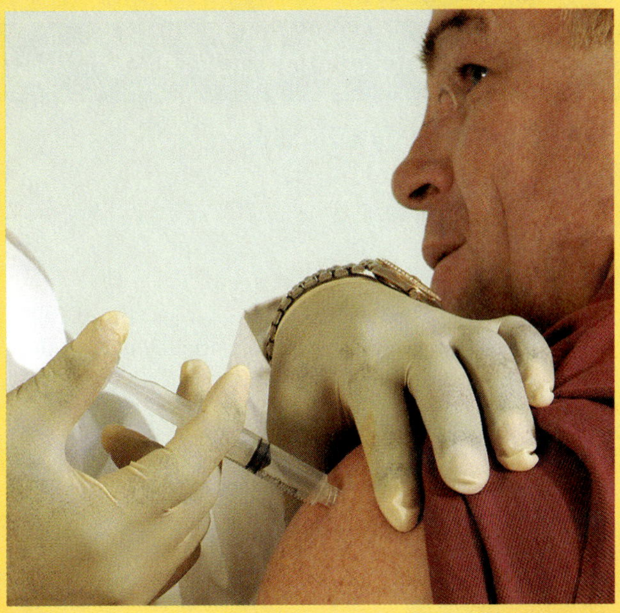

Figure 24-34 Using deltoid muscle, insert needle to the hub at a 90-degree angle.

25. Quickly remove the needle and syringe and activate safety mechanism.
26. Immediately dispose of needle and syringe in a sharps container.
27. Cover site. Massage (unless contraindicated as with insulin, Imferon, and heparin).
28. Dispose of equipment. Remove gloves.
29. Wash hands.
30. Observe the patient for signs of difficulty.
31. Provide for patient's safety. Return medication vial to storage.
32. Document procedure in patient's chart or electronic medical record. Destroy the medication note.

DOCUMENTATION

12/16/20XX 10:00 AM Demerol 75 mg IM (L) deltoid. S. Jones, CMA (AAMA) ———

Procedure 24-7

Administering an Intradermal Injection of Purified Protein Derivative (PPD)

STANDARD PRECAUTIONS:

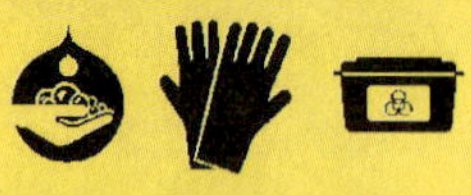

PURPOSE:

Correctly administer an intradermal injection of PPD after receiving a provider's order and assembling the necessary equipment and supplies.

EQUIPMENT/SUPPLIES:

Medication as ordered by provider with medication note
Appropriately sized needle and syringe
Alcohol wipes
Disposable gloves
Sharps container
Medicine tray
Adhesive strip

PROCEDURE STEPS:

1. Verify the provider's order. Write out a medication note.
2. Follow the "Six Rights."
3. Perform medical asepsis handwash. Adhere to OSHA guidelines.
4. Work in a well-lighted, quiet, clean area.
5. Organize the appropriate equipment and supplies.
6. Select the correct medication (PPD).
7. Compare the medication label with the medication note (first time).
8. Check expiration date.
9. Calculate dosage, if necessary.
10. Correctly prepare the parenteral medication.
11. Compare medication label with the medication note (second time).
12. Correctly transport the medication to the patient on tray with medication vial.
13. Identify the patient. Explain the procedure.
14. Assess the patient. Put on gloves.
15. Prepare the patient for the injection (drape, position, allay apprehension).
16. Check medication note with medication (third time).
17. Select an appropriate injection site (see Figure 24-19B).
18. Correctly cleanse the site with an alcohol wipe using a circular motion and covering a 2-inch diameter. Allow the skin to dry (Figure 24-35A).
19. Remove needle guard.
20. Pull the skin tissue taut.
21. Carefully insert the needle at a 10–15-degree angle, bevel upward to about ⅛ inch (Figure 24-35B). Do not aspirate. Release skin.
22. Steadily inject PPD to form a wheal (Figure 24-35C).
23. Correctly remove the needle after a brief delay. RATIONALE: Minimizes leakage.
24. Activate safety mechanism.

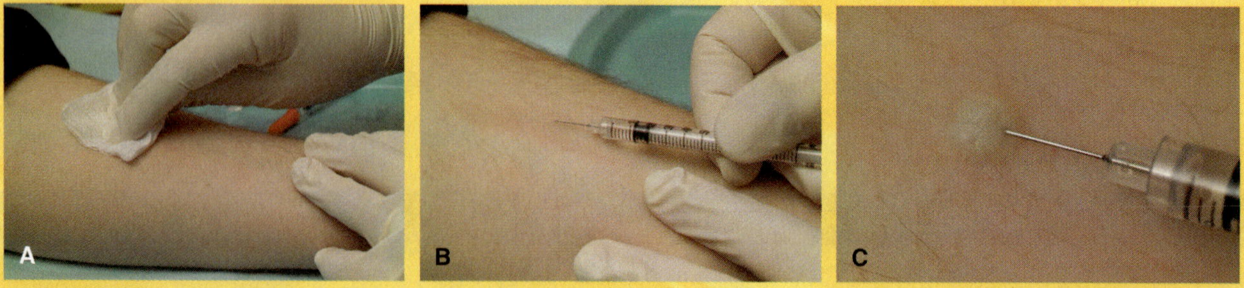

Figure 24-35 (A) Cleanse the injection site with alcohol and allow area to air-dry. (B) Insert the needle at a 10 to 15–degree angle, bevel upward about ⅛ inch. (C) Steadily inject the medicine, allowing a wheal to form.

continues

Procedure 24-7 (continued)

25. Immediately dispose of needle and syringe in a sharps container.
26. Blot site. Do not massage. Remove gloves.
27. Wash hands.
28. Observe the patient for signs of difficulty.
29. Provide for patient's safety.
30. Caution patient not to rub wheal.
31. Return vial to storage and document procedure in patient's chart or electronic medical record. Destroy the medication note.
32. The injected area should be read in 48 to 72 hours for the amount of induration (hardness) to determine tuberculosis exposure. Measure the induration. If injection area is hardened and elevated 10 mm or larger, the test is positive and the provider should be notified.

DOCUMENTATION

10/14/20XX 10:00 AM 0.1 mL PPD intradermally (L) forearm. Pt given appointment to return 10/16/20XX to have PPT read. S. Jones, CMA (AAMA) ——————

Procedure 24-8

Reconstituting a Powder Medication for Administration

STANDARD PRECAUTIONS:

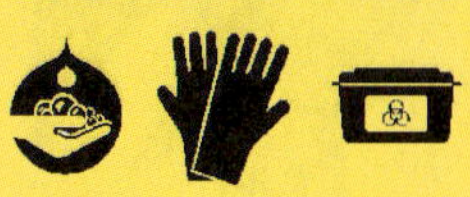

PURPOSE:

Drugs for injection may be supplied in a powdered (dry) form and must be reconstituted to a liquid for injection. A diluent (usually sterile water) is added to the powder, mixed well, and the appropriate dose is drawn up to be administered.

EQUIPMENT/SUPPLIES:

Medication as ordered by the provider and medication note
Diluent
Two appropriately sized needles and syringes
Alcohol wipes
Disposable gloves
Sharps container

PROCEDURE STEPS:

1. Prepare the needle–syringe unit in preparation for reconstituting powder medication.
2. Remove tops from diluent and powder medication containers and wipe with alcohol swabs (Figure 24-36A).
3. Insert the needle through the rubber stopper on the vial of diluent. The syringe should have an amount of air in it equal to the amount of diluent to be withdrawn (Figure 24-36B).
4. Withdraw the appropriate amount of diluent to be added to the powder medication (Figure 24-36C).
5. Inject the diluent into the powder medication vial (Figure 24-36D).
6. Remove needle from vial and discard into sharps container (Figure 24-36E).
7. Roll the vial between the palms of the hands to completely mix together the powder and diluent (Figure 24-36F). Label the multiple-dose vial with the dilution or strength of the medication prepared, the date and time, your initials, and the expiration date.
8. With a second sterile needle and syringe, withdraw the desired amount of medication (Figure 24-36G).
9. Flick away any air bubbles that cling to side of syringe (Figure 24-36H).
10. The medicine tray with reconstituted medication and medication note are ready for transport to the patient.
11. Proceed as in Steps 11 to 32 of Procedure 24-6, Administering an Intramuscular Injection.

continues

Procedure 24-8 (continued)

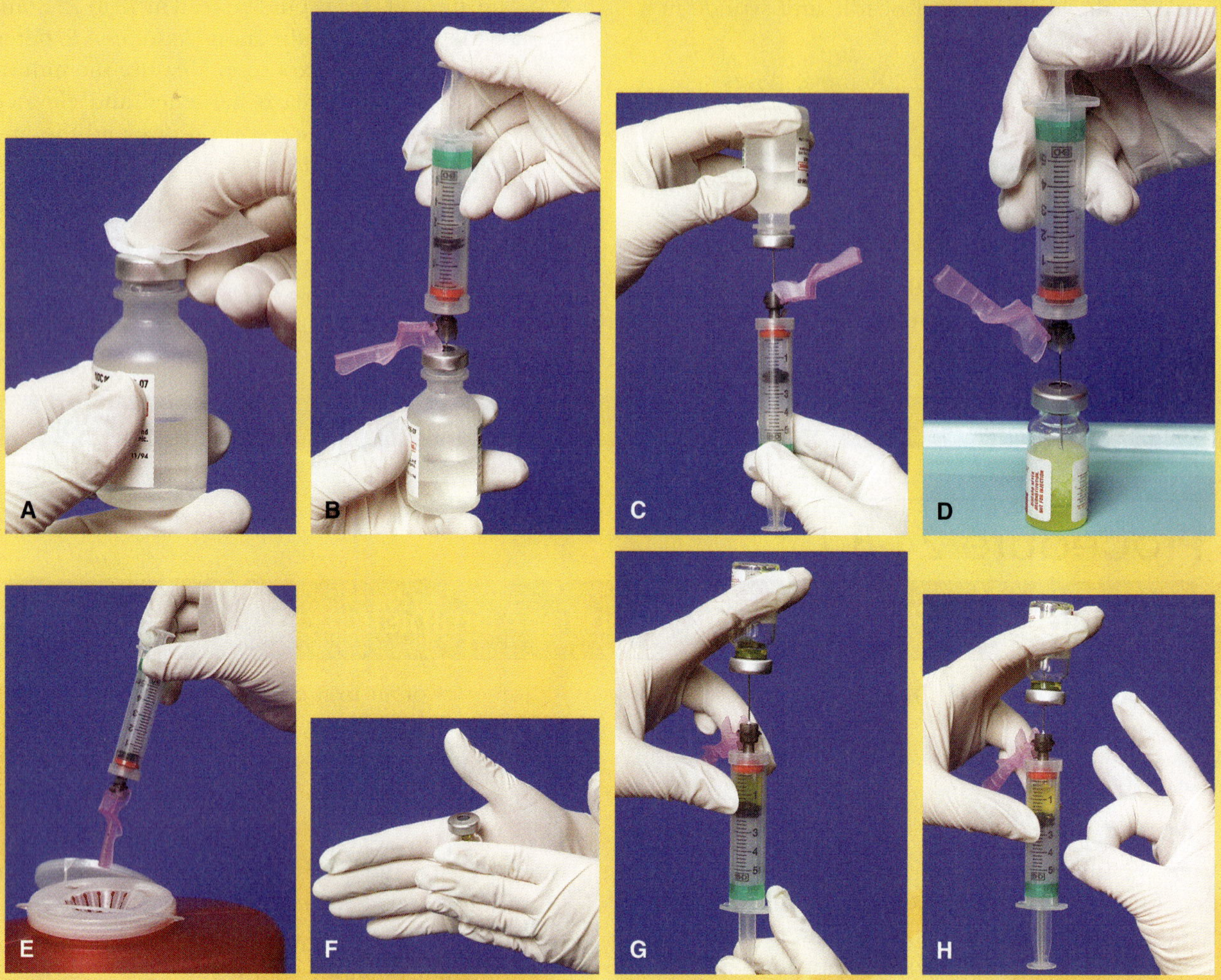

Figure 24-36 (A) Remove top from diluent and powdered medication. Wipe top of each with an alcohol wipe. (B) Inject air in an equal amount to diluent being removed from the vial. (C) Prepare to remove the needle from the vial after withdrawing diluent. (D) Inject diluent into vial containing powdered medication. (E) Discard safety needle–syringe unit. (F) Roll vial of solution medication between palms of hands to mix well. Label vial with date, amount of diluent added, strength of dilution, time mixed, and your initials. (G) Use a second sterile needle–syringe unit to draw the prescribed dose of medication ordered by the provider. (H) Flick away any air bubbles that cling to the side of the syringe. Withdraw more medication if needed. Labeled, reconstituted medication will be taken to the room with the syringe and placed on the shelf or in the refrigerator according to the manufacturer's instructions after the injection is given.

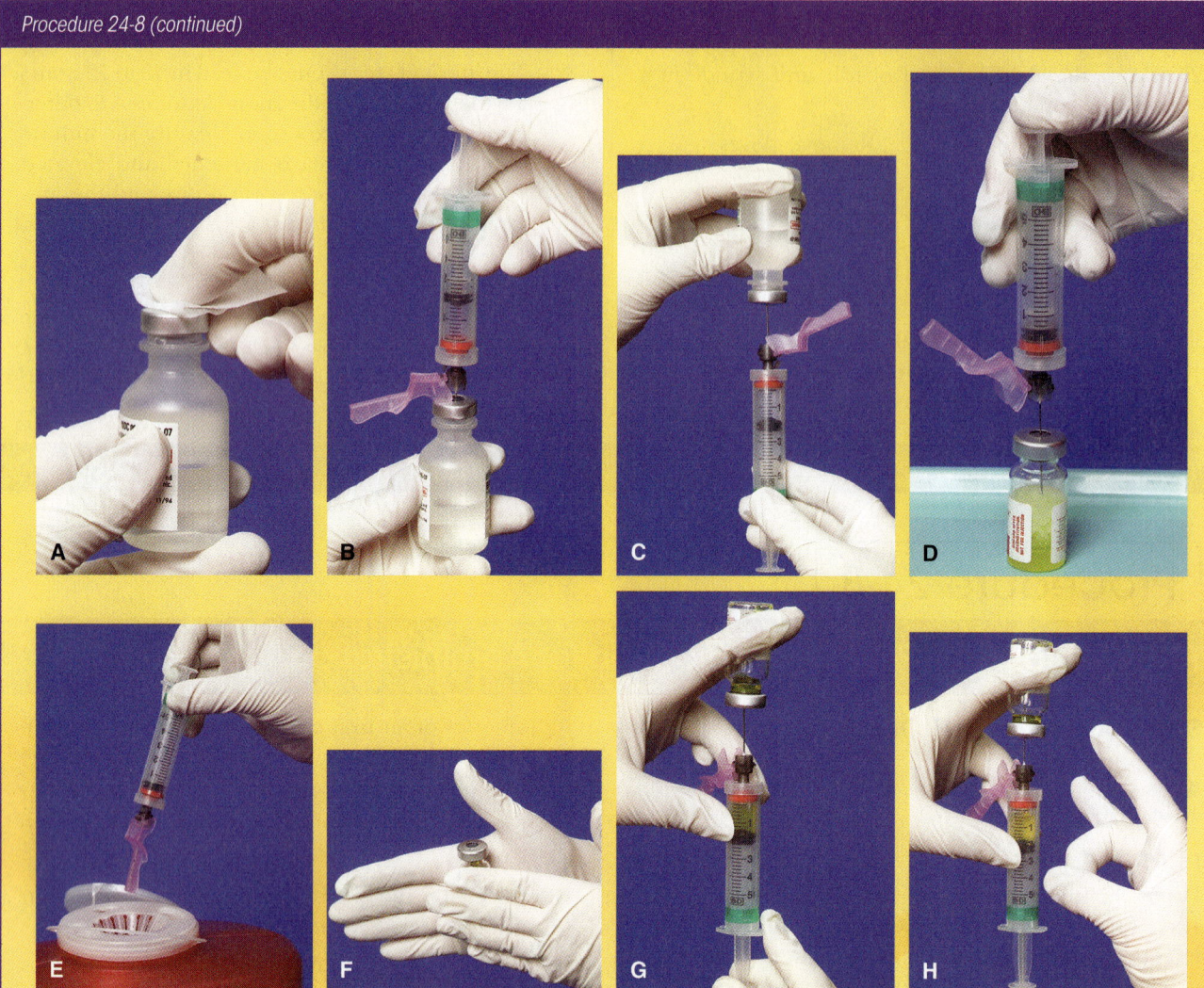

Procedure 24-9

Z-Track Intramuscular Injection Technique

STANDARD PRECAUTIONS:

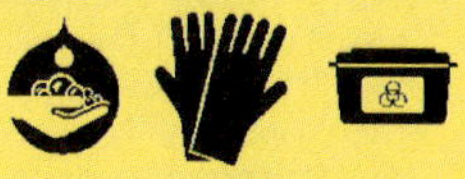

PURPOSE:

Correctly administer a Z-track intramuscular injection after receiving a provider's order and assembling the necessary equipment and supplies.

EQUIPMENT/SUPPLIES:

Medication ordered by provider and medication note
Appropriately sized needle and syringe
Alcohol wipes
Disposable gloves
Sharps container
Medicine tray
Adhesive strip

PROCEDURE STEPS:

1. Verify the provider's order. Write out a medication note.
2. Follow the "Six Rights."
3. Perform medical asepsis hand cleansing. Adhere to OSHA guidelines.
4. Work in a well-lighted, quiet, clean area.
5. Organize the appropriate equipment and supplies.
6. Select the correct medication.
7. Compare the medication label with the medication note (first time).
8. Check expiration date.
9. Calculate dosage, if necessary.
10. Correctly prepare the parenteral medication.
11. Compare medicine label with the medication note (second time).
12. Correctly transport the medicine to the patient.
13. Identify the patient. Explain the procedure.
14. Assess the patient. Put on gloves.
15. Prepare the patient for the injection (drape, position, allay apprehension).
16. Recheck medication note with the order and the syringe (third time).
17. Select an appropriate injection site.
18. Correctly cleanse the site with an alcohol wipe using a circular motion and covering a 6-inch diameter. Allow the skin to dry.
19. Remove needle guard.
20. Pull the skin laterally 1½ inch away from the injection site. RATIONALE: Prevents medication from leaking.
21. Insert needle quickly, using a dartlike motion at a 90-degree angle. Maintain Z position (Figure 24-37).
22. Aspirate to check for blood.
23. Slowly inject medication.
24. Wait 10 seconds before removing needle to allow medication to begin to be absorbed.
25. Remove needle and syringe at same angle of insertion.
26. Immediately release traction of the Z position to seal off the needle track. This prevents medication from reaching the subcutaneous tissues and the surface of the skin.
27. Immediately activate safety mechanism and dispose of needle–syringe unit in a sharps container.
28. Cover site. Do not massage.
29. Remove gloves. Wash hands.
30. Observe patient for signs of difficulty.
31. Provide for patient safety.
32. Return medication vial to storage.
33. Document procedure in patient's chart or electronic medical record.

DOCUMENTATION

12/01/20XX 2:00 PM Interferon 1,000,000 International units IM (R) Dorsogluteal muscle using Z-track technique. J. Guerro, CMA (AAMA) ——————

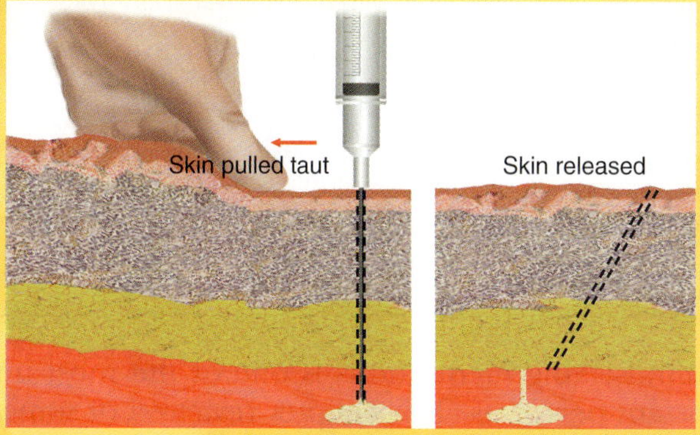

Figure 24-37 With client supine, grasp and pull the muscle laterally before injecting medication. Inject medication. Keep skin pulled taut for 10 seconds. Quickly withdraw the needle and release the skin to seal the site.

Case Study 24-1

Refer to the scenario at the beginning of the chapter.

CASE STUDY REVIEW

1. Explain the consequences of preparing and administering a medication without a medicine card.
2. Is it possible under normal circumstances to commit to memory the medication, dose, route, patient, and documentation?

Case Study 24-2

Abigail Johnson, a patient of Dr. Lewis, has been unable to keep her type 2 noninsulin-dependent diabetes mellitus under control with oral hypoglycemics, and Dr. Lewis has decided that Abigail needs to begin to take insulin injections. Today in the clinic, her fasting blood glucose level is 190 mg/mL. Dr. Lewis prescribes Humulin® insulin 10 units subcutaneously stat.

CASE STUDY REVIEW

1. What size insulin syringe should be used?
2. What does the medication label state are the number of units per milliliter? Show how to calculate the correct dosage.
3. Discuss the route of administration and the specifics about insulin administration that require it to be given slightly differently from other subcutaneous injections.
4. Describe several topics of discussion in which you would engage Abigail to help her learn how to better control her disease.

Case Study 24-3

Alice Chambers weighs 28 pounds and is 33 inches tall. The adult dose of erythromycin is 400 mg every 6 hours by mouth.

CASE STUDY REVIEW

1. Calculate the dose of erythromycin Alice needs.
2. If the provider ordered erythromycin by injection rather than by mouth, how would the dose be calculated if the erythromycin adult dose is 400 mg/mL?
3. What size needle and syringe are appropriate for giving Alice the injection?

SUMMARY

Administering medications is one of the most important and essential responsibilities that the medical assistant performs. This chapter reviewed of some of the fundamental elements of pharmacology, dosage calculations, and medication administration.

Each state has enacted laws governing the practice of medicine, nursing, and pharmacy. These laws vary from state to state; therefore, it is essential that medical assistants become familiar with the laws of the state in which they are employed before administering any medication.

Under the law, those administering medications are expected to be knowledgeable about the drugs that they administer and the effects the drug may or will have on the patient. They are responsible for their own actions.

STUDY FOR SUCCESS

To reinforce your knowledge and skills of information presented in this chapter:

- Review the Key Terms
- Practice the Procedures
- Consider the Case Studies and discuss your conclusions
- Answer the Review Questions
  - Multiple Choice
  - Critical Thinking
- Navigate the Internet by completing the Web Activities
- Practice the StudyWARE activities on your student CD
- Apply your knowledge in the Student Workbook activities
- Complete the Web Tutor sections
- View and discuss the DVD situations

REVIEW QUESTIONS

Multiple Choice

1. A written legal document that gives directions for compounding, dispensing, and administering medication to a patient is a:
   a. medication note
   b. prescription
   c. medication order
   d. subscription
2. An abbreviation symbol that means nothing by mouth is:
   a. non rep
   b. NPO
   c. IM
   d. mm
3. Insulin-dependent diabetes mellitus is:
   a. Type 1
   b. Type 2
   c. Type 3
   d. Type 4
4. Body surface area is used:
   a. when calculating children's dosages
   b. when calculating adult dosages
   c. when determining an injection site
   d. when selecting an appropriately sized needle
5. An injection given just below the surface of the skin at a 15-degree angle is called a(n):
   a. intramuscular injection
   b. intradermal injection
   c. subcutaneous injection
   d. parenteral injection

Critical Thinking

1. Describe the process to follow to determine the state law regarding a medical assistant administering medications.
2. What is a medication order? Describe its purpose.
3. List nine parts of a prescription and define each part.
4. Name and describe factors that can affect medication dosage. Explain why and how the dosage is affected.
5. List the fundamental units of the metric system.
6. Name two methods used to calculate children's dosages of medication.
7. List and describe the "Six Rights."
8. A fellow student tells you that she accidentally gave a patient the incorrect dose of medication. Explain in detail what should be done.
9. You accidentally stick yourself with a used needle. What are the steps to take?
10. Discuss allergenic extracts. What are they? What safeguards are needed after administration?
11. List two reasons for the provider to prescribe oxygen for a patient. Describe how oxygen is administered and oxygen safety.

Calculation Problems

1. Calculate the following dosages according to body surface area (BSA):

   If the adult dose of E.E.S. tabs is 400 mg every 6 hours, what is the dosage for a child who is 35 inches tall and weighs 28 pounds (BSA 0.57)?

   If the adult dose of penicillin V potassium, USP, is 250 mg every 6 to 8 hours, what is the dosage for a child who is 24 inches tall and weighs 35 pounds (BSA 0.56)?
2. Calculate the following dosages according to kilogram of body weight:

   The provider orders Augmentin 20 mg/kg/day for Sally Whitney, who weighs 72 pounds. The dose is to be divided and given every 8 hours. What is the total dose? What is the amount to be given every 8 hours?

   The provider orders Cefadyl 40 mg/kg for George Kipperley, who weighs 78 pounds. The dose is to be divided into four equal doses. What is the total dose? What is the amount to be given in four equal doses?

   The provider orders Garamycin 2.0 mg/kg every 8 hours for a child who weighs 86 pounds. What is the correct dosage?
3. The provider ordered 64 units of U-100 Humulin insulin. Shade the correct dosage on the U-100 syringe pictured.

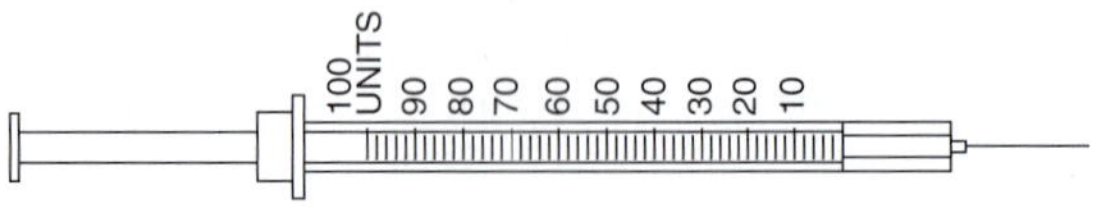

Using the proportional or formula method, calculate the following dosages.

4. The provider orders 125 mg of Diamox. On hand you have 250-mg tablets. You will give ____ tablets to your patient.
5. The provider orders 250 mg of Tagamet liquid. On hand you have 300 mg/5 mL. How many milliliters will you give?

WEB ACTIVITIES

1. Search for a Web site to explore the various types of safety needles available for injection and venipuncture. What is the most recent ruling by OSHA in regard to these types of needles?
2. Check the Web site http://www.cerner.com and search for the following:
   a. What is the most common medication error?
   b. Which group of medical professionals makes the most medication errors?
   c. How can medication errors be prevented?

REFERENCES/BIBLIOGRAPHY

Centers for Disease Control and Prevention, Division of Health Care Quality Promotion (2004, February). *Workbook for designing, implementing, and evaluating a sharps injury prevention program.* Retrieved August 9, 2004, from http://cdc.gov/sharpsafety/wk_info.html.

Centers for Disease Control and Prevention. (2006). *Health care workers and regulations regarding safety needles.* Retrieved October 15, 2008, from http://www.cdc.gov/features/medicationsafety.

Josephson, D. (2004). *Intravenous infusion therapy for nurses principle and practice.* (2nd ed.). Clifton Park, NY: Delmar Cengage Learning.

Keir, L., Wise, B., Krebs, C., & Kelley-Arney, C. (2008). Medical assisting administrative and clinical competencies (6th ed.). Clifton Park, NY: Delmar Cengage Learning.

Prescription for drug safety. (2003, March). *Consumer Reports on Health, 15*(3), 1, 4–6.

Rice, J., (2006). *Principles of pharmacology for medical assisting* (4th ed.). Clifton Park, NY: Delmar Cengage Learning.

Spratto, G., & Woods, A. (2009). *Delmar Nurse's Drug Handbook 2009 Edition.* Clifton Park, NY: Delmar Cengage Learning.

Taber's cyclopedic medical dictionary (22nd ed.). (2005). Philadelphia: F. A. Davis.

To the point. (2004, August 2). *Advance for nursing serving RN's in New England, 4*(17), 30–31.

THE DVD HOOK-UP

This chapter discussed the medical assistant's role in prescription writing, administering nonparenteral medications, and administering parenteral medications.

In one of the first scenes in Program 9, the provider gave Tyrah verbal medication orders for two separate patients. In cases where the provider dictates his or her notes, he or she may not have anything written in the chart so he or she may give a verbal order to save time.

1. What did Tyrah do as soon as the provider gave her the verbal orders?
2. You will notice that the provider used common prescription abbreviations when talking to Tyrah. Do you think that was wise? What are some of the abbreviations that the provider used that are no longer considered acceptable with certain governmental agencies?
3. What did you think of Tyrah's nails when she demonstrated the inhaler?
4. Do you think there was a more sanitary way of demonstrating the inhaler instead of using the patient's inhaler? Should Tyrah have observed Mrs. Edmonson when she practiced her inhaler?

You will notice that the book illustrates the medical assistant wearing gloves when withdrawing medications; however, Program 10 of the DVD program showed the medical assistant without gloves drawing up medication.

1. Why might it be a bit more sanitary to wear gloves when drawing up medications?
2. The medical assistant in the DVD program allowed the alcohol to dry before administering the injection. Is this acceptable with your teacher? What is the purpose of allowing the alcohol to dry before injecting the patient?

DVD Journal Summary

Write a paragraph that summarizes what you learned from watching today's DVD programs. Making a medication error could result in a negative reaction or even death to the patient. Write a paragraph that will reassure your instructors that you will be cautious when drawing up and administering medications.

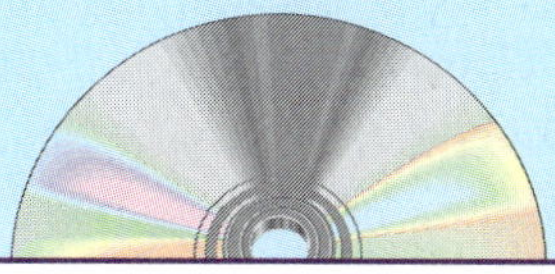

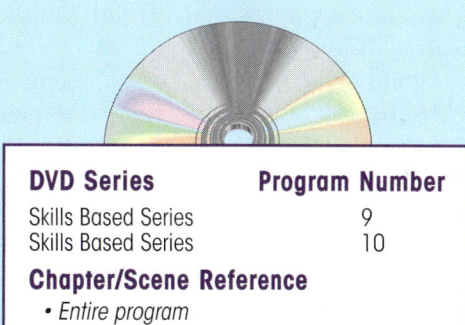

DVD Series	**Program Number**
Skills Based Series	9
Skills Based Series	10

Chapter/Scene Reference

- *Entire program*

Chapter 25

Electrocardiography

OUTLINE

Anatomy of the Heart
Electrical Conduction System of the Heart
The Cardiac Cycle and the ECG Cycle
- Calculation of Heart Rate on ECG Graph Paper

Types of Electrocardiographs
- Single-Channel Electrocardiograph
- Multichannel Electrocardiograph
- Automatic Electrocardiograph Machines
- Electrocardiograph Telephone Transmissions
- Facsimile Electrocardiograph
- Interpretive Electrocardiograph

ECG Equipment
- Electrocardiograph Paper
- Electrolyte
- Sensors or Electrodes
- Lead Wires
- Electrocardiograph Machine
- Care of Equipment

Lead Coding
The Electrocardiograph and Sensor Placement
- Standard Limb or Bipolar Leads
- Augmented Leads
- Chest Leads or Precordial Leads

Standardization and Adjustment of the Electrocardiograph
Standard Resting Electrocardiography
Mounting the ECG Tracing
Interference or Artifacts
- Somatic Tremor Artifacts
- AC Interference
- Wandering Baseline Artifacts
- Interrupted Baseline Artifacts
- Patients with Unique Problems

Myocardial Infarctions (Heart Attacks)
Cardiac Arrhythmias
- Atrial Arrhythmias
- Ventricular Arrhythmias

Defibrillation
Other Cardiac Diagnostic Tests
- Holter Monitor (Portable Ambulatory Electrocardiograph)
- Loop ECG
- Treadmill Stress Test or Exercise Tolerance ECG
- Thallium Stress Test
- Echocardiography/Ultrasonography

Cardiac Procedures
- Procedures for Heart Disease
- Procedures for Arrhythmias

KEY TERMS

Amplified
Amplitude
Angiogram
Arrhythmia
Artifact
Augment
Baseline
Bipolar
Bradycardia, Sinus
Calibration
Cardiac Catheterization
Cardiac Cycle
Cardioversion
Countershock
Defibrillation
Defibrillator
Deoxygenated
Depolarization
Diastole
Electrocardiogram
Electrocardiograph
Electrocardiography
Electrodes
Electrolyte
Galvanometer
Implantable Cardioverter Defibrillator (ICD)
Infarction
Ischemia
Isoelectric
Lead Wires
Mounting
Noninvasive
Normal Sinus Rhythm

OBJECTIVES

The student should strive to meet the following performance objectives and demonstrate an understanding of the facts and principles presented in this chapter through written and oral communication.

1. Define the key terms as presented in the glossary.
2. Follow the circulation of blood through the heart starting at the vena cavae.
3. Describe the electrical conduction system of the heart.
4. State three reasons why patients may need an electrocardiogram (ECG).
5. Identify the various positive and negative deflections and describe what each represents in the cardiac cycle.
6. Explain the purpose of standardization of the ECG.
7. Identify the 12 leads of an ECG and describe what area of the heart each lead represents.
8. State the function of ECG graph paper, electrodes (sensors), and electrolyte.
9. Describe various types of ECGs and their capabilities.
10. Explain each type of artifact and how each can be eliminated.
11. Name and describe the purposes of the various cardiac diagnostic tests and procedures as outlined in this chapter.
12. Identify the placement of Holter monitor electrodes.
13. Describe the reason for a patient activity diary during ambulatory electrocardiography.
14. Identify six arrhythmias and explain the cause of each.
15. Explain how to calculate heart rates from an ECG tracing.
16. Identify a common coding system used to code each lead on an ECG tracing.
17. Describe the procedure for mounting an ECG tracing.

KEY TERMS (continued)

Oscilloscope
Precordial
Repolarization
Rhythm Strip
Sensor
Sonographer
Stylus
Syncope
Systole
Tachycardia, Sinus
Test Cable
Thallium Scan
Tracing
Transducer
Ultrasonography
Unipolar

Scenario

Wanda Slawson, CMA (AAMA), clinical medical assistant at Inner City Health Care, recently had her own physical examination that included her first electrocardiogram (ECG). This is now Wanda's baseline ECG, which provides a basis for future ECG readings to be compared. Because Wanda currently has no heart problems, future tests will indicate differences from her normal baseline ECG. It was different for Wanda to be the patient versus the person performing the ECG. Having the test performed on her, Wanda can now relate to feelings many of her patients must have felt when having an ECG. These included feelings of fear that the test may be abnormal; a cold feeling because even though the room temperature was normal, she was partially uncovered and the pads were cold when applied; and anxiousness because she found it difficult to stay completely still through the entire tracing. Wanda could empathize more with her patients after she had the test than she did before her test. Wanda now makes a more concerted effort to allay patient fears and make patients comfortable during ECGs.

INTRODUCTION

Many providers include an ***electrocardiogram*** *(ECG or EKG) as part of a complete physical examination, especially for patients who are 40 years or older, for patients with a family history of cardiac disease, or for patients who have experienced chest pain. It is a noninvasive, safe, and painless procedure that can provide valuable information about the health of the patient's heart or suspected cardiac symptoms. A graphic representation of the heart's electrical activity, an ECG measures the amount of the electrical activity produced by the heart and the time necessary for the electrical impulses to travel through the heart during each heartbeat.*

Some reasons for ***electrocardiography*** *are to: (1) detect myocardial* ***ischemia,*** *(2) estimate damage to the myocardium caused by a myocardial* ***infarction,*** *(3) detect and evaluate cardiac* ***arrhythmia,*** *(4) assess effects of cardiac medication on the heart, and (5) determine if electrolyte imbalance is present. An ECG cannot always detect impending heart disease or cardiovascular disease. The ECG is used in conjunction with other laboratory and diagnostic tests to assess total cardiac health. An ECG alone cannot diagnose disease.*

In a medical office or ambulatory care setting, it is the medical assistant who records the ECG; therefore, special knowledge and skills are necessary and include these aspects of the correct electrocardiography procedures: patient preparation; operation of the ***electrocardiograph;*** *elimination of* ***artifacts, mounting,*** *and labeling the ECG; and maintenance and care of the instrument.*

Spotlight on Certification

RMA Content Outline

- Body systems
- Disorders and diseases
- Patient education
- Vital signs and mensurations
- Electrocardiography

CMA (AAMA) Content Outline

- Anatomy and physiology
- Communication
- Equipment preparation and operation
- Performing selected tests

CMAS Content Outline

- Anatomy and physiology
- Vital signs and measurements
- Examination preparation
- Medical office emergencies

ANATOMY OF THE HEART

The heart has four chambers: two upper chambers known as atria, and two lower chambers known as ventricles. **Deoxygenated** blood enters the right atrium from the superior and inferior vena cavae and passes through the tricuspid valve into the right ventricle. In a healthy heart, the blood between right and left sides cannot mix together. It then travels to the lungs via the pulmonary arteries. The deoxygenated blood gives off the carbon dioxide and picks up oxygen in the capillary bed of the lungs. Oxygenated blood is pumped through the pulmonary vein into the left atrium, through the mitral valve, into the left ventricle. The oxygenated blood then passes through the aortic valve into the aorta and from the aorta to all cells, tissues, and organs of the body (Figure 25-1). The cycle begins with each heartbeat.

On its external surface, the heart is surrounded by coronary arteries that supply the myocardium with its blood supply, from which oxygen and nutrients are obtained (see the section on the circulatory system in Chapter 18).

ELECTRICAL CONDUCTION SYSTEM OF THE HEART

There are basically two kinds of cardiac cells: electrical cardiac cells and myocardial cells. The electrical cells, which are located in distinct pathways around and through the heart, are sensitive to electrical impulses. Their pathways are referred to as the conduction system of the heart and have specific names.

The body's natural pacemaker, the sinoatrial (SA) node, is located in the upper part of the right atrium. It sends out an electrical impulse that begins and regulates the heartbeat. When the electrical impulses are sent along the pathways or conduction system of the heart (via the electrical cells), the myocardial cells contract, causing the heart muscle to pump the blood from chamber to chamber and through the lungs. The contraction of the cardiac cells is called **depolarization** (from the electrical "discharge"). The first chambers affected (contracted) by the electrical discharge

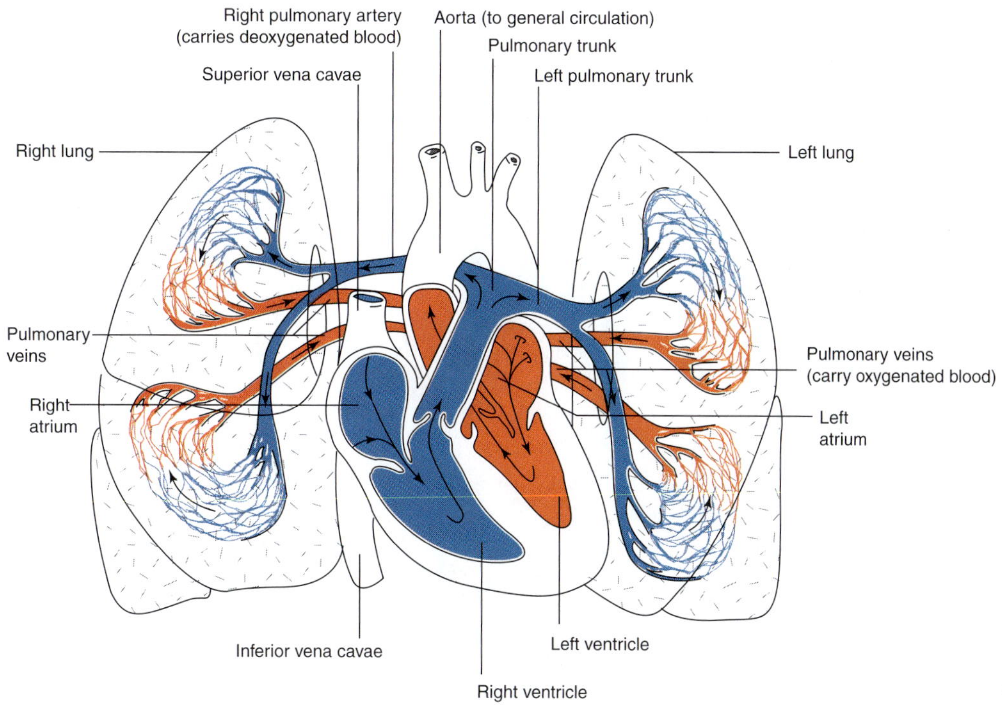

Figure 25-1 Oxygenated blood passing through the heart and then to the rest of the body.

from the SA node are the atria. From the atria, the electrical impulses travel along the conduction system toward the ventricles, to the atrioventricular (AV) node, located at the base of the right atrium. From here, the electrical impulses are transmitted to the bundle of His. The bundle of His divides into right and left bundle branches that continue the electrical impulses on to the Purkinje fibers. These fibers disperse the electrical impulses to the right and left ventricles, causing them to contract. The heart recovers electrically **(repolarization)**, then relaxes briefly (polarization), and then a new impulse is begun by the SA node and the cycle begins again (Figure 25-2). This cycle is known as the **cardiac cycle** and it represents one heartbeat. The electrocardiograph records the electrical activity that causes the contraction **(systole)** and the relaxation **(diastole)** of the atria and ventricles. The ECG cycle is the recording or the graphic representation of the cardiac cycle. These electrical impulses can be recorded on special ECG paper or displayed on an **oscilloscope.**

THE CARDIAC CYCLE AND THE ECG CYCLE

The **baseline,** or **isoelectric,** line is the flat line that separates the various waves. It is present when there is no current flowing in the heart. The waves are either deflecting upward, known as positive deflection, or deflecting downward, known as negative deflection from the baseline.

The P, QRS, and T waves, recorded during the ECG, represent the depolarization (contraction) and repolarization (recovery) of the myocardial cells. The P wave represents atrial depolarization and is recorded as a positive deflection. The QRS complex represents ventricular depolarization and is measured from the beginning of the first wave of the QRS to the end of the last wave of the QRS complex (see Figure 25-2). The T wave represents ventricular repolarization and is a positive deflection. The recovery of the atria is so slight, it is lost behind the QRS complex.

Each complete cardiac cycle takes about 0.8 second, with each wave taking an appropriate amount of time if the heart is healthy. By observing and measuring the size, shape, and location of each wave on an ECG recording, the provider can analyze and interpret the conduction of electricity through the cardiac cells, the heart's rhythm and rate, and the health of the heart in general.

Calculation of Heart Rate on ECG Graph Paper

ECG graph paper is divided into 1-mm squares (small squares) and 5-mm squares (large squares). Each large square consists of 25 small squares and is

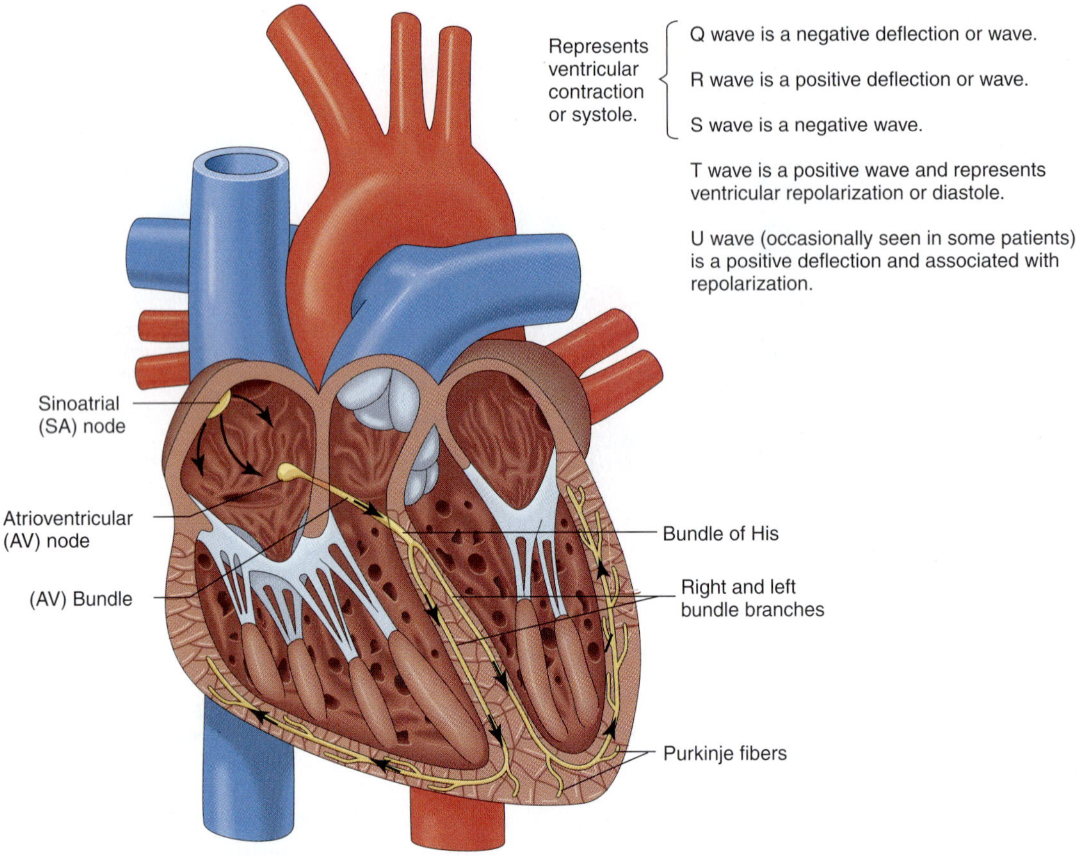

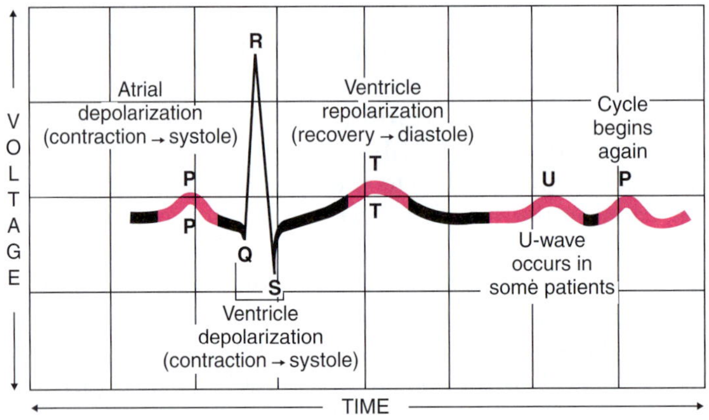

Figure 25-2 The heartbeat is controlled by electrical impulses that comprise the continuous cardiac cycle.

5 mm high and 5 mm wide. On the horizontal line, one small square represents 0.04 second. On the vertical line, one small square represents 1 mm of voltage. Because a large square is five small squares wide and five deep, each small square represents 0.2 second horizontal and 5 mm vertical. *NOTE:* Every fifth line, both horizontally and vertically, is darker than the other lines, making squares that are 5 × 5 mm (Figure 25-3). These measurements are accepted worldwide and enable the provider to interpret the time of each deflection on the horizontal line and cardiac electrical activity (voltage) on the vertical line to help determine cardiac health.

Because all cardiac complexes consist of P, QRS, and T waves, and the electrocardiograph paper measures time on the horizontal line, it is possible to calculate heart rate. Count the number of 5-mm boxes (number within the dark lines) between two R waves. Divide this number into 300. The result is the heart rate in beats per minute.

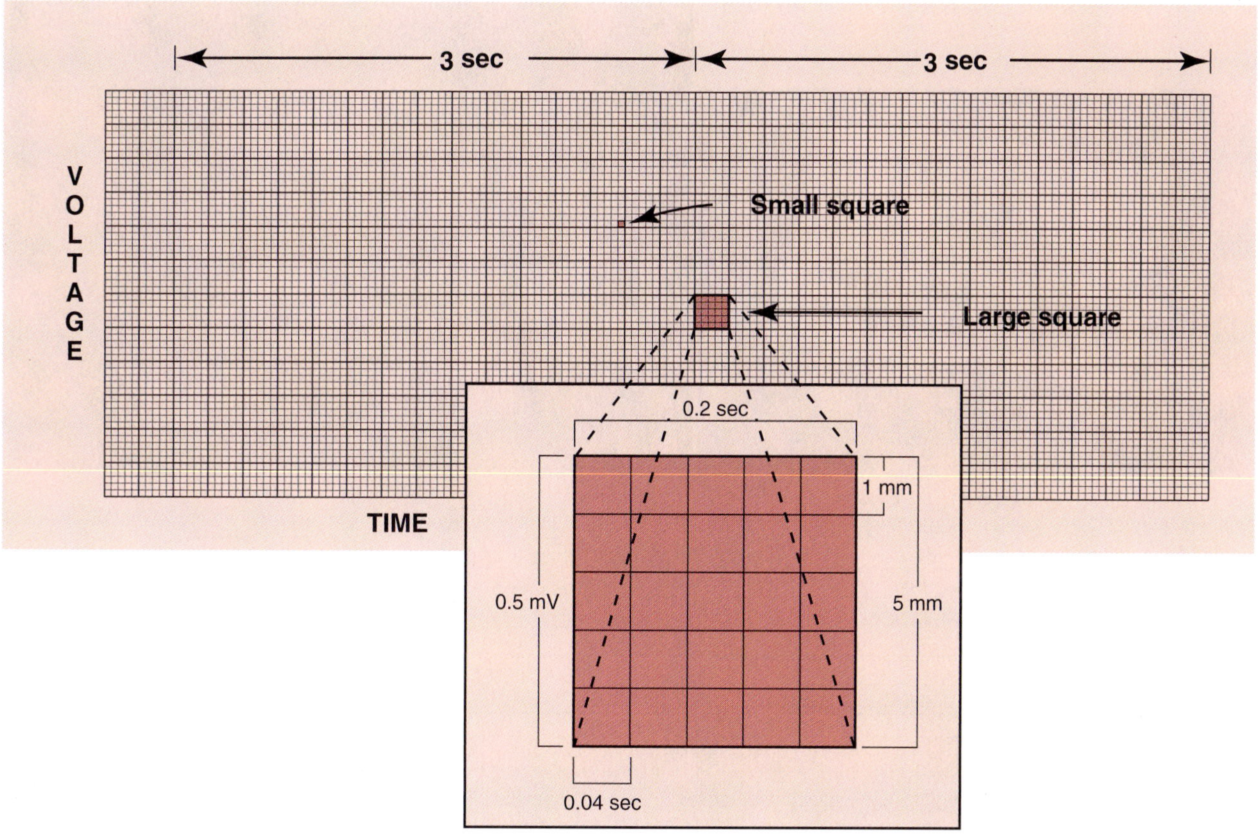

Figure 25-3 Electrocardiogram graph paper measurements allow medical professionals to determine the time and voltage of heartbeats. (A) The small square is 1 mm wide and 1 mm high. One small square = 0.04 second. (B) The large square consists of 25 small squares and measures 5 mm wide and 5 mm high. One large square = 0.04 second × 5, or 0.2 second.

Example:

One small square (1 mm) = 0.04 second in time
One large square (5 mm) = 0.04 × 5 = 0.2 second
Divide 60 seconds (1 minute) by 0.2 second 60 ÷ 0.2 = 300

Example:

There are three large squares between two R waves.

300 ÷ 3 = 100

The heartrate is 100 beats per minute.

Critical Thinking

Explain the significance of the small and large boxes on ECG paper. There are 2.5 large boxes between each cardiac cycle. What is the heart rate in beats per minute?

TYPES OF ELECTROCARDIOGRAPHS

Single-Channel Electrocardiograph

A conventional 12-lead single-channel electrocardiograph can be used in either manual mode or automatic mode. When using automatic mode, the 12-lead ECG tracing is complete in less than 40 seconds. With a single-channel machine, only one lead can be recorded at a time. If not automatic, the single-channel ECG requires manually turning the lead selector on and off between each of the 12 leads. It may also require the leads to be coded so that they can be identified later and properly mounted. Lead coding and mounting are explained more fully later in this chapter. The ECG tracing from a single-channel machine will need to be cut and mounted onto special forms for filing into the patient record. Figure 25-4 shows a sample of a single-channel electrocardiograph machine and tracing.

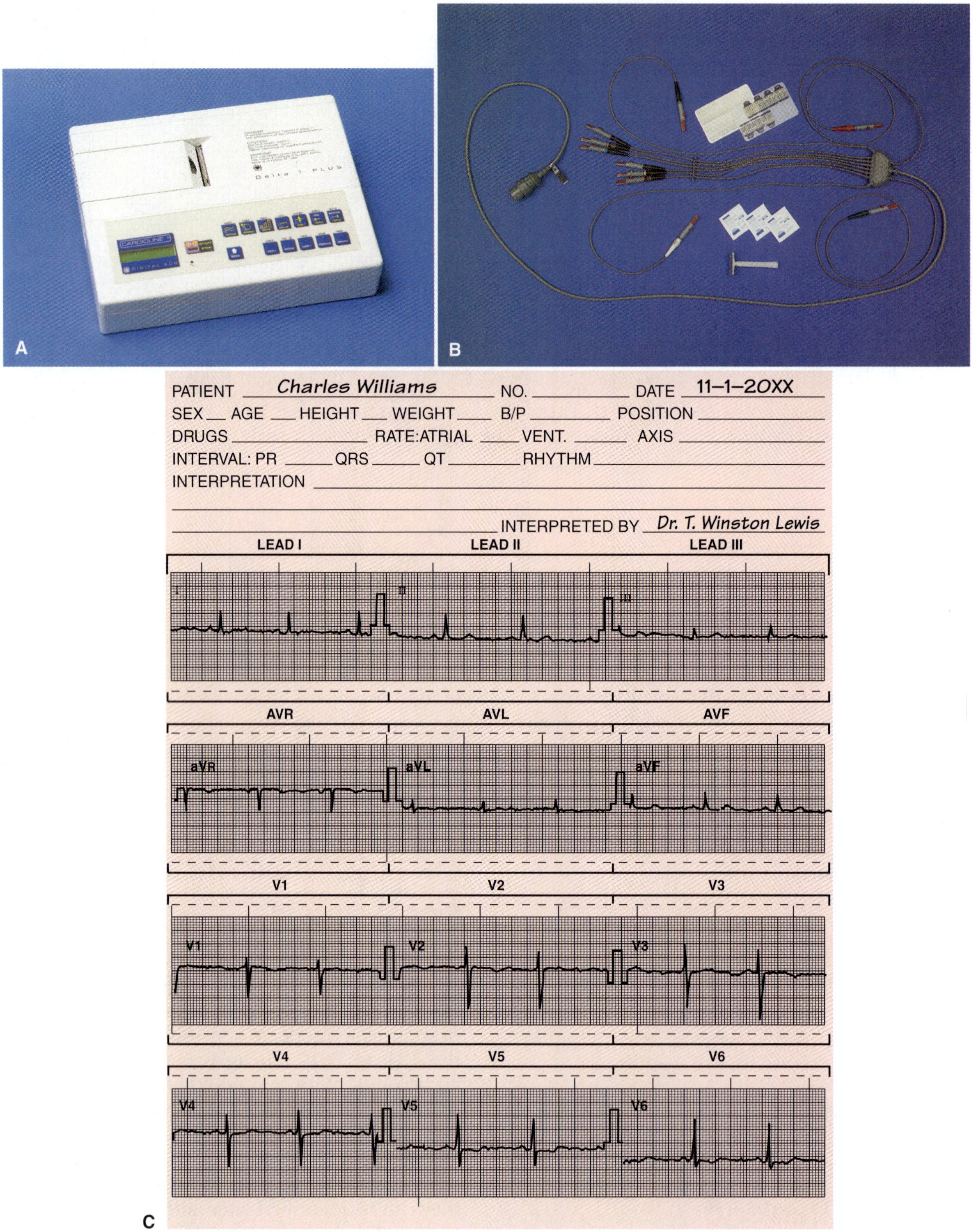

Figure 25-4 (A) Single-channel 12-lead electrocardiograph machine. (B) Supplies for single-channel 12 lead electrocardiograph. (C) Mounted single ECG tracing or recording.

Multichannel Electrocardiograph

An electrocardiograph that can simultaneously record several different leads is known as a multichannel electrocardiograph. The conventional electrocardiograph records one lead at a time. A three-channel machine, one type of multichannel electrocardiograph, records three channels at one time. It records lead I, II, and III, followed by aVR, aVL, and aVF, followed by V_1, V_2, and V_3, followed by V_4, V_5, and V_6. The advantage of the multichannel machine is its speed. The most common multichannel machine used in the provider's office is the three-channel machine. This type of machine requires three-channel recording paper that is 8½ × 11 inches and fits into the patient record with no cutting or mounting. Figure 25-5 shows an example of a multichannel tracing. Other multichannel electrocardiograph machines are available, such as 6- and 12-channel machines. Some have a built-in rechargeable battery, an interpretation software program, a spirometery module, and transmission capability.

Automatic Electrocardiograph Machines

When using an automatic electrocardiograph, the lead length and switching of leads are done automatically by the electrocardiograph and there is no need to advance the control knob. For these reasons, both time and paper can be saved with the automatic machine. The automatic machine also comes equipped with a manual control that can be used if a longer tracing is necessary.

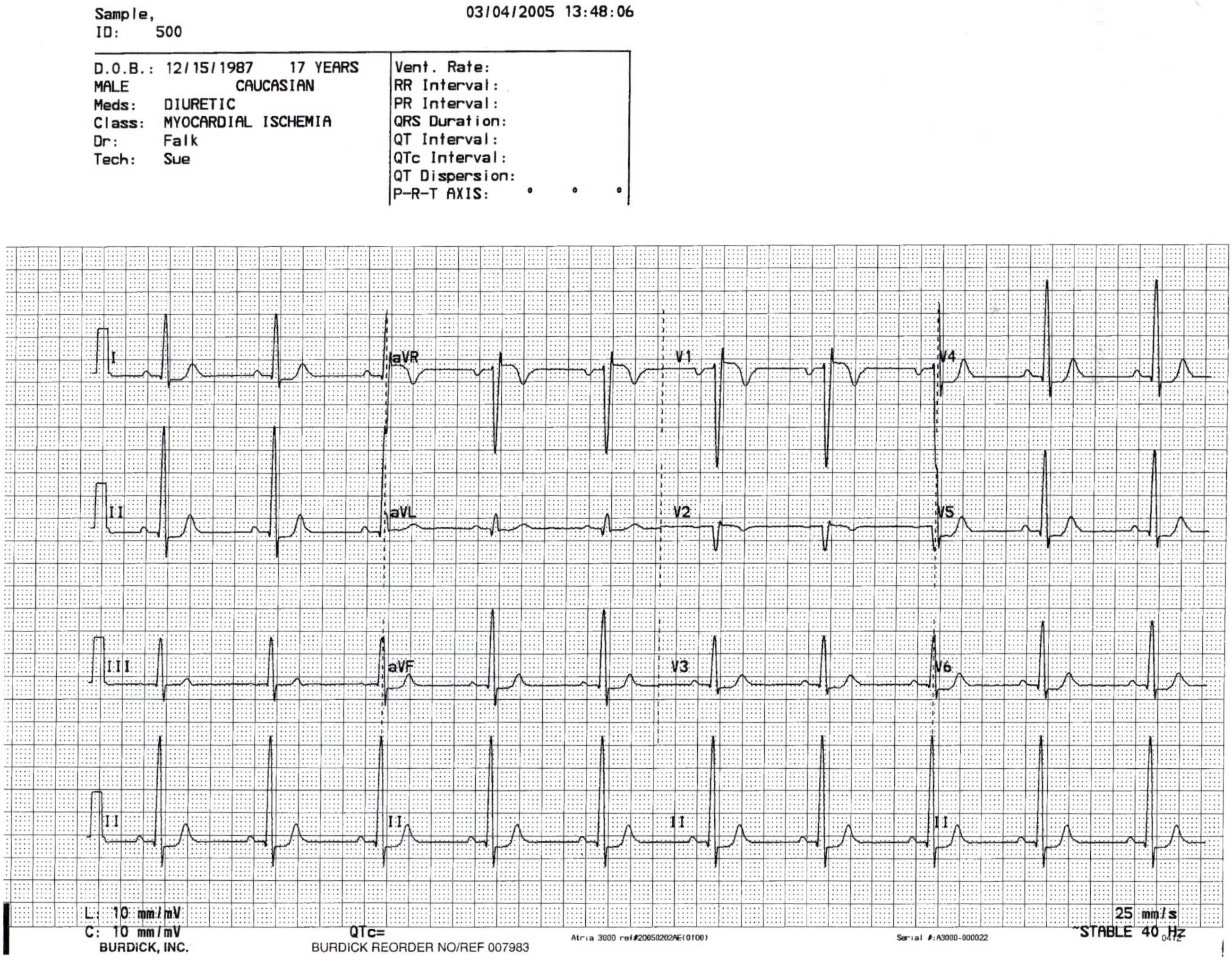

Figure 25-5 Example of three-channel electrocardiogram recording in which three leads are recorded simultaneously. (Courtesy of Quinton Cardiology, Inc.)

Electrocardiograph Telephone Transmissions

An electrocardiogram can be transmitted via a telephone line to an ECG interpretation site when using an electrocardiograph with such capabilities. A recording printout and interpretation (many times interpretation is done by a cardiologist or by a computer) are transmitted automatically on the electrocardiograph. Results of the ECG can be transmitted verbally as well.

Facsimile Electrocardiograph

The provider may need a rapid, expert ECG interpretation from an off-site diagnostician. Direct ECG fax transmits from the electrocardiograph to a fax machine, and a high-quality facsimile is produced and sent to a diagnostician, who calls back with a reading. This saves time by eliminating the step of copying the report and sending it via the traditional fax machine.

Interpretive Electrocardiograph

The interpretive electrocardiograph has a built-in computer program that interprets the ECG tracing while it is being recorded, allowing for faster diagnosis and treatment. The provider in charge will review the tracing before a diagnosis is confirmed and treatment is begun.

ECG EQUIPMENT

Electrocardiograph Paper

ECG paper can be either black or dark blue and is wax or plastic coated with a white or pink background and color lines. The paper is heat and pressure sensitive. As the heated **stylus** of the electrocardiograph moves across the paper, the background coating is melted away, revealing the black or blue color of the paper, and the ECG cycles are recorded or traced. The heat of the stylus can be adjusted to obtain a sharp, clear recording, or **tracing**. Medical assistants should learn how to adjust the proper control using the specific manual or instructions that accompany the electrocardiograph in their facility.

Electrolyte

Because the skin is a poor conductor of electricity, there are various types of conductive **electrolyte** substances applied with each electrode to pick up the electrical current. The impulses are transmitted to the electrocardiograph by metal tips on the patient lead wires or cables that are attached to the sensors. Because electrolyte substances must contain moisture to properly conduct impulses, they are manufactured in the forms of gels, lotions, pastes, presaturated pads, or, more commonly, are contained within adhesive sensors. For our purposes here, we use the disposable self-adhesive electropads/sensors.

Sensors or Electrodes

There are various types of **sensors** or **electrodes** made of metal or other conductive material. The sensors detect the electrical impulses on the body surface and relay them through cables, or lead, wires to the ECG machine.

Disposable Electrodes. Disposable sensors (electrodes) contain a layer of electrolyte gel on their adhesive surface and can be used on both the limbs and chest. They do not require additional electrolytes. These sensors are applied to the skin of the limbs and chest and held in place by the adhesive. The self-adhesive electrodes are discarded after use. They should be kept in an airtight bag because they dry out and will not stick well.

Lead Wires

Once the self-adhesive sensors are placed, a series of lead wires coming from the machine will be connected to them. Small clips, sometimes referred to as alligator clips, will grasp the tabs on the sensors (Figure 25-6). This completes the circuit from the patient to the machine.

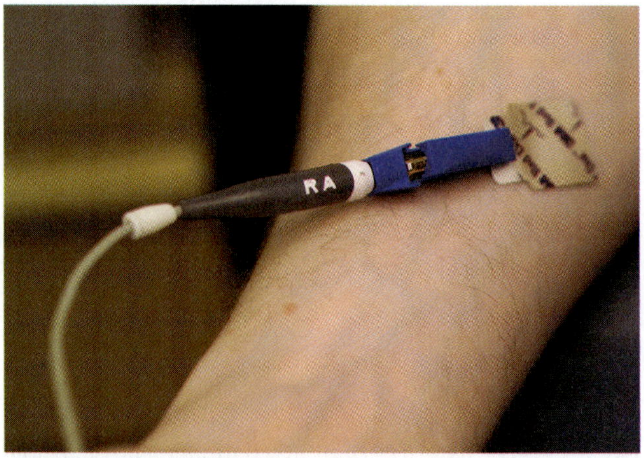

Figure 25-6 Alligator clip and disposable sensor.

THE PROCESS OF RECORDING CARDIAC ELECTRICITY

Skin—Poor conductor
Electrolyte—Must contain moisture to conduct current
Electrodes—Must contain metal to conduct current
Metal clips or tips—To connect the electrodes to the lead wires
Lead wires—To conduct the current from the patient to the machine
Amplifier in the machine—To amplify the electricity enough to measure it
Stylus—An instrument to record the electrical pattern
ECG paper—On which the stylus can record the pattern

Older electrocardiographs may have plain lead wire tips for use with the older metal plates and suction cups. They can easily and inexpensively be converted to use the current self-adhesive sensor electrodes. The only conversion equipment necessary is a set of "alligator" clips that will fit over the end of the lead wire tips. Contact the manufacturer or a medical supplier for conversion sets.

Electrocardiograph Machine

Because the electrical activity that comes from the body is small, it is made larger, or **amplified**, by the amplifier of the electrocardiograph machine. The voltage is changed into a mechanical motion by the **galvanometer** and recorded on the paper by the heated stylus.

Care of Equipment

Once the ECG tracing is complete, remove the lead wires from the sensors, then remove the sensors from the patient. Dispose of the sensors. Check supplies on machine so it is ready for next use. Neatly and loosely place the lead wires on top of or beside the machine. Change the ECG paper when necessary according to manufacturer's suggestions.

LEAD CODING

There are a number of codes used to identify each lead recorded on the ECG reading. There are 12 leads recorded using the 10 lead wires. These codes are necessary for later identification and for mounting purposes. Newer electrocardiographs automatically mark (code) each lead in the upper margin of the ECG paper during the recording. Older electrocardiographs must be manually coded by depressing the lead marker button. Figure 25-7 shows an example of a common coding system.

THE ELECTROCARDIOGRAPH AND SENSOR PLACEMENT

The standard ECG consists of 10 sensors that record 12 leads of the heart's electrical activity from different angles, allowing for a thorough three-dimensional interpretation of its activity. The electrical impulses given off by the heart are picked up by the electrodes and conducted into the machine through **lead wires.**

The electrodes are placed on the patient's four limbs and chest. The four limb leads are right arm (RA), left arm (LA), right leg (RL), and left leg (LL). The right leg electrode is not used as part of the recording. It is an electrical reference point only. The limb leads are placed on the fleshy, nonmuscular area of upper arms and lower legs. The chest leads are known as precordial leads, V leads, or C leads, and use an electrode for each of six areas on the chest wall or one electrode that is moved to six different positions on the chest wall. (This depends on the type of electrocardiograph being used.)

Standard Limb or Bipolar Leads

The first three leads that are recorded on a standard ECG are called leads I, II, and III (Figure 25-8A). These are known as **bipolar** leads because each of them uses two limb electrodes that record simultaneously. Lead I records electrical activity between the right arm (RA) and left arm (LA); lead II records electrical activity between the right arm (RA) and left leg (LL); and lead III records activity between the left arm (LA) and left leg (LL). Lead II is used as a **rhythm strip** because it portrays the heart's rhythm better than the other leads. The rhythm strip is usually a separate longer recording approximately 6 to 12 inches.

Augmented Leads

The next three leads are **augmented** (added to) leads and are designated aVR, aVL, and aVF (Figure 25-8B). The aV stands for augmented voltage; the R, L, and F stand for right, left, and

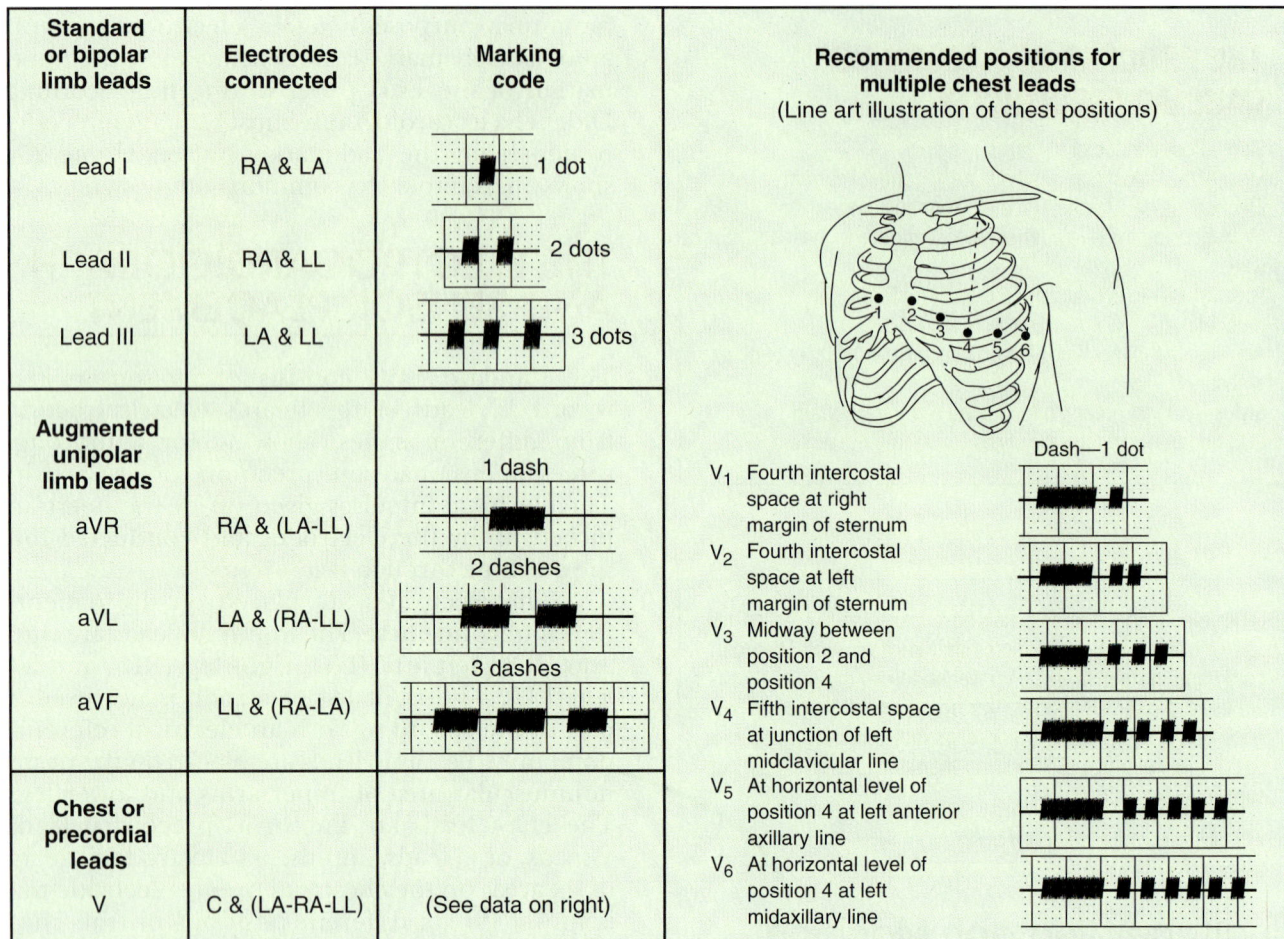

Standard or bipolar limb leads	Electrodes connected	Marking code
Lead I	RA & LA	1 dot
Lead II	RA & LL	2 dots
Lead III	LA & LL	3 dots
Augmented unipolar limb leads		
aVR	RA & (LA-LL)	1 dash
aVL	LA & (RA-LL)	2 dashes
aVF	LL & (RA-LA)	3 dashes
Chest or precordial leads		
V	C & (LA-RA-LL)	(See data on right)

Recommended positions for multiple chest leads
(Line art illustration of chest positions)

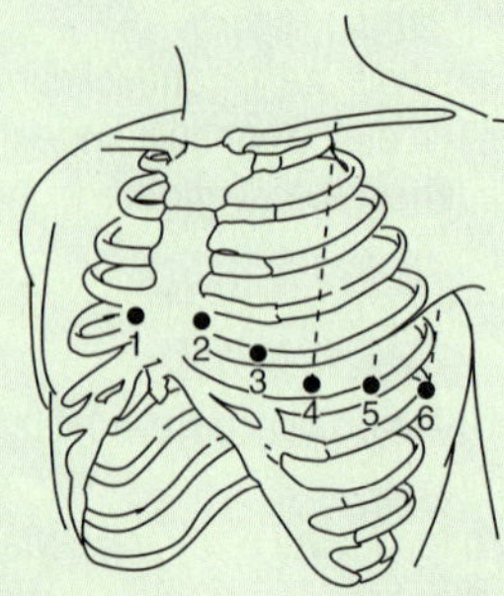

Lead	Position
V_1	Fourth intercostal space at right margin of sternum
V_2	Fourth intercostal space at left margin of sternum
V_3	Midway between position 2 and position 4
V_4	Fifth intercostal space at junction of left midclavicular line
V_5	At horizontal level of position 4 at left anterior axillary line
V_6	At horizontal level of position 4 at left midaxillary line

Dash—1 dot

Figure 25-7 Example of a common coding system for electrocardiogram leads that must be manually coded on older electrocardiographs. Accurate coding is accomplished by pressing the lead marker button appropriately. (Courtesy of Quinton Cardiology, Inc.)

foot (or leg). These are **unipolar** leads. Lead aVR records electrical activity from the midpoint between the left arm added to the left leg, directed to the right arm. Lead aVL records electrical activity from the midpoint between the right arm added to the left leg, directed to the left arm. Lead aVF records electrical activity from the midpoint between the right arm added to the left arm, directed to the left leg. Because these three leads produce such small electrical impulses, the electrocardiograph machine augments, or increases, their size to record them. Figure 25-8B will help you visualize the augmented process.

Chest Leads or Precordial Leads

The remaining six leads of the standard 12-lead ECG are the chest leads or **precordial** leads (Figure 25-8C). These are unipolar leads and are designated V_1, V_2, V_3, V_4, V_5, and V_6. These leads record the heart's electrical impulse from a central point within the heart to one of six predesignated positions on the chest wall where an electrode is attached. The correct position *must* be used for each lead recording.

The anatomic positions for placement of the chest or precordial leads are:

V_1: fourth intercostal space at right margin of sternum
V_2: fourth intercostal space at left margin of sternum
V_4: fifth intercostal space on left midclavicular line
V_3: midway between V2 and V4 (*NOTE:* This is correct order, V3 after V4.)
V_5: horizontal to V4 at left anterior axillary line
V_6: horizontal to V4 at left midaxillary line

When using an electrocardiograph with one chest wire, the chest electrode must be moved manually one by one to each of the six chest lead positions. This necessitates stopping the instrument between each chest lead to move the electrode to the

(A) Standard limb or bipolar leads

	Electrodes Connected
Lead I	LA and RA
Lead II*	LL and RA
Lead III	LL and LA

* Also used for rhythm strip

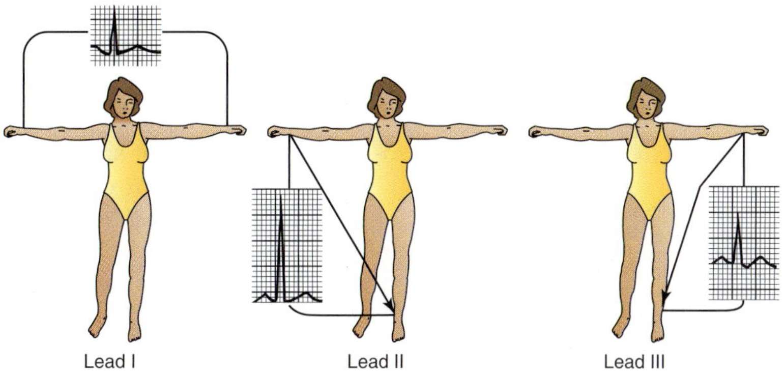

(B) Augmented limb leads

aVR	RA and (LA-LL)
aVL	LA and (RA-LL)
aVF	LL and (RA-LA)

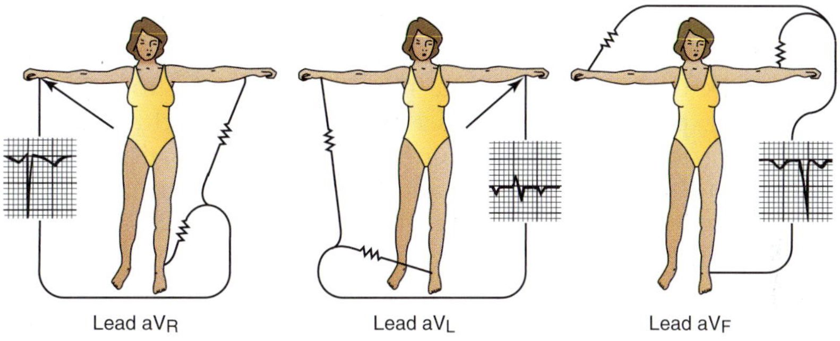

(C) Precordial or chest leads	Electrodes connected	Placement
V_1	V_1 and (LA-RA-LL)	Fourth intercostal space at right margin of sternum
V_2	V_2 and (LA-RA-LL)	Fourth intercostal space at left margin of sternum
V_4	V_4 and (LA-RA-LL)	Fifth intercostal space at junction of left midclavicular line
V_3	V_3 and (LA-RA-LL)	Midway between position 2 and position 4
V_5	V_5 and (LA-RA-LL)	At horizontal level of position 4 at left anterior axillary line
V_6	V_6 and (LA-RA-LL)	At horizontal level of position 4 at left midaxillary line

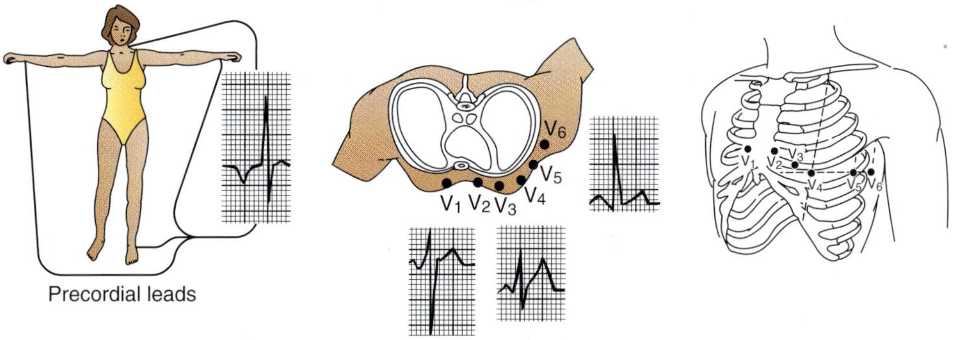

Figure 25-8 Lead types, connections, and placement. (A) Standard limb or bipolar leads. (B) Augmented limb leads. (C) Precordial or chest leads.

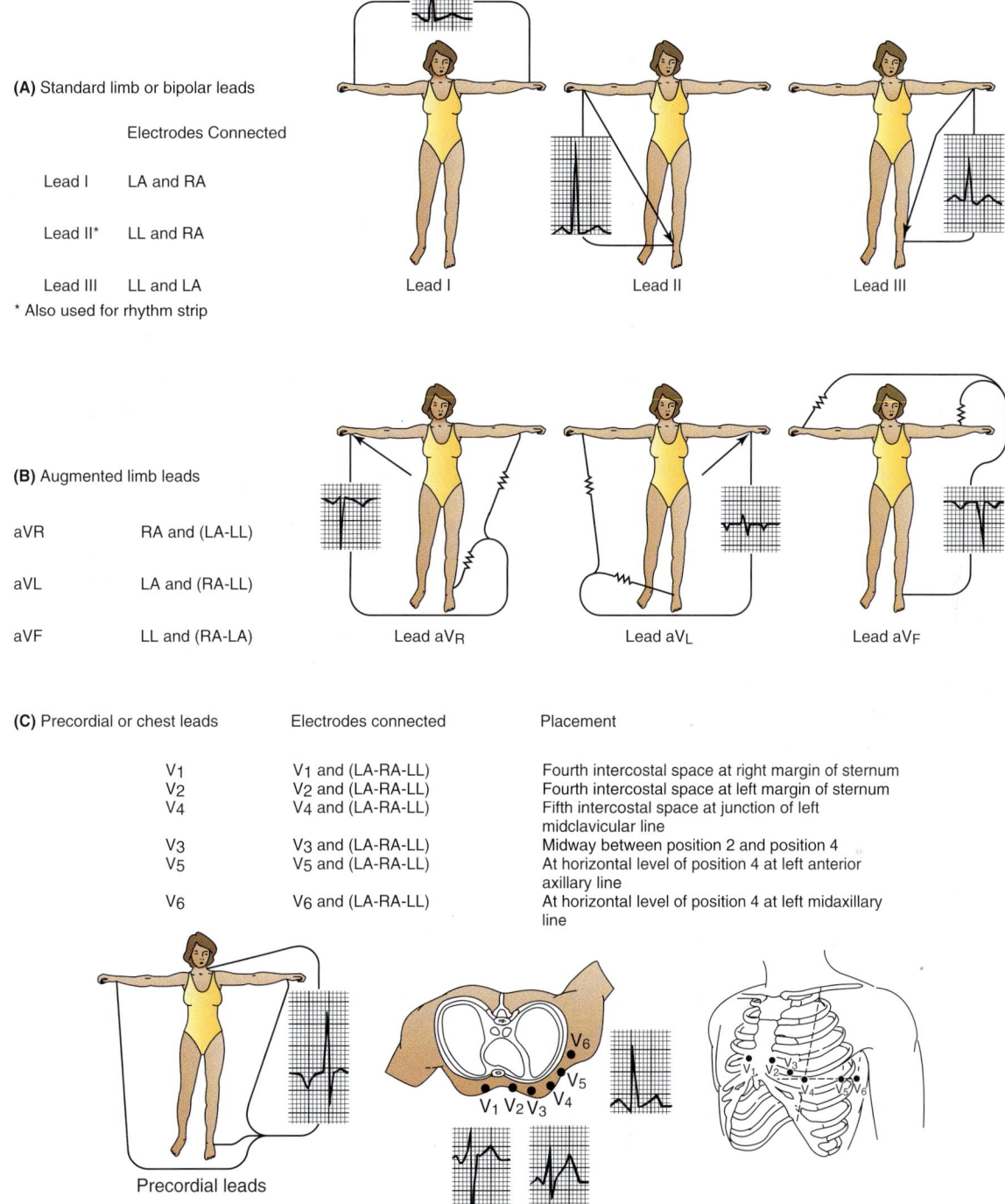

next appropriate position on the chest wall. Some electrocardiographs have six lead wires allowing all six chest leads to be applied at one time; therefore, there is no interruption between chest lead recordings (see Figure 25-18C in Procedure 25-1).

STANDARDIZATION AND ADJUSTMENT OF THE ELECTROCARDIOGRAPH

The value of an ECG recording depends on it being performed accurately. To ensure a precise and reliable recording, you must standardize the ECG instrument before every ECG performed. The standardization of the machine is a quality-assurance check to determine if the machine is set and working properly. Standardization measurements have been adopted internationally as a means of accurate **calibration** according to universal measurements. The universal standard is that 1 mV (millivolt) of cardiac electrical activity will deflect the stylus exactly 10 mm high. This is the equivalent of 10 small squares on the ECG paper. Figure 25-9 shows an example of the 10-mm standardization at the beginning of each row.

On occasion, R waves may be large and go off the paper. Repositioning the stylus may not correct the situation. In such instances, the medical assistant can record the lead(s) in which the R wave is large at one-half sensitivity. This action will record all ECG cycles at half their normal **amplitude.**

Conversely, the waves of the ECG cycles may be small, making it difficult to interpret. In this circumstance, the medical assistant can record the ECG cycles at twice the normal standard. This action will record ECG cycles at twice their normal amplitude. Whenever a change is made from a normal standardization (10 mm high) to either a one-half standardization (5 mm high) or a double standardization (20 mm high), the medical assistant must include the adjusted standardization mark with that particular lead to alert the provider to the change in standard. The standard must be returned to normal to prevent accidentally running the next lead at a standard other than normal. The paper is usually run at a speed of 25 mm/second. If cycles are too close together, the paper speed can be adjusted to 50 mm/second.

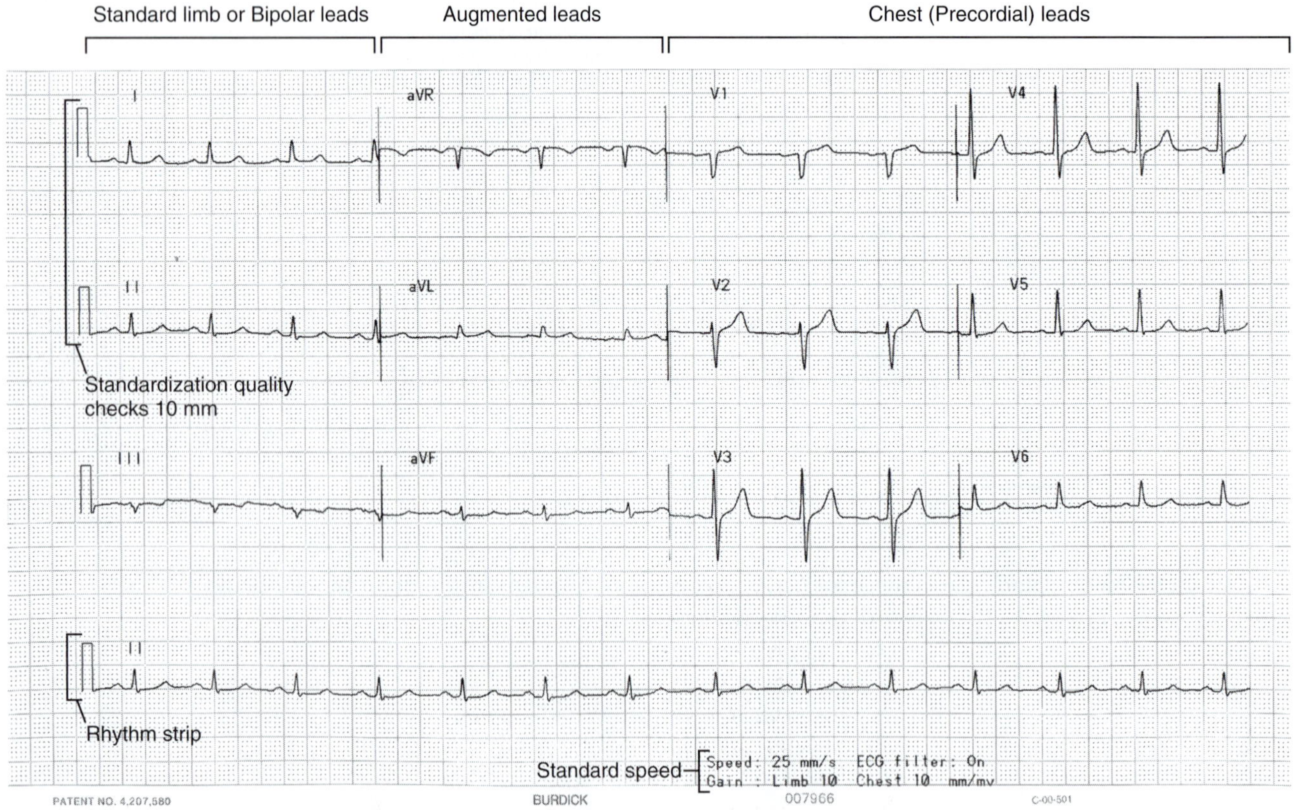

Figure 25-9 An electrocardiogram showing all 12 leads recorded in minutes at one time with no interruption. (Courtesy of Quinton Cardiology, Inc.)

Make a note on the ECG paper if paper speed or amplitude is changed.

STANDARD RESTING ELECTROCARDIOGRAPHY

Regardless of the type of electrocardiograph used, the basic components of the standard electrocardiography procedure remain the same. Patient preparation, placement of limb and chest leads, attachment of lead wires, and elimination of artifacts vary little from one electrocardiograph to another. Procedure 25-1 explains a 12-lead ECG using a multiple-lead channel electrocardiograph. Before performing the procedure, medical assistants must be familiar with the electrocardiograph machine in their facility and should thoroughly review the manufacturer's instruction manual that accompanies the machine. Knowledge of the basic procedures included here can be adapted for all other electrocardiographs.

MOUNTING THE ECG TRACING

Commercially prepared mounting forms are available, and the medical assistant should mount the completed tracing after the provider has reviewed the entire recording. The mounting of the ECG recording depends on the machine. Some machines produce a strip already printed on a durable paper record. Some machines produce a long strip that will need to be cut apart and adhered to a mounting paper or card. There are many options within these two varieties. Included with any ECG recording should be the patient's name, date, address, age, sex, blood pressure, height and weight, and cardiac medications on the mounting form.

INTERFERENCE OR ARTIFACTS

The ECG is a valuable diagnostic aid to the provider and must be performed accurately. The medical assistant is responsible for obtaining a recording that can be easily read and interpreted by the provider.

There can be unusual and unwanted activity in the tracing not caused by the electrical activity of the heart. These defects in the ECG tracing are known as *artifacts,* and their appearance can make the ECG tracing difficult to read and interpret. Four of the more common artifacts are somatic tremor, alternating current (AC) interference, wandering baseline, and interrupted baseline. The medical assistant should understand the causes of each type of artifact and know how to eliminate them. The newer machines have filters, which will automatically filter out the artifact.

Somatic Tremor Artifacts

Somatic tremor artifact is also known as muscle tremor. It is characterized by unnatural baseline deflections such as jagged peaks or irregularity of spacing and height. The tracing appears fuzzy (Figure 25-10A). Somatic tremor occurs when the patient is apprehensive or uncomfortable, resulting in involuntary muscle movement. Voluntary muscle movement occurs when the patient moves, talks, coughs, and so on. Parkinson's disease, a nervous system disorder, is an example of involuntary somatic tremor. It is not possible for the patient to control the muscle tremors. (Often, involuntary somatic tremor can be minimized somewhat by having the patient slide the hands under the buttocks during the recording.)

It is natural for the patient to feel apprehensive before and during the ECG tracing. Reassurance and an explanation of the procedure will allay apprehension and relax muscles. Be certain the patient is comfortable. Use pillows for the head and under the knees; be sure the temperature of the room is comfortable. These simple techniques will help to minimize somatic tremor.

AC Interference

The AC interference artifact is caused by electrical interference and appears as a series of small regular peaks (Figure 25-10B). Electricity present in medical equipment or wires in the area can leak a small amount of energy into the room in which the ECG is being recorded. The current can be picked up by the patient's body and it will be detected by the ECG tracing as an AC artifact.

Common Causes of AC Interference Artifacts.

Some common causes of AC interferences are:

1. Improper grounding of electrocardiograph. The three-pronged plugs in the newer electrocardiographs should be inserted into a properly grounded three-receptacle outlet. This reduces AC interference from improper grounding.
2. Presence of other electrical equipment in the room. Unplug other electrical equipment in the room (electrical examination tables, lamps, autoclaves, and so on).

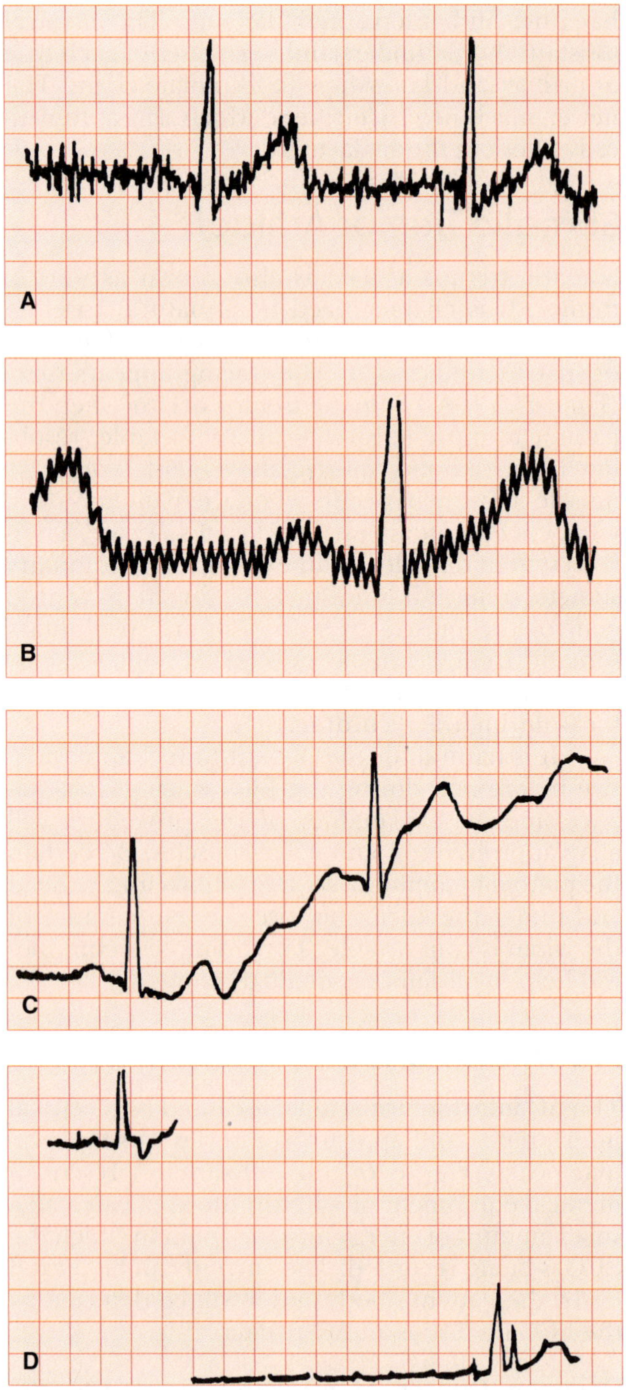

Figure 25-10 Electrocardiogram artifacts. (A) Somatic tremor. (B) Alternating current. (C) Wandering baseline. (D) Interrupted baseline. (Courtesy of Quinton Cardiology, Inc.)

3. Electrical wiring in the floor, ceiling, or walls. Move the ECG table away from walls.
4. Crossed lead wires and lead wires not following body contour. Straighten lead wires and be sure they are positioned to follow the patient's body contour.

Wandering Baseline Artifacts

A wandering baseline occurs when the stylus moves from the center of the ECG paper, resulting in the complexes "wandering" across the ECG paper; for example, from the top of the paper to the bottom, or bottom to top (Figure 25-10C). This makes it difficult to follow the complexes when the provider reads and interprets the recording.

Common Causes of Wandering Baseline Artifacts. Wandering baseline artifacts can be caused by the following conditions:

1. Electrodes applied too loosely or too tightly. There should be equal tension on all four limb leads, metal tips should be firmly attached to the electrodes, and the cable attached to patient should not have tension on it nor be dangling to cause pulling on the electrode.
2. Corroded or dirty electrodes or metal tips of the lead wires. Clean and rinse after each use.
3. Inappropriate amount or poor-quality electrolyte gel or paste. Each electrode should have the same amount of electrolyte gel or paste on it.
4. Lotions, oils, or creams on the patient's skin that interfere with the adhesive sticking well. Remove any of these substances before applying the electrode by cleansing the area with an alcohol wipe.

Wandering baseline artifacts are more often seen in older ECG machines that use metal electrodes and electrolyte. Newer machines use electrodes (sensors) that are disposable and self-adhesive, thereby eliminating the four causes of wandering baseline artifacts.

Interrupted Baseline Artifacts

On occasion, the baseline is interrupted and a break is seen between waves (Figure 25-10D). Possible causes are a broken cable, a lead wire that became detached from an electrode, or an electrode that came completely off.

Patients with Unique Problems

On occasion, the medical assistant performs an ECG on a patient who has unique medical problems. An obese patient, a woman with large breasts, or a patient with thick chest muscles will make it difficult to palpate the intercostal spaces. Place the chest leads on the chest as accurately as you can.

Critical Thinking

Mr. Williams has a diagnosis of Parkinson's disease. The provider requests an ECG. What strategies can you use to ensure an adequate tracing?

For a patient with a limb amputation or a cast, the medical assistant should apply the sensors as close to the preferred site as possible, higher on the limb. Place the sensor in a similar position on the other limb.

Do not place sensors on wounds, open areas, sutures, or staples. Try to situate the sensors as close as possible to the preferred site.

If the patient has dyspnea, the ECG can be taken with the patient in semi-Fowler's position (see Chapter 13 for positions).

If you have difficulty performing an ECG on patients with certain medical problems or conditions, ask for assistance from your supervisor/delegator.

MYOCARDIAL INFARCTIONS (HEART ATTACKS)

Myocardial infarctions (heart attacks) are the number one cause of death in the United States today. With the approval of the employer–provider, medical assistants are in an excellent position to offer healthy tips and suggestions from which patients can benefit. For instance, they can offer patient health tips regarding diet and exercise while applying the ECG equipment and provide handouts and informational Web sites for patients to research (Table 25-1).

Table 25-1 Behaviors to Adopt for a Healthy Heart

The provider may want the medical assistant to remind patients of the following healthy behaviors:
1. Avoid tobacco
2. Take medications as prescribed
3. Report any unusual symptoms or problems to the provider
4. Eat a low-fat, low-cholesterol, low-sodium diet
5. Exercise regularly with provider's permission
6. Get adequate rest
7. Keep weight under control and at an acceptable level
8. Practice stress reduction behaviors

Patient Education

Atherosclerosis is the buildup of fatty deposits on the lining of coronary arteries causing narrowing and obstruction of the arteries. Blood flow to the heart muscle is diminished particularly when the heart is called on to work harder, for example, during increased physical activity, emotional stress, exposure to cold temperatures, and after a heavy meal. The heart's muscle tissue responds to these conditions by symptoms of pain or discomfort beneath the sternum, into the neck, jaw, left arm and shoulder, and throat. Rest usually relieves the pain. This condition is known as angina pectoris.

Treatment of angina consists of rest and medication. Nitroglycerin may be prescribed in tablet or patch form. Change in lifestyle and other suggestions (Table 25-1) may be recommended. Tests that the provider may order include a 12-lead ECG, a stress ECG (stress test), blood tests, chest radiograph, and coronary **angiogram**.

Pain that does not subside after rest may indicate a more serious condition such as a complete obstruction of the coronary arteries and no blood flow to the heart muscle, a myocardial infarction, or heart attack. Seek immediate medical attention if pain persists.

CARDIAC ARRHYTHMIAS

The medical assistant should recognize cardiac arrhythmias that occur during the ECG recording and without alarming the patient make the provider aware of them as soon as they are noticed. The normal, healthy ECG cycle consists of P, QRS, and T waves in a regularly appearing sequence or pattern. The term **normal sinus rhythm** refers to an ECG that is within normal limits (WNL). The normal adult heart rate is 60 to 100 beats/min. A rate less than 60 beats/min is known as **sinus bradycardia** (Figure 25-11A); a rate greater than 100 beats/min is known as **sinus tachycardia** (Figure 25-11B). These two heart rates, although regular in rhythm, are considered cardiac arrhythmias.

Atrial Arrhythmias

Premature Atrial Contractions (PACs). Healthy individuals can experience PACs. They are seen in patients who use tobacco and stimulants such as caffeine, but they can forewarn of more serious cardiac problems. This type of arrhythmia is characterized by a cardiac cycle that occurs before the next cycle is due. The P wave is shaped differently from the P wave of the normal cycle (Figure 25-12A).

Paroxysmal Atrial Tachycardia (PAT). This arrhythmia can be seen in healthy individuals; and in persons with cardiac disease. PAT is characterized by its unprovoked sudden onset and abrupt termination. The heart rate is regular and ranges between 160 to 250 beats/min. The episode usually lasts only a few seconds; the heart rate then returns to its original rate (Figure 25-12B). The patient may describe a fluttering in the chest, apprehension, shortness of breath, and, on occasion, dizziness.

Atrial Fibrillation. This arrhythmia can be seen in healthy individuals or in those with cardiac disease. In younger patients, common causes can be congenital heart disease and mitral valve damage caused by rheumatic heart disease. In older patients, the arrhythmia can be caused by hypertension, coronary

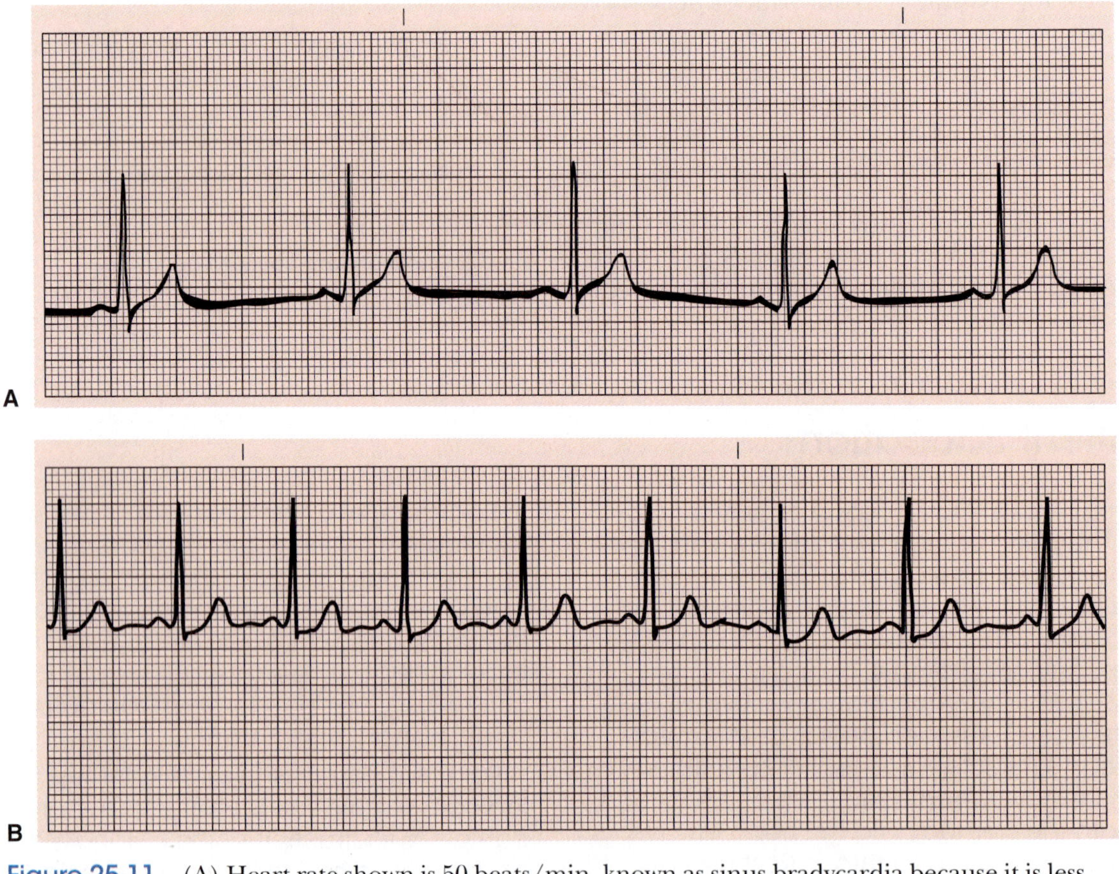

Figure 25-11 (A) Heart rate shown is 50 beats/min, known as sinus bradycardia because it is less than 60 beats/min. One large square = 0.2 second; 1 minute (60 seconds) ÷ 0.2 = 300. There are six large squares between R waves: 300 ÷ 6 = 50 beats/min. (B) Sinus tachycardia is a heart rate faster than 100 beats/min. There are three large squares between R waves: 300 ÷ 3 = 100 beats/min.

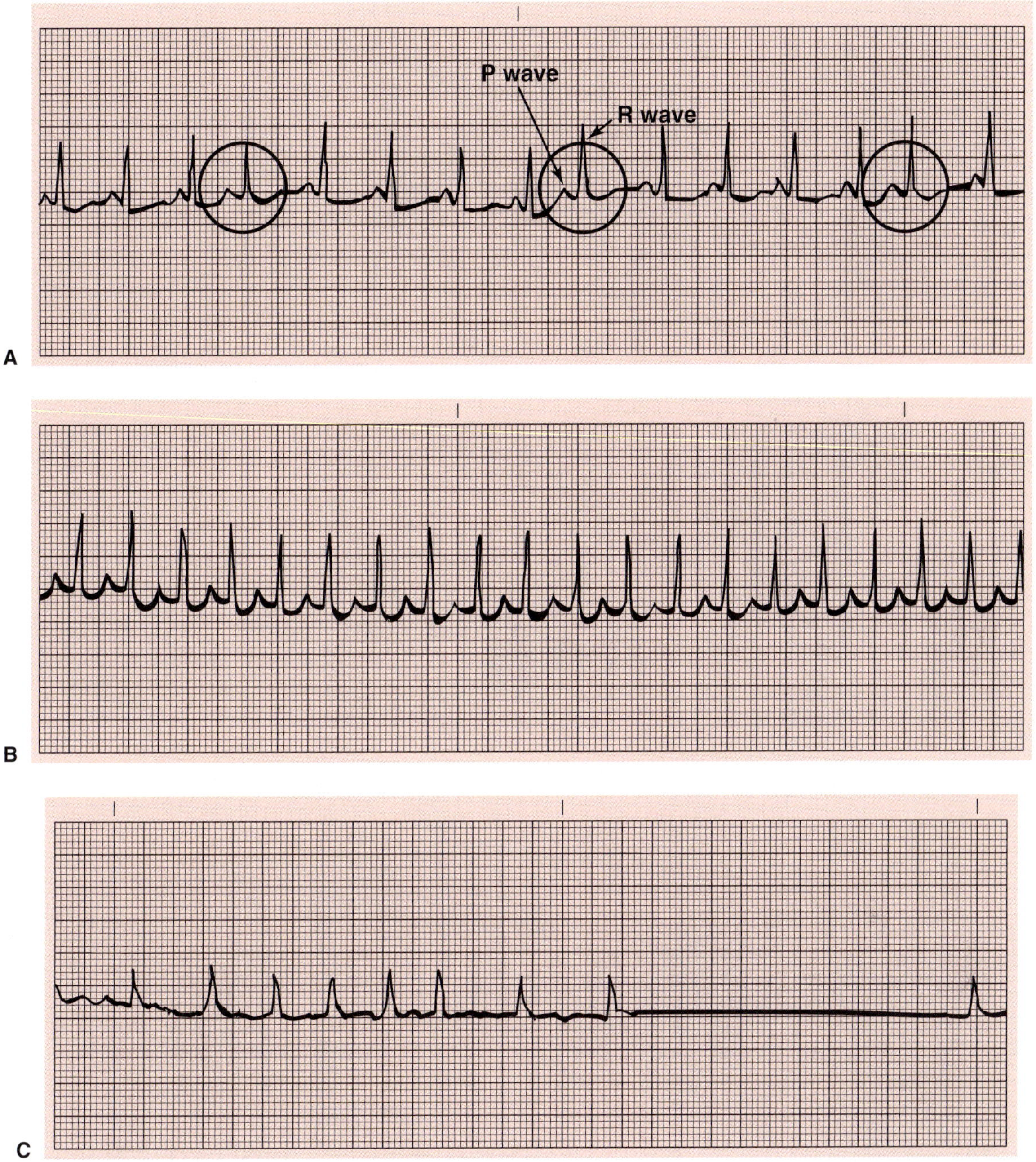

Figure 25-12 Atrial arrhythmias. (A) Premature atrial contractions. (B) Paroxysmal atrial tachycardia. (C) Atrial fibrillation.

artery disease, or mitral valve prolapse. It is characterized by extremely rapid, incomplete contractions 400 to 500 beats/min resulting in small, irregular, and uncoordinated complexes that are difficult to measure accurately because the P waves cannot be distinguished (Figure 25-12C).

Ventricular Arrhythmias

Premature Ventricular Contractions (PVCs). This arrhythmia can be seen in healthy individuals and in patients with hypertension, coronary artery disease, and lung disease. In healthy individuals, PVCs can be caused by tobacco, anxiety, alcohol, and medications that contain epinephrine (Figure 25-13A). PVCs are seen on ECG tracings fairly frequently and are considered common disturbances in the rhythm. They are characterized by a beat that comes early in the cycle, has no P wave, a wide QRS complex, and a different T wave. The PVC is followed by a pause before the occurrence of the next normal cycle.

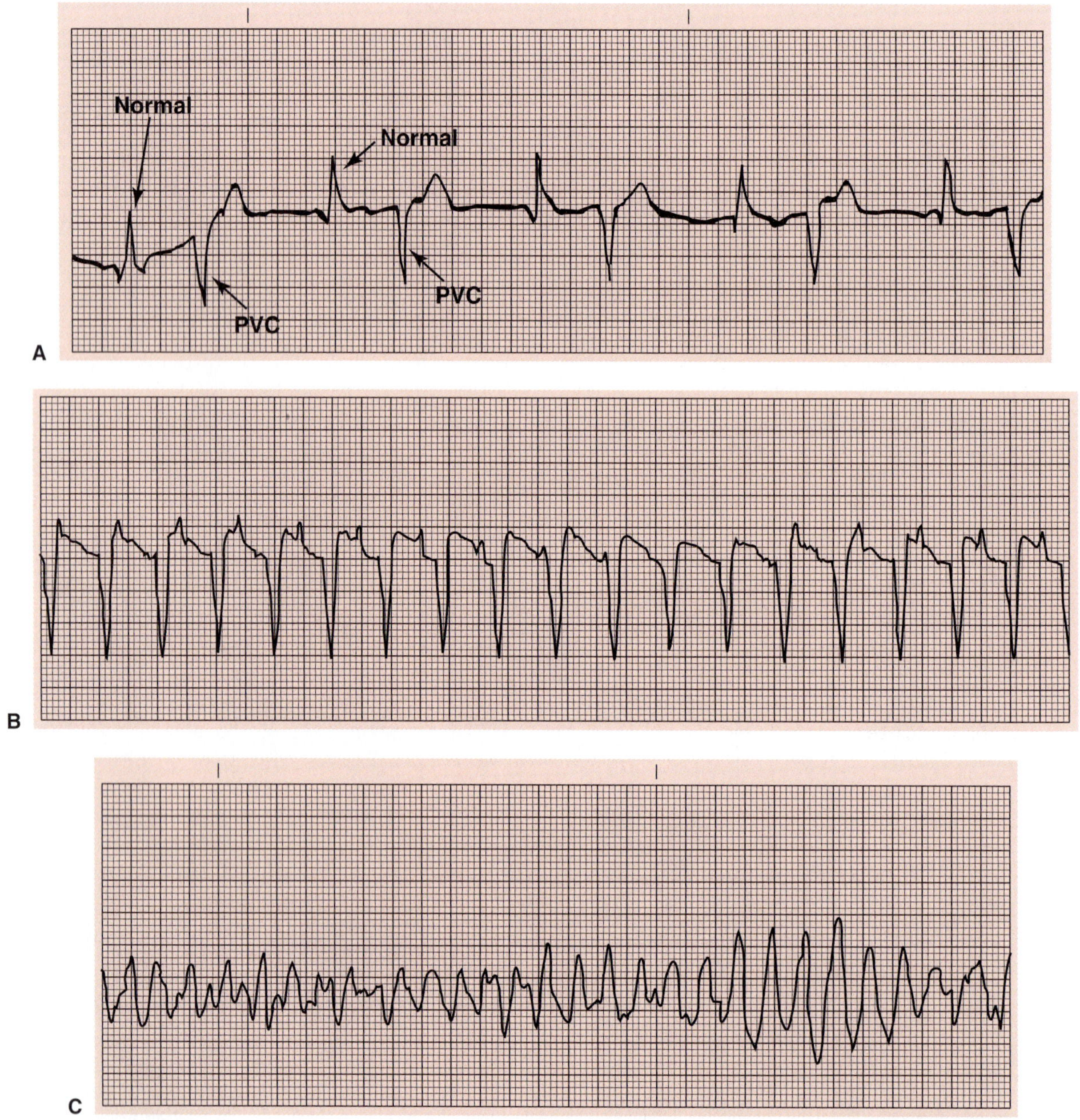

Figure 25-13 Ventricular arrhythmias. (A) Premature ventricular contractions (PVCs). (B) Ventricular tachycardia. (C) Ventricular fibrillation.

Ventricular Tachycardia. This arrhythmia is seen in patients with cardiac disease, both acute and chronic. It is common in patients with coronary artery disease, and frequently the patient experiencing a myocardial infarction will have ventricular tachycardia as a result of the infarction (Figure 25-13B). The arrhythmia is manifested by three or more PVCs that occur at a rate ranging from 150 to 250 beats/min. There are no P waves, and the QRS complexes are distorted. Ventricular tachycardia is life threatening and can rapidly deteriorate into fibrillation and cardiac standstill.

Ventricular Fibrillation. This arrhythmia is seen in patients experiencing a myocardial infarction or in patients with existing cardiac disease. It may be preceded by PVCs or ventricular tachycardia, or it may begin as ventricular fibrillation. It is a life-threatening arrhythmia (Figure 25-13C).

DEFIBRILLATION

A **defibrillator** is an electrical device that applies **countershocks** to the heart through electrodes or pads placed on the chest wall (Figure 25-14). The purpose is to convert cardiac arrhythmia into normal sinus rhythm. This is known as **defibrillation** or **cardioversion.** In most offices and clinics, a defibrillator is kept on a crash cart for quick access in emergency situations. The medical assistant should regularly check the equipment for proper operation and preparedness and assist the provider as needed.

Automated external defibrillators (AEDs) are widely used and are found in places where many people congregate, such as airports and the workplace, and in private homes of individuals at risk for cardiac arrest.

The devices are portable, small, and battery operated. Emergency medical technicians, police, and firefighters trained in defibrillation techniques and who are the first to respond in an emergency were primarily the individuals who used these devices. Now, many citizens are certified to use AEDs (see Figure 25-14).

In an individual experiencing a myocardial infarction, ventricular fibrillation is not uncommon. If the fibrillation can be stopped within the first 5 minutes using a defibrillator, the life can be saved (see Chapter 9 for more about AEDs).

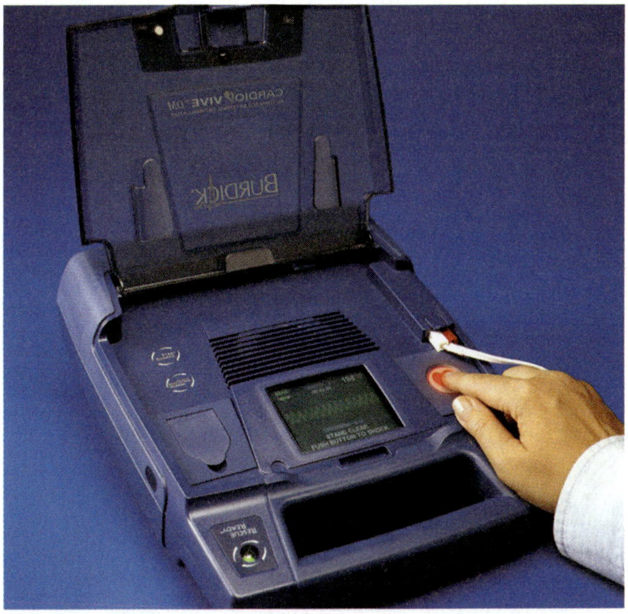

Figure 25-14 The CardioVive DM AED. (Courtesy of Quinton Cardiology, Inc.)

OTHER CARDIAC DIAGNOSTIC TESTS

Holter Monitor (Portable Ambulatory Electrocardiograph)

The Holter monitor is a portable continuous recording of cardiac activity for a 24-hour period (Figure 25-15). The patient is monitored while going about the usual daily activities with no restrictions. This **noninvasive** test helps to diagnose cardiac arrhythmias by correlating them with the patient's symptoms. Some symptoms are **syncope,** fatigue, chest pain, and vertigo. This type of monitoring is useful for patients whose arrhythmias are sporadic and are not found on a 12-lead ECG tracing. Also, ambulatory monitoring helps assess the function of an artificial pacemaker and the effectiveness of antiarrhythmic medications.

Special electrodes attached to lead wires are placed in the appropriate areas of the patient's chest. A special portable tape recorder, either digital or magnetic, computer or magnetic, continually records, the heart's electrical activity for a 24-hour period. The monitor is a battery-operated recorder that is placed in a leather pouch or bag and is worn by the patient either on a belt around the waist or by a strap over the patient's shoulder. Table 25-2 lists locations for placement of electrodes.

One kind of digital Holter monitor is a three-channel (five-lead) ECG that has Windows-based software technology. A keypad is used to enter the patient's information, such as date of recording, patient identification number, etc. There is no need to check the effectiveness of the monitor by attaching it to a test cable and an ECG machine. Some monitors have a removable flash memory card and a

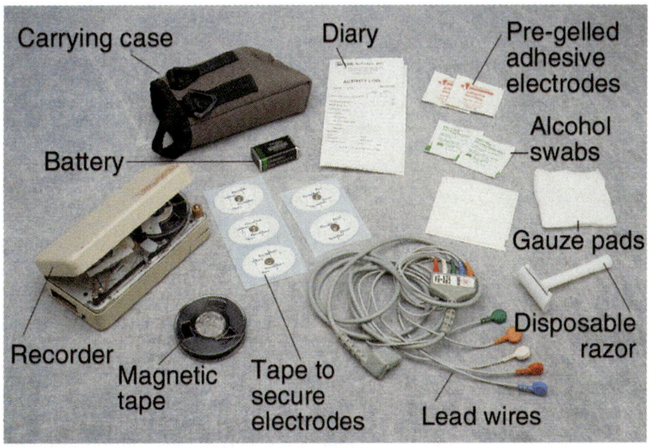

Figure 25-15 Holter monitor and supplies needed for application.

Table 25-2 Holter Monitor Electrode Placement

Electrode	Lead	Location
A (black)	mV_1	Fourth intercostal space at right of the sternal edge
B (white)	mV_5	Right clavicle, just lateral to sternum
C (brown)	mV_1	Left clavicle, just lateral to the sternum
D (red)	mV_5	Fifth intercostal space at left axillary line
E (green)	Ground	Lower right chest wall

flash card reader that can download information in 90 seconds. It can hold up to 48 hours of ECG information. The tracing is interpreted and sent back by computer. It can be accessed and printed. The electrode placement is the same for a digital Holter monitor as it is for a magnetic tape Holter monitor, but both digital and magnetic tape electrode placement is not the same as it is for a standard 12-lead resting ECG.

Other computerized continuous cardiac monitoring devices are available and are prescribed for patients according to the patient's symptoms and the practitioner's preference. The tracing can be read over the telephone or is computerized. Transtelephone monitor devices are frequently used by patients with a pacemaker and or **implantable cardioverter-defibrillator (ICD).** These patients have routine scheduled checks of their devices over the phone.

Some cardiac monitoring devices are sent directly to the patient from the supplier, complete with printed or telephone directions for the patient. When the specific time period has elapsed for the particular monitor being used, the patient is responsible for returning the device to the supplier.

Medical Assistant's Role. The medical assistant is responsible for preparing the patient, instructing the patient, checking and replacing the battery, and applying and removing the monitor.

Holter Monitor Electrode Placement. Special disposable electrodes, which are round plastic and have a strong adhesive backing, are available for the Holter monitor. These disposable electrodes contain an electrolyte gel. There may be either four or five electrodes depending on whether the monitor has a built-in ground. Notice that the leads for the Holter monitor are applied to different locations from the electrodes of a resting ECG. Table 25-2 lists the locations for lead placement.

Holter Monitor Attachment. Once the Holter monitor has been attached to the patient, the monitor should be checked for effectiveness by attaching the **test cable** to the monitor and the other end to an ECG instrument. A baseline strip can be recorded to verify the correct wave activity and lack of artifact. If there are inaccurate readings, the monitor may not have been applied properly. The medical assistant can reconnect the leads to the electrodes or reposition the electrodes and reconnect the leads (see Procedure 25-2). The skin should be cleansed with an alcohol wipe and rubbed with gauze to roughen it. Males should be shaved so that the electrodes adhere well.

Patient Education

When preparing patients to wear a 24-hour Holter monitor, instruct them in the following:

1. Keep a diary of daily activities, symptoms, and emotions, and note the time of occurrence.
2. Depress the event marker only briefly and only when experiencing a significant symptom. Overuse of the marker can mask the ECG tracing.
3. Do not shower, bathe, or swim while wearing the monitor because the recording could be interrupted or the monitor could be damaged.
4. Do not handle the electrodes. Doing so could cause artifacts.
5. Do not remove the recorder from its case.
6. Do not use an electric blanket. This can cause interference.

The following are examples of some of the daily activities that should be recorded by the patient in the patient activity diary:

- Eating meals
- Ascending and descending stairs
- Sexual activity
- Medications taken
- Times of sleep
- Smoking
- Bowel movements
- Physical exercise

Patient Activity Diary. The patient activity diary is an important component of the monitoring procedures. As noted in the Patient Education box, all activities and emotional states, and the time of their occurrence, should be noted during the 24-hour monitoring time. Symptoms such as chest pain, shortness of breath, dizziness, palpitations, and so on, and the time the event occurred should also be noted. Patient symptoms recorded while being monitored can be compared with the patient's notations in the activity diary and correlated to the heart's activity. Symptoms can be further noted by the patient briefly depressing an event marker button located at one end of the monitor. This places an electronic "tag" on the tape. This signal can alert the person interpreting the ECG to look for a significant event or abnormality on the tape.

Holter Monitor Removal. The patient is instructed to return to the office or ambulatory care center 24 hours later to have the monitor removed. Usually no appointment is necessary. The tape is analyzed by a Holter monitor scanner or by a computer. This is usually done in the ECG department of a nearby hospital. The provider can access the report from the computer with samples of any abnormalities that were picked up during the monitoring period. A follow-up appointment is scheduled with the provider to discuss the results.

Critical Thinking

State three purposes for using a Holter monitor and give the instructions that the patient will need to know while wearing the monitor.

Loop ECG

Another type of ambulatory electrocardiography is called *loop ECG*. It uses only two electrodes. It records a few minutes of the ECG at a time on a computer chip. It constantly records new information and discards the oldest information. Thus, the memory contains only the last few minutes of the ECG recording. When a patient has an "episode or event" (symptoms), the patient pushes the "record" button and the recording remains in the device's memory. The recorded event is transmitted (played back) by telephone to the provider. The device then erases the event.

The recorder constantly refreshes its memory. It is suitable for capturing brief events and can be carried for long periods of time. Other types of recorders take a longer period of time, and if a patient is experiencing dizziness, it takes too long to apply a recorder. This may result in not being able to capture episodes associated with syncope.

Treadmill Stress Test or Exercise Tolerance ECG

On occasion patients have symptoms of cardiac problems that do not appear as abnormalities on a resting ECG. The provider may prescribe a treadmill stress test or exercise tolerance test to aid in the determination of the patient's diagnosis and prognosis. The test is done to diagnose heart disorders, to diagnose the probable cause of the patient's chest pain, and to assess the patient's cardiac ability after cardiac surgery. The treadmill stress test is a noninvasive ECG tracing taken under controlled conditions while the patient is closely monitored by the medical assistant and the provider. Frequent blood pressure readings are taken. The patient wears comfortable clothing and flat shoes such as sneakers with rubber soles and exercises on a treadmill at prescribed rates of speed (Figure 25-16). Electrodes are applied to the chest only.

As with the Holter monitor, the patient's skin should be cleansed with an alcohol wipe and rubbed with gauze to roughen it. Male patients should be shaved at the site of the electrodes to ensure electrode adherence.

The myocardium requires extra oxygen during exercise and in the presence of narrowed or obstructed coronary arteries; the additional workload on the myocardium will often be demonstrated as an abnormality on the ECG recording. The patient should have no pain, shortness of breath, or excess fatigue. If any of these or other unusual symptoms occur, the provider may terminate the test because this could indicate cardiac disease.

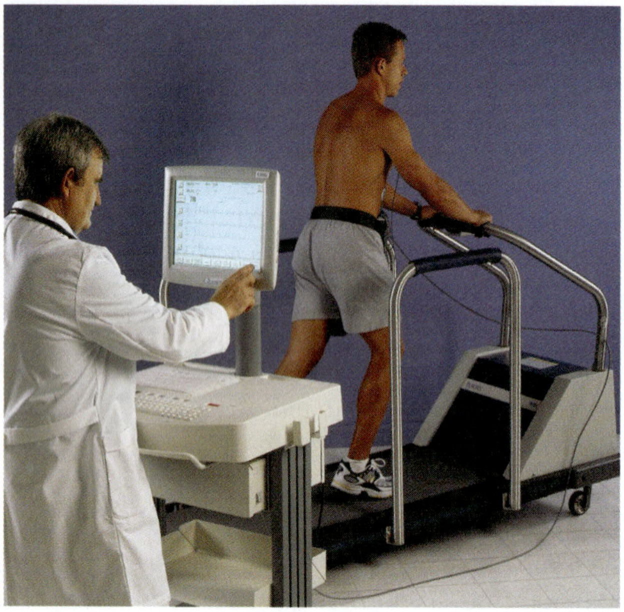

Figure 25-16 The Quest Exercise Stress System. (Courtesy of Quinton Cardiology, Inc.)

At the conclusion of the test, the patient is told to rest. Monitoring continues until the vital signs and heart rate return to normal. Prior to the patient leaving the office, the patient should be instructed to rest, refrain from a hot bath or shower, avoid stimulants such as caffeine, and avoid extreme temperature changes for several hours.

Complications such as a myocardial infarction or a serious arrhythmia can occur during testing. Although these events are unusual, appropriate emergency equipment must be readily available, and the medical assistant should check them frequently for proper functioning. Some equipment to have available on a crash cart for cardiac emergencies include oxygen, antiarrhythmic drugs, an Ambu-bag™, a defibrillator, an endotracheal tube, and a laryngoscope. The medical assistant is responsible for checking the supplies and plugging in the defibrillator.

Further diagnostic tests such as **cardiac catheterization** (angiogram) may be necessary to diagnose the extent of the atherosclerosis buildup and obstruction of the coronary arteries.

Thallium Stress Test

Thallium stress test is similar to a treadmill stress test in that the patient has an ECG tracing while exercising on the treadmill after having been given an injection of a radioactive substance such as thallium. The test shows how well blood flows to the heart muscle. It can help diagnose coronary artery blockage, the cause of a patient's chest pain, cardiac function, post myocardial infarction, and to check the level of exercise a patient can safely engage in.

The thallium is injected intravenously while the patient is being monitored on the treadmill and is exercising. After the stress test, the patient is "scanned" under a machine in the diagnostic imaging department. The patient leaves the department for 3 or 4 hours (rests), then returns, and another scan is done. Therefore, the patient has been "scanned" during exercise and after a rest period of a few hours.

The thallium intravenous injection mixes with blood in the bloodstream and in the arteries and enters the heart muscle cells. If a portion of the heart does not receive a normal blood supply, than a less amount of thallium will be present in the heart muscle cells. To the cardiologist this finding indicates a degree of block in the heart's blood supply. The patient most likely has ischemia of the heart muscle or an infarct of the heart muscle.

Patients who can not tolerate an exercise stress test because of serious heart disease or patients with special needs, such as wheelchair-bound patients, can be given a vasodilator and the undergo ECG test seated in a chair or wheelchair. The medication will cause an increase in heart rate, thus simulating the stress of walking on a treadmill. The thallium stress test is performed in the outpatient department of the hospital or in a cardiology office or clinic.

Echocardiography/Ultrasonography

Echocardiography is a noninvasive, diagnostic test that uses ultrasound (ultrahigh-frequency sound waves) to image the internal structures of the heart. X-rays are not useful. General anatomy, myocardial function, valve function, and heart chamber size can be evaluated. Echocardiography may be performed in a cardiologist's office.

During **ultrasonography,** a handheld **transducer** acts as a transmitter and receiver of the high-frequency sound waves as it is held against the chest wall and moved over the heart area. As the sound waves go through the skin and hit internal structures, echoes are sent back to the transducer. A machine converts the images when the various structures provide different echoes. The images can then be examined by a computer and converted into photographs and films of structures and blood flow.

There is little patient preparation other than to have the patient lie on the examination table with the four-limb leads of a 12-lead electrocardiograph attached. The test is usually performed by a

sonographer. The provider views the results later and informs the patient.

CARDIAC PROCEDURES

The following section discusses cardiac procedures performed for heart disease and arrhythmias. Some cardiac procedures for diagnosing diseases of the heart are computerized (Figure 25-17), and the results are stored in the patient's electronic medical record. The data are accessible on demand.

Procedures for Heart Disease

Percutaneous transluminal coronary angioplasty (PTCA) is a procedure that widens a narrowed or blocked coronary artery. One type of PTCA is balloon angioplasty. A catheter with a deflated balloon is inserted into the patient's femoral artery and threaded up into the heart. The small balloon is inflated inside the blocked coronary artery and opens the blocked area. A stent is often placed within the artery to increase blood flow to the myocardium. The stent remains in the artery permanently, keeping the artery open.

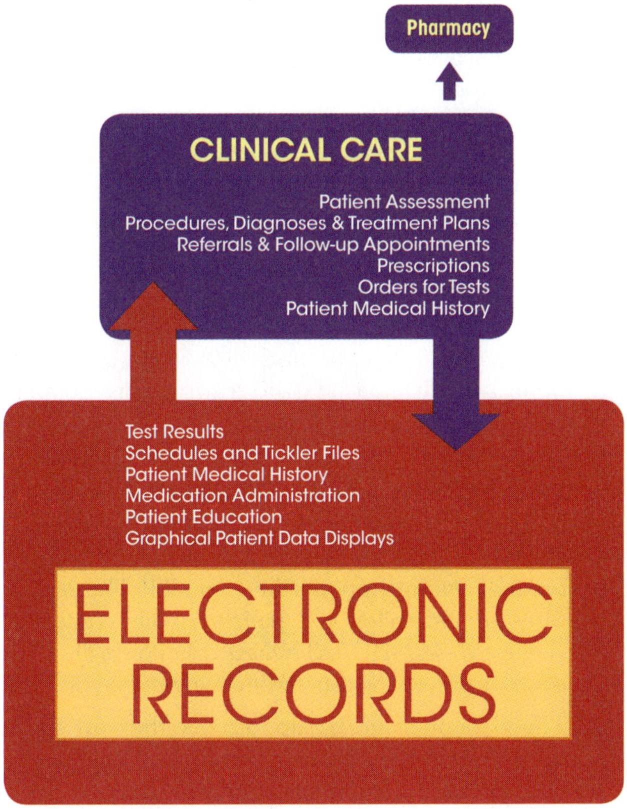

Figure 25-17 Total practice management system (TPMS) data flow.

Other cardiac procedures that can be performed for heart disease are atherectomy and laser angioplasty. In atherectomy, the provider uses a very small device on the end of the catheter to cut away the blocked area inside the coronary artery. In laser angioplasty, the provider uses a laser beam to destroy the blockage in the artery.

Coronary artery bypass is a procedure in which a portion of a vein (typically the saphenous) transplanted into one or more of the heart's coronary arteries. The transplanted vein circumvents or bypasses the blocked coronary artery, thus reestablishing blood supply to that portion of the heart.

A catheter with a large balloon can be used to open a standard (normal) valve. The balloon is inflated and, as in the angioplasty, the valve can be loosened. The catheter with balloon is removed after the procedure.

A heart valve can be repaired or replaced. In a replacement procedure, a tissue or mechanical valve replaces the heart's damaged valve.

Procedures for Arrhythmias

A cardiac electrophysiologist is a specialist who provides care to patients with arrhythmias. After a study by the cardiac electrophysiologist determines the source of the patient's arrhythmia within the electrical conduction system of the heart, a catheter is inserted into the femoral artery and a special device with radio waves is "aimed" at the source of the abnormal heart rhythm. This is known as *cardiac ablation*. The tiny scar produced prevents the electrical conduction system from traveling through the scarred area, resulting in normal rhythm.

A permanent battery-operated pacemaker can be surgically implanted into the patient's chest wall for treatment of certain types of arrhythmias. Wires from the pacemaker are inserted into the heart to provide a steady, regular heartbeat.

An implantable cardioverter defibrillator (ICD) is a device surgically implanted into the patient's chest wall with wires leading into the heart. When the patient's heart rate is extremely low or the patient's heart stops beating, the defibrillator delivers a small electric shock to jar the heart back into a normal rhythm (works like the AED; see section on defibrillation and Chapter 9).

Two other diagnostic tools for cardiac disease are cardiac computerized tomography (CCT) and cardiac magnetic resonance (CMR). Both are very useful tools, but they expose the patient to radiation and they are very expensive. Some cardiologists believe echocardiography (no radiation exposure) is just as useful in diagnosing heart disease.

Procedure 25-1

Perform Single-Channel or Multichannel Electrocardiogram

STANDARD PRECAUTIONS:

PURPOSE:

To obtain an accurate, graphic, artifact-free reading of the electrical activity of the patient's heart to identify arrhythmias, estimate damage caused by myocardial infarction, assess effects of cardiac medication, determine if electrolyte imbalance is present, identify cardiac ischemia, and determine the effects of hypertension or other disorders on the heart.

EQUIPMENT/SUPPLIES:

Examination or ECG table with pillow and sheet or blanket
Patient gown (open in front)
Automated electrocardiograph with patient cable wires
Alligator clips
Electropads (sensors)
ECG paper
Alcohol wipes
Gauze squares
Mounting form/card
Razor

PROCEDURE STEPS:

1. Perform tracing in a quiet, warm, and comfortable room away from electrical equipment that may cause artifacts. RATIONALE: Patient is less apprehensive in a quiet atmosphere. AC interference is minimized when ECG is performed away from other electrical equipment.
2. Wash hands, gather equipment, identify the patient, and explain the procedure to the patient. RATIONALE: Following these universal steps minimizes transmission of microorganisms and reassures patient.
3. Have the patient remove clothing from the waist up and uncover lower legs; nylon stockings must be removed; socks can be worn. RATIONALE: Electropads must be placed on bare skin for optimum conductivity of electricity. Provide a sheet or blanket for privacy and warmth. Place the patient in supine position on the examination table with arms and legs supported. Pillows can be used under the knees and head. RATIONALE: All four limbs and chest must be uncovered for proper electrode placement.
4. Explain that the procedure is painless and why it is necessary not to move or talk during the procedure. RATIONALE: Patient cooperation ensures good quality tracing.
5. Place the electrocardiograph with the power cord pointing away from the patient. Do not allow the cable to go underneath the table. RATIONALE: Helps reduce AC interference.
6. Apply the limb electropads (sensors) first. Apply the sensors to the fleshy parts of the four limbs. If the sensor does not adhere well, use an alcohol wipe on the skin, let it dry, and apply a new sensor. Shave sites if necessary. RATIONALE: Skin oils can be removed by alcohol, thus improving the adherence of the sensor. By removing excess hair on the chest, the sensor will adhere better. Place sensors on a nonbony, nonmuscular (fleshy) area of the upper arms and lower legs. Arm sensors should have tab pointing down, leg sensors point upward. RATIONALE: Artifact can be reduced if sensors are placed on nonbony, nonmuscular areas of the limbs. Directing tabs properly reduces tension on the electrodes.
7. Place the sensors on the chest wall on the appropriate intercostal spaces with sensors pointing downward. Shave chest sites if necessary.
8. Attach lead wires from the ECG machine to each sensor using alligator clips, special clips applied to the ends of the lead wires (Figure 25-18 A and B). Be sure to connect lead wires to the correct sensors. Lead wires are labeled with abbreviations (RA, LA, RL, LL, and V or C) and are color-coded as follows: RA = white; LA = black; RL = green; LL = red, V or C = (chest) = brown or multicolored depending on machine model. The lead wires should follow the patient's body contour (Figure 25-18C–D). RATIONALE: Following body contour prevents sensors from being pulled off.
9. The patient cable is supported either on the table or on the patient's abdomen. Plug the patient cable into the electrocardiograph.

continues

Procedure 25-1 (continued)

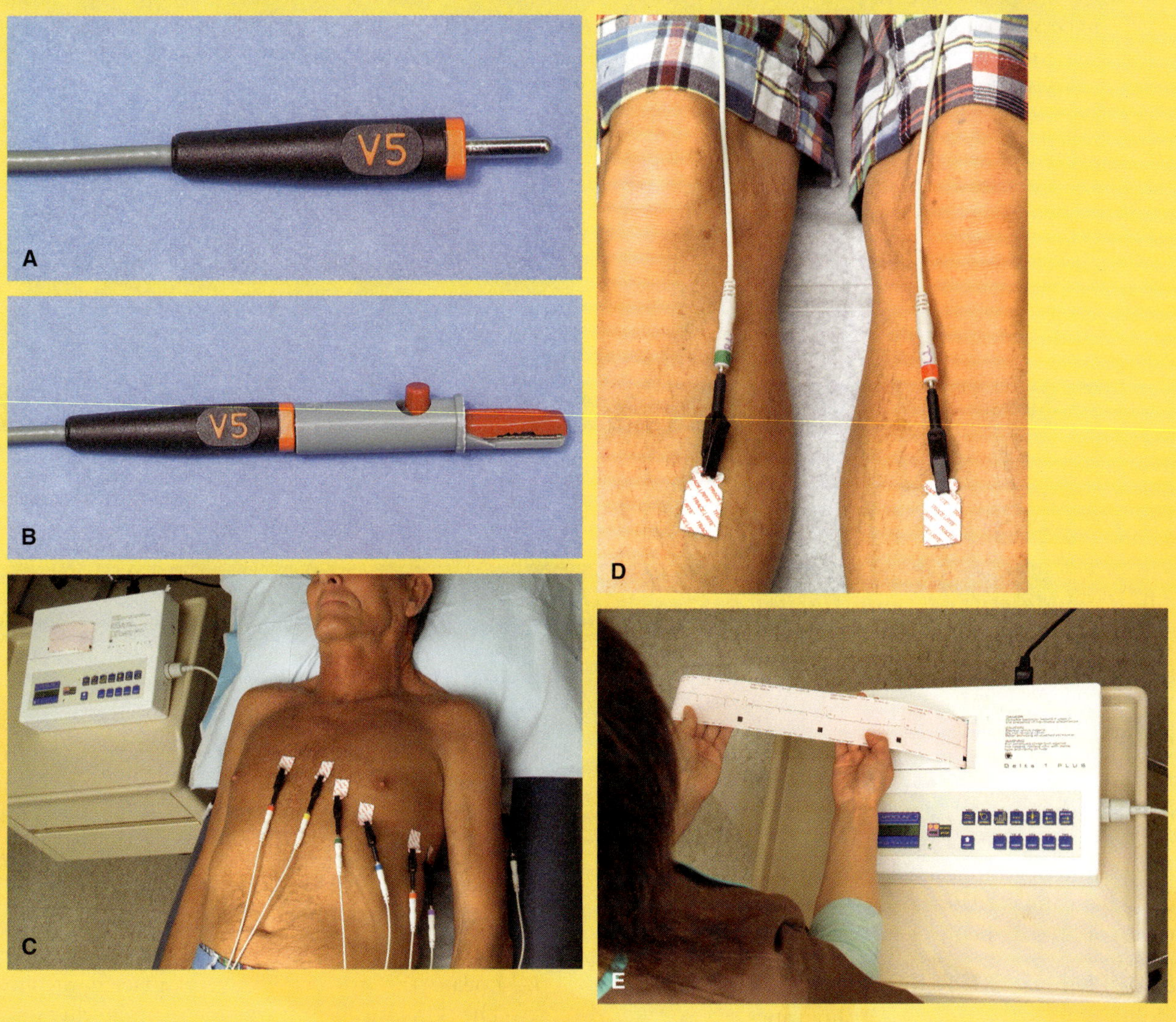

Figure 25-18 (A) Lead wires with nothing attached. (B) Alligator clip attached to top of lead wires. (C) Lead wires attached to the patient's chest and arms. (D) Lead wires attached to the patient's legs. (E) The machine prints each lead sequentially on a strip of ECG paper.

10. Turn the instrument to ON.
11. Enter information (patient name, date of birth, age, height, weight, sex, identification number, and cardiac medications the patient is presently taking). RATIONALE: The ECG machine automatically prints the information entered onto the ECG printout.
12. Remind the patient not to talk and to try not to move. (If the patient has a neuromuscular condition such as Parkinson's disease and cannot remain still, try having the patient slide his or her hands under the buttocks.) RATIONALE: Somatic tremor artifact may be lessened when the patient's hands are slid under the buttocks.
13. Press AUTO and the machine will automatically record and standardize the tracing. RATIONALE: Standardization ensures a dependable and accurate ECG.
14. The single-channel machine prints each lead sequentially on a strip of ECG paper (Figure 25-18E). A multichannel machine prints the tracing on an 8 ½- × 11-inch sheet of paper.
15. Check the quality of the tracing (artifacts, low voltage) before disconnecting lead wires. If it

continues

Procedure 25-1 (continued)

is necessary to repeat the tracing, first correct the problem that is causing a poor quality tracing. RATIONALE: Checking the tracing before removing the electropad sensors will save time if the ECG must be repeated.

16. Disconnect lead wires and remove the electropad sensor from the patient.
17. Assist patient as needed.
18. Be certain the patient information is on the tracing before giving it to the provider to read.
19. If the tracing is a single-channel tracing, cut and mount it, remembering to handle it carefully. Place in patient's record.
20. Document procedure in patient's chart or electronic medical record.

DOCUMENTATION

4/19/20XX 2:00 PM Twelve-lead ECG completed. Tracing given to Dr. Woo. Patient cooperative and seemed comfortable throughout procedure and says she "feels fine" after tracing. W. Slawson, CMA (AAMA) ——————

Procedure 25-2

Holter Monitor Application (Cassette and Digital)

STANDARD PRECAUTIONS:

PURPOSE:

To detect sporadic cardiac arrhythmias, to determine correlation of symptoms with activity, and to evaluate chest pain and cardiac status after pacemaker implantation or after acute myocardial infarction.

EQUIPMENT/SUPPLIES:

Holter monitor
Patient activity diary
Blank magnetic tape or flash memory card
Disposable electrodes
Razor
Alcohol wipes
Gauze
Carrying case
Belt or shoulder strap

PROCEDURE STEPS:

1. Wash hands and assemble equipment.
2. Prepare the equipment by removing old (used) battery from the monitor and replacing it with a new battery. Insert a blank magnetic tape or flash card into the monitor. RATIONALE: Installing a new battery each 24-hour period will ensure the monitor will function because it will have sufficient power.
3. Wash hands.
4. Identify the patient and explain the procedure. RATIONALE: Adherence to patient guidelines helps ensure an accurate tracing.
5. Have patient remove clothing from the waist up.
6. Have patient sit on the examination table or chair. RATIONALE: This allows for patient comfort and relaxation and for the medical assistant to place the electrodes appropriately.
7. Locate the correct electrode placement sites. The skin must be prepared in the following way:
   a. Dry shave patient's chest at each electrode site if chest is hairy.
   b. Cleanse the shaved area with an alcohol wipe. Let area dry.
   c. Abrade the skin slightly with a dry 4 × 4 gauze. Areas should be red. RATIONALE: Shaved site and abraded skin help the electrodes to adhere better to the skin and facilitate easier removal.
8. Take the electrodes from the package and peel away the backing from one of them (electrode should be moist). Continue to remove electrodes one by one and attach as in Step 9.

continues

Procedure 25-2 (continued)

9. Apply adhesive-backed electrode to the appropriate sites by applying firm pressure at the center of the electrode and moving outward toward the edges. Run your fingers along the outer rim to ensure firm attachment. Avoid moving from one side of electrode to the other. Gel could be forced out and could cause interference. RATIONALE: Firmly attached electrodes ensure a good quality tracing.
10. Attach the lead wires to the electrodes. Connect them to the patient cable.
11. Plug the monitor into the electrocardiograph with the test cable. Run a baseline tracing (not necessary with digital monitor). RATIONALE: Running a baseline tracing will validate proper setup of electrodes and confirm there is no malfunction of the leads or cable.
12. Place the electrode cable so that it extends from between the buttons of the patient's shirt or from below the bottom of the shirt.
13. Place the recorder into its carrying case and either attach it to the patient's belt or over the patient's shoulder. Be certain there is no pulling on the lead wires (Figure 25-19). RATIONALE: Pulling on electrodes could cause them to become detached.
14. Plug the electrode cable into the monitor. Record the starting time in the patient activity log (diary). These data will already be recorded in a digital monitor. RATIONALE: The beginning time is noted to correlate cardiac activity with the patient activity log.
15. Help patient get dressed.
16. Give the activity log to the patient, being certain that the patient information is completed. RATIONALE: The activity log helps correlate cardiac activity with patient symptoms.
17. Inform patient what time the following day the monitor will be removed. Remind the patient to bring along the activity log/diary.
18. Wash hands.
19. Document procedure in patient's record or electronic medical record.

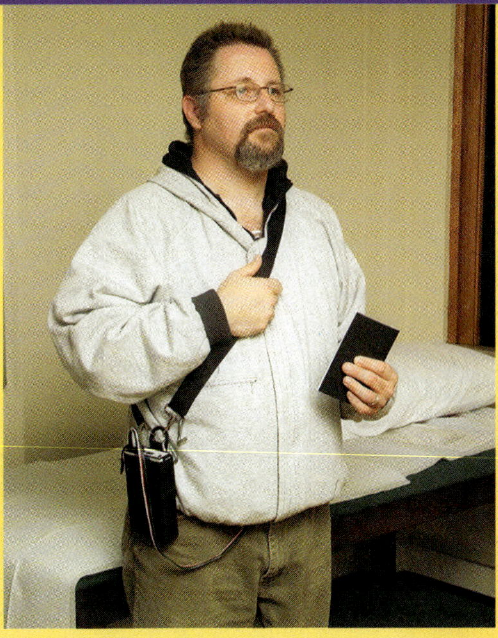

Figure 25-19 Correct placement of Holter monitor on patient.

20. Upon the patient's return 24 hours later, take the patient's electrodes off, remove flash memory card, accept cassette, remove battery.
21. Document patient returned with equipment.

DOCUMENTATION

3/2/20XX 10:00 AM Holter monitor applied. Patient given complete written instructions and restrictions and seems to understand them well. Time and date noted on activity log. Patient reminded to return to cardiac clinic at the same time tomorrow (10:15 AM) to have monitor removed and also to bring the activity diary. Patient given after-hours number if he needs assistance. J. Guerro, CMA (AAMA) ————————

3/3/20XX 10:00 AM Holter monitor electrodes removed from patient. Cassette and activity log returned/or flash memory card removed for later analysis on the computer analysis system. J. Guerro, CMA (AAMA) ————————

Case Study 25-1

Refer to the scenario at the beginning of the chapter. Wanda can empathize better with her patients now that she herself has had a baseline ECG.

CASE STUDY REVIEW

1. The feelings Wanda had while having her tracing are experienced by many patients. Explain what you can do for your patients to allay their fears when they are getting ready for an ECG and dur-

Case Study 25-2

Abigail Johnson, who is in her mid-70s, arrives at the urgent care center reporting chest pain. She has been seen on two other occasions for similar pain and has a history of diabetes, hypertension, arteriosclerotic heart disease, and angina pectoris. Medical assistant Wanda Slawson immediately alerts Dr. Rice of Mrs. Johnson's chest pain and then takes her into the cardiac examination and treatment room. Dr. Rice tells Wanda to have Mrs. Johnson take one of her nitroglycerin tablets and to perform an ECG on her. Mrs. Johnson is restless and anxious as Wanda prepares for the ECG and while the tracing is in progress. There is significant somatic tremor. Wanda attempts to allay Mrs. Johnson's apprehension to obtain a good quality ECG. The patient's pain subsides within a few minutes and she begins to feel better.

CASE STUDY REVIEW

1. What immediate action could Wanda have taken if Mrs. Johnson's pain had not subsided?
2. Mrs. Johnson tells Wanda that Dr. Rice explained arteriosclerotic heart disease and angina pectoris to her, but that she was nervous and understood little and that she is embarrassed to admit that to Dr. Rice. How can Wanda explain, in language that the patient can comprehend, what causes arteriosclerotic heart disease and angina, and what Mrs. Johnson experiences during an attack of angina? What strategies can Wanda teach Mrs. Johnson to promote healthier habits and prevent more serious heart problems?
3. Research community resources are available for persons with Mrs. Johnson's heart condition. Explain how Mrs. Johnson can locate them and how she could benefit from them.

Case Study 25-3

George Matthews, a 79-year-old patient of Dr. Abbott, has a history of cardiovascular heart disease. He tells Dr. Abbott that today he has been experiencing "palpitations and slow and fast heartbeats and sometimes dizziness." Dr. Abbott orders a resting ECG that shows no evidence of arrhythmia and decides that a Holter monitor electrocardiograph for Mr. Matthews might be helpful in diagnosing a cardiac arrhythmia.

CASE STUDY REVIEW

1. Describe why Dr. Abbott ordered Holter monitor electrocardiography for Mr. Matthews.
2. What instructions will you give to Mr. Matthews about wearing the monitor?
3. Mr. Matthews says he is not certain what activities should be recorded in the patient activity diary. Explain what they are and the reason for their importance.

SUMMARY

Electrocardiography is a noninvasive, painless procedure that is helpful in diagnosing heart arrhythmias, ischemia, and effects of cardiac medications. Wires with sensors are attached to the patient's arms, legs, and chest. The electrocardiograph amplifies the electrical currents generated by the electrical cells of the heart. A series of deflections (waves) is recorded on special ECG paper when a heated stylus on the electrocardiograph moves across the paper. The cardiac cycles that appear are then interpreted by the provider. The recording or tracing, known as an ECG, represents the heart's rate, rhythm, and other myocardial actions. Each of the 12 leads of the recording becomes part of the patient's permanent record.

In addition to a resting ECG, other types of electrocardiography can be done. Cardiac stress testing is done while the patient is physically challenged to perform increasingly strenuous exercises. The heart's tolerance to the increased demands placed on it during exercise can be observed and recorded while the patient is being closely monitored. This type of electrocardiography helps determine cardiac health and arrhythmias that would not be evident if a resting ECG were done.

Holter electrocardiography or ambulatory cardiac monitoring is an ECG test done as the patient goes about normal daily activities. The patient wears chest leads and carries a small recording device on a belt or on a strap over the shoulder for a period of 24 hours and documents activities in the patient activity diary. This type of electrocardiography helps diagnose cardiac arrhythmias that occur sporadically and may be difficult to capture on a resting ECG because of their unpredictability. Echocardiography is a diagnostic test that uses ultrasound to image the internal structures of the heart. Myocardial function, valvular function or defects, and chamber size can be determined.

In most cases, the medical assistant is responsible for patient preparation; patient education; operation of the electrocardiograph; elimination of artifacts; mounting, labeling, and placing ECG readings into the patient's file; and maintenance and care of the equipment. The diagnostic value of the test depends on the medical assistant's accuracy and skill.

STUDY FOR SUCCESS

To reinforce your knowledge and skills of information presented in this chapter:

- Review the Key Terms
- Practice the Procedures
- Consider the Case Studies and discuss your conclusions
- Answer the Review Questions
  - Multiple Choice
  - Critical Thinking
- Navigate the Internet by completing the Web Activities
- Practice the StudyWARE activities on your student CD
- Apply your knowledge in the Student Workbook activities
- Complete the Web Tutor sections
- View and discuss the DVD situations

REVIEW QUESTIONS

Multiple Choice

1. Which of the following is the most common type of artifact?
   a. somatic tremor
   b. AC interference
   c. wandering baseline
   d. interrupted baseline

2. Which of the following may cause somatic tremor?
   a. too much electrolyte
   b. cable across patient's lap
   c. corroded sensors
   d. Parkinson's disease

3. One cardiac cycle (heartbeat) takes approximately how long?
   a. 0.2 second
   b. 0.4 second
   c. 0.6 second
   d. 0.8 second
4. Which of the following indicates ventricular depolarization?
   a. QRS complex
   b. P wave
   c. T wave
   d. S-T segment
5. Another name for V leads is:
   a. precordial
   b. augmented
   c. standard
   d. limb

Critical Thinking

1. The provider wants you to explain to Mrs. Johnson (see Case Study 2) what behaviors she can adopt to have a healthy heart. With a partner, role-play medical assistant and patient and explain to the patient what she can do to improve her heart's health.
2. During the ECG, the equipment malfunctions. What options are available to the medical assistant?
3. Name four cardiac abnormalities that can be detected on an ECG.
4. Identify the placement of the 12 leads of the ECG.
5. The patient coughs and moves during the ECG. How can this affect the ECG tracing?
6. Explain standardization and why it is important.
7. What causes AC interference, wandering baseline, and interrupted baseline and how can they be eliminated?

WEB ACTIVITIES

Search on the Internet for a national organization that focuses on heart and blood vessel disorders such as the American Heart Association or the American College of Cardiology.

1. Print information about risk factors for cardiovascular heart disease.
2. What is the mortality rate for first-time myocardial infarctions for men versus women? Is there any difference in the mortality rate?
3. Are the symptoms identical in male and female patients when they are experiencing a myocardial infarction? Explain the similarities/differences between them.
4. Determine if there are newer types of 24-hour cardiac monitoring devices. How are they the same as or different from the Holter monitor?

REFERENCES/BIBLIOGRAPHY

Delaune, S. C., & Ladner, P. (2002). *Fundamentals of nursing standards and practice* (2nd ed.). Clifton Park, NY: Delmar Cengage Learning.

Heartsaver AED. Retrieved September 18, 2009, from http://www.americanheart.org.

Passanisi, C. (2001). *Electrocardiology essentials.* Clifton Park, NY: Delmar Cengage Learning.

Taber's cyclopedic medical dictionary. (20th ed.). (2005). Philadelphia: F. A. Davis.

THE DVD HOOK-UP

This chapter discusses the proper techniques for performing electrocardiographic procedures.

In the first scene, the student extern prepared Mr. Byrne for his ECG. Typically, men do not wear gowns when exposing only the chest. Mr. Byrne, however, has a little more breast tissue than most men.

1. Do you think that the extern should have offered him a gown for modesty purposes?

Things do not always go as planned. In the majority of cases, the patient is placed in a supine position for an ECG. In today's program, the patient was unable to lie down for the ECG because of a neck and back injury.

1. What are some other obstacles that may interfere with the way you would normally attach or run an ECG?

DVD Journal Summary

Write a paragraph that summarizes what you learned from watching today's DVD program. What steps could you take to help a patient relax who is anxious about having an ECG?

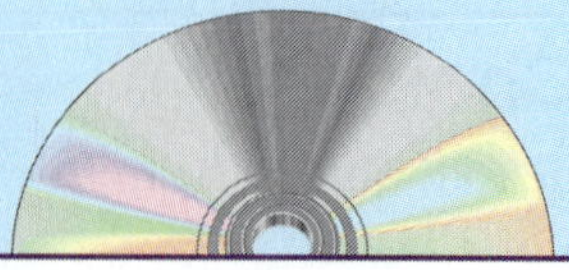

DVD Series Skills Based Series
Program Number 13
Chapter/Scene Reference
- *Entire program*

UNIT 7

Laboratory Procedures

Chapter 26

Safety and Regulatory Guidelines in the Medical Laboratory

OUTLINE

OBJECTIVES

The student should strive to meet the following performance objectives and demonstrate an understanding of the facts and principles presented in this chapter through written and oral communication.

1. Define the key terms as presented in the glossary.
2. Identify the governmental agency that regulates procedures performed on patients and describe the agency's main concerns.
3. List the types of human specimens that CLIA regulates.
4. Name two performance requirements CLIA imposes on all laboratories.
5. Describe how CLIA '88 regulates the use of quality control in automated hematology instruments.
6. Recall the three categories of testing and list several from the waived category.
7. Discuss the importance of CLIA to the medical assistant.
8. Identify and discuss the contents of the law of CLIA '88.
9. Describe CMS form 116 and explain its purpose.
10. Identify two OSHA standards that seek to safeguard employees.
11. Describe MSDS manuals and their purpose.
12. Differentiate among the four colors and five numbers of the National Fire Protection Association.

KEY TERMS

Acetone
Aegis
Body Fluid
Calibration
Chemotherapeutic Agents
Communicable
Ethyl Alcohol
Excretion
Formaldehyde
Fume Hood
Mandate
Medical Asepsis
Proficiency Testing
Provider Performed Microscopy Procedure (PPMP)
Pulmonary Edema
Quality Assurance
Quality Control
Reimbursement
Requisition
Secretion
Suppressed Immune System
Waived

Scenario

At Inner City Health Care, Dr. Susan Rice ordered a complete urinalysis for patient May Pankey. Dr. Rice's medical assistant, Wanda Slawson, CMA (AAMA), has obtained the specimen from the patient, has performed the physical examination and the chemical examination of the urine, and has documented her findings on the lab report form. She has also spun a test tube of urine in the centrifuge and has prepared a slide of the sediment for Dr. Rice to examine under the microscope. While Wanda is waiting for the doctor, she examines the slide to see if she can identify any abnormalities. She will compare her findings with Dr. Rice's findings to see how closely she comes to correctly identifying the cellular components in the urine sediment. This is one way for Wanda to continue her education on a daily basis while performing her clinical duties.

INTRODUCTION

Laboratory safety is a concern for all—management, staff, and patients. An unsafe work environment and work practices can threaten the emotional and physical health of the health care worker, as well as the patient. Injuries are costly on many levels: personally to the injured individual, lost work days, workers' compensation, medical treatment, potential legal action, and potential fines from regulatory agencies. These situations have a direct effect on the individuals involved, but they also have an indirect effect by lowering staff morale, ultimately resulting in less productivity. Management's response to safety is the key. Appropriate orientation, annual reviews, periodic drills, and consistent enforcement of staff adherence to policy are all part of a successful laboratory safety program.

All health care providers continually come into contact with patients who are ill. Some patients have ***communicable*** *or contagious diseases; others may have a* ***suppressed immune system*** *that does not protect them from infection. In the course of performing your duties as a medical assistant, you will be in contact with blood and* ***body fluids*** *that may be highly infectious. It is of extreme importance that your health and safety, as well as the health and safety of your patients, be protected.*

There are a number of infection control measures that can be used to reduce the transmission of bloodborne and other pathogens. ***Medical asepsis,*** *also known as infection control, consists of procedures and practices that health care professionals use to prevent the spread of infection (see Chapter 10). State and federal agencies also have established policies, procedures, and guidelines for health care providers and employers to follow to reduce the risk for transmission of infectious diseases. This chapter, as well as Chapter 10, examines the major guidelines.*

The Centers for Disease Control and Prevention (CDC) in Atlanta, Georgia, a division of the United States Public Health Service, is an agency that investigates various diseases in an attempt to control them and makes recommendations on how to prevent the spread of disease. The CDC issued the system of seven isolation categories for patients with infectious diseases and recommended the guidelines known as Universal Precautions. In 1996, the CDC released Standard Precautions, which represent the most current and comprehensive approach to infection control. The CDC Guidelines for Standard Precautions and Universal Precautions are covered thoroughly in Chapter 10. This chapter focuses on the federal regulations of the Clinical Laboratory Improvement Amendments of 1988 (CLIA '88) and the Occupational Safety and Health Administration (OSHA) in relation to the providers' office laboratory (POL).

CLIA '88 and OSHA, together with the CDC, regulate the safety of patients and health care workers. CLIA '88 comes under the ***aegis,*** *or protection, of the Centers for Medicare & Medicaid Services (CMS), formerly known as the Health Care Financing Administration (HCFA) of the U.S. Department of Health and Human Services (DHHS) of the federal government. OSHA comes under the U.S. Department of Labor. Both agencies require that health care settings, including clinical laboratories, adhere to the strict regulations that they set forth.*

The purpose of CLIA '88 is to safeguard the public by regulating all testing of specimens taken from the human body. The purpose of OSHA is to require employers to ensure employee safety in regard to occupational exposure to potentially harmful substances.

CLIA '88 and OSHA guidelines are discussed separately in this chapter. Keep in mind as you go through this chapter that CLIA '88 is designed to protect patients, and OSHA regulations are designed to protect workers. Table 26-1 summarizes the guidelines and purposes of CDC, CLIA '88, and OSHA.

Table 26-1 Federal Health and Safety Guidelines

Guidelines	Issuing Agency	Purpose
Standard Precautions	Centers for Disease Control and Prevention (CDC), U.S. Public Health Service	Issued in 1996 to augment and synthesize Universal Precautions and techniques known as body substance isolation (BSI). Standard Precautions contain measures intended to protect all health care providers, patients, and visitors from infectious diseases.
Transmission-Based Precautions	CDC	Designed to reduce the risk for airborne, droplet, and contact transmission of pathogens. These are used in addition to Standard Precautions and are intended for specific categories of patients.
Universal Blood and Body Fluid Precautions (Universal Precautions)	CDC	Released in 1985 to assist health care providers to greatly reduce the risk for contracting or transmitting infectious diseases, particularly AIDS and hepatitis B.
Clinical Laboratory Improvement Amendments of 1988 (CLIA '88)	Centers for Medicare & Medicaid Services (CMS), U.S. Department of Health and Human Services (DHHS)	Safeguards the public by regulating all testing of specimens taken from the body.
Occupational Safety and Health Administration (OSHA) Guidelines	OSHA, U.S. Department of Labor	Requires employers to ensure employee safety in regard to occupational exposure to potentially harmful substances.

Spotlight on Certification

RMA Content Outline

- Medical law
- Asepsis
- Laboratory procedures (safety)
- First aid

CMA (AAMA) Content Outline

- Medicolegal guidelines and requirements
- Principles of infection control
- Processing specimens
- Quality control
- Preplanned action

CMAS Content Outline

- Legal and ethical considerations
- Asepsis in the medical office
- Medical office emergencies
- Safety
- Supplies and equipment

CLINICAL LABORATORY IMPROVEMENT AMENDMENTS OF 1988

CLIA '88 was designed to set safety policies and procedures that protect patients.

In 1988, there was a public outcry as a result of articles published in the *Washington Post* and the *Wall Street Journal* and televised reports of deaths that were attributed to misread Pap smears. The public wanted action taken to ensure its safety, particularly in regard to laboratory testing. The outcry prompted the federal government to become more involved in regulating laboratories.

Although CLIA had been enacted into law in 1967, the issue of the misread Pap smears caused Congress to reexamine the regulations it had set forth in 1967. Thus, CLIA '88 was passed and included amendments to the original law. The amended regulations took effect on September 1, 1992.

States can seek exemptions from the CLIA standards if they have regulations that are comparable to those imposed by CLIA. If the federal government grants the state an exemption, laboratories in that state are under the control of state standards and applicable fees, not federal standards and fees. Few states have exempt status.

The Intention of CLIA '88

The intent of CLIA '88 is to protect the public by regulating all laboratory tests performed on specimens taken from the human body, that is, tissue, blood, and body **secretions** and **excretions,** which are used in the diagnosis, treatment, and prevention of disease. Previous regulations (Medicare, Medicaid, and CLIA '67) were based on the site and scope of the laboratory testing. CLIA '88 regulates laboratory testing regardless of site, scope, volume, or frequency. As of June 2007, registered CLIA laboratories total more than 200,600, with POL making up more than 50% of the total. The regulations require that all laboratories in the United States and its territories meet performance requirements that are based on how complex a test is and the risk factors that are associated with incorrect test results. Laboratories must comply with the requirements to be certified by the DHHS.

It is necessary to understand what the CLIA '88 regulations encompass and how they impact medical assistants and other health care workers who participate in testing human specimens. It is important because all laboratories, including POLs, must abide by the CLIA law.

CLIA '88 regulations are based on the complexity of tests performed and they affect all aspects of the laboratory. They specify the type of test performed, personnel involved in testing, and **quality control.**

General Program Description

Congress passed CLIA in 1988, establishing quality standards for all laboratory testing to ensure the accuracy, reliability, and timeliness of patient test results regardless of where the test was performed. A laboratory is defined as any facility that performs laboratory testing on specimens derived from humans for the purpose of providing information for the diagnosis, prevention, or treatment of disease, or impairment or assessment of health. CLIA is user-fee funded; therefore, all costs of administering the program must be covered by the regulated facilities.

The final CLIA regulations were published on February 28, 1992, and are based on the complexity of the test method; thus, the more complicated the test, the more stringent the requirements. Three categories of tests have been established: waived; moderate complexity, including the subcategory of **Provider-Performed Microscopy Procedure (PPMP);** and high complexity. CLIA specifies quality standards for proficiency testing (PT), patient test management, quality control, personnel qualifications, and quality assurance as applicable. Because problems in cytology laboratories were the impetus for CLIA, there are also specific cytology requirements.

CMS is charged with the implementation of CLIA, including laboratory registration, fee collection, surveys, surveyor guidelines and training, enforcement, approvals of PT providers, accrediting organizations, and exempt states. The CDC is responsible for test categorization and CLIA studies.

To enroll in the CLIA program, laboratories must first register by completing an application, pay fees, be surveyed if applicable, and become certified. CLIA fees are based on the certificate requested by the laboratory (i.e., waived, PPMP, accreditation, or compliance) and the annual volume and types of testing performed. Waived and PPMP laboratories may apply directly for their certificate because they are not subject to routine inspections. Those laboratories that must be surveyed routinely—that is, those performing moderate- or high-complexity testing—can choose whether they wish to be surveyed by CMS or by a private accrediting organization. The CMS survey process is outcome-oriented and uses a quality assurance focus and an educational approach to assess compliance (Table 26-2).

Table 26-2 How to Tell What Level of CLIA Is Required

If these tests are performed	This type of certificate and/or survey is needed
Waived tests only	Certificate of Waiver
PPMP	Certificate of PPMP
Tests of moderate complexity	Certificate of Registration, CLIA survey, and Certificate of Compliance
Tests of high complexity	Certificate of Registration, survey by an accrediting agency, and Certificate of Accreditation

Data indicate that CLIA has helped to improve the quality of testing in the United States. The total number of quality deficiencies has decreased significantly from the first laboratory survey to the second.

Work is currently in progress with the CDC and CMS to develop a final CLIA rule that will reflect all comments received and new technologies.

Categories of Testing

CLIA '88, under the aegis of the CMS of the DHHS, has designated three categories of testing:

1. Waived tests
2. Moderate-complexity tests, including PPMP
3. High-complexity tests

Each of these categories has different requirements for personnel and quality control.

Waived tests are simple, are unvarying, and require a minimum of judgment and interpretation. Test error carries minimal hazard to the patient. Waived tests represent the lowest percentage of the total number of tests performed.

PPMP tests are moderate-complexity tests but represent a subcategory that was added at the request of providers.

The following criteria are used to categorize moderate- and high-complexity tests.

- The degree of operator intervention needed
- The necessary knowledge and experience the operator possesses
- The degree of maintenance and troubleshooting needed to perform the tests

Even though most of the tests medical assistants perform fall into the waived category, POLs will often perform moderate tests, including the PPMP tests. POLs are not limited to any category as long as they have sufficiently trained and credentialed personnel, equipment, and approval.

Manufacturers of self-contained test kits apply for and receive Food and Drug Administration (FDA) approval for their particular test to be on the CLIA waived list. To find out if your particular brand of self-contained test kit is on the CLIA waived list, access an up-to-date listing at the FDA Web site http://www.fda.gov and use the key search term "currently waived analytes" (be forewarned, though, the list is very long). You can obtain a list of categories and the complete CLIA '88 guidelines from the CDC Web site (http://www.cdc.gov and use key search term "CLIA").

Contents of the Law

1. All laboratories are required to register with CLIA '88 even if just one test is performed, regardless of whether there is Medicare and Medicaid **reimbursement** and regardless in which of the categories the test is found.
2. The regulations apply to all laboratories.
3. The regulations are specific to the complexity of the test. The waived tests are the simplest with the fewest regulations. Standards become more stringent as the complexity of the test increases.
4. A laboratory must obtain a certificate to perform tests. An initial filing for a certificate is made on CMS form 116. One of five certificates can be obtained. (There can be a state exemption as previously mentioned.)
   a. *Certificate of Waiver.* This certificate is issued to a laboratory to perform only waived tests.
   b. *Certificate for PPMP.* This certificate is issued to a laboratory in which a provider, midlevel practitioner, or dentist performs no moderate complexity tests other than the PPMP procedures (Table 26-3). This certificate permits the laboratory to also perform waived tests.
   c. *Certificate of Registration.* This certificate enables the entity to conduct moderate- and high-complexity laboratory testing until the entity is determined by survey to be in compliance with CLIA regulations.
   d. *Certificate of Compliance.* This certificate is issued to a laboratory after an inspection finds the laboratory to be in compliance with all applicable CLIA requirements.

Table 26-3 Examples of Provider-Performed Microscopy Procedures

All direct wet-mount preparations for the presence or absence of bacteria, fungi, parasites, and human cellular elements
All potassium hydroxide (KOH) preparations
Pinworm examinations
Fern tests
Postcoital direct, qualitative examinations of vaginal or cervical mucus
Urine sediment examinations
Nasal smears for granulocytes
Fecal leukocyte examinations
Qualitative semen analysis (limited to the presence or absence of sperm and detection of motility)

e. *Certificate of Accreditation.* This is a certificate that is issued to a laboratory on the basis of the laboratory's accreditation by an organization approved by CMS.

To date, more than 200,600 CLIA certifications have been issued, more than half being Certificates of Waiver or PPMP.

5. All five certificates require renewal every 2 years.
6. After a laboratory has been certified, it must notify CMS within 6 months if it changes the type of tests it performs. Changing the tests performed may change the laboratory's classification.
7. Some examples of sanctions or penalties imposed by CMS for noncompliance with CLIA law are:

Infraction	***Penalty***
Failure to enroll with CMS	Denial or revocation of certificate
Nonparticipation in proficiency testing	A score of zero (a score of 80% is required)
Failure to return the proficiency testing result	A score of zero

In addition, Medicare and Medicaid payments may be suspended or terminated and civil penalties of up to a $10,000 fine per violation or per day of noncompliance may be imposed.

For CLIA '88 conditions other than proficiency testing, newly regulated laboratories will not be subjected to penalties during the first inspection cycle unless it is determined that the laboratories' inadequacies pose immediate patient danger.

8. The law **mandates quality assurance** for nonwaived tests. Laboratories are required to establish policies and procedures through programs that assess test quality; identify problems and correct them; ensure precise, dependable, and punctual reporting of test results; and guarantee sufficient competent staff. In addition, laboratories must ensure that all quality-control data are studied, and if there is a complaint, an investigation must be undertaken and appropriate action taken and recorded. It is a requirement that quality-assurance records be maintained.
9. The law mandates quality control for nonwaived tests. Laboratories are required to have an adequate supply of equipment to perform the number and types of tests that they offer. A procedures manual must be available in the testing area and must include complete testing instructions. Documentation of maintenance programs for instruments, equipment, and test systems must be evident.
10. The law establishes requirements for the correct collection, transportation, and storage of specimens and the reporting of results (see No. 16, Patient Test Management).
11. The law mandates maintenance of records, equipment, and facilities of laboratories performing nonwaived tests (see No. 17, Documentation).
12. The law mandates personnel standards. There are requirements for personnel who perform nonwaived tests and they spell out the necessary qualifications and responsibilities required of them. Each person who takes the tests must be licensed by the state if required, have a high school diploma or equivalent, have adequate training, and be able to demonstrate an understanding of laboratory procedures; **calibration,** or standardization of instruments; specimen collection; and quality control. Personnel must report test results accurately and with dependability. All high-complexity tests must be done by technologists and technicians except for cytology, which requires more stringent qualifications.
13. The law mandates **proficiency testing** for nonwaived tests. The procedures and tests found in the waived category are exempt from proficiency testing, regardless of the type of laboratory in which the tests are performed. Moderate- and high-complexity test laboratories must enroll in proficiency testing programs that are approved by the DHHS. The proficiency testing samples are checked in the same manner as patient specimens. Unsatisfactory performance on a proficiency testing check can result in various penalties ranging from termination of the laboratory's license to operate to the termination of reimbursement from Medicare and Medicaid.
14. The law mandates unannounced on-site inspection. All laboratories in the moderate- and high-complexity category are subject to unannounced inspections by DHHS or an agency assigned to the task by DHHS. Laboratories that perform only waived tests must prove that tests are being

CMS FORM 116

CMS form 116 for the clinical laboratory application for CLIA, CMS-116, must be completed and returned to the CMS within 30 days of receipt. The form collects information regarding a laboratory's operation and is needed to evaluate fees, to determine baseline data, to update existing data, and to fulfill legal requirements. The information obtained from the application will give the surveyor of the laboratory a perspective of the laboratory's operation and if it will be subject to an on-site inspection.

done according to the manufacturer's directions. Inspections can involve interviewing employees, observation of employees performing tests, analysis of data, and documentation of results. Violations of requirements by any laboratory can result in penalties. The cost of inspection will be billed to the laboratory.

15. The law mandates an annual listing of laboratories that have had action taken against them.
16. The law mandates patient test management. All laboratories must have a strategy for properly receiving and processing specimens and for the precise reporting of the results. Written instructions regarding collection, safeguarding of specimens, and labeling of specimens must be available for patients. There must be a specific procedure for the reporting of life-threatening results and a follow-through to the person requesting the test. Test records must be kept for 2 years after the reporting of results.
17. The law mandates documentation. The following documentation must be done and be available:

- Specimen
  - Patient preparation
  - Specimen collection procedure
  - Proper labeling technique
  - Preservation of specimen if applicable
- Proficiency testing
  - Corrective action taken
- Quality control and quality assurance
  - Any corrective action taken
- Problem and complaint log
- **Requisitions** or written requests
  - Patient name
  - Name and address of laboratory
  - Date and time of collection
  - Name of test requested
  - Diagnosis
- Results
  - Name and address of laboratory where test is done
  - Test name
  - Test results, including normal ranges listed on test results
  - Disposition of unacceptable specimens must be released to authorized person
- Log of Results
  - Printouts from instruments report must be kept
  - Identification of person performing test
  - Patient identification number
  - Specimen identification
  - Date
  - Time specimen is received in laboratory
  - Specimen rejection log maintained
  - Records and dates of all tests done

Criteria for PPMP

To be categorized as a PPMP, the procedure must meet the following criteria:

1. The examination must be personally performed by one of the following practitioners:
   a. A provider during the patient's visit on a specimen obtained from his or her own patient or from a patient of a group medical practice of which the provider is a member or an employee
   b. A midlevel practitioner, under the supervision of the provider or in independent practice only if authorized by the state, during the patient's visit on a specimen obtained from his or her own patient or from a patient of a clinic, group medical practice, or other health care provider of which the midlevel practitioner is a member or an employee
   c. A dentist during the patient's visit on a specimen obtained from his or her own patient or from a patient of a group dental practice of which the dentist is a member or an employee
2. The procedure must be categorized as moderately complex.
3. The primary instrument for performing the test is the microscope, limited to bright-field or phase-contrast microscopy.
4. The specimen is labile, or a delay in performing the test could compromise the accuracy of the test result.
5. Control materials are not available to monitor the entire testing process.
6. Limited specimen handling or processing is required.

Criteria for CLIA Waived Tests

To be categorized as a laboratory performing waived tests, the procedures must meet the following criteria:

1. The tests must be simple laboratory examinations and procedures that are cleared by the FDA for home use, use methods that are simple and accu-

rate so errors are negligible, or pose no reasonable risk for harm to the patient if performed incorrectly.

2. The tests performed must be on CLIA's waived test list.
3. The manufacturer's instructions for performing the tests must be followed.
4. Minimal scientific and technical knowledge is required to perform the test, or knowledge required to perform the test may be obtained through on-the-job instruction.
5. Minimal training is required for preanalytic, analytic, and postanalytic phases of the testing process, or limited experience is required to perform the test.
6. Reagents and materials are generally stable and reliable, or reagents and materials are prepackaged; premeasured; or require no special handling, precautions, or storage conditions.
7. Operational steps are either automatically executed (such as pipetting, temperature monitoring, or timing of steps) or are easily controlled.
8. Calibration quality-control materials are stable and readily available, and external proficiency testing materials, when available, are stable.
9. Test system troubleshooting is automatic or self-correcting, clearly described, or requires minimal judgment, and equipment maintenance is provided by the manufacturer, is seldom needed, or can be performed easily.
10. Minimal interpretation and judgment are required to perfom preanalytic, analytic, and postanalytic processes, and resolution of problems requires limited independent interpretation and judgment.

CLIA '88 Regulation for Quality Control in Automated Hematology

CLIA '88 regulations require that three different procedures be performed in the quality-control protocol for automated hematology instruments. The procedures are calibration, control sample testing, and proficiency testing. CLIA's regulations require that the automated hematology instrument be calibrated at regularly scheduled intervals with either a calibrator sample or a normal control sample testing. Many manufacturers of automated hematology instruments recommend or may require that the instrument be recalibrated at shorter intervals than are required by CLIA '88. CLIA '88 mandates that two levels of control samples be tested first each day on any parameter that will be performed on a patient's sample. These quality-control checks must be performed before the patient's sample is tested. The results for quality-control samples must fall within two standard deviations of the expected mean value for that sample.

In addition to calibrations and control sample testing, an ambulatory care setting that uses automated hematology instruments must enroll in a proficiency testing program with a reference laboratory that is CLIA '88 approved.

> The findings of errors in processes at Certificate of Waiver (COW) laboratories and PPMP certificate laboratories are of concern. Both COW and PPMP laboratories currently have virtually no oversight. Results of studies indicate that, even though COW laboratories have the least amount of complexity to their tests, there are huge gaps in quality of the tests performed. It was discovered that POLs are lacking in the areas of following instructions, quality assurance, and quality control. PPMP laboratories were lacking in the areas of inappropriate certificates, not documenting personnel competency, and not evaluating test accuracy. Although these findings are of concern to the CLIA program, no patient harm has been documented as a result of these errors. Personnel performing the tests at COW laboratories surveyed were mostly nurses and physicians. The Centers for Medicare & Medicaid Services (CMS) confirmed that lack of routine oversight in COW and PPMP laboratories continues to be a significant challenge to ensuring quality testing. They recommend the following:
>
> - Institute educational programs for COW and PPMP laboratories
> - Validate the effectiveness of this educational program
> - Survey a percentage of COW and PPMP laboratories annually
> - Develop a self-assessment for PPMP laboratories
> - Provide educational material as part of the CLIA enrollment process
> - Have state survey agencies contact COW and PPMP laboratories to verify test menus

Aftermath of CLIA '88

There are many individuals who have serious concerns about whether CLIA has led to improved testing as was intended, or if the law has just produced an overload of paperwork and problems. Some question if the law will be fully implemented or even eliminated altogether.

Important developments help to put the law into perspective. CMS has postponed the date that Medicare payments would be cut off for failure to register. The deadline has been postponed at least three times. The American Medical

Association (AMA) complained that unannounced inspections of POLs would disrupt patient office visits. As a result, the Secretary of DHHS declared that POL inspections would be announced.

The category of PPMP was added as another certificate and testing category because providers argued that the microscopic tests were essential to their practice. Already the PPMP has expanded to include midlevel practitioners such as nurse practitioners, nurse midwives, and physician assistants.

The law states that CLIA must be self-supporting. However, far fewer laboratories registered than was originally anticipated, and the result is a significantly lower amount of revenue than had been expected.

It is interesting to note that the CDC has proposed easing CLIA regulations by adding another category of testing. It would fall between the waived tests and the moderately complex tests. The tests within this new category would be subject to minimal regulation. This proposal is under consideration. Many question whether CLIA will have any value if this event occurs.

Impact of CLIA on Medical Assistants

CLIA '88 requires every facility that tests human specimens for diagnosis, treatment, and prevention of disease to meet specific federal requirements. The law applies to any facility that performs tests for the preceding purposes. This includes any POLs and ambulatory care setting, two typical areas where medical assistants are employed. The law covers all facilities even if only one test or a few basic tests are done and even if there is no charge for the testing.

Medical assistants may be responsible not only for performing the tests but also for maintaining personnel records, including such information as workers' college diplomas, state licenses, national certifications, employees' continuing education, and recredentialing. Employee hepatitis B status must also be on file. Medical assistants may be involved with compiling a procedures manual on how to perform every test done; these must be reviewed every year. An instrument log must be available for each piece of equipment. Systems must be in place for calibration, quality control, quality assurance test recording, and proficiency testing (if higher than waived category tests are performed). Documentation by medical assistants is of utmost importance; for instance, a quality-control plan may be in action, but it may not be written down in detail.

Medical assistants are the only health care professionals trained specifically for the ambulatory setting, including the POL procedures. Lacking a medical laboratory technician or medical technologist in the POL, the burden of quality performance of the waived tests falls to the person specifically trained in that area, the medical assistant. Because laboratory training of the medical assistant focuses primarily on CLIA waived tests, it is of major concern that medical assisting programs offer the best training possible in the areas of quality assurance, quality control, and following manufacturer's instructions. Keep in mind that the medical assistant may be the only health care professional in the POL who has formal training in the performance of the waived laboratory tests. Add that to the received findings of errors in processes at COW and PPMP laboratories and medical assistants are definitely on the front lines of ensuring the best quality for test results performed in the POLs.

Because CMS has received only a fraction of the money that they expected to collect from application fees, there is little money to carry the CLIA '88 program forward. Medical assistants must realize that CLIA '88 is the law even though a number of laboratories have not seen inspectors nor felt any impact from the CLIA '88 regulations. Some laboratories are delaying concern about CLIA '88 rules and do not understand the law and, therefore, have not fully implemented the regulations. Medical assistants must know and comply with the law and be prepared for a CLIA inspection. Penalties are imposed on laboratories that are not in compliance with the law.

Medical assistants who perform clinical laboratory procedures must keep up with government changes.

Where to Find More Information Regarding CLIA '88

The original CLIA '88 guidelines and updates are available from the Federal Register for a fee. See the appendices for ordering information or visit the CMS Web site (http://www.cms.hhs.gov/CLIA).

OSHA REGULATIONS

OSHA regulations are intended to ensure employers have a safe and healthy work environment for their employees. This applies to all workers, not just health care workers. Some of the regulations include hard hats and steel-toed shoes for construction workers, safety switches for machinery, fire prevention equipment in restaurants, and, of course, safety equipment and supplies for health care workers. Two OSHA standards have the greatest impact: *The Occupational Exposure to Hazardous Chemicals* (revised from *The Hazard Communication Standard*) and *The Bloodborne Pathogen Standard. The Bloodborne Pathogen Standards* is reviewed in Chapter 10. This chapter discusses the standard for *Occupational Exposure to Hazardous Chemicals.* It is important to note that states have their own worker safety standards. Those state standards are required to be as strict or greater than the federal OSHA standards.

The Standard for Occupational Exposure to Hazardous Chemicals in the Laboratory

In an effort to reduce the number of chemically related illnesses and injuries in the workplace, OSHA published its *Hazard Communications Standard* in 1983. This led many states to develop *right-to-know* laws. In 1992, OSHA expanded the *Hazard Communications Standard,* and published *The Occupational Exposure to Hazardous Chemicals in the Laboratory Standard,* which specifically addressed clinical laboratories.

The intention of this law is to heighten employee awareness of risks linked with chemical dangers. It serves to improve work practices through employee training and identification of hazardous chemicals that exist in the workplace. The use of protective equipment is utilized to protect employees from harmful chemicals.

Chemical Hygiene Plan

The Chemical Hygiene Plan (CHP) on hazardous chemicals is the core of the OSHA safety standard on hazardous chemicals. A written plan must specify the training and information requirements of the standard. Certain specific control measures such as **fume hoods** and glove boxes must be included in the plan. A designated employee is the chemical hygiene or safety officer. Provisions for housekeeping and maintenance of the facility are included. OSHA standards are not optional, and penalties are imposed for noncompliance with the standard. Employers must meet the requirements not only to be in compliance with the law but to protect employees as well.

All laboratories and ambulatory care settings, including providers' offices, must comply with a chemical hygiene plan to meet the OSHA regulations. The only laboratories exempt from compliance are those that exclusively use methods that do not place employees at risk for exposure to chemicals that are hazardous. For example, some POLs perform only dipstick tests or use other commercially prepared kits in which reagents are not exposed and, as a result, they are exempt from compliance. The primary component of the OSHA standard is that a written chemical hygiene plan and program must be operational if chemicals are stored in a facility and handled by employees. Some examples of chemicals include, but are not limited to, stains, **ethyl alcohol,** sodium hypochlorite (household bleach), **formaldehyde,** fixatives, preservatives, injectables such as **chemotherapeutic agents,** and **acetone.** Many laboratory accidents result in chemical-related illnesses ranging from eye irritations to **pulmonary edema.**

There are three primary goals that an employer must accomplish to be in compliance with the OSHA standard for chemical exposure. The first is that there must be an inventory taken and a list compiled of all chemicals considered hazardous. The following information must be documented (Figure 26-1): the quantity of chemical stored per month or year; whether the substance is gas, liquid, or solid; the manufacturer's name and address; and the chemical hazard classification.

Second, a Material Safety Data Sheet (MSDS) (Figure 26-2) manual must be assembled. The MSDS statements are provided by the manufacturer when the chemicals are purchased and give detailed information about the chemicals and whether they are a health hazard. The MSDS statements should be organized into a notebook for employee use and located in an area of immediate access by employees. Every employee who is exposed to or works with chemicals must read the MSDS about those chemicals and know where the manual is kept. The various chemicals are labeled using the National Fire Protection Association's color and number method (Figure 26-3). There are four colors, each signifying a warning to the person handling the chemical(s) (Figure 26-4). They are:

- Blue signifies a health hazard
- Red signifies a flammability hazard

Critical Thinking

Compare whom CLIA protects with whom OSHA protects. Do they have similar missions?

SAMPLE

CHEMICAL INVENTORY FORM

Office of ______________________________

Date ______________________________

Chemical Name	Catalog #	Quantity Stores L./gm. (monthly)	Physical State	Hazard Class				Manufacturer	Comments
				H	F	R	P		

(H) Health
0 - Minimal
1 - Slightly
2 - Moderate
3 - Serious
4 - Extreme

(F) Fire Hazard
0 - Will not burn
1 - Slight
2 - Moderate
3 - Serious
4 - Extreme

(R) Reactivity
0 - Stable is not reactive with water
1 - Slight
2 - Moderate
3 - Serious
4 - Extreme

(P) Protection
A. - Goggles
B. - Goggles/Gloves
C. - Goggles/Gloves/Apron
D. - Face Shield/Gloves/Apron
E. - Goggles/Gloves/Mask
F. - Goggles/Gloves/Apron/Mask
X. - Gloves

Figure 26-1 Sample chemical inventory form for listing chemicals on the premises, including quantity, physical state, hazard class, manufacturer, and comments. (Courtesy of POL Consultants, 2 Russ Farm, Delanco, NJ 08075.)

- Yellow signifies reactivity or instability hazard
- White signifies a special hazard and the use of personal protective equipment (PPE)

The numbers 0 to 4 are used in conjunction with the colors to indicate the level of risk for each product and are assigned by the manufacturer using the rating system. The numbers can be found on the MSDS (Figure 26-5).

Third, the employer is required to provide a hazard communication educational program to the employee within 30 days of employment and before the employee handles any hazardous chemicals (Figure 26-6A). The training program should consist of the location and identification of hazardous chemicals, how to read and understand the labels on the chemicals, where the MSDS manual is kept, when to use PPE, and procedures to follow for chemical spills. The training sessions must be documented, signed by the employer, and permanently retained in the employee record (Figure 26-6B).

Requirements of Chemical Hygiene Plan (CHP). The requirements for a CHP include:

- Employers must have an operational written plan (a manual) relevant to the safety and health of employees.
- Written instructions on the use of PPE must be available.

MATERIAL SAFETY DATA SHEET

I – PRODUCT IDENTIFICATION

COMPANY NAME: We Wash Inc.

ADDRESS: 5035 Manchester Avenue
Freedom, Texas 79430

Tel No: (314) 621-1818
Nights: (314) 621-1399
CHEMTREC: (800) 424-9343

PRODUCT NAME: Spotfree

Product No.: 2190

Synonyms: Warewashing Detergent

II – HAZARDOUS INGREDIENTS OF MIXTURES

MATERIAL: (CAS#)	% By Wt.	TLV	PEL
According to the OSHA Hazard Communication Standard, 29CFR 1910.1200, this product contains no hazardous ingredients.	N/A	N/A	N/A

III – PHYSICAL DATA

Vapor Pressure, mm Hg: N/A
Evaporation Rate (ether=1): N/A
Solubility in H_2O: Complete
Freezing Point F: N/A
Boiling Point F: N/A
Specific Gravity H_2O=1 @25C: N/A

Vapor Density (Air=1) 60–90F: N/A
% Volatile by wt N/A
pH @ 1% Solution 9.3–9.8
pH as Distributed: N/A
Appearance: Off-White granular powder
Odor: Mild Chemical Odor

IV – FIRE AND EXPLOSION

Flash Point F: N/AV

Flammable Limits: N/A

Extinguishing Media: The product is not flammable or combustible. Use media appropriate for the primary source of fire.

Special Fire Fighting Procedures: Use caution when fighting any fire involving chemicals. A self-contained breathing apparatus is essential.

Unusual Fire and Explosion Hazards: None Known

V – REACTIVITY DATA

Stability - Conditions to avoid: None Known

Incompatibility: Contact of carbonates or bicarbonates with acids can release large quantities of carbon dioxide and heat.

Hazardous Decomposition Products: In fire situations heat decomposition may result in the release of sulfur oxides.

Conditions Contributing to Hazardous Polymerization: N/A

Figure 26-2 Example of a Material Safety Data Sheet (MSDS) listing product name, hazardous ingredients, physical data, fire and explosion data, reactivity data, health hazard data, emergency and first aid procedures, spill or leak procedures, protection information/control measures, and special precautions. (Courtesy of POL Consultants, 2 Russ Farm, Delanco, NJ 08075.)

Spotfree

VI – HEALTH HAZARD DATA

EFFECTS OF OVEREXPOSURE (Medical Conditions Aggravated/Target Organ Effects)

A. ACUTE (Primary Route of Exposure) EYES: Product granules may cause mechanical irritation to eyes.
SKIN (Primary Route of Exposure): Prolonged repeated contact with skin may result in drying of skin.
INGESTION: Not expected to be toxic if swallowed, however, gastrointestinal discomfort may occur.

B. SUBCHRONIC, CHRONIC, OTHER: None known.

VII – EMERGENCY AND FIRST AID PROCEDURES

EYES: In case of contact, flush thoroughly with water for 15 minutes. Get medical attention if irritation persists.
SKIN: Flush any dry Spotfree from skin with flowing water. Always wash hands after use.
INGESTION: If swallowed, drink large quantities of water and call a physician.

VIII – SPILL OR LEAK PROCEDURES

Spill Management: Sweep up material and repackage if possible.
Spill residue may be flushed to the sewer with water.

Waste Disposal Methods: Dispose of in accordance with federal, state and local regulations.

IX – PROTECTION INFORMATION/CONTROL MEASURES

Respiratory: None needed

Eye: Safety glasses

Glove: Not required

Other Clothing and Equipment: None required

Ventilation: Normal

X – SPECIAL PRECAUTIONS

Precautions to be taken in Handling and Storing: Avoid contact with eyes. Avoid prolonged or repeated contact with skin. Wash thoroughly after handling. Keep container closed when not in use.
Additional Information: Store away from acids.

Prepared by: D. Martinez

Revision Date: 04/11/XX

Seller makes no warranty, expressed or implied, concerning the use of this product other than indicated on the label. Buyer assumes all risk of use and/or handling of this material when such use and/or handling is contrary to label instructions.

While Seller believes that the information contained herein is accurate, such information is offered solely for its customers' consideration and verification under their specific use conditions. This information is not to be deemed a warranty or representation of any kind for which Seller assumes legal responsibility.

Figure 26-2 (continued)

CHEMICAL WARNING LABEL DETERMINATION

The Hazard Communication Act contains specific labeling requirements. Labels must be on all hazardous chemicals that are shipped to and used in the workplace. Labels must not be removed. Material safety data sheets for all chemicals will be available to employees.

Manufacturer Requirements: Chemical manufacturers are required to evaluate chemicals, determine status as hazards, provide material safety data sheets (MSDS), and label all shipped chemicals properly. Manufacturer labels must never be removed. The best way to determine the hazards of the chemical is to read the MSDS, obtain an OSHA designated list or State Hazardous Substance list. For most mixed chemicals, it is necessary to contact the manufacturer for MSDS.

Office Chemicals: Search through your office and write down all chemicals you have in the office. Most pharmaceuticals and common household products do not come under this standard. Ingredients can then be compared to a list of regulated substances or MSDS sheets will provide necessary information.

Employer's Responsibility: Any hazardous chemical used in the workplace that is not in its original container must be labeled with the identity of the chemical and hazards. "Target Organ" chemical labels may be used. The label must include the chemical and common name, warnings about physical and health hazards, and the name and address of the manufacturer. The employer is to compile a chemical inventory list that is to be updated as needed. MSDS information should be located in a place where it is accessible to all employees. Label and MSDS information should be provided during the safety training program.

Identity: The term identity can refer to any chemical or common name designation for the individual chemical or mixture, as long as the term used is also used on the list of hazardous chemicals and the MSDS.

NOTE: If a chemical is poured into another container for immediate use, it does not need to be labeled.

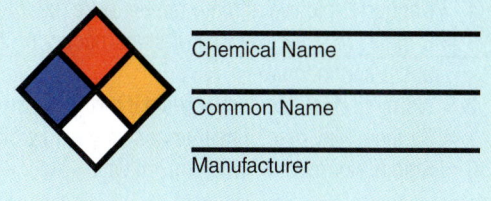

Chemical Name

Common Name

Manufacturer

Figure 26-3 Chemical warning label determination indicates necessary information for labels, including manufacturer's requirements, office chemicals, employer's responsibility, and identity of chemical or its common name. (Courtesy of POL Consultants, 2 Russ Farm, Delanco, NJ 08075.)

- Fume hoods or biohazard hoods must be checked regularly.
- Training sessions must be held for employees regarding their right to know what hazardous chemicals are in their work environment.
- It is the employer's legal responsibility to provide medical attention for an employee should an accidental chemical spill occur.
- The responsibility for executing training sessions, keeping manuals current, and documentation is designated to an employer.
- Instruction must be provided regarding disposal of hazardous waste produced in the workplace. (Usually a hazardous waste company is contracted by the employer.)
- Each employee's record must have a written statement, signed by the employer, stating the employer's responsibility to arrange for employee training and a safe work environment.

Critical Thinking

Name three other professions beside health care that should abide by OSHA regulations. For each profession, list four rules that should be in place. Do you think they are in place?

Importance of Chemical Standard to Medical Assistants. Meeting the requirements set forth by OSHA is not optional. All must comply or face penalties. All employees, including medical assistants, have the right to know and be given information and be educated regarding chemical hazards that they are exposed to in their place of employment. Medical assistants can be exposed to hazardous chemicals through skin contact, injection, or inhalation. Because many laboratory accidents result in chemical-related

BLUE: HEALTH HAZARD

4 = Danger: May be fatal
3 = Warning: Corrosive or toxic
2 = Warning: Harmful if inhaled
1 = Caution: May cause irritation
0 = No unusual hazard

RED: FLAMMABILITY

4 = Danger: Flammable gas or extremely flammable liquid
3 = Warning: Flammable liquid
2 = Caution: Combustible liquid
1 = Caution: Combustible if heated
0 = Noncombustible

YELLOW: REACTIVITY/INSTABILITY

4 = Danger: Explosive at room temperature
3 = Danger: May be explosive if spark occurs or if heated under confinement
2 = Warning: Unstable or may react if mixed with water
1 = Caution: May react if heated or mixed with water
0 = Stable: Nonreactive when mixed with water

WHITE: SPECIAL HAZARD/PROTECTION

A Goggles
B Goggles, gloves
C Goggles, gloves, apron
D Face shields, gloves, apron
E Goggles, gloves, mask
F Goggles, gloves, apron, mask
X Gloves

Figure 26-4 National Fire Protection Association's color and number method.

illnesses, it is important for medical assistants to understand how the law affects them, their place of employment, and their employer. Medical assistants and other health care providers should know what hazards they face, and know the proper technique for handling, storing, and disposing of hazardous chemicals. Medical assistants in administrative positions must use their knowledge and skills to provide a safe work environment for themselves and their staff.

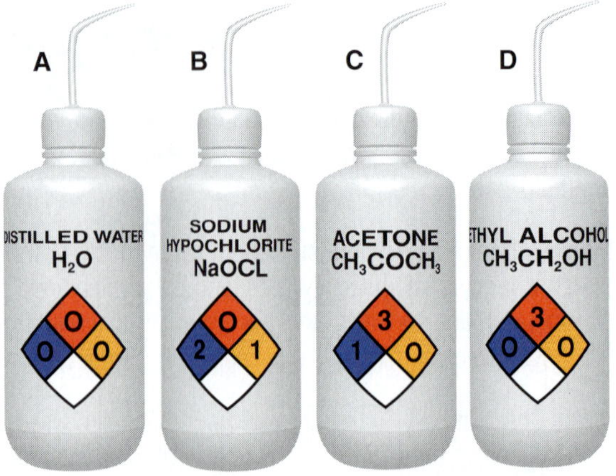

Figure 26-5 Four containers are marked using the National Fire Protection Association's color and number method for identifying and warning of chemical hazards. (A) Distilled water: Presents no health, flammability, or reactivity/instability hazard and requires no PPE when used (all areas are zero). (B) Sodium hypochlorite: Does not promote a flammability hazard (red is zero), is harmful if inhaled (blue is 2), and may react or become unstable if heated or mixed with water (yellow is 1). (C) Acetone: Flammable (red is 3), may cause irritation (blue is 1), and is stable/nonreactive when mixed with water (yellow is zero). (D) Ethyl alcohol: Flammable (red is 3), no unusual health hazards (blue is zero), and is stable/nonreactive when mixed with water (yellow is zero).

OSHA REGULATIONS AND STUDENTS

With the passage of the OSHA laws, all students with potential exposure to chemicals and bloodborne pathogens should follow all safety procedures as outlined by OSHA. Because students are not considered employees of a health care facility and are attending an educational institution, they do not fall under the OSHA guidelines. They should, however, take precautions to avoid contact with potentially infectious materials and toxic chemicals wherever learning is taking place.

Avoiding Exposure to Chemicals

Students may come into contact with harmful chemicals when doing procedures that can cause such problems as burns to the skin and eyes. Students will be made aware of these through information packaged with kits and the MSDS. As a

SAFETY TRAINING CRITERIA

Safety training will be offered to all employees within 30 days of employment or before the employee assumes responsibilities that involve exposure to body fluids or chemicals.

Items to be covered in training session:

- General explanation of OSHA laws
- General explanation of the epidemiology and symptoms of HBV and HIV
- Who is at risk in office
- Modes of transmission of HBV and HIV
- Method of control in workplace
- Universal Precautions
- Handwashing
- Personal protective equipment
- How to clean up spills
- What to do after a needlestick injury
- Medical follow-up after an exposure
- Cleaning protocol for office
- Hazardous Communication Standard
- Types of chemical labels
- How to read MSDS and NFPA signs
- Warning signs
- How to get MSDS
- Location of MSDS
- How to store chemicals
- How to record chemical inventory
- Hazardous Waste laws
- How to comply with laws
- How to use and label bio-bins and sharps containers
- How to keep records
- Who keeps the records
- Medical consent forms
- HBV forms
- Safety training certificate
- Engineering control records

Figure 26-6A Safety Training Form lists the items to be covered by the employer during OSHA training sessions. (Courtesy of POL Consultants, 2 Russ Farm Way, Delanco, NJ 08075.)

SAMPLE

CERTIFICATE OF TRAINING

____

First Name Middle Initial Last Name

has completed the

OSHA HAZARD COMMUNICATION
INFORMATION TRAINING PROGRAM

This certificate indicates your successful participation in a program instructing you of your rights as a worker and the proper handling of hazardous substances in the workplace.

__________________ __________________

Date Employee Signature

____

Instructor's Signature

____

Employer's Signature

Figure 26-6B Sample Certificate of Training shows that the employee has completed an OSHA Hazard Communication Information Training Program. (Courtesy of POL Consultants, 2 Russ Farm Way, Delanco, NJ 08075.)

general rule, if the chemical comes in contact with the skin, it must be flushed with water immediately and continued for five minutes. Chemicals that get into the eye must be flushed for 15 minutes (unless contradicted on the label). Refer to the MSDS for specific postexposure procotol. Eyewash stations and showers should be available in case of accidental exposure to hazardous chemicals with a follow-up in the emergency department.

Chemical spills should be carefully cleaned following the procedure for the particular chemical. The same chemical biohazard spill cleanup kits used in POLs can be used in school laboratories. Students should familiarize themselves with the contents of the kits and the instructions for use before an actual spill occurs.

Toxic fumes can occur with certain chemicals and certain tests can cause lung irritation and damage. This type of chemical should be handled under a fume hood that will take the fumes away by means of a ventilation mechanism.

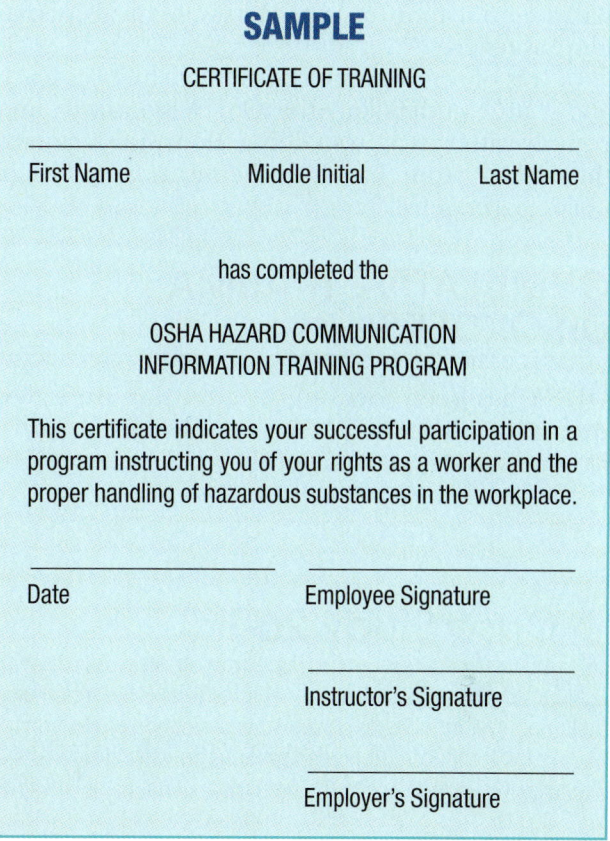

A student safety laboratory manual outlining an exposure control plan with emphasis on Standard Precautions, PPE, work practice controls, lists of hazardous chemicals, and MSDS should be compiled and accessible. Students should be thoroughly familiar with its contents. In addition, students should be educated as to the location and identification of hazardous chemicals just as employees are.

It is of utmost importance that students learn about and understand the OSHA standards and comply with them. In so doing, they will safeguard themselves from harmful chemicals and bloodborne pathogens.

CUMULATIVE TRAUMA DISORDERS

OHSA has been focusing its attention on a new threat to the workplace: ergonomic hazards. Ergonomics is the study of the workplace. OSHA published its first standard, *Ergonomic Hazards,* in 1991. At the heart of these guidelines is the prevention of cumulative trauma disorders. Cumulative trauma disorders are injuries involving the musculoskeletal or nervous system, such as carpal tunnel syndrome and trigger finger. They are the result of long-term, repetitive work actions, such as gripping, keyboard use, pipetting, and microscopy. Limiting or preventing repetitive work actions is the key to minimizing cumulative trauma disorders. Use of ergonomically correct equipment and supplies, proper work site design, staff training, and job rotation are essential in creating an ergonomically sound workplace.

Case Study 26-1

Refer to the scenario at the beginning of the chapter. Wanda performs the microscopic examination of the urine slide even though the procedure is not a waived test. She compares her findings to Dr. Rice's assessment.

CASE STUDY REVIEW

1. Besides learning more about urine components and continuing her education, what benefit does Wanda obtain by putting forth this extra effort?
2. Do you think Dr. Rice will appreciate her extra effort?

Case Study 26-2

Marie Tyndall is a student in the Jackson Heights Community College Medical Assisting Program. She and two other classmates have been assigned the project of creating a plan for cleaning up spills that might occur in the classroom laboratory and ensuring that all students using the laboratory have been trained in the proper procedure.

CASE STUDY REVIEW

1. What materials would her group need?
2. How would her group go about learning the proper steps in the clean-up process?
3. How would her group ensure that all other students in the laboratory also have the proper training?

SUMMARY

Infectious diseases and accidents occur through lack of education and carelessness. Medical assistants must understand the importance of the regulations and guidelines set forth by the federal government and follow through by helping employers implement them. In doing so, the health and safety of patients and health care workers will be protected, the spread of infectious diseases can be kept under control, and the risk for contracting an infectious disease such as AIDS or hepatitis B will be greatly minimized.

Every medical office and ambulatory care setting must, by law, have clearly written and readily available manuals containing information about Standard Precautions, CLIA '88, and OSHA for the safe handling, storage, and disposal of blood, body fluids, and chemicals.

Through consistent use of Standard Precautions and adherence to the CLIA and OSHA laws, health care providers can acquire the behaviors and techniques needed to safeguard themselves and their patients.

Because of frequent changes in the laws, it is necessary for medical assistants and all other health care providers to keep abreast of the government mandates.

STUDY FOR SUCCESS

To reinforce your knowledge and skills of information presented in this chapter:

- Review the Key Terms
- Consider the Case Study and discuss your conclusions
- Answer the Review Questions
  - Multiple Choice
  - Critical Thinking
- Navigate the Internet by completing the Web Activities
- Practice the StudyWARE activities on the CD
- Apply your knowledge in the Student Workbook activities
- Complete the Web Tutor sections
- View and discuss the DVD situations

REVIEW QUESTIONS

Multiple Choice

1. Standard Precautions were issued by:
   a. DHHS
   b. CDC
   c. CMS
   d. OSHA
2. CLIA '88 was made law to regulate:
   a. the disposal of infectious waste
   b. the use of chemicals in the workplace
   c. laboratory tests performed on specimens taken from the human body
   d. the transmission of the human immunodeficiency virus (HIV)
3. The core of the OSHA safety standard for chemical exposure is:
   a. the dipstick test
   b. the chemical hygiene plan
   c. the quantity of chemical stored per month
   d. the MSDS manual
4. The agency that requires employers to ensure employee safety concerning occupational exposure to potentially harmful substances is:
   a. CDC
   b. U.S. Public Health Service
   c. CMS
   d. OSHA
5. Successful laboratory safety programs include:
   a. threats to the emotional and physical health of health care workers
   b. lost workdays and increased workers' compensation claims
   c. orientation, periodic drills, and consistent enforcement of policy
   d. potential fines from regulatory agencies
6. CLIA regulations specify all the following except:
   a. the type of test performed
   b. the personnel involved in testing
   c. quality control
   d. the methods used in testing
7. The agency charged with implementing CLIA is:
   a. CDC
   b. United States Public Health Service
   c. CMS
   d. OSHA
8. Which is not an approved provider for PPMP?
   a. a physician
   b. a nurse practitioner
   c. a dentist
   d. a medical assistant
9. The standard published by OSHA to prevent cumulative trauma disorders is:
   a. *Workplace Standard*
   b. *Standard for Prevention of Cumulative Trauma*
   c. *Ergonomic Hazards*
   d. *Ergonomic Standard*
10. Match the chemical warning color with the hazard represented.

1. Blue	a. Reactivity or instability
2. Red	b. Use PPE
3. Yellow	c. Health
4. White	d. Flammability
	e. Disaster

Critical Thinking

1. Explain the purpose of CLIA '88 and why the law was amended.
2. Name three categories of testing and explain each category.
3. Discuss the 17 major components of CLIA '88.
4. Describe quality control and quality assurance. Why are they important?
5. What is CMS Form 116? Explain its use.
6. You have been asked to develop a manual for your provider–employer. The manual is to detail a chemical hygiene plan (CHP) for all employees in the office. How would you proceed? What should be included in the plan? In the CHP include three major goals that will ensure the provider–employer's compliance with the hazard standard. You have been asked to compile a manual of the MSDSs. What must be included in the manual and from where does the information come?

WEB ACTIVITIES

1. Using the Internet, go to http://www.cms.hhs.gov and search for the list of CLIA waived tests. Is this list extensive/brand specific or general?
2. Go into the FDA's Web site at http://www.fda.gov and see if the list of CLIA waived tests on that site differs. What do you think is the reason for the lists being different or the same?
3. While you are searching those two Web sites, find out what language(s) is acceptable for labels on hazardous chemicals.
4. Go to the CDC Web site at http://www.cdc.gov/mmwr and find the report on Good Laboratory Practices. Find the seven important criteria to be considered before introducing a new waived test.

REFERENCES/BIBLIOGRAPHY

Centers for Disease Control and Prevention. (2007). *Good laboratory practices for waived testing report.* Retrieved December 2008, from http://www.cdc.gov/mmwr.

Centers for Medicare & Medicaid Services. Retrieved October 2008, from http://www.cms.hhs.gov.

U.S. Food and Drug Administration. (2004). *Databases on the FDA web site.* Retrieved October 2008, from http://www.fda.gov/search/databases.html.

THE DVD HOOK-UP

This chapter discusses safety and regulatory guidelines for the medical office.

Both the chapter and selected DVD scene discuss the three major categories for testing.

1. What is the most common category that medical offices fall into for laboratory testing? Why?
2. In a waived laboratory, which personnel have the authority to perform microscopy?
3. What does CLIA stand for and who oversees CLIA?

DVD Journal Summary

Write a paragraph that summarizes what you learned from watching the selected scene from today's DVD program.

What would you do if you found out that your employer was running tests that he should not, based on the office's CLIA classification?

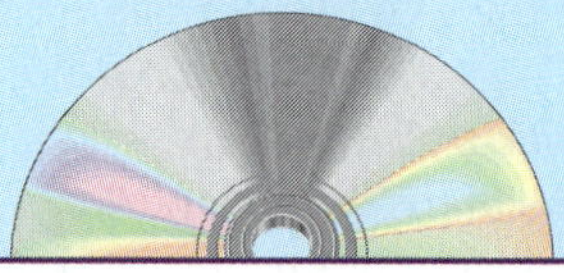

DVD Series	**Program Number**
Skills Based Series	11

Chapter/Scene Reference

- *Introduction to Venipuncture, Hematology, and Immunology Procedures*

Introduction to the Medical Laboratory

Chapter 27

KEY TERMS

Assay
Asymptomatic
Baseline Values
Biopsy
Clinical Chemistry
Clinical Diagnosis
Condenser
Control Test
Culture and Sensitivity (C&S)
Cytology
Diagnosis
Diaphragm
Differential Diagnosis
DNA
Electrolyte
Glucose
Hematology
Histology
Hormone Replacement Therapy (HRT)
Hospital-Based Laboratories
Immunohematology
Immunology
Invasive
Microbiology
Mycology
Objective
Panel
Parasitology
Patient Service Centers
Peak
Physician's Office Laboratory (POL)

OUTLINE

- The Laboratory
  - Purposes of Laboratory Testing
  - Types of Laboratories
  - Laboratory Personnel
  - Laboratory Departments
  - Panels of Laboratory Tests
- Billing for Laboratory Services
- Quality Controls/Assurances in the Laboratory
  - Control Tests
  - Proficiency Testing
  - Preventative Maintenance
  - Instrument Validations
  - The Medical Assistant's Role
- Laboratory Requisitions and Reports
- Specimen Collection
  - Proper Procurement, Storage, and Handling
  - Processing and Sending Specimens to a Laboratory
- Microscopes
  - Types of Microscopes
  - How to Use a Microscope
  - How to Care for a Microscope

OBJECTIVES

The student should strive to meet the following performance objectives and demonstrate an understanding of the facts and principles presented in this chapter through written and oral communication.

1. Define the key terms as presented in the glossary.
2. Explain the purposes of laboratory testing.
3. Describe the main similarities and differences between independent laboratories and physicians' office laboratories.
4. Explain the levels of laboratory personnel in relation to their education, skills, and duties.
5. List eight different departments within the medical laboratory and list at least two types of testing performed within each of those departments.
6. Name nine of the most common laboratory panels and explain the body system or function being surveyed.
7. Explain the concepts of quality control and quality assurance in the medical laboratory.
8. Describe at least three methods of ensuring quality in the medical laboratory.
9. Demonstrate how to correctly complete a laboratory requisition.

OBJECTIVES (continued)

10. List 10 pieces of information required on a written laboratory requisition.
11. Explain the rationale behind proper patient preparation before laboratory testing.
12. Explain where accurate and reliable information might be obtained about proper procurement, storage, and handling of laboratory specimens.
13. On a diagram, label the parts of a compound microscope.
14. Explain the function of a compound microscope.
15. Demonstrate the proper use of a compound microscope.
16. List six rules to ensure proper care of a compound microscope.

KEY TERMS (continued)

Qualitative Test
Quantitative Test
Reagent
Reference Laboratories
Reference Values
Requisition
Serum
Therapeutic Drug Monitoring (TDM)
Toxicology
Trough
Urinalysis
Virology

Scenario

Dr. Susan Rice's patient, Annette Samuels, has come into the Inner City Health Care clinic complaining of lower abdominal cramps and burning when she urinates. After discussion of her symptoms and a brief examination, Dr. Rice's clinical diagnosis is urinary tract infection. She asks Wanda Slawson, CMA (AAMA), to obtain a urine sample for a urinalysis and culture with sensitivity. The urinalysis is to be performed in the physician's office laboratory (POL) within the Inner City Health Care clinic, and a portion of the sample will be sent to an outside independent lab for the culture and sensitivity testing. Wanda gives Annette specific instructions on how to prepare for the urine test and how to collect the urine. She asks Annette if she has any questions and she has Annette repeat the instructions to be sure she understands them. When Annette returns with the specimen, Wanda immediately labels it, transfers a portion of the urine into a urine transport tube, places the tube into a biohazard transport bag, and completes a lab requisition for a culture and sensitivity test. The requisition and lab specimen are then ready to be sent to the outside lab for testing. Wanda performs a urinalysis on the remaining urine sample, and the test confirms Dr. Rice's clinical diagnosis of a urinary tract infection. Dr. Rice is able to prescribe an antibiotic for Annette while waiting for the culture results. The culture will determine what type of bacteria is in the urine, and the sensitivity will assure Dr. Rice that the proper antibiotic was prescribed. The culture will take 24 to 48 hours, so Wanda assures Annette that she will contact her the next day when the report is received. A return appointment is made for Annette for a follow-up check and urinalysis in about 10 days.

INTRODUCTION

Providers use laboratory tests to diagnose illnesses, assess patients' health, and manage chronic diseases such as diabetes and arthritis. Medical assistants in providers' offices, clinics, and laboratories may be responsible for patient preparation, obtaining specimens, and testing or sending specimens to an independent laboratory. It is important for medical assistants to be aware of laboratory procedures to ensure accurate testing.

Spotlight on Certification

RMA Content Outline

- Medical law
- Laboratory procedures

CMA (AAMA) Content Outline

- Medicolegal guidelines and requirements
- Principles of infection control
- Principles of operation
- Processing specimens
- Quality control

CMAS Content Outline

- Legal and ethical considerations
- Asepsis in the medical office
- Supplies and equipment

THE LABORATORY

The current health care environment offers numerous options in the methods used to process laboratory tests.

- The specimen may be obtained and the test performed within the **physician's office laboratory (POL).**
- The specimen may be procured and packaged for transport to a separate laboratory.
- The patient may be referred to a separate laboratory for collection and testing of the specimen.

Each laboratory setting has specific requirements for the training and qualifications of the health care personnel who work in that setting. The equipment, supplies, and paperwork, as well as the instructions given to the patient, are also determined by the type of laboratory. Whichever laboratory setting is selected, the focus should be on the safety of the public, the patient, and the health care personnel, while always maintaining quality testing to ensure accurate results.

Purposes of Laboratory Testing

Physicians depend on the ability of medical laboratories to help in determining a patient's state of health or disease in some of the following ways.

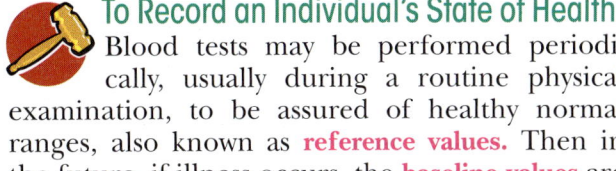

To Record an Individual's State of Health. Blood tests may be performed periodically, usually during a routine physical examination, to be assured of healthy normal ranges, also known as **reference values.** Then in the future, if illness occurs, the **baseline values** are available for comparison.

To Satisfy Employment, Insurance, or Legal Requirements. If an accident occurs, quite often blood is tested for the presence of drugs and alcohol. Such a determination can prove a person guilty or innocent of a crime. Sometimes, places of employment or life insurance companies request laboratory tests to be assured that their employees or clients are free of illegal or dangerous drugs. Employment-required drug and alcohol testing is a classic example of this reason for testing.

To Gain Statistics for Research and Clinical Trials. Laboratory tests are sometimes a part of the data gathered for research and for clinical trials information. When we read about the relation between osteoporosis and **hormone replacement therapy (HRT),** the information is gathered through research. Clinical trials might address the efficacy of certain medications, vitamins, and minerals on osteoporosis in women receiving HRT.

To Detect Asymptomatic Conditions or Diseases. Occasionally, a patient has no complaints of illness and is **asymptomatic**—that is, exhibits no symptoms that might be associated with a disease process—but during routine screening or testing in another, perhaps unrelated, area, a disorder may be discovered. An example is a young man presenting at the office for an athletic physical. Routine urinalysis reveals he has a mild bladder infection.

To Confirm a Clinical Diagnosis. When a patient reports specific symptoms and describes a particular condition (subjective information), and data are compiled through a clinical examination (objective information), the provider may be able to determine a **diagnosis** without the aid of laboratory tests. This is referred to as a **clinical diagnosis.** To confirm a clinical diagnosis, the provider orders laboratory tests. For example, a child has symptoms of a strep throat infection such as sudden onset of sore throat, fever, headache, and upset stomach. On visual examination, the provider discovers small abscesses on the child's tonsils. The provider is almost certain that the diagnosis will be strep throat, but a quick and simple strep test is performed to confirm the clinical diagnosis.

To Differentiate between Two or More Diseases. Sometimes, a patient presents with a combination of symptoms that can be related to more than one condition. For the provider to diagnose accurately, a laboratory test is performed. In situations such as these, the provider chooses to perform the simplest and least **invasive** laboratory test to rule out a particular disease before requiring more extensive testing. This is known as a **differential diagnosis.** For example, if the child in the preceding case had a negative strep test but perhaps exhibited other more systemic symptoms, a blood test might confirm mononucleosis or another condition. The provider is then able to differentiate between the two diagnoses—strep throat and mononucleosis.

To Diagnose. If symptoms are vague, thereby making the clinical diagnosis difficult for the provider, a series of laboratory tests may be required. Sometimes a **panel,** or group of related tests, is ordered. This helps narrow the field for diagnosis. For example, a patient presents with reports of severe fatigue, but preliminary testing does not indicate a diagnosis. Further testing will eventually either lead the provider in a specific direction or at least eliminate a wide variety of conditions.

To Determine the Effectiveness of Treatments. After a patient has been diagnosed and has begun treatment, the provider monitors the patient's health to be sure that the treatment is therapeutic. For example, a patient diagnosed with epilepsy must take an effective amount of antiseizure medication. A blood test is used to check the level of medication in the patient's system. Sometimes the provider wants to know the highest and lowest ranges of medication in the patient's blood to determine if the levels are within a therapeutic range, called **therapeutic drug monitoring (TDM),** and to check for drug toxicity (if the drug level is too high). To measure the highest level of medication in the patient's blood serum (called the **peak**), the specimen is taken about a half hour after the patient has taken his or her regular dose of medicine. To measure the lowest level (called the **trough**), the specimen is taken just before the patient takes his or her next scheduled dose of medicine. A periodic blood test can also be used to determine the effectiveness of dietary and lifestyle changes in reducing blood cholesterol levels.

To Prevent Diseases/Disorders. Protection of the public, families, and coworkers can warrant laboratory tests. An example is protecting an unborn child from contracting genital herpes through the birthing process. A culture of the mother's cervical and vaginal mucosa helps to determine if the child is at risk. If the culture is positive, performing a caesarean section is the treatment of choice to protect the newborn from contracting herpes. Because a newborn's immune system is not fully developed, contracting herpes can cause serious illness and even death.

To Prevent the Exacerbation of Diseases. Patients with chronic conditions require regular blood tests to prevent exacerbation of the disease. When the results of the blood test are obtained, the provider or patient determines whether it is necessary to adjust the diet or medication. For example, a patient with diabetes tests his or her blood regularly to measure the blood sugar, or **glucose,** level. If the blood sugar level is too high or too low, the patient may adjust the insulin dosage or have something to eat to return the blood sugar level to normal.

Types of Laboratories

There are many different types and locations of medical laboratories. They are identified by their size, capabilities, and affiliations. Independent laboratories may be located within medical centers or large clinics. They often have small satellite **patient service centers** located near more isolated medical facilities or in areas of convenience to patients. Satellite laboratories facilitate patients' specimens being obtained closer to their neighborhoods and ambulatory care settings. The specimens are usually couriered back to the independent central laboratory for processing.

Hospital-based laboratories perform most of the tests required by that hospital area, but even large hospitals use reference laboratories for specialized testing. **Reference laboratories** are independent, regionally located laboratories that service larger areas. Reference laboratories are used by hospitals and providers for complex, expensive, or specialized tests.

In a business sense, medical laboratories are quickly becoming more and more competitive. Growth and profitability depend on community relations and service, convenience, efficiency, cost, location, and even reputation. Competition often places the medical assistant and other medical personnel in a position of being asked to recommend a particular medical laboratory over another. Unless the provider has a valid reason for using a particular laboratory or not referring to a particular laboratory, the patient should choose the laboratory. The patient's insurance plan may also be a factor in determining which laboratory is used. Many insurance plans require the patient to use a particular laboratory or to choose a laboratory from those participating in the plan to guarantee payment for the tests. The medical assistant is then a resource for options rather than a referral service. The law is clear that a provider may not have a financial interest in the laboratory to which he or she refers patients.

Point-of-Care Testing (POCT). With the many changes in health care delivery and managed care, the clinical laboratory is also experiencing changes to improve clinical services in the laboratory area. On the forefront of change in the laboratory is POCT, also referred to as near-patient testing or bedside testing. Medical conditions, location of the patient, and treatment methods often require laboratory results as quickly as possible so proper medical care can be administered without delay. POCT uses small instruments that provide rapid, accurate results when used correctly.

Medical personnel can be trained to do laboratory tests of moderate complexity (as defined by CLIA '88) during POCT. The laboratory staff, because of their education, knowledge, and experience in this area, are responsible for advice and management of the quality control and various aspects of this new area of testing. The extension of this laboratory service demands cooperation and cross-departmental efforts from all nontraditional personnel in the health care facility. POCT also has provided new career tracks for the laboratorian, together with multiple skills for several disciplines of health care providers.

POLs. POLs are those laboratories physically set within the office. Some of the more commonly performed medical laboratory tests can easily and inexpensively be performed in the office by the medical assistant. With a simple fingerstick and a few readily available medical supplies, a patient's blood glucose levels can be determined. Another commonly performed test in the ambulatory care setting is **urinalysis,** in which urine is physically, chemically, and microscopically examined for irregularities. With the availability of the many varieties of self-contained kits, tests for strep throat, pregnancy, blood sugar (serum glucose) levels, and hidden (occult) blood in stool can be performed quickly. Other kits are being developed daily. Patients may use a kit that can be purchased without a prescription at home. Some of the home kits available to the general public are "just as accurate" as the kits used in medical offices. The major difference is that the person performing the test may not be trained, which may affect the accuracy of the test results. Consistent quality control measures might not be used by the nonmedical person (see Quality Control/Assurances in the Laboratory section). For example, a pregnancy test kit may be exposed to extreme temperatures while in the patient's care, on a grocer's shelf, or in the patient's home. These extreme temperatures may invalidate the chemical reaction in the test kit. More training, education, and credentialing are required as the complexity of the testing and equipment increases. (See CLIA '88 in Chapter 26 for specific testing parameters.) If the results are not within normal limits, the provider needs to be consulted for confirmation and diagnosis/treatment.

Laboratory Personnel

All independent medical laboratories must be managed by a pathologist, a physician who specializes in disease processes. Additional staffing consists of clinical laboratory scientists, technicians, clinical laboratory assistants, phlebotomists, and medical assistants. Many agencies certify laboratory personnel.

Table 27-1 gives specific information about laboratory personnel, their titles, training required, and duties performed within the clinical lab.

Laboratory Departments

Laboratories are usually divided into departments and may even be subdivided, depending on the size and specialties within the laboratory (Figure 27-1). The various departments perform special tests categorized within their expertise (Table 27-2). Categorization becomes evident when test results are requested over the telephone or whenever there is a need to converse with laboratory personnel. Through knowledge of the various departments within the laboratory, information can be more readily obtained.

Hematology Department. The **hematology** department tests the formed (cellular) elements of the

Table 27-1 Laboratory Personnel

Credential/Title	Education Required	Duties Performed
Physician Pathologist (MD) or Scientist (PhD)	Board-certified medical doctor or PhD scientist (either must be CAP accredited)	Director of the lab Manages the laboratory Interprets biology results, Pap smears, and other cytology samples
Clinical Laboratory Scientist (CLS) or Medical Technologist (MT) or Registered Medical Technologist (RMT) Clinical Laboratory Technologist (CLT)	Bachelor's degree in life sciences or medical technology, including 3 years of course work and 1 year of clinical experience. Must be certified by ASCP, AMT, DHHS, ISCLT, NCA, or NRM	Qualified to perform analysis testing in all departments of the lab Has leadership role; often trains, manages, and supervises other lab personnel May perform routine lab tests as well as highly specialized lab tests Troubleshoots problems with results, specimens, and/or instruments Works directly with the lab director/manager Performs quality control checks Evaluates new instruments Implements new test procedures Often specializes in one area within the lab
Medical Laboratory Technician (MLT) Clinical Laboratory Technician (CLT)	Usually has associate's degree or certificate from an accredited MLT/CLT program May be certified by ASCP or NCA	Performs routine tests Performs microscopic exams and utilizes other lab equipment May specialize in one area in the lab
Phlebotomist/Phlebotomy Technician (PBT)-ASCP Registered Phlebotomy Technician (RPT)-AMT Certified Phlebotomy Technician (CPT)-ASPT Clinical Laboratory Phlebotomist (CLP)-AMT	High school and additional phlebotomy training through a certificate program or on-the-job training May be certified through ASCP, AMT, ASPT, or NCA, and registered under state law	Performs venipuncture and skin puncture May perform CLIA waived testing Collects specimens Processes specimens for transport
Certified Medical Assistant (CMA)-AAMA Registered Medical Assistant (RMA)-AMT	Generally an associate's degree or certificate from an ABHES- or CAAHEP-accredited program in a community college, technical school, or proprietary school May be certified through AAMA or AMT May be registered under state law	May perform routine specimen procurement and waived testing as well as administrative duties, receptioning, computerized record keeping, and billing Often works in POL

Credentialing Associations: AAMA: American Association of Medical Assistants; ABHES: Accrediting Bureau of Health Education Schools; ASCP: American Society of Clinical Pathologists; ASPT: American Society for Phlebotomy Technicians; AMT: American Medical Technologists; CAAHEP: Commission on Accreditation of Allied Health Education Programs; CAP: College of American Pathologists; DHHS: Department of Health and Human Services; ISCLT: International Society of Clinical Laboratory Technology; NCA: National Credentialing Agency for Medical Laboratory Personnel; NRM: National Registry of Microbiologists.

blood. These tests may be quantitative or qualitative. The **quantitative tests** involve actual number counts such as counting the number of white blood cells (WBC), red blood cells (RBC), or platelets. The **qualitative tests** focus on the quality or characteristics of the components, such as the size, shape, and maturity of the cells. In addition, the hematology department tests the ability of the blood components to perform their individual tasks correctly. An example is testing the coagulation ability of clotting factors in blood.

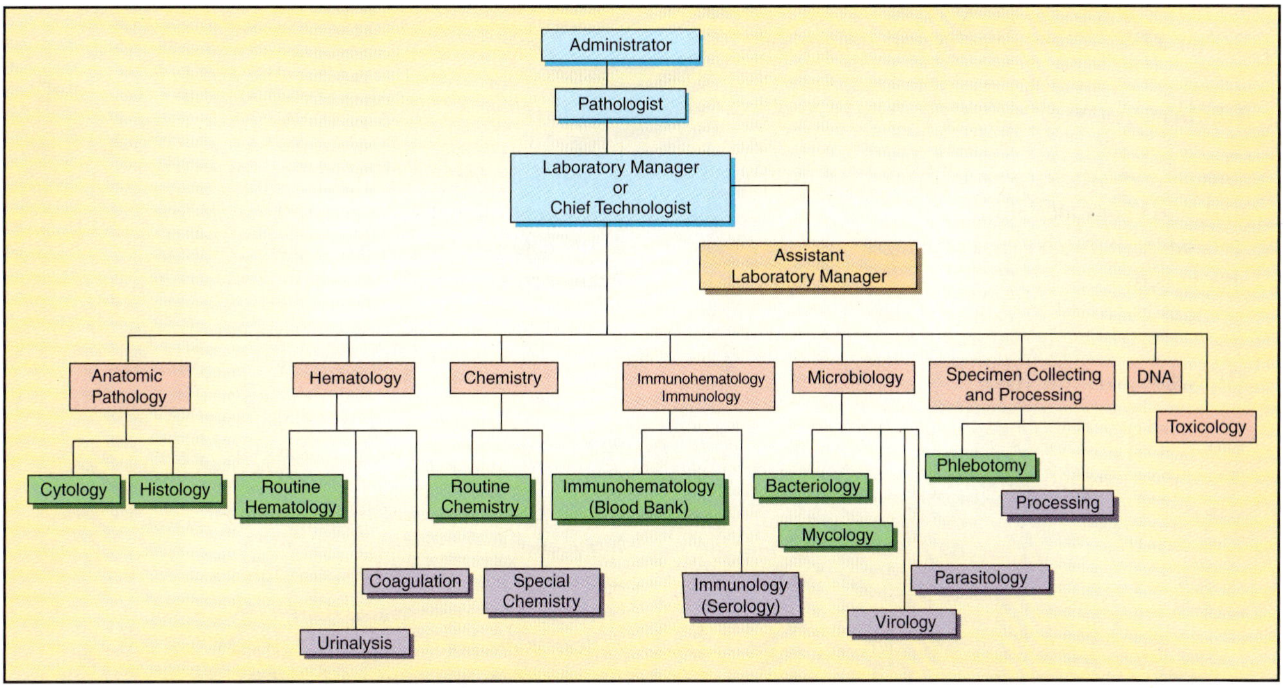

Figure 27-1 Departments of a typical medical laboratory.

Urinalysis Department. Urinalysis is the physical, chemical, and microscopic examination of urine. Required cultures are sent to the microbiology or bacteriology department. In a large laboratory, the urinalysis department is often located under hematology because of the microscopic examinations performed on urine (Figure 27-2).

Clinical Chemistry Department. The **clinical chemistry** department analyzes the chemical composition of blood, cerebrospinal fluid, and joint fluid. Some of the procedures within this department include **assay** of enzymes in the **serum,** serum glucose, or **electrolyte** levels. Toxicology, including TDM and identification of drugs of abuse, is also performed in this department.

Immunohematology (Blood Bank) Department. **Immunohematology** is a special area that deals with blood typing procedures, cross-matching, and the separation and storage of blood components for transfusion, as well as antibody-antigen reactions.

Serology (Immunology) Department. The serology **(immunology)** department is the area of the laboratory that performs tests to evaluate the body's immune response, both production of antibodies and the cellular immune response. Procedures in this area include the detection of antibodies to bacteria and viruses, as well as antibodies produced against one's own body (autoimmune), as in rheumatic diseases such as rheumatoid arthritis and lupus erythematosus. Diseases such as AIDS have helped move laboratory evaluation of the cellular immune system out of the research setting and into the diagnostic setting of the medical laboratory. Molecular biology and flow cytometry are becoming commonplace in today's medical laboratory. Traditionally, serology has been an area within the microbiology department, but with the introduction of many new immunologic techniques, most medical laboratories now include a separate immunology department.

Toxicology. The **toxicology** department tests for toxic substances in a person's blood and monitors any drug usage, therapeutic levels of medication prescribed, or toxicity to the drugs being used. Medications commonly monitored for toxicity are digoxin, phenobarbital, lithium, and pain management drugs. Blood tests also determine levels of occupational exposure to metals and chemicals in the course of one's employment. Testing for drug usage/toxicity is now required in a growing number of pre-employment physical examinations. Toxicity levels for chemicals and metals include lead, zinc, iron, copper, arsenic, and carbon dioxide. The Department of Social and Health Services requires toxicology tests in child protection cases. Drug testing is often required for special assistance

Table 27-2 Categories of Laboratory Tests

HEMATOLOGY	
White blood cell (WBC) count	Hematocrit (Hct)
Red blood cell (RBC) count	Prothrombin time (PT)
Differential white blood cell count (Diff)	Erythrocyte sedimentation rate (ESR)
RBC indices	Platelet count
Hemoglobin (Hgb)	
CLINICAL CHEMISTRY	
Glucose	Potassium
Blood urea nitrogen (BUN)	Bilirubin
Creatinine	Cholesterol
Total protein	Triglycerides
Albumin	Uric acid
Globulin	Lactate dehydrogenase, LD (LDH)
Calcium	Aspartate aminotransferase, AST (SGOT)
Inorganic phosphorus	Alanine aminotransferase, ALT (SGPT)
Chloride	Alkaline phosphatase
Sodium	Phospholipids
SEROLOGY (IMMUNOLOGY/IMMUNOHEMATOLOGY) AND BLOOD BANKING	
Syphilis detection tests (VDRL, RPR)	Rheumatoid Arthritis factor (RA factor)
C-reactive protein test (CRP)	Mono test
ABO blood typing	Heterophil antibody titer test
Rh typing	Hepatitis tests
Rh antibody titer test	HIV tests: ELISA and Western blot
Cross-match	Antistreptolysin O (ASO) titer
Direct Coombs' test	Pregnancy tests
Cold agglutinins	
URINALYSIS	
Physical analysis of urine:	Bilirubin
Color	Urobilinogen
Clarity	Nitrite
Specific gravity	Leukocyte esterase
Chemical analysis of urine:	Microscopic analysis of urine:
pH	Red blood cells
Glucose	White blood cells
Protein	Epithelial cells
Ketones	Casts
Blood	Crystals

(continues)

Table 27-2 (continued)

MICROBIOLOGY	
Candidiasis Chlamydia Diphtheria Gonorrhea Meningitis Pertussis Pharyngitis	Pneumonia Streptococcal sore throat Tetanus Tonsillitis Tuberculosis Urinary tract infection
PARASITOLOGY	
Amebiasis Ascariasis Hookworm disease Malaria Pinworm disease (enterobiasis)	Scabies Tapeworm disease (cestodiasis) Toxoplasmosis Trichinosis Trichomoniasis
CYTOLOGY	
Chromosome studies Pap test	
HISTOLOGY	
Tissue analysis Biopsy studies	
DNA	
DNA tests compare individuals according to their individual genotype	
TOXICOLOGY	
Tests for chemicals, specifically for drugs and other toxins in blood	

in low-income housing and other public financial assistance programs. The reasons for drug testing are wide and varied and are growing every year, making this department larger than in the past.

DNA. The second area within the medical laboratory growing larger each year is the **DNA** department. With the advent of DNA tests for proving paternity and maternity of children and the growing use of DNA testing for criminal cases, DNA testing is quickly becoming a major focus in many laboratories.

Microbiology Department. The **microbiology** department is the area in the laboratory where microorganisms such as bacteria and fungi are grown in an appropriate medium, cultured, and then identified. Sensitivity tests are then performed to identify which antibiotics can effectively eradicate the pathogenic organisms. The combination of culturing and identifying the best antibiotic is called **culture and sensitivity (C&S). Mycology** is an area within the microbiology department where fungi are studied. **Virology** is an area within the

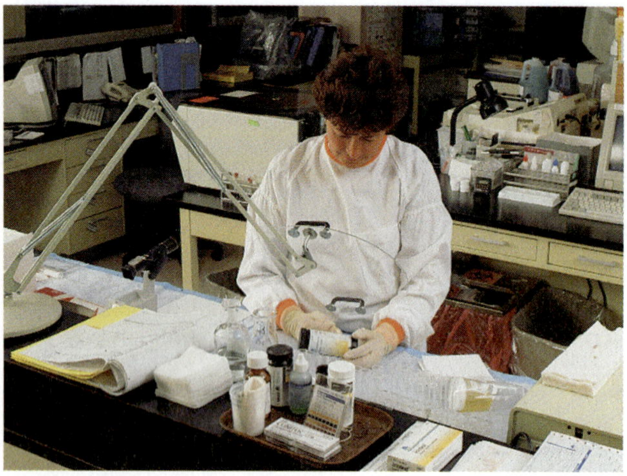

Figure 27-2 Clinical reference laboratories may have a separate urinalysis department where the laboratory professional tests urine for physical, chemical, and microbiological properties.

microbiology department where viruses are studied.

Parasitology Department. **Parasitology** is a subdivision of the microbiology department where ova and parasite (O&P) tests are performed on specimens such as feces. The specimens are examined for the presence of parasites or their eggs.

Cytology Department. The **cytology** department is the area in which microscopic examinations of cells are performed to detect early signs of cancer and other diseases. The Papanicolaou test, known as the Pap smear, for irregular cervical cells is an example of a test performed in the cytology department.

Histology Department. **Histology** is the study of tissue sample biopsies for the determination of disease. Frozen samples or **biopsies** are sliced/stained and then microscopically examined for cancer and other anomalies.

Panels of Laboratory Tests

Laboratory tests are often categorized into related groups to provide information about a particular body system or related bodily function. The groups are usually referred to as panels, formerly called "profiles." In addition, laboratory tests are organized into panels for ease of ordering. For a current list of CMS-approved organ- and disease-oriented panels, see Table 27-3.

Medicare requires that providers order tests under their approved panels. Providers may not refer to panels under other names such as the previously named Chem Screen, SMAC, Chem 7, and so on. The panels listed in Table 27-3 are the only panels allowed. If a provider would like a specific series or combinations of tests under a special panel, he or she must apply to the CMS for the approval to design their own panel.

BILLING FOR LABORATORY SERVICES

Providers must justify which lab tests are ordered by using the correct diagnosis code. For example, if the diagnosis is pneumonia, a urinalysis would not be justified and would not be covered. If a provider wants to order a test that probably will not be covered by insurance under CMS guidelines, the patient should sign a waiver. Medicare patients would sign an Advance Beneficiary Notice (ABN). The waiver/ABN notifies the patient that the test might not be covered and that the patient will have to pay for it. If the clinic fails to notify the patient, the patient does not have to pay for the test, and the provider is liable for the charges.

QUALITY CONTROLS/ ASSURANCES IN THE LABORATORY

The accuracy of any laboratory test result depends on all safeguards being followed. These standards ensure the quality of the testing equipment, supplies, personnel, and the accuracy of the test results. Many factors can compromise the accuracy of laboratory test results. Among these factors are collection of specimen, temperature, amount or age of specimen, time limits of test, and using chemicals or reagents past their expiration dates. Even when laboratory guidelines are strictly followed, inaccurate results may be obtained by using test kits that have been exposed to extreme heat or cold, or using chemicals or reagents after their expiration. It is important to follow all laboratory guidelines, but the medical assistant must also confirm that the specimen, chemicals, and test kits are handled and processed properly.

Table 27-3 Centers for Medicare and Medicaid Services (CMS) Approved Organ- and Disease-Oriented Panels (with Current Procedural Terminology [CPT] Codes), Updated October 2008

BASIC METABOLIC PANEL (CPT CODE 80048)	
BUN (84520) Calcium, total (82310) Carbon dioxide (82374) Chloride (82435)	Creatinine (82565) Glucose (82947) Potassium (84132) Sodium (84295)
GENERAL HEALTH PANEL (CPT CODE 80050)	
Comprehensive metabolic panel (CPT code 80053) TSH (84443)	CBC w/manual differential (80054) or CBC w/automated differential (85025)
ELECTROLYTE PANEL (CPT CODE 80051)	
Carbon dioxide (82374) Potassium (84132)	Chloride (82435) Sodium (84295)
COMPREHENSIVE METABOLIC PANEL (CPT CODE 80053)	
Albumin (82040) Alkaline phosphatase (84075) Bilirubin, total (82247) BUN (84520) Calcium, total (82310) Carbon dioxide (82374) Chloride (82435)	Creatinine (82565) Glucose (82947) Potassium (84132) Protein, total (84155) Sodium (84295) SGOT (AST) (84450) SGPT (ALT) (84460)
OBSTETRIC PANEL (CPT CODE 80055)	
CBC w/manual differential (80054) or CBC w/automated differential (85025) Hepatitis B surface antigen (87340) Rubella antibody (86762)	Syphilis test, qualitative (e.g., VDRL, RPR) (86592) Antibody screen, RBC (86850) Blood typing, ABO (86900) and Rh (D) (86901)
LIPID PANEL (CPT CODE 80061)	
Cholesterol (82465) HDL cholesterol (83718) and LDL cholesterol, calculated	Triglyceride (84478)
RENAL FUNCTION PANEL (CPT CODE 80069)	
ALBUMIN (82040) BUN (84520) Calcium, total (82310) Carbon dioxide (82374) Chloride (82435)	Creatinine (82565) Glucose (82947) Phosphorous (84100) Potassium (84132) Sodium (84295)
ARTHRITIS PANEL (CPT CODE 80072)	
Uric acid (84550) ESR, erythrocyte sedimentation rate (85651)	Fluorescent noninfectious agent, screen (86255) Rheumatoid factor, qualitative (86430)
ACUTE HEPATITIS PANEL (CPT CODE 80074)	
Hepatitis A antibody, IgM (86709) Hepatitis B core antibody, IgM (86705)	Hepatitis B surface antigen (87340) Hepatitis C antibody (86803)
HEPATIC FUNCTION PANEL (CPT CODE 80076)	
Albumin (82040) Alkaline phosphatase (84075) Bilirubin, direct (82248) Bilirubin, total (82247)	Protein, total (84155) SGOT (AST) (84450) SGPT (ALT) (84460)
TORCH ANTIBODY PANEL (CPT CODE 80090)	
Cytomegalovirus antibody, IgG (86644) Herpes simplex (1 & 2) antibody, IgG (86694/86695)	Rubella antibody, IgG (86762) Toxoplasmosis antibody (86677)

Control Tests

To further ensure accurate test results, **control test** samples are tested together with the patient's sample. The control samples have a known value, negative or positive result, or abnormal or normal result, which is compared with the results of the patient's test. One of the purposes of this control measure is to minimize human error. By being able to compare a sample of known value or positive or negative test result with the patient's test, the health care worker performing the test can accurately determine the result. An error in the testing method may be discovered if the control sample does not test accurately.

Another purpose of the control test is to check the **reagents** or chemicals. If the control sample is not showing accurate results, it may be determined that the chemicals (reagents) are faulty or have expired. On receiving any test in the POL, the person responsible for quality assurance and quality control (probably the medical assistant performing the tests) should perform the calibration or control test provided by and as directed by the manufacturer. This ensures proper test function.

Proficiency Testing

CLIA '88 requires laboratories to participate in an accredited proficiency program for certain identified tests (see Chapter 26 for CLIA '88 requirements). Proficiency testing is similar to quality control in that "known" proficiency samples are tested the same as patient samples. The difference is an approved outside agency evaluates the accuracy of the testing and submits the performance records to CMS for CLIA '88 compliance.

Preventative Maintenance

Preventative maintenance helps identify potential problems before they actually occur. Procedures include manufacturer-recommended maintenance on equipment; daily temperature checks on refrigerators, freezers, and incubators; daily checks on expiration dates of reagents and supplies; and instrument log and centrifuge checks.

Instrument Validations

The quality of test results can be ensured by consistently checking the calibration and linear range of the instruments and machines. If the equipment is not maintained or is functioning improperly, accurate test results cannot be ensured.

The Medical Assistant's Role

Medical assistants are educated to perform administrative office duties, prepare patients, collect specimens, and perform waived tests in such a manner that patients and health care personnel are safe from contamination, patients are not harmed, samples are reliable, and tests are accurate. These four aspects of quality laboratory testing are critical for accuracy. When the patient is prepared properly, the specimen is obtained as expertly as possible, the reagents and equipment are in the best condition and calibration possible, and the test is performed by a trained professional, the test results will be accurate.

LABORATORY REQUISITIONS AND REPORTS

A written **requisition** for laboratory work must be sent to the laboratory with the patient or with the specimen (Figure 27-3). These forms are preprinted with the most commonly requested tests separated into logical categories. Additional space is provided for writing special requests. The laboratories that patients use can provide your medical agency with these forms. Laboratory requisition forms are computer generated, and the provider's name, address, and other information necessary for proper reporting and recordkeeping are often pre-printed on the forms. If the requisitions are not preprinted, spaces are provided for the information to be written in. The information must be complete, accurate, and clearly legible. A properly completed requisition contains the following data:

- *Provider's name, account number, address, and telephone number.* This information is necessary to contact the office for any clarification or further information and to report the results.
- *Patient's name, address, and telephone number.* Be sure the name is complete and spelled correctly. Avoid using alternate versions of the patient's name without also including the proper, legal name. Make certain to include apartment numbers and zip codes. This information will be used for billing purposes, as well as medical records. Social Security numbers and middle initials are helpful when it is necessary to differentiate between patients.
- *Patient's billing information, insurance, and identification number.* Because the patient is often not the person who is the subscriber to the insurance, the subscriber's name, address, telephone number, and insurance identification numbers

Requested By	
	Courtesy Copy/Comments

Patient Information (REQUIRED)

Chart Number	Pre-Op? ☐Y ☐N	Surgery Date
Social Security Number	Sex	Date of Birth (required)
Patient Name		
Mailing Address	City	
State Zip	Patient Phone	

Insurance Information (REQUIRED)

Insurance Company (Name/Billing Address)
Guarantor (Responsible Party)
Insurance Number
Medicare Number

ICD.9 Diagnosis Code(s) (REQUIRED)

Physician Notice: For reimbursement, Medicare **requires ABN signature** review (see reverse side) be made for the following tests in **bold,** that may NOT be covered under "Medical Necessity".

☐ **STAT** ☐ **ASAP** ☐ **ROUTINE**	Phone Results ☐ # ______ FAX Report ☐ # ______	Fasting ____ hrs	**Last Dose** Medication ______ Date/Time ______	**Collected By** ID ______ Date ______ Time ______ (REQUIRED)

Comments/Additional Tests

SS = SST | L = LAV | B = BLUE | R = RED | G = GRAY | GN = GREEN | PK = PINK | U = URINE | C = CULTURE | S = SERUM | FROZEN | BIOPSY | SLIDES

Alphabetical Test Listing	COLL CODE	Alphabetical Test Listing	COLL CODE	Alphabetical Test Listing	COLL CODE	Alphabetical Test Listing	COLL CODE	Microbiology
☐ ABO 50100 ☐ Rh 50200	R	☐ Creatinine 30570	S	☐ **Hepatitis Panel, Acute 40781**	S	☐ Prolactin 40450	S	Indicate Exact Specimen Source
☐ Albumin 30590	S	☐ Creatinine, Urine, 24hr 32100	U	**• Hep A Ab (IgM) • HBcAb (IgM)**		☐ Protein, Urine	U	______
☐ Alkaline Phosphatase 30670	S	☐ Creatinine, Urine, Ran 32081	U	**• HBsAg • Hep C Ab**		☐ RAN 32180 ☐ 24hr 32200		☐ AFB Culture with Smear 64450
☐ **Alpha-fetoprotein 41150**	S	☐ Creatinine Clearance 32240	S,U	☐ **HIV-1 & -2 Antibody 42007**	S	☐ **PSA, Diagnostic 42158**	S	☐ C. difficile Toxin 68016
☐ ALT (SGPT) 30680	S	☐ C-Reactive Protein (CRP) 58200	S	☐ **HIV-1 RNA, PCR, Quant 42015**	L	☐ **PSA, Screen 41954**	S	☐ Chlamydia Only, Amplified 68361
☐ Amylase 31710	S	☐ CRP, Cardiac Risk 43575	S	☐ Homocysteine 43600	L	☐ **PSA Ratio, Free & Total 42147**	S	☐ Chlamydia/GC, Amplified 68395
☐ ANA (with Reflex) 69107	S	☐ **Digoxin 33060**	S	☐ **Iron 30720**	S	☐ **PT (Protime w/INR) 25000**	B	☐ Fungal Culture 64300
☐ Anitbody Screen 50500	R	☐ Electrolytes 31310	S	☐ **Iron, TRF Sat., (TIBC) 44210**	S	☐ PTH (Whole Molecule) 40571	L	☐ Giardia Antigen 67031
☐ AST (SGOT) 30700	S	• Na • K • Cl • CO_2		☐ LDH 30710	S	☐ **PTT, Activated 25100**	B	☐ Gram Stain, Direct 60050
☐ **B_{12} 41250**	S	☐ Electrophoresis, Serum 48010	S	☐ **LDL Direct 43571**	S	☐ **Reticulocyte Count 21150**	L	☐ Herpes simplex Virus Culture 68263
☐ B_{12}/Folate 41311	S	☐ Electrophoresis, Urine 48310	U	☐ LH 40500	S	☐ **Rheumatoid Factor 44480**	S	☐ Herpes/Varicella Virus Culture 68277
☐ Basic Metabolic Panel 31307	S	☐ **ESR (Sed Rate) 21050**	L	☐ Lipase 31740	S	☐ **RPR 58800**	S	☐ Influenza A & B, Direct Exam 65092
• Na • K • Cl • CO_2		☐ Estradiol 41600	S	☐ **Lipid Panel 1 43560**	S	☐ Rubella 58681	S	☐ KOH Prep 64200
• BUN • Creat • Gluc • Ca		☐ **Ferritin 41350**	S	**• Chol • HDL • Trig • LDL**		☐ Semen, Post Vasectomy 23540	Se	☐ Ova & Parasite 67002
☐ BNP 31379	L	☐ Folate 41300	S	**• Chol/HDL • LDL/HDL**		☐ T3, Free 40070	S	☐ Pinworm Prep 67200
☐ BUN 30560	S	☐ FSH 40400	S	☐ **Rflx Direct LDL, Trig> 400 43562**		☐ T3, Total 40200	S	☐ Polys (WBC's) 67455
☐ Bilirubin, Total 30640	S	☐ **GGT 30690**	S	☐ **Lithium 33320**	S	☐ **T4 (Thyroxine) 40000**	S	☐ Rapid Strep-A Antigen,
☐ Bilirubin, Direct 30650	S	☐ **Glucose 30550**	S	☐ Lymphocyte T-Cell Subsets 29100	LGN	☐ **T4, Free 40050**	S	Culture if Negative 65100
☐ **CA 125 41050**	S	☐ **Glucose Tolerance Test ___ hrs**	S	☐ Lymphocytes, T-Helper 29150	LGN	☐ **Free Thyroxine Index,**	S	☐ Rotavirus 68073
☐ **CA 19.9 42900**	S	☐ **Glucose 2hr PP 31820**	S	☐ **Magnesium 31280**	SS	**FTI (T4 + TU) 40025**		☐ Trichomonas Wet Mount 60103
☐ **CA 27.29 41061**	S	☐ **hCG-beta, Quantitative 41100**	S	☐ Microalbumin, Urine	U	☐ Thyroid Peroxidase Ab 34720	S	**Culture, Bacterial**
☐ Calcium 30610	S	☐ **hCG-beta, Tumor Marker 41110**	S	☐ Ran 43980 ☐ 24hr 42101		☐ **Theophylline 33430**	S	☐ Anaerobic 61653
☐ Carbamazepine (Tegretol) 33050	S	☐ **HCV RNA, PCR, Quant 40738**	L	☐ Timed ___hrs___min 42100		☐ Total Protein 30580	S	☐ Blood 60250
☐ Cardiolipin Abs, IgG, IgM 27500	S	☐ H. pylori, IgG 58322	S	☐ Microalbumin/Creat Ratio 43985	U	☐ **Triglycerides 30730**	S	☐ CSF 60450
☐ **CBC w/auto differential 20000**	L	☐ **Hemoglobin AIC (Glycol) 42550**	L	☐ Monotest 58550	S	☐ **Troponin I 31378**	S	☐ Catheter Tip 60420
☐ **Hemogram Only 20150**		☐ **Hepatic Function Panel 31306**	S	☐ **Occult Blood Screen 67100**	F	☐ **TSH 40250**	S	☐ E. coli – 0157, Only 61227
☐ **CEA 41000**	S	**• Alk Phos • Alb • DBil • TBil • TP**		☐ **Occult Blood Diagnostic 67105**	F	☐ **TSH with Reflex 40012**	S	☐ GC Only 60750
☐ **Cholesterol 30740**	S	**• ALT (SGPT) • AST (SGOT)**		☐ Phenytoin (Dilantin) 33360	S	☐ **Testosterone 40550**	S	☐ Genital, Full Culture 60800
☐ CK, Total 31350	S	☐ Hep A Ab, IgM 42114	S	☐ Phenytoin, Free & Total 87060	R	☐ Uric Acid 30630	S	☐ Group-B Strep Only, Genital 60217
☐ Comp Metabolic Panel 31305	S	☐ Hep B Core Ab, IgM 42141	S	☐ Phosphorus 30620	S	☐ **UA & Microscopic 24080**	U	☐ MRSA Screen, Nares 60867
• Na • K • Cl • CO_2 • Gluc		☐ Hep C Ab 40711	S	☐ **Potassium/NA 30510**	S	☐ **UA & Microscopic, Reflex**	U	☐ Sputum/Trach/Bronch 61100
• BUN • Creat • Ca • AST • ALT		☐ Hepatitis B Immunity Scrn 40770	S	☐ Prealbumin 44470	S	**with C&S if Indicated 11850**		☐ Stool, Full Culture 61150
• TP • Alb • A/G • Alk Phos • TBil		☐ HBsAg 42127	S	☐ Progesterone 41750	S			☐ Strep-A Screen, Throat 60207
								☐ Throat Culture 61350
								☐ **Urine Culture 61500**
						Lab Use Only		☐ Wound, 61657
						Veni ☐ A 95370 ☐ C 95372 ☐ NH 99561		source: ______
						Hfee ☐1 ☐2 ☐3		

Many payors (including Medicare and Medicaid) have a necessity requirement for the diagnosis and treatment of the patient, therefore, only those tests which are medically necessary should be ordered.

Figure 27-3 Sample laboratory requisition form.

are extremely important, especially if the patient does not live with the subscriber. Some patients have secondary insurance coverage. Be sure to include that data also. The laboratory would prefer to receive an additional sheet of information than to have incomplete insurance records in its business office.

- *Unique patient identifier.* This can be an identification number that is hospital or laboratory generated. In the outpatient setting, this can be the patient's Social Security number or date of birth.
- *Patient's age/date of birth and sex.* Age and sex both influence the results of some tests and should not be assumed.
- *Source of specimen.* This information is especially important when dealing with tests such as cultures and biopsies. In the case of cultures, knowing the source of the specimen aids the laboratory in determining whether the specimen contains normal flora or is abnormal for that area of the body.
- *Time and date of the specimen collection.* Some tests require that the specimen be tested fairly quickly after leaving the body; other tests must be performed after a certain period has elapsed. The time and date of the specimen collection are important because accuracy can be compromised if the specimen is not sent to the laboratory in a reasonable amount of time.
- *Test requested.* This is usually a matter of putting a check mark in the appropriate box on the requisition, but it is surprising how often laboratories receive specimens with nicely completed requisitions and no indication of the test desired.
- *Medications the patient is taking.* Because medication can influence some test results, it is important that the laboratory be provided this information. Patients are often asked to refrain from taking certain medications before testing. Be sure to consult with the provider to verify orders. If a medication is not discontinued before testing, the type of medication, the dosage amount, and the time of the last dose must be included on the requisition.
- *Clinical diagnosis.* The provider's tentative diagnosis is useful to the laboratory in helping to differentiate between diagnoses or confirm a diagnosis. The clinical diagnosis may also alert the laboratory personnel to any possible special considerations of which to be aware. For example, if diabetes is suspected, the laboratory will give special consideration to the glucose value. The diagnosis or preferably the ICD-9 code is also necessary for billing.
- *Urgency of results.* Sometimes the provider needs a test to be performed immediately (STAT) or would like a result as soon as possible (ASAP). The provider's orders need to be clearly stated on the requisition. Additional space is also provided for other special instructions if necessary.
- *Special collection/patient instructions.* Examples include fasting specimens, timed collections, and "do not collect from a specific area" instructions.
- If copies of the results are to be sent to a second provider, the medical assistant must include the provider's full name, address, and fax number. Be careful to print the fax number clearly so that the patient's results are not sent to the wrong place in error.

> Many offices copy both sides of the patient's insurance card and attach the copies to the laboratory requisition. This ensures the laboratory will have all the insurance information it needs to bill for its services.

The laboratory will send back a written report (Figure 27-4) that will contain the following information:

- Name, address, and telephone number of the laboratory
- Referring provider's name, address, and identification numbers
- Patient's name, identification number, age, and sex
- Date the specimen was received by the laboratory
- Date and time the specimen was collected
- Date the laboratory reported the results
- The test name, results, and normal reference ranges if applicable

EHR Lab requisitions may be electronically generated using an electronic health record (EHR) program and completed on screen and then either printed for the patient to take to the outside lab or sent electronically to the lab. Occasionally a requisition will be faxed to a lab if the EHR is not available. Interestingly, today's medical clinic staff may perform a combination of electronic and manual communication with outside labs. Eventually the electronic format will replace all manual methods.

Reports are sent to the provider by fax (Figure 27-5), manually delivered to the clinic, or sent electronically using EHR software (Figure 27-6).

Patient Name: FAKEY FAKERSON
Note: All result statuses are Final unless otherwise noted.

Tests (1) BASIC METABOLIC PANEL (31308)

SODIUM	[H]	155 mmol/L	136-145
POTASSIUM	[H]	5.7 mmol/L	3.5-5.1
CHLORIDE	[H]	115 mEq/L	96-108
TOTAL CO2		25 mmol/L	22-29
GLUCOSE	[H]	200 mg/dL	70-109
UREA NITROGEN (BUN)		15 mg/dL	5-20
CREATININE		1.1 mg/dL	0.6-1.3
CALCIUM	[H]	10.5 mg/dL	8.4-10.2

Test Performed at Northwest Regional Laboratories

Note: An exclamation mark (!) indicates a result that was not dispersed into the flowsheet.
Document Creation Date: 09/18/2008 2:33 PM

---

(1) Order result status: Final
Collection or observation date-time: 09/18/2008 14:12
Requested date-time: 09/18/2008 14:12
Receipt date-time: 09/18/2008 14:12
Reported date-time: 09/18/2008 14:16
Referring Physician:
Ordering Physician: MARK SMITH (17006)
Specimen Source:
Producer ID: SMSLIS
Filler Order Number: NZ80009408
Lab site:

Signed by: Mary L Ponder on 09/23/2008 at 10:14 AM

Figure 27-4 Sample computerized laboratory report.

Abnormal test results are always flagged in some way, either in a different color, a different column, or perhaps designated by a star or simply by *H* (for high) or *L* (for low). Critical values (results that may indicate serious medical conditions) are alerted to the provider by a phone call from the laboratory.

When the results are received, the medical assistant should attach them to the patient's chart for the provider to review and initial before filing them. The provider should be alerted to any abnormal test results as soon as possible. Laboratories often send results via computer-generated reports directly to the provider's office or hospital.

HIPAA

If a patient wants a copy of the results for his or her own records, the provider must send permission or the patient will need to sign a release form. This is required by HIPAA.

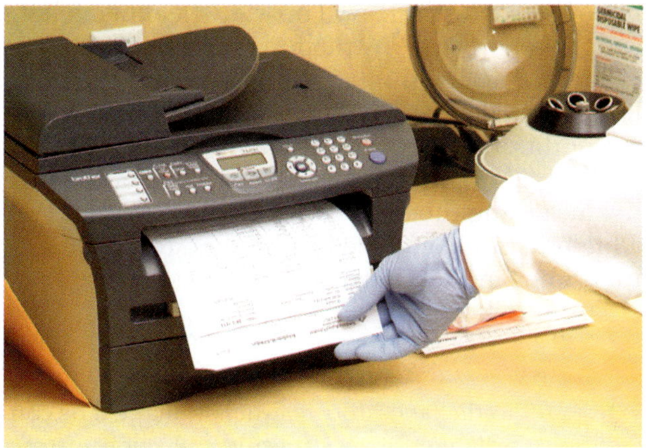

Figure 27-5 The computerized laboratory report is transmitted directly from the reference lab to the provider's office.

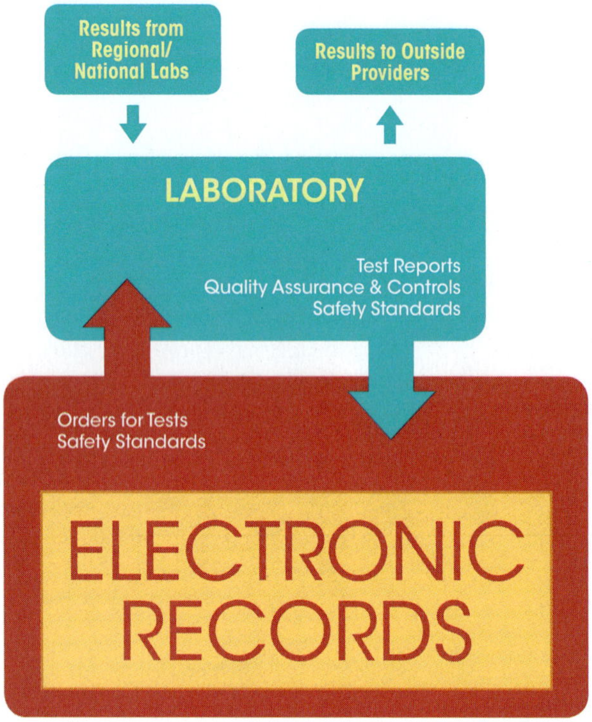

Figure 27-6 The laboratory arm of the total practice management system (TPMS). Lab requisitions may be electronically generated and completed on screen, then sent directly to an outside lab.

SPECIMEN COLLECTION

Proper Procurement, Storage, and Handling

Instructions for procuring, storing, and handling and transporting laboratory specimens properly can be obtained from the independent laboratories. Most laboratories will provide the office/clinic with a step-by-step instruction manual, sometimes called a compendium, a laboratory manual, or a user manual and will also be available to answer any additional questions by telephone.

Obtaining the specimen in the proper manner and using the right equipment will ensure that a high-quality specimen is submitted to the laboratory. Some guidelines are as follows:

- Check the provider's orders and identify the patient.
- Refer to the laboratory instruction manual or consult the laboratory for specific collection instructions.
- Instruct the patient on any necessary dietary restriction.
- Instruct the patient to ingest special food or take other substances if required.
- Select or provide to the patient appropriate containers with the proper preservatives in them, if required.
- Be certain to label the specimen with the patient's name, identification number, date, type of specimen, time of collection, and provider's name. Label the container, not the lid, because the lid will be removed during testing. Label the container, not the wrapping, because the wrapping will be separated from the container when testing is performed, for example, throat swabs.
- Obtain the specimen or instruct the patient to provide the specimen according to the directions given by the laboratory.
- Follow applicable OSHA bloodborne pathogens guidelines (see Chapter 10) when packaging the specimen for transport so it will not leak or contaminate the courier or other office staff and so that it will safely arrive at the laboratory without being damaged or destroyed (Figure 27-7).
- Place any biological specimen to be sent to an outside laboratory into an approved biological transport bag (Figure 27-8A–C). These bags, which have the universal symbol for biohazard caution stamped on them, contain two sections: one for the specimen and one for the requisition. The requisition and specimen are placed in the proper areas within the transport bag, and the bag is sealed. When the testing laboratory receives the bag, the other end is torn open so that the specimen and requisitions can be removed without contaminating the receiver.

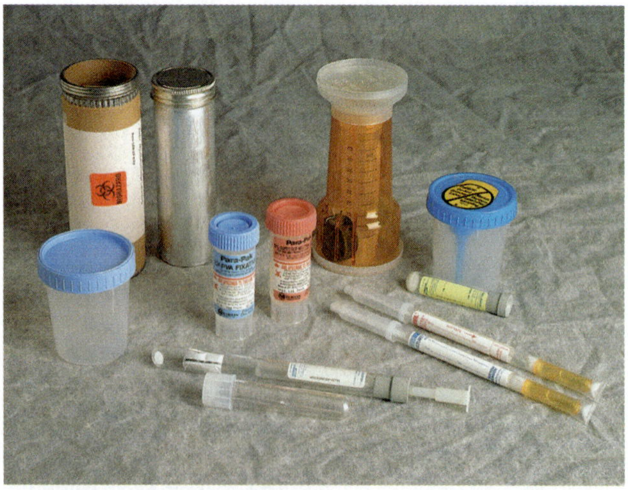

Figure 27-7 Various types of collection and transportation containers for laboratory specimens.

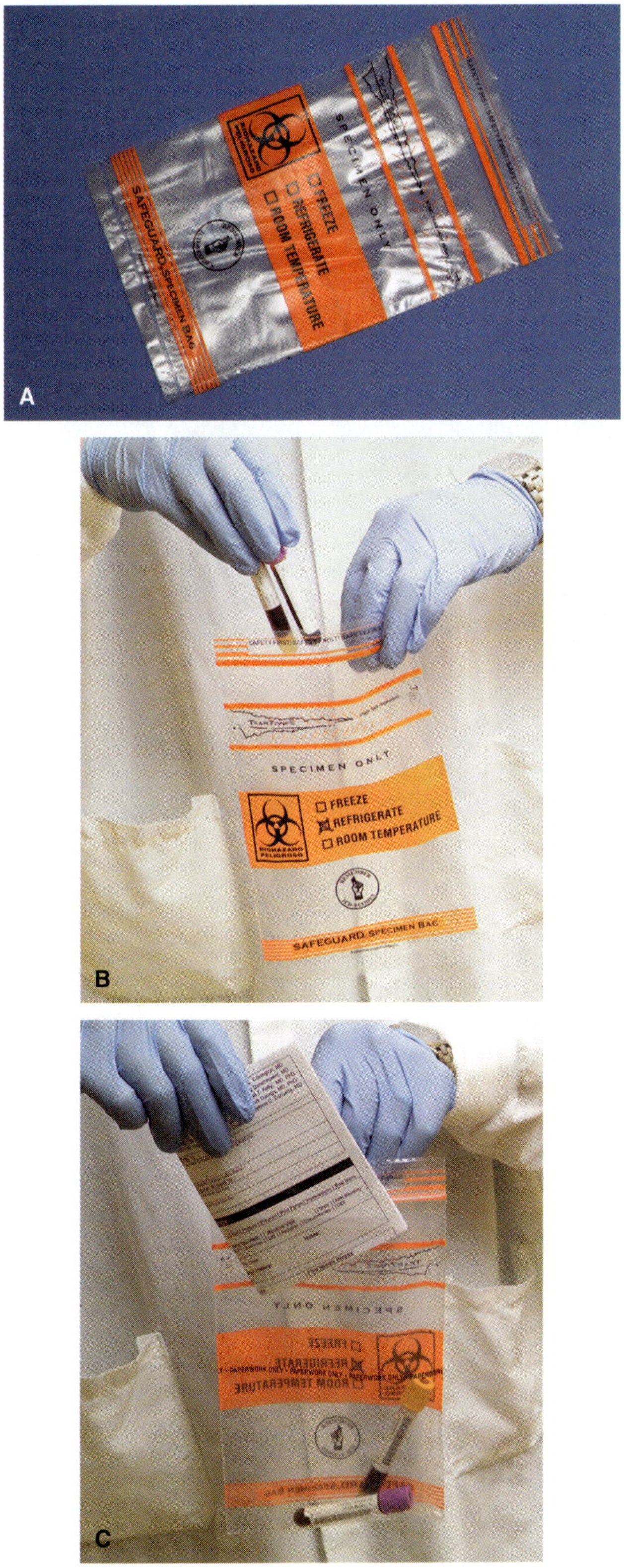

Figure 27-8 Preparing a biological specimen to be sent to an outside laboratory. (A) Laboratory specimen transport bag. (B) The medical assistant places the specimen into the transport bag and seals that part of the bag. (C) The medical assistant places the requisition into a separate compartment of the bag.

- Document in the patient's chart or electronic medical record the type of specimen collected, the tests ordered, which laboratory the specimen is being sent to (even if it is being tested in your POL), how the patient tolerated the procedure (including any complications), and other pertinent information according to your office policy. Many offices also keep a copy of the laboratory requisition in the patient's chart for later reference. If the testing is performed in your POL, the results of the test should be recorded on a laboratory report form and, after the provider has initialed it, filed in the laboratory section of the chart.

EHR If the clinic is using EHRs, lab requisitions often stay in a "pending" file until the results are reported from the laboratory. The medical assistant may be responsible for tracking pending lab tests until the reports are received.

If the medical clinic and lab both are using EHRs, they may share an interface software program that allows the report to be imported onto the provider's desktop as an "unsigned" document. Many clinics have policies in place that require the provider to electronically "sign" lab reports within 36 or 48 hours of receipt.

Processing and Sending Specimens to a Laboratory

Specimens collected by the medical assistant are often sent from the office to a laboratory many miles away or are picked up by a courier representing the outside laboratory. These are often large commercial laboratories that are not associated with a local hospital laboratory. The patient's insurance often dictates the laboratory contracted to perform the patient's testing. It is not unusual for several different laboratories to pick up at one location. A situation could be that the blood work from patient Jones would go to laboratory A, the blood work from patient Smith would go to laboratory B, and a urine sample from patient Doe would be tested in the laboratory within the building. It sometimes can be confusing as to where to send the specimen.

All laboratory test results are dependent on the quality of the specimen submitted. The quality of the specimen depends on patient preparation, proper collection, correct patient identification, and transportation of the specimen. If there is any doubt or question regarding the type of specimen to be collected, it is imperative that the appropriate laboratory be called to clarify the specimen

Patient Education

The patient will often need to be instructed on a specific preparation before a specimen is taken. Because food and medication can greatly influence test results, a patient may need to be instructed not to eat for several hours before having the specimen taken or drawn. Fasting means the patient may not have anything except water for the 12 hours before the test. NPO means the patient may not have even water. The patient may need to refrain from taking a routine dosage of medication before the test is performed. Sometimes the patient preparation instructions will include a special diet for a few days. Regardless of how simple instructions may seem, it is important to give the patient clear, written directions. Take the time to go over any instructions with the patient (and sometimes other family members). Your patients will welcome the opportunity to ask questions and to have a written set of instructions to take home.

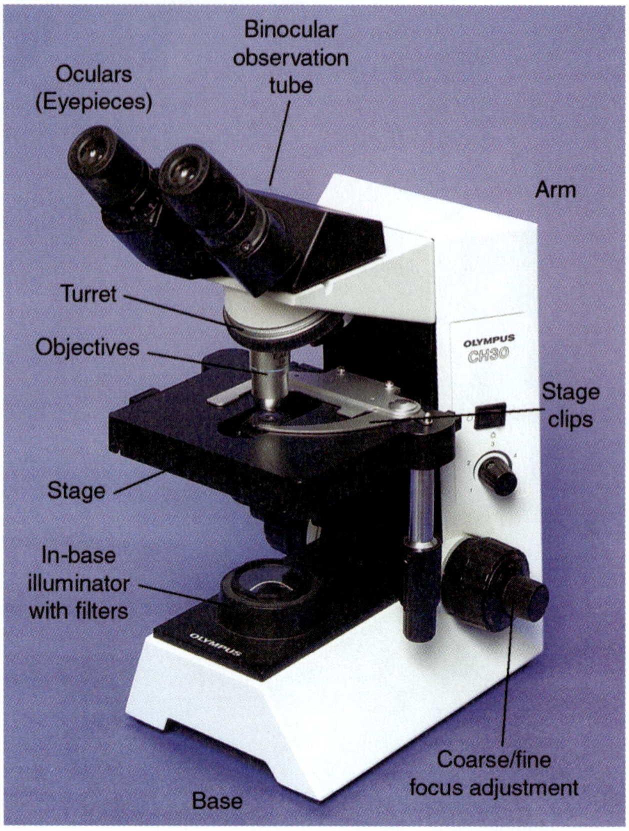

Figure 27-9 Basic compound microscope.

needed. There are often differences between laboratories; the type of specimen acceptable for one laboratory is not necessarily the acceptable specimen for another laboratory.

MICROSCOPES

One of the most used pieces of equipment in the medical laboratory is the microscope. Consisting of a light source, eyepieces, objectives, **condenser,** and **diaphragm,** the microscope enables us to see bacteria and other microorganisms that are much too small to be seen without magnification.

Types of Microscopes

The most commonly used microscope in the clinic is the compound microscope (Figure 27-9). As the name indicates, the image is compounded by the use of two different lenses. One lens compounds or increases the magnification produced by the other lens. The first lens system is located in the **objectives,** and the second lens system is in the eyepiece (ocular). The light source is a bulb in the base. The light is directed up through the specimen on the slide and into the objective lenses. The light, or image, is then reflected by the condenser onto the specimen to the ocular lenses for visualization.

The eyepiece may have a single (monocular) lens, or there may be two (binocular) lenses. This lens is not adjustable or changeable. The magnification in the eyepiece is usually 10 times (10x) the normal size of the object being viewed.

The objective lenses are adjustable between low power, high power, and oil immersion. When viewing through the microscope under low power, more of the slide can be seen but with less detail than when using high power. When viewing under high power, a smaller portion of the field can be seen but with greater detail. The low-power objective lens allows the item being viewed to be magnified 10 times larger than life. This magnification combined with the 10 times magnification of the ocular lens gives the ability to see microscopically 100 times the normal size (10x × 10x = 100x).

Combining the 10-power (10x) ocular lens with the high-power objective lens, which has the magnification power of forty times life (40x), increases magnification vision to 400 times the normal size (10x × 40x = 400x). This is enough magnification to see large microorganisms but is still not enough to see smaller organisms, such as bacteria, clearly. An oil-immersion lens is needed to view bacteria closely.

The oil-immersion lens give the ability to multiply the ocular lens magnification (10x) by one hundred (100x) to reach a possible total magnification of one thousand times normal life size (10x × 100x = 1,000x). Because more light is needed to actually see this amount of magnification, the lens is immersed in oil. This prevents the scattering and loss of light rays, which naturally occurs when light travels through air, consequently increasing the efficiency of the magnification.

Other types of microscopes have been developed especially for specific uses. The phase-contrast microscope is specifically designed for viewing specimens that are transparent and unstained. Some microscopic specimens must be stained with a fluorescent dye to be examined in detail (e.g., when detecting specific bacteria). A fluorescent microscope is the instrument best suited for viewing those specimens. In dark-field microscopy, the light is reflected from an angle, which causes the specimen to appear as a bright object on a dark field.

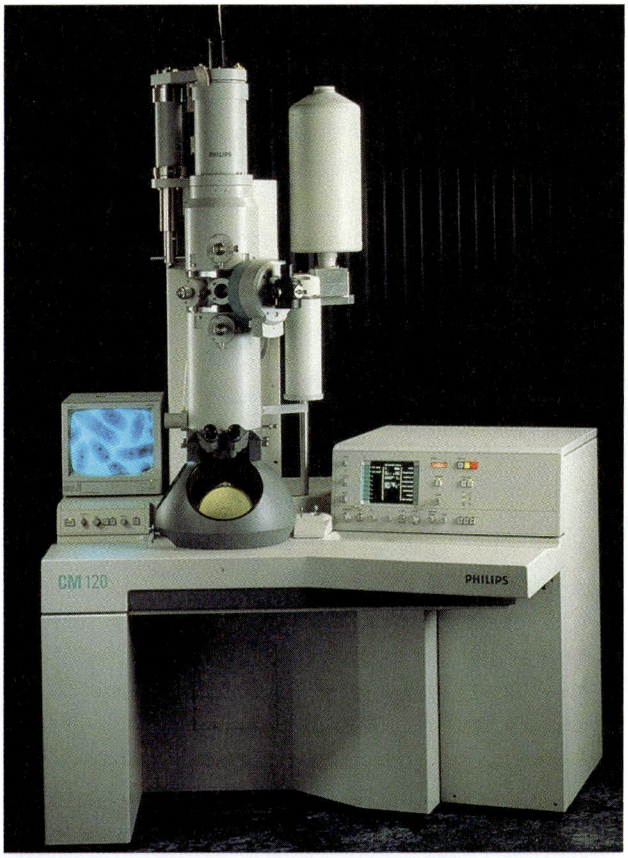

Figure 27-10 S440 scanning electron microscope.

Another type of microscope is the electron microscope (Figure 27-10). Special training is required to operate this sophisticated instrument. The electron microscope is large (several feet tall) and expensive; therefore, it is only found in larger regional and hospital laboratories. An electronic beam, rather than light, is passed through the specimen. The image is projected onto a fluorescent screen and may then be photographed and enlarged. The electron microscope provides views of extremely small organisms, such as viruses, in great detail and in three dimensions. Figure 27-11 shows blood cells seen using an electron microscope.

How to Use a Microscope

Besides being able to adjust a microscope's magnification, it may be necessary to adjust focus. The microscope contains a coarse adjustment and a fine adjustment. The coarse adjustment is to be used with the low-power (short) objective only. The coarse adjustment is used to bring the object into view. The fine adjustment may then be used to sharpen the image. Depending on the individual microscope, the coarse and fine adjustments may raise and lower the nosepiece, which houses the objectives, or they may raise and lower the stage, or platform, on which the slide rests.

It is important always to remember to raise the platform of the lower objectives using the coarse adjustment and the low-power objective *while viewing the slide from the side.* This allows the lens to come close to the slide without actually touching it. If the slide is not viewed from the side

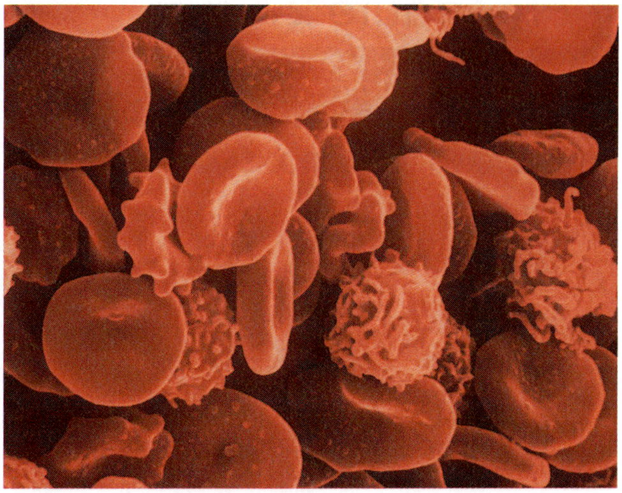

Figure 27-11 Blood cells as seen under an electron microscope.

for the coarse adjustment, there is the possibility of running the objective through the slide and seriously damaging the lens and the microscope, or of breaking the slide. After bringing the slide and objective together, the adjustments may be made through the ocular, always moving away from the slide. Once the item is in view, the fine adjustment may be used for clarity.

The bulb in the base directs light through the slide. The light first goes through a condenser and then through an iris diaphragm. The condenser is used to control the intensity of the light, and the iris diaphragm may be adjusted to control the amount of light.

To use the oil-immersion lens, place a drop of cedar or mineral oil on top of the coverslip directly over the specimen on the slide. Then carefully lower the oil-immersion lens into the oil, making sure that the lens never actually touches the slide.

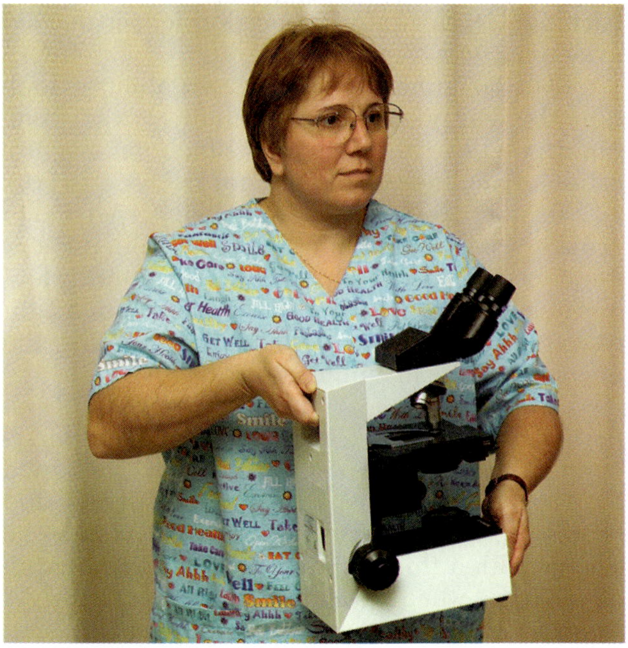

Figure 27-12 The proper way to carry a microscope.

How to Care for a Microscope

Microscopes can be expensive and, like any precision instrument, should be treated with care. Some practices that will extend the life of a microscope and maintain the quality of its performance are:

- Always follow the manufacturer's and clinic's rules for the care and maintenance of the microscope.
- Carry the microscope with one hand securely supporting the base and the other hand holding the arm (Figure 27-12).
- Keep the microscope covered when it is not being used.
- Clean the lenses with special lens paper and lens cleaner after each use. Using standard tissue can scratch the lenses.
- When looking through the eyepiece and focusing, always move the platform away from, never toward, the eyepiece to prevent the objective from coming into contact with the slide. If you are actually looking at the platform, then you can move it closer to the eyepiece without coming into contact with the slide.
- Use oil only with the oil-immersion lens.

Procedure 27-1

Using the Microscope

STANDARD PRECAUTIONS:

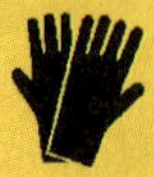

PURPOSE:

To properly use a microscope to view microscopic organisms using the coarse and fine adjustments, as well as the low- and high-power and oil-immersion objectives.

EQUIPMENT/SUPPLIES:

Hand disinfectant
Microscope (monocular or binocular)
Lens paper
Lens cleaner
Prepared slides (commercially available)
Immersion oil
Surface disinfectant

NOTE: Procedure will vary slightly according to microscope design. Consult the operating procedure in the microscope manual for specific instructions.

continues

Procedure 27-1 (continued)

PROCEDURE STEPS:

1. Wash hands.
2. Assemble equipment and materials.
3. Clean the ocular(s) and objectives with lens paper.
4. Use the coarse adjustment to raise the eyepiece or lens unit.
5. Rotate the 10x, or low-power, objective into position so that it is directly over the opening in the stage.
6. Turn on the microscope light.
7. Open the diaphragm until maximum light comes up through the condenser.
8. Place the slide on the stage (specimen side up).
9. Locate the coarse adjustment.
10. Look directly at the stage and 10x objective and turn the coarse adjustment until the objective is as close to the slide as it will go.

    NOTE: Do not lower any objective toward a slide while looking through the ocular(s).
11. Look into the ocular(s) and slowly turn the coarse adjustment in the opposite direction (as in Step 10) to raise the objective (or lower the stage) until the object on the slide comes into view.
12. Locate the fine adjustment.
13. Turn the fine adjustment to sharpen the image.

    NOTE: If a binocular microscope is used, the oculars must be adjusted for each individual's eyes.

    a. Adjust the distance between the oculars so that one image is seen (as when using binoculars).

    b. Use the coarse and fine adjustments to bring the object into focus while looking through the right ocular with the right eye.

    c. Close the right eye, look into the left ocular with the left eye, and *use the knurled collar on the left ocular* to bring the object into sharp focus. (Do not turn the coarse or fine adjustment at this time.)

    d. Look into the oculars with both eyes to observe that the object is in clear focus. If it is not, repeat the procedure.
14. Scan the slide by either method:

    a. Use the stage knobs to move the slide left and right and backward and forward while looking through the ocular(s),

    or

    b. Move the slide with the fingers while looking through the ocular(s) (for microscope without movable stage).
15. Rotate the high-power (40x) objective into position while observing the objective and the slide to see that the objective does not strike the slide.
16. Look through the ocular(s) to view the object on the slide; it should be almost in focus.
17. Locate the fine adjustment.
18. Look through the ocular(s) and turn the fine adjustment until the object is in focus. Do not use the coarse adjustment.
19. Adjust the amount of light. This can be done by closing the diaphragm, lowering the condenser, or adjusting the light at the source.
20. Scan the slide as in Step 14, using the fine adjustment if necessary to keep the object in focus.
21. Rotate the oil-immersion objective to the side slightly (so that no objective is in position).
22. Place one drop of immersion oil on the portion of the slide that is directly over the condenser.
23. Rotate the oil-immersion objective into position, being careful not to rotate the 40x objective through the oil.
24. Look to see that the oil-immersion objective is touching the drop of oil.
25. Look through the ocular(s) and slowly turn the fine adjustment until the image is clear. Use only the fine adjustment to focus the oil-immersion objective.
26. Adjust the amount of light using the procedure in Step 19.
27. Scan the slide using the procedure in Step 14.
28. Rotate the 10x objective into position (do not allow the 40x objective to touch the oil).
29. Remove the slide from the microscope stage and gently clean the oil from the slide with lens paper. A copeland jar containing a solvent cleaner, such as xylene, can be used to remove excess oil from the slide.

continues

Procedure 27-1 (continued)

30. Clean the oculars, 10x objective, and 403 objective with clean lens paper and lens cleaner.
31. Clean the 100x objective with lens paper and lens cleaner to remove all oil.
32. Clean any oil from the microscope stage and - condenser.
33. Turn off the microscope light and disconnect.
34. Position the eyepiece in the lowest position using the coarse adjustment.
35. Center the stage so that it does not project from either side of the microscope.
36. Cover the microscope and return it to storage.
37. Clean the work area; return slides to storage.
38. Wash hands.

Case Study 27-1

Refer to the scenario at the beginning of the chapter. Now imagine that Wanda sent Annette to the lab for the urinalysis rather than performing the test in the POL.

CASE STUDY REVIEW

1. What was the advantage of Wanda performing the urinalysis in the POL rather than sending Annette to the lab for the urinalysis?
2. What would have been an advantage of sending Annette to the outside lab for the urinalysis?

Case Study 27-2

Edith Leonard came to Inner City Health Care because she was experiencing sight disturbances, constant thirst, and fainting spells. After examining Edith, Dr. Ray Reynolds ordered a glucose tolerance test. Certified medical assistant Wanda Slawson gave Edith a special diet that she was to follow for the 3 days preceding the test and instructions regarding fasting before the test.

Edith has returned to the clinic to have the test. "Did you follow the diet I gave you, Mrs. Leonard?" Wanda asks. "Yes, I did." "Did you have anything to eat this morning?" "No, but I did have a cup of coffee. I thought it would be all right because I drink it black. I can't start the day without my coffee."

CASE STUDY REVIEW

1. Should Wanda perform the test? Explain your answer.
2. How can Wanda emphasize the importance of following the diet, fasting, and test instructions?
3. What can Wanda do to try to ensure Edith's cooperation?

SUMMARY

If disease did not exist, we would have little need for clinical laboratories. If we were not susceptible to viral illnesses, if bacteria never infected our bodies, if our bodies always operated in their healthiest state regardless of what we did to them, and, perhaps most important of all, if we chose our parents wisely, there would be little that a clinical laboratory would be asked to do. The fact that our bodies are susceptible to disease necessitates the existence of clinical laboratories.

Together with clinical laboratory personnel, medical assistants play an important role in laboratory testing. They prepare patients for tests, obtain specimens, and perform simple, routine tests or send specimens to the appropriate laboratory. Medical assistants are educated to perform these tasks in a manner that ensures the accuracy of the test and safeguards the health of patients and health care personnel.

STUDY FOR SUCCESS

To reinforce your knowledge and skills of information presented in this chapter:

- Review the Key Terms
- Practice the Procedure
- Consider the Case Study and discuss your conclusions
- Answer the Review Questions
  - Multiple Choice
  - Critical Thinking
- Navigate the Internet by completing the Web Activities
- Practice the StudyWARE activities on the textbook CD
- Apply your knowledge in the Student Workbook activities
- Complete the Web Tutor sections

REVIEW QUESTIONS

Multiple Choice

1. All of the following statements concerning point-of-care testing are true *except:*
   a. performed at the patient's bedside
   b. must be performed by certified laboratory professionals
   c. provides for rapid, accurate results
   d. the medical laboratory's role includes training and management of quality control
2. Independent medical laboratories must be managed by a:
   a. clinical laboratory technologist
   b. pathologist
   c. clinical laboratory technician
   d. medical assistant
3. The hematology department of a laboratory:
   a. studies microorganisms and their activities
   b. studies blood and blood-forming tissues
   c. detects the presence of disease-producing human parasites or eggs present in specimens taken from the body
   d. detects the presence of abnormal tissues
4. The quality of patient test results is maintained by:
   a. instrument calibration procedures
   b. preventative maintenance procedures
   c. quality control testing
   d. all of the above
5. When a patient or specimen is sent to a laboratory for testing, the medical assistant also sends:
   a. a written requisition
   b. a report
   c. the patient's file
   d. an insurance form
6. The most commonly used microscope in the clinic is the:
   a. fluorescent microscope
   b. electron microscope
   c. phase-contrast microscope
   d. compound microscope

Critical Thinking

1. A patient asks you to recommend a laboratory for the tests ordered by the provider. How will you respond to the request? What are some factors that will influence your response?
2. A patient performed a pregnancy test at home, but her provider has requested a pregnancy test in the office. Explain to the patient why the home test may not be as accurate as the test performed in the office.
3. The provider has ordered a metabolic panel for a patient. What is a panel, and how will it help the provider to diagnose the patient's condition?
4. Explain why it is important to handle and process specimens, test kits, and chemicals properly.
5. The time and date of specimen collection were not included on the requisition form. Why are these data always important to the laboratory?
6. Explain how a compound microscope is able to magnify.

WEB ACTIVITIES

1. For each group of laboratory personnel discussed in this chapter, search the Internet for a Web site that pertains to it. What kind of information does it offer?
2. Locate a local hospital's Web site. Does it outline all the specialty departments described in this chapter? What unique services do they offer?
3. Visit your insurance company's Web site. Does it specify which laboratories must be used?

REFERENCES/BIBLIOGRAPHY

American Medical Technologists. (2004). Retrieved October 2008, from http://www.amt1.com.

American Society for Clinical Laboratory Science. Retrieved October 2008, from http://www.ascls.org.

American Society for Clinical Pathology. Retrieved October 2008, from http://www.ascp.org.

National Accrediting Agency for Clinical Laboratory Sciences. Retrieved October 2008, from http://www.naacls.org.

National Credentialing Agency for Laboratory Personnel. Retrieved October 2008, from http://www.nca-info.org.

Phlebotomy: Venipuncture and Capillary Puncture

Chapter 28

KEY TERMS

Additive
Aliquot
Anticoagulant
Buffy Coat
Cannula
Centrifuge
Constrict
Dilate
Edematous
Erythrocyte
Hematology
Hematoma
Hemoconcentration
Hemolysis
Hypoglycemia
Leukocyte
Lipemia
Luer-Lok
Oxygenated
Palpate
Phlebotomy
Plasma
Primary Container
Serum
Thixotropic Separator Gel
Thrombocyte
Tourniquet
Venipuncture
Viscosity

OUTLINE

OBJECTIVES

The student should strive to meet the following performance objectives and demonstrate an understanding of the facts and principles presented in this chapter through written and oral communication.

1. Define the key terms as presented in the glossary.
2. Explain the medical assistant's responsibility to the patient in terms of quality of care and respect for the patient as a human being.

OBJECTIVES (continued)

3. Explain why the medical assistant has a special responsibility to present a neat, pleasant, and competent demeanor.
4. Differentiate between serum and plasma.
5. State the relationship between diameter and the gauge of the needle.
6. Explain the principle of the vacuum tube system.
7. State the manner in which anticoagulants prevent coagulation.
8. Name the anticoagulant associated with the various color-coded vacuum tubes.
9. State the purpose of additives to vacuum tubes.
10. Explain the three skills used in collecting blood specimens.
11. Explain the importance of correct patient identification; complete specimen labeling; and proper handling, storage, and delivery.
12. Describe the step-by-step procedure for drawing blood with a syringe, vacuum tube system, butterfly, or capillary puncture.
13. Explain how to handle the various reactions a patient might have to venipuncture.
14. List two items commonly used in phlebotomy that may cause a problem with a patient who has a latex sensitivity or allergy.

Scenario

At Inner City Health Care, medical assistant Bruce Goldman often performs venipunctures. Bruce is personable and has an easy-going manner that makes patients feel comfortable with him. He takes time to talk to patients before performing a venipuncture to determine their feelings about the procedure and to learn about their previous experiences. Bruce is confident and professional in his interactions with patients. He is always well-groomed, and he treats patients with respect. Using his social, technical, and administrative skills, Bruce is usually able to collect the necessary blood samples while providing a positive experience for patients.

INTRODUCTION

The task of collecting blood samples from patients for diagnostic testing is known as phlebotomy. The health care professional who performs this duty varies at each health care setting. The task of phlebotomy is not restricted to one individual. A variety of individuals are cross trained to do phlebotomy and other tasks. Many health care settings do not have enough patients to justify having a phlebotomist available at all times. Therefore, the medical assistant may be designated to perform phlebotomy procedures.

Spotlight on Certification

RMA Content Outline

- Anatomy and physiology
- Human relations
- Asepsis
- Laboratory procedures

CMA (AAMA) Content Outline

- Systems, including structure, function related conditions, and diseases
- Maintaining confidentiality
- Medical records
- Principles of infection control
- Equipment preparation and operation
- Safety precautions
- Collecting and processing specimens; diagnostic testing

CMAS Content Outline

- Anatomy and physiology
- Professionalism
- Asepsis in the medical office
- Communication

WHY COLLECT BLOOD?

Hematology is the study of blood and its components, fluids, and cells. Hematology also includes the study of blood- forming organs and blood diseases.

Phlebotomy is the process of collecting blood for diagnostic purposes or bloodletting as a therapeutic measure. The history of bloodletting dates back to the early Egyptians and continues into modern times. Phlebotomy in the past was a method to cure individuals with "bad" blood. The blood was drained out of individuals as a treatment, thereby alleviating the patient's symptoms. Phlebotomy, also called **venipuncture,** is now used to help determine the disease process taking place and to determine the method of treatment. Testing blood samples give the provider more tools for gathering diagnostic information.

THE MEDICAL ASSISTANT'S ROLE IN PHLEBOTOMY

A phlebotomist is a person trained to obtain blood specimens by venipuncture and capillary puncture techniques. The phlebotomist's primary role is to collect blood as efficiently as possible for accurate and reliable test results. How the medical assistant will be involved in phlebotomy will vary greatly from one health care environment to another. The medical assistant performing venipuncture will have direct contact with the patient and perform tasks that are critical to the patient's diagnosis and care. During the direct contact with the patient, the medical assistant will leave an impression with the patient. It can be positive or negative depending on the skill with which the medical assistant performs the venipuncture.

It is the medical assistant's responsibility to provide high-quality care to patients. The medical assistant must act professionally when working with patients. Professionalism is displayed by performing tasks in an efficient, competent manner; wearing clean, neat attire; and showing concern for patients and their feelings.

Patients will not tell family and friends that their blood was run through expensive state-of-the-art instruments but rather that the person drawing their blood sample was friendly and skilled. A smile and a kind word can allay a patient's fear and ensure a more satisfied and loyal patient.

ANATOMY AND PHYSIOLOGY OF THE CIRCULATORY SYSTEM

To be prepared to collect blood, the medical assistant must understand the system that carries the blood and the composition of the blood. The system in which the blood is transported is the circulatory system. Blood forms in the organs of the body. The bone marrow is the primary factory for production of blood cells. The lymph nodes, thymus, and spleen are also sites for the production of blood cells. The function of blood is to carry oxygen to body tissues and to remove the waste product, carbon dioxide. The blood also carries nutrients to all parts of the body and moves the waste products to the lungs, kidneys, liver, and skin for elimination.

The circulatory system consists of the heart, which pumps blood through the body by way of tubing called arteries, veins, and capillaries. When blood flows away from the heart, it flows in arteries; blood flowing back to the heart flows through the veins. Connecting most of the arteries and veins are the capillaries (Figure 28-1).

Arteries have a thick wall that helps them withstand the pressure of the pumping action of the heart. The arteries branch to form arterioles, which branch again to become capillaries. The

ARTERIES TO VEINS	
Arteries	**Veins**
1. Carry blood from the heart, carry oxygenated blood (except pulmonary artery)	1. Carry blood to the heart, carry deoxygenated blood (except pulmonary vein)
2. Normally bright red in color	2. Normally dark red in color
3. Elastic walls that expand with surge of blood	3. Thin walls/less elastic
4. No valves	4. Valves
5. Can feel a pulse	5. No pulse

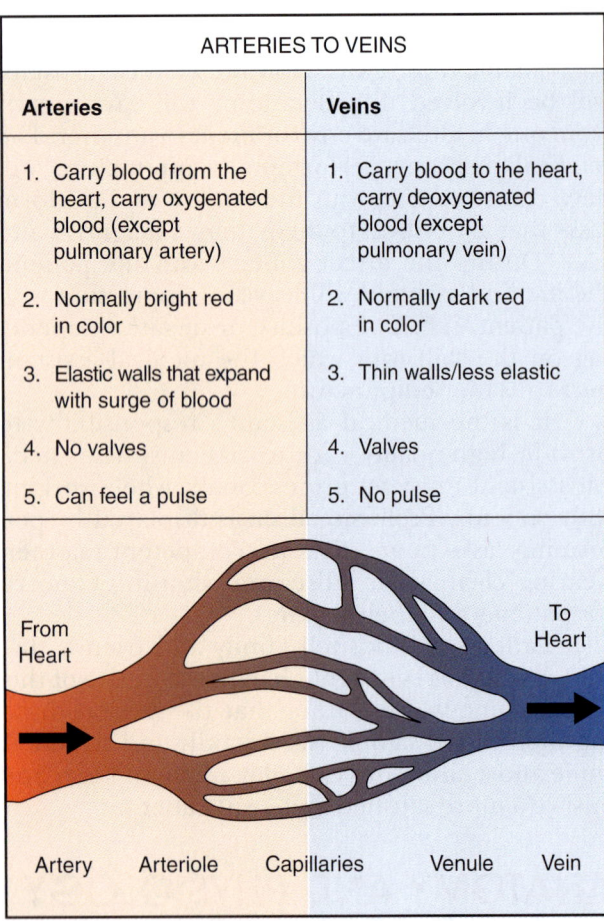

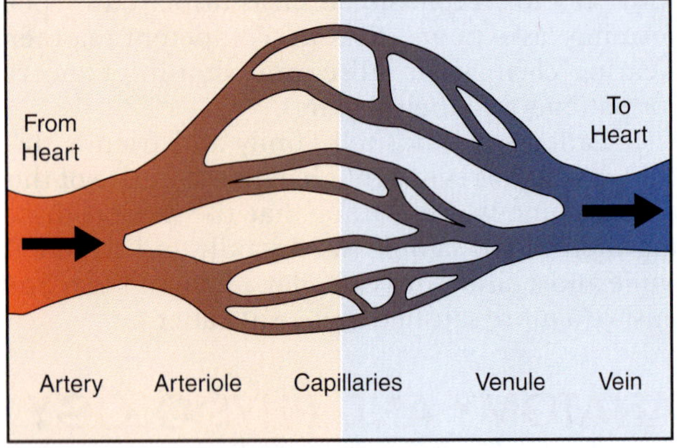

Figure 28-1 Blood flows from the heart through the larger arteries to arterioles to arterial capillary beds at the cellular level, then back to the heart through venous capillary beds into venules and finally larger veins.

capillaries then begin coming together to form venules, and the venules then become veins. As blood flows through the body, it follows this path of artery-arteriole-capillary-venule-vein. **Oxygenated** arterial blood, which contains a high level of oxygen, leaves the heart and carries the oxygen to the tissue by releasing the oxygen through the cell walls of the capillaries. At the same time, carbon dioxide is being absorbed by the blood, and then is transported to the lungs to be exhaled as a waste product. The flow of the blood also regulates body temperature. When the body gets warm, the capillaries in the extremities **dilate** and let off heat. This process then cools the body. If the body becomes cold, the capillaries **constrict** and less blood flows through, thereby conserving heat for the rest of the body.

The body contains approximately 6 liters (L) of blood, 45% of which is formed elements. The formed cellular elements consist of **erythrocytes, leukocytes,** and **thrombocytes** (Figure 28-2). The remaining 55% of the blood is liquid. Generally 2.5 milliliters (mL) blood will yield about 1 mL serum. The liquid portion of uncoagulated blood is known as plasma. Plasma is the fluid that provides a matrix for blood cells, electrolytes, proteins, and chemicals to travel throughout the body via the blood vessels. Blood flowing through the body contains a substance called fibrinogen. The clotting process converts the fibrinogen into fibrin. The fibrin is like a sticky spider web that traps the formed elements into the fibrin mass called a clot. The clot then contracts and the liquid **(serum)** portion is extracted. The serum is a clear, straw-colored liquid that is used for many of the tests done in the laboratory. The main difference between serum and plasma is that plasma contains fibrinogen, and serum does not.

The formed elements and the liquid portion of the blood are often separated for laboratory testing. To speed the removal of the serum from a tube of blood, an instrument called a **centrifuge** spins the blood. A carrier holds the tubes of blood, and when the centrifuge is activated, the carrier spins. The spinning action of the carrier pushes the blood cells to the bottom of the tube. The blood separates according to weight. The clot goes to the bottom of the tube and the serum goes to the top.

To produce a plasma specimen, the blood must be prevented from clotting by the use of a chemical anticoagulant. Blood collected in a tube containing an anticoagulant can be centrifuged to separate the formed elements (cells) from the plasma. The bottom layer will contain the erythrocytes, then there will be a thin layer called the **buffy coat.** The buffy coat contains a mixture of leukocytes and thrombocytes, which are lighter and less numerous than the red blood cells (RBCs). On top of all these layers is the plasma layer. The plasma will contain fibrinogen and usually is slightly hazy (Figure 28-3).

BLOOD COLLECTION

Most laboratory tests are performed on serum, plasma, or whole blood. Generally, when a serum sample is needed, a serum separator vacuum tube with thixotropic gel is used. The purpose of the thixotropic gel is to create a barrier between the clotted cells and the serum during centrifugation. This protects the serum from contamination from any hemolyzed RBCs. There will be certain restrictions in some cases; refer to the laboratory user manual to verify tube requirements. When a serum separator tube is used, several steps must be followed:

1. Perform venipuncture by the preferred method.
2. Invert the tube five times to activate the clotting.

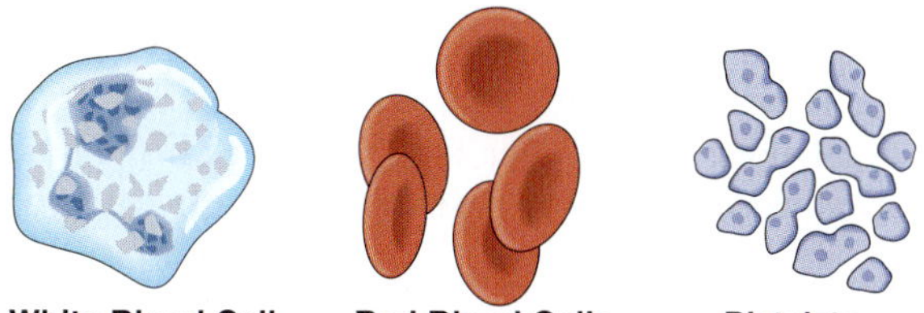

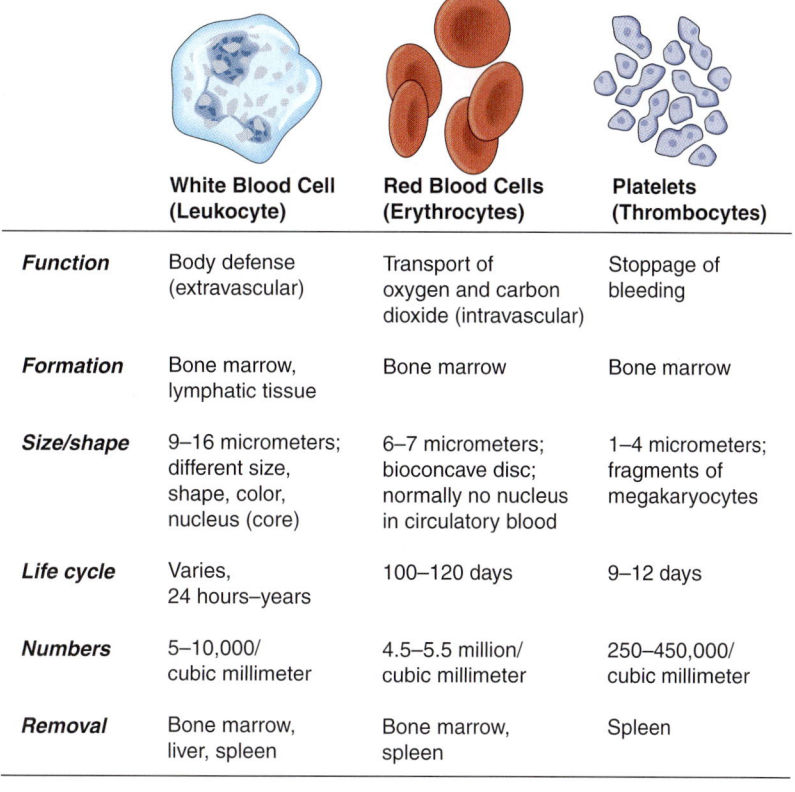

	White Blood Cell (Leukocyte)	Red Blood Cells (Erythrocytes)	Platelets (Thrombocytes)
Function	Body defense (extravascular)	Transport of oxygen and carbon dioxide (intravascular)	Stoppage of bleeding
Formation	Bone marrow, lymphatic tissue	Bone marrow	Bone marrow
Size/shape	9–16 micrometers; different size, shape, color, nucleus (core)	6–7 micrometers; bioconcave disc; normally no nucleus in circulatory blood	1–4 micrometers; fragments of megakaryocytes
Life cycle	Varies, 24 hours–years	100–120 days	9–12 days
Numbers	5–10,000/ cubic millimeter	4.5–5.5 million/ cubic millimeter	250–450,000/ cubic millimeter
Removal	Bone marrow, liver, spleen	Bone marrow, spleen	Spleen

Figure 28-2 Cellular components of blood.

3. Allow the specimen to clot with the tube in the upright position in a rack for at least 30 minutes but no longer than an hour.
4. Centrifuge the tube at 2,500 g for 15 minutes.
5. Store the tube upright or transfer the serum to a plastic transport vial for pickup by the laboratory. These are usually frozen specimens and require a stat pickup. Check the manual to see indications.

There will be different requirements for different laboratories. *NOTE:* Do not use serum separator tubes for therapeutic drug monitoring (TDM) or toxicology studies. The gel has a tendency to absorb the drugs, thereby decreasing the accuracy of the test results. Collect these samples in a plain red-top vacuum tube. Remove the serum immediately (if indicated in the test requirements) after centrifugation and place it in a plastic transport vial. Indicate if the specimen is a serum specimen or for type and cross match.

Plasma and Whole-Blood Collection

Tubes containing anticoagulants are used to collect plasma and whole-blood samples. There are a variety of different anticoagulant tubes that can be used. The anticoagulant needed in the tube will be specified by the laboratory or testing requirements. Preparing the plasma specimen for transport or testing is similar to serum preparation:

1. Perform venipuncture by the preferred method.
2. Invert the tube 8 to 10 times to mix the blood with the anticoagulant.
3. Centrifuge the tube at 2,500 g for 10 minutes.
4. Transfer the plasma to a plastic transport vial for pickup by the laboratory. Do not allow any blood cells to mix with the plasma specimen. Indicate

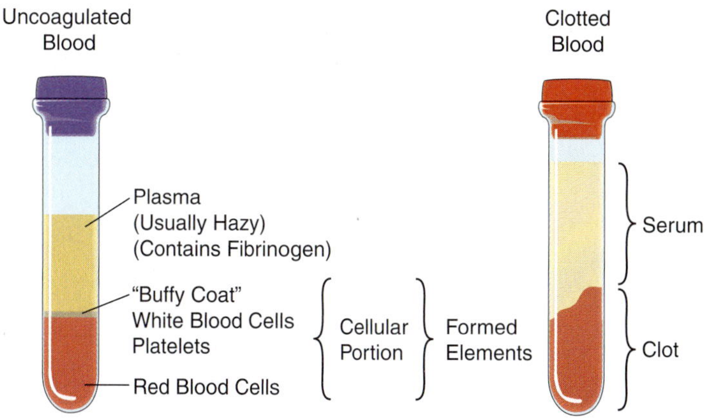

Figure 28-3 Vacuum collection tubes showing serum and plasma.

the specimen as a plasma specimen and what type of anticoagulant was used. There will be different requirements for different laboratories. Refer to your laboratory user manual for the appropriate test requirements.

To prepare whole blood specimens for transport or testing:

1. Perform venipuncture by the preferred method.
2. Invert the tube 8 to 10 times to mix the blood with the anticoagulant.
3. Maintain the tube at room temperature unless otherwise instructed. Never freeze a whole-blood sample unless specifically instructed to do so.

Collection of Blood Specimens

The most commonly used method for blood collection is venipuncture. To obtain a blood sample, the medical assistant must locate a vein that is acceptable for blood collection. The preferred site for venipuncture is the antecubital space, which is located anterior to the elbow on the inside of the arm. The veins are near the surface and are large enough to give access to the blood (Figure 28-4). The median cubital vein is the vein that is used the majority of the time. When this vein is not available, any of the other veins that can be felt may be used. These veins include the basilic, cephalic, and median veins. When necessary, veins on the dorsal surface of the hand or wrist may be used for venipuncture, but they are more painful for the patient and may require a smaller needle or the use of a butterfly apparatus.

The veins of the feet are an alternative when the arms are not available. The provider's permission is needed before drawing blood from the veins of the legs and feet. The provider may not want the patient's leg or foot veins punctured because the act of drawing blood may cause clots to form. These clots then have the possibility of dislodging and causing a blockage elsewhere in the body. It would be extremely rare for a medical assistant

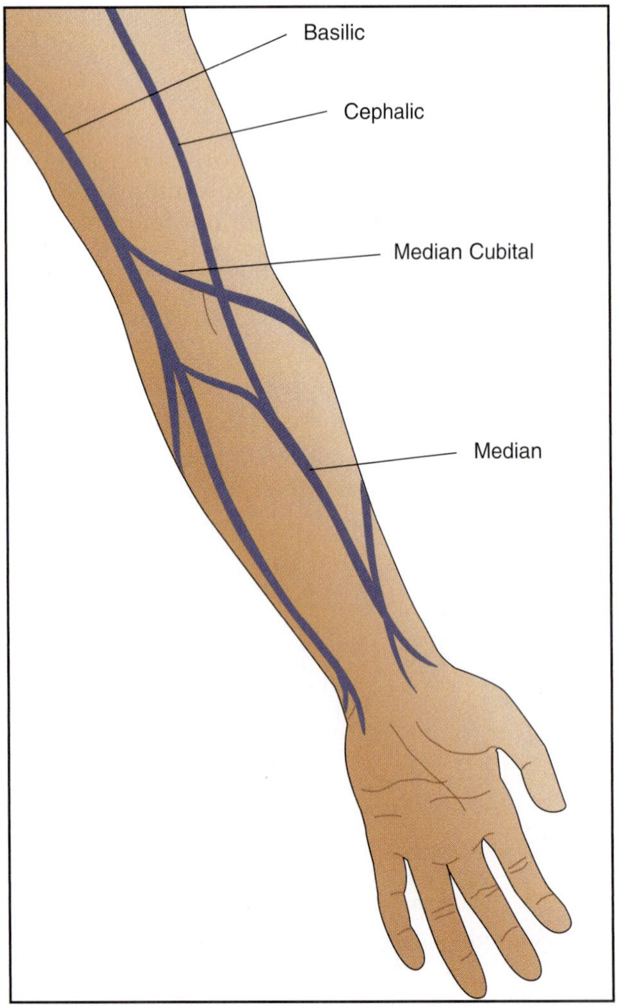

Figure 28-4 Superficial veins of the arm.

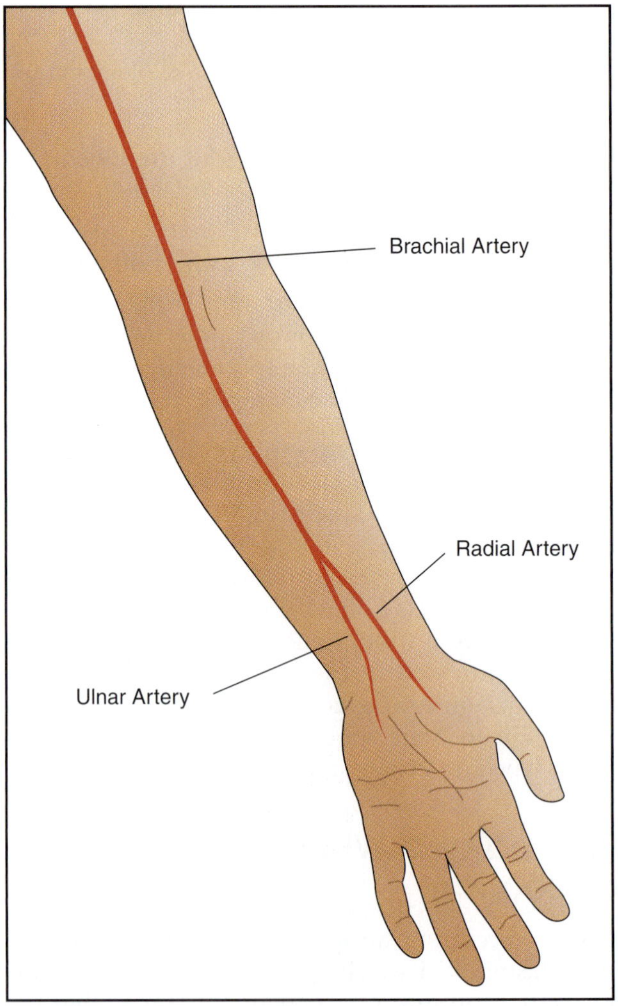

Figure 28-5 Arteries of the arm.

to use this location. The provider should be consulted before a foot puncture is considered. The person performing a foot draw must be specially trained for that procedure.

The arteries in the arm consist of the brachial artery in the brachial region of the arm and the radial and ulnar arteries in the wrist (Figure 28-5). Special techniques are necessary to puncture arteries to obtain a blood specimen for the examination of gases absorbed by the blood. Arterial punctures and the techniques used to draw blood from these locations for blood gas testing are not generally done by a medical assistant. Refer to individual state laws for specific training and certification/registration requirements.

VENIPUNCTURE EQUIPMENT

All methods of venipuncture require the invasive procedure of punturing into a vein to obtain a blood sample. The three methods used to perform venipuncture are the syringe method, the vacuum tube method, and the butterfly method. Each method has advantages and disadvantages (Table 28-1). It is important that the well-trained medical assistant have options when attempting to draw blood from a wide range of patients in a variety of situations. There will be times in one's career when one method will be preferred over another. Regardless of which method is chosen to perform the blood draw, the blood will probably be transferred into a vacuum tube eventually. This is because vacuum tubes contain the chemicals and substances necessary for the blood tests to be performed.

Syringes and Needles

Syringes used in venipuncture are usually made of plastic (Figure 28-6). They come in a variety of sizes. Each manufacturer has their own packaging

Table 28-1 Comparison of Blood Collection Methods

Method	Indications for Use	Advantages	Disadvantages
Vacuum tube	Routine collection Multiple tubes are needed Whenever possible	Fast Relatively safe Best specimen quality Large collection amount possible	May not work with: Small veins Fragile veins Difficult draws Small children Hand or feet draws
Butterfly assembly	Small or fragile veins Difficult draws Small children or older adult patients	Least likely to collapse vein Less painful to patient Can attach syringe Can attach tube adapter Least likely to pass through small veins Good specimen quality	Syringe not as safe because tube transfer is necessary Specimen may be hemolyzed Not good for large amounts of blood
Syringe	Children Infants Older adult patients Onocology patients Severely burned patients Obese patients Inaccessible veins Extremely fragile veins Home testing by patient Procedure requires capillary specimen	Easier to perform Allows for smaller amount of specimen	Not good for dehydrated patients Not good for patient with poor circulation Cannot be used for: Blood cultures Erythrocyte sedimentation rate

Source: Courtesy of Sheri R. Greimes, CMA (AAMA), PBT (ASCP).

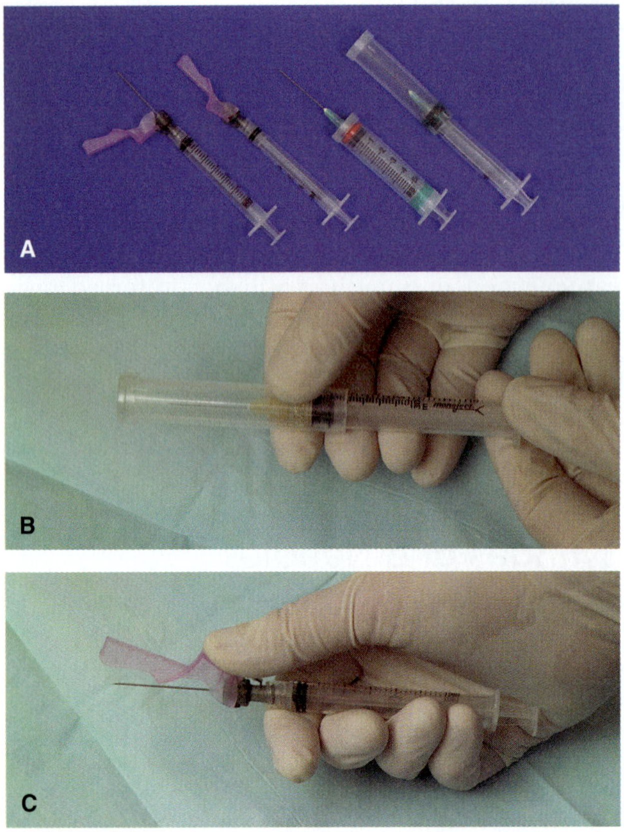

Figure 28-6 (A) Safety syringes with needles, before and after safety mechanisms are engaged. (B) Pull entire casing over the needle to engage this type of safety mechanism. Once engaged, it is locked into place. (C) With the thumb and forefinger, press the safety mechanism over the needle; or, an even safer technique is to press it against a hard surface such as the edge of the counter. Be sure to listen for the click. Once engaged, the safety mechanism should be firmly locked in place.

and coloring, thus there is really no significance related to the color and design of syringes. Most syringes used in venipuncture will be 5 and 10 mL in size. Some syringes are designed with a **Luer-Lok** tip. This tip allows the needle to be securely twisted onto the syringe. The Luer-Lok tip may be preferred to the push-on tip for additional safety for the user.

Needles attached to syringes and used for venipuncture do not necessarily differ in function and design from needles used for injections (Figure 28-6). They come in a wide variety of lengths and gauges. Most common sizes for venipuncture are 20, 21, and 22 gauges and about 1 or 1.5 inches in length (Table 28-2). Sixteen-gauge needles are often used for blood banking procedures. Remember, the larger the number, the smaller the gauge.

Table 28-2 Needle Gauges Used in Phlebotomy

Gauge Size	Comments
23	Often considered too small, can cause hemolysis of blood cells; used sometimes with butterfly system
22	Preferred for pediatric phlebotomy or very small veins of the hands or feet
21	Most common size used with vacuum tubes
20	Appropriate, but large for common phlebotomy
18	Not used for phlebotomy, but sometimes used in blood banking/donations
16	Most commonly used in blood banking/donations

Another type of needle used in venipuncture is the special needle, designed for use with the vacuum tube method. This needle has a double end—the longer needle to puncture the vein and the shorter needle to puncture into the vacuum tube (Figure 28-7). These needles also come in a variety of gauges and lengths; the most common is the same as the standard needle described previously: 20, 21, and 22 gauge, 1 to 1.5 inches in length. When selecting a double-ended needle for use with the vacuum tube, you will use a multidraw needle, which enables drawing of more than one tube of blood. The multidraw needles come with a rubber sheath over the shorter needle, which goes into the vacuum tube. This rubber sheath prevents blood from leaking out of the needle during tube changes. Multidraw needles are sometimes referred to as multisample or multiple sample needles.

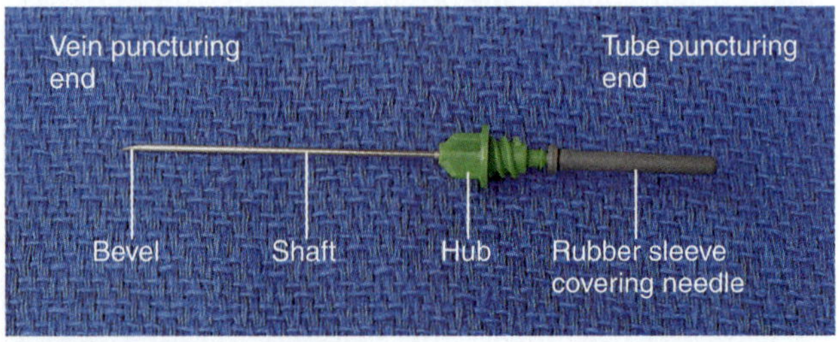

Figure 28-7 Multidraw needle for vacuum tube blood collection system.

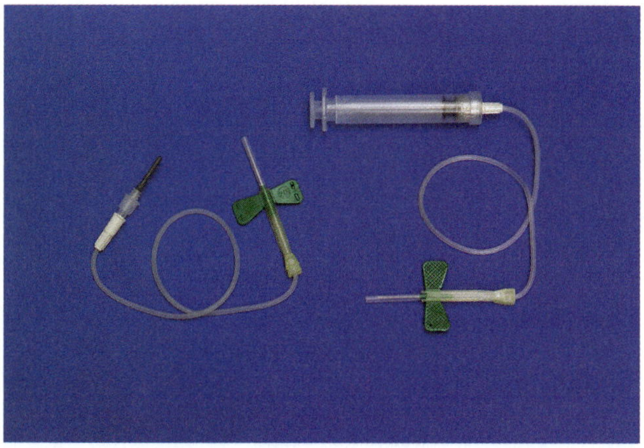

Figure 28-8 (A) Winged infusion set (butterfly) with safety needle. (B) Butterfly attached to syringe.

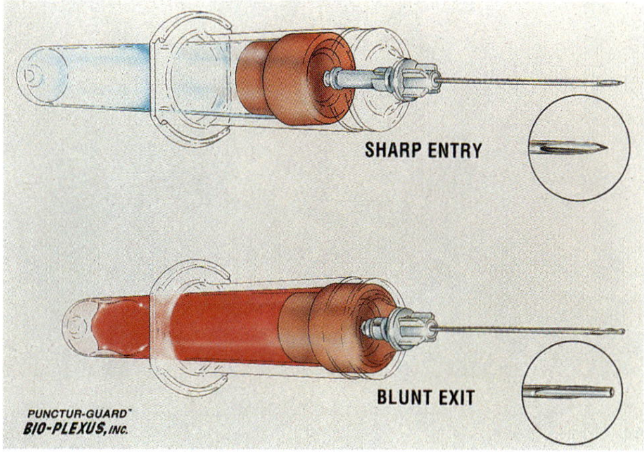

Figure 28-9 Puncture Guard is one type of safety needle. (Courtesy of BioPlexus, Inc., Tolland, CT)

Another type of needle used in venipuncture is on a "winged" infusion set called the butterfly collection system (Figure 28-8). Because of the reasons for using the butterfly collection system, the needles are smaller, usually 21 or 23 gauge.

More details about each collection method are discussed later in this chapter.

Safety Needles and Blood Collection Systems

The Occupational Safety and Health Administration (OSHA) requires that safety needles be made available to employees to prevent on-the-job needlestick injuries. The huge variety of safety needles and blood collection systems currently available greatly reduces the risks for accidental needlesticks. The main issue is deciding which to select for use in your clinic based on personal preferences. OSHA requires that employers make purchasing decisions based on formal feedback from front-line employees rather than costs and administrative contracts. This means that you have a great deal of choice about what systems you select to use. It is recommended that you examine a variety of safety systems on a regular basis to determine which one gives you the greatest protection from accidental needlestick injury. These systems are often referred to as needlestick prevention devices (NPDs). Among the available systems are passive systems in which the needle is automatically covered when withdrawn and systems that require the medical assistant to activate a mechanism of covering the needle. Within each type are many options and brands. This chapter discusses and shows a few currently available options in no particular order. The first is the Plexus Puncture Guard system (Figure 28-9). Before withdrawing the needle from the patient's vein, a **cannula** is clicked into place. The cannula fills the inside of the needle, virtually blunting the tip. Another option is the Eclipse system by Becton-Dickinson (Figure 28-10), which requires the medical assistant to snap a cover over the needle after it is removed from the vein. A third option, called the Safety-Lok, also manufactured by Becton-Dickinson, requires the medical assistant to slide the cover over the needle until it locks into place. Whichever system you choose, always combine the safest equipment with the safest practices for the best all-around benefit for you, your coworkers, and your patients. Many accidents occur when we become distracted or hurried in our tasks.

Vacuum Tubes and Adapters/Holders

The vacuum tube system is often called the Vacutainer system. Vacutainer can be a misnomer because the term *Vacutainer*® is a brand name for the vacuum tube system manufactured by Becton-Dickinson. Medical assistants often say Vacutainer when they are using another company's product.

Vacuum tubes are vacuum-packed test tubes with rubber stoppers. The safest ones are made of plastic and have screw-on caps. They are available in a variety of sizes for a variety of uses (Figure 28-11). Vacuum tubes come plain or with added chemicals or substances necessary for the appropriate test to be run. The color of the rubber stopper designates the additive inside the tube. Although most colors are universal regardless of manufacturer, the shades may vary and can be confusing

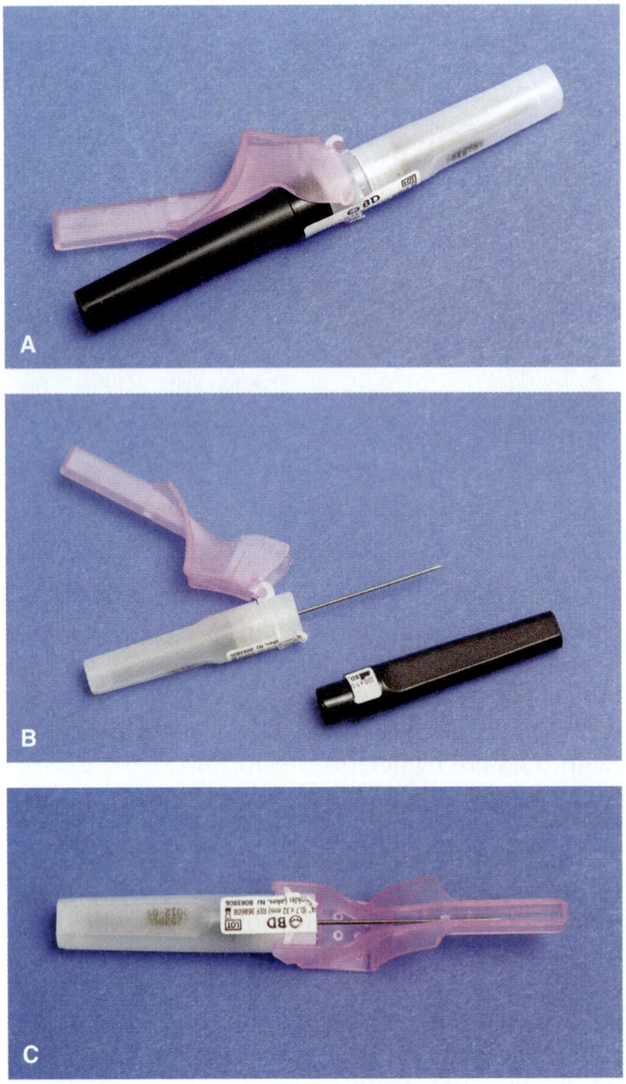

Figure 28-10 Three Eclipse safety needles for use with vacuum tubes. (A) Needle capped, safety mechanism not engaged. (B) Needle exposed, safety mechanism not engaged. (C) Safety mechanism engaged.

to beginners. It is always best to read the label to determine the additive if the shade is different.

Plastic holders or tube adapters (Figure 28-12) are used in conjunction with the vacuum tubes. Figure 28-13 shows safety holders developed to minimize the risk for accidental needlesticks. Some plastic holders are reusable, but there is much debate about the appropriateness of reusing them, even after disinfection. They are fairly inexpensive and the inner threads will eventually wear out, therefore replacing them frequently is always good practice. The holders with the safety mechanisms shown in Figure 28-13 are not reusable.

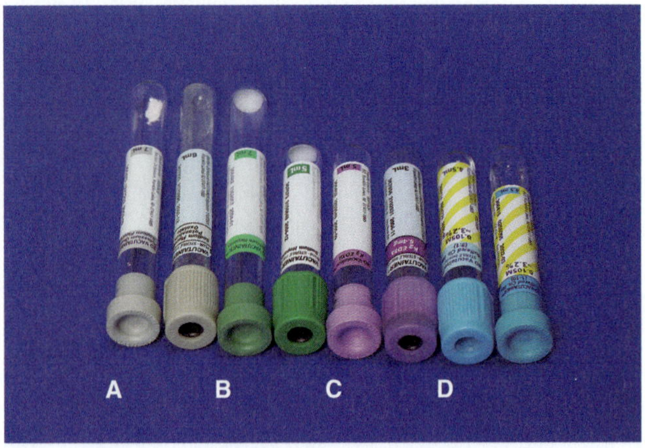

Figure 28-11 Standard anticoagulant tubes with conventional rubber stopper and Hemogard twist off closures. (A) Gray top, tube contains antiglycocytic agent; left tube with rubber stopper, right tube with twist off Hemogard top. (B) Green top, tube contains heparin anticoagulant; left tube with rubber stopper, right tube with twist off Hemogard top. (C) Lavender top, tube contains EDTA anticoagulant; left tube with rubber stopper, right tube with twist off Hemogard top. (D) Light blue top, tube contains sodium citrate; left tube with twist off Hemogard top, right tube with rubber stopper.

Anticoagulants, Additives, and Gels

Different tests require different types of blood specimens. Some specimens require a serum sample and need to be drawn in a tube that allows the blood to clot. Others require a whole-blood or plasma specimen and need to be drawn in a tube that does not allow the blood to clot. **Additives** are put into the tubes during manufacturing.

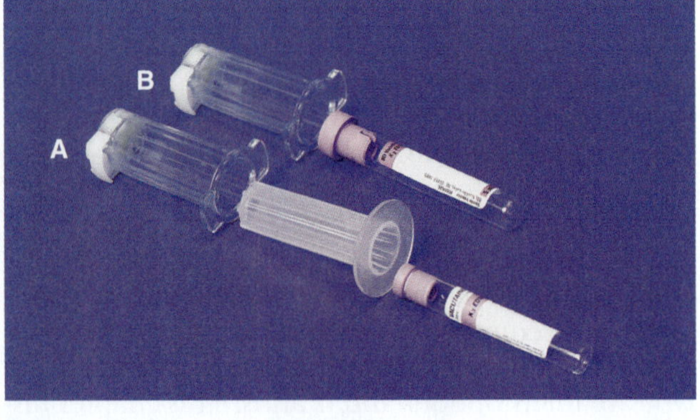

Figure 28-12 Holders for vacuum tube system. (A) Adult holder. (B) Pediatric tube using an adapter.

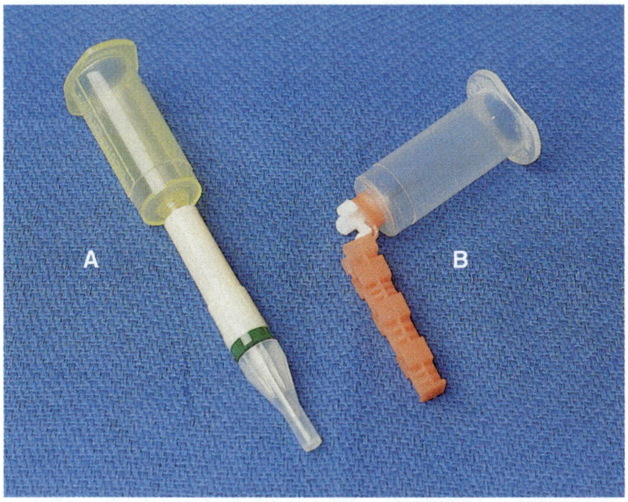

Figure 28-13 Safety tube holders. (A) Safety needle and holder. (B) Locking cover.

The additive may be an anticoagulant to prevent clotting of the blood, a chemical to help preserve the blood, or a substance to accelerate the clotting process (called a clot activator). Some tubes also contain gel plugs, which act as separators between the blood cells/clot and the serum/plasma. An anticoagulant is a chemical substance that prevents the clotting by removing calcium in the form of calcium salts or by inhibiting the conversion of prothrombin to thrombin. Coagulation occurs naturally according to the steps in Table 28-3. If a step is prevented, the blood does not clot.

Table 28-3 Steps to Blood Clotting

1. Uncoagulated blood
2. Calcium utilized
3. Prothrombin converts to thrombin
4. Fibrinogen converts to fibrin
5. Clot forms

A tube containing an anticoagulant removes one of the steps in the process, preventing the blood from clotting. The step removed depends on the anticoagulant used. The basic anticoagulants used consist of oxalates, citrates, ethylenediaminetetraacetic acid (EDTA), or heparin (Figure 28-14). Anticoagulants are identified by tube color. It is important to use the correct anticoagulant for the test because the improper anticoagulant can alter test results.

Red Top

Contains:	None
Effects on Specimen:	Blood clots, and the serum is separated by centrifugation
Uses:	Chemistries, Immunology and Serology, Blood Bank (Crossmatch)

Red-Gray Mottled Top ("Tiger top")

Contains:	Serum Separating Tube (SST) with clot activator
Effects on Specimen:	Forms clot quickly and separates the serum with SST gel at the bottom of the tube
Uses:	Blood type screening and chemistries

Gold Top

Contains:	Separating gel and clot activator
Effects on Specimen:	Serum separator tube (SST) contains a gel at the bottom to separate the blood from serum on centrifugation
Uses:	Serology, endocrine, immunology, including HIV

Light Green Top

Contains:	Plasma Separating Tube (Na Heparin)
Effects on Specimen:	Anticoagulants with lithium heparin: plasma is separated with PST gel at the bottom of the tube
Uses:	Chemistries

Lavender/Purple Top

Contains:	EDTA (liquid form)
Effects on Specimen:	Forms calcium salts to remove calcium
Uses:	Hematology (CBC) and Blood Bank (Crossmatch); requires a full draw—invert 8 times to prevent clotting and platelet clumping

Light Blue Top

Contains:	Sodium citrate (Na Citrate)
Effects on Specimen:	Forms calcium salts to remove calcium
Uses:	Coagulation tests (PT, PTT, TCT, CMV), tube must be filled 100%

Figure 28-14 Collection tubes and their additives for phlebotomy (continues).

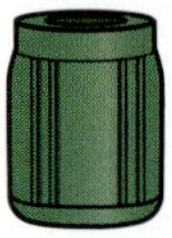

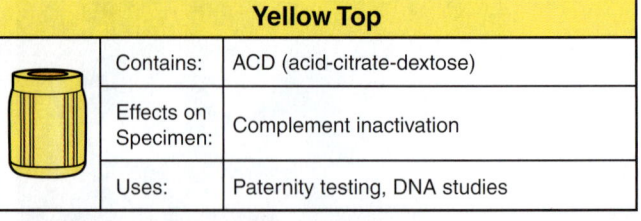

Dark Green Top	
Contains:	Sodium heparin or lithium heparin
Effects on Specimen:	Inactivates thrombin and thromboplastin
Uses:	Ammonia, lactate, HLA typing For lithium level, use sodium heparin For ammonia level, use sodium or lithium heparin

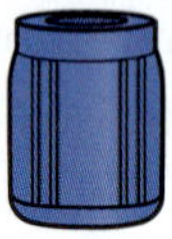

Dark Blue/Royal Blue Top	
Contains:	Sodium heparin or Na_2 EDTA
Effects on Specimen:	Forms calcium salts Tube is designed to contain no contaminating metals
Uses:	Toxicology and trace element testing (zinc, copper, lead, mercury) and drug level testing

Light Gray Top	
Contains:	Sodium fluoride and potassium oxalate
Effects on Specimen:	Antiglycolytic agent preserves glucose up to 5 days
Uses:	For lithium level, use sodium heparin Glucoses requires a full draw (may cause hemolysis if short draw)

Yellow Top	
Contains:	ACD (acid-citrate-dextose)
Effects on Specimen:	Complement inactivation
Uses:	Paternity testing, DNA studies

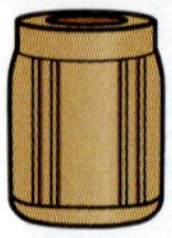

Tan/Brown Top	
Contains:	Sodium heparin
Effects on Specimen:	Inactivates thrombin and thromboplastin
Uses:	Serum lead determination

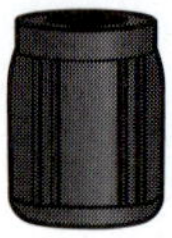

Black Top	
Contains:	Sodium citrate (buffered)
Effects on Specimen:	Forms calcium salts to remove calcium
Uses:	Westergren Sedimentation Rate; requires a full draw

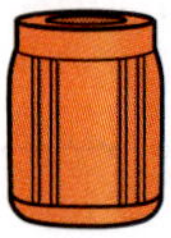

Orange Top	
Contains:	Thrombin
Effects on Specimen:	Quickly clots blood
Uses:	STAT serum chemistries

Figure 28-14 (continued)

Clot activators consists of silica (small glass) particles on the sides of the tubes that initiate the clotting process. The silica particles work as a catalyst for the clotting process by promoting the clotting process. The plastic vacuum tubes with the red tops have clot activators in them. The glass red top vacuum tubes do not.

Serum and plasma tubes can also be purchased with a **thixotropic separator gel** (Figure 28-15). The gel is an inert material that undergoes a temporary change in **viscosity** during centrifugation. When centrifuged, the gel changes to a liquid and moves up the sides of the tube to create a barrier between the blood cells or clot and the liquid portion of the blood. The gel then forms a solid plug and separates the cells/clot from the plasma/serum (Figure 28-16).

Actions of Additives

Potassium oxalate	Binds calcium
Sodium fluoride	Inhibits glycolysis
Sodium citrate	Binds calcium
EDTA	Binds calcium
Lithium heparin	Inhibits prothrombin to thrombin
No additive	Clot naturally forms
Sodium polyanetholesulfonate (SPS)	Binds calcium
Glass particles/silica	Promotes clotting
Ammonium heparin	Inhibits prothrombin to thrombin

Order of Draw

The order in which blood is drawn or mixed with the additives is important. Sterile collection bottles (for blood cultures) need to be filled first to prevent any contamination. After the sterile culture tubes are drawn, the order for the other tubes is related to the additives in them. It does not matter whether

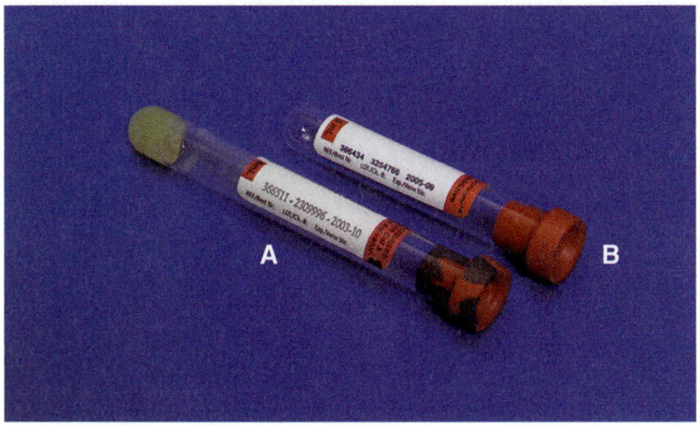

Figure 28-15 Standard vacuum tubes. (A) SST (red/gray or "speckled top") top tube contains clot activators and thixotropic gel. (B) Standard red top (glass) tube contains no anticoagulant but might contain glass particles/silica on the inside walls to irritate the thrombocytes to promote clotting.

Table 28-4 Standard Order of Draw—CLSI Guidelines as of December 2008

Blood culture tubes or vials	Yellow top or culture bottles
Sodium citrate	Light blue top
Serum tubes	Red top and red/gray top (SST)
Heparin tubes	Green tops, light and dark
EDTA tubes	Lavender top, then pink, white, or royal blue
Glycolytic inhibitor	Gray top
FDP	Dark blue

the blood is drawn directly into a vacuum tube or into a syringe, then transferred to the vacuum tube. The order of the tubes remains the same for either method. Table 28-4 also lists the order of draw.

Tourniquets

The **tourniquet,** when applied to the arm, constricts the flow of blood in the arm and makes the veins more prominent. The tourniquet is a soft, pliable, rubber or elastic strip approximately 1 inch wide by 15 to 18 inches long (Figure 28-17). The elastic strip serves as the best tourniquet for all conditions. The elastic strip can easily be released with one hand. Being about 1 inch wide, it does not cut into the patient's arm but distributes the pressure. The tourniquet can easily be disinfected but is inexpensive enough that it should be replaced often. If the tourniquet is obviously contaminated, it should be discarded into biohazard waste. If a patient has been identified as having a latex hypersensitivity, you must use a nonlatex tourniquet. Latex-free tourniquets are readily available and inexpensive, so they can be used for all patients regardless of latex allergy or hypersensitivity.

A blood pressure cuff can also be used as a tourniquet. Its use is primarily for veins that are difficult to locate using a standard tourniquet. The

Critical Thinking

Which vacuum tube would you use to draw a serum specimen: lavender or red top? Why did you choose that tube? What differentiates the two tubes?

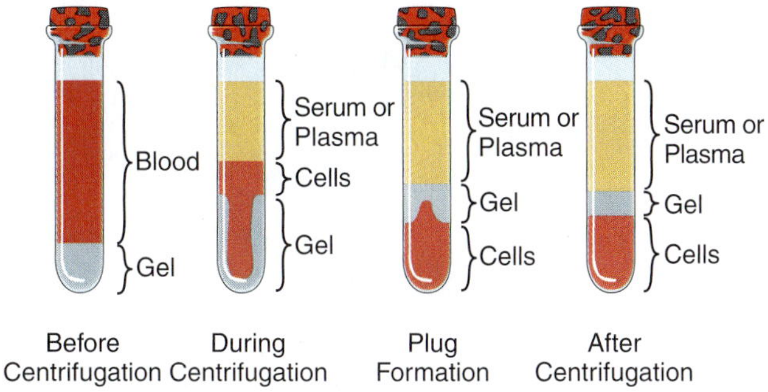

Figure 28-16 Separator thixotropic gel tube showing how the centrifugation process works.

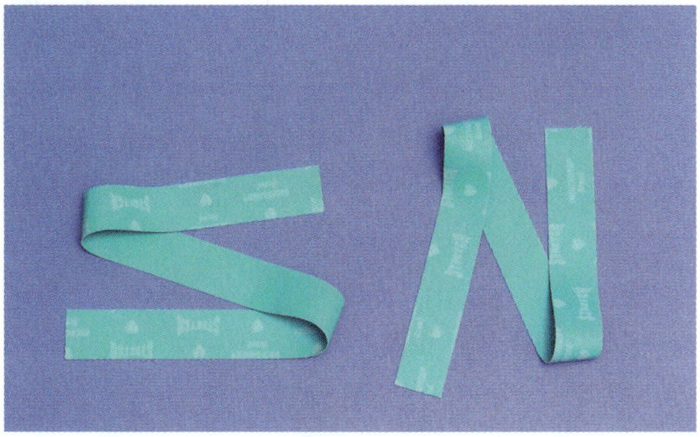

Figure 28-17 One kind of tourniquet.

blood pressure should be taken first, and then the cuff should be maintained slightly below the diastolic pressure (average: 40 mm Hg).

Specimen Collection Trays

The medical assistant may need a specimen collection tray to hold all the equipment necessary for proper specimen collection. The tray can be taken to the patient in the examination room so that whatever procedure is performed the phlebotomy can be conducted without searching for the proper equipment. The trays vary depending on the type of collections done. Because the tray is also used to transport blood specimens, the OSHA *Bloodborne Pathogen Standard* requires the tray be all red or prominently labeled with an approved biohazard symbol. The tray is usually preferred because it is more portable and can easily be taken to the patient. The trays come in a variety of sizes and shapes to better fit the preference and needs of the individual collecting the blood sample (Figure 28-18). Sometimes the equipment is stored in a special drawer for venipuncture equipment in each examination room or in a central laboratory area.

VENIPUNCTURE TECHNIQUE

Venipuncture is a detailed process that consists of many steps (Table 28-5).

Table 28-5 Steps in Venipuncture

1. Identify the patient.
2. Verify test ordered.
3. Verify diet/drug restrictions, e.g., fasting vs. nonfasting.
4. Wash hands. Put on gloves, as well as safety glasses and mask, if there is a potential for blood splatter
5. Assemble supplies and inspect equipment.
6. Reassure the patient and explain the procedure.
7. Position the patient.
8. Verify paperwork and tubes.
9. Perform venipuncture
10. Fill the tubes.
11. Bandage the patient's arm.
12. Dispose of sharps in the proper container.
13. Label the tubes.
14. Remove gloves and other PPE. Dispose of properly. Wash hands.
15. Chill specimen (only for certain tests).
16. Process paperwork. Complete laboratory requisition.
17. Send correctly labeled tubes to the office laboratory or prepare them to be sent to a reference laboratory.
18. Document procedure.

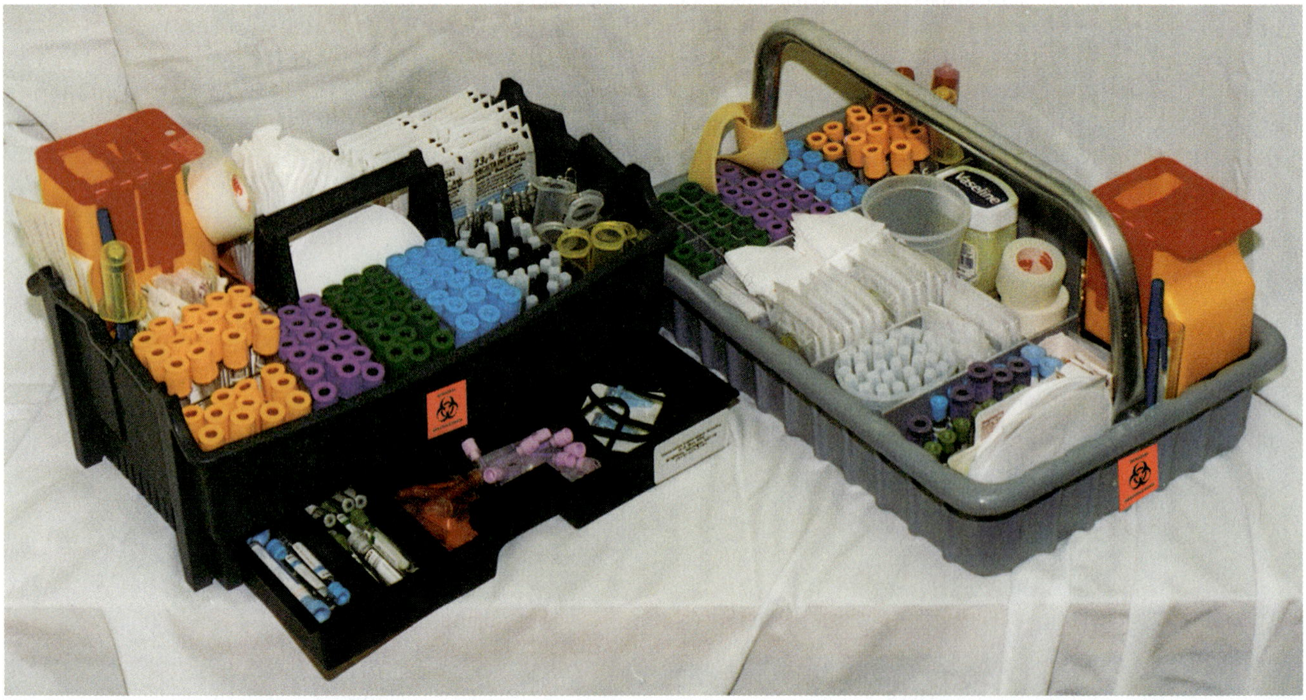

Figure 28-18 Two types of well-stocked phlebotomy trays.

Approaching the Patient

The first step to a successful venipuncture is to put the patient at ease. The medical assistant uses many skills when interacting with patients during phlebotomy. Three of the skills used are:

1. Social skills
2. Technical skills
3. Administrative skills

Social skills are used by the medical assistant to obtain cooperation from the patient. Some patients will be calm, whereas others may be extremely frightened. The nicest patient may be irritable and may even become physically or emotionally abusive when placed in the unfamiliar health care setting. The medical assistant uses social skills to put the patient at ease, allay the patient's fears, and persuade the patient to allow blood to be drawn.

After calming the patient and explaining the procedure, the medical assistant uses technical skills to perform the phlebotomy with a minimum of pain to the patient. As important as it is to obtain a good specimen, it is equally important to treat the patient with empathy. Using social and technical skills, the medical assistant can provide a positive experience for the patient. A patient who has had a positive experience will talk with friends and neighbors about that experience, which could result in new patients for the physician's office, the clinic, or the laboratory.

For the medical assistant, administrative skills involve drawing the correct patient's blood and correctly labeling the specimen. Incorrect labeling constitutes the greatest number of errors in phlebotomy. All patient specimens must be positively identified on the **primary container,** the container that holds the specimen, to avoid any errors in reporting of results, thereby affecting patient diagnosis or treatment.

Greeting the Patient

1. Reassure the patient that the procedure is going to be simple and there will only be a slight inconvenience.
2. Be friendly and outgoing and talk to the patient, explaining the procedure. Polite conversation with all patients gives them the feeling someone cares about them.
3. Do not tell the patient that the procedure will not be painful. Explain that the procedure can be slightly uncomfortable but you will take care to cause the least discomfort possible. If the patient seems overly concerned about pain, check frequently with him or her to see how he or she is doing. If the patient seems extremely apprehensive, ask if he or she would prefer to lie down during the procedure. This may prevent further problems if the patient faints.
4. Exhibit concern for patients, because this will result in more satisfied patients who will return in the future for care from the same provider.

Preparing Supplies and Greeting the Patient

Prepare all supplies and equipment before the venipuncture. Place all tubes within easy reach to avoid crossing over the patient and possibly moving the needle after it is in the patient. Remember that occasionally a tube will not fill completely; therefore, it is best to keep a few spare tubes or have the phlebotomy tray within reach.

Patient and Specimen Identification

Proper patient and specimen identification is essential to accurate patient testing. The results of specimen testing will be incorrect if the specimen is not accurately identified. When entering the room, do not say, "Mr. Jones, I'm here to draw your blood," assuming if the patient says "Yes" this is Mr. Jones. The patient may not have been paying attention and may answer yes even if it is not his name. Ask the patient to state his or her full name. If the patient is unable to communicate with you, or if you are in an inpatient environment such as a hospital or extended care facility, always check the patient's identification wristband or check with the caretaker. In the ambulatory setting, a good policy is to ask for picture identification from non-English-speaking patients.

Once the medical assistant has identified the patient and the blood is drawn, the specimen needs proper identification. The patient's first and last name, middle initial, date of birth, any assigned identification number, the date, the time, and the initials of the person collecting the specimen must be written on the tube immediately after drawing the patient's blood. Label the tubes clearly, using a permanent marker, before leaving the patient's presence. By doing so, if the tubes are taken to the physician's office laboratory or an outside reference laboratory, the specimens will be properly identified. Any paperwork or forms accompanying the specimens must be checked with the blood tubes to verify that names and numbers match.

EHR Many offices are using various types of computer systems for test ordering and result reporting (Figure 28-19). The computer label has several advantages in that it lists the

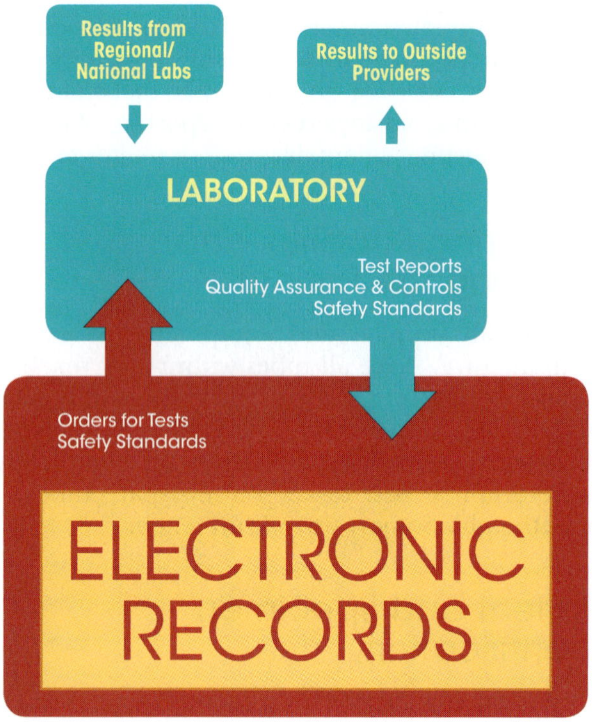

Figure 28-19 Laboratory arm of a total practice management system (TPMS). Test ordering and result reporting are capabilities of a TPMS.

specific tests that are ordered and the required specimen and specimen requirements. The label can also be adhesive so it can be attached directly to the tube. Smaller labels can also be printed at the same time for smaller aliquot specimens. An **aliquot** specimen is a portion of a specimen that has been taken for use or storage. The computer has multiple advantages in timing the printing of orders, sorting lists of orders for one patient at one time, and speeding entry of draw times and test results. The computer labels print off in a roll with one label following the other. Two attached labels (Figure 28-20A and B) require special attention. One label must be checked carefully with the other to ensure that each label is for the same person, date, and time. Labels may also contain bar codes to assist in electronic patient and specimen identification. With computerized systems, the medical assistant will verify by entering information into the computer when the blood is drawn.

Positioning the Patient

The position of the patient is critical for proper patient blood collection. The best position is the position that is comfortable for the patient and the health care professional. Proper positioning of the

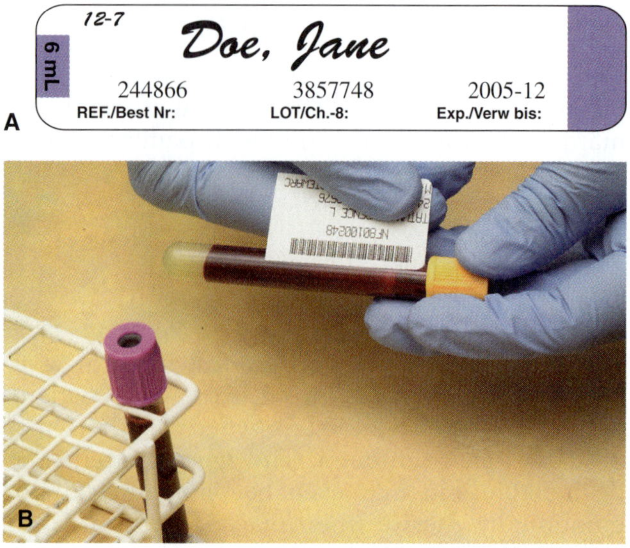

Figure 28-20 (A) Adhesive computer-generated labels for identifying specimen tubes from one patient. (B) The medical assistant applies a computer-generated label to the patient's specimen tube.

patient will make the patient feel more at ease and facilitate the performance of the venipuncture.

Selecting the Appropriate Venipuncture Site

The appropriate venipuncture site can vary depending on the patient. The usual site that is first checked is the antecubital region of the arm.

Positioning the Patient

Before a patient's blood is drawn, discuss with the patient any previous problems with blood being taken. Usually one of two situations must be addressed:

1. Patients who do not have a problem with having blood drawn.
   a. The patient must be in a seated or reclining position before any attempt is made to draw blood.
   b. Do not allow the patient to sit on a tall stool or stand while drawing blood. There is always the possibility that the patient will faint (syncope) and be injured.
   c. The sitting position requires a chair with adequate arm supports that are adjustable for the best venipuncture position.
2. Patients who will faint (syncope).
   a. Apprehensive patients and patients who indicate they have fainted in the past when having blood drawn should be instructed to lie down.
   b. The reclining position is the ideal position from which to draw a blood sample from the patient.
   c. A pillow may be required to help support the patient's arm by keeping it straight for easier venous access.

Patient Safety

- Question the patient about his or her past experiences with venipuncture.
- Position the patient properly to avoid injury.
- Do not attempt to draw blood from a combative patient.
- Restrain uncooperative children.
- Note allergies or sensitivities to latex, alcohol, and tape adhesives.

The primary vein used in the antecubital region of the arm is the median cubital vein. This is usually the prominent vein in the middle of the bend of the arm (see Figure 28-4). The basilic or cephalic vein can be used as an alternative. These veins may not be accessible or may not be prominent enough to obtain a blood sample. The next step is to go to the back of the hand to determine other possibilities. The veins in the back of the hand have the tendency to "roll" more than the arm veins because they are not supported by as much tissue and are closer to the surface. To avoid this, the vein will have to be held in place securely while a smaller gauge needle or a butterfly is used. The hand veins are ideal for a 3- to 5-cc syringe with a 22 gauge needle. Careful, slow pulling on the syringe will obtain the blood sample without collapsing the vein or hemolyzing the blood. The veins at the back of the wrist are also an alternative, but they are generally much more painful than the other sites. The foot and ankle veins may also be used if the patient's provider gives permission to use them and the medical assistant is properly trained to perform venipuncture on the lower extremities. The veins in the foot or ankle will also have the tendency to "roll." The medical assistant will in all likelihood never draw from the foot or ankle, but this is an area that will give an acceptable blood sample when all other attempts have failed.

The order for checking for the best available site is: (1) antecubital region of the arm, (2) back of hand, (3) back of wrist, and (4) ankle or foot. The next alternative is to have a more experienced medical assistant check. If venous access is not possible, draw the sample by capillary puncture if the test can be performed on a capillary specimen. Check the laboratory manual for criteria.

Applying the Tourniquet

A tourniquet must be used to assist the medical assistant in feeling a vein. The tourniquet is applied 3 to 4 inches above the intended puncture site. It is applied tightly enough to slow the flow of blood in the veins but not so tightly as to prevent the flow of blood in the arteries (Figures 28-21A–D). This is similar to damming a small stream. When a stream is dammed, the water forms a pond in front of the dam. With the tourniquet applied, the veins fill with blood, pooling in the veins below the tourniquet. This pooling of blood makes the veins more prominent. The veins can then be **palpated** (examined with the fingertips) to determine their direction, depth, and size. The tourniquet should be on the arm no longer than one minute. A stream will become stagnant when it no longer flows. A tourniquet that is left on too long will cause **hemoconcentration** of the blood, an increased concentration of constituents in the blood sample that may lead to inaccurate test results. If the patient has sensitive skin or a skin problem, the tourniquet should be applied over the patient's upper arm clothing or a piece of gauze pad. This will minimize the discomfort felt by the patient.

The tourniquet often causes greater discomfort for patients than the venipuncture itself. The tourniquet should ideally be removed as soon as blood flow is established. This is not practical for the novice medical assistant. The act of removing the tourniquet may move the needle or vein just enough so that no more blood can be obtained and a second venipuncture must be performed. It is recommended to wait until just before the needle is removed from the patient to remove the tourniquet. If the tourniquet is not removed before the needle is removed, the patient will bleed heavily. Blood will be forced out of the needle hole and into the surrounding tissue, resulting in a **hematoma** (an accumulation of blood around the venipuncture site).

Performing a Safe Venipuncture

The first step in actual collection of a venous blood specimen is to find the site that will give the best blood return. The vein must be palpated with the tip of the index finger. Feel for and trace the path

Critical Thinking

You are having a difficult time getting the needle to cooperate when putting together a butterfly system and you accidentally contaminate it. The patient has the tourniquet already on her arm. What do you do? Why? Is there something else you could have done?

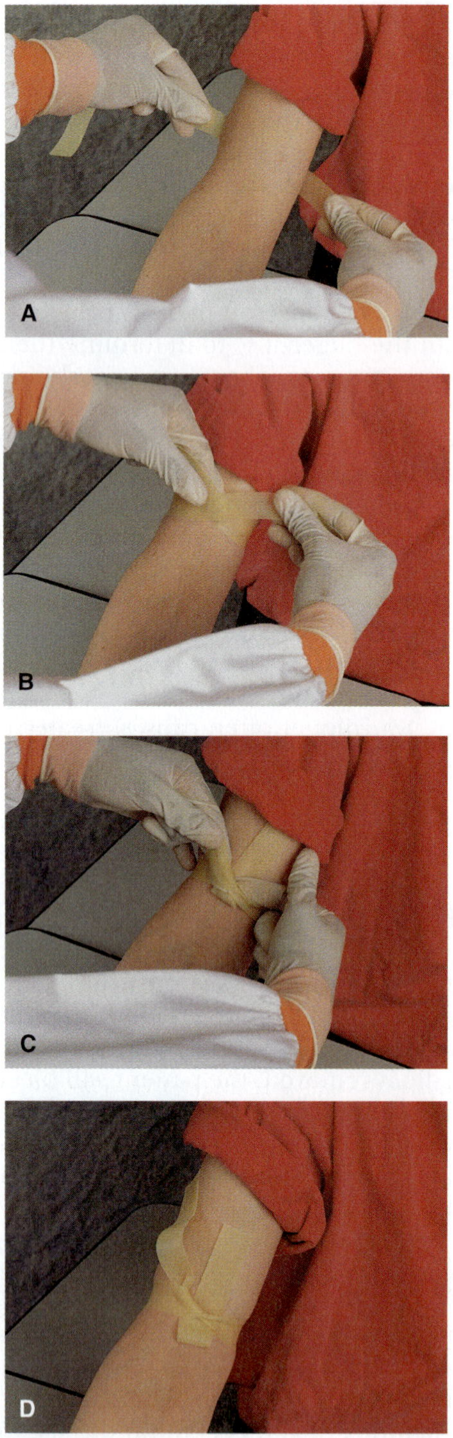

Figure 28-21 Applying a tourniquet. (A) Wrap the tourniquet around the arm 3 to 4 inches above the venipuncture site. Keeping the tourniquet flat to the skin will help minimize the discomfort felt by the patient. (B) Stretch the tourniquet tight and cross the ends. (C) While holding the ends tight, tuck one portion of the tourniquet under the other. (D) The tourniquet should not be loose and the ends should be secure. The ends of the tourniquet should be pointed upward and not hanging into the intended venipuncture site.

of the vein several times. Avoid using the thumb because it has a pulse and is not as sensitive as the rest of the fingers. The vein will feel soft and bouncy to the touch. The roundness of the vein and the direction it follows may be determined. All veins are not straight up and down the arm. If no veins become prominent, retie the tourniquet tighter but not so tightly as to stop the flow of arterial blood into the arm. If the tourniquet is tied tightly enough to stop arterial blood flow, the patient will no longer have a pulse in the wrist. If this occurs, immediately remove the tourniquet because this indicates that blood has ceased flowing below the tourniquet.

If the "vein" that is felt has a pulsing action to it, it is an artery, not a vein, and the vessel should not be punctured (see safety box). Tendons can be deceptive and give the appearance of veins. They do not have the soft, bouncy feel and will be hard to the touch. Puncturing a tendon will give no blood return and will be painful to the patient. Nerves also run the length of the arm. The nerves cannot be seen or felt, but by avoiding deep, probing venipunctures, the chance of puncturing a nerve will be diminished. If the patient complains that the venipuncture is extremely painful, it is best to stop and try another site.

Veins of **edematous** arms, which are swollen because of fluid in the tissue, will not be prominent and the tourniquet will not be effective because of the swelling. Using the tourniquet in this instance may cause tissue damage. Areas of scarring should also be avoided because of possible injury or excessive pain to the patient. Specimens collected from an area of a hematoma may cause erroneous test results. If another vein site is not available, the specimen is collected distal from the hematoma. Because of the potential for harm to the patient due to lymphostasis (the stoppage of the flow of lymph), the arm on the side of a mastectomy or any

Safety Box

If you accidentally puncture an artery, you will see that the blood is a brighter color. This is due to the oxygenation of arterial blood versus venous blood. Go ahead and calmly fill the tubes. Often the laboratory can run the blood tests on arterial blood just as with venous blood. After the needle is removed, pressure needs to be held for a full 3 minutes (longer if the patient is taking a blood thinner such as Coumadin). As with any phlebotomy procedure, make sure the bleeding has stopped before the patient leaves your care. While the patient is still there, check with the lab. If the test requires venous blood, you will need to repeat the procedure.

Correct Hand Position to Hold a Syringe

1. The needle is attached to the syringe.
2. Hold the syringe and needle system in your dominant hand, cradling it on your four fingers. A right-handed person would hold the syringe in the right hand, leaving the left hand to pull on the plunger. A left-handed person would do the opposite.
3. Place the thumb on top of the syringe (Figure 28-22).
4. With the syringe held in this position, turn it slightly so the bevel of the needle is facing up.
5. Hold the hand in such a position that by tilting the point of the needle down slightly the needle will enter the skin at a 15-degree angle and about 0.5 cm below the point where the vein was felt.

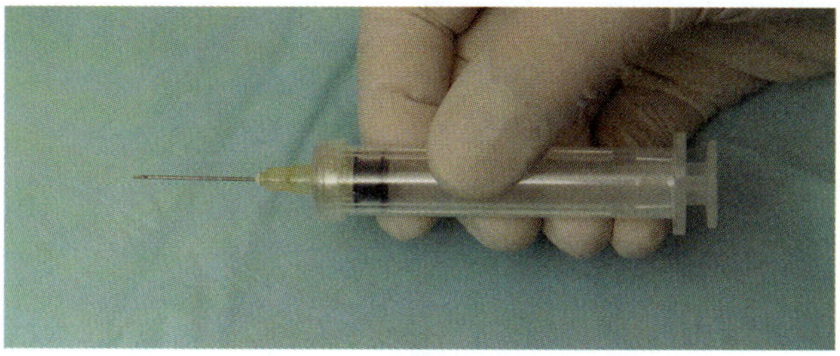

Figure 28-22 Proper hand position to hold a syringe for blood collection.

lymphatic compromise should be avoided. If the patient has had a double mastectomy, a physician should be consulted before drawing the blood.

SPECIMEN COLLECTION

The patient has been identified, paperwork and tubes have been verified, equipment has been assembled, and the patient is in a comfortable position. Hand washing is the most critical step to preventing the spread of infection. Before touching the patient, medical assistants should wash their hands. It is good practice to wash your hands in view of the patient to give the patient confidence in your technique. The next step is to tie the tourniquet. Have the patient close the hand, and then select a vein. If possible, place the patient's arm in a downward position. After locating an acceptable vein, mentally map the location. Set mental sites on the vein by visualizing the puncture site as the target for an accurate puncture. Cleanse the site with a gauze pad wet with 70% isopropyl alcohol solution. A commercially prepared alcohol pad or one with 0.5% chlorhexidine in alcohol may also be used. Wipe the skin firmly with an alcohol pad. This removes any oil, sweat, perfume, lotions, and skin contaminations. This process is often referred to as "defatting" the skin. Allow the area to air dry, or you may dry it with a clean cotton ball or gauze pad. Puncturing the skin through wet alcohol can cause hemolysis of the specimen and give the patient a stinging sensation. Residual alcohol can also contaminate the specimen.

Some authorities suggest putting on gloves first and then palpating for the vein. This technique is required for the patient who is isolated because of a communicable disease and is good practice for all patients. Standard Precautions require that personal protective equipment be worn when there is a chance of coming in contact with blood and body fluid. If the patient has veins that are difficult to palpate, the gloves can be put on after the site has been palpated and before the cleansing. To avoid forgetting where the collection site is, palpate the vein 1 to 2 inches above and below the intended puncture site. It helps the medical assistant feel that the vein is located in a straight line and these points can be used to "reset" the mental crosshairs without contaminating the venipuncture site. Safety glasses and a mask must be worn if there is a potential for blood spatter.

The Syringe Technique

The syringe technique is used less often than the vacuum tube method. The syringe is ideal for collecting small volumes of blood from fragile, thin, or "rolling" veins or veins on the back of the hand or from the foot. Pulling on the plunger of the syringe creates suction; the larger the syringe, the greater the suction that can be obtained. Too great a suction might cause the vein to collapse. Vein collapse can be avoided by pulling the plunger slowly and by resting between pulls to allow the vein to refill. Because pediatric and geriatric patients often have thin and fragile veins, the syringe is the preferred method of venipuncture for them. The use of a syringe larger than 15 mL is not recommended. If more than 12 mL is needed, the butterfly collection method should be considered. Syringe draws are also ideal in special procedures when the blood must be transferred to a different container. Procedure 28-2 gives detailed instructions for venipuncture with syringe.

When a syringe is used, the blood obtained must be placed in appropriate containers. The order of filling the tubes is important.

The use of a needle to transfer blood from a syringe to a vacuum tube or culture bottle is unsafe

Correct Needle Position

The patient will experience the least amount of pain if the bevel of the needle is facing upward when the needle is inserted into the vein. The bevel of the needle is upward when the opening in the needle is visible when you look straight down on the needle as it is inserted. This position also helps prevent the suction from causing the inside wall of the vein to adhere to the needle bevel, thus occluding the needle.

The needle should be inserted at a 15-degree angle to the surface of the skin (Figure 28-23).

The skin should be held taut until the needle has been inserted. This technique allows the point of the needle to enter the skin with little drag or bunching of the skin, thereby reducing the discomfort of the puncture.

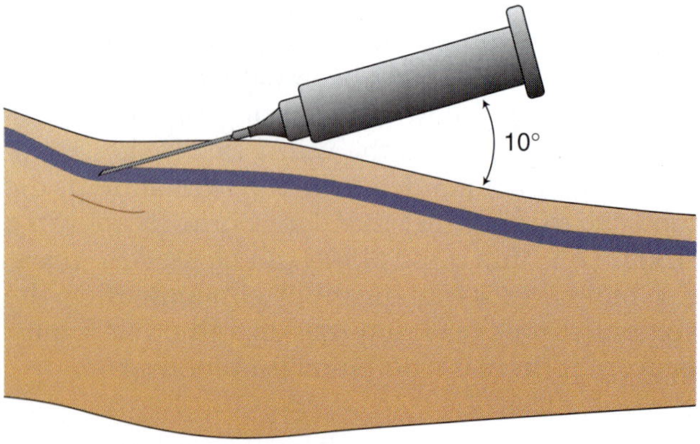

Figure 28-23 Proper angle of needle insertion for venipuncture.

and prohibited by OSHA. The use of a safety system such as the BD Vacutainer Blood Transfer Device is recommended (Figure 28-24). After drawing the blood into the syringe, activate the needle's safety mechanism, then remove the needle and dispose of it. Connect the needleless syringe to the transfer device. Insert a vacuum tube to the device and allow the blood to transfer from the syringe to the tube using the tube's vacuum. Never push on the syringe plunger or force the blood into the tube. This could cause the tube's stopper to pop off. When the appropriate tubes have been filled, dispose of the entire syringe and transfer assembly as one unit according to your clinic policies.

When transferring blood from a syringe to a vacuum tube, keep these safety features in mind:

- Never transfer to a vacuum tube using a needle. When transferring from a syringe to a vacuum tube, use a needleless transfer device.
- Never push the blood into the vacuum tube. It will fill on its own.
- Always wear gloves, goggles, and face guard when performing this procedure.

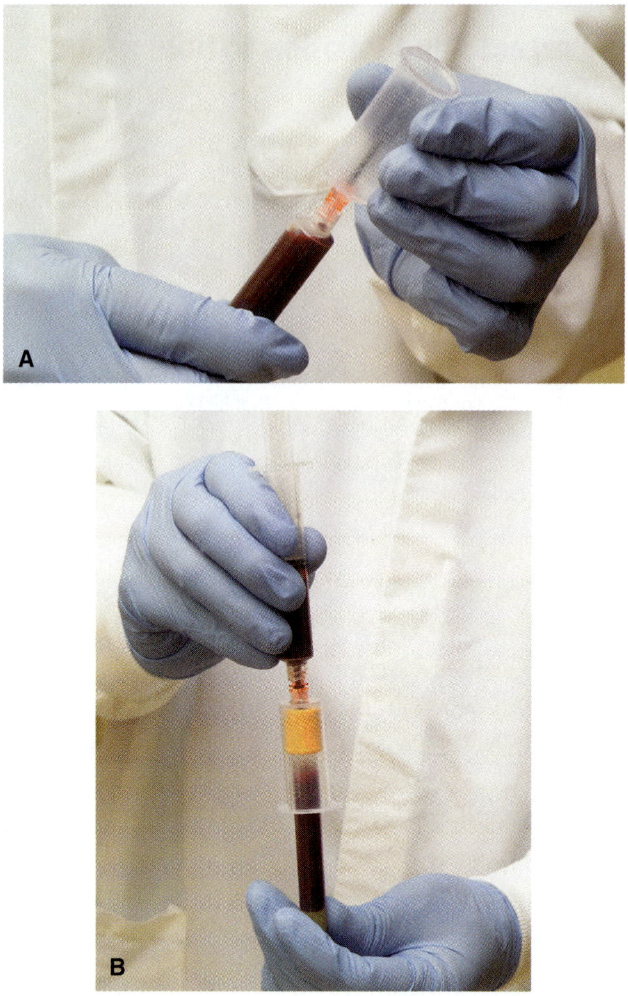

Figure 28-24 (A) The medical assistant attaches the BD Vacutainer Blood Transfer Device. (B) The device is used to safely transfer blood from a syringe to a vacuum tube.

Immediately after filling, mix any tubes containing additives (Figure 28-25).

Vacuum Tube Specimen Collection

The vacuum tube system is an improvement over the syringe method yet maintains many similarities. When the syringe method is used, a vacuum is created as the medical assistant pulls on the syringe plunger. The vacuum tube method has the vacuum already in the tube. Another advantage of the vacuum tube system is that with multiple blood

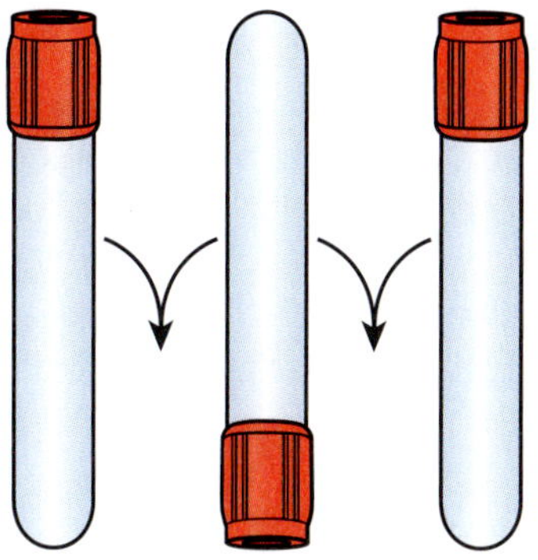

BD Vacutainer™ Tube Type	Closure Color	Number of Inversions
EDTA	Lavender	8–10
Sodium citrate	Light Blue	3–4
SST with gel	Tiger (Red Gray) or Gold	5
Serum	Red	5
Sodium fluoride	Gray	8–10
Heparin	Green	8–10

Figure 28-25 Vacuum tubes should be inverted several times (not shaken) to mix the additives well.

samples, syringes do not need to be changed; only the tubes need to be changed.

The similarity between the vacuum tube system and the syringe system is that the holder and needle are held in the same manner (Figure 28-26). The syringe is held in a manner that allows the medical assistant access to pull on the plunger. Access must be left in the vacuum tube system for one tube to be pulled out and another inserted. The hand that pulled on the plunger of the syringe is the hand that changes tubes with the vacuum tube system.

The procedure for venipuncture with the vacuum tube system follows the same steps as the syringe method with only slight variations.

Butterfly Needle Collection System

The butterfly collection system combines the benefits of the syringe system and the vacuum tube system. The butterfly collection system has on one end a 21- or 23-gauge needle with attached plastic wings. Six or twelve inches of tubing leads from the needle. On the other end of this tubing is a hub that can attach to a syringe. A needle covered by a rubber sleeve can also be attached to the tubing. The covered needle screws into an evacuated tube holder (Figure 28-27).

The butterfly system is used for small veins that are difficult to puncture with the vacuum tube system and standard vacuum tube system needle. The system also facilitates drawing from veins that have a tendency to collapse. The winged needle of the butterfly needle will slide into a small surface vein in the back of the hand, wrist, or foot. Instead of entering the vein at the usual 15-degree angle, the winged needle is inserted at a 5- to 10-degree angle, and then threaded into the vein. This procedure anchors the needle in the center of a small vein that is inaccessible by other methods. If the patient moves, the tubing gives flexibility so the needle will stay anchored

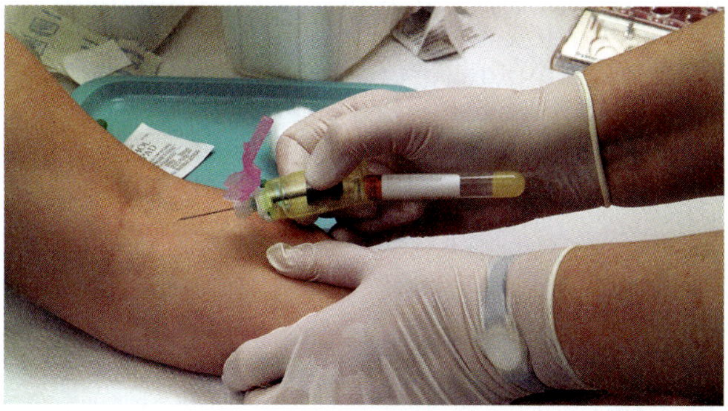

Figure 28-26 Proper hand position to hold a vacuum tube system.

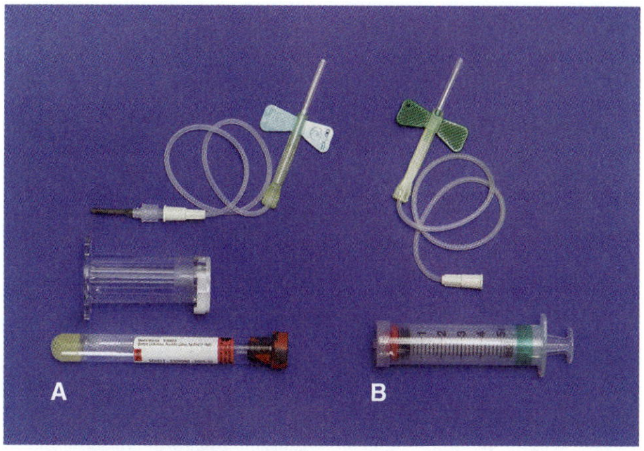

Figure 28-27 Butterfly needle sets with connections for either a (A) vacuum tube or (B) a Luer-Lok tipped syringe.

and not pull out of the vein. The butterfly collection set works well on children who have small veins and the tendency to move while blood is being collected.

The system also gives the adaptability of initiating a draw with a syringe and then finishing it with the evacuated tube system. A syringe can be filled for procedures that require a syringe sample. It can then be removed, and the vacuum tube system can be attached for multiple tube collection. Remember to draw into or transfer into the vacuum tubes in the proper order (see Table 28-4). Although the butterfly collection system has many benefits, it is not used for all collections. It is more expensive than the needle system. The additional expense is unnecessary for the majority of venipunctures.

Blood Cultures

Occasionally a patient will need to have blood collected for culture. The culture will determine if the patient has pathogens in the blood. Normally blood is sterile. When drawing blood for cultures, use a surgical solution (often Betadine) rather than alcohol and sterile rather than clean procedure. This means using sterile gloves; do not wipe away the surgical solution, touch the puncture site, or in any way compromise the sterile process. The blood is collected into special transport bottles, which are like vacuum tubes but shaped differently (Figure 28-28). The blood culture bottle contains transport media to preserve any microorganisms present while they are transported to the laboratory for culture. Because it is unknown whether the pathogen is anaerobic (living without oxygen) or aerobic (living with oxygen), blood is collected to test for both. The aerobic bottle is filled first, then the anaerobic bottle is filled.

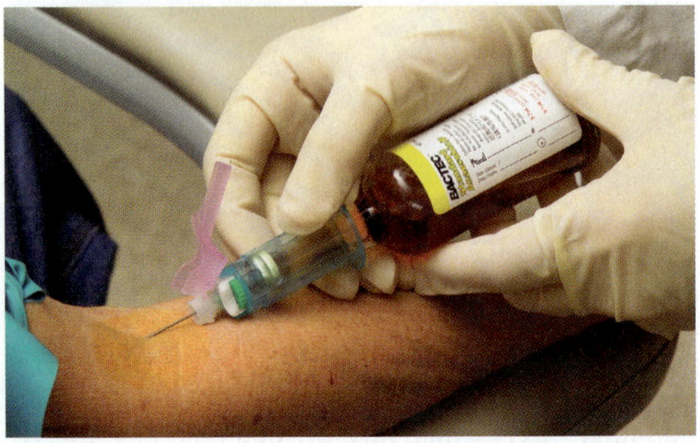

Figure 28-28 Blood being drawn for cultures.

Critical Thinking

You are preparing to perform a venipuncture on a geriatric patient who has fragile veins. Which system would you use: a syringe or a vacuum tube system? What makes one technique more successful in this case?

Patient Reactions

Patients can have a variety of reactions to having their blood drawn. The medical assistant must anticipate these reactions and respond appropriately as quickly as possible. The most common patient reaction is pain. The patient will indicate that the venipuncture is painful. Slightly reposition the needle, and then loosen the tourniquet. Loosening the tourniquet often helps because the tourniquet may be pinching the arm and causing discomfort rather than the needle. Avoid deep, probing venipunctures because they may go deeply into the arm and get too close to the nerves. If the pain persists, discontinue the venipuncture.

Other possible patient reactions and the medical assistant's appropriate responses are listed in Table 28-6.

The Unsuccessful Venipuncture

Methods of vein stimulation are shown in Table 28-7. When a blood sample cannot be obtained, it may be necessary to change the position of the needle. Rotate the needle half a turn. The bevel of the needle may be against the wall of the vein. If the needle has not penetrated the vein far enough, advance it further into the vein. Advance it only slightly; a small change may mean the difference between a failed and a successful venipuncture. If the needle has penetrated too far into the vein, pull back a little. Always withdraw the needle slowly when the venipuncture has been unsuccessful. The blood often may start coming just as it seems the needle is ready to come out of the skin. The tube used may not have sufficient vacuum. Try another tube before withdrawing the needle.

Probing the site is not recommended. Probing is painful to the patient and may cause a hematoma. Never attempt a venipuncture more than two times. If a blood sample cannot be obtained after two attempts, have another person attempt the draw. Notify the patient's provider if two medical assistants have been unsuccessful.

Table 28-6 Patient Reactions to Blood Draws

Patient Reaction	Medical Assistant Response
Syncope (fainting)	Immediately remove the tourniquet, then the needle, and stop the patient from falling. Lower the patient's head and arms. Wipe the patient's forehead and back of the neck with a cold compress if necessary. If the patient does not respond, notify the provider, move the patient to the floor, and place a pillow under the patient's legs
Nausea	If a patient becomes nauseated, apply cold compresses to the patient's forehead. Give the patient an emesis basin, and have facial tissues ready if the nausea does not diminish. Deep, slow breathing through the mouth may help
Insulin shock or hypoglycemia	The first signs of insulin shock are a cold sweat and pallor similar to the signs of syncope. The patient becomes weak and shaky, sudden mental confusion may follow, and it appears as though the patient's personality changes instantly. Call the provider if the patient loses consciousness. This can happen especially to patients having a fasting blood sugar test
Convulsions	The patient loses consciousness and exhibits violent or mild convulsive motions. Do not try to restrain the patient. Move objects or furniture out of the way to prevent the patient from striking objects and being hurt. Help the patient to the floor and into a reclining position. The patient usually recovers within a few minutes. Notify the provider about the patient's reaction. The provider will determine when to release the patient

Criteria for Rejection of a Specimen

The primary goal of the medical assistant is to provide an acceptable specimen for laboratory testing as required by the provider. Certain general criteria must be met for a specimen to be acceptable. If the criteria are not met, the specimen is rejected and another venipuncture of the patient must be performed.

Table 28-8 lists quality-assurance controls for specimen collection and processing. The list is not all inclusive. The type of specimen that is acceptable and the volume required are determined by the procedure ordered. The quality-control checks done by the laboratory may indicate the results are valid. If the results do not agree with what the provider believes is the patient's diagnosis, the blood specimen may need to be redrawn to confirm the results. This is accomplished by either retesting the specimen or collecting another sample. This will either reconfirm that blood was drawn from the correct patient or that the patient's test results changed significantly.

Table 28-7 Methods of Vein Stimulation

1. Position the patient's arm lower than his or her heart.
2. Reapply the tourniquet; it may not be tight enough.
3. Massage the arm from the wrist to the elbow to encourage venous return.
4. Tap sharply at the venipuncture site with your fingertips. This can cause the veins to dilate.
5. Use a blood pressure cuff in place of the tourniquet. Pump it to about 40–60 mm Hg.
6. Warm the venipuncture site with a warming device or a warm washcloth (not hotter than 100°F.)
7. Have the patient make a fist. Do not have the patient pump his or her fist; that can cause a false high level of potassium in the specimen.

Factors Affecting Laboratory Values

Numerous variables can affect laboratory test results. The specimens are tested by analytic instruments that give accurate and precise results. These results will accurately reflect what is wrong with the patient only if the specimen is collected correctly. The medical assistant is responsible for collecting and caring for the specimen properly. When in doubt of how to care for a specimen, refer to the manual supplied by the laboratory or contact the laboratory for specific instructions. It is always better to ask the question and perform the proper procedure than not to ask and have to repeat the venipuncture. In addition, if you ever do need to repeat a venipuncture because of improper collection or handling of the specimen,

Table 28-8 Quality Assurance for Specimen Collection and Processing

1. Each specimen must have its own label attached to the specimen's primary container.
2. Each specimen must have a laboratory requisition label.
3. Labels must have the patient's complete name and identification number, date of birth, date and time, and your signature.
4. Specimens in syringes with needles still attached are unacceptable.
5. All specimens must be in the appropriate anticoagulant.
6. Blood collection tubes with anticoagulant must be at least 75% full. All blood collection tubes for coagulation testing must be at least 90% full.
7. Uncoagulated blood specimens must be free of clots.
8. Certain tests require specimens to be free of hemolysis and lipemia, a milky appearance due to lipids.
9. The specimen may need to be recollected if the results do not agree with what the provider believes is the diagnosis of the patient.
10. Do not combine partially filled tubes.
11. Do not mix tubes of different additives.
12 As soon as possible, invert tubes 8 to 10 times to prevent microclots from forming (see Figure 28-25).
13. Mix tubes gently to prevent hemolysis of specimen.

the patient should not be billed for the second collection. Patient physiologic factors may also contribute to inaccurate results. Other factors that can alter results are listed in Table 28-9.

Occasionally, a specimen requires protection from light, incubation, refrigeration, or chilling immediately after collection. Any delay in these requirements will alter the results. The laboratory manual will direct you as to which specimens need to be chilled. See Table 28-10 for examples of special handling requirements.

The medical assistant is not the only person who can affect test results. The patient can knowingly or unknowingly alter the results by certain actions. For example, a patient has consumed a cup of coffee but claims not to have had anything to eat or drink. The patient is often under the misconception that black coffee without sugar will not be a problem. Caffeine and smoking affect the metabolism and can affect the test results.

Table 28-9 Factors Affecting Laboratory Results

Factor	Effect
Blood alcohol	When drawing a specimen for blood alcohol testing, a nonalcohol-based antiseptic should be used to clean the venipuncture site. The cleansing alcohol may falsely elevate the test result.
Diurnal rhythm	Some specimens must be drawn at timed intervals because of medication or diurnal (daily) rhythm. The exact time of collection must be noted on the specimen.
Exercise	Strenuous short-term exercise can make the heart work harder and increase the heart enzymes. Long-term exercise such as that performed by highly trained runners can cause erroneous results due to runner's anemia.
Fasting	Patient not in fasting state when fasting is required. Results of tests will not be accurate.
Hemolysis	Destruction of red blood cell membrane and release of intercellular contents into serum/plasma can be caused by not allowing alcohol to air-dry at venipuncture site, using a needle that is too small (less than 22 gauge), forcing the blood into a vacutainer tube from a syringe, or shaking the vacutainer tube instead of mixing by gentle inversion when mixing tubes with additives.
Heparin	Incorrect heparin used that interferes with tests being run on patient.
Stress	In children, violent crying before a specimen is collected can increase the white blood cell count.
Tourniquet on too long	Hemoconcentration, change in chemical concentration.
Volume	Not enough blood will cause a dilution factor, which can change the size of the cells and therefore produce a variation in test results.

Table 28-10 Common Laboratory Tests that Require Special Handling

Laboratory Test	Special Handling
A, vitamin	Protect from light by wrapping tube in foil
Acid phosphatase	Deliver to laboratory within 1 hour. Separate, freeze serum after clotting
Adrenocorticotropic hormone (ACTH)	Place in ice slurry
Alcohol, blood	Do NOT use alcohol pad to clean site
Ammonia	Place in ice slurry
B6, vitamin	Protect from light by wrapping tube in foil
B12, vitamin	Protect from light by wrapping tube in foil
Beta-carotene	Protect from light by wrapping tube in foil
Bilirubin, total or direct	Protect from light by wrapping tube in foil
Catecholamines	Place in ice slurry
Clot retraction	Incubate in 37°C until clotted
Cold agglutinins	Warm tube, incubate in 37°C
Complement C4	Separate and freeze serum after clotting
Complement, total (CH50)	Let clot in refrigerator, separate immediately and freeze immediately
Complement, total (CH100)	Let clot in refrigerator, separate immediately and freeze immediately
Cryofibrinogen	Warm tube, incubate in 37°C
Gastrin	Place in ice slurry
Gentamicin	Label peak or trough and time of last medication
Glucose tolerance	Label tubes with time intervals of draw specimens
Human leukocyte antigen (HLA-B27)	Do NOT refrigerate or freeze, record date and time collected
Lactic acid	Place in ice slurry
Parathyroid hormone (PTH)	Place in ice slurry
Partial thromboplastin time (PTT)	Refrigerate, test within 4 hours of drawing specimen
pH / blood gas	Place in ice slurry
Porphyrins	Protect from light by wrapping tube in foil
Prostate-specific antigen	Deliver to laboratory within 1 hour, separate, freeze serum after clotting
Prostatic acid phosphatase	Deliver to laboratory within 1 hour, separate, freeze serum after clotting
Prothrombin time (PT)	Refrigerate
Pyruvate	Place in ice slurry
Red cell folate	Protect from light by wrapping tube in foil
Renin	Place in ice slurry
Thioridazine (Mellaril)	Protect from light by wrapping tube in foil
Tobramycin	Label peak or trough and time of last medication

Source: Courtesy of Sheri R. Greimes, CMA (AAMA), PBT (ASCP).

CAPILLARY PUNCTURE

Venipuncture is the most frequently performed phlebotomy procedure, but it is not the procedure of choice in all circumstances. An alternative to venipuncture is capillary puncture, also known as dermal puncture or skin puncture.

Capillary puncture is a method of obtaining one to several drops of blood for a variety of tests. With proper instruments, tests such as a complete blood count, RBC count, white blood cell (WBC) count, hemoglobin, and hematocrit can be run. One drop of blood can be used to test glucose blood levels, a few drops of blood can fill capillary tubes, and several drops can complete a phenylketonuria (PKU) test card. Tests that cannot be run on capillary blood specimens are sedimentation rates, blood cultures, coagulation studies, and any other tests requiring large amounts of serum or plasma.

Capillary puncture is the method of choice with two types of patients: when patient blood volume is a concern, such as with infants, and when vein access is difficult, such as with burned or scarred patients. Capillary puncture should not be used when a patient is edematous, dehydrated, or has poor peripheral circulation.

Composition of Capillary Blood

Blood obtained via capillary puncture is a mixture of blood from arterioles, venules, capillaries, and interstitial fluid. In most instances, a capillary puncture specimen most resembles arterial blood. There may be significant differences between specimens obtained by capillary puncture and those collected by venipuncture. For example, the glucose level may be increased in capillary blood, whereas the potassium, calcium, and total protein levels may be decreased. It is therefore important to always note on the specimen when capillary blood has been obtained.

Capillary Puncture Sites

The usual site for capillary puncture in adults and children is the fingertip (Figure 28-29). In adults, the ring finger is often selected because it usually is not callused. In infants, the lateral or medial plantar surface of the heel pad is usually used, and the procedure is often called a heelstick. The heelstick is most often performed when testing for PKU, which is covered in detail in Chapter 32.

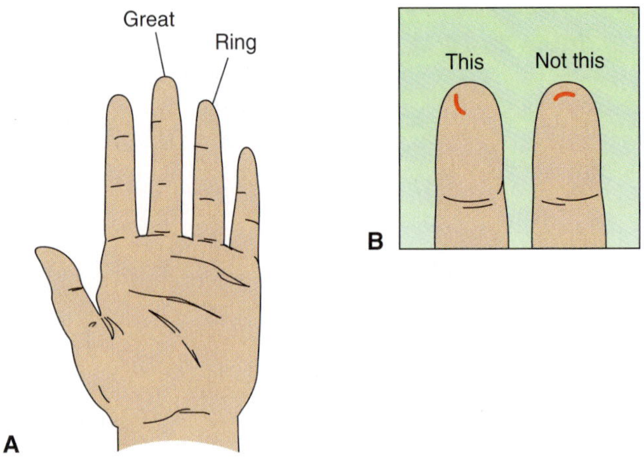

Figure 28-29 (A) Capillary blood collection sites. (B) Correct direction of capillary puncture.

Preparing the Capillary Puncture Site

The area selected for a capillary puncture must be carefully prepared. The puncture site will be warm if blood circulation is adequate. Coolness of the skin indicates decreased circulation. To increase circulation, the site can be gently massaged, or a warm, moist towel, face cloth, or warm pack (at a temperature not higher than 100°F) can be placed on the site for 3 to 5 minutes.

Alcohol-soaked gauze or cotton should be used to cleanse and disinfect the puncture site. The site should then be allowed to air-dry, or dry with a gauze pad. A cotton ball is not recommended because the tiny cotton fibers can stay on the puncture site, assisting in clotting, which is not desirable at this point. When the puncture is complete, a cotton ball can be used as a compress. Residual alcohol at the puncture site results in hemolysis of the specimen, which may affect test results, as well as cause a burning sensation to the patient. Betadine® (povidone-iodine) should not be used to clean the puncture site. Blood contaminated with iodine may falsely increase certain blood chemistries.

Performing the Puncture

Safety glasses, a mask, and gloves should be worn by the medical assistant while performing capillary puncture. Some patients bleed quite readily from the puncture, so be sure to have extra gauze on hand. The patient's hand and finger should be held so the puncture site is readily accessible. The puncture is made at the tip of the fleshy pad and slightly to the side (see Figure 28-29). The skin near the chosen site should be pulled taut. If the tips of the fingers are heavily callused or thickened, a lancet with a longer point may be used. Capillary punctures are performed using semiautomated devices such as the disposable Microtainer® Brand Safety Flow Lancet®.

The BD Microtainer® Genie Lancet is shown in Figure 28-30. After cleansing the puncture site, twist off the indicator as directed on the tab. Press the safety lancet firmly against the puncture site. Hold the lancet between your fingers and press the white button with your thumb. The lancet should not bounce off the skin. The puncture should be performed in one quick, steady movement. Once you have depressed the plunger, the button will lock into the housing and the needle will be permanently encapsulated. Practice working the lancets until you are comfortable with the action.

Collecting the Blood Sample

The first drop of blood is wiped away with dry, sterile gauze because it contains tissue fluid, which dilutes the blood drop and can also activate clotting. The second and following drops of blood are used for test samples. Depending on the tests to be performed, the blood may be collected in capillary tubes or other capillary collecting devices. Capillary tubes are small-diameter glass or plastic tubes that are open at both ends. Capillary tubes are extremely fragile and care should be taken to prevent breakage. The tubes have a colored line around one end. A red or black line indicates that the tube contains heparin, an anticoagulant, and will yield a nonclotted specimen. A blue line indicates that the tube contains no anticoagulant and will yield a clotted specimen. When taking the blood sample directly from the puncture site, a capillary tube that contains anticoagulant would be used; when taking blood from a vacuum tube that already has anticoagulant in it, the plain capillary tube would be used. Capillary tubes are used for many tests, depending on the equipment available. Chapter 29 explains how to use capillary tubes to check hematocrit levels. When capillary tubes are used for hematocrit tests, they are called microhematocrit tubes.

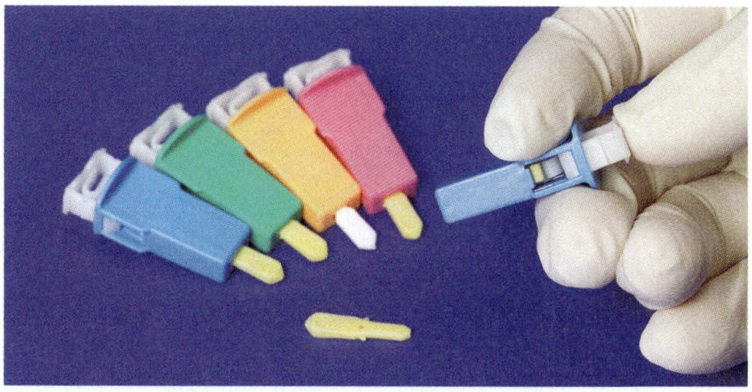

Figure 28-30 Microtainer brand lancets are available in different types for various purposes. They are color coded and have specific information on their packaging.

It may be necessary to massage the finger to increase the blood flow. It is best to massage the whole hand, taking care not to apply direct pressure near the puncture site. Squeezing the fingertip should be avoided; this forces tissue fluid into the blood sample and dilutes it or may cause hemolysis. Do not use a scooping technique when collecting blood from the puncture site. Scooping can break the RBC membranes, leading to hemolysis.

Figure 28-31 shows the basic steps to follow when filling a capillary tube. Allow well-rounded drops of blood to form at the puncture site. Holding the capillary tube at a horizontal position, gently touch the tip of tube to the top of the blood drop. The blood will enter the tube through "capillary action" caused by surface tension. Take care to not tilt the tube downward, which can cause air to enter the tube, nor upward, which can cause blood to come out of the tube. Continue to fill the tube until it is two-thirds to three-quarters full. When the tube is sufficiently filled, remove it from the drop and, at the same time, place your gloved finger over the opposite end of the tube. This will prevent the blood from flowing out of the tube. Keep your gloved finger over the end of the tube and, using your other hand, wipe off any residue blood from the outside of the tube with a gauze pad. Gently place the end of the tube into the sealing clay. Sealing clay trays are specially made for this purpose. They have numbered sections to help identify the samples. Some capillary tubes have plastic caps. Carefully follow the manufacturer's instructions for the type of tube you are using.

During the filling of the tubes, if the flow of blood begins to slow, rewipe the puncture site firmly with dry gauze (not a cotton ball). This action will dislodge the platelet plug and allow the blood to flow freely. Be sure the patient is relaxed. Have the patient take a deep breath. After filling the required number of tubes, apply a cotton ball compress to the puncture site. The patient can usually help hold the compress. The compression should be held in place for 1 to 3 minutes, depending on the patient. If the patient taking aspirin, Coumadin, or other anticoagulants, compression should be for at least 5 minutes.

In many ways the procedure for capillary puncture is similar to the other collection procedures discussed in this chapter (e.g., patient identification, safety precautions, specimen labeling). Procedure 28-5 provides a detailed description of capillary puncture.

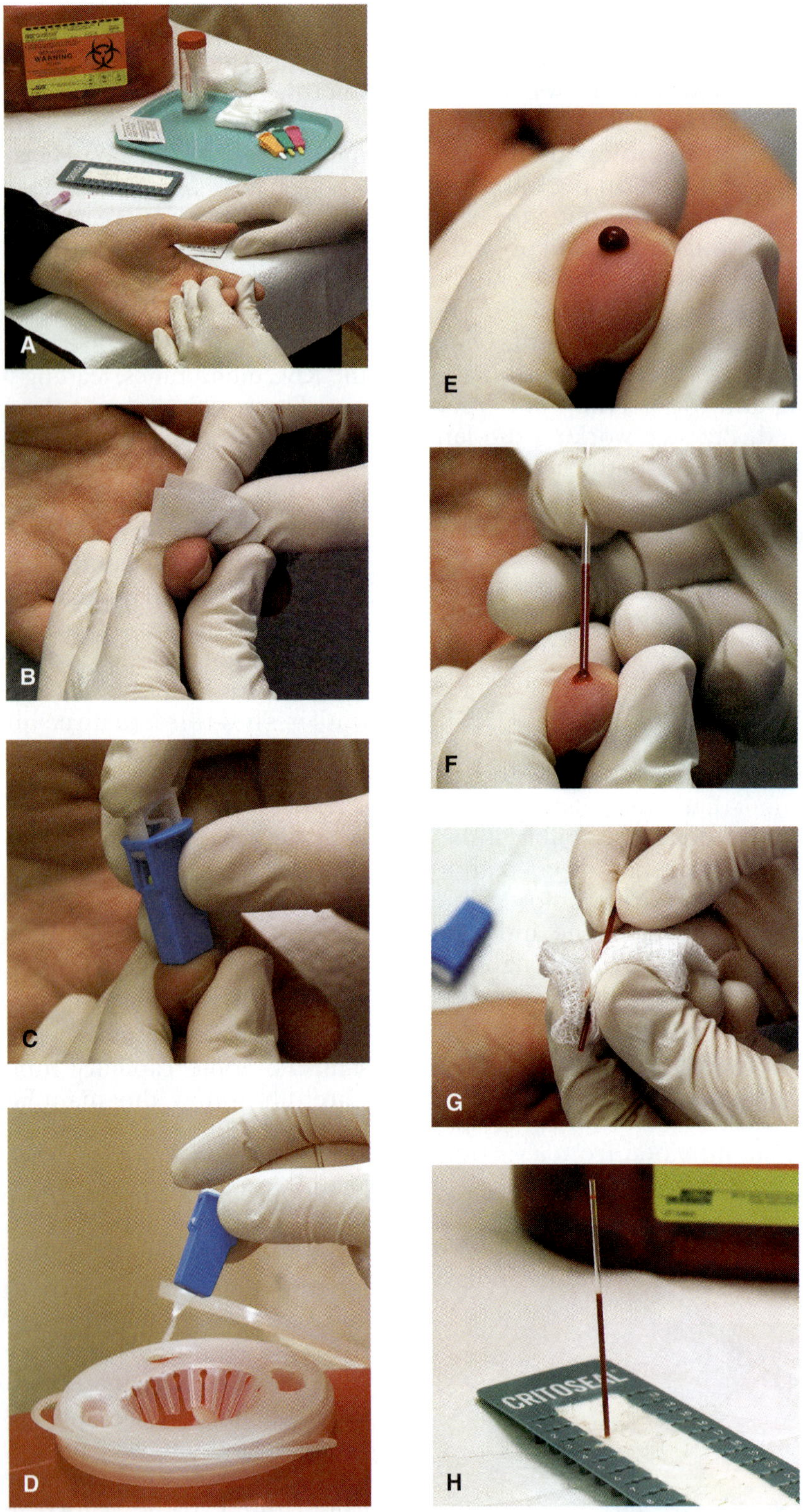

Figure 28-31 Collecting a specimen into a capillary tube through capillary puncture. (A) Assemble the necessary equipment and supplies and examine the finger for the best puncture site. (B) Clean the site with alcohol and allow the area to dry. (C) Perform the puncture. (D) Discard the lancet into a nearby sharps container. (E) Wipe off the first drop (not shown) and allow a well-rounded drop to form. (F) Holding the capillary tube horizontally, touch the end to the drop and allow the tube to fill. (G) Carefully wipe the residue blood off the tube. (H) Gently place the end of the tube into the sealing clay. Repeat to collect a second tube. Draw at least two tubes; some laboratories require three. Follow your laboratory manual instructions.

Procedure 28-1

Palpating a Vein and Preparing a Patient for Venipuncture

STANDARD PRECAUTIONS:

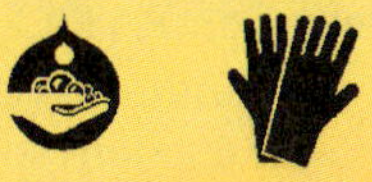

PURPOSE:

To palpate a vein and assess patient preparation prior to performing venipuncture.

EQUIPMENT/SUPPLIES:

Gloves
Tourniquet

PROCEDURE STEPS:

1. Identify the patient and explain the procedure. Ask the patient's name and verify it with the computer label or identification number. If a fasting specimen is required, verify that the patient has not had anything to eat or drink except water for 12 hours. RATIONALE: Proper identification of the patient and specimen and ensuring that the patient has properly prepared for the blood tests are quality-control and quality-assurance measures.
2. Wash hands. Put on gloves.
3. Apply tourniquet 3 to 4 inches above the venipuncture site. Apply tightly enough to slow venous blood flow but not so tight that blood flow in arteries is stopped (see Figure 28-21). RATIONALE: Applying the tourniquet too tightly can lead to excessive engorgement of the veins, causing blood to enter the tissues during puncture, further causing a hematoma.
4. Have the patient close the hand and place the patient's arm in a downward position. Do not allow the patient to pump his or her hand. RATIONALE: Having the patient close his or her hand and positioning the arm below the heart causes enlargement of the vein, allowing for an easier, more successful puncture. Pumping of the hand can lead to excessive engorgement of the vein, causing blood to leak into surrounding tissue during the puncture, which will cause a hematoma to occur.
5. Palpate the antecubital space of the arm, feeling for the basilic or cephalic vein with the tip of your middle or ring finger. Feel for a soft bounce and a roundness to the vein. RATIONALE: The tip of the middle or ring finger is less callused and more sensitive than the tip of the index finger. Veins will have a soft round feel.
6. After locating an acceptable vein, mentally map the location. Visualize the puncture site. Follow the direction of the vein with your finger tip, making a mental note of any turns, dips, and twists. RATIONALE: Mentally mapping the location and visualizing the puncture site will help in planning a successful direction.
7. If a vein cannot be found in the antecubital space of either arm, then the hand veins must be checked following the same procedure. The butterfly technique is more successful for hand venipuncture. RATIONALE: Butterfly is more successful because the hand veins have a greater tendency to roll and are smaller than the veins in the arm.

Procedure 28-2

Venipuncture by Syringe

STANDARD PRECAUTIONS:

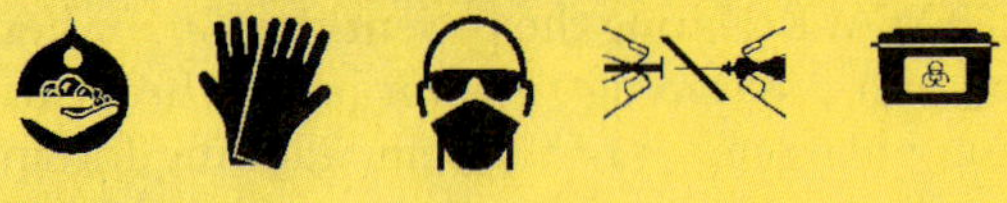

PURPOSE:

To obtain venous blood acceptable for laboratory testing as requested by the provider.

EQUIPMENT/SUPPLIES:

- Gloves
- Goggles and mask
- 10 mL syringe, 21-gauge needle
- Vacuum tube(s) or special collection tube(s)
- Tourniquet
- 70% isopropyl alcohol swab
- Cotton balls
- Adhesive bandage or tape
- Sharps container and biohazard red bag
- Test tube rack
- Biohazard transport bag (optional)
- Lab requisition (optional)

PROCEDURE STEPS:

1. Assemble the supplies. RATIONALE: Organizing supplies before the procedure ensures a more timely and professional process.
2. Position and identify the patient. Ask the patient's name and verify it with the tests ordered and the computer label or identification number. If a fasting specimen is required, verify that the patient has not had anything to eat or drink except water for 12 hours. RATIONALE: Proper identification of the patient and the tests ordered and ensuring that the patient is properly prepared for the blood tests are all quality-control and quality-assurance measures.
3. Wash hands and apply gloves and goggles/mask. RATIONALE: Clean hands further protect the patient. Gloves protect you. Goggles/mask should be worn if there is a possibility of blood splatter.
4. Open the sterile needle and sterile syringe packages and assemble if necessary. Pull the plunger halfway out and push it all the way in again. RATIONALE: Preparing the equipment ahead of time ensures a smoother process. Syringes can stick when new, so pulling once on the plunger prevents it from sticking during the venipuncture.
5. Select the proper vacuum tubes for later transfer of the specimen; tap all tubes containing anticoagulants and check the expiration dates. Arrange them in a holding rack in proper order. RATIONALE: Having the supplies ready and in the rack saves confusion later. The rack is a safety item so you are not holding the tube while transferring the specimen. Tapping the tubes ensures that all the additive is dislodged from the stopper and wall of the tubes. Checking expiration dates is a quality-assurance measure.
6. Apply the tourniquet (Figure 28-32A) and select a site. See Procedure 28-1. RATIONALE: Applying the tourniquet causes the vein to enlarge for easier venipuncture.
7. Ask the patient to close the hand. The patient must not pump the hand. Place the hand in a downward position. RATIONALE: Closing the hand and placing the arm in a downward position further enlarges the vein, allowing for easier venipuncture. Pumping the hand can damage the quality of the specimen collected.
8. Select a vein, noting the location and direction of the vein. RATIONALE: This allows you to prepare mentally for the venipuncture.
9. Cleanse the site with an alcohol swab with one firm swipe (Figure 28-32B). Avoid touching the site after cleansing. RATIONALE: Alcohol removes body oils, sweat, and other contaminants. The site should stay as clean as possible.
10. Draw the skin taut with your thumb by placing it 1 to 2 inches below the puncture site. RATIONALE: This will anchor the vein.
11. With the bevel up, line up the needle with the direction of the vein and perform the puncture (Figure 28-32C). The point of the needle should enter the skin about ¼ inch below where the vein was palpated. With experience, a sensation of entering the vein can be felt. Once the vein has been entered, do not move the needle from side to side. Do not push down or pull up the needle. The needle can be moved in or out gently if needed to locate the vein. RATIONALE: Lining up the needle with the vein is a mental exercise to help enter the vein in the proper direction. Entering the skin a fraction of an inch below the palpated site will aid in entering the vein at the correct site. This will align the needle so that it will enter the vein.

continues

Procedure 28-2 (continued)

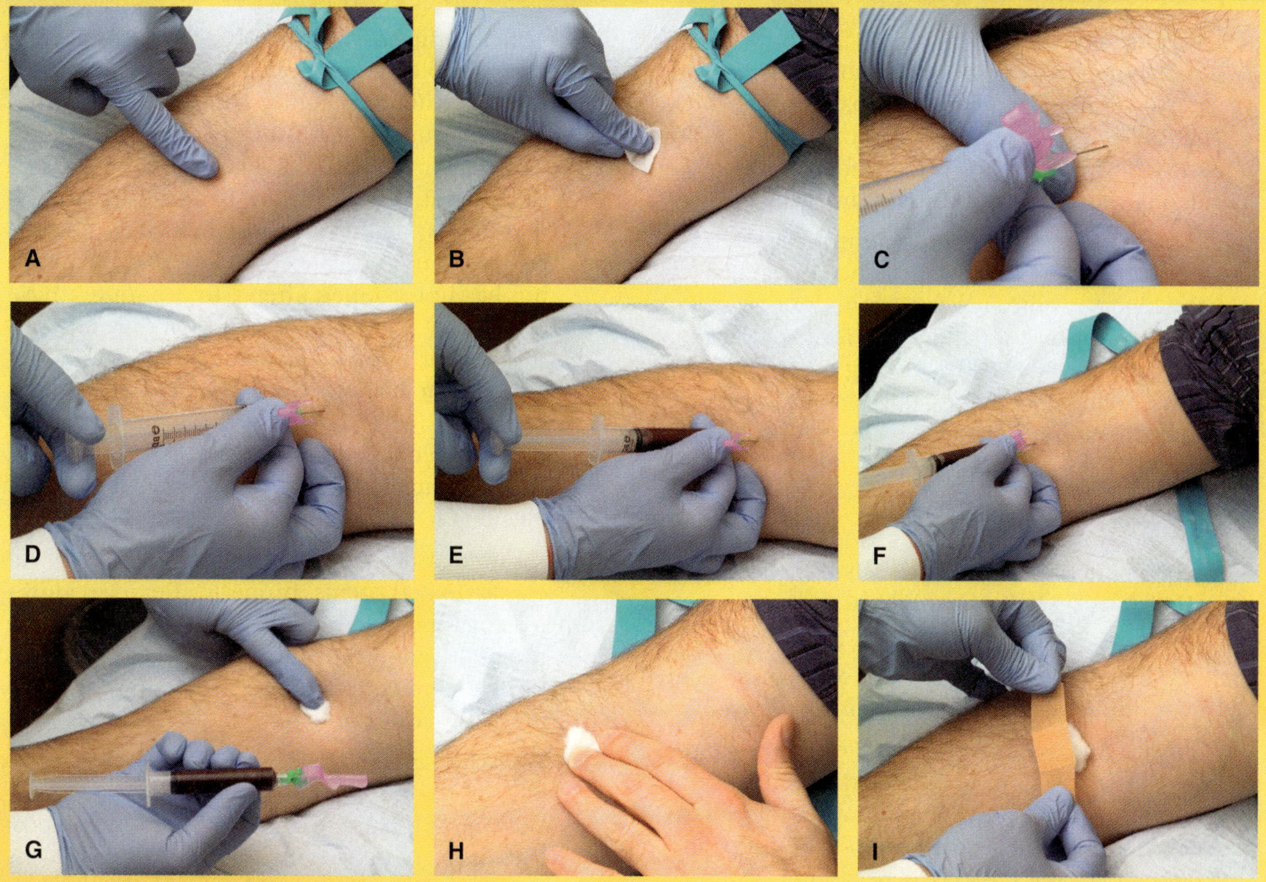

Figure 28-32 Performing a venipuncture with the syringe method. (A) Apply tourniquet and find vein. (B) Apply alcohol in one with motion and allow with to dry. Area can be wiped with a clean 2 × 2 gauze (do not use a cotton ball). (C) Draw skin taut (not shown) and insert needle. (D) Let go of skin and use that hand to pull back on the plunger. (E) Withdraw blood slowly, until the syringe is full. (F) Release tourniquet. (G) Apply a clean cotton ball immediately after withdrawing needle. (H) Have patient apply pressure to the site until a clot forms. (I) Apply a bandage over the site.

12. Let go of the skin and use that hand to pull back on the plunger (Figure 28-32D). Pull gently and only as fast as the syringe fills (Figure 28-32E). If the vein collapses, stop pulling on the plunger and let the vein refill. RATIONALE: Pulling too rapidly or too hard can cause the vein to collapse.
13. When the syringe is full, have the patient open the hand. Remove the tourniquet (Figure 28-32F). RATIONALE: Opening the hand and removing the tourniquet releases the pressure so the needle can be removed.
14. Lightly place a cotton ball above the puncture site and remove the needle in the same direction as inserted (Figure 28-32G). RATIONALE: Holding the cotton ball above the site allows for immediate pressure to be applied once the needle is removed.
15. Apply pressure to the site for 2 to 3 minutes, or longer if the patient is taking prescribed anticoagulants (blood thinners) such as warfarin (Coumadin) or is taking aspirin or an herbal blood thinner such as ginkgo biloba. Let the patient assist by holding the pressure if desired (Figure 28-32H). The patient can elevate the arm but should be instructed not to bend the elbow. RATIONALE: Two to three minutes is usually enough time for the bleeding to stop. Elevating the arm while holding pressure aids in the clotting. Bending the elbow can cause a hematoma to form.

continues

Procedure 28-2 (continued)

16. Aliquot blood into the appropriate tubes in the rack in the proper order (see Table 28-4). During transfer, hold each tube at the base only. RATIONALE: Having the tubes in the rack and holding the tubes at the base protects your hand from accidental needlestick during the transfer process.
17. Puncture the vacuum tube through the rubber stopper with the syringe needle and allow the blood to enter the tube until the flow stops. Never push on the plunger or force blood into the tube. RATIONALE: Pushing on the plunger and forcing blood into the vacuum tube can cause the rubber stopper to pop off, splashing blood.
18. Implement safety mechanism or devices on the needle immediately. RATIONALE: Immediate implementation of safety mechanisms will protect from accidental needlesticks.
19. Mix any anticoagulant tubes immediately. RATIONALE: Mixing the anticoagulants right away minimizes the chance of miniclots forming.
20. Discard the syringe and needle into a sharps container and the contaminated cotton ball and other contaminated waste into a red biohazard bag. RATIONALE: Proper disposal of sharps and biohazard waste protects all personnel.
21. Label all tubes before leaving the room. If any special treatment is required for the specimens, institute the handling protocol right away. RATIONALE: Labeling the tubes right away lessens the chances of a mix-up error. Proper handling of specimens ensures an accurate test result.
22. Check the patient. Observe him or her for signs of stress. RATIONALE: Venipuncture can be stressful for some patients.
23. When sufficient pressure has been applied to stop the bleeding, apply a small pressure bandage by pulling a cotton ball in half, applying it to the puncture site, and placing an adhesive bandage or tape over it (Figure 28-32I). Instruct the patient to remove the bandage in 20 minutes. If the patient is sensitive or allergic to latex, be sure to use nonlatex paper tape. If the bleeding has not stopped after 2 to 3 minutes, have the patient continue to hold direct pressure on the site for another 5 minutes with his or her arm elevated above the heart. He or she can do this by lying down with his or her arm on a pillow. Recheck after 5 minutes. RATIONALE: The patient should not leave your care until the bleeding has stopped.
24. Disinfect tray and supplies and dispose of all contaminated items properly. Remove gloves using proper technique. RATIONALE: Proper disposal and disinfection of all contaminated supplies and equipment protects from exposure to biohazardous substances.
25. Wash hands, record the procedure, and complete the laboratory requisition. RATIONALE: Washing hands after removing gloves further protects from biohazardous substances and lessens the chance of cross contamination to the patient's chart and the laboratory requisition. Completing the documentation and requisition as soon as possible after the procedure improves accuracy.

DOCUMENTATION

11/13/XX 2:54 PM Venipuncture performed right arm for CBC and sed rate. Specimen sent to Inner City Lab. Identification #987654321. Patient tolerated the procedure well and will call back tomorrow for the test results. Joe Guerrero, CMA (AAMA) ______

Procedure 28-3

Venipuncture by Vacuum Tube System

STANDARD PRECAUTIONS:

PURPOSE:

To obtain venous blood acceptable for laboratory testing as requested by a provider.

EQUIPMENT/SUPPLIES:

Gloves
Goggles and mask
Vacuum tube adapter/holder
Lab requisition (optional)
70% isopropyl alcohol swab
Cotton balls
21-gauge multidraw needle
Vacuum tube(s) or special collection tube(s)
Tourniquet
Adhesive bandage or tape
Sharps container and biohazard red bag
Biohazard transport bag (optional)

PROCEDURE STEPS:

1. Place specimen and requisition into biohazard transfer bag.
2. Position and identify the patient. Ask the patient's name and verify it with the tests ordered and the computer label or identification number. If a fasting specimen is required, verify that the patient has not had anything to eat or drink except water for 12 hours. RATIONALE: Proper identification of the patient and the tests ordered and ensuring that the patient is properly prepared for the blood tests are all quality-control and quality-assurance measures.
3. Wash hands and apply gloves and goggles/mask. RATIONALE: Clean hands further protect the patient. Gloves protect you. Goggles/mask should be worn if there is a possibility of blood splatter.
4. Break the seal on the shorter needle; thread the shorter needle into the holder/adapter. Select the first tube and gently place it into the holder/adapter (do not puncture the tube yet). RATIONALE: Preparing the equipment ahead of time ensures a smoother process.
5. Tap all tubes containing anticoagulants and check the expiration dates. RATIONALE: Tapping the tubes ensures that all the additive is dislodged from the stopper and wall of the tubes. Checking expiration dates is a quality-assurance measure.
6. Select a site and apply the tourniquet (see Procedure 28-1). RATIONALE: Applying the tourniquet causes the vein to enlarge for easier venipuncture.
7. Ask the patient to close the hand. The patient must not pump the hand. Place the hand in a downward position. RATIONALE: Closing the hand and placing the arm in a downward position further enlarges the vein, allowing for easier venipuncture. Pumping the hand can damage the quality of the specimen collected.
8. Select a vein, noting the location and direction of the vein. RATIONALE: This allows you to prepare mentally for the venipuncture (Figure 28-33A).
9. Cleanse the site with an alcohol swab with one firm swipe. RATIONALE: Alcohol removes body oils and contamination (Figure 28-33B).
10. Avoid touching the site after cleansing. RATIONALE: The site should stay as clean as possible.
11. Draw the skin taut with your thumb by placing it 1 to 2 inches below the puncture site. RATIONALE: This will anchor the vein.
12. With the bevel up, line up the needle with the direction of the vein and perform the puncture. The point of the needle should enter the skin about ¼ inch below where the vein was palpated. With experience, a sensation of entering the vein can be felt. Once the vein has been entered, do not move the needle. RATIONALE: Lining up the needle with the vein is a mental exercise to help enter the vein in the proper direction. Entering the skin a fraction of an inch below the palpated site will aid in entering the vein at the palpated site (Figure 28-33C).
13. Let go of the skin and use that hand to grasp the flange of the vacuum tube holder and push the tube forward until the needle has completely entered the tube (Figure 28-33D). Do not change hands while performing venipuncture. The hand performing the venipuncture is the hand that is holding the vacuum tube holder. The other hand is free for tube insertion and removal. RATIONALE: Using the flange of the adapter helps you hold the needle steady while changing tubes. Changing hands while performing venipuncture could cause the needle to move.

continues

Procedure 28-3 (continued)

14. Fill the tube until the vacuum is exhausted and the blood flow stops. Rotate tubes so the label is down. RATIONALE: Letting the tubes completely fill will ensure the right ratio of blood to additive. Positioning the label down enables you to see the tube filling.
15. When the blood ceases, gently remove the vacuum tube from the needle and holder. Do this by grasping the tube with the fingers and palm of your spare hand and using your thumb to push off from the flange of the holder (Figure 28-33E). RATIONALE: Using the flange will help steady the needle.
16. Immediately mix the blood in the anticoagulant tubes by gently inverting them several times. RATIONALE: Mixing the anticoagulant tubes right away minimizes the chance of miniclots forming.
17. Insert the second tube onto the needle by using the same motion as the first tube (Figure 28-33F). Let it fill; then remove it with the same motion as the first tube. Invert it several times if it contains anticoagulants. RATIONALE: Mixing the additives prevents the blood from coagulating.
18. When the last tube has filled, remove it from the needle. Ask the patient to open his or her

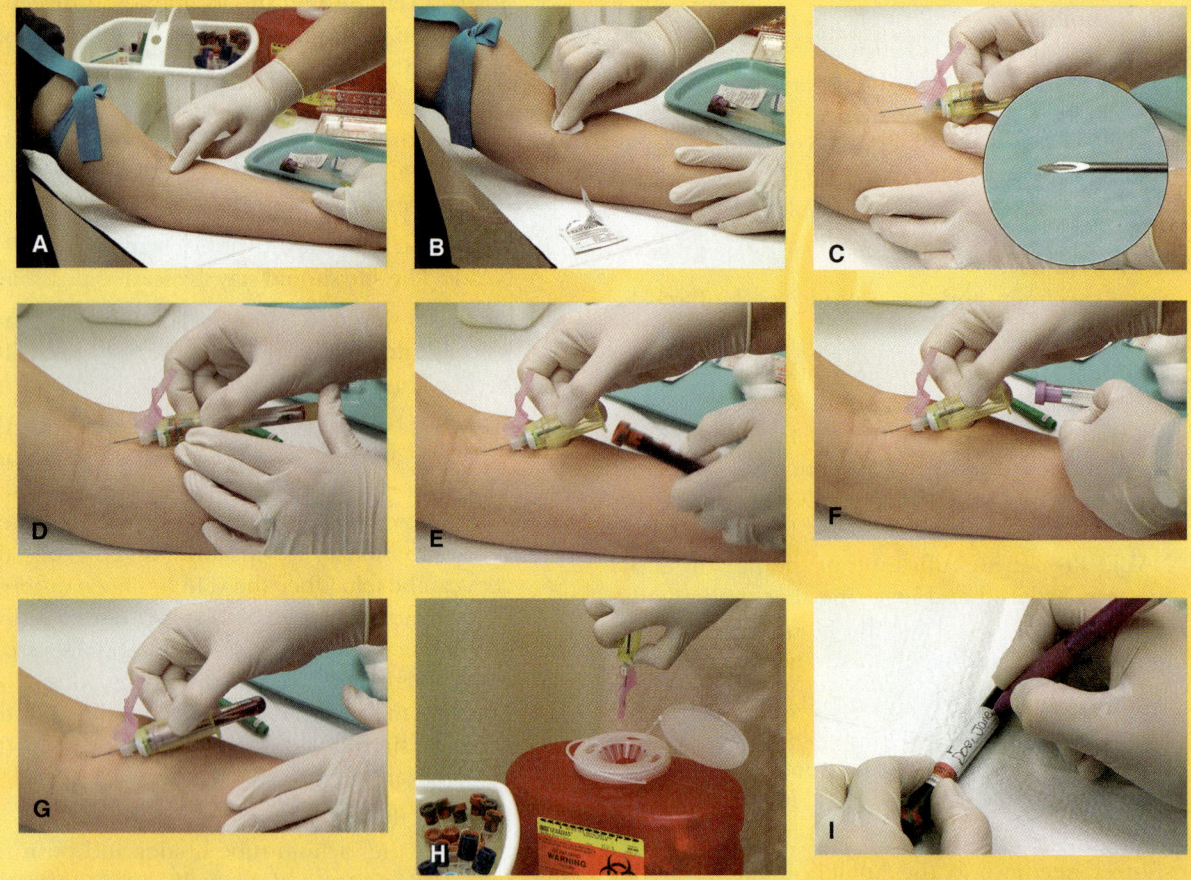

Figure 28-33 Performing a venipuncture with a vacuum tube assembly. (A) After tying the tourniquet, palpate the vein. (B) Cleanse the site with alcohol. Allow area to dry or wipe with a clean 2 × 2 gauze. (C) While holding the skin taut, hold needle with bevel up and penetrate the vein with a smooth rapid movement. (D) Grasp the flange of the vacuum tube holder to push the vacuum tube onto the needle. (E) When the tube has stopped filling, remove it gently from the needle and holder using the flange to push from. Invert it several times to mix the additives. (F) Place another tube onto the needle and let it fill. (G) When the last tube has filled, gently remove it from the holder. Release the tourniquet (not shown) and smoothly remove the needle from the vein, immediately applying pressure with the cotton ball. Mix well by inverting several times. (H) Dispose of the needle and holder into a nearby sharps container. (I) Properly label the tubes.

continues

Procedure 28-3 (continued)

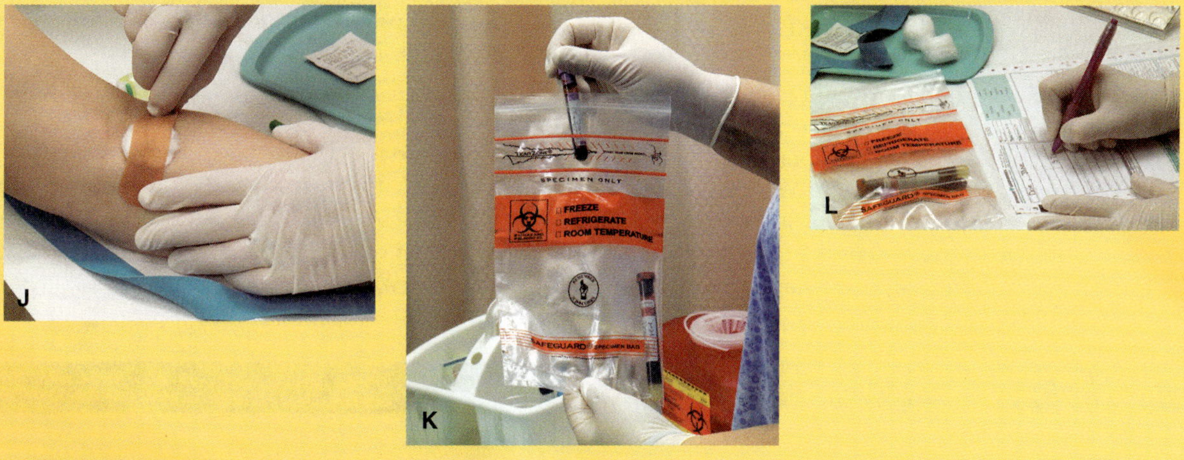

Figure 28-33 (continued) (J) Check the patient, apply a bandage. (K) Package the specimens properly for transport (be aware of special storage or treatment needed, such as centrifugation or refrigeration). (L) Complete the laboratory requsition and document the procedure in the patient's chart or electronic medical record.

hand and release the tourniquet. RATIONALE: Removing the last tube from the needle prevents any residual suction from drawing blood through the tissues when the needle is removed from the vein. Opening the hand and removing the tourniquet relieves pressure so the needle can be removed without causing excessive blood loss through the puncture site.

19. Lightly place the cotton ball above the puncture site and smoothly remove the needle from the arm in the same direction of insertion. RATIONALE: Holding the cotton ball above the site allows for immediate pressure to be applied once the needle is removed.
20. Immediately activate the safety device. RATIONALE: Activating the safety device protects you from accidental needlesticks (Figure 28-33H).
21. Apply pressure on the site for 2 to 3 minutes. Let the patient assist by holding the pressure. Ask him or her not the bend his or her arm, but he or she can elevate his or her arm while applying pressure. RATIONALE: Two to three minutes is usually enough time for bleeding to stop. Hold pressure for longer if the patient is taking prescribed anticoagulants (blood thinners) such as warfarin (Coumadin) or taking aspirin or an herbal blood thinner such as ginkgo biloba. Elevating the arm while holding pressure aids in the clotting. Bending the elbow can cause a hematoma to form.
22. Dispose of the needle into a sharps container and the contaminated cotton ball and other contaminated waste into a biohazard red bag. RATIONALE: Proper disposal of sharps and biohazard waste protects all personnel.
23. Label all the tubes before leaving the patient (Figure 28-33I). If any special treatment is required for the specimens, institute the handling protocol right away. RATIONALE: Labeling the tubes right away lessens the chances of a mix-up error. Proper handling of the specimens ensures accurate test results.
24. Check the patient. Observe him or her for signs of stress. He or she should stop bleeding within 2 to 3 minutes. If the bleeding has stopped, apply a small pressure bandage by pulling a cotton ball in half, applying it to the site, and placing an adhesive bandage or tape over it (Figure 28-33J). The patient should be instructed to remove the bandage in about 20 minutes. If the patient is sensitive to latex, be sure to use a nonlatex paper tape. If the bleeding has not stopped, have the patient continue to hold direct pressure another 5 minutes with his or her arm elevated above his or her heart level. Have him or her lie down with his or her arm up on a pillow. Recheck the site after 5 minutes of additional direct pressure. RATIONALE: Check the patient for signs of distress because venipuncture can be stressful for some people. The patient should not leave your care until the bleeding has stopped.
25. Disinfect all surfaces and supplies/equipment. Remove gloves using proper technique. Dispose of contaminated items appropriately. RATIONALE: Proper disposal and disinfection of all

continues

Procedure 28-3 (continued)

contaminated supplies and equipment protects from exposure to dangerous biohazard substances.

26. Wash hands, record the procedure, and complete the laboratory requisition. Place specimen and requisition into biohazard transport bag (Figures 28-33K and L). RATIONALE: Washing hands after removing gloves further protects from biohazard substances and lessens the chance of cross contamination to the patient's chart and the laboratory requisition. Completing the documentation and requisition as soon as possible after the procedure improves accuracy.

DOCUMENTATION

4/27/XX 8:36 AM Venipuncture performed left arm for CBC, Hgb & Hct, and thyroid panel. Specimen sent to Inner City Lab. Patient ID # 56776523. Patient tolerated the procedure well and will return on 4/30/XX for a recheck. Joe Guerrero, CMA (AAMA) ____________________

Procedure 28-4

Venipuncture by Butterfly Needle System

STANDARD PRECAUTIONS:

PURPOSE:

To obtain venous blood acceptable for laboratory testing as requested by a provider.

EQUIPMENT/SUPPLIES:

Gloves
Goggles and mask
Vacuum tube holder if using a vacuum tube connection
A 10- to 15-mL/cc syringe if using a syringe connection
Butterfly needle system with 21-gauge needle (use a multisample needle system with a Luer-lok adapter for attaching to the vacuum tube and a hypodermic needle for syringe attachment)
Vacuum tubes if appropriate
Tourniquet
70% isopropyl alcohol swab
Gauze
Adhesive bandage or tape
Sharps container and biohazard red bag
Lab requisition (optional)

PROCEDURE STEPS:

1. Assemble the supplies. RATIONALE: Organizing supplies before the procedure ensures a more timely and professional process.
2. Position and identify the patient. Ask the patient's name and verify it with the computer label or identification number. If a fasting specimen is required, verify that the patient has not had anything to eat or drink except water for 12 hours. RATIONALE: Proper identification of the patient and the tests ordered and verifying that the patient is properly prepared are quality-control and quality-assurance measures.
3. Wash hands. Put on gloves, as well as goggles and mask if there is a potential for blood splatter. RATIONALE: Clean hands further protect the patient. Gloves and goggles/face shield protect you from any potential splatters.
4. Open the package of butterfly needle system. If using the multisample needle, connect the needle to the vacuum tube holder/adapter. If using the hypodermic needle and syringe, connect the needle to the syringe (Figure 28-34A). If using a syringe, set the vacuum tubes in a rack for later use. RATIONALE: The more organized you are before the venipuncture; the smoother the procedure will go.
5. Tap the vacuum tubes to be sure any additive is dislodged from the stopper and sides of the tube. Check the expiration dates. RATIONALE: Dislodging the additive will ensure proper ratio in the specimen. The tubes should not be older than their expiration date.

continues

Procedure 28-4 (continued)

6. Apply the tourniquet. Select a vein. RATIONALE: Applying a tourniquet enlarges the vein, making it more accessible.
7. Ask the patient to close his or her hand (Figure 28-34B). The patient should not pump his or her hand. If possible, place the arm in a downward position. RATIONALE: Pumping of hand can lead to excessive engorgement of the vein, which can cause blood to enter the tissues during the puncture, causing a hematoma.
8. Select the vein, noting the direction and location of the vein. RATIONALE: You will want to enter the vein in the same direction it is going.
9. Cleanse the site with an alcohol swab using one swift firm swipe and allow to dry (Figure 28-34C). RATIONALE: Alcohol removes body oils and other contaminations. Puncturing the skin through wet alcohol can cause stinging and hemolysis of the specimen and will contaminate the specimen.
10. Avoid touching the site after cleansing. RATIONALE: Touching the skin will recontaminate it.
11. Draw the skin taut by placing your thumb 1 to 2 inches below the site and pulling down firmly. RATIONALE: This will anchor the vein.
12. Hold the wings of the butterfly together with the bevel up, line up the needle with the vein, and smoothly insert it into the vein at about a 5- to 10-degree angle (Figure 28-34D). RATIONALE: This process will cause the least amount of discomfort and provide the greatest success.
13. Remove your hand from holding the skin taut. RATIONALE: You will need one hand free to handle the other equipment.
14. If you are connected to a vacuum tube holder, grasp the flange of the vacuum tube holder and push the tube forward until the needle has completely entered the tube. RATIONALE: Using the flange when inserting and removing vacuum tubes will help the needle stay in position.
15. If you are connected to a syringe, pull gently on the syringe (Figure 28-34E). RATIONALE: Pulling too rapidly can cause the vein to collapse.
16. Do not change hands while performing venipuncture. The hand performing the venipuncture is the hand that is holding the vacuum tube holder. The other hand is for inserting and removing the vacuum tubes. RATIONALE: Changing hands can cause the needle to change position.
17. If you are collecting directly into vacuum tubes, remove and replace the vacuum tubes as explained in Procedure 28-3 until you have drawn the necessary amounts. If you are drawing into a syringe, you will be limited to the size of the syringe being used. RATIONALE: You do not have the option of removing and replacing the syringe during a draw.
18. When the syringe is filled, ask the patient to open his or her hand and release the tourniquet. RATIONALE: Opening of the hand and releasing the tourniquet takes the pressure off the vein and allows the blood to flow freely through the arm.
19. Lightly place a cotton ball above the puncture site and smoothly remove the needle from the arm in the same direction of insertion (Figure 28-34F). RATIONALE: You are getting the cotton ball ready so you can apply pressure on the puncture site immediately on removing the needle.
20. Activate the safety device of the butterfly needle immediately (Figure 28-34G). RATIONALE: The safety devices are better able to protect if activated immediately.
21. Apply pressure on the site. Let the patient assist by holding the pressure (Figure 28-34H). Ask him or her not the bend his or her arm. He or she can elevate his or her arm while applying pressure though. RATIONALE: Applying pressure and elevating the arm lessens the chance of bruising, whereas bending the elbow increases the chance of the patient forming a hematoma.
22. If using a syringe, aliquot blood into the appropriate tubes as outlined in Procedure 28-2. RATIONALE: Following proper procedure when transferring blood from the syringe into the vacuum tubes ensures the best specimens for testing.
23. Dispose of the needle into a sharps container (Figure 28-34I). RATIONALE: Immediate disposal of contaminated needles is the safest practice.
24. Label all the tubes. RATIONALE: Not labeling the tubes right away increases the likelihood of a mix-up error.
25. Check the patient. Observe him or her for signs of stress. RATIONALE: Patient safety is a primary concern. Venipuncture can be difficult for some patients.

continues

Procedure 28-4 (continued)

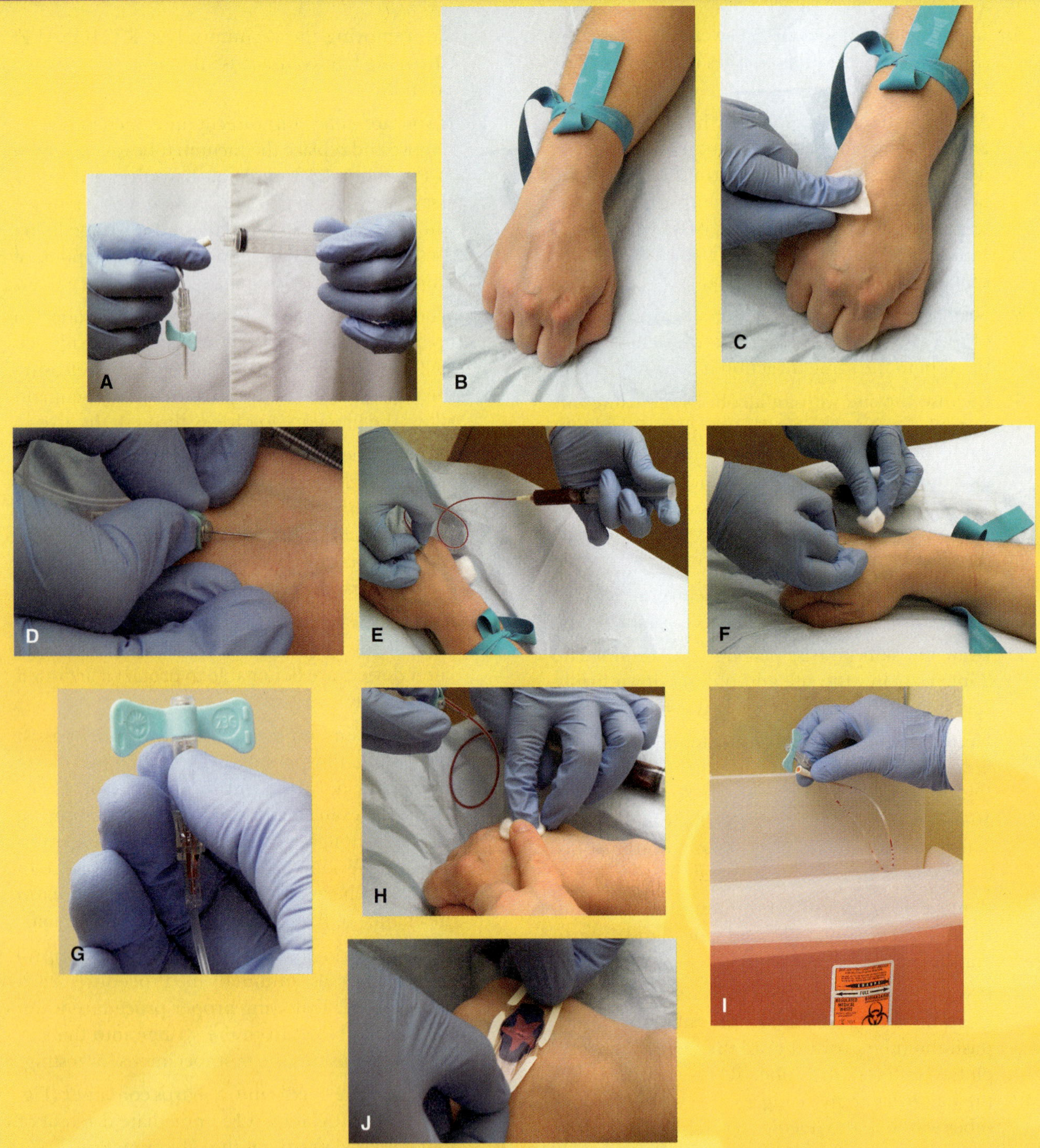

Figure 28-34 Performing a venipuncture with the butterfly needle system. (A) Open the package with the butterfly needle system and assemble the needle. In this case, the needle is connected to the syringe. (B) Apply the tourniquet and ask the patient to close his hand. (C) Cleanse the site with using one swift wipe and allow to air dry. (D) Draw skin taut. While holding the wings of the butterly together, line up the needle with the vein, and insert at a 5- to 10-degree angle. (E) Pull gently on the syringe, allowing it to fill. (F) When filled, have the patient open his hand, and release the tourniquet. Place a cotton ball above the puncture site and remove the needle. (G) Activate the safety device of the butterfly needle. (H) Apply pressure on the site, and ask the patient to continue holding the pressure. (I) Dispose of the needle into a sharps container. (J) Apply a bandage to the site.

continues

Procedure 28-4 (continued)

26. The patient should stop bleeding within 2 to 3 minutes. If the bleeding has stopped, apply a small pressure bandage by pulling a cotton ball in half, applying it to the site, and placing an adhesive bandage or tape over it (Figure 28-34J). The patient should be instructed to remove the bandage in about 20 minutes. If the patient is sensitive to latex, be sure to use a nonlatex paper tape. If the bleeding has not stopped, have the patient continue to hold pressure another 5 minutes with his or her arm elevated above his or her heart level, then recheck. RATIONALE: The patient should not be released from your care until the bleeding has stopped.
27. Clean up tray and supplies; dispose of contaminated cotton ball. Remove gloves using proper technique. Discard gloves into biohazard container and disinfect goggles. RATIONALE: Proper disposal and disinfection of contaminated supplies and equipment protects from exposure to biohazard substances.
28. Wash hands, record the procedure, and complete the laboratory requisition. Place specimen and requisition into biohazard transfer bag. RATIONALE: Washing hands after removing the gloves further protects from biohazard substances and lessens the chance of cross contamination to the patient's chart and laboratory requisition. Completing the documentation and requisition as soon as possible after the procedure improves accuracy.

DOCUMENTATION

11/13/XX 2:54 PM Venipuncture performed right arm for CBC and sed rate. Specimen sent to Inner City Lab. Identification #987654321. Patient tolerated the procedure well and will call back tomorrow for the test results. Joe Guerrero, CMA (AAMA) ____________

Procedure 28-5

Capillary Puncture

STANDARD PRECAUTIONS:

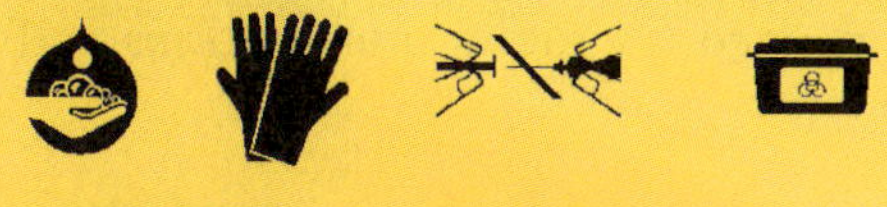

PURPOSE:

To obtain capillary blood acceptable for laboratory testing as requested by a provider.

EQUIPMENT/SUPPLIES:

Gloves
70% isopropyl alcohol swab
Microcollection tubes or capillary tubes
Safety lancet
Gauze 2 × 2
Adhesive bandage or tape
Sharps container
Cotton balls
Biohazard red bag
Laboratory requisition (optional)
Biohazard transport bag (optional)

PROCEDURE STEPS:

1. Assemble the supplies. RATIONALE: Organizing the supplies before the procedure ensures a more timely and professional process.
2. Identify the patient, introduce yourself, explain the procedure, and recheck the provider's orders. RATIONALE: Introducing yourself and explaining the procedure will establish a professional relationship with the patient and might help put him or her at ease. Identifying the patient and rechecking the provider's orders will ensure the proper tests will be performed on the right patient.
3. Wash hands and apply gloves. RATIONALE: Washing your hands protects the patient, and applying gloves protects you.
4. Select the puncture site on the fleshy part of the ring or middle finger, avoiding the very tip and the extreme sides. RATIONALE: The ring and

continues

Procedure 28-5 (continued)

middle fingers generally will have fewer calluses and less scarring. The tip and sides are more sensitive than the fleshy part.

5. Have the patient wash his or her hands in very warm water; if necessary, apply a warming pack to the fingertip, encourage the patient to relax, and provide a comfortable, professional atmosphere. RATIONALE: The patient washing his or her hands in very warm water provides two benefits: his or her hands will be cleaner and warmer, which encourages better blood to the area. Appling a warming pack to the fingertips will further encourage blood flow. A relaxed patient in a comfortable, professional atmosphere is more likely to provide a better sample.
6. Clean the selected puncture site with alcohol swab and allow it to air dry or dry it with a gauze pad. RATIONALE: Alcohol will remove any residue soap or debris. Allowing the alcohol to dry will prevent irritation and stinging. If the site is wiped dry, the irritation of the gauze pad will further encourage blood to the area.
7. Holding the distal phalange firmly, perform the puncture across the lines of the fingerprint rather than along the lines. RATIONALE: Holding the distal phalange firmly will add support to the finger and prevent the patient from pulling back on the finger during the puncture. Puncturing across the fingerprint will assist the blood to form a drop rather than flow across the fingertip.
8. Using a gauze pad, wipe away the first drop. RATIONALE: The first drop usually contains contamination from the alcohol and tissue fluid and would not be a good representation of the blood sample needed. Using gauze rather than cotton to wipe it away lessens the likelihood of it clotting too quickly.
9. Collect the specimen according to the test being performed (see Chapter 29 for hemoglobin and hematocrit; see Chapter 32 for PKU, glucose, and other specialty tests performed on capillary blood).
10. Have patient hold firm, direct pressure on the site with a cotton ball for at least 2 minutes. If the bleeding has stopped, an adhesive strip can be applied. If the bleeding has not stopped yet, hold firm, direct pressure on the site for another 5 minutes and then recheck. Adhesive strips are not recommended for patients younger than 2 years. RATIONALE: A cotton ball is used because the cotton fibers further encourage clotting at the puncture site. The bleeding should be stopped before the patient leaves your care. Adhesive strips for children younger than 2 years are not recommended because they are a choking hazard.
11. Disinfect the area and equipment, remove gloves, and dispose of them into a biohazard waste container/red bag. Wash hands. RATIONALE: Biohazard waste should be controlled for everyone's protection. Hand washing after removing gloves further protects you.
12. Record the procedure and complete the laboratory requisition or test. The laboratory requisition is completed in the presence of the patient if possible. RATIONALE: Documentation is critical for good patient records. Completing the laboratory requisition in the presence of the patient provides accurate insurance and personal information if needed for the insurance forms and for your medical records.

DOCUMENTATION

4/27/XX 8:15 AM Capillary puncture performed left ring finger for Hgb A1c. Patient tolerated the procedure well. Dr. Lewis is scheduled to see the patient today to discuss progress. Joe Guerrero, CMA (AAMA)

Procedure 28-6

Obtaining a Capillary Specimen for Transport Using a Microtainer Transport Unit

STANDARD PRECAUTIONS:

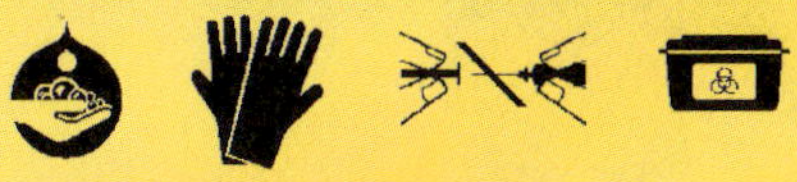

PURPOSE:

To obtain a specimen of capillary blood for transport to a laboratory for testing, using a Microtainer.

EQUIPMENT/SUPPLIES:

Capillary puncture supplies:
- Gloves
- 70% isopropyl alcohol swab
- Gauze
- Safety lancet
- Cotton balls
- Adhesive bandage
- Sharps container and biohazard waste receptacle

Microtainer transport unit
Laboratory requisition
Small sturdy container with a tightly fitting lid (such as a urine specimen cup or red top vacuum tube)
Biohazard specimen transport bag

PROCEDURE STEPS:

1. Determine the appropriateness of submitting a capillary specimen for the specific test you are performing. RATIONALE: Not all tests can be performed on capillary specimens.
2. Assemble the supplies. RATIONALE: Organizing the supplies before the procedure ensures a more timely and professional process.
3. Identify the patient, introduce yourself, explain the procedure, and recheck the provider's orders. RATIONALE: Introducing yourself and explaining the procedure will establish a professional relationship with the patient and might help put him or her at ease. Identifying the patient and rechecking the provider's orders will ensure the proper tests will be performed on the right patient.
4. Wash hands, apply gloves, and perform the capillary puncture according to Procedure 28-5. RATIONALE: Washing your hands protects the patient, and applying gloves protects you.
5. Discard the first drop of blood. Wipe it away with a gauze square. RATIONALE: The first drop can contain mostly alcohol residue and tissue fluid and would not be a good representation of the blood sample needed. Using gauze rather than cotton to wipe it away lessens the likelihood of it clotting too quickly.
6. Allow a good size drop to form. RATIONALE: Allowing a good size drop to form is a good idea with any capillary specimen; the blood is more likely to stay in a drop and not flow over the finger.
7. Scoop the drop into the Microtainer (Figure 28-35A). RATIONALE: This is the method used to get the specimen into the tip of the Microtainer.
8. Tip the Microtainer, allowing the drop to slide into the tube (Figure 28-35B). RATIONALE: As soon as a drop is obtained on the scoop it should be moved into the tube where it can mix with the additive.
9. Gently agitate the tube. RATIONALE: Agitating the tube allows the additive to mix with the blood.
10. Continue collection of blood until the tube is filled (Figure 28-35C). RATIONALE: The tube must be filled to the fill line to ensure the proper ratio of blood to additive.
11. Provide the patient with a cotton ball and ask him or her to hold pressure on the puncture site. RATIONALE: The pressure with a cotton ball will encourage the wound to clot.
12. Remove the scoop from the Microtainer and discard the scoop into the sharps container (Figure 28-35D). RATIONALE: The scoop is contaminated with blood and therefore is considered to be biohazard waste. Being hard plastic, it is capable of scratching someone, so the sharps container is safer than the red bag waste receptacle.
13. Remove the colored cap from the back of the Microtainer and place it securely onto the opening. RATIONALE: Placing the cap securely onto the Microtainer will ensure the specimen will stay in the Microtainer during handling and transport.

continues

Procedure 28-6 (continued)

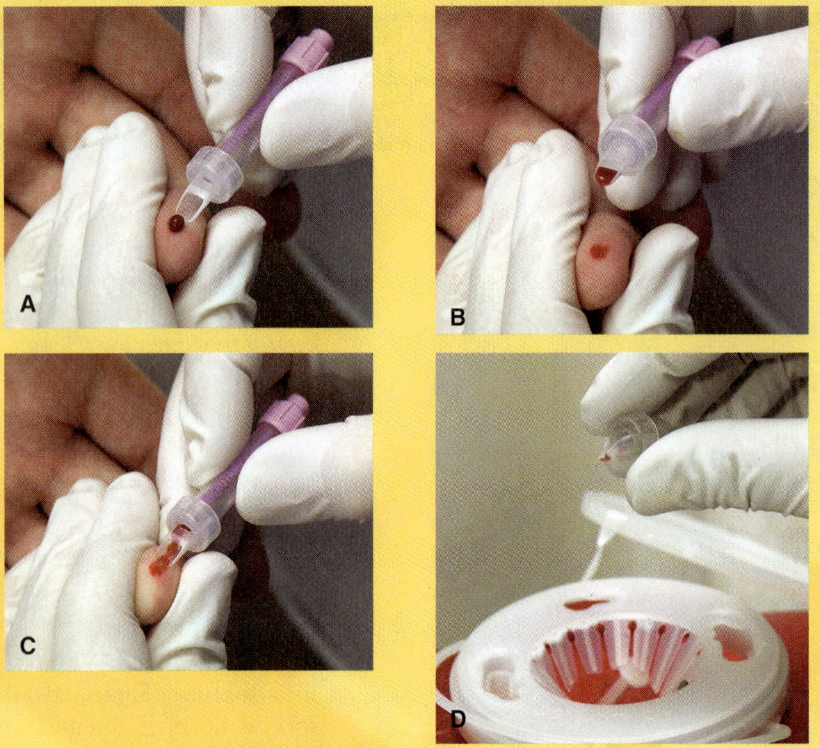

Figure 28-35 Collecting a capillary specimen for transport. (A) After wiping away the first drop (not shown), allow drop to form. Touch the scoop on the collection Microtainer tube to the blood droplet. (B) Tip the collection Microtainer tube up so that the blood flows into the tube. Agitate it gently to mix the anticoagulant with the blood. (C) Continue collecting the blood until the collection Microtainer tube is filled to the marked level. (D) Remove the scoop from the collection Microtainer tube and dispose of the scoop into a nearby sharps container.

14. Place the capped Microtainer into a small sturdy container with a tight-fitting lid. RATIONALE: Placing the Microtainer in another container protects it from being uncapped and (because of its small size) lost in transport. The Microtainer is also not large enough for adequate labeling.
15. Label the container. RATIONALE: Proper labeling ensures the proper tests on the right specimen.
16. Fill out the laboratory requisition while the patient is present. Place the specimen and the requisition into the biohazard transport bag in their separate compartments. RATIONALE: Any questions about the patient's address and insurance can be answered immediately if the patient is present while you complete the form.
17. Check the patient's puncture site. If bleeding has stopped, apply an adhesive strip, answer any questions the patient has, and release the patient. RATIONALE: Caring for the patient both physically and emotionally shows a professional dedication to your job.
18. Document procedure in patient's chart or electronic medical record. RATIONALE: Documentation ensures that the proper information is recorded into the patient's chart or electronic medical record.

DOCUMENTATION

3/3/XX 4:15 PM Capillary puncture was performed for a CBC. Specimen (Microtainer) sent to Inner City Laboratory. Patient tolerated the procedure well and will call in on Friday (3/6/XX) for the results. No return appointment scheduled. W. Slawson, CMA (AAMA)

Procedure 28-7

Obtaining Blood for Blood Culture

STANDARD PRECAUTIONS:

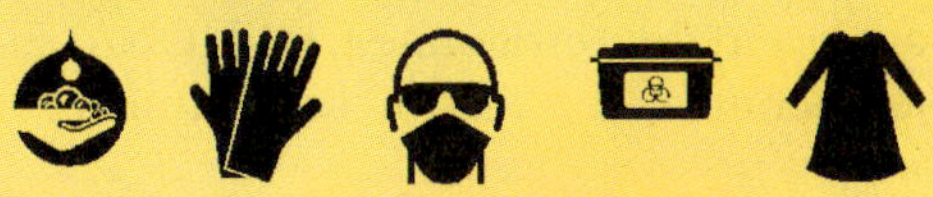

PURPOSE:

While performing venipuncture from two separate sites, prepare two culture bottles of blood from each site for culture (four total).

EQUIPMENT/SUPPLIES:

Nonsterile gloves for use with povidone-iodine solution
Sterile gloves
Laboratory requisition
Blood culture bottles, anaerobic and aerobic (usually four: two bottles each for two sets of cultures)
70% isopropyl alcohol
Povidone-iodine solution swabs or towelettes
Venipuncture supplies (according to method used) for two separate sites
Biohazard red bag
Sharps container
Labeling pen

PROCEDURE STEPS:

1. Identify the patient, introduce yourself, and explain the procedure.
2. Ensure that the patient has not initiated antimicrobial therapy. RATIONALE: Antibiotic therapy can interfere with the culture results. If the patient has started antibiotics, the name and strength of the antibiotic, dosage, duration, and last dose must be documented clearly on the laboratory report.
3. Wash hands and put on gloves. RATIONALE: Washing hands before any laboratory process prevents contamination of the specimen. Gloving provides personal protection.
4. Assemble equipment and supplies according to the venipuncture procedure being used and the laboratory requirements (Figure 28-36A). Check expiration dates on all collection and culture supplies. RATIONALE: Organizing your work area prevents confusion and error due to missing supplies. Usually two separate sites are used for collection, with two bottles (one aerobe and one anaerobe) from each site. Occasionally, three sites will be necessary. Expired supplies and culture bottles must not be used.
5. Place the culture bottles on a flat surface within reach during the procedure. Mark the correct fill line on both bottles at 10 mL per bottle (1–3 mL per bottle for pediatric patients). RATIONALE: Marking the fill line helps in viewing the proper amount during the procedure.
6. Prepare the venipuncture site with isopropyl alcohol and allow to dry, then apply povidone-iodine in progressively larger concentric circles from the inside outward (Figure 28-36B). The iodine must remain on the skin for 1 full minute and be allowed to dry naturally. The venipuncture site should not be touched after the skin is disinfected. RATIONALE: Alcohol removes oils and other debris, the povidone-iodine is a more thorough antiseptic. One full minute is required to ensure antisepsis. Touching the site may recontaminate it.
7. Cleanse the bottle tops with alcohol and povidone-iodine solution. RATIONALE: The bottle tops need to be disinfected to remove contamination. *NOTE:* Some laboratory guidelines state that iodine can disintegrate the rubber stopper and therefore should not be used. Follow your laboratory guidelines as stated in your laboratory manual.
8. Remove the preparation gloves and apply the sterile gloves using sterile procedure. RATIONALE: Sterile gloves will ensure the procedure will be as sterile as possible.
9. Perform venipuncture according to method used. Insert the aerobic culture bottle onto the needle (Figure 28-36C). Fill to the appropriate line, usually 10 mL per bottle (1–3 for pediatric patients). Remove the first bottle, invert 8 to 10 times, and apply the second (anaerobic) bottle. Fill. Remove the second bottle and invert 8 to 10 times. RATIONALE: Follow your laboratory manual guidelines. The aerobic bottle should be filled first because there will be some residual air in the needle. The anaerobic bottle will then collect only blood. Inverting the bottles ensures the culture media will be well mixed with the blood.

continues

Procedure 28-7 (continued)

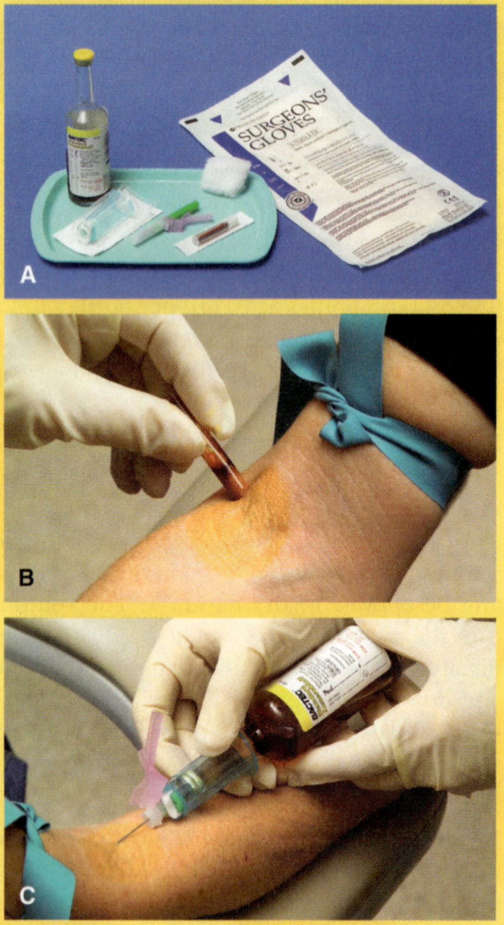

Figure 28-36 Obtaining blood for blood culture. (A) Assemble equipment and supplies (only one culture bottle shown). (B) Prepare the venipuncture site with alcohol and allow to dry, then apply povidone-iodine in concentric circles from the inside outward. Allow the iodine to dry naturally. (C) Perform venipuncture. Insert the aerobic culture bottle onto the needle and fill to the appropriate line.

10. Complete the venipuncture procedure as determined by the method used. Remove the remaining iodine from the skin with isopropyl alcohol. RATIONALE: The next two bottles will be filled from a different site. The iodine solution can irritate the skin and should be removed.
11. Perform venipuncture at the second site, repeating the process as stated above. The second and subsequent culture bottles must be collected within 30 minutes of the first. RATIONALE: The 30-minute time frame rules out the possibility of transient bacteria coming into the blood (such as through teeth brushing or scratching a skin lesion, and so on).
12. The culture bottles should be stored at room temperature and not refrigerated. RATIONALE: Room temperature is ideal for the cultures so organisms are not destroyed.
13. Label the bottles with the patient's name, date, time, and other required information. RATIONALE: Labeling with the required information prevents mix-ups of specimens and ensures a quality timeline. Specimens will be rejected if not labeled properly.
14. Dispose of all contaminated supplies, disinfect all surfaces, remove gloves, and wash hands. RATIONALE: Using appropriate disposal techniques and disinfecting all surfaces according to Standard Precautions safely control biohazard substances.
15. Complete the laboratory requisition including the date and time of each specimen collected, any antibiotic therapy the patient is on, the name and strength of the antibiotic, as well as the dosage, duration, and the last dose taken. Include the clinical diagnosis and any special organisms suspected or to rule out. The laboratory requisition must indicate if the culture is for *brucella* or *francisella.* The information on the laboratory requisition should match exactly the information given on the bottles. RATIONALE: Labeling with the required information prevents mix-ups of specimens, ensures a quality timeline, and ensures the laboratory will have the necessary information. Specimens will be rejected if there is a discrepancy between the information on the bottle and the information on the laboratory requisition.
16. Document the procedure in the laboratory section of the patient's chart or electronic medical record. RATIONALE: Necessary information and the patient's chart or electronic medical record will be accurate and complete.

DOCUMENTATION

08/06/20XX Venipuncture performed left arm for blood culture. Specimen sent to Inner City Lab. Patient ID #56776533. Patient tolerated procedure well and instructed to call us on Wednesday for the results. Joe Guerrero, CMA (AAMA) ———

Case Study 28-1

Refer to the scenario at the beginning of the chapter.

CASE STUDY REVIEW

1. What types of information will patients be able to share with Bruce about their previous venipuncture experiences?
2. How can Bruce use that information to better serve the patients?
3. Do you think patients are a good source of information about their bodies and their reactions to past experiences?

Case Study 28-2

Inner City Health Care is short-staffed today, and medical assistant Liz Corbin is feeling pressed for time. She has many tasks to complete, but first she must perform a venipuncture. She greets the patient, Wayne Elder, in a perfunctory manner, discouraging time-wasting conversation. Although Wayne appears apprehensive, he is not resistant, so Liz quickly assembles the necessary supplies, applies the tourniquet, and inserts the needle. While she is drawing his blood, Wayne faints.

CASE STUDY REVIEW

1. What should Liz do now?
2. What could Liz have done to prevent this situation from occurring?
3. In the future, what are some steps Liz can take to provide a positive experience for venipuncture patients?

SUMMARY

With a little practice, the medical assistant will become an expert at phlebotomy. The skills of phlebotomy cannot be learned primarily from a textbook; continuous practice will develop the skill to perfection. It may take months before the medical assistant feels comfortable and is able to obtain a sample without difficulty.

In all phlebotomy, safety is of the utmost consideration. Dispose of all sharps properly and separately from the noncontaminated trash. Proper hand cleansing between patients and wearing gloves, goggles, and masks with each phlebotomy will ensure safety for both the patient and the medical assistant.

Proper specimen collection and handling of the specimen after collection by the medical assistant will ensure that the patient obtains the most accurate result. The specimen must be treated in such a way that the integrity of the specimen is maintained. The quality of the sample must be the same when collected as when tested. Correct method of draw, order of draw, and the correct handling of the sample after collection will reduce the number of factors affecting the sample and give the most accurate result possible.

STUDY FOR SUCCESS

To reinforce your knowledge and skills of information presented in this chapter:

- Review the Key Terms
- Practice the Procedures
- Consider the Case Study and discuss your conclusions
- Answer the Review Questions
  - Multiple Choice
  - Critical Thinking
- Navigate the Internet by completing the Web Activities
- Practice the StudyWARE activities on the CD
- Apply your knowledge in the Student Workbook activities
- Complete the Web Tutor sections
- View and discuss the DVD situations

REVIEW QUESTIONS

Multiple Choice

1. Drawing blood with a 25-gauge needle increases the chance for:
   a. vein collapse
   b. hematomas
   c. hemoconcentration
   d. hemolysis
2. An anticoagulant is an additive placed in vacuum tubes to:
   a. dilute the blood before testing
   b. ensure the sterility of the tube
   c. make the blood clot faster
   d. prevent the blood from clotting
3. When collecting a blood sample with a vacuum tube system, the last tube drawn is withdrawn from the holder before removing the needle from the patient to:
   a. avoid hematoma at the venipuncture site
   b. avoid dripping blood out the end of the needle
   c. prevent clotting of the blood
   d. cause the blood to clot
4. Leaving the tourniquet on a patient's arm for an extended length of time before drawing blood may cause:
   a. hemoconcentration
   b. specimen hemolysis
   c. stress
   d. bruising
5. The single most important way to prevent the spread of infection from patient to patient is:
   a. gowning and gloving
   b. hand washing
   c. always wearing masks
   d. avoid breathing on clients
6. Under Standard Precautions, all used needles are to be disposed of in the following manner:
   a. recapped
   b. discarded intact in a sharps container
   c. bent
   d. broken or cut off
7. When drawing multiple specimens in vacuum tubes, it is important to fill which of the following color-stoppered tubes first?
   a. light blue
   b. green
   c. lavender
   d. red
8. The anticoagulant of choice when drawing coagulation studies such as PT and APTT is:
   a. (red) no anticoagulant
   b. (light blue) sodium citrate
   c. (lavender) EDTA
   d. (green) heparin
9. When the medical assistant cannot perform a venipuncture successfully after two attempts, the medical assistant should:
   a. try at least two more times
   b. notify the provider
   c. ask another medical assistant to try
   d. request the test for the next day

10. If the blood is drawn too quickly from a small vein, the vein has a tendency to:
    a. collapse
    b. bruise
    c. disintegrate
    d. roll
11. What is OSHA's policy about choosing the safest needle systems to prevent accidental needlestick injuries?
    a. The clinic administrators can choose whatever is most cost effective.
    b. The clinic administrators should carefully choose the safest system for their staff.
    c. The clinic administrators must select the safest equipment based on feedback from the people who are using the needles.
    d. OSHA is not interfering with the clinics' rights to use any system they choose.

Critical Thinking

1. A frightened patient begins crying when you enter the room to perform a venipuncture. How will you handle the situation? What is your responsibility to the patient? Why are your demeanor and appearance important in this type of situation?
2. Explain the difference between serum and plasma. Describe how serum and plasma samples are collected.
3. How can vein collapse be avoided in a geriatric patient?
4. Discuss how clots are formed and what can be done to stop the clotting process.
5. You have calmed the crying patient and successfully drawn the patient's blood. What will you do next? Why is this step important? Describe the skills you have used.
6. The patient cries out in pain when you insert the needle into the vein. What will you do to make the patient more comfortable? If you decide to try another site, how will you locate it?

WEB ACTIVITIES

1. Visit the CDC and other government Web sites for the most current information on Standard Precautions and proper protection during blood draws.
2. Search the keywords "phlebotomy" and "puncture" on the Web. What organizations can you find that offer information for medical assistants?
3. Search the Internet for the laws in your state governing phlebotomy training.

REFERENCES/BIBLIOGRAPHY

Walters, N. J., Estridge, B. H., & Reynold, A. P. (2008). *Basic medical laboratory techniques* (5th ed.). Clifton Park, NY: Delmar Cengage Learning.

THE DVD HOOK-UP

This chapter discusses the various techniques for obtaining blood specimens from patients.

Today's designated scenes illustrate three various methods that are used to collect blood samples. The first method was the vacuum tube system. There was a special order for filling the blood tubes. The order of draw was slightly different between the DVD program and the text in this chapter. This is because both projects were written at different time intervals and the tube order changed between the projects. The information in this chapter has the latest information for the correct order of draw.

1. What is the order of draw according to this chapter? Does the order change when using a syringe? How about the capillary method? What will you do to make certain that you stay up to date with the latest information regarding tube orders and other important laboratory information once you graduate?
2. This chapter states that you should label the tubes immediately after the blood draw, but the DVD program states that you should label the tube before drawing the blood. Which technique does your instructor want you to follow?
3. Why is it important to determine if the patient followed all the fasting instructions before taking the patient's blood?

DVD Journal Summary

Write a paragraph that summarizes what you learned from watching the selected scenes from today's DVD program. Lori, the medical assistant, spoke about a patient who had a syncope episode while performing a phlebotomy. The patient fell back, hitting his head on the floor, and he immediately went into convulsions. The convulsions eventually stopped and the patient underwent X-rays. Fortunately, the patient had no damage as a result of the fall. How will you ascertain that your patients are safe during and after a blood draw? What are some signs that could indicate that the patient may faint? How would you feel if the patient did injure himself or herself while under your care?

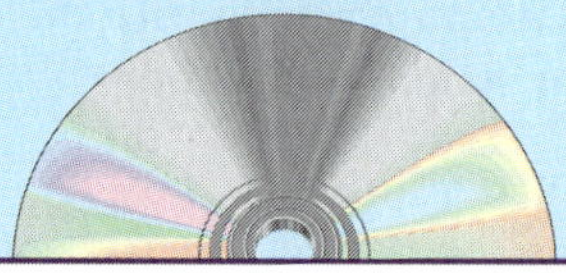

DVD Series Skills Based Series

Program Number 11

Chapter/Scene Reference

- *Administer Venipuncture, Vacuum Tube, and Syringe Method*
- *Preparing Slides for a Differential*
- *Administering Capillary Puncture and Performing Hematocrit Testing*

Chapter 29

Hematology

KEY TERMS

- Anisocytosis
- Basophil
- C-Reactive Protein (CRP)
- Complete Blood Count (CBC)
- Eosinophil (ESP)
- Erythrocyte
- Erythrocyte Indices
- Erythrocyte Sedimentation Rate (ESR)
- Erythropoietin
- Hematocrit
- Hematology
- Hematopoiesis
- Hemoglobin
- Hemoglobinopathy
- Hypochromic
- Leukocyte
- Lymphocyte
- Macrocytic
- Microcytic
- Monocyte
- Neutrophil
- Normochromic
- Normocytic
- Protime
- Reticulocyte (Retic)
- Thrombocyte

OUTLINE

- Hematologic Tests
- Hemoglobin and Hematocrit Tests
  - Hemoglobin
  - Hematocrit
- White and Red Blood Cell Counts
  - White Blood Cells and Differential
  - Red Blood Cells
- Platelets
- Erythrocyte Indices
  - Understanding RBC Indices
  - Using Erythrocyte Indices to Diagnose
- Erythrocyte Sedimentation Rates (ESR or SED Rate)
  - Wintrobe Method
  - Westergren Method
  - Using the ESR to Screen
- C-Reactive Proteins
- Coagulation Studies
- Automated Hematology

OBJECTIVES

The student should strive to meet the following performance objectives and demonstrate an understanding of the facts and principles presented in this chapter through written and oral communication.

1. Define the key terms as presented in the glossary.
2. Describe the process of hematopoiesis.
3. Discuss how the clinical science of hematology and the complete blood count (CBC) are used in the diagnosis and treatment of disease.
4. Compare the normal versus abnormal values of the CBC parameters.
5. Describe which blood tests and methods are within the scope of practice and training of the medical assistant performing under a CLIA Waived Test Certificate.
6. Discuss how the hemoglobin and hematocrit are used to diagnose anemia.
7. Describe how the erythrocyte indices are used in the differential diagnosis of anemias.
8. Perform the calculations necessary to derive the erythrocyte indices mean corpuscular cell volume, mean corpuscular hemoglobin, and mean corpuscular hemoglobin concentration.
9. List the five types of normal white blood cells and give the identifying characteristics of each.

OBJECTIVES (continued)

10. Describe the differences in the procedures for the Wintrobe and Westergren erythrocyte sedimentation rates.
11. Recognize the physiologic reasons why the erythrocyte sedimentation rate varies with different states of health and disease.
12. Describe CRP and its uses as a screening test for general infection and inflammation.
13. List the two general types of automated hematology instruments used in the ambulatory care setting and describe their technology.
14. Perform the laboratory procedures included in this chapter in a manner acceptable for entry-level employment.

Scenario

The providers in the office of Drs. Lewis and King often order hematologic tests to assist them in diagnosing and treating patients. As she performs the tests in the physician's office laboratory, medical assistant Audrey Jones uses her knowledge of hematology every day. Audrey is comfortable using an automated hematology analyzer or performing tests manually because she understands the purposes and procedures of the tests. She always follows all safety and quality-control guidelines to protect herself and others and to ensure the accuracy of test results.

INTRODUCTION

Hematology *is the study of the blood cells and coagulation in both normal and diseased states. The two main components of the blood are plasma (the liquid portion) and cells. Cells of the blood are also known as the formed elements of the blood. The study of hematology is usually limited to the cellular components of the blood and does not include the chemistry of the blood. See Chapter 32 for the chemistry of blood and tests related to blood chemistry.*

The cellular components of blood include ***erythrocytes*** *(red blood cells [RBCs]),* ***leukocytes*** *(white blood cells [WBCs]), and* ***thrombocytes*** *(platelets). Blood has many different functions. RBCs are responsible for supplying oxygen to all the cells of the body and removing the waste products of the cells: carbon dioxide. WBCs are involved in fighting infection, as well as producing antibodies for the immune system to defend against foreign antigens. There are five basic types of WBCs and they all have specific disease-fighting functions. Platelets are involved in homeostasis, the control of bleeding. Figure 28-2 shows the cellular elements of blood.*

Hematopoiesis *is defined as the formation of blood cells (Figure 29-1). The process of hematopoiesis, as well as the blood-forming tissues of the body, is included in the study of hematology. In the embryo, hematopoiesis occurs in the yolk sac, liver, and spleen. After we are born, the primary site for the production of erythrocytes, granulocytes, and platelets is the bone marrow. Lymphocytes are also produced in the bone marrow, as well as in the lymph nodes. At birth, most of the bone marrow in the body is capable of producing blood cells. This process is confined*

Spotlight on Certification

RMA Content Outline

- Asepsis
- Laboratory procedures

CMA (AAMA) Content Outline

- Principles of infection control
- Processing specimens
- Quality control
- Performing selected tests

CMAS Content Outline

- Asepsis in the medical office

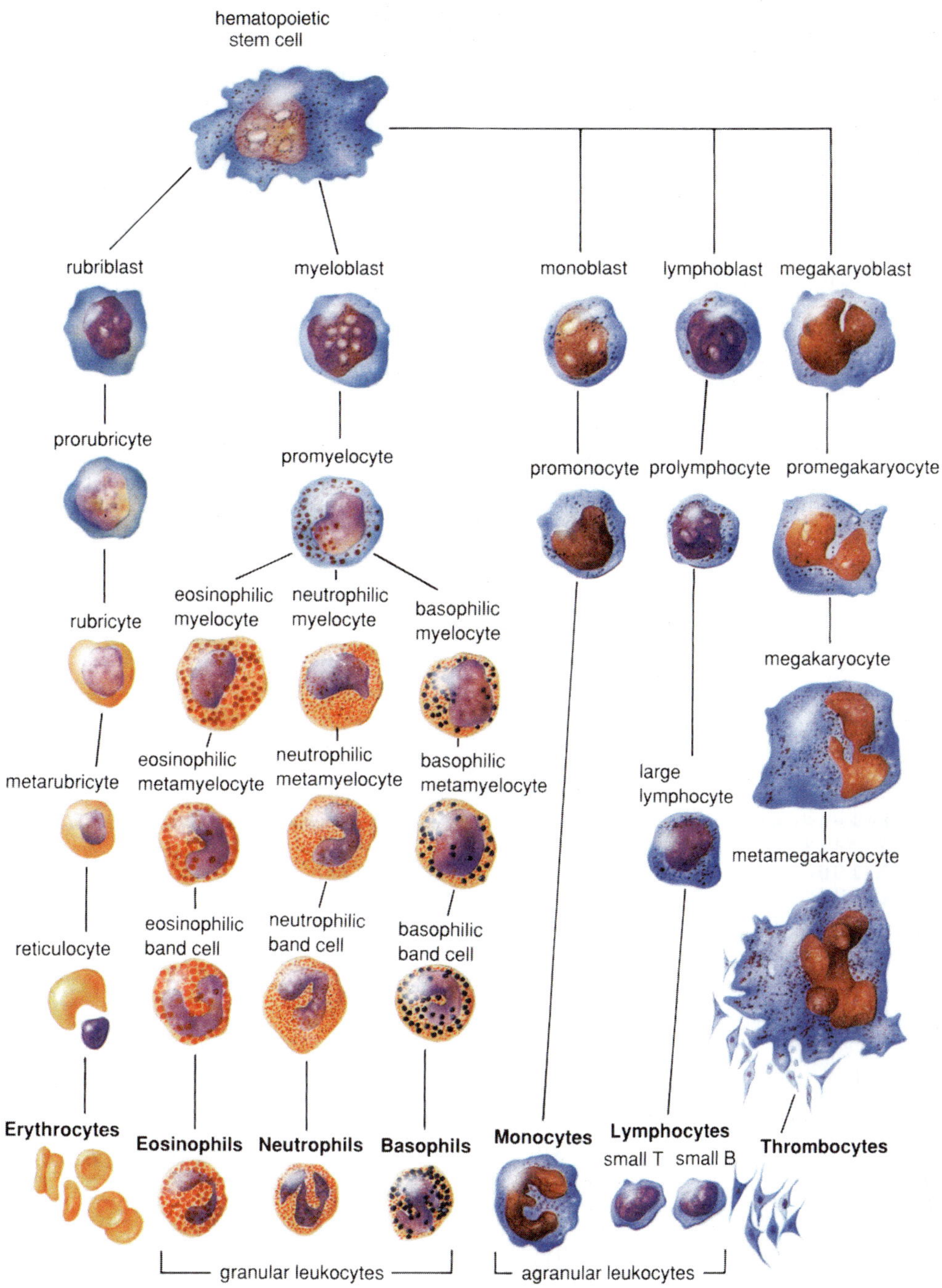

Figure 29-1 Hematopoiesis showing blood cells and platelet formation starting with hematopoietic stem cell.

to the bone marrow of the ribs, vertebrae, sternum, and iliac crest by the age of 20 years. Bone marrow that is producing cells is known as red marrow. As the area for hematopoiesis is reduced, the red bone marrow is replaced by yellow marrow, which is stored fat. When a provider collects a bone marrow sample in an adult, the site chosen for sampling is the sternum or the iliac crest because this is where the blood cells are still being produced.

Critical Thinking

What do you think would happen if you did not have any leukocytes? What would your symptoms be?

HEMATOLOGIC TESTS

Hematologic tests are the second most common tests performed in the physician's office laboratory (POL). The most common test is the urinalysis. The cellular components of the blood may be affected by changes in either the blood-forming organs or in other tissues of the body. The study of these changes forms the basis of hematologic tests performed in the POL.

Hematologic tests performed in the clinical laboratory include:

- Hemoglobin
- Hematocrit
- WBC count
- Differential WBC count
- RBC count
- RBC indices
- Platelet count
- Erythrocyte sedimentation rate (ESR)
- Prothrombin time (PT)

The results of these hematologic tests provide valuable information used by the provider in making a diagnosis, evaluating a patient's progress, and regulating further treatment.

The laboratory test ordered most frequently on blood in the ambulatory care setting is the **complete blood count (CBC).** The exact number of parameters included in the CBC will vary from laboratory to laboratory (Figure 29-2). The CBC generally includes:

- Hemoglobin determination
- Hematocrit determination
- RBC count (and indices)
- WBC count (and differential)
- Platelet count

Pat Name: Page: 1
Unit #/Acct #:
Loc:
Phys-Service:

In: 11/12/XX 0843
Out: 11/12/XX 1002
Coll Time: 11/12/XX 0840
Order Phys:

CBC WITH DIFFERENTIAL

Spec: Blood
Techs: V185 T180*
[A9331600017/4590]

Result Name	Result		Reference Range
WBC(10*3/ul):	12.6	H	4.8-10.8
RBC(10*6/ul):	4.51		4.2-5.4
Hgb(gm/dl):	12.8		12.0-16.0
Hct(%):	37.9		37.0-47.0
MCV(fl):	84.1		81.0-99.0
MCH(pg):	28.4		27.0-31.0
MCHC(gm/dl):	33.8		32.0-36.0
RDW(%):	13.6		11.5-14.5
Plt Cnt(X(10)3):	303		130-450
Neutrophil(%):	62.0		43-75
Lymph(%):	29.7		20-51
Mono (%):	5.9		2-11
Eos(%):	2.0		0-7.5
Basos(%):	0.4		0-2
Neutrophil(X(10)3):	9.3	H	1.5-6.6
Lymph (X(10)3):	2	L	1.5-3.5
Mono(X(10)3):	0.4		0-1.0
Eos (X(10)3):	0.1		0-0.7
Baso(X(10)3):	0.0		0-0.1

End of Report - 03/09/XX 15:34

Single Test Report-HEMATOLOGY

Figure 29-2 Hematology report form.

All these tests can be performed by manual testing procedures or with an automated hematology analyzer. Manual blood cell counts are considered by the Clinical Laboratory Improvement Act (CLIA) to be of moderate to high complexity, whereas the automated tests are considered to be moderately complex; therefore, neither are within the medical assistant's scope of practice. The manual blood cell counts are performed only at reference laboratories by medical technicians. The automated analyzers may be located in the POL, but the testing and interpretation of the tests, the maintenance of the analyzers, as well as training and supervision of laboratory personnel is performed by the medical technician.

Test results are recorded in the patient's medical record in the progress notes section and a lab report is completed. The lab report is filed in the lab section of the patient record. Accurate and timely documentation are important in medical laboratory procedures.

A total practice management system (TPMS) allows test results to be recorded in the patient's medical record as well as documentation of quality controls performed prior to patient test results (Figure 29-3).

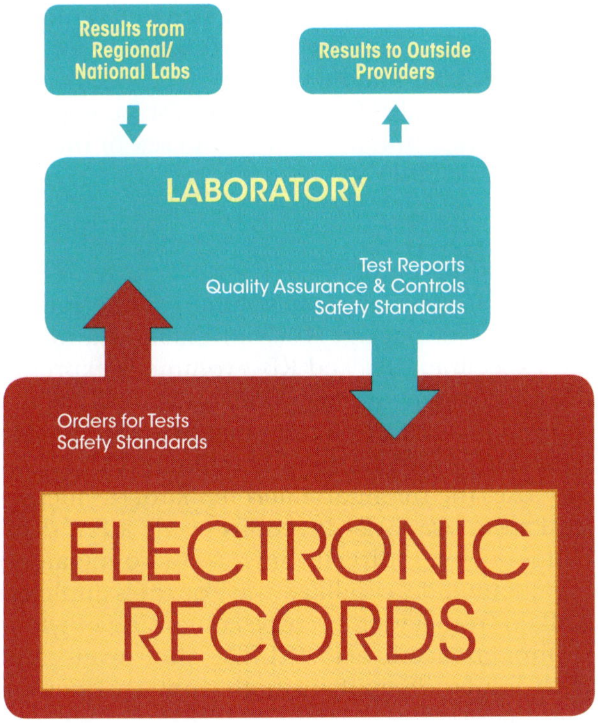

Figure 29-3 The laboratory arm of the total practice management system (TPMS). Quality controls and test results are easily recorded in a TPMS.

HEMOGLOBIN AND HEMATOCRIT TESTS

Hemoglobin and **hematocrit** tests are part of the CBC; however, they are frequently individually ordered by the provider rather than a CBC. The abbreviations for hemoglobin and hematocrit are Hgb and Hct, respectively. Although they are separate tests, they have a unique relationship with each other but may be performed individually. Both the hemoglobin and the hematocrit are performed to obtain similar information about RBCs in relation to the rest of the blood sample, but they also give decidedly different information. In normal results, the hemoglobin often will be about one third the number of the hematocrit.

Hemoglobin

Hemoglobin is the major component of the RBC and serves to transport oxygen and carbon dioxide through the body. Hemoglobin, which is responsible for about 85% of the dry weight of the RBC, is a conjugated (combined) protein composed of heme and globin. A single hemoglobin molecule consists of four globin chains with a heme group attached to each globin (Figure 29-4). The central component of each heme group is an iron molecule. One oxygen molecule can be transported to each heme group; therefore, each RBC can carry four oxygen molecules.

Synthesis of the heme portion of the hemoglobin molecule requires iron, which is usually obtained through our diets. The daily iron

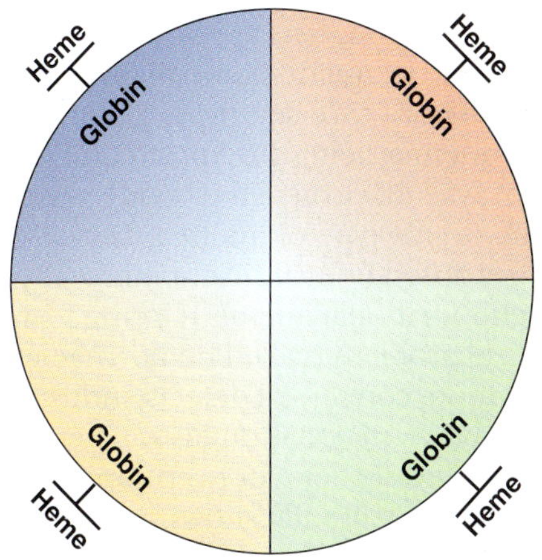

Figure 29-4 A normal hemoglobin molecule containing four globin chains with a heme group attached to each globin. One oxygen molecule can be transported by each heme group.

requirement for an adult man is about 0.5 mg/day, whereas a menstruating woman requires about four times that much, or 2 mg/day.

Hemoglobin carries about 95% of the oxygen to the body cells and carries away about 27% of the carbon dioxide. The RBCs pick up the oxygen in the lungs from when we breathe in, and they drop off the carbon dioxide in the lungs to be expelled when we breathe out. The rest of the carbon dioxide is removed through other processes. Oxygenated hemoglobin is bright red, and hemoglobin unbound to oxygen is darker. This explains the bright red color of arterial blood (going from the lungs and to the cells) and the darker color of venous blood (going back to the lungs).

A second function of hemoglobin is as a blood buffer; that is, hemoglobin helps maintain the proper pH balance of the blood as it picks up and drops off oxygen and carbon dioxide.

The production of new RBCs and consequently the formation of new hemoglobin is triggered by a hormone called **erythropoietin,** which is produced in the kidney. The erythropoietin process is activated when the body cells sense a low oxygen level.

There are several forms of hemoglobin. Hemoglobin A (Hgb A) is the most common form found in adults. The other hemoglobin types are abnormal and are responsible for a group of diseases known as **hemoglobinopathies.** These abnormal forms of hemoglobin include hemoglobin S (Hgb S), hemoglobin C, and hemoglobin E. Hgb S is the most common abnormal form of hemoglobin observed in the laboratory. It is the form of hemoglobin that causes sickle cell anemia. When Hgb S molecules are subjected to certain conditions, they alter the physical structure of the RBCs. The RBCs assume a sickle shape, which makes it difficult, if not impossible, for the cell to pass through a capillary bed.

The most frequent hemoglobin disease seen in the ambulatory care setting is anemia, with iron deficiency anemia being the most common type. A decrease of available iron in the body is the most common cause of this type of anemia. Lack of available iron can be caused by insufficient intake through the diet (called nutritional anemia); losing iron because of a bleeding problem (called hemorrhagic anemia); or less common, congenital defects, industrial toxins, diseases of bone marrow (aplastic anemia), and a variety of other disorders. In nutritional anemia, the laboratory finding usually shows a normal or near-normal hematocrit (because these patients have the right percentage of RBCs) but a low hemoglobin. Their RBCs are hypochromic (pale) because they lack oxygen. The main symptom of anemia, fatigue, is also caused by lack of oxygen.

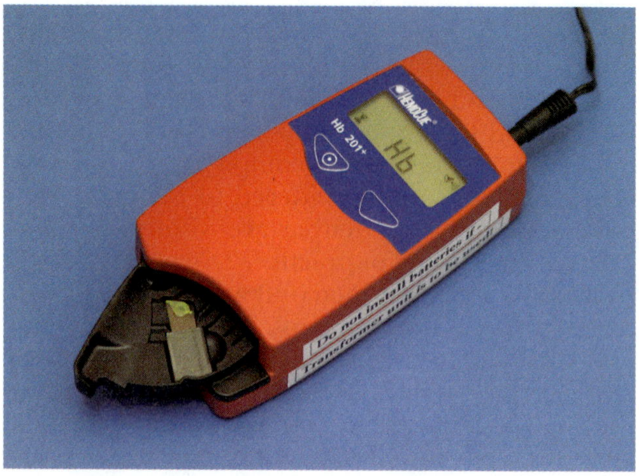

Figure 29-5 HemoCue instrument used for automated test.

Hemoglobin is measured in the POL using an automated device called the HemoCue (Figure 29-5). The HemoCue is an infrared analyzer that measures the density of the hemoglobin pigment by light refraction. The more hemoglobin present in the sample, the more light is refracted. This is a quick method, uses only a small drop of blood, and gives immediate results (see Procedure 29-1).

CAUTION: The solution within the HemoCue is poisonous. Precautions to observe when working with any reagents includes wearing gloves, working in a well-ventilated area, properly disposing of used reagents, wiping up all spills, and hand washing.

The normal reference values for hemoglobin vary according to both the age and sex of the individual (Table 29-1).

Hematocrit

Hematocrit (packed RBC volume) is the ratio of the volume of packed RBCs to that of the whole-blood specimen. Packed RBC volume is expressed as a percentage of the whole specimen. This is achieved manually or by automated methods. Most medical assistants working in ambulatory care settings use the manual microhematocrit method (see Procedure 29-2) It requires only a few drops of blood either directly into a microhematocrit tube obtained by capillary draw, or the sample can be taken from a vacuum tube containing ethylenediaminetetraacetic acid (EDTA) after a venipuncture. Chapter 28 explains both capillary draw and venipuncture.

The cellular components of the blood sample separate into layers when they are centrifuged at high speeds (Figures 29-6 and 29-7). The cellular layers

Table 29-1 Normal Hemoglobin Values or Reference Ranges by Age and/or Sex

Newborn	15–20 g/dL
Age 3 months	9–14 g/dL
Age 10 months	12–14.5 g/dL
Adult woman	12–16 g/dL
Adult man	13–18 g/dL

Table 29-2 Normal Hematocrit Values or Reference Ranges by Age and/or Sex

Newborn	45–60%
1-year-old child	27–44%
Adult female	36–46%
Adult male	40–55%

Table 29-3 Normal Leukocyte Counts

	Leukocyte Count (cells/mm³)	
Age	**Average**	**Reference Range**
Newborn	18,000	9,000–30,000
1-year-old toddler	11,000	6,000–14,000
6-year-old child	8,000	4,500–12,000
Adult	7,000	4,500–11,000

Table 29-4 Normal Values for a Differential Leukocyte Count in Adults

Neutrophil Bands: 3–5% Neutrophil bands increase in appendicitis and many other diseases.
Neutrophil Segs: 54–62% Segmented neutrophils increase in appendicitis and many other diseases. An elevation in neutrophils usually is indicative of an infectious disease.
Lymphocytes: 25–33% Lymphocytes increase with infectious mononucleosis, lymphocytic leukemia, and many diseases of viral origin.
Monocytes: 3–7% Monocytes increase in tuberculosis and monocytic leukemia.
Eosinophils: 1–3% Eosinophils increase with allergic reactions, hay fever, and parasitic infections.
Basophils: 0–1% Basophils increase in polycythemia vera, chicken pox, and ulcerative colitis.

Table 29-5 Normal Erythrocyte Counts

Age	Reference Range
Newborn	$5.0–6.5 \times 10^6/mm^3$
1-year-old child	$4.0–5.0 \times 10^6/mm^3$
Adult woman	$4.0–5.5 \times 10^6/mm^3$
Adult man	$4.5–6.0 \times 10^6/mm^3$

Table 29-6 Normal Values for the Erythrocyte Indices

MCV	80–100 fL
MCH	27–33 pg
MCHC	32–36 g/dL

Table 29-7 Normal Values for the Wintrobe Method of ESR

Male patients	0–9 mm/hr
Female patients	0–20 mm/hr

Table 29-8 Normal Values for the Westergren Method of ESR

Male patients younger than 50 years	0–15 mm/hr
Male patients older than 50 years	0–20 mm/hr
Female patients younger than 50 years	0–20 mm/hr
Female patients older than 50 years	0–30 mm/hr

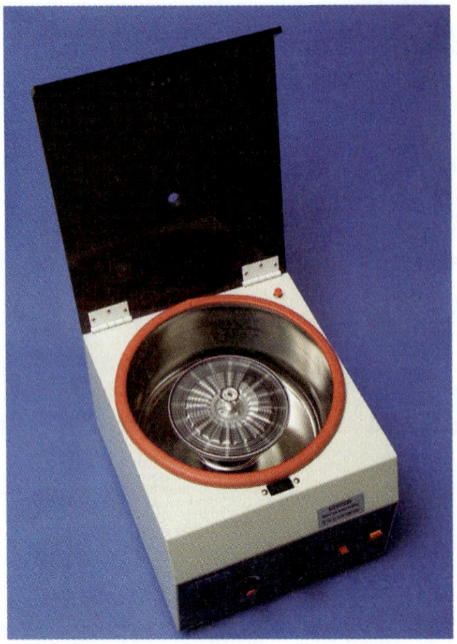

Figure 29-6 Microhematocrit centrifuge.

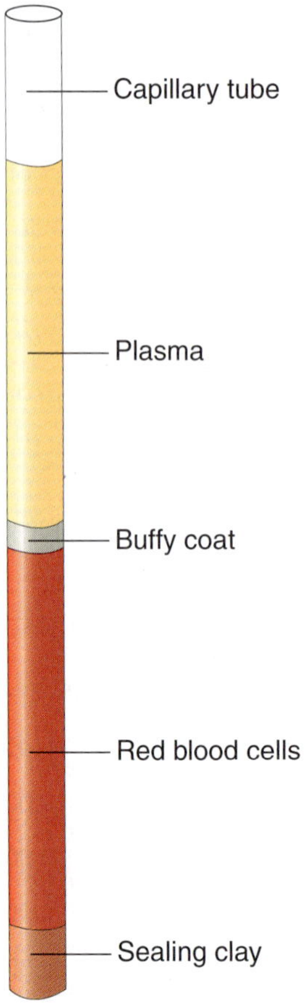

Figure 29-7 Diagram of packed cell column in the hematocrit tube showing separation of cellular components after centrifugation.

arrange themselves with the RBCs at the bottom of the tube. RBCs are the most numerous and the heaviest of the cellular components. WBCs and platelets form a thin layer called the buffy coat on top of the erythrocytes. The buffy coat has a whitish tan appearance. The plasma often is so clear it is difficult to see.

The WBC count of the sample can be estimated by measuring the buffy coat thickness. Each 0.1 mm of the buffy coat equals approximately 1,000 WBC/mm^3. Therefore, a buffy coat of 1 mm would equal a leukocyte count of approximately 10,000 WBCs/mm^3, and a 0.5 mm reading would equal 5,000 WBCs/mm^3. The cell counts may be reported in units of microliters (mcL), which are equivalent to cubic millimeters.

The normal values of hematocrit vary according to the age and sex of the individual (Table 29-2).

Sources of error associated with the microhematocrit method include improper centrifugation, resulting in increased trapped plasma, and improper reading of the packed RBC volume, such as including the buffy coat layer.

Procedure 29-2 explains the microhematocrit method of determining blood hematocrit levels. Review Chapter 28 sections on capillary tubes and capillary draw together with Procedure 28-5.

WHITE AND RED BLOOD CELL COUNTS

WBC and RBC counts can be performed using either a manual or automated method. Because neither method is considered CLIA waived, neither is within the scope of practice for the medical assistant. The Introduction discusses the functions of blood cells, and you will learn much more in your anatomy and physiology course. The formation of blood cells was shown in Figure 29-1. Because blood cell counts are not performed by medical assistants, this section does not discuss the test process itself but rather the diagnostic implications of the leukocyte count with the differential.

White Blood Cells and Differential

WBCs do not necessarily remain within the blood vessels like RBCs do. They leave the blood vessels and travel to the tissues of the body to find and destroy pathogens. When a "bacterial battle" is fought in an area and many WBCs have died, the "battlefield" may be too large for the body to clean up. In these cases, pus can occur. A localized accumulation of pus is called an abscess and often must be incised (lanced) to aid in the removal of the pus. Chapter 19 discusses incision and drainage surgery for the purpose of incising and draining an abscess. Antibiotics are useful in some cases to help the leukocytes fight off the bacteria and remove the infection. When leukocytes travel into the tissues, most of them do not return to the bloodstream. The **lymphocyte** is the only type that does; it travels to the lymphatic system where it is specialized and matured (hence, its name), then returns to the bloodstream to await a mission. The normal values for white blood cells vary with age. Babies need more, because they have not yet built up antibody protections (Table 29-3).

WBCs or leukocytes can be divided into two basic groups: granulocytes, which contain granules within their cytoplasm, and agranulocytes, which do not contain granules. The presence of granules can be visualized by the trained eye after a staining process during the manual WBC count. Even during the automated method, the leukocyte is identified by the contents of the cytoplasm and the shape of their nuclei. The granulocytes are the **neutrophils, basophils,** and **eosinophils** (notice they all end in *-phil,* which will help you remember their cytoplasm is "filled" with granules). The agranulocytes are the lymphocytes and the monocytes.

The nuclei of the leukocytes differ from each other, as well as the cytoplasm. All three of the granulocytes contain nuclei that are multilobed or segmented (sometimes they are even called segs). They are described as being polymorphonuclear cells (*poly* means "many," *morpho* means "shape," and *nuclear* means "nucleus"). The immature neutrophil has a nucleus that has not yet formed lobes and is called a band cell (or stab cell) because its nucleus looks sort of like a comma. The agranulocytes do not form lobed nuclei; their nuclei are rounded in a single mass. Because of their single nuclei, the aganulocytes are sometimes called mononuclear (meaning one nucleus). Because so many different names can be confusing, this chapter provides an identification guide and pictures for you (see Table 29-4, Leukocyte Identification Guide box, and Figure 29-8).

Each of the five types provide specialized protection. Some of their methods include phagocytosis, detoxification, inflammation, and immune response.

Phagocytosis is an engulfing process performed by all leukocytes, but especially the neutrophils and the monocytes. Once the bacteria or particles are engulfed, the material is destroyed by enzymes present in the leukocyte. Phagocytosis is so important as a means of protection, we would die if our leukocytes lost their ability to perform this process.

Detoxification is a neutralizing process that is effective against poisons and other harmful substances. Eosinophils use detoxification to control allergic reactions and histamine production.

Inflammation is a general process that occurs as a sequence of events. Chapter 10 explains the inflammatory process in more detail. The leukocyte most actively involved in inflammation is the basophil, which releases histamine into injured tissue to increase inflammation (antihistamines work to reduce inflammation). Basophils also contain the anticoagulant heparin. The basophil synchronizes the entire inflammatory process; thus, the poison is rendered harmless, the offending agents are eliminated, and the area is cleaned up of all the necrotic tissue and is ready for repair.

Immune response is a series of complicated and involved specific antigen–antibody reactions. Simply stated, when a harmful substance enters the human body, the adaptive immune response provided by the lymphocyte destroys the harmful substance. A "memory" is created so that the next time the body is exposed, it recognizes the intruder and is better able to prevent the illness again. This is called immunity. Immunity can be permanent or temporary, passively acquired or actively acquired. Passively acquired immunity is

LEUKOCYTE IDENTIFICATION GUIDE

Cell Types	Functions
Granulocytes	
Neutrophils	Phagocytosis of bacteria
Mature are segmented cells/segs	Destruction by enzymes
Immature are bands or stabs	
Eosinophils	Detoxification of toxins and harmful substances
	Neutralize histamine
	Destroy parasitic worms
Basophils	Mediate inflammation
	Release histamine to increase inflammation
	Release heparin to inhibit blood clotting
Agranulocytes	
Monocytes	Phagocytosis to clean up
Lymphocytes	Destruction of viruses
	Immune response

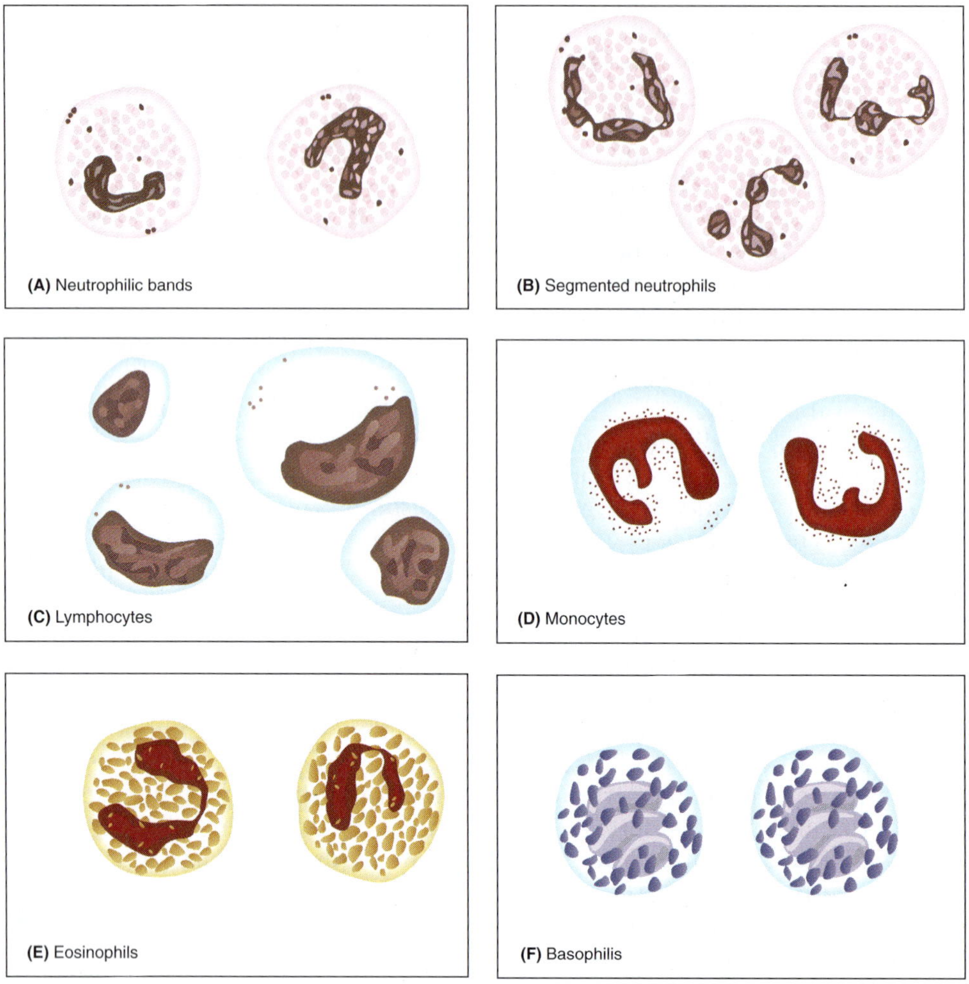

Figure 29-8 Various types of leukocytes from a stained blood smear.

gifted to us either in utero (congenital or natural) or through an injection (artificial). Actively acquired immunity requires us to actively fight off a disease, and because we take active part in creating the immunity, it is usually permanent. Passively acquired immunities do not make us sick, but they usually do not last longer than 6 months.

Not only do the leukocytes fight off pathogens/toxins in a variety of ways, they also are fairly specific in the types of pathogens they do battle with (see Table 29-4). Neutrophils are the most numerous of all leukocytes and for good reason. They are there to destroy bacteria, which is our most common enemy. The second largest group is the lymphocytes, and they fight our second most common enemy: viruses. Lymphocytes are also involved in immune responses, which explains why we have immunity to viruses and not to other substances or microbes. Basophils release histamine to increase inflammation into injured tissues. Inflammation usually is our friend, but sometimes the inflammation is too severe.

This is what can happen in an allergic reaction. Eosinophils are especially well suited to battle the inflammation accompanying allergic-type reactions

Some examples of blood cell changes associated with disease states are:

1. When a patient is experiencing an acute appendicitis, the white blood cell count increases rapidly with a high percentage of neutrophils. There is also an increase in the number of early or younger forms of these cells.
2. Patients who are suffering from a viral infection, especially adults, frequently experience a reduction in white blood cells and an increase in the percentage of lymphocytes. Patients with infectious mononucleosis have increased numbers of lymphocytes, many of which are atypical.
3. When patients have iron deficiency anemia, their indices demonstrate red blood cells that show marked reduction in hemoglobin content. Their erythrocytes appear hypochromic, lacking or low in color, because they lack the normal amount of hemoglobin in the red blood cells.

because they neutralize the histamines. **Monocytes** can be likened to the "cleanup crew" because these "big eaters" come in later to clean up the battlefield of the cellular debris and other substances.

Red Blood Cells

RBCs (erythrocytes) are very different from WBCs in composition, function, and numbers (Table 29-5). Remember from the Introduction that erythrocytes are responsible for carrying oxygen to the body's cells and bringing back the carbon dioxide. To have room to carry the oxygen and carbon dioxide molecules, the erythrocyte leaves its nucleus in the bone marrow where it is formed. The nucleus is used again and again to create other erythrocytes. Our bodies are efficient at recycling raw materials. If an erythrocyte is released from the bone marrow before it is mature, it may retain some of its nucleus material. It is then called a **reticulocyte (retic).** About 1% of the circulating erythrocytes are reticulocytes, and an increase in the number of circulating reticulocytes is an indication that the body needs more erythrocytes. This can occur in cases of hemorrhage and anemia. Erythrocytes can be of varying sizes. When erythrocytes are of normal size, they are called **normocytic.** Those that are larger are called **macrocytic,** and those that are smaller are called **microcytic.** When the erythrocytes show marked variation in size, the condition is called **anisocytosis.** The normal erythrocyte has a round or slightly oval shape. If the shape of the erythrocytes show marked variation, the condition is known as poikilocytosis.

The RBC should contain hemoglobin that fills about half of the cell. The RBC is biconcave, so most of the hemoglobin is seen around the outer part of the cell. The central area of the RBC is pale. RBCs with the proper amount of hemoglobin are called **normochromic.** Those that do not have enough hemoglobin, that demonstrate too large of a pale central area, are called **hypochromic.**

Clinical Laboratory Improvement Amendment, 1988 (CLIA '88) Regulation Regarding WBC Differential Counts

- Laboratories that are certified for waiver-level testing only are not permitted to perform manual WBC differential counts.
- Laboratories with a moderate-complexity certification can perform a manual differential WBC count but may only identify and report normal cells.
- Laboratories certified to perform tests of high complexity can perform a manual differential WBC count and are permitted to identify and report both abnormal and normal cells.
- Laboratories with moderate to complex certification can perform automated WBC counts including the reporting of abnormal results. Only qualified medical technicians and higher personnel may use and maintain the machines.

See Chapter 26 for details on CLIA '88 regulations.

PLATELETS

The normal number of platelets (thrombocytes) is 140,000 to 400,000 per microliter of blood. Thrombocytes are actually fragments of cells. Like mature erythrocytes, thrombocytes have no nuclei. Thrombocytes are involved in the clotting of blood, or coagulation. Coagulation is a complex series of events that contains 13 distinct steps. A brief overview is provided here. When the body is physically injured, chemicals are released. Included in these chemicals are thromboplastin from injured tissues and plasma proteins and factors released from platelets. These chemicals form prothrombin activator. Prothrombin activator (with calcium) converts (activates) a blood protein called prothrombin into thrombin. Thrombin converts another blood protein called fibrinogen into fibrin. Fibrin is stringy and traps the sticky blood cells in a web at the site of injury, forming a plug of sorts. Eventually, the plug starts drying up, shrinks (pulling the edges of a wound together), and forms a scab.

What is really fascinating about the clotting of blood is why blood does not normally clot inside the blood vessels. Two chemicals made in the human body prevent that from happening. One is heparin, which is released from basophils and endothelial cells, and the other is antithrombin, which is released by the liver. The body needs blood to clot to stop bleeding, but it is important that blood not clot inside the body where it can cause problems and even death.

ERYTHROCYTE INDICES

The **erythrocyte indices** include the mean corpuscular (cell) volume (MCV), the mean corpuscular hemoglobin (MCH), and the mean corpuscular hemoglobin concentration (MCHC). These indices (plural for index) are calculations that provide information about the size of the RBCs and the hemoglobin content. The blood parameters needed to calculate all three indices are the RBC count, the hematocrit, and the hemoglobin. The erythrocyte indices values are important in the diagnosis or classification and treatment of different types of anemia. Table 29-6 shows normal values for the erythrocyte indices.

Before the automated hematology instrument became commonly used in the ambulatory care setting, the erythrocyte indices were not included as a part of the CBC because the RBC count was not an accurate measurement.

The following formulas are used to calculate the erythrocyte indices:

$$\text{MCV} = \frac{\text{Hematocrit}}{\text{RBC (in millions)}} \times 10$$

The result is reported in femtoliters (fL), a unit of volume 10^{-15} L, formerly reported in cubic microns (μm^3). This index gives the average volume of RBCs in the sample.

$$\text{MCH} = \frac{\text{Hemoglobin (in grams)}}{\text{RBC (in millions)}} \times 10$$

The result is expressed in picograms (pg), a micro microgram, or 1×10^{-12} g. This index estimates the weight of hemoglobin in RBCs of the sample.

$$\text{MCHC} = \frac{\text{Hemoglobin (in grams)}}{\text{Hematocrit}} \times 10$$

This result is expressed in grams/deciliter (g/dL). The MCHC is the average concentration of hemoglobin in a given volume of packed RBCs (hematocrit).

Understanding RBC Indices

If we think of the red blood cells as water balloons filled with red-colored water, we might better understand the indices: The red-colored water signifies the hemoglobin inside the red blood cell. We have a basket of water balloons to signify our blood sample.

Because each water balloon is a different size (as are our red blood cells), we would need to measure the size of all of them to get the average volume or mass. We would add together the size/mass of all the balloons in our basket, then divide that number by the number of balloons in the basket. This gives us the average (mean) mass (volume), or MCV.

If we use MCH in the above example, we are measuring the average amount/concentration of water in the balloons. To measure this, we would pop each balloon, measure the total amount of water, and then divide by how many balloons there were. This would give us the average (mean) amount of red water (hemoglobin), or MCH.

Using the same water balloon comparison for explaining the MCHC, it would be the intensity of the red water within all the balloons. Some of the balloons might contain light red water, some might contain dark red water. The average of the intensity would give us the average (mean) intensity (concentration), or the MCHC.

All of these numbers together tell us about how many balloons (RBC) there are in the basket/sample, their average size (volume), how much they contain (amount hemoglobin/water), and the average concentration/intensity of the red water (hemoglobin) within all of them.

Understanding the relationship between the MCV, MCH, and MCHC helps to better understand what is happening when a patient is anemic due to low hemoglobin within each RBC versus a patient who is anemic due to low RBC count and so forth.

Critical Thinking

If the patient's hematocrit is 37 and the RBC count is 5 million, what would the MCV be?

Using Erythrocyte Indices to Diagnose

The MCH and MCV are increased in megaloblastic anemias such as vitamin B_{12} and folate deficiency anemias. They also are increased in acute blood loss anemia, chronic hemolytic anemias, aplastic anemias, hypothyroidism, and liver disease. The MCH and MCV are decreased in hypochromic and microcytic anemias, including iron deficiency anemia, thalassemias, and occasionally in hyperthyroidism.

The MCHC is increased in hereditary spherocytosis. It is normal in macrocytosis. The MCHC is decreased in iron deficiency anemia. The stained blood smear of a person with iron deficiency anemia demonstrates RBCs that are both hypochromic and microcytic.

ERYTHROCYTE SEDIMENTATION RATES (ESR OR SED RATE)

The **erythrocyte sedimentation rate (ESR),** as the name implies, is a measurement of the rate at which the RBCs in a well-mixed, anticoagulated blood sample will fall, or settle, toward the bottom when it is placed in a vertical tube. This test is commonly referred to in the laboratory as a "sed rate" (see Procedure 29-3). The ESR has been used for many years in the diagnosis and treatment of many disease states of the body. It is an inexpensive, accurate, and easy test to perform. Two factors that influence the sedimentation rate are the condition of the surface membrane of the RBC and changes in the level of fibrinogen in the plasma of the blood. During disease conditions in the body, the surface membrane of the RBC is altered, as well as the levels of fibrinogen, and this affects the rate at which the RBCs fall in the tube. RBCs will demonstrate this change even after the disease has subsided because RBCs have an average life of 120 days. For this reason, the ESR is a more accurate tool in diagnosing the onset of a disease than in checking the progress of treatment.

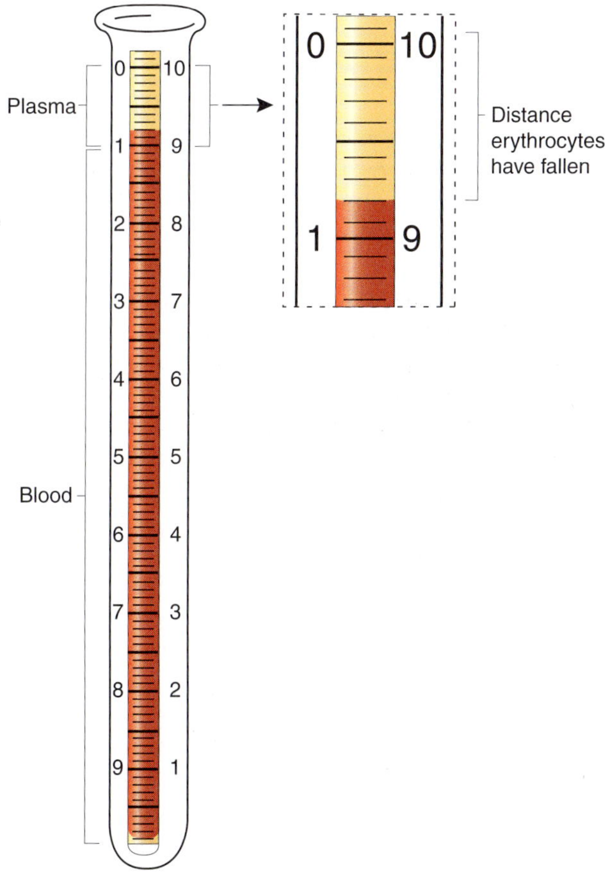

Figure 29-9 Wintrobe sedimentation tube showing settling of cells. The example shows a sedimentation of 8 mm.

Two ways to perform an ESR test are the Wintrobe method and the Westergren method. Both methods will provide the same information. Because of the simplicity in setting up the Westergren ESR, it has become the more widely used method in the ambulatory care setting's POL.

Wintrobe Method

An EDTA venous blood sample is thoroughly mixed. With the use of a Pasteur pipette, the blood is transferred to a Wintrobe tube. The blood is added to the left zero mark at the top of the tube. It is important that no air bubbles are present in the blood column. The tube is placed exactly vertical in a rack and allowed to stand for exactly 60 minutes. The test is read by determining the number of millimeters (mm) the red cells have settled. The tube has a total capacity of 100 mm. The test is reported in millimeters per hour (Figure 29-9). Table 29-7 lists normal values for the Wintrobe method of ESR.

Westergren Method

The Westergren method differs from the Wintrobe method in that the blood sample is mixed with 3.8% sodium citrate solution before the tube is filled. The blood and sodium citrate are mixed and the tube is filled to the zero mark and placed exactly vertical in a rack. The tube is read after exactly 60 minutes, and the test is reported in millimeters per hour. Table 29-8 gives normal values for the Westergren method of ESR.

The Polymedco company produces a Sediplast® system to perform a Westergren ESR that is self-filling. It is a completely closed system that protects laboratory personnel from the risks associated with blood handling. The Sediplast® ESR System is shown in Figure 29-10.

The following guidelines should be followed when performing Wintrobe and Westergren ESR procedures to ensure accurate test results:

1. The tube must remain exactly vertical during the 1-hour test time.
2. The test must be read at exactly 60 minutes (1 hour).
3. The counter on which the rack is placed must be free of vibrations.
4. The test should be set up within 2 hours after the blood is drawn.
5. The test should be conducted at room temperature.

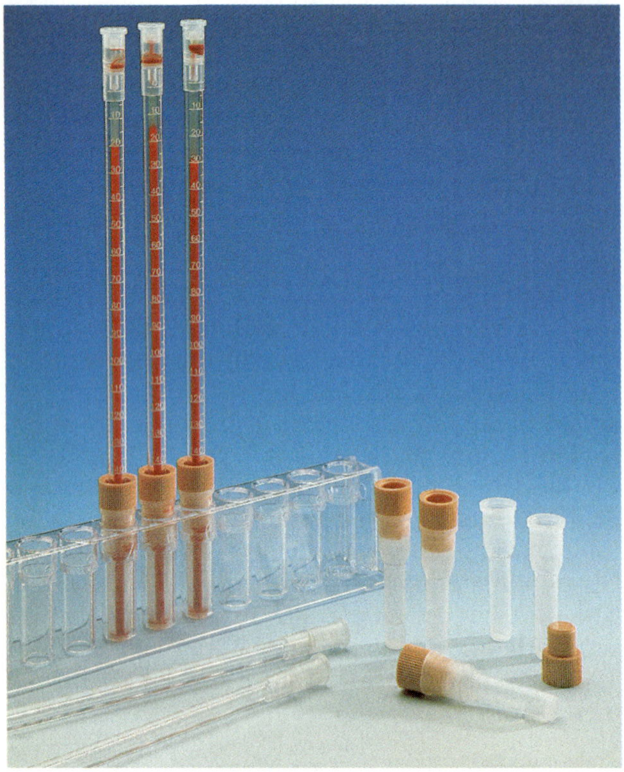

Figure 29-10 Westergren method using Sediplast® ESR System. Three filled tubes are standing in the rack. Note the diluting vials with sodium citrate solution (right). (Courtesy of Polymedco, Inc., Cortlandt Manor, NY.)

6. The tube should not be placed in a draft, and it should not be exposed to direct sunlight.
7. The column of blood must be free of bubbles.

The erythrocytes in normal, nondiseased blood tend to remain suspended in the plasma. They do not aggregate (clump) together to form rouleaux. Rouleaux is a phenomenon where RBCs form aggregates that look like rolls or stacks of coins (Figure 29-11).

This aggregate form causes the rate of sedimentation to increase. RBCs have membrane properties that tend to make them remain separated in the plasma. During certain diseased states, this repelling property is lost and the RBCs tend to aggregate.

Using the ESR to Screen

ESRs are increased in infections, acute stress, and inflammatory diseases, tissue destruction, and other conditions that lead to an increase in plasma fibrinogen. They are also increased with menstruation, pregnancy, lupus, malignant neoplasms, and multiple myeloma. With anemia, the ESR increases according to the severity of the condition.

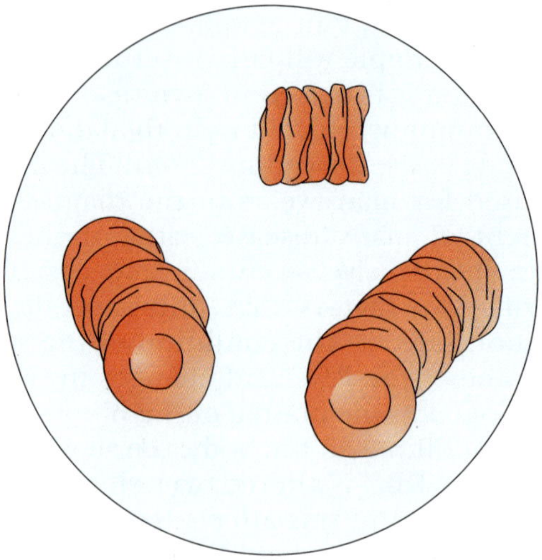

Figure 29-11 Erythrocytes forming rouleaux.

The ESR may be normal in osteoarthritis and in some cases of cirrhosis and malaria. ESR values are decreased in polycythemia, spherocytosis, and sickle cell anemia.

C-REACTIVE PROTEINS

Another screening blood test for inflammation is **C-reactive protein** or **CRP.** The CRP level will rise and drop quicker than the ESR, giving the provider more timely information about the effectiveness of treatment.

Like the ESR, CRP is helpful in determining systemic inflammatory conditions such as autoimmune diseases, inflammatory bowel conditions, and some forms of arthritis. While it is not specifically diagnostic for any one disease, it can serve as a marker for general infection and inflammation, and, once the disease or condition is diagnosed, it can help determine the effectiveness of treatment.

CRP is made by the liver and released into the bloodstream. It increases when infection and inflammation are present. It has been used for many years as an indicator of bacterial and viral infections.

Due to the more recent studies showing the correlation between vascular inflammation and heart disease, a more sensitive CRP-related test called hsCRP (highly sensitive C-reactive protein) has gained popularity in detecting vascular inflammation that can indicate coronary artery disease and cardiovascular disease. The hsCRP is used in conjunction with the traditional lipid profile and cardiac risk assessment.

COAGULATION STUDIES

Persons prone to forming blood clots often are medicated with anticoagulants (blood thinners) such as Coumadin or heparin. While a patient is taking an anticoagulant, it is important to determine the blood is able to clot within a reasonable amount of time, which ensures that the patient is taking the correct dosage. The method of monitoring coagulation time is called the prothrombin time (PT), or, more commonly the **protime.** The protime is reported in the time (seconds) it takes for the patient's blood to clot and in the international normalized ratio (INR). We still refer to both tests as protime. Currently the INR is more useful because it is standardized, that is, it can be universally applied, in contrast to the timing test, which can vary quite a bit from facility to facility. Normal blood will clot in about 11 to 13 seconds. The provider will want the patient taking anticoagulant medication to have a protime of approximately 16 to 18 seconds and INR of 2.0 to 2.6 (sometimes higher). If blood clots too soon, the anticoagulant medication is not at a therapeutic level. If the blood clotting takes too long (prolonged clotting), then the patient is taking too much medication. An INR of 1.0 is considered ineffective; 5.0 is considered dangerous.

Because activities of daily living, such as diet, can interfere with clotting factors, the protime usually is tested on a regular basis, weekly at the beginning of treatment, then monthly or less frequently as treatment progresses. If the patient experiences frequent unusual bruising or bleeding that might indicate an imbalance in clotting ability, then the protime test can be run "on demand." Some foods rich in vitamin K (e.g., dark leafy vegetables), alcohol, vitamins and supplements, aspirin, and many other medications can interfere with anticoagulant therapy. Health care professionals must interview the patient carefully about what is being taken. Patient education and patient compliance both are important components of effective treatment with anticoagulants.

The protime test is also used as a screening test for people who have liver disease or clotting factor disease or who are vitamin K deficient.

The protime is a simple CLIA waived test that is performed on a drop of blood (Figure 29-12). Procedure 29-4 describes the step-by-step process.

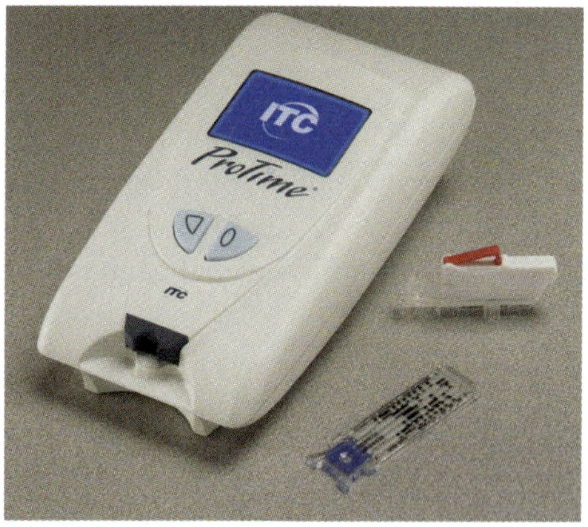

Figure 29-12 ProTime coagulation analyzer. (Courtesy of ITC, Edison, NJ.)

AUTOMATED HEMATOLOGY

Use of the automated or semiautomated hematology instruments is not categorized as waived testing under CLIA and therefore is not within the medical assistant's scope of practice without further education and training. Many medical assistants have obtained additional education and training and are performing moderately complex tests under additional credentials. All procedures performed with automated instrumentation are modifications of manual methods. Automated hematology procedures have many advantages over the manual methods. They are faster, less expensive, simple to operate, and accurate. The instruments can be calibrated and lend themselves to control testing. Most are equipped with printers that produce hard copy results. Many can store quality-control results and print out quality-control data summary sheets.

In addition to performing a wide variety of hematologic tests, many automated hematology instruments also calculate part or all of the RBC indices and print the results. Some automated hematology instruments can be connected to other computers in the medical facility.

The hematologic parameters that are available on different automated office hematology instruments are:

- RBC count
- WBC count
- Hemoglobin
- Hematocrit
- Platelet count
- MCV
- MCH
- MCHC
- Percentage of granulocytes

- Granulocyte count (neutrophils, eosinophils, basophils)
- Percentage of lymphocytes/monocytes
- Non granulocyte count (lymphocytes and monocytes)
- Mid-cell count (monocytes and band neutrophils)
- Percentage of mid-cells
- Lymphocyte count
- Percentage of lymphocytes
- RBC distribution width (RDW)

Procedure 29-1

Hemoglobin Determination Using a CLIA Waived Hemoglobin Analyzer

STANDARD PRECAUTIONS

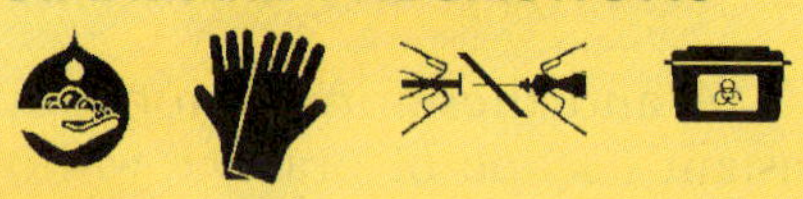

PURPOSE

Properly and safely perform an automated hemoglobin determination to evaluate the oxygen-carrying capacity of the blood.

EQUIPMENT/SUPPLIES

Gloves
Biohazard container
Sharps container
Capillary puncture equipment
  70% isopropyl alcohol
  Safety lancet
  Cotton ball
  Gauze 2 × 2
  Adhesive bandage
CLIA waived hemoglobin analyzer with test slides

PROCEDURE STEPS

1. Assemble and organize equipment and supplies. RATIONALE: Being organized helps the process go more smoothly and professionally.
2. Wash hands and put on gloves. RATIONALE: Hand washing and gloving protects the patient and you.
3. Turn on the analyzer and calibrate or standardize according to the manufacturer's instructions (Figure 29-13A). RATIONALE: Turn on analyzer to warm machine up, calibrate to maintain quality controls.
4. Identify the patient and explain the procedure. RATIONALE: Identifying the patient ensures that you have the right patient. Explaining the procedure reassures the patient and gains his or her cooperation with the procedure.
5. Select the site, prepare the site, and perform the capillary puncture (see Chapter 28). Wipe away the first drop with gauze. RATIONALE: The first drop may be contaminated with tissue fluid. Using gauze rather than a cotton ball will discourage a clot from forming.
6. Apply the second drop of blood into the slide reservoir using the appropriate technique for the analyzer (Figure 29-13B). RATIONALE: Each machine has a slightly different applicator device and technique.
7. Apply a cotton ball to the puncture site and ask the patient to hold pressure for 2 minutes. RATIONALE: Cotton will assist the site to clot during the 2 minutes the pressure is held.
8. Place the slide into the analyzer and perform appropriate steps as required by the manufacturer's instructions. RATIONALE: Each manufacturer has specific processes for use with its analyzer.
9. Read and make a note of the test results (Figure 29-13C). RATIONALE: Making a note helps you retain the results until they can be charted in the patient's medical record.
10. Assess the patient and apply a bandage strip to the puncture site. RATIONALE: The patient should not leave your care until the bleeding has stopped. Do not apply a fingertip bandage to an infant or young child because it could pose a choking hazard.
11. Disinfect analyzer according to manufacturer's instructions. Discard all contaminated equip-

continues

Procedure 29-1 (continued)

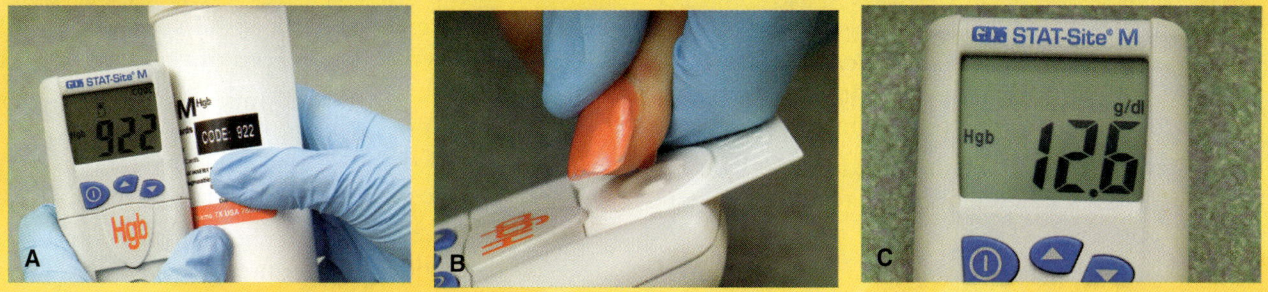

Figure 29-13 (A) Turn on the machine and perform control testing if necessary. Always follow the manufacturer's instructions. (B) Place the patient's drop of blood into the slide reservoir. (C) Read and record the hemoglobin value.

ment and supplies into appropriate biohazard waste receptacles. Disinfect counter space. RATIONALE: Using disinfectants not recommended by the manufacturer could harm the analyzer. Use sharps containers for sharp supplies and red bags for contaminated cotton ball and gloves.

12. Discard note, remove gloves and discard into biohazard container, and wash hands. RATIONALE: Washing hands removes residual contamination.
13. Document the procedure in the patient's medical record in the progress notes charting section and complete a lab report. File the lab report in the lab section of the patient record. RATIONALE: Accurate and timely documentation are important in medical laboratory procedures.

DOCUMENTATION

08/06/20XX Capillary puncture performed for hemoglobin determination. Specimen tested in our lab. Results lab report filed. Patient tolerated the procedure well and Dr. Rice discussed results with her. Joe Guerrero, CMA (AAMA)

Laboratory Report

Patient Name Diane Pankey *Date* 08-06-20XX

Hematocrit — % *Hemoglobin* 14.5 gm/dL

Joe Guerrero, CMA (AAMA)
MA signature

Procedure 29-2

Microhematocrit Determination

STANDARD PRECAUTIONS

PURPOSE

Properly and safely perform a microhematocrit determination.

EQUIPMENT/SUPPLIES

Gloves
Biohazard container
Sharps container
Capillary puncture equipment
- 70% isopropyl alcohol
- Safety lancet
- Cotton ball
- Gauze 2 × 2
- Adhesive bandage

Microhematocrit tubes (heparinized, plastic, self-sealing or use sealing clay)
Microhematocrit centrifuge and reader

continues

Procedure 29-2 (continued)

PROCEDURE STEPS

1. Assemble and organize equipment and supplies. RATIONALE: Being organized helps the process go more smoothly and professionally.
2. Wash hands and put on gloves. RATIONALE: Hand washing and gloving protects the patient and you.
3. Identify the patient and explain the procedure. RATIONALE: Identifying the patient ensures that you have the right patient. Explaining the procedure reassures the patient and gains his or her cooperation with the procedure.
4. Select the site, prepare the site, and perform the capillary puncture (see Chapter 28). Wipe away the first drop with gauze. RATIONALE: The first drop may be contaminated with tissue fluid. Using gauze rather than a cotton ball will discourage a clot from forming.
5. Allow the second drop of blood to form on the patient's finger. Holding the microhematocrit tube horizontally, touch the end onto the top of the blood drop and let the tube fill by capillary action until the tube is approximately ¾ full (Figures 29-14A and B).
6. With a 2 × 2 gauze, wipe off the end of the tube. Gently place the tube into clay until a plug is formed or use self-sealing tube (Figure 29-14C). RATIONALE: Wiping the end of the tube of blood lessens contamination to the clay holder. Sealing the tube prevents the specimen from being forced out during centrifugation.
7. Repeat the procedure with one more tube. RATIONALE: The two tubes balance one another in the centrifuge and the amounts are averaged to get the hemotocrit results.
8. Apply a cotton ball to the puncture site and ask the patient to hold pressure for 2 minutes. RATIONALE: Cotton will assist the site to clot during the 2 minutes the pressure is held.
9. Place the tubes into the centrifuge with sealed ends outward against the gasket. Make certain the tubes balance each other across the centrifuge. Fasten the lid securely, lock into place, and turn the centrifuge on. Set the timer and spin for the appropriate amount of time as required by the manufacturer's instructions. RATIONALE: Centrifugal force requires that the outside ends of the tubes be plugged to prevent the specimen from leaking out. Balancing the tubes and locking the lid ensure laboratory safety and prevents breakage.
10. Assess the patient and apply a bandage strip to the puncture site. RATIONALE: The patient should not leave your care until the bleeding has stopped. Do not apply a fingertip bandage to an infant or young child because it could pose a choking hazard.
11. Allow the centrifuge to come to a complete stop before touching it. Remove the tubes. Using a

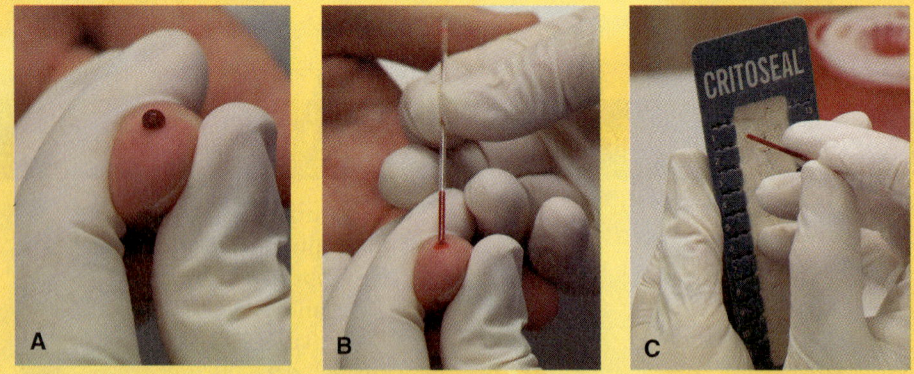

Figure 29-14 (A) Perform the capillary puncture, and wipe away the first drop with gauze. Allow the second drop of blood to form on the patient's finger. (B) Holding the microhematocrit tube horizontally, touch the end onto the top of the blood drop and let the tube fill by capillary action until it is approximately ¾ full. (C) Seal the microhematocrit tube with sealing clay.

continues

Procedure 29-2 (continued)

reader or accompanying graph, determine the hematocrit level. Read and make a note of the test results. RATIONALE: A spinning centrifuge is very dangerous and can cause a friction burn if touched. Making a note helps you retain the results until they can be charted in the patient's medical record.

12. Discard all contaminated equipment and supplies into appropriate biohazard waste receptacles. Disinfect counter space and centrifuge according to manufacturer's instructions. RATIONALE: Using disinfectants not recommended by the manufacturer could harm the analyzer. Use sharps containers for sharp supplies and red bags for contaminated cotton ball and gloves.
13. Discard note, remove gloves and discard into biohazard container, and wash hands. RATIONALE: Washing hands removes residual contamination.
14. Document the procedure in the patient's medical record in the progress notes charting section and complete a lab report. File the lab report in the lab section of the patient record. RATIONALE: Accurate and timely documentation are important in medical laboratory procedures.

DOCUMENTATION

08/06/20XX Capillary puncture performed for hematocrit determination. Specimen tested in our labs. Results in lab report filed. Patient tolerated the procedure well and Dr. Rice discussed results with her. Joe Guerrero, CMA (AAMA)——

Laboratory Report

Patient Name Diane Pankey *Date* 08-06-20XX

Hematocrit 38 % *Hemoglobin* — *gm/dL*

Joe Guerrero, CMA (AAMA)
MA signature

Procedure 29-3

Erythrocyte Sedimentation Rate

STANDARD PRECAUTIONS:

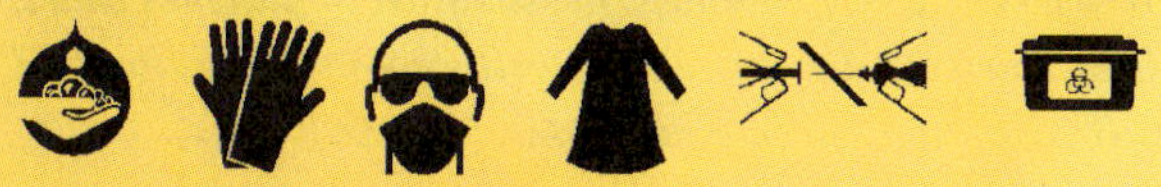

PURPOSE:

Properly and safely examine a blood sample by using either the Sediplast® (Westergren) or Wintrobe method to record the ESR.

EQUIPMENT/SUPPLIES:

Gloves
Sample of venous blood collected in EDTA
Sediplast® kit (or other ESR kit):
  Sedivial and sedirack
  Sediplast® autozeroing pipette
  Pipette capable of delivering up to 1.0 mL
Wintrobe method:
  Wintrobe sedimentation tube (disposable or reusable)
  Wintrobe sedimentation rack
  Long-stem Pasteur-type pipette with rubber bulb
Timer
Disinfectant
Biohazard disposal container
Acrylic face shield or goggles and mask
Sharps container

NOTE: Consult the manufacturer's package insert for specific instructions for the ESR kit being used.

PROCEDURE STEPS:

1. Wash hands and put on gloves.
2. Assemble equipment and materials.
3. Gently mix blood sample for 2 minutes.
4. Perform either method a (Sediplast® ESR) or method b (Wintrobe):
   a. Sediplast® ESR (modified Westergren) method:
      (1) Remove stopper on sedivial and fill to the indicated mark with 0.8 mL blood.

continues

Procedure 29-3 (continued)

Replace stopper and invert vial several times to mix (or mix using pipette).

(2) Place sedivial in Sediplast® rack on a level surface.

(3) Gently insert the disposable Sediplast® pipette through the pierceable stopper with a twisting motion and push down until the pipette rests on the bottom of the vial. The pipette will autozero the blood and any excess will flow into the sealed reservoir compartment.

(4) Set timer for 1 hour.

(5) Return blood sample to proper storage. (If no laboratory work will be performed during the incubation, remove gloves, discard appropriately, and wash hands. Reglove before handling test materials.)

(6) Let the pipette stand undisturbed for exactly 1 hour, and then read the results of the ESR: Use the scale on the tube to measure the distance from the top of the plasma to the top of the RBCs.

(7) Record the sedimentation rate:
ESR (Mod. Westergren, 1 hr) = ___ mm

(8) Dispose of tube and vial in appropriate biohazard container.

b. Wintrobe method:

(1) Place tube in Wintrobe sedimentation rack.

(2) Check the leveling bubble to ensure that the Wintrobe rack is level.

(3) Fill Wintrobe tube to the zero mark with well-mixed blood using the Pasteur pipette and being careful not to overfill. *NOTE:* Tube must be filled from the bottom to avoid getting air bubbles in the tube.

(4) Set timer for 1 hour. Be certain the tube is vertical and left undisturbed for the entire hour.

(5) Return blood sample to proper storage. (If no other laboratory work is scheduled, remove gloves, discard appropriately, and wash hands. Reglove before handling test materials.)

(6) Measure the distance the erythrocytes have fallen (in mm): after exactly 1 hour, use the scale on the tube to measure the distance from the top of the plasma to the top of the RBCs.

(7) Record the sedimentation rate:
ESR (Wintrobe, 1 hr) = ___ mm

(8) Disinfect and clean equipment and return to storage.

NOTE: If disposable equipment is used, dispose of in biohazard container.

5. Clean work area with surface disinfectant.
6. Remove gloves and discard into biohazard container.
7. Wash hands.
8. Document the procedure in the patient's medical record in the progress notes charting section and complete a lab report. File the lab report in the lab section of the patient record. RATIONALE: Accurate and timely documentation are important in medical laboratory procedures.

DOCUMENTATION

08/06/20XX ESR performed. Results filed in patient's chart. Patient tolerated the procedure well and Dr. Rice discussed results with him. Joe Guerrero, CMA (AAMA) ——————

Laboratory Report

Patient Name George Pankey *Date* 08-06-20XX

Erythrocyte Sedimentation Rate 17 *mm/hr*

Joe Guerrero, CMA (AAMA)
MA signature

Procedure 29-4

Prothrombin Time (Using CLIA Waived ProTime Analyzer)

STANDARD PRECAUTIONS

PURPOSE

Properly and safely perform an automated prothrombin time determination to evaluate the clotting time of a drop of blood.

EQUIPMENT/SUPPLIES

Gloves
Biohazard container
Sharps container
Capillary puncture equipment
- 70% isopropyl alcohol
- Safety lancet
- Cotton ball
- Gauze 2 × 2
- Adhesive bandage

CLIA Waived ProTime Analyzer (ITC ProTime-3) with accessories

PROCEDURE STEPS

1. Assemble and organize equipment and supplies. Check expiration dates. RATIONALE: Being organized helps the process go more smoothly and professionally.
2. Wash hands and put on gloves. RATIONALE: Hand washing and gloving protects the patient and you.
3. Turn on the ProTime-3 and follow the prompts. Insert the test cuvette into the analyzer. RATIONALE: Turn on analyzer to warm up machine, calibrate to maintain quality controls.
4. Identify the patient and explain the procedure. RATIONALE: Identifying the patient ensures that you have the right patient. Explaining the procedure reassures the patient and gains his or her cooperation with the procedure.
5. Select the site, prepare the site, and perform the capillary puncture using the Tenderlett lancet. Remember to use gauze to wipe away the first drop. RATIONALE: The Tenderlett lancet contains the reservoir required for use with the ProTime-3.
6. Fill the Tenderlett lancet cup to the fill line then place it onto the cuvette, which was placed into the machine in Step 3. Be sure it is snapped into place. Press the start button. RATIONALE: The Tenderlett cup is calibrated for the analyzer and must be properly placed for the test to run correctly.
7. Apply a cotton ball and ask the patient to hold pressure for 3 to 5 minutes. RATIONALE: A patient having this test performed usually has a delayed clotting time. Assess that the bleeding has stopped and apply bandage. RATIONALE: A patient should never leave your care until the bleeding has stopped.
8. Stay by the analyzer and await a prompt to remove the Tenderlett lancet device. When prompted, immediately remove the device and discard it into a nearby sharps container. RATIONALE: The device must be removed as soon as the clot has formed. This must be done very quickly, within seconds. The Tenderlett device contains a lancet and must be discarded into a sharps container.
9. Read the clotting time in seconds and the INR. Record the results. RATIONALE: Results should be recorded as soon as possible to decrease the chance of error.
10. Notify the provider immediately if the results fall within a critical range. RATIONALE: If the patient has a seriously delayed clotting time, the risk of serious event occurring (such as a stroke) is greater. The provider must be notified immediately in order to adjust the anticoagulant dosage and/or prescribe other treatment.
11. Disinfect analyzer according to manufacturer's instructions, discard all contaminated equipment and supplies into appropriate biohazard waste receptacles, and disinfect counter space. Remove gloves and wash hands. RATIONALE: Using disinfectants not recommended by the manufacturer could harm the analyzer. Use sharps containers for sharp supplies and red bags for contaminated cotton ball and gloves. Washing hands removes residual contamination.

continues

Procedure 29-4 (continued)

12. Document the procedure in the patient's medical record in the progress notes charting section and complete a lab report. File the lab report in the lab section of the patient record. RATIONALE: Accurate and timely documentation are important in medical laboratory procedures.

DOCUMENTATION

08/06/20XX Capillary puncture performed for protime determination. Specimen tested in our lab. Results in lab report filed. Patient tolerated the procedure well and Dr. Rice discussed results with her. Joe Guerrero, CMA (AAMA)

Laboratory Report

Patient Name Cynthia Januszewski Date 08-06-20XX

Protime 16 seconds INR 2.0

Joe Guerrero, CMA (AAMA)

MA signature

Case Study 29-1

Refer to the scenario at the beginning of the chapter.

CASE STUDY REVIEW

1. What should Audrey do if the clinic buys a new machine for laboratory analysis that she is not familiar with?
2. How can Audrey be sure that she is using the laboratory analyzers properly and that the patient test results are accurate?
3. Who should Audrey consult if she has questions about how to perform a test using an analyzer?

Case Study 29-2

Today is busier than usual at Drs. Lewis and King. While she is performing an ESR for Jim Marshal, a patient in his late 30s, medical assistant Audrey Jones is called on to help with another patient. She hurriedly places the sedimentation rack on top of an incubator in the sunlight by an open window and leaves to assist Dr. King.

CASE STUDY REVIEW

1. List two ways in which the test results may be affected.
2. What are the normal Westergren ESR values for male and female patients younger than 50 years?
3. What are the best conditions for an accurate test?

SUMMARY

Hematology tests are the second most frequently performed tests in the ambulatory care setting. Only urinalysis is performed more frequently. Medical assistants must have a knowledge of hematology to accurately and efficiently perform the tests. The study of hematology includes hematopoiesis, which is the formation of the blood elements, as well as the hematologic tests and their relation to the pathology of the body.

This chapter introduced the more common hematologic tests that are performed in the ambulatory care setting, including all the parts of the CBC, the ESR methods, and the erythrocyte indices. All of these tests are used by the provider in the diagnosis and treatment of disease.

Most of the hematology procedures performed in today's ambulatory care setting use some type of automated instrumentation. Some automated hematology instruments require a diluted blood sample, whereas others do not. Both methods of automated instrumentation are discussed in this chapter.

Blood specimens used in the sampling of hematologic procedures are biohazardous material. Be sure to follow Universal and Standard Precautions when you work with these specimens (see Chapter 10).

STUDY FOR SUCCESS

To reinforce your knowledge and skills of information presented in this chapter:

- Review the Key Terms
- Practice the Procedures
- Consider the Case Studies and discuss your conclusions
- Answer the Review Questions
  - Multiple Choice
  - Critical Thinking
- Navigate the Internet by completing the Web Activities
- Practice the StudyWARE activities on the CD
- Apply your knowledge in the Student Workbook activities
- Complete the Web Tutor sections
- View and discuss the DVD situations

REVIEW QUESTIONS

Multiple Choice

1. Which of the following is *not* a cellular component of blood?
   a. erythrocytes
   b. leukocytes
   c. thrombocytes
   d. erythropoietin
2. The formation of blood cells is defined as:
   a. erythropoietin
   b. hematopoiesis
   c. mean corpuscular volume
   d. hemoglobinopathy
3. Sickle cell anemia, a hereditary disease, has which type of hemoglobin?
   a. hemoglobin S
   b. hemoglobin A
   c. hemoglobin E
   d. hemoglobin C
4. The volume of packed red cells compared with the total volume of the sample is calculated for which test?
   a. hematocrit
   b. hemoglobin
   c. MCH
   d. MCV
5. The most common white cell type found in the granulocytic series is the:
   a. lymphocyte
   b. monocyte
   c. neutrophil
   d. basophil
6. The erythrocyte indices are used for the diagnosis, classification, and treatment of different:
   a. infections
   b. anemias
   c. inflammatory diseases
   d. neoplasms
7. Which hematologic test result shows an increase with infections, inflammatory disease, acute stress, and tissue destruction?
   a. hemoglobin
   b. MCV
   c. hematocrit
   d. ESR
8. The most frequent hemoglobin disease seen in the ambulatory care setting is:
   a. iron deficiency anemia
   b. sickle cell anemia
   c. leukemia
   d. anisocytosis
9. Which test within a CBC is within the scope of practice of a medical assistant under CLIA's waived test category?
   a. Using a HemoCue® to determine a hemoglobin level
   b. Using a hemacytometer to count WBCs manually
   c. Using the Unopette system to count RBCs manually
   d. Using an automated blood analyzer that requires calculations and mixing of reagents

10. The highly sensitive C-reactive protein (hsCRP) test is used for detecting:
    a. any type of protein in the blood
    b. vascular inflammation
    c. very specific diseases such as lupus
    d. anemia and leukemia

Critical Thinking

1. What hematologic factors do the erythrocyte indices provide information about? List one example for each index in which a disease causes an elevation or decrease.
2. You are serving your practicum in a local clinic. A provider has made a tentative diagnosis of appendicitis for a patient. In addition to the urinalysis, what single hematologic test is most likely to confirm the diagnosis?
3. List the guidelines that must be followed to ensure accurate sed rate results.
4. How does aspirin interfere with clotting?
5. What test would have elevated results if a patient had systemic arthritis? Why?

WEB ACTIVITIES

1. Visit the CDC's Web site to review Standard Precautions required during blood collection.
2. Does the American Heart Association's Web site offer parameters for different blood counts and hematology values? Are guidelines and tips on specimen collection outlined?

REFERENCE/BIBLIOGRAPHY

Walters, N. J., Estridge, B. H., & Reynolds, A. P. (2008). *Basic medical laboratory techniques* (5th ed.). Clifton Park, NY: Delmar Cengage Learning.

THE DVD HOOK-UP

This chapter discusses common hematologic procedures that are performed in the medical office.

The selected scenes in this program taught you how to perform a hematocrit, hemoglobin, and ESR test. Procedures will vary depending on the equipment used.

1. The selected clip for performing a hematocrit test stated that you may test one or two tubes, depending on equipment used and the policy of your office. Why is it best to run two tubes when measuring a patient's hematocrit?
2. How can you make certain that you are performing waived tests when working in a waived laboratory?
3. What tube color should you use for hematologic testing? Is the ESR considered a hematologic test?

DVD Journal Summary

Write a paragraph that summarizes what you learned from watching the selected scenes from today's DVD program. It is important to make certain that test results are accurate. What would you do if your controls do not match what is listed on the control bottle and the office supervisor tells you to ignore the control values?

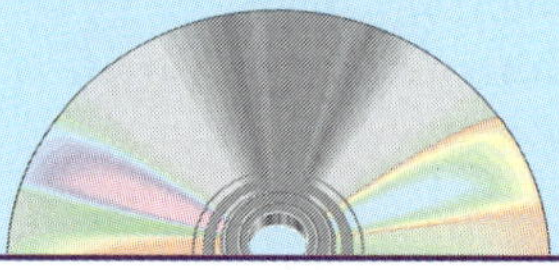

DVD Series Skills Based Series

Program Number 11

Chapter/Scene Reference

- *Administering Capillary Puncture and Performing Hematocrit Test*
- *Performing Automated Hemoglobin*
- *Performing ESR Test*

Chapter 30

Urinalysis

KEY TERMS

Acid/Base Balance
Amorphous
Bilirubin
Bilirubinuria
Casts
Chain of Custody
Circadian Rhythm
Creatinine
Critical Values
Crystals
Culture and Sensitivity (C&S)
Cultures
Glucose
Glucosuria
Hematuria
Hyaline
Ketoacidosis
Ketone
Ketonuria
Ketosis
Leukocyte Esterase
Midstream Collection
pH
Quality Control (QC)
Reagent
Reagent Test Strip
Refractometer
Sediment
Specific Gravity
Supernatant
Turbid
Urea
Urinalysis
Urinary Tract Infection (UTI)
Urobilinogen

OUTLINE

OBJECTIVES

The student should strive to meet the following performance objectives and demonstrate an understanding of the facts and principles presented in this chapter through written and oral communication.

1. Define the key terms as presented in the glossary.
2. Explain the process of urine formation.
3. Discuss the importance of safety procedures and quality control when working with urine.
4. Describe the importance of proper collection and preservation of 24-hour urine specimens.
5. Identify the proper technique for examining the physical characteristics of a urine specimen.
6. Explain pathologic and nonpathologic causes of abnormal physical characteristics of urine.
7. Describe methods for chemical examination of a urine specimen.
8. Identify the proper method of preparing urine sediment for microscopic examination.
9. Identify normal and abnormal structures found during the microscopic examination of urine sediment.

Scenario

At Inner City Health Care, clinical medical assistant Wanda Slawson performs many urinalyses. Although urinalysis is a routine procedure, Wanda recognizes its importance as a diagnostic tool, and she performs each test carefully to ensure accurate results. Wanda takes time to instruct patients in the proper collection procedures. She encourages patients to ask questions before collecting the urine sample, and she provides written instructions for easy reference. When she performs the urinalysis, Wanda follows safety and quality-control guidelines. By paying attention to the details of the procedure, Wanda does her best to ensure the quality of the urinalysis results.

INTRODUCTION

*Examination of the urine (**urinalysis**) as a diagnostic tool for many diseases has been performed for centuries by medical practitioners. Urinalysis refers to the study of urine as an aid in patient diagnosis or to follow the course of disease. The urine examination is a routine part of most physical examinations.*

The routine urinalysis is one of the most frequently performed procedures in the medical office laboratory. Many tests can be performed on one urine sample. This procedure is often ordered because urine is easily obtained, and much information about the body's metabolism may be gained from the results of this testing.

When providers order a "routine urinalysis," they expect timely and accurate results. Results can indicate a systemic disease process or renal (kidney) or urinary tract disease.

Practice, experience, and attention to detail are the most important tools in achieving quality results. Following Standard Precautions when working with any body fluid is mandatory.

URINE FORMATION

Before discussing the analysis of urine, it is helpful to understand how urine is formed in the human body. The formation and excretion of urine is the principal way the body excretes water and gets rid of waste. These waste products, if not removed, rapidly can become toxic.

The kidney is a highly specialized organ that eliminates soluble (dissolved in water) waste products of metabolism. Urine is formed in the kidney and is excreted from the body by way of the urinary tract system (Figure 30-1). The kidney also regulates the fluid outside the cells of the body by eliminating certain fluids and returning other fluids, maintaining a careful balance (homeostasis). In this manner, the body is protected from dramatic changes in fluid volume, acidity and alkalinity **(acid/base balance),** composition, and pressure.

There are two kidneys, one on each side of the body. They are about 11 to 12 cm long and 5 to 6 cm wide. Kidneys are shaped like a lima bean with their concave border directed toward the midline of the body. The left kidney is slightly higher than the right.

Filtration

The kidney filters waste products, salts, and excess fluid from the blood. The filtering unit of the kidney is called the glomerulus. The part of the kidney

Spotlight on Certification

RMA Content Outline

- Anatomy and physiology
- Patient education
- Asepsis
- Laboratory procedures

CMA (AAMA) Content Outline

- Systems, including structure, function, related conditions and diseases
- Patient instruction
- Legislation
- Principles of infection control
- Collecting and processing specimens; diagnostic testing

CMAS Content Outline

- Asepsis in the medical office
- Communication

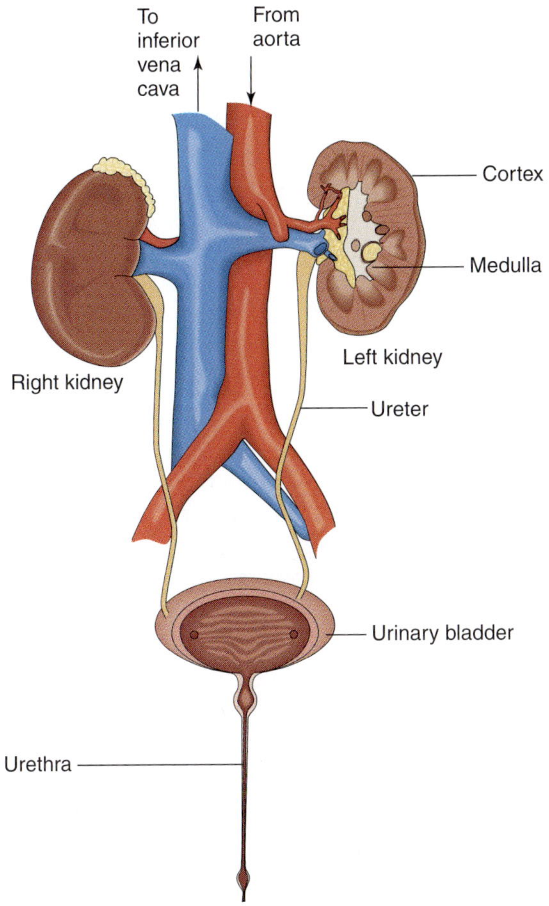

Figure 30-1 The urinary system.

that concentrates the filtered material is called the tubule. Together, the glomerulus and the tubule combine to form the nephron (Figure 30-2).

Most of the work of the kidney is done by the nephrons. There are approximately one million nephrons in each kidney. Each minute, more than 1,000 mL of blood flows through the kidney to be cleansed. In the glomerulus, certain substances are filtered out of the blood. The remaining filtrate then passes into the tubule where various changes occur. Substances filtered out from the body can include water, ammonia, electrolytes, **glucose,** amino acids, **creatinine,** and **urea.** These wastes leave the body in the eliminated urine.

For example, when diabetics have excess sugar in their blood, the body attempts to eliminate the excess glucose through the urine. Routine urinalysis testing will reveal the excess glucose, alerting the provider to the presence of too much glucose. In this manner, diabetes can be diagnosed, and it can be determined that a patient with diabetes is not taking enough insulin to control the glucose in the blood.

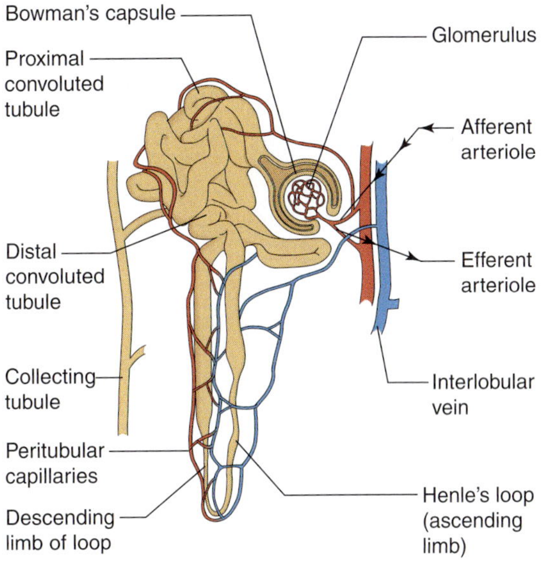

Figure 30-2 Parts of the nephron, including the glomerulus.

Reabsorption

While passing through the kidney, some substances may need to be reabsorbed by the blood. Approximately 180 L of filtrate is produced daily by the body, but only 1 to 2 L of urine is eliminated from the normally functioning human body. Therefore, much of the filtrate, including water, sodium, chloride, potassium, bicarbonate, glucose, calcium, and amino acids, is reabsorbed into the body.

Under normal conditions, blood cells and most proteins stay in the blood plasma because they are too large to pass through the walls of the capillaries of the glomerulus. If blood cells and excess protein are found in the urine, the provider is alerted that the kidney is not filtering properly due to an irregular condition affecting the urinary tract.

As long as the concentration of glucose in the blood is less than 180 mg/dL (milligrams per deciliter), the glucose will be completely reabsorbed. If the level increases to more than 180 mg/dL, the glucose is not reabsorbed. Substances such as glucose that are reabsorbed in relation to their concentration in the blood are known as threshold substances. The needs of homeostasis call for sugar and protein to be almost completely reabsorbed, whereas other threshold substances such as creatinine, amino acids, potassium, sodium, and chloride are only partially reabsorbed.

Secretion

Near the end of the blood's journey through the kidney, specifically in the distal convoluted tubule,

Critical Thinking

1. What are the three actions that take place in the formation of urine?
2. Why do you suppose we test for sugar in urine but not salt/sodium?

other substances that have not already been filtered are secreted into the urine. Such substances as hydrogen and ammonium ions may be secreted into the urine in exchange for sodium. Certain drugs in the blood at this point may also be secreted into the urine.

URINE COMPOSITION

After urine progresses through a healthy kidney, it is approximately 96% water and 4% dissolved substances, most of which come from either dietary intake or metabolic waste products. These substances are primarily urea, salt, sulfates, and phosphates. Abnormal constituents of urine include red and white blood cells, fat, glucose, casts, bile, acetone, and hemoglobin (Table 30-1).

When certain disease processes occur in the human body, the following changes in urine production and composition can occur:

- The amount of urine excreted can increase or decrease
- Urine color can change
- Urine appearance can vary
- Urine odor can change
- Cells can be present in urine
- Chemical constituents in urine can change
- Urine concentration (specific gravity) may vary

Table 30-1 Normal and Abnormal Substances in Urine

Normal	Abnormal
Urea	Bile
Uric acid	Blood
Creatinine	Fat
Sodium	Glucose
Potassium	Protein
Ammonium	White blood cells
Sulfate	Urobilinogen
Chloride	Microorganisms (bacteria, parasites)

SAFETY

Chapter 26 discusses the guidelines set up by government agencies to ensure the safety of everyone working in the health care field and for the protection of our environment. These guidelines are now referred to as Standard Precautions. Other terms used to describe care when handling infectious materials are Transmission-Based Precautions and biohazard precautions.

QUALITY CONTROL

As in every area of the laboratory, every effort must be made by health care professionals to produce test results free from error. Much pressure is placed by regulatory agencies on facilities that perform laboratory tests such as urinalysis to maintain standards that will ensure reliable results. **Quality control (QC)** programs are an important part of urine testing to ensure accurate and reliable results for the patient. QC programs must be incorporated into every urine testing procedure. Because many of the tests are interpreted by visual examination, the QC procedures are dependent on the expertise of the person performing the examination.

Testing protocols must be written out and available to personnel. Records of testing must

Precautions To Use When Handling Urine Specimens

- Treat all specimens as if they were infectious, handling them with gloved hands.
- Avoid splashes or creation of aerosols when handling or disposing of urine specimens. Wearing face shields will prevent splashes from getting into the eyes, nose, or mouth.
- Process urine specimens as soon as possible.
- Store urine specimens appropriately in a designated refrigerator that contains no food or drink items.
- Dispose of urine appropriately, possibly in a designated sink (run water to wash the specimen into the drain) or toilet.

be maintained. Equipment and instruments used for urine testing must be maintained and checked daily for proper calibration. If the instrument should require recalibration, the manufacturer's instructions are provided with the instrument.

Always be careful to perform the QC procedures *exactly* as you perform the procedures on actual patient samples. Documentation of the performance of daily control testing must be kept for at least 3 years. With computer storage, the data can be stored indefinitely. Commercially available urine control samples can be purchased from a number of manufacturers. Positive and negative controls should be run each day on all tests to be performed. Control results should be recorded on a daily log for easy access. The control samples should be stored as directed by the manufacturer.

CLINICAL LABORATORY IMPROVEMENT AMENDMENTS OF 1988 (CLIA '88)

The regulations under the new CLIA are discussed in Chapter 26. Several CLIA '88 regulations apply to the medical assistant performing urine testing. They include:

- Appropriate training in the methodology of the test being performed
- Understanding of urine-testing QC procedures
- Proficiency in the use of instrumentation, being able to troubleshoot problems
- Knowledge of the stability and proper storage of **reagents** (substances involved in urine testing)
- Awareness of factors that influence test results
- Knowledge of how to verify test results
- The microscopic examination of urine is designated by CLIA to be a PPMP (provider-performed microscopy procedure) and therefore must be performed by a provider. The medical assistant is trained and able to prepare the slide for viewing and reading by the provider. The medical assistant should always take the opportunity to view the slide and discuss the finding with the provider as part of professional development and continued education.

Critical Thinking

1. What criteria does CLIA use to determine which tests are in each category?
2. In a urinalysis, which part is not in CLIA's waived category?

Critical Thinking

1. Is there any test that can be performed on urine that is not in a sterile container?
2. If a patient brings in a urine specimen from home in a clean baby food jar, can it be used for any testing or any part of a urinalysis?

URINE CONTAINERS

The first step toward achieving proper results during laboratory testing is proper collection of the specimen to be tested. There are a variety of containers (Figure 30-3) used for urine collection, including nonsterile containers for random specimens (urinalysis), sterile containers for **cultures** (testing specimens for growth of bacteria), and 24-hour collection containers with added preservatives.

Just before handing the urine specimen cup to the patient, label the cup with the patient's name, the date, and the time. Some facilities require more information, so follow the protocol of your facility. Always use a permanent marker so the information stays clear. Always label the cup, not the lid. This practice ensures that the specimen will not be separated from the label if the lid is removed. If the patient is unable to procure a specimen, discard the cup and give the patient a new cup if the patient is later able to give a specimen.

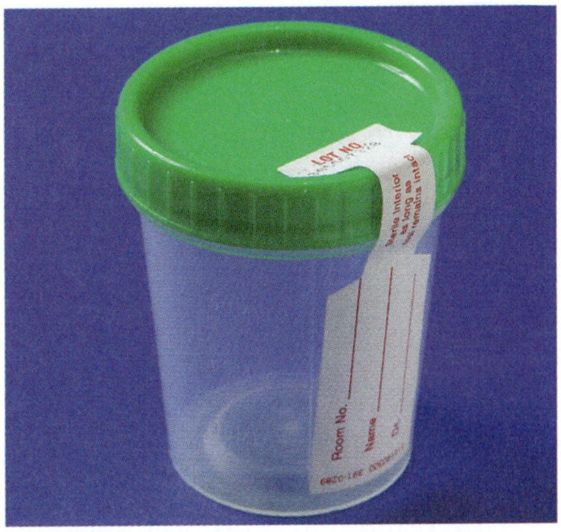

Figure 30-3 Urine collection containers should be calibrated, clear, and have a secure lid.

EHR When using electronic medical records, computer-generated labels can be printed. One label can be applied to the cup and other labels used for additional tests ordered, if appropriate. An example of an additional lab test is a culture and sensitivity of the urine as explained later in this chapter.

Occasionally, a patient will bring a sample with him or her in a generic container from home. General recommendations are to provide the patient with a new urine specimen cup and request a fresh sample. The exception to this rule would be if the patient has brought a "first morning void" specimen in an appropriate container.

URINE COLLECTION

Urine Specimen Types

Patients may have questions about how a specimen should be collected. The medical assistant must be able to give proper instructions using common terms that the patient will be able to understand. Following are common types of urine specimens that might be ordered frequently by providers.

Random (Spot) Specimen. Random (spot) urine samples are specimens that can be obtained at any time and are the most common collection performed in the outpatient setting. Random simply means that there is no particular time placed on the collection. Patients are requested to give a specimen whenever they are present for their appointment. If the patient has already voided, not knowing a specimen would be required, the medical assistant may offer the patient several cups of water in an attempt to procure another specimen. Because the kidneys constantly produce urine, the patient should be able to provide another specimen within 15 to 20 minutes of drinking several cups of water.

First Morning Void Specimen. The first morning void is typically the most concentrated specimen and has a higher acid pH (which helps preserve the cellular components). It is preferred, but because it is less convenient, it is seldom ordered unless the patient is an inpatient or is in a controlled setting.

Fasting/Timed Specimens. A fasting (going without food and drink except water) urine specimen is ordered less often than a random specimen. The provider may want to measure a urinary substance without interference from food intake. Some providers may require an overnight fast. Others may ask the patient to have a meal and then urinate four hours later.

It is up to the medical assistant to give the patient proper instruction as to how to collect a fasting, or timed, specimen. Written directions given to the patient in addition to oral instructions are best. A regular urinalysis container can be used for a fasting specimen. It does not require a sterile container.

Twenty-Four-Hour Specimen. Urine varies in its concentration of certain substances at different times during any 24-hour period because of **circadian rhythm** and the intake of food and water. For instance, the amount of water excreted is greatest from 10 AM to noon and 4 to 6 PM. Chloride is in its highest concentration from noon to 2 PM. Therefore, a 24-hour specimen is sometimes requested when quantitative tests (measuring the amount) for different substances are desired. The results of this type of collection then will be expressed in *units per 24 hours.* Some commonly tested substances include sodium, potassium, calcium, and creatinine.

The container used to collect this amount of urine should be of adequate size. Usually a one-gallon, dark-colored plastic bottle is used. For measuring urine constituents, preservatives need to be added to the bottle before the collection begins. Without the preservative, these substances may break down and be impossible to quantify. Preservatives include thymol, toluene, and certain acids.

Urine collected over a 24-hour period may be refrigerated between collections. After the collection is complete, it must be returned to the medical laboratory as soon as possible.

Many 24-hour urine bottles contain preservatives. Some preservatives are strong acids or bases. As with all laboratory chemicals, the medical assistant and the patient should avoid contact between the preservative and the skin. The urine specimen should be collected into a smaller container and then poured carefully into the main container. Vapors must not be inhaled when adding the specimen to the container. The patient's written instructions should contain a warning about avoiding contact with preservatives.

Providers sometimes choose to have a 2-hour or a 12-hour specimen instead of the usual 24-hour collection. All of the collection steps for a 24-hour specimen apply. Recording the time of day is important.

Collection Methods

In addition to ordering the type of urine specimen desired (random, fasting, 24-hour), the provider might also order a certain type of collection method to collect the specific sample. These methods include clean-catch midstream and catheterized collection.

Clean-Catch Midstream Collection. To avoid as much contamination as possible when collecting a specimen, providers prefer that the patient cleanse the genital area before collection. The clean-catch order means that cleansing towelettes are provided in addition to a urine container. Male patients are directed to cleanse the urethral opening twice with cleansing towelettes, and female patients are directed to cleanse the urethral area with three swipes, using three separate towelettes. (See Patient Education box and Procedure 30-7 for complete instructions.) Female patients should also be instructed to notify the medical assistant if they are menstruating during the collection.

After cleansing, the patient should begin to urinate into the toilet. The patient begins urinating, pulls the cup into the urine stream and collects the sample, then removes the cup from the stream and voids the rest of the urine into the toilet. This is called a midstream specimen. The midstream urine should be as free of contamination as possible.

Catheterized Collection. Urinary catheterization involves insertion of a sterile flexible tube into the urinary bladder through the urethra. Although urinary catheterization is performed for many reasons, this section discusses only the use of catheterization as a way to obtain a urinary sample (see Procedures 18-2 and 18-3).

Obtaining a urine specimen by catheterization is required when a completely sterile specimen is needed or when the patient is unable to follow cleansing instructions. The patient may not understand the language, may be mentally unable to comprehend the instructions, or may be physically unable to perform the process. It is the medical assistant's responsibility to determine if the patient understands the instructions for obtaining a clean-catch midstream urine sample and is able to perform the process.

Catheterization is a sterile procedure and is only performed under a provider's order and only by health care professionals who have been adequately trained. Because the urinary bladder is considered a sterile environment, if the catheterization is not performed properly, bacteria may be introduced into the patient's bladder, which can cause a bladder infection.

Patient Education

24-Hour Urine Collection

1. When giving a patient any type of instructions, make sure that the patient understands the importance of each step. Always provide written instructions as well. Emphasize that failing to follow the instructions will cause the results to be invalid, requiring another collection.
2. The patient begins a 24-hour collection by emptying the bladder and not keeping the specimen. The container is then labeled with the time of bladder emptying. Patients generally start the collection between 6 and 8 PM, but any 24-hour period is acceptable.
3. Explain that each time the patient urinates within the 24-hour period, the urine is transferred into the collection container.
4. Instruct the patient to refrigerate the container between urinations if required.
5. Explain that at the end of the 24-hour period, the patient should urinate and transfer the urine into the container. The exact time should be written on the label as the "ended" or "completed" time.
6. The most common errors in the 24-hour urine specimen collection are the inclusion of the first voided specimen and the discarding of one or more of the voided specimens during the 24-hour period. Be sure the patient understands these steps.

Culture and Sensitivity of Urine. Occasionally, the provider orders a **culture and sensitivity (C&S)** of a urine specimen. The medical assistant is responsible for preparing the sample for transport. A commonly used system is the Urine Culture and Sensitivity Transport kit (see Procedure 30-6).

EXAMINATION OF URINE

Urine should be examined in a fresh state, preferably while still warm if possible. However, on rare occasion the urine sample cannot be tested immediately. If immediate testing is not possible, the urine should be refrigerated at about 4°C (39°F) or stored on ice. The urinalysis should be performed as soon as possible, preferably within 2 hours. **Crystals** and **casts** begin to break down after 2 hours. Any time delay allows bacteria to multiply and can lead to inaccurate microbiology results.

Patient Education

Clean-Catch, Midstream Urine Specimen Collection Instructions

1. The patient should be provided with a clean or sterile covered urine cup, a pair of gloves, and adequate cleansing towelettes (three for female patients, two for male patients). The cup should be labeled with the patient's name and the date. Caution the patient not to contaminate the inside of the cup. A shelf near the toilet is extremely helpful for patients, allowing them to have the towelettes and cup within reach during collection of the specimen.
2. Instruct the patient in proper cleansing of the genital area. It is best to give the patient written instructions as well. Men and women should have separate instructions. The written instructions should be posted next to the toilet for reference by the patient during the procedure. Logically, the female instructions should be posted on the wall beside the toilet at reading level while she is sitting, and the male instructions should be posted on the wall behind the toilet at reading level while he is standing. Laminating the instruction documents protects the writing from any sprays or splashes.
    - *Men:* After thoroughly washing his hands, the male patient should retract the foreskin on the penis (if not circumcised). A cleansing towelette should be used to cleanse the urethral opening with a single stroke directed from the tip of the penis toward the ring of the glans. The cleansing procedure should be repeated again using a new towelette.
    - *Women:* After thoroughly washing her hands, the female patient should position herself comfortably on the toilet seat and spread her knees as far apart as she can. She should spread the outer vulval folds and hold them open with one hand. With the other hand, using the first towelette, the patient should cleanse on one side from front to back with one swipe, disposing of the towelette into the toilet. With the second towelette, she should wipe on the other side front to back with one swipe, disposing of that towelette into the toilet. While still holding the vulval folds open, she should use the third towelette to wipe the urethral opening front to back with one swipe. She may dispose of that towelette into the toilet, too. She should continue to hold the vulval folds open until she has completed the collection of the urine specimen.
3. Instruct the patient also about the midstream collection technique. Explain why it is necessary. These instructions should also be written and included with the clean-catch written directions.
    - After cleansing the area using the clean-catch directions, the patient should begin to void into the toilet. The specimen cup should then be held into the stream until it is about half full, then the cup should be removed from the stream. Assure the patient that urinalysis can be performed on a small amount of urine if they are unable to give half a cup. The patient may finish urinating into the toilet. Only the middle portion of the urine flow is included in the sample. After the specimen has been collected, the container should be capped. After securely capping the urine cup, the patient may cleanse the outside of the cup if desired. The patient should always avoid touching the inside of both the container and the lid.
4. The patient should be instructed on where/how to return the specimen to the medical assistant. Some physicians' office laboratories (POLs) have a special shelf with a small door opening into the laboratory, whereas other offices prefer the patient actually hand the specimen to the medical assistant directly. Either way, the specimen should be taken immediately into the laboratory by the medical assistant.
5. All surface areas in the restroom should be immediately decontaminated in preparation for the next patient.

The routine urinalysis procedure is composed of three parts:

- *Physical* examination of the urine
- *Chemical* examination of the urine
- *Microscopic* examination of urine sediment

The medical assistant should wash hands, put on gloves, and follow all the safety guidelines when performing any of the following procedures. Some facilities require eye protection when pouring urine or performing any procedure where splashing of urine into the eye could occur. All surface areas in the restroom should be decontaminated immediately after procuring or testing urine specimens.

Physical Examination of Urine

When the medical assistant begins the process of performing a urinalysis, the first step is performing the physical examination. This examination consists of:

- Assessing the volume of the urine specimen, making sure that the amount is sufficient for testing
- Observing and recording the color, appearance, and transparency of the specimen
- Noting any unusual urine odor
- Measuring the specific gravity of the specimen

Procedure 30-1 describes how to assess the volume, color, appearance, transparency, and odor of urine. Procedure 30-2 discribes testing for the specific gravity.

Specimen Volume. The first step in performing a urinalysis is to determine if the sample's volume is adequate for testing.

The medical assistant must have enough urine to fill a test tube with at least 10 mL (about two teaspoons) of urine with enough leftover in the specimen cup to completely insert and wet a chemical reagent strip and to culture if ordered.

The volume usually requested of the patient is a half cup, but patients should be assured that samples of much less volume can be tested. If the patient is only able to submit a small volume of urine, which tests can be performed are determined, depending on the priority set by the provider according to the patient's suspected diagnosis. For example, if only a test for protein and glucose is requested, then only enough urine to process the chemical reagent strip portion is needed. However, if a test for microscopic examination of the urine, such as to diagnose a bladder infection, is requested, then a full test tube is needed as well as some extra urine for a culture. These tests are thoroughly discussed later in this chapter.

The provider should be consulted for further direction if the amount of urine submitted is less than needed for the complete urinalysis. The urinalysis report should reflect that the quantity was not sufficient for complete testing. The medical assistant should write "QNS" (quantity not sufficient) where applicable or follow clinic protocol.

If the patient is able to give less than 10 mL of urine for the test tube, the medical assistant should make a note of the amount of urine used. For example, if the patient provides 5 mL, the medical assistant may go ahead with the microscopic examination of urine but should note on the report that the specimen was only 5 mL. The rationale for this notation becomes clear when you understand that the amount of a substance found in 10 mL of urine will be less in a smaller sample. In other words, if the patient has five white blood cells in 10 mL of urine, he or she might only have two to three white blood cells in 5 mL of urine. Unless the notation is made that the sample was smaller, the provider may diagnose incorrectly.

Most clinics/POLs do not require that the urine volume be noted unless it is less than adequate for a complete urinalysis.

Urine Color. There is a wide range of color in normal urine, usually ranging from a pale yellow to a dark yellow or amber (Figure 30-4). The range of color usually is the result of the concentration of the urine. A darker color generally indicates a more concentrated urine. The color of urine

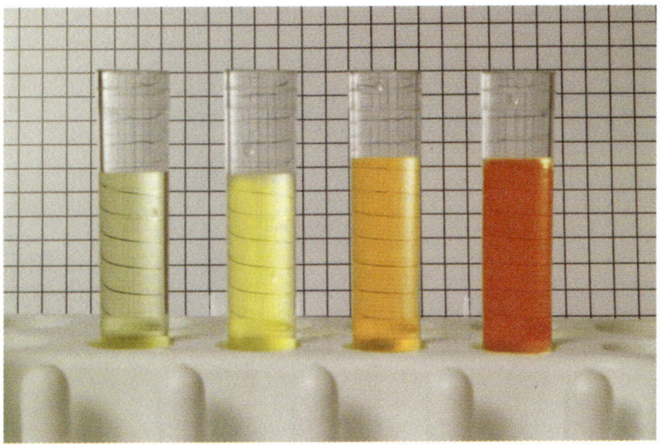

Figure 30-4 Normal urine can range in color from straw and yellow, to amber. Abnormal urine (depending on it constituents) can be red, brown, fluorescent orange, and more.

comes from normal metabolic processes, the end products of which are deposited in the urine.

After assessing the adequacy of the urine volume, the medical assistant then observes and records the color of the urine (see Procedure 30-1).

The diet and certain drugs can add substances to the urine that give it a specific color. The medical assistant should be familiar with common reasons for abnormally colored urine and whether they are pathologic (due to a disease process) or nonpathologic abnormalities. For example, the most common pathologic cause of red urine is the presence of red blood cells, known as **hematuria.** Red blood cells in urine may indicate bleeding in the urinary tract either because of a bladder infection or a kidney stone. A nonpathologic example of abnormally colored urine is the medication phenazopyridine (Pyridium), which can turn the urine bright orange. Table 30-2 lists several urine color variations and possible causes.

Urine Transparency. In order to assess transparency, the urine should be viewed through a clear cup or tube. Urine is considered clear if a line of print can be read through it. Urine transparency normally is not significant by itself. However, it may be helpful when included with the rest of the urinalysis information. Transparency of urine usually is recorded as clear, cloudy, hazy, or **turbid** (opaque) (Procedure 30-1). These descriptive terms may vary in different facilities.

There are many causes of cloudy urine, most of which are considered normal. Cloudiness could be contributed to contamination from vaginal discharges, white blood cells, bacteria, or yeast. As urine cools, sometimes crystals form that may give urine a cloudy appearance.

Table 30-2 Urine Colors and Possible Causes

Color	Possible Cause
Straw to yellow	Normal
Orange to amber	Concentrated urine
Colorless	Dilute urine
Deep yellow	Vitamin intake
Bright orange	Drugs, usually phenazopyridine (Pyridium)
Orange-brown	Urobilin
Greenish orange	Bilirubin
Smokey	Red blood cells
Wine red/reddish brown	Hemoglobin pigments
Green or blue	Methylene blue

Urine Odor. With experience, the medical assistant will recognize certain odors in the urine that can indicate specific conditions. Odors, though not recorded on the final laboratory urinalysis report, should not be disregarded. For example, the urine of a diabetic patient who may have a condition known as **ketoacidosis** may have a sweet odor. Urine full of bacteria will have a foul odor that is easily recognized.

Urine Specific Gravity. **Specific gravity** is defined as the ratio of the weight of a given volume of a substance to the weight of the same volume of distilled water at the same temperature. Distilled water used as the reference point has been given the specific gravity value of 1.000. The specific gravity of urine indicates the concentrations of solids such as phosphates, chlorides, proteins, sugars, and urea that are dissolved in urine.

Variations in urine specific gravity can give the provider diagnostic information. In uncontrolled diabetes, glucose in released into the patient's urine. Glucose molecules are dense and may give the urine a high specific gravity. Another reason for high specific gravity readings is dehydration, because less fluid is being released by the body in relation to whatever chemicals are in the urine. The color of this urine will also probably be darker. In a well-hydrated patient, the specific gravity is low, meaning that the urine is mostly water. The normal range of specific gravity for urine is from 1.005 to 1.030. Specific gravity is highest in the first morning samples because the urine is more concentrated.

Specific gravity is often tested by using either a test strip, urinometer, or refractometer. A urinometer is a calibrated, floating device. A **refractometer** measures the amount of light that is bent by particles suspended in a liquid. A specific gravity reading is also available in conjunction with chemical testing on some reagent strips. The urinometer is the least accurate method and perhaps the most difficult; therefore, it is being replaced by the refractometer or reagent test strips in most POLs.

Urinometer. A urinometer is made from a small glass tube weighted to float in a sample of urine (usually 15 mL). The glass tube has been calibrated, and the stem of the tube has been marked accordingly to read 1.000 at the bottom of the meniscus in distilled water at room temperature. The meniscus is the curvature that appears in a liquid's upper surface when the liquid is placed in a container. The medical assistant reads the specific gravity of the urine from the stem at the meniscus. However, the temperature of the urine must be taken into account if it differs from 70°F, which is normal room temperature. The buoyancy of a liquid changes with the temperature. If the urine is allowed to come to room temperature, the medical assistant risks the physical and chemical changes that can occur to urine when left for more than 20 minutes. It is because of these and other conflicting processes (such as human error) that the urinometer is not recommended as the best option for measuring the weight (specific gravity) of urine.

Refractometer. The most common tool for determining the specific gravity of liquids is the refractometer (Figures 30-5A and B). This instrument measures the refractive index of urine, which is the speed at which light travels through the air as compared with the speed at which it passes through urine. Light is slowed, and therefore bent, as it encounters particles—the more particles, the more bend. The bend can be used to determine the total number of particles and is not affected by the weight of the particles.

The refractometer reading is about 0.002 less than that of the true specific gravity. This slight difference is more than made up for by the ease of using the instrument and the instrument's reliability. This instrument only needs a drop or two of urine, and the result does not have to be adjusted for temperature as long as the temperature is between 60° and 100°F (see Procedure 30-2).

Reagent Test Strips. Reagent test strips that include specific gravity are available through many medical laboratory supply companies. Look for SG in the name, such as brands MultiStix 10 SG or Chemstrip 10 SG (the "10" designates there are 10 tests included on those particular test strips). Keep in mind that the more tests available on the reagent test strips, the more expensive the product will be.

Chemical Examination of Urine

After the physical testing of a urine specimen, the next step in urinalysis testing is chemical testing. This procedure once was complex, but today many manufacturers have made the task simple through a wide range of ready-to-use reagents and the reagent test strip (Figure 30-6).

A **reagent test strip** is a narrow strip of plastic on which pads containing reagents for different reactions are attached. The pads have reagents to test for many metabolic processes, including kidney and liver functions, **urinary tract infection (UTI),** and **pH** balance. The reagent test strip is the primary tool used for chemical examination of urine. Specific confirmatory tests or methods may

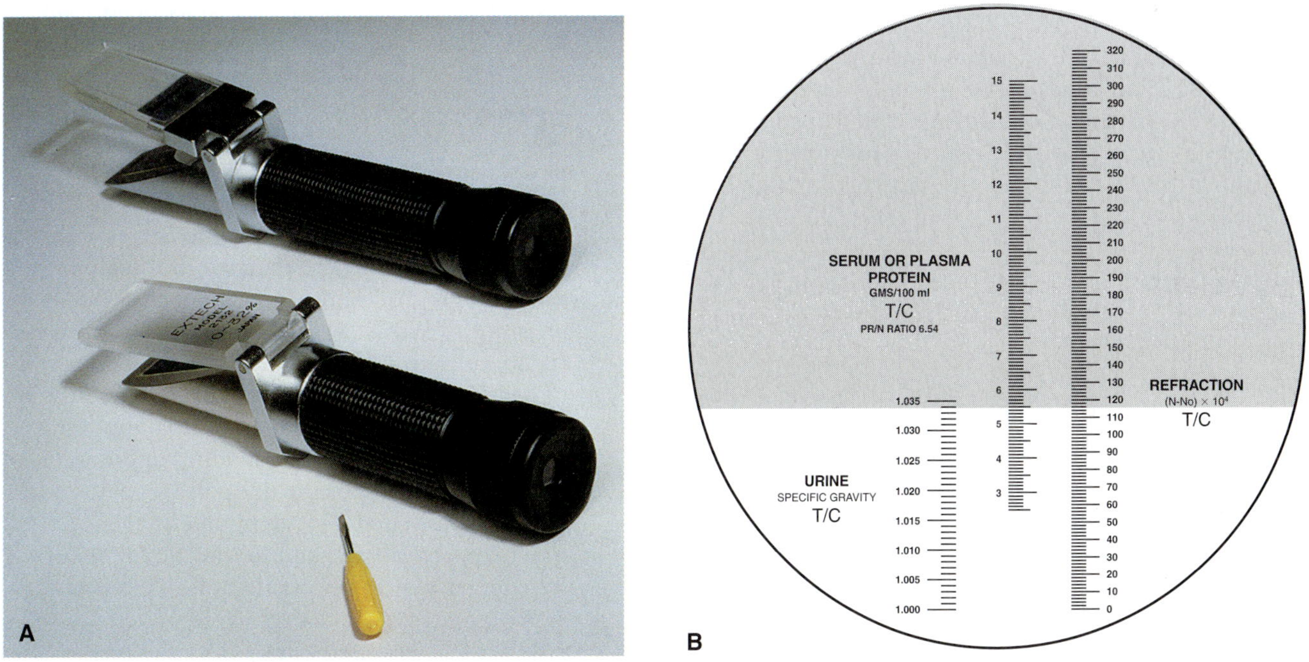

Figure 30-5 (A) Refractometers. (B) Specific gravity as viewed through a refractometer.

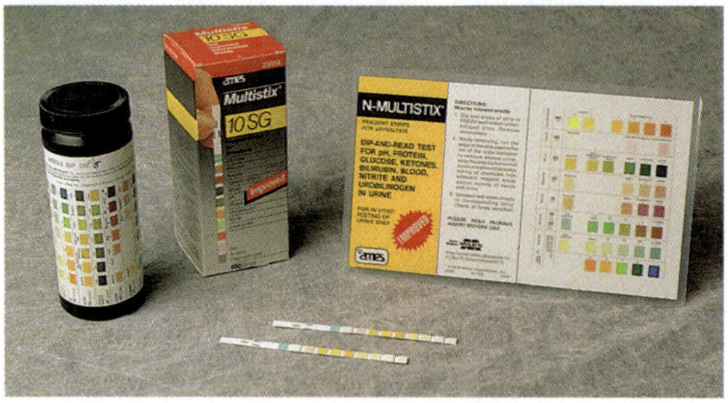

Figure 30-6 Chemical reagent test strips with color-coded chart.

be necessary based on the result of the reagent test strip. Table 30-3 lists some tests available on urine reagent strips.

Specific Reagent Test Strips. *Glucose* is the sugar most commonly found in urine. Glycosuria and **glucosuria** both are terms that describe the condition of having glucose in urine. Sugar is normally filtered out of urine in the glomerulus of the kidney and is reabsorbed in the renal tubules. If the body has too much glucose in the blood, the extra will not be reabsorbed and instead will "spill" into the urine. Reagent test strips are embedded with an enzyme called glucose oxidase, which detects glucose. Of course the first pathological condition we think of for glucosuria is diabetes, but other nonpathological conditions can cause some glucose to spill into the urine. Glucose is stored by the liver and used for energy. Although unusual, conditions such as extreme physical or emotional stress can cause the liver to put a lot of glucose into the blood. Eating an unusual amount of sugar can also cause high amounts of glucose in the blood and either of these conditions can cause excess glucose to be lost in the urine. These nonpathological causes are some of the reasons further testing is required before a diagnosis of diabetes can be made.

Table 30-3 Chemical Testing Available on Urine Reagent Test Strips

pH	Blood
Protein	Urobilinogen
Glucose	Nitrite
Ketones	Leukocyte esterase
Bilirubin	Specific gravity

- *pH* is the abbreviation for potential hydrogen ion concentration. The pH test determines if the urine is alkaline or acidic. The scale for pH runs from 0 for the most acidic to 14 for the most alkaline or base. Neutral pH, of course, is 7. The pH of urine varies from 4.5 to 8. The kidneys and lungs are responsible for helping the blood stay at its perfect pH (7.35 to 7.45). The kidneys do this by adjusting the substances they secrete. A person can die if the blood is too acidic (acidosis) or too alkaline (alkalosis). Because there is so little room for deviation in the pH of blood, the kidneys and lungs are constantly adjusting secretions. Many things affect the pH of the urine, from medication and diets to pathological conditions. Diets high in protein, some medications, renal tuberculosis, high fevers, and uncontrolled diabetes can cause acidic urine, whereas alkaline urine can be caused by diets high in vegetables, citrus fruits, dairy products, some medications, and UTIs. Letting a urine specimen sit at room temperature for too long can cause a false high-pH reading.
- *Protein* (albumin) may be secreted in very small (trace) amounts by the kidneys. The presence of protein in urine (proteinuria) occasionally has a nonpathological basis such as excessive exercise, exposure to extreme heat or cold, or acute emotional stress. Any substantial and/or consistent presence of protein in urine is of concern for renal disease. Proteins are large compounds and can only get through the filtering system (glomerulus) of the kidney if there has been damage to the glomeruli. Think of a volleyball net that a small golf ball could pass through but not a larger basketball, unless there are holes (damage) to the net. Damage can be caused by many things: diseases, toxins, or systemic conditions, such as diabetes and uncontrolled hypertension. Any condition that causes the blood pressure to increase in the nephron can also cause damage to the glomeruli. A false high-protein reading can occur when large amounts of WBCs, RBCs, epithelial cells, or bacteria are present in the urine. When these four types of cells rupture in urine, they can release protein, causing a false-positive reading. It is important to note, too, that any protein reading in dilute urine is of concern because a normal SG in the same patient would show a much higher level of proteinuria. Thus, it is important to look at the SG of the specimen whenever protein is found in urine.
- **Ketones** are formed whenever the body uses fat/fatty acids for energy rather than carbohydrates/

sugars. This can happen whenever there is a low intake of carbohydrates/sugars such as in dieting and in certain metabolic disorders such as diabetes. In diabetes, the body lacks insulin or is unable to use sugar properly for energy, so it uses fatty acids. Insulin is a chemical that helps the body use sugar for energy, so some diabetics replace their insulin. As fats are broken down, ketone bodies form and "spill" into the urine. The presence of ketones in urine is called **ketonuria.** The burning of fats for energy is called *ketosis* or sometimes *lipolysis.* Persons on carbohydrate-careful diets often use chemical reagent test strips to check if their urine contains ketones, thus indicating that their bodies are burning fats. **Ketosis** should not be confused with ketoacidosis, which is a dangerous condition for diabetics and alcoholics.

- **Bilirubin** is a yellow-orange substance that comes from the breakdown of hemoglobin. Hemoglobin is contained within the red blood cells. Because individual RBCs live for only 120 days, they are constantly breaking down and being replaced. When the RBCs "die," the "heme" part of the hemoglobin circulates in the blood until the liver filters it out. The liver is responsible for changing the heme into a water-soluble substance called bilirubin. Before it gets to the liver, it is called "indirect" or "free" bilirubin. After it leaves the liver, it is called direct or conjugated bilirubin. The liver sends the conjugated bilirubin to the gall bladder where it is released with bile into the small intestine. When there is a blockage in the liver or gall bladder ducts or when there is a disorder or disease of the liver, the bilirubin cannot get past the gall bladder to the small intestine, so it continues to circulate in the blood. This excess of bilirubin in the blood can lead to yellow-orange skin called *jaundice.* The body will try to get rid of extra bilirubin through the urine. Hence, any detection of bilirubin in the urine **(bilirubinuria)** can be indicative of a problem in the liver and/or gall bladder. Newborn babies can be jaundiced because their systems are not mature enough to rid the bile. Because bilirubin breaks down in sunlight, we treat jaundiced babies with special "bili-lights" to help them break down the bilirubin in their skin. Knowing that bilirubin is so unstable, we need to protect it from light in our urine samples, another good reason to test urine samples immediately. Keep in mind that further testing is required before a diagnosis can be made, because bilirubinuria is a symptom, not a disease.
- *Blood* in urine is called *hematuria.* If the blood in the urine is not from a nonpathogenic source, such as a contaminate from menstruation, it is indicative of a bladder infection (often called a *urinary tract infection* [UTI]), irritation of the urinary tract from a kidney stone, or, rarely, a neoplasm. Many chemical reagent test strips differentiate between hemoglobin and intact red blood cells. Hemoglobin in urine is called *hemoglobinuria* and can indicate pathogenic conditions such as severe infectious diseases, transfusion reactions, and hemolytic anemias. A nonpathogenic cause of hemoglobinuria occurs when the urine is allowed to sit too long, so any RBCs present start breaking down, thus releasing their hemoglobin. Sometimes the chemical reagent test strips indicate the presence of blood in the urine, but no blood cells are seen during the microscopic examination. This is an example of hemoglobin being present rather than the intact RBCs. The presence of blood in urine is combined with the patient symptoms and other tests to arrive at a diagnosis.
- *Urobilinogen* is a substance formed when bacteria in the digestive tract breaks down bilirubin. A very small percentage is excreted in the urine and is increased in liver disease. Urobilinogen gives color to feces.
- *Nitrite* forms in urine when certain pathogenic bacteria are present. These specific bacteria convert normal nitrate in urine to abnormal nitrite; thus, nitrite in urine is always indicative of the presence of these pathogenic bacteria in sufficient quantities to cause a bladder infection. Whenever nitrite is positive in a urine sample, white blood cells, bacteria, and often red blood cells also will be seen. The provider often orders a urine culture to determine the type of bacteria and the best medication to eradicate it.
- *Leukocytes* are white blood cells. They may be either granulocytes or agranulocytes. Either type can fight urinary tract infectious bacteria, and either type may be present in infected urine. You will learn more about specific WBCs in another chapter. The chemical reagent test strips will only detect esterase from granulocytes and will not detect the presence of agranulocytes, so a microscopic examination is still important as well as a urine culture and sensitivity. These results along with the patient's symptoms will help the provider diagnose and treat the UTI.
- *Specific gravity* (SG) has been discussed previously in this chapter and is available as a test option on many brands of chemical reagent test strips. The normal SG for urine is between 1.005 (very dilute urine) to 1.030 (concentrated urine).

Reagent Test Strip Quality Control. Reagent test strips are easy to use, but the complexity of the chemical testing should not be overlooked. As with any chemical reaction, each test involves multiple steps that are sensitive to temperature, time, dilution, and other factors. Outdated strips or reagents should never be used, so be sure to check the expiration date every time. To get optimum results, a certain amount of care must be taken when handling and storing the reagent strips. They must not be exposed to moisture, volatile substances, direct sunlight, or excess heat. The strips should not be removed from their original container except at the time of use. Always follow the manufacturer's instructions for storage. Test results are represented by a color change. The test result is compared with a color chart on the label of the reagent test strip container. Employees performing this test should be tested for color blindness as many of the color changes are subtle.

Reagent test strips are ready to use directly from their container. Correct QC procedures should be followed as required by CLIA '88 and the facility where the testing is performed. This usually includes using a QC urine sample (with predetermined results). All that is needed for this testing are the strips, QC specimen, and patient specimens. Procedure 30-5 explains how to perform a urinalysis chemical examination.

Automated urine analyzers (Figure 30-7) capable of timing and reading the test strip are

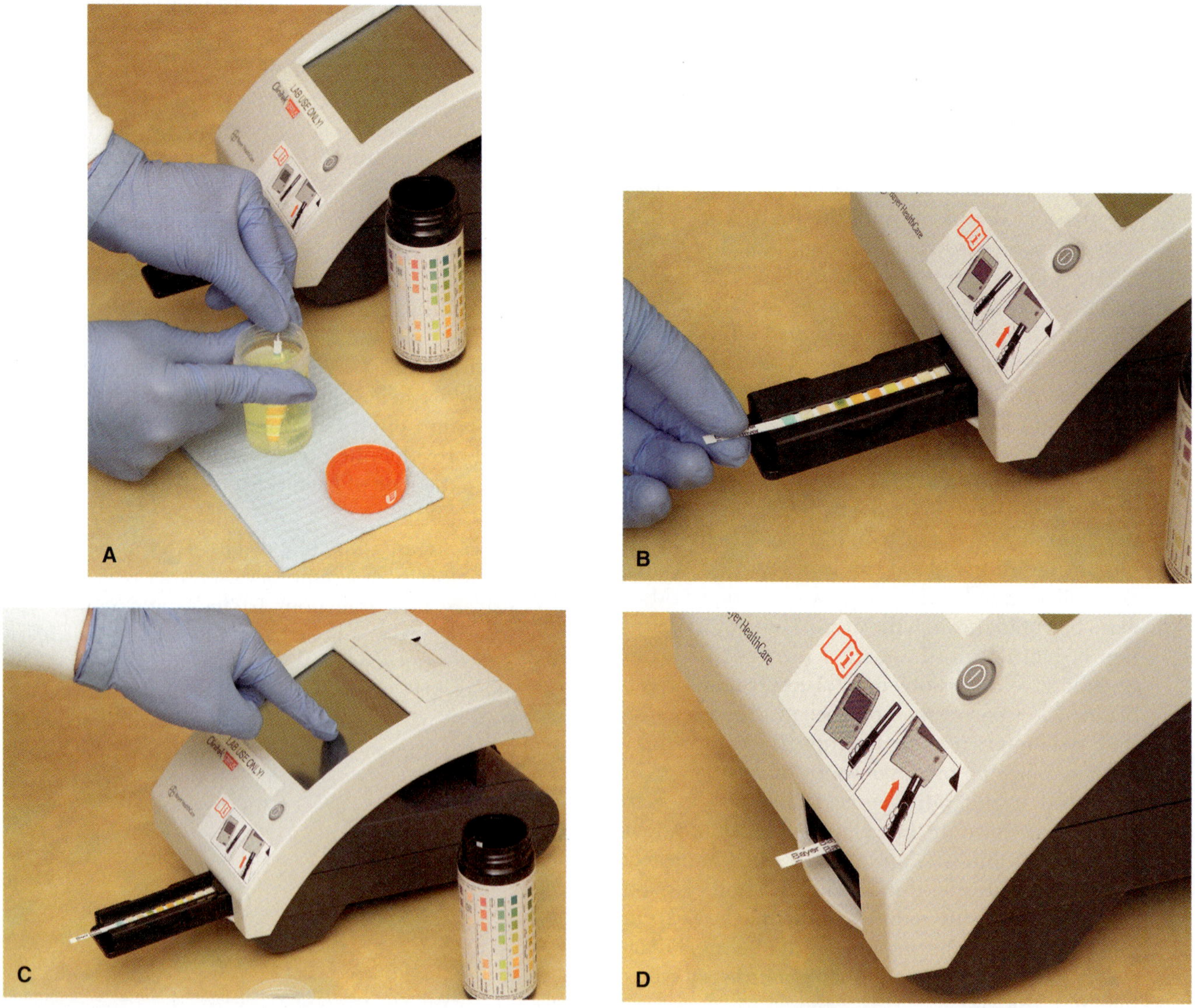

Figure 30-7 Automated urine analyzers are used frequently because of their accuracy. (A) The reagent strip is immersed in the urine specimen and then tapped lightly on a paper towel to remove excess urine. (B) The strip is placed into the machine. (C, D) The test is selected, and the machine pulls the strip into the machine to be analyzed.

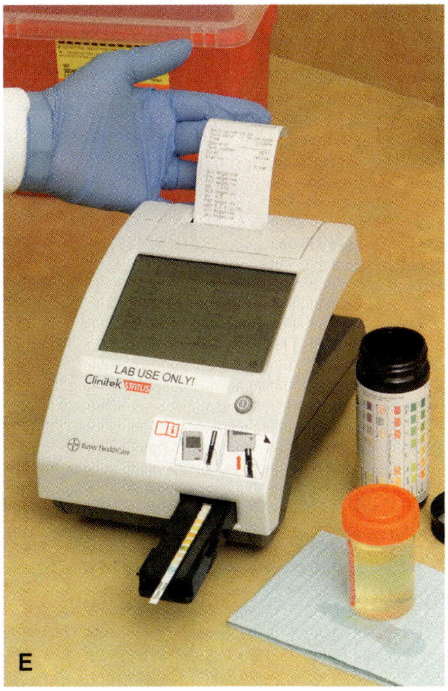

Figure 30-7 (continued) (E) Results are printed from the machine.

available. These instruments can be expensive and are not available in small laboratories. Currently, automated urine analyzers are used more frequently because they are more accurate and reduce human error.

When reporting results, it is important to use the proper units and terms as directed by your laboratory. An example of the sensitivity of the reagent strips is shown in Table 30-4 (there is variation in sensitivity among manufacturers).

Microscopic Examination of Urine Sediment

In addition to the physical and chemical examination of urine, the medical assistant should be familiar with the microscopic examination of urine. CLIA '88 considers the microscopic examination of urine to be a PPMP and not within the category of waived tests. Nevertheless, the medical assistant must be able to properly centrifuge the specimen and set up a slide of the urine sediment for the provider to examine. It is recommended that the medical assistant have a working knowledge of all urine sediment, the pathologic significance of the components, and how to report the presence of sediment components. The **sediment** (insoluble material) at the bottom of the centrifuge tube is used for the microscopic examination (see Chapter 27 for proper use of the microscope). The microscopic examination is helpful in determining kidney disease, disorders of the urinary tract, and systemic disease. It is particularly important that urine be freshly voided and examined as soon as possible to prevent deterioration of sediment components.

One of the most important items to have on hand when performing a microscopic urine examination is a urine color atlas. It takes years to be able to correctly identify abnormal components of urine. A color atlas should always be available to the medical assistant to help with identification.

Some laboratories make use of urine stains to add color to certain structures in the urine sediment. Sedi-Stain® is an example of such a stain (Figure 30-8).

Table 30-4 Reagent Strip Sensitivity

Test	Range	Normal Value
pH	5–9	5–8
Protein	Negative to positive*	Negative
Glucose	Negative to >1,000 mg/dL	Negative
Ketone	Negative to >80 mg/dL	Negative
Bilirubin	Negative to large	Negative
Blood	Negative to large	Negative
Leukocyte esterase	Negative to large	Negative
Nitrites	Negative to positive	Negative
Urobilinogen	0.2–8.0 mg/dL	2.0 mg/dL
Specific gravity	1.000–1.035	Varies greatly

*Note that positive results in a newborn for glucose, ketone, and protein are considered **critical values** and should be reported to the provider immediately.

Critical Thinking

If a medical assistant is color blind, does that mean she/he cannot perform the chemical testing of urine? What (if any) accommodations can be made for her/him?

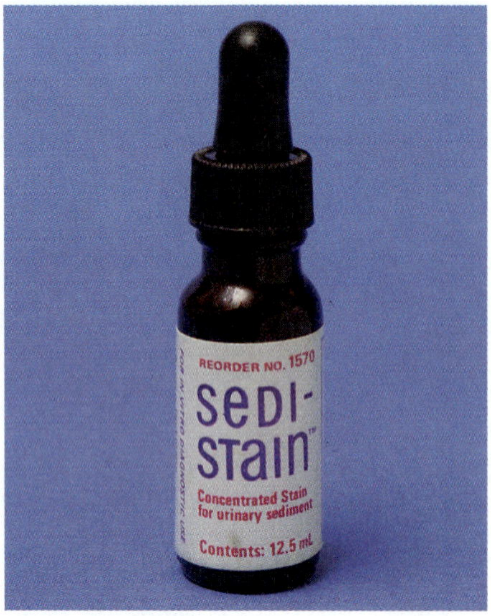

Figure 30-8 Sedi-Stain® is an example of a stain used in laboratories.

Sediment Components. Sediment is obtained by centrifugation of 10 to 15 mL of urine. The solid substances, such as cells and crystals, are forced to the bottom of the test tube, leaving clear fluid called supernatant on the top. The **supernatant** urine is carefully poured off. Most urine test tubes are specifically formed to assist in the process of pouring off all but 1 mL of the supernatant fluid. This is accomplished by quickly inverting the tube completely upside down (do not shake the tube in this position). When returned to the upright position, the 1 mL of fluid will be present in the bottom of the tube, together with the urine sediment. This is the perfect amount of supernatant fluid needed to resuspend the sediment. Try the inversion process first with plain water until you are able to perform it easily. After the supernatant has been poured off, the sediment needs to be resuspended or mixed back into the 1 mL of fluid. This mixing can be accomplished by gently tapping the tube on the counter or flicking it with your finger until the sediment and cellular components have all been mixed and resupended in the fluid. A drop of sediment is then placed on a slide and examined microscopically.

When viewing a normal urine specimen, the medical assistant may see very little under the microscope. Squamous epithelial cells (Figure 30-9A) may be seen, especially in women. These cells have no medical significance because they are skin cells continuously sloughed off into the urine. They are generally reported as few, moderate, or many. If the provider sees many epithelial cells in the urine specimen, it is indicative that the specimen is contaminated with skin cells. Better education of the patient of the reasons for and the technique of a clean-catch midstream collection should result in a less contaminated specimen.

Abnormal Urine Sediment Cells and Microorganisms. The methods of reporting abnormal urine sediment may vary among health facilities. Microscopic examination of the urine sediment may show one or more of the following cells and microorganisms:

- *Red blood cells.* Red blood cells appear as pale, light-refractive disks when seen under high power. Large amounts of red blood cells in urine (hematuria) indicate disease or trauma. These cells are counted in a microscopic field (high-power field, or HPF) and reported as cells counted per HPF (e.g., 10/HPF).
- *White blood cells.* A few white blood cells can appear in normal urine. More than four white blood cells in urine often indicate a UTI. White blood cells are slightly larger than red blood cells, may appear granular, and have a visible nucleus (the red blood cell has no nucleus). Figure 30-9B shows white blood cells in urine. White blood cells are reported in the same manner as red blood cells.
- *Renal tubular epithelial cells.* Renal tubular epithelial cells (Figure 30-9C) can indicate kidney disease if they are present in large numbers. They can be confused with both white blood cells and other epithelial cells. Renal and vaginal epithelial cells are smaller than squamous epithelial cells. Renal epithelia are rounder and vaginal epithelia are more oblong with pointed ends. They are also reported in the same manner as white and red blood cells.
- *Bacteria.* Bacteria can appear as tiny round or rod-shaped objects (Figure 30-9D). Rod-shaped bacteria are generally easier to see because round bacteria may appear as **amorphous,** or shapeless, material. Bacteria often seem to be shaking or vibrating. This is called Brownian movement and is caused by the molecules of water bumping against the bacteria. Bacteria can be very active, actually moving across the microscopic field. If many bacteria are seen and the specimen is not an obviously contaminated specimen, the indication is usually a UTI. The provider will consider the patient's symptoms in addition to the results of the urinalysis to make a diagnosis and will often order a C&S of the urine. Bacteria can be reported as few, moder-

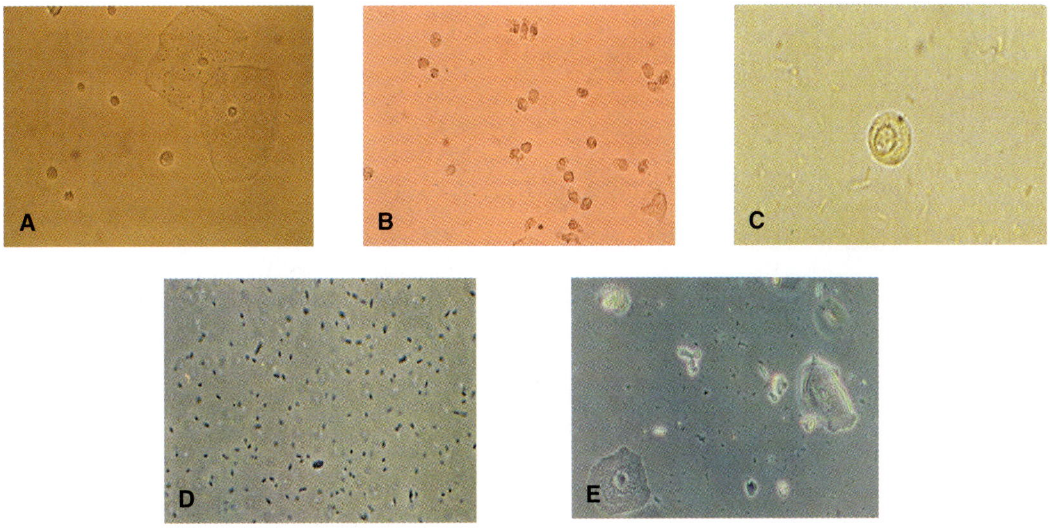

Figure 30-9 (A) Squamous epithelial cells. (B) White blood cells. (C) Renal epithelial cells. (D) Bacteria in urine sediment. (E) Yeasts and squamous epithelial cells. (Courtesy of Bayer Healthcare.)

ate, or many. If both rod-shaped and round bacteria are seen in the same specimen, they may be reported as mixed bacteria. Mixed bacteria more often indicate a contaminated specimen rather than an infection.

- *Yeast.* Yeast cells (Figure 30-9E) may be present in urine, possibly indicating a yeast infection in the urinary tract. Yeast cells are smaller than red blood cells but may appear similar to them. Yeasts are round and can be observed to be budding. To distinguish between yeast and red blood cells, a drop of dilute acetic acid is added to the urine sediment. The red blood cells will lyse, but the yeast will not. The most common yeast found is *Candida albicans.* Yeasts are reported as the amount per HPF.
- *Parasites.* The most frequently seen parasite in urine is *Trichomonas vaginalis* (Figure 30-10). *Trichomonas* is a parasite that can infect the urinary tract. It is often recognized by the movement of its tail (flagella). Always check with a provider or someone more familiar with these organisms before reporting this organism.
- *Sperm.* Sperm is reported when seen in male and female urine. Sperm have oval bodies with one long, thin flagella (Figure 30-11A).
- *Artifacts.* Hair, fibers, powder, and oil are among the substances that may appear in urine sediment as a result of contamination during collection or later. If a structure cannot be identified using a good urine atlas, it probably is an artifact. A urine atlas will show illustrations of artifacts. If in doubt, get an expert opinion (Figures 30-11B and C).

Crystals in Urinary Sediment. Crystals make up unorganized urine sediment. Because crystals are big, the tendency of the novice examiner is

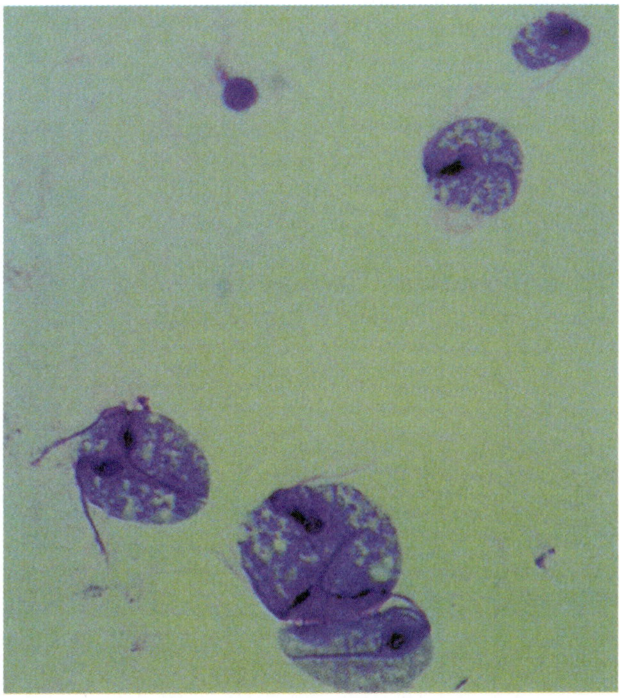

Figure 30-10 *Trichomonas* in stained urine sediment.

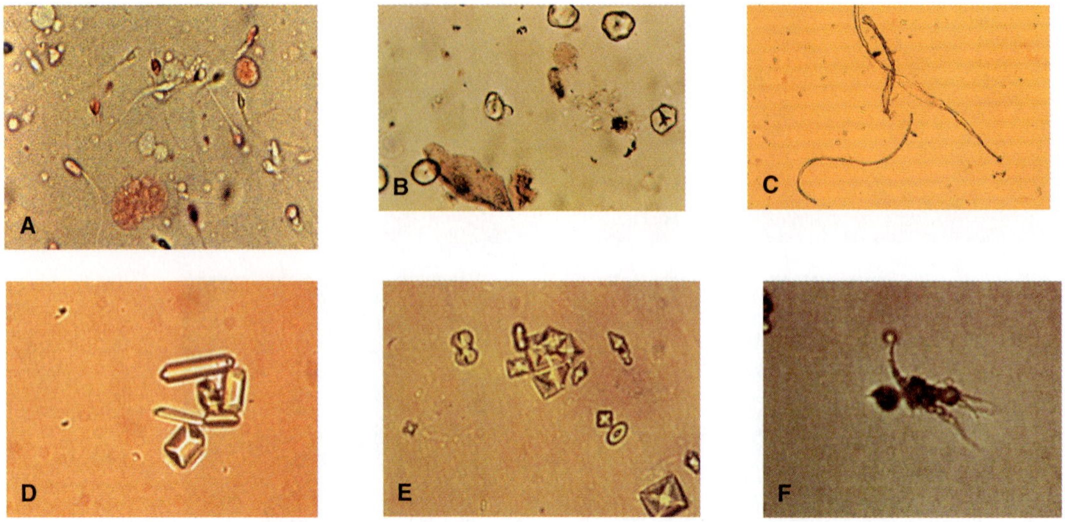

Figure 30-11 Crystals and miscellaneous structures that can appear in urine. (A) Spermatazoa. (B) Starch granules. (C) Cotton fibers. (D) Triple phosphate. (E) Calcium oxalate. (F) Ammonium biurate. (Courtesy of Bayer Healthcare.)

to pay attention to them. However, they are the most insignificant part of the urinary sediment. These crystals include calcium phosphate, triple phosphate, calcium oxalate, amorphous phosphates and urates, and calcium carbonate. These crystals generally form as urine specimens stand, especially when refrigerated. Many laboratories do report these crystals. Refer to a urine color atlas to identify crystals. Figures 30-11D–F illustrates several kinds of crystals that can be found in urine.

Some specific crystals in urine that should be particularly noted if seen because they may indicate disease states are uric acid, cystine, and sulfa drug crystals. Refer to a urine atlas for the shape of these crystals.

Casts in Urinary Sediment. Casts are important to see and identify in urine sediment. It takes a great deal of experience and expertise to recognize the many different kinds of casts that can be in sediment.

Casts are formed when protein accumulates and precipitates in the kidney tubules. The casts are then washed into the urine. Most casts are made from a particular type of protein called Tamm-Horsfall mucoprotein. Other proteins can also form casts. Serum proteins can form waxy casts. The presence of casts in the urine may indicate kidney disease.

Casts are cylindrical with rounded or flat ends. They are classified according to the substances observed inside them. Some casts include debris as they are forming and may appear cellular or granular.

The most common cast seen in urine sediment is the **hyaline** cast. Rare hyaline casts can be seen in normal urine but increase with any kidney disease. They can also be seen as a result of fever, emotional stress, or strenuous exercise. Hyaline casts are nearly transparent and can be difficult to see under the microscope without some light adjustment.

Other types of casts include granular casts, containing remnants of disintegrated cells that appear as fine or coarse granules. Cellular casts may contain epithelial cells, red blood cells, or white blood cells. Figure 30-12 illustrates hyaline, granular, and cellular casts.

Identification of casts in urine requires an experienced eye (see Procedures 30-4 and 30-5).

Urinalysis Report

When reporting the results of a urinalysis, you may use a ready-made form, or your clinic may create a form specifically for your practice. When using electronic medical records, test results are entered directly into the patient's medical record on the computer (Figure 30-13). No printed report is needed unless the patient requires a hard copy (printed document). The report should contain the patient's name, the type of urine specimen (voided or catheterized and if it was a clean-catch midstream

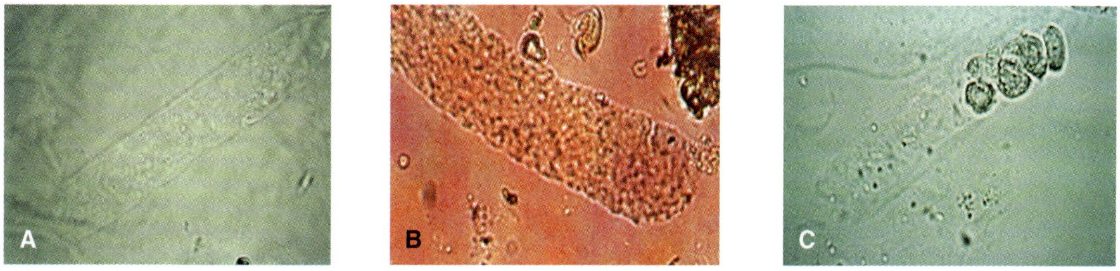

Figure 30-12 Casts in urine sediment. (A) Hyaline. (B) Granular. (C) Cellular. (Courtesy of Hycor Biomedical Inc., Garden Grove, CA.)

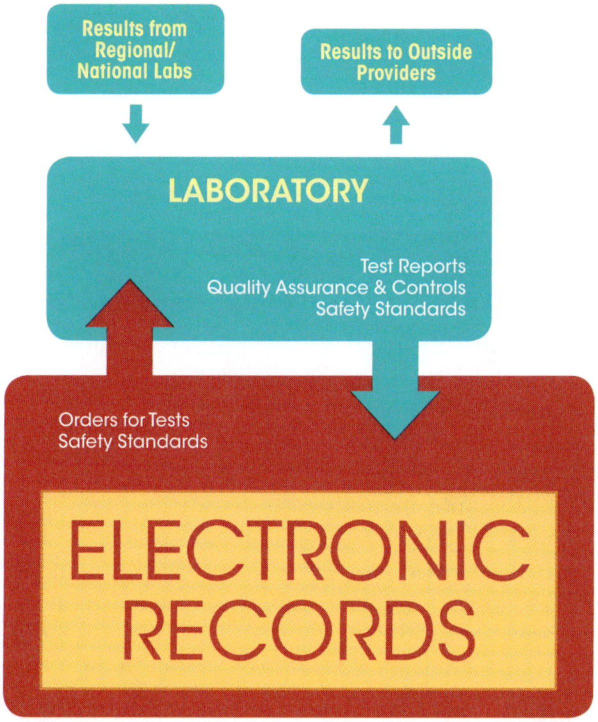

Figure 30-13 The laboratory arm of the total practice management system (TPMS). The patient's urinalysis results are entered directly into the electronic medical record, which automatically compares the data to normal values.

specimen), the provider who ordered the urinalysis, the medical assistant performing the physical and chemical portions of the urinalysis, the date and time the specimen was obtained and the date and time it was tested, and the findings (see Figure 30-14 for an example of a urinalysis report).

DRUG SCREENING

Testing for drugs is becoming more common during the job interview process. Some clinics specialize in occupational health, offering pre-employment physicals including drug screening. The actual test is simple and is CLIA waived, but there are detailed protocols and legal documentations that need to be strictly adhered to. The POL should be certified to perform drug testing, and all clinical personnel should receive special training. A **chain of custody** must take place so that the specimen is guarded against tampering and to guarantee the integrity of the specimen.

Some basic criteria in the process are as follows:

- When the patient arrives, he or she must show photo ID, which is copied. The copy is signed
- The patient signs a consent form for the testing and completes a questionnaire.

Patient: May Pankey Chart # 567-89 MA: W. Slawson, CMA (AAMA) **URINALYSIS**

Req. by: Dr. Rice Date/Time Spec. Rec'd: 3-3-XX 10:15 AM Date Test Completed: 3-3-XX 10:18 AM

	TEST	NORM	RESULT	TEST	NORM	RESULT	MICRO TEST	NORM	RESULT	TEST	NORM	RESULT
☒ VOID	Color	Yellow	lt yellow	Protein	Neg	neg.	WBC	0 – 2	-0-	Bact.	Trace	tr.
☒ CC	Glucose	Neg	neg.	Nitrite	Neg	neg.	RBC	0 – 2	-0-	Mucus	None	-0-
☐ CATH	Ketone	Neg	neg.	Leuk	Neg	neg.	Epith.	Few	rare	Casts	Occ	-0-
☐ TURBID	Sp. Gr.	1.005-1.030	1.010				Cryst.	None	-0-			
☐ HAZY	Blood	Neg	neg.				OTHER:					
☒ CLEAR	Ph	5 – 8	6.0									

City Health Care

Figure 30-14 A sample of a completed urinalysis report.

- The urine collection cup has a built in thermometer to ensure the urine is fresh and is at body temperature.
- The patient is asked to leave coats and bags with the clinic personnel, and these items should be secured.
- The bathroom and patient are inspected for chemicals and/or urine samples that do not belong to the patient.
- In the case of a legal court ordered drug test, the donation of the urine is monitored. Monitoring may occur in all drug testing, depending on clinic policy.
- After the sample is collected, the temperature is recorded and the sample is sealed and secured for transport to a testing facility. The patient signs to verify that the sample is his or hers.
- If a CLIA waived test kit is used in the POL, a test strip is dipped into the urine, and the reagent will react qualitatively (positive, negative, or sometimes inconclusive) for various substances during a specific amount of time. Inconclusive samples must be tested further.

Procedure 30-1

Assessing Urine Volume, Color, and Clarity

STANDARD PRECAUTIONS:

PURPOSE:

Determine and document the volume of a urine sample.

EQUIPMENT/SUPPLIES:

Gloves
Urine container
Laboratory report form
Biohazard container
Disinfectant cleaner

PROCEDURE STEPS:

1. Wash hands and put on gloves. RATIONALE: Washing hands before any laboratory process prevents contamination of the specimen. Gloving provides personal protection.
2. Assemble equipment and supplies. RATIONALE: Organizing your work area prevents confusion and error caused by missing supplies.
3. Follow all safety guidelines, being careful not to splash the urine specimen. Wipe up all spills immediately with disinfectant cleaner. RATIONALE: Preventing splashes and spills will prevent exposure to biohazardous substances. Cleaning any spill immediately prevents further contamination and risk for exposure.
4. Examine the specimen for proper labeling. Any unlabeled specimen is not to be tested. If the missing, unlabeled specimen cannot be identified, the patient should be notified to submit a new specimen. The provider ordering the test should be notified of the delay. The specimen should be labeled on the cup, not the lid. RATIONALE: An unlabeled specimen cannot be proven to come from any particular patient and we should never guess or assume whose specimen it is. The provider should be notified so that he or she is kept informed about the processing of laboratory tests he or she orders. The specimen should be labeled on the cup rather than the lid, because the lid can be removed from the specimen and mixed up with other lids.
5. Ensure the lid is securely tightened and mix the urine thoroughly. RATIONALE: Securing the lid will prevent leaking of urine while mixing. Mixing the specimen will suspend all particles and cellular components in the specimen so that the urine that is poured into the centrifuge tube contains a good sampling of the specimen.
6. Measure and note the amount of urine in the specimen if it is less than 10 mL. The amount of the specimen does not have to be noted if it is more

continues

Procedure 30-1 (continued)

than 10 mL. RATIONALE: If the sample is less than 10 mL, the sample is considered an inadequate amount. If unable to obtain an adequate amount, the testing may still be run on the sample, but the exact amount of the specimen should be well noted on the laboratory report form, and the test should be run according to the priority set by the provider. For example, he or she may request only a C&S be performed or only chemical testing using chemical reagent test strips rather than a complete urinalysis. Samples that are not of adequate quantity to perform the test ordered should be marked as QNS (quantity not sufficient).

7. Note and assess the urine color. Many medical assistants find it helpful to assess the color against a white background. Be sure to have good lighting. In the practice setting, comparing a variety of urine specimens with each other will help with learning about color assessment (see Table 30-2 for appropriate urine color descriptors). RATIONALE: The color of urine is helpful in predicting the concentration of the specimen. The white background helps with assessment of the color; good lighting also is helpful. Urine color names should come only from accepted color descriptors, not from arbitrary names.
8. After the volume and color have been assessed and recorded, assess the clarity of the urine. Holding the urine against a white background with good lighting, observe it for cloudiness. If you can clearly see print through the urine, it is said to be clear. If the urine appears cloudy, it is said to be slightly cloudy, cloudy, or very cloudy/turbid. Record the description on the report form. RATIONALE: The clarity of the urine is useful in predicting the presence of contaminants such as skin cells, mucus, and other debris.
9. Dispose of the specimen into the toilet or designated sink and all supplies into appropriate biohazard containers. Disinfect all reusable equipment and all surfaces. RATIONALE: Using appropriate disposal techniques and disinfecting all surfaces according to Standard Precautions safely controls all biohazard substances.
10. Remove gloves. Wash hands.
11. Document procedure in patient's chart or electonic medical record.

Procedure 30-2

Using the Refractometer to Measure Specific Gravity

STANDARD PRECAUTIONS:

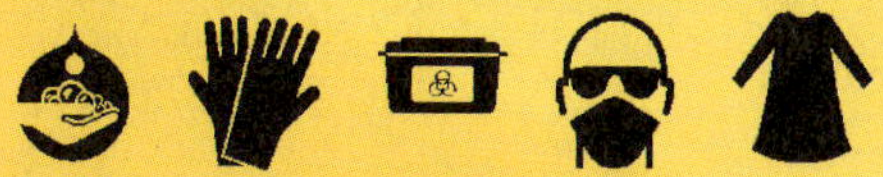

PURPOSE:

Measure and record the specific gravity of a urine specimen.

EQUIPMENT/SUPPLIES:

Refractometer
Urine sample
Gloves
Pipettes
Distilled water
Lint-free tissues
Biohazard container
Disinfectant cleaners
Laboratory report form

PROCEDURE STEPS:

1. Wash hands and put on gloves. RATIONALE: Washing hands before any laboratory process prevents contamination of the specimen. Gloving provides personal protection.
2. Assemble equipment and supplies. RATIONALE: Organizing your work area prevents confusion and error caused by missing supplies.
3. Follow all safety guidelines, being careful not to splash the urine specimen. Wipe up all spills immediately with disinfectant cleaner. RATIONALE: Preventing splashes and spills will prevent exposure to biohazardous substances. Cleaning any spill immediately prevents further contamination and risk for exposure.

continues

Procedure 30-2 (continued)

4. QC must be performed on the refractometer before every use. This is accomplished by checking the specific gravity of a drop of distilled water:
   a. Clean the surface of the prism and the cover with lint-free tissue and distilled water. Wipe dry.
   b. Depending on the type of refractometer used, you may either apply the drop and then close the cover, or close the cover and apply the drop of distilled water to the notched portion of the cover so it flows over the prism. (Figure 30-15A).
   c. With the instrument tilted to allow light to enter, view the scale and read the specific gravity number (Figure 30-15B). It should be exactly 1.000.
   d. If the QC test shows the refractometer to be calibrated properly, you may record the results on your QC sheet and proceed to test the urine specimen (Step 5). If the QC test shows the refractometer to be inaccurate (the refractometer does not measure the second sample of distilled water accurately), the instrument is not calibrated properly. Use the small screwdriver to adjust the calibration. Do this adjustment using distilled water until the gauge reads 1.000.
5. Test the urine specimen exactly as the distilled water was tested and record the specific gravity on the urinalysis report form (Figure 30-15C).
6. Dispose of the specimen into the toilet or designated sink and all supplies into appropriate biohazard containers. Disinfect all reusable equipment and all surfaces. RATIONALE: Using appropriate disposal techniques and disinfecting all surfaces according to Standard Precautions safely controls all biohazard substances.
7. Remove gloves. Wash hands.
8. Document procedure in patient's chart or electronic medical record.

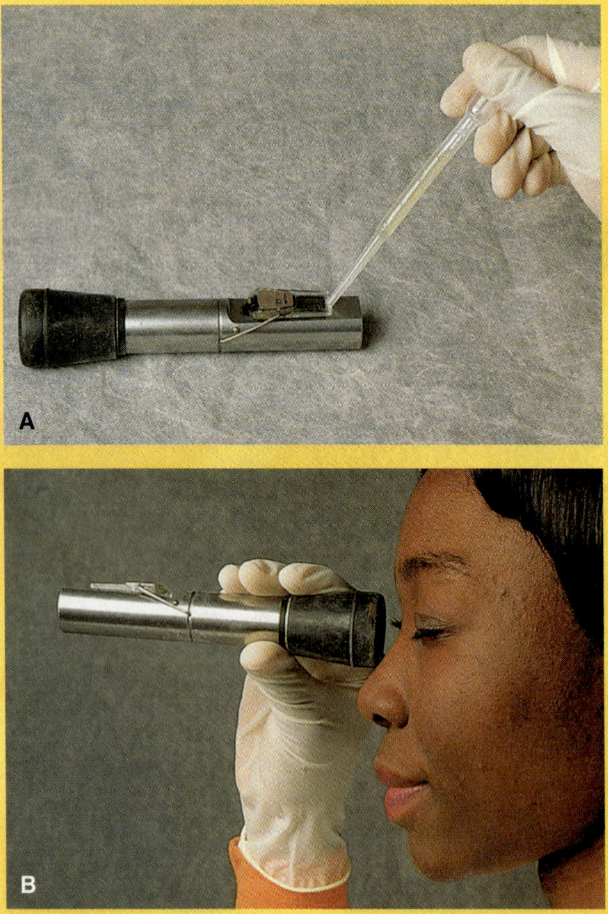

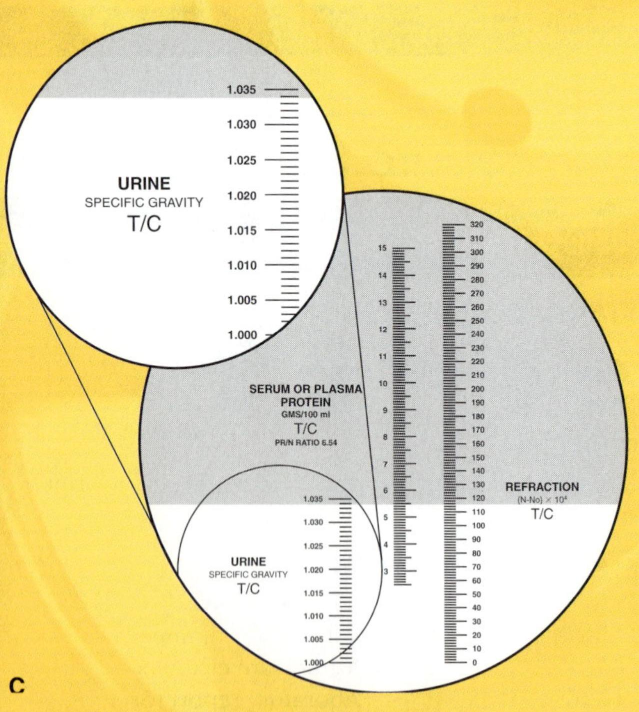

Figure 30-15 (A) A pipette or dropper may be used to fill the refractometer with urine. (B) The medical assistant looks through the refractometer. The instrument is held toward a light source. (C) The specific gravity readout.

Procedure 30-3

Performing a Urinalysis Chemical Examination

STANDARD PRECAUTIONS:

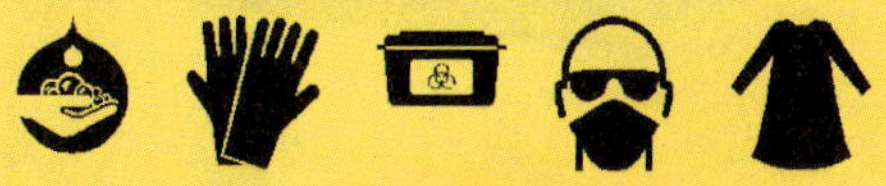

PURPOSE:

Detect any abnormal chemical constituents of a urine specimen.

EQUIPMENT/SUPPLIES:

Gloves
Urine test strips
Urine specimen
Biohazard container
Disinfectant cleaner
Laboratory report form

PROCEDURE STEPS:

1. Wash hands and put on gloves. RATIONALE: Washing hands before any laboratory process prevents contamination of the specimen. Gloving provides personal protection.
2. Assemble equipment and supplies. RATIONALE: Organizing your work area prevents confusion and error caused by missing supplies.
3. Follow all safety guidelines, being careful not to splash the urine specimen. Wipe up all spills immediately with disinfectant cleaner. RATIONALE: Preventing splashes and spills will prevent exposure to biohazardous substances. Cleaning any spill immediately prevents further contamination and risk for exposure.
4. Examine the specimen for proper labeling. Any unlabeled specimen is not to be tested. If the missing, unlabeled specimen cannot be identified, the patient should be notified to submit a new specimen. The provider ordering the test should be notified of the delay. The specimen should be labeled on the cup, not the lid. RATIONALE: An unlabeled specimen cannot be proven to come from any particular patient and we should never guess or assume whose specimen it is. The provider should be notified so that he or she is kept informed about the processing of laboratory tests he or she orders. The cup should be labeled on the cup rather than the lid, because the lid can be removed from the specimen and mixed up with other lids.
5. Ensure the lid is securely tightened and mix the urine thoroughly. RATIONALE: Securing the lid will prevent leaking of urine while mixing. Mixing the specimen will suspend all particles and cellular components in the specimen so that the urine that is poured into the centrifuge tube contains a good sampling of the specimen.
6. If you are planning to perform a complete urinalysis, label a urine centrifuge tube with the patient's name and pour 10 mL into the tube for the microscopic examination. Set aside in the centrifuge. RATIONALE: Setting this portion of the sample aside ensures that it is not contaminated by the chemicals of the test strips or the process of the chemical examination.
7. Read and follow the manufacturer's instructions exactly. The following procedure is a basic guideline. RATIONALE: Each manufacturer will provide specific instructions related to their product. Even manufacturers whose test strips you are already familiar with could change their instructions. The package insert should be read carefully every time a new package is used.
8. Remove a test strip from the container and replace the cap tightly. RATIONALE: Strips are adversely affected by light and moisture and should always be kept sterile in the original container with the lid securely on.
9. Immerse the test strip completely in the well-mixed urine and remove it immediately (Figure 30-16A). While removing the test strip from the cup, tap it gently onto a paper towel to remove excess urine (Figure 30-16B). RATIONALE: Removing the excess urine prevents the specimen from cross contamination of adjacent chemical pads on the strip, which can cause inaccurate results.
10. Properly time the test for each test pad. RATIONALE: Proper timing is essential for accurate results. The manufacturer's instructions will clearly list the proper time for each test.
11. Holding the test strip close to the container (or chart) but not touching it, compare the color of

continues

Procedure 30-3 (continued)

the pads on the test strip with the color guides on the container (or chart) (Figure 30-16C). RATIONALE: Touching the chart or container with the wet test strip will contaminate the chart/container with urine. If this accidentally happens, be sure to disinfect the surface well.

12. Record the results on the laboratory report form.
13. Dispose of the specimen into the toilet or designated sink and all supplies into appropriate biohazard containers. Disinfect all reusable equipment and all surfaces. RATIONALE: Using appropriate disposal techniques and disinfecting all surfaces according to Standard Precautions safely controls all biohazard substances.
14. Remove gloves. Wash hands.
15. Document procedure in patient's chart or electronic medical record.

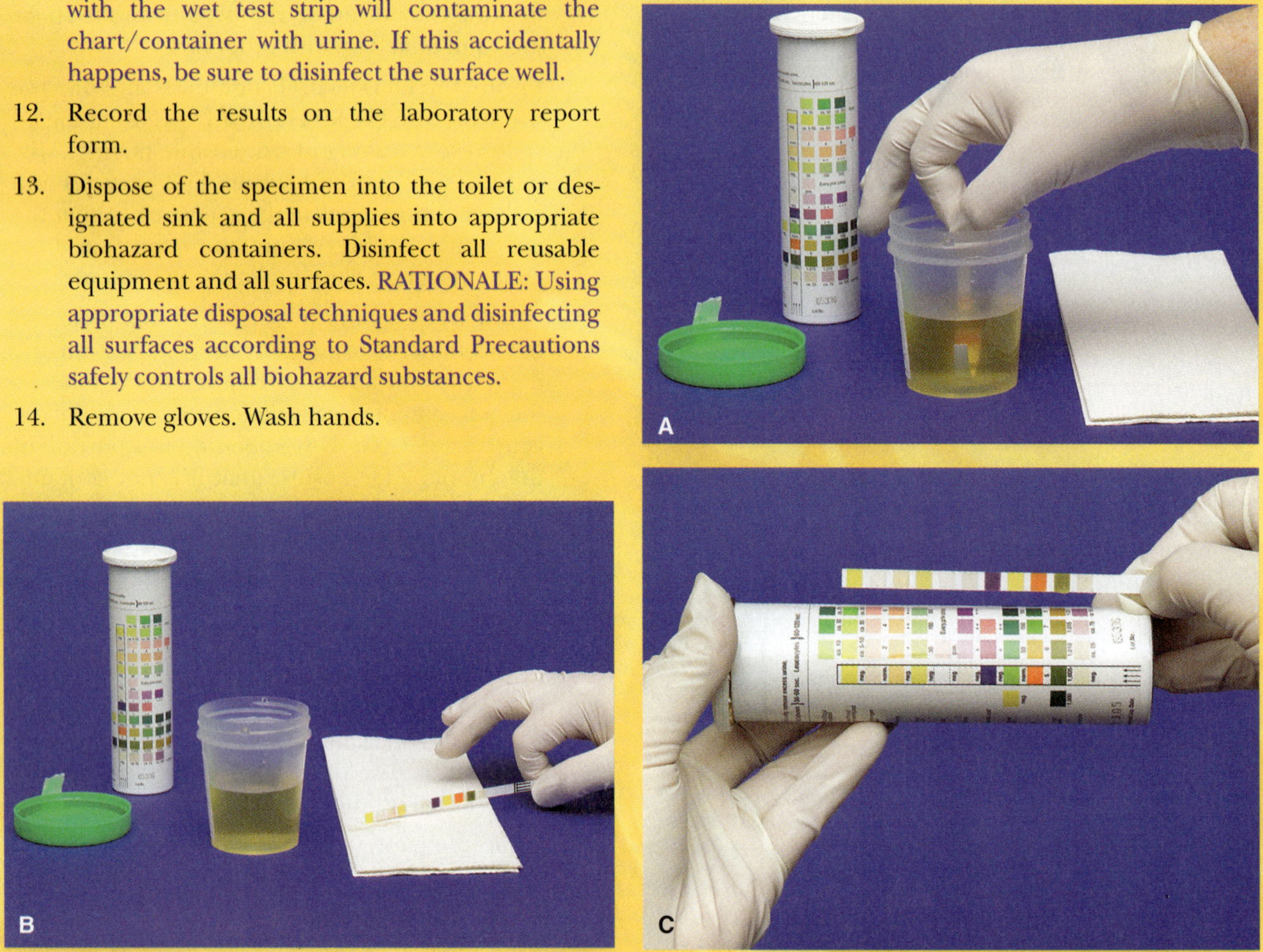

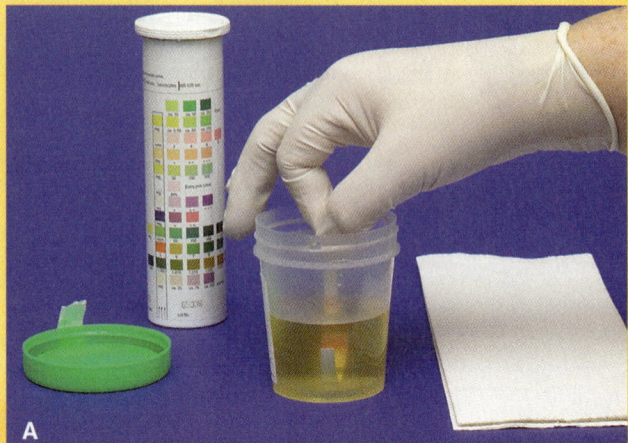

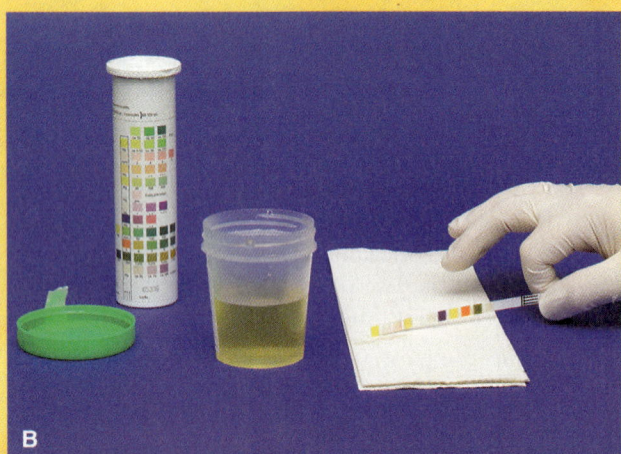

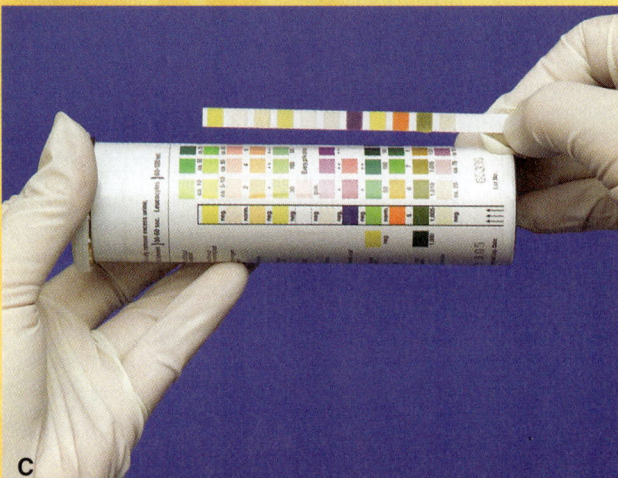

Figure 30-16 Performing a chemical examination of urine. (A) Immerse the reagent strip into the urine. (B) Remove the strip and tap it lightly on a paper towel to remove excess urine. (C) Read the strip by matching the color on the strip to the color chart. Take care not to touch the strip onto the color chart.

Procedure 30-4

Preparing Slide for Microscopic Examination of Urine Sediment

STANDARD PRECAUTIONS:

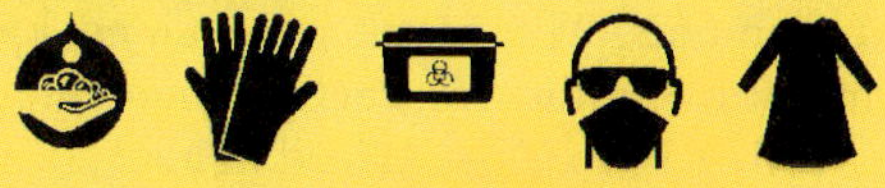

PURPOSE:

Prepare slide for a microscopic examination of urine sediment.

EQUIPMENT/SUPPLIES:

Gloves	Sharps container
Microscope	Centrifuge tubes and holder
Centrifuge	Urine atlas guide
Microscope slides	Disinfectant cleaner
Coverslips	Biohazard container
Disposable pipettes	Sedi-Stain® (optional)

PROCEDURE STEPS:

1. Wash hands and put on gloves. RATIONALE: Washing hands before any laboratory process prevents contamination of the specimen. Gloving provides personal protection.
2. Assemble equipment and supplies. RATIONALE: Organizing your work area prevents confusion and error caused by missing supplies.
3. Follow all safety guidelines, being careful not to splash the urine specimen. Wipe up all spills immediately with disinfectant cleaner. RATIONALE: Preventing splashes and spills will prevent exposure to biohazardous substances. Cleaning any spill immediately prevents further contamination and risk for exposure.
4. Examine the specimen for proper labeling. Any unlabeled specimen is not to be tested. If the missing, unlabeled specimen cannot be identified, the patient should be notified to submit a new specimen. The provider ordering the test should be notified of the delay. The specimen should be labeled on the cup, not the lid. RATIONALE: An unlabeled specimen cannot be proven to come from any particular patient and we should never guess or assume whose specimen it is. The provider should be notified so that he or she is kept informed about the processing of laboratory tests she or he orders. The cup should be labeled on the cup rather than the lid, because the lid can be removed from the specimen and mixed up with other lids.
5. Ensure the lid is securely tightened and mix the urine thoroughly. RATIONALE: Securing the lid will prevent leaking of urine while mixing. Mixing the specimen will suspend all particles and cellular components in the specimen so that the urine poured into the centrifuge tube contains a good sampling of the specimen.
6. Label a urine centrifuge tube with the patient's name and pour 10 mL into the tube. Set into the centrifuge. Balance the centrifuge, securely close and lock the lid, and spin at 1,500 *g* (revolutions per minute) for 5 minutes. RATIONALE: The urine sediment will be forced to the bottom of the test tube and then will be placed on a slide for microscopic examination.
7. After centrifugation, pour off the supernatant, leaving about 1 mL in the bottom of the tube. Add two drops of Sedi-Stain® if desired. Remix the sediment by tapping gently on the counter or with your fingernail. RATIONALE: The test will be performed on the sediment only so the excess supernatant is not needed. Sedi-Stain® colors the cells and other elements for easier viewing.
8. Place a drop of the well-mixed sediment onto a clean microscope slide. Cover with a coverslip by holding the coverslip at an angle to the drop, bringing the edge close to the drop until the urine spreads along the edge of the coverslip, and then gently lower the coverslip onto the drop. Keep the tube. RATIONALE: Using this technique to place the coverslip onto the specimen will prevent air pockets from forming. Keep the tube in the event that a fresh slide needs to be prepared.
9. Place the slide onto the microscope stage but do not leave the light on. RATIONALE: Do not leave the light on because this will heat the slide and destroy the specimen.
10. Alert the provider that the slide is ready for viewing. RATIONALE: The microscopic examination is considered by CLIA to be in the moderately complex test category of PPMP. You are encouraged to view and discuss the microscopic examination with the provider as part of your professional development and continuing education. If you do view the slide

continues

Procedure 30-4 (continued)

before the provider views it, do not leave on the light. If the slide dries before the provider can view it, prepare a fresh slide.

11. *NOTE:* The following steps are included so the medical assistant can learn to examine urine microscopically even though the provider must perform the actual assessment.
    a. When examining urine sediment, it is important to keep the light subdued by lowering the condenser and to constantly vary the fine focus adjustment to view the structures that are faint. Proper lighting and focus adjustments take a great deal of practice.
    b. Scan the sediment using a 100× (low-power) magnification. A 100× magnification is achieved by using the 10× objective lens (10× × 10× = 100×).
    c. View 10 to 15 fields and around the edges of the slide for casts. Casts are often forced to the edges. It may be necessary to use the 40× objective (400× magnification) to identify the casts.
    d. Scan the slide using the 40× objective (400× 5 high magnification) for other cells and formed elements. The count is obtained by averaging the number of each formed element or cell in 10 to 15 visualized fields.
12. After the provider is finished with the specimen and the patient has left the clinic, dispose of the specimen into the toilet or designated sink and all used supplies into appropriate biohazard containers. Disinfect all reusable equipment and all surfaces. Remove gloves and wash hands. RATIONALE: Using appropriate disposal techniques and disinfecting all surfaces according to Standard Precautions safely controls all biohazard substances. Remember that microscopic slides and coverslips are glass and should be placed into an appropriate biohazard sharps container.

Procedure 30-5

Performing a Complete Urinalysis

STANDARD PRECAUTIONS:

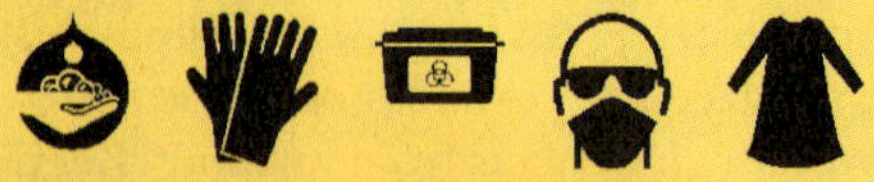

PURPOSE:

Perform a complete urinalysis, including the physical, chemical, and microscopic examination within 30 minutes of obtaining the specimen.

EQUIPMENT/SUPPLIES:

Gloves	Reagent test strips
Urine specimen	Urine atlas
Pipettes	Refractometer
Centrifuge tube	Distilled water
Centrifuge	Lint-free tissues
Microscope	Biohazard container
Microscope slides	Sharps container
Coverslip	Disinfectant cleaner
Permanent marker	Laboratory report form
Sedi-Stain® (optional)	

PROCEDURE STEPS:

NOTE: The following procedure is a compilation and summary of the physical, chemical, and microscopic examination of urine (see Procedures 30-1, 30-2, 30-3, and 30-4). For details within each step, refer to the specific procedure as referenced.

1. Wash hands and put on gloves.
2. Assemble equipment and supplies.
3. Follow all safety guidelines.
4. Examine the specimen for proper labeling.
5. Ensure the lid is securely tightened and mix the urine thoroughly.
6. Label a urine centrifuge tube with the patient's name, pour 10 mL into the tube and set it into the centrifuge. Balance the centrifuge, securely close and lock the lid, and spin at 1,500 *g* (revolutions per minute) for 5 minutes.

continues

Procedure 30-5 (continued)

7. While the sample is being centrifuged, assess and record the color and clarity.
8. Perform the specific gravity test using a refractometer if specific gravity is not included in the chemical test strip.
9. Perform the chemical examination following the manufacturer's instructions. Record the results.
10. After centrifugation, pour off the supernatant, leaving about 1 mL in the bottom of the tube. Add two drops of Sedi-Stain® if desired. Remix the sediment by tapping gently on the counter or with your fingernail.
11. Place a drop of the well-mixed sediment onto a clean microscope slide. Cover with a coverslip.
12. Place the slide onto the microscope stage and alert the provider that the slide is ready for viewing.
13. Dispose of the specimen into the toilet or designated sink and all supplies into appropriate biohazard containers. Disinfect all reusable equipment and all surfaces. Remember that microscopic slides and coverslips are glass and should be placed into an appropriate biohazard sharps container. Remove gloves and wash hands.
14. File the completed laboratory report form into the laboratory section of the patient's chart or electronic medical record and document the procedure.

DOCUMENTATION

11/13/XX 4:15 PM Complete urinalysis performed on random voided specimen. Report filed. Joe Guerrero, CMA (AAMA)—

Procedure 30-6

Utilizing a Urine Transport System for C&S

STANDARD PRECAUTIONS:

PURPOSE:

Prepare a urine specimen for transport using a Culture and Sensitivity Transport Kit.

EQUIPMENT/SUPPLIES:

Gloves
Sterile urine cup and specimen
Urine Culture and Sensitivity Transport kit
Laboratory requisition
Paper towel

PROCEDURE STEPS:

1. Wash hands and put on gloves. RATIONALE: Washing hands before any laboratory process prevents contamination of the specimen. Gloving provides personal protection.
2. Assemble equipment and supplies (Figure 30-17A shows one type of system). RATIONALE: Organizing your work area prevents confusion and error caused by missing supplies.
3. Follow all safety guidelines, being careful not to splash the urine specimen. Wipe up all spills immediately with disinfectant cleaner. RATIONALE: Preventing splashes and spills will prevent exposure to biohazardous substances. Cleaning any spill immediately prevents further contamination and risk for exposure.
4. Examine the specimen for proper labeling. RATIONALE: The specimen cup must be properly labeled to ensure QC.
5. Check the urine C&S Transport kit expiration date. RATIONALE: If the kit has expired, the contents cannot be guaranteed sterile.
6. Open the urine C&S Transport kit package (Figure 30-17B). Remove the cap from the specimen cup, placing the lid upside down on the paper towel. RATIONALE: The cap must be placed upside down to maintain the sterile inner surface.
7. Follow the manufacturer's instructions exactly:
   a. Place the urine tube in the tube adapter (Figure 30-17C) and the specimen straw into the

continues

Procedure 30-6 (continued)

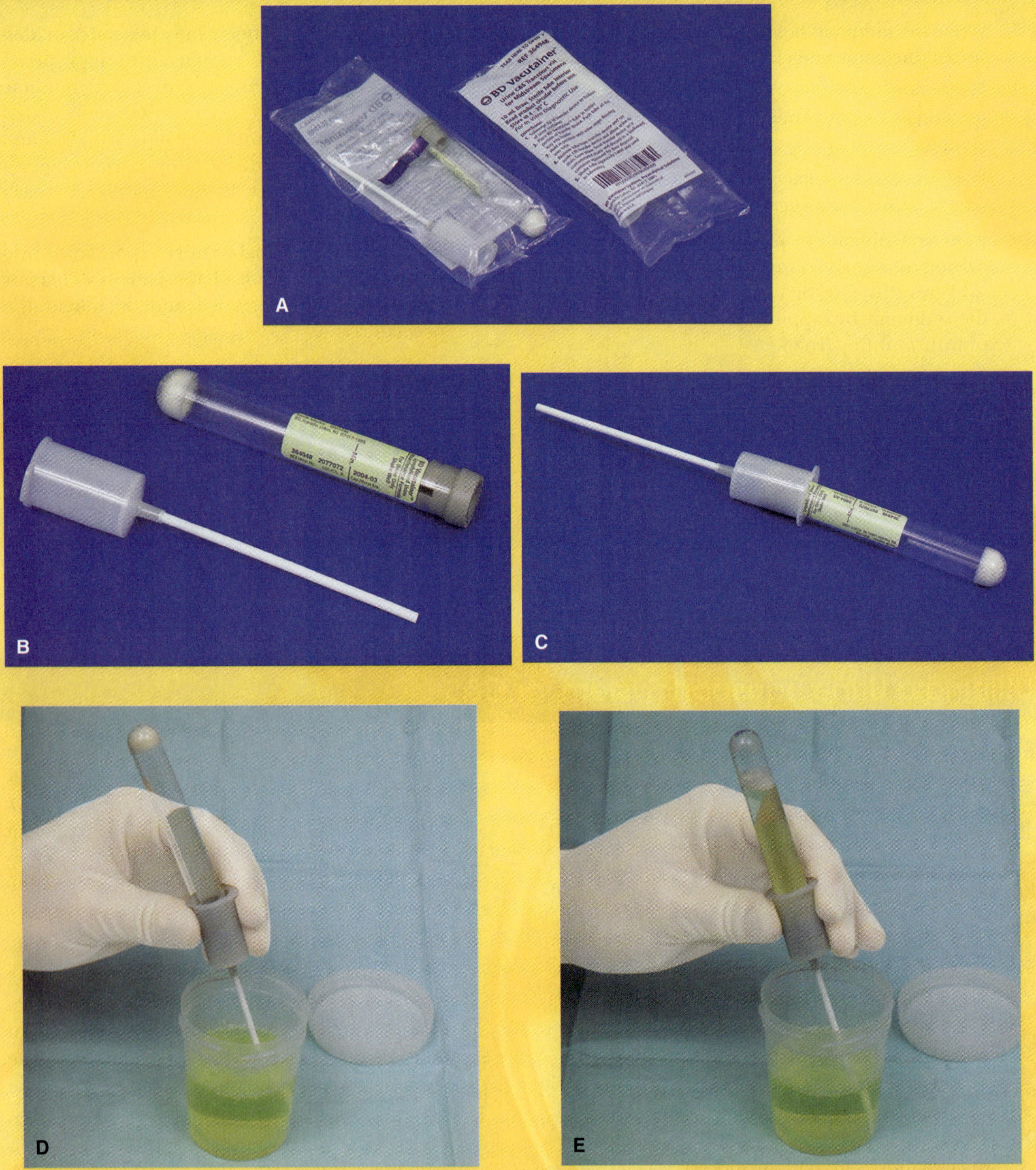

Figure 30-17 The urine transport kit for culture and sensitivity. (A) Packaged as a kit. (B) The components of the kit. (C) The tube is connected to the straw and adapter. (D) The end of the straw is placed in the urine (the vacuum tube is not pushed completely onto the adapter until the straw is submerged in the urine). (E) The vacuum in the tube draws up the urine.

continues

Procedure 30-6 (continued)

urine within the specimen cup (Figure 30-17D).

b. Advance urine tube into the adapter, pushing the tube onto the needle while keeping the specimen straw submerged in the urine.

c. Allow the vacuum in the urine tube to draw up the urine. Fill to the exhaustion of the vacuum within the tube (Figure 30-17E).

d. Remove the tube and the specimen straw/adapter unit and dispose of it into a biohazard container.

e. Gently invert the tube 8 to 10 times to mix the preservative within the tube.

8. Label the tube with patient's name, date, time, and other required information. RATIONALE: Labeling with the required information prevents mix-ups of specimens and ensures a quality timeline.

9. Dispose of all contaminated supplies, disinfect all surfaces, remove gloves, and wash hands. RATIONALE: Using appropriate disposal techniques and disinfecting all surfaces according to Standard Precautions safely controls biohazard substances.

10. Complete the laboratory requisition and document procedure in patient's chart or electronic medical record. RATIONALE: Proper documentation ensures the laboratory will have the necessary information and the patient's medical record will be accurate and complete.

Procedure 30-7

Instructing a Patient in the Collection of a Clean-Catch, Midstream Urine Specimen

PURPOSE:

To instruct a patient on the proper technique of collecting a urine specimen suitable for urinalysis testing.

EQUIPMENT/SUPPLIES:

Gloves
Urine cup with a secure lid
Cleansing towelettes (two for males, three for females)
Marking pen

PROCEDURE STEPS:

1. Wash hands and assemble the supplies. RATIONALE: Always wash hands before working with each patient as a means of preventing disease transmission. Being organized ensures that the procedure will be performed in a professional manner.

2. Identify the patient, introduce yourself, and provide for a private area free from distractions. RATIONALE: Identifying the patient ensures that the right patient will have the right procedure. Intoducing yourself provides for a professional rapport with the patient. Providing for a private area ensures that the patient will have the freedom to ask questions and that confidentiality will be maintained. Being in an area that is free from distractions allows you to use a moderate voice volume and still be heard and understood by the patient.

3. Provide the patient with a capped urine cup labeled with his/her name, a pair of gloves, and the cleansing towelettes. RATIONALE: The cup should be labeled (not the cap) prior to giving it to the patient so there is not a chance of a mixup. Gloves will protect the patient's hand from contamination from the urine and from the genital area. The towelettes will be used for cleansing the area prior to obtaining the sample.

continues

Procedure 30-7 (continued)

4. Show the patient the written instructions posted in the bathroom. RATIONALE: The patient should always have written instructions in case he or she forgets a step. The instructions should be posted at a level that can be read by the female patient while sitting and by the male patient while standing.
5. Explain to the patient why the urine sample should be a clean-catch midstream sample and what that means. RATIONALE: When the patient understands the reasons behind the instructions, he or she is much more likely to follow the steps completely.
6. Ask the patient to first wash his or her hands and apply the gloves. RATIONALE: Gloves are worn to protect the patient's hands from contamination.
7. Explain the cleansing process for a clean-catch: For the male patient, explain that he is to cleanse the urethral opening twice, using two separate towelettes before he begins to urinate. For the female patient, explain that she will need to spread her labia and cleanse from front to back first on one side, then the other, and lastly, in the middle. Explain that she is to hold her labia apart until the urine sample is obtained. RATIONALE: Cleansing the urethral opening ensures that the sample will have no or few epithelial cells from the skin. Epithelial cells are quite large and can make the urine difficult to evaluate microscopically because the bacteria and other cells can be hidden behind them.
8. Explain the process of obtaining the midstream specimen: For both the male and the female patient, he or she is to bring the cup into the stream and obtain about half a cup before removing the cup from the stream. RATIONALE: The mid-stream catch is used to further prevent epithelial cells from entering the sample. If the patient were to stop and start the urine flow, the chances of epithelial contamination increases.
9. Explain to the patient that he or she should secure the cap onto the cup. RATIONALE: The secure lid will prevent spillage.
10. The patient may rinse the outside of the capped cup if needed and towel dry it. RATIONALE: Rinsing and drying the outside of the cup will remove any urine that may be present.
11. The patient is to then remove the gloves, dispose of them into the red bag waste recepticle, and wash his or her hands. RATIONALE: Contaminated waste should always go into red bag recepticles. Hands should be washed to remove any residual powder from the gloves and/or contamination that may have touched the hands.
12. Using a paper towel as a barrier, the cup may be returned to the medical assistant or placed in the lab recepticle as directed. RATIONALE: The POL often has a shelf or designated area for the patient to place the urine sample onto. If not, the sample may be handed to the medical assistant. The paper towel creates a barrier between the specimen and the hand.

Case Study 30-1

Refer to the scenario at the beginning of the chapter. Wanda is careful to prepare her patient properly, so she gets a good sample, she pays attention to the details so that the test is run properly, and she cares about the quality of the results.

CASE STUDY REVIEW

1. What is the worst that can happen if the patient does not give a good clean-catch midstream urine sample?
2. What might happen if the reagents Wanda uses are outdated or have not been stored properly?
3. If Wanda does not care about the quality of the urine tests, how does that reflect on the rest of Wanda's work?

Case Study 30-2

Annette Samuels came to Inner City Health Care today because she is experiencing frequent urination, itching, and burning when urinating. Dr. Rice ordered a urinalysis, which clinical medical assistant Wanda Slawson is performing. Wanda notes that the urine has a cloudy appearance and the chemical reagent test strip tests positive for nitrites. Wanda confers with Dr. Rice, who instructs her to prepare a slide for a microscopic examination of the specimen.

CASE STUDY REVIEW

1. Why might Dr. Rice want to examine this specimen microscopically?
2. How would the findings be reported?

SUMMARY

This chapter summarizes the basics of the urinalysis. Providers order a variety of tests on urine to help them determine or rule out certain abnormalities to make a correct diagnosis and prescribe treatment.

Urine is formed as blood is filtered through the kidney. Substances such as by-products of metabolism, mineral excesses, cells, bacteria, parasites, crystals, and casts can be found in the urine during examination.

It is important for the medical assistant to:

- Understand the proper collection techniques for urine specimens. Medical assistants often are called on to instruct patients on the proper collection procedures.
- Understand the safety guidelines involved with collecting and handling specimens, preservatives, and reagents. These guidelines must *always* be observed.
- Understand the importance of and the procedures for maintaining a consistent quality-control program.
- Understand how to properly perform the urinalysis, following up with proper confirmatory tests when necessary.
- Understand and be constantly aware of factors that may interfere with the accuracy of a urinalysis.

STUDY FOR SUCCESS

To reinforce your knowledge and skills of information presented in this chapter:

- Review the Key Terms
- Practice the Procedures
- Consider the Case Study and discuss your conclusions
- Answer the Review Questions
  - Multiple Choice
  - Critical Thinking
- Navigate the Internet by completing the Web Activities
- Practice the StudyWARE activities on the CD
- Apply your knowledge in the Student Workbook activities
- Complete the Web Tutor sections
- View and discuss the DVD situations

REVIEW QUESTIONS

Multiple Choice

1. What safety guideline is important to follow during a routine urinalysis?
   a. use the same pipette for all patients' urine samples
   b. allow urine to sit at room temperature to ferment the urine properties
   c. once tested, urine can be disposed of by the janitorial service
   d. treat all specimens as if they were infectious
2. What are the three basic parts of a typical urine examination?
   a. volumetric, chemical, and macroscopic
   b. pathologic, chemical, and confirmatory
   c. physical, chemical, and microscopic
   d. random, 24-hour, and catheterized
3. What is the specimen of choice for routine urinalysis?
   a. sterile
   b. clean-catch
   c. catheterized
   d. timed
4. A diabetic patient will normally have an excess of what substance in the urine?
   a. hemoglobin
   b. glucose
   c. insulin
   d. sodium
5. What is the most common way of doing a chemical analysis of urine in a provider's office?
   a. reagent test strip
   b. microscopic examination
   c. culture test
6. Which substance or structure is automatically considered abnormal when found in urine?
   a. phosphates
   b. urea
   c. blood
   d. salt

Critical Thinking

1. What is the importance of proper urine collection?
2. When is a urine preservative necessary?
3. Why is the first morning specimen preferred for routine urinalysis?
4. What would give a urine sample a cloudy appearance?

WEB ACTIVITIES

1. Search for CLIA information on the Internet. Are guidelines posted for specimen collection? When were these guidelines last updated?
2. According to CLIA, which tests are waived in regard to urinalysis and which tests are not?

3. Visit the CDC's Web site and review the Standard Precautions that apply to urine collection and analysis.
4. Using your favorite search engine, search for images that show specific cells and bacteria in urine. You might even find some video clips that show cells or bacteria in action.

REFERENCE/BIBLIOGRAPHY

Walters, N. J., Estridge, B. H., & Reynold, A. P. (2008). *Basic medical laboratory techniques* (5th ed.). Clifton Park, NY: Delmar Cengage Learning.

THE DVD HOOK-UP

This chapter discusses common urologic procedures that are performed in the medical office.

In one of the first scenes, Dr. Rao's medical assistant Shannon explains to Mr. Bean how to collect a clean-catch urine sample.

1. What do you think about the chemistry between Shannon and Mr. Bean?
2. This chapter states that you should not touch the test strip against the bottle when performing a chemical analysis of the urine. Did Shannon follow those guidelines? What should you do if you accidentally touch the bottle with the contaminated test strip?
3. Today's program stated that you should not insert the test strip into the original specimen container. Why?

DVD Journal Summary

Write a paragraph that summarizes what you learned from watching the selected scenes from today's DVD program.

Mr. Bean and Shannon really struggled to connect. What could Shannon have done differently to improve her encounter with Mr. Bean? Do you think that Mr. Bean was trying to hide something?

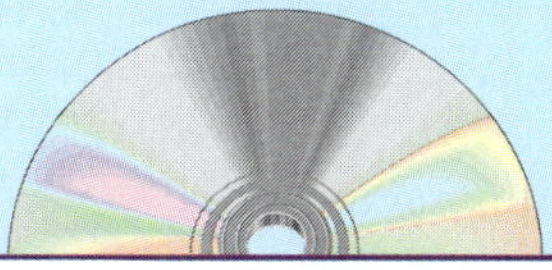

DVD Series	**Program Number**
Skills Based Series	12

Chapter/Scene Reference

- *Introduction to Specimen Collection and Processing Procedures*
- *Administering and Performing Urinalysis*
- *Administering 24-Hour Urine Test*

Chapter 31

Basic Microbiology

OUTLINE

OBJECTIVES

The student should strive to meet the following performance objectives and demonstrate an understanding of the facts and principles presented in this chapter through written and oral communication.

1. Define the key terms as presented in the glossary.
2. Define microbiology, discussing classifications and nomenclature relevant to the microbiology laboratory.
3. Describe bacterial cell structure.

KEY TERMS

Aerobic
Aerosols
Agar
Anaerobic
Biochemical Tests
Broth Tubes
Culture
Dermatophytes
DNA
Expectorate
Genus
Gram Stain
Holding Media
Immunosuppressed
Inoculate
Lumbar Puncture
Microbiology
Mordant
Morphology
Mycology
Nematode
Normal Flora
Nosocomial
Ova
Parasitology
Pathogen
Petri Dish
Potassium Hydroxide (KOH)
Protozoa
Quality Control
Reagents
Sensitivity
Species
Spores

OBJECTIVES (continued)

4. List and describe the equipment used in the physicians' office laboratory (POL).
5. Explain how to safely handle microbiology specimens.
6. Describe the importance of and steps involved in quality control in the POL.
7. Explain the types of microbiology specimens collected in the POL and how they are collected.
8. List different types of stains used to microscopically observe microorganisms.
9. List the different classifications of media used in the POL and microbiology laboratory.
10. Describe how organisms are inoculated onto various media.
11. Describe the significance of sensitivity testing.
12. List two parasites and two fungi that can be observed in the POL.

KEY TERMS (continued)

Stab Culture
Taxonomy
Virology
Wet Mount
Wood's Lamp

Scenario

To aid in diagnosing and treating patients, the providers at Drs. Lewis and King's office order tests to identify disease-causing bacteria, fungi, viruses, and parasites. Some of these tests, such as the quick tests for group A *Streptococcus*, are performed in the office laboratory, whereas other tests are sent to a reference laboratory. Regardless of where the test will be performed, medical assistant Joe Guerrero follows all Safety Precautions when handling specimens. He checks the test manufacturer's or laboratory's procedures and carefully completes each step. By following all safety guidelines and test procedures, Joe ensures his and others' safety. He also obtains a high-quality specimen for testing.

INTRODUCTION

The field of **microbiology** *encompasses the study of all microorganisms, living structures that can be seen only with the powerful magnification of a microscope. The word microbiology comes from the Greek words* micro *("small") and* bios *("living"). The field of microbiology includes the study of such organisms as bacteria, fungi, viruses, parasites, and algae (Table 31-1).*

Many medical textbooks in microbiology include extensive study of all of the preceding organisms, including lesser known species in each category. It is the goal of this chapter to introduce the student to the field of microbiology with emphasis on bacteria, fungi, and parasites. Safety while working with microorganisms in the laboratory is emphasized. The relation of bacteria to diseases also is explored.

THE MEDICAL ASSISTANT'S ROLE IN THE MICROBIOLOGY LABORATORY

The role of the medical assistant in microbiology within the physicians' office laboratory (POL) is to obtain specimens, test specimens within the Clinical Laboratory Improvement Act (CLIA) waived categories, and prepare slides and **cultures** for microscopic examination by the provider or for transport to an outside laboratory.

This chapter discusses cultures in detail. Simply put, a culture is a sample of a body secretion that is placed on special media to allow the bacteria to

Spotlight on Certification

RMA Content Outline

- Medical law
- Asepsis
- Laboratory procedures

CMA (AAMA) Content Outline

- Equipment preparation and operation
- Principles of operation
- Principles of infection control
- Collecting and processing specimens and diagnostic testing

CMAS Content Outline

- Legal considerations
- Asepsis in the medical office

grow. Some samples of cultures discussed in this chapter are throat, sputum, urine, blood, vaginal and penile, and wound cultures. Cultures are usually allowed to grow in optimum temperatures and environments for at least 12 hours before they are examined for identification.

In certain situations, a provider may request a **sensitivity** in addition to the culture. This test will identify which antibiotic(s) will effectively kill the microorganism identified as causing the infection.

In healthy individuals, several types of bacteria are found naturally in various parts of the body. These natural bacteria are called **normal flora.** These organisms are always present and help with the body's immune system. In disease, the causative microorganism is called a **pathogen** because it causes harm to the body.

The medical assistant's technique must be exact to avoid laboratory error. The medical assistant also must ensure that the specimen for culture was taken with sterile supplies and delivered to the laboratory in a reasonable amount of time. Delivery time of the specimen or culture may vary depending on the type of specimen collected for culture. Some specimens may be refrigerated without harm. Some may be kept in **holding media**—media that will keep a specimen on a swab moist until it is cultured. These variations are discussed later in specimen processing.

By doing the smear, culture, and identification through biochemical tests, the microbiologist can identify the organism and aid the provider in diagnosing and treating the patient. Most identification of organisms can be done successfully within 12 to 24 hours. Some organisms may take longer to grow.

Many test kits are currently available to test for microbiologic pathogens; these kits are quick and fairly simple to perform. CLIA has identified

Table 31-1 Biologic Sciences

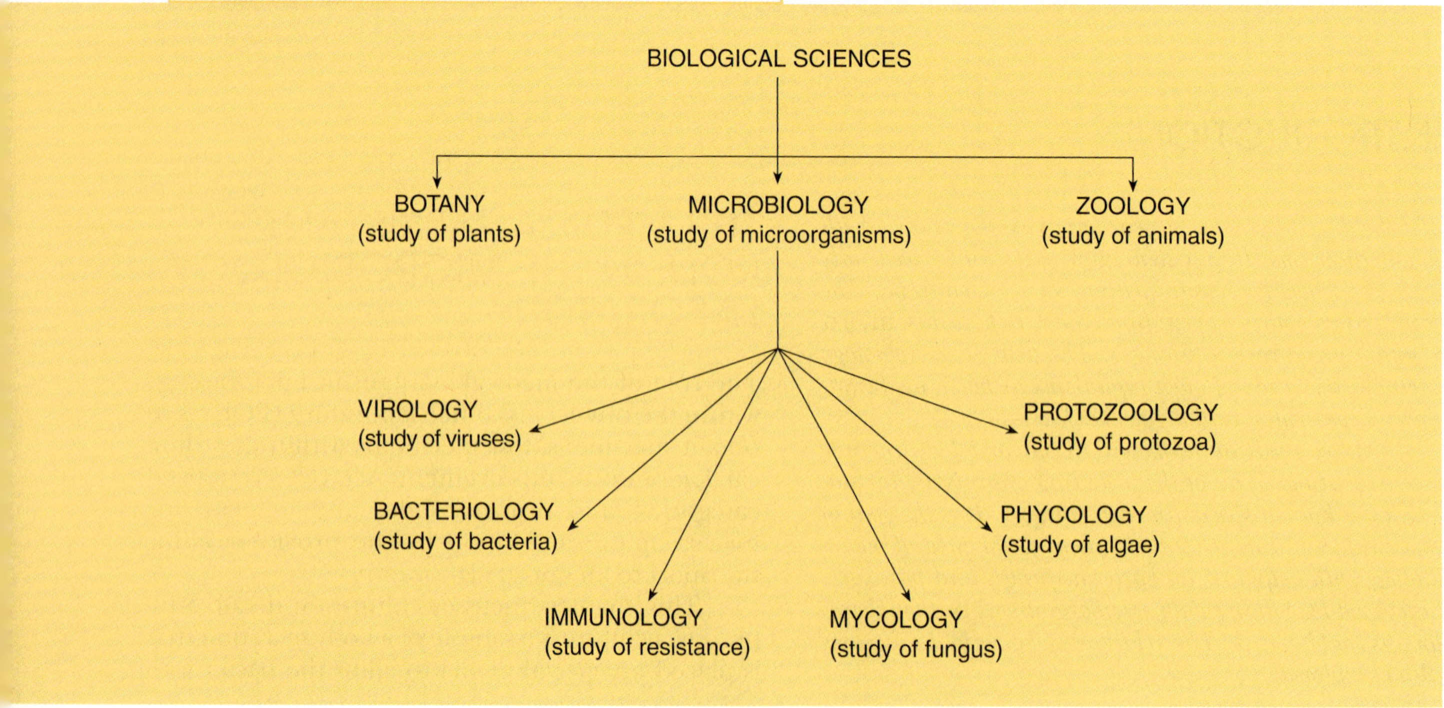

which test kits are within their waived category and therefore appropriate for the medical assistant and other nonlaboratory medical personnel to perform. What used to take days and required the expertise of a laboratory technologist now takes minutes and can be performed within the POL and sometimes even within patients' homes. The at-home pregnancy tests were probably the first test kits available over the counter, but now there are literally hundreds. The test kits range from urine testing for cocaine and other drugs to cholesterol and cancer screening tests.

MICROBIOLOGY

Classification

Taxonomy deals with the classification of living organisms.

A common system divides living organisms into kingdoms. Before the discovery of the microscope in the sixteenth century, there were two known kingdoms, animal and plant. A new kingdom of microscopic organisms, the *Protista,* was developed because most microbes are neither plant nor animal. The members of this kingdom are called *protists* and are one-celled organisms (Table 31-2).

The microorganisms of importance in medical microbiology are divided into two groups: the lower protists, or *prokaryotes* (including blue-green algae and bacteria), and the higher protists, or *eukaryotes* (including **protozoa,** algae, and fungi).

Nomenclature

The system used for naming bacteria is a two-part system of names. Two Greek or Latin names are used, the first name being a **genus,** which is capitalized. The second name is the **species** name, which is not capitalized. These names may reflect a characteristic of a bacterium or names of places or persons associated with the discovery of the microorganism. For example, *Salmonella typhi* was discovered by an American microbiologist named Salmon. The bacterium causes typhoid fever.

Individuals who study bacteria are referred to as bacteriologists or microbiologists. These individuals have taken extensive courses in the field of microbiology. In most laboratories, clinical laboratory scientists or assistants help perform microbiology procedures. The job of these individuals is to quickly and efficiently identify the organism in a given culture that has been properly obtained and brought to the laboratory within a reasonable time frame.

Together with routine bacteriologic cultures, many microbiology departments, especially in larger health care facilities, perform **parasitology** procedures for the identification of parasites; **virology** procedures for the identification of viruses; and **mycology** procedures for the identification of fungi. If an institution such as a clinic or POL is too small to properly identify many microorganisms, cultures often are sent to a reference laboratory. These laboratories are specialized laboratories with up-to-date equipment to handle large amounts of complex tests. In today's health care environment, it is cost-effective to centralize expensive and complex procedures. Instead of 10 small laboratories each having their own specialized equipment, one laboratory buys the equipment and runs the specialized test for all 10 laboratories.

The microbiology department works closely with the infection control department of a hospital to determine if certain organisms are causing infections throughout the hospital. These infections can be acquired by an **immunosuppressed** patient and become a serious problem. Infections acquired in hospitals are referred to as **nosocomial** infections and should be closely monitored. Some common nosocomial infections are caused by bacteria such as Staphylococcus, Serratia, and Candida (a yeast).

Certain types of bacteria and yeasts that are identified and grown in the laboratory must be reported to the Department of Public Health in your county or state because they are communicable diseases. These diseases vary from city to city and state to state. Some of the common bacteria that are reported are Salmonella; Shigella; and those organisms that cause sexually transmitted diseases (STDs), such as gonorrhea, syphilis, chlamydia, and herpes. The state and county you work in will have a list of reportable diseases that the clinic or POL will have posted.

Table 31-2 Kingdom Protista

I. Lower protists
 1. Prokaryotic—nuclear material not organized
  A. Bacteria
  B. Blue-green algae

II. Higher protists
 1. Eukaryotic—true nucleus
  A. Algae
  B. Slime molds
  C. Fungus
  D. Protozoa

Cell Structure

All living forms are alike in that their cells contain a nuclear material referred to as **DNA** (deoxyribonucleic acid), which carries special genetic information. The main structural difference of eukaryotes and prokaryotes is the arrangement of the nucleus. A eukaryote has a well-defined or true nucleus and is a higher form of microorganism. The prokaryote is a lower form of microorganism and has a simple nucleus that is not well-defined.

The bacterial cell, classified as a lower protist, is a single-celled organism with a cytoplasmic cell membrane, cell wall, and nucleus. The nucleus is not well-defined. The cell grows by taking in materials from the environment. After a certain amount of growth, the bacteria reproduce by division of the cell. Certain conditions are required for this reproduction to take place.

Figure 31-1 illustrates a basic bacterial cell. Not all bacteria possess flagella for motility, as some are not motile. Some bacteria can encapsulate themselves in protein, providing protection from antibiotic penetration and white blood cell attack. Once encapsulated they are called **spores,** an inactive state that can help bacteria resist chemicals, freezing, drying, radiation, and heating. Bacterial spores are so resistant they can live 150,000 years and can survive in dust. Tetanus is an example of bacteria that create spores.

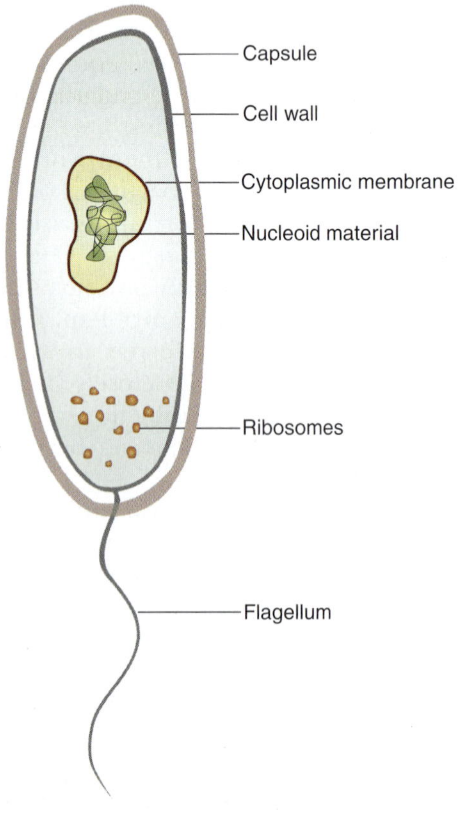

Figure 31-1 Basic bacterial cell.

EQUIPMENT

Basic equipment needed in a microbiology department of a clinic or a POL varies depending on the size of the facility. Most laboratories have some of the following equipment.

Autoclave

An autoclave (Figure 31-2) is used in the laboratory to sterilize equipment that may have been contaminated while processing specimens. It can be used to sterilize contaminated materials as well. The setting of 15 pounds per square inch and a temperature of 121°C for 15 to 20 minutes is sufficient to kill infectious agents, spores, viruses, and contaminants. Many laboratories no longer use autoclaves because of the use of presterilized and disposable equipment. (See Chapter 10 for more information on the autoclave.)

Microscope

An important piece of equipment for the POL or clinic is the microscope. This instrument is used to view organisms that cannot be seen with the naked eye on a prepared slide. Skill in using the microscope is necessary to gain information from studying the slide. The microscope is a delicate instrument and should be cared for properly as stated by the manufacturer (see Chapter 27 for more information on the microscope).

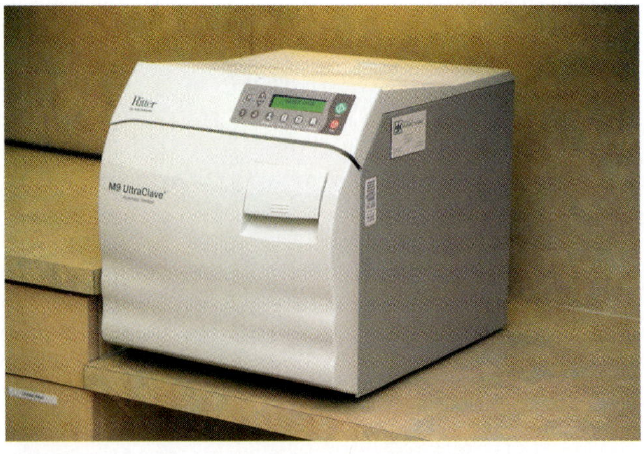

Figure 31-2 Small laboratory autoclave.

Safety Hood

Some laboratories, especially if they are culturing specimens with aerosols, will have a safety hood (Figure 31-3). **Aerosols** are airborne particles that can be released into the air when culturing. They are potentially dangerous if inhaled. By using the safety hood, the health care worker is separated from the specimen by a glass in front of the face, with fumes and aerosols suctioned into the hood. The use of a safety hood is mandatory when performing a culture on a specimen with a potential aerosol. Aerosols are particularly dangerous in fungus and mycobacterium cultures. It is a good idea to use the safety hood with foul-smelling specimens to minimize odors. Tuberculosis is an example of bacteria that travels by aerosol from person to person.

Incubator

The incubator is a cabinet that has a constant temperature of 35 to 37°C. Most organisms, whether **aerobic** (grow well in oxygen) or **anaerobic** (will not grow well or at all in oxygen), grow at these temperatures. Some bacteria, such as Yersina, grow at a lower temperature (26°C). A bacterium called Campylobacter requires a higher temperature (42°C). When working with these organisms, temperature requirements must be met for adequate growth.

Anaerobic Equipment

Certain types of cultures, such as deep-wound cultures, could contain anaerobic pathogens. At the time of culturing, the medical assistant sets up some cultures in an oxygenated environment, as well as an oxygen-reduced environment. Most laboratories post lists of cultures that need an anaerobic setup.

To grow anaerobic bacteria, the absence of oxygen is achieved by using something as simple as a candle jar (Figure 31-4) containing a lighted candle into which the inoculated petri dish is placed. When the cover is put on the jar, the burning of the candle will use up the available oxygen and generate carbon dioxide. Organisms such as *Neisseria gonorrhoeae,* which causes gonorrhea, need a high carbon dioxide atmosphere to survive. The use of a candle jar allows an easy collection and transport system that maximizes the recovery rate of certain microorganisms.

Another method of maintaining an anaerobic condition is a specialized jar called a gas pack jar (Figure 31-5). This jar contains a foil pack that, when activated, gives off carbon dioxide, decreasing the oxygen in the jar. Extensive culturing of anaerobes often is not performed by smaller laboratories. Anaerobic specimens are sent to reference laboratories better equipped to process them. Some small laboratories will perform a Gram stain on the suspected anaerobic cultures. The **Gram stain** is the most common stain used to observe the gross morphologic features of bacteria and is discussed later in this chapter.

Inoculating Equipment

An *inoculating loop* (Figure 31-6) is a piece of wire with a rounded end and a handle at the other end. The loop is used to **inoculate** organisms onto a

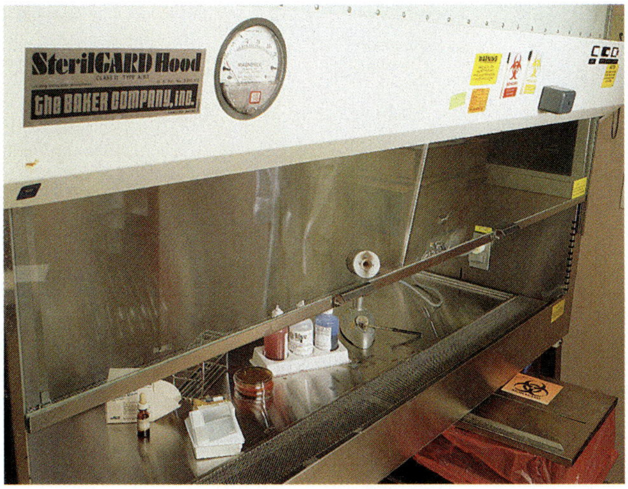

Figure 31-3 Laboratory safety hood.

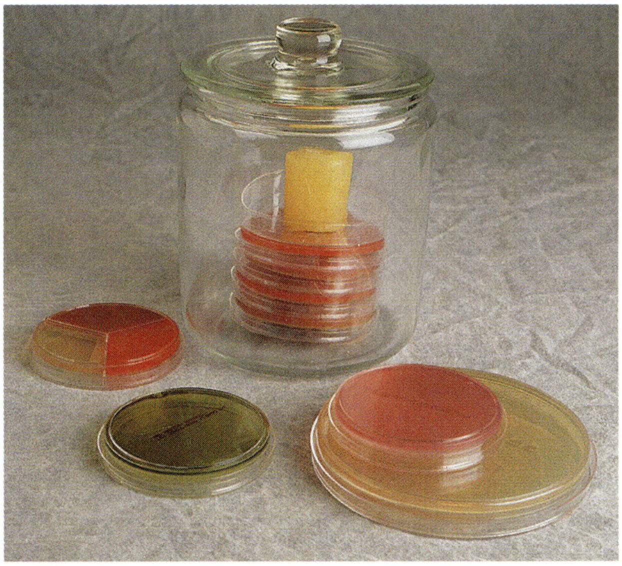

Figure 31-4 Candle jar with media for high CO_2 conditions.

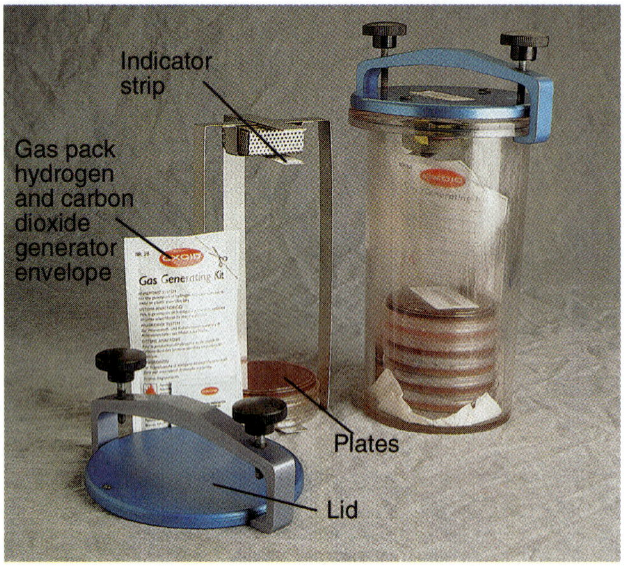

Figure 31-5 Gas pack anaerobic system.

culture medium in a plate or broth. If it is made of wire, the loop can be flamed to sterilize it before and after use. As an alternative, sterile plastic disposable loops can be used. These are one-time use and are disposed of in the biohazardous waste.

An *inoculating needle* (Figure 31-7) is similar to the loop but has a straight end. The needle is used when performing a **stab culture,** also known as "deep" inoculation. The needle is flamed, and the culture material is "stabbed" on the needle into medium in a tube. This technique is used for certain **biochemical tests** used for identification.

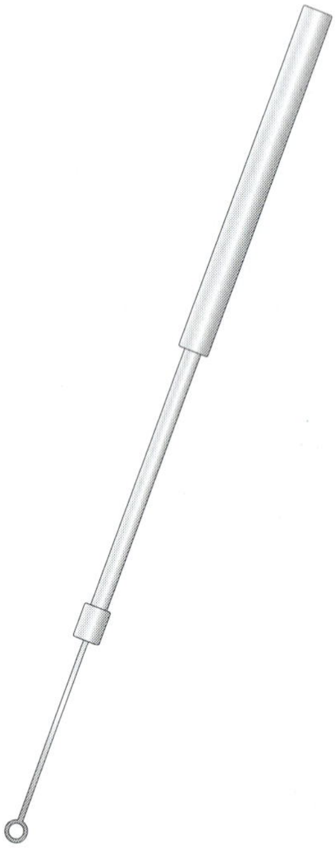

Figure 31-6 Inoculating loop.

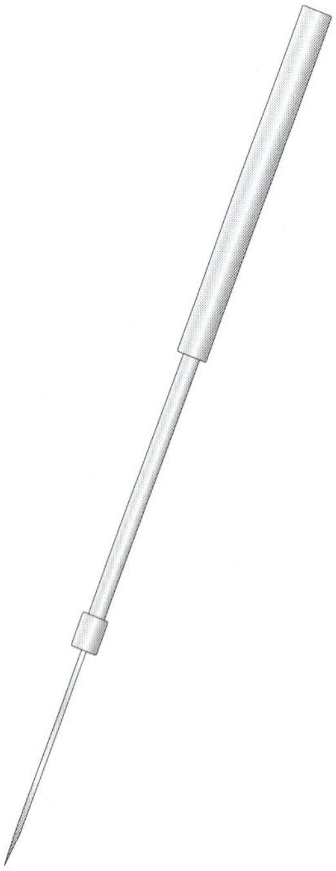

Figure 31-7 Inoculating needle.

Incinerator

Incineration is the quickest method of sterilizing the inoculating loop and needle. This can be accomplished by using an electrical incinerator (Figure 31-8) or a Bunsen burner (less popular today because of the open flame danger). When doing cultures, the inoculating needle or loop must be sterilized before and after it is used. This is done by placing the loop in the incinerator or passing through the flame of the Bunsen burner.

Media

Media in the microbiology laboratory refers to a host of substances used to foster the growth of bacteria. It is listed in this section of basic equipment (Figure 31-9) but is explained in detail in the section about media.

Refrigerator

A refrigerator is needed to store certain materials, such as media and testing kits that need a temperature of 2 to 8°C. Food or drink should never be stored in the refrigerator with any specimens, kits, or media.

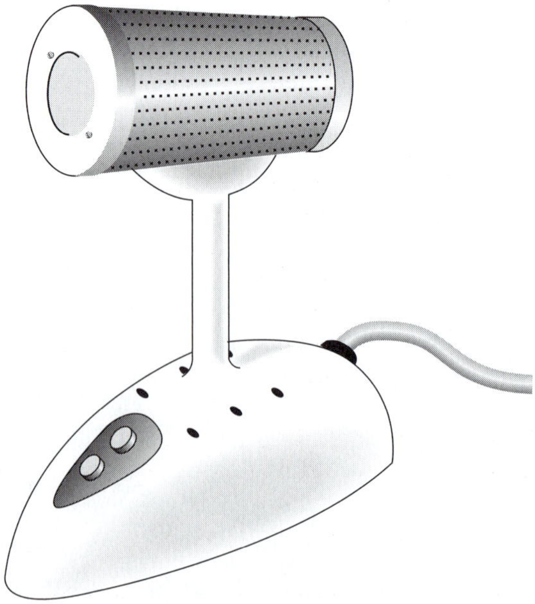

Figure 31-8 Electrical incinerator.

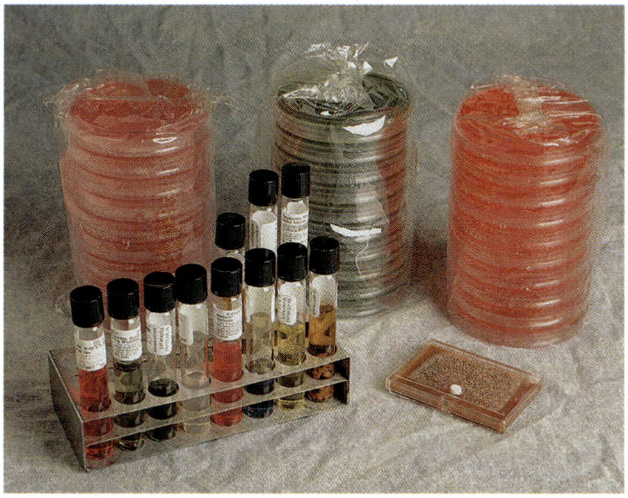

Figure 31-9 Various types of media tubes and plates.

SAFETY WHEN HANDLING MICROBIOLOGY SPECIMENS

Safety should be practiced in every area of the clinical laboratory at all times. Microbiology specimens can be dangerous because of potential pathogens. Following safety rules will reduce danger to all personnel concerned. Some important safety measures follow. Detailed discussions can be found in Chapters 10 and 26.

Personal Protective Equipment

Personal protective equipment should be worn at all times when processing microbiology specimens. It should be removed when leaving the work area. When processing microbiology specimens, the medical assistant wears a buttoned laboratory coat or apron, safety goggles, and gloves. At times, personnel performing microbiology testing work behind a shield or use a safety hood to avoid inhalation of aerosol pathogens and to avoid splashes and spatters of blood and body fluids.

There is never any eating, smoking, drinking, or putting objects into the mouth while working with microbiology specimens or in the laboratory area itself. Contact lenses should not be touched, nor should makeup be applied. The practice of washing hands several times should be a habit. Washing hands after glove removal is important.

Work Area

The counters where specimens are processed and set up should be cleaned with a strong germicide before and after daily use or immediately after a spill. Pathogens could be present where microbiology specimens are cultivated. This area should be dust-free and clean at all times.

Care should be taken not to have a cluttered work area. If using burners or incinerators, caution should be practiced to avoid body burns or fires.

Specimen Handling

Some microbiology specimens will be brought to the POL or clinic to be processed, so the medical assistant should look for leaks and contamination on the outside of the transporting containers. It is a good practice always to wear gloves when receiving specimens. Most specimens will arrive in an "outside" plastic bag to avoid danger to laboratory personnel. When sending specimens to an outside laboratory to be cultured, it is important to use the appropriate container to avoid contamination of others. Remember, if there is a possibility of an aerosol specimen, the specimen must be cultured under a safety hood. All specimens should be handled as if they were contaminated (see Chapter 10 for more information on Standard Precautions).

Disposal of Waste and Spills

Most facilities have a plan for disposal of dangerous biohazardous waste that should be strictly followed. Biohazardous waste generally is placed in red bags marked with the universal biohazard symbol (Figure 31-10). Most clinics or POLs employ an outside agency to dispose of waste. It is extremely important that biohazardous waste is not placed with the regular waste and disposal guidelines are followed.

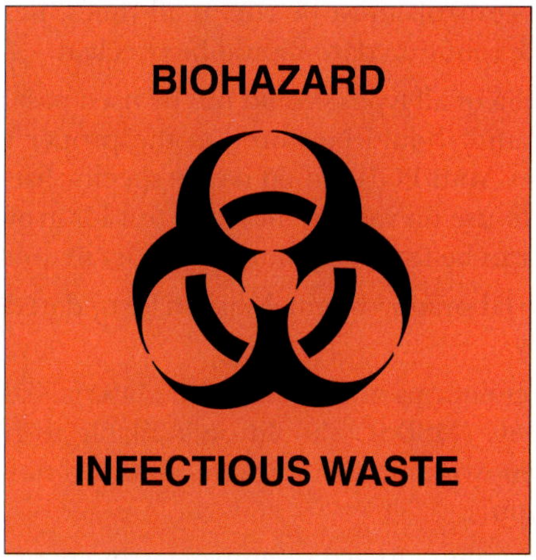

Figure 31-10 Biohazard symbol.

A
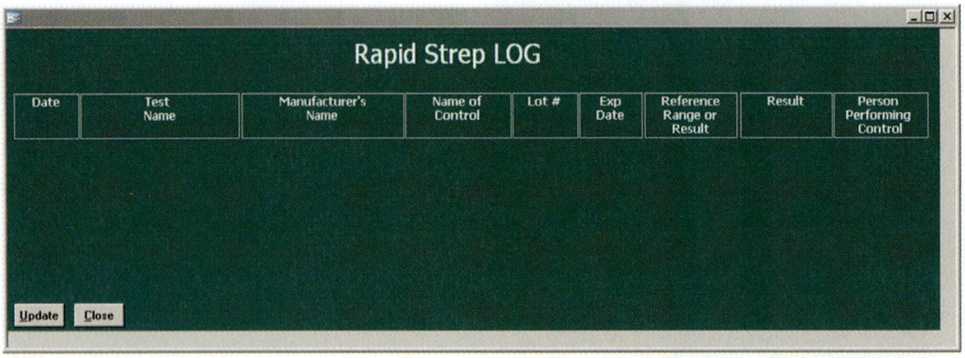

Figure 31-11A In a total practice management system (TPMS), quality control documentation can be entered into electronic logs. (SynapseEHR screen shot courtesy of E.S. Butler.)

If a spill should occur, follow the agency's or employer's rules. Remember to disinfect with a 5% phenol or a 10% bleach solution.

QUALITY CONTROL

Although **quality control** is practiced in all areas of the clinical laboratory, the microbiology department has equipment, media, and reagents that need quality-control checks with almost every test. The following list details some measures that are a part of a quality-control program in microbiology:

- All equipment with temperature controls should be monitored daily.
- The microscopes should be cleaned and kept dust-free.
- Testing for microorganism identification is often accomplished with the use of a special kit. When using kits for different tests, the positive and negative controls must be run at all times. Before use, the expiration date should be checked.
- Media of all types should not be used past the shelf life and should be stored at the proper temperatures. Your POL should have a specific list of bacteria to use on various media to test for growth. This list can be found in your laboratory manual.
- The laboratory manual should be updated periodically.
- All chemicals or reagents with Material Safety Data Sheets (MSDSs) should be available to reference when working with a chemical that is not familiar to you.
- Document all quality control testing in proper laboratory logs (Figure 31-11).

COLLECTION PROCEDURES

When a provider needs identification of an organism that is causing infection, he or she orders a culture from that site. The culture specimen should be collected properly, delivered within a reasonable period, and collected in sufficient quantity. The results of the culture will depend on the quality of the original specimen. All specimens obtained for identification of infectious organisms must be

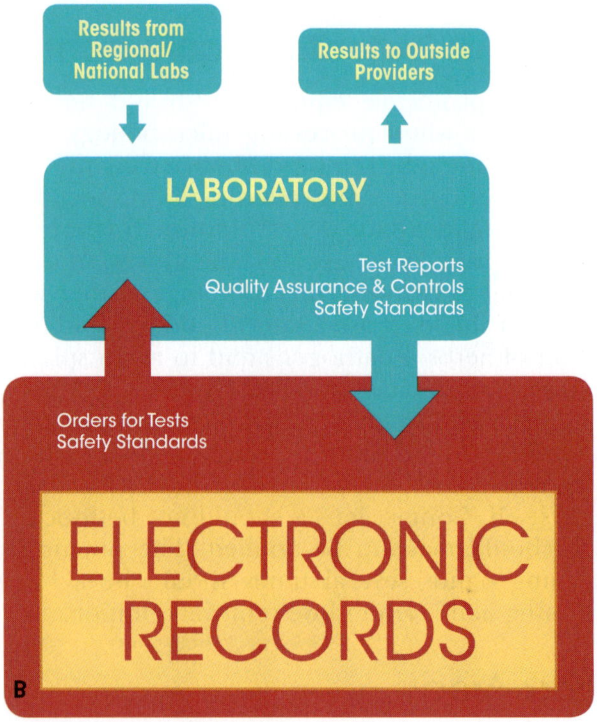

B

Figure 31-11B The laboratory arm of the total practice management system (TPMS).

taken from the site of the infection, not the surrounding area.

Once the specimen is collected correctly, it should be placed in the appropriate container and delivered to the laboratory soon after collection. Many organisms will die if not kept moist. Transport media can have a moistening agent to keep the specimen from drying out.

If a specimen comes into the laboratory in an improper container or has not been delivered within a reasonable period soon after collection, it must be rejected and another specimen obtained. The container in which the specimen has been placed should be sterile, and the right type should be used for a specific culture (Figure 31-12). Sterile containers are used for most collections, with the exception of stool collection containers, which do not have to be sterile. Culturette cultures are from swabs and should be kept moist. This system is a plastic tube that has a sterile swab used to collect the specimen and then is placed back into the tube. The tube contains a medium which keeps the swab moist and preserves the specimen.

The laboratory's success in isolating the causative pathogens depends on the following factors:

1. Proper collection from infection site
2. Collection of specimen during infectious period
3. Sufficient amount of specimen
4. Appropriate specimen container
5. Appropriate transport medium
6. Specimen labeled properly
7. Specimen delivered to the laboratory in a minimal amount of time
8. Specimen collected before the administration of antibiotics
9. Specimen inoculated onto proper media and placed in correct atmosphere to ensure growth

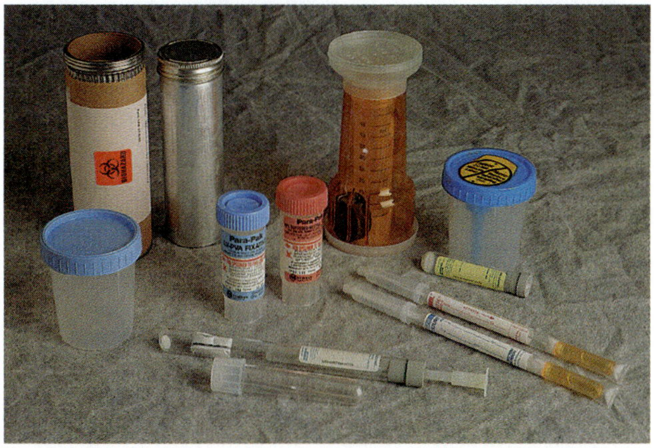

Figure 31-12 Various collection and transport containers for bacteriologic specimens.

When collecting specimens, it is important that the medical assistant carefully follow the instructions as designated in the laboratory manual. Standard Precautions must be strictly adhered to while obtaining and processing specimens and everyone (including couriers, receptionists, and laboratory assistants) handling specimens should wear gloves to protect themselves from leakage of the container and contamination with a pathogenic organism.

Specific Collection Requirements for Cultures

Urine. Patients should be instructed to obtain a clean-catch urine specimen in a sterile container. A clean-catch midstream specimen is obtained by first cleaning the genital area and then urinating midstream into a specimen container. Details of this procedure are found in Chapter 30. Patients should be given strict instructions so that a quality specimen for culturing can be obtained.

Sometimes a catheterization is done to collect a sterile urine specimen for culture. The urine must be collected into a sterile container.

Throat. When taking a throat specimen for culture, explain to the patient that a throat culture is necessary to identify certain organisms. Be sure to tell the patient that there may be some momentary discomfort in obtaining the specimen, especially if his or her throat is sore. Answer all questions about the process of obtaining the specimen. Throat culture specimens are taken using the culturette. As mentioned in the previous section, the culturette contains a sterile swab and growth medium for moisture to keep the bacteria viable.

Once you have gathered all the necessary supplies (see Procedure 31-1) and put on gloves and a face shield, have the patient open his or her mouth and say "ah." This will lower the back of the tongue for better viewing (Figure 31-13A). Be sure to have a good light source available. Use a sterile tongue depressor to help hold the tongue down. While avoiding the tongue and inside of the cheeks, take the specimen directly from the affected area with the sterile swab. Once the specimen is obtained on the swab, place the swab back into the culturette (Figure 31-13B). The culturette is now ready for labeling and transport to the laboratory for testing (Figure 31-13C). As with any culture test ordered,

Patient Education

As you obtain throat cultures from patients, you may want to give them some helpful advice concerning their condition. Generally when a person has a sore throat, it is associated with other respiratory symptoms as well. The following suggestions may provide some relief from discomfort and help patients toward better health.

1. Advise patients to drink plenty of liquids, especially water, and to eat sensibly from the basic food groups.
2. Urge patients to get extra rest and dress comfortably (according to the weather/temperature outside).
3. Suggest use of gargles or throat lozenges (or both) to relieve painful sore throat.
4. Remind patients to avoid tobacco/smoking.
5. Instruct patients to cough/sneeze into tissue and discard into proper waste container wherever they are to prevent the spread of microorganisms. Because sewer waste is treated and disinfected, flushing a contaminated tissue is an effective method of disposal.
6. Remind patients to refrain from sharing drinking glasses and tableware and from intimate contact such as kissing while they are infected and still contagious. All eating utensils should be sanitized in hot water after use to avoid the spread of contagious diseases. Perhaps the most important educational advice is reminding patients to wash their hands frequently.

a requisition stating the site from which the specimen was obtained is required.

Throat swabs for the detection of group A Streptococcus infection (strep throat) usually are tested in the POL using a self-contained kit that produces quick results (see Procedure 31-3). Performing the rapid strep tests are well within the medical assistant's scope under CLIA's waived test category. More information about performing rapid strep tests is provided later in this chapter in the section on Streptococcus Screening.

Nose. A nasopharyngeal swab may be requested with a throat culture. This is collected with a swab

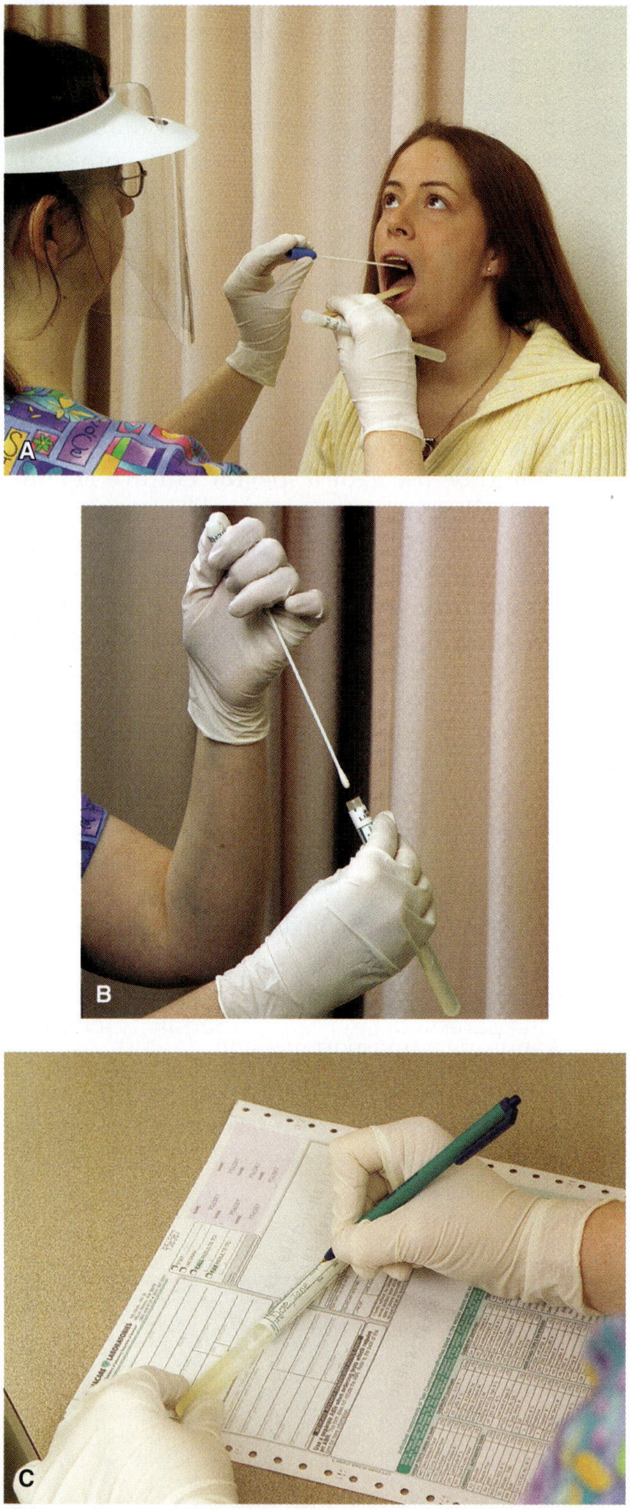

Figure 31-13 (A) The medical assistant obtains a throat culture using a culturette, taking care to not touch the cheeks or tongue. (B) After swabbing the patient's throat, the medical assistant returns the swab to the culturette, which contains the moist media. (C) The culturette is labeled, and a requisition is completed in preparation for transport to the regional laboratory for testing.

on a thin wire. A separate swab may be used for each nostril. The patient tilts back the head, and each swab is gently inserted into each of the nostrils. The swab is then placed into a sterile tube and kept at room temperature for transport to the laboratory.

Wound. When culturing a wound, a sterile needle might be used to aspirate pus-filled fluid from the wound, or a swab is used. It is important to get the swab deep into the wound without touching the surrounding skin. Specimens for wound cultures often are placed in anaerobic transport medium, especially if the wound is not superficial.

Sputum. To collect this specimen correctly, the patient should cough deeply and **expectorate** into the sterile container (Figure 31-14). The specimen should be a first morning specimen and placed into a sterile container designed to protect all who handle the specimen from contamination.

Stool. Stool specimens are brought to the laboratory for various tests. If the stool is to be examined for **ova** (eggs) or parasites, the specimen should be as fresh as possible. Special containers often are used for ova and parasites. Stool specimens must be kept at between room temperature and body temperature. Refrigeration may destroy the parasites within the specimen.

For bacterial cultures of stool (as well as for ova and parasites), several different specimens may be sent for testing at different times. The collection containers for stool cultures do not have to be sterile, but they must be clean and have a tight-fitting lid (see Procedure 31-4).

Cerebrospinal Fluid (CSF). The provider obtains CSF by doing a **lumbar puncture** (see Procedure 18-22). The fluid generally is dispersed in several departments of the clinical laboratory. Generally, the fluid goes first to the microbiology laboratory for a culture before it becomes contaminated by doing other tests. Before the culture set up, the tube should be placed in an incubator or left at room temperature. Refrigeration of spinal fluid can kill two common meningitis-causing bacteria, *Haemophilus influenzae* and *Neisseria meningitidis.* CSF culture is a STAT order for processing, and the medical assistant is responsible for calling the laboratory for immediate pickup.

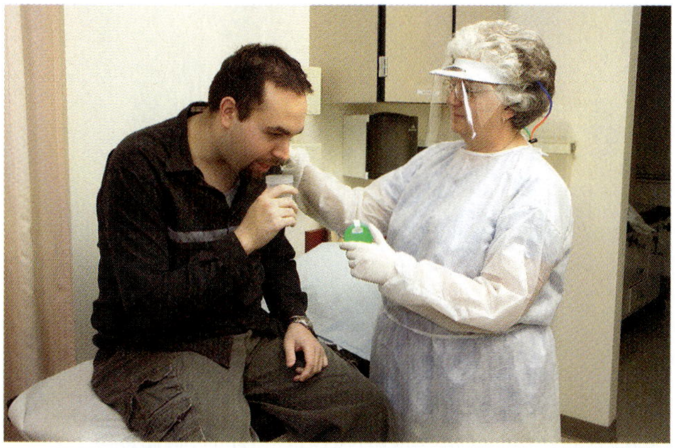

Figure 31-14 A patient gives a sputum sample.

Blood. Human blood is free from bacteria in a healthy human. If blood does become contaminated with bacteria, septicemia (septic blood infection) can result. Blood cultures are collected by the same means as regular blood collection, with special considerations to avoid any contamination of the blood. A variety of collection devices are available for collecting blood cultures, all requiring careful sterile techniques (see Procedure 29-4 for blood culture).

MICROSCOPIC EXAMINATION OF BACTERIA

There are usually two procedures involved in properly identifying bacteria: the microscopic examination and the culture. The microscopic examination involves viewing stained or unstained bacteria through the microscope.

Culturing is a means of isolating a disease-causing microorganism for identification. A specimen is obtained and placed in a culture medium, which contains nutrients comparable to human tissue to encourage growth of microorganisms. The medium is **agar,** a gelatin-like substance, mixed with nutrients. The nutrients mixed in the agar will vary according to what each particular bacterium prefers. The section on Culture Media later discusses in detail the types of nutrients each type of bacterium prefers. Table 31-4 lists the more common bacteria and their growth requirements.

Microscopically identifying bacteria is not in CLIA's waived categories; therefore, although the medical assistant will not actually perform these tests, the staining information is included here to aid in understanding the staining and examination processes that culture specimens go through. It is important for medical assistants to be familiar with the processes and the terminology related to staining and microscopic identification of bacteria to better serve their patients, employer, and colleagues.

Bacterial Shapes

Each genus of bacteria has a characteristic shape. A knowledge of the shapes of bacteria helps in identification. Bacteria have three basic shapes:

1. *Cocci.* Cocci (Figure 31-15) are round in shape, occurring in clusters, pairs, singles, and tetrads (groups of three). They are nonmotile microorganisms. (They do not move on their own accord.)
2. *Bacilli.* Bacilli are rod-shaped and can have rounded, straight, or pointed ends (Figure 31-16). Some bacilli have flagella that give bacteria motility (movement). Most bacteria are the shape of bacilli.
3. *Spirilla.* Spirilla are spiral-shaped bacteria that have one too many turns (Figure 31-17). Most spirilla are motile.

The microscopic examination produces information that is often needed to identify bacteria. However, biochemical reactions and the sensitivity pattern (how the organisms respond to antibiotics) are also needed to make the full identification.

Dyes (Stains)

The dyes used in microbiology are derived from coal tar. These dyes are acidic or basic and impart a color to the microorganism. Basic dyes carry a positive ion and stain structures that are acidic in nature. An acid dye carries a negative ion and stains structures that are basic (alkaline) in nature such as cytoplasmic structures. Several different types of stains are used depending on what test is ordered. (Table 31-3 lists stains and their uses.)

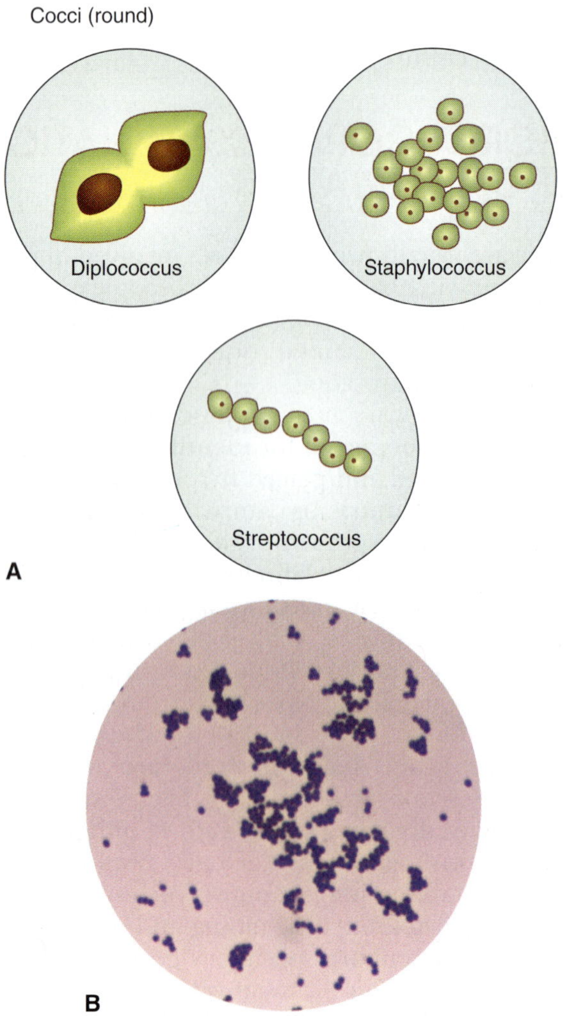

Figure 31-15 (A) *Cocci* (round). (B) *Cocci*, as seen through a microscope.

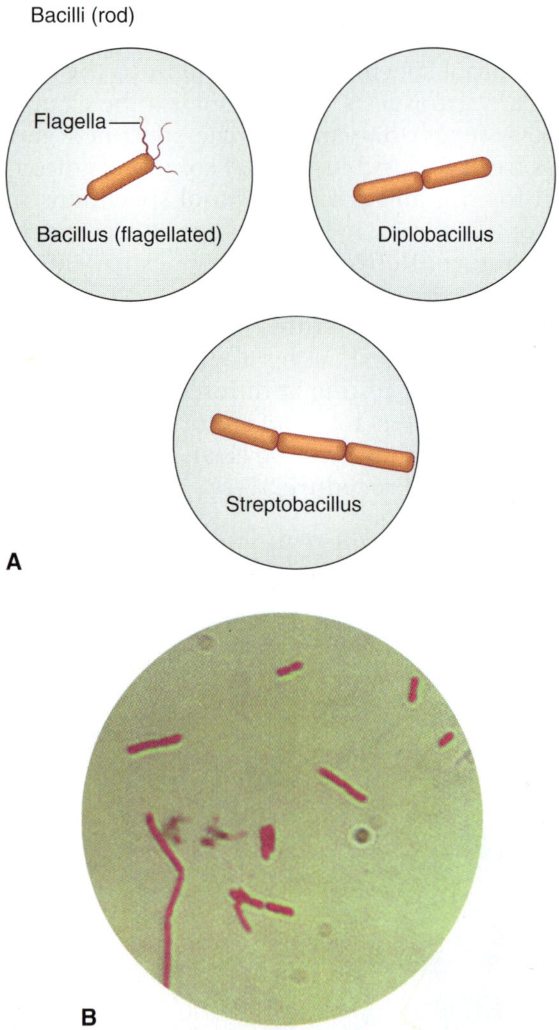

Figure 31-16 (A) *Bacilli* (rod). (B) *Bacilli*, as seen through a microscope.

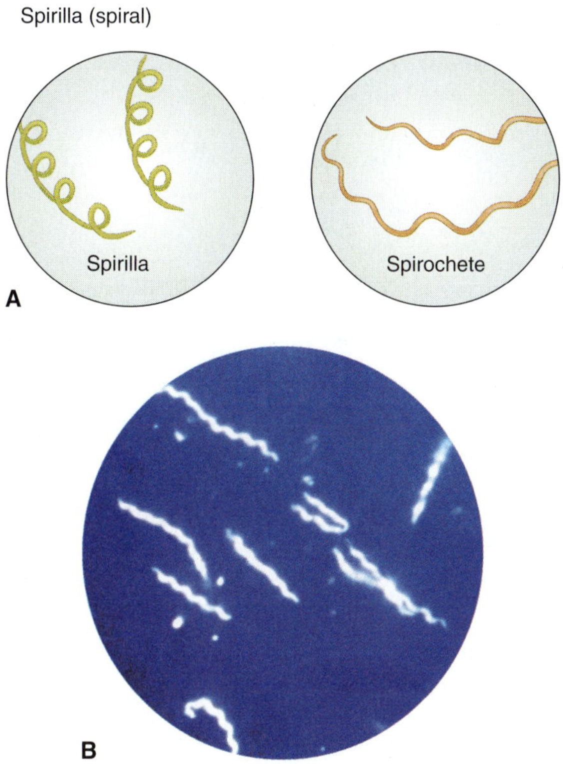

Figure 31-17 (A) *Spirilla* (spiral). (B) *Spirilla*, as seen through a microscope.

Simple Stain

A simple stain uses a single stain on a fixed slide for a given period of time. A simple stain shows the arrangement and structure of the bacterial cell. It is fast, taking no more than 3 minutes to stain, but it does not give much information.

Table 31-3 Stains and Their Uses

Stain	Example
Simple	Carbolfuchsin Gentian violet Methylene blue Safranin
Differential	Gram Acid-fast (Ziehl-Neelsen, Kinyoun)
Special	Capsule (Welch negative) Flagella (Leifson) Nuclei (Feulgen) Spore (Doerner)

Differential Stain

A differential stain is more complex than a simple stain. It is known as a differential stain because the stain result varies. A common differential stain is the Gram stain.

The Gram stain was developed in 1884 by Dr. Hans Christian Gram. More than 100 years later, this famous stain is still in use with little variation. This staining procedure differentiates bacteria by their Gram stain ability of being either negative or positive. A bacterium is Gram negative or positive by the nature of the cell wall and the ability of it either to retain or lose color through decolorization. This identification of Gram-positive or Gram-negative bacteria aids in identification of an organism. Gram-positive bacteria have a lower lipid (fat) content and are not decolorized as compared with Gram-negative bacteria, which have a higher lipid content and are readily decolorized.

The **reagents** used in the Gram stain are gentian or crystal violet, a purple stain that is the primary stain. Iodine, which acts as a **mordant,** holds the purple stain. Alcohol-acetone is the decolorizer that removes the purple color. Safranin is the red counterstain. When stained according to the manufacturer's directions, the Gram-positive bacteria stain purple, and the Gram-negative bacteria stain pink. Sometimes an organism will appear Gram-variable. This is found with Gram-positive organisms that have been exposed to acidic media, that are often old and lose their ability to retain the gentian violet, or the proper procedure has not been followed (Figure 31-18).

The Gram stain is one of the most important procedures in the microbiology laboratory, giving valuable information by identifying Gram-positive bacteria such as *Staphylococcus* and *Streptococcus* or Gram-negative bacteria such as *Escherichia coli* and Proteus.

The morphologic arrangement, shape, and Gram stain characteristic will begin to help identify the bacteria. Sometimes this is all the physician needs to know to start treatment for a pathogenic organism. For example, the bacteria causing gonorrhea (*Neisseria gonorrhoeae*) is a distinctive organism, having a characteristic diplococci shape that resembles a coffee or kidney bean. These organisms are found in and outside of white blood cells and can be identified by a Gram stain.

Acid-Fast Stain

Another differential stain, which is often referred to as a specific stain, is the acid-fast stain. This stain is either differential or specific in that it allows

Step	Time	Procedure	Result
1	1 minute	Primary stain: Apply crystal violet stain (purple) ↓ Rinse slide	All bacteria stain purple 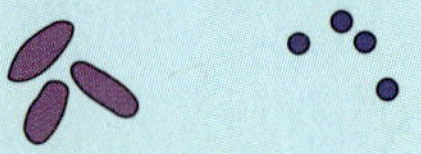
2	1 minute	Mordant: Apply Gram's iodine ↓ Rinse slide	All bacteria remain purple 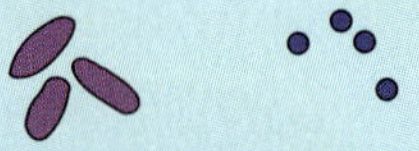
3	3 to 5 seconds	Decolorize: Apply alcohol ↓ Rinse slide	Purple stain is removed from Gram-negative cells 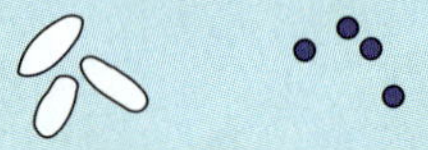
4	1 minute	Counterstain: Apply safranin stain (red) ↓ Rinse slide	Gram-negative cells appear pink-red; Gram-positive cells appear purple 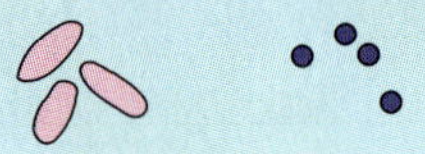

Figure 31-18 Steps in the Gram stain procedure.

microscopic examination of acid-fast organisms. This group of organisms does not respond well to the Gram stain and is difficult to stain under ordinary circumstances because of a waxy capsule cell wall that resists staining.

To stain these organisms, heat or a powerful dye is used in the procedure to stain the bacteria. The bacteria, once stained, resist decolorization with an acid alcohol, giving them the acid-fast name. The bacteria that causes tuberculosis is an acid-fast organism.

Two methods commonly used to stain acid-fast organisms are the Ziehl–Neelsen stain, which uses heat, and the Kinyoun stain, a cold method that does not include a heating process. Either of these stains is satisfactory.

Special Techniques

There are several special situations when more than the Gram stain or the shape and arrangement of an organism is needed to aid in the identification. Such situations would be the demonstration of the presence of flagella, spore, capsule, or nuclei of cells.

There also are microscopic examinations of organisms in a living state, without staining. Characteristics that can be studied by this method include motility, shape, and arrangement of organisms. This technique requires the microorganisms to be in a liquid suspension. The medical assistant often is responsible for setting up the slide for microscopic examination by the provider. Although microscopy is not a CLIA waived test, the medical assistant can certainly view the slides microscopically and discuss the finding with the provider as a learning exercise.

For vaginal secretions, a swab of the vaginal discharge is placed in a sterile tube containing 1 mL normal saline and mixed. Then the suspension is viewed under a microscope. For stool or other bacterial specimens, a small amount of specimen is mixed with a drop of normal saline, then viewed under a microscope. These methods are known as the **wet-mount** preparation and the hanging drop preparation (see Procedure 31-2).

The wet-mount preparation is a valuable diagnostic tool in determining the cause of vaginosis. Bacterial vaginosis is identified by the presence of "clue cells," epithelial cells covered by coccobacillary bacteria. Motile trichomonads are seen with *Trichomonas vaginalis*. The presence of pseudohyphae indicates a yeast infection. In many cases, an accurate diagnosis can be made from the wet-mount preparation, thus making more complex techniques unnecessary.

Potassium Hydroxide Preparation

Another type of wet preparation is using 10% solution of **potassium hydroxide (KOH)** in a wet preparation for the study of fungi and spores. The slide is prepared by using fragments of human hair, skin, or nails that could have fungus. KOH wet mounts are also useful for examining other body fluids such as vaginal swabs. These specimens are placed on a slide with a drop of 10% KOH and a coverslip on top. The KOH will clear debris. The slide should sit at room temperature for about a half hour before examination for debris settlement.

The direct examination of specimens is best viewed with a phase or dark-field microscope rather than a bright-field microscope because of reduced illumination. If using a bright-field microscope, lower the condenser to reduce transmitted light. Proper disposal of these specimens is important because the organisms are alive and possibly pathogenic.

CULTURE MEDIA

After the proper collection of the specimen, the material collected must be inoculated on a proper culture medium. This is necessary for growth and eventual identification of an organism.

The results of culture, the growing of an organism on special media in the laboratory, are only as reliable as the method used in collecting the specimen. In addition, growth requirements of different organisms must be considered, such as moisture, temperature, oxygen, carbon dioxide, and essential nutrients. Organisms that are sensitive to drying must be put into transport medium immediately after collection to prevent loss of viability. Some bacteria require a specialized medium to grow and multiply. Aerobic bacteria grow only in the presence of oxygen. Anaerobic bacteria live and grow in the absence of oxygen. Examples of common bacteria and their growth requirements are listed in Table 31-4.

When specimens are collected for the laboratory, the microorganism's growth requirements must be considered. No matter how good the specimen, if an anaerobic organism is kept in an aerobic atmosphere while being transported to the reference laboratory, it will probably not survive. Special anaerobic transport systems must be used.

Neisseria gonorrhoeae, the causative agent of the STD gonorrhea, requires special media and an atmosphere of reduced oxygen and increased carbon dioxide. Therefore, the specimen must be collected from the patient and immediately placed on a special media in a reduced oxygen atmosphere.

Medical assistants who send bacterial specimens to a reference laboratory must be familiar with the transport media the reference laboratory provides. Your laboratory manual explains how and when to use the various microbiology transport systems.

Media can be a solid, liquid, or semisolid substance that has the required nutrients to support the growth of bacteria. Such ingredients include vitamins, sugar, salt, minerals, and amino acids. Some media have the addition of special products such as egg, potato, meat, milk, blood, and dyes.

The solid form of media is called agar. Agar has an appearance similar to gelatin and is made of seaweed. When heated, agar is a liquid; when cooled, it solidifies. Agar is poured into a **petri dish** (a plastic dish used to grow bacteria) so the bacteria can be studied for gross **morphology** (form and structure). Agar can also be placed in tubes.

Semisolid media is made by adding less agar. Media in a liquid broth form is stored in tubes

Table 31-4 Common Bacteria and Their Growth Requirements

Organism	Disease	Medium	Oxygen Requirements
Streptococcus	Strep throat	Blood agar	$\downarrow O_2$, $\uparrow CO_2$
Neisseria gonorrhoeae	Gonorrhea	Chocolate agar, modified Thayer-Martin (MTM)	$\downarrow O_2$, $\uparrow CO_2$
Staphylococcus	Infections, boils	Blood agar	O_2
Escherichia coli	Urinary tract infection	Blood agar, eosin methylene blue (EMB), MacConkey	O_2

called **broth tubes** and allows for the observation of gas production, change in pH, and odor. Figure 31-9 shows many different types of media that can be used to identify bacteria. Media can be purchased already prepared, or it can be produced from ingredients in the laboratory. Charts listing the proper media to set up for specific types of cultures generally are prominently displayed in the setup area of most microbiology laboratories.

Media Classification

There are several classifications of media, including:

- *Basic.* Basic media are used for general purposes and do not contain added nutrients. They will support the growth of many Gram-negative and Gram-positive organisms.
- *Differential.* Differential media contain substances that alter the appearance of some types of organisms and not other types. An eosin methylene blue (EMB) plate for lactose and nonlactose fermenters is an example of differential media. The lactose fermenter can use lactose and looks different on the agar.
- *Selective.* Selective media support the growth of one type of organism while inhibiting the growth of another. This is done by the addition of a salt, dye, chemical, or antibiotic. A hektoen enteric (HE) plate for the growth of salmonella and shigella is a selective type of medium.
- *Enriched.* This type of medium contains substances that inhibit certain bacteria from growing. These media work well with cultures from sites that possess normal flora, such as the throat. The normal flora is inhibited and pathogenic bacteria are encouraged to grow. Blood agar and chocolate agar are examples of enriched media.

All media that are used should first be checked with known organisms for quality control and for contaminants. The manufacturer will usually suggest a list of organisms for a quality-control check. A check for contaminants involves a thorough visual check of the plate before using it. It is also important to store media according to the manufacturer's direction. *Never use outdated media.*

Table 31-5 lists common media by classification and use. Table 31-6 lists media that might be selected for specific sources. All laboratories vary slightly in their recommendations of media to set up on specimens.

MICROBIOLOGY CULTURE

Inoculating the Media

After selecting the correct medium for the culture and observing the specimen to make sure it is properly collected, the specimen is inoculated onto the medium. If the specimen is on a swab, the swab is rolled directly onto the upper quadrant of the agar

Table 31-5 Common Microbiology Media by Classification and Use

Type	Name	Use
Basic	Trypticase agar Trypticase broth	Supports the growth of most organisms
Differential	Blood agar MacConkey Eosin methylene blue (EMB)	Supports the growth of *Streptococcus* and *Staphylococcus;* demonstrates hemolysis Certain Gram-negative organisms *Escherichia coli*
Selective	Salmonella and Shigella (SS) Hektoen Phenylethyl alcohol Mannitol salt Selenite (GN) broth Thayer-Martin Thioglycollate broth	Gram-negative Salmonella and Shigella Enteric organisms Inhibits Gram-negative growth Promotes growth of *Staphylococcus* Promotes growth of enteric organisms Promotes growth of *Neisseria* species Promotes growth of anaerobes
Enriched	Loefflers Chocolate Lowenstein-Jensen	Promotes growth of *Corynebacterium* Promotes growth of *Haemophilus* species Promotes growth of mycobacteria

Table 31-6 Common Specimens, Suspected Pathogens, and Media Recommendations

Specimen Source	Potential Pathogens	Blood agar	Chocolate	Eosin Methylene Blue	MacConkey	Salmonella and Shigella Hektoen Enteric	Selenite	Thayer–Martin	Thioglycollate	CO_2
Eye/Ear	*Neisseria gonorrhoeae* *Haemophilus species* *Staphylococcus aureus* *Streptococcus pyogenes* *Pseudomonas aeruginosa* *Moraxella species*	x	x	x	x			x	x	x
Cerebrospinal fluid	*Neisseria meningitidis* *Streptococcus pneumoniae* *Haemophilus influenzae*	x	x						x	x
Throat	*Streptococcus pyogenes*	x								x
Sputum	*Streptococcus pneumoniae*	x								
Urine	*Escherichia coli* *Klebsiella* *Proteus* *Pseudomonas aeruginosa* *Enterococcus*	x		x	x					
Wounds	*Staphylococcus* *Streptococcus* *Enterobactericae* Anaerobic bacteria	x	x	x	x				x	x
Stool	*Salmonella* *Shigella*			x	x	x	x			
Stool	Pathogenic *E. coli* *Yersinia* species									
Vaginal	*Neisseria gonorrhoeae*	x	x					x		x

plate. If the specimen is a sputum or liquid, it is inoculated onto the plate with a loop.

The inoculum is spread back and forth in a sweeping motion with a flamed loop or needle.

After the agar plate has been inoculated and properly labeled, it should be turned upside down and placed in the proper environment for growth. By turning the agar upside down, any condensation that forms from bacterial growth will be on the inside lid.

Liquid broths and agar slant tubes have screw caps. These caps must not be screwed on too tightly because of gas production by some organisms that can break the tube.

Other Types of Streaking

Other types of streaking include the lawn streak. This streaking technique is used to place an organism over an entire area of an agar plate for sensitivity testing. The bacteria is spread over the entire plate using a swab (Figure 31-19), streaking over the entire area several times from different angles. After the streaking has been completed, disks saturated

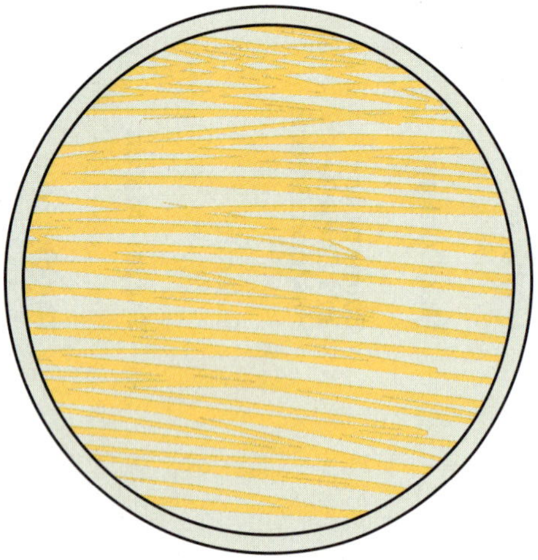

Figure 31-19 Lawn or spread streak.

with different antibiotics are placed equidistant throughout the streaked area (Figure 31-20B).

The colony count is a streaking technique much like the lawn technique. This technique is used to plate urine cultures. A special calibrated urine loop is used to make the first streak, followed by a second streak that goes across the entire length of the initial streak. Then another complete streaking is placed over the original streaks after rotating the plate (Figure 31-20A). This method of using a calibrated loop to get a more accurate inoculation gives the provider an idea of how many colonies of bacteria are present.

Every laboratory will use slightly different ways of performing the basic streaks. The important factor is to use good aseptic techniques so there is no contamination from outside organisms, and all organisms that are streaked out are isolated enough to test further if necessary.

Primary Culture

After the media has been incubated for 24 to 48 hours, the initial or primary culture is read.

Subculture

When working with bacterial cultures, there can be more than one pathogen growing in the culture. For instance, a wound culture may have both Gram-positive and Gram-negative organisms growing. To identify each organism, you must separate these bacteria to other media (Figure 31-21). It is also necessary at times to separate the pathogenic bacteria from the normal flora, as in the throat and sputum cultures. Some initial cultures do achieve excellent isolation without having to subculture.

RAPID IDENTIFICATION SYSTEMS

The age of high technology and computerized equipment has also made inroads into microbiology laboratories, clinics, and POLs. Many traditional methods of identifying bacteria have been replaced by rapid identification test kits.

Rapid test systems, which are CLIA waived, give a quick identification, are economical, and allow the provider to start treatment sooner. Rapid tests allow the provider to receive results while the patient is still in the office.

Streptococcus Screening (Rapid Strep Testing)

A number of instant or rapid test kits identify group A *Streptococcus* (also known as beta-hemolytic *Strepto-*

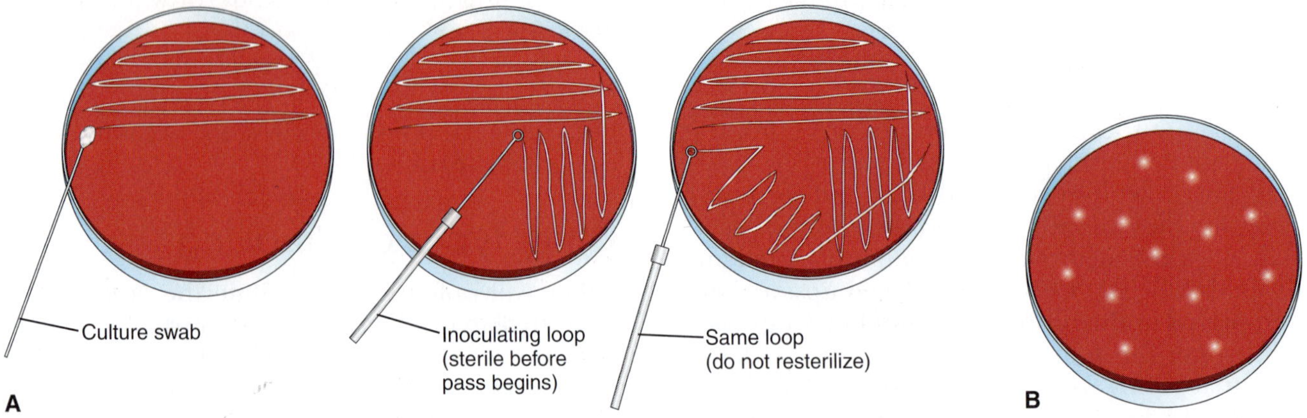

Figure 31-20 Colony count streak.

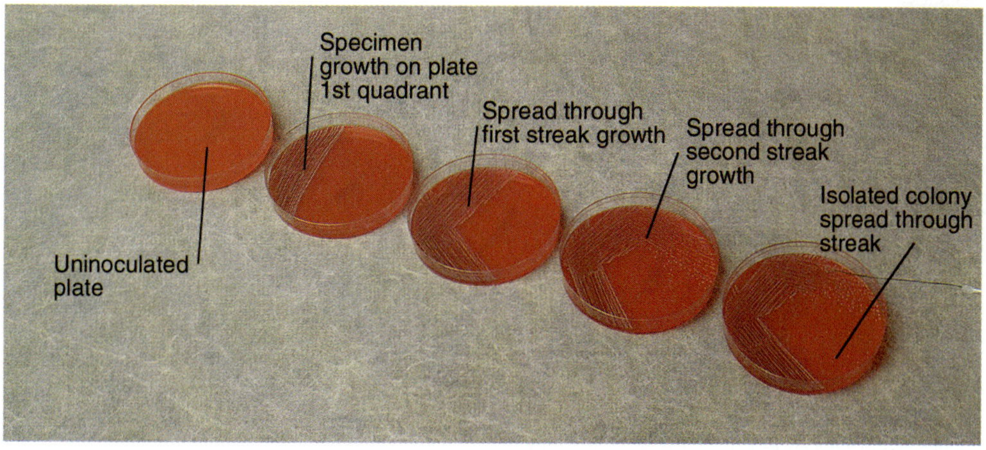

Figure 31-21 Stages of spreading out the bacteria to isolate colonies.

coccus group A), the causative agent of a serious sore (strep) throat. It is important to identify this Gram-positive *Streptococcus* as soon as possible because the bacteria can cause serious damage (i.e., kidney and heart valve damage) if not treated immediately with antibiotics.

This test is sensitive and eliminates false-positive results. The directions should be followed strictly to produce an accurate test result. The results are based on color development of a spot on the test filter. Test results are available in minutes.

A latex agglutination test for group A Streptococcus is based on an antigen and antibody agglutination. A throat swab is placed directly on the antibody-coated slide, and the presence of a positive test is seen by the appearance of agglutination (clumping). Although these tests are quick and convenient, the following rules should be followed strictly:

- Read and understand the manufacturer's instructions and directions before starting the test.
- Never use outdated materials.
- Observe all safety guidelines and precautions.
- Use the correct swab in taking the throat culture. Some cottons and chemicals on swab will interfere with the test reagents. If possible, use the swabs provided with the kit.
- Always run the positive and negative control together with the patient's actual test.

If a patient has symptoms of an infected throat and the slide test is negative, the provider will also order a regular throat culture to make sure there is no infection present. Latex agglutination kits can give false readings, and it is best to follow up with the throat culture. A list of all the CLIA waived rapid tests is available at the CDC Web site (http://www.cdc.gov) using the search words Waived Tests.

SENSITIVITY TESTING

Antibiotic sensitivity testing often is ordered on the pathogenic organisms recovered from the culturing process. By setting up an antibiotic sensitivity test, the laboratory can identify which antibiotics destroy the pathogen, and the provider will be able to set up antibiotic treatment for the patient. Today's health care environment demands that this information be made available to the provider as soon as possible.

When a patient has had multiple bacterial infections and the provider is concerned with prescribing an ineffective antibiotic, or when the bacterial infection is not responding to the currently prescribed antibiotic, the provider will order a culture and sensitivity (C&S). The antibiotic that is effective against the culture bacteria is reported as "sensitive to," and the antibiotics that are not effective will be reported as "resistant to," meaning that the bacteria will be sensitive to some antibiotics and resistant to others.

To determine which antibiotic will destroy the culture bacteria, the technician places small discs on the culture plate. The discs contain various antibiotics. The antibiotic to which the bacteria is sensitive will eventually become surrounded by an area of no growth (Figure 31-22).

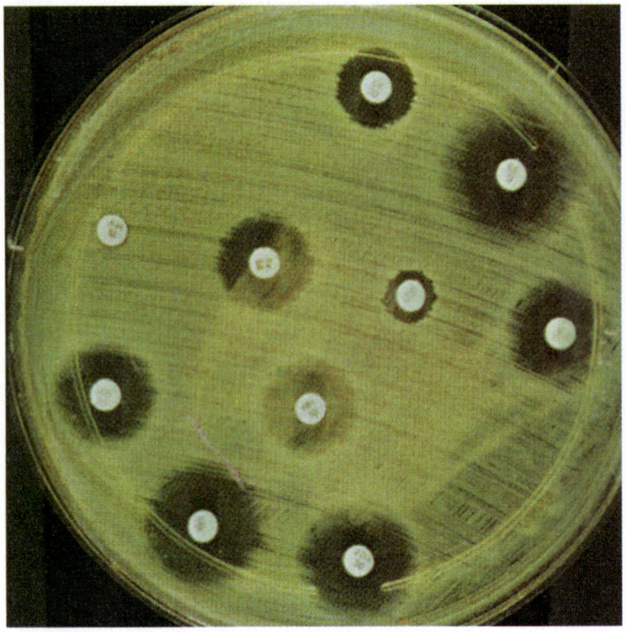

Figure 31-22 Culture plate showing antibiotic discs on bacteria. Note the one antibiotic disc in the top left area that the bacteria are totally "resistant to." Most of the other antibiotics have carrying degrees of effectiveness and would be labeled "sensitive to." The one just right of the center area is barely effective and would be reported as "intermediate."

PARASITOLOGY

With the age of travel and more public awareness, we are beginning to see more parasitic infections. The field of parasitology is a vast one with many different types of parasites. They range from extremely small microscopic ones to those that are large and macroscopic in size. Parasites have varying life cycles. The degree of severity of illness depends on which parasite enters the human body and infects it. Parasites can be found in the blood, urine, or feces. The more common ones are found in the feces.

Different geographic areas have different types of parasites that are seen. Resettled immigrant populations may be infected with a parasite previously unseen in a geographic area. World travelers can also bring back rare parasitic infections from their adventures.

Even though parasitology tests are performed by medical technologists rather than medical assistants, the medical assistant must be able to properly obtain the sample (such as a throat culture or wound culture), instruct the patient on how to properly obtain the sample (such as a stool sample), and make sure the patient is prepared properly, understands how and where to transport the specimen, how to maintain the proper temperature of the specimen, and even how quickly the specimen must be returned to the laboratory.

Examination Methods

The most common methods of fecal specimen examination for parasitic identification in a clinic or POL is the direct wet-mount slide.

Specimen Collection

Fecal specimens for identification of ova and parasites should be collected in wide-mouth containers with a tight lid to prevent leakage. The container should be put in a biohazard transport bag to avoid contamination and sent for examination immediately. The patient should be instructed not to contaminate the specimen with urine because it could interfere with testing. Special vials containing formalin are also available for ova and parasite testing that are preferred by some laboratories. Refer to the laboratory user's manual for specific instructions.

The laboratory procedure for collection and processing of the parasite specimen should be strictly followed to provide an accurate testing of the specimen. The collection time of the specimen should be followed as directed by the provider. Three specimens may be ordered over a specified period. Provider's offices will have specific instructions and containers with a preservative in them when an ova and parasite examination is requested.

When the specimen is sent for testing, it should be labeled correctly with the patient's name, date, and time of the specimen. It is important to know if the patient has been traveling, to what area of the world, and what is suspected by the provider to help aid in identification (see Procedure 31-4).

Common Parasites

Some of the more common parasites identified in the POL are *Enterobius vermicularis,* the causative organism of pinworm infection, and *Trichomonas vaginalis,* a parasite that infects the urogenital tracts of men and women.

Enterobius vermicularis. This **nematode** (round worm) is found worldwide, predominantly in children. The adult worm is shaped like a pin, wide at one end and pointed at the other end. The female worm is larger than the male. Infection with pinworm can cause severe itching, irritability, and insomnia, depending on the severity of the infection. The adult female worm migrates to the anus at night, depositing ova (eggs) that cause itching during hatching. At times, the adult worm can be found around the anus and on the stool. The adult worm measures approximately 7 to 12 mm long. The egg is the infectious stage of the parasite (Figure 31-23).

To diagnose the presence of the parasite, either the adult worm or ova has to be located in the specimen. A negative test should be confirmed by as many as six negative tests performed. The test is performed by taking a cellophane tape swab and placing the sticky side down to the skin around the anal area. The tape is placed on a slide and brought to the laboratory for examination (Figure 31-24).

Trichomonas vaginalis. This parasite is found in both men and women, but its presence is five times higher in women (men can harbor the organism for years without symptoms). Because men can harbor this parasite and have no symptoms, it is recommended that both partners be treated. This will prevent the ongoing reinfection of the female patient. The organism belongs to the flagellate (possesses flagella) class and is extremely motile. Infection with this flagellate causes a purulent yellowish green discharge and dysuria. The organism is recovered from the discharge or urine and is transmitted sexually.

The trichomonad is recovered in a wet preparation slide of spun urine or vaginal secretion mixed with a drop of saline (see Procedure 31-2.) The specimen should not be contaminated with fecal material, which could contain *Trichomonas hominis,* another flagellate. The prepared slide is

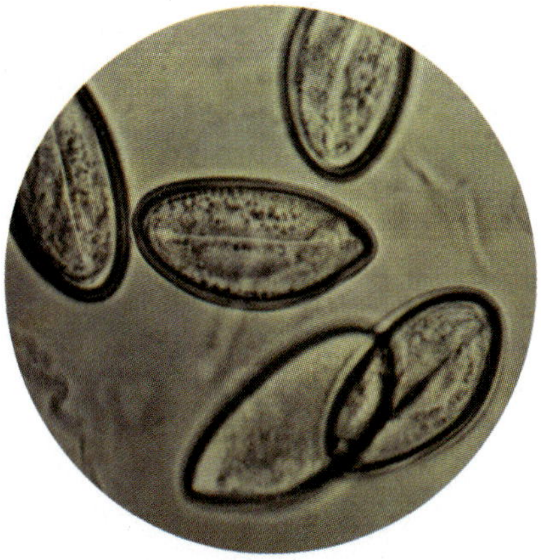

Figure 31-23 Pinworm ova, as seen through a microscope. (From CDC, Atlanta, GA.)

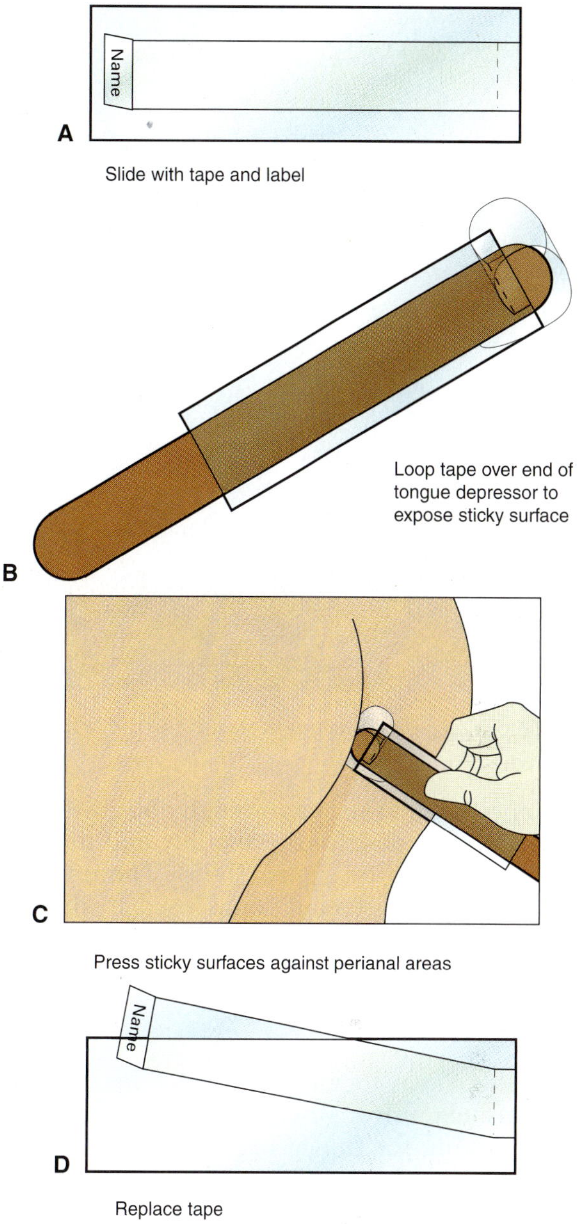

Figure 31-24 Technique for preparing and using a cellophane tape swab.

Online Images and Information about Parasites

The Centers for Disease Control and Prevention (CDC) has an extensive Web site with a wealth of information about many health issues. Of particular interest to medical assistants and other health care professionals interested in parasites is the DPDx, a Web site that is maintained by the CDC's Division of Parasitic Diseases. Go to http://www.dpd.cdc.gov/dpdx and click on Image Library for a great college-level epidemiology image library.

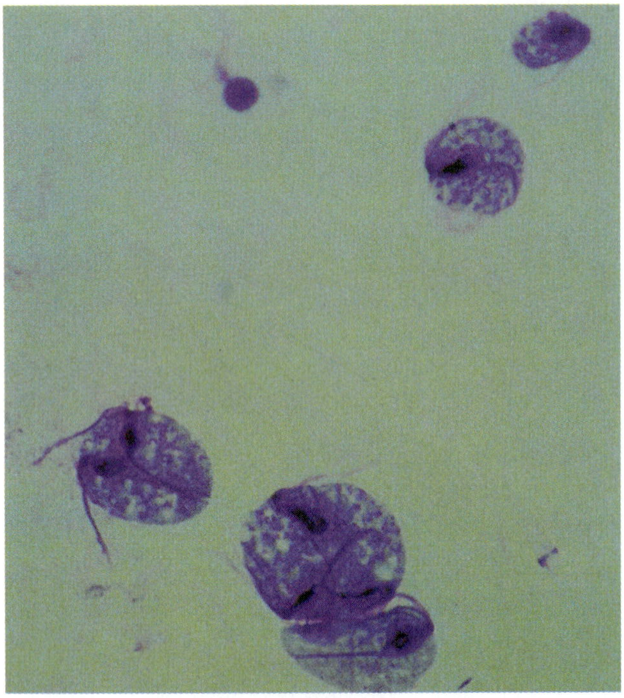

Figure 31-25 *Trichomonas* in stained urine sediment.

examined under the low and high objectives of the microscope to observe the motility and morphology of the parasite (Figure 31-25). There are also test kits and fluorescent stains used to diagnose this parasite.

MYCOLOGY

The field of mycology and the infections that cause fungi are extensive. Most identification and sensitivities testing for fungal organisms take place in larger laboratories and specific reference laboratories. Identification of two of the common fungal infections can be made quickly in the clinic or POL.

The genus *Candida* has several species that cause yeast infections in the body. *Candida* species are also present in the environment around us. They present a particular problem in the health care setting where they can cause serious nosocomial infections. Equipment can be easily contaminated with *Candida* organisms.

Yeast infections commonly are found on the moist areas of the body and in the subcutaneous tissue. An infection with yeast can range from mild to serious. *Candida albicans* is the causative agent of vaginal yeast infections. The specimen is examined microscopically for the characteristic budding yeast forms (see Procedure 31-2). If the specimen is fluid and clear, it is placed on a slide with a drop of saline. If the specimen is thick, it should be mixed with 10% KOH (one drop) on the slide to clear away debris. Once the specimen is prepared, it is examined microscopically.

Another group of significant fungi that sometimes can be generally identified are the **dermatophytes.** These fungi cause infections on the hair, skin, and nails. The microscopic structure of these fungi is detailed. Some of the fungi that cause dermatophytic infections can be diagnosed using a **Wood's lamp.** This is a lamp with an ultraviolet light. Some dermatophytes will fluoresce (glow brightly) under this light.

Mycotic infections can also be identified through culture and kit identification systems. Fungi can produce heavy aerosols and should be processed and observed under a safety hood.

Procedure 31-1

Procedure for Obtaining a Throat Specimen for Culture

STANDARD PRECAUTIONS:

PURPOSE:

To obtain secretions from the nasopharynx and tonsillar area for means of identifying a pathogenic microorganism.

EQUIPMENT/SUPPLIES:

Tongue depressor
Culture tube with applicator stick or commercially prepared culture collection system (culturette)
Label and requisition form
Gloves and face shield
Good light source

continues

Procedure 31-1 (continued)

PROCEDURE STEPS:

1. Identify yourself and explain the procedure to the patient. RATIONALE: Identifying yourself helps establish professional trust and rapport with the patient. Explaining the procedure allows the patient to understand the process and encourages cooperation.
2. Have an emesis basin and tissues ready. RATIONALE: You will want to be prepared in case the patient spits up or vomits.
3. Have the patient in a sitting position. RATIONALE: The patient in a sitting position will facilitate better visualization of the throat area.
4. Wash hands, gather supplies, and apply gloves and face shield. RATIONALE: Washing hands before any patient contact will eliminate contamination. Gathering equipment before beginning the procedure ensures less chance of errors caused by missing supplies. Gloves and a face shield will offer personal protection in case the patient coughs, spits up, or vomits.
5. Ask the patient to open his or her mouth wide and then adjust the light source. RATIONALE: A widely opened mouth and properly adjusted light source will facilitate better visualization of the throat area.
6. Remove the swab from the culturette using sterile technique. RATIONALE: Using sterile technique maintains the sterility of the swab, which results in a quality specimen for culture.
7. Ask the patient to say "ah." Depress the tongue with the tongue depressor and swab the back of the throat and tonsillar area. Concentrate primarily on any red, raw areas and pustules. Take care to not touch the swab on the inside of the cheeks or on the tongue. RATIONALE: Having the patient say "ah" lowers the back of the tongue. Depressing the tongue reminds the patient to keep the mouth opened and assists in keeping the back of the tongue down. Swabbing only the tonsillar area and the back of the throat without touching the inside of the cheeks or the tongue ensures that the specimen will contain mostly the bacterial infectious agent (streptococci), if present, and not normal mouth flora or other contaminants. The red, raw areas and pustules will most likely contain the greatest concentration of streptococci.
8. Place the swab back into the culturette using sterile technique and crush the glass capsule containing the culture media. (*NOTE:* Some culturettes require a puncturing action to release the media. Follow the manufacturer's instructions.) RATIONALE: Using sterile technique avoids contaminating the specimen and having the specimen contaminate any other area. Crushing the glass capsule (or piercing the culture membrane) releases the culture medium, which will maintain the optimum environment for the specimen until it is tested at the regional laboratory.
9. Label the culturette according to the POL policy and requirements. RATIONALE: Proper and timely labeling of all specimens ensures that samples will not be mixed up with other patient samples.
10. Ensure patient comfort and answer any questions related to the testing. RATIONALE: Ensuring patient comfort and answering questions will establish professional rapport.
11. Discard contaminated supplies into a biohazard waste container. Disinfect all work surfaces. Remove gloves and face shield and discard appropriately. RATIONALE: Following Standard Precautions when disposing of contaminated supplies and disinfecting work surfaces will eliminate biohazard contaminations.
12. Wash hands. RATIONALE: Gloves protect hands from most but not all infectious microorganisms. Washing hands will remove residual powders and latex.
13. Complete the laboratory requisition and record procedure in patient's chart or electronic medical record. RATIONALE: Completing the laboratory requisition properly and in a timely manner will give the regional laboratory accurate information regarding the patient and the specimen. Charting the procedure will establish a timeline and document the procedure.

DOCUMENTATION

1/12/20XX 10:11 AM Throat culture specimen obtained and sent to Inner City Laboratory for C&S. Patient tolerated the procedure well and will return for a follow-up visit and medication reevaluation in 2 days per Dr. King's request. Appt scheduled 1/14 at 3:30 PM. Joe Guerrero, CMA (AAMA)——

Procedure 31-2

Wet Mount and Hanging Drop Slide Preparations

STANDARD PRECAUTIONS:

PURPOSE:
Prepare a slide for viewing live organisms for motility and identifying characteristics.

EQUIPMENT/SUPPLIES:

Gloves	Coverslips
Laboratory coat	Petroleum jelly
Clean glass slide	Dropper
Glass slide with concave well	Bacterial suspension

PROCEDURE STEPS:

1. Wash hands and apply gloves. RATIONALE: Washing hands before any procedure helps to eliminate contamination. Gloves will offer personal protection.
2. Assemble equipment and supplies. RATIONALE: Gathering equipment before beginning the procedure ensures less chance of errors caused by missing supplies.

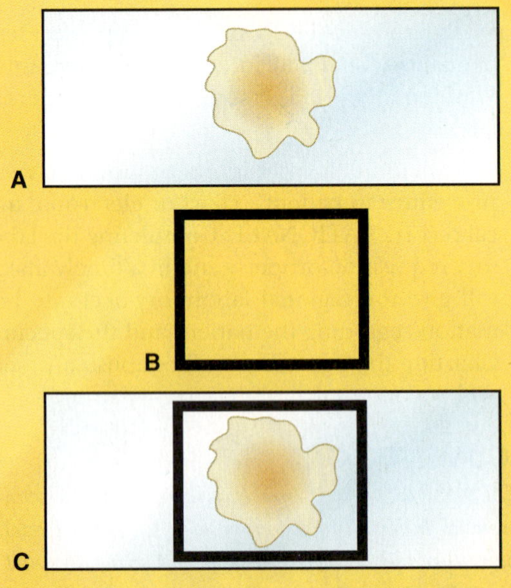

Figure 31-26 Wet-mount slide. (A) Specimen placed on a glass slide. (B) Coverslip with petroleum jelly on edges. (C) Coverslip placed directly on top of slide with specimen.

3. For wet-mount slide preparation:
   a. Place a drop of the bacterial suspension onto a clean glass slide (Figure 31-26A). RATIONALE: The suspension of bacteria in a drop facilitates viewing.
   b. Place petroleum jelly around the edges of the coverslip (Figure 31-26B) and place the coverslip on top of the bacterial suspension (Figure 31-26C). RATIONALE: The petroleum jelly cuts down on air currents and keeps the slide from drying out.
4. For hanging drop slide preparation:
   a. Place the bacterial specimen (in suspension) in the center of the coverslip with petroleum jelly around the edges (Figure 31-27A). RATIONALE: For the suspended drop to be formed properly, this technique is used.
   b. Invert the slide and place the concave well of the slide over the specimen drop on the cover slip (Figure 31-27B). RATIONALE: This method allows the slide well to protect the drop.
   c. The slide is then carefully turned right side up for microscopic examination (Figure 31-27C). RATIONALE: The slide must be handled carefully to avoid slippage and disruption of the drop.

NOTE: After the smear is prepared properly, it can be observed microscopically at any power. Viewing the slide is considered by CLIA to be a provider-performed microscopy procedure.

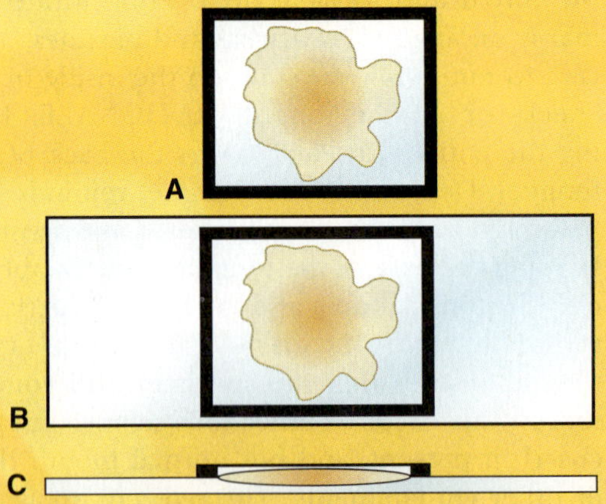

Figure 31-27 Hanging drop slide. (A) Specimen placed on coverslip. (B) Slide placed over coverslip. (C) Slide turned right side up for examination.

Procedure 31-3

Performing Strep Throat Testing

STANDARD PRECAUTIONS:

PURPOSE:

To test for streptococcus infection of the throat for diagnostic purposes. The following steps are intentionally general, so a variety of kits can be used.

EQUIPMENT/SUPPLIES:

Gloves
Commercial (CLIA waived) strep throat testing kit:
- Controls and reagents
- Sterile cotton-tipped swabs
- Test tubes and holder or receptacles (depending on the kit used)

Tongue blade
Adjustable light source

PROCEDURE STEPS:

1. Wash hands and apply personal protective equipment (PPE). RATIONALE: Hands should always be washed prior to working with patients to avoid transferring pathogens. PPEs protects you from the patient in case he or she coughs or vomits during the procedure.
2. Assemble and organize equipment and supplies. RATIONALE: Organization presents a more professional image.
3. Introduce yourself, identify the patient, and explain the procedure. RATIONALE: Introducing yourself and explaining the procedure to the patient will gain his or her cooperation and establish a good rapport. Identifying the patient ensures that the right patient will receive the test.
4. Using the tongue blade and light source, obtain the specimen from the patient's throat on the cotton-tipped applicator. RATIONALE: The tongue blade will assist in keeping the mouth opened for ease in obtaining the specimen without contaminating it on the tongue, cheek, or roof of the mouth.
5. Follow the manufacturer's instructions exactly to perform the strep throat test. Be sure to also run the controls tests. RATIONALE: Each manufacturer's kit varies slightly in the method used. The controls are to ensure quality results.
6. Properly dispose of all waste in biohazard container. Disinfect the equipment and the area. RATIONALE: Standard precautions are used to prevent disease transmission.
7. Complete the laboratory report form and notify the provider of the results. RATIONALE: The provider will treat the disease as soon as it is confirmed.
8. Document procedure in patient's chart or electronic medical record. RATIONALE: Proper documentation ensures good recordkeeping.

DOCUMENTATION

04/27/20XX Strep throat test performed in office. Patient tolerated procedure well. Dr. Lewis notified of results. Initialed report on file. Joe Guerrero, CMA (AAMA) ________

Laboratory Report

Patient Name Lisa Carter *Date* 04-27-20XX

Strep Throat Test negative

Joe Guerrero, CMA (AAMA)
MA signature

Procedure 31-4

Instructing a Patient on Obtaining a Fecal Specimen

STANDARD PRECAUTIONS:

PURPOSE:

To instruct a patient in the correct collection of a fecal sample.

EQUIPMENT/SUPPLIES:

Gloves
Biohazard container
Sturdy, opaque, waterproof specimen container with a securely fitting lid
Special laboratory manual instructions if needed (depending on the test being performed)

PROCEDURE STEPS:

1. Assemble and organize equipment and supplies. RATIONALE: Being organized helps the process go more smoothly and professionally.
2. Identify the patient and explain the procedure. Give the patient written instructions as well. RATIONALE: Identifying the patient ensures that you have the right patient. Explaining the procedures reassures the patient and gains his or her cooperation with the procedure. Written instructions helps the patient to remember better.
3. Hand the patient the labeled specimen container, instructing him or her to deposit a sample of stool into the cup then securely set the lid onto it. RATIONALE: Labeling the container rather than the lid will ensure that the specimen will not be mixed up with another patient's sample in the laboratory. The sturdy lid will prevent leakage of the specimen during transport.
4. Caution the patient to avoid contaminating the stool specimen with urine. RATIONALE: Urine may interfere with the test.
5. Give the patient a biohazard transport bag and instructions on which pocket to put the specimen into and how to secure the bag. The medical assistant can place the laboratory requisition into the other pocket. RATIONALE: Using a biohazard transport bag and properly sealing it will prevent contamination during transport to the laboratory. Keeping the requisition in a separate pocket from the specimen further prevents contamination of the paperwork.
6. The patient should be prepared to transport the specimen to the laboratory as soon as possible while keeping the specimen at or just below body temperature. RATIONALE: If the stool is being tested for parasites and their eggs (ova and parasite, commonly called O&P), the laboratory will want to test the parasites while they are still viable.
7. Document that the instructions were given to the patient, both orally and written. RATIONALE: Proper documentation serves as a record for future reference.

Case Study 31-1

Refer to the scenario at the beginning of the chapter. You can see that Joe is very careful with all safety precautions when handling specimens.

CASE STUDY REVEIW

1. Name a few diseases Joe could contract from the specimens he handles.
2. Discuss the methods of transfer those diseases would take during transmission.

Case Study 31-2

Mary O'Keefe has brought her 3-year-old son Chris to the office of Drs. Lewis and King with a temperature of 102°F and an extremely sore and red throat. He is irritable and crying. After examining Chris, Dr. King orders a quick test for group A Streptococcus. Medical assistant Joe Guerrero has a difficult time acquiring the throat swab for the test because of Chris's condition. The test is run, and the results are negative.

CASE STUDY REVIEW

1. What could be some reasons the test result is negative?
2. What other procedure can be done to diagnose strep throat?
3. How would the test in question 2 be set up?

SUMMARY

The field of microbiology is vast. Many microorganisms are pathogenic and can cause serious infection in patients. The successful culturing and identification of such organisms is an important aspect of the successful treatment of patients. All specimens that are processed in the POL should be handled carefully, and all safety guidelines should be followed.

For the pathogen to be identified correctly, the utmost care must be taken in obtaining the culture. Sterile equipment must be used. When the culture is processed, the correct microscopic examination, media, incubation, and confirmatory tests must be used correctly to identify the pathogen.

Often a sensitivity test will be requested together with the culture. The information from this test will guide the physician in selecting the appropriate treatment for the patient.

POLs vary in the type and number of cultures that are performed on the premises and those that are sent out to be performed in a reference laboratory. It is important to provide the best care for the patient by doing only those tests that a POL can reasonably handle given equipment, personnel limitations, and CLIA regulations.

In addition to performing bacterial identification, some POLs perform parasitology and mycology tests on a limited basis. When performing parasitology tests, it is important to obtain the proper specimen in the correct manner. When performing mycology tests, it is important to work under a safety hood to minimize the risk for exposure to spores from the fungal specimens.

Of utmost importance is the careful adherence to Quality Control guidelines. These procedures ensure the integrity of test results.

STUDY FOR SUCCESS

To reinforce your knowledge and skills of information presented in this chapter:

- Review the Key Terms
- Practice the Procedures
- Consider the Case Study and discuss your conclusions
- Answer the Review Questions
    - Multiple Choice
    - Critical Thinking
- Navigate the Internet by completing the Web Activities
- Practice the StudyWARE activities on the CD
- Apply your knowledge in the Student Workbook activities
- Complete the Web Tutor sections
- View and discuss the DVD situations

REVIEW QUESTIONS

Multiple Choice

1. A structure that is *not* part of all bacterial cells is the:
   a. nucleus
   b. ribosome
   c. spore
   d. cell wall

2. An example of nonselective media would be media that:
   a. contain a substance that alters the appearance of some organisms
   b. will support the growth of all organisms and does not alter their appearance
   c. support the growth of one type of organism and inhibit the growth of other types of organisms
   d. identify the biochemical activity of some organisms

3. When a CSF culture cannot be set up immediately, it should be placed in the incubator or remain at room temperature as opposed to being placed in the refrigerator because some organisms are affected by a low temperature. An example of this type of organism would be:
   a. *Beta streptococci*
   b. *Neisseria meningitidis*
   c. *Streptococcus pneumoniae*
   d. *Staphylococcus aureus*
4. The best method of taking a specimen for the recovery of anaerobic organisms is to:
   a. swab deep and place into an anaerobic container
   b. aspirate purulent fluid and place into a test tube
   c. swab around the wound and place into an anaerobic container
   d. take as any other specimen for culture

Critical Thinking

1. Name two ways to identify whether an organism is motile.
2. Define an aerosol and explain how protection is provided when working with an aerosol.
3. Identify one potential pathogen and list the specimen source, media for culture, microscopic appearance, and the disease it causes.
4. A patient is given a requisition slip for a stool culture, ova, and parasite examination. How would you instruct this patient to collect the specimen?
5. Explain why pinworm specimens are collected at a certain time of the day.

WEB ACTIVITIES

Visit the Centers for Disease Control and Prevention's Web site and other Web sites to review guidelines on reportable diseases for your state.

REFERENCES/BIBLIOGRAPHY

Department of Health and Human Services, Centers for Disease Control and Prevention. (2008). Diseases and Conditions. Retrieved October 2008, from http://www.cdc.gov.

U.S. Food and Drug Administration. (2008). Databases on the FDA Website. Retrieved October 2008, from http://www.fda.gov/search/databases.html.

Walters, N. J., Estridge, B. H., & Reynold, A. P. (2008). *Basic medical laboratory techniques* (5th ed.). Clifton Park, NY: Delmar Cengage Learning.

THE DVD HOOK-UP

This chapter discusses basic microbiology procedures. The selected scenes in this program demonstrate how to educate patients in collecting more sensitive specimens.

1. Do you think that Mr. Turell was a little embarrassed about discussing the proper technique for collecting a stool sample with the medical assistant? Why?
2. In the scene about collecting a sputum specimen, the medical assistant waited in the room while the patient collected the specimen. Did that scene bother you? Do you think that you will be able to stay in the room with the patient when you are responsible for collecting a sputum sample?
3. Why should you not touch the tongue when collecting a throat specimen?

DVD Journal Summary

Write a paragraph that summarizes what you learned from watching the selected scenes from today's DVD program.

Are you worried about collecting specimens that may cause you or the patient to gag? What if you suddenly become sick yourself and have to run out of the patient's room? How would you handle such an episode with the patient?

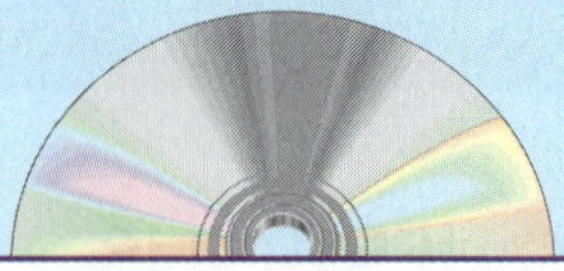

DVD Series — Skills Based Series
Program Number — 12

Chapter/Scene Reference
- *Administer Fecal Collection and Performing Occult Blood Test*
- *Administering Sputum Collection*
- *Administering Throat Culture and Performing Rapid Strep Test*

Chapter 32

Specialty Laboratory Tests

KEY TERMS

ABO Blood Group
Agglutination
Antibody
Antigen
Antiserum
Bilirubin
Blood Urea Nitrogen (BUN)
Cholesterol
Choriocarcinoma
Cushing's Syndrome
Diabetes Mellitus
Ectopic Pregnancy
Enzyme Immunoassay
Epstein–Barr Virus (EBV)
Guthrie Screening Test
Heterophile Antibodies
High-Density Lipoprotein (HDL)
Human Chorionic Gonadotropin (hCG)
Hydatidiform Mole
Hyperglycemia
Hypoglycemia
Infectious Mononucleosis
Insulin
Latex Beads
Low-Density Lipoprotein (LDL)
Mantoux Test
Phenylketonuria (PKU)
Purified Protein Derivative (PPD)

OUTLINE

Urine Pregnancy Tests
- Commercial/Home Urine Pregnancy Tests
- Testing Methods
- Slide Test or Agglutination Inhibition Test
- Enzyme Immunoassay Test

Infectious Mononucleosis
- Transmission of EBV
- Symptoms of IM
- Treatment of IM
- Diagnosis of IM
- CLIA Waived IM Tests
- Prothrombin Time/ProTime/INR

Blood Typing
- ABO Blood Typing
- Rh Blood Typing

Semen Analysis
- Semen Composition
- Altering Factors in Semen Analysis

Phenylketonuria Test
- Blood Testing for PKU

Tuberculosis
- Cause of TB
- Resistance in Mycobacteria
- Transmission of Infectious TB
- Diagnosis of TB
- Screening for TB: Skin Testing
- The Mantoux Test

Blood Glucose
- Fasting Blood Glucose
- Two-Hour Postprandial Blood Glucose
- Glucose Tolerance Test
- Automated Methods of Glucose Analysis
- Testing Panels
- Glycosylated Hemoglobin

Cholesterol and Lipids
- The Chemistry of Cholesterol
- Functions of Cholesterol
- Lipoproteins and Cholesterol Transport
- Triglycerides

Blood Chemistry Tests
- Alanine Aminotransferase (ALT)
- Albumin
- Alkaline Phosphatase (ALP)
- Aspartate Aminotransferase (AST)
- Bilirubin, Total and Direct
- Blood Urea Nitrogen Test
- Calcium
- Chloride
- Carbon Dioxide (CO_2)
- Creatinine
- Gamma Glutamyltransferase (GGT)
- Lactate Dehydrogenase (LDH)
- Phosphorus (Phosphate)
- Potassium (K)
- Sodium
- Total Protein
- Uric Acid

OBJECTIVES

The student should strive to meet the following performance objectives and demonstrate an understanding of the facts and principles presented in this chapter through written and oral communication.

1. Define the key terms as presented in the glossary.
2. List the three main precautions to be observed during all tests and the collection of samples included in this chapter.
3. Collect samples and perform and interpret all tests included in this chapter.
4. Discuss factors to be considered when evaluating test results.
5. Discuss transmission, incubation period, and symptoms of Epstein–Barr virus/infectious mononucleosis.
6. List the blood group antigens and antibodies found in each of the four ABO groups and the Rh factors.
7. Explain the cause of phenylketonuria (PKU) and the symptoms caused by untreated PKU.
8. Indicate normal and increased levels of phenylalanine and the dietary restrictions to be observed by PKU patients.
9. Discuss the cause of tuberculosis and some major characteristics of *Mycobacterium tuberculosis.*
10. Discuss the role of insulin in the regulation of blood glucose levels.
11. List and discuss differences among the normal values for fasting blood glucose, 2-hour postprandial glucose, and the glucose tolerance test.
12. Explain the importance of cholesterol and triglyceride testing to identify patients at high risk for coronary heart disease.
13. Give the desirable values of cholesterol for adults.
14. Give the acceptable level of low-density lipoprotein (LDL) in persons with or without coronary heart disease, and discuss the role of high-density lipoprotein and LDL in coronary heart disease.
15. Give the normal values of urea nitrogen for adults, children, infants, and newborns, and discuss the significance of increased blood urea levels.

KEY TERMS (continued)

Rh Factor
Semen
Triglycerides
Tuberculosis (TB)
Wheal

Scenario

Audrey Jones, CMA (AAMA), has worked at Drs. Lewis and King's office for more than 5 years. In that time, Audrey has become proficient in obtaining specimens from patients for various laboratory tests. Audrey enjoys the work and finds it extremely challenging. She also realizes that communicating with patients to help them understand why their specimens are necessary for testing is just as important as being skillful in collecting and testing the specimens. Audrey has found that when she explains the reason the specimen is needed in terms patients can understand, they are often less fearful, which helps them relax. This can be especially helpful when collecting blood specimens.

INTRODUCTION

An increasing number of tests are performed in the ambulatory care setting, many of them by the medical assistant. To meet these new demands, the medical assistant must have a strong background in a variety of areas including medical terminology, Clinical Laboratory Improvement Amendments (CLIA) regulations, laboratory safety procedures, and specimen collection. Because many procedures require collection of a blood specimen, the medical assistant must also be an excellent phlebotomist. Good recordkeeping and communications skills round out the requirements. A quality-control program is necessary to ensure that the results are accurate and reliable (Figure 32-1). This will require a commitment on the part of the medical assistant to maintain the highest standards throughout the process.

A variety of specialty tests are covered in this chapter, including testing for pregnancy, infectious mononucleosis, tuberculosis (TB), and phenylketonuria (PKU), as well as blood types, hemoglobin A1c, and protime. This chapter also discusses the chemistry of blood, including chemistry panels, blood glucose, cholesterol, triglycerides, and other specialty laboratory tests such as semen analysis.

URINE PREGNANCY TESTS

Pregnancy tests are used when pregnancy is suspected. Pregnancy tests may also be used to rule out pregnancy before prescribing birth control pills, radiograph studies, certain antibiotics or other drugs, and for female patients who are to undergo surgery.

Pregnancy testing is based on detection of **human chorionic gonadotropin (hCG),** a hormone secreted by the placenta that can be detected in the serum or urine of pregnant women as early as 5 days after conception. During pregnancy, hCG levels peak at about 8 weeks, then decrease to lower but detectable levels for the remainder of the pregnancy.

Commercial/Home Urine Pregnancy Tests

A variety of accurate and easy-to-use commercial tests are available for use in the medical office. Manufacturers of pregnancy test kits have designed them to be sensitive, to be easy to perform and interpret, and to give rapid results. Pregnancy tests are one of many tests available for purchase as an over-the-counter product. However, results of tests performed at home should be confirmed by a laboratory test using appropriate quality-control measures and properly trained personnel. CLIA has

Spotlight on Certification

RMA Content Outline

- Medical law
- Patient education
- Laboratory procedures

CMA (AAMA) Content Outline

- Patient instruction
- Medicolegal guidelines and requirements
- Collecting and processing specimens; diagnostic testing

CMAS Content Outline

- Legal and ethical considerations
- Communication

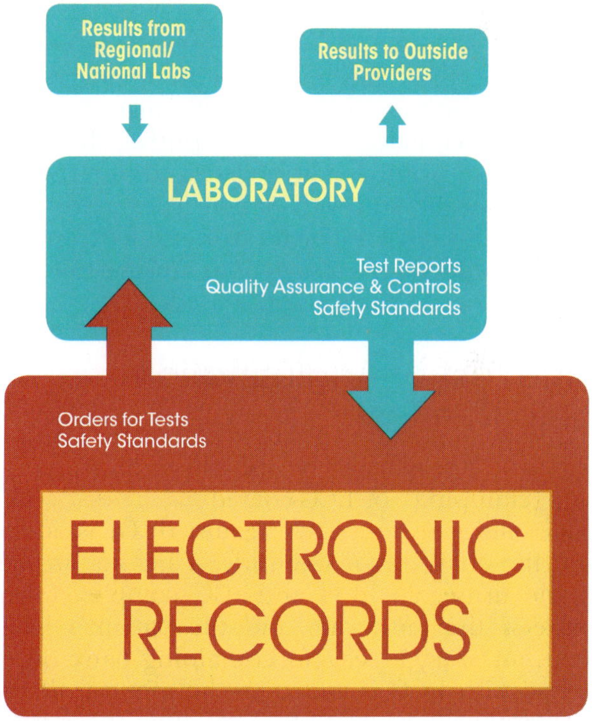

Figure 32-1 The laboratory arm of the total practice management system (TPMS). When tests are ordered, the medical assistant performs these procedures and records the results directly in the lab and progress notes sections of the patient's electronic medical record. The medical assistant can check to see whether controls have been performed in the lab's global electronic log to ensure the highest degree of patient care. Finally, the medical assistant can print patient education materials and follow-up instructions contained in the TPMS.

granted waived status to all urine pregnancy tests that use visual color comparison and specifically to the Bayer Corporations Clinitek 50 Urine Chemistry Analyzer for hCG in urine. Medical assistants qualify for the waived test category within the physicians' office laboratory (POL).

Testing Methods

Two testing methods using urine are discussed in this section: the slide test or agglutination inhibition test and the modified enzyme immunoassay. Diagnosis of pregnancy is made using these test results in conjunction with a physical examination including a pelvic examination by the provider.

A positive reaction to any pregnancy test does not necessarily indicate a normal pregnancy. Detection of hCG can also indicate such abnormal conditions as an **ectopic pregnancy,** a developing **hydatidiform mole** of the uterus, **choriocarcinoma,** or cancer of the lung, stomach, pancreas, colon, or breast.

Quality Control. Kits must be stored and used at the temperature directed by the manufacturer. Most kits contain a built-in control; however, appropriate positive and negative urine controls must always be run with patient specimens. Kits and reagents must not be used after the expiration date. Manufacturer's instructions must be followed precisely for the particular test used.

Precautions for Pregnancy Testing

1. Use a clean container for collection of the urine specimen. Disposable containers are preferred. Detergent residue on nondisposable containers may interfere with test results.
2. The first-voided morning urine has the highest concentration of hCG and is the preferred specimen. If this is not available, a urine specimen with a specific gravity of at least 1.010 is acceptable.
3. Although it is always best to run tests on fresh specimens, if the urine specimen cannot be tested immediately, it may be stored at 4°C for up to 24 hours. Both urine and serum specimens may be used with some test kits; other kits use only one or the other.
4. Allow refrigerated urine specimens and test reagents to come to room temperature before starting test procedures.
5. If using the slide test procedure:
   a. Avoid cross contamination with other urine specimens.
   b. Use a new stirrer for each test.

Slide Test or Agglutination Inhibition Test

The slide test is based on inhibition of **agglutination** (clumping) of hCG-coated **latex beads.** The hCG **antiserum** (**antibody** against hCG) is added to urine on a microscope slide. If hCG is present in the urine, an hCG/anti-hCG complex forms between the antiserum and the patient's hCG. Next, an **antigen** reagent containing latex beads coated with hCG is added to the mixture. If the hcG/anti-hCG complex formed, then there is no hCG antiserum available to react with the latex beads, and agglutination will *not* occur. No agglutination indicates positive pregnancy. Agglutination of the latex beads indicates negative pregnancy.

Enzyme Immunoassay Test

The **enzyme immunoassay** (EIA) is a more complex procedure than agglutination. The test can be designed in several different ways, but it always involves an antigen, an antibody specific for the antigen, and a second antibody. The test may be designed to detect a particular antibody in a patient's serum or to detect an antigen in a patient specimen.

Numerous tests are based on variations of the EIA. New technologies have been developed called membrane EIAs. In these tests, most of the reagents are incorporated into an absorbent membrane, which is enclosed in plastic. When the sample (serum or urine) is added, it migrates through the membrane, reacting with the reagents and forming a color. Many of these tests are simple to set up and interpret even though the technology is complex. Examples of membrane EIAs include over-the-counter pregnancy test kits and tests for group A *Streptococcus.*

Enzyme immunoassays for hCG vary in design but have some features in common. Most have the reagents incorporated into an absorbent membrane within a self-contained test unit, which may look like a plastic slide, a reagent strip, or a test cylinder. Tests may require the addition of the sample only or the addition of the sample and reagents to the test unit. Procedure 32-1 describes the general steps for pregnancy testing.

INFECTIOUS MONONUCLEOSIS

Infectious mononucleosis (IM) is a contagious disease that may have vague clinical symptoms and can mimic other diseases. Serologic tests are often the basis for an early diagnosis of the disease and may also be used to follow the course of the disease.

IM is commonly called "mono" or "kissing disease." The disease is a result of infection of the lymphocytes by the **Epstein-Barr virus (EBV).** EBV is common in our population. By 5 years of age, approximately 50% of the population is infected, increasing to 90% to 95% in adults. After the primary infection, the virus establishes a lifelong latency. The infectious virus may be isolated from saliva for several months, whereas antigens may be detected for life. In addition to causing IM, EBV has been implicated in other diseases such as nasopharyngeal carcinoma (NPC) and chronic fatigue syndrome.

Transmission of EBV

Transmission of EBV IM is primarily by saliva, which is why it is often referred to as "the kissing disease." EBV may also be spread by the sharing of drinking glasses and less often by blood transfusion. The disease is moderately contagious and is transmitted approximately 10% to 38% of the time in close social groups. In the home or in the hospital, careful handwashing will help prevent transmission of the virus.

Symptoms of IM

Mononucleosis is seen most often in children and young adults. Incubation may vary from 4 to 50 days; however, 7 to 14 days is the average. Infection in younger children is usually asymptomatic or manifests minor symptoms such as pharyngitis, otitis media, bronchitis, and other upper respiratory discomforts.

Classic symptoms usually occur when the primary infection is delayed until the second decade of life. IM is most often observed in the 15- to 25-year-old age group. Symptoms usually begin with a fever and swollen glands lasting for 3 to 5 days. Over the next 7 to 20 days, the patient may develop a headache; malaise; chest pain; a cough; tonsillitis; a rash; soft, swollen lymph nodes; and a swollen spleen. While the spleen is enlarged, the patient is advised to curtail activity, especially contact sports and rough activities, to prevent the rare, but serious, rupture of the spleen. Symptoms usually persist for 2 to 4 weeks and in more serious cases may last for more than 1 month.

Treatment of IM

Because there are currently no effective drugs available for EBV IM, treatment is primarily palative, or supportive. Although a vaccine is not yet available, some important work in that direction is ongoing.

Diagnosis of IM

To properly diagnose IM, the provider must consider blood and serology test results together with the patient's symptoms.

Blood Test for IM. The hematologic tests for IM include white blood cell count and evaluation of the patient's lymphocytes. In IM, lymphocytosis, or increase in lymphocytes, usually occurs, and large numbers of lymphocytes (greater than 20%) have an unusual or atypical appearance.

Serologic Test for IM. Persons with IM produce antibodies called **heterophile antibodies** by the sixth to tenth day of the illness. Heterophile antibodies are antibodies that react with similar antigens in more than one species. They are usually of the IgM class.

Detection of heterophile antibodies combined with the blood tests and patient symptoms provide the basis for the diagnosis of IM. The serologic test is usually positive after the first week of illness. However, if test results are negative, the test should be repeated after 1 week if clinical symptoms are still present.

CLIA Waived IM Tests

Several manufacturers have produced CLIA waived test kits suitable for use by the medical assistant in the POL.

Kits for IM usually provide all the necessary reagents, materials, and controls. The laboratory must obtain only the specimen to be tested, which is usually a small sample of the patient's plasma or serum or a drop of capillary blood.

Prothrombin Time/ProTime/INR

Prothrombin time, which is also called protime, PT, and international normalized ratio (INR), is a test for blood's clotting ability. It is used often for people who are taking anticoagulant medications such as Coumadin (warfarin). Monitoring is needed to maintain a careful balance that must be monitored between the blood clotting too readily and the blood being so thin it will not clot. The desired levels of INR are 2.0 to 3.0. Refer to Chapter 28 for more information on coagulation tests and Procedure 28-4 for the process of running a protime test.

BLOOD TYPING

Blood typing is based on the presence or absence of certain antigens on the surface of red blood cells (RBCs). These antigens are carbohydrate molecules that react with antibodies specific to them to cause agglutination of the RBCs. Antibodies are protein molecules that are found in serum; they are also referred to as immunoglobulins (Ig). When RBC antigens and antibodies react, they cause the RBCs to agglutinate. This process is called hemagglutination. Hemagglutination reactions are used in the typing of blood. The two major categories of blood typing are for the **ABO blood group** and the **Rh factor.** The ABO blood group consists of type A, type B, type AB, and type O. Within each of these types are the Rh factors, either Rh-positive (factor present) or Rh-negative (no factor). Figure 32-2 illustrates how RBCs are tested for blood type. In the example, type O blood would have no reaction to either anti-A or anti-B, whereas type AB blood would have a reaction to both. By process of elimination, one can determine which type the specimen is.

The ABO and Rh systems place certain restrictions on how blood can be transfused from one individual to another. Depending on their blood type, individuals with a particular RBC antigen may have antibodies against the other types (Table 32-1). An incompatible blood transfusion results when the antigens of the donor RBCs react with the antibodies of the recipient RBCs. This is a potentially life-threatening situation that varies in severity from mild fever to anaphylaxis with severe intravascular hemolysis. Although ABO and Rh typing does not completely rule out the possibility of reaction, it greatly reduces the chances.

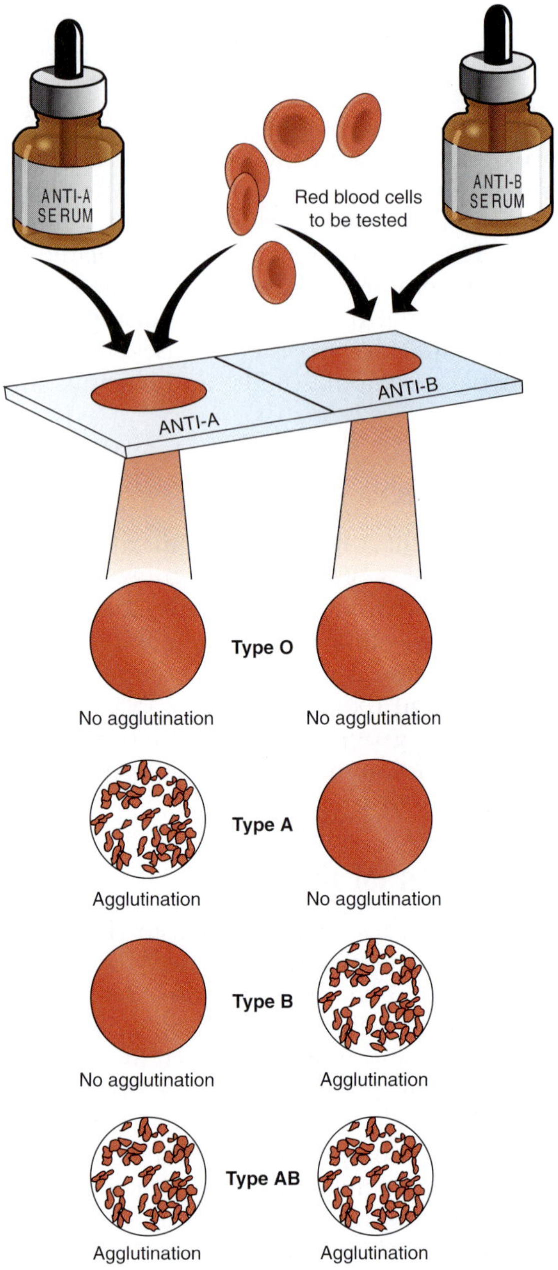

Figure 32-2 Blood typing the ABO groups.

ABO Blood Typing

ABO blood typing is determined by the presence or absence of two major antigens, A and B. All people have one of the four blood group categories: A, B, AB, or O. People with group A RBCs have A antigens, group B RBCs have B antigens, group AB RBCs have antigens for both A and B, and group O RBCs lack both A and B antigens. Naturally occurring antibodies to the other antigen types are found in the serum.

ABO type can be determined by the slide or tube method. The tube method is now most often used for blood typing. Because neither method is considered in the waived category by CLIA, they usually are not performed in the POL. Even if the patient carries a card listing his or her blood type, the patient's blood will be retested as a precaution. This is called a "blood cross and match" test. Nevertheless, it is a good idea to know your individual blood type and Rh factor.

Rh Blood Typing

Rh typing is routinely performed together with ABO typing. The Rh system is named for the rhesus monkey used in experiments that led to its dis-

Table 32-1 Antigens and Antibodies in ABO and Rh Blood Systems

Blood Group/Type	Antigen on RBC	Serum Antibodies
O (universal donor)	None	Anti-A and Anti-B
A	A	Anti-B
B	B	Anti-A
AB	A and B	None
Rh+	D	No anti-D*
Rh−	None	No anti-D*

*There are no naturally occurring antibodies to the Rh system.

covery. The Rh factor is found on the surface of RBCs. People possessing the Rh factor are said to have Rh-positive (Rh+) blood. Those without the Rh factor have Rh-negative (Rh−) blood.

About 85% of North Americans are Rh-positive; 15% are Rh-negative. Neither Rh-negative nor Rh-positive people have naturally occuring Rh antibodies in their blood. However, if an Rh-negative individual receives a transfusion of Rh-positive blood, he or she will develop antibodies to it. The antibodies take 2 weeks to develop. Both blood type and Rh factor must be taken into account for safe and successful transfusions.

Rh blood typing is also performed on pregnant women to determine the mother's Rh blood type. During the patient's initial prenatal care examination, blood typing is usually performed as part of the prenatal panel. In situations where the mother is Rh-negative, the mother's blood is tested for the presence of Rh antibodies. If the test is negative, then there is no risk to the fetus. A negative test should be repeated at weeks 30 and 36. If the test is positive, then the mother has been exposed to Rh-positive blood and has produced antibodies. A positive reaction also means that maternal hemolysis of fetal RBCs can occur. This condition is also called hemolytic disease of the newborn (HDN, also known as erythroblastosis fetalis). When the mother's antibodies attack the baby's RBCs, the RBCs are destroyed. This will make the baby anemic, which limits the amount of oxygen to his or her tissues and organs. The baby responds by trying to make more RBCs in his or her liver and spleen. This overuse can cause these two organs to become enlarged. The new RBCs are usually immature (called erythroblasts) and are not able to do the work of the mature RBC. Also, when the RBCs are destroyed, **bilirubin** is formed. Babies cannot rid the body of bilirubin, which can builds up in the blood, tissues, and body fluids of the baby. This condition is called hyperbilirubinuremia (too much bilirubin in the blood). Bilirubin is pigmented and causes a yellowing or jaundice of the newborn's skin and tissues.

This jaundice is not to be confused with the jaundice many newborns have, which is caused by a similar process but to a much less degree and with mild consequences. Hemolytic disease can be determined by evaluating the quantity of bilirubin in the amniotic fluid and in the newborn's blood.

HDN can cause severe complications for the newborn, ranging from the enlarged liver and anemia to seizures, brain damage, and even death.

Treatment before the baby is born can include intrauterine blood transfusions and early delivery if the baby is mature enough to survive. After the baby is born, blood transfusions, intravenous fluids, and help with respiration and oxygen intake may be necessary.

Patient Education

When a woman gives birth (or has a miscarriage or abortion), some of the fetal blood can mix with the mother's as the placenta tears away from the uterus. When the Rh-negative woman is exposed to the baby's Rh-positive blood (there is an 85% chance that the baby is Rh-positive), she builds antibodies against the Rh factor. Consequently, during the next pregnancy, her antibodies (which cross the placental barrier) would attack the next Rh-positive baby's RBCs. Giving the woman an injection of RhoGAM after each exposure to the Rh antigens prevents her from building the antibodies. Rh-negative women will need RhoGAM each time they are exposed to the Rh factor.

Fortunately, most cases of HDN can be prevented by administering RhoGAM to the Rh-negative mother. When injected into the mother, RhoGAM will prevent her from producing the RhD antibody. The injection must be administered at the 28th week of pregnancy and within 72 hours after delivery of an Rh-positive baby, miscarriage, or termination of pregnancy.

SEMEN ANALYSIS

With the progression of managed health care, more primary care providers are performing **semen** analysis in their offices to determine sperm cell counts before referring patients to fertility specialists. Examination of semen is also performed as part of a complete fertility work-up, to evaluate the effectiveness of a vasectomy, to determine paternity, and to substantiate rape cases.

When semen analysis is performed as part of a fertility work-up, the procedure involves macroscopic and microscopic analysis of seminal fluid for determination of total sperm count, percentage of motility, presence of agglutination, and percentage of normally formed sperm cells (Table 32-2). All male individuals will have variable sperm counts; therefore, a single analysis is insufficient. To achieve a reasonable estimate of these factors, the seminal analysis should be repeated at least three times over a 2-month period. A complete analysis will also include an evaluation of the partner's cervical secretions and sperm survival. This involves determining the ability of sperm to penetrate the mucus and maintain motility.

Postvasectomy semen analysis is evaluated a few weeks after surgery. If sperm are seen at that time, then follow-up analysis is required. The patient is not considered sterile until he has returned *two* samples, at least 1 week apart, that demonstrate no sperm, viable or dead. This typically will take several weeks. Until that time, an alternative method of birth control must be used.

Semen Composition

Semen is a composite solution produced by the testes and the accessory male reproductive organs. It consists primarily of spermatozoa suspended in seminal plasma. Because there is considerable variation in composition between different portions of the fluid as ejaculated, it is important to collect the entire sample. Refer to the Patient Education box for instructions to give to the male patient before semen analysis.

Table 32-2 Reference Values for Semen Analysis

Parameter	Normal Range
Appearance	White, viscid, opaque
Volume	1.5–5 mL
pH	7.12–8.00
Total count	50–200 million
% normal sperm	At least 80%
% motility	At least 60%

Altering Factors in Semen Analysis

Many factors can alter the results of semen analysis. Several drugs such as cyclophosphamide (Cytoxan) and nitrogen mustard reduce sperm count, as well as certain conditions such as orchitis (inflammation of the testes), testicular atrophy, testicular failure, and obstruction of the vas deferens. Cigarette smoking is associated with a decrease in the volume of semen, whereas coffee drinking results in increased sperm density and an increase in the percentage of cells with abnormal morphology. Fever may temporarily suppress the count. Although research suggests that consumption of alcohol does not affect sperm function as measured by semen analysis, the patient is instructed to avoid alcohol for several days before testing as a precaution.

Although research suggests that fertility is most closely correlated with motility and morphology, men with very high (>200 million/mL) or very low (≤20 million/mL) counts are likely to be infertile. Patients with aspermia (no sperm) or oligospermia (low sperm count, ≤20 million/mL) should be endocrinologically evaluated for pituitary, testicular, adrenal, or thyroid abnormalities.

PHENYLKETONURIA TEST

Phenylketonuria (PKU) is an inherited condition in which the baby cannot metabolize protein

Patient Education

The following instructions should be given to male patients when a semen sample is required for analysis:

1. Advise the patient to avoid consumption of alcohol for several days before the test. He should also avoid ejaculation for 3 days before collection of the semen sample.
2. Provide the patient with instructions and a container. The entire sample should be collected in a clean, dry, glass bottle that has been labeled, dated, and timed. The sample is collected by masturbation or interrupted coitus at home, or it may be collected at the medical office of the laboratory. A condom should never be used to collect a semen specimen due to the spermide content.
3. Specimens for complete fertility analysis collected outside the laboratory must be brought to the laboratory within 30 minutes. Postvasectomy specimens should be brought to the laboratory within 1 hour of collection.
4. The sample must be transported to the laboratory at 37°C (98.6°F). Low temperature during transport will decrease the motility of sperm. Temperature that is too warm could destroy the sperm. Keeping the sample close to his body during transport might be the best advice.

properly. Phenylalanine is present in milk and other dairy proteins. If the baby has PKU, phenylalanine can build up in his or her brain and other organs and cause irreversible mental retardation, loss of muscle coordination, and other serious disorders. Diagnosis should be made early so that the baby can be put on a diet low in proteins. The baby should be tested at about 2 days old and again at 7 to 14 days old. Although a phenylalanine-restricted diet will prevent mental retardation, it will not cure the underlying condition. Routine screening of newborns for PKU is mandatory in all states and may be performed in the hospital or the medical office. The medical assistant's role is to properly explain the procedure to the infant's parents and to collect the blood specimen for analysis.

Many other tests can be performed using the blood sample sent on the PKU card, including tests for congenital hypothyroidism (CH), congenital adrenal hyperplasia (CAH), galactosemia, sickle cell disease, and others. The tests that are performed depend on individual state requirements.

Excess phenylalanine can be detected in blood or in urine. Normal levels of phenylalanine are less than 2 mg/deciliter (dL); more than 4 mg/dL is considered elevated. The **Guthrie screening test** is used to evaluate blood and is considered more accurate than urine tests. Phenylalanine can be detected in the blood of infants with PKU after 3 to 4 days on a breast milk or formula milk diet. Testing of breast-fed infants is delayed a few days because of the lack of phenylalanine in colostrum, the first breast milk. Colostrum is produced for the first 2 to 3 days after birth and is rich in antibodies, protein, and calories. True breast milk production begins after this time. Positive results from blood testing are confirmed by measuring serum phenylalanine and tyrosine levels. Infants with PKU have increasing phenylalanine levels (>4 mg/dL) and decreasing tyrosine levels (<0.6 mg/dL).

Blood Testing for PKU

The Guthrie test was developed to screen for phenylalanine in the blood, and the first test is usually performed before the discharge of infants from the hospital. However, with managed care and the trend toward very short hospital stays for newborns, many pediatrician offices are now performing this first test. Capillary blood is collected from

Patient Education

Infants who test positive for PKU require a restricted phenylalanine diet for normal development to occur. Parents will need to have an appointment with a dietician to understand fully what foods the baby can and cannot eat. The diet will include a suitable milk substitute such as Lofenalac. Blood and urine tests will be necessary periodically to monitor the special diet.

Women who have PKU and become pregnant must be especially careful to avoid phenylalanines during pregnancy.

a heel stick onto a "filter paper" test card and sent to the laboratory for testing. Patient, provider, and test information, together with the blood samples, are placed directly on the laboratory test card, which is typically provided by most state Departments of Health (Figure 32-3). (See Procedure 32-3 and Chapter 28 for proper capillary puncture technique.)

Factors That May Influence the Guthrie Test. The following factors may influence the Guthrie test:

- Feeding problems such as vomiting may result in a false-negative reaction.
- Failure to ingest sufficient phenylalanine—testing before 3 to 4 days of the beginning of a milk diet—will result in a false-negative reaction.
- Premature infants may give false-positive test results because of a delay in the development of certain liver enzymes.
- Drugs such as salicylates, aspirin, or antibiotics taken by the mother (if breast-feeding) or the child may interfere with test results.

TUBERCULOSIS

Despite efforts to control its spread, **tuberculosis (TB)** infections are on the increase in the United States and around the world. Because tuberculosis morbidity is on the rise, increasing 14% from 1985 to 1997, more patients are screened now for the disease than ever before. The Advisory Council for Elimination of Tuberculosis, an independent group of TB-control experts, recommends screening all patients who fall into high-risk groups, or those who associate with high-risk groups, such as health care workers, including medical assistants. See the Current Family Practice Recommendations for TB Testing for a more complete list.

Cause of TB

Infectious TB is caused by the small, rod-shaped bacterium *Mycobacterium tuberculosis.* This aerobic bacterium is nonmotile and has a high content of lipid in its cell wall, making it difficult to stain using basic aniline dyes. For this reason, the Ziehl-Neelsen method was developed and is used as a tool for identification of mycobacteria. Mycobacteria will retain the red stain in the presence of acid alcohol and are therefore referred to as acid-fast. Other bacterial species stain blue.

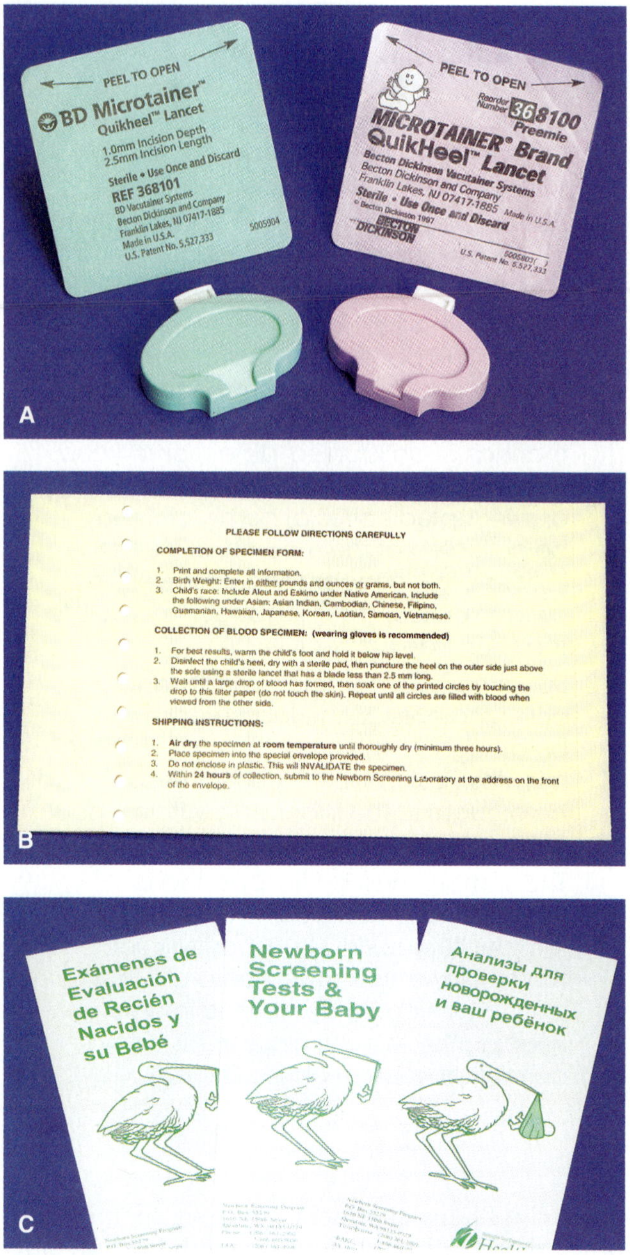

Figure 32-3 (A) Pediatric-sized safety lancets are available to vary the depth of the puncture. (B) The back of the PKU test card provides detailed instructions on performing the test and completing the card correctly. (C) Patient information and permission forms are available in a variety of languages.

Resistance in Mycobacteria

Mycobacteria exhibit an unusual degree of resistance on many fronts. They are able to tolerate drying and the effects of many disinfectants. Mycobacteria also show resistance to most antibiotics, making these infections difficult to treat. To help overcome bacterial resistance to antimicro-

Patient Education

Current Family Practice Recommendations for TB Testing

TB screening is recommended for:

- Close contacts of those with known or suspected TB.
- Persons infected with HIV.
- Intravenous drug users or users of other illicit drugs.
- Chronically ill patients with conditions or diseases that increase the risk for progressing from latent to active TB. Risk factors include diabetes, high-dose steroids, immunosuppressive therapy, chronic renal failure, lymphoma, leukemia, other cancer, weight loss to more than 10% below ideal weight, silicosis, gastrectomy, and jejunoileal bypass.
- Foreign-born persons and those arriving within the last 5 years from countries that have had a high incidence of TB.
- Residents and employees of high-risk institutions, such as correctional facilities, nursing homes, mental institutions, and homeless shelters.
- Health care workers, especially those caring for patients at high risk.
- Medically underserved and low-income populations.
- Infants, children, and adolescents exposed to adults at high risk.

bial agents, patients take two or three drugs for a period of 6 to 9 months. The most common drug used to fight TB is isoniazid (INH). Other drugs used are rifampin, pyrazinamide, ethambutol, and streptomycin.

Transmission of Infectious TB

Infectious TB is highly contagious. Seventy-five percent of new cases occur by inhalation of cough-produced airborne droplets from symptomatic or asymptomatic persons. Crowded conditions contribute to this transmission. TB often is associated with poverty, poor nutrition, and crowded conditions such as what is often seen in prisons and mental health hospitals. A recent increase in TB is related to the increase in AIDS cases.

Diagnosis of TB

TB diagnosis differentiates between active and inactive TB, and the treatments differ. Active TB is a serious and contagious condition that requires isolation of the patient and aggressive treatment with several drugs over several months.

Patients exhibiting a positive or questionable **purified protein derivative (PPD)** reaction should have a chest X-ray to examine for tubercles, and a sputum sample should be stained to search for acid-fast rods. The presence of acid-fast rods in the sputum confirms active TB. Reasons for a positive reaction to PPD are varied. First and most obvious is that the patient has been exposed to TB or has an active case of TB. Persons with an old, inactive case will also give a positive skin test, as will persons who have been vaccinated with BCG. BCG (the bacille of Calmette and Guerin) is a vaccine made from live, avirulent *Mycobacterium bovis.* The vaccine is used in Europe and South America to help prevent childhood cases of TB. Persons who receive BCG will give a positive skin reaction for a minimum of 4 years and much longer in many cases. Many immigrants will show positive PPD because of a BCG vaccination. The chest X-ray is an important second step for those individuals.

Screening for TB: Skin Testing

Screening for TB may be performed as part of a routine medical examination or as a prerequisite for school or employment. In states where medical assistants can legally perform injections, they may be responsible for administration and interpretation of the skin test. The most accurate method used is the **Mantoux test.** The tine test, which is a multiple-puncture test, may still be used in some areas but is no longer recommended by the American Academy of Pediatrics. Both the Mantoux and the tine methods use tuberculin, also referred to as PPD, which is a filtrate of tuberculin cultures that are used for skin testing. Persons who have been exposed to TB will develop a hypersensitive response to PPD resulting in the formation of an induration. An induration is a hard, red spot on the skin that is the result of sensitized lymphocytes migrating to the site of the injection. It is important to keep in mind that a positive skin test does not distinguish between active or inactive cases of TB. Again, a positive skin test will require further diagnostic testing including an X-ray for lung lesions and an acid-fast stain of sputum to examine for the presence of *Mycobacterium tuberculosis.* Because of the severity of the reaction, do not administer the skin test to persons who have had a positive reaction in the past.

The Mantoux Test

In the Mantoux test, 0.1 mL of 5 TU (toxin unit) strength PPD is injected intradermally using a 1 mL tuberculin syringe. A short (⅜–½ inch), 26 or 27 gauge needle is used. Care must be taken to inject the PPD so that a **wheal** forms (Figure 32-4). If the injection is too deep, it will be impossible to form the wheal. If the injection is too shallow, the PPD may leak onto the skin. Either of these two errors would invalidate the test results. It is also important to draw exactly 0.1 mL of the PPD, because too much or too little will lead to erroneous test results.

Choosing a Site to Administer the Mantoux Test. To select a site for the Mantoux test, locate a site approximately 3 to 4 inches down from the bend of the arm on the anterior side. Avoid areas with excess hair, visible blood vessels, or scar tissue. The chosen site should be cleaned with alcohol and allowed to dry before administering the PPD. The left arm is the standard arm.

Reading the Results of the Mantoux TB Test. Have the patient return in 48 to 72 hours for examination of the injection site. Gently feel the induration—the hard, raised area. Do not include the area of redness or erythema in your assessment. See Procedure 24-7 for the complete injection procedure and Figures 32-5 and 32-6 for measuring the induration.

Proper patient instructions should be given both verbally and in written form to help ensure patient compliance. If the patient delays more

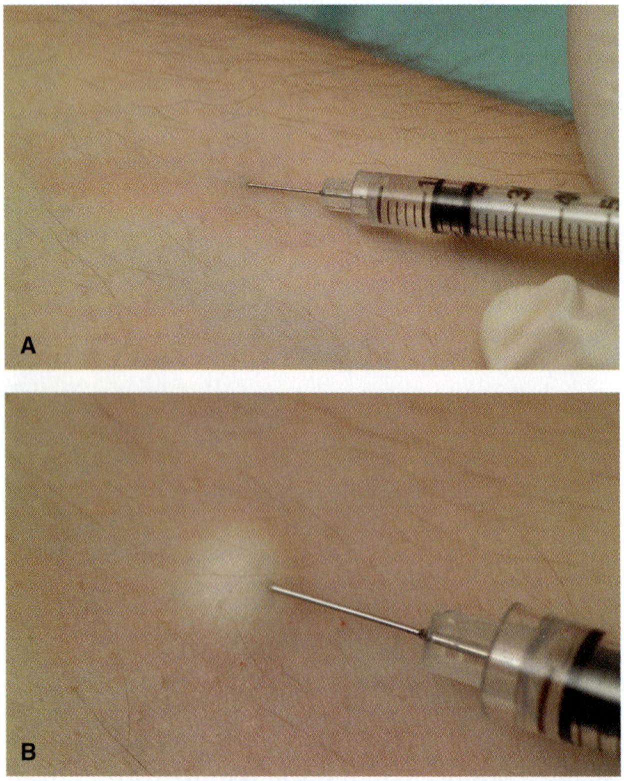

Figure 32-4 (A) Gently insert the needle just under the skin surface at about a 5-degree angle. Imbed the entire bevel. Slowly and carefully inject the medication. (B) A wheal should appear as a whitish raised bump.

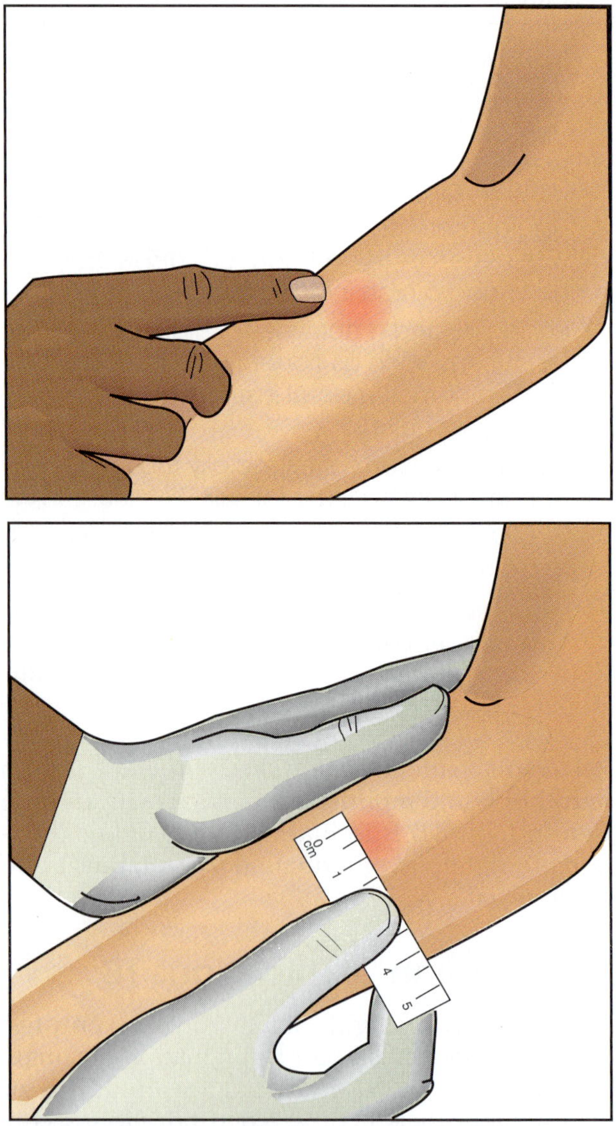

Figure 32-5 Gently inspect and measure the induration (the elevated firm area, not the area of redness or erythema) in response to the tuberculin test within 48 to 72 hours after administration. Some patients will have no induration.

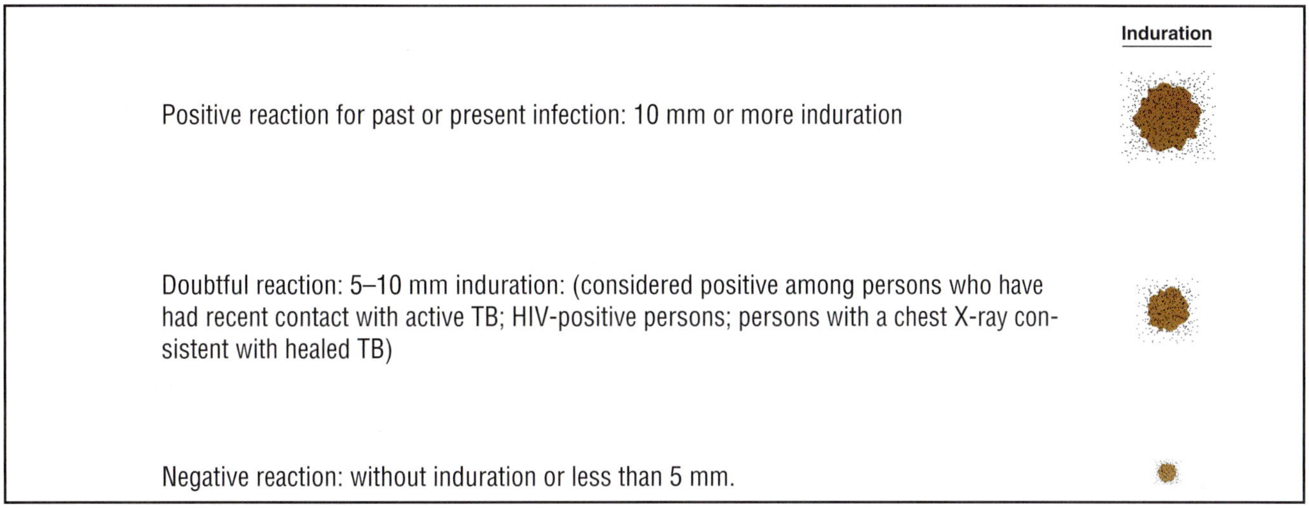
Induration
Positive reaction for past or present infection: 10 mm or more induration
Doubtful reaction: 5–10 mm induration: (considered positive among persons who have had recent contact with active TB; HIV-positive persons; persons with a chest X-ray consistent with healed TB)
Negative reaction: without induration or less than 5 mm.

Figure 32-6 The size of the induration (raised and firm area, not the redness) is measured and recorded as shown.

than 72 hours in returning to the clinic for the test reading, the test cannot be accepted.

Some patients may show swelling, itching, or localized, raised hives when injected with the PPD. This is not a true induration but rather an allergic reaction to the protein derivative, and should not be misinterpreted as a positive response. Do not repeat the Mantoux test if an allergic reaction occurs. If you are unable to get a wheal, repeat the test at least 2 inches from the first attempt.

BLOOD GLUCOSE

Glucose is the principal and almost exclusive carbohydrate found circulating in blood. It may also be detected in urine, cerebrospinal fluid, and semen. Glucose serves as an energy source for the body. Excess glucose is converted into glycogen for short-term storage in the liver and muscle cells, and as adipose tissue for long-term storage. Tests for blood glucose levels are commonly performed in the medical office. The results are used to screen for carbohydrate disorders such as **hypoglycemia** (low blood glucose level), **hyperglycemia** (high blood glucose level, which occurs in **diabetes mellitus**), and liver dysfunction. A variety of testing methods have been developed to diagnose, evaluate, and monitor abnormalities in carbohydrate metabolism. They include the fasting blood glucose (FBG), the 2-hour postprandial blood glucose, and the glucose tolerance test (GTT). All tests are discussed here, but the FBG is preferred as the first step in the clinical setting because it is easier and faster to perform, more convenient and acceptable to patients, and less expensive.

Blood glucose concentrations rise after a meal and are regulated by the action of several hormones including **insulin** and glucagon. Both insulin and glucagon are produced by the pancreas. Insulin is secreted by pancreatic cells in response to increased glucose levels and aids with the entry of glucose into cells for conversion into energy. Insulin is also required for proper storage of glucose (which is first converted into glycogen) in the liver and in muscle cells. Glucagon is secreted by the pancreas when blood sugar levels decrease and triggers the breakdown of glycogen to help increase and regulate blood sugar levels.

Fasting Blood Glucose

Evaluation of FBG levels is commonly used to screen for diabetes mellitus. Diabetes mellitus is a type of carbohydrate disorder characterized

Patient Education

In preparation for the test, the patient should be instructed to fast for 12 hours (except for water). A fasting blood sample is usually collected in the morning to minimize inconvenience to the patient. Certain drugs such as oral contraceptives, salicylates, diuretics, and steroids may alter the results, so the provider may restrict their use for 2 to 3 days before the test. The patient should receive both verbal and written instructions for the testing requirements and preparation.

by insulin deficiency (or no insulin) and a state of hyperglycemia (*hyper* means "too much," *glyc* means "sugar," and *emia* means "blood").

The normal fasting value of glucose ranges from 70 to 110 mg/100 mL (mg/dL). Table 32-3 lists reference glucose values. A value of 120 mg/dL glucose is the dividing point between healthy and hyperglycemic individuals. Generally, truly increased glucose levels indicate diabetes mellitus. Other causes of hyperglycemia include **Cushing's syndrome** and acute stress response. Increased blood glucose levels should be further evaluated using the glucose tolerance test.

Two-Hour Postprandial Blood Glucose

The 2-hour postprandial (after eating) evaluation of blood glucose levels is used to screen for diabetes and to monitor insulin dosage. After fasting from midnight the night before, the patient eats a prescribed meal containing 75 to 100 g carbohy-

Table 32-3 Reference Values For Blood Glucose Level

Test	Glucose Concentration (mg/dL)
Fasting	
Serum	70–110
Whole blood	60–100
Two-hour postprandial	≤110
Glucose tolerance (oral, serum)	
Fasting	70–110
1 hour	20–50 above fasting
2 hour	5–15 above fasting
3 hour	Fasting level or below

Values vary slightly between laboratories depending on testing method used.

Patient Education

Let your patient know there are more than 25 glucose meters available for them to choose from. All of them use the typical process of a drop of blood applied to a disposable "test strip" and inserted into the meter. The unit measures how much glucose is in the sample. All the meters display the result. Some meters allow a much smaller sample to be used and allow the sample to be taken from sites other than the fingertip (alternate site testing). Some meters record and store a number of test results, and some meters can connect to a personal computer to store results and print them out. Some new models have automatic timing, error codes and signals, or barcode readers to help with calibration. Some meters have a large display screen or spoken instructions for people with visual impairments. In choosing a meter, the patient should consider the following:

- Cost per strip
- Number of tests required per day
- Amount of blood needed for testing
- Testing speed
- Overall size and portability
- Cost of the meter
- Ability to store test results in memory
- Ability to test sites other than fingertip
- Other personal preferences

Many manufacturers offer free meters with the purchase of the test strips. Your clinic may be given free meters to give to patients together with a few sample strips in hopes the patient will continue to use that meter and purchase the strips. Unfortunately, the meters given to patients might not be the best choice for them, but they will continue to use it because their doctor gave it to them. Be sure to let patients know that there are many choices, and that the free meter you are giving them is *not necessarily an endorsement* of one meter over another.

drate or consumes a 75 to 100-gram glucose test load solution such as Glucola®. Two hours later, a blood specimen is collected and tested for glucose concentration. Glucose levels will return to or fall below the fasting level within 2 hours in individuals without diabetes. Increased glucose levels should be further examined using the GTT.

According to the standards of the American Diabetes Association, a normal blood glucose is defined as less than 100 mg/dL in a fasting plasma glucose test and a 2-hour postload (75 g glucose load solution) value of less than 140 mg/dL.

A fasting plasma glucose test of 126 mg/dL or greater indicates a need for further testing, and a 2-hour postload value of 140 mg/dL or greater is a diagnosis of having "prediabetes" indicating a relatively high risk for development of diabetes.

A 2-hour postload value of 200 mg/dL or greater is a positive test for diabetes and should be confirmed on another day.

Glucose Tolerance Test

The GTT provides more detailed information used to assess insulin response to glucose and to diagnose diabetes.

When the patient arrives, he or she should be fasting (nothing but water) for at least 10 hours. A capillary specimen is drawn to determine the fasting blood sugar (FBS) level. If the FBS level is less than 200 mg/dL, then a venous specimen and urine specimen are obtained. These are labeled as fasting specimens with the date and time noted. If the results of the capillary test shows the FBS level greater than 200 mg/dL, the provider should be notified immediately. Hyperglycemia after fasting is abnormal and not an appropriate condition for further loading with additional glucose and may be dangerous to the patient.

After providing the fasting urine and blood specimens, the patient consumes a glucose test solution containing 1.75 g glucose/kilogram of body weight, or the standard adult dose of 75 to 100 g. The patient must consume the entire glucose solution within a 5-minute time frame. The test timing starts immediately after the patient has finished drinking the solution. If the patient should vomit within the first 30 minutes after drinking the solution, the test will be stopped and rescheduled on a different day. It is probably best not to mention this to the patient, though, because it is a rare occurrence and it is best not to have the patient worried about the possibility of vomiting. Blood and urine specimens are typically collected at 30 minutes, 1 hour, 2 hours, and 3 hours (and sometimes 6 hours) after ingestion of the glucose solution and are tested for glucose level. These measurements help determine the patient's ability to deal with increased glucose. During the test, the patient must not ingest anything (other than the solution) except water. The patient must also abstain from smoking, because smoking acts as a stimulant and increases blood glucose levels. The patient must also refrain from chewing gum, which stimulates the digestive process and also may add sugar to his or her system. Physical activity should be strongly discouraged because activity can activate sugar utilization in the body and affect the test results. Sedentary activity level is suggested.

During the second and third hours of the test, the patient may experience weakness, slight faintness, and perspire. These are all normal symptoms. If, however, the patient develops a headache, faints, or displays irrational speech or behavior, he or she may be experiencing hypoglycemic shock and the provider should be notified immediately.

The blood glucose level of patients without diabetes usually peaks 30 to 60 minutes after consumption of the test load at 160 to 180 mg/dL and returns to the fasting level after 2 to 3 hours. Patients with diabetes will still have increased glucose levels at the end of the test.

Automated Methods of Glucose Analysis

Several types of glucose analyzers are available that are suitable for POLs or small clinical laboratories. Many of these operate on the principle of reflectance photometry and use adaptations of the enzymatic methods of glucose analysis. One example of an instrument suitable for small laboratories is the HemoCue® blood glucose analyzer.

Dozens of small, inexpensive, handheld glucose meters are also made and are designed for home use by patients with diabetes. See the Patient Education box for some criteria for patients to consider when purchasing an at-home testing method. Most of these are suitable for use in point-of-care (POC) testing or in the provider's office (Figure 32-7).

Glucose controls can be purchased to check instrument performance. It is always necessary to use test materials that are made for a particular instrument only with that instrument.

All of these analyzers are designed to be easy to use and to give rapid results. With all instruments, it is necessary to use consistent proper specimen collection and testing technique to avoid variations in results.

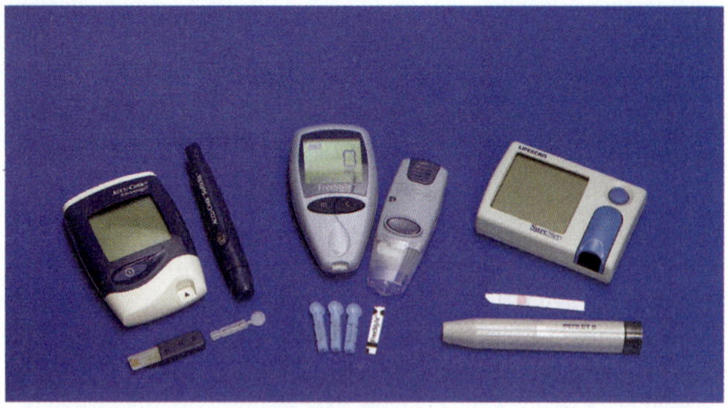

Figure 32-7 A variety of hand-held glucose analyzers (commonly called glucometers) are available for home or clinic use.

The medical assistant often is responsible for providing education to patients on how to use glucometers, including maintenance and calibration of the meter. It is important that the medical assistant who works with patients with diabetes become familiar with a variety of meters and their differences and similarities.

Photometry Analyzers. The HemoCue® blood glucose system is a compact glucose analyzer based on the principle of photometry. The system consists of a compact photometer and disposable microcuvettes. The self-filling microcuvette automatically draws up 5 mcL blood from a capillary puncture into its reaction chamber. The microcuvette is then placed into the holder and pushed into the photometer. The glucose concentration in milligrams per deciliter (mg/dL) is displayed within 45 to 240 seconds (Figure 32-8). This system is ideal for POLs and POC testing because of the stability of calibration and the minimum operator training required.

Reflectance Photometry Analyzers. Several glucose analyzers are available that are based on reflectance photometry. Blood from a fingerstick, serum, or plasma is applied to the reagent area of a test strip. The glucose in the sample reacts with the reagents in the pad(s), causing a color to form. The more glucose present in the sample, the darker or more intense the color. At the appropriate time, the strip is inserted into the test chamber and light is directed onto the test area. The amount of light reflected from the colored test area is measured by the photometer and converted to a digital readout showing the glucose concentration in milligrams per deciliter (or mmol/L). Most instruments give results in 1 to 3 minutes. Instructions included with the test strips must be followed carefully for reliable test results (see Procedure 32-5).

Testing Panels

Glucose testing may be part of a general chemistry panel test that can be useful in giving an overall view of an individual's state of health, especially when used in conjunction with other tests. Glucose testing may also be performed as part of a specific chemistry panel such as a glucose panel. Glucose serum levels are included in both the Basic Metabolic Panel (BMP) and the Comprehensive Metabolic Panel (CMP).

Glycosylated Hemoglobin

Glycosylated hemoglobin or hemoglobin A1c (Hb A1c) determination is a blood test that measures how well the glucose level has been controlled over the past 2 to 3 months versus the conventional blood test that shows only current day status. Pro-

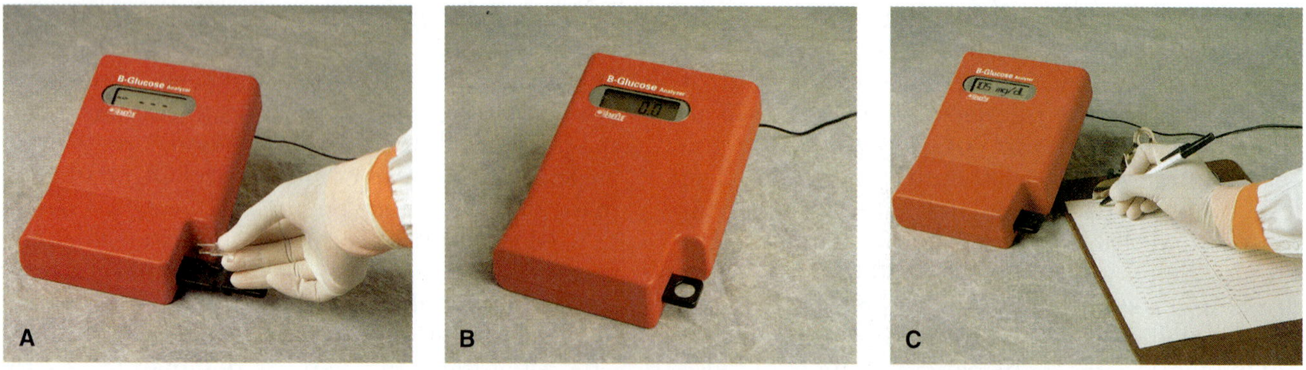

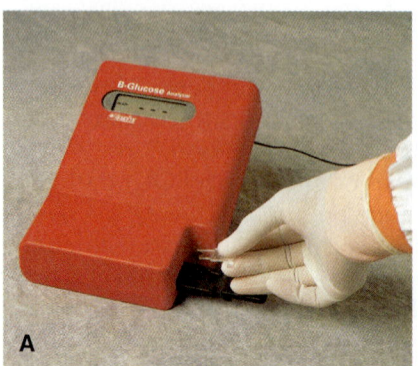

Figure 32-8 The HemoCue Blood Glucose System. (A) The patient's blood specimen in placed on the microcuvette. The microcuvette is inserted into its holder and pushed into the photometer. (B) Specimen is allowed to remain in the analyzer until test is completed. (C) When the analyzer has completed the testing, the results are displayed and recorded.

ORGAN OR DISEASE PANELS
See reverse for components

Test #	Test		Code	Tube
322744	Acute Hepatitis Panel	@	80074	SST
322758	Basic Metabolic Panel (8)		80048	SST
322000	Comp Metabolic Panel (14)		80053	SST
303754	Electrolyte Panel		80051	SST
322755	Hepatic Function Panel (7)	@	80076	SST
303756	Lipid Panel	% @	80061	SST
322777	Renal Function Panel		80069	SST

HEMATOLOGY

Test #	Test		Code	Tube
005009	CBC w Diff w Plt	@	85025	LAV
115907	CBC w Diff w/o Plt	@	~	LAV
028142	CBC w/o Diff w Plt	@	85027	LAV
005017	CBC w/o Diff w/o Plt	@	~	LAV
005058	Hematocrit	@	85014	LAV
005041	Hemoglobin	@	85018	LAV
005249	Platelet Count	@	85049	LAV
005033	RBC Count		85041	LAV
005025	WBC Count	@	85048	LAV
005090	WBC Differential	@	85004	LAV

ALPHABETICAL/COMBINATION TESTS

Test #	Test		Code	Tube
006049	ABO and Rh		86900 86901	LAV
001081	Albumin		82040	SST
001107	Alkaline Phosphatase		84075	SST
001545	ALT (SGPT)		84460	SST
001396	Amylase		82150	SST
006254	Antinuclear Antibodies		86038	SST
001123	AST (SGOT)		84450	SST
000810	B_{12} and Folate	@	82607 82746	SST
001099	Bilirubin, Total		82247	SST
001040	BUN		84520	SST

ALPHABETICAL TESTS CON'T

Test #	Test		Code	Tube
001016	Calcium		82310	SST
007419	Carbamazepine (Tegretol®)		80156	SER
002139	CEA	% @	82378	SST
001065	Cholesterol, Total	% @	82465	SST
001370	Creatinine		82565	SST
007385	Digoxin (Lanoxin®)	% @	80162	SER
004515	Estradiol		82670	SST
004309	FSH		83001	SST
001958	GGTP	% @	82977	SST
001818	Glucose, Plasma	% @	82947	GRY
001032	Glucose, Serum	% @	82947	SER
004556	hCG, Beta Subunit, Qual	@	84703	SST
004416	hCG, Beta Subunit, Quant	% @	84702	SST
004036	hCG, Qualitative, Urine	@	81025	URN
001925	HDL Cholesterol	% @	83718	SST
162289	*Helicobacter pylori*, IgG		86677	SST
006395	Hep B Surface Antibody		86706	SST
006510	Hep B Surface Antigen		87340	SST
140608	Hep C Antibody		86803	SST
001453	Hemoglobin A_{1c}	% @	83036	LAV
083824	HIV-1 Antibodies *	% @	86701	SST
001321	Iron and IBC	@	83540 83550	SST
001115	LDH		83615	SST
004283	LH		83002	SST
001404	Lipase		83690	SER
007708	Lithium (Eskalith®)	% @	80178	SER
001537	Magnesium	@	83735	SST
007401	Phenytoin (Dilantin®)	% @	80185	RED
001180	Potassium	@	84132	SST

ALPHABETICAL TESTS CON'T

Test #	Test		Code	Tube
512094	PreGen-Plus™	#		
202945	Prenatal Profile 1	@		
004465	Prolactin		84146	SST
010322	PSA	% @	84153 / % G0103	SST
001073	Protein, Total		84155	SST
005199	Prothrombin Time (PT)	% @	85610	BLU
020321	PT and PTT Activated	% @	85610 85730	BLU
005207	PTT Activated	@	85730	BLU
006502	Rheumatoid Arthritis Factor	@	86431	SST
006072	RPR	@	86592	SST
006197	Rubella Antibodies, IgG		86762	SST
005215	Sed Rate, Westergren	@	85651	LAV
004226	Testosterone		84403	SST
001156	T3 Uptake	% @	84479	SST
330015	Thyroid Cascade Profile	% @		SST
001149	Thyroxine (T_4)	% @	84436	SST
001974	Thyroxine (T_4) Free	% @	84439	SST
001172	Triglycerides	% @	84478	SST
002188	Triiodothyronine (T_3)		84480	SST
004259	TSH, 3rd generation	% @	84443	SST
001057	Uric Acid		84550	SST
003038	Urinalysis Microscopic on Positives	@	81003	URN
003772	Urinalysis with Microscopic	@	81001	URN

MATERNAL SERUM TESTING

017319 AFP Tetra @ % 017335 AFP X-tra @ %

GA: ___wks___ days on ___/___/___ by: LMP US EDD
DOB: _____/_____/_____ Maternal Wt: _______
Insulin Dependent: Yes No Repeat Test: Yes No
Type: Single Twins Other Race: Cau Blk Other
NTD History: __________________
Other Indications: __________________

MICROBIOLOGY - See Reverse Side
ENDOCERVICAL THROAT URINE
STOOL URETHRAL INDICATE SOURCE

OTHER

Test #	Test	Code	Transport
008847	Urine Culture, Routine† @	87086	Urn Cul Trnspt
008169	Throat, *Beta-Hemolytic Strep Cult, Group A*	87081	Bact Trnspt
008342	Upper Respiratory Culture, Routine †	87070	Bact Trnspt
180810	Lower Respiratory Culture †	87070	Steril Trnspt
008334	Genital Culture, Routine †	87070	Bact Trnspt
188128	Group B Strep Colonization Detection Cult/DNA Probe	87081 87149	Bact Trnspt
008144	Stool Culture †	87045 87046 X 2	Fecal Trnspt
008649	Aerobic †	87070	Bact Trnspt
008623	Ova and Parasites	87177 88312	O & P Kit
164202	Chlamydia DNA Probe *	87490	Probe Trnspt
164210	*N. gonorrhoeae* DNA Probe *	87590	Probe Trnspt
164160	*Chlamydia/GC* DNA Probe w/Confirmation on positives *	PENDING	Probe Trnspt
096479	*Chlamydia/GC* DNA Probe without Confirmation	PENDING	Probe Trnspt
008904	Anaerobic Culture	87075	Anaer Trnspt

† = ID / Susceptibility at Additional Charge
* = Confirmation at Additional Charge

OTHER TESTS / INDIVIDUAL PROFILE COMPONENTS

TEST #	TEST NAMES

Figure 32-9 Laboratory panels are combinations of tests related to a specific function, body organ, or organ system.

viders can use this test to determine if patients with diabetes are consistently adhering to their diet and health guidelines or are adhering to their diet only for a day before their office visit.

Glycosylated hemoglobin is a stable molecule formed when sugar and hemoglobin bind together on the RBC. An increased finding of glycosylated hemoglobin indicates poor glucose control in the assessment of the diabetic patient.

When the RBC is first formed, it contains no glucose. If glucose is present at increased levels in the blood, the excess enters the RBC and attaches (glycates) to the hemoglobin. The more glucose is present, the more hemoglobin becomes glycated.

The A1c measures the percentage of the glycated hemoglobin. This offers us an average of the glucose in the blood over about 3 months. Most RBCs live about 120 days and maintain the glycated state.

What hemoglobin A1c does not do is indicate whether the patient has experienced hyperglycemia or hypoglycemia over that time frame because day-to-day readings of glucose levels are not provided; thus, it is not useful in adjusting insulin. Having the patient monitor his or her blood glucose level with a meter and keep a daily diary is a good way to look at his or her day-to-day blood glucose levels. Both tests are useful tools in helping manage diabetes.

The advantage of hemoglobin A1c not being affected by day-to-day variations in blood glucose levels is that the patient does not need to be fasting for this test.

CHOLESTEROL AND LIPIDS

Cholesterol is a fatty compound that is essential for many vital life functions and is a normal constituent of blood. Although it is required for life, excess cholesterol is not a necessary part of the diet, except in babies and children. Sufficient quantities are manufactured by the body from carbohydrates and other fats. Cholesterol has been linked to coronary artery disease. According to the American Heart Association and the National Institutes of Health, cholesterol should not be restricted in babies and toddlers. Fats and cholesterol are important for normal growth and development. Babies and very young children should be on healthy diets, though, containing unsaturated and polyunsaturated oils and fats. From about 4 or 5 years old, they can be transitioned to heart-healthy foods such as nonfat milk. To help reduce the risk for coronary artery disease, nutritionists and agencies such as the American Heart Association and the National Cholesterol Education Program advise that fats make up no more than 30% of the total intake of calories daily, and that the concentration of cholesterol in blood not exceed 200 mg/dL. Cholesterol of 240 mg/dL or greater is considered to present a high risk for heart disease. Cholesterol levels between 200 and 239 mg/dL are considered borderline (see Procedure 32-6).

The Chemistry of Cholesterol

The cholesterol molecule consists of carbon, hydrogen, and oxygen. Cholesterol is a saturated, fatty acid. Saturated refers to the number of hydrogen atoms attached to the molecule. The more saturated the fat, the harder it is at room temperature. Fats of animal origin, for example, butter and animal fat, are saturated and are solid at room temperature. Monounsaturated and polyunsaturated fats are liquid at room temperature. Research into coronary artery disease has shown that saturated fats tend to increase levels of blood cholesterol. Monounsaturated fats (olive and peanut oils) do not change blood cholesterol levels, and polyunsaturated fats (corn, safflower, sunflower, and many fish oils) tend to reduce those levels.

Functions of Cholesterol

The human body is efficient at manufacturing cholesterol. Most cells are capable of doing so, espe-

Patient Education

Let your patients know that several factors can influence their blood cholesterol levels:

- *Age and sex:* Cholesterol levels naturally increase as we age, and women experiencing menopause often will experience an increase in their LDL levels.
- *Heredity and family history:* High cholesterol often runs in families. Studies are still in process about the role genetics play in cholesterol levels.
- *Weight:* Gaining weight increases cholesterol levels in the blood, and losing weight helps to reduce cholesterol levels.
- *Exercise:* Regular physical exercise may reduce the LDL level, as well as increase the HDL levels.

cially the liver, the adrenal cortex, the testes, and the ovaries. All of the preceding cells, with the exception of the liver, use cholesterol to manufacture steroid hormones. In addition, cholesterol is an important component of bile and cellular membranes. Although the body is efficient at making cholesterol, it is not as easily degraded and may accumulate in the body and reach dangerous levels.

In addition to what the body produces, humans take in additional cholesterol through the ingestion of meat, eggs, and dairy products (Figure 32-10). The liver metabolizes cholesterol to its free form, which is then bound to lipoprotein and transported through the blood. Over time, excess cholesterol in the diet can result in a gradual increase of cholesterol concentration in the plasma. Increased concentrations of cholesterol in the plasma can increase to pathogenic levels. Some of the excess is stored in the liver, whereas some is deposited on the walls of blood vessels (atherosclerosis). Atherosclerosis of the coronary arteries is the most common cause of acute myocardial infarction (heart attack).

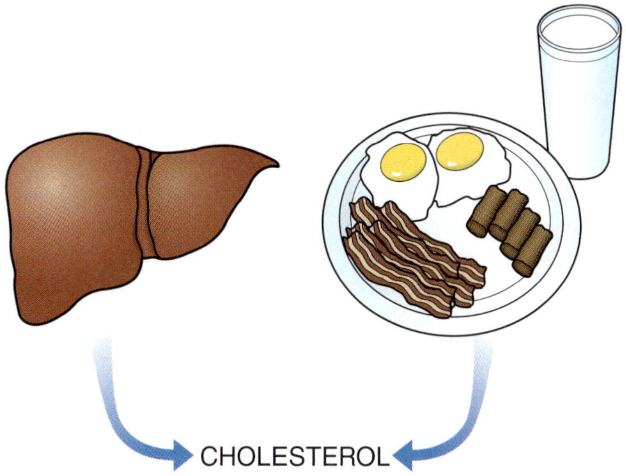

Figure 32-10 Cholesterol is created by the liver or obtained through animal sources of food such as meat, eggs, and dairy products.

Lipoproteins and Cholesterol Transport

Two kinds of lipoprotein are involved in the transport of cholesterol through the body: **high-density**

Patient Education

The Simple Scoop on Cholesterol

Cholesterol can be a confusing subject to try to explain to patients. Here is a very basic explanation that may help them:

Our bodies need cholesterol and we get it in two ways. We eat it and our liver manufactures it. Our liver manufactures plenty of cholesterol, so we do not need to eat it (except as babies and young children). There is only one source of cholesterol in our food: animal products (meat, eggs, and dairy). Vegetables, fruits, and grains naturally contain no cholesterol, although they may contain oils.

Our bodies have cholesterol transporters called high-density lipoproteins (HDLs) and low-density lipoproteins (LDLs).

HDLs (sometimes called "healthy lipoprotein") carry cholesterol to the liver where it can be released into the stool as bile. We want high levels of HDLs so we can get rid of excess cholesterol.

LDLs (sometimes referred to as the "lousy lipoprotein") carry cholesterol to our tissues and blood vessels where it is stored and can cause problems such as blocked arteries, fatty liver, and obesity. We want low levels of the LDLs so we can have less risk for heart disease and arterial disease.

Fats and oils can also be confusing. Saturated fats are solid at room temperature and come from animal fats and butter and from manufactured products such as hydrogenated fats. These are the worst fats. Unsaturated fats, which are liquid at room temperature, may be in two forms: monounsaturated fats (*mono* means "single") and polyunsaturated fats (*poly* means "many"). Monounsaturated fats such as olive and peanut oils do not affect blood cholesterol levels, whereas polyunsaturated fats such as corn, safflower, sunflower, and fish oils will actually reduce blood cholesterol levels.

Triglycerides are a type of lipid found in our blood that provides energy. If we have too much in our blood, it is also stored in our tissues as fat. The liver converts some of our foods (fatty acids and glycerol) into triglycerides.

lipoprotein (HDL) and **low-density lipoprotein (LDL).** Cholesterol bound to HDL is transported to the liver where it is excreted in the form of bile. HDL is sometimes referred to as good cholesterol. LDL cholesterol is deposited in the tissues as fat and inside the walls of blood vessels, and it is referred to as bad cholesterol. High levels of LDL are associated with an increased risk for coronary artery disease. Persons with coronary artery disease should have levels of less than 100 mg/dL LDL, whereas those without the disease should have levels of less than 160 mg/dL. Desirable values for HDL and LDL are shown in Table 32-4. Levels of HDL and LDL are influenced by many factors, both genetic and environmental. It is possible to increase HDL levels through a combination of weight loss, a diet low in saturated fats, exercise, and cessation of smoking.

Blood cholesterol may be reported as total cholesterol or as total cholesterol and the HDL and LDL fractions. Cholesterol screening is used to help identify patients who are at a high risk for heart disease.

Cholesterol testing is part of a lipid profile that also evaluates lipoproteins and triglycerides to help identify patients at a high risk for heart disease. Figure 32-9 shows tests performed for lipid profiles on the laboratory form.

Triglycerides

Triglycerides are a type of lipid found in the blood that serve as a source of energy. Fatty acids and glycerol from the diet are converted into triglycerides by the liver. When triglyceride levels in the blood are excessive, they are deposited in tissues as adipose tissue. Triglycerides are transported within the bloodstream by LDL and very low-density lipoproteins (VLDLs).

Many factors influence serum triglyceride levels. Serum triglyceride concentration will increase moderately after ingesting a meal containing fat, peaking 4 to 5 hours later. Increased concentrations of triglycerides are associated with an increased risk for coronary and vascular disease.

Table 32-4 Values for Cholesterol, HDL, LDL, and Triglycerides

	Total
Cholesterol (with no other risk factors such as hypertension and/or diabetes)	
Desirable	<200
Less desirable	200–239
At risk	>240
HDL (good cholesterol)	
Desirable	>60
At risk for women	<50
At risk for men	<40
LDL (bad cholesterol)	
Optimal	<100
Borderline risk	130–160
High risk	>190

All values are measured in milligrams per deciliter (mg/dL).

BLOOD CHEMISTRY TESTS

There are many natural chemicals in blood. The amounts of those chemicals are controlled by the efficiency of the body's organs and organ systems and certainly by environmental factors such as diet, smoking, drugs, and activity, as well as genetic composition.

The provider can order a general chemistry panel (BMP or CMP) or specific panels. A panel is a series of tests related to a body system, organ, or function. In interpreting a chemistry panel, the provider can determine pathology within the organ or malfunctions.

This chapter discusses each of the components briefly and explains some of the conditions and diseases that can cause these chemical tests to be abnormal. Keep in mind that all laboratory chemistry tests can vary slightly from laboratory to laboratory. Also remember that no one test, just like no one symptom, will make a diagnosis independent of other clues. The provider is considering laboratory tests together with the clinical picture, patient symptoms, and many other data in finalizing a diagnosis or diagnoses.

Alanine Aminotransferase (ALT)

ALT is an enzyme found in liver tissue. A high level indicates liver damage. A normal ALT level is less than 45 units/L.

Albumin

Most of the protein in plasma is albumin. It is responsible for transporting many small molecules (such as calcium, drugs, and bilirubin). It is synthesized in the liver; thus, low levels of albumin may indicate liver disease. It may also result from kidney disease, because the kidney is allowing too much albumin to spill into the urine. Low albumin may also be caused by malnutrition or a low-protein diet. A normal albumin level is 3.4 to 5.4 mg/dL.

Alkaline Phosphatase (ALP)

ALP is an enzyme. It is present in all our body tissues but mostly in the liver and bone. When levels are high in the blood, liver or bone disease must be suspected. A normal ALP level is 44 to 147 International Units/L.

Aspartate Aminotransferase (AST)

AST is found in the muscle cells (heart and skeletal muscles) and in the liver. High levels cannot indicate specifically liver disease, but it is considered together with other liver enzymes. It is also used to monitor patients who have had heart muscle damage (such as heart attacks), but it is not the best or only enzyme tested for that purpose. A normal AST level is 10 to 34 International Units/L.

Bilirubin, Total and Direct

Bilirubin is a yellow-orange substance that comes from the breakdown of hemoglobin. Hemoglobin is contained within the RBCs. Because individual RBCs live for only 120 days, they are constantly breaking down and being replaced. When the RBCs "die," the "heme" part of the hemoglobin circulates in the blood until the liver filters it out. The liver is responsible for changing the "heme" into a water-soluble substance called bilirubin. Before it reaches the liver, it is called "indirect" or "free" bilirubin. After it leaves the liver, it is called "direct" or "conjugated" bilirubin. The liver sends the conjugated bilirubin to the gall bladder where it is released with bile into the small intestine. When there is a blockage in the liver/gall bladder ducts or a disorder/disease of the liver, the bilirubin cannot get past the gall bladder to the small intestine, so it continues to circulate in the blood. This excess of bilirubin in the blood can lead to a yellow-orange coloring of the skin called jaundice. The body will try to get rid of extra bilirubin through the urine. Hence, any detection of bilirubin in the urine (bilirubinuria) can be indicative of a problem in the liver or gall bladder. When the bilirubin level increases, it causes the skin and whites of the eyes to become yellow. This change to yellow is called jaundice. Newborn babies can be jaundiced because their systems are not sophisticated enough to get rid of the bile. Because bilirubin breaks down in sunlight, babies with jaundice are treated with special "bili-lights" to help them break down the bilirubin in their skin. The total bilirubin test will indicate problems in the liver and the hepatic system. Notice the total bilirubin test is in the general panel and the direct bilirubin test is part of the hepatic panel. Some types of general blood problems can cause high levels of bilirubin because more blood cells are breaking down than usual. Normal bilirubin ranges are as follows:

Total bilirubin	0.1–0.2 mg/dL
Indirect bilirubin	0.1–0.7 mg/dL
Direct bilirubin	0.1–0.3 mg/dL
Newborn total bilirubin	1–12 mg/dL

Blood Urea Nitrogen Test

The **blood urea nitrogen (BUN)** test measures the concentration of urea in blood. The amount of urea in blood reflects the metabolic function of the liver and the excretory function of the kidneys. Most renal diseases result in inadequate excretion of urea from the body; therefore, increased concentrations of urea appear in the blood. BUN is one of several tests, including creatinine, that are used to screen for renal disease and is especially useful for evaluating glomerular function.

Excess protein in the diet is not stored in the body but is metabolized (catalyzed) for energy production. Urea is the nitrogenous end product of protein catabolism and is produced in the liver. It is deposited in the blood and carried to the kidneys for excretion. Surplus urea is measured as BUN. Normal values of urea vary but in adults range between 8 and 25 mg/dL; concentrations greater than 100 mg/dL indicate serious impairment of renal function. A slightly elevated BUN can indicate dehydration.

Calcium

All the cells in the human body need calcium for many functions. It is a critical element for bones, muscles, and the nervous system. Too much calcium can cause the muscles and nerves to become hyperactive, whereas too little calcium can cause the muscles and nerves not to function at all.

Muscle cramps (Charlie Horses) are often caused by low calcium. Calcium needs to be maintained within certain levels in the blood. If we eat more calcium than we need, the excess is stored in the bones. If our diets are low in calcium, the needed amount is pulled from the bones. The storage of excess calcium becomes less efficient as women lose estrogen, hence the need to take in adequate daily calcium to prevent osteoporosis as we age. A normal calcium level is 8.5 to 10.2 mg/dL.

Chloride

Chloride is an electrolyte. Its main function is to help with the electrical impulses of the cells. Chloride works closely with sodium. Changes in either sodium or chloride levels usually affect each other. A normal chloride level is 96 to 106 mEq/L.

Carbon Dioxide (CO_2)

Measuring CO_2 actually is measuring bicarbonate. This test is part of an arterial blood gas analysis. The kidneys are the main organs responsible for balancing CO_2. Anything that throws off the body's metabolic balance (excessive vomiting and diarrhea) can affect the CO_2 levels. The CO_2 levels in the blood are influenced by kidney and lung function. Normal CO_2 is 20 to 29 mEq/L.

Creatinine

Creatinine forms when muscle (creatine) breaks down. Logically, these levels will vary depending on the patient's size and muscularity. This test is used to determine kidney function, and is especially important for patients on diabetic or hypertension medications. A normal creatinine level is 0.8 to 1.4 mg/dL.

Gamma Glutamyltransferase (GGT)

The highest concentrations of GGT are in the liver and kidney. Abnormal levels usually indicate diseases of the liver, kidney, or bone. It is used in conjunction with other enzymes, especially ALP, to diagnose diseases. A normal GGT level is 0 to 51 International Units/L.

Lactate Dehydrogenase (LDH)

LDH is an enzyme found in many organs, especially the liver, heart, kidneys, brain, skeletal muscles, and lungs. Abnormal levels indicate tissue damage but are not specific by themselves. Like all enzymes, LDH is examined in conjunction with other tests. A normal LDH level is 105 to 133 International Units/L.

Phosphorus (Phosphate)

Phosphorus works closely with calcium, another electrolyte. It is used to assist in the proper assessment of calcium levels and to detect endocrine and kidney disorders. Phosphorus levels are related to uncontrolled diabetes and malnourished conditions. A normal phosphorus level is 2.4 to 4.1 mg/dL.

Potassium (K)

K is an electrolyte and is critical to muscle and nerve function and for the transportation of nutrients and cellular wastes across cellular membranes. Abnormal levels of K can cause heart muscle irregularities and, if severe, can lead to cardiac arrest. K is controlled by aldosterone, a hormone. Uncontrolled diabetes or excessive vomiting/diarrhea can cause abnormal K levels. Patients taking certain diuretics (such as Lasix) should be observed for low K. A normal K level is 3.7 to 5.2 mEq/L.

Sodium

Sodium is an electrolyte and works closely with chloride. Dietary intake of sodium is usually sufficient, and the kidney can excrete the excess. Sodium is closely related to fluid balance and retention. Normal sodium is 135 to 145 mEq/L.

Total Protein

Total protein is a measurement of protein in the blood serum and can reflect the nutritional state of the body, liver, kidneys, and many other conditions. If the total protein is abnormal, then further, more specific tests will need to be performed to find out exactly the source of the problem. Of course, if the total protein is abnormal, other tests might show some abnormal levels, too. A normal total protein level is 6.0 to 8.3 mg/dL.

Uric Acid

Uric acid is created when purine is metabolized. It is usually secreted by the kidneys, but too much can build up as crystals in the body and seem to settle in the largest dependent joint, the great toe. This is known as gout. A normal uric acid level is 3.0 to 7.0 mg/dL.

Procedure 32-1

Pregnancy Test

STANDARD PRECAUTIONS:

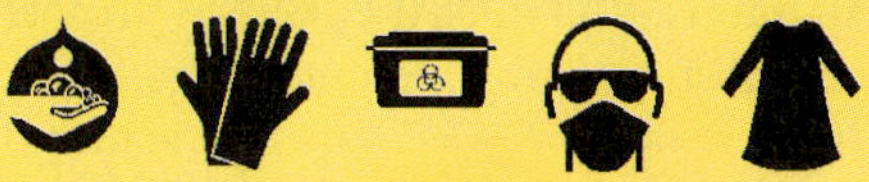

PURPOSE:

To perform the enzyme immunoassay or agglutination inhibition test to detect hCG in urine to determine positive or negative pregnancy results.

EQUIPMENT/SUPPLIES:

Gloves
Urine specimen
Stopwatch
Disinfectant (10% chlorine bleach solution)
Biohazard container
hCG negative and positive urine control
Pregnancy test kit

PROCEDURE STEPS:

1. Wash hands and put on gloves. RATIONALE: While working with body fluids, such as urine, gloves should be worn as personal protection.
2. Assemble all equipment and supplies. RATIONALE: Organizing all equipment and supplies before running the test will eliminate errors caused by missing supplies.
3. Perform the test following the manufacturer's instructions. The following steps are intentionally general so a variety of kits can be used. RATIONALE: The manufacturer's instructions will differ from kit to kit. It is important, as a quality-assurance measure, for the instructions to be read and understood thoroughly. Any questions must be directed to the manufacturer.
   a. Determine materials are at room temperature.
   b. Apply urine to the test unit using dispenser provided (Figure 32-11A).
   c. Wait appropriate time interval (use stopwatch to time test).
   d. Apply first reagent/antibody to test unit using dispenser provided.
   e. Observe color development after appropriate time interval.
   f. Stop reaction.
   g. Consult manufacturer's package insert to interpret test results (Figure 32-11B).
4. Record the results of the test on a laboratory report form following laboratory policy. RATIONALE: Interpretation of results may differ from kit to kit according to the manufacturer's design, and even though laboratory processes are the same, policies and forms will differ from laboratory to laboratory.

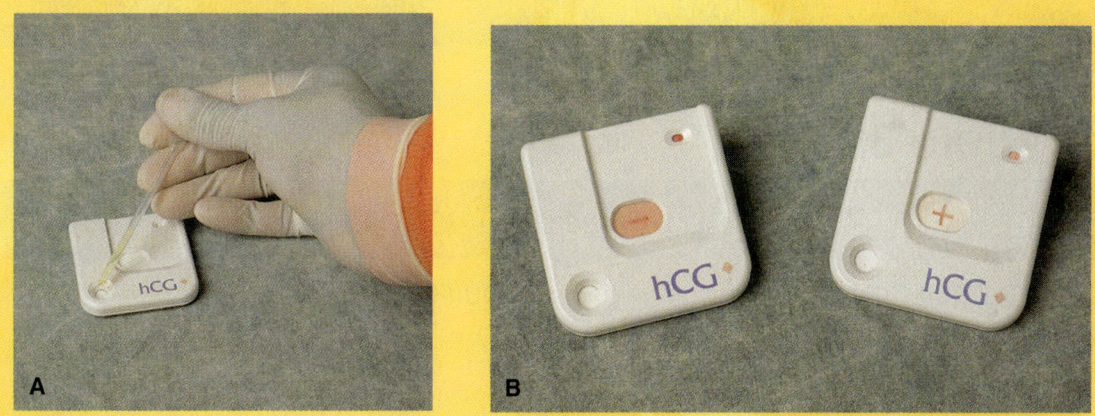

Figure 32-11 (A) Urine is place in the test unit according to the manufacturer's instructions. (B) The package instructions specify how the test is to be interpreted. A common interpretation is with a negative sign (left) and a positive sign (right).

continues

Procedure 32-1 (continued)

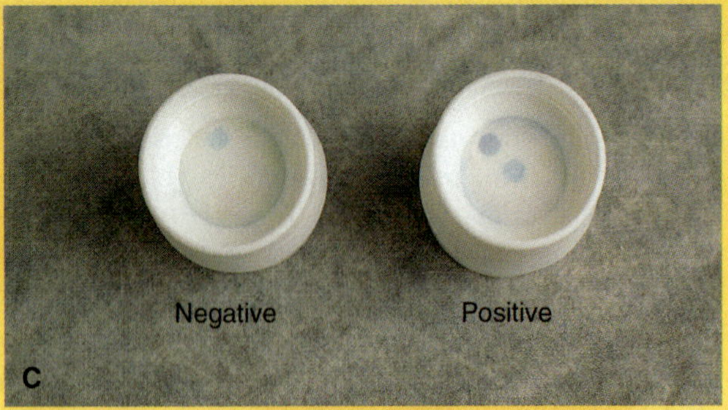

Figure 32-11 (C) Control tests must be performed according to the manufacturer's instructions. The results of the positive and negative controls test are shown.

5. Repeat steps with both positive and negative urine controls (Figure 32-11C). RATIONALE: Controls are performed to ensure the quality of the reagents and testing supplies. If a positive control test does not show a positive result, then something is wrong with the reagent or the testing supplies. If the control test is not accurate, the patient's test will not be accurate either.
6. Disinfect reusable equipment. Discard disposable supplies into biohazard container. Dispose of specimen per laboratory policy. Clean work area with disinfectant. RATIONALE: Follow Standard Precautions and laboratory policies for disposal of biohazard substances and disinfection of supplies/equipment.
7. Remove gloves and discard into biohazard container. Wash hands. RATIONALE: Gloves protect hands from most but not all microorganisms. Hands should always be washed after removal of gloves to ensure complete protection and to remove glove powders and latex residue.
8. Document procedure in patient's chart in the progress notes. Complete a lab report. After the provider has initialed the report, it should be filed in the lab section of the patient's chart.. RATIONALE: Documentation should refer the reader to the test result in the laboratory section of patient's chart.

DOCUMENTATION

08/06/20XX Urine HCG test performed for pregnancy determination. Specimen tested in our lab. Results filed in lab section. Patient tolerated the procedure well and Dr. Rice discussed results with her. Audrey Jones, CMA (AAMA)———

Laboratory Report

Patient Name Lynn Engle *Date* 08-06-20XX

Urine Pregnancy Test negative

Audrey Jones, CMA (AAMA)

MA signature

Procedure 32-2

Performing Infectious Mononucleosis Test

STANDARD PRECAUTIONS:

PURPOSE:

To perform an accurate test of serum or plasma to detect the presence or absence of antibodies of infectious mononucleosis (IM).

EQUIPMENT/SUPPLIES:

Gloves
Serum or plasma specimen
Stopwatch or lab timer
Surface disinfectant (10% chlorine bleach solution)
Test kit for IM
Biohazard container

continues

Procedure 32-2 (continued)

PROCEDURE STEPS:

NOTE: These instructions are intentionally general so a variety of test kits may be used. The manufacturer's instructions will differ from kit to kit. It is important, as a quality-assurance measure, for the instructions to be thoroughly read and understood before performing the test. Any instructions not clearly understood should be clarified with the manufacturer.

1. Wash hands and put on gloves. RATIONALE: While working with body fluids, such as urine, gloves should be worn as personal protection.
2. Assemble all equipment and supplies. RATIONALE: Organizing all equipment and supplies before running the test will eliminate errors caused by missing supplies.
3. Perform the test according to the manufacturer's instructions exactly. RATIONALE: The manufacturer's instructions will vary with each specific kit. Quality results are assured only when instructions are followed precisely.
4. Record the results on a laboratory report form following laboratory policy. RATIONALE: Even though laboratory processes are the same, policies and forms will differ from laboratory to laboratory.
5. Repeat the test procedure using positive and negative controls. RATIONALE: Controls are performed to ensure the quality of the reagents and testing supplies. If a positive control test does not show a positive result, then something is wrong with the reagent or the testing supplies. If the control test is not accurate, the patient's test will not be accurate either.
6. Discard contaminated materials into biohazard container. Dispose of specimen appropriately and disinfect reusable materials. Clean work area with disinfectant. RATIONALE: Follow Standard Precautions and laboratory policies for disposal of biohazard substances and disinfection of supplies/equipment.
7. Remove gloves and discard into biohazard container. Wash hands. RATIONALE: Gloves protect hands from most but not all microorganisms. Hands should always be washed after removal of gloves to ensure complete protection and to remove glove powders and latex residue.
8. Document results in the progress notes. Complete a lab report. After the provider has initialed the report, it should be filed in the lab section of patient's chart. RATIONALE: Documentation should refer the reader to the test result in the laboratory section of patient's chart .

DOCUMENTATION

4/27/20XX 2:54 PM Mononucleosis test performed. Results forwarded to provider and initialed. Form filed in laboratory section of medical record. Joe Guerrero, CMA (AAMA) ———

DOCUMENTATION

08/06/20XX Venipuncture performed for infectious mononucleosis test. Specimen tested in our lab. Results in lab report filed. Patient tolerated the procedure well and Dr. Rice discussed results with her. Audrey Jones, CMA (AAMA) ———

Laboratory Report

Patient Name <u>*Carolyn Siderland*</u> *Date* <u>*08-06-20XX*</u>

Infectious Mononucleosesis Test <u>*negative*</u>

<u>*Audrey Jones, CMA (AAMA)*</u>
MA signature

Procedure 32-3

Obtaining Blood Specimen for Phenylketonuria (PKU) Test

STANDARD PRECAUTIONS:

PURPOSE:

To obtain a blood specimen using a PKU test card or "filter paper" to determine phenylalanine levels in newborns who are at least 3 days old.

continues

Procedure 32-3 (continued)

EQUIPMENT/SUPPLIES:

Gloves
PKU filter paper test card and mailing envelope
Alcohol swabs
Cotton balls/gauze pad
Sterile pediatric-sized lancet
Biohazard waste container

PROCEDURE STEPS:

1. Wash hands and put on gloves. RATIONALE: While working with body fluids, gloves should be worn as personal protection.
2. Identify the infant. Explain the purpose of the test and the procedure to the parents. Discuss the current health of the infant before beginning the procedure. RATIONALE: Certain antibiotics, medications, or vomiting problems may cause false results.
3. Select and clean an appropriate puncture site (Figure 32-12A). Allow the alcohol to dry before the puncture. RATIONALE: Cleaning the site before puncture will remove any powders, oils, lotions, and contaminates. Allowing the alcohol to dry prevents the stick from stinging.
4. Grasp the infant's foot, taking care not to touch the cleansed area. Make a puncture approximately 2 to 3 mm deep in the infant's heel, making sure the infant's lateral, or side, portion of the heel pad is used. A pediatric-sized lancet, which limits the depth of puncture, should be used (Figure 32-12B). If possible, recent puncture sites should always be avoided (see Procedure 28-5, Capillary Puncture).
5. Wipe away the first drop of blood with a gauze pad. RATIONALE: The first drop is diluted with alcohol and should not be collected for the test. Using a gauze pad rather than a cotton ball is preferred because the cotton ball may leave tiny fibers on the puncture site. The fibers may encourage clotting, which will interfere with obtaining sufficient specimen for the test.
6. To collect blood for the test, press the back side of the filter paper test card against the infant's

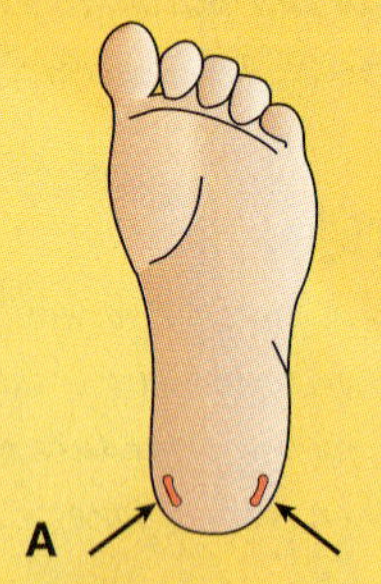

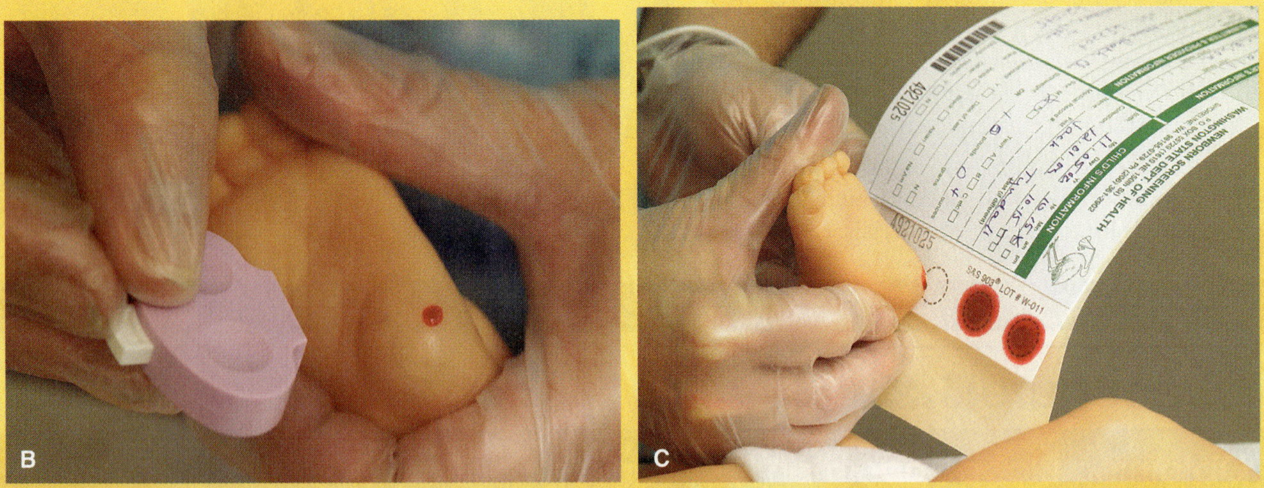

Figure 32-12 (A) Capillary blood collections sites on an infant's heel. (B) The infant's foot should be held securely with the nondominant hand while the dominant hand uses the pediatric lancet to perform the capillary heelstick. (C) Drops of blood are transferred from the capillary heelstick puncture site to the PKU filter card, completely filling all the circles.

continues

Procedure 32-3 (continued)

heel while exerting gentle pressure on the heel (Figure 32-12C). The drop of blood should be large enough to completely fill and soak through the circle. *Do not* layer the multiple blood drops within a single circle. Completely fill all of the circles on the test card. RATIONALE: Failure to do so will require a retest.

7. Hold a cotton ball over the puncture and apply gentle pressure until the bleeding stops. Do not apply a bandage. RATIONALE: The bleeding should be stopped before the patient is released from your care. Bandages are discouraged because they can be a choking hazard for infants and toddlers.
8. Properly dispose of all waste in biohazard container. RATIONALE: Follow Standard Precautions and laboratory policies for disposal of biohazard substances and disinfection of supplies/equipment.
9. Remove the gloves and wash hands. RATIONALE: Gloves protect hands from most but not all microorganisms. Hands should always be washed after removal of gloves to ensure complete protection and to remove glove powders and latex residue.
10. Allow the PKU test card to completely dry on a nonabsorbent surface at room temperature. This will take about 2 hours. If collecting more than one card, *do not* lay one card on another when drying. RATIONALE: This could cause cross contamination of blood between the cards.
11. After the test card is dry, complete the PKU test card with all patient and provider information. RATIONALE: Allowing the blood to dry thoroughly before further handling lessens the chances of contaminating other parts of the form.
12. Place the test card in the mailer envelope and send it to the laboratory within 2 days. RATIONALE: It is important that the completed card be mailed as soon as possible to eliminate the breakdown of the contents within the specimen and to obtain the results as soon as possible to begin treatment if necessary.
13. Document the procedure in patient's chart. When test results are returned, they should be initialed by the provider and be placed in the lab section of patient's chart. RATIONALE: Documentation should refer the reader to the test result in the laboratory section of patient's chart.

DOCUMENTATION

6/27/20XX 10:54 AM Capillary puncture performed on lateral aspect of left heel for PKU testing. Patient is 12 days old, currently taking no medication, and is not ill. Patient tolerated the procedure well and adequate specimen was obtained. PKU card completed and mailed. Audrey Jones, CMA (AAMA)

7/10/20XX PKU test results received and initialed by Dr. King and filed in the laboratory section of the patient's medical record. The patient's parents were notified of the negative results per Dr. King's instructions. Audrey Jones, CMA (AAMA)

Procedure 32-4

Screening Test for PKU

STANDARD PRECAUTIONS:

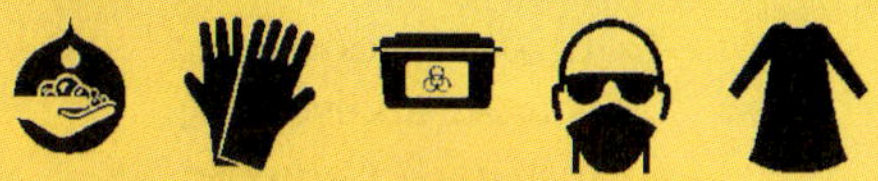

PURPOSE:

Test a urine specimen using the diaper test or the Phenistik test to determine phenylalanine levels in newborns who are at least 6 weeks old. This is a quick screening test only.

EQUIPMENT/SUPPLIES:

Gloves
10% ferric chloride for the diaper test
or
Phenistik for the Phenistik Method Test
Biohazard waste container

continues

Procedure 32-4 (continued)

PROCEDURE STEPS:

1. Assemble and organize equipment and supplies. RATIONALE: Being organized helps the process go more smoothly and professionally.
2. Identify the infant. Verify that the infant is at least 6 weeks of age. Explain the purpose of the test and the procedure to the parents. RATIONALE: Explaining the procedure helps the parents understand and the process usually goes more smoothly.
3. Wash hands and apply gloves. RATIONALE: Because biohazard body fluids will be tested, personal protective equipment is required for safety.
4. Follow one of the two following procedures after removing the diaper away from the infant. RATIONALE: Always follow manufacturer's instructions for assuring test accuracy. The diaper is remove away from the infant to ensure that no chemical comes in contact with the infant.
   a. *Diaper test:* Apply several drops of 10% ferric chloride to a diaper that contains fresh urine. Development of a green color indicates a positive test.
   b. *Phenistik test:* Dip the Phenistik test strip into fresh urine or press it against a diaper containing fresh urine. Development of a green color indicates a positive test.
5. A positive urine test should be followed up with a blood test. RATIONALE: This is a screening test only and should be followed up with the more accurate blood test.
6. Properly dispose of all waste in a biohazard waste container. RATIONALE: Follow Standard Precautions and laboratory policies for disposal of biohazard substances and disinfection of supplies/equipment.
7. Remove gloves and wash hands. RATIONALE: Gloves protect hands from most but not all microorganisms. Hands should always be washed after removal of glove to ensure complete protection and to remove glove powders and latex residue.
8. Document the procedure in the progress notes. Complete a lab report. After the provider has initialed the report, it should be filed in the lab section of patient's chart. RATIONALE: The documentation should refer the reader to the laboratory section of patient's chart.

DOCUMENTATION

08/06/20XX Phenistik test performed in urine for PKU screening. Specimen tested in our lab. Results filed in lab section. Dr. Rice discussed results with the patient's parents. Audrey Jones, CMA (AAMA)

Laboratory Report

Patient Name *Pedro Gonzalas* *Date* *08-06-20XX*

Screening PKU (Urine) *negative*

Audrey Jones, CMA (AAMA)
MA signature

Procedure 32-5

Measurement of Blood Glucose Using an Automated Analyzer

STANDARD PRECAUTIONS:

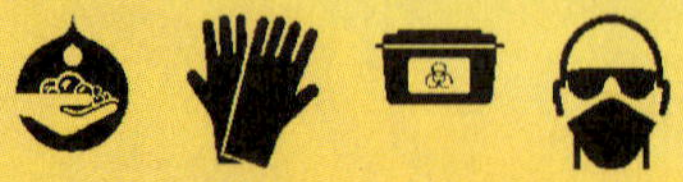

PURPOSE:

To measure blood glucose.

EQUIPMENT/SUPPLIES:

Gloves
Goggles
Safety lancet
Alcohol swabs
Glucose analyzer
Adhesive strip
Gauze
Control solutions for glucose analyzer
Test strips for glucose analyzer
Laboratory tissue
Cotton balls

continues

Procedure 32-5 (continued)

PROCEDURE STEPS:

1. Review the manufacturer's manual for the specific glucose analyzer being used. Turn on the analyzer. RATIONALE: Always read and follow the manufacturer's instructions exactly for your particular analyzer to ensure accurate results.
2. Clean the work area and assemble all materials and supplies. RATIONALE: Organizing all equipment and supplies before running the test will eliminate errors caused by missing supplies.
3. Wash hands. Put on gloves and goggles. RATIONALE: Washing your hands ensures that your skin is clean before gloving and decreases contaminants. Applying personal protection equipment when working with body fluids will lessen the chances of exposure to dangerous biohazard substances.
4. Record the control ranges, control lot number, and test strip lot number. RATIONALE: Recording the lot numbers and control ranges is another type of quality-assurance measure and is required by CLIA for many automated tests.
5. Perform the check test and the control test according to the manufacturer's instructions. If both tests are within range, proceed to the glucose test. Repeat both tests if either is out of acceptable range. RATIONALE: Controls are performed to ensure the quality of the reagents and testing supplies. If a positive control test does not show a positive result, then something is wrong with the reagent or the testing supplies. If the control test is not accurate, the patient's test will not be accurate either.

To perform the glucose test:

1. Remove a test strip from the bottle and replace the lid. RATIONALE: Replacing the lid securely ensures that the reagents are protected from light and moisture.
2. Insert the test strip into the test chamber. RATIONALE: Follow the manufacturer's instructions for proper use of test kits.
3. Perform a capillary puncture (see Procedure 28-5). Wipe first drop with gauze. RATIONALE: Wiping the first drop away lessens the amount of tissue fluid in the specimen.
4. Apply a large drop of blood to the test strip. RATIONALE: The test requires a large drop of blood for accurate results. Let a large drop form before applying it to the test device.
5. While the test is running, check the puncture site. If the bleeding has stopped, apply an adhesive strip. RATIONALE: The test will take time to compute, allowing you time to treat the patient.
6. After the appropriate time interval has passed, read the glucose concentration. RATIONALE: The test requires an appropriate amount of time for accurate results.
7. Properly dispose of all waste in a biohazard waste container. RATIONALE: Follow Standard Precautions and laboratory policies for disposal of biohazard substances and disinfection of supplies/equipment.
8. Remove gloves and wash hands. RATIONALE: Gloves protect hands from most but not all microorganisms. Hands should always be washed after removal of gloves to ensure complete protection and to remove glove powders and latex residue.
9. Document the procedure in the progress notes. Complete a lab report. After the provider has initialed the report, it should be filed in the lab section of patient's chart. RATIONALE: The documentation should refer the reader to the laboratory section of patient's chart.

DOCUMENTATION

08/06/20XX Fingerstick performed for blood glucose. Specimen tested in our lab. Results filed in lab section. Patient tolerated the procedure well and Dr. Rice discussed results with her. Audrey Jones, CMA (AAMA) ____________________

Laboratory Report

Patient Name _Veronica Hernandez_ *Date* _08-06-20XX_

Blood Glucose ___108___ *mg/dL*

Audrey Jones, CMA (AAMA)
MA signature

Procedure 32-6

Cholesterol Testing

STANDARD PRECAUTIONS:

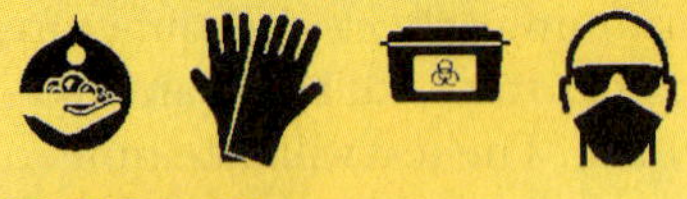

PURPOSE:

To measure cholesterol and triglyceride for monitoring purposes. For cholesterol, HDL, LDL, or triglyceride monitoring. *NOTE:* The following steps are intentionally general so a variety of kits can be used. The manufacturer's instructions will differ from kit to kit. It is important, as a quality-assurance measure, for the instructions to be read and understood thoroughly. Any questions must be directed to the manufacturer.

EQUIPMENT/SUPPLIES:

Gloves
Blood collecting equipment
Pipettes with disposable tips
Chlorine bleach
Commercial kit for manual determination of cholesterol
Controls and standards
Marking pen
Biohazard container

PROCEDURE STEPS:

1. Assemble all necessary equipment and materials. RATIONALE: Organizing all equipment and supplies before running the test will eliminate errors caused by missing supplies and will show the patient a more professional process.
2. Wash hands; apply gloves. RATIONALE: Washing your hands ensures that your skin is clean before gloving and decreases contaminants. Applying personal protection equipment when working with body fluids will lessen the chances of exposure to dangerous biohazard substances.
3. Obtain a blood sample from the patient, either by fingerstick or venipuncture, depending on the manufacturer's instructions (see Chapter 28). RATIONALE: Always read and follow the manufacturer's instructions to ensure accurate results.
4. Follow the manufacturer's instructions to perform the cholesterol test. Be sure to run the controls also. RATIONALE: Following all manufacturer's instructions will assure accurate test results. Controls are performed to ensure the quality of the reagents and testing supplies. If the control test is not accurate, the patient's test will not be accurate either.
5. Properly dispose of all waste in biohazard container. RATIONALE: Follow Standard Precautions when disposing of sharps and biohazard and contaminated waste.
6. Record the results of the test on a laboratory report form and document the procedure in the patient's chart. After the provider has initialed the report, file it in the patient's chart. RATIONALE: The chart note should refer the reader to the laboratory section of the patient's chart.

DOCUMENTATION

08/06/20XX Fingerstick performed for serum cholesterol. Specimen tested in our lab. Initialed results filed in the lab section of the chart. Dr. Rice discussed the results with the patient. Audrey Jones, CMA (AAMA) ——————

Laboratory Report

Patient Name *Jennifer Yu* *Date* *08-06-20XX*

Serum Cholesterol *150* *mg/dL*

Audrey Jones, CMA (AAMA)
MA signature

Case Study 32-1

Refer to the scenario at the beginning of the chapter.

Audrey takes pride in paying attention to every detail when performing lab tests. She is also committed to explaining processes to her patients and increasing their comfort level.

CASE STUDY REVIEW

1. What are some key points to adhere to when performing testing using a CLIA waived test kit to ensure accuracy?
2. What are some specific ways you can reassure a patient to have confidence in your ability?

Case Study 32-2

Anna Preciado, CMA (AAMA), a clinical medical assistant with Drs. Lewis and King, has performed many venipunctures during her training at college, throughout her practicum, and since her employment with Drs. Lewis and King. She has not, however, performed a heelstick capillary draw since she was in college and even then she practiced on a doll. Until now another medical assistant in the clinic was doing all the heelstick capillary draws for PKU testing, but Anna is ready to start performing them herself. She is concerned and understandably nervous about performing this procedure on an infant.

CASE STUDY REVIEW

1. What course of action should Anna take to prepare herself for performing a procedure that she has not done in several years?
2. Once Anna feels she is technically ready to perform the PKU blood test, what should she do to ensure that the procedure goes well?

SUMMARY

CLIA has identified many rapid test kits and automated methods for use in the ambulatory care setting in the waived category. For all of the tests discussed in this chapter, it is important for the medical assistant to have a basic understanding of the principles involved and the proper sampling procedures required. Safety procedures and Standard Precautions must be observed at all times and include the proper disposal of infectious materials and reagents. Gloves and goggles are always used when obtaining samples and while performing the actual test. Careful documentation by the medical assistant will help the provider in the diagnosis of the patient.

STUDY FOR SUCCESS

To reinforce your knowledge and skills of information presented in this chapter:

- Review the Key Terms
- Practice the Procedures
- Consider the Case Studies and discuss your conclusions
- Answer the Review Questions
  - Multiple Choice
  - Critical Thinking
- Navigate the Internet by completing the Web Activities
- Practice the StudyWARE activities on the CD
- Apply your knowledge in the Student Workbook activities
- Complete the Web Tutor sections
- View and discuss the DVD situations

REVIEW QUESTIONS

Multiple Choice

1. In addition to pregnancy, a positive hCG test can be found in the following pathologic conditions *except:*
   a. ectopic pregnancy
   b. hydatidiform mole of the uterus
   c. pelvic inflammatory disease
   d. cancer of the lung
2. If a urine sample for a pregnancy test cannot be tested immediately, it may be stored in the following way for 24 hours:
   a. room temperature, 25°C
   b. body temperature, 37°C
   c. frozen
   d. refrigerated at 4°C
3. The kissing disease is synonymous with the disease:
   a. tuberculosis
   b. infectious mononucleosis
   c. hemolytic anemia
   d. hypoglycemia
4. Serum or blood would be the specimen for all but the following test:
   a. ABO typing
   b. testing for EBV
   c. cholesterol
   d. hCG hormone
   e. all of the above
5. Which of the following statements is incorrect regarding blood type:
   a. Type A RBCs have A antigens on the cell.
   b. Type B RBCs have B antigens on the cell.
   c. Type O RBCs have A and B antigens on the cell.
   d. Type AB RBCs have both A and B antigens on the cell.
6. Which of the following is a *true* statement about the Rh factor?
   a. Rh factor is a rare blood type.
   b. Rh factor is present on all RBCs.
   c. Rh factor was discovered by experiments on rhesus monkeys.
   d. People without the Rh factor on their RBCs have naturally occurring antibodies called anti-D in their plasma.
7. When instructing a patient in the correct collection of a specimen for semen analysis, all of the following should be considered *except:*
   a. avoid the consumption of alcohol several days before the test
   b. collection of semen into a condom is unacceptable
   c. specimen should be transported to the laboratory at 37°C within 30 minutes of collection
   d. avoid the consumption of fats several days before the test
8. Testing for PKU is done on:
   a. newborns
   b. children 1 to 3 years of age
   c. teenagers
   d. adults older than 40 years
9. The best site location for a tuberculin Mantoux test is:
   a. back of the hand
   b. forearm 3 to 4 inches from bend of arm
   c. ½ inch above the back of the knee
   d. upper part of the arm in the deltoid muscle

10. A patient with hypoglycemia would have a blood glucose level of:
    a. 50–70 mg/dL
    b. 70–110 mg/dL
    c. 110–150 mg/dL
    d. 150–200 mg/dL

Critical Thinking

1. Why is the first-voided morning urine the preferred specimen for a pregnancy test?
2. Why is it necessary to repeat the seminal sperm count analysis three times over a 2-month period?
3. What factors may alter the results of a blood glucose measurement?
4. How can you distinguish between the diabetic and nondiabetic patient based on the results of the 2-hour postprandial glucose evaluation?
5. Discuss the relation between saturated fats and coronary artery disease.
6. What is the function of triglycerides in the body?
7. What instructions should the patient be given in preparation for a triglyceride evaluation?
8. What is the source of urea in the blood?

WEB ACTIVITIES

1. Search the CDC's and other government Web sites for information on infectious diseases such as mononucleosis.
2. Use search engines to research some of the conditions discussed in this chapter, such as PKU and TB.

REFERENCES/BIBLIOGRAPHY

Department of Health and Human Services, Centers for Disease Control and Prevention. (2008). *Epstein-Barr virus and infectious mononucleosis.* Retrieved November 2008, from http://www.cdc.gov.

U.S. Food and Drug Administration. (2007). *Databases on the FDA Website.* Retrieved October 2008, from http://www.fda.gov/search/databases.html.

Walters, N. J., Estridge, B. H., & Reynold, A. P. (2008). *Basic medical laboratory techniques* (5th ed.). Clifton Park, NY: Delmar Cengage Learning.

THE DVD HOOK-UP

This chapter discusses specialty tests that may be performed in the medical office.

1. This program illustrated the technique for performing a blood glucose test. The medical assistant ran a control before performing the test. Why is it important to run a control before performing the test?
2. What should you do if a patient asks you for his or her laboratory results before the doctor has had a chance to review them?

DVD Journal Summary

Write a paragraph that summarizes what you learned from watching the selected scenes from today's DVD programs. When viewing the scene from program 12, you saw a medical assistant give a testimonial about giving out a test result without checking with the provider first. The patient was traumatized and the provider was furious with the medical assistant for giving out the test results without checking with him first. Why is it best for the provider to communicate test results to the patient? Is it ever acceptable for the medical assistant to communicate test results to a patient?

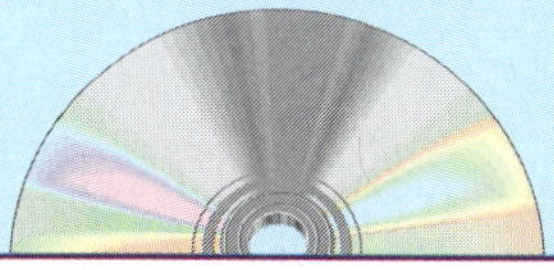

DVD Series Skills Based Series
Program Number 11, 12

Chapter/Scene Reference
- *Performing Blood Sugar Test*
- *Performing Mononucleosis Test*
- *Performing Pregnancy Test*

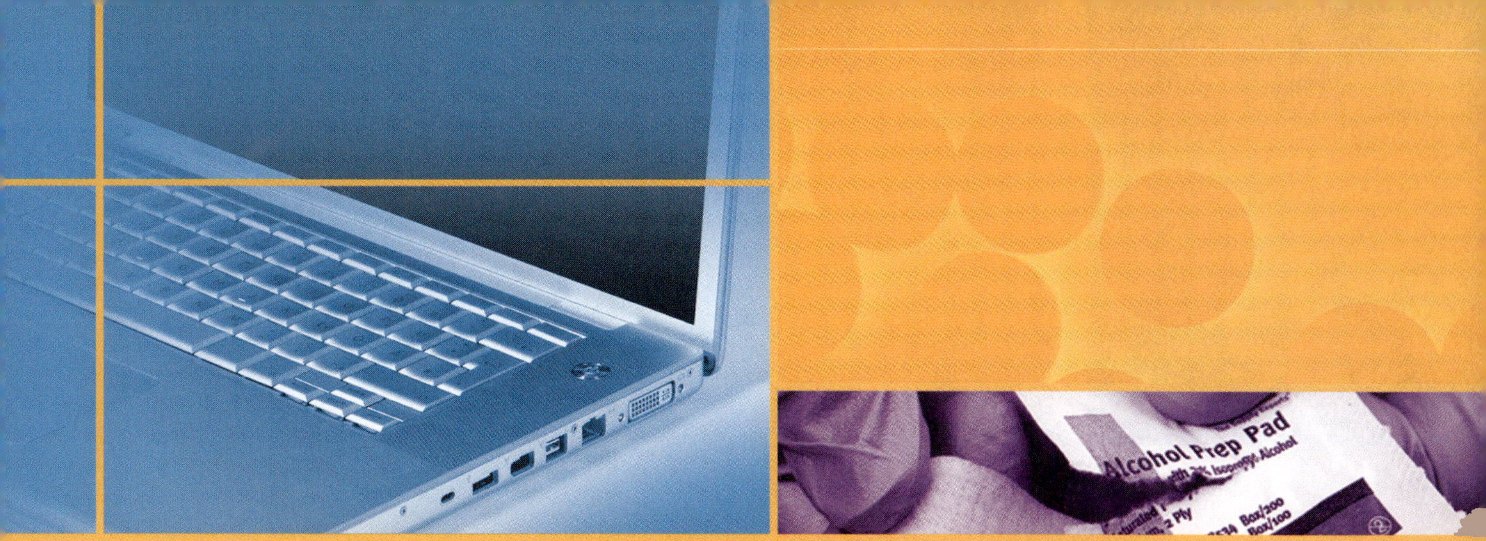

SECTION III Professional Procedures

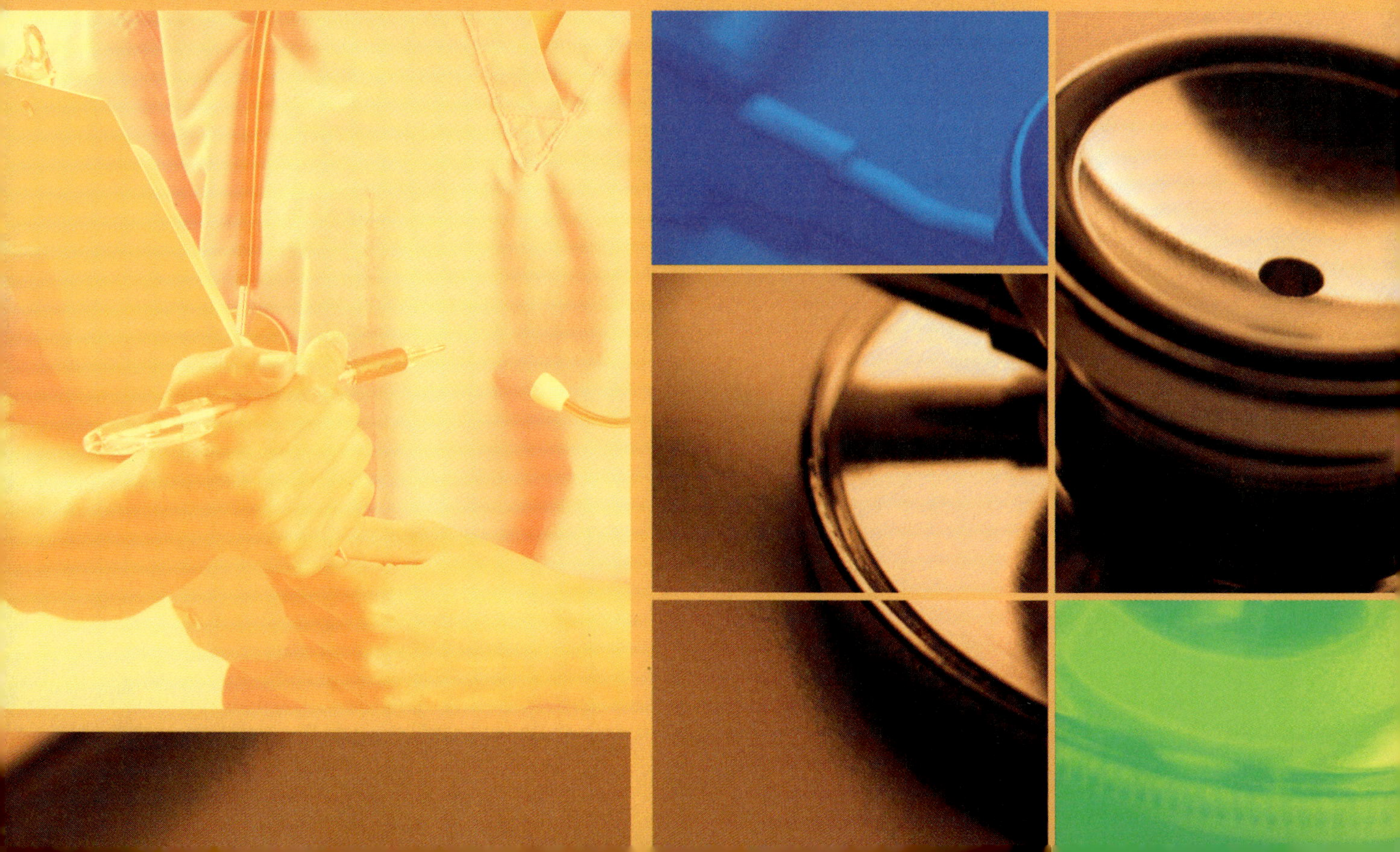

UNIT 8

Office and Human Resources Management

Chapter 33

The Medical Assistant as Office Manager

KEY TERMS

Agenda
Ancillary Services
Authoritarian Manager
Benchmark
Benefit
Bond
Brainstorming
Conflict Resolution
Embezzle
Fringe Benefit
"Going Bare"
Itinerary
Liability
Malpractice
Management by Walking Around (MBWA)
Marketing
Mentor
Minutes
Negligence
Participatory Manager
Practicum
Procedure Manual
Professional Liability Insurance
Profit Sharing
Risk Management
Salary Review
Self-actualization
Shadow
Subordinate
Teamwork
Work Statement

OUTLINE

- The Medical Assistant as Office Manager
- Qualities of a Manager
  - Office Manager Attitude
  - Professionalism
- Management Styles
  - Authoritarian Style
  - Participatory Style
  - Management by Walking Around
- Risk Management
- Importance of Teamwork
  - Getting the Team Started
  - Using a Team to Solve a Problem
  - Planning and Implementing a Solution
  - Recognition
- Supervising Personnel
  - Staff and Team Meetings
  - Conflict Resolution
- Harassment in the Workplace
  - Assimilating New Personnel
  - Employees with Chemical Dependencies or Emotional Problems
  - Evaluating Employees and Planning Salary Review
  - Dismissing Employees
- Procedure Manual
  - Organization of the Procedure Manual
  - Updating and Reviewing the Procedure Manual
- HIPAA Implications
- Travel Arrangements
  - Itinerary
- Time Management
- Marketing Functions
  - Seminars
  - Brochures
  - Newsletters
  - Press Releases
  - Special Events
- Records and Financial Management
  - Electronic Health Records and the Office Manager
  - Payroll Processing
- Facility and Equipment Management
  - Administrative and Clinical Inventory of Supplies and Equipment
  - Administrative and Clinical Equipment Calibration and Maintenance
- Liability Coverage and Bonding
- Legal Issues

OBJECTIVES

The student should strive to meet the following performance objectives and demonstrate an understanding of the facts and principles presented in this chapter through written and oral communication.

1. Define the key terms as presented in the glossary.
2. Describe the qualities of a manager.

OBJECTIVES (continued)

3. Discuss characteristics of managers and leaders.
4. Differentiate between authoritarian and participatory management styles.
5. Describe management by walking around and its usefulness in ambulatory care settings.
6. Recall a minimum of four common risks and risk-control measures.
7. List three benefits of a teamwork approach.
8. Discuss the importance of a meeting agenda.
9. Describe appropriate evaluation tools for employees.
10. Recall effective methods of resolving conflict.
11. Identify the steps required to make travel arrangements.
12. Define the term itinerary and list important information the itinerary should contain.
13. List three methods of increasing productivity and efficient time management.
14. Describe the purpose of a procedure manual.
15. Discuss the impact of HIPAA's privacy policy in ambulatory care settings.
16. Describe the general concept of marketing and recall at least three marketing tools.
17. Describe the purpose and benefit of marketing.
18. Discuss the steps involved in the inventory of administrative and clinical supplies and equipment.
19. Discuss the steps involved in administrative and clinical equipment calibration and maintenance.

Scenario

Marilyn Johnson has been employed by Drs. Lewis and King's office for the past 8 years. Three years ago, she was promoted to the position of office manager when the facility added the second office for its associates in a nearby suburb. Marilyn has a baccalaureate degree in business administration. Her responsibilities at Drs. Lewis and King's office include various duties involving personnel, finances, and office efficiency.

INTRODUCTION

The drive to improve the productivity of the medical office, precipitated by managed care, Medicare, and insurance limits placed on fees, have broadened the scope of employment options and job marketability for medical assistants. This has created an opportunity for medical assistants to advance to the position of office manager.

In small offices, the position of office manager may include the duties of the human resources (HR) representative; in larger clinics, these positions will be inde-

Spotlight on Certification

RMA Content Outline

- Medical law
- Medical ethics
- Human relations

CMA (AAMA) Content Outline

- Basic principles (psychology)
- Working as a team member to achieve goals
- Evaluating and understanding communication
- Medicolegal guidelines & requirements
- Computer applications
- Records management
- Resource information and community services
- Managing physician's professional schedule and travel
- Managing the office
- Office policies and procedures
- Manage practice finances
- Employee payroll

CMAS Content Outline

- Legal and ethical considerations
- Professionalism
- Patient information and community resources
- Medical records management
- Medical office financial management
- Medical office management

pendent. This book treats them as separate positions (see Chapter 34). In the larger facilities, the office manager and HR representative must coordinate their personnel-related functions into a seamless organization.

THE MEDICAL ASSISTANT AS OFFICE MANAGER

The manager of a medical office or ambulatory care facility can have vast and diverse responsibilities. This chapter covers the following office manager duties:

1. Make travel arrangements and prepare an itinerary
2. Arrange and maintain practice insurance and develop risk management strategies
3. Supervise office personnel
4. Approve financial transactions and account disposition; generate financial reports as needed
5. Supervise the purchase and storage of office supplies
6. Prepare staff meeting agenda, conduct the meeting, and record minutes
7. Supervise the purchase, repair, and maintenance of office equipment
8. Assist in improving work flow and office efficiencies (time management)
9. Create and update the office procedure manual, Material Safety Data Sheets (MSDSs), and Health Insurance Portability and Accountability Act (HIPAA) manual.
10. Prepare patient education materials and arrange patient/community education workshops as needed

QUALITIES OF A MANAGER

An office manager should not feel the need to be superior to employees but should strive to develop a synergistic organization. The best manager is like an orchestra conductor. He or she constructively blends together the skills and abilities of diverse people to produce a smooth and efficient team. The result is an organization having greater capability than would be achievable by the individuals acting independently.

The office manager should have two overarching goals:

- Get the job done.
- Make the process enjoyable.

This does not mean work should be one big party. It means developing ownership for the work, pride in doing the job well, and a sense of teamwork. There will be times when employees will not like having to stay late to meet important deadlines, but through developed self-actualization, they will take enjoyment from even the most undesirable task.

A good office manager needs to be two persons in one body: leader and manager. The two functions are different, and the good manager will use some of each characteristic in meeting objectives. Table 33-1 lists the differences between an authoritarian style manager and a leader/manager.

Good managers are leaders, providing their coworkers with vision, guidance, and a feeling of ownership in the process. They do these things without threats, usually through the power of their

Table 33-1 Differences Between an Authoritarian Style Manager and a Leader/Manager

Authoritarian	Leader
• Establishes and adheres to written procedures	• Empower people
• Focused on short-range goals	• Inspires by example
• Authoritarian style of management	• Vision and long range goals
• Bottom line all important	• Consensus or team style of management
• Does things right	• Does the right thing
• Annual raises	• Pay for performance
• Reluctant to change	• Not afraid of change

personal charisma. It is also important that managers clearly convey their expectations to their employees. Possibly nothing leads to ill feeling between the manager and an employee more than failure to let the employee know what is expected of him or her. Furthermore, a lack of expectations stifles career growth and organizational vitality. Good leaders need to blend many admirable personality traits of leadership to be successful and still control the resources entrusted to them.

Before proceeding with a listing of qualities of a leader/manager, a rule that defines almost all of the ethical qualities needs to be mentioned (Figure 33-1). Some texts call it the Golden Rule; this rule will make the difference between a manager who is successful and one who fails miserably. The rule needs no explanation and will serve any manager well in any circumstance.

Qualities needed by a leader/manager include the following:

- *Effective communication skills.* Communication skills include written and oral methods. The manager must communicate clearly, diplomatically, tactfully, and with respect for the feelings of others.
- *Fairmindedness.* It is important to always be fair with coworkers. Decisions that impact one fellow employee create a ripple effect. That is, you may have to make the same decision for another employee at another time. Decisions should be based, as much as possible, on the assumption that what is granted to one employee will be granted to others in similar situations. This approach will decrease the risk for being accused of playing favorites or being unfair.
- *Objectivity.* The office manager must be able to view challenges without bias or prejudice. For example, when promotions are made, the office manager must be able to focus on the job description criteria and individual qualifications without introducing personal preference.
- *Organizational skills.* Being organized includes being able to prioritize tasks, working efficiently and methodically. Know when and be willing to delegate tasks when others have the expertise and time to complete the task within the time lines.
- *People skills.* The office manager must like people in general and enjoy working with them. Building confidence and self-esteem in others and being interested in promoting constructive relationships are essential qualities of the office manager. The ability to function as an effective team leader provides a role model for other staff members to emulate.
- *Problem-solving skills.* The office manager must be a problem solver. This may include being creative and doing away with old paradigms and traditional approaches to solving a problem. When difficult issues arise, focus on the situation, issue, or behavior, not on the person. A discussion about solving the problem without laying blame is much more productive. Positive solutions may be more readily attained when discussing what was observed rather than what was told by someone else.
- *Technical expertise.* Have a working knowledge of each procedure performed in the office, although it is not necessary to be the acknowledged technical expert. A good office manager is continually learning and encourages **subordinates** to seek opportunities to continue their education and advance their technical skills.
- *Truthfulness.* Lead by example! If an honest mistake is made, be the first to admit to the error and seek the best solution for preventing it from happening again. Respond honestly to requests. For example, two staff members ask for the same day off. The office manager will make the decision that only one member may have the day off and will review the policy manual to determine the appropriate criteria for designating who will have the request granted.

TREAT OTHERS AS YOU WOULD LIKE TO BE TREATED!

Figure 33-1 The Golden Rule.

Office Manager Attitude

Many managers share a common enemy—themselves. The part of ourselves that is our enemy is our mind and the outlook we have on the world. People who succeed attribute positive results to their own actions. People who underachieve or fail usually attribute negative results to someone else or to chance, over which they have no control. Because underachievers feel helpless to affect results, psychologists conclude that their motivation to succeed is diminished. A low achiever would be unlikely to have a personal risk management system in place. They would feel they could not affect events. The more positive person could easily take steps to avoid these problems.

The effect of a negative mindset does not stop with failure to accept responsibility for the things that happen to each of us, it continues on. Unless we change our outlook, we lower our expectations and begin accepting the mediocre. Individuals who feel they are helpless to affect events become afraid of success as well as failure, and they subconsciously find a way to fail to avoid the challenges success will bring.

How do you change your mindset? The following are a few suggestions considered helpful:

- Come to terms with what you would have to change if you are to be successful and be ready for the change.
- Identify what you really want to achieve.
- Put your goals in writing using positive terms (say "I will" not "I'll try").
- Begin with small, achievable goals.
- Eliminate poor habits such as procrastination.
- Tune out negative thoughts and focus on positive thoughts.

We are what we think we are. Be careful of your mindset, it can derail you and your job as a manager.

Professionalism

The medical assistant as office manager must exhibit professional behavior at all times. He or she must be courteous and diplomatic and demonstrate a responsible and positive attitude. All verbal and written communications should be accurate and correct and should follow appropriate guidelines. The office manager should demonstrate knowledge of federal and state health care legislation and regulations and must perform within legal and ethical boundaries. All documentation must be performed appropriately.

Critical Thinking

How does the office manager begin to develop good working relationships with other community service organizations to better serve and provide for the patient's health care needs? How would this improve the quality of public relations?

The office manager serves as a liaison between the provider, patient, and other professionals. Therefore, professional demeanor in all respects must be followed. It is not uncommon to be called on to locate community resources and information for patients and employers. A good working relationship with other community service organizations fosters the sharing of information vital to your patient's health care needs and promotes quality public relations. Review Procedure 4-1 for specific information on how this is done.

MANAGEMENT STYLES

There are many books written on management styles; however, it is possible to break all of them down into only two basic styles, each with an infinite number of variations. Because this is not a management text, we take a simplistic view and look at only the fundamental styles: authoritarian and participatory. We also examine a third management style, managing by walking around, which, although not a people interaction style, is an effective management technique for keeping abreast of what is going on in an organization.

HIPAA

In many offices, the office manager is also designated to fill the role of Security Officer. The responsibilities of the Security Officer include coordinating and overseeing the various impacts of HIPAA on each department and assisting with compliance issues related to HIPAA regulations. The Security Officer must also keep abreast of any changes and rulings and how they may apply to their particular office environment. Some online resources are available at http://www.cms.hhs.gov; or e-mail questions to askhipaa@cms.hhs.gov.

Authoritarian Style

Authoritarian managers operate on the premise that most workers cannot make a contribution without being directed, sometimes in the minutest detail, and even if they could, they would not be inclined to do so. This type of manager believes in the carrot and stick approach to motivate people to work. The carrot is monetary reward, and the stick is docked pay or being reprimanded or fired. The personality of the manager tends to influence natural tendencies of style. Individuals who are task or procedure oriented tend to be authoritarian. Authority control is easily accomplished in the case of simple tasks that can readily be structured and defined. Authoritarian managers try to control work to the maximum extent possible, for example, micro-management. Complex jobs, however, are difficult for the authoritarian manager to control.

Sometimes a manager needs to use the authoritarian style. It should be used quite sparingly because it may destroy morale and personal incentive. An assumption regarding the character of an employee frequently becomes a self-fulfilling prophecy. Workers with an authoritarian manager either give up and quit, or they become mindless robots asking "how high" when told to jump. As a manager, you use the authoritarian style in the case of new employees until you have a chance to determine their capabilities, in the case of a worker who has proved to be without self-motivation, or in supervising short-term temporary labor.

Can an authoritarian manager style work in the twenty-first century? Yes. It has worked for a few well-respected, large companies in the United States, but this occurred only because management had unlimited resources to use as a carrot for rewarding employees. Most managers will not have these resources.

Participatory Style

The **participatory management** style is based on the premise that the worker is capable and wants to do a good job. The best known form of participatory management is the use of teams to do work tasks. This type of management is well suited to complex tasks where each member can contribute his specialty to the job at hand. The manager's function in this type of system is communicating direction and vision to the team and selling the team on the importance of the task. Providing the team with the necessary resources required is an important managerial function. Managers using this type of style need to be comfortable teaching, coaching, communicating, inspiring, and motivating. Workers engaged in a participatory management style are motivated by much more than monetary reward and develop an ownership for the work in which they are involved. Although the carrot is still important, their reward comes from teamwork, peer recognition, and self-actualization, that is, the pleasure derived from doing a job well and being recognized for it. Competition between teams is sometimes used as a motivation technique.

Management by Walking Around

Management by walking around (MBWA) is not really a management style but rather a technique for keeping the manager informed about the health of his or her organization. This style consists of just what the title says, the manager walks around looking at what is going on in the organization and talks with employees to get their opinion on how things could be done better. The manager collects data on new ideas; in a participatory system, a team is assigned to study and come up with a better way of doing the work. The manager must be careful to make sure his or her motives are not to micromanage and to convey this to the workers.

Critical Thinking

How would you make the medical office (front- and back-office space) safe for employees and nonemployees (e.g., patients, venders, visitors)? List as many considerations as possible.

RISK MANAGEMENT

The office manager should formulate a **risk management** procedure that assesses risks to which he or she and the organization is exposed and takes steps to develop contingencies that minimize probable risks. Some common risks and risk-control measures are:

- *Loss of a critical employee.* Have cross training of employees to permit them to assume the duties of an employee who is ill or terminates his or her employment.
- *Failure of a supplier or contractor.* Maintain sufficient inventory to permit contracting with a secondary supplier before critical shortages occur. Monitor the status of orders so that you are aware of any

failures in delivery before they have a negative impact and supplies can be obtained from a second source. Have a list of secondary sources.

- *Accidental disclosure of confidential information through error or unauthorized entry.* Have protocols in place regarding breach of confidentiality and defining steps to be taken in the event information is compromised. Define protocols to patients alerting them to the unlikely but potential possibility of accidental disclosure. Notify patients immediately if confidential information is compromised and work with them for resolution.
- *Computer failure.* Back up the system regularly. Have a secondary system that permits the office to operate until repairs are effected. Have a maintenance contract in place with a reputable firm permitting overnight repair.
- *Injury to a staff member or nonemployee.* Continually review safety procedures and conduct safety surveys. Have adequate liability insurance for the medical office.
- *Managerial position change.* Continuously network with friends and associates to permit you to rapidly seek a new position before experiencing a job loss. It's always easier to get a job while you still have a job.

Incident reports are required to notify managers of events involving injuries to patients, visitors, or staff, medical errors or omissions, breech of confidential information, and potentially dangerous conditions associated with facilities or equipment. This report signals the risk manager to implement existing protocols to minimize risk. Medical incident reports are confidential and cannot be released to anyone without a signed release of information agreement. The medical incident report form is an administrative document and is not considered part of the medical record. Procedure 33-1 provides steps for completing a medical incident report.

IMPORTANCE OF TEAMWORK

The use of **teamwork** to improve the efficiency of the office at first may seem incongruent to your desire to improve office efficiency, because it seems that several people are now involved in solving a problem that you as the manager should solve and explain. Teamwork builds morale and actually results in getting more accomplished with the resources you have because the team members develop ownership of the solution to a problem and want to make it work. When it works, it flatters them and builds their esteem.

Efficiency of a team results from collectively working together to plan how to "work smarter" and how to dovetail tasks and support each other so that wasted effort is avoided. To achieve all of these things, a team not only must be given the responsibility and the authority to plan and execute their plan to solve a problem, but they must know your expectations for them. Sometimes this means that you, the office manager, must stick your neck out for them. They will reward you handsomely for doing so.

Getting the Team Started

A successful teamwork approach is not a mysterious event that just happens; it is the result of clear vision, specific goals, and a well-planned strategy on the part of the team leader. For teamwork to be successful, individual team members must understand and support the specifics of the problem they are being asked to solve. This is probably the most significant task of the team leader or the office manager. It is helpful in taking this important step to let the team develop its own **work statement,** for in this way they assume ownership of the goals and objectives you want them to achieve. The work statement frequently outlines specific tasks and their sequential order of accomplishment. Its purpose is to ensure that everyone is working toward the team goals and objectives.

A major pitfall at this stage may be diverse opinions that can lead to a work statement that does not meet the manager's goals and objectives for the team. It is your job as office manager to try to direct the team back to what you want them to work on without undermining their team spirit. Take care at this stage not to begin making assignments or to let team members start solving the problem until the work statement is complete. Under some circumstances, it may be necessary for you, the office manager, to exercise your authority in defining the work statement, but be careful, because this approach could harm the team's collective spirit.

The next step in team development is to establish a timetable for achieving results and identifying the standards that must be maintained. Without a timetable a team feels no sense of urgency and tends to lose direction. You also have to paint a clear picture of the standards that must be maintained as you attempt to solve the problem. You should let the team develop both the standards and the timetable, but with your leadership and support.

Using a Team to Solve a Problem

Problem solution is the next step in team development. Some people call this stage **brainstorming** a solution. Brainstorming is fun, but unless it is controlled by the leader, it will bog down into needless arguments and hurt feelings. In a successful brainstorming session, everyone feels free to contribute solutions to the problem without any consideration for practicality or flaws in the proposal. Only after everyone has had a chance to speak are the solutions looked at in terms of practicality and for technical correctness. At this point the team should not look at what is wrong with the solution, but what needs to be done to make it a workable solution.

Prioritization of the solutions comes next. To do this, it is helpful to assign scores for impact on solving the problem and for changeability, or the difficulty in implementing a particular solution in your office environment. The result is a list of solutions to the problem in descending order from the greatest impact on the problem with the least cost or difficulty in implementation. Do a needs assessment, remove yourself from the issue, and look at it from a different perspective. **Benchmark** (compare) your facility to other facilities and organizations to see how they accomplish tasks, compensate employees, and so on.

Planning and Implementing a Solution

The team should work out a detailed plan for implementation of the solution selected, including a schedule. Assignments should be made, resources of equipment and funds available to the team should be defined, and any remaining problems should be assigned to subteams that will function just as the primary team did in solving them. The team should continue to meet to discuss progress and to resolve additional problems that may occur.

Recognition

A successful team should not be disbanded until it is acknowledged for its efforts and physical recognition is given in the case of an important problem that was solved. In some cases, a dinner or luncheon is in order. This is the most important phase of team development, because it is responsible for developing a team spirit or sense of **self-actualization** within the organization. Once this spirit is implanted into an organization, it becomes infectious.

SUPERVISING PERSONNEL

Creating an atmosphere in which open and honest communication can take place is critical to supervising personnel. This type of communication may be encouraged through the establishment of regular staff meetings, with each staff member sharing ideas for improvement and areas of concern. Eliciting the help of others in problem-solving strategies promotes harmony (Figure 33-2).

Staff and Team Meetings

The office manager usually initiates the staff and team meeting idea and should officiate at such meetings. Failure of the office manager to be present may convey a message that the meeting is an event not worthy of attention. It is important that the office manager be familiar with basic parliamentary procedures. The purchase of books such as *Robert's Rules of Order* or *Parliamentary Procedure at a Glance* is an excellent investment.

Successful staff and team meetings are announced well in advance or on established time lines to enable the majority of office personnel to attend. An **agenda** identifying the subjects to be covered during a given meeting should be issued before the meeting so that each attendee arrives prepared with input or questions relevant to the topics. Procedure 33-2 outlines the procedural steps for creating a meeting agenda. Figure 33-3 shows a sample agenda. Each meeting should end with opportunity for nonagenda items to be discussed or suggested for inclusion in the next meeting. The meeting should have a fixed time to end.

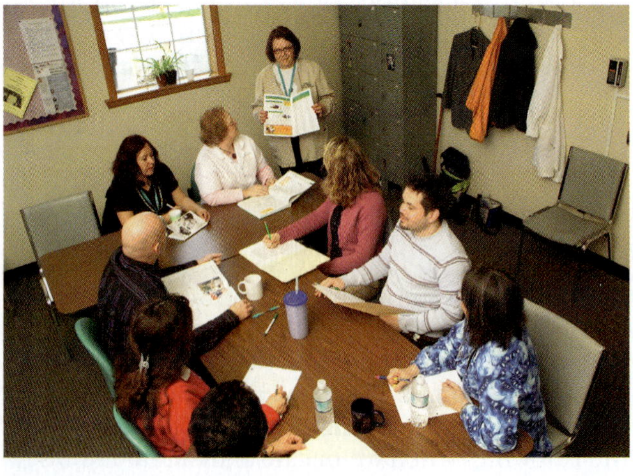

Figure 33-2 Consistently scheduled staff meetings promote communication and harmony among the health care team.

AGENDA

STAFF MEETING Wednesday, February 16, 20XX
2:00 PM — Conference Room

1. Read and approve minutes of last meeting
2. Reports
   A. Satellite facility — Marilyn Johnson
   B. Patient flow — Joe Guerrero
   C.
3. Discussion of new telephone system
4. Unfinished Business
   A. Review new procedure manual pages
   B.
5. New Business
   A. Appoint committee for design of new marketing brochure
   B.
6. Open discussion and/or topics for next meeting's agenda
7. Set next meeting time
8. Adjourn

Figure 33-3 Sample meeting agenda.

A written record in the form of **minutes** should be maintained and sent to all team members regardless of whether they attended the meeting. This policy keeps all members informed about policy changes and decisions that impact the office operations. The minutes also trigger a reminder for any new procedures or revisions to be made in the procedure manual.

The minutes for a staff and team meeting should record action plans under each agenda topic. Summarize all action items agreed to in the meeting in one section of the minutes. This facilitates easy access to information at a later date should it be required.

The date, time, and place of the next meeting should be included. The person preparing the minutes should always sign them. A copy of the minutes should always be maintained in a book for easy reference.

Conflict Resolution

A good human resources manager is a master at **conflict resolution,** solving problems between any two parties. The most difficult task is to prevent or solve conflicts that occur between employees and supervisors or providers. Most conflict occurs because of poor communication or a misunderstanding; thus effective communication is a goal for any manager.

Volumes of materials have been written about successful conflict management. One can probably never get enough material on the subject. Some guidelines that may be helpful in preventing conflicts include the following:

- Listen to your employees. What do they say? What do they communicate nonverbally?
- Manage by walking around and talking to your employees.
- Do not tolerate negative comments or actions among employees.
- Encourage an open-door policy for concerns and complaints.
- Be a role model for all employees.
- Keep confidences.

An office manager who cares about each employee, who "carries water for the workers in the trenches," and who administers fairly and honestly creates an environment where conflict is at a minimum.

When conflicts arise, do not avoid taking immediate action to resolve the issue even if it appears to be superficially resolved. It will resurface at the first instance of stress between the individuals. Conflicts usually are the result of misunderstanding. In some cases the manager can mediate the issue and resolve the contentious behavior, but this places you with the role of judge and jury, and one party will feel injured or abused regardless of the outcome. Mediation is the only approach when the conflict is between a provider or supervisor and an employee. In all other instances the best approach is to use a confrontational approach. The two persons having a conflict are brought together and asked to express their conflicting opinions without interruption. The purpose is to communicate what each perceives to be the problem. If an obvious solution that is acceptable to both parties does not appear, the manager must insist that the parties come up with an acceptable solution to the conflict. (This latter step is not appropriate for conflicts between an employee and a superior in the organization.) In doing so both parties have ownership of the resolution.

HARASSMENT IN THE WORKPLACE

Harassment consists of verbal or physical behavior/conduct that is (a) unwelcome, (b) based on a protected class (e.g., race, sex, age, national origin, veteran status, or sexual orientation), (c) severe or pervasive, and (d) has a negative impact or creates a hostile environment. As a manager, you are legally responsible for ensuring nondiscrimination and preventing harassment. You, as a manager, may be innocent of any kind of sexual harassment yourself, but if the workplace you manage is construed as hostile by any one of your employees and you do not take appropriate action, you and your company can be held liable in a court of law.

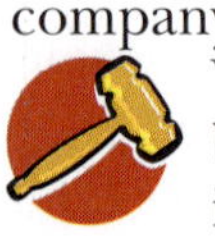

When an employee contacts you or you become aware of harassment, you should immediately contact your Human Resources Equal Opportunity Office (EOO). If your facility does not have an EOO, you should collect facts and confront the offending individuals or group, clearly notifying them that the offensive behavior must stop immediately. A report of the incident should be placed in the file of the offending individuals, with a written warning that a future incident will result in termination.

The manager must carefully evaluate the facts surrounding an incident. It is not uncommon for innocent events to be perceived as harassment. When there is conflict between people who are in some way different from each other, simple misunderstandings can be perceived as harassment. Blatant harassment is far less common than this kind of muddled interaction. Although some situations do involve malicious intent, many are largely the result of poor communication, and it is the manager's responsibility to differentiate between the two.

Every employer needs a comprehensive policy that prohibits all types of harassment. The policy needs to include a definition of what could constitute harassment or create a hostile work environment, information on who to report to, and a nonretaliation provision. This policy must be made available to all employees.

Assimilating New Personnel

The goal in the assimilation of new personnel into the workplace is to make it happen as seamlessly as possible. The office manager and HR representative usually assume this task jointly, with the office manager being responsible for orientation in medical protocols and procedures, and the HR representative handling orientation regarding medical practice rules and regulations and any legal implications.

New Personnel Orientation. The new personnel orientation process consists of orienting and training new employees in the medical protocols and procedures unique to the practice. If the procedure manual is detailed and accurate, this manual now becomes a guide for new employees.

It is important to introduce new employees to other staff members and to assign a **mentor** who can respond to questions that new employees may raise. Sometimes the individual leaving a position still is present and is asked to assist in the orientation process. This is especially beneficial if there is a good working relationship between the employee who is leaving and the management of the practice. Depending on the responsibilities of the new employee, a supervisor may be asked to monitor all procedures for a period for accuracy, safety, and patient protection.

The orientation should clearly present what is expected of new employees and explain that, at the end of their probationary period, their performance will be evaluated to determine if full-time employment will be offered. The same procedures followed for new employees should be followed for student practicums, with the exception that expectations and the evaluation process may vary.

Probation and Evaluation. It is common for a new employee to be placed on probation for 60 to 90 days. During this period, both the employee and supervisory personnel determine if the position is a suitable match for both employer and employee. Near the end of the probation period, the employee should be officially evaluated to determine how competently he or she is performing the assigned tasks/duties. The employee should also be given an opportunity to express their personal thoughts relative to job satisfaction. Figure 33-4 shows a sample probationary employee evaluation form. The evaluation becomes part of the employee's personnel record at the end of the probation period.

Supervising Student Practicums. The student **practicum** is a transitional stage that provides opportunity for the student to apply theory learned in the classroom to a health care setting through practical, hands-on experience. Some institutions use the term *externship* or *internship,* and still oth-

PROBATIONARY EMPLOYEE EVALUATION FORM

Name ____________________

Hire Date ____________________

Job Title ____________________

Pay Rate __________ Supervisor __________

Do you recommend the employee continue in employment?

_______ Yes _______ No

Please state your reasons for whatever action you recommend. Use the guidelines below to make your decision.

1. Has the employee required more training than is normally needed for the job?
2. Has the employee grasped this job with very little training?
3. Is the employee performing at, above, or below (circle one) the standard for this job?
4. If below, when do you expect the employee to reach the standard?
5. Does the employee get along well with all staff members?
6. Has the employee maintained a good attendance record and a good work attitude?
7. Has the employee expressed any dissatisfactions?

____________________ __________

Supervisor's Signature Date

Figure 33-4 Sample probationary employee evaluation.

ers operate through a cooperative education program. The number of hours for the practicum are predetermined together with criteria for site selection and tasks to be performed by the student.

The office manager should schedule an information interview with the student before the practicum begins. During this time, the expectations of the office manager and the student may be established. A tour of the facility and introductions to key personnel aid the student in feeling more comfortable the first day of "work."

Because the student will be writing in medical records where correct spelling is mandatory or may be scheduling appointments and must write telephone numbers without transposition, some pretesting may be offered. By giving a spelling test of 10 commonly used medical terms or verbally stating five telephone numbers for the student to write down, an immediate evaluation is attained.

The office manager should directly supervise or identify someone else to supervise the student. During the first few days of the practicum, the student may simply **shadow** the supervisor, learning the routine, provider preference, and protocols for that particular office. As the student begins to feel comfortable in the new environment, minimal tasks should be assigned. Based on the student's ability to follow directions and perform tasks, increased skill-level tasks may be added.

The supervisor will direct and evaluate the student's progress; schedule activities that will provide experience in all aspects of medical assisting, including administrative, clinical, and laboratory procedures; maintain accurate records of attendance and hours "worked"; and communicate the student's progress to the medical assisting supervisor from the educational institution. Procedure 33-3 provides steps for supervising a student practicum.

When working with students, it is important to remember that they still have much to learn and will need lots of reassuring guidance. When you take time to explain each step and to provide the rationale for each, students will learn more quickly. Demonstrating new or different techniques and approaches helps students by providing them with options that they may find more comfortable.

Remember that this type of learning is stressful. The student is not yet accustomed to communication with a "real" patient, let alone working with a provider. Your role as office manager is to reduce as much stress as possible for everyone concerned. Introduce the student to the patient and ask the patient's permission to allow the student to perform a procedure. Many patients will be tolerant when they realize the circumstances and will be quite cooperative.

Employees with Chemical Dependencies or Emotional Problems

Employees with chemical dependencies or emotional problems are ill and are to be treated as such. Approach the situation constructively rather than punitively. Make a commitment to the employee, to the rest of the staff, and to the patients that at no time will patient care be put at risk. Help an employee with a problem to find the support and counseling necessary. No staff member should be permitted to remain on the premise with impaired judgment while under the influence of alcohol or controlled substances. If chemical dependency treatment is necessary, make accommodation as seems appropriate or is warranted. Everyone occasionally feels discouraged and distressed. Hopefully, the provider–employer and the manager are able to recognize problems before they become too serious.

It has been said that one in four individuals will experience some form of mental health problem during the course of a year. Work-related stress is the base cause of a significant degree of mental ill health. Plan for and create a work environment that reduces as much stress as possible. Actions to consider may include the following:

1. Properly educate and train all employees for their positions.
2. Encourage teamwork and reward those who help each other.
3. Mandate "break periods" in the day for each employee.
4. Create a pleasant work environment (plants, water, music, and so on).
5. Establish a blowing off steam place for when employees are especially frustrated.
6. Take everyone out for lunch at least once a quarter.
7. Have regular staff meetings to discuss employee concerns and office improvements.
8. Celebrate birthdays and special occasions (i.e., length of service).

Keep in mind that a happy employee who feels valued in his or her position will stay much longer than someone who is unhappy and does not feel valued.

Evaluating Employees and Planning Salary Review

It is important that all employees know whether they are performing their job as expected and know how they can improve their performance if necessary.

Performance Evaluation. Not only is evaluation of employees necessary during the probation period, but it is necessary for current employees as well. Evaluations should be performed no less than once a year on the anniversary of the hire date. Some office managers may wish to evaluate an employee more often, especially if a problem has surfaced in an evaluation.

The evaluation may take many forms; it can be formal or informal; it may involve more than one person. The results of the evaluation, however, must be a part of the employee's personnel record. For that reason, a formal evaluation is preferred. Many practices use a written evaluation that requires that the employee evaluate himself before meeting with the office manager (Figure 33-5). The office manager uses the same form for evaluation. During the meeting, notes are compared as the evaluation is conducted.

The climate of the performance evaluation should be comfortable and provide privacy (Figure 33-6). The meeting should be friendly, but the employee must sense the importance of the evaluation. Do not allow any disagreements to escalate into arguments during the evaluation. Without reading the employee's self-evaluation, ask the employee to tell about the self-assessment. Acknowledge the employee's point of view and identify when you agree or differ from the self-assessment. Be prepared to describe specific examples of positive performance and negative performance.

When negative performance is identified, ask the employee for possible solutions. Then a plan can be determined to alter the negative performance. In this way, a trusting atmosphere is established in that both of you are working together for a solution that will benefit the medical practice. Always look for and seek a win-win situation whenever possible. The action plan determined should then be evaluated at the next performance evaluation.

At the close of the evaluation, always express your confidence in the individual to make any changes necessary, offer assistance where needed, and thank the employee for participating. End any evaluation with a positive statement about some portion of the employee's performance.

There are occasions when reviews are performed more frequently than annually. A review would occur 2 to 3 months after a significant promotion to measure how things are progressing. Reviews occur more often when general performance falls well short of past efforts or a serious error in judgment has been made. This type of review may end with a reprimand, a warning to correct the problem by a given date, or possibly, immediate dismissal. Document any steps to be taken to correct a problem and any reason that is cause for dismissal.

Salary Review. Although the practice is common in some areas, it may be better not to tie salary increases or bonuses with the annual performance evaluation. Conduct the **salary review** at the beginning

PERFORMANCE REVIEW FORM

Employee Name ________________	Title ________________
Supervisor ________________	Department ________________

TYPE OF REVIEW (Check One)

_______ Quarterly

_______ Annual

_______ Probation

_______ Other _______________

Review Period Covered _____________ to _____________

PERFORMANCE DEFINITIONS

5 = Outstanding	Performance that is clearly superior, beyond the call of duty, or substantially above standard level. Seldom attained level of performance but achievable.
4 = Above Standard	Very commendable performance; exceeds the norm for the job.
3 = Standard	Competent and consistent performance; expected level of activity and performance for the job. Most often rating received.
2 = Below Standard	Performance needs improvement. This level of performance is unacceptable; needs improvement to meet the standards for the job.
	Employee new to the job: Performance might receive below standard rating due to lack of job knowledge and is expected to improve with experience.
	Experienced Employee: Performance is below acceptable level and requires direction and/or counsel.
1 = Unsatisfactory	Performance is unacceptable. Job activity is clearly and substantially lacking in quality, quantity, or timeliness. May also not be meeting cost or budget constraints. Needs much improvement to meet the standards for the job.

(office use only)	FINAL RATING: CHECK ONE (office use only)
EVALUATION SUMMARY	_______ Merit Increase Recommended
Total I _______	_______ No Merit Increase—Satisfactory Performance/No Growth
+ Total II _____	_______ No Merit Increase (Probationary/Special Evaluation)
	_______ No Merit Increase (Performance Probation)
	Re-evaluate in 90 Days for Unsatisfactory or in 180 Days for Needed Improvement

GENERAL PERFORMANCE RATING (PART I)

General Criteria	*Rating*	*Comments Supporting Rating*
1. **Patient Relations:** How well does the employee communicate a "we care" image to the patients, visitors, providers, and fellow employees?		
2. **Work Responsibilities:** What is the quality of the employee's work relative to quality, quantity, and timeliness?		
3. **Teamwork:** Does the employee have a team spirit? Does the employee interact well with co-workers/supervisor/manager?		

(continues)

Figure 33-5 Sample performance review form.

General Criteria	*Rating*	*Comments Supporting Rating*
4. Adaptability: Is the employee open to change and new ideas? Does the employee remain flexible to changes in routine, workload, and assignments?		
5. Personal Appearance: How well does the employee maintain appropriate personal appearance, including proper attire, hygiene?		
6. Communication: Does the employee communicate well? Is information given and received clearly? Does he/she have good verbal and written skills?		
7. Dependability: Can the employee be relied upon for good attendance? Does the employee perform and follow through on work without supervisory intervention or assistance?		

Subtotal I ____________ ÷ 7 General Criteria = ____________

JOB-SPECIFIC CRITERIA RATING (PART II) (To be used with Job Description attached)

Responsibility and Standard	*Rating*	*Comments Supporting Rating*
Complete a section for each responsibility listed on the employee's job description.		

Subtotal II ____________ ÷ ____________ = ____________
\# job duties

Contributions made since last review:

____

____

____

Education or training received since last review:

____

____

____

Action to be taken based on performance:

____

____

____

Comments:

____

____

____

______________________ Employee Signature	____________ Date
______________________ Supervisor Signature	____________ Date
______________________ Provider Signature	____________ Date

Figure 33-5 (continued)

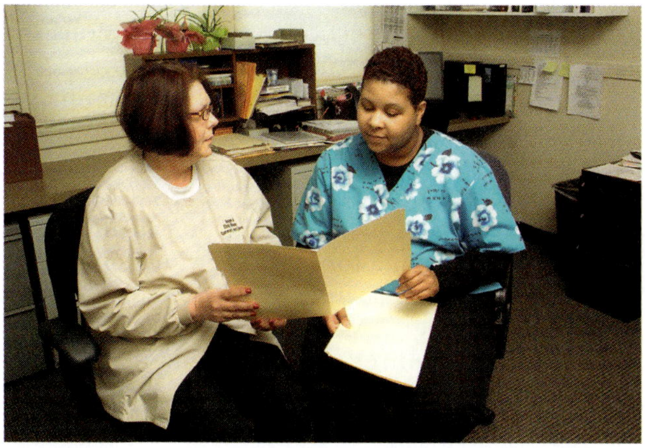

Figure 33-6 A comfortable, private setting encourages discussions during an employee performance review.

of the new year separate from performance evaluations.

Salary review is important. Unfortunately, in smaller medical offices and ambulatory care settings, the review of salary may have to be raised by the employee. Provider–employers tend to forget that their employees have been with them for over a year without a raise or a discussion of financial reimbursement. If this is the case, it is perfectly acceptable for the employee to raise the issue on a yearly basis. However, the best approach is for the office manager to conduct salary reviews at the beginning or end of each calendar year.

Data should be collected before a salary review. The office manager should network with other office managers to determine wages and salaries for comparable individuals with comparable skills. Remember, also, that it is far more cost-effective to reward good employees with a salary increase than it is to train a new employee who commands a lesser salary than current employees. Reward employees well and provide benefits that encourage them to stay with the practice. Employees who stay with the practice for a long time not only fully understand how best to serve their provider–employers, they have established a relationship with patients that is beneficial.

How much of a raise is to be awarded at the time of salary review is difficult to determine and depends on many factors that might include the profits of the year, the patient load, the workload, and the current cost of living.

The critical shortage of health care employees today is reflected in the shortage of medical assistants across the country. Newspapers advertising for individuals to work in the ambulatory care setting tell the story. A consideration worth mentioning is that often the salary does not match the education, experience, and special training required of someone working in the health care field. Educators often hear, "Why would I spend a year or more in education to be paid what I would make working in a fast food restaurant?" Because it is costly in time and resources to replace employees, it is best to invest that cost into a fair and just salary increase for valued employees.

Dismissing Employees

Most human resources managers do not enjoy rating the performance of other employees, particularly when difficult topics are involved and it may be necessary to dismiss an employee. However, the written performance evaluation actually establishes the format for such a dismissal when necessary and is more likely to remove the emotion from the situation. Involuntary dismissal is still difficult when it is necessary.

Involuntary Dismissal. Involuntary dismissal results from two primary causes: poor performance or serious violation of office policies or job descriptions. When it becomes apparent to the office manager that the effectiveness of an employee is dropping well below expectations, it will be known in the review or a performance review may be called. The review allows the employee to be informed of the shortcomings, to explain any reasons for the present situation, and to determine a plan to alleviate the problem. If the problem is a serious one, probation is usually invoked and any lack of significant improvement in the time provided results in immediate dismissal.

When the problem is a violation of either office policy or procedures, both a verbal and a written warning are given to the employee. Involuntary dismissal follows if the situation persists. Dismissal may be immediate if the action is a serious violation of policy. Serious violations depend on the office practice, but some causes for immediate dismissal include theft, making fraudulent claims against insurance, placing the patient in jeopardy by not practicing safe techniques, and breach of patient confidentiality.

Some key points to keep in mind when dismissal is necessary are:

1. The dismissal should be made in privacy.
2. Take no longer than 10 minutes for the dismissal.
3. Be direct, firm, and to the point in identifying reasons.

4. Do not engage in an in-depth discussion of performance.
5. Explain terms of dismissal (keys, clearing out area of personal items, final paperwork).
6. Listen to employee's opinion and emotions; it is not necessary to agree.
7. Accompany the employee to his or her desk to pack his or her belongings.
8. Escort the employee out of the facility; do not allow him or her to finish the work of the day.

Voluntary Dismissal. Other reasons for dismissal may be more pleasant. Changes in personnel occur for many good reasons, and people voluntarily leave their jobs. They may relocate, seek advancement in another facility, or simply have personal reasons for leaving. These employees will give their manager proper notice and will be able to turn their current projects and duties over to their replacements. They have time to say good-bye to their friends and leave with a good feeling about their employment.

PROCEDURE MANUAL

The **procedure manual** provides detailed information relative to the performance of tasks within the facility in which one is employed. Each procedure manual should be designed for that specific office setting and should satisfy its requirements.

The procedure manual serves as a guide to the employee assigned a specific task and may also be useful in evaluating the employee's performance. If a temporary employee is assigned the task, the procedure manual will be invaluable in assuring that each procedure is completed as outlined.

The provider(s) and the office manager should have copies of the procedure manual, and all employees should have access to the procedure manual. Copies of individual sections may be given to the employee responsible for the task; the employee should be instructed to follow these guidelines and told that they may be used as employee evaluation tools. If all employees have access to the office computer system, the procedures manual can be made available in electronic format.

Organization of the Procedure Manual

It is best to use a loose-leaf binder with separator pages denoting each procedure. Many office managers find it helpful to divide the binder into administrative and clinical sections with subdivisions for each primary task performed (Figure 33-7).

To facilitate using the procedure manual, a consistent format should be developed and used throughout the manual. Each procedure should be a step-by-step outline or list of steps to be taken to complete a task as desired in that facility. Providing the rationale for a step, when appropriate, enhances the learning process, especially for new staff members. Material Safety Data Sheets (MSDSs) are required to be maintained in the clinic and available for personnel to reference at any time. MSDS must be compiled for all chemicals considered hazardous and maintained in an appropriate manual. Some offices opt to maintain these records in a separate tabbed section of the procedure manual. Others choose to maintain a separate MSDS manual. The information must be reviewed and updated on a regular basis. See Chapter 26 for detailed information regarding MSDS. Procedure 33-4 provides steps for developing and maintaining a procedure manual.

Updating and Reviewing the Procedure Manual

When new procedures are added to the office routine, a new procedure page should be developed immediately. The new page is useful as an educational tool or job aid while team members are learning new techniques.

An annual page-by-page review should be done to ascertain if each procedure is still being used and to ensure that each page is correct in each detail and satisfies all criteria established by the staff personnel. This contributes to an efficient

Administrative Section	Clinical Section
Personnel Management	Physical Examinations
Communication (oral and written)	Infection Control
Patient Scheduling	Collecting Specimens
Records Management	Laboratory Procedures
Financial Management	Surgical Asepsis
Facility and Equipment Management	Emergencies
	Material Safety Data Sheets (MSDS)
	OSHA
	CLIA '88

Figure 33-7 Many offices find that dividing the procedure manual into tabular sections helps organize the material. A table of contents with page numbers helps locate information easily.

office and gives all employees a sense of pride and satisfaction that they are performing within the scope of their training and to their greatest potential. The procedure manual should be reviewed by personnel performing the various tasks, and their suggestions should be evaluated and incorporated into the revisions when appropriate. All new procedure pages and revisions should be dated (Rev. 02/15/XX).

HIPAA IMPLICATIONS

HIPAA regulations require each office to develop a separate HIPAA manual that is in either an electronic form or a paper manual. The manual spells out all policies and procedures of the practice and security management measures; identifies the security officer; addresses workforce security issues, information access concerns, security awareness and training, security incidents, and contingency plans; evaluates security effectiveness; and contains copies of all business associate contracts.

The HIPAA manual must be available to all employees and updated on a regular basis. During an audit, the office manager will be asked to produce the HIPAA manual for review and to establish compliance with all regulations. All documentation of policies and procedures are to be kept for 6 years even though the wording has changed or been eliminated. If an incident is under investigation, this allows an investigator to go back to what a policy said 6 years ago.

TRAVEL ARRANGEMENTS

The office manager may be asked to make travel arrangements for providers going on vacation or to conventions, symposiums, or out-of-town seminars and continuing medical education (CME) courses. If the providers do a fair amount of travel or if they live in a metropolitan area, they may use the services of a travel agent. Attention to detail is extremely important in preventing travel disruptions.

Read carefully the instructions for completing registration forms, complete them, and mail them as quickly as possible to secure reservations to conventions and so forth. Next make hotel and travel arrangements. General information regarding the provider's travel preferences should be maintained in a file folder and referred to when making travel arrangements. Helpful information to maintain in this file includes:

- Name of travel agents used in the past (ranked by reputation and recommendation)
- Provider's or office credit card numbers
- Car rental preference
- Preferred airline, class of travel, seating choice
- Hotel/motel accommodations (bed size, suite, studio, connecting rooms, price range, amenities)
- Shuttle service

Next, contact the travel agent and identify the destination, date and time for departure and return, number traveling in party, and seating preference. A travel agent can assist with rental car and hotel accommodations if needed. Take your time and pay attention to details. When tickets are received, always check to see that all departure and arrival times match what is needed and that a confirmation number has been provided for car rentals and hotel arrangements. Procedure 33-5 outlines the procedural steps involved in making travel arrangements through a travel agent.

The Internet can be used to search for the lowest-cost air, auto, and lodging reservations. The procedures do not require extensive knowledge of travel and airline reservation protocols. Searching for information on the Internet requires the use of a search engine if you do not already have a list of favorite travel Web sites. A search engine is a special computer program available through your Internet service provider. With a search engine, you enter only the subject of your search, and the Web provides a list of Web sites related to your subject. For example, if you are making travel arrangements, you might access a search engine such as Google.com and enter the key words "air fares." The engine returns either a list of Web sites or asks you to further refine your subject, with suggestions such as cheap air fares, international travel, and so on. Once you refine your search, you may have choices such as Travelocity.com, Expedia.com, or Priceline.com. Select the appropriate Web site and follow its instructions.

Priceline.com and similar Web sites are services that allow you to name the price you want to pay; Priceline finds a major airline willing to release seats on flights where they have unsold space. You need to have a reasonable idea of the price of the service you are trying to purchase; unreasonably low bids will just waste your time and effort. Procedure 33-6 outlines the steps for making travel arrangements via the Internet.

Itinerary

If you have used a travel agent in making the travel arrangements, the agency most likely will provide several copies of the **itinerary.** An itinerary is a detailed plan for a proposed trip. The office should maintain one copy of the itinerary in case the provider must be reached for emergencies. The provider should have one copy to carry with him or her and a copy to leave with family members. You may need to develop the itinerary if you have made the travel arrangements via computer. Figure 33-8 shows a sample travel itinerary.

Important information to be included on any itinerary includes:

- *Air travel:* departure and arrival date and time, meals, airline name and telephone number, airport
- *Car rental:* name of provider, telephone number, confirmation number
- *Hotel/motel:* name, confirmation number, dates, telephone number
- *Meeting location:* name, address, room number, telephone number

TRAVEL ITINERARY

James Whitney, MD
Inner City Health Care
400 Inner City Way
Seattle, WA 98400

15 Sept 20XX   INVOICE: 880133795

29 Sept Friday					
USAIR	630	Coach Class	Equip-Boeing 757 Jet		
LV: Seattle		11:55P	Nonstop	Miles-2125	Confirmed
AR: Pittsburgh		7:23A	Elapsed time-4:28	Arrival Date-30Sept	
			Seat-31C		

30 Sept-Saturday					
Alamo			1 Compact 2/4 DR	Drop-101CT	Confirmed
Pickup-Pittsburgh			Pittsburgh Airport	Chg-USD .00	
Rate-	59.98	Baserate	Guaranteed		Extra Hr 10.00-UN
Phone-412-472-5060					
		Confirmation-1870649			

01 Oct Sunday				
USAIR	1419 Coach Class	Equip-Boeing 737 Jet		
LV: Pittsburgh	3:05P	Nonstop	Miles-2125	Confirmed
AR: Seattle	5:27P	Elapsed time-5:22		
Lunch		Seat-20A		

Ticket Number/s:					
Whitney/James	3570933		BA Card		$461.00
Air Transportation	$416.36	Tax	44.64	TOTAL	$461.00
		Sub Total			$461.00
		Credit Card Payment			$461.00-
		Amount Due			0.00

TICKET IS NON REFUNDABLE. TRIP INSURANCE IS AVAILABLE. RECONFIRM ALL FLTS 24 HRS PRIOR TO DEPARTURE

Figure 33-8 Sample travel itinerary.

TIME MANAGEMENT

Time management is an item of critical importance to the manager. You may have upward of 20 staff members putting demands on your time, and added to this are vendors, your superiors, business associates, and a host of others. A manager has not a moment to lose in the day, so managing time makes the difference between a normal 8- or 10-hour day and a 15-hour or more day. The following suggestions are some proven means of managing your time whether in management or as a salaried employee.

- *Handle items once.* Once the mail is opened, sorted, and prioritized, try to handle it only once more, when action is taken with it. Picking it up, reading it, and setting it down again without taking action is a real waste of time.
- *Develop a to-do list.* At the end of each day prepare a list of things you plan to complete the next day and try to work down this list. Prioritize the list by importance or by practical order.
- *Guard your time.* Schedule meetings with personnel and vendors so that they do not fragment your time, making you have to restart a task and get up to speed over and over again. Although modern management practice is to have an open-door policy with employees, this does not mean you should allow them to come into your office whenever they think about it. Have them schedule time with you. Make them think about what they want to discuss and do not let them monopolize your time. This is also true of meeting with vendors; require vendors to schedule ahead a time to meet with you.
- *Delegate work.* Assign others or a team to perform some of the functions discussed in this chapter. Having a team prepare weekly work schedules and vacation schedules results in less bickering and feelings of favoritism that you would have to spend time defusing if you made the schedules yourself. This does not mean that you do not have to approve them and, in some instances, make the hard decisions, but it results in your people having ownership in the decisions.

MARKETING FUNCTIONS

Effective communication skills are essential in the management of the ambulatory care setting. These skills are used by the office manager inside the ambulatory care setting to establish friendly, professional relationships with colleagues and patients. Communication is just as critical when relating to external audiences, such as other organizations, potential new patients, and community members. Developing relationships outside the office is often called marketing, a concept that office managers may use to enhance the image and visibility of an ambulatory care setting while also providing benefits to patients, potential patients, and the neighboring community.

In its broadest sense, **marketing** can be defined as the process by which the provider of services makes the consumer aware of the scope and quality of these services. Although marketing is a tool traditionally used by for-profit organizations to promote and sell products and services, it has become increasingly acceptable among health care organizations, whether they are for- or not-for-profit.

Marketing functions and materials are diverse and can include seminars and workshops, patient education brochures, brochures that describe the ambulatory care setting and its scope of services, HIPAA policies, newsletters, press releases, and special events such as open houses or participation in community health care events. Depending on the size and resources of the medical office, the manager may choose to use all or some of these tools (Figure 33-9).

When producing written material and organizing events, it is essential that ethical guidelines be respected at all times. Marketing tools should be appropriate, in good taste, and designed to quietly enhance the reputation of the office. Cultural issues should always be considered. For example, patient education brochures for a practice with many Spanish-speaking patients should be produced in bilingual editions, with English on one side and Spanish on the other. Legal issues are important as well; when presenting material of a medical nature, it is extremely important that information be accurate and up to date.

Effective marketing is a valuable tool for the office manager, especially as managed care calls on all health care professionals to become more competitive to survive. Marketing can increase visibility and credibility. The effective manager enlists the talents and skills of the entire team in developing a marketing plan.

Seminars

As consumers become increasingly aware of lifestyle choices, they look to health care professionals for information and guidance. Seminars and workshops are useful vehicles for presenting health-related

Marketing Tool	Potential Uses and Value
Seminars	Can educate patients and provide good will in the community. All staff—administrative and clinical—can work as a team to organize, publicize, and deliver the seminars.
Brochures	Brochures are typically of two types: patient education brochures and brochures on office services. Can be simple 8-1/2" x 11" fact sheets, with text only, or more elaborate brochures folded to 4" x 9" that incorporate both text and graphics or photos. Both types of brochures are informative for patients and present a professional image of the ambulatory care setting.
Practice Web site and E-zines	The practice Web site is an excellent means of promoting the practice. Personnel can be introduced, and procedures and technologies can be discussed. The E-zine approach is rapidly catching on as a promotional tool. It can be e-mailed to patients so it saves time and money. The patient may choose to view, delete, or save to read at a later time.
Newsletters	Newsletters can be produced on a biannual or quarterly basis and can form the nucleus of a marketing program. Because they are versatile tools, they can include a wide range of information from health-related articles to staff introductions to insurance updates. They should be sent to individuals on the office's mailing list and be available in the reception area.
Press Releases	Periodic press releases on new equipment, new staff, and expanded or remodeled office space can be a vital link to the local community.
Special Events	Special events are an effective way to join with other community organizations to promote wellness. They can include participation in health fairs, cosponsorship of a charity event, or an open house on the premises to acquaint the community with new services or equipment.

Figure 33-9 Marketing tools and their use in a medical environment.

information; while expert advice can be given, there is also the opportunity for patients and health care professionals to interact.

Seminars can be organized to meet patient and community needs. Some popular seminar topics include hypertension, diabetes, eating disorders, and exercise and weight management programs.

No matter what the topic area, the content should be oriented to the lay person's level of understanding, with a focused message and a delivery designed to maintain attention. Interactive seminars, which encourage audience participation, can be productive and enjoyable. Audiovisuals, such as PowerPoint™ slides, provide visual reinforcement. Handouts, either from professional organizations or those produced by office staff, can elaborate on seminar content and help the participant review and remember what was said.

Brochures

Despite the promise of a paperless society, brochures continue to be valuable sources of information. In the health care setting, patients welcome a rack of brochures as a source of current, accurate background on medical issues. New patients also find that a brochure on office services answers many questions about the practice, its philosophy, and its scope of services and gives provider profiles.

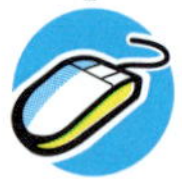

Today, it is possible to produce a professional-looking brochure in the office using a computer program that integrates text and graphics. If a brochure is produced in-house, it is important to consider writing, design, and production. Writing should be clear, to the point, and grammatically correct. Always proofread carefully before printing. Design should be kept simple. Avoid the use of too many typefaces; choose a typeface and size for readability, and, if using artwork or photography, consider its reproduction qualities. Black or another dark ink against a light background is best for readability.

Often, a local printer can advise the office manager on how to prepare a brochure or handout for printing. The simplest handouts can be quick-copied (a high-speed photocopy) on a white or lightly colored or textured stock. After printing, brochures should be made accessible to patients and other visitors in a rack or neatly arranged in piles (Figure 33-10). Occasionally, a brochure is mailed; one that folds to 4 × 9 inches fits into a standard #10 business envelope.

Patient Education Brochures. Like seminars, patient education brochures can address a variety of topics, including hypertension, diabetes, eating disorders, and exercise and weight management

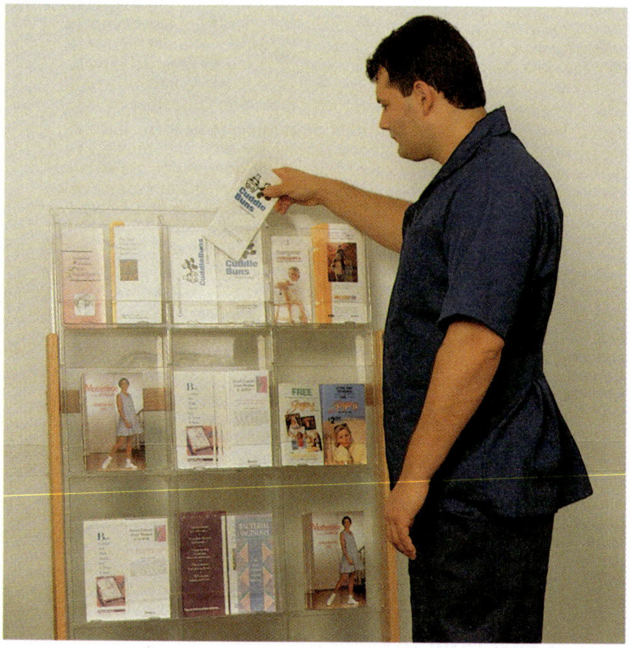

Figure 33-10 Brochures and handouts should be accessible and inviting to patients and office visitors.

programs. When writing these brochures, always research material carefully, request permission for copyrighted materials, and present the information in a manner that is accessible to your patient population.

Office Brochures. A brochure on the practice can provide a wide range of information and orient the new patient to the practice. One way to determine what information to include is to develop a list of frequently asked patient questions. Once this list is compiled, it can serve as the beginning of the brochure outline. Issues to consider might include:

- Brief history of the practice
- Brief résumés or credentials of providers
- Philosophy of the practice
- Scope of services
- How to reach the practice in case of emergency
- Insurances accepted
- Rights of patients
- Policies regarding the release of information
- Scheduling information: how to schedule an appointment, cancellation policies
- Amenities on the premises, such as parking, pharmacy, laboratory
- Location, map if necessary, and location of satellite offices

Newsletters

Newsletters are effective communication tools because they encourage regular contact with patients and other readers. Newsletters are a versatile medium; they can contain patient education articles, updates on staff changes, awards, information on insurance carriers, calendars of events, and even recipes that are consistent with a healthful lifestyle.

Most newsletters can be written and produced in the office. Like brochures, they should be simple in design and format. An additional factor in newsletter production is mailing; an up-to-date database must be maintained, postal regulations followed, and costs of mailing considered.

Press Releases

Press releases are simple, inexpensive marketing tools. Use them to announce new staff, promote a new service, or publicize a series of seminars. If a professional, courteous relationship is developed with the local press, most will be happy to receive and publish releases. When writing releases, always follow proper format, which includes a date of release, a contact person's name and telephone number, and a short headline. Releases are best kept to one double-spaced typed page. At the end of the release, type "30" or a number sign (#). Maintain an active list of local newspapers and editors' names so that you can mail or fax the release to the appropriate editor.

Special Events

Although they can be time-consuming to organize and participate in, special events are rewarding because they present an opportunity to interact with the community. They have high visibility; often a group of community organizations collaborate to cosponsor an event such as a walk-a-thon, blood pressure clinic, health fair for seniors, or wellness day for children and families. Sponsorship can be as simple as a donation to the cause; other times, staffing a booth or offering a service such as blood pressure checks is appropriate.

Like all marketing efforts, special events require organizational skills and teamwork, but they often result in heightened communication with the community and provide an educational service to patients and their families.

Form W-4 (2008)

Purpose. Complete Form W-4 so that your employer can withhold the correct federal income tax from your pay. Consider completing a new Form W-4 each year and when your personal or financial situation changes.

Exemption from withholding. If you are exempt, complete **only** lines 1, 2, 3, 4, and 7 and sign the form to validate it. Your exemption for 2008 expires February 16, 2009. See Pub. 505, Tax Withholding and Estimated Tax.

Note. You cannot claim exemption from withholding if (a) your income exceeds $900 and includes more than $300 of unearned income (for example, interest and dividends) and (b) another person can claim you as a dependent on their tax return.

Basic instructions. If you are not exempt, complete the **Personal Allowances Worksheet** below. The worksheets on page 2 adjust your withholding allowances based on itemized deductions, certain credits, adjustments to income, or two-earner/multiple job situations. Complete all worksheets that apply. However, you may claim fewer (or zero) allowances.

Head of household. Generally, you may claim head of household filing status on your tax return only if you are unmarried and pay more than 50% of the costs of keeping up a home for yourself and your dependent(s) or other qualifying individuals. See Pub. 501, Exemptions, Standard Deduction, and Filing Information, for information.

Tax credits. You can take projected tax credits into account in figuring your allowable number of withholding allowances. Credits for child or dependent care expenses and the child tax credit may be claimed using the **Personal Allowances Worksheet** below. See Pub. 919, How Do I Adjust My Tax Withholding, for information on converting your other credits into withholding allowances.

Nonwage income. If you have a large amount of nonwage income, such as interest or dividends, consider making estimated tax payments using Form 1040-ES, Estimated Tax for Individuals. Otherwise, you may owe additional tax. If you have pension or annuity income, see Pub. 919 to find out if you should adjust your withholding on Form W-4 or W-4P.

Two earners or multiple jobs. If you have a working spouse or more than one job, figure the total number of allowances you are entitled to claim on all jobs using worksheets from only one Form W-4. Your withholding usually will be most accurate when all allowances are claimed on the Form W-4 for the highest paying job and zero allowances are claimed on the others. See Pub. 919 for details.

Nonresident alien. If you are a nonresident alien, see the Instructions for Form 8233 before completing this Form W-4.

Check your withholding. After your Form W-4 takes effect, use Pub. 919 to see how the dollar amount you are having withheld compares to your projected total tax for 2008. See Pub. 919, especially if your earnings exceed $130,000 (Single) or $180,000 (Married).

Personal Allowances Worksheet (Keep for your records.)

A Enter "1" for **yourself** if no one else can claim you as a dependent . . . . **A** ______

B Enter "1" if:
- You are single and have only one job; or
- You are married, have only one job, and your spouse does not work; or
- Your wages from a second job or your spouse's wages (or the total of both) are $1,500 or less.

. **B** ______

C Enter "1" for your **spouse.** But, you may choose to enter "-0-" if you are married and have either a working spouse or more than one job. (Entering "-0-" may help you avoid having too little tax withheld.) . . . . **C** ______

D Enter number of **dependents** (other than your spouse or yourself) you will claim on your tax return . . . . . **D** ______

E Enter "1" if you will file as **head of household** on your tax return (see conditions under **Head of household** above) . **E** ______

F Enter "1" if you have at least $1,500 of **child or dependent care expenses** for which you plan to claim a credit . **F** ______
(**Note.** Do **not** include child support payments. See Pub. 503, Child and Dependent Care Expenses, for details.)

G **Child Tax Credit** (including additional child tax credit). See Pub. 972, Child Tax Credit, for more information.
- If your total income will be less than $58,000 ($86,000 if married), enter "2" for each eligible child.
- If your total income will be between $58,000 and $84,000 ($86,000 and $119,000 if married), enter "1" for each eligible child plus "1" **additional** if you have 4 or more eligible children. **G** ______

H Add lines A through G and enter total here. (**Note.** This may be different from the number of exemptions you claim on your tax return.) ▶ **H** ______

For accuracy, **complete all worksheets that apply.**
- If you plan to **itemize or claim adjustments to income** and want to reduce your withholding, see the **Deductions and Adjustments Worksheet** on page 2.
- If you have **more than one job** or are **married and you and your spouse both work** and the combined earnings from all jobs exceed $40,000 ($25,000 if married), see the **Two-Earners/Multiple Jobs Worksheet** on page 2 to avoid having too little tax withheld.
- If **neither** of the above situations applies, **stop here** and enter the number from line H on line 5 of Form W-4 below.

Cut here and give Form W-4 to your employer. Keep the top part for your records.

Form **W-4** — Department of the Treasury, Internal Revenue Service

Employee's Withholding Allowance Certificate

▶ **Whether you are entitled to claim a certain number of allowances or exemption from withholding is subject to review by the IRS. Your employer may be required to send a copy of this form to the IRS.**

OMB No. 1545-0074 — **2008**

1 Type or print your first name and middle initial.	Last name	2 Your social security number
Home address (number and street or rural route)	3 ☐ Single ☐ Married ☐ Married, but withhold at higher Single rate. **Note.** If married, but legally separated, or spouse is a nonresident alien, check the "Single" box.	
City or town, state, and ZIP code	4 **If your last name differs from that shown on your social security card, check here. You must call 1-800-772-1213 for a replacement card.** ▶ ☐	

5 Total number of allowances you are claiming (from line **H** above **or** from the applicable worksheet on page 2) **5** ______

6 Additional amount, if any, you want withheld from each paycheck . . . . **6** $ ______

7 I claim exemption from withholding for 2008, and I certify that I meet **both** of the following conditions for exemption.
- Last year I had a right to a refund of **all** federal income tax withheld because I had **no** tax liability **and**
- This year I expect a refund of **all** federal income tax withheld because I expect to have **no** tax liability.

If you meet both conditions, write "Exempt" here . . . . ▶ **7** ______

Under penalties of perjury, I declare that I have examined this certificate and to the best of my knowledge and belief, it is true, correct, and complete.

Employee's signature
(Form is not valid unless you sign it.) ▶ **Date** ▶

8 Employer's name and address (Employer: Complete lines 8 and 10 only if sending to the IRS.)	9 Office code (optional)	10 Employer identification number (EIN)

For Privacy Act and Paperwork Reduction Act Notice, see page 2. Cat. No. 10220Q Form **W-4** (2008)

Figure 33-11 Form W-4 indicates the number of exemptions claimed by the employee for income tax purposes.

RECORDS AND FINANCIAL MANAGEMENT

Providers entrust a great deal of responsibility to their medical office managers. The daily payments received through the mail and office visits must be processed and prepared for banking. Office expenses must be processed and paid in a timely fashion to capitalize on any discounts available. Employee requirements and records such as Social Security records; Withholding Allowance Certificates (W-4 forms) (Figure 33-11) indicating the number of exemptions claimed; and Employment Eligibility Verification Forms (I-9) ensuring that all persons employed are either United States citizens, lawfully admitted aliens, or aliens authorized to work in the United States must be completed and filed with the appropriate federal agencies. Also, state and local tax records must be maintained for each employee.

Electronic Health Records and the Office Manager

EHR The Total Practice Management System (TPMS) is the nerve center for the office manager as he or she orchestrates a smooth-running organization. It provides all of the data needed by the office manager at the click of a mouse or a few keystrokes. Figure 33-12 graphically shows the most significant types of data flowing between the TPMS and the office manager. Table 33-2 lists sample data types and the resulting actions by the manager.

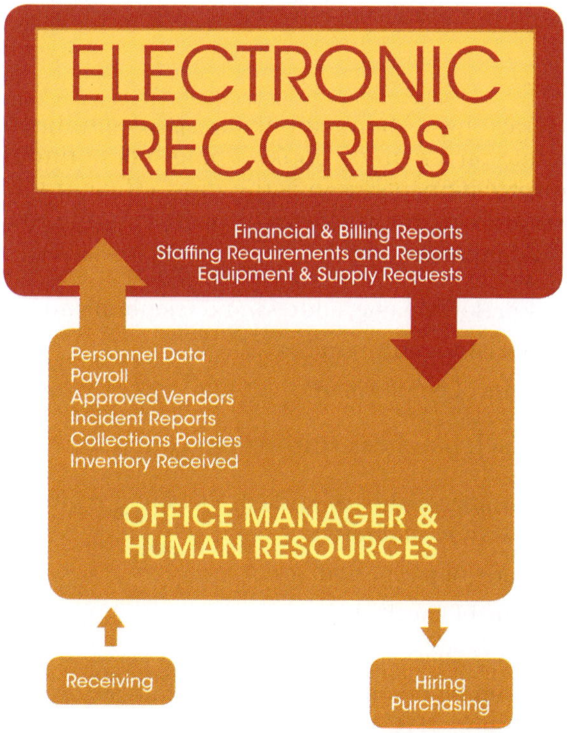

Figure 33-12 Data flow between the total practice management system and the office manager.

Payroll Processing

In some cases, it is the office manager's responsibility to prepare payroll checks for each employee and record all deductions withheld. A W-2 form (Figure 33-13) summarizing all earnings and deductions for the year must be prepared for each employee by January 31 of each year. The Social Security Administration must receive a summary report of W-2 forms each year.

To comply with all governmental regulations, federal, state, and local, it is important that the office manager who processes payroll maintain complete, up-to-date records on every employee. This information should be gathered from new employees and updated every year and with any change in employee status. For more specific information

Table 33-2 Office Manager Actions in Response to TPMS Data

Data	Action by Office Manager
Staffing requirements and appointment schedules	Hire or terminate employees, obtain additional office space and equipment, adjust vacation schedules
Equipment and supplies requests, and inventory data	Issue purchase orders, authorize payment of invoices, secure vendors and suppliers, negotiate maintenance contracts
Financial and billing reports	Practice financial status reports, instructions for coding and billing on past due accounts, actions on billing denied due to coding errors
Employee time sheets	Payroll authorization, corrective actions for missed work
Medical records	Review if patient demographics and HIPAA requirements are current
Personnel data	Progress reviews, salary reviews, W-4 forms, corrective actions, licenses, malpractice insurance contracts

22222	Void ☐	a Employee's social security number
For Official Use Only ▶ OMB No. 1545-0008		
b Employer identification number (EIN)	1 Wages, tips, other compensation	2 Federal income tax withheld
c Employer's name, address, and ZIP code	3 Social security wages	4 Social security tax withheld
	5 Medicare wages and tips	6 Medicare tax withheld
	7 Social security tips	8 Allocated tips
d Control number	9 Advance EIC payment	10 Dependent care benefits
e Employee's first name and initial / Last name / Suff.	11 Nonqualified plans	12a See instructions for box 12 (Code)
	13 Statutory employee ☐ / Retirement plan ☐ / Third-party sick pay ☐	12b (Code)
	14 Other	12c (Code)
f Employee's address and ZIP code		12d (Code)

15 State	Employer's state ID number	16 State wages, tips, etc.	17 State income tax	18 Local wages, tips, etc.	19 Local income tax	20 Locality name

Form **W-2** Wage and Tax Statement **2008**

Department of the Treasury—Internal Revenue Service

For Privacy Act and Paperwork Reduction Act Notice, see back of Copy D.

Cat. No. 10134D

Copy A For Social Security Administration — Send this entire page with Form W-3 to the Social Security Administration; photocopies are **not** acceptable.

Do Not Cut, Fold, or Staple Forms on This Page — Do Not Cut, Fold, or Staple Forms on This Page

Figure 33-13 Form W-2 summarizes all earnings and deductions for the year and must be prepared for each employee by January 31.

regarding printed and electronic filing forms, go to the Internal Revenue Service Web site (http://www.irs.gov) for detailed instructions. It is a good idea to have employees update their W-4 form each year in case they want to adjust their deductions or make any other change. To accomplish this, many payroll managers include a new W-4 form with the first paycheck at the beginning of each year. Every employee file should contain Social Security number, number of exemptions claimed on the W-4 Form, employee's gross salary, and all deductions withheld for all taxes, including Social Security, federal, state, local, and unemployment tax (where applicable), and disability insurance (where applicable).

To process payroll, the provider's office must have a federal tax reporting number, obtained from the Internal Revenue Service. In some states, a state employer number also is needed.

Preparing Payroll Checks. When preparing payroll checks, it is important to keep a record of all tax and insurance amounts deducted from an employee's earnings. Many ambulatory care settings that operate on a manual bookkeeping system find that the write-it-once system is the most efficient way to accurately maintain these records. Payroll records should include:

- Employee name, address, and telephone number
- Social Security number
- Date of employment

Each paycheck stub should contain:

- Number of hours worked, including regular and overtime (if hourly)
- Dates of pay period
- Date of check
- Gross salary
- Itemized deductions for federal income tax, Social Security (FICA) tax, state tax, city or local tax
- Itemized deductions for health insurance and disability insurance

- Other deductions such as uniforms, loan payments, and so on
- Net salary (gross earnings minus taxes and deductions)

Procedure 33-7 provides steps for processing payroll.

Figuring Employee Taxes. When figuring federal income taxes and Social Security taxes, use the "Circular E" tables provided by the Internal Revenue Service. Federal tax is based on amount earned, marital status, number of exemptions claimed, and length of pay period. State and city or local taxes are typically a percentage of the gross earnings.

All federal and state taxes withheld must be paid on a quarterly basis to the appropriate government offices. These monies should be accompanied by the required reporting forms. It is important to observe deposit requirements for withheld income tax and Social Security and Medicare taxes. These requirements, which change frequently, are listed in the Federal Employer's Tax Guide, available from the U.S. Government Printing Office, Internal Revenue Service (or online at http://www.irs.gov).

Managing Benefits and Other Responsibilities. **Benefits,** or additional remuneration to the salary earned by full-time employees, must be managed and records maintained for each employee. Examples of benefits include paid vacation, paid holidays, health/dental insurance, disability, **profit-sharing** options, and complimentary health care. Some ambulatory care settings may refer to all or some of these benefits as **fringe benefits.**

Other responsibilities of the office manager include maintaining a personnel file for each employee providing his or her history with the facility, application for the current position, evaluations, promotions, problems, awards, entitlements, legal forms required by state and federal agencies, and so on. All Occupational Safety and Health Administration (OSHA) data, hazard material training and documentation, HIPAA training documentation, cardiopulmonary resuscitation (CPR) certifications, immunization records, AIDS education, and confidentiality agreement must be recorded and maintained.

FACILITY AND EQUIPMENT MANAGEMENT

The physical plant or building must be observed and maintained with safety being a key ingredient. It should be the responsibility of each staff member to report to the office manager any facility repairs that require attention and suggest replacement or recommend new pieces of equipment as required by the practice to support the health care needs of its population.

The office manager usually is responsible for maintenance of the office and may hire **ancillary services** to provide janitorial and laundry services, dispose of hazardous materials, and maintain aquariums or plants that may enhance the environment of the facility. The office manager must be cognitive of the importance of patient confidentiality when ancillary services are present. Ancillary services must not view confidential material. A signed Business Associate agreement must be on file for each ancillary service contracted.

Magazine subscriptions and health-related literature for the reception area are the responsibility of the office manager. Selections should be made carefully, keeping in mind the interests of the patients and their cultures. These materials should not be kept once they become dog-eared, torn, and outdated. The use of plastic protectors and appropriate storage shelving aid in keeping the area and materials tidy.

The office manager, together with the provider, is responsible for facility improvements, including any necessary repairs, decorating and color scheme, and floor plan suggestions. The wise office manager does not make these decisions independently but asks for suggestions from staff members. Remember, the team-building approach adds a cohesive element to any office environment.

Administrative and Clinical Inventory of Supplies and Equipment

All administrative and clinical supplies and equipment in the facility must be inventoried. Maintaining a sufficient inventory of administrative and medical supplies requires implementation of a system for taking inventory of supplies frequently enough to permit placing and receiving an order before a shortage occurs. Large facilities frequently use the TPMS to inventory items that normally would be billed as part of a procedure, but this will not identify routinely used medical and administrative supplies.

Medical offices operate on a budget, so comparison shopping is prudent. Many companies have online catalogs with full descriptions and prices of their products. The cost of an item is not the only consideration when purchasing inventory. Consider the following:

- Warranties
- Bulk orders
- Maintenance agreements
- Quality and durability
- Personal preferences
- Cost factors

Online ordering via the Internet can save time and money. When placing orders, select those with secure Web sites; it is generally safe to use credit cards with these vendors. Supplies also can be ordered through hardcopy catalogs. Benchmarking with other medical offices nets valuable information in determining reputable vendors.

When an order is received, it must be opened and checked properly. Look first for the packing slip, which lists the items ordered and the items shipped. Verify that no items have been substituted or backordered. Each item unpacked must be checked with the packing slip to be sure there are no discrepancies. Write the date the shipment was received, who verified it, and any follow-up information. The new stock should be stored appropriately.

Some items purchased come with a warranty. A warranty usually is activated online at the vendor's Web site or by using a warranty card packaged with the purchased item. Warranty cards are similar to postcards and establish the purchase date and name and address of the purchaser. The returned warranty information provides the vendor with information should it be necessary to notify the buyer of recalls or defective parts. It is also proof of purchase and gives the length of time the warranty is in effect.

It is important to create a file for each piece of equipment in the medical office. Information in this file should include:

- Date of purchase and original receipt
- Manufacturer name, address, and telephone number
- Model number and owner's manual
- Technical support information and telephone number
- Warranty information
- Service agreement
- Date last serviced
- Routine maintenance or calibration information

The steps for inventorying supplies and equipment for administrative and clinical needs are given in Procedure 33-8.

Administrative and Clinical Equipment Calibration and Maintenance

Administrative and clinical equipment must be cleaned, calibrated, and maintained on a regular basis. Most offices use a computer spreadsheet or relational-type database, depending on the size of the facility. The database identifies the equipment by name or type, its assigned facility identification number, location in the facility, warranty expiration date, service period, dates when service and calibration were last performed, and when the next service or calibration will be required. The database also may identify service contracts for equipment not maintained or calibrated by facility personnel and information on service contractors of equipment, such as contacts, phone numbers, and addresses. The database is backed up by a paper file containing operation manuals, warranty information, and service contracts.

Administrative equipment such as the computer should be cleaned and maintained regularly. Telephones as well as any other pieces of equipment should be cleaned and working order checked.

Laboratory and clinical equipment must be maintained and quality-control measures utilized. Calibration checks are required for a number of pieces of equipment: sphygmomanometers and centrifuges to name two. Microscopes and various types of scopes used during physical examinations and specialty procedures contain light sources that must be checked before each use. A replacement supply of bulbs should be available. See Chapter 26 for more information on quality control and safety in the medical laboratory. Assigning a clinical laboratory manager to oversee the equipment is a good idea. Procedure 33-9 provides steps for routine maintenance or calibration of administrative and clinical equipment.

The office storage areas should be well maintained, and each item should always be put back in its place with lids replaced properly to prevent any accidents. Medication storage requires special attention. Many medications must be stored at certain temperatures, kept dry, or stored in dark, airtight containers. All medications, including samples, must be kept out of patient access areas. Narcotics should always be stored in a separate locked cabinet. Dispensing requires two individuals to sign off when narcotic supplies are used. A daily inventory should be maintained.

LIABILITY COVERAGE AND BONDING

Negligence is performing an act that a reasonable and prudent provider would not perform or failure to perform an act that a reasonable and prudent provider would perform. The common term used to describe professional **liability** or legal responsibility today is **malpractice.** It is much easier to prevent malpractice than to defend it in litigation; therefore every effort should be taken to prevent negligence. Events that could result in a malpractice litigation invariably will occur from time to time in even the best of medical offices. When such an incident occurs, complete honesty with the patient and insurance carrier is the best policy. Protocols should be implemented or existing ones revised to prevent any future occurrences, and all steps necessary to minimize risk to the patient should be taken.

Insurance policies specifically designed to protect the provider's assets in the event a liability claim is filed and awarded in the patient's favor are available. Any provider not carrying such insurance is said to be **"going bare"** and would personally be responsible for any court costs, damages, and attorney fees if a malpractice suit were lost.

Practicing medical assistants should carry **professional liability insurance** for protection. Medical assistants who are members of the American Association of Medical Assistants (AAMA) have the option of purchasing personal and professional insurance through the organization at corporate rates.

Some providers carry the names of their employees on their policies. If this is the case, always ask to see the policy and verify that your name is printed on the policy—no name indicates no coverage. The manager may need to see that professional liability insurance has been purchased, all appropriate names are listed, and the premiums are paid in a timely fashion.

Professional liability insurance is important if the provider–employer is sued. In this event, the provider and the medical assistant could be named in the suit. If the case were lost, both the provider and the medical assistant could be liable.

Individuals who are responsible for handling financial records and money in the medical office may be bonded. A **bond** is purchased for a cash value in an employee's name that ensures that the provider will recover the amount of loss in the event that an employee **embezzles** funds. It is the office manager or the HR manager's responsibility to ask prospective employees if they are bondable. Individuals who are not bondable may not be the best candidates for the position.

LEGAL ISSUES

The office manager must be aware of and follow all state and federal regulations impacting the practice. Information related to Clinical Laboratory Improvement Amendments of 1988 (CLIA '88) and Occupational Safety and Health Administration (OSHA) can be found in Chapter 26. Federal regulations related to provider office laboratories (POLs) are discussed in Chapter 26. The Centers for Medicare and Medicaid Services Web site also is helpful (http://www.cms.hhs.gov).

Procedure 33-1

Completing a Medical Incident Report

PURPOSE:
To complete a medical incident report and submit it in a timely manner.

EQUIPMENT/SUPPLIES:
Appropriate medical incident report form
Computer with Incident Report Software

PROCEDURE STEPS:

1. Complete the office-approved Medical Incident Report form. A single-sheet, multiple-copy form is best. The form should contain basic patient identification data, a checklist of different incidents, and a space for written comments. RATIONALE: Ensures that all information needed is documented.
2. The person completing the incident report form should be the individual who witnessed the incident, first discovered the incident, or is most familiar with the incident. RATIONALE: This ensures the most accurate recording of the incident.
3. Each section of the form must be completed. The incident description should be a brief narrative consisting of an objective description of the facts but should not draw any conclusions. Quotes should be used when appropriate with any unwitnessed incidents (e.g., "Patient states..."). The name(s) of any witnesses should be included on the report as well as employees directly involved in the incident. RATIONALE: To provide unbiased information without making judgments.
4. Incident reports must be submitted in a timely manner to the appropriate administrator or office following protocol identified in the Procedure Manual for the office. RATIONALE: Ensures that appropriate documentation and action is taken for follow-up.

Procedure 33-2

Preparing a Meeting Agenda

PURPOSE:
To prepare a meeting agenda, a list of specific items to be discussed or acted on, to maintain the focus of the group and allow business to be transacted in a timely fashion.

EQUIPMENT/SUPPLIES:
List of participants
Order of business
Names of individuals giving reports
Names of any guest speakers
Computer and paper to print agendas

PROCEDURE STEPS:

1. Reserve proposed date, time, and place of meeting. RATIONALE: Ensures that the facilities are available for the meeting.
2. Collect information for meeting agenda by previewing the previous meeting's minutes for old business items, checking with others for report items, and determining any new business items. RATIONALE: Ensures that all old and new business items have been identified.
3. Prepare a hard copy of the agenda and have it approved by chair of the meeting. RATIONALE: Confirmation by the chair of the agenda content ensures that agenda is correct and complete.
4. Send agenda to meeting participants a few days in advance of the meeting. RATIONALE: Permits participants to prepare for the meeting by completing any tasks required and preparing any necessary documentation.

Procedure 33-3

Supervising a Student Practicum

PURPOSE:

To prepare a training path for a student extern being assigned to the office. To make the involved office personnel aware of their responsibilities. To preplan which jobs the student extern performs and in what sequence they will be assigned. To make the practicum successful by providing as much supervision and assistance as necessary.

EQUIPMENT/SUPPLIES:

None needed

PROCEDURE STEPS:

1. Review the clinical practicum contract or agreement between your agency and the educational institution. RATIONALE: Guidelines and procedures are reviewed and refreshed in your mind.
2. Determine the amount of supervision the student will require. RATIONALE: Prepares you to speak with the student and site supervisor regarding supervision.
3. Identify the supervisor who will be immediately responsible for the student. RATIONALE: Establishes a person who knows he or she is to supervise the student and be responsible for the practicum procedures.
4. Plan what tasks the student will be allowed or encouraged to perform. RATIONALE: The office may or may not permit the student to perform invasive procedures. Determining tasks the student can and cannot perform beforehand promotes a better relationship.
5. Create a schedule outlining the time the student will be assigned to each unit. RATIONALE: Establishing a schedule keeps everyone appraised of what is happening and when.
6. Begin orientation for the student as soon as he or she arrives at the office. Include a tour of the office and introduction to the staff. RATIONALE: Orients student and staff to each other and establishes guidelines for procedures.
7. Give the student a copy of the Office Policy Manual and the work schedule for the entire practicum. Answer any questions the student might have. RATIONALE: Orients student and staff to each other and establishes guidelines for procedures.
8. Maintain an accurate record of the hours the student works. Also log the date and reason for any missed days, late arrivals, or early dismissals. RATIONALE: Provides necessary documentation for the hours completed by the student.
9. Check with the student frequently to be sure the student is receiving meaningful training from the work experience. RATIONALE: Verifies that necessary training is being provided.
10. Consult providers and staff members with whom the student has worked for their opinion of the student's capabilities. Follow up on any problems that might be identified. RATIONALE: Verifies that necessary training is being provided.
11. Report the student's progress to the medical assisting supervisor from the educational institution. This person usually visits once or twice each rotation. RATIONALE: Verifies that necessary training is being provided.
12. Prepare the student evaluation report from comments provided by the supervisor assigned and each employee who worked with the student. RATIONALE: Provides necessary documentation for the practicum experience.

Procedure 33-4

Developing and Maintaining a Procedure Manual

PURPOSE:

To develop and maintain a comprehensive, up-to-date procedure manual covering each medical, technical, and administrative procedure in the office, with step-by-step directions and rationale for performing each task.

EQUIPMENT/SUPPLIES:

Computer or electronic typewriter (electronic storage allows changes and revisions to be made easily)
Binder, such as a three-ring binder
Paper
Standard procedure manual format

PROCEDURE STEPS:

1. Write detailed, step-by-step procedures and rationales for each medical, technical, and administrative function. Each procedure is written by experienced employees close to the function and then reviewed by a supervisor and office manager. Rationales help employees understand *why* something is done. RATIONALE: Establishes consistent guidelines to be followed.
2. Include regular maintenance instructions and flow sheets for cleaning, servicing, and calibrating of all office equipment, both in the clinical area and in the office/business areas. RATIONALE: Equipment needs to be cleaned and maintained on a regular basis to ensure it is working properly and that it lasts as long as needed. Some manufacturer guarantees and service contracts require regular cleaning and maintenance, especially on new and leased equipment. Instructions are necessary so that the task can be performed properly. The flow sheets provide documentation of dates the equipment was cleaned, serviced, and/or calibrated and the person who performed the task.
3. Include step-by-step instructions on how to accomplish each task in the office/clinic in both the clinical area and in the office/business areas. RATIONALE: Clear and concise instructions ensure that each task is consistently performed to the clinic standards.
4. Include local and out-of-the-area resources for clinical staff, office/business staff, providers, and patients. Provide a listing in each area with contact information and services provided. RATIONALE: The procedures and instructions listed in the Procedure Manual should provide supporting documentation needed for accomplishing each task. For example, if the clinic requires that local public transportation resources be given to each patient who needs transportation, the Procedure Manual has a listing of all transportation available in the area with telephone numbers and schedules. This document could either be printed from the computer or photocopied from the manual and provided to the patient.
5. Include basic rules and regulations, state and federal, which are related to processes performed in both clinical and office/business areas. RATIONALE: Having a listing of the rules and regulations assists in performing those regulated duties correctly and legally.
6. Include the clinic procedures and flow sheets for taking inventory in each of the areas and instructions on ordering procedures. RATIONALE: When a clinic has processes clearly written for managing inventory and ordering of equipment and supplies, the clinic is less likely to run out of needed items and may even be able to take advantage of discounts offered by manufacturers.
7. Collect the procedures into the Office Procedure Manual. RATIONALE: Provides a reference guide with step-by-step instructions and examples where appropriate.
8. Store one complete manual in a common library area. Provide a completed copy to the provider–employer and the office manager. Distribute appropriate sections to the various departments. RATIONALE: Provides a reference guide with step-by-step instructions and examples where appropriate.
9. Review the procedure manual annually and add any new procedures, delete or modify as necessary, and indicate the revision date (Rev. 10/12/XX). RATIONALE: Maintains current office protocols.

Procedure 33-5

Making Travel Arrangements with a Travel Agent

PURPOSE:

To make travel arrangements for the provider.

EQUIPMENT/SUPPLIES:

Travel plan
Telephone and telephone directory
Computer
Provider's or office credit card to pay for reservations

PROCEDURE STEPS:

1. Confirm the details of the planned trip: dates, time, and place for departure and arrival; preferred mode of transportation (plane, train, bus, car); number of travelers; preferred lodging type and price range; and whether travelers checks are required. RATIONALE: Confirming pertinent travel details ensures that correct arrangements will be made.
2. Make travel and lodging reservations by calling travel agent or using the computer for online ticket services. RATIONALE: Ensure that space for provider is reserved at desired times.
3. Pick up tickets or arrange for their delivery.
4. Check to see that ticket arrangements are accurate (dates, times, places).
5. Check to see that car rental and lodging accommodations are accurate and confirmed. RATIONALE: Avoid inaccuracies and confusion with schedule.
6. Make additional copies of the itinerary or create the itinerary if making arrangements via computer. The itinerary should list date and time of departures and arrivals, including flight numbers and seat assignments. Note mode of transportation to lodging (shuttle, bus, car, taxi). Include name, address, and telephone number of lodgings and meeting places.
7. Maintain one copy of the itinerary in the office file.
8. Give several copies of the itinerary to the provider. RATIONALE: Ensure that a copy is on file with the office and that there are sufficient copies for the traveler(s) and their families.

Procedure 33-6

Making Travel Arrangements via the Internet

PURPOSE:

To make travel arrangements for the provider using the Internet.

EQUIPMENT/SUPPLIES:

Travel plan
Computer
Provider's or office credit card to pay for reservations.

PROCEDURE STEPS:

1. Confirm the details of the planned trip: dates, time, and place for departure and arrival; preferred mode of transportation (plane, train, bus, car); number of travelers; preferred lodging type and price range; and whether travelers checks are required. RATIONALE: Confirming pertinent travel details ensures that correct arrangements will be made.
2. Go to the computer and access the Internet.
3. Select a search engine to locate Web pages using the key term "air fares." Web pages may provide links to air fares, auto reservations, and hotel/motel reservations. Follow Web page instructions for making arrangements. Review and copy confirmation of your transaction. RATIONALE: The Internet can be a time saver and a cost-effective way of securing travel arrangements.
4. Pick up tickets or arrange for their delivery, if necessary. Tickets purchased on the Internet can

continues

Procedure 33-6 (continued)

be mailed or picked up at an airport, or they can be electronic tickets.

5. Make additional copies of the itinerary or create the itinerary. The itinerary should list date and time of departures and arrivals, including flight numbers and seat assignments. Note the mode of transportation to lodging (shuttle, bus, car, taxi). Include name, address, and telephone number of lodgings and meeting places.
6. Maintain one copy of the itinerary in the office file.
7. Give several copies of the itinerary to the provider. RATIONALE: Ensure that a copy is on file with the office and that there are sufficient copies for the traveler(s) and their families.

Procedure 33-7

Processing Employee Payroll

PURPOSE:

To process payroll compensating employees, calculating all deductions accurately.

EQUIPMENT/SUPPLIES:

Computer and payroll software or checkbook
Tax withholding tables
Federal Employers Tax Guide

PROCEDURE STEPS:

1. Verify copies of the employee's Social Security card and current I-9 and W-4 forms are in each employee file. RATIONALE: Provides verification that employee is eligible to work in the United States and to calculate withholding amounts that should be deducted from paychecks.
2. Review time cards looking for any tardiness, early dismissals, or absences. RATIONALE: To access any problems that could lead to termination. Be sure to document any that may be found and action taken.
3. Calculate the salary or hourly wages due the employee for the work period. RATIONALE: To determine the amount owed each employee.
4. Calculate any deductions that must be withheld from the paycheck. These may include federal, state, and local taxes; Social Security withholdings; Medicare withholdings; insurance; savings; or donations. RATIONALE: To ensure compliance with all federal, state, and local laws and satisfy all proper deductions are made.
5. Use computer and payroll software or hand write the payroll check and explanation of deductions.
6. Distribute individual payroll checks in envelopes according to office protocol. RATIONALE: Ensures compliance and confidentiality issues are maintained.

Procedure 33-8

Perform an Inventory of Equipment and Supplies

PURPOSE:

To develop an inventory of expendable administrative and clinical supplies in a medical office.

EQUIPMENT/SUPPLIES:

Printout of most recent inventory spreadsheet, listing items by storage location, name and identification code, number of items, minimum quantity requiring reorder, date and quantity of last reorder, and expiration date of items if any.

Clipboard, pad of reorder forms, pen or pencil.

PROCEDURE STEPS:

1. Compare number of items on hand corresponding to each name or code identification number with the printout, and write in the new inventory number on the printout. RATIONALE: To determine what is on hand and what needs to be ordered.
2. If the number of any item is less than the minimum quantity, fill out a reorder form listing completely the name, identification number, and quantity required.
3. Repeat the previous step for each storage location on the inventory printout sheet.
4. After completing the inventory, enter the new inventory information, including date of inventory, quantity, and date of reorder request, into the computer database. RATIONALE: To determine what needs to be ordered.
5. Forward the reorder forms to the person responsible for purchasing. RATIONALE: To forward information to the person responsible for reordering supplies and equipment.

NOTE: If the office or clinic uses handheld computers on a wireless network, all of the printouts and reorder forms can be entered directly into the computer record while doing the inventory, making unnecessary the reentry and preparation of reorder forms. If the handheld computer is not networked, it will be necessary to download or sync the data after completing the inventory.

Procedure 33-9

Perform Routine Maintenance or Calibration of Administrative and Clinical Equipment

PURPOSE:

To ensure the operability and calibration of administrative and clinical equipment.

EQUIPMENT/SUPPLIES:

Equipment list with maintenance or calibration requirements

Clipboard, pen, maintenance record sheets, and deficiency tags

Access to operation and service manuals of equipment to be serviced

Access to any necessary maintenance tools and supplies

PROCEDURE STEPS:

1. Date the maintenance record. RATIONALE: Documents when equipment was last checked and serviced.
2. Check equipment for cleanliness and clean thoroughly if required. RATIONALE: Equipment works more efficiently when clean; this is a safety issue as well.
3. Perform visual safety check for electrical and mechanical integrity. RATIONALE: Visual inspection quickly determines deficiencies.
4. Tag any equipment with safety hazards and report the deficiency. RATIONALE: Equipment with safety hazards should not be used until repaired to protect operators.
5. Check for operability using procedures defined in the operation manual.
6. Check to ensure the equipment meets operational/calibration standards as defined in the

continues

Procedure 33-9 (continued)

operation and service manual. Recalibrate the equipment following the instructions in the manual if required. RATIONALE: Calibration standards must be maintained for correct results.

7. Tag any equipment not meeting operational standards and report the deficiency. RATIONALE: Equipment must be either replaced or repaired to ensure proper results.
8. Fill out and sign the maintenance record sheet if the equipment meets operations standards. RATIONALE: Documents routine maintenance was performed.

NOTE: The equipment list, maintenance records, and deficiency reports may be included in the TPMS of many practices.

Case Study 33-1

Review the scenario at the beginning of the chapter.

Drs. Lewis and King have requested sigmoidoscopy procedures to be scheduled for two different patients. The patients are scheduled. Both patients are put on a strict diet and pretest protocol for several days to prepare for the procedures. The day of the appointments, Marilyn Johnson, CMA (AAMA), and office manager, discovers that the two sigmoidoscopy procedures have been scheduled at the same time. The problem is that the office has only one sigmoidoscope available.

CASE STUDY REVIEW

1. Divide the class into two groups to discuss problem-solving solutions. Assume that rescheduling a patient is not an acceptable solution because of the patient's pretest protocol. The patients would be upset if the procedure could not be performed due to a scheduling problem.
2. How could this problem have been avoided?
3. Both patients have been told about the scheduling problem and one is upset and argumentative. What role should the office manager assume in this predicament?

Case Study 33-2

Anita Juarez, the office administrative medical assistant, speaks privately with Jane O'Hara, the office manager and the person responsible for personnel. Anita has a suspicious lump in her breast. She has seen both her internist and a surgeon for evaluation. Next week, she will have the lump removed, perhaps even a complete mastectomy. Anita is concerned about the time she will need to be away from the office.

CASE STUDY REVIEW

1. Identify the first and immediate concerns to be addressed.
2. What action might be taken to help both Anita and the office manager address these concerns?
3. Is it helpful to plan for the best results, the worst results, or both?

SUMMARY

The office manager is the glue that holds the office together and keeps it running smoothly. When the manager sets a positive example for others and is considerate and aware of the diversity of others, a positive environment is created for teamwork. A teamwork approach enables the entire office to be more productive, provide the best health care, and foster an enjoyable work relationship.

The role of office manager varies greatly depending on the size of the medical practice, the provider's trust in the manager's competency level, and the provider's comfort in delegating authority to others. An effective office manager is a tremendous asset to providers. The personal and financial rewards are worthwhile to the medical assistant who desires a new dimension to explore and enjoys a challenge.

STUDY FOR SUCCESS

To reinforce your knowledge and skills of information presented in this chapter:

- Review the Key Terms
- Practice the Procedures
- Consider the Case Studies and discuss your conclusions
- Answer the Review Questions
    - Multiple Choice
    - Critical Thinking
- Navigate the Internet by completing the Web Activities
- Practice the StudyWARE activities on the textbook CD
- Apply your knowledge in the Student Workbook activities
- Complete the Web Tutor sections

REVIEW QUESTIONS

Multiple Choice

1. For teamwork to be successful, individual team members must:
    a. do as they are told by the office manager
    b. not ask why they are doing something a certain way
    c. understand and support the task
    d. think independently and solve the problem on their own
2. Meeting minutes:
    a. should address each agenda topic and include a brief summary of discussions, actions taken, name of each person making a motion, the exact wording of motions, and motion approval or defeat
    b. are a detailed plan for a proposed trip
    c. include information regarding mode of transportation and lodging reservations
    d. must follow parliamentary procedures
3. When working with practicum students, it is important to remember that:
    a. they should have expert knowledge about their field
    b. they do not need supervision when working with a patient
    c. they are experienced with working on real patients
    d. they have much to learn
4. Which of the following statements is *not* correct regarding a student practicum?
    a. It is a transitional stage that provides opportunity for students to apply theory learned in the classroom to a health care setting through hands-on experience.
    b. It assumes that the student is an employee who does not need to be introduced to patients.
    c. It may require the student to shadow another medical assistant for a few days.
    d. It involves an evaluation of the student's progress.
5. The procedure manual:
    a. is a detailed plan for a proposed trip
    b. provides detailed information regarding mode of transportation and lodging reservations
    c. provides detailed information relative to the performance of tasks within the health care facility
    d. summarizes action details of staff meetings

6. Developing relationships outside the office is often called:
   a. marketing
   b. benchmarking
   c. advertising
   d. sales
7. Record and financial management involves all of the following *except:*
   a. payroll processing
   b. preparing payroll checks
   c. figuring taxes
   d. equipment and supplies maintenance
8. Controlled substances must:
   a. be kept separate from other drugs
   b. be stored in a separate locked cabinet
   c. be recorded in a book that is maintained daily
   d. all of the above

Critical Thinking

1. How would you, as the office manager, handle someone who is spreading a harmful rumor about another employee in the office?
2. How can the office manager promote open and honest communication?
3. The student practicum can be a stressful time for the extern. As an office manager, how can you help the extern feel more at ease the first day of "work"?
4. Describe how a procedure manual for a single-provider practice would differ from a procedure manual for a multiprovider practice.
5. Describe how a procedure manual could become outdated and need revision.

WEB ACTIVITIES

Use the Web sites given in the text or alternative sites you know about to plan a trip between two cities within the United States. Compare the fares for Sunday departure and Friday return dates with the fares for low-volume days as obtained from the Priceline.com site. Also compare fares on flights purchased within 1 week of departure with fares on flights purchased 1 month before departure. Follow the instructor's instructions on completing and turning in your results.

REFERENCES/BIBLIOGRAPHY

Colbert, B. J. (2000). *Workplace readiness for health occupations.* Clifton Park, NY: Delmar Cengage Learning.

ingenix. (2003). *HIPAA tool kit.* Salt Lake City, UT: St. Anthony Publishing/Medicode.

Krager, D., & Krager, C. (2005). *HIPAA for medical office personnel.* Clifton Park, NY: Delmar Cengage Learning.

The Medical Assistant as Human Resources Manager

Chapter 34

KEY TERMS

Exit Interview
Involuntary Dismissal
Job Description
Letter of Reference
Letter of Resignation
Overtime
Probation

OUTLINE

OBJECTIVES

The student should strive to meet the following performance objectives and demonstrate an understanding of the facts and principles presented in this chapter through written and oral communication.

1. Define the key terms as presented in the glossary.
2. Describe the role of the human resources manager.
3. Explain the function of the office policy manual.
4. Identify methods of recruiting employees for a medical practice.
5. Discuss the interview process.
6. Identify items to keep in an employee's personnel record.
7. List and define a minimum of four laws related to personnel management.
8. Compare and contrast voluntary and involuntary separations.
9. Recall continuing education possibilities for employees.

Scenario

Jane O'Hara, CMA (AAMA), is the office manager at Inner City Health Care. She also functions in the role of the human resources manager. Part of her responsibilities includes recruiting, hiring, and orienting employees.

In one day Jane may meet with Dr. Rice to update the policy manual; begin the hiring process for a new medical assistant; welcome a new provider to the practice, being sure she completes all the necessary employment forms; and meet with another staff member to evaluate her continuing education.

INTRODUCTION

The medical assistant's employment responsibilities are many and varied. As you learned in Chapter 33, often they become office managers and assume a quite different function in the medical setting. The size of the ambulatory care setting and the number of employees likely determines if a human resources (HR) manager is a part of the practice. Whether the HR manager heads an HR department in a large, corporate medical setting with the title Human Resources Manager or is a medical assistant/office manager who serves as the HR representative, there are some common tasks assigned as specific HR duties.

TASKS PERFORMED BY THE HUMAN RESOURCES MANAGER

Tasks usually assigned to the HR manager include determining job descriptions for, hiring, and orienting employees; maintaining employee personnel records that include credentials and continuing education units (CEUs); and managing employee separations. With today's quest for greater office efficiency and the tremendous increase in federal and state regulatory requirements, the skills required of an HR manager have greatly broadened. Former responsibilities have been expanded to include preparing the policy manual, scheduling employee evaluations, preventing and investigating discrimination and harassment claims, and complying with regulatory agencies. The HR manager also assists in providing training and educational opportunities for employees so they are up to date in all aspects of quality patient care.

Increasingly, HR managers are expected to be able to support the organization's efforts that focus on productivity, service, and quality. In a climate in which there are too few persons for the positions to be filled and the delivery methods for health care are changing almost daily, productivity, service, and quality are essential to a successful practice. It becomes the responsibility of the HR manager to see that every employee's productivity level is high, that the service is A+, and that quality is at the highest level. Today's customers, the patients, often choose their health care provider on the basis of service and quality.

The position of HR manager now requires a higher level of education and experience to better grasp the legal and regulatory aspects of personnel management. The HR manager also must have excellent people skills, a

Spotlight on Certification

RMA Content Outline

- Medical law
- Medical ethics
- Human relations

CMA (AAMA) Content Outline

- Basic principles (psychology)
- Interview techniques
- Medicolegal guidelines and requirements
- Maintaining the physical plant
- Office policies and procedures

CMAS Content Outline

- Legal and ethical considerations
- Professionalism
- Human resources

strong sense of fairness, and the ability to resolve conflicts. None of this is accomplished in a vacuum. It requires working in close cooperation with the office manager and the employer(s).

This chapter discusses these responsibilities in the following separate but overlapping functions:

1. Creating and updating the office policy manual
2. Recruiting and hiring office personnel
3. Orienting new personnel
4. Scheduling salary reviews
5. Conducting exit interviews
6. Maintaining personnel records
7. Complying with all state and federal regulations regarding personnel
8. Planning/providing employee training and education
9. Maintaining records of credentials, licensure, certifications, and CEUs such as cardiopulmonary resuscitation (CPR)

THE OFFICE POLICY MANUAL

The procedure manual described in Chapter 33 identifies specific methods of performing tasks. The policy manual provides more general guidelines for office practices (Table 34-1).

Table 34-1 Possible Content of Policy and Procedure Manuals

Policy Manual	Procedure Manual
Mission statement	Details of procedures performed
Employer(s) biographic data	Administrative procedures
Employment issues	Clinical procedures
Wages, salaries, and benefits	Safety issues
Employee conduct	Asepsis
Confidentiality guidelines	Material Safety Data Sheets
HIPAA compliance	Emergency protocol

The policy manual identifies clear guidelines and directions required of all employees. It also defines appropriate expectations and boundaries of the employment relationship. Having written policies means not having to determine a policy on a case-by-case basis. Policy manuals will vary by the size of the practice or problems to be addressed, but some topics include the mission statement of the practice, biographic data on each provider, employment policies, wage and salary policies, benefits to be awarded, and employee conduct expectations.

Establishing and stating the mission of the practice clearly identifies the goals and objectives to be sought by each employee. Having biographic data of each provider helps employees to respond to queries from patients about a provider's experience, education, and interests.

Employment policies might include statements on equal employment opportunity, job requirements for particular positions and to whom the person reports, recruitment and selection procedures, orientation of new employees, probation, and dismissal. Wage and salary policies should be in writing. How are employees classified, what are the working hours, how is overtime compensated, how are salary increases determined, what benefits (medical, retirement, vacation, holidays, sick leave, profit sharing) does the practice have? The answers to such questions are part of the policy manual. Employee conduct is another piece of the policy manual. A statement regarding the confidentiality of all information received in the practice is essential in this area of the policy manual. Guidelines should be established about uniforms, dress codes, appearance, and personal hygiene. Can an employee hold a second job outside the practice? Is smoking allowed? Are staff members responsible for housekeeping duties?

When the policy manual is computerized, changes and updates are easily made (Figure 34-1). Any changes made are to be shared with employees so that everyone is up to date on policies. Having a policy manual with clearly written directives helps employees understand the expectations and boundaries of the employment relationship. The policy manual is reviewed with each new employee and updated on a regular basis. Procedure 34-1 provides details on developing and maintaining a policy manual.

RECRUITING AND HIRING OFFICE PERSONNEL

The majority of employees in the ambulatory care center are full-time, part-time, or occasional

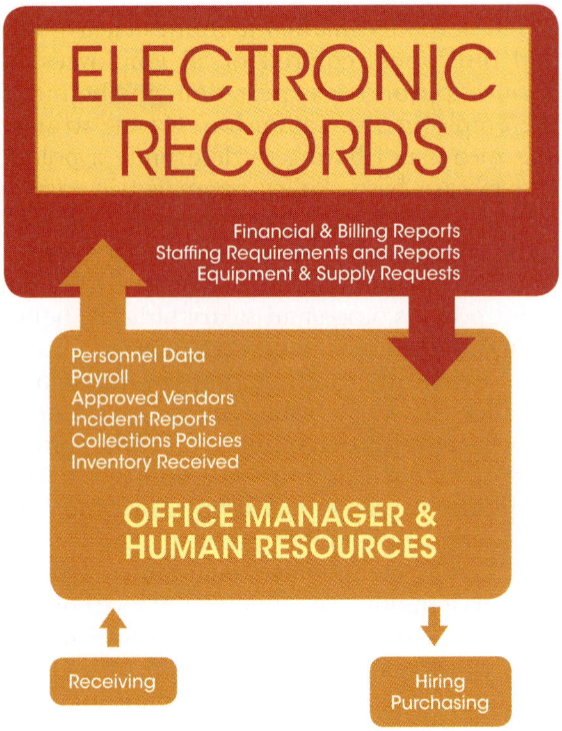
ELECTRONIC RECORDS
Financial & Billing Reports
Staffing Requirements and Reports
Equipment & Supply Requests
Personnel Data
Payroll
Approved Vendors
Incident Reports
Collections Policies
Inventory Received
OFFICE MANAGER & HUMAN RESOURCES
Receiving
Hiring
Purchasing

Figure 34-1 A total practice management system (TPMS) includes management and human resources functions.

independent contracted employees. Full-time employees generally work 30 hours or more per week; part-time employees work less than 30 hours per week. Either may be paid by the hour. Full-time employees may be salaried and are exempt from overtime regulations. Most part-time employees are paid by the hour. Benefits are often different between full- and part-time employees. Independent contractors usually work with the facility to perform specific predetermined tasks at a predetermined rate of pay for the services provided.

Before recruiting and hiring personnel to fill positions within the medical facility, the HR manager and employers must understand exactly what the role and responsibilities of the position are by having a current job description for the position and following a recruiting policy that is effective, fair, and observes all appropriate laws and regulations.

Job Descriptions

Before any position is filled, a **job description** must be in place. This usually is created cooperatively by the office manager and the employer(s). Once the job qualifications are defined, the lead personnel and HR manager can begin efforts to fill the position.

In daily operations most job descriptions are on file, but if the situation involves a new or greatly expanded office, a complete set of job descriptions is needed before recruiting can begin. Even when a written description is on file, it should be reviewed when a new employee is to be hired. The person who is leaving the position is often an excellent resource for the accuracy of the current job description and any changes that should be made.

The job description must include basic qualifications for the position and have enough information to provide both the supervisor and the employee with a clear outline of what the job entails (Figure 34-2). Necessary work experience, skills, education, and any special certification or licensure that is expected is to be identified in the job description. Procedure 34-2 provides details on preparing job descriptions.

Another important point with respect to the job description is that a review and update of the description should be done every year. Most jobs change constantly whether from a minor shifting of duties or the addition of some new technical procedure or device. Without updating a job description, a person with the wrong qualifications may be recruited to fill a vacancy.

Recruiting

A major challenge facing the HR manager today is recruitment. Medical assistants are listed in the top 10 occupations with employment growth much faster than average through 2014 according to the U.S. Department of Labor, Bureau of Labor Statistics. One reason for this demand is the aging of the U.S. population. It is estimated that more than 80% of jobs are in the service industry, and all health care positions fit into that category. When employers have been unsuccessful in recruiting qualified medical assistants, they have turned to contracting out some work, such as transcription and billing.

Once the hiring need is determined, the HR manager begins the recruitment process. Often a process called networking is a highly effective

Critical Thinking

Identify proper qualifications for an administrative medical assistant in a fairly large ambulatory care setting. Determine what work experience might qualify versus what work experience is preferred. Would certification be helpful? Explain.

JOB DESCRIPTION

POSITION TITLE:
Administrative Medical Assistant

REPORTS TO:
Office Manager and Provider–Employer(s)

RESPONSIBILITIES AND DUTIES:

- Being a therapeutic and helpful receptionist
  1. Answer telephone as quickly as possible, hopefully by the second ring
  2. Greet all patients warmly and with a helpful attitude
- Manage time efficiently with appropriate scheduling for patients and professional staff
  1. Schedule patients according to their needs, scheduling guidelines, staff availability, and equipment readiness
  2. Call to remind patients of their visit the day before appointment
- Responding to patient requests on the telephone and in person
  1. Ascertain reason for request
  2. Satisfy patient request or refer patient to one who can
- Preparing patient charts for professional staff
  1. Print schedules and encounter forms
  2. Pull patient charts late afternoon the day before appointment; print as necessary
  3. Check charts for completeness
  4. Attach encounter form when patient arrives to check in

AUTHORITY BOUNDARIES:
The office manager will assist in answering questions. Remember that it is better to ask than to make an error. Screening concerns not identified in a policy/procedure manual also can be directed to the clinical medical assisting staff.

POSITION REQUIREMENTS:
Two years experience and/or graduate of a medical assistant program. CMA (AAMA), RMA, or CMAS preferred.

Figure 34-2 Sample job description for administrative medical assistant.

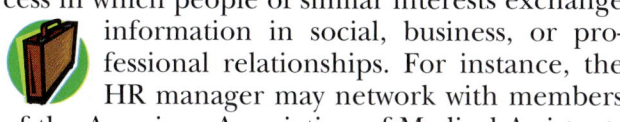

method of finding employees. Networking is a process in which people of similar interests exchange information in social, business, or professional relationships. For instance, the HR manager may network with members of the American Association of Medical Assistants and express an interest in a new employee for an open position. Current employees are often an excellent resource because they may know of a qualified person who is looking for a position.

Critical Thinking

Is there ever a time when providers are considered recruiters for their medical practice's personnel? When and how?

Checking with nearby colleges' medical assistant departments is another good resource. Employing a private or state placement agency is another possibility. Although newspaper advertisements may generate many résumés, they are only marginally effective as a search tool. It is often far too time consuming to review the large volume of applications generated by this approach. Online options may be beneficial. There are a number of medical employment Internet sites that identify positions for medical assistant personnel, often in specific localities.

Preparing to Interview Applicants

Once several applicants have expressed interest in the position, preparation for the interview begins. The HR manager should have a number of résumés to consider. Some may have already filled out a job application when they dropped off a résumé. The résumés and applications can be reviewed together. Some important points to remember in reading résumés and applications follow.

When considering education, look beyond the degree earned. Look for a good performance record at school and the kinds of supplemental education achieved. Does attendance at seminars and short-course training programs relate to your position needs? When reading a person's work history, make note of unexplained gaps in employment. You may want to ask specific questions in the interview. Has advancement been gained in each new position? Are the responsibilities and duties of the applicant's positions explained, or will questions need to be asked of the prospective employee?

Look for information that indicates if this candidate really enjoys the kind of work setting you have. Is the applicant comfortable serving the infirm? Can you truly identify the level of skill from the descriptions, or are the skills vague? The cover letter, if one is included, should address the specifics required of your position. Does the person display a negative or a positive attitude? Do not excuse any errors or unprofessional appearance in the job application or the résumé. Each should be letter perfect. An individual who is careless in this respect is likely to be careless on the job.

Some applications will be discarded when compared to the preceding guidelines. With the remaining candidates, determine who is to be interviewed and make telephone calls to establish interviews. You may make note of the quality of speaking skills, especially if this person will be using the telephone on the job. Make an interview appointment date with only those who seem truly interested in the position during your telephone conversation.

The Employment Interview

The employment interview is usually conducted by only one person if second interviews are anticipated. The provider–employer, office manager, or another employee may be present in either the first or the second interview, however (Figure 34-3). The interviewer(s) will want to review the application and résumé before the interview for particular points to ask the candidate. Before the interview, those doing the interviews should establish a set of questions for the applicants. These predetermined questions will help alleviate one applicant being given privileges over another and will help ensure continuity throughout all the interviews. An interview worksheet is an excellent tool to use to make certain that you are fair and equitable with each candidate. The worksheet should provide enough room for notes taken during the interview.

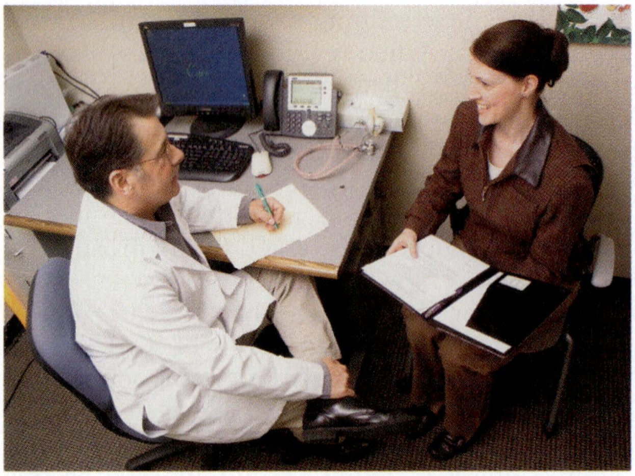

Figure 34-3 The interview can be conducted on a one-to-one basis with only the applicant and one staff member or with several staff members meeting with the applicant at once.

Suggested items for the interview worksheet are:

- Applicant's name
- Telephone number
- Education and training
- Work experience
- Special skills
- Professional demeanor
- Voice and mannerisms specific to position
- Questions and responses
- Ability to problem solve when given a scenario
- Any health-related or work-related problems applicant discloses
- Interviewer's personal impressions and recommendations

Conduct interviews in a quiet and private setting. Do not schedule interviews back to back without time to collect your thoughts or to allow you to compare notes with others participating in the interview. Ask job-related questions. For example, Describe your last job. What did you like best about it? What did you like least? What is most important to you about a job? Describe your administrative and clinical skills. Figure 34-4 shows some sample questions. Let the applicant do the most of the talking.

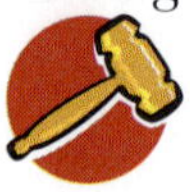

Any questions related to age, sex, race, religion, or national origin are inappropriate. Inquiries about medical history, drug use, or arrest records may not be made (see Chapter 7). Keep your questions related to performance on the job. If you may want to bond this employee, you may ask candidates if they have been bonded before or are willing to be bonded. It may be best to leave salary discussions for a second interview, but it can also be helpful to determine if applicants' salary expectations are in line with what you can offer. A question such as "What salary are you expecting?" is appropriate. Do not make a job offer until all the candidates selected for interview have been interviewed, and do not prejudge someone on any factor during or after the interview, except the person's qualifications.

At the close of the interview, let the applicant know when a decision will be made or whether a second interview will be conducted and how notification will be made. A tour of the facility and introduction to key staff members may be offered but are not necessary at the time of the first interview. Finally, thank the applicant for participating in the interview and being interested in the position.

General Questions

- What are your strengths and weaknesses?
- Why did you leave your last job?
- Identify what is most important to you in a job.

Questions Related to Work Relationships

- Describe an individual you have enjoyed working with.
- Explain how a conflict with a coworker was resolved.
- How would a coworker describe you?

Questions Related to Problem Solving

- Describe a work-related decision that made you very proud.
- Identify a task/procedure/assignment you could not do, and explain why.
- How do you approach a task when it seems mundane or boring?

Questions Related to Integrity

- If asked to do something you believe is illegal or unethical, what would you do?
- Tell us about a time when you broke a confidence.
- If you saw a coworker put a patient at risk, what would you do?

Figure 34-4 Common interview questions.

Selecting the Finalists

Shortly after the final interview is completed, the HR manager should compare notes with all the others involved in the interviews to select the top candidates. This is done by comparing notes and impressions from the interviews and by taking into consideration the ability of a candidate to work with patients and colleagues who might have a variety of problems and cultural backgrounds. The next step is to check references from former employers, supervisors, coworkers, and instructors. A large corporate medical practice may even have a consent form each candidate is asked to sign that gives permission to check references and call former employers and instructors. You may need to recognize, however, that even with a release from a potential new employee, many organizations and businesses restrict the release of reference information to only name, dates of employment, and title of position served. Telephone checks for references are an excellent strategy before you receive an immediate response. If you stress confidentiality when you make the contact, it will be easier for the person to respond to your questions. When possible, always check with more than one reference and former employer to get an accurate assessment of the candidate. All reference information is to be kept confidential. A sample telephone reference check form is shown in Figure 34-5.

TELEPHONE REFERENCE

Name of Applicant ____________________

Person Contacted ____________________

Position and Name of Business ____________________

____

Telephone Number ____________________

Relationship to Applicant ____________________

- May I verify the employment history of (applicant's name) who is applying for a position with our medical clinic?
  __________, 20____ to __________, 20____
- Describe the responsibilities held by this individual.
- Identify the salary ____________________
- What are this individual's strong points?
- What are this individual's weak points?
- Describe this individual's overall attitude toward the job and toward patients.
- Please comment on dependability and attendance.
- Given the opportunity, would you rehire? Why or why not?
- Why did this individual leave the job?
- Describe personal and professional growth this individual made while in your firm.
- Is there anything else you would like to tell us?

Reference call made by ____________________

Date ____________________

Figure 34-5 Sample form to use for telephone references.

A checklist of questions to ask might include:

1. What were the dates of employment of (name of applicant) in your firm?

2. Describe the job performed.
3. Reason for leaving the job?
4. Strong points of the employee?
5. Limitations of the employee?
6. Can you comment on attendance and dependability?
7. Would you rehire?
8. Anything else we should know about this candidate?

Offer the position when a first-choice candidate has been determined and indicate when a response is needed. Be prepared with a second-choice candidate should the preferred candidate respond negatively. At the time of the offer, the candidate should understand the salary offered, the starting date, the practice policies, and the benefits. When a candidate has accepted the position, a confirmation letter should be written that clearly spells out details discussed earlier. Give specific instructions on when and where the new employee should report the first day on the job. If practical, the employee should be given the policy and procedure manuals to read. Employers are required by federal law to verify that all employees are authorized to work. This is done by having the candidate complete an Eligibility Verification (I-9) form (see Case Study 34-2).

For the unsuccessful applicants, send a letter explaining that "we have selected another candidate whose qualifications and experience more closely meet our needs at this time. We would like to keep your résumé on file should another suitable position become available." Copies of these letters, as well as the interview checklists, should be kept for a minimum of 6 months should any questions arise regarding your choice of candidates. Procedure 34-3 provides details on interviewing.

ORIENTING NEW PERSONNEL

Orienting new employees is usually the responsibility of both the office manager and lead personnel who are most likely to work the closest with the new employee. It is common for a new employee to be placed on **probation** for 60 to 90 days, during which time both the employee and supervisory personnel may determine if the environment and the position are satisfactory for the employee. Procedure 34-4 outlines how to orient personnel.

Important elements to orientation include the introduction of the new employee to other staff members, assigning a mentor who can respond to questions, and making the employee aware of the procedures to be performed in this new position. If the procedure manual is detailed and accurate, this manual now becomes the daily guide for the new employee. Sometimes the individual leaving a position may still be present and is asked to assist in the orientation process. This is especially beneficial if there is a good working relationship between the employee who is leaving and the management of the practice. Depending on the responsibilities of the new employee, a supervisor may be asked to monitor all procedures for a period for accuracy, safety, and patient protection. During the probation period, the employee should be officially evaluated by the office manager.

DISMISSING EMPLOYEES

The function of employee dismissal or separation falls mostly to the office manager; however, in a large facility with an HR representative, discussing dismissal or separation with that individual can be quite beneficial. Such a discussion ensures that all the information necessary is in place before a separation. There are voluntary and involuntary dismissals or separations.

Voluntary separations usually occur when an employee is relocating, advancing to another position elsewhere, retiring, or leaving for personal reasons. A letter of resignation is usually submitted to both the office manager and the HR representative. These employees will give their manager proper notice and may be able to turn current projects and duties over to their replacement. There is also time to say good-bye to their colleagues and have a good feeling about their employment.

Involuntary dismissals or separations usually occur when an employee's performance is poor or there has been a serious violation of the office policies or job description. The office manager is aware of poor performance through the probationary reviews. Verbal and written warnings must be given to the employee and are to be well documented. Dismissal can be immediate if there is a serious breach of office policy. The HR director can provide necessary detail to the office manager regarding when and if immediate dismissal is recommended. If an office manager expects any serious difficulties with an employee during an immediate dismissal, the HR director should be present when the employee is notified. (see Chapter 33 for a more detailed discussion).

Exit Interview

An **exit interview** is an excellent opportunity for the employee who voluntarily leaves a practice and the HR manager to discuss the positive and negative aspects of the job and what changes might be made for a new person coming into the facility. A sample exit interview form is shown in Figure 34-6. It also allows the opportunity for the employee to ask for a **letter of reference** or to view the personnel file before leaving. In a voluntary dismissal, a **letter of resignation** for the personnel file is necessary.

Any dismissal process, voluntary or involuntary, must include a statement in the personnel file. For involuntary dismissal, be certain that the reasons for the dismissal are well documented in an honest, nonjudgmental statement. State only the facts in the personnel file; do not state opinion. Remember that employees have the right to view their personnel file at any time.

EXIT INTERVIEW FORM

1. What did you like and dislike about the work you have been doing?
   (Including: support on the job; opportunity for personal growth; recognition and rewards)
2. What kind of people have you found the providers, your immediate supervisor, and co-workers to be?
   (Including: attitude; fairness; scheduling and assignment of work; work expectations; technical competence; assistance and guidance available; team spirit)
3. What is your view of our management practices and policies?
   (Including: clarity and fairness of practice policies; communications; management and staff)
4. How have you felt about performance appraisals, your salary and benefits?
   (Including: adequacy of salary; regularity and fairness of appraisals)
5. What are your principal reasons for leaving the practice?
   (Including: primary dissatisfactions; job or personal changes)
6. In what areas do you feel we need to improve?

Interviewer signature: _______________ Date ________

Employee signature: _______________ Date ________

Figure 34-6 Sample exit interview form. (From Ricardo, M. (1992). *Personnel management handbook* [2nd ed.]. New York: The McGraw-Hill Companies, Inc. Copyright 1992. Reprinted with permission.)

Employers should always be informed of any dismissal as quickly as possible. Some may be involved in the actual dismissal process.

MAINTAINING PERSONNEL RECORDS

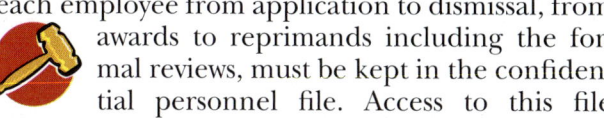

An important aspect of the responsibilities of the HR manager is maintaining personnel records. All documentation and correspondence related to each employee from application to dismissal, from awards to reprimands including the formal reviews, must be kept in the confidential personnel file. Access to this file is limited to certain management personnel and the employee. Not all of these people are allowed to see the entire file. These files are usually kept for a period of 3 to 5 years after employees leave the practice. Some of the personnel files may be maintained electronically on the computer. However, access to those files must be protected so that only those with authorized access are able to open the files or make changes to them.

This file also includes the kind of information normally maintained for payroll and business practices. That information includes name, address, and sex of employee. The position title, date of beginning employment, rate of pay (hourly or otherwise), total overtime pay, deductions or additions to wages, wages paid each pay period, and date employee leaves the practice also are included.

COMPLYING WITH PERSONNEL LAWS

This text is not meant to be a legal guide for an HR manager. The practice attorney should always be contacted if there is any question regarding personnel laws, which may vary in some states depending on the size of the practice. Only a brief introduction of the laws related to the ambulatory care setting are given.

Overtime must be addressed in each practice. Who is reimbursed for overtime and how is that reimbursement determined? Typically, administrative medical assistants, insurance billers, medical transcriptionists, and clinical medical assistants are likely to be paid overtime. Overtime pay at a rate of not less than one and one-half times the regular rate of pay after a 40-hour work week is standard. Each week stands alone and one week cannot compensate for another. If the practice does not want to be involved in overtime situations, require that any overtime be preauthorized in advance.

The Equal Pay Act of 1963 prevents wage discrimination for jobs that require equal skill, effort, and responsibility. The Civil Rights Act of 1964 prevents employers from discriminating against individuals on the basis of race, color, religion, sex, age, or national origin (see Chapter 7).

Sexual harassment violates Title VII of the Civil Rights Act. Steps must be taken to ensure that all employees are working in an atmosphere that is not hostile, where sexual gestures, the presence of pornographic or offensive materials, or obscene language are not allowed (see Chapter 7).

Employees have a right to expect safe working conditions. The Occupational Safety and Health Act (OSHA) was established to prevent injuries and illnesses resulting from unsafe or unhealthy working conditions (see Chapter 10 for detailed discussion of the standards and requirements, especially the section on bloodborne pathogens, which went into effect in 1992.) Compliance with this law requires that each employee be aware of possible risks associated with chemical hazards and how to protect themselves. Because there are many of these hazards in a medical practice, compliance and protection for employees are extremely important, and training sessions should be held in this area.

The Immigration Reform Act requires employers to verify the right of employees to work in the United States. Documentation acceptable for verification is a Social Security card or birth certificate. The U.S. Department of Justice Immigration and Naturalization Service will provide instructions and a form for employees and employers to complete, commonly referred to as the I-9 or Employment Eligibility Verification form.

Employers cannot discriminate against or condemn any full-time employee for jury duty. Although the employer does not have to continue pay during jury duty, the employee cannot lose seniority, insurance, or other benefits. Many employers continue an employee's full pay during the time of service on a jury because the reimbursement for jury service is minimal. This is a way to benefit employees and encourage good citizenship.

This list is by no means comprehensive but does include personnel regulations most likely to affect the medical practice. Any concerns should be directed to the practice's attorney.

SPECIAL POLICY CONSIDERATIONS

Several other managerial issues may arise in a medical setting for which the office manager and the HR manager will have to plan. These can include policies for temporary employees, rules of conduct, avoiding discrimination, and having a support system in place for employees who need physical or emotional help.

Temporary Employees

Temporary employees who may be employed for 90 days or less include students who are serving an internship or externship from a local college practicing their skills for when they will be on the job. They should be reviewed on a regular basis in cooperation with their college supervisor. Give them as much actual hands-on experience as possible; they are future employees. Accommodating students in the practice is a two-way benefit. Students learn what reality is in the ambulatory care setting and are able to practice newly developed skills. Current staff members in the facility are "sharpened" by the students' presence. Teaching and monitoring someone's actions always results in sharpening and rethinking the skills of the current staff. Many HR directors and managers depend on these programs for future job applicants.

Smoking Policy

Smoking on the premises, especially a health care facility, is a concern. Many places of employment do not allow smoking at all. Additionally, some states and cities have laws that govern this issue. When a policy is established, it should cover everyone—employers, employees, and patients. The objective is to have a policy that is workable and enforceable, promotes health, encourages employee morale and productivity, and sets examples for patients.

Discrimination

The Americans with Disabilities Act (ADA) prohibits discrimination by all private employers with 15 or more employees. Some states may further prohibit discrimination in facilities regardless of the size of their workforce. *All* public entities are prohibited from discrimination against qualified individuals with disabilities. The ADA establishes guidelines prohibiting discrimination against a "qualified individual with a disability" in regard to employment. Someone with a disability who satisfies the skills necessary for the job; has the experience, education, and any other job requirements; and who, with reasonable accommodation, can perform the job cannot be discriminated against. Employers often find that persons with disabilities are their finest employees.

Persons who are HIV-positive or have AIDS are included in the guidelines set forth by the ADA. Persons with HIV/AIDS cannot be discriminated against. It can be assumed that if a safe working environment is provided when all employees follow the rules for Standard Precautions; then reasonable accommodation has been made for the person with HIV or AIDS.

An employer cannot refuse the job to a qualified person based on the belief that in the future the employee may become too ill to work. The hiring decision must be based on the individual's ability to perform the functions of the position at the present time. If a current employee reveals to the manager that he or she is HIV positive or has AIDS, that information must be kept confidential and must be kept apart from the general personnel file. The manager may choose to hold a discussion at that time of what accommodations might be needed in the future.

PROVIDING/PLANNING EMPLOYEE TRAINING AND EDUCATION

Health care changes daily; new procedures are established, a better technique is discovered for performing a particular task. Major changes regularly occur in medical insurance. Computer systems are updated or new software is added. A more sophisticated telephone system is installed to make certain patients are responded to promptly. New state or federal regulations mandate additional training or compliance in safety. New medications become available that providers may prescribe and employees must understand. All this demands that employees receive a continuing and constant update in their area of employment.

Training and education may be accomplished within the practice or outside the practice. When an employee is a member of a professional organization such as the American Association of Medical Assistants, many monthly meetings include continuing education opportunities. Numerous seminars and conferences held throughout the country may be beneficial to employees. Local hospitals often have continuing education opportunities that may be beneficial. Managers will keep abreast of these opportunities and encourage employees to attend. Any continuing education opportunity that may benefit the employee on the job and the medical practice itself should ideally be paid for by the employer(s). Credentialed employees will always need to update skills and earn CEUs to maintain their credentials in active status. An important function of HR is to make CEU opportunities available to employees.

It is often best to provide training and education within the facility when the training necessary is specific to the medical practice. For instance, training on new computer software is apt to be specific to the particular setting. When sophisticated new equipment is purchased, companies often provide in-house training for the individuals who will be using the equipment. Take advantage of as many of those opportunities as are available and for as many of your employees as possible. When the training is quite expensive or time consuming, make certain one person receives the training. Then have that individual train others. Whenever possible, provide training outside of regular hours when patients are not being seen—before the office opens or after the office closes or during a lunch period. Always pay employees for any time served over their regular working hours. Offer certificates for any inservices.

Careful attention to continuing education and training for employees will pay for itself many times over again. The more confident and secure employees feel in the skills they are expected to perform, the more satisfied the practice's patients will be.

Procedure 34-1

Develop and Maintain a Policy Manual

PURPOSE:

To develop and maintain a comprehensive, up-to-date policy manual of all office policies relating to employee practices, benefits, office conduct, and so on.

EQUIPMENT/SUPPLIES:

Computer
Binder, such as a three-ring
Paper
Standard policy manual format

PROCEDURE STEPS:

1. Develop precise, written office policies detailing all necessary information pertaining to the staff and their positions. The information should include benefits, vacation, sick leave, hours, dress codes, evaluations, rules of conduct, and grounds for dismissal. RATIONALE: Well-defined policies clearly outlined for each employee are necessary for efficient and effective staff operations.
2. Identify procedures for reimbursing overtime, preventing discrimination and harassment, creating a safe working environment, and allowing for jury duty.
3. Include a policy statement related to rules of conduct.
4. Identify steps to follow should an employee become disabled during employment.
5. Determine what employee opportunities for continuing education, if any, will be reimbursed; include requirements for recertification or licensure.
6. Provide a copy of the policy manual for each employee. RATIONALE: Each employee is made aware of facility policies.
7. Review and update the policy manual regularly. Add or delete items as necessary, dating each revised page. RATIONALE: Policy manual will always be current.

Procedure 34-2

Prepare a Job Description

PURPOSE:

To provide a precise definition of the tasks assigned to a job, to determine the expectations and level of competency required, and to specify the experience, training, and education needed to perform the job for purposes of recruiting and performance evaluation.

EQUIPMENT/SUPPLIES:

Computer
Paper
Standard job description format

PROCEDURE STEPS:

1. Detail each task that creates the job. RATIONALE: A detailed job description identifies clear expectations for each employee.
2. List special medical, technical, or clerical skills required.
3. Determine the level of education, training, and experience required for the position.
4. Determine where the job fits in the overall structure of the practice.
5. Specify any unusual working conditions (hours, locations, and so on) that may apply.
6. Describe career path opportunities.

Procedure 34-3

Conduct Interviews

PURPOSE:

To screen applicants for training, experience, and characteristics to select the best candidate to fill the position vacancy.

PROCEDURE STEPS:

1. Review résumés and applications received.
2. Select candidates who most closely match the education and experience being sought.
3. Create an interview worksheet for each candidate listing points to cover.
4. Select an interview team; this team should always include the HR or office manager and the immediate supervisor to whom the candidate will report.
5. Call personally to schedule interviews. RATIONALE: This allows you to judge the applicant's telephone manners and voice.
6. Remind the interviewers of various legal restrictions concerning questions to be asked.
7. Conduct interviews in a private, quiet setting. RATIONALE: Careful interviewing of potential employees is an important step in hiring the best candidate for the position.
8. Put the applicant at ease by beginning with an overview about the practice and staff, briefly describing the job, and answering preliminary questions.
9. Ask questions about the applicant's work experience and educational background using the résumé and interview worksheet as a guide.
10. Provide the most promising applicants additional information on benefits and a tour of the office if practical.
11. Applicant's general salary requirements may be discussed, but avoid discussion of a specific salary until a formal offer is tendered.
12. Inform the applicants when a decision will be made and thank each for participating in the interview.
13. Do not make a job offer until all the candidates have been interviewed.
14. Check references of all prospective employees.
15. Establish a second interview between the provider–employer(s) and the qualified candidate if necessary.
16. Confirm accepted job offers in writing, specifying details of the offer and acceptance. RATIONALE: Written document provides proof of hiring and employment details.
17. Notify all unsuccessful applicants by letter when the position has been filled. RATIONALE: Makes a positive statement to those not hired and keeps the doors open for future employment possibilities.

Procedure 34-4

Orient Personnel

PURPOSE:

To acquaint new employees with office policies, staff, what the job encompasses, procedures to be performed, and job performance expectations.

PROCEDURE STEPS:

1. Tour the facilities and introduce the office staff.
2. Complete employee-related documents and explain their purpose.
3. Explain the benefits programs.
4. Present the office policy manual and discuss its key elements.
5. Review federal and state regulatory precautions for medical facilities.

continues

Procedure 34-4 (continued)

6. Review the job description.
7. Explain and demonstrate procedures to be performed and the use of procedure manuals supporting these procedures.
8. Demonstrate the use of any specialized equipment.
9. Assign a mentor from the staff to help with the orientation. RATIONALE: Without proper orientation and training, the best new employee can fail.

Case Study 34-1

Refer to the scenario at the beginning of the chapter.

It is sometimes difficult for Jane O'Hara to complete her responsibilities as both the office manager and the human resources manager.

CASE STUDY REVIEW

1. What steps might Jane take to manage her many and time-consuming tasks comfortably?
2. What responsibilities, if any, that normally fall to the human resources manager could be assigned to other staff members?

Case Study 34-2

Daly Jacobsen, RMA, is an administrative medical assistant at Inner City Health Care. The HR manager has suggested that she might expand her skills and learn some of the procedures in the hiring process. A new medical assistant who specializes in nutrition is coming on board. Daly has been asked to make certain the I-9 form is completed appropriately. The HR manager tells Daly that she will need to download the latest form before completion.

CASE STUDY REVIEW

1. Daly knows that the I-9 is a government form verifying employment eligibility. What keywords might she use in her Internet search to find the form?
2. Once the form has been located, identify the specific rules necessary in completion of the form. What document in List A might a number of prospective employees likely have?
3. In what area of the office might you post the lists of acceptable documents for the I-9 form?
4. With what agency is the form filed on successful completion?

Case Study 34-3

Charles Kensington has just been hired as the HR manager in a large metropolitan clinic. In studying the policy manual, he notes that there is no defined policy for sick leave or bereavement leave. Describe the steps he might take to write such a policy.

CASE STUDY REVIEW

1. To whom should he speak regarding what currently occurs when an employee is ill or when there is a death in the family?
2. What might Charles consider in writing this policy?
3. How should a policy be approved once it is written?
4. What parameters would you suggest for the policy?

SUMMARY

As shown in this discussion, HR management is a challenge. It is, however, a rewarding one. While provider–employers are responsible for patients' physical care, the management team is responsible for hiring and maintaining the employees in the organization. The HR manager who is successful will hire the right people for the jobs and monitor employees in a way that enables and encourages them to give the best patient care possible. The medical assistant who has good communication skills and acquires additional training in HR management will always have variety on the job and will have the satisfaction of watching a health care team run smoothly and efficiently.

STUDY FOR SUCCESS

To reinforce your knowledge and skills of information presented in this chapter:

- Review the Key Terms
- Practice the Procedures
- Consider the Case Studies and discuss your conclusions
- Answer the Review Questions
  - Multiple Choice
  - Critical Thinking
- Navigate the Internet and complete the Web Activities
- Practice the StudyWARE activities on the textbook CD
- Apply your knowledge in the Student Workbook activities
- Complete the Web Tutor sections

REVIEW QUESTIONS

Multiple Choice

1. HR managers:
   a. need no special training for the job
   b. are responsible for hiring and orienting personnel
   c. often work longer hours than other employees
   d. both b and c
2. The following questions may be asked in an interview:
   a. How old are you?
   b. Have you ever been arrested?
   c. Can you supply a birth certificate or a Social Security card?
   d. Do you plan to start a family soon?
3. When a candidate has been accepted for a position, the HR manager should:
   a. call the candidate to determine what salary is preferred
   b. write a letter defining the position details
   c. check references listed by the candidate
   d. notify patients of a staff change
4. Overtime hours in the medical facility:
   a. are to be expected as part of the job
   b. do not require prior authorization
   c. are usually paid at no less than one and one-half times the regular pay rate
   d. are paid only to managers
5. The HR manager will work closely with:
   a. the provider–employer(s)
   b. the office manager
   c. all employees
   d. all of the above
6. OSHA:
   a. requires employers to verify an employee's right to work in the United States
   b. protects employees who have disabilities from employment discrimination
   c. protects employees with chemical dependencies or emotional problems
   d. protects employees from unsafe or unhealthy working conditions

7. The best area for hiring medical employees comes from:
   a. students in a business college
   b. newspaper advertisements
   c. networking sources
   d. the state's unemployment office
8. Employees receiving training or education necessary to the job:
   a. will seek that training after hours and not expect reimbursement
   b. will be current and up to date in the health care field
   c. should always be paid for any time served over regular working hours
   d. both b and c
9. Personnel records:
   a. are usually kept for 3 to 5 years after employment ends and may include payroll data
   b. are not available for everyone to view and must be kept confidential
   c. include all papers related to employment and personal data
   d. all of the above
10. Dismissal:
   a. may be voluntary or involuntary
   b. should always be documented
   c. is a good time for an exit interview
   d. all of the above

Critical Thinking

1. You have just accepted a position to work in a larger, more specialized clinic where you will be able to use skills you are not currently able to exercise. Identify two or three main points for a letter of resignation you will prepare.
2. An employee approaches you, the HR manager, identifying that he or she has just become responsible for the care of an aging parent and may require occasional time away from work. You have no policy about how this absence should be treated. What kind of policy might be helpful? Where would you look for suggestions?
3. An exit interview form has been introduced in this chapter. Another simple form for an exit interview is to use the ABCs. *A* stands for "awesome." What do we do that is awesome? *B* stands for "better." What could we do better in our organization? *C* stands for "change." What would you recommend we change? Discuss the merits of both forms for an exit interview.
4. Do a simple comparison of salaries in your community. Compare the hourly wages of a secretary, a medical assistant, a plumber, your automobile mechanic, and a person working in a fast-food restaurant. How might you use this material when seeking salary increases?
5. What might employers and HR managers do to make certain they keep valued employees? Is salary really the most important issue?

WEB ACTIVITIES

1. Research the Centers for Medicare & Medicaid Services Web site (http://www.cms.hhs.gov) for information related to the prohibition of discrimination on the basis of sexual orientation. What do you find? Are there other sources on this subject that are helpful? Can the manager choose not to hire a person who is otherwise qualified on the basis that he or she is gay? Why or why not?
2. "NOLO Law for All" has a helpful Web site with many topics in their directory. Research the area related to personnel policies and practices. What suggestions do they make for establishing goals and standards for employee evaluations? Do they identify any helpful evaluation tips? If so, outline them for your instructor.
3. Research the ADA Web site to determine if there are any examples of accommodations made in the medical setting. If yes, describe them. Are all provider–employers covered by the ADA? If not, how might discrimination be prevented?

REFERENCES/BIBLIOGRAPHY

Fallon, Jr., F. L. (2007). *Human resource management in health care: Principles and practice.* Bowling Green, OH: Bowling Green State University.

Mathis, R. L., & Jackson, J. H. (2004). *Healthcare human resource management* (10th ed.). Cincinnati, OH: South-Western College Publishing.

McWay, D. C. (2008). *Today's health information management.* Clifton Park, NY: Delmar Cengage Learning.

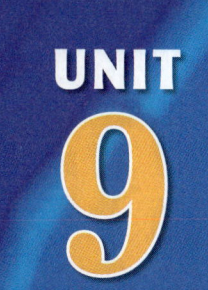

Entry into the Profession

UNIT 9

Chapter 35

Preparing for Medical Assisting Credentials

OUTLINE

Purpose of Certification
- Certification Agencies

Preparing for Certification Examinations

American Association of Medical Assistants (AAMA)
- Certified Medical Assistant (AAMA) Examination Format and Content
- Certified Medical Assistant (AAMA) Application Process
- Certified Medical Assistant (AAMA) Examination Scheduling and Administration
- Certified Medical Assistant (AAMA) Recertification

American Medical Technologists (AMT)
- Registered Medical Assistant (RMA) Examination Format and Content
- Registered Medical Assistant (RMA) Application Process
- Registered Medical Assistant (RMA) Examination Scheduling and Administration
- Registered Medical Assistant (RMA) Recertification

National Healthcareer Association (NHA)
- Certified Clinical Medical Assistant and Certified Medical Administrative Assistant Examination Format and Content
- Certified Clinical Medical Assistant and Certified Medical Administrative Assistant Application Process
- Certified Clinical Medical Assistant and Certified Medical Administrative Assistant Examination Scheduling and Administration
- Certified Clinical Medical Assistant and Certified Medical Administrative Assistant Recertification

Professional Organizations
- American Association of Medical Assistants (AAMA)
- American Medical Technologists (AMT)
- National Healthcareer Association

KEY TERMS

Accrediting Bureau of Health Education Schools (ABHES)

American Association of Medical Assistants (AAMA)

American Medical Technologists (AMT)

Certification Examination

Certified Clinical Medical Assistant (CCMA)

Certified Medical Administrative Assistant (CMAA)

Certified Medical Administrative Specialist (CMAS)

Certified Medical Assistant (CMA [AAMA])

Commission on Accreditation of Allied Health Education Programs (CAAHEP)

Continuing Education Units (CEUs)

National Healthcareer Association (NHA)

Recertification

Registered Medical Assistant (RMA)

Task Force for Test Construction (TFTC)

OBJECTIVES

The student should strive to meet the following performance objectives and demonstrate an understanding of the facts and principles presented in this chapter through written and oral communication.

1. Define the key terms as presented in the glossary.
2. List the necessary qualifications to sit for the certified medical assistant (AAMA) certification examination.

OBJECTIVES (continued)

3. State when the certified medical assistant (AAMA) certification examination is offered and the registration deadlines.
4. List the necessary qualifications to sit for the registered medical assistant examination.
5. State when the registered medical assistant examination is offered and the registration protocols.
6. Differentiate between being certified and being registered.
7. Discuss the National Healthcareer Association and its options for medical assisting certification.
8. Identify the benefits of certification and registration.
9. Describe several methods for continuing education opportunities.
10. Explain when recertification must take place for the CMA (AAMA).
11. Describe the procedure for recertification for the registered medical assistant.

Scenario

Dr. Ray Reynolds currently is the senior provider at Inner City Health Care, a multiprovider urgent care center. When he began his practice 32 years ago, however, he had a private practice and employed one full-time and two part-time medical assistants. Dr. Reynolds felt the office ran smoothly, except when an assistant had to be replaced. Retraining a new person consumed a great deal of valuable time. Even if the new employee came with experience from another medical office, the procedures still required retraining.

Dr. Reynolds finds that when he needs to replace a medical assistant now, he looks at the applicants' résumés and interviews only those candidates who are Certified Medical Assistants or Registered Medical Assistants. The office is too busy to spend time training and retraining new people.

INTRODUCTION

Forty years ago, medical assistants were trained on the job by the practitioner with whom they were employed. Quality control of training varied because there were no established criteria for evaluating such training. This chapter will present the purpose of certification, certifying agencies, and preparation for certification examinations.

PURPOSE OF CERTIFICATION

Certification is intended to set a consistent minimum standard for evaluating an individual's professional competence as a medical assistant. The medical assisting profession continues to be one of the fastest growing in the U.S. economy. Because of the demand for skilled medical assistants, increasing numbers of career-oriented candidates enter this profession annually. Certification acknowledges the professional has standard entry-level knowledge and skills. Successfully passing a **certification examination** also builds personal self-esteem and confidence in performing the responsibilities assigned.

Other reasons for certification include help in your career advancement and compensation. Hiring providers view these credentials as professional and an indication of proficiency in entry-level skills. Individuals who are competent and interested in continued learning experiences are more apt to be rewarded with promotions and salary increases. Maintaining the credential demonstrates a life-long commitment to professional development. The graduate medical assistant has a goal and challenge

Critical Thinking

Take time to think through your personal medical assisting career goals. Will credentialing be an important consideration? Why or why not?

Spotlight on Certification

RMA Content Outline

- Medical law
- Oral and written communication

CMA (AAMA) Content Outline

- Displaying a professional attitude
- Professional communication and behavior

CMAS Content Outline

- Legal and ethical considerations
- Professionalism
- Communication

to which to aspire, first by earning the credential and second by maintaining the credential through continued education and recertification.

Some certifying agencies offer membership into their organizations. This avenue provides excellent opportunities to network and be mentored by fellow professionals, to enroll in continuing education programs, and to receive many other membership perks.

Certification Agencies

Agencies such as the **Commission of Accreditation of Allied Health Education Programs (CAAHEP)** certifies the **Certified Medical Assistant (CMA [AAMA])**. The **American Medical Technologists (AMT)** offers examinations to certify the **Registered Medical Assistant (RMA)** and the **Certified Medical Administrative Specialist (CMAS)**. The **National Healthcareer Association (NHA)** is another agency offering certification to healthcare professionals. These professionals include the **Certified Clinical Medical Assistant (CCMA)** and the **Certified Medical Administrative Assistant (CMAA)**. Figure 35-1 illustrates a comparison of agencies providing certification for medical assistants.

Effective January 1, 2008, medical assistants certified through AAMA use the title Certified Medical Assistant or the abbreviation CMA (AAMA). This title indicates that a person whose services are competent, having graduated from a Commission of Accreditation of Allied Health Education Programs (CAAHEP) or an Accrediting Bureau of Health Education Schools (ABHES)

Certification Details			
Certifying Agency	American Association of Medical Assistants (AAMA)	American Medical Technologists (AMT)	National Healthcareer Association (NHA)
Credential	CMA (AAMA)	RMA or CMAS	CCMA or CMAA
Certification Exam	Computer-based national exam, offered at Prometric testing centers (www.prometric.com)	Computer-based national exam offered at PearsonVue testing centers (www.pearsonvue.com), or paper exam by appointment	National exam taken by online or paper exam
Number of Questions and Make-up of Exam	200 multiple choice questions Topics from the Content Outline for the CMA (AAMA)	200–210 multiple choice questions Clinical, Administrative, and General questions	200 mutiple choice questions Separate tests for CCMA and CMAA (exam completing time approximately 90 minutes)
Continuing Education	AAMA Approved CEUs 60 points every 5 years 10 Clinical 10 Administrative 10 General 30 Discretionary	Certification Continuation Program (CCP) 30 points every 3 years AMT and AMTIE* offer several CE options for credits	Continuing education (CE) program 5 credits per year Home study program taken online, downloaded, or using printed copies

*American Technologists Institute For Education

Figure 35-1 Comparison of agencies providing certification.

accredited program and having successfully passed the AAMA certification examination, will perform medical assisting services.

RMA certificants may use the term "certified medical assistant" in a descriptive sense to describe the credentialing services offered by AMT's Registered Medical Assistant program or to describe individuals who have been awarded the RMA certification. When responding to advertisements or during the interview process, "certified medical assistants" who are AMT certificants must make clear to the prospective employer that they are certified by AMT as a Registered Medical Assistant.

PREPARING FOR CERTIFICATION EXAMINATIONS

Preparation for the examination requires planning, scheduling, and discipline. It is important to plan well in advance to ensure confidence and a passing score to earn your credential. If you are sitting for the examination immediately on graduation, your preparation time for the examination may only allow 2 to 3 months. If you have been out of school for some time or your work experience has been very specialized, you may need longer to prepare for the examination.

During the planning stage, determine the date you want to sit for the examination. Check with the appropriate Web site or call the appropriate examination department to obtain the current application form. The application form contains information such as dates, times, and locations of test sites; policies regarding deadlines; incomplete applications; examination verification information; and information regarding study guides.

It is important to consider having a study group or partner. The right study environment can be invaluable to your success for several reasons. First, it is important to select a study partner or group who shares your commitment to a successful outcome and who plans to sit for the examination on or near the same date you have selected. A study partner can also give you some accountability for keeping to the planned schedule.

Once it has been determined when and where you will sit for the examination and who your study partner(s), if any, will be, a meeting should be scheduled to discuss the review/study approach. It may be that your group will decide to review/study each subject provided in the Curriculum Content Outline accompanying the application. Other groups review/study only those areas in which they feel less confident. A plan that meets the needs of each group member and that all can agree to works best.

Meeting once or twice a week helps the group stay focused and on task. Independent study should be done throughout the week. During the independent study time, each group member may be asked to write 10 multiple choice questions relevant to the weeks' study topic. Answers to these questions should be on a separate page. Some find it helpful to also provide the rationale or textbook page number that supports their answer. When the group meets, a discussion of the study topic could take place and copies of the questions could be distributed for answering. The questions could then be corrected and discussion of any questionable or missed answers could take place.

Once a schedule has been established and agreed on, discipline is required. It is critical that each group member spend time individually preparing for the next group meeting. Someone should be put in charge of each group meeting to keep the event from turning into a social time. To help with this, it is a good idea to set a specific time limit for the study/review session. If individuals want to visit after the session, they are free to do that without disrupting the purpose of the session. All members should be committed to being prepared and attending each scheduled review/study session.

AMERICAN ASSOCIATION OF MEDICAL ASSISTANTS (AAMA)

The AAMA is an organization whose objective is to promote skills and professionalism, protect the medical assistants' right to practice, and encourage consistent health care delivery through professional certification. The AAMA is a sponsoring member of the Commission on Accreditation of Allied Health Education Programs (CAAHEP). CAAHEP establishes the standards for medical assisting programs and is the issuing body of the accreditation for AAMA.

Only graduates of CAAHEP- and **Allied Bureau of Health Education Schools (ABHES)**-accredited medical assistant programs may sit for the Certified Medical Assistant exam. To locate either CAAHEP or ABHES medical assisting programs, go to http://www.aama-ntl.org and click on *About AAMA*. Follow the drop-down menu for specific information.

Eligibility categories and documentation requirements to sit for the Certified Medical Assistant exam include the following:

- *Category 1:* The candidate must be a CAAHEP or ABHES graduating student or recent graduate. A transcript-to-date with the institution's seal or registrar's signature, or an official transcript and verification of graduation date, are required as documentation.
- *Category 2:* The candidate may be a CAAHEP or ABHES nonrecent graduate. A nonrecent graduate is one with a graduation date more than 12 months prior to the examination date. An official transcript and verification of graduation date are required documentation.
- *Category 3:* The candidate may be a recertificant, a Certified Medical Assistant® applying for the CMA Examination to recertify his or her credential.

The AAMA Endowment is a not-for-profit corporation that provides funding for two purposes:

- Awarding of scholarships to students in CAAHEP-accredited medical assisting education programs
- Accreditation of medical assisting education programs through CAAHEP

The Medical Assisting Education Review Board (MAERB) operates under the authority of the endowment and evaluates medical assisting programs according to standards adopted by the endowment and the CAAHEP. The MAERB recommends programs to CAAHEP for accreditation. The MAERB also reviews standards for medical assisting curricula, conducts accreditation workshops for educators, and provides medical assisting educators with current information about CAAHEP, accreditation laws, policies, and practices. CAAHEP's purpose is to accredit entry-level, allied health education programs.

Certified Medical Assistant (AAMA) Examination Format and Content

The AAMA certification examination is a comprehensive test of the knowledge actually used in today's medical office. The content is drawn from an in-depth analysis of the numerous tasks medical assistants perform on a daily basis.

Examination questions are formulated by the Certifying Board's **Task Force for Test Construction (TFTC).** This group is composed of practicing medical assistants, providers, and medical assisting educators from across the United States. The TFTC updates the examination annually to reflect changes in medical assistants' day-to-day responsibilities, as well as the latest developments in medical knowledge and technology.

The three major areas tested include:

1. *General:* Medical Terminology, Anatomy and Physiology, Psychology, Professionalism, Communication, and Medicolegal Guidelines and Requirements
2. *Administrative:* Data Entry, Equipment, Records Management, Screening and Processing Mail, Scheduling and Monitoring Appointments, Resource Information and Community Services, Managing the Office, Office Policies and Procedures, and Practice Finances
3. *Clinical:* Principles of Infection Control, Treatment Area, Patient Preparation and Assisting the Provider, Patient History Interview, Collecting and Processing Specimens; Diagnostic Testing, Preparing and Administering Medications, Emergencies, First Aid, and Nutrition

Students must enroll as an AAMA member before their graduation date to be eligible for the reduced student rate. Once they are a student member they may stay at the student rate for 1 year after graduation if they do not choose to be an active or associate member and pay the higher dues amount. The additional year of membership at the reduced rate helps the recent graduate maintain membership while finding a job and becoming established in a career.

Certified Medical Assistant (AAMA) Application Process

Candidates should read all instructions carefully before completing the application form. Incomplete or incorrect applications will not be processed and will be returned to the candidate. Postmark deadlines for applications, cancellations, and examination location changes are strictly enforced.

Applications are available from the AAMA Certification Department, 7999 Eagle Way, Chicago, IL 60678-1079. The application may also be downloaded from the AAMA Web site (http://www.aama-ntl.org).

It is recommended that the application be sent by certified mail, return receipt requested to verify delivery. The application must be typewritten or printed using black ink only. Be sure the application is signed and dated properly and the eligibility category section is completed appropriately. Applications take up to 45 days after the postmark date to process.

Tear off the application page from the instruction pamphlet. Do not mail the instructions back with the application. Keep this information for future reference together with a copy of everything submitted, including a copy of your completed payment check or money order. If you are paying by VISA or MasterCard, provide the requested information at the top of the application.

A guide for the certification examination entitled *A Candidate's Guide to the AAMA Certification Examination* provides explanations of how to approach the types of questions used on the examination and tips on how to study for the content that will be tested. A sample 120-question examination is included to help assess your knowledge of the categories tested and the format used to formulate the questions.

Certified Medical Assistant (AAMA) Examination Scheduling and Administration

The AAMA certification examination is made up of 200 multiple choice questions, covering topics listed on the Content Outline for the CMA (AAMA) Certification/Recertification Examination. As of January 2009, the CMA (AAMA) certification examination is now offered via computer-based testing (CBT). Candidates whose applications are accepted will receive a Scheduling Permit containing instructions for making a testing appointment, and are able to select locations and flexible testing times at Prometric test centers throughout the United States. To schedule examination appointments, candidates may call 800-853-6761 or go to www.prometric.com and select a test center and appointment test time. Centers are open 9:00 AM to 5:00 PM Monday through Saturday. An email confirming your appointment will be sent to you.

Critical Thinking

You will graduate from a CAAHEP-accredited program in June and want to sit for the CMA examination the last Saturday of June (the same month in which you graduate). Go to the AAMA web site and determine when your application must be postmarked for acceptance for this test date.

Photo identification is required for admission to the examination. Candidates are not permitted to bring any items except identification in the examination area. Candidates are allowed 3 hours and 15 minutes to complete the exam, which includes a 15 minute tutorial.

All exam candidates will receive an unofficial pass/fail result immediately upon completion of the exam. An official report of your scores will be mailed within 6 to 10 weeks after the exam date.

Certified Medical Assistant (AAMA) Recertification

Effective January 2005, all newly certified and recertifying CMAs (AAMA) will be current through the last day of their birth month in the sixth calendar year following their last certification/recertification. In other words, if you were born on August 6th and certified in June 2004, you would be due to recertify by the end of August 2010.

Recertification can be achieved either by reexamination or by the continuing education method. Recertification credits are evaluated on supportive documentation and on their relevancy to medical assisting as defined by the AAMA Medical Assistant Role Delineation Study or the Content Outline for the Certification/Recertification Examination.

A total of 60 points is necessary to recertify the CMA (AAMA) credential. A minimum of 10 points is required in each category: general, administrative, and clinical. The remaining 30 points can be accumulated in any of the three content areas or from any combination of the three categories. At least 30 of the required 60 recertification points must be accumulated from AAMA-approved **continuing education units (CEUs).** If desired, all 60 points may be AAMA CEUs.

CMAs (AAMA) applying for recertification must also provide documentation of current

On successfully passing the Certification Examination and earning the CMA (AAMA) credential, one should begin to document all CEUs earned. It is important to have the following information for CEU documentation:

- Complete date of the activity
- Sponsor (group or organization issuing the credit for the continuing education activity)
- Program title
- Amount and type of credit earned (e.g., CEU, CME, contact hour or college credit)
- Recertification points (AAMA CEUs or other credit)
- Points per content area (general, administrative, clinical)

cardiopulmonary resuscitation (CPR) certification for health care professionals or providers. Acceptable courses of CPR include the American Red Cross and the American Heart Association. The components of certification must include adult and pediatric CPR and obstructed airway training and Automated External Defibrillator (AED) instruction.

Applicants who accumulate all 60 points through AAMA CEUs, and in the correct content areas, can order a recertification over the telephone. Application fees still apply; however, an application form is not required. All CMAs employed or seeking employment must have current certified status to use the CMA (AAMA) credential.

Continuing education courses are offered by local, state, and national AAMA groups. Guided study programs are also available through AAMA's "Quest for Excellence" program. *CMA Today,* the official bimonthly publication of AAMA, provides articles designated for CEUs.

A CMA (AAMA) need not be a member of the AAMA nor currently employed to recertify. The entire recertification by continuing education instructions and application can be downloaded from AAMA's Web site (http://www.aama-ntl.org). Review of recertification applications can take up to 90 days. If all criteria are met, recertification is granted. The date that the application is postmarked to the AAMA Executive Office will be the date of recertification.

On meeting recertification requirements, the applicant receives an identification card, which indicate the year of recertification and the expiration date.

AMERICAN MEDICAL TECHNOLOGISTS (AMT)

The American Medical Technologists (AMT) awards the registered medical assistant (RMA) credential to individuals graduating from an ABHES-accredited medical assisting program who successfully passes their examination. ABHES is recognized by the U.S. Department of Education for accreditation of post-secondary schools offering traditional instruction as well as instruction by distance delivery.

The AMT also offers certification for the certified medical administrative specialist (CMAS). The CMAS is employed primarily in the "front office" of provider offices, clinics, or hospitals. They must understand and use medical terminology properly and be skilled in all administrative tasks performed in health care settings. Each individual state decides the scope of practice for the CMAS, with most states not requiring licensure.

Additional information regarding CMAS education requirements, duties performed, working conditions, employment outlook, and estimated earnings can be found online at http://www.amt1.com. Simply click on Certified Medical Administrative Specialist to access the information.

Registered Medical Assistant (RMA) Examination Format and Content

AMT certification examinations are intended to evaluate the competence of entry-level practitioners. The Education, Qualifications, and Standards Committee of American Medical Technologists develop registered medical assistant (RMA) examinations. The medical assistant committee writes test questions and reviews questions submitted from other sources (e.g., instructors, experts, practitioners, and other individuals associated with the medical assistant profession). The medical assistant committee also determines certification requirements and addresses standard-setting issues related to the credential. Once test construction has been completed, the examination is reviewed and approved by the AMT Board of Directors.

The AMT registration examination consists of 200 to 210 four-option multiple-choice questions. Examinees are required to select the single best answer; multiple answers for a single item are scored as incorrect. Test questions may require examinees to recall facts, interpret graphic illustrations, interpret information presented in case studies, analyze situations, or solve problems. The approximate percentages of questions in content areas are as follows:

1. General Medical Assisting Knowledge—41.0%
   - Anatomy and physiology
   - Medical terminology
   - Medical law
   - Medical ethics
   - Human relations
   - Patient education
2. Administrative Medical Assisting—24.0%
   - Insurance
   - Financial bookkeeping
   - Medical secretarial-administrative medical assistant

3. Clinical Medical Assisting—35.0%
   - Asepsis
   - Sterilization
   - Instruments
   - Vital signs
   - Physical examinations
   - Clinical pharmacology
   - Minor surgery
   - Therapeutic modalities
   - Laboratory procedures
   - Electrocardiography
   - First aid

Registered Medical Assistant (RMA) Application Process

The following criteria have been established for applicants sitting for the RMA examination:

1. Applicant shall be of good moral character and at least 18 years of age.
2. Applicant shall be a graduate of an accredited high school or acceptable equivalent.
3. Applicant must meet one of the following requirements:
   a. Applicant shall be a graduate of a(n):
      - Medical assisting program that holds programmatic accreditation by (or is in a postsecondary school or college that holds institutional accredition by) the ABHES or the CAAHEP.
      - Medical assisting program in a postsecondary school or college that has institutional accreditation by a Regional Accrediting Commission or by a national accrediting organization approved by the U.S. Department of Education. That program must include a minimum of 720 clock hours (or equivalent) of training in medical assisting skills (including a clinical externship).
      - Formal medical services training program of the U.S. Armed Forces.

   b. Applicant shall have been employed in the profession of medical assisting for a minimum of five years, no more than two years of which may have been as an instructor in a postsecondary medical assisting program.
4. Applicants applying under 3 A or B *must* take and pass the AMT certification examination for RMA.
5. The AMT Board of Directors has further determined that applicants who have passed generalist medical assistant certification examination offered by another medical assisting certification body (provided that examination has been approved for this purpose by the AMT Board of Directors), who have been working in the medical assisting field for the past 3 of 5 years, and who meet all other AMT training and experience requirements may be considered for RMA (AMT) certification without further examination.

Applications can be downloaded from AMT's Web site (http://www.amt1.com) either in print and fill-in format or as online fill-in format.

Registered Medical Assistant (RMA) Examination Scheduling and Administration

All applications must be completed online or printed clearly except for the signatures required. All ancillary documentation must also be submitted (e.g., application fee; proof of high school graduation or equivalent; official final transcripts stating graduation from medical assistant school, college, or training program [with school seal affixed or notarized]).

When the AMT Registrar has received the application and all required information, an authorization letter containing a toll-free number is mailed to you. You can then contact Pearson Vue locations at http://www.pearsonvue.com/amt to schedule a date and time to take the examination. Two forms of valid identification are required, both bearing your signature and at least one bearing your photo. Photo identification is limited to a driver's license, state-issued identification card, military identification, or passport.

All AMT registration examination tests are available in paper-and-pencil format or in computerized formats at over 200 locations in the United States, its territories, and Canada. Tests can be scheduled daily except Sundays and holidays. Both formats are identical in length; however, experience has shown the computerized test takes less time to complete. Your computerized test score is displayed moments after you complete your test. A paper copy of your result letter is provided to you before you leave the testing center.

Registered Medical Assistant (RMA) Recertification

The AMT has established the Certification Continuation Program (CCP) for continuing education points. Certification will be suspended following a 30-day grace period if proper documentation is not submitted.

Each RMA is required to accumulate 30 points, which must be turned in every 3 years for recertification. A Compliance Evaluation Worksheet and Attestation will be mailed close to the 3-year mark. This worksheet must be completed, signed, and returned to AMT by the due date. Retaking the RMA examination is not an option for reinstatement or recertification.

NATIONAL HEALTHCAREER ASSOCIATION (NHA)

The National Healthcareer Association (NHA) also offers national certification examinations for health care professionals. NHA works with educational institutions throughout the country on curriculum development, competency testing, and preparation and administration of their examination and offers a continuing education (CE) program. The NHA is dedicated to the following:

- Set guidelines for national certification competencies/standards
- Ensure a high level of performance among healthcare professionals
- Establish educational/continuing education requirements
- Adhere to the highest ethical standards

Certified Clinical Medical Assistant and Certified Medical Administrative Assistant Examination Format and Content

The NHA certifies the Certified Clinical Medical Assistant (CCMA) and the Certified Medical Administrative Assistant (CMAA) among other health career professions. Criteria for taking the NHA certification examinations include one of the following: The applicant must have a high school diploma and have recently successfully completed an NHA-approved training program, or the applicant must have either a high school diploma or equivalency and have recently worked in the field of certification for a minimum of 1 year as a full-time employee. Work experience must be documented in writing and signed by the director or employer.

The NHA offers several methods to help prepare candidates for their national certification examination. All students applying for NHA certification examination receive NHA Study Guides. Separate tests are taken for each healthcareer certification. The CCMA and the CMAA test is composed of multiple choice questions and takes approximately 90 minutes to complete.

The examination is offered in traditional pencil-and-paper formats or can be taken online at any of the specified approved locations. For details regarding testing, contact the NHA by telephone at 1-800-499-9092 or email them at http://www.nhanow.com. You will receive a confirmation notice of your seating including the date and location of the examination.

Certified Clinical Medical Assistant and Certified Medical Administrative Assistant Application Process

There are four ways to apply or register for the NHA national certification examination.

- Online using http://www.nhanow.com. Go directly to the secured registration page and submit the registration form using Visa, MasterCard, Discover, American Express, or school voucher.
- The registration form can be downloaded and printed. Once it is filled out completely, it can be mailed along with payment. Address and mail to:

  National Healthcareer Association

  7 Ridgedale Ave, Suite 203

  Cedar Knolls, NJ 07927
- The completed registration form can be faxed to NHA with credit card information or school voucher. The fax number is 1-973-644-4797.
- Telephone the Customer Service Department at 1-800-449-9092. You can then complete the registration over the phone. You will need your credit card number and expiration date or school voucher accessible for payment information.

Certified Clinical Medical Assistant and Certified Medical Administrative Assistant Examination Scheduling and Administration

The NHA examination can be scheduled at any of the specified approved locations:

- Training Schools/Colleges—Check with your school for details

- Testing Sites—Over 950 NHA testing sites nationwide
- Experienced individuals can take examinations at their place of employment

NOTE: All examinations are required to have an exam proctor present.

Certified Clinical Medical Assistant and Certified Medical Administrative Assistant Recertification

NHA offers a Continuing Education (CE) Program to make the process of continuing education more convenient for the health care professional. Courses in this program can be taken at your convenience at home.

New industry standards require that each NHA-certified health care professional complete at least 5.0 CE credits per year to keep certification current. These CE credits are obtained by completing three of the six minor topics at 1.0 credit each and one of two major topics worth 2.0 credits each from the NHA curriculum, which is updated annually.

If certification has expired, the entire program must be completed; all six CE minor topics and two CE major topics. Candidates are required to pay the cost of the 10 credits plus a reinstatement fee.

Applicants who pass the examination will be nationally certified as recognized by the NHA. They will receive a certification certificate suitable for framing and a wallet-size ID certification card containing their national certification number. CE credits will be reviewed by NHA, and a sticker to apply to the certification ID card will be mailed if the credits are accepted.

PROFESSIONAL ORGANIZATIONS

Professional organizations have evolved to establish standards by which medical assistants and medical assisting programs are evaluated. Programs accredited by agencies must meet certain criteria, and students must pass national examinations to become certified. Medical assistants are not licensed and need not be certified to meet employment requirements; however, those certified are viewed as professionals with entry-level skills and a commitment to continued education.

American Association of Medical Assistants (AAMA)

The AAMA was instrumental in defining the scope of training required for the profession and developed standards and guidelines by which programs could become accredited and the medical assistant credentialed. Membership in the AAMA offers many benefits, which include, but are not limited to, the following:

- Medical assisting news and health care information through the bimonthly magazine *CMA Today*
- CEUs for AAMA activities entered in the Continuing Education Registry and access to your transcript online
- Educational events provided by local chapters, state societies, and national meetings
- Answers to legal questions regarding job-related issues
- If eligible, application for the prestigious CMA examination at a reduced fee
- Discounts on car rentals, conventions, workshop and seminar fees, and self-study courses
- Opportunity to network with other practicing medical assistants

American Medical Technologists (AMT)

The AMT is another nonprofit certification agency and professional membership association representing allied health care individuals. It certifies medical assistants by awarding the RMA national credential to those candidates successfully satisfying requirements. AMT has many local chapters, 38 state societies, and a Uniform Services Committee. Each of these societies meets regularly and annually for a national convention.

AMT benefits and services include:

- Continuing education through the *Journal of Continuing Education Topics & Issues* published three times a year
- AMT's Institute for Education (AMTIE), which monitors continued education credits and sends a "report card" each year
- Four scholarships available to members who want to return to school and five scholarships for current students enrolled in allied health care programs
- State societies that offer opportunities for continued education, activities, and networking

- Peer recognition through AMT's prestigious RMA credential
- Personal discount programs

National Healthcareer Association

The NHA serves as a reliable resource for up-to-date information on health career opportunities, training programs, education opportunities, and industry forecasts. The NHA newsletter *The NHA Today* is well respected and provides current trends and information regarding the health care field.

NHA benefits and services include:

- National certification
- Continuing education opportunities
- Collaboration with educational institutions in curriculum development and competency testing
- Annual Continuing Education Program
- Elite Membership Program that puts you in touch with a team of placement specialists to expand job opportunities

Case Study 35-1

Review the scenario at the beginning of the chapter.

CASE STUDY REVIEW

1. Discuss the advantages of certification to the medical assistant.
2. Discuss the advantages of certification to the provider.
3. How does certification set a consistent minimum standard for evaluating professional competence as a medical assistant?

Case Study 35-2

It is May, and Nancy McFarland, who graduated from an ABHES-accredited program 4.5 years ago, is beginning to research the procedures and requirements for taking the RMA examination. Nancy completed her internship at Inner City Health Care and was hired to work there full time (35 hours per week) when she graduated.

CASE STUDY REVIEW

1. If Nancy wants to take the examination in January, what is the procedure for applying?
2. Nancy is setting up a study schedule. She plans to review course textbooks and tests, purchase a study guide, and set up a study group. Develop a simple study schedule.
3. What criteria should Nancy use when asking people to join her study group?

SUMMARY

Many advantages for certification/recertification and registration have been discussed in this chapter. Although certification examinations are not legally required for practicing medical assistants, it is the goal of CAAHEP- and ABHES-accredited institutions to encourage graduates to sit for and maintain their credentials. Membership in the AAMA or in the AMT is also encouraged.

With nearly 400 local AAMA chapters and 51 affiliate state societies, there is the benefit of networking with others in the profession. As an information source for both professional and association issues, the executive staff at the AAMA's national headquarters is available to answer questions at a toll-free number (1-800-228-2262).

AMT currently has 38 chapters that meet regularly and allow networking with other RMAs plus other allied health professionals registered through the AMT, including phlebotomists, medical laboratory technicians, and dental assistants.

The NHA offers national certification examinations for CMAAs and CCMAs among other health care professionals. NHA offers CE programs and encourages recertification.

STUDY FOR SUCCESS

To reinforce your knowledge and skills of information presented in this chapter:

- Review the Key Terms
- Consider the Case Studies and discuss your conclusions
- Answer the Review Questions
  - Multiple Choice
  - Critical Thinking
- Navigate the Internet and complete the Web Activities
- Practice the StudyWARE activities on the textbook CD
- Apply your knowledge in the Student Workbook activities
- Complete the Web Tutor sections
- View and discuss the DVD situations

REVIEW QUESTIONS

Multiple Choice

1. The goal and challenge of each graduating medical assistant should be to:
   a. find employment
   b. have a good benefit package
   c. possess entry-level skills
   d. earn the CMA/RMA credential and maintain it
2. The certification examination is:
   a. a comprehensive test based on tasks medical assistants perform daily
   b. all true/false questions
   c. developed by the AMTIE
   d. developed by the NBME
3. Benefits of membership in a professional organization such as AAMA or AMT include all of the following *except:*
   a. discounted rates on legal representation
   b. legal advice
   c. nationwide networking opportunities
   d. professional journal publications
4. Recertification of the CMA (AAMA) credential options include:
   a. submit work experience
   b. reexamination or CEU method
   c. submit on-the-job training
   d. submit military training
5. To keep the RMA credential current, an individual must earn:
   a. 5 credits each year
   b. 30 points every three years
   c. 30 points every five years
   d. 60 points every five years
6. The RMA was established by the:
   a. ABHES
   b. CAAHEP
   c. AMT
   d. AAMA
7. The NHA offers medical assisting certification for which of the following:
   a. CMA
   b. RMA
   c. CCMA and CMAA
   d. CMAS
8. RMA examinations:
   a. are offered at Pearson Vue locations
   b. are offered twice a year
   c. are offered three times a year
   d. are offered six times a year

Critical Thinking

1. You are a recent high school graduate and have decided to pursue medical assisting as a career. What will you do to find a school offering an accredited program? Is accreditation important? How might your school selection impact your future as a professional medical assistant?
2. After graduation you plan to sit for the certification examination. How will you prepare for the examination to ensure a positive outcome and earn your CMA/RMA credential?
3. After graduating from an accredited program, you immediately went to work as an medical assistant. Now that you have been working several years

you decide to become credentialed. How will you achieve this?

WEB ACTIVITIES

Using the Internet, search your local and state AAMA or AMT Web sites. Print and turn in to your instructor the location, meeting schedules, and any upcoming events planned for your state. Review the certification process that applies to your program.

REFERENCES/BIBLIOGRAPHY

American Association of Medical Assistants. (2008). *AAMA certification/recertification examination for medical assistants.* Retrieved February 10, 2008, from http://www.aama-ntl.org.

American Association of Medical Assistants. (n.d.). *FAQs on CMA (AAMA) certification.* Retrieved January 29, 2009, from http://www.aama-ntl.org.

American Medical Technologists. Allied Health Professionals Association for Certification as a Registered Medical Assistant. (n.d.). Retrieved February 10, 2008, from http://www.amt1.com.

National Healthcareer Association. (n.d.). *NHA national certification examination.* Retrieved September 9, 2007, from http://www.NHAnow.com.

Simmers, L. (2004). *Diversified health occupations* (6th ed.). Clifton Park: NY: Delmar Cengage Learning.

THE DVD HOOK-UP

This chapter discussed credentialing opportunities for the medical assistant.

This program discussed the importance of critical thinking when working in the medical industry.

1. How does good critical thinking apply to your goal of becoming a Certified or Registered Medical Assistant?
2. What credentials are you able to attain as a graduate of your Medical Assistant institution?

DVD Journal Summary

Write a paragraph that summarizes what you learned from watching today's DVD program. Why is becoming credentialed an important goal for you? What will you do to stay current once you graduate from your medical assistant program?

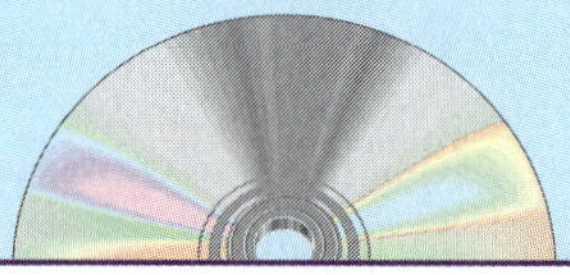

DVD Series | **Program Number**
Critical Thinking | 1

Chapter/Scene Reference
- *Introduction*

Chapter 36

Employment Strategies

KEY TERMS

Accomplishment Statements
Application/Cover Letter
Application Form
Benefits
Bullet Point
Career Objective
Chronologic Résumé
Contact Tracker
Direct Skills
E-résumé
Functional Résumé
Interview
Keywords
Power Verbs
References
Résumé
Targeted Résumé
Transferable Skills

OUTLINE

Developing a Strategy
- Attitude and Mindset
- Self-Assessment

Job Search Analysis and Research

Résumé Preparation
- Résumé Specifications
- Clear and Concise Résumés
- Accomplishments
- References
- Accuracy
- Résumé Styles
- Vital Résumé Information

Application/Cover Letters

Completing the Application Form

The Interview Process
- The Look of Success
- Preparing for the Interview
- The Actual Interview
- Interviewing the Employer
- Closing the Interview

Interview Follow-Up
- Follow-Up Letter
- Follow Up by Telephone

After You Are Employed
- Dealing with Difficult People
- Getting a Raise

Professionalism

OBJECTIVES

The student should strive to meet the following performance objectives and demonstrate an understanding of the facts and principles presented in this chapter through written and oral communication.

1. Define the key terms as presented in the glossary.
2. List the steps involved in job analysis and research.
3. Describe a contact tracker and its usefulness.
4. Give three examples of accomplishment statements.
5. Differentiate chronologic, functional, and targeted résumés.
6. Identify the purpose and content of a cover letter.
7. Demonstrate effective ways to anticipate and respond to an interviewer's questions.
8. Describe appropriate overall appearance and dress for an interview.
9. Identify the benefits of writing a follow-up letter.
10. Discuss professionalism as it relates to employment strategies.

Scenario

Eun Mee Soo is a graduate of an accredited medical assisting program and recently passed the certification examination. While attending school, Eun Mee was employed part-time as a sales representative (clerk) in one of the city's prestigious clothing stores. She has no medical work experience except her practicum at Inner City Health Care. She is now preparing her résumé and beginning her job search. Eun Mee plans to move out of state (she always dreamed of moving north), so she will also be looking for a new apartment. All of these changes are a bit unsettling for Eun Mee. She is beginning to wonder if she should defer relocating at this time and stay close to home until she feels more secure.

INTRODUCTION

So you are about to graduate from the medical assistant program! This time is often unsettling because many changes are occurring; the loss of security the classroom environment provided, loss of contact with fellow classmates, and loss of a structured schedule are just a few changes. Questions such as: Am I ready for my first job? How do I find a job? What do I say at the interview? begin to surface.

The focus on employment may represent apprehension and doubt or be sparked with anticipation and a sense of fulfillment. This chapter provides direction and answers some of the questions related to the job search.

DEVELOPING A STRATEGY

It is best to begin developing your job search strategy early in your training as a medical assistant. If you have not started this phase, determine to begin today.

The first step in developing a strategy is to look at reality. You and maybe a hundred other medical assistants may be applying for the same job position. How are *you* different from every other person applying for this job? The following sections will help make *you* stand out, be different, and hopefully be successful in your job search.

Attitude and Mindset

One important quality an employer looks for in employees is their attitude. Your attitude is not something you turn on and off or learn in school. It is the result of your innate personality combined with the events that mold you during your life. Your instructors and acquaintances have a significant impact over who you are. Your attitude is reflected by how you react to:

1. Taking direction
2. Seeking excellence or doing just enough to get by
3. Meeting employer's needs, not just looking forward to payday
4. Assuming responsibility for your actions versus considering your problems to be someone else's fault

If you find yourself having a negative attitude in any of the ways mentioned in the preceding list, you need to make an effort to change while you are still in training. An employer will zero in on a negative attitude and eliminate you as a candidate almost immediately. Your formal training is important and you can be retrained to do things the way a new employer desires, but your attitude takes time to change and requires a willingness to make the change. Develop a strategy to evolve a positive attitude while you are still in school because this is a time when you will have professional guidance and resources, as well as excellent models.

Spotlight on Certification

RMA Content Outline

- Medical law
- Human relations
- Oral and written communications

CMA (AAMA) Content Outline

- Displaying professional attitude
- Job readiness and seeking employment

CMAS Content Outline

- Legal and ethical considerations
- Professionalism
- Communication

Beyond a positive attitude, being successful in your search for a job requires positive thinking on your part. There is a good position out there for you. Finding it is your first job. Those individuals who are successful at finding that first job devote many hours per week at job strategy tactics. You should not become discouraged by rejection but learn from it and apply what you have learned to the next interview opportunity.

Self-Assessment

As you begin your job search campaign, you should identify what you want in a job. It is always better to do work you enjoy in the type of practice you find most interesting. Take a moment now to complete the self-evaluation work sheet shown in Figure 36-1. When you have finished, you will have some idea of the type of practice you would

SELF-EVALUATION WORK SHEET

Respond to the following questions honestly and sincerely. They are meant to assist you in self-assessment.

1. List your three strongest attributes as related to people, data, or things.
   i.e., Interpersonal skills related to people
   Accuracy related to data
   Mechanical ability related to things
   ____________________ related to ____________________
   ____________________ related to ____________________
   ____________________ related to ____________________
2. List your three weakest attributes as related to people, data, or things.
   ____________________ related to ____________________
   ____________________ related to ____________________
   ____________________ related to ____________________
3. How do you express yourself? Excellent, Good, Fair, Poor
   Orally ____________________ In writing ____________________
4. Do you work well as a leader of a group or team? Yes _____ No _____
5. Do you prefer to work alone? Yes _____ No _____
6. Can you work under stress/pressure? Yes _____ No _____
7. Do you enjoy new ideas and situations? Yes _____ No _____
8. Are you comfortable with routines/schedules? Yes _____ No _____
9. Which work environment do you prefer?
   Single-provider setting _____ Multiple-provider setting _____
   Small clinic setting _____ Large clinic setting _____
10. Which type of practice do you prefer?
    Pediatrics _____ Obstetrics/Gynecology _____
    Geriatrics _____ General Medicine _____
    Internal Medicine _____ Other ____________
11. Which work setting do you prefer?
    Front office (reception) _____ Back office (assisting provider) _____
    Laboratory (phlebotomy) _____ Administrative (coding/billing) _____

Figure 36-1 Self-evaluation work sheets can help determine a person's strengths, weaknesses, and preferences before the job search begins.

like to work in and what position you would find most satisfying.

Before you begin a self-assessment, review what a medical assistant does, determine what level pay can be expected, and compare that with your personal skills and financial requirements. In some practices you may specialize in administrative or clinical duties: in others you may be expected to function in both specialties.

A medical assistant is salaried, with yearly earnings varying between $20,160 and $38,800, inflation adjusted to 2008. Entry-level salaries will be closer to the lower figure but will vary depending on credentials, practicum performance, and geographic location. Medical assistants who can show proficiency in both administrative and clinical capability command higher salaries in some medical settings.

As part of the self-assessment you should evaluate what direct and transferable skills you have that will make you a contributing member of the medical team. **Direct skills** are the medical procedures you have acquired in school and in which you are proficient. **Transferable skills** are those skills that would be useful in a wide variety of professions and may have been perfected during the education process or learned in other employment settings. Leadership, communication, writing, computer literacy, keyboarding, linguistics, and spelling are some examples of transferable skills.

When you have completed this portion of the self-assessment, you will be in a better position to determine what type of job to seek. You will also have identified the skills that you can highlight as you prepare your application/cover letter and résumé.

The final part of your self-assessment is conducting a budgetary need analysis to determine how much income you need to make per month to meet your living expenses.

The budgetary analysis should include a list of the **benefits** you find necessary, such as medical, dental, and vision insurance, 401k program, and stock options. You also might need to consider work schedule, location/travel, and childcare leave policies.

To accomplish this, begin to keep a diary of all purchases and payments. By reviewing your checkbook register, you should be able to itemize basic expenditures, such as rent, utilities, payments (car, credit card), food, clothing, insurance, and taxes. Once a monthly expenditure record is established the amount of money needed to meet living expenses can be calculated.

JOB SEARCH ANALYSIS AND RESEARCH

The job analysis and research phase of your job search should start before graduation. Telephoning or visiting various clinics and asking questions to determine what the duties of a medical assistant are in different types of practices will help to further clarify where you would like to work and will help you become acquainted with a potential employer or identify a possible site for practicum experience. If you visit the facility, dress appropriately just as you would for an interview. You want to impress the clinic personnel just as if it were a formal interview. Remember to send a letter thanking the person taking time on the telephone or authorizing the visit.

Based on the self-assessment you completed and the preliminary job analysis, you know what type of clinic or practice you want to work in, so now is the time to compile a list of potential employers in the geographic area where you want to work. Begin your job search by networking with students who have graduated before you and are successfully employed. Statistics tell us that 80% of positions are filled through networking contacts. Next compile a list from the Yellow Pages, Job Expositions, the Internet, Want Ads for your specialty in the local papers, American Association of Medical Assistants (AAMA) or American Medical Technologists (AMT) publications, and contacts acquired through attending state and local meetings. Other sources are your program director and instructors and the network of contacts at the site where you did your practicum. A practicum site is frequently your best prospect because they will know your capabilities and your attitude and have expended time and resources in your training. If the site is hiring and you performed well, experience has shown that most sites will frequently hire the extern.

Candidate job sites can also be found through employment agencies. These agencies usually charge a fee, although sometimes the employer pays the fee. Extreme caution should be exercised in dealing with agencies because fees are sometimes excessive. Fees should only be paid after successfully obtaining a job and never for getting an interview.

Prioritize the list based on your assessment of chances of employment. Sites where you have personal contacts or where you have done your practicum should be at the top of the list, with sites advertising for help wanted next. Further down the list should be sites that, in sales parlance, would be called cold prospecting. You can further prioritize the list by putting your personal choices at the top each category.

Now is the time to complete detailed homework or research on each prospective employer. Start collecting information on each prospective site, identifying their services, policies, fees and insurance protocol, hours of service, number of providers, and very importantly their mission statement and philosophy of practice criteria. Brochures may be available in their offices, on the Internet, and in wellness publications for patients. Pamphlets on new procedures are other sources of this information. You can use this information to prepare the cover letter for your résumé and to brief yourself should you be invited for an interview.

As part of a serious job search, you should contact many individuals and will need some means of recording the contacts, their responses, and your actions. Figure 36-2 shows a helpful sample **contact tracker.** It should be used to prevent confusion and to keep track of valuable information and action items.

RÉSUMÉ PREPARATION

A **résumé** is a summary data sheet or a brief account of your qualifications and progress in the career you have chosen and should include both direct and transferable skills. The purpose of your résumé is to sell you. It provides an opportunity to describe your education, what you have done, and what you can do, and it lists those who can vouch for your integrity and experience. A résumé that is well thought out and written in such a way as to create interest in what you have to contribute to the employer may reward you with many interviews. During the interview your résumé serves as a reference from which the interviewer may be prompted to ask questions.

> Copy or design your own contact tracker form and document all pertinent information regarding your job search contacts.

Résumé Specifications

The résumé should be limited to one page in length whenever possible. Each page should contain your name and the page number. Keep a 1- to 1½-inch margin on all four sides of the page to create a picture-like frame. Capitalize major headings and single space between lines. Double space between sections. The use of **bullet point** lists instead of paragraphs aids the interviewer in gleaning key points quickly.

Select a high-quality bond stationery that is standard 8½ × 11 inches with a weight between 16 and 25 pounds. This paper weight provides aesthetic benefit and accepts the ink better, resulting in a clean, sharp print resolution. Buff or ivory paper with matching envelope has great eye appeal and helps distinguish your résumé from others.

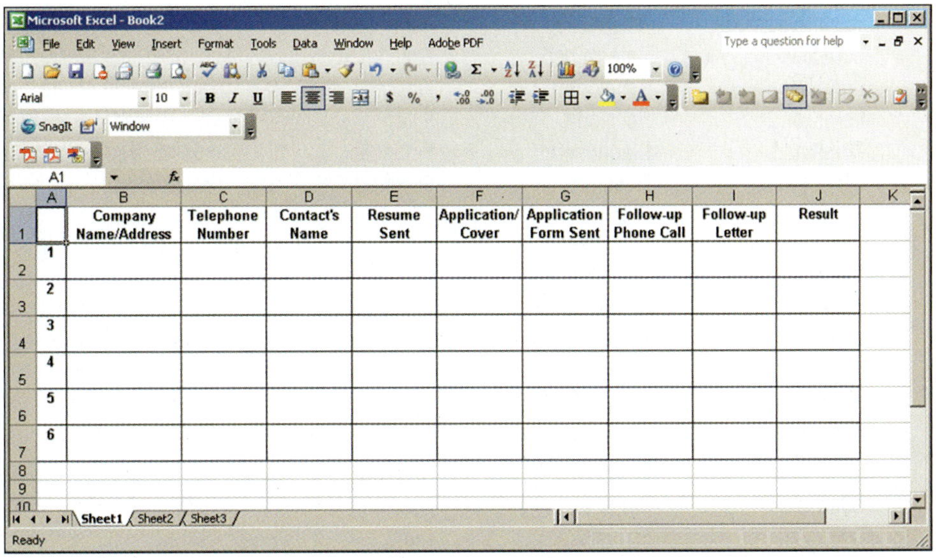

Figure 36-2 A simple contact tracker such as this can help organize all communication you have with potential employers.

Use a word processing program to produce your résumé. It allows you the freedom to experiment with placement and create a picture-perfect résumé or to individualize the résumé for a particular position or facility.

Clear and Concise Résumés

Your résumé must be concise and easy to read and understand. Use statements that are positive, reflect confidence, and portray you as a problem solver. Be sure that any information given within your résumé or application form is not misleading or exaggerated. Leave out the word *I* when writing your résumé. This is your personal résumé, and it is understood that you are referring to yourself.

Accomplishments

Use **accomplishment statements** if you have them from your practicum or work experience. Accomplishment statements begin with **power verbs** and give a brief description of what you did and the demonstrable results that were produced. Figure 36-3 provides a list of sample power verbs. Some accomplishment statement examples are "Utilized computer skills to schedule and reschedule patient appointments" and "Demonstrated skills in setting up sterile trays and assisting with sterile procedures."

References

Select a variety of **references** to be included with your résumé. References should be listed on a separate sheet of paper that matches your résumé. Remember to include the same letterhead as on your résumé on the references page. An individual who knows you or has worked with you long enough to make an honest assessment and recommendation regarding your background history is an excellent reference person. Use only nonre-

Accompanied	Changed	Corrected	Entertained	Implemented	Listed
Accumulated	Charged	Corresponded	Enumerated	Improved	Listened
Achieved	Charted	Counseled	Established	Improvised	Loaded
Acquired	Classified	Created	Estimated	Increased	Located
Administered	Cleaned	Debated	Evaluated	Indexed	Logged
Admitted	Cleared	Decided	Examined	Indicated	Mailed
Advised	Closed	Delegated	Exchanged	Influenced	Maintained
Allowed	Coded	Delivered	Exhibited	Informed	Managed
Analyzed	Collated	Demonstrated	Expanded	Initiated	Manufactured
Answered	Collected	Deposited	Expedited	Inspected	Marked
Applied	Commanded	Described	Experienced	Installed	Marketed
Appointed	Communicated	Detailed	Fabricated	Instructed	Measured
Appraised	Compiled	Determined	Facilitated	Insured	Met
Arranged	Completed	Developed	Figured	Integrated	Modified
Assembled	Composed	Devised	Filled	Interpreted	Monitored
Assessed	Computed	Diagnosed	Financed	Interviewed	Motivated
Assigned	Conducted	Directed	Finished	Introduced	Negotiated
Attached	Conferred	Discovered	Fitted	Inspected	Nominated
Attained	Constructed	Dismantled	Fixed	Inventoried	Noted
Attended	Consulted	Dispatched	Formalized	Investigated	Notified
Authorized	Contacted	Distributed	Formulated	Invoiced	Observed
Balanced	Contracted	Documented	Fulfilled	Issued	Obtained
Billed	Contrasted	Drew	Generated	Judged	Opened
Bought	Contributed	Drove	Graded	Justified	Operated
Budgeted	Controlled	Earned	Graphed	Kept	Ordered
Built	Converted	Educated	Greeted	Learned	Organized
Calculated	Convinced	Employed	Headed	Lectured	Outlined
Cashed	Coordinated	Encouraged	Hired	Led	
Catalogued	Copied	Engineered	Identified	Licensed	(continues)

Figure 36-3 These sample power verbs may help you define your previous job responsibilities.

Overcame	Priced	Ran	Related	Secured	Summarized
Packaged	Printed	Rated	Relayed	Selected	Supervised
Packed	Processed	Read	Renewed	Sent	Supplied
Paid	Procured	Rearranged	Reorganized	Separated	Taught
Participated	Produced	Rebuilt	Repaired	Served as	Telephoned
Patrolled	Programmed	Recalled	Replaced	Serviced	Tested
Perfected	Promoted	Received	Reported	Set up	Trained
Piloted	Prompted	Recommended	Requested	Showed	Transferred
Placed	Proofread	Reconciled	Researched	Sold	Transported
Planned	Proposed	Recorded	Responsible for	Solicited	Typed
Posted	Proved	Reduced	Retrieved	Sorted	Verified
Prepared	Provided	Referred	Revised	Stocked	
Prescribed	Published	Registered	Routed	Stored	
Presented	Purchased	Regulated	Scheduled	Straightened	

Figure 36-3 (continued)

lated persons as references unless the work relationship has been formalized.

Choose references who are well respected and are clear speakers and writers. No matter how much someone likes you and your work, they may not be helpful to you if they cannot convey the information in a business-like manner. Professional references such as a former instructor, provider, practicum supervisor, or fellow coworker are excellent choices.

Always ask permission to use someone as a reference *before* the name is printed on the reference list. Verify the correct spelling of the reference's name, title, place of employment and position, and telephone number for prospective employers.

Help your references aid you in obtaining an interview and employment. A personal visit or telephone call to discuss your career objectives and how you plan to conduct your job search will be helpful. Ask for any suggestions they may have to offer. Provide them with a copy of your résumé and cover letter. This helps them visualize the position for which you are applying and picture how you may benefit that employer.

Keep in touch with references. Check back to see who has called and how things went. Knowing what employers ask may produce some valuable pointers for your next letter, résumé, or interview.

Finally, thank your references. They will appreciate knowing how you are doing and that you value their assistance.

Leave out "References Upon Request" if necessary to shorten your résumé to save space. Employers know they can ask for references at a later date.

Accuracy

Proofread, proofread, and proofread your résumé. Ask someone who is a good speller or one of your references to edit your résumé. Then proofread it again yourself. Do not rely on your computer spell check; it does not differentiate between words such as to, too, two or here and hear. Eliminate repetition of information such as task descriptions. Summarize employment before 10 years ago or leave it off entirely if not relevant to the position you are seeking.

Résumé Styles

Various résumé styles have been developed, each having specific advantages and disadvantages. Choose the style or combination of styles that best describes your strengths and ability to do the job. It may be advantageous to check with the human resources department of the facility to which you are applying to determine if they have a résumé style preference.

Chronologic Résumé. Your **chronologic résumé** should be organized so that the most important information you want to share is the first thing the reader sees. If your job experience is your greatest asset and may set you apart from other applicants, put your work history and job skills first. If your education and training is your best professional feature, put your education and training first. Some medical managers and human resources directors take only 10 seconds to scan a résumé. You want them to see clearly and quickly what you have to offer.

ASHLEY JACKSON, CMA (AAMA)
2031 Craig Street ~ Renton, Washington 98055

Work: 206-878-1545 Cell: 206-835-9879
Home: 253-838-6690 email: asjack@pinetree.com

WORK EXPERIENCE

September, 1999-Present GROUP HEALTH COOPERATIVE
Directed support for a dermatology/surgery practice.
Patient preparation.
Medical and surgical asepsis.
Assist with sterile procedures.
Patient follow-up.

June, 1997-August, 1999 VALLEY INTERNAL MEDICINE
Clinical responsibilities.
Assisted with surgeries in ambulatory care setting.
Patient preparation.
Medical and surgical asepsis.
Assisted with sterile procedures.

March, 1997-June, 1997 VALLEY INTERNAL MEDICINE
Medical Assistant Practicum
Administrative duties and clinical responsibilities utilizing all medical assisting skills, including patient induction, chief complaint, vital signs, patient preparation, EKGs, medical and surgical asepsis, and sterile procedures.

EDUCATION/CERTIFICATION

Associate in Applied Science degree, June, 1997, Highline Community College, Des Moines, Washington, 98198-9800.

Certified Medical Assistant (AAMA), June, 1997.

Figure 36-4 Sample chronologic résumé.

The chronologic résumé is advantageous when:

- The position is in a highly traditional field, such as teaching, law, or health care, where specific employers are of paramount interest
- You are staying in the same field as prior jobs
- Job history shows real growth and development
- Prior titles are impressive

The chronologic résumé is *not* advantageous when:

- Your work history is spotty
- You are changing career goals
- You have been in the same job for many years
- You are looking for your first job

Figure 36-4 illustrates a chronologic résumé.

Functional Résumé. The **functional résumé** highlights specialty areas of accomplishment and strengths. It allows you to organize them in an order that supports your work objective.

The functional résumé is advantageous when:

- Your experience can be sorted into areas of function, i.e., administrative, clinical, supervisory
- You are changing careers

- You are reentering the job market after an absence
- Your career path or growth is not clear from a chronologic listing
- You have had a variety of different, apparently unconnected work experiences
- Much of your work has been volunteer, freelance, or temporary
- You want to eliminate repetition of descriptions of job duties
- You have extensive specialized experience

The functional résumé is *not* advantageous when:

- You want to emphasize a management growth pattern
- Your most recent employers are highly prestigious and the specific employers are of paramount interest

A sample of a functional résumé for a person reentering the job market is shown in Figure 36-5.

JOAN BISHOP, RMA
4320 Sprig Street
Renton, Washington 98055

Work: 206-878-1545 Cell: 206-835-9879
Home: 253-838-6690 email: jbishop@abc.net

TEACHING:

Instructed community groups on issues related to child abuse.

Taught volunteers how to set up community program for victims of domestic violence.

Conducted workshops for parents of abused children.

Instructed public school teachers on signs and symptoms of potential and actual child abuse.

COUNSELING:

Consulted with parents for probable child abuse and suggested courses of action.

Worked with social workers on individual cases, in both urban and suburban settings.

Counseled single parents on appropriate coping behaviors.

Handled pre-take interviewing of many individual abused children.

ORGANIZATION/COORDINATION:

Coordinated transition of children between original home and foster home.

Served as liaison between community health agencies and schools.

Wrote proposal to state for county funds to educate single parents and teachers.

WORK HISTORY:

1998–2000 Community Mental Health Center, Tacoma, Washington
Volunteer Coordinator—Child Abuse Program

2000–2003 C.A.R.E.—Child-Abuse Rescue-Education, Trenton, New Jersey
County Representative

EDUCATION:

1998 B.S. Sociology, Douglass College, New Brunswick, New Jersey

Figure 36-5 Sample functional résumé. This style is useful for a person reentering the job market.

Targeted Résumé. The **targeted résumé** is best for focusing on a clear, specific job target. It should contain a **career objective** and list your skills, capabilities, and any supporting accomplishments related to that objective. This résumé style enables graduating students to list classes related to their career objective, grade point average, student awards, and achievements. This information adds substance to a résumé when work experience is minimal and should be at the beginning of the résumé because it is your most significant asset.

The targeted résumé is advantageous when:

- You are very clear about your job target
- You have had a variety of experiences that appear unrelated to each other but that include skills that you can use in a skills list related to your job target
- You can go in several directions and want a different résumé for each
- You are just starting your career and have little experience but know what you want and are clear about your capabilities
- You are able to keep your résumé on a computer disk

The targeted résumé is *not* advantageous when:

- You want to use one résumé for several different applications
- You are not clear about your abilities and accomplishments

Figure 36-6 shows a sample targeted résumé.

E-Résumé. An electronic résumé, also known as an **e-résumé,** is electronically delivered via email, submitted to Internet job boards, or placed on Web pages. When employers post jobs on their own Web sites, they generally expect job seekers to respond electronically.

Special care must be taken when preparing the e-résumé because many employers place résumés directly into searchable databases. The following points should be considered:

- Formatting must be removed before the résumé can be placed in a database. Submitting a formatted résumé may cause it to be eliminated.
- Submit a text résumé, also known as a text-based résumé, plain-text résumé, or ASCII text résumé. These variations are preferred when submitting résumés electronically.
- The e-résumé is not visually appealing. Eye appeal is not required because its main purpose is to be placed into one of the keyword-searchable databases.
- The text résumé is not vulnerable to viruses and is compatible across computer programs and platforms.
- The text résumé is versatile and can be used for:
  - Posting on job boards
  - Pasting piece-by-piece into the profile forms of job boards, such as Monster.com
  - Pasting into the body of an email to be sent to prospective employers
  - Converting to a Web-based HTML résumé
  - Sending as an attachment to prospective employers
  - Conversion to a scannable résumé

Employers are often inundated with résumés from job seekers each time they advertise a position opening. Therefore, in an effort to save time and to determine the best-qualified candidates for the position, employers digitize the résumés to create an electronic résumé. Using software to search for specific **keywords** that relate to the position, the numbers of candidates can quickly be narrowed. If you apply for a job with a company that searches databases for keywords and your résumé does not conform, you may not be considered for the position.

How do you determine keywords? Begin scrutinizing employment ads and list keywords repeatedly mentioned in association with jobs that interest you. Nouns that relate to the skills and experience the employer is looking for will quickly surface. Keywords may include:

- Job-specific skills/profession-specific words (e.g., specialty experience, bilingual, scheduling, data entry, insurance verification, telephone and communication skills, laboratory/X-ray experience)
- Technologic terms and descriptions of technical expertise (including hardware and software in which you are proficient, e.g., PRISM, DEXA experience)
- Job titles, certifications (e.g., MA, CMA [AAMA], RMA, CMAS, Biller, Coder)
- Types of degrees, names of colleges (e.g., AAS, BA)
- Awards received, professional organization memberships (e.g., Dean's list, scholarships, certificates, AAMA or AMT member)

Keywords should be used throughout the résumé, but they should be front loaded. Front loaded means to use as many keywords as possible in the first 100 words of the résumé. A good goal is to aim for 25 to 35 keywords. This may be achieved by using synonyms, various forms of the keyword, and using both the spelled-out and acronym versions of common terms. If a person reviews the

ASHLEY JACKSON, CMA (AAMA)
2031 Craig Street ~ Renton, Washington 98055

Work: 206-878-1545 — Cell: 206-835-9879
Home: 253-838-6690 — email: asjack@pinetree.com

CAREER OBJECTIVES: To obtain a position as a medical assistant in an ambulatory care/surgery facility that allows use and development of clinical skills.

ACHIEVEMENTS:

Certified Medical Assistant.
Graduate of an Accredited Medical Assistant Program accredited by the Commission on Accreditation of Allied Health Education Programs (CAAHEP).
Experienced in providing assistance with surgeries in an ambulatory care setting.
Excellent communication and interpersonal skills.

SKILLS AND CAPABILITIES:

Post-surgery patient follow-up.
Patient induction.
Vital signs.
Patient preparation.
EKGs.
Medical and surgical asepsis.
Sterile procedures.

WORK HISTORY:

September, 1996 to present	Group Health Cooperative, Seattle, WA Surgical Medical Assistant.
June, 1994-August, 1996	Valley Internal Medicine, Renton, WA Clinical Medical Assistant.
March 1994-June, 1994	Valley Internal Medicine, Renton, WA Practicum Student/Trainee.

EDUCATION/CERTIFICATION:

Associate in Applied Science Degree, Highline Community College.
Certified Medical Assistant (AAMA).

AFFILIATIONS:

American Association of Medical Assistants.

Figure 36-6 Sample targeted résumé. This style is useful when focusing on a specific job target.

résumé, he or she will see enough keywords to process it through the software search.

Vital Résumé Information

All résumé styles must contain certain vital information about the job applicant. Essential information includes:

- Your full name and credential, address including street number, city, state, and zip code.
- Your telephone number or a number where a message can be left. The telephone selected should be one you are confident will be answered in a professional manner. Always include the area code with the number.
- Your email address.
- Your education. Begin with the most recent school attended and include the name, address, and graduation date with the diploma, certificate, or degree earned.
- Work experience. List company name and address. Do not underestimate the value of any job; relate transferable skills to your career objective.

- Skills that are necessary for the job. The list can be completed from your program curriculum. Be careful not to list course titles that have no meaning to the reader. It is much better to list the skills obtained in courses.

The following are the top errors found in résumés:

- Typographical and grammatical errors
- Lack of specifics on work training or history
- Use of same résumé for all job applications (résumé should be tailored to specific job)
- Emphasizing what you did instead of highlighting your accomplishments
- Stating objectives that do not focus on the needs of the employer
- Lack of power verbs and keywords
- Not mentioning jobs that gave you transferable skills
- Lying or exaggerating about skills and experience
- Eliminating key accomplishments in order to meet a one-page goal

APPLICATION/COVER LETTERS

The **application/cover letter** is a means of introducing yourself and submitting your résumé to a potential employer with the goal of obtaining an interview. A well-written cover letter highlights your qualifications and experience for employment and enhances the information contained within your résumé. It should reflect how your skills satisfy the employer's needs. The letter should follow a standard business style and should not be more than one page in length. It should be printed on the same paper as the résumé.

Because this may be your first contact with a potential employer, the letter should sell you and describe your intentions regarding employment, display your personality, and create an interest in reading your enclosed résumé.

Some guidelines to follow in writing the application/cover letter include:

1. Address your letter to a specific individual whenever possible. You may need to make a telephone call to obtain the name, title, and correct spelling.
2. Keep the letter concise, use correct grammar and spelling, and follow standard business letter format (formality is key).
3. The first paragraph should state your reason for writing and focus the reader's attention. It should not give as a reason "in response to a help wanted ad."
4. The second paragraph should identify how your education, experience, and qualifications relate to the job and refer to the enclosed résumé.
5. The last paragraph should close with a request for an interview.
6. Have someone with management experience review your cover letter. This could be your practicum supervisor, an instructor, a friend, or an acquaintance who is in a supervisory position.
7. Do not reproduce cover letters. An original letter should be sent to each individual.
8. The cover letter should be placed on top of the résumé and mailed in a business size envelope that matches its contents or in an 8½ × 11 manila envelope containing your return address.
9. Do not staple the cover letter to the résumé.

A sample of an application/cover letter is shown in Figure 36-7A.

An alternate example of an application/cover letter using Information Mapping® to highlight and draw attention to specific information in your letter is shown in Figure 36-7B. This format is considered easier to read because the focus is on specific blocks of information. In addition, its uniqueness draws attention to your letter and may result in your being selected when competition is keen.

COMPLETING THE APPLICATION FORM

Sooner or later during the job search you will be asked to complete an **application form.** How well you complete this task may be a key factor in obtaining an interview and that first job.

Reading through the application form questions, you may be tempted to write in "See résumé" rather than repeat pertinent information already contained within your résumé. Do not fall into this pitfall. Answer every item completely. The application is organized in the manner that suits the clinic, whereas individual résumés are organized in a variety of ways. Finding specific information on a résumé is more time consuming for the clinic, whereas finding the same information on the job application is easy and quick because they know where to look for it. Read all the directions carefully. Look for seemingly insignificant directions placed at the top or bottom of the page that state "Print Carefully," "Complete in Your Own Hand-

2031 Craig Street
Renton, Washington 98055
August 22, 20XX

Sarah Molles, Manager
Seattle Group Health Cooperative
304 Fourth Avenue
Seattle, Washington 98124-1716

Dear Ms. Molles:

I am interested in the medical assistant position to assist in a dermatology surgery practice. I meet the qualifications and would like to be considered for the position.

I am currently a certified medical assistant certified through the National Healthcareer Association (NHA). I have experience as a clinical assistant in an internal medicine clinic and have excellent communication and interpersonal skills.

I will be available Tuesday and Thursday afternoon from 1:00 p.m. to 4:00 p.m. I will call you next Thursday to set up an appointment for an interview.

Yours truly,

Porscha Dolan, CMA (AAMA)

Enclosure, Résumé

Figure 36-7A Sample application/cover letter.

writing," or "Please Type." Employers may use this to assess your ability to read and follow directions and pay attention to detail.

If the application is to be handwritten, use black ink to complete the form. Black ink is considered legal and often is an indelible (permanent) ink and is more legible if the form must be duplicated. Concentrate when completing the form and be sure to print clearly and make no errors. When possible, copy the application before beginning in case an error is made.

The current trend is toward online application forms. These forms are prepared by keying information into the appropriate spaces or blocks by using a computer. The completed forms are printed and mailed to the perspective employer or sent electronically. Sending electronically is increasingly the preferred method. All of the concerns relative to care in following instructions, providing complete and accurate information, and proofreading the application for any errors before sending are applicable.

If you are asked to list experience but the application does not specify "paid experience," be sure to list any volunteer or practicum experience that relates to the position you are seeking. Part-time employment can be important as an indicator of your willingness to work, your ability to serve the public, and your organizational skills.

You may be asked to complete the application form "on the spot." Plan ahead for this event and carry a completed copy of your résumé, reference list, and application/cover letter with you. Also carry with you information not included in

2031 Craig Street
Renton, Washington 98055
August 22, 20XX

Sarah Molles, Manager
Seattle Group Health Cooperative
304 Fourth Avenue
Seattle, Washington 98124-1716

SUBJECT: SURGICAL MEDICAL ASSISTANT POSITION

Background	I am interested in the medical assistant position to assist in a dermatology surgery practice. I meet the qualifications and would like to be considered for the position.
Qualifications	I am currently a certified medical assistant graduated from a 2-year program accredited by the Commission on Accreditation of Allied Health Education Programs (CAAHEP). I have experience as a clinical assistant in an internal medicine clinic and have excellent communication and interpersonal skills.
Requested Action	I will be available Tuesday and Thursday afternoon from 1:00 p.m. to 4:00 p.m. I will call you next Thursday to set up an appointment for an interview.

Yours truly,

Ashley Jackson, CMA (AAMA)

Enclosure, Résumé

Figure 36-7B Sample information mapped letter.

your résumé, such as which years you attended high school and your salary history. A pocket spelling wordbook or dictionary may be a useful tool to carry for those who find spelling challenging. These documents should provide all the information needed to complete the application form and may be submitted with the application form. This demonstrates to the potential employer your seriousness and preparedness for finding a job.

THE INTERVIEW PROCESS

If your application/cover letter, résumé, and application form have made a favorable impression with the organization, you may be invited for an interview. An **interview** is a meeting in which you and the interviewer discuss the employment opportunities within that particular organization. It is the interviewer's responsibility to determine if you have the personality, education, and skills to perform the job. The interviewer uses the interview process to assess appearance, attitude, and dependability. The interviewer also tries to verify that you have been honest in the skills you claim to have mastered. You, on the other hand, are selling your qualifications and assessing if this is an organization in which you want to be employed.

Being well prepared for the interview will increase your self-confidence and ability to focus during the actual interview. Knowing that your application/cover letter, résumé, and references all support your career goal and objectives allows you time to concentrate on interview preparation and presentation.

The Look of Success

The look of success begins with the outward appearance. First impressions are lasting, so strive for a favorable, professional look from head to toe. Appropriate conservative attire is important. Remember, your goal is to sell your professional abilities.

Hair should be clean and healthy looking, and worn in an appropriate style for the ambulatory care setting. Long hair should be worn off the collar in perhaps a French braid or twist. Strive for a neat, professional style.

The skin should have a healthy glow. Consultation with a cosmetician may prove helpful in solving skin problems or provide opportunity for trying new products. A basic understanding of your personal skin type and selection of cosmetics that complement your skin tone aid in the presentation of a professional appearance. The natural look is most appropriate for the medical office.

A daily shower and use of personal hygiene products is advised. Remember to use caution where perfumes and scents are concerned because many magnify when the body is under stress and the scent may be offensive or cause allergic reactions in others. Smokers should be aware that smoke odor carries in their hair, skin, and clothing. This odor may not be acceptable in health care settings.

Fingernails should be short and oval shaped or have rounded corners. Only clear nail polish should be worn in the ambulatory care setting if you are not working in the clinical area. Nail polish that is chipped or cracked must be removed or replaced immediately because it creates crevices in which pathogens may hide, multiply, and spread.

First impressions are lasting, so make yours professional in all respects. Conservative business attire is appropriate. Smart casual attire is appropriate for both men and women. This consists of a skirt and blouse or a tailored pantsuit for women and slacks and dress shirt with or without a tie for men. Pay attention to details such as your accessories and shoe selection. Accessories should be small and tasteful. Shoes should be clean, polished, and in good repair. They should fit properly and be comfortable and easy to walk in (Figure 36-8).

Women may carry a small purse if necessary. A portfolio is recommended in which to keep an extra copy of your résumé, reference list, application, and cover letter. A pen should be handy. Do

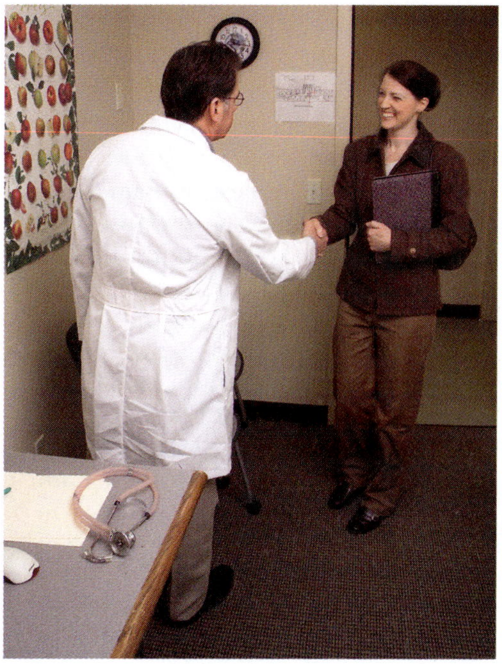

Figure 36-8 Medical assistant appropriately dressed and prepared for the interview.

not plan to search in either a purse or a portfolio for a pen or papers, keys, and so forth. Be sure that your cell phone is turned off before entering the clinic.

When you feel well and know that you look good, you project a confident and professional appearance. In other words, you are professionally poised. *Webster's Dictionary* defines *poise* as balance and stability; ease and dignity of manner. Personal poise combines all of the previously mentioned body appearances plus smoothness of movement and physical flexibility.

Preparing for the Interview

Before the interview takes place, carefully research the organization offering the position. Study the organization's mission statement, financial reports, future projections, and any other information available. Be prepared to relate your skills and interests

Critical Thinking

If you are a smoker, how can you minimize the smoke odor carried on your person before you go on a job interview? Make a list and prioritize each suggestion into a plan of action.

to the needs of this organization. In other words, what can you contribute and why should they hire you? The interview is your opportunity to sell yourself and identify ways in which you can benefit the employer.

Bring a copy of your résumé and cover letter to the interview just in case the interviewer cannot locate the original or wants another copy. You should also have copies of letters of recommendation, a list of references, a copy of your transcript from the schools you attended, and copies of any certificates such as AIDS training, First Aid, and CPR. These items should not be presented unless dictated by events that take place during the interview. You might also have with you the name of the interviewer and a copy of any questions you plan to ask the interviewer. A last-minute review will refocus your thoughts before you go into the interview. Keep your list available for quick reference in the event your mind goes blank when you are asked if you have questions.

To arrive 5 to 10 minutes early, check a map for directions or make a trip the day before your interview. Try to travel about the same time as you would for the interview so you have an idea of the time it takes, traffic flow, construction areas encountered, and parking availability. Plan for inclement weather (raincoat, umbrella, shoes). It is a good idea to make a quick trip to the restroom on arrival to change shoes or recheck your appearance.

Introduce yourself confidently to the administrative medical assistant and identify by name the person you wish to see and the time of your appointment. Always arrive alone. The employer wants to see you and sense your self-reliance and responsibility. While you wait, try to relax and observe the office setting, other employees, what they are wearing, and their manner of conducting business. This may be helpful to you during the interview and in making a decision to work there.

Figure 36-9 lists reasons why employers do not hire applicants.

REASONS FOR EMPLOYERS NOT HIRING

Employers in business were asked to list reasons for not hiring a job seeker. Given in rank order (from most unwanted to least unwanted), the 15 biggest gripes are as follows:

1. Poor appearance (not dressed properly, poorly groomed).
2. Acting like a know-it-all.
3. Cannot express self clearly; poor voice, diction, grammar.
4. Lack of planning for work—no purpose or goals.
5. Lack of confidence or poise.
6. No interest in or enthusiasm for the job.
7. Not active in school extracurricular programs.
8. Interested only in the best dollar offer.
9. Poor school record (academic, attendance).
10. Unwilling to start at the bottom.
11. Making excuses, hedges on unfavorable record.
12. No tact.
13. Not mature.
14. No curiosity about the job.
15. Critical of past employers.

Figure 36-9 Reasons for employers not hiring. (Courtesy of Highline Community College, Counseling/Career Center, Des Moines, WA.)

The Actual Interview

When you enter an interviewer's office, think of yourself as a guest and take your cues from him or her. Most interviewers will introduce themselves and extend a hand. A firm handshake, responding by introducing yourself, and smiling confidently convey a positive professional image. Remain standing until you are invited to be seated. Keep your personal items on your lap or place them on the floor near your chair. Do not invade the interviewer's territory by placing your things on the desk.

Sit erect in the chair with your feet flat on the floor or cross only your ankles. Avoid nervous mannerisms while you speak and maintain good eye contact, but do not stare the interviewer down. Be natural and positive about the position, organization, and yourself. Present a professional image by using medical terminology when responding to questions or providing information. Observe the interviewer carefully for cues. Respond to questions completely, trying not to repeat yourself or give more information than was requested.

Be prepared for the kinds of questions that may be asked during the interview process. Ask yourself, "If I were the employer, what would I want to know about the applicant?" Figure 36-10 gives examples of standard questions asked by most employers. Consider how you would respond to each question.

TYPICAL QUESTIONS ASKED DURING AN INTERVIEW

1. I see from your résumé you graduated from ____________ college. What did that college have to offer that others didn't?
2. What subjects did you enjoy the most and why?
3. What do you see yourself doing 5 years from now?
4. What salary do you expect and what do you think it will be in 5 or 10 years?
5. What do you consider to be your greatest strengths and weaknesses?
6. How do you think a friend or professor who knows you well would describe you?
7. What qualifications do you have that make you think you would be successful in this position?
8. In what ways do you think you can make a contribution to our organization?
9. What two or three accomplishments have given you the most satisfaction?
10. What didn't you like about your last employer?
11. How well do you work under pressure?
12. Will you be able to work overtime occasionally?
13. How do you respond to criticism?
14. How would you respond if a patient or coworker made advances toward you?
15. How would you handle following procedures with which you do not agree?
16. Describe a specific medical procedure.
17. Do you have any questions you would like to ask?
18. How would you establish credibility quickly with our team?
19. What attracted you to this clinic?
20. What is the last book you read?
21. Why should we hire you?
22. What is your personal mission statement?

Figure 36-10 Knowing how you would answer some of these typical questions can prepare you for your interview.

Remember that the interviewer is asking questions to determine if you are qualified for the position and if you are the kind of person who will fit into the organization. *Think* before answering questions; try to provide the information requested in a positive and professional manner. Do not respond with slang terms. *Listen* carefully so that you understand what information the question is requesting. *Ask* for clarification if you are uncertain. This demonstrates your ability to be open enough to ask questions when in doubt.

Interviewing the Employer

The worst thing that can happen to an entry-level employee is to be hired and then have to quit or be fired because of a conflict with the employer. The interview process is a two-way street. You, the interviewee, should also interview the potential employer. The following are danger signs of an employer who could make your work life very difficult:

- Disrespectful behavior during the interview toward other staff members or to you
- Signs of insecurity by the manager
- Lack of enthusiasm toward the organization
- Shows signs of being highly stressed
- Negative attitude in statements
- Arrogance or answers own questions
- Uses the pronoun "I" excessively

You have to read the interviewer because some of the signs listed could be attributed to a "bad day." If too many signals are showing or, after prudent questioning on your part, you still have concerns, perhaps you should look for employment elsewhere to avoid the possibility of damaging your future career.

Following are a few questions you might ask the interviewer to resolve some of these concerns raised by observations:

- How would you describe the clinic culture?
- How do you handle differing opinions on how best to accomplish tasks?
- How are employee accomplishments recognized?
- What is the leadership style at the clinic?
- What is the attitude toward professional growth and educational opportunities?

Answers to these questions will help you determine if the clinic culture is one you can embrace.

Closing the Interview

By observing the interviewer and listening carefully, you will be able to determine when the interviewer feels he or she has enough information about you to make a decision. Usually during the closing the interviewer asks if you have any additional questions. This is your opportunity to collect information helpful in making a decision to accept or decline an offer. Your questions provide another opportunity to sell yourself, show that you have done your homework about the organization, and have listened carefully during the interview.

Select three or four questions that will help you the most.

Questions about the organization are excellent choices. Examples are:

- "What are the opportunities for advancement with this organization?"
- "I read that your organization has educational benefits. Could you explain briefly how that program works?"
- "You mentioned in-house training programs for employees. Could you give one or two examples?"

You may also have some questions about the job itself. Examples of these types of questions are:

- "Is this a newly created position? If so, what results are you hoping to see?"
- "Was the last person in this position promoted? What contributed to their advancement?"
- "What do you consider the most difficult task on this job?"
- "What are the lines of authority for this position?"

Do not use this question time to ask about salary, sick leave, vacations, or retirement benefits. At this point, your focus should be on the value and skills you can contribute to the organization. These questions may be asked during a second interview or when a position is offered.

Before you leave, thank the interviewer for taking time to discuss the position with you. If you definitely are interested in the position, ask to be considered as a candidate for the position. If follow-up procedures have not been explained, now is the time to ask when the final selection will be made and how you will be notified. A firm handshake as you leave, a pleasant smile, and confidence as you exit will leave a professional picture in the interviewer's mind.

INTERVIEW FOLLOW-UP

Following up after the interview is essential. This is the time to telephone your references to let them know the name of the organization and the person's name with whom you interviewed, something about the position, and your qualifications. Share any information that will help your references support you in obtaining the position.

Follow-Up Letter

Take time to write a follow-up letter or handwritten note to the interviewer a day or two after your interview to thank him or her for the time spent interviewing you. The letter should be written in standard business format and printed on the same paper as your application/cover letter and résumé. Be sure that all spelling and grammar are correct.

The follow-up letter provides another opportunity to express your interest in the organization and the position. You can briefly emphasize the experience and skills you have to offer and again request being considered a candidate for the position.

Record the mailing date on your contact tracker and keep a copy of the letter in a file with other information about the organization. Figure 36-11 shows a sample follow-up letter.

Follow Up by Telephone

Allow a few days for your follow-up letter to reach the interviewer. If you do not hear from the interviewer within a week or by the designated time established during the interview, you may call to ask if you are still being considered for the position or if a decision has been made.

Speak directly into the mouthpiece of the telephone using good diction and voice volume. Identify yourself and provide some information to aid the interviewer in recalling who you are. Perhaps mentioning the date you interviewed will suffice. Be polite and professional, and remember to thank the individual for speaking with you. At the end of the conversation say good-bye and wait until the other person hangs up before you break the connection. Log the telephone call and its response on your contact tracker for future reference.

AFTER YOU ARE EMPLOYED

You are now a newly employed medical assistant. What do you do now to advance your career? Following are some suggestions:

- Make sure your workstation is set up and you have what you need to do the job
- Practice good time management skills
- Try to allow time for emergencies, which will occur
- Do not be a know-it-all; ask other employees how they do things around here
- Get to know colleagues and be part of the team
- Seek feedback on how you are doing your job
- Create a professional image

Dealing with Difficult People

Sooner or later you will encounter coworkers who could be described as just plain "jerks." Jerks may

2031 Craig Street
Renton, Washington 98055
August 28, 20XX

Sarah Molles, Manager
Seattle Group Health Cooperative
304 Fourth Avenue
Seattle, Washington 98124-1716

Dear Ms. Molles,

Thank you for scheduling a personal interview with me last Wednesday, August 26, at 9:45 AM. I enjoyed discussing the medical assistant position open in one of your dermatology surgery practices. I would like to be considered for the position.

After talking with you, I feel my qualifications match closely with those you requested. My communication and interpersonal skills are excellent and a necessary ingredient for any medical assistant.

I look forward to hearing from you September 5 as you mentioned during the interview. If there are any questions I may answer, please telephone me.

Sincerely,

Ashley Jackson

Ashley Jackson, CMA (AAMA)
(206) 255-1365

Figure 36-11 Sample follow-up letter.

be defined as persons who use power to belittle and ridicule people who work under them. These people may be foul-mouthed, power hungry, bullies, uncouth, or unethical. There are several ways to free yourself from jerks.

- Check out emotionally (attempt to ignore the comments); indifference is an underrated virtue
- Try to move to a different position within the organization
- If all else fails, change jobs

Getting a Raise

One of the main reasons people do not get a raise is because they do not ask. This is particularly true of professional women. It has been reported that less than half ask for a raise or promotion within a 12-month period. Of those that did ask, almost three quarters received a raise or promotion. After taking into consideration the wages of persons with similar job descriptions and experience, if your salary appears to be lagging you should not feel uncomfortable asking for a raise at your next favorable performance review.

Critical Thinking

As you begin to prepare for a job interview, how can you prepare yourself to reflect a professional image, attitude, demeanor, verbal and nonverbal communication skills, as well as articulately describe your skills and abilities to fit the position to which you are applying? Develop a complete written checklist and review it before each interview.

PROFESSIONALISM

Areas of professionalism directly related to the medical office may include:

- Display a professional manner and image. The chapter content stresses the importance of having a positive attitude, taking pride in doing the best you can, being prepared, and dressing appropriately for job interviews.
- Promote your CMA (AAMA), RMA, CMAS, or other credential. On graduation from an accredited school, you will be ready to sit for the national certification examination. On notification of passing the examination, you will be awarded the appropriate credential. When signing your name, include your credential and educate others regarding its significance.

Case Study 36-1

Review the scenario at the beginning of the chapter.

CASE STUDY REVIEW

1. Which résumé style represents Eun Mee best and why?
2. List transferable skills that Eun Mee may want to include in her résumé.
3. What is the purpose of an accomplishment statement? Provide examples Eun Mee might use.

Case Study 36-2

Drs. Lewis and King maintain a two-provider family practitioner office. They are in need of a new medical assistant to take the place of one who will be leaving at the end of the month. They have scheduled interviews with five applicants. Eun Mee Soo is the first candidate to be interviewed.

CASE STUDY REVIEW

1. Eun Mee enters the interview with some papers in her hand. What paperwork should she have brought with her?
2. Why should Eun Mee arrive 5 to 10 minutes early for the interview?
3. How should Eun Mee enter the room?

SUMMARY

Finding your first job is your first job. How well you research, plan, prepare, and implement your tasks will make the difference between being hired and not being hired. Learn from each interview session. Recall the questions that were asked and formulate answers that you feel would be appropriate for your next interview. Tell everyone you are looking for a job and solicit their help. Follow up on all leads and do not become discouraged.

Once you have been hired at that first job, continue your learning experience. Ask appropriate questions and try not to ask the same question a second or third time. Pay attention to details and learn individual preferences. Become a team player and look for ways you can help others. Carry your share of responsibility and do not be afraid to admit you are unfamiliar with certain aspects of the office. Employers need to know you can be trusted to work within the scope of your education and not beyond. Practice being an asset to your employer.

STUDY FOR SUCCESS

To reinforce your knowledge and skills of information presented in this chapter:

- Review the Key Terms
- Consider the Case Studies and discuss your conclusions
- Answer the Review Questions
  - Multiple Choice
  - Critical Thinking
- Navigate the Internet by completing the Web Activities
- Practice the StudyWARE activities on the textbook CD
- Apply your knowledge in the Student Workbook activities
- Complete the Web Tutor sections
- View and discuss the DVD situations

REVIEW QUESTIONS

Multiple Choice

1. The résumé:
   a. is a summary data sheet or brief account of your qualifications and progress in your career
   b. is also known as a contact tracker
   c. always includes references
   d. is used to introduce yourself and identify qualifications
2. References:
   a. must always be listed on the résumé
   b. should be a relative
   c. should be someone who likes you and your work but may not be a good communicator
   d. should be someone who knows you or has worked with you long enough to make an honest assessment of your capabilities and integrity
3. The targeted résumé is advantageous:
   a. when prior titles are impressive
   b. when reentering the job market after an absence
   c. when you are just starting your career and have little experience
   d. when you have extensive specialized experience
4. The application/cover letter:
   a. is a detailed data sheet describing your vital information, education, and experience
   b. introduces you to a prospective employer and captures their interest in you as a candidate for the position
   c. lists individuals who can vouch for you
   d. should be lengthy and detailed
5. The interview:
   a. does not require much thought or preparation
   b. requires you to think before answering questions, listen carefully, and ask for clarification if uncertain of the question
   c. provides time to ask questions about salary, vacation, and benefits
   d. does not require any follow-up
6. Preparing for the interview:
   a. bathe yourself, groom your hair and fingernails, and wear clean and pressed conservative business attire
   b. allow adequate time to get to the interview
   c. prepare a packet to give the interviewer containing certificates, letters of recommendation, a list of references, and your list of questions
   d. all of the above
7. Job analysis should include:
   a. compiling a list of potential employers
   b. gathering information about employers in whom you have interest
   c. preparing a budgetary needs analysis
   d. all of the above
8. The best source for job search data is:
   a. the Internet
   b. friends and acquaintances
   c. the Yellow Pages and classified ads
   d. all of the above

Critical Thinking

1. Discuss the various résumé styles with a classmate and how to determine which style best presents your knowledge and skills to a prospective employer.

2. After reading the section discussing methods of researching a prospective employer, how will you proceed with your research?
3. Review Figure 36-9, which lists reasons for employers not hiring, with a classmate. How will you prevent the 15 biggest gripes from being an employment stumbling block for you personally?
4. How will you prepare a budget for living expenses to determine job salary requirements?
5. Sometimes employers may ask illegal or inappropriate questions during an interview in true innocence, or true ignorance. Give a legal reason why an employer might need the following information once you have been hired.
   a. Are you married?
   b. How many kids do you have?
   c. How old are you?
   d. Where were you born?

WEB ACTIVITIES

1. Being prepared to answer and discuss interview questions is critical in the selection for the position opening. Using Google.com, or your favorite search engine, search job interview questions. Many sites provide sample questions and appropriate answers. Study them and prepare a list of questions with personal responses you feel are appropriate.
2. There are some illegal interview questions based on Federal Discrimination Laws enforced by the Equal Employment Opportunity Commission. They are questions that specifically discriminate against you on the basis of:
   - Age
   - Color
   - Disability
   - Sex
   - National origin
   - Race, religion, or creed

Using your favorite search engine, research these inappropriate questions and ways in which you might handle them appropriately. Compile a list of questions and your personal appropriate response to each. Discuss these with a classmate and role-play responding to the questions.

REFERENCES/BIBLIOGRAPHY

Farr, M. (2000). *Quick resume & cover letter book.* Indianapolis, IN: JIST Works, Inc.

Keir, L., Wise, B. A., Krebs, C., Kelley-Arney, C. (2008). *Medical assisting: Administrative and clinical competencies* (6th ed.). Clifton Park, NY: Delmar Cengage Learning.

Nobel, D. F. (2000). *Gallary of best resumes for people without a four-year degree.* Indianapolis, IN: JIST Works, Inc.

Sindell, M., & Sindell, T. (2006). *Sink or swim.* Avon, MA: Adams Media Publishing.

Washington, T. (2000). *Resume power selling yourself on paper in the new millennium.* Indianapolis, IN: JIST Works, Inc.

Zedlitz, R. H. (2003). *How to get a job in health care.* Clifton Park, NY: Delmar Cengage Learning.

THE DVD HOOK-UP

This chapter discusses strategies that you can use to help gain employment.

One of the first testimonials in this scene showed Paula talking about the fact that she can determine a person's professionalism within 5 minutes of the interview.

1. Do you really think that it is possible to gauge a person's professionalism within 5 minutes of an interview?
2. What do you think about the outfit that Dee was wearing for her interview? Do you think it was professional?
3. What will you wear for your interviews when you apply for a medical assisting position?

DVD Journal Summary

Write a paragraph that summarizes what you learned from watching the selected scenes from today's DVD program.

Using a scale of 1 to 10, how would you have rated your professionalism skills when you started the program? How would you rate your professional skills now that you have almost completed with the program? What improvements do you need to make to be the best possible medical assistant you can be?

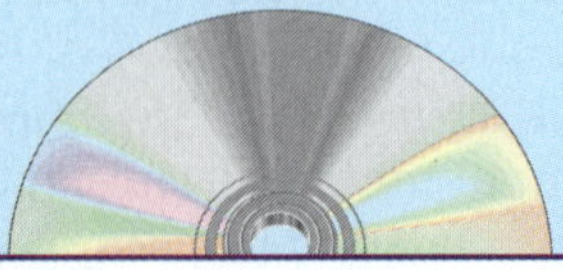

DVD Series Critical Thinking

Program Number 1

Chapter/Scene Reference
- *Preparing for a Job*

Common Medical Abbreviations and Symbols

Appendix A

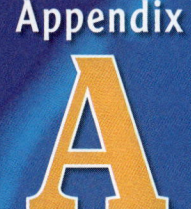

āā	of each
AAMA	American Association of Medical Assistants
AAP	American Academy of Pediatricians
AAPC	American Academy of Professional Coders
ab	abortion
abd	abdomen
ABE	acute bacterial endocarditis
ABG	arterial blood gases
ABHES	Accrediting Bureau of Health Education Schools
ABO	blood groups
abs	absent
ac	before meals (ante cibum)
	acute
ACAP	Alliance of Claims Assistance Professionals
ACIP	Advisory Committee on Immunization Practices
ACOG	American College of Obstetricians and Gynecologists
ACTH	adrenocorticotropic hormone
ADA	Americans with Disabilities Act
ADHD	attention deficit hyperactivity disorder
ADL	activities of daily living
ad lib	as desired
adm	admission
AED	automated external defibrillator
AFP	alpha fetal protein
AHD	arteriosclerotic heart disease
	atherosclerotic heart disease
AHDI	Association for Healthcare Documentation Integrity
AHIMA	American Health Information Management Association
AIDS	acquired immunodeficiency syndrome
alb	albumin
AM	before noon (ante meridiem)
AMA	against medical advice
	American Medical Association
AMBA	American Medical Billing Association
AMI	acute myocardial infarction
amt	amount
AMT	American Medical Technologists
AMTIE	American Medical Technologists Institute for Education
ant	anterior
ante	before
A&P	anterior and posterior
	auscultation and palpation
	auscultation and percussion
APC	ambulatory payment classifications
aq	water
A/R	accounts receivable
ARDS	acute (or adult) respiratory distress syndrome
ARU	automated routing unit
ASA	acetylsalicylic acid
ASAP	as soon as possible
ASC	atypical squamous cell
ASCAD	arteriosclerotic coronary artery disease
ASC US	atypical squamous cell of uncertain significance
ASCVD	arteriosclerotic cardiovascular disease
	atherosclerotic cardiovascular disease
A&W	alive and well
Ba	barium
BaE	barium enema
BBB	bundle branch block
BC	birth control
BCP	birth control pills
BC/BS	Blue Cross/Blue Shield
BE	bacterial endocarditis
bid	twice a day
bil	bilateral
BM	basal metabolism
	bowel movement
BMI	body mass index
BMR	basal metabolism rate
BNA	budget neutrality adjuster
BP	blood pressure
BPH	benign prostatic hypertrophy
BS	blood sugar
	bowel sounds
	breath sounds
BSA	body surface area
BSL	blood sugar level
BSN	bowel sounds normal
BSO	bilateral salpingo-oophorectomy
BSR	blood sedimentation rate
BUN	blood urea nitrogen
BW	below waist
	birth weight
	body weight
Bx	biopsy
C	Celsius
	centigrade
c̄	with

C1	first cervical vertebra
CA	cancer
	carcinoma
Ca	calcium
CAAHEP	Commission on Accreditation of Allied Health Education Programs
CAD	coronary artery disease
CAHD	coronary arteriosclerotic heart disease
caps	capsules
CAM	complementary and alternative medicine
CAT	computerized axial tomography
CBC	complete blood count
CC	chief complaint
CCA	Certified Coding Associate
CCMA	Certified Clinical Medical Assistant
CCP	Certification Continuation Program
CCR	continuity of care record
CCS	Certified Coding Specialist
CCS-P	Certified Coding Specialist-Physician-Based
CCT	cardiac computerized tomography
CCU	coronary care unit
C&D	cystoscopy and dilation
CDC	U.S. Centers for Disease Control and Prevention
CE	continuing education
cerv	cervical
	cervix
CEU	continuing education unit
CF	conversion factor
CHAMPVA	Civilian Health and Medical Program of the Veterans Administration
CHD	childhood disease
	congenital heart disease
	congestive heart disease
	coronary heart disease
CHEDDAR	chief complaint, history, examination, details of problems, drugs and dosages, assessment, return visit if applicable
CHF	congestive heart failure
CHO	carbohydrate
CIN	cervical intraepithelial neoplasia
ck	check
Cl	chlorine
cldy	cloudy
CLIA	Clinical Laboratory Improvement Amendments
cm	centimeter
CMA (AAMA)	Certified Medical Assistant through the American Association of Medical Assistants
CMAA	Certified Medical Administrative Assistant
CMAS	Certified Medical Administrative Specialist
CME	continuing medical education
CMR	cardiac magnetic resonance
CMS	Centers for Medicare and Medicaid Services
CMT	Certified Medical Transcriptionist
CNS	central nervous system
C/O	complains of
CO_2	carbon dioxide
COB	coordination of benefits
COPD	chronic obstructive pulmonary disease
CPC	Certified Professional Coders
CPC-A	Certified Professional Coders-Apprentice
CPC-H	Certified Professional Coders-Hospital
CPC-HA	Certified Professional Coders-Hospital Apprentice
CPR	cardiopulmonary resuscitation
CPT	Current Procedural Terminology
CPU	central processing unit
CRB	Curriculum Review Board
crit	hematocrit
CS	cerebrospinal
	cesarean section
C&S	culture and sensitivity
CSF	cerebrospinal fluid
CT	computerized tomography
CVA	cerebrovascular accident
CVE	capsule video endoscopy
CVP	central venous pressure
CVS	chorionic villus sampling
cx	cervix
CXR	chest X-ray
cysto	cystoscopic examination
	cystoscopy
DACUM	developing a curriculum
DC	doctor of chiropracty
D&C	dilation and curettage
DDS	doctor of dentistry
DEA	U.S. Drug Enforcement Agency
dec	decrease
DEERS	Defense Enrollment Eligible Reporting System
del	delivery
DES	diethylstilbestrol
DHHS	U.S. Department of Health and Human Services
diab	diabetic
diag	diagnosis
diff	differential white blood cell count
dil	dilute
disc	discontinue
disp	dispense
DM	diabetes mellitus
DNA	deoxyribonucleic acid
	does not apply
DNR	do not resuscitate
DO	doctor of osteopathy
DOA	dead on arrival
DOB	date of birth
DOD	date of death
DOE	dyspnea on exertion
dos	dosage
DPI	dry powder inhaler

DPM	doctor of podiatric medicine
DPT	diphtheria, pertussis, and tetanus
DR	delivery room
Dr	doctor
DRGs	diagnosis-related groups
DS	discharge summary
DSD	dry sterile dressing
dsg	dressing
DT	delirium tremens
DTR	deep tendon reflex
D&V	diarrhea and vomiting
DW	distilled water
D/W	dextrose in water
dx	diagnosis
ea	each
EBV	Epstein–Barr virus
ECG	electrocardiogram
echo	echocardiogram echoencephalogram
E. coli	*Escherichia coli*
ECT	electroconvulsive therapy electronic claims transmission
EDC	estimated date of confinement or expected date of confinement
EDD	estimated date of delivery or expected date of delivery
EEG	electroencephalogram
EENT	eyes, ears, nose, and throat
e.g.	for example
EHR	electronic health record
EKG	electrocardiogram
elix	elixir
Email	electronic mail
EMG	electromyography
EMR	electronic medical record
EMS	emergency medical service
ENT	ear, nose, and throat
EOB	explanation of benefits
eos	eosinophil
EPA	Environmental Protection Agency
EPCA-2	early prostate cancer antigen-2
EPO	exclusive provider organization
eq	equivalent
ER	emergency room
ERT	estrogen replacement therapy
ESR	erythrocyte sedimentation rate
EST	electroshock therapy
exam	examination
ext	extract
F	Fahrenheit female
FAS	fetal alcohol syndrome
fax	facsimile
FBS	fasting blood sugar
FDA	U.S. Food and Drug Administration
FECA	Federal Employees Compensation Act Program
FH	family history
FHR	fetal heart rate
FHS	fetal heart sound
fl	fluid
fl oz	fluid ounce
FMP	first menstrual period
FP	family practice
freq	frequent
FSH	follicle-stimulating hormone
ft	foot
FTA	fluorescent treponemal antibody
FTP	file transfer protocol
fx	fracture
G	gravida
g	gram
GB	gallbladder
GC	gonococcus gonorrhea
GERD	gastroesophageal reflux disease
GI	gastrointestinal
gm	gram
GP	general practice
GPCI	Geographic Practice Cost Index
gr	grain
grav	pregnancy
GTH	gonadotropic hormone
GTT	glucose tolerance test
gtt(s)	drop (drops)
GU	genitourinary
GYN	gynecology
h	hour
HAI	healthcare–associated infection
HBP	high blood pressure
HCFA	U.S. Health Care Financing Administration
hCG	human chorionic gonadotropin
HCl	hydrochloric acid
HCPCS	Healthcare Common Procedure Coding System
Hct	hematocrit
HCVD	hypertensive cardiovascular disease
HEENT	head, eyes, ears, nose, and throat
HEPA	high-efficiency particulate air
Hgb	hemoglobin
H&H	hemoglobin and hematocrit
HIPAA	Health Insurance Portability and Accountability Act
HMO	health maintenance organization
H/O	history of
H_2O	water
H&P	history and physical
HPI	history of present illness
HPV	human papillomavirus
HR	human resources
HRS	Healthcare Reimbursement Specialist

HRT	hormone replacement therapy
HSV1	herpes simplex virus 1
HSV2	herpes simplex virus 2
HT	hormone therapy
ht	height
hx	history
Hz	hertz
ICCU	intensive coronary care unit
ICD-9-CM	International Classification of Diseases, 9th revision, Clinical Modification
ICU	intensive care unit
ID	intradermal
I&D	incision and drainage
IDS	integrated delivery system
IM	internal medicine
	intramuscular
imp	impression
inf	infusion
inj	injection
I&O	intake and output
IOM	Institute of Medicine
IPA	independent physician association
IPV	intimate partner violence
IPPB	intermittent positive pressure breathing
IPPS	inpatient prospective payment systems
ISP	Internet service provider
IUD	intrauterine device
IV	intravenous
IVF	in vitro fertilization
IVP	intravenous pyelogram
JAAMT	*Journal of the American Association for Medical Transcription*
JAMA	*Journal of the American Medical Association*
jt	joint
K	potassium
kg	kilogram
KOH	potassium hydroxide
KUB	kidney, ureter, and bladder
kV	kilovolt
L	left
	liter
l	length
LA	left atrium
	lactic acid
L&A	light and accommodation
lab	laboratory
lac	laceration
LAN	local area network
lap	laparotomy
lat	lateral
lb	pound
LBBB	left bundle branch block
LDL	low-density lipoprotein
LE	lupus erythematosus
LEEP	loop electrosurgical excision procedure
liq	liquid
LLQ	lower left quadrant
LMP	last menstrual period
LP	lumbar puncture
LRQ	lower right quadrant
LUQ	left upper quadrant
L&W	living and well
lymphs	lymphocytes
M	male
m	meter
MA	medical allowable
MBCD	management by coaching and development
MBCE	management by competitive edge
MBDM	management by decision models
MBP	management by performance
MBS	management by styles
MBWA	management by wandering around
MBWS	management by work simplification
MCHC	mean corpuscular hemoglobin and red cell indices
MCO	managed care organization
MCV	mean corpuscular volume and red cell indices
MD	doctor of medicine
	muscular dystrophy
MDI	metered dose inhaler
MDR	minimum daily requirement
med	medicine
mEq/L	milliequivalents per liter
MFS	Medicare fee schedule
mg	milligram
MH	marital history
	medical history
	menstrual history
MHx	medical history
MI	maturation index
	myocardial infarction
mL	milliliter
mm	millimeter
mm^3	cubic millimeter
mm Hg	millimeters of mercury
MMR	measles, mumps, and rubella
MOM	milk of magnesia
mono	mononucleosis
MP	menstrual period
MRC	Medical Reserve Corps
MRI	magnetic resonance imaging
MRIA	magnetic resonance imaging angiography
MRSA	methicillin resistant *Staphylococcus aureus*
MS	mitral stenosis
	multiple sclerosis
MSDS	material safety data sheets
MSHA	Mine Safety and Health Administration
MT	medical technologist
	medical transcriptionist

multip	multipara
MVP	mitral valve prolapse
NA	not applicable
NaCl	sodium chloride
NACP	National Association of Claims Assistance Professionals
narc	narcotic
NB	newborn
NCAI	National Coalition for Adult Immunization
N/C	no complaints
ND	doctor of naturopathy
NEBA	National Electronic Billers Alliance
NEC	not elsewhere classified
neg	negative
NG	nasogastric
NGU	nongonococcal urethritis
NHA	National Healthcareer Association
NIDDM	noninsulin–dependent diabetes mellitus
NL	normal limits
NMP	normal menstrual period
noct	at night
Non-PAR	nonparticipating provider
non rep	do not repeat
NOS	not otherwise specified
NPI	national provider identification
NPO	nothing by mouth
NR	no refill
	nonreactive
	normal range
NS	nonspecific
	normal saline
	not significant
	not sufficient
N&T	nose and throat
N&V	nausea and vomiting
NVD	nausea, vomiting, and diarrhea
O	oral
	oxygen
O_2	oxygen
OB	obstetrics
OB-GYN	obstetrics-gynecology
OC	office call
	on call
	oral contraceptive
occ	occasionally
OCR	Office of Civil Rights
	optical character reader
OGTT	oral glucose tolerance test
OM	office manager
OOB	out of bed
OP	outpatient
O&P	ova and parasites
OPIM	other potentially infectious material
OPPS	outpatient prospective payment systems
OPV	oral poliovaccine
OR	operating room
	operative report
ortho	orthopedics
os	mouth
OSHA	U.S. Occupational Safety and Health Administration
OT	occupational therapist
	occupational therapy
OTC	over the counter
OURQ	outer upper right quadrant
OV	office visit
OWCP	Office Workers' Compensation Programs
oz	ounce
P	phosphorus
	pulse
P&A	percussion and auscultation
PA	physician's assistant
	posteroanterior
PAC	phenacetin, aspirin, and codeine
	premature atrial contraction
PACS	picture archiving and communications systems
Pap	Papanicolaou (smear, test)
PAR	participating provider
para	number of pregnancies
para I	primipara
PAT	paroxysmal atrial tachycardia
path	pathology
PBI	protein-bound iodine
pc	after meals
PC	personal computer
PCA	patient-controlled analgesic
PCC	Poison Control Center
PCN	penicillin
PCP	primary care physician
PCR	polymerase chain reaction
PCV	packed cell volume
PDA	personal digital assistant
PDR	*Physician's Desk Reference*
PE	physical examination
peds	pediatrics
PEG	pneumoencephalography
PERRLA	pupils equal, round, regular, react to light, and accommodation
PET	positron emission transmission or tomography
PH	past history
	personal history
	public health
pH	hydrogen in concentration
PHI	protected health information
PHO	physician-hospital organization
PI	present illness
	pulmonary infarction
PID	pelvic inflammatory disease
PKU	phenylketonuria

PM	after noon (post meridiem)
	post mortem (after death)
PMN	polymorphonuclear neutrophils
PMP	past menstrual period
PMS	premenstrual syndrome
PNC	penicillin
PO	postoperative
po	by mouth
POB	place of birth
POLST	physician orders for life-sustaining treatment
POMR	problem-oriented medical record
POS	point-of-service plan
pos	positive
poss	possible
postop	postoperative
PP	present problem
	postprandial
PPB	positive pressure breathing
PPBS	postprandial blood sugar
PPD	purified protein derivative
PPO	preferred provider organization
preop	preoperative
primip	woman bearing first child
prn	as the occasion arises, as necessary
procto	proctoscopy
prog	prognosis
PROM	premature rupture of membranes
pro-time	prothrombin time
PRSP	penicillin-resistant *Streptococcus* pneumonia
PSA	prostate-specific antigen
PSRO	Professional Standards Review Organization
PT	physical therapy
	prothrombin time
pt	patient
PTA	prior to admission
PTT	partial thromboplastin time
pulv	powder
PVC	premature ventricular contraction
px	physical examination
	prognosis
q	each; every
q AM	every morning
QA	quality assurance
qh	every hour
q (2, 3, 4)h	every 2, 3, or 4 hours
qid	four times a day
QISMC	Quality Improvement System for Managed Care
qns	quantity not sufficient
qs	of sufficient quantity
qt	quart
R	registration
	right
RAM	random access memory
RBC	red blood cell
RBC/hpf	red blood cells per high power field
RBCM	red blood cell mass
RBCV	red blood cell volume
RBRVS	Resource-Based Relative Value Scale
REM	rapid eye movement
resp	respiration
Rh	rhesus (factor)
Rh-	rhesus negative
Rh+	rhesus positive
RHD	rheumatic heart disease
RLQ	right lower quadrant
RMA	Registered Medical Assistant
RNA	ribonucleic acid
R/O	rule out
ROA	received on account
ROM	range of motion
	read-only memory
ROS	review of systems
ROTA	rotavirus
RT	radiation therapy
RUQ	right upper quadrant
RVUs	relative value units
Rx	prescription
S	subjective data (POMR)
s̄	without
S&A	sugar and acetone (urine)
SA	sinoatrial
SARS	severe acute respiratory syndrome
SBE	shortness of breath on exertion
	subacute bacterial endocarditis
SE	standard error
sed rate	sedimentation rate
segs	segmented neutrophils
seq	sequela
SF	scarlet fever
	spinal fluid
SG	specific gravity
SH	social history
SIDS	sudden infant death syndrome
sig	instructions, directions
sigmoid	sigmoidoscopy
SIL	squamous interepithelial lesion
SMA 12/60	Sequential Multiple Analyzer (12-test serum profile)
SOAP	subjective data, objective data, assessment, and plan
SOAPER	subjective, objective, assessment, plan, education, response
SOB	shortness of breath
SOF	signature on file
sol	solution
solv	solvent
SOMR	source-oriented medical record
SOP	standard operating procedure
SOS	if necessary
spec	specimen

sp gr	secific gravity
spont ab	spontaneous abortion
SR	sedimentation rate
SS	signs and symptoms
$\overline{ss}$	one-half
SSI	Supplemental Security Income
Staph	Staphylococcus
stat	immediately
STD	sexually transmitted disease
Strep	Streptococcus
subq	subcutaneous
supp	suppository
surg	surgery
sx	signs
	symptoms
sym	symptoms
syr	syrup
T	temperature
T_3	tri-iodothyronine
T_4	thyroxine
T&A	tonsillectomy and adenoidectomy
tab	tablet
TAT	temporal artery thermometer
TB	tuberculin
	tuberculosis
TBS	The Bethesda System
tbs	tablespoon
TC	throat culture
	tissue culture
	total capacity
	total cholesterol
TENS	transcutaneous electrical nerve stimulator
TFTC	Task Force for Test Construction
ther	therapy
therap	therapeutic
TIA	transient ischemic attack
tid	three times a day
tinct	tincture
TLC	tender loving care
TMJ	temporomandibular joint
top	topically
TOPV	trivalent oral poliovirus vaccine
TP	total protein
TPI	treponema pallidum immobilization test
TPMS	Total Practice Management System
TPN	total parenteral nutrition
TPR	temperature, pulse, and respiration
tr	tincture
trig	triglycerides
TSH	thyroid-stimulating hormone
tsp	teaspoon
TSS	toxic shock syndrome
TUR	transurethral resection
tus	cough
T&X	type and cross match
UA	urinalysis
UB04	Uniform Bill 04
UCG	urinary chorionic gonadotropin
UCHD	usual childhood diseases
UCR	usual, customary, reasonable
ULQ	upper left quadrant
ung	ointment
UNICEF	United Nations International Children's Emergency Fund
UR	utilization review
urg	urgent
URI	upper respiratory infection
URL	Uniform Resource Locator
urol	urology
URQ	upper right quadrant
URT	upper respiratory tract
URTI	upper respiratory tract infection
USB	universal system bus port
USMLE	United States Medical Licensing Examination
USP	United States Pharmacopoeia
UT	urinary tract
UTI	urinary tract infection
UV	ultraviolet
vac	vaccine
vag	vagina
	vaginal
VD	venereal disease
VDRL	Venereal Disease Research Laboratory
VIS	vaccine information statement
vit	vitamin
vit cap	vital capacity
vol	volume
VoIP	voice over Internet protocol
VRE	vancomycin-resistant enterococcus
VRS	voice recognition software
VS	vital signs
WAN	wide area network
WBC	white blood cell
WC	white cell
WDWN	well developed, well nourished
WHO	World Health Organization
WN	well nourished
WNF	well-nourished female
WNL	within normal limits
WNM	well-nourished male
WO	written order
w/o	without
wt	weight
WVE	wireless video endoscopy
x	multiply by
XDR TB	extensively drug-resistant tuberculosis
XR	X-ray

YOB	year of birth
yr	year

Symbols

*	birth
†	death
♂	male
♀	female
+	positive
–	negative
±	positive or negative, indefinite
÷	divide by
=	equal to
>	greater than
<	less than
×	multiply by
#	number, pound
′	foot, minute
″	inch, second

Top 50 Brand Drugs for 2007 by Number of U.S. Prescriptions Dispensed

Appendix B

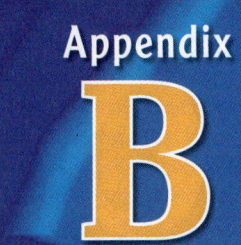

1. Lipitor
2. Nexium
3. Advair Diskus
4. Prevacid
5. Plavix
6. Singulair
7. Seroquel
8. Effexor
9. Lexapro
10. Actos
11. Protonix
12. Vytorin
13. Topamax
14. Risperdal
15. Abilify
16. Cymbalta
17. Lamictal
18. Zyprexa
19. Levaquin
20. Celebrex
21. Zetia
22. Valtrex
23. Crestor
24. Fosamax
25. Zyrtec
26. Lantus
27. Adderall XR
28. Diovan
29. Avandia
30. Tricor
31. AcipHex
32. Diovan HCT
33. OxyContin
34. Concerta
35. Coreg
36. Flomax
37. Lyrica
38. Wellbutrin XL
39. Aricept 9
40. Imitrex Oral
41. Ambien
42. Lotrel
43. Nasonex
44. Toprol XL
45. Ambien CR
46. Enbrel
47. Spiriva
48. Viagra
49. Lidoderm
50. Actonel

Drug Topics. (2008). *Top 200 brand-name drugs by retail dollars in 2007.* Retrieved July 24, 2008, from http://drugtopics.modernmedicine.com/drugtopics/data/articlestandard//drugtopics/102008/500221/article.pdf.

Appendix C

AAMA 2007–2008 Occupational Analysis of the CMA (AAMA)*

In furtherance of its leadership role in the profession, the American Association of Medical Assistants (AAMA) has completed the following *2007–2008 Occupational Analysis of the CMA (AAMA)*. In previous years, this document was titled *AAMA Role Delineation Study: Occupational Analysis of the Medical Assisting Profession.*

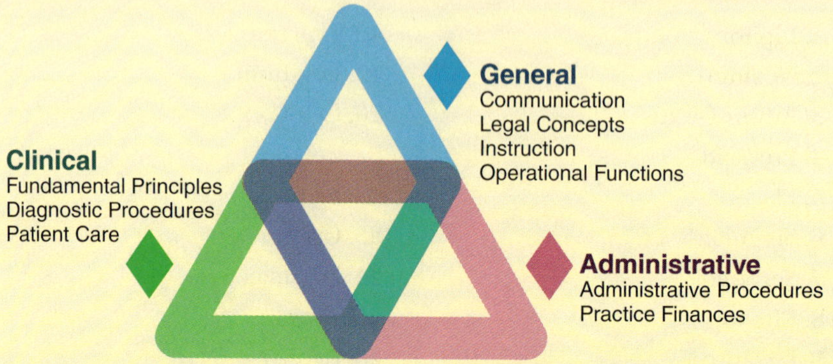
General
Communication
Legal Concepts
Instruction
Operational Functions
Clinical
Fundamental Principles
Diagnostic Procedures
Patient Care
Administrative
Administrative Procedures
Practice Finances

A Necessary Distinction

A professional's skills are largely determined by professional education. The CMA (AAMA) is the only credential that requires candidates to be graduates of a programmatically accredited medical assisting program. Therefore, it is appropriate and necessary that the qualifying language "of the CMA (AAMA)" be incorporated into this document's title.

About the Survey

A survey was sent to a random sample of CMAs (AAMA)—AAMA members and nonmembers. The CMA (AAMA) represents a medical assistant who has been certified by the Certifying Board of the AAMA. Of the 15,500 surveys distributed, 3,658 were collected and analyzed, resulting in a 95 percent confidence level. The results obtained from the sample are within ±1.6 percent of the results if all 15,500 individuals had responded.

Analysis Highlights

Today's CMA (AAMA) is expected not only to master the body of knowledge of the profession, but also to apply this knowledge in the complex and fast-paced world of ambulatory health care. Thus, critical thinking is emphasized in this *Occupational Analysis.*

Another dimension in the *Occupational Analysis* reflects the growing awareness that the CMA (AAMA) is uniquely qualified to "speak the patient's language" and serve as a "communication liaison" between the busy physician and patients. The roles of the CMA (AAMA) as "patient advocate" and "health coach," as well as "communication liaison," are given appropriate prominence in this document.

All health professionals have been expected to refine their knowledge and skills in responding to natural and manmade emergencies, and the vital roles of CMAs (AAMA) have come into increasing focus in recent years. In keeping with this priority, the *Occupational Analysis* includes emergency-related functions under Communication, Instruction, and Patient Care.

Uses of the Study

This document provides valuable data to the Certifying Board (CB) and the Continuing Education Board (CEB) of the AAMA, as well as to the Medical Assistant Education Review Board (MAERB). However, the *Occupational Analysis* should not be confused with the following documents:

- *Content Outline of the CMA (AAMA) Certification/Recertification Examination,* published by the CB
- *Advanced Practice of Medical Assisting,* published by the CEB
- *Standards and Guidelines for Medical Assisting Educational Programs,* published by CAAHEP
- *Curriculum Content and Competencies,* published by the CRB

*Permission is granted from the American Association of Medical Assistants.

Legal Scope of Practice

This *Occupational Analysis* does not delineate the legal scope of medical assisting practice. Legally delegable responsibilities vary from state to state. Scope of practice questions should be directed to AAMA Executive Director and Legal Counsel Donald A. Balasa, JD, MBA, at dbalasa@aama-ntl.org.

Occupational Analysis Committee

Chair: Charlene Couch, CMA (AAMA)

Karen Minchella, CMA (AAMA), PhD

Rebecca Walker, CMA (AAMA), CP

Nina Watson, CMA (AAMA), CPC, COS

Ex officio

Linda Brown, CMA (AAMA), 2007-2008 President

Kathryn Panagiotacos, CMA (AAMA), 2007-2008 Vice President

Donald A. Balasa, JD, MBA, Executive Director

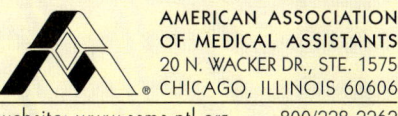

AMERICAN ASSOCIATION OF MEDICAL ASSISTANTS®
20 N. WACKER DR., STE. 1575
CHICAGO, ILLINOIS 60606
website: www.aama-ntl.org 800/228-2262

General, Clinical, and Administrative Skills* of the CMA (AAMA)

General Skills

Communication
- Recognize and respect cultural diversity
- Adapt communications to individual's understanding
- Employ professional telephone and interpersonal techniques
- Recognize and respond effectively to verbal, nonverbal, and written communications
- Utilize and apply medical terminology appropriately
- Receive, organize, prioritize, store, and maintain transmittable information utilizing electronic technology
- Serve as "communication liaison" between the physician and patient
- Serve as patient advocate professional and health coach in a team approach in health care
- Identify basics of office emergency preparedness

Legal Concepts
- Perform within legal (including federal and state statutes, regulations, opinions, and rulings) and ethical boundaries
- Document patient communication and clinical treatments accurately and appropriately
- Maintain medical records
- Follow employer's established policies dealing with the health care contract
- Comply with established risk management and safety procedures
- Recognize professional credentialing criteria
- Identify and respond to issues of confidentiality

Instruction
- Function as a health care advocate to meet individual's needs
- Educate individuals in office policies and procedures
- Educate the patient within the scope of practice and as directed by supervising physician in health maintenance, disease prevention, and compliance with patient's treatment plan
- Identify community resources for health maintenance and disease prevention to meet individual patient needs
- Maintain current list of community resources, including those for emergency preparedness and other patient care needs
- Collaborate with local community resources for emergency preparedness
- Educate patients in their responsibilities relating to third-party reimbursements

Operational Functions
- Perform inventory of supplies and equipment
- Perform routine maintenance of administrative and clinical equipment
- Apply computer and other electronic equipment techniques to support office operations
- Perform methods of quality control

Clinical Skills

Fundamental Principles
- Identify the roles and responsibilities of the medical assistant in the clinical setting
- Identify the roles and responsibilities of other team members in the medical office
- Apply principles of aseptic technique and infection control
- Practice Standard Precautions, including handwashing and disposal of biohazardous materials
- Perform sterilization techniques
- Comply with quality assurance practices

Diagnostic Procedures
- Collect and process specimens
- Perform CLIA-waived tests
- Perform electrocardiography and respiratory testing
- Perform phlebotomy, including venipuncture and capillary puncture
- Utilize knowledge of principles of radiology

Patient Care
- Perform initial-response screening following protocols approved by supervising physician
- Obtain, evaluate, and record patient history employing critical thinking skills
- Obtain vital signs
- Prepare and maintain examination and treatment areas
- Prepare patient for examinations, procedures and treatments
- Assist with examinations, procedures, and treatments
- Maintain examination/treatment rooms, including inventory of supplies and equipment
- Prepare and administer oral and parenteral (excluding IV) medications and immunizations *(as directed by supervising physician and as permitted by state law)*
- Utilize knowledge of principles of IV therapy
- Maintain medication and immunization records
- Screen and follow up test results
- Recognize and respond to emergencies

Administrative Skills

Administrative Procedures
- Schedule, coordinate, and monitor appointments
- Schedule inpatient/outpatient admissions and procedures
- Apply third-party and managed care policies, procedures, and guidelines
- Establish, organize, and maintain patient medical record
- File medical records appropriately

Practice Finances
- Perform procedural and diagnostic coding for reimbursement
- Perform billing and collection procedures
- Perform administrative functions, including bookkeeping and financial procedures
- Prepare submittable ("clean") insurance forms

Appendix D

Medical Assisting Task List

The various tasks that medical assistants perform include, but are not necessarily limited to, those on the following list.

The tasks presented in this inventory are considered by American Medical Technologists to be representative of the medical assisting job role. This document should be considered dynamic, to reflect the medical assistant's evolving role with respect to contemporary health care. Therefore, tasks may be added, removed, or modified on an on-going basis.

Medical Assistants that meet AMT's qualifications and pass a certification examination are certified as a Registered Medical Assistant (RMA).

I. GENERAL MEDICAL ASSISTING KNOWLEDGE

A. Anatomy and Physiology

1. Body systems
2. Disorders and diseases of the body

B. Medical Terminology

1. Word parts
2. Medical terms
3. Common abbreviations and symbols
4. Spelling

C. Medical Law

1. Medical law
2. Licensure, certification, and registration

D. Medical Ethics

1. Principles of medical ethics
2. Ethical conduct
3. Professional development

E. Human Relations

1. Patient relations
2. Interpersonal skills
3. Cultural diversity

F. Patient Education

1. Identify and apply proper communication methods in patient instruction
2. Develop, assemble, and maintain patient resource materials

II. ADMINISTRATIVE MEDICAL ASSISTING

A. Insurance

1. Medical insurance terminology
2. Various insurance plans
3. Claim forms
4. Electronic insurance claims
5. ICD-9CM/CPT Coding applications
6. HIPAA mandated coding systems
7. Financial applications of medical insurance

AMT American Medical Technologists
Allied Health Professionals

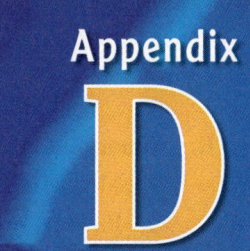

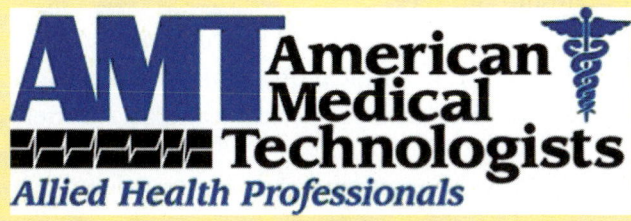

B. Financial Bookkeeping

1. Medical finance terminology
2. Patient billing procedures
3. Collection procedures
4. Fundamental medical office accounting procedures
5. Office banking procedures
6. Employee payroll
7. Financial calculations and accounting procedures

C. Medical Secretarial—Receptionist

1. Medical terminology associated with receptionist duties
2. General reception of patients and visitors
3. Appointment scheduling systems
4. Oral and written communications
5. Medical records management
6. Charting guidelines and regulations
7. Protect, store, and retain medical records according to HIPAA regulations
8. Release of protected health information adhering to HIPAA regulations
9. Transcription of dictation
10. Supplies and equipment management
11. Medical office computer applications
12. Compliance with OSHA guidelines and regulations of office safety

III. CLINICAL MEDICAL ASSISTING

A. Asepsis

1. Medical terminology
2. State/Federal universal bloodborne pathogen/body fluid precautions
3. Medical/surgical asepsis procedure

B. Sterilization

1. Medical terminology associated with sterilization
2. Sanitization, disinfection, and sterilization procedures
3. Record keeping procedures

C. Instruments

1. Specialty instruments and parts
2. Usage of common instruments
3. Care and handling of disposable and reusable instruments

D. Vital Signs/Mensurations

1. Blood pressure, pulse, respiration measurements
2. Height, weight, circumference measurements
3. Various temperature measurements
4. Recognize normal and abnormal measurement results

E. Physical Examinations

1. Patient history information
2. Proper charting procedures
3. Patient positions for examinations
4. Methods of examinations
5. Specialty examinations
6. Visual acuity/Ishihara (color blindness) measurements
7. Allergy testing procedures
8. Normal/abnormal results

F. Clinical Pharmacology

1. Medical terminology associated with pharmacology
2. Commonly used drugs and their categories
3. Various routes of medication administration
4. Parenteral administration of medications (subcutaneous, intramuscular, intradermal, ZTract)
5. Classes or drug schedules and legal prescriptions requirements for each
6. Drug Enforcement Agency regulations for ordering, dispensing, storage, and documentation of medication use
7. Drug Reference books (PDR, Pharmacopeia, Facts and Comparisons, Nurses Handbook)

G. Minor Surgery

1. Surgical supplies and instruments
2. Asepsis in surgical procedures
3. Surgical tray preparation and sterile field respect
4. Prevention of pathogen transmission

5. Patient surgical preparation procedures
6. Assisting physician with minor surgery including set-up
7. Dressing and bandaging techniques
8. Suture and staple removal
9. Biohazard waste disposal procedures
10. Instruct patient in pre- and postsurgical care

H. Therapeutic Modalities

1. Various standard therapeutic modalities
2. Alternative/complementary therapies
3. Instruct patient in assistive devices, body mechanics, and home care

I. Laboratory Procedures

1. Medical laboratory terminology
2. OSHA safety guidelines
3. Quality control and assessment regulations
4. Operate and maintain laboratory equipment
5. CLIA waived laboratory testing procedures
6. Capillary, dermal, and venipuncture procedures
7. Office specimen collection such as: urine, throat, vaginal, wound cultures – stool, sputum, etc
8. Specimen handling and preparation
9. Laboratory recording according to state and federal guidelines
10. Adhere to the MA Scope of Practice in the laboratory

J. Electrocardiography

1. Standard, 12 lead ECG testing
2. Mounting techniques for permanent record
3. Rhythm strip ECG monitoring on lead II

K. First Aid

1. Emergencies and first aid procedures
2. Emergency crash cart supplies
3. Legal responsibilities as a first responder

American Medical Technologists
10700 W. Higgins Road
Rosemont, Illinois 60018
Phone: (847) 823-5169 – Fax: (847) 823-0458
Website: www.amt1.com

Appendix E

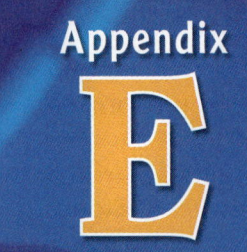

Software Support: The Critical Thinking Challenge

TECHNICAL SUPPORT INFORMATION

Technical Support at Delmar Cengage Learning is available from 8:30 AM to 6:30 PM, Eastern Standard Time.

- Telephone: 1-800-648-7450
- Email: delmar.help@cengage.com

ABOUT THE CRITICAL THINKING CHALLENGE 2.0

The new Critical Thinking Challenge (CTC) 2.0 is a game that simulates a 3-month practicum in Dr. Connor's medical office. In this game, you'll be confronted with a series of situations in which you have to use critical thinking skills to select the most correct action in response to the situation. Your actions will be evaluated by how the decision has affected the practice, the patient, and your career. You will also be awarded points for your overall decision-making. The 2.0 version includes 10 all-new video-based scenarios that include more follow-on scenarios, depending on the decisions made. After successfully completing the program, print out a Certification of Completion.

Setup and Time Requirements

The program automatically starts when you put the CD into your computer. Completion of the game requires about 30 minutes of your time.

After watching the Overview video, you must **set up your character as male or female** by clicking the appropriate button. You can turn on Subtitles by clicking the buttons in the bottom left corner of the game window. You can **turn Subtitles on or off** at any point in the game.

To **adjust the volume level,** click on the Volume button at the lower right side of the game window. Then, move the fader to the desired setting. Click Close in the volume window to return to the game.

To exit the Critical Thinking Challenge, click on the Quit button in the bottom right corner of the game window. Your score will not be saved. The next time you enter the Critical Thinking Challenge, you will have to start from the beginning.

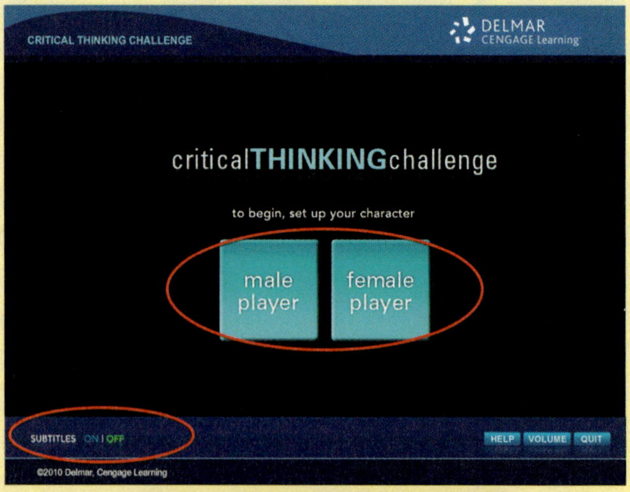

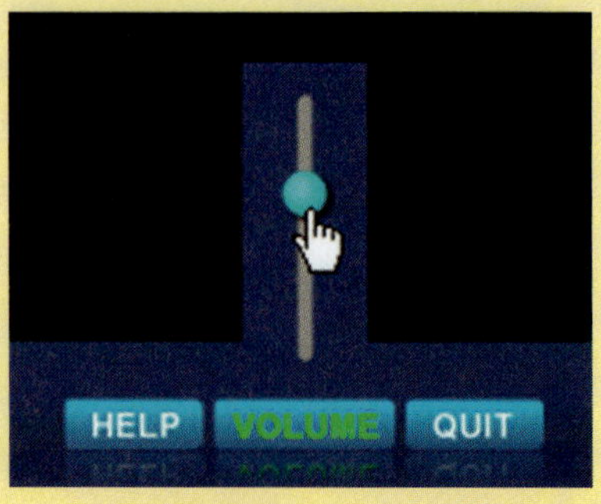

Playing the Game

You are a character in each situation in the game. Each situation is a video presented from your point of view. In some cases, you will be directly involved in the situation, interacting with other staff members or patients; in other instances, you will be a witness to the situation. However, in every situation presented, you must use your critical thinking skills to respond.

The object of the game is to receive an offer of employment from the medical practice.

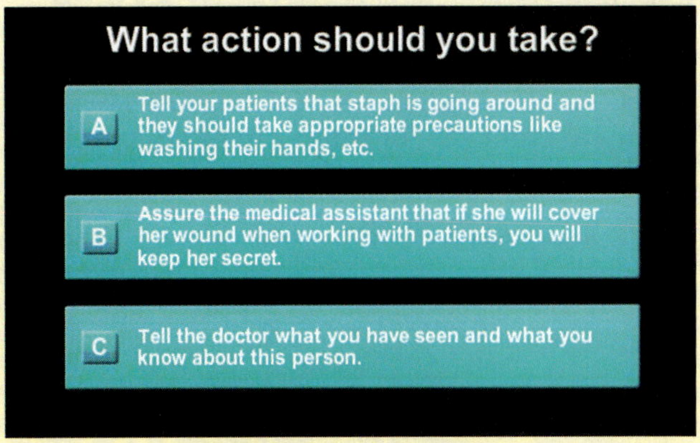

The Situations. You will need to view each video situation **to determine the best action** to take. To control the pace of the narrative, use the video buttons at the bottom of the game window. These allow you to play, pause, forward, and reverse the narration. After you view the video scenario, you are presented with three possible actions that you can take.

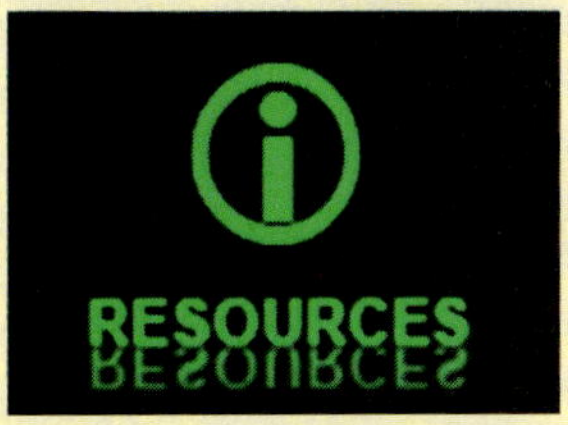

Using Resources. To help you choose the most correct action, you may **consult your Resources Panel** by clicking the Resources button on the lower left side of the game window. The Resources Panel allows you to access People and Documents resources and the Available Time clock.

The **People resources** allow you to interact with individuals in the medical office who may be able to assist you in choosing the appropriate action. Click on the staff member with whom you would like to speak.

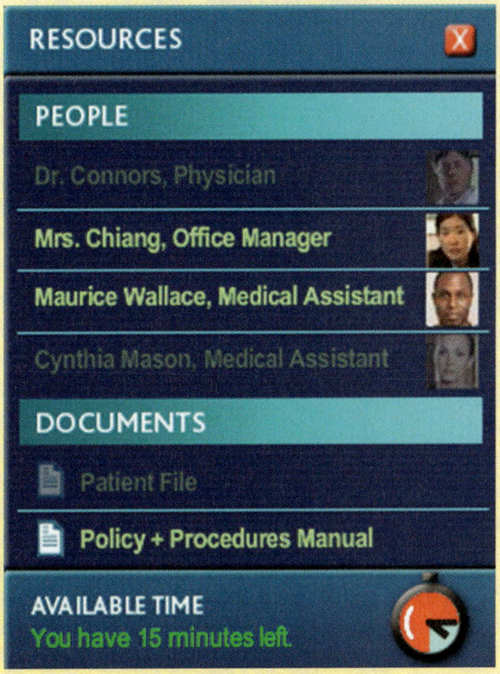

The **Documents resources** represent files that would be found in the medical office and that may be able to help you. Keep in mind that not all the resources may be available when you need them or helpful to you, depending on the situation. Always use your critical thinking skills!

Available Time Clock. Each time you consult with a resource, you use up 5 minutes of **the scenario clock.** Most of the time you'll be able to check with up to four resources; however, some situations are more time-sensitive than others, so you'll have to choose your resources carefully. Don't worry about using up time while you're thinking about what to do; the clock only moves ahead each time you consult a resource.

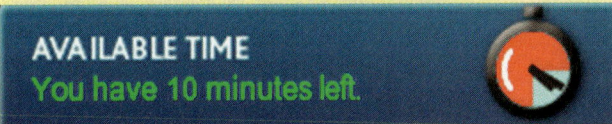

Evaluation and Points Awarded

When you have finished consulting your resources, select one of the actions presented. Your decisions are then **evaluated in three categories:** practice, patient, and career.

- *Practice* means how your decisions affect the medical office—reputation, patient retention, ethical and legal compliance, or medical malpractice liability.
- *Patient* means how your decision affects the patient—sensitivity, privacy, health, convenience, and satisfaction.
- *Career* means how your decisions affect your career as a medical assistant—employability, professionalism, effectiveness, reputation, ethical and legal compliance, or medical malpractice liability.

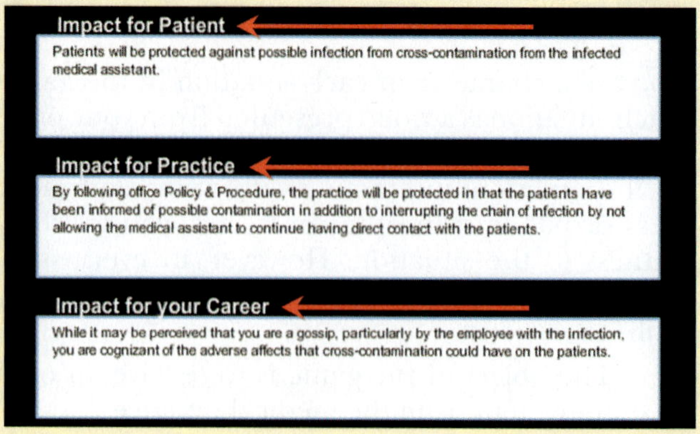

You will receive positive and negative feedback discussing the merits of your decision and the outcome of the situation, and then you are awarded points for your overall decision-making skills.

You will **receive points according to the merits of the action** chosen:

- You will receive 10 points for selecting the best action.
- You will receive 5 points for selecting a good action to take, but not the best action.
- You will not receive any points for selecting the least desirable action.

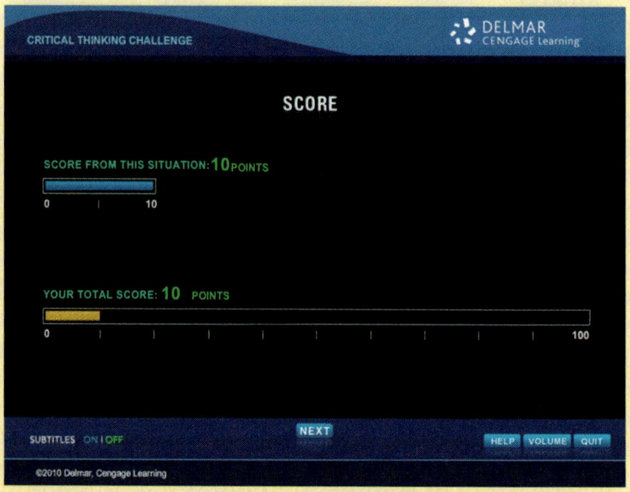

Follow-on Situations

In some cases, if you do not select the best decision in the first instance, you will be presented with a follow-on situation that directly resulted from the action (or lack of action) that you chose.

In these situations, the maximum point value you are awarded is less than what you would have received in the original scenario. Remember, these situations could have been avoided if you had taken the most appropriate action at first, even if it seemed difficult to do.

Points are awarded in follow-on situations as follows:

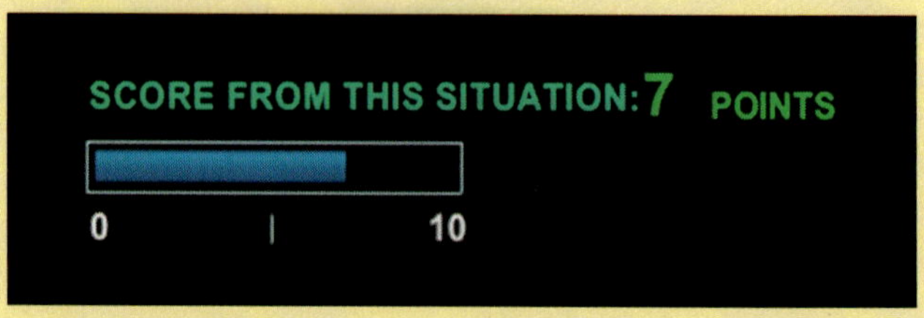

- You will receive 7 points for selecting the best action.
- You will receive 3 points for selecting the next-best action.
- You will not receive any points for selecting the least desirable solution.

Scoring the Game

Your goal is to be hired by Dr. Connor's office as a full-time medical assistant. On the other hand, if you show a serious lack of critical thinking skills that threatens the well-being of the medical office or the patients, Dr. Connor's office will terminate your practicum and you'll have to start over.

- You will receive a job offer to work in the office if you score above 85 points in the game. At the end of game play, you will receive a Certificate of Completion that you can print out.
- If you score between 70 and 85 points, you will receive a letter of recommendation from Dr. Connor's office. At the end of game play, you will receive a Certificate of Completion that you can print out.
- If you score below 70 points, your practicum is terminated, and you'll need to start over.
- Your practicum also can be terminated early if you choose the least desirable action three times in a row at any point during game play.

Glossary of Terms

Note: The equivalent Spanish word follows in parentheses in green.

A

abduction (abducción) motion away from the midline of the body (Ch. 33).

ABO blood group (grupo sanguíneo ABO) genetically determined system of antigens found on the surface of erythrocytes. The population can be divided into four ABO blood groups: A, B, AB, and O (Ch. 44).

abortion (aborto) expulsion of the products of conception before viability (Ch. 26).

abuse (abuso) misuse; excessive or improper use, especially of narcotics or psychoactive drugs (Ch. 17, 35).

accession record (numeric system) (registro de entrada [sistema de ordenación por número]) logbook used to assign numbers to correspondence or patients (Ch. 14).

accomplishment statements (declaraciones de logros) statements that begin with a power verb and give a brief description of what you did, and the demonstrable results that were produced (Ch. 48).

accounting (contabilidad) system of monitoring the financial status of a facility and the financial results of its activities, providing information for decision making (Ch. 21).

accounts payable (cuentas por pagar) sum owed by a business for services or goods received (Ch. 19); also unwritten promise to pay a supplier for property or merchandise purchased on credit or for a service rendered (Ch. 21).

accounts receivable (cuentas por cobrar) amount owed to a business for services or goods supplied (Ch. 19).

accounts receivable (A/R) ratio assets (relación de cuentas por cobrar a activos) outstanding accounts receivable divided by the average monthly gross income for the past 12 months (Ch. 20, 21).

accreditation (acreditación) process whereby recognition is granted to an educational program for maintaining standards that qualify its graduates for professional practice; to provide with credentials (Ch. 1).

Accrediting Bureau of Health Education Schools (ABHES) (Junta de Acreditación de Escuelas de Educación en Salud [ABHES]) entity accrediting private, postsecondary institutions in the U.S. which offer allied health education programs as well as programmatic accreditation of medical assistant, medical laboratory technician and surgical technology programs (Ch. 1, 47).

accrual basis accounting (contabilidad según el principio del devengo) reports income at the time charges are generated (Ch. 21).

acetone (acetona) colorless, inflammable liquid. Found in the blood and urine of diabetics as a result of the breakdown of fatty acids (Ch. 38).

acid/base balance (equilibrio ácido-básico) condition that occurs when the net rate at which the body produces acids or bases is equal to the net rate at which acids or bases are excreted (Ch. 42).

acquired immunodeficiency syndrome (AIDS) (síndrome de inmunodeficiencia adquirida [SIDA]) disorder of the immune system caused by a human immunodeficiency virus (HIV), a retrovirus that destroys the body's ability to fight infection. As the disease progresses, the individual becomes overcome by disorders, including cancers and opportunistic infections. There is no known cure for AIDS (Ch. 22).

active listening (escucha activa) received message is paraphrased back to the sender to verify the correct message was decoded (Ch. 4).

activities of daily living (ADL) (actividades de la vida diaria [AVD]) activities usually performed during a typical day that involve caring for oneself, such as eating and brushing teeth (Ch. 33).

acupuncture (acupuntura) treatment to relieve pain and disease by puncturing the skin with thin needles at specific points (Ch. 2).

acyclovir (aciclovir) antiviral drug used in some herpes infections (Ch. 22).

additive (aditivo) any material placed in a tube that maintains or facilitates the integrity and function of the specimen (Ch. 40).

adduction (aducción) motion toward the midline of the body (Ch. 33).

adjustments (ajustes) increases or decreases to patient accounts not due to charges incurred or payments received (Ch. 17, 19).

administer (administrar) to give a medication (Ch. 7, 35, 36).

administrative law (derecho administrativo) establishes agencies that are given the power to make laws and enact regulations (Ch. 7).

aegis (auspicio) sponsorship or protection (Ch. 38).

aerobic (aerobio) organism that requires oxygen for growth (Ch. 43).

aerosolyzed (aerosolizado) dispensed by means of a mist (Ch. 27).

aerosols (aerosoles) particles from potentially infectious materials that may be released in the air (Ch. 22, 43).

afebrile (afebril) without fever (Ch. 24).

agar (agar) a gelatin-like substance extracted from red algae that contains nutrients and moisture for bacteria growth (Ch. 43).

agenda (orden del día) printed list of topics to be discussed during a meeting, sometimes giving time allocation (Ch. 15, 45).

agent (agente) person representing another (Ch. 7).

agglutination (aglutinación) antigen–antibody reaction in which a solid antigen clumps with a solid antibody (Ch. 44).

airborne transmission (transmisión por aire) spread of disease-causing microorganisms over long distances through the air (Ch. 22).

algorithm (algoritmo) a special method for solving a specific kind of problem (Ch. 11).

aliquot (alícuota) part of the whole specimen that has been taken off for use or storage (Ch. 40).

allergen (alérgeno) any substance that causes signs of allergy; examples are inhalants such as dust and pollen, foods such as wheat and strawberries, drugs, penicillin, chemicals, heat, bacteria (Ch. 30).

allergy (alergia) acquired hypersensitivity to a substance (allergen) that does not normally cause a reaction (Ch. 23, 31).

allopathic (alopático) method of treating disease with remedies that produce effects different from those caused by the disease itself. Most traditional practitioners today are considered allopathic practitioners (Ch. 3).

alternative dispute resolution (ADR) (resolución alternativa de conflictos [RAC]) an alternative to trial that encourages the parties to settle their differences out of court (Ch. 7).

amblyopia (ambliopía) disorder of the eye characterized by dimness of vision (Ch. 30).

Ambu Bag™ (Ambu Bag™) a brand name for a bag placed over nose and mouth to assist in providing artificial ventilation to the lungs (Ch. 9).

ambulation (ambulación) ability to walk (Ch. 33).

ambulatory care setting (entorno de atención ambulatoria) health care environment where services are provided on an outpatient basis. *Ambulatory* is from the Latin and means "capable of walking." Examples include the solo-provider's office, the group practice, the urgent care center, and the health maintenance organization (Ch. 1, 2).

American Association of Medical Assistants (AAMA) (Asociación Estadounidense de Asistentes Médicos [AAMA]) professional organization dedicated to serving the interests of Certified Medical Assistants (Ch. 47).

American Medical Technologists (AMT) (Tecnólogos Médicos Estadounidenses [AMT]) national organization which credentials health care professionals, including Registered Medical Assistants (RMA) and Certified Medical Administrative Specialists (CMAS) (Ch. 1, 47).

amino acid (aminoácido) basic structural unit of protein (Ch. 34).

amniocentesis (amniocentesis) surgical puncture of the amniotic sac to remove fluid for laboratory analysis (Ch. 22, 26).

amniotomy (amniotomía) artificial rupture of the amniotic sac (Ch. 26).

amoebic dysentery (disentería amébica) infectious intestinal disease caused by amoebas and characterized by inflammation of the mucous membrane of the colon (Ch. 22).

amorphous (amorfo) shapeless; possessing no definite form (Ch. 42).

amplified (amplificado) made larger or enlarged. The amplifier of the electrocardiograph enlarges the electrical impulse activity and the recording can be read more easily (Ch. 37).

amplitude (amplitud) amount, extent, size, abundance, or fullness (Ch. 37).

Amsler grid (cuadrícula de Amsler) a grid of lines used in testing for macular degeneration (Ch. 30).

anaerobic (anaerobio) organism that needs little or no oxygen for growth (Ch. 43).

anaphylaxis (anafilaxia) hypersensitive state of the body to a foreign protein or drug (Ch. 9, 35).

ancillary services (servicios auxiliares) professional occupational companies hired to complete a specific job (Ch. 45).

andropause (andropausia) midlife changes in a male (Ch. 29).

anesthesia (anestesia) loss of feeling or sensation; an anesthetic is any mechanism that causes anesthesia (Ch. 31).

angiogram (angiograma) series of X-rays of a blood vessel(s) after injection of a radiopaque substance (Ch. 37).

anisocytosis (anisocitosis) marked variation in the size of cells (Ch. 41).

anorexia (anorexia) loss of appetite (Ch. 22).

answering services (servicios de respuesta) services employed to answer the calls of an ambulatory care setting after hours; unlike an answering machine, a live operator answers the call and forwards it appropriately (Ch. 12).

antibacterial (antibacteriano) capable of destroying bacteria, often applied to a wound in the form of an ointment or cream (Ch. 31).

antibody (anticuerpo) specific chemical produced by B cells of the immune system in response to an antigen (Ch. 22, 44).

anticoagulant (anticoagulante) chemical in a blood tube that prevents the clotting of the blood by removing the calcium from the blood or by stopping the formation of thrombin (Ch. 40).

antigen (antígeno) substance such as bacteria or other agents that the body recognizes as foreign; the stimulus for antibody production (Ch. 22, 44).

antiglare screen (pantalla antirreflejo) a filter put over the screen of a computer monitor to reduce glare (Ch. 11).

antioxidant (antioxidante) something that prevents oxidation (Ch. 34).

antiserum (antisuero) serum containing antibodies (Ch. 44).

apical (apical) pertaining to the apex of the heart. A site for measuring heart rate with a stethoscope (Ch. 24).

apnea (apnea) cessation or absence of normal spontaneous breathing (Ch. 24, 36).

appendicular skeleton (esqueleto apendicular) skeleton that consists of the pectoral and pelvic girdles and the upper and lower extremities. The pelvic girdle attaches the upper extremities to the trunk (Ch. 30).

application/cover letter (solicitud/carta de presentación) letter used to introduce yourself and your résumé to a prospective employer with the goal of obtaining an interview (Ch. 48).

application form (formulario de solicitud) form devised by a prospective employer to collect information relative to qualifications, education, and experience in employment (Ch. 48).

application software (software de aplicación) software that performs a specific data-processing function (Ch. 11).

approximate (aproximar) to bring together the edges of a wound (Ch. 31).

arbitration (arbitraje) a form of dispute resolution that allows a neutral party to settle the dispute (Ch. 7).

arrhythmia (arritmia) deviation from the normal pattern or rhythm of the heartbeat (Ch. 24, 37).

arteriosclerosis (arteriosclerosis) hardening of the arteries caused by buildup of plaque, a deposit of fatty substances on the artery lining (Ch. 29).

articulating (elocuente) expressing oneself clearly and distinctly (Ch. 12).

artifact (artefacto) anything artificially produced (Ch. 37).

ascorbic acid (ácido ascórbico) vitamin C (Ch. 34).

asepsis (asepsia) protecting against infection caused by pathogenic microorganisms (Ch. 3).

aseptic (aséptico) freedom from any infectious material; absence of microorganisms (Ch. 22, 30).

aspirate (aséptico) to remove by suction (Ch. 22).

assay (ensayo) analysis of a substance to determine constituents and relative proportion of each (Ch. 39).

assets (activos) properties of value that are owned by a business entity (Ch. 21).

assignment of benefits (asignación de beneficios) signing over of benefits by the beneficiary to another party (Ch. 17).

Association for Healthcare Documentation Integrity (AHDI) (Asociación para la Integridad de la Documentación del Cuidado de la Salud [AHDI]) professional organization in the field of medical transcription/editing (Ch. 16).

asymptomatic (asintomático) without symptoms (Ch. 39).

ataxia (ataxia) defective muscular coordination, primarily seen when attempting voluntary muscular movements (Ch. 25).

atherosclerosis (aterosclerosis) a form of arteriosclerosis marked by calcium deposits in the arterial linings (ch. 24).

attribute (atributo) inherent characteristic (Ch. 1).

auditor (auditor) a person responsible for determining the final content of a document and the document's correctness in every aspect (Ch. 16).

augment (aumentar) to add or increase (Ch. 37).

auscultatory gap (brecha auscultatoria) while measuring blood pressure, the tapping sounds heard may disappear between the Korotkoff phases of sound (Ch. 24).

auricle (aurícula) the external ear, also called pinna (Ch. 30).

authentication (autenticación) dictating provider signs or authenticates the document indicating that the information was accurate and complete at the time of signing (Ch. 16).

authoritarian manager (gerente autoritario) operates on the premise that most workers cannot make a contribution without being directed (Ch. 45).

automated external defibrillator (AED) (desfibrilador externo automatizado [DEA]) portable, self-contained, automatic device with voice instructions on use for individuals in cardiac arrest. It is used externally to electronically "shock" the myocardium into contracting again. Same as cardioversion (Ch. 9).

automated routing unit (ARU) (enrutador automático [ARU]) telephone system that answers a call and uses a recorded voice to identify departments or services (Ch. 12).

autopsy report (informe de autopsia) also called an autopsy protocol, a necropsy report, or a medical examiner report. Autopsies are performed to determine the cause of death or to ascertain and confirm disease presence (Ch. 16).

avascularization (avascularización) expulsions of blood from tissues. Leaves the tissues with no blood supply (Ch. 31).

axial skeleton (esqueleto axial) consists of bones that lie around the center of the body (Ch. 30).

B

bachelor's degree (licenciatura) four-year academic degree conferred by colleges and universities (Ch. 1).

backup (hacer una copia de seguridad) copying or saving data to a secure location to prevent loss of data in the event of a disaster (Ch. 11).

balance (balancear) amount owed (N); to verify posting accuracy (V); records difference between debit and credit columns (Ch. 19).

balance sheet (balance general) itemized statement of assets, liabilities, and equity; a statement of financial condition (Ch. 21).

bandage (venda) nonsterile gauze or other material applied over a sterile dressing to protect and immobilize (Ch. 9, 31).

bariatrics (bariátrica) the branch of medicine that deals with prevention, control, and treatment of obesity (Ch. 30).

barrier (barrera) obstacle that exists to protect an individual from contact with blood or other potentially infected materials. Called personal protective equipment (PPE), barriers include gloves, masks, face shields, laboratory coats, protective eyewear, and gowns (Ch. 22).

Bartholin gland (glándula de Bartolino) one of two small mucous glands located at the vaginal opening at the base of the labia majora (Ch. 26).

basal metabolic rate (BMR) (índice metabólico basal [IMB]) level of energy required when the body is at rest (Ch. 34).

baseline (valor de referencia) known or initial measurement against which future measurements are compared (Ch. 24, 39); also, flat, horizontal line that separates the various waves of the ECG cycle (Ch. 37).

basophil (basófilo) granulocytic white blood cell with dark purple cytoplasmic granules. It is the least common of the white blood cells (Ch. 41).

benchmark (comparador de rendimiento) making a comparison among different organizations relative to how they accomplish tasks, such as office computerization, organizing file systems, and employee remuneration (Ch. 11, 45).

beneficiary (beneficiario) person under a policy eligible to receive benefits (Ch. 17).

benefit (beneficio) remuneration that is in addition to the salary (Ch. 45, 48).

benefit period (período de beneficios) the specified time during which benefits will be paid under certain types of health insurance coverages (Ch. 17).

beriberi (beriberi) disease caused by a deficiency in vitamin B (thiamin), characterized by headaches, depression, anorexia, constipation, tachycardia, edema, and heart failure (Ch. 34).

Betadine® (Betadine®) brand of povidone-iodine solution used as a skin antiseptic. Betadine® is also available in a scrub (soap) solution (Ch. 31).

bias (sesgo) slant toward a particular belief (Ch. 4).

bilirubin (bilirrubina) orange–yellow pigment that forms from the breakdown of hemoglobin in damaged red blood cells. Bilirubin usually travels in the bloodstream to the liver, where it is converted to a water-soluble form and is excreted into the bile (Ch. 42, 44).

bilirubinuria (bilirrubinuria) the presence of bilirubin in urine (Ch. 42).

bimanual examination (examen bimanual) an examination performed by the provider using two hands to examine the internal pelvic organs. Two fingers of one hand are inserted into the vagina and the other hand presses on the outside of the abdominal wall. Shape, consistency, and position of the pelvic organs can be determined (Ch. 26).

biochemical tests (análisis bioquímicos) tests that show biochemical properties and reactions of bacteria to achieve identification of microorganisms; often performed in solid and liquid media (Ch. 43).

bioethics (bioética) branch of medical ethics concerned with moral issues resulting from high technology and sophisticated medical research. Social issues such as genetic engineering, abortion, and fetal tissue research raise important bioethical questions (Ch. 8).

biohazard (riesgo biológico) material that has been in contact with body fluid and is capable of transmitting disease (Ch. 22).

biometric (biometría) a type of electronic signature that may use alphanumeric computer key entries as identification; an electronic writing device; or a biometric system using voice, fingerprints, or the retina of the eye (Ch. 16).

biopsy (biopsia) removal of a small piece of living tissue from an organ or other part of the body for microscopic examination to confirm or establish a diagnosis (Ch. 30, 39).

bipolar (bipolar) having two poles or processes (Ch. 37).

birthday rule (regla del cumpleaños) method to determine which of two or more policies covering a dependent child will be primary; that parent with the birthday falling first in the calendar year has the primary policy (Ch. 17).

blind copy (copia oculta) protects the privacy of email. Other recipients cannot identify who else may have received the transmitted message (Ch. 15).

bloodborne (transmisión sanguínea) means of transmission of an infectious disease (such as HIV and HBV) via human blood (Ch. 22).

bloodborne pathogen (patógeno transmitido por la sangre) microorganism capable of causing disease found in blood or components of blood (Ch. 22).

blood urea nitrogen (BUN) (nitrógeno ureico en sangre [BUN]) nitrogen in the blood in the form of urea. The level of nitrogen in the blood is an indicator of kidney function (Ch. 44).

Bluetooth® (Bluetooth®) a technical industry standard that facilitates communication between wireless devices such as personal digital assistants, handheld computers, and wireless-enabled laptop computers or desktop computers (Ch. 11).

body fluid (líquido corporal) any secretion or excretion from the human body such as vaginal, cerebrospinal, synovial, pleural, pericardial, peritoneal, amniotic, sputum, and saliva (Ch. 38).

body language (lenguaje corporal) nonverbal communication that includes unconscious body movements, gestures, and facial expressions that accompany verbal messages (Ch. 4).

body mechanics (mecánica corporal) practice of using certain key muscle groups together with correct body alignment to avoid injury when lifting or moving heavy or awkward objects (Ch. 33).

body surface area (BSA) (área de superficie corporal [ASC]) a highly accurate method for calculating medication dosages for infants and children up to 12 years of age (Ch. 36).

bond (fianza) binding agreement with an employee ensuring recovery of financial loss should funds be stolen or embezzled (Ch. 45).

bond paper (papel bond) durable, strong paper usually used for correspondence (Ch. 15).

booting (arranque) everything that happens between the time the computer is turned on, performs the operations necessary to get all components functioning, and the operating system loaded (Ch. 11).

bradycardia (sinus) (bradicardia [sinusal]) slow (less than 60 beats per minute), but regular heartbeat (Ch. 24, 37).

bradypnea (bradipnea) abnormally slowed respiratory rate (Ch. 24).

brainstorming (tormenta de ideas) process of developing ideas through a synergistic interaction among participants in an environment free of criticism (Ch. 45).

Braxton–Hicks (Braxton–Hicks) irregular, intermittent, and painless uterine contractions; also known as false labor (Ch. 26).

bronchi (bronquios) bifurcates from the trachea into each lung that terminate in the bronchial tubes (Ch. 30).

bronchodilator (broncodilatador) a drug that expands the bronchial tubes (Ch. 30).

broth tubes (tubos de caldo) tubes filled with a broth substance that will support the growth of certain microorganisms (Ch. 43).

bruits (ruidos) sound of venous or arterial origin heard on auscultation (Ch. 25).

bubonic plague (peste bubónica) infectious disease with a high fatality rate transmitted to humans from infected rats and ground squirrels by the bite of the rat flea (Ch. 3).

buffer words (palabras de relleno) expendable words used while answering the telephone (Ch. 12).

buffy coat (capa leucocitaria) layer of white blood cells and platelets that forms at the interface between the plasma and red blood cells in a tube of blood containing an anticoagulant (Ch. 40).

bullet point (viñeta) asterisk or dot followed by a descriptive phrase; helps the reader identify important points easily (Ch. 48).

bundled codes (códigos agrupados) a grouping of several services that are directly related to a specific procedure and are paid as one (Ch. 18).

burnout (agotamiento profesional) a state of fatigue or frustration brought about by a devotion to a cause, a way of life, or a relationship that failed to produce the expected reward (Ch. 5).

C

cachectic (caquéctico) describes a state of ill health, malnutrition, and wasting (Ch. 34).

calibration (calibración) determination of the accuracy of an instrument by comparing the information provided with an accepted standard known to be accurate (Ch. 37, 38).

calorie (caloría) unit of heat. The large Calorie (which is always capitalized) is used in discussion of human nutrition. The large Calorie is also expressed as the kilogram calorie (kcal), equal to 1,000 small calories (Ch. 34).

candidiasis (candidiasis) infection of the skin or mucous membrane with any species of *Candida* (Ch. 26).

cannula (nasal) tubing (cánula) used to deliver oxygen (Ch. 36); also, the blunting member in a Bio-Plexus Punctur-Guard® needle (Ch. 40).

capitation (capitación) use of the number of members enrolled in a plan to determine salary of the provider; the provider is paid a fixed fee for each member no matter how many times that member is seen by the provider (Ch. 17).

caption (leyenda) method of designation used on file guides (Ch. 14).

carbuncle (ántrax) necrotizing infection of skin and tissue composed of a cluster of boils (Ch. 30).

carcinoma in situ (carcinoma in situ) cancer that does not extend beyond the basement membrane (Ch. 26).

cardiac catheterization (cateterismo cardíaco) passage of a catheter into the heart through an arm or leg vein and blood vessels leading into the heart. The purpose is to obtain cardiac blood samples, detect abnormalities, and determine intracardiac pressure. Contrast medium can be injected and a coronary artery angiogram can be performed (Ch. 37).

cardiac cycle (ciclo cardíaco) period from the beginning of one heartbeat to the beginning of the next succeeding beat, including systole and diastole. One complete heartbeat (Ch. 37).

cardiopulmonary resuscitation (CPR) (reanimación cardiopulmonar [RCP]) combination of rescue breathing and chest compressions performed by a trained individual on a patient experiencing cardiac arrest (Ch. 9).

cardioversion (cardioversión) conversion of a pathological cardiac rhythm (arrhythmia), such as ventricular fibrillation, to normal sinus rhythm (Ch. 9, 37).

cardioverter/defibrillator (cardioversor/desfibrilador) an implantable device used for life-threatening arrhythmias.Its purpose is to shock the heart out of the arrhythmia and into a more normal sinus rhythm (Ch. 37).

career objective (objetivo profesional) expresses your career goal and the position for which you are applying (Ch. 48).

carotene (caroteno) vitamin A (Ch. 34).

carrier (portador) person who harbors a pathogenic organism and who is capable of transmitting the organism to others (Ch. 22).

cash basis accounting (contabilidad de caja) reports income at the time money is collected (Ch. 21).

cashier's check (cheque de caja) bank's own check drawn against the bank's account (Ch. 19).

casts (cilindros) tiny structures usually formed by deposits of protein or other substances on the walls of renal tubules; in urine, they can indicate kidney disease (Ch. 42).

catalyst (catalizador) substance that allows a chemical reaction to proceed at a much quicker rate and without as much energy input (Ch. 34).

catheterization (cateterismo) insertion of a catheter tube into the body for evacuating fluids or injecting fluids into body cavities. In urinary catheterization, the tube is inserted through the urethra into the bladder for withdrawal of urine (Ch. 25).

cathode (cátodo) a negative electrode from which electrons are emitted (Ch. 32).

caustic (cáustico) corrosive and burning; destructive to living tissue (Ch. 22, 31).

cauterize (cauterizar) to destroy tissue through application of a caustic agent, a hot instrument, an electric current, or other agent (Ch. 9).

cautery (cauterio) destruction of tissue by burning (Ch. 31).

cell-mediated immunity (inmunidad mediada por células) the regulatory activities of T cells during the specific immune response (Ch. 22).

cellular telephones (teléfonos celulares) a short range portable device used for voice or data communication over a network of base stations known as cell sites. The cell sites are interconnected to the public switched telephone network (Ch. 12).

cellulose (celulosa) type of indigestible fiber made of carbohydrates found in plants (Ch. 34).

Centers for Medicare and Medicaid Services (CMS) (Centros de Servicios de Medicare y Medicaid [CMS]) formerly known as HCFA. CMS is a federal agency within the U.S. Department of Health and Human Services (DHHS). The agency administers Medicare, Medicaid, and the State Children's Health Insurance Program (SCHIP). CMS also administers the Health Insurance Portability and Accountability Act of 1996 (HIPAA) and Clinical Laboratory Improvement Act of 1988 (CLIA '88) (Ch. 17).

central processing unit (CPU) (unidad de procesamiento central [CPU]) brain of the computer that performs instructions defined by software (Ch. 11).

centrifuge (centrifugador) device that spins tubes using centrifugal force to separate the fluid portion of blood from the formed elements (Ch. 40).

certification (certificación) guarantees as being true or as represented by or as meeting a standard (Ch. 1).

certification examination (examen de certificación) standardized means of evaluating medical assistant competency (Ch. 47).

certified check (cheque certificado) depositor's own check that the bank has indicated with a date and signature to be good for the amount written (Ch. 19).

Certified Clinical Medical Assistant (CCMA) (Asistente Clínico Médico Certificado [CCMA]) an NHA certification for a clinical medical assistant. (Ch. 47).

Certified Medical Administrative Assistant (CMAA) (Asistente Administrativo Médico Certificado [CMAA]) an NHA certification for a medical administrative assistant (Ch. 47).

Certified Medical Administrative Specialist (CMAS) (Especialista Administrativo Médico Certificado [CMAS]) an AMT certification for a medical administrative specialist (Ch. 47).

Certified Medical Assistant (CMA [AAMA]) (Asistente Médico Certificado [CMA (AAMA)]) a certified medical assistant who has successfully completed the AAMA's national certification examination (Ch. 1, 47).

Certified Medical Transcriptionist (CMT) (Transcriptor Médico Certificado [CMT]) completion of a two-part certification examination administered by the Association for Healthcare Documentation Integrity (AHDI) (Ch. 16).

cervical punch biopsy (biopsia cervical en sacabocados) a biopsy of the uterine cervix using an instrument, the end of which is a punch (Ch. 26).

cesarean section (operación cesárea) delivery of fetus through surgical incision into the uterus (Ch. 26).

chart notes (notas clínicas) (also called progress notes) provider's formal or informal notes about presenting problem, physical findings, and plan for treatment for a patient examined in the office, clinic, acute care center, or emergency department (Ch. 16).

check register (registro de cheques) record of checks written; categorized into separate and identified columns (Ch. 21).

cheilosis (queilosis) caused by a deficiency of vitamin B_2 (riboflavin) and characterized by sores on the lips and cracks in the corners of the mouth (Ch. 34).

chemotherapeutic agents (agentes quimioterapéuticos) agents used in the treatment of diseases; the application of chemical reagents that are toxic to pathogenic microorganisms. Commonly used to describe agents (chemicals) used in the treatment of certain malignancies (Ch. 38).

Cheyne–Stokes (Cheyne–Stoke) regular pattern of irregular breathing rate often seen in children and that may be seen in brain dysfunction (Ch. 24).

chief complaint (CC) (queja principal [QP]) specific symptom or problem for which the patient is seeing the provider today (Ch. 16, 23).

chlamydia (clamidia) a bacterium that causes one of the most prevalent sexually transmitted diseases (Ch. 26).

cholecalciferol (colecalciferol) vitamin D (Ch. 34).

cholesterol (colesterol) sterol lipid that is widely distributed in animal tissues. Cholesterol is produced in the liver and is a component of bile (Ch. 44).

choriocarcinoma (coriocarcinoma) rare malignant neoplasm, usually of the uterus or of an ectopic pregnancy. The exact cause is unknown (Ch. 34, 37, 44).

chronologic résumé (curriculum vitae cronológico) résumé format used when you have employment experience (Ch. 48).

circadian rhythm (ritmo circadiano) pattern based on a 24-hour cycle emphasizing the repetition of certain physiologic phenomena such as eating and sleeping (Ch. 42).

circumduction (circunducción) circular motion of a body part (Ch. 33).

cirrhosis (cirrosis) a chronic liver disease in which normal functioning liver tissue is replaced with nonfunctioning scar tissue (Ch. 22).

civil law (derecho civil) law related to actions between individuals (Ch. 7).

clinical email (correo electrónico clínico) type of email established using defined protocols as a means of communication between providers and established patients (Ch. 12).

claim register (registro de reclamaciones) diary or register of claims submitted to each insurance carrier. When payment is received, the date and amount of payment is entered in the register (Ch. 18).

claustrophobia (claustrofobia) fear of being confined in any space (Ch. 32).

clinical chemistry (química clínica) analysis and study of blood, body fluids, excreta, and tissues in the diagnosis and treatment of disease (Ch. 39).

clinical diagnosis (diagnóstico clínico) identification of a disease by history, laboratory studies, and symptoms (Ch. 23, 39).

closed fracture (fractura cerrada) uncomplicated fracture in which the bone does not break the skin (Ch. 30).

closed questions (preguntas cerradas) questions answered with a yes or no (Ch. 4).

clustering (agrupación) a grouping together of nonverbal messages into statements or conclusions. Can also be used to describe a scheduling system where patients with similar complaint/conditions are scheduled consecutively (example is scheduling all the allergy injections for 3:00 PM to 4:00 PM every Tuesday and Thursday) (Ch. 4).

CMS 1500 (08/05) (CMS 1500 [08/05]) formerly known as the HCFA 1500 form that is the office health insurance claim form for Medicare and Medicaid (Ch. 18).

cobalamina (cobalamina) vitamin B_{12} (Ch. 34).

cochlear implantation (implante coclear) an electrical device that receives sounds and transmits the resulting signal to electrodes implanted in the cochlea. The signal stimulates the cochlea and the individual is able to perceive sound (Ch. 27).

coenzyme (coenzima) substance that enhances a catalyst (Ch. 34).

cognitive functioning (funcionamiento cognitivo) awareness with perception, reasoning, judgment, intuition, and memory (Ch. 29).

coinsurance (coseguro) that percentage paid by the company or that paid by the insured (Ch. 17).

collection ratio (relación de cobranza) gross income divided by the amount that could have been collected less disallowances (Ch. 20, 21).

colonoscopy (colonoscopia) visual examination of the colon with a lighted scope (Ch. 30).

colposcopy (colposcopia) visual examination of vaginal and cervical tissues using a colposcope following abnormal Pap smear. A magnifying lens and powerful lights are used (Ch. 26).

comedone (comedón) blackhead; usually the result of blocked sebaceous glands caused by acne (Ch. 30).

Commission on Accreditation of Allied Health Education Programs (CAAHEP) (Comisión de Acreditación de Programas Educativos Asociados a la Salud [CAAHEP]) entity accrediting over 2,000 educational programs in 20 health sciences professions (Ch. 1, 47).

common law (derecho consuetudinario) refers to laws developed in England and France and brought to the United States by the early settlers; sometimes referred to as judge-made law (Ch. 7).

communicable (transmisible) contagious. Capable of being transmitted from one person to another either directly or indirectly (Ch. 22, 38).

compact disk (CD) (disco compacto [CD]) see **optical disk** (Ch. 11).

compensation (compensación) overemphasizing of characteristics to make up for a real or imagined failure or handicap (Ch. 4).

competency (competencia) legally qualified or adequate (Ch. 1).

complete blood count (CBC) (recuento sanguíneo completo [RSC]) battery of hematologic tests consisting of hemoglobin, hematocrit, total white blood cell count including differential, total red blood cell count, including indices, and platelets (Ch. 41).

compliance (cumplimiento) conformity in fulfilling official requirements (Ch. 1).

compounding (composición) combining two or more substances in definite proportions (Ch. 36).

condenser (condensador) in a microscope, directs a beam of light from the source to the specimen (Ch. 39).

condylomata (condiloma) a wartlike lesion of viral origin found on external genitalia or perianal region (Ch. 26).

confidentiality (confidencialidad) ethical and legal rules in regard to patient privacy (Ch. 16).

confidentiality agreement (acuerdo de confidencialidad) when signed, the agreement signifies that the medical transcriptionist is committed to keep all patient information confidential (Ch. 16).

conflict resolution (resolución de conflictos) solving problems between coworkers or any two parties (Ch. 45).

congenital anomalies (anomalías congénitas) being born with; existing at time of birth (Ch. 26).

congruency (congruencia) the verbal message and the nonverbal message must agree (Ch. 4).

consecutive or serial filing (archivado consecutivo o en serie) numeric filing method where numbers are considered in ascending order using the entire set of figures (Ch. 14).

constitutional law (derecho constitucional) consists of laws that are made by constitutions of the United States or individual states (Ch. 7).

constrict (constreñirse) to become smaller in diameter (Ch. 40).

constriction band (banda de constricción) term used to replace tourniquet (no longer used) in emergencies. A band of material used to control severe bleeding in an extremity that has been injured due to trauma. The band is applied above the source of bleeding, but not so tight that it restricts the flow of blood completely. Some slight trickling of blood should be evident. This action avoids loss of an extremity because of complete blood flow restriction. Complete blood flow restriction results in no blood flow to the extremity's cells and tissues; therefore, the cells, tissues and body part receive no oxygen and die (Ch. 9).

consultation report (informe de consulta) document that reports the findings and advice of another provider requested to see a patient by the attending provider (Ch. 16).

contact tracker (seguidor de contactos) form used to keep track of employment contact information such as name of employer, name of contact person, address and telephone number, date of first contact, résumé sent, interview date, follow-up information, and dates (Ch. 48).

contact transmission (transmisión por contacto) spread of disease-causing microorganisms by directly or indirectly touching the source of the infection or by touching an object or environmental surface (Ch. 22).

contaminate (contaminar) to make something unclean; often used to describe a sterile area being made "unsterile" or exposing a clean area to a pathogenic substance (Ch. 22, 31).

continuing education units (CEU) (unidades de educación continua [UEC]) method for earning points toward recertification (Ch. 47).

contract law (derecho contractual) law that refers to agreements between individuals and entities that are binding (Ch. 7).

contracting (contraer) acquiring an infection from pathogens (Ch. 22).

contraindication (contraindicación) any symptom or circumstance indicating that the use of a particular drug is inappropriate when it would otherwise be advisable. For example, the use of alcoholic beverages is a contraindication when the drug Flagyl® is prescribed (Ch. 35).

control test (prueba de control) test of a sample of known results used to compare with the results of a patient's sample (Ch. 39).

coordination of benefits (COB) (coordinación de beneficios [COB]) the provision of an insurance contract that limits benefits to 100% of the cost (Ch. 17).

co-payment (copago) payment required when seen by the provider (Ch. 17).

coryza (coriza) acute inflammation of the membranes of the nose accompanied by profuse drainage (Ch. 22).

cost analysis (análisis de costos) procedure that determines the costs of each service (Ch. 21).

cost ratio (relación de costos) formula that shows the cost of a procedure or service and helps determine the financial value of maintaining certain services (Ch. 21).

cough etiquette (protocolo de manejo de la tos) coughing/sneezing into a tissue to prevent microorganisms from spreading to others. Includes properly disposing of tissue into a waste receptacle and washing hands as soon as possible (Ch. 22).

countershock (contrachoque) application of an electric current to the heart directly or indirectly to alter a disturbance in cardiac rhythm (Ch. 37).

coupling agent (agente de acoplamiento) an agent used when ultrasonography is used; enhances penetration of sound waves through tissue (Ch. 26).

crash tray or cart (bandeja o carro de parada) tray or portable cart that contains medications and supplies needed for emergency and first aid procedures (Ch. 9).

creatinine (creatinina) waste product formed in muscle that is excreted by the kidneys; increased in blood and urine when kidney function is abnormal (Ch. 42).

credentialed (acreditado) testimonials showing that a person is entitled to credit or has a right to exercise official power (Ch. 1).

credit (crédito) decreases balance due; column used for entering payments (Ch. 19).

crepitation (crepitación) grating sound heard on movement of ends of a broken bone (Ch. 9).

criminal law (derecho penal) law related to wrongs committed against the welfare and safety of society as a whole (Ch. 7).

critical values (valores críticos) test results that indicate a potentially life-threatening or greatly debilitating situation that must be reported to the provider immediately (Ch. 42).

cross-reference (referencia cruzada) notation in a file to direct the reader to a specific record that may be filed under more than one name/subject (e.g., married name/maiden name or foreign names) where the surname is not easily recognizable (Ch. 14).

cryopreservation (crioconservación) storage of biologic materials (sperm, embryo, tissue, plasma) at extremely cold temperature for use at a later time (Ch. 8).

cryosurgery (criocirugía) the destruction of tissue by application of extreme cold, silver nitrate, and carbon dioxide (Ch. 26).

cryotherapy (crioterapia) use of cold to treat a physical condition (Ch. 33).

cryptorchidism (criptorquidia) undescended testicle (Ch. 28).

crystals (crystals) found in normal urine sediment having no particular significance; should be noted because they may indicate disease states (Ch. 42).

cultivate (cultivar) to foster the growth of (Ch. 1).

cultural brokering (intermediación cultural) the act of bridging, linking, or mediating between groups or persons through the process of reducing conflict or producing change (Ch. 4).

culture (cultura) the attitudes and behavior that are characteristic of a particular social group or organization (Ch. 4).

culture and sensitivity (cultivo y sensibilidad) often referred to as C&S. The sample is cultured for bacteria and then is exposed to various antibiotics to determine what the bacteria is sensitive (and resistant) to (Ch. 39, 42).

cultures (cultivos) microorganisms cultivated in a nutrient medium (Ch. 42, 43).

Current Procedural Terminology (CPT) (Terminología Actual sobre Procedimientos [TAP]) standard codes for procedures and services. Used by most ambulatory care settings in encoding the claim form and recognized by most insurance carriers (Ch. 19).

current reports (informes actuales) reports such as history and physical examinations that should be complete within 24 hours (Ch. 16).

Cushing's syndrome (síndrome de Cushing) hypersecretion of the adrenal cortex producing excessive glucocorticoids. The condition may be caused by a tumor or hyperfunction of the anterior pituitary (Ch. 44).

cyanosis (cianosis) discoloration of the skin due to abnormal amounts of reduced hemoglobin in the blood caused by decreased oxygen and increased carbon dioxide in the blood (Ch. 25).

cyberspace (ciberespacio) reference to the nonphysical space of binary computer communication (Ch. 11).

cystitis (cistitis) inflammation of the bladder (Ch. 29).

cytology (citología) science that deals with the formation, structure, and function of cells (Ch. 39).

D

data storage device (dispositivo de almacenamiento de datos) device capable of permanently or temporarily storing digital data (Ch. 11).

data storage memory (memoria de almacenamiento de datos) permanent memory not part of the motherboard. Uses any suitable data storage device. Can be read-only or read-write type of memory (Ch. 11).

day sheet (hoja diaria) form used with pegboard system to record daily patient transactions (Ch. 19).

debit (debe) used for entering charges and description of services; column is on the left (Ch. 19).

debris (detritos) remains of broken down or damaged cells or tissues (Ch. 22).

declination form (formulario de rechazo) written formal refusal (Ch. 22).

decode (decodificar) to translate into language that is easily understood; to interpret (Ch. 4).

deductible (deducible) that amount of incurred medical expenses that must be met before the insurance policy will begin to pay (Ch. 17).

defendant (demandado) person who defends action brought in litigation (Ch. 7).

Defense Enrollment Eligible Reporting System (DEERS) (Sistema de Informes de Elegibilidad para la Inscripción en Defensa [DEERS]) a system operated by the Department of Defense and used by TRICARE contractors to determine and confirm the eligibility of beneficiaries (Ch. 17).

defense mechanism (mecanismo de defensa) behavior that protects the psyche from guilt, anxiety, or shame (Ch. 4).

defibrillation (desfibrilación) stopping fibrillation of the heart by use of drugs or by physical means (Ch. 37).

defibrillator (desfibrilador) a machine that delivers an electric current to alter a disturbance in cardiac rhythm (Ch. 37).

defragmentation (desfragmentación) reorganization of information on a hard disk to store files as continuous units rather than as small packets. A computer with little fragmentation of files will operate at a higher speed (Ch. 11).

dementia (demencia) impairment of intellectual function that is progressive and interferes with normal activities (Ch. 29).

demyelination (desmielinización) destruction of the myelin sheath; often a factor in multiple sclerosis (Ch. 30).

denial (rechazo) rejection of or refusal to acknowledge (Ch. 4).

deoxygenated (desoxigenada) blood that is high in carbon dioxide, low in oxygen, and pumped through the heart to the lungs where the carbon dioxide is exchanged for oxygen (Ch. 37).

depolarize (despolarizar) process of reducing to a nonpolarized condition. Generation of an electrical current is enhanced. Electrical activity generated when the atria or ventricles contract (Ch. 37).

deposition (declaración) oral testimony given by an individual with a court reporter and attorneys for both sides present; often used as part of the discovery process (Ch. 7).

dermatophytes (dermatofitos) category of fungi causing infections of hair, skin, and nails (Ch. 43).

dexterity (destreza) skill and ease in using the hands (Ch. 1).

diabetes mellitus (diabetes mellitus) chronic disorder of carbohydrate metabolism characterized by hyperglycemia and resulting from inadequate production or utilization of insulin (Ch. 44).

diagnosis (diagnóstico) determination of disease or condition (Ch. 39).

diaphragm (diafragma) a lens or other object that opens and closes to increase or decrease the amount of light on the object being illuminated. This refers to optic diaphragm such as in a microscope (diaphragms are used in birth control and also the large respiratory muscle) (Ch. 39).

diastole (diástole) one component of blood pressure measurement representing the lowest amount of pressure exerted during the cardiac cycle; the force exerted on the arterial walls during cardiac relaxation (Ch. 24, 37).

diathermy (diatermia) the therapeutic use of high-frequency current to generate heat within some part of the body without damaging tissues (Ch. 33).

diethylstilbestrol (DES) (dietilestilbestrol [DES]) a synthetic hormone used therapeutically in menopausal disturbances. It should not be given during pregnancy. It has been related to cervicovaginal malignances in daughters of mothers who had it prescribed for them to treat a threatened abortion. DES has been related to reproductive disorders in males whose mothers took it during pregnancy (Ch. 26).

differential diagnosis (diagnóstico diferencial) diagnosis based on comparison of symptoms of similar diseases (Ch. 39).

digestion (digestión) breaking down of food into smaller particles. It can be either physical or chemical (Ch. 34).

digital video disk/digital versatile disk (DVD) (disco de video digital/disco versátil digital [DVD]) an optical disk that holds 4.7 to 9.0 gigabytes of data depending on format (Ch. 11).

dilate (dilatarse) to enlarge in diameter (Ch. 40).

dilation (dilatación) expansion of an orifice or organ (Ch. 26).

diploma (diploma) a document bearing record of graduation from or of a degree conferred by an educational institution (Ch. 1).

direct skills (habilidades directas) skills that are job specific. Skill in taking a blood pressure reading would be specific to the medical field (Ch. 48).

discharge summary (DS) (resumen de alta médica [DS]) medical reports that document the hospitalization history of a patient (Ch. 16).

discovery (exhibición de pruebas) the time in which both parties are allowed access to all information and evidence related to a case; follows the subpoena process (Ch. 7).

disinfection (desinfección) use of chemicals or boiling water to free an item from infectious materials but not its spores (Ch. 22).

dislocation (luxación) displacement of a bone or joint from its normal position (Ch. 30).

dispense (dosificar) prepare and give out a medication to be taken at a later time (Ch. 7, 35, 36).

displacement (desplazamiento) displacing negative feelings onto something or someone else with no significance to the situation (Ch. 4).

disposition (temperamento) temperament, character, personality (Ch. 1).

diuretic (diurético) substance that causes less water to be reabsorbed by the kidney and therefore causes water to be excreted from the body (Ch. 34).

DNA (ADN) deoxyribonucleic acid; important nuclear material that carries genetic codes (Ch. 39, 43).

doctrine (doctrina) principle of law established through past decisions (Ch. 7).

documentation (documentación) written material that accompanies purchased software containing the information necessary for using the software appropriately; sometimes known as the manual (Ch. 11, 22); also, providing factual support through written information (Ch. 22).

Doppler (doppler) a noninvasive technique used with ultrasonography to evaluate blood flow through major arteries and veins of the arms, legs, and neck. It can reveal blood clots or blockages (Ch. 32).

dorsiflexion (dorsiflexión) moving the foot upward at the ankle joint (Ch. 33).

dosimeter (dosímetro) a device for measuring X-ray output (Ch. 32).

down-coding (baja de codificación) insurance carriers downcode if documentation or codes are ambiguous and reimburse for the lowest possible fee (Ch. 18).

donut hole (período sin cobertura) within the Medicare Part D prescription drug program, the donut hole is the phase of coverage in which all costs are covered by the enrollee rather than CMS (Ch. 17).

dressing (apósito) sterile gauze or other material applied directly to a wound to absorb secretions and to protect (Ch. 9, 31).

driver (controlador) computer program designed to convert data output from one device to a format compatible with another device (Ch. 11).

droplet transmission (transmisión por gotitas) method of spreading disease from respiratory secretions through the air. Spread is usually confined to within 3 feet of the infected patient (Ch. 22).

durable power of attorney for health care (poder legal duradero para atención médica) legal form that allows a designated person to act on another's behalf in regard to health care choices (Ch. 6, 7).

dysmenorrhea (dismenorrea) painful menses (Ch. 26).

dyspareunia (dispareunia) painful intercourse (Ch. 26).

dysplasia (displasia) abnormal development of tissue (Ch. 26).

dyspnea (disnea) shortness of breath or labored/difficult breathing (Ch. 24).

dysuria (disuria) painful or difficult urination (Ch. 30).

E

E codes (códigos E) ICD-9-CM codes for the external causes of injury, poisoning, or other adverse reactions that explain how the injury occurred (Ch. 18).

echocardiogram (ecocardiograma) noninvasive diagnostic method that uses ultrasound to visualize internal cardiac structure, including valves (Ch. 32).

eclampsia (eclampsia) complication of pregnancy that includes general edema, hypertension, proteinuria, and convulsions (Ch. 26).

ectopic pregnancy (embarazo ectópico) implementation of the fertilized ovum outside of the uterine cavity (Ch. 26, 44).

edematous (edematoso) abnormal accumulation of fluid in the tissues resulting in swelling (Ch. 40).

editing (corrección) the process of manipulating text to avoid inaccuracies and inconsistencies within a document (Ch. 16).

editor (corrector) see auditor (Ch. 16).

effacement (borramiento) thinning and shortening of the cervical canal during labor to permit passage of fetus (Ch. 26).

effleurage (effleurage) deep or gentle stroking massage (Ch. 33).

EHR (RSE) see **electronic health record** (Ch. 11).

electrocardiogram (electrocardiograma) record of the electrical activity of the heart; showing P, QRS, and T waves (Ch. 37).

electrocardiograph (electrocardiografío) instrument for recording the electrical activity of the heart (Ch. 37).

electrocardiography (electrocardiografía) process of recording the electrical activity originating in the heart (Ch. 37).

electrode (electrodo) also known as a sensor. Used to conduct electricity from the body to the electrocardiograph (Ch. 37).

electrolyte (electrolito) substances that conduct electricity whose components are important in maintaining fluid and acid–base balance (Ch. 34, 37, 39).

electrocochleography (electrococleografía) diagnostic tool used to help diagnose Meniere's disease. It records the electrical activity of the inner ear in response to sound (Ch. 30).

electronic health record (EHR) (registro de salud electrónico [RSE]) a patients' electronic medical records from multiple sources combined into one master database (Ch. 11).

electronic medical record (EMR) (registro médico electrónico [RME]) patient medical record from a single medical practice, hospital, or pharmacy (Ch. 11, 16).

emaciation (emaciación) state of being extremely lean (Ch. 30).

emancipated minor (menor emancipado) persons under age 18 years who are financially responsible for themselves and free of parental care (Ch. 7).

embezzle (malversar) to appropriate fraudulently to one's own use (Ch. 45).

Emergency Medical Services (EMS) (Servicios Médicos de Emergencia [SME]) a local network of police, fire, and medical personnel trained to respond to emergency situations. In many communities, the system is activated by calling 911 (Ch. 9).

empathy (empatía) ability to be objectively aware of and have insight into another's feelings, emotions, and behaviors, and to be aware of the significance and meaning of these to the other person (Ch. 1, 29).

emphysema (enfisema) chronic pulmonary disease characterized by dilated and damaged alveoli (Ch. 24).

EMR (RME) see **electronic medical record** (Ch. 11).

encode (encoding) (codificar [codificación]) creating a message to be sent (Ch. 4).

encounter form (formulario de visita) formerly known as a charge slip or superbill. A copy of the encounter form is given to the patient after seeing the provider. It identifies the procedures performed, diagnoses, charges, and when to return (Ch. 18, 19).

encrypted email (correo electrónico cifrado) the process of coding email to render the transmission essentially secure (Ch. 12).

encryption technology (tecnología de cifrado) converts information into code; used to protect privacy and confidentiality of individuals in computer software (Ch. 13).

endemic (enfermedad endémica) disease that occurs continuously or in cycles with a certain number of cases expected for a given period (Ch. 22).

endometriosis (endometriosis) tissue that resembles the endometrium invades various locations in the pelvic cavity and elsewhere (Ch. 26).

endoscopy (endoscopia) visual examination of body cavities with a lighted scope (Ch. 22).

engineering controls (controles de ingeniería) physical or mechanical devices that isolate or remove health hazards from the workplace (Ch. 22).

enunciation (dicción) speaking clearly; articulating (Ch. 12).

enzyme immunoassay (inmunoensayo enzimático) measurement of reaction of antigen with specific antibody (Ch. 44).

eosinophil (eosinófilos) granulocytic white blood cell with red eosin-stained granules in the cytoplasm. It is elevated in cases of allergies (Ch. 41).

epidemic (epidemia) an infectious disease that attacks many persons at the same time in the same location (Ch. 22).

epidemiology (epidemiología) field of science that studies the history, cause, and patterns of infectious diseases (Ch. 22).

epinephrine (epinefrina) used to treat allergic reactions (Ch. 9); also, hormone also known as adrenaline. Epinephrine is manufactured as a chemical (pharmaceutical preparation) and is often mixed with local anesthetics for use as a vasoconstrictor in minor surgery (Ch. 31).

epistaxis (epistaxis) nosebleed (Ch. 22).

Epstein–Barr virus (EBV) (virus de Epstein-Barr [VEB]) virus that is believed to be the cause of infectious mononucleosis and is implicated in such conditions as African Burkitt's lymphoma and nasopharyngeal carcinoma (Ch. 44).

e-résumé (curriculum vitae electrónico) electronic résumés may be delivered electronically via e-mail, submitted to Internet job boards, or placed on Web pages (Ch. 48).

ergonomics (ergonomía) scientific study of work and space, including factors that influence worker productivity and that affect workers' health (Ch. 11).

erythema (eritema) redness or inflammation of the skin or mucous membranes that is the result of dilatation and congestion of superficial capillaries (Ch. 30).

erythrocyte (eritrocito) red blood cell, one of the formed elements of the blood (Ch. 40, 41).

erythrocyte indices (índices de eritrocitos) three equations that provide information about the sizes and hemoglobin content of red blood cells. These include the mean corpuscular cell volume, mean corpuscular hemoglobin, and mean corpuscular hemoglobin volume (Ch. 41).

erythrocyte sedimentation rate (velocidad de eritrosedimentación) measurement of how far the red cells in a sample of blood settle in one hour (Ch. 41).

erythropoietin (eritropoyetina) hormone that causes production of new red blood cells (Ch. 41).

esophageal varices (várices esofágicas) tortuous dilation of the esophageal vein associated with any condition that causes obstruction of drainage from the esophageal veins into the portal vein of the liver. Seen in cirrhosis of the liver and alcoholism (Ch. 32).

Ethernet (Ethernet) references the networking of computers using metallic conductors or hard wires (Ch. 11).

ethics (ética) defined in terms of what is morally right and wrong; ethics will differ from person to person; often defined by a code or creed as in the Code of Ethics from the American Association of Medical Assistants (AAMA) (Ch. 8).

ethyl alcohol (alcohol etílico) alcohol, used to make a solution (Ch. 38).

etiquette (etiqueta) manners, politeness, proper behavior (Ch. 12).

eupnea (eupnea) normal breathing (Ch. 24).

evaluation (evaluación) assessment of an employee's job performance (Ch. 46).

eversion (eversión) moving a body part outward (Ch. 33).

exclusion (exclusión) specific disease or condition listed in an insurance policy for which the policy will not pay (Ch. 17).

exclusive provider organization (EPO) (organización de proveedor exclusivo [EPO]) a closed-panel preferred organization (PPO) plan where enrollees receive no benefits if they opt to receive care from a provider who is not in the EPO (Ch. 17).

excoriated (excoriación) abrasion of the epidermis by trauma, chemicals, burns, or other causes (Ch. 22).

excretion (excreción) waste matter. The elimination of waste products from the body (Ch. 22, 38).

exfoliated (exfoliación) the shedding of something such as cervical cells (Ch. 26).

exit interview (entrevista de salida) opportunity for departing employees to provide their positive and negative opinions of the position and facility (Ch. 46).

expectorate (expectorar) act of coughing up material from airways that lead to the lungs (Ch. 22, 43).

expert witness (testigo experto) individual with highly specialized knowledge and skills in a particular area who testifies to a standard of care (Ch. 7).

explanation of benefits (EOB) (explicación de beneficios [EDB]) insurance report that is sent with claim payments explaining the reimbursement of the insurance carrier (Ch. 18).

explicit (explícito) fully revealed or expressed without ambiguity or vagueness, leaving no question as to intent (Ch. 9).

expressed contract (contrato explícito) written or verbal contract that specifically describes what each party in the contract will do (Ch. 7).

extension (extensión) straightening of a body part (Ch. 33).

external respiration (respiración externa) ventilation of the lungs when the exchange of oxygen and carbon dioxide takes place (Ch. 30).

externship (práctica laboral) transition stage between the classroom and actual employment; may also be referred to as internship or practicum (Ch. 1, 24, 45).

extracellular (extracelular) pertaining to the environment outside of a body cell (Ch. 34).

exudate (exudado) accumulated fluid in a cavity; an oozing of pus; matter that penetrates through vessel walls into adjoining tissue (Ch. 22, 27, 31).

F

facilitate (facilitar) to make an action or process easier (Ch. 1).

Fair Debt Collection Practice Act (Ley sobre Prácticas Justas para el Cobro de Deudas) 1977 federal law that outlines collection practices (Ch. 20).

fat-soluble (soluble en lípidos) pertaining to substances that are hydrophobic and therefore dissolve better in fat (Ch. 34).

fax (facsimile) (fax [facsímilx]) machine that sends documents from one location to another by way of telephone lines (Ch. 12).

febrile (febril) having a fever (Ch. 24).

Federal Register (Registro Federal) federal government agency from which written CLIA '88 documents may be obtained (Ch. 38).

felony (delito mayor) a serious crime such as murder, larceny (thefts of large sums of money), assault, and rape (Ch. 7).

fenestrated (fenestrado) having openings. A sterile, fenestrated drape is used in surgery. It has an opening (round) in it to expose only the operative site. The remainder of the drape covers the patient and is a sterile area (Ch. 31).

fenestrated drape (paño fenestrado) a type of drape with an opening, usually round, that can be placed with the opening over a particular body area; used in surgery and for proctologic examinations (Ch. 25).

firewall (cortafuegos) hardware device or software program designed to prevent unauthorized access to a computer system (Ch. 11).

first aid (primeros auxilios) immediate (or first) care provided to persons who are suddenly ill or injured; first aid is typically followed by more comprehensive care and treatment (Ch. 9).

fiscal intermediary (intermediario fiscal) local administrator for Medicare (Ch. 17).

fixed cost (costo fijo) cost that does not vary in total as the number of patients vary (Ch. 21).

flag (indicador de mensaje) method of identifying a blank space or a question regarding dictator's meaning by attaching a note or marker to indicate the question (Ch. 16).

flash drive (unidad flash) solid-state data storage device (Ch. 11).

flexion (flexión) bending of a body part (Ch. 33).

fluent (fluido) able to write or speak easily or flowing smoothly (Ch. 12).

fluoroscope (fluoroscope) a device consisting of a screen; mounts separately or with an X-ray tube that shows the images of objects interposed between the table and the screen (Ch. 32).

folic acid (ácido fólico) one of the B-complex vitamins (Ch. 34).

fomite (fómite) substance that absorbs and transmits infectious material; for example, contaminated items such as equipment (Ch. 22).

fontanel (fontanela) soft spot lying between the cranial bones of the skull of a fetus, newborn, and infant (Ch. 27).

forensic (forense) applying scientific knowledge to legal issues (Ch. 38).

form letter (carta tipo) letter containing the same content in the body but sent to different individuals (Ch. 15).

formaldehyde (formaldehído) colorless gas combined with methanol and used as a solution, such as a disinfectant, astringent, or a preservative for histologic specimen (Ch. 38).

formalin (formalina) an aqueous solution of 37% formaldehyde (Ch. 26).

fracture (fractura) break in a bone. There are several types of fractures, but all are classified as either open or closed fractures (Ch. 9).

fraud (fraude) deliberate misrepresentation of facts (Ch. 17).

frenulum (frenillo) of the tongue, a fold of mucous membrane located under the tongue attaching the tongue to the floor of the mouth (Ch. 24).

frequency (frecuencia) urinating frequently (Ch. 30).

friable (friable) easily broken (Ch. 31).

fringe benefit (beneficio complementario) benefit above and beyond salary to which an employee may be entitled. Examples include health and life insurance, paid vacation, sick days, personal days, and tuition reimbursement for courses related to employment (Ch. 2, 45).

fulgarated (fulgurado) destroyed by electric current (Ch. 26).

full block letter (carta de bloque completo) major letter style in which all lines begin flush with the left margin. This style is suggested for offices desiring a contemporary-looking, efficient letter (Ch. 15).

fume hood (campana de humo) type of hood or barrier used in the laboratory to capture chemical vapors and fumes and move them away from health care workers and into a building's exhaust fan system (Ch. 38).

functional résumé (curriculum vitae funcional) résumé format used to highlight specialty areas of accomplishment and strengths (Ch. 48).

furuncle (forúnculo) localized, suppurative staphylococcal skin infection originating in a gland or hair follicle (Ch. 30).

G

gait (marcha) manner or style of walking including rhythm and speed (Ch. 33).

gait belt (cinturón de marcha) safety belt worn by the patient around the waist that provides a firm handhold for the caregiver when transferring the patient or when assisting in ambulation (Ch. 33).

gallium (galio) a nontoxic metal, similar to mercury in appearance, that can be used in place of mercury for fever thermometers. It is not yet widely available for use (Ch. 24).

galvanometer (galvanómetro) mechanism in the electrocardiograph that changes the voltage into a mechanical motion for recording purposes (Ch. 37).

genetic engineering (ingeniería genética) alteration, manipulation, replacement, or repair of genetic material (Ch. 8).

genitalia (genitales) the reproductive organs, internal and external (Ch. 26).

genus (género) first Greek or Latin name given to a microorganism; always capitalized (Ch. 43).

geriatrics (geriatría) the branch of medicine concerned with the problems of aging (Ch. 29).

gerontology (gerontología) the scientific study of the problems associated with aging (Ch. 29).

gestation (gestación) period of development from fertilization to birth (Ch. 26).

gestational diabetes (diabetes gestacional) diabetes that first manifests clinically during pregnancy. It usually subsides after delivery (Ch. 26).

gestures/mannerisms (gestos/ademanes) movement of various body parts while communicating (Ch. 4).

glucose (glucosa) simple sugar that is a major source of energy in the human body; monitoring of blood glucose levels in urine and blood is a vital diagnostic test in diabetes and other disorders; also a test on a reagent strip (Ch. 39, 42).

glucosuria (glucosuria) the presence of glucose in urine (also correct is glycosuria) (Ch. 42).

glycogen (glicógeno) carbohydrate form used for storage of sugar in the body (Ch. 34).

goal (meta) result or achievement toward which effort is directed (Ch. 5).

"going bare" ("estar desprotegido") said of a provider who does not carry professional liability insurance (Ch. 45).

goniometer (goniómetro) instrument used to measure the angle of a joint's range of motion (Ch. 33).

goniometry (goniometría) measurement of joint motion (Ch. 33).

Good Samaritan laws (leyes del Buen Samaritano) laws designed to protect individuals from legal action when rendering emergency medical aid, without compensation, within the areas of their training and expertise (Ch. 12).

Gram stain (tinción de Gram) named for its inventor, Hans Christian Gram, and is, therefore, always capitalized; most common stain used in microbiology to observe gross morphologic features of bacteria; a differential stain, allowing differentiation between Gram-negative and Gram-positive organisms (Ch. 43).

gravidity (gravidez) total number of pregnancies a woman has had regardless of duration, including a present one (Ch. 26).

gross contamination (contaminación importante) highly infectious material present (Ch. 22).

gross examination (examen macroscópico) viewing specimens with the naked eye (Ch. 16).

guarantor (garante) the person identified as responsible for payment of the bill (Ch. 19).

Guthrie screening test (prueba de detección de Guthrie) also known as newborn screening test; diagnostic test for the detection of phenylketonuria (PKU) (Ch. 44).

H

hard drive (disco duro) a nonvolatile storage device that stores digitally encoded data on rapidly rotating rigid disks with magnetic surfaces. The capacity is approximately 100 GB. The device is either permanently installed within the computer case or can be portable (Ch. 11).

hardware (hardware) physical equipment used by the computer system to process data (Ch. 11).

hard-wired networks (redes con cableado físico) networks connected by metallic conductors or cables; under some circumstances, optical cables could be used (Ch. 11).

Health Insurance Portability and Accountability Act (HIPAA) (Ley de Portabilidad y Responsabilidad de Seguros de Salud [HIPAA]) government rules, regulations, and procedures resulting from legislation designed to protect the confidentiality of patient information (Ch. 16).

health maintenance organization (HMO) (organización de mantenimiento de la salud [HMO]) type of managed care operation that is typically set up as a for-profit corporation with salaried employees. HMOs "with walls" offer a range of medical services under one roof; HMOs "without walls" typically contract with providers in the community to provide patient services for an agreed-upon fee (Ch. 2, 17).

Healthcare Common Procedure Coding System (HCPCS) (Sistema de Códigos de Procedimientos Comunes de la Atención Médica [HCPCS]) a coding system consisting of the CPT, national codes (level II), and local codes (level III); previously known as HCFA Common Procedure Coding System (Ch. 18).

Heimlich maneuver (maniobra de Heimlich) abdominal thrusts designed to overcome breathing difficulties in individuals who are choking (Ch. 9).

hematocrit (hematocrito) percentage of red blood cells within a specimen of anticoagulated whole blood (Ch. 41).

hematology (hematología) study of blood and the blood-forming tissues (Ch. 39, 41).

hematoma (hematoma) a large bruise, accumulation of blood around the venipuncture site during or after venipuncture caused by the leakage of blood from where the needle punctured the vein (Ch. 31, 40).

hematopoiesis (hematopoyesis) formation of blood cells (Ch. 41).

hematuria (hematuria) abnormal presence of blood in urine, symptomatic of many disorders of the genitourinary system and renal diseases (Ch. 30, 42).

hemiplegia (hemiplejía) paralysis of one side of the body (Ch. 33).

hemoconcentration (hemoconcentración) pooling of blood at the location of the venipuncture caused by leaving the tourniquet on the arm longer than one minute, resulting in inaccurate blood samples (Ch. 40).

hemoglobin (hemoglobina) molecule within the red blood cell that transports oxygen (Ch. 41).

hemoglobinopathy (hemoglobinopatía) inherited disease resulting from the formation of an abnormal hemoglobin molecule (Ch. 41).

hemolysis (hemólisis) rupturing of the red blood cells during the process of blood collection. The serum or plasma becomes contaminated and has a reddish color (Ch. 40).

hemoptysis (hemoptisis) spitting up of blood arising from the mouth, larynx, trachea, bronchi, or lungs characterized by a sudden attack of coughing with production of bloody sputum (Ch. 30).

heterophile antibody (anticuerpo heterófilo) antibody that reacts with other than the specific antigens as seen in infectious mononucleosis (Ch. 44).

Hibeclens® (Hibeclens®) brand of antiseptic soap solution (Ch. 31).

hierarchy of needs (jerarquía de necesidades) needs that are arranged in a specific order or rank; sequential arrangement. Associated with Abraham Maslow (Ch. 4).

high-context communication (comunicación de alto contexto) communication style that involves great reliance on body language, reference to objects in the environment, and culturally relevant phraseology to convey an idea. Relies on the listener knowing related events through close association with the speaker or culture (Ch. 4).

high-density lipoprotein (HDL) (lipoproteína de alta densidad [HDL]) lipoprotein in the blood composed primarily of protein; removes cholesterol from peripheral tissues and transports them to the liver for excretion (Ch. 44).

histology (histología) study of a tissue biopsy sample for the determination of disease (Ch. 39).

history and physical examination report (H&P) (informe de historia clínica y examen físico [H&P]) report of patient's history and physical examination to document reason for visit (Ch. 16).

history of present illness (HPI) (antecedentes de enfermedad actual [AEA]) the chronologic description of the development of the patient's illness (Ch. 16).

holding media (medios de sostén) specific media used in the transport of microorganisms to support the life of the organisms until they can be put on nutrient medium in the laboratory (Ch. 43).

homeopathy (homeopatía) a healing modality that uses diluted doses of certain substances to create an "energy imprint" in the body to bring about a cure (Ch. 2).

homeostasis (homeostasia) state of equilibrium of internal environment (Ch. 34).

hormone replacement therapy (HRT) (terapia de reemplazo hormonal [TRH]) the replacement of hormones lacking from the patient's system. In this case, HRT refers to the replacement of varying levels of estrogen and progesterone in perimenopausal or postmenopausal women (Ch. 26, 39).

hospital-based laboratories (laboratorios con base en el hospital) hospital-owned laboratories that perform most tests required by the hospital and local communities (Ch. 39).

human chorionic gonadotropin (hCG) (gonadotropina coriónica humana [hCG]) hormone secreted by the trophoblast after fertilization of the ovum. It may be detected in the blood and urine of pregnant women (Ch. 26, 44).

human immunodeficiency virus (HIV) (virus de la inmunodeficiencia humana [VIH]) virus causing AIDS; it is a retrovirus that ultimately destroys immune system cells (Ch. 22).

humoral immunity (inmunidad humoral) immunity mediated by antibodies in body fluids such as plasma and lymph (Ch. 22).

hyaline (hialino) transparent, clear; hyaline casts consist of mucuprotein, they are transparent and often difficult to see in urine (Ch. 42).

hydatidiform mole (mola hidatidiforme) development of cysts and rapid growth of the uterus with bleeding (Ch. 44).

hydrocollator pack (paquete de hidrocolator) pack filled with gel that is warmed in a water bath (Ch. 33).

hydrogen peroxide (peróxido de hidrógeno) antibacterial solution that has a mechanical cleansing action (Ch. 31).

hyperemesis gravidarum (hiperemesis gravídica) severe nausea and vomiting during pregnancy with inability to eat; may lead to severe dehydration (Ch. 26).

hyperextension (hiperextensión) position of maximum extension, or extending a body part beyond its normal limits (Ch. 33).

hyperglycemia (hiperglucemia) increased levels of blood glucose. Hyperglycemia does not necessarily mean that the patient is diabetic but may be an indication of prediabetes (Ch. 44).

hyperpnea (hiperpnea) increased respiratory rate and depth as seen in exercise, pain, fever, and hysteria (Ch. 24).

hypertension (hipertensión) blood pressure that is consistently greater than 140/90 mm Hg (Ch. 24).

hyperthermia (hipertermia) body temperature above normal range; an unusually high fever (Ch. 29).

hyperventilation (hiperventilación) ventilation rate that is greater than metabolically necessary, potentially leading to alkalosis (Ch. 24).

hypochromic (hipocrómico) less color than normal (Ch. 41).

hypoglycemia (hipoglucemia) state of having a lower than normal blood glucose level (Ch. 40, 44).

hypotension (hipotensión) abnormally low blood pressure resulting in inadequate tissue profusion and oxygenation (Ch. 24).

hypothermia (hipotermia) extremely dangerous cold-related condition that can result in death if the individual does not receive care and if the progression of hypothermia is not reversed. Symptoms include shivering, cold skin, and confusion (Ch. 9, 29).

hypoventilation (hipoventilación) decrease in respiration rate with shallow depth of respiration (Ch. 24).

hypoxemia (hipoxemia) lack of oxygen in the blood (Ch. 36).

hypoxia (hypoxia) oxygen deficiency (Ch. 26).

hysterosalpingogram (histerosalpingograma) X-ray of uterus and fallopian tubes using a contrast medium (Ch. 26).

I

immune system (sistema inmunitario) body's strong line of defense against invading microorganisms. The body recognizes foreign substances such as microorganisms and produces substances to fight them off. Antibodies, white blood cells, digestive enzymes, and resistance of the skin are some examples (Ch. 22).

immunity (inmunidad) ability of the body to resist specific pathogens and their toxins (Ch. 22).

immunoglobulins (inmunoglobulinas) family of proteins capable of acting as antibodies, thereby protecting individuals from pathogenic microorganisms; also, antibodies produced by the cells of the immune response system (Ch. 22, 30).

immunohematology (inmunohematología) study of blood group antigens and antibodies; blood banking (Ch. 39).

immunology (inmunología) the study of the components of the immune system and their function (Ch. 39).

immunomodulator (inmunomodulador) a substance that has the ability to change immune responses (Ch. 22, 43).

immunosuppressed (inmunosuprimido) referring to a patient whose immune system is unhealthy because of disease, medication, and genetics; these patients can be particularly susceptible to attack by microorganisms (Ch. 22, 43).

implicit (implícito) capable of being understood from something else though unexpressed; implied (Ch. 9).

implied consent (consentimiento implícito) consent assumed by the health care provider, typically in an emergency that threatens the patient's life. Implied consent also occurs in more subtle ways in the health care environment; for example, when a patient willingly rolls up the sleeve to receive an injection (Ch. 7).

implied contract (contrato implícito) contract indicated by actions rather than words (Ch. 7).

improvise (improvisar) to make, invent, or arrange in an unplanned or spontaneous manner (Ch. 1).

incinerate (incinerar) to destroy by fire (Ch. 22).

income statement (estado de resultados) financial statement showing net profit or loss (Ch. 21).

incompetence (incompetencia) legally, a person who is insane, inadequate, or not an adult (Ch. 7).

incontinence (incontinencia) uncontrollable loss of urine or feces (Ch. 29).

increment (incremento) an increase or addition in number, size, or extent (Ch. 24).

independent physician association (IPA) (Asociación Independiente de Médicos [IPA]) independent network of physicians in private practice who contract with the association to treat patients for an agreed-upon fee (Ch. 2).

indexing (indexar) selecting the name, subject, or number under which to file a record and determining the order in which the units should be considered (Ch. 14).

indirect statements (declaraciones indirectas) means of eliciting a response from a patient by turning a question into a statement of interest (Ch. 4).

infarction (infarto) area of tissue in an organ or part that becomes necrotic (dead) after cessation of blood supply (Ch. 37).

infection (infección) invasion of pathogens into living tissue (Ch. 31).

infection control (control de infecciones) methods to eliminate or reduce the transmission of infectious microorganisms (Ch. 22).

infectious agent (agente infeccioso) pathogen responsible for a specific infectious disease (Ch. 22).

infectious mononucleosis (mononucleosis infecciosa) acute infectious disease primarily affecting the lymphoid tissue, caused by the Epstein–Barr virus (Ch. 44).

infectious waste (residuos patógenos) items that have come in contact with patient blood or body fluids. Contaminated items (Ch. 22).

inflammation (inflamación) the normal nonspecific immune response by the body to any type of injury (trauma, bacterial, viral, and temperature extremes) (Ch. 31).

inflammatory response (respuesta inflamatoria) body's defense against the threat of infection or trauma. Characterized by redness, pain, heat, and swelling (Ch. 22).

informed consent (consentimiento informado) consent given by the patient who is made aware of any procedure to be performed, its risks, expected outcomes, and alternatives (Ch. 7, 31).

inner-directed people (personas con autodeterminación) people who decide for themselves what they want to do with their lives (Ch. 5).

inoculate (inocular) to place colonies of microorganisms onto nutrient media (Ch. 43).

inoculation (inoculación) injection (Ch. 22).

input device (dispositivo de entrada) a device used to input data into a computer (Ch. 11).

instrument tray (bandeja de instrumentos) see **Mayo stand** (Ch. 31).

insulin (insulina) hormone secreted by beta cells of the islets of Langerhans of the pancreas essential for the proper metabolism of glucose (Ch. 44).

integrate (integrar) to incorporate into a larger unit; to form or blend into a whole (Ch. 1).

integrated delivery system (IDS) (sistema de prestación de servicios médicos integrado [IDS]) a health care organization of affiliated provider sites combined under a single ownership that offers the full spectrum of managed health care (Ch. 17).

integrative medicine (medicina integradora) bringing together of two or more treatment modalities so they function as a harmonious whole, as seen in alternative forms of health care (Ch. 2).

internal respiration (respiración interna) passage of oxygen from the blood into the cells (Ch. 30).

***International Classification of Diseases, 9th Revision, Clinical Modification* (ICD-9-CM) (*Clasificación Internacional de Enfermedades, 9.ª Revisión, Modificación Clínica* [CIE-9-MC])** standard diagnosis codes used to identify a patient's medical problem. Used by most ambulatory care settings in encoding the claim form and recognized by most insurance carriers (Ch. 18).

internship (pasantía) transition stage between classroom and employment (Ch. 1).

interrogatory (interrogatorio) a written set of questions that must be answered, under oath, within a specific time period; part of the discovery process (Ch. 7).

interview (entrevista) meeting in which you and the interviewer discuss employment opportunities and strengths you can contribute to the organization (Ch. 48).

interview techniques (técnicas de entrevista) methods of encouraging the best communication between the applicant and the interviewer (Ch. 4).

intraepithelium (intraepitelial) within the epithelium (Ch. 26).

intravenous pyelogram (pielograma intravenoso) radiographic studies of the kidneys, ureters, and bladder using a contrast medium (Ch. 28).

invasive procedure (procedimiento invasivo) surgical technique or a procedure that requires penetration of the skin or a body opening. The potential for pathogenic microorganisms to enter the body exists (Ch. 22, 39).

inversion (inversión) moving a body part inward (Ch. 33).

involuntary dismissal (despido involuntario) termination of employment based on poor job performance or violation of office policies (Ch. 46).

involution (involución) return of the uterus to normal size and shape after childbirth (Ch. 26).

ionizing radiation (radiación ionizante) X-ray beams (Ch. 32).

ischemia (isquemia) local and temporary lack of blood to an organ or part caused by obstruction of circulation (Ch. 37).

isoelectric (isoeléctrico) having equal electrical potentials. It is represented on the ECG as the flat horizontal line, the baseline (Ch. 37).

isolation (aislamiento) separating a patient with certain infections or communicable diseases from other individuals (Ch. 22).

isolation categories (categorías de aislamiento) system of seven categories developed by the Centers for Disease Control (CDC) that isolates patients according to known infections. These categories have been condensed into three Transmission-Based Precautions based on air, contact, and droplet routes of transmission (Ch. 22).

isopropyl alcohol (alcohol isopropílico) commonly called rubbing alcohol; 70% alcohol solution commonly used as a cleaner (Ch. 31).

isotope (isótopo) a chemical element (Ch. 32).

itinerary (itinerario) detailed written plan of a proposed trip (Ch. 45).

J

jargon (jerga) words, phrases, or terminology specific to a profession (Ch. 12).

jaundice (ictericia) yellow discolorization of the skin and sclera caused by excess bilirubin in the blood (Ch. 22, 25).

jet injection (inyección a chorro) an injection given under the skin without a needle, using the force of the liquid under pressure to pierce the skin (Ch. 22).

job description (descripción del trabajo) outline of tasks, duties, and responsibilities for every position in the office (Ch. 46).

Joint Commission (Comisión Conjunta) formerly the Joint Commision on Accreditation of Healthcare Organizations, a commission established to improve the quality of care and services provided in organized health care setting, through a voluntary accreditation process (Ch. 16).

K

keratitis (queratitis) inflammation of the cornea (Ch.22).

ketoacidosis (cetoacidosis) accumulation of ketones in the body, occurring primarily as a complication of diabetes mellitus; if left untreated, it could cause coma (Ch. 42).

ketone (cetona) chemical compound produced during an increased metabolism of fat; also, test on a reagent strip (Ch. 42).

ketonuria (cetonuria) having ketones in urine (Ch. 42).

ketosis (cetosis) a condition of the body burning fatty acids for energy in the absence of appropriate glucose/carbohydrates; may be referred to as lipolysis (Ch. 42).

key (keyed) (mecanografiar) to input data by keystrokes on a computer keyboard (Ch. 15).

key unit (unidad clave) first indexing unit of the filing segment (Ch. 14).

keywords (palabras clave) words that relate to a job-specific position. Keywords may be job-specific skills or profession-specific words (Ch. 48).

kinesics (cinésica) study of body language (Ch. 4).

L

labyrinthitis (laberintitis) inflammation of inner ear or labyrinth (Ch. 25).

lackluster (deslucido) dull, lacking in sheen (Ch. 9).

Lamaze (Lamaze) technique consisting of breathing exercises to facilitate delivery (Ch. 26).

latex beads (perlas de látex) tiny latex beads coated with antibodies or antigens that react with antigens or antibodies in the test sample in an agglutination reaction. The latex beads may be colored to make the reaction easier to visualize (Ch. 44).

lead wire (alambre guía) a conductor attached to an electrocardiograph. Consists of limb leads and chest leads (Ch. 37).

ledger (libro mayor) record of charges, payments, and adjustments for individual patient or family (Ch. 19).

lesion (lesión) injury or wound. A circumscribed area of tissue that has been altered pathologically (Ch. 22, 30).

letter of reference (carta de referencia) letter usually written by an employee's past employer describing the employee's performance, attitude, or qualifications. This letter is presented to a potential employer when applying for a new job (Ch. 46).

letter of resignation (carta de renuncia) letter informing the current employer of the employee's decision to resign from a current position (Ch. 46).

leukocyte (leucocito) white blood cell, one of the formed elements of blood (Ch. 40, 41).

leukocyte esterase (esterasa leucocitaria) test on a reagent strip that indicates the presence of white blood cells in the urinary tract (Ch. 42).

leukorrhea (leucorrea) whitish or yellowish mucus discharged from the cervical canal or vagina. Usually normal unless there is an increase in amount or variation in color (Ch. 22).

liability (pasivo) debts and financial obligations for which one is responsible (Ch. 21); legal responsibility (Ch. 45).

libel (calumnia) false and malicious writing about another constituting a defamation of character (Ch. 7).

libido (libido) sexual drive (Ch. 28).

license (licencia) permission by competent authority (the state) to engage in a profession; permission to act (Ch. 1); permission statement authorizing the use of copyrighted computer software (Ch. 11).

license (matrícula) granting of licenses to practice a profession (Ch. 1).

ligature (ligadura) length of suture thread without a needle, used for tying off vessels during surgery (Ch. 31).

lipemia (lipemia) excessive amount of fat (lipids) in the blood, resulting in a blood sample that has a milky appearance (Ch. 40).

liquid nitrogen (nitrógeno líquido) commonly and incorrectly referred to as dry ice, liquid nitrogen is a volatile freezing agent used to destroy unwanted tissue such as warts (Ch. 31).

lithotripsy (litotricia) procedure using shock waves directed at calculi to crush them (Ch. 30).

litigation (litigio) court action (Ch. 7).

litigious (pleiteador) prone to engage in lawsuits (Ch. 1).

living will (testamento en vida) document allowing a person to make choices related to treatment in a life-threatening illness (Ch. 6).

local area network (LAN) (red de área local [LAN]) network of computers usually in one office or building (Ch. 11).

lochia (loquios) discharge from the uterus of blood, mucus, and tissue during the period after childbirth (Ch. 22, 26).

long-range goals (metas a largo plazo) achievements that may take three to five years to accomplish (Ch. 5).

low-context communication (comunicación de bajo contexto) communication style that uses few environmental or cultural idioms to convey an idea or concept. Ideas are spelled out explicitly (Ch. 4).

low-density lipoprotein (LDL) (lipoproteína de baja densidad [LDL]) lipoprotein in the blood composed primarily of cholesterol. The cholesterol carried by LDL may be deposited in peripheral tissues and is associated with an increased risk for heart disease (Ch. 44).

lumbar puncture (punción lumbar) surgical puncture of the lumbar area of the intervertebral spaces to aspirate cerebrospinal fluid for laboratory analysis (Ch. 22, 43).

lumen (luz) the space within an artery, vein, intestine, needles, and catheter or tube (Ch. 24).

lymphadenopathy (linfadenopatía) a disease of the lymph nodes (Ch. 22).

lymphocyte (linfocito) white blood cell with a dense nonsegmented nucleus and lacking granules in the cytoplasm (Ch. 41).

lyophilized (liofilizado) the process of rapidly freezing a substance at extremely low temperatures and then dehydrating the substance in a high vacuum (freeze drying) (Ch. 27).

M

M codes (morphology codes) (códigos M [códigos morfológicos]) found in the ICD-9-CM and used primarily with cancer registries. M codes further identify behavior and the cell type of a neoplasm (Ch. 18).

macroallocation (macroasignación) of scarce medical resources; decisions are made by Congress, health systems agencies, and insurance companies (Ch. 8).

macrocytic (macrocítico) term that describes a larger than normal cell (Ch. 41).

macular (macular) pertaining to a discoloration of a patch of skin, neither elevated nor depressed, of various colors, sizes, and shapes (Ch. 22).

macular degeneration (degeneración macular) degeneration of the macula area of the retina caused by aging; a leading cause of visual impairment in people older than 50 years, making it difficult to do fine work (Ch. 29).

magnetic drive (disco magnético) memory storage device that uses the magnetic state of a ferrous coating to record data (Ch. 11).

mainframe computer (computadora central) large computer system capable of processing massive volumes of data (Ch. 11).

major mineral (mineral principal) mineral that is required in large amounts by the body (Ch. 34).

malabsorption (malabsorción) inadequate absorption of nutrients from the intestinal tract (Ch. 30).

malaise (malestar) discomfort, uneasiness, or indisposition, often indicative of infection (Ch. 22, 30).

malaria (paludismo) acute infectious disease caused by the presence of protozoan parasites within the red blood cells; usually comes from the bite of a female mosquito (Ch. 3, 22).

malfeasance (fechoría) conduct that is illegal or contrary to an official's obligations (Ch. 7).

malpractice (mala praxis) professional negligence (Ch. 7, 45).

managed care operation (establecimiento de atención administrada) any health care setting or delivery system that is designed to reduce the cost of care while still providing access to care (Ch. 2).

managed care organization (MCO) (organización de atención administrada [MCO]) a health insurance organization that adheres to the principles of strong dependence on selective contracting with providers, the use of primary care physicians, prospective and retrospective utilization management, use of treatment guidelines for high cost chronic disorders, and an emphasis on preventive care, education, and patient compliance with treatment plans (Ch. 17).

management by walking around (MBWA) (gestión itinerante [MBWA]) a technique for keeping managers informed about the health of their organization (Ch. 45).

mandate (mandato) formal order to obey certain rules and regulations (Ch. 38).

manifest (manifestar) to reveal in an obvious way (Ch. 22).

manometer (manómetro) device for measuring a liquid or gaseous pressure. The measurement is expressed in millimeters of mercury or water (Ch. 24).

Mantoux test (prueba de Mantoux) test for tuberculosis involving the intracutaneous injection of purified protein derivative (see PPD) (Ch. 44).

marketing (comercialización) process by which the provider of services makes the consumer aware of the scope and quality of those services. Marketing tools might include public relations, brochures, patient education seminars, and newsletters (Ch. 45).

masking (ocultamiento) attempt to conceal or repress true feelings or the message (Ch. 4).

matrix (matriz) to establish an appointment matrix, a provider's unavailable time slots are marked with an *X*. Patients are not scheduled during those times (Ch. 13).

mature minor (menor maduro) a person, usually younger than 18 years, who is able to understand and appreciate the consequences of treatment despite their young age (Ch. 7).

Mayo stand (mesa de Mayo) portable metal tray table used for setting up small sterile fields for minor surgery and procedures (Ch. 31).

meconium (meconio) first feces of newborn (Ch. 26).

mediation (mediación) dispute resolution that allows a facilitator to help the two parties settle their differences and come to an acceptable solution (Ch. 7).

medical asepsis (asepsia médica) clean and free from infection (Ch. 22, 38).

medically indigent (médicamente indigente) refers to those individuals unable to pay for their own medical coverage (Ch. 7).

Medicare Part A (Medicare Parte A) benefits covering inpatient hospital and skilled nursing facilities, hospice care, and blood transfusion (Ch. 17).

Medicare Part B (Medicare Parte B) benefits covering outpatient hospital and health care provider services (Ch. 17).

Medicare Part C (Medicare Parte C) commonly referred to as Medicare advantage plans. These plans are approved by Medicare and are run by private companies (Ch. 17).

Medicare Part D (Medicare Parte D) prescription drug coverage by Medicare (Ch. 17).

Medigap policy (póliza de Medigap) an individual plan covering the patient's Medicare deductible and co-pay obligations that fulfills the federal government standards for Medicare supplemental insurance (Ch. 17).

memorandum (memorándum) interoffice correspondence, usually referred to as a memo (Ch. 15).

memory (memoria) refers to storage of computer data. Memory can be volatile (lost when computer is turned off) or nonvolatile (permanently written to storage device) (Ch. 11).

meniscus (menisco) curvature appearing in a liquid's upper surface when a liquid is placed in a container (Ch. 24, 36).

menses (menstruación) menstruation (Ch. 22).

mentor (mentor) person assigned or requested to assist in training, guiding, or coaching another (Ch. 45).

metabolism (metabolismo) total of all changes, chemical and physical, that take place in the body (Ch. 34).

metastasis (metástasis) in cancer, malignant cells spread from the primary growth to a new location (Ch. 28).

metered dose inhaler (inhalador de dosis medida) a device used to deliver a prescribed amount of medication to the respiratory tract, especially the lungs (Ch. 30).

metrorrhagia (metrorragia) uterine bleeding at irregular intervals (Ch. 26).

microallocation (microasignación) of scarce medical resources; decisions are made by providers and individual members of the health care team (Ch. 8).

microbiology (microbiología) branch of biology dealing with the study of microscopic forms of life (Ch. 39, 43).

microcomputer (microcomputadora) personal or desktop computer. Also, a handheld or laptop model (Ch. 11).

microcytic (microcítico) term describing a smaller than normal cell (Ch. 41).

microorganism (microorganismo) microscopic living creature capable of transmission and reproduction in specific circumstances (Ch. 22).

microscopic examination (examen microscópico) viewing a specimen with the aid of a microscope (Ch. 16).

microscopy (microscopia) inspection with a microscope (Ch. 38).

midstream collection (recolección de mitad de micción) urine sample collected in the middle of a flow of urine (Ch. 42).

minicomputer (minicomputadora) one of the four categories of computers based on size: larger than a microcomputer and smaller than a mainframe (Ch. 11).

minor (menor) person who has not reached the age of majority, usually 18 years (Ch. 7).

minutes (actas) written record of topics discussed and actions taken during meeting sessions (Ch. 15, 45).

misdemeanor (contravención) a lesser crime; misdemeanors vary from state to state in their definition. Punishment is usually probation or a time of public service and a fine (Ch. 7).

misfeasance (irregularidad) a civil law term referring to a lawful act that is improperly or unlawfully executed (Ch. 7).

modalities (modalidades) physical agents such as heat, cold, light, water, and electricity used to treat muscular or joint malfunction (Ch. 33).

modified block letter, indented (carta estilo bloque modificado, con sangría) modified letter style with indented paragraphs. Paragraphs in this style of letter may be indented five spaces (Ch. 15).

modified block letter, standard (carta estilo bloque modificado, estándar) major letter style where all lines begin at the left margin with the exception of the date line, complimentary closure, and keyed signature. The exceptions usually begin at the center position or a few spaces to the right of center (Ch. 15).

modified wave scheduling (planificación en olas modificada) system where multiple patients are scheduled at the beginning of each hour, followed by single appointments every 10 to 20 minutes the rest of the hour (Ch. 13).

modifier (modificador) an additional code that may be added to a five-digit CPT code to further explain the service provided (Ch. 18).

modulated (modulado) speech that varies in pitch and intensity (Ch. 12).

money market savings accounts (cuentas de ahorro del mercado monetario) bank accounts that pay a higher interest rate (money market rate) than standard savings accounts and permit writing a limited number of checks (Ch. 17).

monocyte (monocito) white blood cell without cytoplasmic granules that has a large convoluted nonsegmented nucleus (Ch. 41).

morbid obesity (obesidad mórbida) obesity so severe that it can result in serious diseases (Ch. 30).

morbidity (morbilidad) number of cases of disease in a specific population (Ch. 22).

mordant (mordiente) substance that causes dye to adhere to an object; iodine is a mordant in Gram stain (Ch. 43).

morphology (morfología) form and structure of an organism (Ch. 22, 43).

mortality (mortalidad) the ratio of the number of deaths to a given population (Ch. 22).

motherboard (placa madre) printed circuit board on which the CPU, ROM, and RAM chips and other electronic circuit elements of a digital computer are frequently located (Ch. 11).

mounting (montaje) process of applying in sequence a portion of each of the 12 leads of the ECG recording onto a commercially prepared mounting form or plain sheet of paper as part of the patient's permanent record (Ch. 37).

moxibustion (moxibustión) ancient Chinese method of treatment that uses a powdered plant substance on the skin to raise a blister (Ch. 3).

multigravida (multigrávida) a woman who has been pregnant more than once (Ch. 26).

mycology (micología) study of fungi (Ch. 39, 43).

myringotomy (miringotomía) incision into the tympanic membrane; part of the treatment for otitis media (Ch. 27).

N

Nägele's rule (regla de Nägele) usual method for calculating expected date of birth (Ch. 26).

National Healthcareer Association (NHA) (Asociación Nacional de Profesiones de Salud [NHA]) an association that offers national certification examinations for health care professionals. NHA works with educational institutions on curriculum development, competency testing, and preparation and administration of their examination for certification (Ch. 47).

negligence (negligencia) failure to exercise a certain standard of care (Ch. 7, 45).

nematode (nematodo) round worm (Ch. 43).

neonatal (neonatal) pertaining to newborn (Ch. 26).

neonate (neonato) newborn.

nephrolithotomy (nefrolitotomía) incision into the kidney to remove stones (Ch. 30).

network interface (interfaz de red) software, servers, and cable connections used to link computers (Ch. 11).

networking (conexión en red) connecting two or more computers together to share files and hardware. The system is called a network (Ch. 11); process in which people of similar interests exchange information in social, business, or professional relationships (Ch. 46).

neutrophil (neutrófilo) the most common type of granulocytic white blood cell (Ch. 41).

nevus (nevo) a mole (Ch. 29).

niacin (niacina) one of the B-complex vitamins (Ch. 34).

nitrogenous (nitrogenoso) pertaining to waste products in the blood indicating kidney disease (Ch. 30).

nocturia (nocturia) excessive urination during the night (Ch. 28, 30).

nomogram (nomograma) graph that shows the relation among numeric values. Body surface area (BSA) of a patient can be estimated by its use (Ch. 36).

noncompliant (inobservancia) failure to follow a required command or instruction (Ch. 7).

nonconsecutive filing (archivado no consecutivo) numeric filing method where numbers are considered in ascending order using subsets of figures within a number; for example, in the number 574 19 2863: 2863 is unit 1, 19 is unit 2, 574 is unit 3 (Ch. 14).

nonfeasance (omisión) a civil law term referring to the failure to perform an act, official duty, or legal requirement (Ch. 7).

noninvasive procedure (procedimiento no invasivo) a procedure that does require penetrating the skin or a body opening (Ch. 37).

normal flora (flora normal) microorganisms that are normally present in a specific site (Ch. 22, 43).

normal saline (solución salina normal) a solution of sodium chloride (salt) and distilled water. It has the same osmotic pressure as blood serum. It is also known as isotonic or physiologic saline (Ch. 9).

normal sinus rhythm (ritmo sinusal normal) term used to describe the heart's rhythm when it is within the normal range (Ch. 37).

normochromic (normocrómico) of normal color, in this case, when referring to red blood cells (Ch. 41).

normocytic (normocítico) term that describes a normal-sized cell (Ch. 41).

nosocomial (intrahospitalaria) infection acquired in a health care setting (hospital, clinic, nursing home) (Ch. 22).

notary (notary public) (escribano público) someone with the legal capacity to witness and certify documents; can take depositions (Ch. 19).

nullipara (nulípara) a woman who has not carried a pregnancy to the stage of viability (Ch. 26).

nutrient (nutriente) ingested substance that helps the body stay in its homeostatic state (Ch. 34).

nutrition (nutrición) study of the bringing of nutrients into the body and how the body uses these nutrients (Ch. 34).

nystagmus (nistagmo) continuous involuntary movement of the eyes (Ch. 30).

O

obfuscation (ofuscación) making things clouded or confused (Ch. 12).

objective (objetivo) a patient sign that is visible, palpable, or measurable by an observer (Ch. 23); also, magnifying lens that is closest to the object being viewed with a microscope (Ch. 39).

obturator (obturador) tool that obstructs or closes a cavity or opening. The internal portion of an examination instrument that facilitates the entry of the instrument into the body; it is then withdrawn, permitting visualization of the internal area (Ch. 30).

occluder (oclusor) instrument used to obstruct or close off vision or light (Ch. 30).

occlusion (oclusión) closure of a passage (Ch. 9).

old reports (informes anteriores) reports such as a discharge summary that should be completed within 71 hours (Ch. 16).

oliguria (oliguria) decrease in urine output (Ch. 30).

open-ended questions (preguntas abiertas) questions that encourage verbalization and response; questions that seek a response beyond a simple yes or no (Ch. 4).

operating system (OS) (sistema operativo [SO]) software used to control the computer and its peripheral equipment. Also referred to as system software (Ch. 11).

operative report (OR) (informe quirúrgico [OR]) medical report that chronicles the details of a surgical procedure (Ch. 16).

opportunistic infection (infección oportunista) an infection that results from a defective immune system that cannot defend itself from pathogens normally found in the environment (Ch. 22).

optical character reader (OCR) (lector óptico de caracteres [OCR]) U.S. Postal Service's computerized scanner that reads addresses printed on letter mail. If the information is properly formatted, then the OCR will find a match in its address files and print a bar code on the lower right edge of the envelope (Ch. 15).

optical disk (disco óptico) portable and transferable read-write or read-only data storage device. Sometimes called a CD-ROM, CD-RW, or compact disk. Capacity is 1 to 8 gigabytes of data. Optical drive unit is required to read-write data from the disk (Ch. 11).

opticokinetic drum test (prueba del tambor optocinético) test used to help diagnose nystagmus (Ch. 30).

orchidectomy (orquidectomía) surgical excision of a testicle (Ch. 28).

organomercurial (compuestos organomercuriales) any mercury-containing organic compound (Ch. 27).

orthopnea (ortopnea) difficulty breathing in any position other than an upright position (Ch. 24).

oscilloscope (osciloscopio) an electronic device used for recording electrical activity of the heart, brain, and muscular tissues (Ch. 32, 37).

otoscope (otoscopio) instrument used to examine the external ear canal and tympanic membrane (Ch. 30).

out guide or sheet (señalador o marcador) card, folder, or slip of paper inserted temporarily in the files to replace a record that has been retrieved from the files (Ch. 14).

outer-directed people (personas influenciables) people who let events, other people, or environmental factors dictate their behavior (Ch. 5).

output device (dispositivo de salida) a device used to output data from a computer. Includes printers, faxes, data storage drivers, screens, and plotters (Ch. 11).

ova (óvulos) eggs, in this case, eggs of a parasite (Ch. 43).

overtime (horas extra) money paid at a rate of not less than one and one-half times the regular rate of pay after a 40-hour work week is completed (Ch. 46).

owner's equity (patrimonio neto) amount by which business assets exceed business liabilities. Also called net worth, proprietorship, and capital (Ch. 21).

oxidation (oxidación) process of a substance combining with oxygen (Ch. 34).

oxygenated (oxigenado) containing high levels of oxygen (Ch. 40).

oxytocin (oxitocina) a pituitary hormone that stimulates the muscles of the uterus to contract, thus inducing labor (Ch. 26).

P

pagers (localizadores) also known as beepers. One-way paging systems often used inside hospitals and by providers on call. Pagers only receive signals (Ch. 12).

palliative (paliativa) measures taken to relieve symptoms of disease (Ch. 22, 32).

pallor (palidez) lack of color, paleness (Ch. 25).

palpate (palpar) to feel with fingertips, to search for a vein with a pressure and release touch (Ch. 40).

pandemic (pandemia) a disease affecting the majority of the population of a large region; is epidemic at same time in many parts of the world (Ch. 22).

panel (panel) a series of tests related to a particular organ or organ system of body function. For example, a liver panel would check many different functions of the liver. Previously called a "profile" (Ch. 39).

papular (papular) pertaining to a small, red, elevated area of the skin, solid and circumscribed (Ch. 22).

paracentesis (paracentesis) puncture of a cavity for removal of fluid (Ch. 22).

parasitology (parasitología) study of organisms (parasites and their eggs) that live within or on another organism and at the expense of that organism (Ch. 39, 43).

parasympathetic nervous system (sistema nervioso parasimpático) part of the autonomic nervous system that returns the body to its normal state after stress has subsided (Ch. 5).

parenteral (parenteral) injection of a liquid substance into the body via a route other than the alimentary canal (Ch. 22, 36).

paresthesia (parestesia) a sensation of numbness, prickling, or heightened sensitivity (Ch. 30).

parity (paridad) carrying a pregnancy to the point of viability regardless of the outcome (Ch. 26).

participatory manager (gerente participativo) operates on the premise that the worker is capable and wants to do a good job (Ch. 45).

parturition (parir) the process of giving birth (Ch. 26).

patch (parche) modification to software to fix deficiencies in the software. Frequently downloaded from the software supplier's Web site or from floppy disks provided by the supplier (Ch. 11).

patent (permeable) open, not blocked (Ch. 26).

pathogen (patógeno) disease-producing microorganism (Ch. 22, 43).

pathology report (informe de patología) medical reports generated to describe the gross and microscopic examinations performed during a surgical procedure (Ch. 16, 31).

Patient Self-Determination Act (PSDA) (Ley de Autodeterminación del Paciente [PSDA]) the Act that includes the Advance Directive giving patients the right to be involved in their health care decisions (Ch. 7).

patient service centers (centros de servicio al paciente) satellite laboratory facilities located in convenient areas for patients where specimens can be collected or dropped off (Ch. 39).

payee (beneficiario) person named on check who is to receive the amount indicated (Ch. 19).

peak (pico) the opposite of "trough," this is the point at which a drug is at its highest level in the body, usually about 30 minutes after administration. In lab tests, the peak would tell the provider the strongest influence the drug would have on the body at that particular dose (Ch. 39).

pegboard system (sistema de tablero de clavijas) most commonly used manual medical accounts receivable system (Ch. 19).

pellagra (pelagra) disease caused by a deficiency in vitamin B_3 (nicotinic acid) characterized by sores on the skin, diarrhea, anxiety, confusion, and death if not treated (Ch. 34).

pelvic inflammatory disease (enfermedad inflamatoria pélvica) infection of uterus, fallopian tubes, and adjacent pelvic structures; most common causes are gonorrhea and chlamydia, spread as sexually transmitted diseases (Ch. 26).

perception (percepción) conscious awareness of one's own feelings and the feelings of others (Ch. 4).

peripheral (periférico) away from the center of the body (Ch. 24).

pernicious anemia (anemia perniciosa) chronic anemia caused by lack of hydrochloric acid in the stomach; weakness, fatigue, tingling of extremities, and even heart failure can result; vitamin B_{12} injections are the treatment for this condition (Ch. 29).

personal computer (PC) (computadora personal [PC]) any computer whose price, size, and capabilities make it useful for individuals to use with no intervening computer operator. Also known as a microcomputer (Ch. 11).

personal digital assistant (PDA) (asistente personal digital [PDA]) an electronic tool for organizing data, a handheld computerized personal organizer device (Ch. 11).

petri dish (placa de Petri) plastic dish into which agar is placed for the purpose of growing bacteria (Ch. 43).

petrissage (petrissage) a kneading movement in massage (Ch. 33).

petty cash (caja chica) small sum kept on hand for minor or unexpected expenses (Ch. 19).

pH (pH) scale that indicates the relative alkalinity or acidity of a solution; measurement of hydrogen ion concentration (Ch. 42).

phacoemulsification (facoemulsificación) treatment for cataracts. An ultrasonic device is used to disintegrate the cataract of the lens of the eye, which is then aspirated and removed (Ch. 30).

pharmacology (farmacología) study of drugs; the science concerned with the history, origin, sources, physical and chemical properties, and uses of drugs and their effects on living organisms (Ch. 35).

pharmacopoeia (farmacopea) book describing drugs and their preparation or a collection or stock of drugs (Ch. 3).

phenylketonuria (PKU) (fenilcetonuria [FCU]) a hereditary disease caused by the body's inability to oxidize the amino acid phenylalanine. If not discovered and treated early, brain damage can occur, causing severe mental retardation (Ch. 27, 44).

phlebotomy (flebotomía) process of collecting blood (Ch. 22, 40).

physician's directive (directiva a los médicos) another name for a living will (Ch. 6).

physicians' office laboratories (POL) (laboratorios del consultorio de los médicos [POL]) laboratories within physicians' offices where common office laboratory tests are performed (Ch. 39).

phytomedicines (fitomedicinas) herbs used as medicinal plants. They contain plant material as their active ingredient (Ch. 36).

placenta abruptio (desprendimiento de la placenta) sudden and abrupt separation of the placenta from uterine wall (Ch. 26).

placenta previa (placenta previa) placenta lies low in uterus and can partially or completely cover the cervical os (Ch. 26).

plaintiff (demandante) person bringing charges in litigation (Ch. 7).

plantar flexion (flexión plantar) moving the foot downward at the ankle (Ch. 33).

plasma (plasma) fluid portion of blood from a tube containing anticoagulant. This fluid contains fibrinogen (Ch. 40).

pluralistic (pluralism) (pluralista [pluralismo]) society where there are several distinct ethnic, religious, or cultural groups that coexist with one another (Ch. 3).

point-of-service (POS) device (dispositivo de punto de servicio [POS]) device allowing direct communication between a medical office and the health care plan's computer (Ch. 18).

point-of-service (POS) plan (plan de punto de servicio [POS]) a plan that allows direct communication between a medical office and the health insurance company (Ch. 17).

polyp (pólipo) tumor with a stem found in nose, uterus, bladder, colon, or rectum (Ch. 30).

port (puerto) shortened term for portal—an entry way. When related to intravenous therapy, it is a type of adapter that can serve as additional means for infusing fluids or medications. The port can be attached to the primary tubing. The port has a needleless entry site (Ch. 36).

portfolio (cartera) notebook or file containing examples of materials commonly used (Ch. 15).

postcoital (poscoital) period of time following (after) intercourse (Ch. 26).

posting (asiento) recording financial transactions into a bookkeeping or accounting system (Ch. 19).

potassium hydroxide (KOH) (hidróxido de potasio [KOH]) 10% solution placed on vaginal smears, as well as skin scrapings, hair, and other dry substances, to dissolve excess debris. This clears the vision field for better viewing of fungi and spores (Ch. 26, 43).

power verbs (verbos de acción) action words used to describe your attributes and strengths (Ch. 48).

practicum (práctica) transitional stage providing opportunity to apply theory learned in the classroom to a health care setting through practical, hands-on experience (Ch. 1, 45).

preauthorization (autorización previa) obtaining an insurance carrier's consent to proceed with patient care and treatment. Unless authorization is obtained, insurance carriers may not pay benefits for specific problems (Ch. 17).

precedents (precedentes) refers to rulings made at an earlier time and include decisions made in a court, interpretations of a constitution, and statutory law decisions (Ch. 7).

precipitate (precipitado) substance in the form of fine particles that separates from a solution if allowed to stand for a time (Ch. 36).

precordial (precordial) pertaining to the area on the anterior surface of the body overlying the heart (Ch. 37).

preeclampsia (preeclampsia) a complication of pregnancy characterized by generalized edema, hypertension, and proteinuria (Ch. 26).

preexisting (preexistente) injury or disease that occurs before a certain date (Ch. 22).

preferred provider organization (PPO) (organización de proveedor preferido [PPO]) organization of providers who network together to offer discounts to purchasers of heath care insurance (Ch. 2, 17).

prejudice (prejuicio) opinion or judgment that is formed before all the facts are known (Ch. 4).

prenatal (prenatal) time period between fertilization and birth (Ch. 26).

presbycusis (presbiacusia) progressive loss of hearing caused by the normal aging process (Ch. 29).

present problem (PP) (problema presente [PP]) see **chief complaint (CC)** (Ch. 16).

prescribe (recetar) to order or recommend the use of a drug, diet, or other form of therapy (Ch. 7, 35).

preservative (conservante) chemical added to food to keep it fresh longer or added to urine to preserve it for testing (Ch. 34, 42).

primary care physician (PCP) (médico de atención primaria [PCP]) primary care physician for a patient; all care is coordinated through the PCP (Ch. 17).

primary container (recipiente principal) container that directly contains the specimen (Ch. 40).

primigravida (primigrávida) a woman pregnant for the first time (Ch. 26).

privileged (privilegiada) confidential information that may only be communicated with the patient's permission or by court order (Ch. 16).

probate court (tribunal sucesorio) court that administers estates and validates wills (Ch. 20).

probation (período de prueba) period during which the employee and supervisory personnel may determine if both the environment and the position are satisfactory for the employee (Ch. 46).

problem-oriented medical record (POMR) (historia clínica orientada al problema [POMR]) a type of patient chart recordkeeping that uses a sheet at a prominent location in the chart to list vital identification data. Patient medical problems are identified by a number that corresponds to the charting; for example, bronchitis is #1, a broken wrist is #2, and so forth (Ch. 14, 23).

procedure manual (manual de procedimientos) manual providing detailed information relative to the performance of tasks within the job description (Ch. 45).

processed food (alimentos procesados) food that is no longer in a whole, natural state; cooked or packaged with parts removed or ingredients added (Ch. 34).

professional liability insurance (seguro de responsabilidad profesional) insurance policy designed to protect assets in the event a claim for damages resulting from negligence is filed and awarded (Ch. 45).

professionalism (profesionalismo) the qualities that characterize or distinguish a professional person who conforms to the technical and ethical standards of the profession (Ch. 1).

proficiency testing (prueba de aptitud) sample tests performed in a clinical laboratory to determine with what degree of accuracy tests are being performed. Testing samples are checked in the same manner as patient specimens (Ch. 38).

profit sharing (participación en las ganancias) sharing in the financial profits, gains, and benefits of an organization (Ch. 45).

progress notes (notas de evolución) also called chart notes. Provider's formal or informal notes about presenting problem, physical findings, and plan for treatment for a patient examined in the office, clinic, acute care center, or emergency department (Ch. 16).

projection (proyección) act of placing one's own feelings on another (Ch. 4).

pronation (pronación) moving the arm so the palm is down (Ch. 33).

pronunciation (pronunciación) saying words correctly (Ch. 12).

proofread (revisar) to read a document to verify the accuracy of content and that correct grammar, spelling, punctuation, and capitalization were used (Ch. 15, 16).

proprietary (empresa de propiedad privada) privately owned and managed facility, a profit-making organization (Ch. 1).

prostaglandin (prostaglandina) modulator of biochemical activity in tissues (Ch. 26).

proteinuria (proteinuria) protein in the urine (Ch. 30).

protozoa (protozoos) one-celled animals divided into four groups: amoebae, flagellates, ciliates, and coccidia (Ch. 43).

provider performed microscopy procedure (PPMP) (procedimiento de microscopia realizada por el proveedor [PPM]) a CLIA term for those microscopic examinations that require the expertise of a physician or mid-level provider qualified in microscopic examinations. The PPMP is part of the CLIA's moderately complex category of tests (Ch. 38).

pruritus (prurito) itchiness (Ch. 22, 35).

psychomotor retardation (retraso psicomotor) slowing of physical and mental responses; may be seen in depression (Ch. 6).

puerperium (puerperio) the period from the end of the third stage of labor until involution of uterus is complete, usually three to six weeks (Ch. 26).

pulmonary edema (edema pulmonar) accumulation of serous fluid in the air vesicles and interstitial tissues of the lungs (Ch. 38).

pulse oximeter (oxímetro de pulso) a device (similar to a clip) that can be attached to a finger or bridge of the nose. It measures oxygen concentration in the blood (Ch. 24).

purging (purga) method of maintaining order in the files by separating active from inactive and closed files (Ch. 14).

purified protein derivative (PPD) (derivado proteico purificado [DPP]) filtrate obtained from *Mycobacterium* cultures used for intradermal testing for tuberculosis (Ch. 44).

purulent (purulento) forming or containing pus (Ch. 22).

pyorrhea (piorrea) discharge of pus from the gums, around the teeth (Ch. 25).

pyrexia (pirexia) fever (Ch. 24).

pyridoxine (piridoxina) vitamin B_6 (Ch. 34).

pyuria (piuria) pus in the urine (Ch. 30).

Q

qualitative test (prueba cualitativa) analysis to identify quality or characteristics of components, such as size, shape, and maturity of cells (Ch. 39).

quality assurance (QA) (aseguramiento de calidad [QA]) process to provide accurate, complete, consistent health care documentation in a timely manner while making every reasonable effort to resolve inconsistencies, inaccuracies, risk management issues, and other problems (Ch. 16, 38).

quality control (control de calidad) measures used to monitor the processing of laboratory specimens. Includes proper use, storage, handling, stability, expiration dates, and indications for measuring precision and accuracy of analytic processes (Ch. 38, 42, 43).

quantitative test (prueba cuantitativa) analysis that can identify quantity or actual number counts such as counting the number of blood cells (Ch. 39).

R

radioactive (radioactivo) emits rays or particles from nucleus (Ch. 32).

radiograph (radiografía) the film on which an image is produced through exposure to X-rays (Ch. 32).

radiology and imaging reports (informes de radiología y de diagnóstico por imágenes) medical reports that describe the findings and interpretations of the radiologist (Ch. 16).

radiolucent (radiolúcido) allowing X-rays to pass through. A dark area appears on the radiograph (Ch. 32).

radionuclides (radionúclidos) atoms that disintegrate by emitting electromagnetic radiation (Ch. 32).

radiopaque (radiopaco) impenetrable to X-rays. A light area appears on the radiograph (Ch. 32).

radiopharmaceuticals (sustancias radiofarmacéuticas) radioactive chemicals used in testing the location, size, outline, or function of tissue, organs, vessels, or body fluids (Ch. 32).

rales (estertores) abnormal bubbling or crackling sound heard by auscultation during the inspiratory phase of respiration (Ch. 24).

random access memory (RAM) (memoria de acceso aleatorio [RAM]) a type of computer memory that can be written to and read from. The word *random* means that any one location can be read at any time. RAM commonly refers to the internal memory of a computer. RAM is usually a fast, temporary memory area where data and programs reside until saved or until the power is turned off (Ch. 11).

range of motion (ROM) (amplitud de movimiento [ROM]) amount of movement that is present in a joint (Ch. 33).

ratchets (trinquetes) locking mechanisms on the handles of many surgical instruments (Ch. 31).

rationalization (racionalización) act of justification, usually illogically, that one uses to keep from facing the truth of the situation (Ch. 4).

read-only memory (ROM) (memoria de sólo lectura [ROM]) permanently stored computer data that cannot be overwritten without special devices. Stores instructions required to start up the computer. Located on the motherboard (Ch. 11).

reagent (reactivo) chemical substance that detects or synthesizes other substances in a chemical reaction; used in laboratory analyses because it is known to react in a specific way (Ch. 39, 42, 43).

reagent test strip (tira de prueba reactiva) narrow strip of plastic on which pads containing reagents are attached; used in the urinalysis chemical examination to detect glucose, bilirubin, ketones, specific gravity, blood, pH, urobilinogen, nitrites, and leukocyte esterase (Ch. 42).

recertification (nueva certificación) documentation admitted to support continued education for maintaining a professional credential (Ch. 47).

redundant array of independent disk (RAID) (matriz redundante de discos independientes [RAID]) a data storage scheme that uses multiple hard drives to share or replicate data among the drives (Ch. 11).

reference laboratories (laboratorios de referencia) independent, regionally located laboratories used by hospitals for complex, expensive, or specialized tests (Ch. 39).

reference values (valores de referencia) also referred to as normal value, normal range, or reference range; range of values that includes 95% of test results for a normal healthy population (Ch. 39).

references (referencias) individuals who have known or worked with a person long enough to make an honest assessment and recommendation regarding the person's background history (Ch. 48).

referral (remisión) term used by managed care facilities for authorization for someone other than the patient's primary care provider to treat the patient (Ch. 17).

refractometer (refractómetro) instrument that measures the refractive index of a substance or solution; used in the urinalysis physical examination to measure the urine specimen's specific gravity (Ch. 42).

Registered Medical Assistant (RMA) (Asistente Médico Matriculado [RMA]) credential awarded for successfully passing the AMT examination (Ch. 1, 47).

regression (regresión) moving back to a former stage to escape conflict or fear (Ch. 4).

regulated waste (residuos regulados) any waste that contains infectious material that would pose a threat due to possible transmission of pathogenic microorganisms (Ch. 22).

rehabilitation medicine (medicina de rehabilitación) field of medical disciplines that seeks to restore an individual or body part to normal or near-normal function after an illness or injury using physical and mechanical agents (Ch. 33).

reimbursement (reembolso) payment (Ch. 38).

repolarization (repolarización) reestablishment of a polarized state in a muscle after contraction (Ch. 37).

repression (represión) coping with an overwhelming situation by temporarily forgetting it; temporary amnesia (Ch. 4).

requisition (solicitud) request form sent with a specimen specifying tests to be performed on the specimen; most common tests are separated into logical categories with additional space for writing special requests (Ch. 38, 39).

rescue breathing (respiración de rescate) performed on individuals in respiratory arrest, rescue breathing is a mouth-to-mouth (using appropriate protective equipment) or mouth-to-nose procedure that provides oxygen to the patient until emergency personnel arrive (Ch. 9).

residual urine (orina residual) amount of urine remaining in bladder immediately after voiding; seen with hyperplasia of prostate (Ch. 28, 29).

resistance (resistencia) ability of the immune system to resist or withstand an infectious disease (Ch. 22).

resource-based relative value scale (RBRVS) (escala de valores relativos basada en recursos [RBRVS]) basis for the Medicare fee schedule (Ch. 17).

résumé (curriculum vitae) written summary data sheet or brief account of qualifications and progress in your chosen career (Ch. 48).

retention (retención) urine held in the bladder; inability to empty the bladder (Ch. 28).

retrolental fibroplasia (fibroplasia retrolenticular) disease of blood vessels of retina in newborns (Ch. 36).

review of systems (ROS) (revisión de sistemas [ROS]) inquires about the system directly related to the problems identified in the history of the present illness (Ch. 16).

Rh factor (factor Rh) blood factor indicating the presence or absence of the Rh antigen on the surface of human erythrocytes (Ch. 44).

rhythm strip (tira de ritmo) ECG recording of a single lead, usually lead II, that is used to determine the rhythm of the heart beat. An arrhythmia can more easily be seen in a rhythm strip because it is run longer per provider's request (Ch. 37).

riboflavin (riboflavina) vitamin B_2 (Ch. 34).

risk management (gestión de riesgos) techniques adhered to in the ambulatory care setting that keep the practice, its environment, and its procedures as safe for the patient as possible. Proper risk management also reduces the possibility of negligence that leads to torts and malpractice suits (Ch. 7, 9, 16, 45).

roadblocks (obstáculos) verbal or nonverbal messages that block communication (Ch. 4).

rosacea (rosácea) a chronic skin condition characterized by pustules, papules, erythema, and hyperplasia. Its cause is unknown (Ch. 30).

rotation (rotación) turning a body part around its axis (Ch. 33); also, opportunity to spend 2 or 3 weeks in a variety of health care settings (Ch. 40).

S

salary review (revisión de salario) informing the employee of his or her revised base pay rate (Ch. 45).

salicylates (salicilatos) aspirin-type drugs that can cause ulcers because of their irritation to the gastrointestinal tract (Ch. 30).

sanitization (higienización) cleaning or scrubbing contaminated instruments or fomites to remove tissue, debris, or other contaminants (Ch. 22).

saturated fat (grasa saturada) fats that are typically solid at room temperature, most commonly found in animal products, such as butter, milk, cream, and eggs as well as coconut and palm oils (Ch. 34).

scabies (sarna) infectious skin disease caused by the itch mite *(Sarcoptes scabiei)*, which is transmitted by direct contact with infected persons (Ch. 22).

scleroderma (esclerodermia) slowly progressing disease characterized by deposition of fibrous connective tissue in the skin and in internal organs (Ch. 25).

scoop technique (técnica de una sola mano) a one-handed technique used to "scoop" up and cover a used needle only if a sharp's container is not immediately available, the covering (cap) over the needle is not manipulated in any way; it is then disposed of in the nearest sharps container (Ch. 22).

scope of practice (ámbito de práctica) the range of clinical procedures and activities that are allowed by law for a profession (Ch. 1).

screening (prueba de detección) evaluating patient symptoms to determine emergent needs. Sometimes used to determine the next best course of action when assisting a provider in giving appropriate patient care (Ch. 42).

scurvy (escorbuto) a deficiency in vitamin C characterized by the abnormal formation of bones and teeth. Signs of hemorrhage can appear, such as bruising (Ch. 34).

secretion (secreción) substance produced by the cells of glandular organs from materials in the blood (Ch. 22, 38).

sediment (sedimento) insoluble material that settles to the bottom of a liquid; material examined in the urinalysis microscopic examination (Ch. 42).

self-actualization (autorealización) being all that you can be; developing your full potential and experiencing fulfillment (Ch. 5, 45).

self-insurance (autoseguro) insurance carried by large companies, nonprofit organizations, and government to reduce costs and gain more control of their finances. Each plan differs in coverage and claim filing requirements (Ch. 17).

semen (semen) thick, viscid secretion discharged from the urethra of males at orgasm. It is a mixed product containing various fluids and spermatozoa. In postvasectomy males, spermatozoa is absent in semen (Ch. 44).

senile (senil) mental and physical weakness sometimes associated with aging (Ch. 29).

sensitivity (sensibilidad) test in which an organism is placed with antibiotics to determine which antibiotic will effectively kill the organism with the smallest dose (see also culture and sensitivity) (Ch. 43).

sensor (sensor) term used to describe a metallic-coated paper tab that is applied to the patient's body in preparation for an ECG (also known as electrode). Sensors are placed on specific locations on the skin, then attached to the ECG with wires. The sensors conduct electricity from the patient to the ECG machine (Ch. 37).

sensorineural (neurosensorial) permanent hearing loss that results from damage or malformation of the middle ear and auditory nerve (Ch. 27).

septicemia (septicemia) invasion of pathogenic bacteria into the bloodstream (Ch. 3).

serum (suero) liquid portion of blood obtained after blood has been allowed to clot (Ch. 39, 40).

server (servidor) computer with massive hard drive capacity that is used to link other computers together so that data can be shared by multiple users. A computer system in an ambulatory care facility is likely to be linked or networked with a central server (Ch. 11).

severe acute respiratory syndrome (SARS) (síndrome respiratorio agudo y grave [SARS]) a viral outbreak of a respiratory illness first reported in Asia in 2003; spread by close person-to-person contact and characterized by fever and respiratory symptoms (Ch. 22).

shadow (aprendizaje por observación) follow a supervisor or delegated subordinate to learn facility protocol (Ch. 45).

sharps (objetos filosos) needles or scalpels or other sharp instruments that are capable of causing a penetrating or puncture wound of the skin (Ch. 22).

shock (shock) potentially serious condition in which the circulatory system is not providing enough blood to all parts of the body, causing the body's organs to fail to function properly (Ch. 9).

short-range goals (metas a corto plazo) long-range goals are dissected and reassembled into smaller, more manageable time segments (Ch. 5).

sickle cell anemia (anemia drepanocítica) an inherited blood disorder that may shorten life span (Ch. 26).

silver nitrate (nitrato de plata) caustic astringent antiseptic. As a weak liquid, it is applied to the eyes of newborns to prevent infections at birth. In the medical office, it is most often seen as a solid substance impregnated onto the end of a wooden applicator. Silver nitrate applicator sticks contain hydrochloric acid and other chemicals and are commonly used to cauterize small blood vessels in the nose or other mucous membranes (Ch. 31).

simplified letter (carta simplificada) major letter style recommended by the Administrative Management Society that omits the salutation and complimentary closure. All lines are keyed flush with the left margin. In medical offices, this style is most often used when sending a form letter (Ch. 15).

sitz bath (baño de asiento) a warm water bath, in which only the hips and buttocks are immersed (Ch. 31).

slander (calumnia) false and malicious words about another constituting a defamation of character (Ch. 7).

SOAP (SOAP) acronym for patient progress notes based on subjective impressions (S), objective clinical evidence (O), assessment or diagnosis (A), and plans for further studies (P) (Ch. 14, 23).

sodium hydroxide (hidróxido de sodio) chemical used to chemically burn and destroy tissue; usually in a liquid state when used in minor surgery (Ch. 31).

sodium hypochlorite (hipoclorito de sodio) household bleach (Ch. 22).

software (software) equivalent of a computer program or programs (Ch. 11).

solvent (solvente) producing a solution, dissolving (Ch. 22).

sonographer (ecografista) professionally trained individual capable of performing the ultrasound examination (Ch. 37).

source-oriented medical record (SOMR) (historia clínica orientada a la fuente [SOMR]) a type of patient chart record keeping that includes separate sections for different sources of patient information, such as laboratory reports, pathology reports, and progress notes (Ch. 14, 23).

species (especie) second Greek or Latin name given to microorganisms; the species name is not capitalized (Ch. 43).

specific gravity (densidad específica) ratio of weight of a given volume of a substance to the weight of the same volume of distilled water at the same temperature; test often performed during the urinalysis physical examination (can also appear on the reagent strip) (Ch. 42).

spermatogenesis (espermatogénesis) the formation of mature sperm (Ch. 28).

spill kit (kit para derrames) commercially packaged materials containing supplies and equipment needed to clean up a spill of a biohazardous substance (Ch. 22).

spirometry (espirometría) test to measure the air capacity of the lungs (Ch. 30).

splint (férula) any device used to immobilize a body part. Often used by EMS personnel (Ch. 9).

spores (esporas) an inactive state of some bacteria in which they are capsulated in protein. The encapsulation protects them from heat, chemicals, freezing, desiccation, and radiation. Spores can live for tens of thousands of years with no nutrient. When they are placed onto fertile soil (such as human tissue), they can become activated and grow. Tetanus is one type of bacteria that creates spores (Ch. 43).

sprain (esguince) injury to a joint, often an ankle, knee, or wrist, that involves a tearing of the ligaments. Most sprains are minor and heal quickly; others are more severe, include swelling, and may not heal properly if the patient continues to put stress on the sprained joint (Ch. 9).

sputum (esputo) substance from the respiratory tract expelled by coughing (Ch. 22).

stab culture (cultivo por punción) culture where the microorganism is stabbed for deep penetration into tubed solid media (Ch. 43).

standard (patrón) rules established to measure quality, weight, extent, or value (Ch. 22, 38).

Standard Precautions (Precauciones Estándar) precautions developed in 1996 by the Centers for Disease Control and Prevention (CDC) that augment universal precautions and body substance isolation practices. They provide a wider range of protection and are used any time there is contact with blood, moist body fluid (except perspiration), mucous membranes, or nonintact skin. They are designed to protect all health care providers, patients, and visitors (Ch. 9, 22).

status asthmaticus (estado asmático) severe episode of asthma that does not respond to ordinary treatment (Ch. 36).

statute of limitations (ley de prescripción) statute that defines the period in which legal action can take place (Ch. 20).

statutory law (derecho estatutario) refers to the body of laws established by states (Ch. 7).

sterile field (campo estéril) an area that is considered sterile, usually designated by a sterile drape. The area contains sterile supplies and instruments needed for a particular sterile procedure or surgery (Ch. 31).

stertorous (estertoroso) snoring sound heard with labored breathing (Ch. 24).

stigma (estigma) a social condition marked by attitudinal devaluing or demeaning of persons who, because of disfigurement or disability, are not viewed as being capable of fulfilling valued social roles (Ch. 26).

stomatitis (estomatitis) inflammation of the mouth associated with chemotherapy. Can include swelling, redness, halitosis, ulcerations (Ch. 32).

strabismus (estrabismo) disorder of the eye in which optic axes cannot be directed to the same object (cross-eye) (Ch. 30).

strain (distensión) injury to the soft tissue between joints that involves the tearing of muscles or tendons. Strains often occur in the neck, back, or thigh muscles (Ch. 9).

stream scheduling (programación ininterrumpida) system where patients are seen on a continuous basis throughout the day; for example, at 15-, 30-, or 60-minute intervals, each patient having a distinct appointment time (Ch. 13).

stress (estrés) body's response to change; can be manifested in a variety of ways, including changes in blood pressure, heart rate, and onset of headache (Ch. 5).

stressors (factores estresantes) demands to change that cause stress (Ch. 5).

strictures (estenosis) narrowing of a tubelike structure such as the esophagus or urethra (Ch. 31).

stridor (estridor) crowing sound heard on inspiration, the result of an upper airway obstruction (Ch. 24).

stylus (estilete) heated slender wire of the electrocardiograph that melts the wax off of the ECG paper during the recording (Ch. 37).

subjective (subjetivo) symptom that is felt by the patient but not observable by others (Ch. 23).

sublimation (sublimación) redirecting a socially unacceptable impulse into one that is socially acceptable (Ch. 4).

subordinate (subordinado) in an organization, a person under the direction of (reporting to) a person of greater authority (Ch. 45).

subpoena (citación) written command designating a person to appear in court under penalty for failure to appear (Ch. 7).

supercomputer (supercomputadora) fastest, largest, and most expensive of the four classes of computers currently being manufactured (Ch. 11).

supernatant (sobrenadante) urine that appears above the sediment when centrifuged; poured off before sediment is examined in the urinalysis microscopic examination (Ch. 42).

supination (supinación) moving the arm so the palm is up (Ch. 33).

suppressed immune system (sistema inmunitario con inmunosupresión) term used to describe an immune system unable to function normally due to the presence of a disease such as AIDS (Ch. 38).

suppurant (supurante) an agent causing pus formation (Ch. 31).

suppurative (supurativo) producing or associated with the generation of pus (Ch. 27).

surge protection (protección contra sobretensiones) protection of the fragile electronics from spikes in electrical voltage that occur on electric distribution lines (Ch. 11).

surgery cards (tarjetas de cirugía) written reference for surgeries and procedures (Ch. 31).

surgical asepsis (asepsia quirúrgica) procedures that render objects sterile; techniques to maintain sterile conditions during invasive procedures (Ch. 22, 31).

surrogate (sustituto) substitute; someone who substitutes for another (Ch. 8).

suture (sutura) surgical material or thread; may describe the act of sewing with the surgical thread and needle (Ch. 31).

swaged (estampada) a surgical needle attached, during manufacturing, to a length of suture material (Ch. 31).

symmetry (simetría) correspondence in shape, size, and position of body parts on opposite sides of the body (Ch. 25).

sympathetic nervous system (sistema nervioso simpático) large part of the autonomic nervous system that prepares the body for fight-or-flight (Ch. 5).

syncope (síncope) fainting (Ch. 9, 37).

system software (software de sistema) see **operating system** (Ch. 11).

systemic (sistémico) pertaining to the whole body (Ch. 9).

systole (sístole) one component of blood pressure measurement representing the highest amount of pressure exerted during the cardiac cycle; the force exerted on the arterial walls during cardiac contraction (Ch. 24, 37).

T

tachycardia, sinus (taquicardia sinusal) abnormally rapid heartbeat greater than 100 beats/minute. A type of cardiac arrhythmia (Ch. 24, 37).

tachypnea (taquipnea) abnormal increased rate of breathing (Ch. 24).

tape drive (unidad de cinta) data storage device that uses magnetic tape as the storage media (Ch. 11).

targeted résumé (curriculum vitae dirigido al objetivo) résumé format utilized when focusing on a clear, specific job target (Ch. 48).

Task Force for Test Construction (TFTC) (Fuerza de Tareas para la Elaboración de Exámenes [TFTC]) committee of professionals whose responsibility is to update the CMA examination annually to reflect changes in medical assistants' responsibilities and to include new developments in medical knowledge and technology (Ch. 47).

taut (tirante) to pull or draw tight a surface, such as skin (Ch. 36).

taxonomy (taxonomía) classification of organisms into appropriate categories (Ch. 43).

Tay–Sachs (Tay–Sachs) an inherited disease that is usually fatal (Ch. 26).

teamwork (trabajo en equipo) persons synergistically working together (Ch. 45).

test cable (cable de prueba) accessory device that attaches between the Holter monitor and the electrocardiograph to check for correct waveform and lack of artifact (Ch. 37).

thalassemia (talasemia) a hereditary anemia that may be fatal (Ch. 26).

thallium scan (gammagrafía con talio) chemical element given intravenously and used in cardiac stress tests. The radioisotope localizes in the myocardium, and a scanning device picks up the distribution of the thallium and can identify blockages in the coronary arteries. An accurate test for coronary artery disease (Ch. 37).

therapeutic communication (comunicación terapéutica) use of specific and well-defined professional communication skills to create a feeling of comfort for patients even when difficult or unpleasant information must be exchanged (Ch. 4).

therapeutic drug monitoring (TDM) (monitoreo de fármacos terapéuticos [TDM]) periodic blood tests to determine the effectiveness of a particular drug. Drugs will have a therapeutic level that must be attained in order for the drug to be therapeutic or effective. If the blood level of the drug is below the range of therapeutic effectiveness, the provider will probably increase the dosage. Likewise, if the drug is above the therapeutic range, the provider will probably lower it (Ch. 39).

thermolabile (termolábil) easily affected by heat (Ch. 22).

thermophile (termófilo) resistant to destruction by heat. Characteristic of some bacteria (Ch. 31).

thermotherapy (termoterapia) use of heat to treat a physical condition (Ch. 33).

thiamin (tiamina) vitamin B_1 (Ch. 34).

thixotropic separator gel (gel separador tixotrópico) gel material capable of forming an interface between the cells and fluid portion of the blood as a result of centrifugation (Ch. 40).

thoracentesis (toracentesis) surgical puncture of the thoracic cavity to aspirate fluid (Ch. 22).

thrombocyte (trombocito) (platelet) cellular fragment of megataryocyte; plays an important role in blood coagulation, hemostasis, and clot formation (Ch. 40, 41).

tickler file (archivo de recordatorios) system to remind of action to be taken on a certain date (Ch. 14).

time focus (enfoque en el tiempo) defines the period of time that is important and to which an individual's actions are directed or oriented (Ch. 4).

tinnitus (tinnitus) ringing or buzzing sound in the ear (Ch. 25).

titer (título) measurement of amount of antibody present against a particular antigen (Ch. 26).

tocopherol (tocoferol) vitamin E (Ch. 34).

tort (agravio) wrongful act that results in injury to one person by another (Ch. 7).

tort law (derecho de responsabilidad civil) laws that stem from torts, or wrongful acts that cause harm to one person, by another (Ch. 7).

Total Practice Management System (TPMS) (Sistema de Gestión de Prácticas Total [TPMS]) a category of software that deals with all the day-to-day operations of a medical practice (Ch. 11).

tourniquet (torniquete) device used to facilitate vein prominence (Ch. 40).

toxicity (toxicidad) the level at which a drug or chemical becomes poisonous or toxic. Some substances, such as certain metals, are considered toxic at any level of accidental exposure (Ch. 39).

trace mineral (oligomineral) mineral required by the body in small amounts (Ch. 34).

tracing (trazado) graphic record usually of an event that changes with time, as with the electrical activity of the heart (Ch. 37).

transcriber (transcriptor) device that makes it possible to transform voice recordings into a transcript or printed documents (Ch. 16).

transducer (transductor) device that converts one form of energy to another. During an ultrasound procedure, the transducer picks up echoes and converts them to electrical energy. The energy is transformed into digitalized images that can be viewed and printed. Photographs of the image can be taken (Ch. 32, 37).

transferable skills (habilidades transferibles) skills that would be used in a host of different and unrelated occupations. Keyboarding skill is an example of a transferable skill. It could be used by a secretary, data entry clerk, medical assistant, or clothing manufacturer (Ch. 48).

transient ischemic attack (ataque isquémico transitorio) temporary interference with blood flow to brain; may last only a few moments or several hours; neurologic symptoms occur (Ch. 29).

transilluminator (transiluminador) instrument used to inspect a cavity or organ by passing a light through the walls (Ch. 28).

transmission (transmisión) spread of infectious disease by direct contact, indirect contact, inhalation, ingestion, or bloodborne contact (Ch. 22).

Transmission-Based Precautions (Precauciones Basadas en la Transmisión) second tier of Centers for Disease Control and Prevention (CDC) guidelines that applies to specific categories of patients and that include air, contact, and droplet precautions. Transmission-Based Precautions are always used in addition to Standard Precautions (Ch. 22).

transurethral resection (resección transuretral) removal of prostate tissue using a device inserted through the urethra (Ch. 28).

traveler's check (cheque de viajero) often used in place of cash when traveling; available in denominations of $20 to $100; requires a signature at place of purchase as well as signature at the time the check is used (Ch. 19).

TRICARE (TRICARE) formerly the Civilian Health and Medical Program for Uniformed Services (CHAMPUS). TRICARE offers HMO, PPO, and fee-for-service medical insurance for dependents of active duty and retired military personnel and dependents of personnel who died while on active duty (Ch. 17).

trichomoniasis (tricomoniasis) infestation with a *Trichomonas* parasite, which may be transmitted through sexual intercourse (Ch. 22, 26).

triglycerides (triglicéridos) form of fat in the bloodstream that functions to store energy (Ch. 44).

trimester (trimestre) three months; one third of the gestational period of pregnancy (Ch. 26).

triple option plan (plan de opción triple) a managed care model allowing enrollees the option of traditional, HMO, or PPO health plans (Ch. 17).

trough (valle) the opposite of "peak," this is the point at which the drug is at its lowest level in the body. Usually this occurs just before the next dose is administered. In lab tests, the trough will tell the physician the weakest influence the drug would have on the body at that particular dose (Ch. 39).

Truth-in-Lending Act (Ley de Veracidad en los Préstamos) also known as the Consumer Credit Protection Act of 1968; an act requiring providers of installment credit to state the charges in writing and to express the interest as an annual rate (Ch. 20).

tuberculosis (TB) (tuberculosis [TB]) infectious disease caused by the bacterium *Mycobacterium tuberculosis* (Ch. 44).

turbid (turbio) opaque, not clear. Used to describe urine that is cloudy (Ch. 42).

turnaround time (plazo de entrega) specific time limits established for completion of medical reports (Ch. 16).

tympanostomy (timpanostomía) placement of a tube through the tympanic membrane to allow ventilation of the middle ear; part of the treatment for otitis media (Ch. 27).

typhus (typhoid) (tifus [tifoide]) acute infectious disease that causes severe headache, rash, high fever, and progressive neurologic involvement. Prevalent where conditions are unsanitary and congested (Ch. 3).

U

ultrasonic cleaner (limpiador ultrasónico) machine that uses the energy of high-frequency sound waves that agitate to sanitize instruments before sterilization (Ch. 22).

ultrasonography (ecografía) process of placing a handheld transducer against a body area to be tested. The transducer sends sound waves through the skin and the various internal organs. When echoes are formed and sent back the transducer converts them into electrical energy. This energy is transformed into a picture on a monitor or printed on paper. Photographs of the images can be taken and become part of the patient's permanent record (Ch. 26, 37).

ultrasound (ultrasonido) use of high-frequency sound waves for therapeutic reasons to generate heat in deep tissue (Ch. 33).

unbundling codes (códigos de desagregación) refers to separating the components of a procedure and reporting them as billable codes with charges to increase reimbursement rates (Ch. 18).

undifferentiated (no diferenciada) a change in the character of a cell(s) toward a malignant state (Ch. 22).

undoing (reparación) actions designed to make amends to cancel out inappropriate behavior (Ch. 4).

Uniform Bill 04 (UB04) (Factura Uniforme 04 [UB04]) unique billing form used extensively by acute care facilities for processing inpatient and outpatient claims (Ch. 18).

uniform resource locater (URL) (localizador uniforme de recursos [URL]) the address that defines the route to a file on the Web or any other Internet facility (Ch. 12).

unipolar (unipolar) having or pertaining to one pole process (Ch. 37).

unit (unidad) each part of a name (business or person), words, or numbers that will be indexed and coded for filing (Ch. 14).

unit dose (dosis unitaria) premeasured amount of medication, individually packaged on a per-dose basis (Ch. 36).

universal emergency medical identification symbol (símbolo universal de identificación médica para emergencias) identification sometimes carried by individuals to identify health problems they may have (Ch. 9).

Universal Precautions (Precauciones Universales) guidelines established by the Centers for Disease Control and Prevention (CDC) for the protection of health care workers from infectious diseases (Ch. 22).

universal serial bus (USB) port (puerto de bus universal en serie [USB]) a type of data entry portal or bus for computer data (Ch. 11).

unsterile field (campo no estéril) area that is adjacent to the sterile field where items needed can be accessed, opened, and supplied by an individual who does not wear sterile garb (Ch. 31).

up-coding (sobrecodificación) also known as code creep, overcoding, and overbilling. Up-coding occurs when the insurance carrier deliberately bills a higher rate service than what was performed to obtain greater reimbursements (Ch. 18).

urea (urea) principal end product of protein metabolism (Ch. 42).

urgency (urgencia) the need to urinate immediately (Ch. 30).

urinalysis (análisis de orina) examination of the physical, chemical, and microscopic properties of urine (Ch. 39, 42).

urinary tract infection (UTI) (infección del tracto urinario [ITU]) also referred to as a bladder infection (Ch. 42).

urobilinogen (urobilinógeno) colorless compound produced in the intestine after the breakdown by bacteria of bilirubin (Ch. 42).

urticaria (urticaria) hives (Ch. 35).

usual, customary, and reasonable (UCR) (usual, acostumbrado y razonable [UCR]) fee schedule often used by Medicare and some insurance carriers. *Usual* refers to the fee typically charged by a provider for certain procedures; *customary* is based on the average charge for a specific procedure by all provider practicing the same specialty in a defined geographic region; and *reasonable* refers to the midrange of fees charged for this procedure (Ch. 17).

utilization review (UR) (revisión de utilización [RU]) review of medical services before they can be performed (Ch. 21).

V

V codes (códigos V) ICD-9-CM codes representing either factors that influence a person's health status or legitimate reasons for contacting the health facility when the patient has no definitive diagnosis or active symptom of any disorder (Ch. 17).

vaccine (vacuna) pharmacologic agent capable of producing artificial active immunity (Ch. 22).

variable cost (costo variable) cost that varies in direct proportion to volume (Ch. 21).

vasoconstriction (vasoconstricción) narrowing or constricting of blood vessels (Ch. 33).

vasovagal syncope (síncope vasovagal) sudden faint due to hypotension induced by response of the autonomic nervous system to abrupt emotional stress, pain, or trauma (Ch. 9).

vector (vector) a carrier of disease, usually an insect, that is the causative organism of disease from infected to noninfected individuals (Ch. 22).

venipuncture (venopunción) puncturing into a vein with a needle to obtain a blood sample (Ch. 40).

vertigo (vértigo) the sensation of moving around in space; dizziness, lightheadedness (Ch. 25).

vesicular (vesicular) characterized by the presence of vesicles. Vesicles are blisters or other elevations on the skin (Ch. 22, 26).

viable (viable) able to live, grow, and develop after birth; usually 24 weeks or greater than 1 pound (Ch. 26).

virology (virología) study of viruses (Ch. 39, 43).

virulence (virulencia) an organism's relative power and degree of pathogenicity (Ch. 22).

viscosity (viscosidad) degree of thickness of a liquid (Ch. 40).

vitiligo (vitíligo) skin disorder characterized by smooth white spots on various areas of the body (Ch. 25).

voice over Internet protocol (VoIP) (protocolo de voz por Internet [VoIP]) the real-time transmission of voice signals over the Internet or Internet Protocol (IP) network (Ch. 12).

voice recognition software (VRS) (software de reconocimiento de voz) software that translates voice commands and is used in place of a mouse and keyboard (Ch. 16).

volatile (volátil) easily evaporated (Ch. 31).

voucher check (cheque con comprobante) check with detachable form used to detail reason check is drawn; commonly used in payroll checks (Ch. 19).

W

waived (prueba de baja complejidad) used to describe a category of clinical laboratory tests that are simple, unvarying, and require a minimum of judgment and interpretation (Ch. 38).

watermark (sello de agua) design incorporated in paper during the papermaking process that is visible when the paper is held up to the light (Ch. 15).

water-soluble (soluble en agua) pertaining to substances that are hydrophilic and therefore dissolve better in water (Ch. 34).

wave scheduling (planificación en olas) system where patients are scheduled for the first half hour of every hour and then are seen throughout the hour (Ch. 13).

wet mount (preparación en fresco) a method of adding liquid, usually saline or potassium hydrochloride, to a specimen on a slide for examination and preservation. The specimen is placed on a slide and one drop of saline (for diagnosis of trichomonas vaginalis) or potassium hydroxide (for diagnosis of vaginal yeast infections) is applied and mixes with the specimen. It is then covered with a coverslip and examined microscopically (Ch. 26, 43).

wheal (roncha) slight elevation of skin that can be produced as a result of an intradermal injection such as the Mantoux/PPD test for TB (Ch. 44).

wheezes (sibilancia) high-pitched musical sound heard on expiration, often the result of an obstruction or narrowing of respiratory passages (Ch. 24).

wide area network (WAN) (red de área amplia [WAN]) connecting together of computers on a large area for the purpose of sharing data (Ch. 11).

WiFi connection (conexión WiFi) connection via a universal wireless network standard that uses radio waves (Ch. 11).

wireless local area network (WLAN) (red de área local inalámbrica [LAN]) a type of local area network that uses high-frequency radio waves rather than wires to communicate between nodes (Ch. 11).

Wood's lamp (lámpara de Wood) special lights used to detect organisms that fluoresce such as certain fungi, bacteria, and parasites. Scabies and ringworm are two examples. Scratches in the eye may be detected using a Woods lamp after the eye has been stained with a fluorescent dye. Also used in determining margin dissection of melanoma (Ch. 43).

work practice controls (controles de prácticas laborales) measures used in the workplace that consist of physical equipment and mechanical devices to control employee exposure to bloodborne pathogens and other potentially infectious materials. Examples are sharps disposal containers, handwashing facilities, personal protective equipment, and eyewash stations (Ch. 22).

work statement (declaración de trabajo) concise description of the work you plan to accomplish (Ch. 45).

Workers' Compensation insurance (seguro de indemnización por accidentes de trabajo) medical and paycheck insurance for workers who sustain injuries associated with their employment (Ch. 17).

wound (herida) a break in the continuity of soft parts of body structures caused by violence or trauma to tissues. In an open wound, skin is broken as in a laceration, abrasion, avulsion, or incision. In a closed wound, skin is not broken as in contusion, ecchymosis, or hematoma (Ch. 9).

X

xerophthalmia (xeroftalmía) dry, lusterless mucous membranes of the eyes (Ch. 34).

Y

yellow fever (fiebre amarilla) acute infectious disease where a person develops jaundice, vomits, hemorrhages, and has a fever; caused mostly by mosquitoes (Ch. 3).

Z

ZIP+4 (ZIP+4) standard zip code including four additional digits that identify a postal delivery area. Mail will be processed more efficiently and effectively with the use of the ZIP+4 code in the address (Ch. 15).

Glosario de términos

Note: The equivalent English word follows in parentheses in green.

A

abducción (abduction) movimiento que consiste en alejarse de la línea media del cuerpo (Ch. 33).

aborto (abortion) expulsión de los productos de la concepción antes de llegar a la viabilidad (Ch. 26).

abuso (abuse) mal uso, uso excesivo o inadecuado, especialmente de fármacos narcóticos o psicofármacos (Ch. 17, 35).

acetona (acetone) líquido incoloro e inflamable. Se encuentra en la sangre y en la orina de las personas diabéticas como resultado de la descomposición de ácidos grasos (Ch. 38).

aciclovir (acyclovir) fármaco antivírico usado en algunas infecciones por herpes (Ch. 22).

ácido ascórbico (ascorbic acid) vitamina C (Ch. 34).

ácido fólico (folic acid) una de las vitaminas del complejo B (Ch. 34).

acreditación (accreditation) proceso por el cual se otorga reconocimiento a un programa educativo por cumplir las normas que califican a sus graduados para el ejercicio de la profesión; proporcionar credenciales (Ch. 1).

acreditado (credentialed) pruebas que demuestran que una persona tiene derecho a un crédito o a ejercer su facultad oficial (Ch. 1).

actas (minutes) registro escrito de los temas tratados y las medidas adoptadas durante las sesiones de reuniones (Ch. 15, 45).

actividades de la vida diaria (AVD) (activities of daily living [ADL]) actividades que generalmente se realizan durante un día típico que incluyen el cuidado propio, por ejemplo, comer y cepillarse los dientes (Ch. 33).

activos (assets) bienes de valor que posee una entidad comercial (Ch. 21).

acuerdo de confidencialidad (confidentiality agreement) cuando se firma este acuerdo, significa que el transcriptor médico se compromete a mantener la confidencialidad de toda la información de los pacientes (Ch. 16).

acupuntura (acupuncture) tratamiento para aliviar el dolor y las enfermedades mediante la inserción en la piel de agujas finas en puntos específicos (Ch. 2).

aditivo (additive) cualquier material que se coloca en un tubo que mantiene o facilita la integridad y la función de la muestra para análisis (Ch. 40).

administrar (administer) dar un medicamento (Ch. 7, 35, 36).

ADN (DNA) ácido desoxirribonucleico; material nuclear importante que contiene códigos genéticos (Ch. 39, 43).

aducción (adduction) movimiento que consiste en acercarse a la línea media del cuerpo (Ch. 33).

aerobio (aerobic) organismo que requiere oxígeno para crecer (Ch. 43).

aerosoles (aerosols) partículas de materiales potencialmente infecciosos que puedan liberarse a la atmósfera (Ch. 22, 43).

aerosolizado (aerosolized) aplicado por medio de un atomizador (Ch. 27).

afebril (afebrile) sin fiebre (Ch. 24).

agar (agar) sustancia gelatinosa extraída de algas rojas que contiene nutrientes y humedad para el crecimiento de bacterias (Ch. 43).

agente (agent) persona que representa a otra (Ch. 7).

agente de acoplamiento (coupling agent) agente usado en una ecografía que mejora la penetración de ondas sonoras a través de los tejidos (Ch. 26).

agente infeccioso (infectious agent) patógeno responsable de una enfermedad infecciosa específica (Ch. 22).

agentes quimioterapéuticos (chemotherapeutic agents) agentes usados en el tratamiento de enfermedades; la aplicación de reactivos químicos tóxicos para los microorganismos patógenos. Comúnmente se usa para describir agentes (sustancias químicas) usados en el tratamiento de ciertos tumores malignos (Ch. 38).

aglutinación (agglutination) reacción antígeno-anticuerpo en la cual un antígeno sólido se une a un anticuerpo sólido (Ch. 44).

agotamiento profesional (burnout) estado de cansancio o frustración ocasionado por la dedicación a una causa, forma de vida o a una relación que no produjo el resultado esperado (Ch. 5).

agravio (tort) acto ilegítimo en el que una persona provoca una lesión a otra persona (Ch. 7).

agrupación (clustering) unión de mensajes no verbales para formar oraciones o conclusiones. También se puede usar para describir un sistema de programación en el cual los pacientes con quejas o afecciones similares se programan consecutivamente (por ejemplo, la programación de todas las infecciones alérgicas entre las 3:00 p. m. y las 4:00 p. m. todos los martes y los jueves) (Ch. 4).

aislamiento (isolation) separar a un paciente con ciertas infecciones o enfermedades transmisibles de otras personas (Ch. 22).

ajustes (adjustments) aumento o disminución en las cuentas de pacientes que no se deben a los cargos incurridos o a los pagos recibidos (Ch. 17, 19).

alambre guía (lead wire) conductor conectado a un electrocardiógrafo. Tiene derivaciones para las extremidades y para el tórax (Ch. 37).

alcohol etílico (ethyl alcohol) alcohol, usado para preparar una solución (Ch. 38).

alcohol isopropílico (isopropyl alcohol) comúnmente llamado alcohol de botiquín; solución de alcohol al 70% que se usa comúnmente como limpiador (Ch. 31).

alérgeno (allergen) cualquier sustancia que produce signos de alergia, por ejemplo, inhalantes como polvo y polen, alimentos como trigo y fresas, fármacos, penicilina, sustancias químicas, calor, bacterias (Ch. 30).

alergia (allergy) hipersensibilidad adquirida a una sustancia (alérgeno) que normalmente no causa una reacción (Ch. 23, 31).

algoritmo (algorithm) método especial para resolver un tipo específico de problema (Ch. 11).

alícuota (aliquot) parte de la muestra completa que se ha retirado para usarla o almacenarla (Ch. 40).

alimentos procesados (processed food) alimentos que ya no están en su estado íntegro y natural; cocinados o envasados sin algunas partes o con ingredientes agregados (Ch. 34).

alopático (allopathic) método para tratar enfermedades con remedios que producen efectos diferentes a los provocados por la propia enfermedad. La mayoría de los profesionales de la salud tradicionales hoy son considerados profesionales alopáticos (Ch. 3).

ámbito de práctica (scope of practice) campo de aplicación de los procedimientos y las actividades clínicas que se permiten por ley para una profesión (Ch. 1).

ambliopía (amblyopia) trastorno de los ojos caracterizado por disminución de la visión (Ch. 30).

Ambu Bag™ (Ambu Bag™) marca de una bolsa que se coloca sobre la nariz y la boca para ayudar a suministrar ventilación artificial a los pulmones (Ch. 9).

ambulación (ambulation) capacidad para caminar (Ch. 33).

aminoácido (amino acid) unidad estructural básica de la proteína (Ch. 34).

amniocentesis (amniocentesis) punción quirúrgica del saco amniótico para extraer líquido para análisis de laboratorio (Ch. 22, 26).

amniotomía (amniotomy) ruptura artificial del saco amniótico (Ch. 26).

amorfo (amorphous) sin forma; que no posee forma definida (Ch. 42).

amplificado (amplified) agrandado o aumentado. El amplificador del electrocardiógrafo agranda la actividad del impulso cardíaco, por lo que el registro se puede leer más fácilmente (Ch. 37).

amplitud (amplitude) cantidad, extensión, tamaño, abundancia o plenitud (Ch. 37).

amplitud de movimiento (ROM) (range of motion [ROM]) grado de movimiento presente en una articulación (Ch. 33).

anaerobio (anaerobic) organismo que requiere poco oxígeno o que no necesita oxígeno para crecer (Ch. 43).

anafilaxia (anaphylaxis) hipersensibilidad del cuerpo ante una proteína o fármaco extraño (Ch. 9, 35).

análisis bioquímicos (biochemical tests) pruebas que muestran las propiedades bioquímicas y las reacciones de las bacterias con el fin de lograr la identificación de los microorganismos; a menudo se realiza en medios sólidos y líquidos (Ch. 43).

análisis de costos (cost analysis) procedimiento que determina los costos de cada servicio (Ch. 21).

análisis de orina (urinalysis) examen de las propiedades físicas, químicas y microscópicas de la orina (Ch. 39, 42).

andropausia (andropause) cambios que se producen en hombres de mediana edad (Ch. 29).

anemia drepanocítica (sickle cell anemia) trastorno sanguíneo congénito que puede acortar la vida (Ch. 26).

anemia perniciosa (pernicious anemia) anemia crónica causada por la falta de ácido clorhídrico en el estómago; puede provocar debilidad, cansancio, hormigueo en las extremidades y hasta insuficiencia cardíaca; las inyecciones con vitamina B_{12} son el tratamiento usado para esta enfermedad (Ch. 29).

anestesia (anesthesia) insensibilidad o ausencia de sensaciones; un anestésico es cualquier mecanismo que produce anestesia (Ch. 31).

angiograma (angiogram) serie radiográfica de un vaso sanguíneo después de la inyección de una sustancia radiopaca (Ch. 37).

anisocitosis (anisocytosis) variación marcada del tamaño de las células (Ch. 41).

anomalías congénitas (congenital anomalies) anomalías de nacimiento, que existen en el momento del nacimiento (Ch. 26).

anorexia (anorexia) pérdida del apetito (Ch. 22).

antecedentes de enfermedad actual (AEA) (history of present illness [HPI]) descripción cronológica del desarrollo de la enfermedad del paciente (Ch. 16).

antibacteriano (antibacterial) que puede destruir bacterias; a menudo se aplica en una herida en forma de ungüento o crema (Ch. 31).

anticoagulante (anticoagulant) sustancia química en tubos de sangre que impide la coagulación de la sangre al quitar el calcio de la sangre o al detener la formación de trombina (Ch. 40).

anticuerpo (antibody) sustancia química específica producida por las células B del sistema inmunitario como respuesta a un antígeno (Ch. 22, 44).

anticuerpo heterófilo (heterophile antibody) anticuerpo que reacciona con otros que no son los antígenos específicos, como se observa en la mononucleosis infecciosa (Ch. 44).

antígeno (antigen) sustancias, tales como bacterias u otro agentes, que el cuerpo reconoce como extrañas; estímulo para la producción de anticuerpos (Ch. 22, 44).

antioxidante (antioxidant) algo que impide la oxidación (Ch. 34).

antisuero (antiserum) suero que contiene anticuerpos (Ch. 44).

ántrax (carbuncle) infección necrosante de la piel y del tejido formada por un agrupamiento de forúnculos (Ch. 30).

apical (apical) perteneciente al vértice o punta del corazón. Lugar para medir la frecuencia cardíaca con un estetoscopio (Ch. 24).

apnea (apnea) cese o ausencia de respiración espontánea normal (Ch. 24, 36).

apósito (dressing) gasa estéril u otro material que se aplica directamente en una herida para absorber secreciones y como protección (Ch. 9, 31).

aprendizaje por observación (shadow) seguir de cerca a un supervisor o a un subordinado delegado para aprender el protocolo del establecimiento (Ch. 45).

aproximar (approximate) juntar los bordes de una herida (Ch. 31).

arbitraje (arbitration) forma de resolución de conflictos que permite a una parte neutral resolver una disputa (Ch. 7).

archivado consecutivo o en serie (consecutive or serial filing) método de archivado numérico en el que los números se consideran en orden ascendente usando todo el conjunto de cifras (Ch. 14).

archivado no consecutivo (nonconsecutive filing) método de archivado numérico en el cual los números se consideran en orden ascendente usando subconjuntos de cifras dentro de un número; por ejemplo, en el número 574 19 2863: 2863 es la unidad 1, 19 es la unidad 2, 574 es la unidad 3 (Ch. 14).

archivo de recordatorios (tickler file) sistema para recordar que se debe ejecutar una acción en una fecha determinada (Ch. 14).

área de superficie corporal (ASC) (body surface area [BSA]) método sumamente exacto para calcular las dosis de medicamentos para bebés y niños de hasta 12 años (Ch. 36).

arranque (booting) todo lo que sucede desde el momento en que se enciende la computadora, se realizan las operaciones necesarias para que comiencen a funcionar todos los componentes y se cargue el sistema operativo (Ch. 11).

arritmia (arrhythmia) desviación del patrón o ritmo normal del latido cardíaco (Ch. 24, 37).

artefacto (artifact) cualquier cosa que se produce artificialmente (Ch. 37).

arteriosclerosis (arteriosclerosis) endurecimiento de las arterias causado por la acumulación de placa, un depósito de sustancias grasas en las paredes de las arterias (Ch. 29).

aseguramiento de calidad (QA) (quality assurance [QA]) proceso para proporcionar documentación de atención médica exacta, completa y uniforme en forma oportuna a la vez que se toman todas las medidas razonables para resolver incoherencias, imprecisiones, cuestiones de gestión de riesgos y otros problemas (Ch. 16, 38).

asepsia (asepsis) protección contra las infecciones causadas por microorganismos patógenos (Ch. 3).

asepsia médica (medical asepsis) limpio y libre de infecciones (Ch. 22, 38).

asepsia quirúrgica (surgical asepsis) procedimientos para esterilizar los objetos; técnicas para mantener las condiciones estériles durante los procedimientos invasivos (Ch. 22, 31).

aséptico (aseptic) libre de cualquier material infeccioso; ausencia de microorganismos (Ch. 22, 30).

asiento (posting) registro de transacciones financieras en un sistema contable o de teneduría de libros (Ch. 19).

asignación de beneficios (assignment of benefits) cesión de beneficios por parte del beneficiario a un tercero (Ch. 17).

asintomático (asymptomatic) sin síntomas (Ch. 39).

Asistente Administrativo Médico Certificado (CMAA) (Certified Medical Administrative Assistant [CMAA]) certificación de la NHA para asistente administrativo médico (Ch. 47).

Asistente Clínico Médico Certificado (CCMA) (Certified Clinical Medical Assistant [CCMA]) certificación de la NHA para asistente clínico médico (Ch. 47).

Asistente Médico Certificado (CMA [AAMA]) (Certified Medical Assistant [CMA (AAMA)]) asistente médico certificado que ha completado con éxito el examen de certificación nacional de la Asociación Estadounidense de Asistentes Médicos (AAMA, por sus siglas en inglés) (Ch. 1, 47).

Asistente Médico Matriculado (RMA) (Registered Medical Assistant [RMA]) credencial otorgada por aprobar con éxito el examen de los Tecnólogos Médicos Estadounidenses (AMT, por sus siglas en inglés) (Ch. 1, 47).

asistente personal digital (PDA) (personal digital assistant [PDA]) herramienta electrónica para organizar datos, dispositivo organizador personal computarizado de mano (Ch. 11).

Asociación Estadounidense de Asistentes Médicos (AAMA) (American Association of Medical Assistants [AAMA]) organización profesional dedicada a atender los intereses de los Asistentes Médicos Certificados (Ch. 47).

Asociación Independiente de Médicos (IPA) (independent physician association [IPA]) red independiente de médicos en la práctica privada que tienen contrato con la asociación para tratar pacientes a cambio de una tarifa convenida (Ch. 2).

Asociación Nacional de Profesiones de Salud (NHA) (National Healthcareer Association [NHA]) asociación que ofrece exámenes de certificación nacional para profesionales de la atención médica. La NHA trabaja con instituciones educativas en el desarrollo de planes de estudio, pruebas de competencias y preparación y administración de su examen de certificación (Ch. 47).

Asociación para la Integridad de la Documentación del Cuidado de la Salud (AHDI) (Association for Healthcare Documentation Integrity [AHDI]) organización sin fines de lucro fundada por los transcriptores médicos para promover la profesión (Ch. 16).

aspirar (aspirate) eliminar mediante succión (Ch. 22).

ataque isquémico transitorio (transient ischemic attack) interferencia temporal en el flujo sanguíneo que va al cerebro; puede durar sólo unos momentos o varias horas; puede haber síntomas neurológicos (Ch. 29).

ataxia (ataxia) trastorno caracterizado por la alteración de la coordinación muscular que se observa principalmente cuando se intenta hacer movimientos musculares voluntarios (Ch. 25).

aterosclerosis (atherosclerosis) forma de arteriosclerosis marcada por depósitos de calcio en las paredes arteriales (Ch. 24).

atributo (attribute) característica inherente (Ch. 1).

audio de forma de onda (WAV) (waveform audio [WAV]) formato estándar usado para comprimir y almacenar datos digitales de sonido (Ch. 16).

auditor (auditor) persona responsable de determinar el contenido final de un documento y la exactitud en cada aspecto informado (Ch. 16).

aumentar (augment) agregar o incrementar (Ch. 37).

aurícula (auricle) el oído externo, también llamado pabellón auricular (Ch. 30).

auspicio (aegis) patrocinio o protección (Ch. 38).

autenticación (authentication) la persona que dicta la información firma o autentica el documento para indicar que la información era exacta y completa en el momento de firmar (Ch. 16).

autorealización (self-actualization) ser todo lo que se puede ser; desarrollar todo el potencial y experimentar la sensación de logro (Ch. 5, 45).

autorización previa (preauthorization) proceso por el cual se obtiene el consentimiento de la compañía de seguros antes de proceder con la atención y el tratamiento de un paciente. Si no se obtiene la autorización, quizás las compañías de seguros no paguen los beneficios para problemas específicos (Ch. 17).

autoseguro (self-insurance) seguro contratado por las grandes empresas, organizaciones sin fines de lucro y por los gobiernos para reducir los costos y obtener más control de sus finanzas. Cada plan difiere en cuanto a su cobertura y a los requisitos para presentar reclamaciones (Ch. 17).

avascularización (avascularization) expulsión de sangre de los tejidos. Deja los tejidos sin suministro sanguíneo (Ch. 31).

B

baja de codificación (down-coding) las compañías de seguros bajan de codificación si la documentación o los códigos son ambiguos y reembolsan la tarifa más baja posible (Ch. 18).

balance general (balance sheet) estado detallado de los activos, los pasivos y el patrimonio; estado de situación patrimonial (Ch. 21).

balancear (balance) verificar la exactitud de un asiento; registra la diferencia entre las columnas del debe y el haber (Ch. 19).

banda de constricción (constriction band) término usado para reemplazar a torniquete (que ya no se usa) en emergencias. Se usa una banda de material para controlar una hemorragia importante de una extremidad que ha sufrido una lesión por un traumatismo. La banda se aplica por encima del origen de la hemorragia pero no tan ajustada de modo que no restrinja el flujo de sangre completamente. Habrá un ligero goteo de sangre. Esta acción evita la pérdida de una extremidad debido a la restricción completa del flujo sanguíneo. Si esto sucede, no hay flujo sanguíneo hacia las células y los tejidos de la extremidad, por lo que las células, los tejidos y esa parte del cuerpo no reciben oxígeno y se mueren (Ch. 9).

bandeja de instrumentos (instrument tray) ver mesa de Mayo (Ch. 31).

bandeja o carro de parada (crash tray or cart) bandeja o carro portátil que contiene medicamentos y suministros necesarios para urgencias y procedimientos de primeros auxilios (Ch. 9).

baño de asiento (sitz bath) baño con agua tibia, en el que sólo se sumergen las caderas y las nalgas (Ch. 31).

bariátrica (bariatrics) rama de la medicina que se ocupa de la prevención, el control y el tratamiento de la obesidad (Ch. 30).

barrera (barrier) obstáculo que existe para proteger a una persona del contacto con la sangre o con otros materiales posiblemente infectados. Llamado equipo de protección personal (EPP), las barreras incluyen guantes, máscaras, protectores faciales, guardapolvos de laboratorio, gafas de protección y batas (Ch. 22).

basófilo (basophil) glóbulo blanco granulocítico con gránulos citoplásmicos de color púrpura oscuro. Es el menos común de los glóbulos blancos (Ch. 41).

beneficiario (beneficiary) persona que reúne los requisitos para recibir beneficios en virtud de una póliza (Ch. 17).

beneficiario (payee) persona nombrada en el cheque y que recibirá el importe indicado (Ch. 19).

beneficio (benefit) remuneración que se agrega al sueldo (Ch. 45, 48).

beneficio complementario (fringe benefit) beneficio que supera el sueldo que tiene derecho a cobrar un empleado. Los ejemplos incluyen seguro de salud y de vida, vacaciones pagas, licencia por enfermedad, días de licencia por razones particulares y reembolso de matrícula para cursos relacionados con el trabajo (Ch. 2, 45).

beriberi (beriberi) enfermedad causada por una deficiencia de vitamina B (tiamina) y caracterizada por dolor de cabeza, depresión, anorexia, estreñimiento, taquicardia, edema e insuficiencia cardíaca (Ch. 34).

Betadine® (Betadine®) marca de una solución de povidona yodada usada como antiséptico para la piel. Betadine® también está disponible como solución jabonosa (en forma de jabón) (Ch. 31).

bilirrubina (bilirubin) pigmento de color entre amarillento y anaranjado que se forma a partir de la descomposición de la hemoglobina en glóbulos rojos dañados. La bilirrubina generalmente se transporta en el torrente sanguíneo hacia el hígado, donde se convierte en una forma soluble al agua y se excreta en la bilis (Ch. 42, 44).

bilirrubinuria (bilirubinuria) presencia de bilirrubina en la orina (Ch. 42).

bioética (bioethics) rama de la ética médica que se ocupa de las cuestiones morales que surgen de la investigación médica sofisticada y del uso de tecnología avanzada. Las cuestiones sociales como ingeniería genética, aborto e investigación en tejido fetal plantean importantes preguntas bioéticas (Ch. 8).

biometría (biometric) tipo de firma electrónica que puede usar entradas de teclas de computadora alfanuméricas como identificación; dispositivo de escritura electrónico; o sistema biométrico que usa la voz, las huellas digitales o la retina del ojo (Ch. 16).

biopsia (biopsy) extracción de una pequeña parte de tejido vivo de un órgano o de otra parte del cuerpo para examinarla microscópicamente y confirmar o establecer un diagnóstico (Ch. 30, 39).

biopsia cervical en sacabocados (cervical punch biopsy) biopsia del cuello uterino usando un instrumento cuyo extremo es un sacabocados (Ch. 26).

bipolar (bipolar) que tiene dos polos o procesos (Ch. 37).

Bluetooth® (Bluetooth®) estándar de la industria tecnológica que facilita la comunicación entre dispositivos inalámbricos como teléfonos celulares, asistentes personales digitales, computadoras de mano y computadoras portátiles o computadoras de escritorio con conexión inalámbrica (Ch. 11).

borramiento (effacement) adelgazamiento y acortamiento del conducto cervical durante el parto para permitir el paso de feto (Ch. 26).

bradicardia sinusal (bradycardia [sinus]) frecuencia cardíaca lenta (menos de 60 latidos por minuto) pero regular (Ch. 24, 37).

bradipnea (bradypnea) frecuencia respiratoria anormalmente baja (Ch. 24).

Braxton–Hicks (Braxton–Hicks) contracciones irregulares, intermitentes e indoloras del útero; también conocidas como contracciones falsas (Ch. 26).

brecha auscultatoria (ausculatatory gap) mientras se mide la presión arterial, los sonidos de golpeteo que se oyen pueden desaparecer entre las fases de los ruidos de Korotkoff (Ch. 24).

broncodilatador (bronchodilator) fármaco que expande los tubos bronquiales (Ch. 30).

bronquios (bronchi) bifurcaciones de la tráquea que se ramifican hacia cada pulmón y terminan en los tubos bronquiales (Ch. 30).

C

cable de prueba (test cable) dispositivo accesorio que se conecta entre el monitor Holter y el electrocardiógrafo para verificar que la forma de onda sea correcta y que no haya artefactos (Ch. 37).

caja chica (petty cash) pequeña suma que se tiene a mano para gastos menores o imprevistos (Ch. 19).

calibración (calibration) determinación de la exactitud de un instrumento comparando la información suministrada con un patrón aceptado del cual se conoce su exactitud (Ch. 37, 38).

caloría (calorie) unidad de calor. La Caloría grande (que a menudo se escribe con mayúscula) se usa para hablar de la alimentación en seres humanos. La Caloría grande también se expresa como kilocaloría (kcal) y equivale a 1,000 calorías pequeñas (Ch. 34).

calumnia (libel) escrito falso y malicioso sobre otra persona que constituye una difamación de la persona (Ch. 7).

calumnia (slander) dichos falsos y maliciosos sobre otra persona que constituyen una difamación del carácter de una persona (Ch. 7).

campana de humo (fume hood) tipo de campana o barrera que se usa en el laboratorio para atrapar los vapores y los humos químicos y desviarlos lejos de los profesionales de la atención médica por el sistema de extracción de aire del edificio (Ch. 38).

campo estéril (sterile field) área que se considera estéril, usualmente designada por un paño estéril. El área contiene insumos e instrumentos estériles que se usarán en un procedimiento particular o cirugía estérils (Ch. 31).

campo no estéril (unsterile field) área adyacente al campo estéril en la que una persona que no usa vestimenta estéril puede entrar, abrir y suministrar elementos necesarios (Ch. 31).

candidiasis (candidiasis) infección de la piel o de la membrana mucosa con alguna especie de *Candida* (Ch. 26).

capa leucocitaria (buffy coat) capa de glóbulos blancos y plaquetas que se forma en la interfaz entre el plasma y los glóbulos rojos en un tubo de sangre que contiene anticoagulante (Ch. 40).

capitación (capitation) uso de la cantidad de miembros inscritos en un plan para determinar el sueldo del proveedor; el proveedor recibe un pago fijo por cada miembro, independientemente de cuántas veces ese miembro consulte al proveedor (Ch. 17).

caquéctico (cachectic) describe un estado de mala salud, desnutrición y consunción (Ch. 34).

carcinoma in situ (carcinoma in situ) cáncer que no se extiende más allá de la membrana basal (Ch. 26).

cardioversión (cardioversion) conversión de un ritmo cardíaco patológico (arritmia), como fibrilación ventricular, al ritmo sinusal normal (Ch. 9, 37).

cardioversor/desfibrilador (cardioverter/defibrillator) dispositivo implantable usado para arritmias que ponen en riesgo la vida. Su objetivo es aplicar descargas eléctricas para eliminar la arritmia y lograr un ritmo sinusal más normal (Ch. 37).

caroteno (carotene) vitamina A (Ch. 34).

carta de bloque completo (full block letter) estilo de carta principal en el cual todos los renglones de los párrafos comienzan alineados en el margen izquierdo. Este estilo se sugiere para oficinas que desean una carta eficiente y de aspecto contemporáneo (Ch. 15).

carta de referencia (letter of reference) carta generalmente escrita por el ex empleador de un empleado en el que se describe el desempeño, la actitud o las aptitudes del empleado. Esta carta se presenta a un posible empleador cuando el candidato se postula para un nuevo empleo (Ch. 46).

carta de renuncia (letter of resignation) carta en la que se informa al empleador actual sobre la decisión del empleado de renunciar al puesto actual (Ch. 46).

carta estilo bloque modificado, con sangría (modified block letter, indented) estilo de carta modificado con párrafos con sangría. Los párrafos de este estilo de carta pueden tener sangría de cinco espacios (Ch. 15).

carta estilo bloque modificado, estándar (modified block letter, standard) estilo de carta principal en el que todos los renglones comienzan en el margen izquierdo excepto el renglón de la fecha, el cierre de cortesía y la firma mecanografiada. Las excepciones generalmente comienzan en la posición central o a una distancia de unos espacios a la derecha del centro (Ch. 15).

carta simplificada (simplified letter) estilo de carta principal recomendado por la Sociedad de Gestión Administrativa (Administrative Management Society) que omite el saludo y el cierre de cortesía. Todos los renglones se escriben alineados en el margen izquierdo. En los consultorios médicos, este estilo es el más usado para enviar una carta tipo (Ch. 15).

carta tipo (form letter) carta que tiene el mismo contenido en el cuerpo pero que se envía a diferentes personas (Ch. 15).

cartera (portfolio) cuaderno o dossier que contiene ejemplos de materiales que se usan comúnmente (Ch. 15).

catalizador (catalyst) sustancia que permite que una reacción química se desarrolle a un ritmo mucho mayor y sin demasiado ingreso de energía (Ch. 34).

categorías de aislamiento (isolation categories) sistema de siete categorías desarrollado por los Centros para el Control de Enfermedades (CDC, por sus siglas en inglés) que aísla a los pacientes de acuerdo con las infecciones conocidas. Estas categorías se han condensado en tres Precauciones basadas en la transmisión, según si la vía de transmisión es por aire, por contacto o por gotitas (Ch. 22).

cateterismo (catheterization) inserción de un catéter en el cuerpo para evacuar líquidos o inyectarlos en las cavidades corporales. En el cateterismo urinario, el tubo se introduce a través de la uretra hacia la vejiga para extraer orina (Ch. 25).

cateterismo cardíaco (cardiac catheterization) pasaje de un catéter hacia el corazón a través de una vena del brazo o de la pierna y de los vasos sanguíneos que van al corazón. El objetivo es obtener muestras de sangre cardíaca, detectar anormalidades y determinar la presión intracardíaca. Se puede inyectar un medio de contraste y se puede realizar una angiografía coronaria (Ch. 37).

cátodo (cathode) electrodo negativo que emite electrones (Ch. 32).

cáustico (caustic) que quema y corroe, que destruye el tejido humano (Ch. 22, 31).

cauterio (cautery) destrucción de tejido al quemarlo (Ch. 31).

cauterizar (cauterize) destruir tejido a través de la aplicación de un agente cáustico, un instrumento caliente, una corriente eléctrica u otro agente (Ch. 9).

celulosa (cellulose) tipo de fibra no digerible compuesta por los hidratos de carbono que se encuentran en las plantas (Ch. 34).

centrifugador (centrifuge) dispositivo que hace girar tubos usando la fuerza centrífuga para separar la parte líquida de la sangre de los elementos más densos (Ch. 40).

centros de servicio al paciente (patient service centres) instalaciones de laboratorio satélite ubicadas en áreas convenientes para pacientes donde se pueden recolectar y dejar las muestras para análisis (Ch. 39).

Centros de Servicios de Medicare y Medicaid (CMS) (Centers for Medicare and Medicaid Services [CMS]) Antes conocido como Administración para el Financiamiento de la Atención Médica (HCFA, por sus siglas en inglés). CMS es una agencia federal dentro del Departamento de Salud y Servicios Humanos (DHHS, por sus siglas en inglés) de los EE. UU. La agencia administra Medicare, Medicaid y el Programa Estatal de Seguro Médico para Niños (SCHIP, por sus siglas en inglés). CMS también administra la Ley de Portabilidad y Responsabilidad de Seguros de Salud (HIPAA, por sus siglas en inglés) de 1996 y la Ley de Mejoras de Laboratorios Clínicos (CLIA, por sus siglas en inglés) de 1988 (Ch. 17).

certificación (certification) garantía que indica que es verdadero o que se rige por un estándar o que lo cumple (Ch. 1).

cetoacidosis (ketoacidosis) acumulación de cetonas en el cuerpo, que se produce principalmente como complicación de la diabetes mellitus; si no se trata puede provocar coma (Ch. 42).

cetona (ketone) compuesto químico producido durante un aumento del metabolismo de los lípidos; también, prueba con una tira reactiva (Ch. 42).

cetonuria (ketonuria) presencia de cetonas en la orina (Ch. 42).

cetosis (ketosis) afección en la que el cuerpo quema los ácidos grasos para obtener energía en la ausencia de la glucosa o los carbohidratos correspondientes; se puede llamar también lipólisis (Ch. 42).

cheque certificado (certified check) cheque propio del depositante que, según lo indica el banco con fecha y firma, tiene los fondos de respaldo del importe escrito (Ch. 19).

cheque con comprobante (voucher check) cheque con un formulario recortable que se usa para detallar el motivo por el que se libra el cheque; generalmente se usa en los cheques de nómina (Ch. 19).

cheque de caja (cashier's check) cheque propio del banco librado a cargo de la cuenta del banco (Ch. 19).

cheque de viajero (traveler's check) a menudo se usa en lugar de efectivo en los viajes; disponible en denominaciones de $20 a $100; requiere la firma en el lugar de compra y la firma en el momento de usar el cheque (Ch. 19).

Cheyne–Stoke (Cheyne–stroke) patrón regular de frecuencia respiratoria irregular que a menudo se observa en niños y que puede verse en la disfunción cerebral (Ch. 24).

cianosis (cyanosis) decoloración de la piel debido a cantidades anormales de hemoglobina reducida en la sangre, provocada por la disminución del oxígeno y el aumento del dióxido de carbono en la sangre (Ch. 25).

ciberespacio (cyberspace) referencia al espacio no físico de la comunicación en informática con sistema binario (Ch. 11).

ciclo cardíaco (cardiac cycle) período desde el inicio de un latido cardíaco hasta el comienzo del siguiente latido, que incluye la sístole y la diástole. Un latido completo del corazón (Ch. 37).

cilindros (casts) estructuras diminutas que generalmente se forman por depósitos de proteína u otras sustancias en las paredes de los túbulos renales; en la orina, pueden indicar enfermedad renal (Ch. 42).

cinésica (kinesics) estudio de lenguaje corporal (Ch. 4).

cinturón de marcha (gait belt) cinturón de seguridad que usa el paciente alrededor de la cintura y que permite un asimiento firme a la persona que está a cargo de su cuidado al transferir al paciente o al ayudarlo en la ambulación (Ch. 33).

circunducción (circumduction) movimiento circular de una parte del cuerpo (Ch. 33).

cirrosis (cirrhosis) enfermedad hepática crónica en la cual un tejido con cicatrización y funcionamiento deficiente reemplaza al tejido hepático de funcionamiento normal (Ch. 22).

cistitis (cystitis) inflamación de la vejiga (Ch. 29).

citación (subpoena) orden por escrito que designa a una persona para que comparezca ante un tribunal bajo pena de recibir penalización por rebeldía (Ch. 7).

citología (cytology) ciencia que trata sobre la formación, la estructura y la función de las células (Ch. 39).

clamidia (chlamydia) bacteria que causa una de las enfermedades de transmisión sexual más frecuente (Ch. 26).

***Clasificación Internacional de Enfermedades, 9.ª Revisión, Modificación Clínica* (CIE-9-MC) *(International Classification of Diseases, 9th Revision, Clinical Modification* [ICD-9-CM])** códigos de diagnóstico estándar usados para identificar la enfermedad de un paciente. Se usa en la mayoría de los entornos de atención ambulatoria para codificar el formulario de reclamación y es reconocida por la mayoría de las compañías de seguros (Ch. 18).

claustrofobia (claustrophobia) miedo de estar confinado en algún espacio (Ch. 32).

CMS 1500 (08-05) (CMS 1500 [08-05]) antes conocido como el formulario HCFA 1500, que es el formulario de reclamación del seguro de salud para Medicare y Medicaid (Ch. 18).

cobalamina (cobalamina) vitamina B_{12} (Ch. 34).

codificar (codificación) (encode [encoding]) crear un mensaje para enviarlo (Ch. 4).

códigos agrupados (bundled codes) agrupamiento de varios servicios que están directamente relacionados con un procedimiento específico y se pagan como uno solo (Ch. 18).

códigos de desagregación (unbundling codes) se refiere a separar los componentes de un procedimiento e informarlos como códigos facturables con los cargos para aumentar las tasas de reembolso (Ch. 18).

códigos E (E codes) códigos ICD-9-CM para las causas externas de lesiones, intoxicación u otras reacciones adversas que explican cómo se produjo la lesión (Ch. 18).

códigos M (códigos morfológicos) (M codes [morphology codes]) se encuentran en el ICD-9-CM y se usan principalmente con registros de cáncer. Los códigos M identifican el comportamiento y el tipo celular de una neoplasia (Ch. 18).

códigos V (V codes) códigos de la Clasificación Internacional de Enfermedades, 9.ª Revisión, Modificación Clínica (ICD-9-CM, por sus siglas en inglés) que representan factores que influyen en el estado de salud de una persona o razones legítimas para comunicarse con el centro de salud cuando el paciente no tiene un diagnóstico definitivo o un síntoma activo de algún trastorno (Ch. 18).

coenzima (coenzyme) sustancia que potencia un catalizador (Ch. 34).

colecalciferol (cholecalciferol) vitamina D (Ch. 34).

colesterol (cholesterol) lípido esterol ampliamente distribuido en tejidos animales. El colesterol se produce en el hígado y es un componente de la bilis (Ch. 44).

colonoscopia (colonoscopy) examen visual del colon con una sonda con luz (Ch. 30).

colposcopia (colposcopy) examen visual de los tejidos vaginales y cervicales usando un colposcopio e indicado después de un Papanicolaou con resultado anormal. Se usa una lente con aumento y luces potentes (Ch. 26).

comedón (comedone) espinilla, generalmente resultado de glándulas sebáceas obstruidas por el acné (Ch. 30).

comercialización (marketing) proceso por el cual el proveedor de servicios comunica al consumidor el alcance y la calidad de los servicios. Las herramientas de comercialización incluyen relaciones públicas, folletos, seminarios de educación para pacientes y boletines (Ch. 45).

Comisión Conjunta (Joint Commission) anteriormente conocida como Comisión Conjunta para la Acreditación de Organizaciones de Cuidado de la Salud; comisión establecida para mejorar la calidad de la atención y de los servicios provistos en el entorno organizado de la atención médica a través de un proceso de acreditación voluntario (Ch. 16).

Comisión de Acreditación de Programas Educativos Asociados a la Salud (CAAHEP) (Commission on Accreditation of Allied Health Education Programs [CAAHEP]) entidad que acredita más de 2,000 programas educacionales en el campo de las profesiones de las ciencias de la salud (Ch. 1, 47).

comparador de rendimiento (benchmark) comparación entre diferentes organizaciones con respecto a la forma en que realizan las tareas, por ejemplo, informatización de oficinas, organización de sistemas de archivos y remuneración de empleados (Ch. 11, 45).

compensación (compensation) exageración de características para compensar una deficiencia o una desventaja real o imaginada (Ch. 4).

competencia (competency) legalmente apto o adecuado (Ch. 1).

composición (compounding) combinación de dos o más sustancias en proporciones definidas (Ch. 36).

compuestos organomercuriales (organomercurial) cualquier compuesto orgánico que contenga mercurio (Ch. 27).

computadora central (mainframe computer) sistema informático grande capaz de procesar volúmenes masivos de datos (Ch. 11).

computadora personal (PC) (personal computer [PC]) cualquier computadora que por su precio, tamaño y capacidad resulta útil para ser usada por un solo usuario, sin la intervención de operadores de computadora. También conocida como microcomputadora (Ch. 11).

comunicación de alto contexto (high-context communication) estilo de comunicación que depende en gran parte del lenguaje corporal, la referencia a los objetos del entorno y la fraseología culturalmente relevante para transmitir una idea. Depende de que el interlocutor conozca los acontecimientos relacionados a través de una asociación estrecha con el hablante o la cultura (Ch. 4).

comunicación de bajo contexto (low-context communication) estilo de comunicación que usa pocas expresiones idiomáticas del ambiente o cultura para trasmitir una idea o un concepto. Las ideas se explican explícitamente (Ch. 4).

comunicación terapéutica (therapeutic communication) uso de habilidades de comunicación profesionales específicas y bien definidas para crear una sensación de comodidad para los pacientes, aun cuando se debe dar información difícil o desagradable (Ch. 4).

condensador (condenser) en un microscopio, dirige un haz de luz desde la fuente hasta la muestra (Ch. 39).

condiloma (condylomata) lesión verrugosa de origen viral que se presenta en los genitales externos o en la región perianal (Ch. 26).

conexión en red (networking) conectar dos o más computadoras para compartir archivos y hardware. El sistema se llama red (Ch. 11).

confidencialidad (confidentiality) reglas éticas y legales con respecto a la privacidad del paciente (Ch. 16).

congruencia (congruency) cuando deben coincidir el mensaje verbal y el no verbal (Ch. 4).

consentimiento implícito (implied consent) consentimiento sobreentendido por el proveedor de atención médica, generalmente en una emergencia que pone en riesgo la vida del paciente. También ocurre de formas más sutiles en el entorno de atención médica; por ejemplo, cuando un paciente levanta las mangas voluntariamente para recibir una inyección (Ch. 7).

consentimiento informado (informed consent) consentimiento dado por el paciente en el que se le explica el procedimiento que se realizará, sus riesgos, los resultados esperados y las alternativas (Ch. 7, 31).

conservante (preservative) sustancia química que se agrega a los alimentos para mantenerlos frescos durante más tiempo o que se agrega a la orina para conservala para el análisis (Ch. 34, 42).

constreñirse (constrict) achicarse en diámetro (Ch. 40).

contabilidad (accounting) sistema de control de la situación financiera de un establecimiento y de los resultados económicos de sus actividades, que proporciona información para la toma de decisiones (Ch. 21).

contabilidad de caja (cash basis accounting) informa sobre los ingresos en el momento en que se cobra el dinero (Ch. 21).

contabilidad según el principio del devengo (accrual basis accounting) informa sobre los ingresos en el momento en que se generan los cargos (Ch. 21).

contaminación importante (gross contamination) presencia de material marcadamente infeccioso (Ch. 22).

contaminar (contaminate) ensuciar algo; a menudo se usa para describir un área estéril que pasó a ser "no estéril" o la exposición de un área limpia a un agente patógeno (Ch. 22, 31).

contrachoque (countershock) aplicación de una corriente eléctrica en el corazón directa o indirectamente para modificar una alteración en el ritmo cardíaco (Ch. 37).

contraer (contracting) adquirir una infección por patógenos (Ch. 22).

contraindicación (contraindication) cualquier síntoma o circunstancia que indica que el uso de un fármaco en particular es inapropiado cuando sí se recomendaría en otra situación. Por ejemplo, el uso de bebidas alcohólicas es una contraindicación cuando se receta el medicamento Flagyl® (Ch. 35).

contrato explícito (expressed contract) contrato escrito o verbal que describe específicamente lo que hará cada parte del contrato (Ch. 7).

contrato implícito (implied contract) contrato indicado por acciones en lugar de palabras (Ch. 7).

contravención (misdemeanor) delito menor; la definición de contravención varía según el estado. El castigo generalmente es libertad condicional o un tiempo de prestación de un servicio público y una multa (Ch. 7).

control de calidad (quality control) mediciones usadas para verificar el procesamiento de muestras de laboratorio. Incluye el uso correcto, el almacenamiento, la manipulación, la estabilidad, las fechas de vencimiento y las indicaciones para lograr precisión en las mediciones y exactitud en los procesos analíticos (Ch. 38, 42, 43).

control de infecciones (infection control) métodos para eliminar o reducir la transmisión de microorganismos infecciosos (Ch. 22).

controlador (driver) programa informático diseñado para convertir la salida de datos de un dispositivo a un formato compatible con otro dispositivo (Ch. 11).

controles de ingeniería (engineering controls) dispositivos físicos o mecánicos que aíslan o eliminan los riesgos para la salud del lugar de trabajo (Ch. 22).

controles de prácticas laborales (work practice controls) medidas usadas en el lugar de trabajo que constan de equipo físico y dispositivos mecánicos para controlar la exposición de los empleados a los patógenos transmitidos por la sangre y otros materiales potencialmente infecciosos. Algunos ejemplos son recipientes para desechar objetos filosos, instalaciones para lavarse las manos, equipo de protección personal y estaciones para lavarse los ojos (Ch. 22).

coordinación de beneficios (COB) (coordination of benefits [COB]) disposición de un contrato de seguro que limita los beneficios al 100% del costo (Ch. 17).

copago (co-payment) pago que se debe hacer cuando se consulta al proveedor (Ch. 17).

copia oculta (blind copy) protege la privacidad del correo electrónico. Los demás destinatarios no pueden identificar las otras personas que recibieron el mensaje transmitido (Ch. 15).

coriocarcinoma (choriocarcinoma) neoplasia maligna poco frecuente, generalmente del útero o de un embarazo ectópico. Se desconoce su causa exacta (Ch. 34, 37, 44).

coriza (coryza) inflamación aguda de las membranas de la nariz acompañada de secreción abundante (Ch. 22).

corrección (editing) proceso de manipular el texto para evitar imprecisiones e incoherencias dentro de un documento (Ch. 16).

corrector (editor) ver auditor (Ch. 16).

correo electrónico cifrado (encrypted Email) proceso para codificar el correo electrónico de modo de lograr una transmisión esencialmente segura (Ch. 12).

correo electrónico clínico (clinical Email) tipo de correo electrónico establecido usando protocolos definidos como medio de comunicación entre proveedores y pacientes establecidos (Ch. 12).

cortafuegos (firewall) dispositivo de hardware o programa de software diseñado para impedir el acceso no autorizado a un sistema informático (Ch. 11).

coseguro (coinsurance) porcentaje pagado por la empresa o que paga el asegurado (Ch. 17).

costo fijo (fixed cost) costo que no varía en total a medida que varía la cantidad de pacientes (Ch. 21).

costo variable (variable cost) costo que varía en proporción directa al volumen (Ch. 21).

creatinina (creatinine) producto de desecho formado en el músculo que se excreta por los riñones; aumenta en la sangre y la orina cuando la función renal es anormal (Ch. 42).

crédito (credit) reducción de un saldo deudor (Ch. 19).

crepitación (crepitation) sonido rechinante que se escucha al mover los extremos de un hueso fracturado (Ch. 9).

criocirugía (cryosurgery) destrucción de tejido mediante la aplicación de frío extremo, nitrato de plata y dióxido de carbono (Ch. 26).

crioconservación (cryopreservation) almacenamiento de materiales biológicos (esperma, embriones, tejido, plasma) a temperaturas sumamente frías para usarlos en otro momento (Ch. 8).

crioterapia (cryotherapy) uso del frío para tratar un problema físico (Ch. 33).

criptorquidia (cryptorchidism) testículo que no ha descendido (Ch. 28).

cristales (crystals) se encuentran en el sedimento normal de la orina y no tienen importancia en particular; se debe prestar atención a la presencia de cristales ya que pueden indicar estados de enfermedad (Ch. 42).

cuadrícula de Amsler (Amsler grid) cuadrícula de líneas usadas para determinar la degeneración macular (Ch. 30).

cuentas de ahorro del mercado monetario (money market savings accounts) cuentas bancarias que pagan una tasa de interés más alta (tasa del mercado monetario) que las cuentas de ahorros estándar y permiten librar una cantidad limitada de cheques (Ch. 19).

cuentas por cobrar (accounts receivable) importe adeudado a una empresa por servicios o productos suministrados (Ch. 19).

cuentas por pagar (accounts payable) suma adeudada por una empresa por servicios o productos recibidos (Ch. 19); también, compromiso no escrito de pagar a un proveedor por bienes o mercadería comprada a crédito o por un servicio prestado (Ch. 21).

cultivar (cultivate) estimular el crecimiento (Ch. 1).

cultivo por punción (stab culture) cultivo en el cual en el microorganismo es introducido para penetración profunda en medios sólidos en tubos (Ch. 43).

cultivo y sensibilidad (culture and sensitivity) a menudo se conoce por la sigla C&S del inglés. Se cultiva la muestra para que desarrolle bacterias y luego se la expone a diversos antibióticos para determinar a qué son sensibles (y resistentes) las bacterias (Ch. 39, 42).

cultivos (cultures) microorganismos cultivados en un medio de nutrientes (Ch. 42, 43).

cultura (culture) actitudes y comportamientos característicos de un grupo u organización social en particular (Ch. 4).

cumplimiento (compliance) observancia de los requisitos oficiales (Ch. 1).

curriculum vitae (résumé) hoja de datos resumidos escritos o recuento breve de aptitudes y de avance en la profesión elegida (Ch. 48).

curriculum vitae cronológico (chronologic résumé) formato de currículum vitae cuando se tiene experiencia laboral (Ch. 48).

curriculum vitae dirigido al objetivo (targeted résumé) formato de currículum vitae que se usa al concentrarse en un objetivo laboral específico y claro (Ch. 48).

curriculum vitae electrónico (e-résumé) el currículum vitae electrónico se puede enviar electrónicamente por correo electrónico, enviarse a las bolsas de trabajo en Internet o publicarse en páginas web (Ch. 48).

curriculum vitae funcional (functional résumé) formato de currículum vitae usado para destacar áreas de especialidad con sus logros y fortalezas (Ch. 48).

D

debe (debit) columna de la izquierda (Ch. 19).

débito (debit) se usa para asentar los gastos y la descripción de los servicios (Ch. 19).

declaración (deposition) testimonio oral dado por una persona en presencia de un taquígrafo judicial y abogados de ambas partes; a menudo se usa como parte del proceso de exhibición de pruebas (Ch. 7).

declaración de trabajo (work statement) descripción concisa del trabajo que planea realizar (Ch. 45).

declaraciones de logros (accomplishment statements) declaraciones que comienzan con un verbo de acción y describen brevemente lo que usted hizo y los resultados demostrables que se obtuvieron (Ch. 48).

declaraciones indirectas (indirect statements) medio de provocar una respuesta de un paciente transformando una pregunta en una declaración de interés (Ch. 4).

decodificar (decode) traducir a un idioma que sea fácil de entender; interpretar (Ch. 4).

deducible (deductible) importe de gastos médicos incurridos al que se debe llegar antes de que la póliza de seguro comience a pagar (Ch. 17).

degeneración macular (macular degeneration) degeneración de la mácula de la retina debido al envejecimiento; causa principal del deterioro visual en personas mayores de 50 años que dificulta las tareas minuciosas (Ch. 29).

delito mayor (felony) delito grave, como homicidio, hurto (robo de grandes sumas de dinero), agresión violenta y violación (Ch. 7).

demandado (defendant) persona que contesta una demanda presentada en un litigio (Ch. 7).

demandante (plaintiff) persona que presenta cargos en un litigio (Ch. 7).

demencia (dementia) deterioro de la función intelectual que es progresivo e interfiere en las actividades normales (Ch. 29).

densidad específica (specific gravity) relación entre el peso de un volumen dado de una sustancia con el peso del mismo volumen de agua destilada a la misma temperatura; prueba que a menudo se realiza durante el examen físico del análisis de orina (también puede aparecer en la prueba de tira reactiva) (Ch. 42).

derecho administrativo (administrative law) establece los organismos que tienen la facultad de dictar leyes y promulgar reglamentaciones (Ch. 7).

derecho civil (civil law) leyes relacionadas con actos entre personas (Ch. 7).

derecho constitucional (constitutional law) consiste en leyes establecidas por las constituciones de los Estados Unidos o de los estados individuales (Ch. 7).

derecho consuetudinario (common law) referente a las leyes desarrolladas en Inglaterra y Francia e introducidas en los Estados Unidos por los primeros colonos; a veces llamada derecho de creación judicial (Ch. 7).

derecho contractual (contract law) leyes que se refieren a los contratos vinculantes entre personas y entidades (Ch. 7).

derecho de responsabilidad civil (tort law) leyes que se originan en los agravios o en los actos ilegítimos en los que una persona provoca daños a otra persona (Ch. 7).

derecho estatutario (statutory law) se refiere al cuerpo de leyes establecidas por los estados (Ch. 7).

derecho penal (criminal law) leyes relacionadas con los delitos cometidos contra el bienestar y la seguridad de la sociedad en su conjunto (Ch. 7).

derivado proteico purificado (DPP) (purified protein derivative [PPD]) filtrado obtenido de los cultivos de *Mycobacterium* usados para pruebas intradérmicas de tuberculosis (Ch. 44).

dermatofitos (dermatophytes) categoría de hongos que provocan infecciones en el cabello, la piel y las uñas (Ch. 43).

descripción del trabajo (job description) descripción de tareas, obligaciones y responsabilidades para cada cargo en la oficina (Ch. 46).

desfibrilación (defibrillation) detener la fibrilación del corazón usando fármacos o por medios físicos (Ch. 37).

desfibrilador (defibrillator) equipo que aplica una corriente eléctrica para modificar una alteración del ritmo cardíaco (Ch. 37).

desfibrilador externo automatizado (DEA) (automated external defibrillator [AED]) dispositivo automático, portátil y autónomo con instrucciones de voz sobre el uso para personas con paro cardíaco. Se utiliza externamente para aplicar electrónicamente una "descarga eléctrica" al miocardio y hacer que se contraiga nuevamente. Igual que la cardioversión (Ch. 9).

desfragmentación (defragmentation) reorganización de la información en un disco duro para guardar archivos como unidades continuas en vez de paquetes pequeños. Una computadora con poca fragmentación de archivos funcionará a mayor velocidad (Ch. 11).

desinfección (disinfection) uso de productos químicos o agua hirviendo para liberar a un objeto de materiales infecciosos pero no de sus esporas (Ch. 22).

deslucido (lackluster) opaco, que le falta brillo (Ch. 9).

desmielinización (demyelination) destrucción de la vaina de mielina, a menudo un factor observado en la esclerosis múltiple (Ch. 30).

desoxigenada (deoxygenated) sangre con alto contenido de dióxido de carbono y bajo contenido de oxígeno que se bombea del corazón a los pulmones, donde el dióxido de carbono se intercambia por oxígeno (Ch. 37).

despido involuntario (involuntary dismissal) desvinculación del empleo debido a un desempeño laboral deficiente o a la violación de las políticas de la oficina (Ch. 46).

desplazamiento (displacement) trasladar sentimientos negativos a algo o alguien sin tener en cuenta la situación (Ch. 4).

despolarizar (depolarize) proceso para reducir hasta un estado no polarizado. Así, se mejora la generación de una corriente eléctrica. La actividad eléctrica generada cuando se contraen las aurículas o los ventrículos (Ch. 37).

desprendimiento de la placenta (placenta abruptio) separación repentina y abrupta de la placenta de la pared uterina (Ch. 26).

destreza (dexterity) habilidad y facilidad para usar las manos (Ch. 1).

detritos (debris) restos de células o tejidos descompuestos o dañados (Ch. 22).

diabetes gestacional (gestational diabetes) diabetes que se manifiesta clínicamente por primera vez durante el embarazo. Por lo general, desaparece después del parto (Ch. 26).

diabetes mellitus (diabetes mellitus) trastorno crónico del metabolismo de los carbohidratos que se caracteriza por hiperglucemia y que es resultado de la producción o el uso inadecuado de la insulina (Ch. 44).

diafragma (diaphragm) lente u otro objeto que se abre y se cierra para aumentar o disminuir la cantidad de luz sobre el objeto que se ilumina. Se refiere a un diafragma óptico como en un microscopio (el diafragma se usa para el control de natalidad y también es el músculo respiratorio principal) (Ch. 39).

diagnóstico (diagnosis) determinación de una enfermedad o afección (Ch. 39).

diagnóstico clínico (clinical diagnosis) identificación de una enfermedad por antecedentes, estudios de laboratorio y síntomas (Ch. 23, 39).

diagnóstico diferencial (differential diagnosis) diagnóstico basado en la comparación de síntomas de enfermedades similares (Ch. 39).

diástole (diastole) un componente de la medición de la presión arterial que representa la presión más baja durante el ciclo cardíaco; fuerza ejercida sobre las paredes arteriales durante la relajación cardíaca (Ch. 24, 37).

diatermia (diathermy) uso terapéutico de corriente de alta frecuencia para generar calor dentro de una parte del cuerpo sin dañar los tejidos (Ch. 33).

dicción (enunciation) hablar con claridad y buena expresión (Ch. 12).

dietilestilbestrol (DES) (diethylstilbestrol [DES]) hormona sintética usada terapéuticamente en trastornos menopáusicos. No se debe administrar durante el embarazo. Se la ha relacionado con tumores malignos cérvicovaginales en hijas de madres que tomaron la hormona para tratar una amenaza de aborto. DES ha sido relacionado con enfermedades reproductivas en hombres cuyas madres tomaron la hormona durante el embarazo (Ch. 26).

digestión (digestion) descomposición de los alimentos en partículas más pequeñas. Puede ser física o química (Ch. 34).

dilatación (dilation) expansión de un orificio u órgano (Ch. 26).

dilatarse (dilate) agrandarse en diámetro (Ch. 40).

diploma (diploma) documento en el consta la graduación de una institución educativa o el título que ésta otorga (Ch. 1).

directiva a los médicos (physician's directive) otro nombre para indicar el testamento en vida (Ch. 6).

disco compacto (CD) (compact disk [CD]) ver disco óptico (Ch. 11).

disco de video digital/disco versátil digital (DVD) (digital video disk/digital versatile disk [DVD]) disco óptico con capacidad para 4.7 a 9.0 gigabytes de datos, según el formato (Ch. 11).

disco duro (hard drive) dispositivo de almacenamiento no volátil que conserva la información almacenada por medio de un sistema de grabación magnética digital en discos metálicos que giran a gran velocidad. La capacidad es de aproximadamente 100GB. El dispositivo puede estár instalado permanente dentro de la carcasa de la computadora o ser portátil (Ch. 11).

disco magnético (magnetic drive) dispositivo de almacenamiento de memoria que usa un recubrimiento magnético en una capa férrea

disco óptico (optical disk) dispositivo de almacenamiento de datos portátil y transferible de solo lectura o de lectura y escritura. A veces se lo denomina CD-ROM, CD-RW o disco compacto. Tiene capacidad de 1 a 8 gigabytes de datos. Se requiere una unidad óptica para leer y escribir los datos del disco (Ch. 11).

disentería amébica (amoebic dysentery) enfermedad intestinal infecciosa provocada por amebas y caracterizada por inflamación de la membrana mucosa del colon (Ch. 22).

dismenorrea (dysmenorrhea) menstruaciones dolorosas (Ch. 26).

disnea (dyspnea) falta de aire o dificultad para respirar (Ch. 24).

dispareunia (dyspareunia) coito doloroso (Ch. 26).

displasia (dysplasia) desarrollo anormal de tejido (Ch. 26).

dispositivo de almacenamiento de datos (data storage device) dispositivo que puede guardar datos digitales en forma permanente o temporal (Ch. 11).

dispositivo de entrada (input device) dispositivo usado para ingresar datos en una computadora (Ch. 11).

dispositivo de punto de servicio (POS) (point-of-service [POS] device) dispositivo que permite la comunicación directa entre un consultorio médico y la computadora del plan de atención médica (Ch. 18).

dispositivo de salida (output device) dispositivo usado para sacar información de una computadora. Incluye impresoras, faxes, unidades de almacenamiento de datos, pantallas y trazadores (Ch. 11).

distensión (strain) lesión en el tejido blando entre las articulaciones que consiste en el desgarro de músculos o tendones. Las distensiones a menudo se presentan en el cuello, la espalda o los músculos de los muslos (Ch. 9).

disuria (dysuria) dolor o dificultad al orinar (Ch. 30).

diurético (diuretic) sustancia por cuya acción el riñón reabsorbe menos agua y, por lo tanto, el agua se excreta del cuerpo (Ch. 34).

doctrina (doctrine) principio de ley establecido a través de decisiones pasadas (Ch. 7).

documentación (documentation) material escrito que acompaña la compra de software y que incluye la información necesaria para usar el software correctamente; a veces se conoce como manual (Ch. 11, 22); también, que proporciona apoyo exacto a través de información escrita (Ch. 22).

doppler (doppler) técnica no invasiva usada junto con la ecografía para evaluar el flujo sanguíneo a través de las venas y arterias principales de los brazos, las piernas y el cuello. Puede revelar coágulos de sangre u obstrucciones en el flujo sanguíneo (Ch. 32).

dorsiflexión (dorsiflexion) movimiento del pie hacia arriba a la altura de la articulación del tobillo (Ch. 33).

dosificar (dispense) preparar y dar un medicamento para que se tome posteriormente (Ch. 7, 36, 36).

dosímetro (dosimeter) dispositivo para medir la radiación generada (Ch. 32).

dosis unitaria (unit dose) cantidad medida previamente de medicamento, envasada individualmente para cada dosis (Ch. 36).

E

eclampsia (eclampsia) complicación del embarazo que incluye edema general, hipertensión, proteinuria y convulsiones (Ch. 26).

ecocardiograma (echocardiogram) método de diagnóstico no invasivo que usa el ultrasonido para visualizar la estructura cardíaca interna, incluidas las válvulas (Ch. 32).

ecografía (ultrasonography) proceso de colocar un transductor manual contra una parte del cuerpo que se desea examinar. El transductor envía ondas de sonido a través de la piel y de los diversos órganos internos. Cuando se forman los ecos y regresan, el transductor los convierte en energía eléctrica. Esta energía se transforma en una imagen en un monitor o se imprime en papel. Se pueden tomar fotografías de las imágenes que pueden ser parte del registro permanente del paciente (Ch. 26, 37).

ecografista (sonographer) persona capacitada profesionalmente para realizar un examen de ecografía (Ch. 37).

edema pulmonar (pulmonary edema) acumulación de líquido seroso en las vesículas aéreas y los tejidos intersticiales de los pulmones (Ch. 38).

edematoso (edematous) acumulación anormal de líquidos en los tejidos que produce inflamación (Ch. 40).

effleurage (effleurage) masaje que emplea golpes prolongados o suaves (Ch. 33).

electrocardiografía (electrocardiography) proceso para registrar la actividad eléctrica que se origina en el corazón (Ch. 37).

electrocardiógrafo (electrocardiograph) instrumento para registrar la actividad eléctrica del corazón (Ch. 37).

electrocardiograma (electrocardiogram) registro de la actividad cardíaca del corazón que muestra ondas P, QRS y T (Ch. 37).

electrococleografía (electrocochleography) herramienta de diagnóstico de ayuda en el diagnóstico de la enfermedad de Meniere. Registra la actividad eléctrica del oído interno en respuesta al sonido (Ch. 30).

electrodo (electrode) también conocido como sensor. Se usa para conducir electricidad del cuerpo al electrocardiógrafo (Ch. 37).

electrolito (electrolyte) sustancias que conducen electricidad cuyos componentes son importantes para mantener el equilibrio acidobásico y de líquidos (Ch. 34, 37, 39).

elocuente (articulating) que se expresa con claridad y con fluidez (Ch. 12).

emaciación (emaciation) estado de extrema delgadez (Ch. 30).

embarazo ectópico (ectopic pregnancy) implementación del óvulo fecundado fuera de la cavidad uterina (Ch. 26, 44).

empatía (empathy) capacidad de percibir y entender los sentimientos, las emociones y los comportamientos de otra persona, y de percibir la importancia y el significado que tienen para la otra persona (Ch. 1, 29).

empresa de propiedad privada (proprietary) establecimiento de propiedad y administración privada; organización con fines de lucro (Ch. 1).

endometriosis (endometriosis) invasión por parte de tejido similar al endometrio en diversas zonas de la cavidad pélvica y en otras partes (Ch. 26).

endoscopia (endoscopy) examen visual de las cavidades corporales con una sonda con luz (Ch. 22).

enfermedad endémica (endemic) enfermedad que se presenta continuamente o en ciclos con una cierta cantidad de casos previstos durante un período determinado (Ch. 22).

enfermedad inflamatoria pélvica (pelvic inflammatory disease) infección del útero, las trompas de Falopio y las estructuras pélvicas adyacentes; las causas más comunes son gonorrea y clamidia; se propaga como las enfermedades de transmisión sexual (Ch. 26).

enfisema (emphysema) enfermedad pulmonar crónica que se caracteriza por dilatación y daño alveolar (Ch. 24).

enfoque en el tiempo (time focus) define el período de tiempo que es importante para una persona y hacia el cual se dirigen y se orientan las acciones de una persona (Ch. 4).

enrutador automático (ARU) (automated routing unit [ARU]) sistema telefónico que responde a una llamada y usa una voz grabada para identificar departamentos o servicios (Ch. 12).

ensayo (assay) análisis de una sustancia para determinar sus componentes y la proporción relativa de cada uno (Ch. 39).

entorno de atención ambulatoria (ambulatory care setting) entorno de atención de la salud en la que se brindan servicios a personas que no están hospitalizadas. *Ambulatorio* proviene del latín y significa "que puede caminar". Los ejemplos incluyen el consultorio de un proveedor único, el ejercicio profesional grupal, el centro de atención de urgencias y la organización de mantenimiento de la salud (Ch. 1, 2).

entrevista (interview) reunión en la que usted y el entrevistador hablan sobre las oportunidades laborales y las fortalezas que puede aportar a la organización (Ch. 48).

entrevista de salida (exit interview) oportunidad para que los empleados que abandonan la empresa den sus opiniones positivas y negativas del puesto de trabajo y del establecimiento (Ch. 46).

eosinófilos (eosinophil) glóbulo blanco granulocítico con gránulos que se tiñen de rojo con eosina en el citoplasma. Su número es elevado en casos de alergias (Ch. 41).

epidemia (epidemic) enfermedad infecciosa que ataca a muchas personas al mismo tiempo en el mismo lugar geográfico (Ch. 22).

epidemiología (epidemiology) campo de la ciencia que estudia los antecedentes, las causas y los patrones de enfermedades infecciosas (Ch. 22).

epinefrina (epinephrine) usada para tratar reacciones alérgicas (Ch. 9); también, hormona llamada también adrenalina. La epinefrina se fabrica como sustancia química (preparado farmacéutico) y a menudo se mezcla con anestésicos locales para usar como vasoconstrictor en cirugías menores (Ch. 31).

epistaxis (epistaxis) hemorragia nasal (Ch. 22).

equilibrio ácido-básico (acid/base balance) estado que se presenta cuando la tasa neta a la cual el cuerpo produce ácidos o bases es igual a la tasa neta a la cual se excretan los ácidos o las bases (Ch. 42).

ergonomía (ergonomics) estudio científico del trabajo y del espacio, incluidos los factores que afectan la productividad de los empleados y su salud (Ch. 11).

eritema (erythema) enrojecimiento o inflamación de la piel o de las membranas mucosas producto de la dilatación y de la congestión de los capilares superficiales (Ch. 30).

eritrocito (erythrocyte) glóbulo rojo, uno de los componentes de la sangre (Ch. 40, 41).

eritropoyetina (erythropoietin) hormona causante de la producción de nuevos glóbulos rojos (Ch. 41).

escala de valores relativos basada en recursos (RBRVS) (resource-based relative value scale [RBRVS]) base para el esquema de tarifas de Medicare (Ch. 17).

esclerodermia (scleroderma) enfermedad que avanza lentamente y que se caracteriza por el depósito de tejido conectivo fibroso en la piel y los órganos internos (Ch. 25).

escorbuto (scurvy) deficiencia de vitamina C caracterizada por la formación anormal de huesos y dientes. Pueden aparecer signos de hemorragia como hematomas (Ch. 34).

escribano público (notary public) persona con la capacidad legal para dar fe y certificar documentos; puede tomar declaraciones juradas (Ch. 19).

escucha activa (active listening) mensaje recibido que se vuelve a parafrasear al remitente para verificar que se ha decodificado el mensaje correcto (Ch. 4).

esguince (sprain) lesión en una articulación, a menudo el tobillo, la rodilla o la muñeca, en la que se desgarran los ligamentos. La mayoría de los esguinces son menores y se curan rápidamente, pero otros pueden ser más graves, con inflamación, y no curarse adecuadamente si el paciente sigue aplicando presión sobre la articulación desgarrada (Ch. 9).

especie (species) segundo nombre griego o latino dado a los microorganismos; el nombre de la especie no va con mayúscula (Ch. 43).

Especialista Administrativo Médico Certificado (CMAS) (Certified Medical Administrative Specialist [CMAS]) certificación de la AMT para especialista administrativo médico (Ch. 47).

espermatogénesis (spermatogenesis) la formación de esperma maduro (Ch. 28).

espirometría (spirometry) prueba para medir la capacidad respiratoria de los pulmones (Ch. 30).

esporas (spores) estado inactivo de algunas bacterias en el cual se encapsulan en proteínas. El encapsulamiento las protege del calor, de las sustancias químicas, del congelamiento, de la desecación y de la radiación. Las esporas pueden vivir decenas de miles de años sin nutrientes. Cuando se colocan en suelo fértil (como el tejido humano), pueden activarse y crecer. El tétanos es un tipo de bacteria que crea esporas (Ch. 43).

esputo (sputum) sustancia de las vías respiratorias que se expulsa con la tos (Ch. 22).

esqueleto apendicular (appendicular skeleton) esqueleto formado por los cinturones pectoral y pélvico y las extremidades superiores e inferiores. El cinturón pélvico conecta las extremidades superiores con el tronco (Ch. 30).

esqueleto axial (axial skeleton) formado por huesos que se encuentran alrededor del centro del cuerpo (Ch. 30).

establecimiento de atención administrada (managed care operation) cualquier entorno o sistema de prestación de atención médica diseñado para reducir el costo de la atención y, al mismo tiempo, proveer acceso a ella (Ch. 2).

estado asmático (status asthmaticus) episodio severo de asma que no responde al tratamiento común (Ch. 36).

estado de resultados (income statement) estado contable que muestra las ganancias o las pérdidas netas (Ch. 21).

estampada (swaged) aguja quirúrgica adherida a un tramo de material de sutura durante la costura (Ch. 31).

"estar desprotegido" ("going bare") se dice del proveedor que no contrata seguro por responsabilidad profesional (Ch. 45).

estenosis (strictures) estrechamiento de una estructura de forma tubular, como el esófago o la uretra (Ch. 31).

esterasa leucocitaria (leukocyte esterase) prueba sobre una tira reactiva que indica la presencia de glóbulos blancos en las vías urinarias (Ch. 42).

estertores (rales) ruido anormal burbujeante o crujiente que se escucha en la auscultación durante la inspiración (Ch. 24).

estertoroso (stertorous) ruido de ronquido que se escucha cuando la persona tiene dificultad para respirar (Ch. 24).

estigma (stigma) condición social marcada por la subvaloración o la degradación de personas que, por una deformidad o una discapacidad, no son vistas como capaces de cumplir roles sociales valorados (Ch. 26).

estilete (stylus) cable delgado caliente del electrocardiógrafo que derrite la cera del papel del ECG durante el registro (Ch. 37).

estomatitis (stomatitis) inflamación de la boca relacionada con la quimioterapia. Puede incluir hinchazón, enrojecimiento, halitosis y ulceraciones (Ch. 32).

estrabismo (strabismus) trastorno de la vista en el cual los ejes ópticos no se pueden dirigir al mismo objeto (bizquera) (Ch. 30).

estrés (stress) respuesta del cuerpo a los cambios; se puede manifestar en una variedad de formas, incluidos los cambios en la presión arterial, la frecuencia cardíaca y la aparición de dolores de cabeza (Ch. 5).

estridor (stridor) ruido como de graznido que se escucha en la inspiración, resultado de una obstrucción en las vías aéreas superiores (Ch. 24).

Ethernet (Ethernet) se refiere a la conexión en red de computadoras usando conductores metálicos o cables físicos (Ch. 11).

ética (ethics) se define en términos de lo que se considera moralmente bien o mal; la ética varía según la persona y a menudo se define mediante un código o credo como el Código de Ética de la AAMA (Ch. 8).

etiqueta (etiquette) modales, cortesía, comportamiento apropiado (Ch. 12).

eupnea (eupnea) respiración normal (Ch. 24).

evaluación (evaluation) valoración del desempeño laboral de un empleado (Ch. 46).

eversión (eversion) rotación de una parte del cuerpo hacia afuera (Ch. 33).

examen bimanual (bimanual examination) examen realizado por el proveedor usando ambas manos para examinar los órganos pélvicos internos. Se introducen dos dedos de una mano en la vagina y la otra mano presiona el exterior de la pared abdominal. De este modo, se puede determinar la forma, la consistencia y la posición de los órganos pélvicos (Ch. 26).

examen de certificación (certification examination) medio estandarizado de evaluar la competencia del asistente médico (Ch. 47).

examen macroscópico (gross examination) ver muestras a simple vista (Ch. 16).

examen microscópico (microscopic examination) visualizar una muestra con la ayuda del microscopio (Ch. 16).

exclusión (exclusion) enfermedad o afección específica enumerada en una póliza de seguro que no cubre dicha póliza (Ch. 17).

excoriación (excoriated) abrasión de la epidermis por traumatismo, sustancias químicas, quemaduras u otras causas (Ch. 22).

excreción (excretion) sustancia de desecho. La eliminación de los productos de desecho del cuerpo (Ch. 22, 38).

exfoliación (exfoliated) el desprendimiento de algo, por ejemplo células cervicales (Ch. 26).

exhibición de pruebas (discovery) momento en que ambas partes tienen acceso a toda la información y la evidencia relacionada con un caso; después del proceso de citación (Ch. 7).

expectorar (expectorate) acto de toser material y expulsarlo desde las vías aéreas que conducen a los pulmones (Ch. 22, 43).

explicación de beneficios (EDB) (explanation of benefits [EOB]) informe del seguro que se envía con los pagos de reclamaciones para explicar el reembolso de la compañía de seguros (Ch. 19).

explícito (explicit) totalmente revelado o expresado sin ser ambiguo o equívoco, que no deja dudas sobre su intención (Ch. 9).

extensión (extension) enderezamiento de una parte del cuerpo (Ch. 33).

extracelular (extracellular) relacionado con el entorno fuera de una célula del cuerpo (Ch. 34).

exudado (exudate) líquido acumulado en una cavidad; supuración de pus; sustancia que atraviesa las paredes de los vasos hacia el tejido contiguo (Ch. 22, 27, 31).

F

facilitar (facilitate) hacer que una acción o un proceso sean más fáciles (Ch. 1).

facoemulsificación (phacoemulsification) tratamiento para las cataratas. Se usa un dispositivo ultrasónico para desintegrar la catarata del cristalino del ojo, que luego se aspira y se retira (Ch. 30).

factor Rh (Rh factor) factor sanguíneo que indica la presencia o la ausencia del antígeno Rh en la superficie de los eritrocitos humanos (Ch. 44).

factores estresantes (stressors) exigencias de cambio que producen estrés (Ch. 5).

Factura Uniforme 04 (UB04) (Uniform Bill 04 [UB04]) formulario de facturación único que usan ampliamente los centros de cuidados agudos para procesar los reclamos de hospitalización y atención ambulatoria (Ch. 18).

farmacología (pharmacology) estudio de los fármacos; ciencia que se ocupa de la historia, el origen, las fuentes, las propiedades físicas y químicas, y los usos de los fármacos y sus efectos en los organismos vivos (Ch. 35).

farmacopea (pharmacopoeia) libro que describe los fármacos y su preparación, o una recopilación o inventario de fármacos (Ch. 3).

fax (facsímil) (fax [facsimile]) máquina que envía documentos de un lugar a otro a través de líneas telefónicas (Ch. 12).

febril (febrile) que tiene fiebre (Ch. 24).

fechoría (malfeasance) conducta ilegal o contraria a las obligaciones de un funcionario (Ch. 7).

fenestrado (fenestrated) que tiene orificios. Paño fenestrado y estéril que se usa en cirugía. Tiene un orificio (redondo) para exponer solamente la zona quirúrgica. El resto del paño cubre al paciente y es una zona estéril (Ch. 31).

fenilcetonuria (FCU) (phenylketonuria [PKU]) enfermedad hereditaria causada por la incapacidad del cuerpo de oxidar el aminoácido fenilalanina. Si no se descubre y se trata a tiempo, puede producirse daño cerebral y un consecuente retraso mental grave (Ch. 27, 44).

férula (splint) cualquier dispositivo para inmovilizar una parte del cuerpo. Usado con frecuencia por el personal del Servicio de Emergencias Médicas (EMS, por sus siglas en inglés) (Ch. 9).

fianza (bond) acuerdo vinculante con un empleado por el cual se garantiza la recuperación de una pérdida financiera en el caso de que se roben o se malversen fondos (Ch. 45).

fibroplasia retrolenticular (retrolental fibroplasia) enfermedad de los vasos sanguíneos de la retina en el recién nacido (Ch. 36).

fiebre amarilla (yellow fever) enfermedad infecciosa aguda en la que una persona presenta ictericia, vómitos, hemorragias y fiebre; provocada principalmente por los mosquitos (Ch. 3).

fitomedicinas (phytomedicines) hierbas usadas como plantas medicinales. Contienen material derivado de plantas como su principio activo (Ch. 36).

flebotomía (phlebotomy) proceso para recolectar sangre (Ch. 22, 40).

flexión (flexion) acción de doblar una parte del cuerpo (Ch. 33).

flexión plantar (plantar flexion) movimiento descendente del pie a la altura del tobillo (Ch. 33).

flora normal (normal flora) microorganismos que normalmente están presentes en un lugar específico (Ch. 22, 43).

fluido (fluent) capaz de escribir o hablar un idioma en forma fácil o corriente (Ch. 12).

fluoroscopio (fluoroscope) dispositivo que consiste en una pantalla; se monta en forma separada o con un tubo de rayos X que muestra imágenes de objetos interpuestos entre la mesa y la pantalla (Ch. 32).

fómite (fomite) sustancia que absorbe y transmite material infeccioso; por ejemplo, elementos contaminados como los equipos (Ch. 22).

fontanela (fontanel) espacio blando que se encuentra entre los huesos del cráneo del feto, del recién nacido y del bebé (Ch. 27).

forense (forensic) aplicar conocimiento cinetífico a asuntos legales (Ch. 38).

formaldehído (formaldehyde) gas incoloro combinado con metanol y usado como solución, por ejemplo, como desinfectante, astringente o conservante de piezas histológicas (Ch. 38).

formalina (formalin) solución acuosa de formaldehído al 37% (Ch. 26).

formar redes de contactos (networking) proceso por el cual personas de intereses similares intercambian información en relaciones sociales, comerciales o profesionales (Ch. 46).

formulario de rechazo (declination form) negativa formal por escrito (Ch. 22).

formulario de solicitud (application form) formulario diseñado por un posible empleador para recabar información relacionada con las aptitudes, la educación y la experiencia en el empleo (Ch. 48).

formulario de visita (encounter form) antes conocido como comprobante de servicio o superfactura. Se entrega una copia del formulario de visita al paciente después de consultar al proveedor. Este formulario identifica los procedimientos realizados, los diagnósticos, las tarifas y cuándo debe regresar (Ch. 18, 19).

forúnculo (furuncle) infección cutánea, estafilocócica, supurante y localizada que se origina en una glándula o folículo piloso (Ch. 30).

fractura (fracture) rotura de un hueso. Hay varios tipos de fracturas, pero todas se clasifican como fractura abierta o cerrada (Ch. 9).

fractura cerrada (closed fracture) fractura sin complicaciones en la cual el hueso no atraviesa la piel (Ch. 30).

fraude (fraud) tergiversación deliberada de los hechos (Ch. 17).

frecuencia (frequency) que orina a menudo (Ch. 30).

frenillo (frenulum) de la lengua, pliegue de membrana mucosa ubicado debajo de la lengua y que une la lengua a la base de la boca (Ch. 24).

friable (friable) que se quiebra fácilmente (Ch. 31).

Fuerza de Tareas para la Elaboración de Exámenes (TFTC) (Task Force for Test Construction [TFTC]) comisión de profesionales cuya responsabilidad es actualizar el examen de los Asistentes Médicos Certificados (CMA, por sus siglas en inglés) anualmente para reflejar los cambios en las responsabilidades de asistentes médicos y para incluir nuevos desarrollos en la tecnología y los conocimientos médicos (Ch. 47).

fulgurado (fulgarated) destruido por la corriente eléctrica (Ch. 26).

funcionamiento cognitivo (cognitive functioning) conocimiento con percepción, razonamiento, juicio, intuición y memoria (Ch. 29).

G

galio (gallium) metal no tóxico, de aspecto similar al mercurio, que se puede usar en lugar de éste para los termómetros usados para medir la fiebre. Todavía no está ampliamente disponible para su uso (Ch. 24).

galvanómetro (galvanometer) mecanismo del electrocardiógrafo que transforma el voltaje en un movimiento mecánico para poder registrarlo (Ch. 37).

gammagrafía con talio (thallium scan) elemento químico que se administra en forma intravenosa y se usa en las pruebas de esfuerzo cardíaco. El radioisótopo se ubica en el miocardio y un escáner capta la distribución del talio y puede identificar obstrucciones en las arterias coronarias. Prueba exacta para enfermedades de las arterias coronarias (Ch. 37).

garante (guarantor) persona identificada como responsable del pago de la factura (Ch. 19).

gel separador tixotrópico (thixotropic separator gel) gel que puede formar una interfaz entre las células y la parte líquida de la sangre como resultado de la centrifugación (Ch. 40).

género (genus) primer nombre griego o latino dado a un microorganismo; siempre se escribe la primera letra con mayúscula (Ch. 43).

genitales (genitalia) órganos reproductivos, internos y externos (Ch. 26).

gerente autoritario (authoritarian manager) opera bajo la premisa de que la mayoría de los empleados no pueden hacer su aporte sin que se les ordene hacerlo (Ch. 45).

gerente participativo (participatory manager) opera bajo la premisa de que el empleado puede y quiere hacer un buen trabajo (Ch. 45).

geriatría (geriatrics) rama de la medicina que se ocupa de los problemas del envejecimiento (Ch. 29).

gerontología (gerontology) estudio científico de los problemas relacionados con el envejecimiento (Ch. 29).

gestación (gestation) período de desarrollo desde la fertilización al nacimiento (Ch. 26).

gestión de riesgos (risk management) técnicas respetadas en el entorno de atención ambulatoria que mantienen en la mayor medida posible la seguridad para el paciente de la práctica, de su entorno y de los procedimientos. Una gestión de riesgos adecuada también reduce la posibilidad de negligencia y los resultantes juicios por agravios y mala praxis (Ch. 7, 9, 16, 45).

gestión itinerante (MBWA) (management by walking around [MBWA]) técnica para mantener a los gerentes informados sobre el estado de su organización (Ch. 45).

gestos/ademanes (gestures/mannerisms) movimiento de diversas partes del cuerpo durante la comunicación (Ch. 4).

glándula de Bartolino (Bartholin gland) una de dos glándulas mucosas pequeñas ubicadas en el vestíbulo de la vagina en la base de los labios mayores (Ch. 26).

glicógeno (glycogen) forma de hidrato de carbono que se usa para almacenar azúcar en el cuerpo (Ch. 34).

glucosa (glucose) azúcar simple que es la fuente principal de energía del cuerpo humano; el control de los niveles de glucosa en sangre en la orina y la sangre es una prueba de diagnóstico fundamental para la diabetes y otros trastornos; también es una prueba con una tira reactiva (Ch. 39, 42).

glucosuria (glucosuria) presencia de glucosa en la orina (también es correcto decir glicosuria) (Ch. 42).

gonadotropina coriónica humana (hCG) (human chorionic gonadotropin [hCG]) hormona secretada por el trofoblasto después de la fertilización del óvulo. Se puede detectar en la sangre y en la orina de mujeres embarazadas (Ch. 26, 44).

goniometría (goniometry) medición del movimiento articular (Ch. 33).

goniómetro (goniometer) instrumento usado para medir el ángulo de la amplitud de movimiento que tiene una articulación (Ch. 33).

grasa saturada (saturated fat) grasas que se caracterizan por ser sólidas a temperatura ambiente, se encuentran por lo general en productos de origen animal, como la mantequilla, leche, crema y huevos, como también en los aceites de palma y coco (Ch. 34).

gravidez (gravidity) cantidad total de embarazos que ha tenido una mujer, independientemente de la duración, incluido el actual (Ch. 26).

grupo sanguíneo ABO (ABO blood group) sistema de antígenos genéticamente determinados que se encuentra en la superficie de los eritrocitos. La población puede dividirse en cuatro grupos sanguíneos ABO: A, B, AB y O (Ch. 44).

H

haber (credit) columna usada para asentar pagos (Ch. 19).

habilidades directas (direct skills) habilidades específicas del trabajo. La habilidad para tomar una lectura de presión arterial sería específica del campo médico (Ch. 48).

habilidades transferibles (transferable skills) habilidades que se usarían en una serie de ocupaciones diferentes y no relacionadas. Saber mecanografía es un ejemplo de habilidad transferible. Pueden emplearla una secretaria, el empleado que ingresa datos, el asistente médico o el fabricante de ropa (Ch. 48).

hacer una copia de seguridad (backup) copiar o guardar datos en un lugar seguro para evitar perderlos en el caso de un desastre (Ch. 11).

hardware (hardware) equipo físico que usa el sistema informático para procesar los datos (Ch. 11).

hematocrito (hematocrit) porcentaje de glóbulos rojos dentro de una muestra de sangre entera anticoagulada (Ch. 41).

hematología (hematology) estudio de la sangre y de los tejidos que forman la sangre (Ch. 39, 41).

hematoma (hematoma) un moretón de tamaño considerable, acumulación de sangre alrededor de la zona de venopunción, durante o después de ésta, provocada por el derrame de sangre del lugar en donde la aguja penetró la vena (Ch. 31, 40).

hematopoyesis (hematopoiesis) formación de células sanguíneas (Ch. 41).

hematuria (hematuria) presencia anormal de sangre en la orina, síntoma de muchos trastornos del sistema genitourinario y de enfermedades renales (Ch. 30, 42).

hemiplejía (hemiplegia) parálisis de un lado del cuerpo (Ch. 33).

hemoconcentración (hemoconcentration) acumulación de sangre en el lugar de la venopunción provocada al dejar el torniquete del brazo más de un minuto, lo que produce muestras sanguíneas inexactas (Ch. 40).

hemoglobina (hemoglobin) molécula dentro de los glóbulos rojos que transporta oxígeno (Ch. 41).

hemoglobinopatía (hemoglobinopathy) enfermedad heredada producto de la formación de una molécula de hemoglobina anormal (Ch. 41).

hemólisis (hemolysis) ruptura de los glóbulos rojos durante el proceso de recolección de sangre. El suero o el plasma se contaminan y tienen color rojizo (Ch. 40).

hemoptisis (hemoptysis) expectoración de sangre que proviene de la boca, de la laringe, de la tráquea, de los bronquios o de los pulmones, caracterizada por un repentino ataque de tos con producción de esputo sanguinolento (Ch. 30).

herida (wound) ruptura en la continuidad de las partes blandas de las estructuras corporales por violencia o traumatismo en los tejidos. En el caso de una herida abierta, la piel está abierta como en el caso de una laceración, abrasión, avulsión o incisión. En una herida cerrada, la piel no se rompe como en el caso de contusión, equimosis o hematoma (Ch. 9).

hialino (hyaline) transparente, cristalino; los cilindros hialinos están compuestos por mucoproteína, son transparentes y a menudo difíciles de ver en la orina (Ch. 42).

Hibeclens® (Hibeclens®) marca de solución de jabón antiséptico (Ch. 31).

hidróxido de potasio (KOH) (potassium hydroxide [KOH]) la solución al 10% colocada en los frotis vaginales, así como también en las raspaduras de piel, el cabello y otras sustancias secas para disolver el exceso de detritos. Esto despeja el campo visual para visualizar mejor los hongos y las esporas (Ch. 26, 43).

hidróxido de sodio (sodium hydroxide) sustancia química usada para quemar químicamente y destruir el tejido, generalmente en estado líquido cuando se usa en cirugía menor (Ch. 31).

higienización (sanitization) limpieza o fregado de instrumentos o fómites contaminados para eliminar tejidos, detritos u otros contaminantes (Ch. 22).

hiperemesis gravídica (hyperemesis gravidarum) náuseas y vómitos intensos durante el embarazo con imposibilidad de comer; puede provocar deshidratación grave (Ch. 26).

hiperextensión (hyperextension) posición de máxima extensión o extensión de una parte del cuerpo más allá de sus límites normales (Ch. 33).

hiperglucemia (hyperglycemia) aumento de los niveles de glucosa en sangre. La hiperglucemia no significa necesariamente que el paciente sea diabético sino que puede ser indicación de prediabetes (Ch. 44).

hiperpnea (hyperpnea) aumento de la frecuencia y la profundidad respiratoria, como se observa al hacer ejercicio, con el dolor, la fiebre y la histeria (Ch. 24).

hipertensión (hypertension) presión arterial que es regularmente superior a 140/90 mm Hg (Ch. 24).

hipertermia (hyperthermia) temperatura corporal superior al rango normal, fiebre inusualmente alta (Ch. 29).

hiperventilación (hyperventilation) frecuencia de ventilación superior a lo metabólicamente necesario que puede provocar alcalosis (Ch. 24).

hipoclorito de sodio (sodium hypochlorite) lejía de uso doméstico (Ch. 22).

hipocrómico (hypochromic) menos color de lo normal (Ch. 41).

hipoglucemia (hypoglycemia) estado en el cual el nivel de glucosa en sangre es inferior a lo normal (Ch. 40, 44).

hipotensión (hypotension) presión arterial anormalmente baja que produce profusión y oxigenación inadecuada de los tejidos (Ch. 24).

hipotermia (hypothermia) afección sumamente peligrosa relacionada con el frío que puede provocar la muerte si la persona no recibe atención y si no se revierte su avance. Los síntomas incluyen escalofríos, piel fría y confusión (Ch. 9, 29).

hipoventilación (hypoventilation) disminución de la frecuencia respiratoria con respiración superficial o poco profunda (Ch. 24).

hipoxemia (hypoxemia) falta de oxígeno en la sangre (Ch. 36).

hipoxia (hypoxia) deficiencia de oxígeno (Ch. 26).

histerosalpingograma (hysterosalpingogram) radiografía del útero y de las trompas de Falopio usando un medio de contraste (Ch. 26).

histología (histology) estudio de la biopsia de la muestra de tejido para determinar una enfermedad (Ch. 39).

historia clínica orientada a la fuente (SOMR) (source-oriented medical record [SOMR]) tipo de registro de las fichas clínicas que incluye secciones separadas para diferentes fuentes de información de pacientes, como informes de laboratorio, informes de patología y notas de evolución (Ch. 14, 23).

historia clínica orientada al problema (POMR) (problem-oriented medical record [POMR]) forma de documentación de las fichas clínicas que usa una hoja en un lugar visible de la ficha para enumerar los datos de identificación vitales. Los problemas médicos de los pacientes se identifican por un número que corresponde a la ficha; por ejemplo, bronquitis es el N.° 1, fractura de muñeca es el N.° 2 y así sucesivamente (Ch. 14, 23).

hoja diaria (day sheet) formulario usado con el sistema de tablero de clavijas para registrar las transacciones diarias de pacientes (Ch. 19).

homeopatía (homeopathy) modalidad de curación que usa dosis diluidas de ciertas sustancias para crear una "huella de energía" en el cuerpo y dar lugar a la cura (Ch. 2).

homeostasia (homeostasis) estado de equilibrio del entorno interno (Ch. 34).

horas extra (overtime) dinero pagado a una tarifa no inferior a una hora y media de la tarifa habitual de pago después de completar una semana de trabajo de 40 horas (Ch. 46).

I

ictericia (jaundice) coloración amarillenta de la piel y de la esclerótica provocada por el exceso de bilirrubina en la sangre (Ch. 22, 25).

implante coclear (cochlear implantation) dispositivo eléctrico que recibe sonidos y transmite la señal resultante a los electrodos implantados en la cóclea. La señal estimula la cóclea y así la persona puede percibir sonidos (Ch. 27).

implícito (implicit) capaz de ser entendido aunque no esté expresado; tácito (Ch. 9).

improvisar (improvise) hacer, inventar u organizar en forma no planificada o espontánea (Ch. 1).

incinerar (incinerate) quemar algo hasta destruirlo (Ch. 22).

incompetencia (incompetence) legalmente, persona que es demente, inepta o no adulta (Ch. 7).

incontinencia (incontinence) incapacidad para controlar la orina o las heces (Ch. 29).

incremento (increment) aumento o suma en cuanto al número, tamaño o medida (Ch. 24).

indexar (indexing) seleccionar el nombre, el sujeto o el número conforme al cual se archiva un registro y determinar el orden en el cual se deben considerar las unidades (Ch. 14).

indicador de mensaje (flag) método para identificar un espacio en blanco o una pregunta sobre el significado de la persona que dicta; para ello, se agrega una nota o un marcador que indica la pregunta (Ch. 16).

índice metabólico basal (IMB) (basal metabolic rate [BMR]) nivel de energía necesario cuando el cuerpo está en reposo (Ch. 34).

índices de eritrocitos (erythrocyte indices) tres ecuaciones que proporcionan información sobre los tamaños y el contenido de hemoglobina de los glóbulos rojos. Éstos incluyen el volumen celular corpuscular medio, la hemoglobina corpuscular media y el volumen de hemoglobina corpuscular media (Ch. 41).

infarto (infarction) área de tejido de un órgano o de una parte del cuerpo que se necrosa (se muere) después de que se detiene el suministro sanguíneo (Ch. 37).

infección (infection) invasión de patógenos en el tejido vivo (Ch. 31).

infección del tracto urinario (ITU) (urinary tract infection [UTI]) también conocida como infección de la vejiga (Ch. 42).

infección oportunista (opportunistic infection) infección producto de un defecto en el sistema inmunitario que no se puede defender de los patógenos que normalmente se encuentran en el medio ambiente (Ch. 22).

inflamación (inflammation) respuesta inmunitaria no específica normal que tiene el cuerpo ante cualquier tipo de lesión (traumatismo, bacteriana, viral y por temperaturas extremas) (Ch. 31).

informe de autopsia (autopsy report) también llamado protocolo de autopsia, informe de necropsia o informe del médico forense. Las autopsias se realizan para determinar la causa de la muerte o para establecer y confirmar la presencia de enfermedad (Ch. 16).

informe de consulta (consultation report) documento que informa las conclusiones y el consejo de otro proveedor que revisó a un paciente a pedido del proveedor principal que lo atiende (Ch. 16).

informe de historia clínica y examen físico (H&P) (history and physical examination report [H&P]) informe de la historia clínica y examen físico de un paciente para documentar el motivo de la consulta (Ch. 16).

informe de patología (pathology report) informes médicos generados para describir los exámenes macro y microscópicos realizados durante un procedimiento quirúrgico (Ch. 16, 31).

informe quirúrgico (OR) (operative report [OR]) informe médico que documenta los detalles de un procedimiento quirúrgico (Ch. 16).

informes actuales (current reports) informes como antecedentes y exámenes físicos que se deben realizar en el plazo de 24 horas (Ch. 16).

informes anteriores (old reports) informes como el resumen del alta que se deben completar en el plazo de 71 horas (Ch. 16).

informes de radiología y de diagnóstico por imágenes (radiology and imaging reports) informes médicos que describen los resultados y las interpretaciones del radiólogo (Ch. 16).

ingeniería genética (genetic engineering) alteración, manipulación, sustitución o reparación de material genético (Ch. 8).

inhalador de dosis medida (metered dose inhaler) dispositivo usado para aplicar una cantidad recetada de medicamento en las vías respiratorias, especialmente los pulmones (Ch. 30).

inmunidad (immunity) capacidad del cuerpo de resistir patógenos específicos y sus toxinas (Ch. 22).

inmunidad humoral (humoral immunity) inmunidad mediada por anticuerpos en los líquidos corporales, como por ejemplo, el plasma y la linfa (Ch. 22).

inmunidad mediada por células (cell-mediated immunity) actividades reguladoras de las células T durante la respuesta inmunitaria específica (Ch. 22).

inmunoensayo enzimático (enzyme immunoassay) medición de la reacción del antígeno con anticuerpos específicos (Ch. 44).

inmunoglobulinas (immunoglobulins) familia de proteínas capaces de actuar como anticuerpos que, de este modo, protegen a las personas de los microorganismos patógenos; también, anticuerpos producidos por las células del sistema de respuesta inmunitaria (Ch. 30).

inmunohematología (immunohematology) estudio de los antígenos y los anticuerpos del grupo sanguíneo; banco de sangre (Ch. 39).

inmunología (immunology) estudio de los componentes del sistema inmunitario y su función (Ch. 39).

inmunomodulador (immunomodulator) sustancia que tiene la capacidad de modificar las respuestas inmunitarias (Ch. 22, 43).

inmunosuprimido (immunosuppressed) paciente cuyo sistema inmunitario no está sano debido a enfermedad, medicamentos y genética. Estos pacientes pueden ser especialmente susceptibles al ataque de microorganismos (Ch. 22, 43).

inobservancia (noncompliant) no seguir una orden o una instrucción exigida (Ch. 7).

inoculación (inoculation) inyección (Ch. 22).

inocular (inoculate) colocar colonias de microorganismos en medios nutrientes (Ch. 43).

insulina (insulin) hormona segregada por células beta de los islotes de Langerhans del páncreas esencial para el metabolismo correcto de la glucosa (Ch. 44).

integrar (integrate) incorporar a una unidad mayor; formar o mezclarse en un todo (Ch. 1).

interfaz de red (network interface) software, servidores y conexiones de cable usadas para conectar computadoras (Ch. 11).

intermediación cultural (cultural brokering) acto de comunicar, vincular o mediar entre grupos o personas reduciendo los conflictos o produciendo cambios (Ch. 4).

intermediario fiscal (fiscal intermediary) administrador local de Medicare (Ch. 17).

interrogatorio (interrogatory) conjunto de preguntas escritas que se deben responder, bajo juramento, dentro de un período específico de tiempo; parte de un proceso de exhibición de pruebas (Ch. 7).

intraepitelial (intraepithelium) dentro del epitelio (Ch. 26).

intrahospitalaria (nosocomial) infección adquirida en un entorno de atención médica (hospital, clínica, hogar de ancianos) (Ch. 22).

inversión (inversion) movimiento de una parte del cuerpo hacia adentro (Ch. 33).

involución (involution) regreso del útero a su tamaño y forma normales después del parto (Ch. 26).

inyección a chorro (jet injection) inyección administrada debajo de la piel sin aguja, usando la fuerza del líquido bajo presión para atravesar la piel (Ch. 22).

irregularidad (misfeasance) término del derecho civil que se refiere a un acto legal que se ejecuta en forma incorrecta o ilegítima (Ch. 7).

isoeléctrico (isoelectric) que tiene potenciales eléctricos iguales. Se representa en el ECG como la línea horizontal plana de base (Ch. 37).

isótopo (isotope) un elemento químico (Ch. 32).

isquemia (ischemia) falta temporal y local de sangre en un órgano o parte provocada por la obstrucción de la circulación (Ch. 37).

itinerario (itinerary) plan por escrito detallado de un viaje propuesto (Ch. 45).

J

jerarquía de necesidades (hierarchy of needs) necesidades que se organizan en un orden o posicionamiento específico, disposición secuencial. Relacionado con Abraham Maslow (Ch. 4).

jerga (jargon) palabras, frases o terminología específica de una profesión (Ch. 12).

Junta de Acreditación de Escuelas de Educación en Salud (ABHES) (Accrediting Bureau of Health Education Schools [ABHES]) entidad que acredita a las empresas privadas, instituciones de educación superior en los EE.UU. que ofrecen programas de educación de salud auxiliares, como también acreditación programática de asistencia médica, asociado en tecnología médica y programas de enfermería quirúrgica (Ch. 1, 47).

K

kit para derrames (spill kit) materiales envasados comercialmente que contienen insumos y equipos necesarios para limpiar un derrame de una sustancia biológicamente peligrosa (Ch. 22).

L

laberintitis (labyrinthitis) inflamación del oído interno o laberinto (Ch. 25).

laboratorios con base en el hospital (hospital-based laboratorios) laboratorios de propiedad del hospital que realizan la mayoría de las pruebas que requiere el hospital y las comunidades locales (Ch. 39).

laboratorios de referencia (reference laboratories) laboratorios independientes, ubicados por región, que usan los hospitales para pruebas complejas, caras o especializadas (Ch. 39).

laboratorios del consultorio de los médicos (POL) (physicians' office laboratories [POL]) laboratorios dentro de los consultorios de los médicos donde se realizan análisis de laboratorio comunes en el consultorio (Ch. 39).

Lamaze (Lamaze) técnica que consiste en ejercicios de respiración para facilitar el parto (Ch. 26).

lámpara de Wood (Wood's lamp) fuente de iluminación especial usada para detectar organismos que brillan con la luz, como ciertos hongos, bacteria y parásitos. Dos ejemplos son la sarna y la tiña. Con la lámpara de Wood es posible detectar rasguños en el ojo después de que éste ha sido impregnado con colorante fluorescente. También usada para determinar el margen de disección de un melanoma (Ch. 43).

lector óptico de caracteres (OCR) (optical character reader [OCR]) escáner computarizado del Servicio Postal de los EE. UU. que lee las direcciones impresas en la correspondencia. Si la información está correctamente formateada, entonces el OCR encontrará una coincidencia en los archivos de direcciones e imprimirá un código de barra en el margen inferior derecho del sobre (Ch. 15).

lenguaje corporal (body language) comunicación no verbal que incluye movimientos corporales inconscientes, gestos y expresiones faciales que acompañan los mensajes verbales (Ch. 4).

lesión (lesion) lastimadura o herida. Zona limitada de tejido que se ha alterado patológicamente (Ch. 22, 30).

leucocito (leukocyte) glóbulo blanco, uno de los componentes de la sangre (Ch. 40, 41).

leucorrea (leukorrhea) secreción blancuzca o amarillenta del conducto cervical o de la vagina. Generalmente es normal, salvo que haya un aumento en la cantidad o variación en el color (Ch. 22).

Ley de Autodeterminación del Paciente (PSDA) (Patient Self-Determination Act [PSDA]) ley que incluye la Directiva

Avanzada que les otorga a los pacientes el derecho a participar en las decisiones sobre su atención médica (Ch. 7).

Ley de Portabilidad y Responsabilidad de Seguros de Salud (HIPAA) (Health Insurance Portability and Accountability Act [HIPAA]) normas, reglamentaciones y procedimientos gubernamentales producto de la legislación destinada a proteger la confidencialidad de la información de los pacientes (Ch. 16).

ley de prescripción (statute of limitations) ley que define el período durante el cual puede tener lugar la acción legal (Ch. 20).

Ley de Veracidad en los Préstamos (Truth-in-Lending Act) también conocida como Ley de Protección de Créditos del Consumidor de 1968; ley que exige a los proveedores de créditos en cuotas que declaren los cargos por escrito y que expresen el interés en forma de tasa anual (Ch. 20).

Ley sobre Prácticas Justas para el Cobro de Deudas (Fair Debt Collection Practice Act) ley federal de 1977 que establece las prácticas de cobro de deudas (Ch. 20).

leyenda (caption) método de designación usado en guías de archivos (Ch. 14).

leyes del Buen Samaritano (Good Samaritan laws) leyes diseñadas para proteger a las personas contra acciones legales cuando prestan asistencia médica de emergencia, sin retribución, dentro de las áreas de su formación y pericia (Ch. 12).

libido (libido) impulso sexual (Ch. 28).

libro mayor (ledger) registro de gastos, pagos y ajustes relacionados con el paciente o la familia (Ch. 19).

licencia (license) declaración de permiso que autoriza el uso de software informático con derecho de autor (Ch. 11).

licenciatura (bachelor's degree) título académico de cuatro años de estudio conferido por universidades e instituciones de enseñanza superior (Ch. 1).

ligadura (ligature) longitud del hilo de sutura sin aguja, usada para cerrar vasos durante la cirugía (Ch. 31).

limpiador ultrasónico (ultrasonic cleaner) máquina que usa la energía de ondas de sonido de alta frecuencia que se agitan para desinfectar instrumentos antes de la esterilización (Ch. 22).

linfadenopatía (lymphadenopathy) enfermedad de los ganglios linfáticos (Ch. 22).

linfocito (lymphocyte) glóbulo blanco con un núcleo no segmentado denso y que carece de gránulos en el citoplasma (Ch. 41).

liofilizado (lyophilized) proceso por el cual se congela rápidamente una sustancia a temperaturas sumamente bajas y luego se deshidrata la sustancia en alto vacío (secado por congelación) (Ch. 27).

lipemia (lipemia) cantidad excesiva de grasas (lípidos) en la sangre, lo que produce una muestra sanguínea que tiene aspecto lechoso (Ch. 40).

lipoproteína de alta densidad (HDL) (high-density lipoprotein [HDL]) lipoproteína de la sangre compuesta principalmente de proteína; elimina el colesterol de los tejidos periféricos y los transporta al hígado para la excreción (Ch. 44).

lipoproteína de baja densidad (LDL) (low-density lipoprotein [LDL]) lipoproteína de la sangre compuesta principalmente de colesterol. El colesterol que transporta la LDL se puede depositar en los tejidos periféricos y se asocia con un mayor riesgo de enfermedad cardíaca (Ch. 44).

líquido corporal (body fluid) toda secreción o excreción del cuerpo humano, por ejemplo, vaginal, cefalorraquídeo, sinovial, pleural, pericárdico, peritoneal, amniótico, esputo y saliva (Ch. 38).

litigio (litigation) acción judicial (Ch. 7).

litotricia (lithotripsy) procedimiento que usa ondas de choque dirigidas a los cálculos para triturarlos (Ch. 30).

localizador uniforme de recursos (URL) (uniform resource locater [URL]) dirección que define la ruta para llegar a un archivo en la Web o en cualquier otra instalación de Internet (Ch. 12).

localizadores (pagers) también conocidos como bíper. Sistemas de localización de una vía que usan a menudo los proveedores que están de guardia dentro de los hospitales. Los localizadores solamente reciben señales (Ch. 12).

loquios (lochia) secreción uterina de sangre, moco y tejido presente durante el período posterior al parto (Ch. 22, 26).

luxación (dislocation) desplazamiento de un hueso o de una articulación de su posición normal (Ch. 30).

luz (lumen) espacio dentro de una arteria, vena, intestino, agujas y catéter o tubo (Ch. 24).

M

macroasignación (macroallocation) de recursos médicos escasos; decisiones que toma el Congreso, las agencias de sistemas de salud y las compañías de seguro (Ch. 8).

macrocítico (macrocytic) término que describe una célula más grande de lo normal (Ch. 41).

macular (macular) relativo a la decoloración de un parche de piel, ni elevada ni deprimida, de diversos colores, tamaños y formas (Ch. 22).

mala praxis (malpractice) negligencia profesional (Ch. 7, 45).

malabsorción (malabsorption) absorción inadecuada de los nutrientes del tracto intestinal (Ch. 30).

malestar (malaise) molestia, incomodidad o indisposición, a menudo indicador de infección (Ch. 22, 30).

malversar (embezzle) apropiarse fraudulentamente para uso propio (Ch. 45).

mandato (mandate) orden formal de obedecer ciertas normas y reglamentaciones (Ch. 38).

manifestar (manifest) revelar en forma evidente (Ch. 22).

maniobra de Heimlich (Heimlich maneuver) presión abdominal brusca y firme destinada a superar dificultades de respiración en personas que están asfixiándose (Ch. 9).

manómetro (manometer) dispositivo para medir la presión líquida o gaseosa. La medición se expresa en milímetros de mercurio o agua (Ch. 24).

manual de procedimientos (procedure manual) manual que proporciona información detallada relacionada con el desempeño de tareas dentro de la descripción del cargo (Ch. 45).

marcha (gait) manera o estilo de caminar, incluidos el ritmo y la velocidad (Ch. 33).

matrícula (license) permiso expedido por la autoridad competente (el estado) para ejercer una profesión; permiso de actuar (Ch. 1).

matriculación (licensure) otorgamiento de matrículas para ejercer una profesión (Ch. 1).

matriz (matrix) para establecer una matriz de citas, los espacios de tiempo no disponibles del proveedor se marcan con una X. Los pacientes no se programan durante esos horarios (Ch. 13).

matriz redundante de discos independientes (RAID) (redundant array independent disk [RAID]) esquema de almacenamiento de datos que usa múltiples discos duros para compartir o replicar datos entre las unidades (Ch. 11).

mecánica corporal (body mechanics) práctica de uso de ciertos grupos musculares clave junto con una alineación corporal correcta para evitar lesiones al levantar o trasladar objetos pesados o difíciles de trasladar (Ch. 33).

mecanismo de defensa (defense mechanism) comportamiento que protege la psiquis de culpa, ansiedad o vergüenza (Ch. 4).

meconio (meconium) primeras heces del recién nacido (Ch. 26).

mediación (mediation) resolución de conflictos que permite al mediador ayudar a ambas partes a conciliar las diferencias y a llegar a una solución aceptable (Ch. 7).

médicamente indigente (medically indigent) se refiere a las personas que no pueden pagar su propia cobertura médica (Ch. 7).

Medicare Parte A (Medicare Part A) beneficios que cubren la hospitalización en hospitales y en centros de enfermería especializada, la atención en hospicios y transfusiones de sangre (Ch. 17).

Medicare Parte B (Medicare Part B) beneficios que cubren la atención ambulatoria en hospitales y los servicios de proveedores de atención médica (Ch. 17).

Medicare Parte C (Medicare Part C) comúnmente se los llama planes de Medicare Advantage. Estos planes están aprobados por Medicare y son administrados por empresas privadas (Ch. 17).

Medicare Parte D (Medicare Part D) cobertura de medicamentos recetados por parte de Medicare (Ch. 17).

medicina de rehabilitación (rehabilitation medicine) campo de las disciplinas médicas que procura restablecer la función normal, o casi normal, de una persona o de una parte del cuerpo después de una enfermedad o lesión usando agentes físicos y mecánicos (Ch. 33).

medicina integradora (integrative medicine) conjunción de dos o más modalidades de tratamiento para que funcionen como un todo armonioso, como se observa en las formas alternativas de la atención médica (Ch. 2).

médico de atención primaria (PCP) (primary care physician [PCP]) médico de atención primaria de un paciente a través del cual se coordina toda la atención (Ch. 17).

medios de sostén (holding media) medios específicos en el transporte de microorganismos para sustentar la vida de los organismos hasta que se coloquen en un medio nutriente en el laboratorio (Ch. 43).

memorándum (memorandum) correspondencia que se usa dentro de la oficina, comúnmente llamada memorando (Ch. 15).

memoria (memory) se refiere al almacenamiento de datos en la computadora. La memoria puede ser volátil (se pierde cuando se apaga la computadora) o no volátil (escrita permanentemente en un dispositivo de almacenamiento) (Ch. 11).

memoria de acceso aleatorio (RAM) (random access memory [RAM]) tipo de memoria de computadora que se puede escribir y leer. La palabra *aleatorio* significa que se puede leer en cualquier ubicación en cualquier momento. RAM comúnmente se refiere a la memoria interna de una computadora. RAM generalmente es un área de memoria temporal rápida donde residen los datos y los programas hasta que se guardan o hasta que se desconecta la energía (Ch. 11).

memoria de almacenamiento de datos (data storage memory) memoria permanente que no forma parte de la placa madre. Usa cualquier dispositivo de almacenamiento de datos adecuado. Puede ser memoria de sólo lectura o de lectura/escritura (Ch. 11).

memoria de sólo lectura (ROM) (read-only memory [ROM]) datos almacenados permanentemente en la computadora que no se pueden sobrescribir sin dispositivos especiales. Se requieren instrucciones de almacenamiento para iniciar la computadora. Se encuentra en la placa madre (Ch. 11).

menisco (meniscus) curvatura en la superficie de arriba de un líquido cuando se lo coloca en un recipiente (Ch. 24, 36).

menor (minor) persona que no ha alcanzado la mayoría de edad, generalmente 18 años (Ch. 7).

menor emancipado (emancipated minor) personas menores de 18 años que son financieramente responsables de sí mismas y libres del cuidado paterno (Ch. 7).

menor maduro (mature minor) persona, generalmente menor de 18 años, que puede entender y medir las consecuencias del tratamiento a pesar de su corta edad (Ch. 7).

menstruación (menses) período (Ch. 22).

mentor (mentor) persona asignada o solicitada para ayudar en la capacitación, la orientación o la instrucción de otra (Ch. 45).

mesa de Mayo (Mayo stand) mesa con bandeja metálica portátil para establecer pequeños campos estériles para cirugías y procedimientos menores (Ch. 31).

meta (goal) resultado o logro hacia el cual se dirigen todos los esfuerzos (Ch. 5).

metabolismo (metabolism) totalidad de todos los cambios, químicos y físicos, que se producen en el cuerpo (Ch. 34).

metas a corto plazo (short-range goals) las metas a largo plazo se dividen y se reacomodan en segmentos de tiempo más cortos y más manejables (Ch. 5).

metas a largo plazo (long-range goals) logros que pueden tardar de tres a cinco años en concretarse (Ch. 5).

metástasis (metastasis) en cáncer, diseminación de células malignas a partir de un tumor primario a una nueva ubicación (Ch. 28).

metrorragia (metrorrhagia) hemorragia uterina en intervalos irregulares (Ch. 26).

micología (mycology) estudio de los hongos (Ch. 39, 43).

microasignación (microallocation) de recursos médicos escasos; decisiones que toman los proveedores y los miembros individuales del equipo de atención médica (Ch. 8).

microbiología (microbiology) rama de la biología que trata del estudio de formas microscópicas de vida (Ch. 39, 43).

microcítico (microcytic) término que describe una célula más pequeña de lo normal (Ch. 41).

microcomputadora (microcomputer) computadora personal o de escritorio. También, modelo de computadora portátil o de mano (Ch. 11).

microorganismo (microorganism) ser vivo microscópico capaz de transmitirse y reproducirse en circunstancias específicas (Ch. 22).

microscopia (microscopy) inspección con el microscopio (Ch. 38).

mineral principal (major mineral) mineral que el cuerpo requiere en grandes cantidades (Ch. 34).

minicomputadora (minicomputer) una de las cuatro categorías de computadoras según el tamaño: más grande que una microcomputadora y más pequeña que una computadora central (Ch. 11).

miringotomía (myringotomy) incisión en la membrana timpánica; parte del tratamiento para la otitis media (Ch. 27).

modalidades (modalities) agentes físicos como calor, frío, luz, agua y electricidad usados para tratar disfunciones musculares o articulares (Ch. 33).

modificador (modifier) código adicional que se puede agregar a un código CPT de cinco dígitos para explicar el servicio provisto (Ch. 18).

modulado (modulated) habla que varía en tono e intensidad (Ch. 12).

mola hidatidiforme (hydatidiform mole) desarrollo de quistes y crecimiento rápido del útero con sangrado (Ch. 44).

monitoreo de fármacos terapéuticos (TDM) (therapeutic drug monitoring [TDM]) análisis de sangre periódicos para determinar la eficacia de un fármaco en particular. Los fármacos deberán alcanzar un nivel terapéutico para que sean terapéuticos o eficaces. Si el nivel en sangre del fármaco está por debajo del espectro de eficacia terapéutica, el proveedor probablemente aumentará la dosis. Del mismo modo, si el fármaco supera el espectro terapéutico, el proveedor probablemente la reducirá (Ch. 39).

monocito (monocyte) glóbulo blanco sin gránulos citoplasmáticos que tiene un núcleo grande no segmentado y arriñonado (Ch. 41).

mononucleosis infecciosa (infectious mononucleosis) enfermedad infecciosa aguda que afecta principalmente el tejido linfoide, provocada por el virus de Epstein-Barr (Ch. 44).

montaje (mounting) proceso que aplica de manera secuencial una parte de cada una de las 12 derivaciones del registro del ECG en un formulario o planilla de montaje de papel preparada comercialmente, como parte del registro permanente del paciente (Ch. 37).

morbilidad (morbidity) cantidad de casos de enfermedad en una población específica (Ch. 22).

mordiente (mordant) sustancia que fija el colorante a un objeto; el yodo es un mordiente en la tinción de Gram (Ch. 43).

morfología (morphology) forma y estructura de un organismo (Ch. 22, 43).

mortalidad (mortality) la proporción del número de muertes en una población dada (Ch. 22).

moxibustión (moxibustion) antiguo método chino de tratamiento que usa una sustancia de una planta en polvo sobre la piel para provocar una ampolla (Ch. 3).

multigrávida (multigravida) mujer que ha estado embarazada más de una vez (Ch. 26).

N

nefrolitotomía (nephrolithotomy) incisión en el riñón para eliminar cálculos (Ch. 30).

negligencia (negligence) falta de cumplimiento de un determinado estándar de atención (Ch. 7, 45).

nematodo (nematode) gusano redondo (Ch. 43).

neonatal (neonatal) relativo al recién nacido (Ch. 26).

neonato (neonate) recién nacido.

neurosensorial (sensorineural) pérdida permanente de la audición producto del daño o una malformación del oído medio y el nervio auditivo (Ch. 27).

neutrófilo (neutrophil) el tipo más común de glóbulo blanco granulocítico (Ch. 41).

nevo (nevus) lunar (Ch. 29).

niacina (niacin) una de las vitaminas del complejo B (Ch. 34).

nistagmo (nystagmus) movimiento involuntario continuo de los ojos (Ch. 30).

nitrato de plata (silver nitrate) antiséptico astringente cáustico. En su forma de líquido débil, se aplica en los ojos de los recién nacidos para prevenir infecciones en el nacimiento. En el consultorio médico, a menudo se usa como sustancia sólida impregnada en el extremo de un aplicador de madera. Las varillas del aplicador de nitrato de plata contienen ácido clorhídrico y otras sustancias químicas y comúnmente se usan para cauterizar pequeños vasos sanguíneos en la nariz o en otras membranas mucosas (Ch. 31).

nitrógeno líquido (liquid nitrogen) llamado comúnmente, y erróneamente, hielo seco; el nitrógeno líquido es un agente congelante volátil usado para destruir tejido no deseado como las verrugas (Ch. 31).

nitrógeno ureico en sangre (BUN) (blood urea nitrogen [BUN]) nitrógeno en la sangre en forma de urea. El nivel de nitrógeno en la sangre es un indicador de la función renal (Ch. 44).

nitrogenoso (nitrogenous) concerniente a productos de desecho en la sangre que indican enfermedad renal (Ch. 30).

no diferenciada (undifferentiated) degeneración maligna de una célula (Ch. 22).

nocturia (nocturia) micción excesiva durante la noche (Ch. 28, 30).

nomograma (nomogram) gráfico que muestra la relación entre valores numéricos. Con él se puede calcular el área de superficie corporal (ASC) de un paciente (Ch. 36).

normas WiFi (WiFi standards) normas de la industria para dispositivos informáticos inalámbricos cuyo objeto es mantener la interoperabilidad (Ch. 11).

normocítico (normocytic) término que describe una célula de tamaño normal (Ch. 41).

normocrómico (normochromic) de color normal, en este caso, cuando se refiere a glóbulos rojos (Ch. 41).

notas clínicas (chart notes) (también llamadas notas de evolución) observaciones formales o informales del proveedor sobre la presentación de un problema, los resultados físicos y el plan de tratamiento para un paciente examinado en el consultorio, la clínica, el centro de cuidados agudos o el departamento de emergencias (Ch. 16).

notas de evolución (progress notes) también llamadas notas clínicas. Observaciones formales o informales del proveedor sobre la presentación de un problema, los resultados físicos y el plan de tratamiento de un paciente examinado en el consultorio, la clínica, un centro de cuidados agudos o el departamento de emergencias (Ch. 16).

nueva certificación (recertification) documentación admitida como prueba de educación continua para mantener una credencial profesional (Ch. 47).

nulípara (nullipara) mujer que no ha llevado un embarazo hasta el estadio de viabilidad (Ch. 26).

nutrición (nutrition) estudio de cómo se incorporan los nutrientes al cuerpo y cómo éste los usa (Ch. 34).

nutriente (nutrient) sustancia ingerida que ayuda al cuerpo a mantenerse en estado homeostático (Ch. 34).

O

obesidad mórbida (morbid obesity) obesidad tan grave que puede provocar una enfermedad grave (Ch. 30).

objetivo (objective) signo del paciente que es visible, palpable o mensurable para el observador (Ch. 23); también; lente con aumento que es el que está más cerca del objeto cuando se lo observa con un microscopio (Ch. 39).

objetivo profesional (career objective) expresa su objetivo en su profesión y el cargo para el que se postula (Ch. 48).

objetos filosos (sharps) agujas o escalpelos u otros instrumentos con punta que pueden penetrar o perforar una herida en la piel (Ch. 22).

obstáculos (roadblocks) mensajes verbales o no verbales que obstaculizan la comunicación (Ch. 4).

obturador (obturator) herramienta que obstruye o cierra una cavidad o abertura. La parte interna del instrumento de un examen que facilita la entrada del instrumento en el cuerpo; luego se lo retira y así se posibilita la visualización del área interna (Ch. 30).

oclusión (occlusion) cierre de una vía (Ch. 9).

oclusor (occluder) instrumento usado para obstruir o cerrar la visión o la luz (Ch. 30).

ocultamiento (masking) intento de ocultar o reprimir los sentimientos o el mensaje verdaderos (Ch. 4).

ofuscación (obfuscation) enredar o confundir las cosas (Ch. 12).

oligomineral (trace mineral) mineral que el cuerpo necesita en pequeñas cantidades (Ch. 34).

oliguria (oliguria) disminución en la producción de orina (Ch. 30).

omisión (nonfeasance) término del derecho civil que se refiere a la falta de cumplimiento de un acto, una obligación oficial o un requisito legal (Ch. 7).

operación cesárea (cesarean section) nacimiento del feto a través de una incisión quirúrgica en el útero (Ch. 26).

orden del día (agenda) lista impresa de temas que se tratarán durante una reunión, que a veces establece el tiempo asignado (Ch. 15, 45).

organización de atención administrada (MCO) (managed care organization [MCO]) organización de seguros de salud que se rige según los principios de fuerte dependencia en la contratación selectiva de los proveedores, el uso de médicos de atención primaria, gestión de utilización prospectiva y retrospectiva, uso de pautas de tratamiento para trastornos crónicos de alto costo y énfasis en la atención preventiva, la educación y el cumplimiento de los planes de tratamiento por parte del paciente (Ch. 17).

organización de mantenimiento de la salud (HMO) (health maintenance organization [HMO]) tipo de actividad de atención administrada que generalmente se constituye como una empresa con fines de lucro con empleados remunerados. Las HMO "con paredes" ofrecen una variedad de servicios médicos bajo un solo techo; las HMO "sin paredes" por lo general contratan a proveedores de la comunidad para brindar servicios a los pacientes a cambio de una tarifa acordada (Ch. 2, 17).

organización de proveedor exclusivo (EPO) (exclusive provider organization [EPO]) plan de organización de proveedor preferido (PPO, por sus siglas en inglés) de conjunto cerrado en la cual los afiliados no reciben ningún beneficio si optan por recibir atención de un proveedor que no está en la EPO (Ch. 17).

organización de proveedor preferido (PPO) (preferred provider organization [PPO]) organización de proveedores que forman una red para ofrecer descuentos a los compradores de seguros de salud (Ch. 17).

orina residual (residual urine) cantidad de orina que queda en la vejiga inmediatamente después de vaciarla; se observa con la hiperplasia de próstata (Ch. 28, 29).

orquidectomía (orchidectomy) extirpación quirúrgica de un testículo (Ch. 28).

ortopnea (orthopnea) dificultad para respirar en cualquier posición que no sea en posición vertical (Ch. 24).

osciloscopio (oscilloscope) dispositivo electrónico usado para registrar la actividad eléctrica del corazón, el cerebro y los tejidos musculares (Ch. 32, 37).

otoscopio (otoscope) instrumento usado para examinar el conducto auditivo externo y la membrana timpánica (Ch. 30).

óvulos (ova) huevos, en este caso, huevos de parásitos (Ch. 43).

oxidación (oxidation) proceso en el cual una sustancia se combina con el oxígeno (Ch. 34).

oxigenado (oxygenated) que contiene altos niveles de oxígeno (Ch. 40).

oxímetro de pulso (pulse oximeter) dispositivo (similar a un clip) que se puede sujetar al dedo o al puente de la nariz. Mide la concentración de oxígeno en la sangre (Ch. 24).

oxitocina (oxytocin) hormona hipofisaria que estimula la contracción de los músculos del útero y así induce el parto (Ch. 26).

P

palabras clave (keywords) palabras relacionadas con un puesto específico en un trabajo. Las palabras clave pueden ser habilidades específicas de un trabajo o palabras específicas de la profesión (Ch. 48).

palabras de relleno (buffer words) palabras prescindibles que se usan mientras se atiende el teléfono (Ch. 12).

paliativa (palliative) medida adoptada para aliviar los síntomas de la enfermedad (Ch. 22, 32).

palidez (pallor) falta de color, lividez (Ch. 25).

palpar (palpate) sentir con la yema de los dedos, buscar la vena con el tacto presionando y soltando (Ch. 40).

paludismo (malaria) enfermedad infecciosa aguda provocada por la presencia de parásitos protozoarios dentro de los glóbulos rojos; generalmente es consecuencia de la picadura de un mosquito hembra (Ch. 3, 22).

pandemia (pandemic) enfermedad que afecta a la mayoría de la población de una región grande; es una epidemia que se produce al mismo tiempo en muchas partes del mundo (Ch. 22).

panel (panel) serie de pruebas relacionadas con un órgano o sistema de órganos en particular del funcionamiento corporal. Por ejemplo, un panel hepático controla muchas funciones diferentes del hígado. Antes llamado "perfil" (Ch. 39).

pantalla antirreflejo (antiglare screen) filtro que se coloca sobre la pantalla del monitor de un equipo de computación para reducir el reflejo (Ch. 11).

paño fenestrado (fenestrated drape) tipo de paño con un orificio, generalmente redondo, que se puede colocar con el orificio sobre un área particular del cuerpo; se usa en cirugía y para exámenes proctológicos (Ch. 25).

papel bond (bond paper) papel duradero y más resistente que generalmente se usa para correspondencia (Ch. 15).

papular (papular) relativo a un área pequeña, roja y elevada de la piel que es sólida y está circunscrita (Ch. 22).

paquete de hidrocolator (hydrocollator pack) paquete lleno con gel que se calienta a baño María (Ch. 33).

paracentesis (paracentesis) punción de una cavidad para extraer líquido (Ch. 22).

parasitología (parasitology) estudio de organismos (parásitos y los huevos) que viven en o dentro de otro organismo y a costa de él (Ch. 39, 43).

parche (patch) modificación en el software para arreglar deficiencias en él. A menudo se descarga del sitio web del proveedor del software o de disquetes suministrados por el proveedor (Ch. 11).

parenteral (parenteral) inyección de una sustancia líquida en el cuerpo mediante una vía alternativa al canal alimentario (Ch. 22, 36).

parestesia (paresthesia) sensación de entumecimiento, escozor o aumento de sensibilidad (Ch. 30).

paridad (parity) llevar un embarazo hasta el punto de viabilidad independientemente del resultado (Ch. 26).

parir (parturition) proceso de dar a luz (Ch. 26).

participación en las ganancias (profit sharing) compartir las utilidades, las ganancias y los beneficios de una organización (Ch. 45).

pasantía (internship) etapa de transición entre las clases y el empleo (Ch. 1).

pasivo (liability) deudas y obligaciones financieras de las cuales uno es responsable (Ch. 21).

patógeno (pathogen) microorganismo que produce enfermedades (Ch. 22, 43).

patógeno transmitido por la sangre (bloodborne pathogen) microorganismo capaz de producir una enfermedad y que se encuentra en la sangre o en los hemoderivados (Ch. 22).

patrimonio neto (owner's equity) monto en que los activos de la empresa superan los pasivos. También llamado activo neto, patrimonio y capital contable (Ch. 21).

patrón (standard) normas establecidas para medir la calidad, el peso, el alcance o el valor (Ch. 22, 38).

pelagra (pellagra) enfermedad producida por una deficiencia de vitamina B_3 (ácido nicotínico) caracterizada por llagas en la piel, diarrea, ansiedad, confusión y muerte, si no se trata (Ch. 34).

percepción (perception) comprensión consciente de los sentimientos propios y de los demás (Ch. 4).

periférico (peripheral) alejado del centro del cuerpo (Ch. 24).

período de beneficios (benefit period) tiempo especificado durante el cual los beneficios se pagarán en virtud de ciertos tipos de coberturas de seguro médico (Ch. 17).

período de prueba (probation) período durante el cual el empleado y el personal de supervisión pueden determinar si el entorno y el cargo son satisfactorios para el empleado (Ch. 46).

período sin cobertura (donut hole) dentro del programa de medicamentos recetados de la Parte D de Medicare, el período sin cobertura es la etapa en la cual todos los costos son cubiertos por el afiliado en lugar de los CMS (Ch. 17).

perlas de látex (latex beads) perlas de látex diminutas cubiertas de anticuerpos o antígenos que reaccionan con antígenos o anticuerpos en la muestra de prueba en una reacción de aglutinación. Las perlas de látex pueden ser de color para facilitar la visualización de la reacción (Ch. 44).

permeable (patent) abierto, no obstruido (Ch. 26).

peróxido de hidrógeno (hydrogen peroxide) solución antibacteriana que tiene una acción de limpieza mecánica (Ch. 31).

personas con autodeterminación (inner-directed people) personas que deciden por sí mismas lo que quieren hacer con su vida (Ch. 5).

personas influenciables (outer-directed people) personas que permiten que los acontecimientos, que otras personas o que los factores ambientales determinen su comportamiento (Ch. 5).

peste bubónica (bubonic plague) enfermedad infecciosa con alta tasa de mortalidad que es transmitida a los seres humanos a través de ratas y ardillas terrestres infectadas que fueron mordidas por la pulga de las ratas (Ch. 3).

petrissage (petrissage) movimiento de amasamiento en masaje (Ch. 33).

pH (pH) escala que indica la alcalinidad o la acidez relativa de la solución; medición de la concentración de iones de hidrógeno (Ch. 42).

pico (peak) lo opuesto de "valle", es el punto en el cual el fármaco alcanza su mayor nivel en el cuerpo, generalmente tiene lugar aproximadamente a los 30 minutos después de la administración. En las pruebas de laboratorio, el pico indica al proveedor la mayor influencia que tendría el fármaco en el cuerpo con esa dosis en particular (Ch. 38).

pielograma intravenoso (intravenous pyelogram) estudios radiográficos de los riñones, uréter y vejiga usando un medio de contraste (Ch. 28).

piorrea (pyorrhea) secreción de pus de las encías, alrededor de los dientes (Ch. 25).

pirexia (pyrexia) fiebre (Ch. 24).

piridoxina (pyridoxine) vitamina B_6 (Ch. 34).

piuria (pyuria) pus en la orina (Ch. 30).

placa de Petri (petri dish) placa plástica en la que se coloca el agar para el crecimiento de bacterias (Ch. 43).

placa madre (motherboard) tablero de circuito impreso en el cual a menudo se encuentran los chips de CPU, ROM y RAM y otros elementos del circuito electrónico de una computadora digital (Ch. 11).

placenta previa (placenta previa) la placenta se implanta en la parte inferior del útero y puede cubrir parcial o completamente el orificio cervical (Ch. 26).

plan de opción triple (triple option plan) modelo de atención administrada que permite a los afiliados la opción de elegir planes de salud tradicionales, HMO o PPO (Ch. 17).

plan de punto de servicio (POS) (point-of-service [POS] plan) plan que permite la comunicación directa entre un consultorio médico y la compañía de seguros de salud (Ch. 17).

planificación en olas (wave scheduling) sistema en el que los pacientes se programan para la primera media hora de cada hora y luego se atienden durante toda la hora (Ch. 13).

planificación en olas modificada (modified wave scheduling) sistema en el que se programan varios pacientes al comienzo de cada hora, seguidos de citas individuales cada 10 a 20 minutos el resto de la hora (Ch. 13).

plasma (plasma) parte líquida de la sangre de un tubo que contiene anticoagulante. Este líquido contiene fibrinógeno (Ch. 40).

plazo de entrega (turnaround time) límite de tiempo específico establecido para terminar los informes médicos (Ch. 16).

pleiteador (litigious) propenso a involucrarse en demandas judiciales (Ch. 1).

pluralista (pluralismo) (pluralistic [pluralism]) sociedad en la que coexisten distintos grupos étnicos, religiosos o culturales diferentes (Ch. 3).

poder legal duradero para atención médica (durable power of attorney for health care) formulario legal que permite a una persona designada actuar en nombre de otra con respecto a las opciones de atención médica (Ch. 6, 7).

pólipo (polyp) tumor pediculado que se presenta en la nariz, el útero, la vejiga, el colon o el recto (Ch. 30).

póliza de Medigap (Medigap policy) plan individual que cubre el deducible de Medicare del paciente y las obligaciones de copago que cumple con las normas del gobierno federal en cuanto al seguro complementario de Medicare (Ch. 17).

portador (carrier) persona que aloja un agente patógeno y que puede transmitirlo a otras personas (Ch. 22).

poscoital (postcoital) período de tiempo que le sigue al (después) coito (Ch. 26).

práctica (practicum) etapa de transición que brinda la oportunidad de aplicar la teoría aprendida en el aula en un entorno de atención médica a través de experiencia práctica y activa (Ch. 1, 45).

práctica laboral (externship) etapa de transición entre los estudios y el empleo real; también se conoce como pasantía o práctica (Ch. 1, 24, 45).

Precauciones Basadas en la Transmisión (Transmission-Based Precautions) segundo nivel de las pautas de los Centros para el Control y la Prevención de Enfermedades (CDC, por sus siglas en inglés) que se aplica a categorías específicas de pacientes y que incluyen precauciones para transmisión por aire, por contacto y por gotitas. Se usan siempre en conjunto con las Precauciones Estándar (Ch. 22).

Precauciones Estándar (Standard Precautions) precauciones desarrolladas en 1996 por los Centros para el Control y la Prevención de Enfermedades (CDC, por sus siglas en inglés) que amplían las precauciones universales y las prácticas de aislamiento de sustancias corporales. Proporcionan una variedad más amplia de protección y se usan en cualquier momento que exista contacto con la sangre, los líquidos corporales húmedos (excepto la sudoración), las membranas mucosas o la piel no intacta. Tienen como objetivo proteger a todos los proveedores de atención médica, los pacientes y los visitantes (Ch. 9, 22).

Precauciones Universales (Universal Precautions) pautas establecidas por los Centros para el Control y la Prevención de Enfermedades (CDC, por sus siglas en inglés) para proteger a los profesionales de la atención médica de las enfermedades infecciosas (Ch. 22).

precedentes (precedents) se refiere a los fallos dictados anteriormente e incluyen decisiones tomadas en el tribunal, interpretaciones de una constitución y decisiones del derecho estatutario (Ch. 7).

precipitado (precipitate) sustancia en forma de partículas finas que se separa de una solución si se deja reposar durante un tiempo (Ch. 36).

precordial (precordial) perteneciente al área de la superficie anterior del cuerpo situada sobre el corazón (Ch. 37).

preeclampsia (preeclampsia) complicación del embarazo que se caracteriza por edema generalizado, hipertensión y proteinuria (Ch. 26).

preexistente (preexisting) lesión o enfermedad que se presenta antes de una fecha determinada (Ch. 22).

preguntas abiertas (open-ended questions) preguntas que incentivan la verbalización y la respuesta; preguntas que buscan obtener una respuesta que va más allá del simple sí o no (Ch. 4).

preguntas cerradas (closed questions) preguntas cuya respuesta es sí o no (Ch. 4).

prejuicio (prejudice) opinión o juicio que se forma antes de conocer los hechos (Ch. 4).

prenatal (prenatal) período de tiempo entre la fertilización y el nacimiento (Ch. 26).

preparación en fresco (wet mount) método para agregar líquido, generalmente solución salina o hidrocloruro de potasio a una muestra en un portaobjetos para examinarla y conservarla. La muestra se coloca en un portaobjetos y se aplica una gota de solución salina (para diagnóstico de *Trichomonas vaginalis*) o hidróxido de potasio (para diagnóstico de infecciones vaginales por hongos) y se mezcla con la muestra. Luego se tapa con un cubreobjeto y se examina microscópicamente (Ch. 26, 43).

presbiacusia (presbycusis) pérdida progresiva de la audición provocada por el proceso normal de envejecimiento (Ch. 29).

primeros auxilios (first aid) cuidados inmediatos (o primeros cuidados) que se brindan a personas que se enferman o se lesionan repentinamente; en general, después de los primeros auxilios se brinda atención y tratamiento integrales (Ch. 9).

primigrávida (primigravida) mujer embarazada por primera vez (Ch. 26).

privilegiada (privileged) información confidencial sobre la cual sólo se puede informar con el permiso del paciente o por orden judicial (Ch. 16).

problema presente (PP) (present problem [PP]) ver **queja principal (QP)** (Ch. 16).

procedimiento de microscopia realizada por el proveedor (PPMP) (provider performed microscopy procedure [PPMP]) término de la Ley de Mejoras de Laboratorios Clínicos (CLIA, por sus siglas en inglés) para aquellos exámenes microscópicos que requieren la pericia de un médico o de un proveedor de nivel medio calificado en exámenes microscópicos. El PPMP es parte de la categoría de pruebas moderadamente complejas de la ley CLIA (Ch. 38).

procedimiento invasivo (invasive procedure) procedimiento que requiere atravesar la piel o hacer una incisión en el cuerpo (Ch. 22, 39).

procedimiento no invasivo (noninvasive procedure) procedimiento que no requiere atravesar la piel o hacer una incisión en el cuerpo (Ch. 37).

profesionalismo (professionalism) cualidades que caracterizan o distinguen a un profesional que cumple con las normas técnicas y éticas de la profesión (Ch. 1).

programación ininterrumpida (stream scheduling) sistema en el que se atiende a los pacientes en forma continua durante el día; por ejemplo, a intervalos de 15, 30 ó 60 minutos, en el cual cada paciente tiene un horario de cita definido (Ch. 13).

pronación (pronation) movimiento del brazo de modo que la palma quede hacia abajo (Ch. 33).

pronunciación (pronunciation) decir las palabras correctamente (Ch. 12).

prostaglandina (prostaglandin) modulador de la actividad bioquímica en los tejidos (Ch. 26).

protección contra sobretensiones (surge protection) protección de los componentes electrónicos frágiles contra las corrientes de fuga en el voltaje eléctrico que se producen en las líneas de distribución de energía (Ch. 11).

proteinuria (proteinuria) proteína en la orina (Ch. 30).

protocolo de manejo de la tos (cough etiquette) toser/estornudar en un pañuelo de papel tisú para impedir que los microorganismos se transmitan a otras personas. Incluye saber cómo desechar correctamente el pañuelo en un recipiente de residuos y lavarse las manos lo antes posible (Ch. 22).

protocolo de voz por Internet (VoIP) (voice over Internet protocol [VoIP]) transmisión en tiempo real de señales de voz a través de Internet o de la red del protocolo de Internet (IP) (Ch. 12).

protozoos (protozoa) animales unicelulares que se dividen en cuatro grupos: amebas, flagelados, ciliados y coccidios (Ch. 43).

proyección (projection) acto de atribuir sentimientos propios a otra persona (Ch. 4).

prueba cualitativa (qualitative test) análisis para identificar las cualidades o las características de los componentes, como tamaño, forma y madurez de las células (Ch. 39).

prueba cuantitativa (quantitative test) análisis que puede identificar la cantidad o el recuento de cantidades reales como el recuento de la cantidad de células sanguíneas (Ch. 39).

prueba de aptitud (proficiency testing) pruebas de muestras realizadas en un laboratorio clínico para determinar con qué grado de exactitud se realizan las pruebas. Las muestras de prueba se verifican del mismo modo que las muestras de los pacientes (Ch. 38).

prueba de baja complejidad (waived) se usa para describir una categoría de pruebas de laboratorio clínico que son simples, invariables y que requieren un mínimo de criterio e interpretación (Ch. 38).

prueba de control (control test) prueba de una muestra de resultados conocidos usados para compararlos con los resultados de la muestra de un paciente (Ch. 39).

prueba de detección (screening) evaluación de los síntomas del paciente para detectar necesidades emergentes. Algunas veces se realizan como ayuda al proveedor de salud para determinar las mejores medidas a tomar en cuanto al cuidado más apropiado para el paciente (Ch. 42).

prueba de detección de Guthrie (Guthrie screening test) también conocida como prueba del talón; prueba de diagnóstico para la detección de fenilcetonuria (FCU) (Ch. 44).

prueba de Mantoux (Mantoux test) prueba para determinar la presencia de tuberculosis que consiste en la inyección intradérmica de derivado proteico purificado (ver DPP) (Ch. 44).

prueba del tambor optocinético (opticokinetic drum test) estudio usado para ayudar a diagnosticar el nistagmo (Ch. 30).

prurito (pruritus) picazón (Ch. 22, 35).

puerperio (puerperium) período desde el final de la tercera etapa del parto hasta que se completa la involución del útero, generalmente de tres a seis semanas (Ch. 26).

puerto (port) término abreviado de portal, vía de ingreso. Cuando se refiere a la terapia intravenosa, es un tipo de adaptador que puede servir como medio adicional para infundir líquidos o medicamentos. El puerto se puede conectar al tubo principal. Tiene un lugar de entrada sin aguja (Ch. 36).

puerto de bus universal en serie (USB) (universal serial bus [USB] port) tipo de portal o bus de entrada de datos para datos informáticos (Ch. 11).

punción lumbar (lumbar puncture) punción quirúrgica del área lumbar de los espacios intervertebrales para aspirar el líquido cefalorraquídeo para análisis de laboratorio (Ch. 22, 43).

purga (purging) método para mantener ordenados los archivos separando los archivos activos de los inactivos y cerrados (Ch. 14).

purulento (purulent) que produce o contiene pus (Ch. 22).

Q

queilosis (cheilosis) trastorno provocado por una deficiencia de vitamina B_2 (riboflavina) y caracterizado por llagas en los labios y grietas en las comisuras de la boca (Ch. 34).

queja principal (QP) (chief complaint [CC]) síntoma o problema específico por el cual el paciente consulta al proveedor hoy (Ch. 16, 23).

queratitis (keratitis) inflamación de la córnea (Ch. 22).

química clínica (clinical chemistry) análisis y estudio de la sangre, los líquidos corporales, los excrementos y los tejidos en el diagnóstico y el tratamiento de enfermedades (Ch. 39).

R

racionalización (rationalization) acto de justificación, generalmente ilógico, que se usa para no enfrentar la verdad de la situación (Ch. 4).

radiación ionizante (ionizing radiation) haces de rayos X (Ch. 32).

radioactivo (radioactive) emite rayos o partículas desde el núcleo (Ch. 32).

radiografía (radiograph) placa en la cual se produce una imagen a través de la exposición a los rayos X (Ch. 32).

radiolúcido (radiolucent) que permite que lo atraviesen los rayos X. Aparece un área oscura en la radiografía (Ch. 32).

radionúclidos (radionuclides) átomos que se desintegran emitiendo radiación electromagnética (Ch. 32).

radiopaco (radiopaque) impenetrable para los rayos X. Aparece un área clara en la radiografía (Ch. 32).

reactivo (reagent) sustancia química que detecta o sintetiza otras sustancias en una reacción química; se usa en los análisis de laboratorio porque se conoce su reacción de una forma específica (Ch. 39, 42, 43).

reanimación cardiopulmonar (RCP) (cardiopulmonary resuscitation [CPR]) combinación de respiración artificial de rescate y compresiones torácicas realizada por una persona capacitada a un paciente que presenta paro cardíaco (Ch. 9).

recetar (prescribe) indicar o recomendar el uso de un fármaco, una dieta u otra forma de terapia (Ch. 7, 35).

rechazo (denial) renuencia o negativa a aceptar algo (Ch. 4).

recipiente principal (primary container) recipiente que contiene directamente a la muestra (Ch. 40).

recolección de mitad de micción (midstream Collection) muestra de orina recogida a la mitad de la micción (Ch. 42).

recuento sanguíneo completo (RSC) (complete blood count [CBC]) batería de análisis hematológicos que consisten en hemoglobina, hematocrito, recuento total de glóbulos blancos que incluye diferencial, recuento total de glóbulos rojos, que incluye índices y plaquetas (Ch. 41).

red de área amplia (WAN) (wide area network [WAN]) conexión de múltiples computadoras juntas en un área grande con el fin de compartir datos (Ch. 11).

red de área local (LAN) (local area network [LAN]) red de computadoras generalmente en una oficina o edificio (Ch. 11).

red de área local inalámbrica (WLAN) (wireless local area network [LAN]) tipo de red de área local que usa ondas de radio de alta frecuencia en lugar de cables para comunicarse entre los nodos (Ch. 11).

redes con cableado físico (hard-wired networks) redes conectadas por conductores metálicos o cables; en algunas circunstancias, se pueden usar cables ópticos (Ch. 11).

reembolso (reimbursement) pago (Ch. 38).

referencia cruzada (cross-reference) anotación en un expediente para guiar al lector hacia un registro específico que puede estar archivado bajo más de un nombre/sujeto (p. ej., nombre de casado/nombre de soltera o nombres extranjeros) cuando el apellido no es fácilmente reconocible (Ch. 14).

referencias (references) personas que conocen a otra persona o han trabajado con ella el tiempo suficiente para hacer una evaluación sincera y una recomendación con respecto a los antecedentes de la persona (Ch. 48).

refractómetro (refractometer) instrumento que mide el índice de refracción de una sustancia o solución; se usa en el examen físico del análisis de orina para medir la densidad urinaria de una muestra de orina (Ch. 42).

registro de cheques (check register) registro de los cheques emitidos, categorizados en columnas separadas e identificadas (Ch. 21).

registro de entrada (sistema de ordenación por número) (accession record [numeric system]) libro de registro usado para asignar números a la correspondencia o a los pacientes (Ch. 14).

registro de reclamaciones (claim register) diario o registro de reclamaciones presentado a cada aseguradora. Cuando se recibe el pago, se escribe la fecha y el importe del pago en el registro (Ch. 18).

registro de salud electrónico (RSE) (electronic health record [EHR]) registros médicos electrónicos de un paciente de varias fuentes combinados en una base de datos principal (Ch. 11).

Registro Federal (Federal Register) agencia federal del gobierno de la cual se pueden obtener los documentos CLIA '88 escritos (Ch. 38).

registro médico electrónico (RME) (electronic medical record [EMR]) registro médico del paciente de una única práctica médica, hospital o farmacia (Ch. 11, 16).

regla de Nägele (Nägele's rule) método habitual para calcular la fecha prevista del parto (Ch. 26).

regla del cumpleaños (birthday rule) método para determinar cuál de dos o más pólizas que cubren a un niño dependiente será la principal, es decir, la póliza del padre o de la madre que cumpla años primero en el año calendario será la póliza principal (Ch. 17).

regresión (regression) movimiento hacia atrás hasta una etapa anterior para escapar del conflicto o de los miedos (Ch. 4).

relación de cobranza (collection ratio) ingresos brutos divididos por el importe que se podría haber cobrado menos los rechazos (Ch. 20, 21).

relación de costos (cost ratio) fórmula que muestra el costo de un procedimiento o servicio y ayuda a determinar el valor financiero de mantener determinados servicios (Ch. 21).

relación de cuentas por cobrar a activos (accounts receivable [A/R]) (accounts receivable [A/R] ratio assets) cuentas por cobrar pendientes de pago divididas por los ingresos brutos mensuales promedio durante los últimos 12 meses (Ch. 20, 21).

remisión (referral) término usado por los centros de atención administrada para autorizar a otro proveedor, que no sea el proveedor de atención primaria, para que atienda al paciente (Ch. 17).

reparación (undoing) acciones destinadas a subsanar y anular un comportamiento inapropiado (Ch. 4).

repolarización (repolarization) restitución de un estado polarizado en un músculo después de una contracción (Ch. 37).

represión (repression) forma de sobrellevar una situación abrumadora olvidándola temporalmente; amnesia temporal (Ch. 4).

resección transuretral (transurethral resection) extirpación de tejido de la próstata usando un dispositivo que se introduce a través de la uretra (Ch. 28).

residuos patógenos (infectious waste) elementos que han estado en contacto con la sangre o los líquidos corporales del paciente. Elementos contaminados (Ch. 22).

residuos regulados (regulated waste) residuos que contienen material infeccioso que representaría una amenaza debido a la posible transmisión de microorganismos patógenos (Ch. 22).

resistencia (resistance) capacidad del sistema inmunitario para resistir o enfrentar las enfermedades infecciosas (Ch. 22).

resolución alternativa de conflictos (RAC) (alternative dispute resolution [ADR]) una alternativa al juicio que alienta a las partes a resolver sus diferencias fuera de un tribunal (Ch. 7).

resolución de conflictos (conflict resolution) solución de problemas entre compañeros de trabajo o entre dos partes dadas (Ch. 45).

respiración de rescate (rescue breathing) realizada en personas con paro respiratorio, la respiración de rescate es un procedimiento boca a boca (usando equipo de protección apropiado) o boca a nariz que proporciona oxígeno al paciente hasta que llegue el personal de emergencia (Ch. 9).

respiración externa (external respiration) ventilación de los pulmones cuando se produce el intercambio de oxígeno y dióxido de carbono (Ch. 30).

respiración interna (internal respiration) paso de oxígeno de la sangre a las células (Ch. 30).

responsabilidad (liability) responsabilidad legal (Ch. 45).

respuesta inflamatoria (inflammatory response) defensa del cuerpo contra la amenaza de infección o traumatismo. Se caracteriza por enrojecimiento, dolor, calor e hinchazón (Ch. 22).

resumen de alta médica (DS) (discharge summary [DS]) informes médicos que documentan el historial de hospitalización de un paciente (Ch. 16).

retención (retention) orina que se retiene en la vejiga; incapacidad de vaciar la vejiga (Ch. 28).

retraso psicomotor (psychomotor retardation) disminución de las respuestas físicas y mentales; se puede observar en la depresión (Ch. 6).

revisar (proofread) leer un documento para verificar que el contenido sea exacto y que se hayan usado correctamente las normas de gramática, ortografía, puntuación y uso de mayúsculas (Ch. 15, 16).

revisión de salario (salary review) informar al empleado sobre su sueldo base por hora revisado (Ch. 45).

revisión de sistemas (ROS) (review of systems [ROS]) consultas sobre el sistema directamente relacionadas con problemas identificados en la historia de la enfermedad presente (Ch. 16).

revisión de utilización (RU) (utilization review [UR]) revisión de los servicios médicos antes de que se brinden (Ch. 21).

riboflavina (riboflavin) vitamina B_2 (Ch. 34).

riesgo biológico (biohazard) material que ha estado en contacto con líquidos corporales y puede transmitir enfermedades (Ch. 22).

ritmo circadiano (circadian rhythm) patrón que se basa en un ciclo de 24 horas y que remarca la repetición de ciertos fenómenos fisiológicos como comer y dormir (Ch. 42).

ritmo sinusal normal (normal sinus rhythm) término usado para describir el ritmo cardíaco cuando está dentro del intervalo normal (Ch. 37).

RME (EMR) ver **registros médicos electrónicos** (Ch. 11).

roncha (wheal) ligera elevación de la piel que se puede producir al aplicar una inyección intradérmica, como la prueba de Mantoux para la tuberculosis (Ch. 44).

rosácea (rosacea) enfermedad crónica de la piel caracterizada por pústulas, pápulas, eritema e hiperplasia. Se desconoce su causa (Ch. 30).

rotación (rotation) giro de una parte del cuerpo alrededor de su eje (Ch. 33); también, oportunidad para pasar 2 o 3 semanas en una variedad de entornos de atención médica (Ch. 40).

RSE (HER) ver registros de salud electrónicos (Ch. 11).

ruidos (bruits) sonido de origen venoso o arterial que se escucha en la auscultación (Ch. 25).

S

saldo (balance) monto adeudado (Ch. 19).

salicilatos (salicylates) fármacos similares a las aspirinas que pueden producir úlceras porque irritan el tracto gastrointestinal (Ch. 30).

sarna (scabies) enfermedad infecciosa de la piel provocada por ácaros *(Sarcoptes scabiei)*, que se transmite por contacto directo con las personas infectadas (Ch. 22).

secreción (secretion) sustancia producida por las células de los órganos glandulares a partir de materiales en la sangre (Ch. 22, 38).

sedimento (sediment) material insoluble que se deposita en el fondo de un líquido; material examinado en el examen microscópico de análisis de orina (Ch. 42).

seguidor de contactos (contact tracker) formulario usado para realizar el seguimiento de la información de contacto laboral, como nombre del empleador, nombre de la persona de contacto, dirección y número telefónico, fecha del primer contacto, currículum vitae enviado, fecha de la entrevista, información de seguimiento y fechas (Ch. 48).

seguro de indemnización por accidentes de trabajo (Workers' Compensation insurance) seguro médico y salarial para los trabajadores que sufren lesiones relacionadas con el empleo (Ch. 17).

seguro de responsabilidad profesional (professional liability insurance) póliza de seguro cuyo objetivo es proteger los activos en el caso en que se presente o se dé lugar a una reclamación por daños y perjuicios producto de la negligencia.

sello de agua (watermark) diseño incorporado al papel durante el proceso de fabricación del papel que es visible cuando se sostiene el papel ante la luz (Ch. 15).

semen (semen) secreción espesa y viscosa segregada por la uretra de los hombres en el orgasmo. Es un producto mixto que contiene distintos líquidos y espermatozoides. El esperma está ausente en el semen de los hombres que se han practicado la vasectomía (Ch. 44).

senil (senile) debilidad mental y física a veces relacionada con el envejecimiento (Ch. 29).

sensibilidad (sensitivity) prueba en la cual se coloca un antibiótico en un organismo para determinar cuál antibiótico eliminará eficazmente el organismo con la menor dosis (ver también cultivo y sensibilidad) (Ch. 43).

sensor (sensor) término usado para describir una lengüeta de papel recubierta en metal que se aplica en el cuerpo del paciente como preparación para un ECG (también conocido como electrodo). Los sensores se colocan en lugares específicos de la piel y luego se conectan al ECG con cables. Los sensores conducen la electricidad desde el paciente hasta el equipo de electrocardiografía (Ch. 37).

señalador o marcador (out guide or sheet) tarjeta, carpeta o tira de papel insertada provisoriamente en los archivos para reemplazar un registro que fue retirado de allí (Ch. 14).

septicemia (septicemia) invasión de bacterias patógenas en el torrente sanguíneo (Ch. 3).

servicios auxiliares (ancillary services) empresas ocupacionales profesionales contratadas para completar un trabajo específico (Ch. 45).

servicios de respuesta (answering services) servicios empleados para responder a las llamadas de entornos de atención ambulatoria después del horario de atención; a diferencia de un contestador automático, un operador en vivo responde a la llamada y la deriva según corresponda (Ch. 12).

Servicios Médicos de Emergencia (SME) (Emergency Medical Services [EMS]) red local de policía, bomberos y personal médico capacitado para responder a situaciones de emergencia. En muchas comunidades, el sistema se activa llamando al 911 (Ch. 9).

servidor (server) computadora con capacidad de disco duro masiva que se usa para conectar otras computadoras entre sí de modo que múltiples usuarios puedan compartir los datos. Probablemente un sistema informático de un centro de atención ambulatoria estará vinculado o conectado en red con un servidor central (Ch. 11).

sesgo (bias) tendencia hacia una creencia en particular (Ch. 4).

shock (shock) afección potencialmente grave en la que el sistema circulatorio no suministra sangre suficiente a todas las partes del cuerpo y que provoca que los órganos del cuerpo no funcionen correctamente (Ch. 9).

sibilancia (wheezes) ruido de tono alto que se escucha en la expiración, a menudo resultado de una obstrucción o estrechamiento de las vías respiratorias (Ch. 24).

símbolo universal de identificación médica para emergencias (universal emergency medical identification symbol) identificación que a veces llevan puesta las personas para identificar los problemas de salud que tienen (Ch. 9).

simetría (symmetry) correspondencia de forma, tamaño y posición de las partes del cuerpo en lados contrarios del cuerpo (Ch. 25).

síncope (syncope) desmayo (Ch. 9, 37).

síncope vasovagal (vasovagal syncope) desmayo repentino debido a la hipotensión inducida por la respuesta del sistema nervioso autónomo al estrés emocional, al dolor o a un traumatismo abrupto (Ch. 9).

síndrome de Cushing (Cushing's syndrome) hipersecreción de la corteza suprarrenal que produce exceso de glucocorticoides. La causa de esta afección puede ser un tumor o la hiperfunción de la hipófisis anterior (Ch. 44).

síndrome de inmunodeficiencia adquirida (SIDA) (acquired immunodeficiency syndrome [AIDS]) trastorno del sistema inmunitario causado por el virus de inmunodeficiencia humana (VIH), un retrovirus que destruye la capacidad del cuerpo para combatir las infecciones. A medida que la enfermedad avanza, los trastornos, que incluyen cáncer e infecciones oportunistas, van doblegando a la persona. No existe cura conocida para el SIDA (Ch. 22).

síndrome respiratorio agudo y grave (SARS) (severe acute respiratory syndrome [SARS]) brote viral de una enfermedad respiratoria que se informó en Asia por primera vez en 2003; se contagia por contacto estrecho de persona a persona y se caracteriza por fiebre y síntomas respiratorios (Ch. 22).

Sistema de Códigos de Procedimientos Comunes de la Atención Médica (HCPCS) (Healthcare Common Procedure Coding System [HCPCS]) sistema de códigos que consta de la Terminología Actual de Procedimientos (CPT, por sus siglas en inglés), códigos nacionales (nivel II) y códigos locales (nivel III); antes conocido como Sistema de Códigos de Procedimientos Comunes HCFA (Ch. 18).

Sistema de Gestión de Prácticas Total (TPMS) (Total Practice Management System [TPMS]) categoría de software que maneja todas las operaciones diarias de la práctica médica (Ch. 11).

Sistema de Informes de Elegibilidad para la Inscripción en Defensa (DEERS) (Defense Enrollment Eligible Reporting System [DEERS]) sistema operado por el Departamento de Defensa y usado por los contratistas de TRICARE para determinar y confirmar la elegibilidad de los beneficiarios (Ch. 17).

sistema de prestación de servicios médicos integrado (IDS) (integrated delivery system [IDS]) organización de atención médica de centros de proveedores afiliados combinados bajo una única propiedad que ofrece el espectro completo de atención médica administrada (Ch. 17).

sistema de tablero de clavijas (pegboard system) sistema manual de cuentas médicas por cobrar que se usa con más frecuencia (Ch. 19).

sistema inmunitario (immune system) mecanismo de defensa del cuerpo contra los microorganismos invasores. El cuerpo reconoce las sustancias extrañas, como los microorganismos, y produce sustancias para combatirlos. Algunos ejemplos son los anticuerpos, los glóbulos blancos, las enzimas digestivas y la resistencia de la piel (Ch. 22).

sistema inmunitario con inmunosupresión (suppressed immune system) término usado para describir un sistema inmunitario que no puede funcionar normalmente debido a la presencia de una enfermedad como el SIDA (Ch. 38).

sistema nervioso parasimpático (parasympathetic nervous system) parte del sistema nervioso autónomo que hace que el cuerpo vuelva a su estado normal después de que diminuye el estrés (Ch. 5).

sistema nervioso simpático (sympathetic nervous system) gran parte del sistema nervioso autónomo que prepara el cuerpo para la reacción de lucha o huída (Ch. 5).

sistema operativo (SO) (operating system [OS]) software usado para controlar la computadora y su equipo periférico. También se lo conoce como software de sistema (Ch. 11).

sistémico (systemic) relativo a todo el cuerpo (Ch. 9).

sístole (systole) un componente de la medición de presión arterial que representa la presión más alta durante el ciclo cardíaco; fuerza ejercida sobre las paredes arteriales durante la contracción cardíaca (Ch. 24, 37).

SOAP (SOAP) sigla de las notas de evolución del paciente basadas en las impresiones subjetivas (S), la evidencia clínica objetiva (O), análisis o diagnóstico (A) y planes para estudios adicionales (P) (Ch. 14, 23).

sobrecodificación (up-coding) también conocido como incremento de códigos y sobrefacturación. La sobrecodificación ocurre cuando la compañía de seguros intencionalmente factura un servicio que tiene una tarifa mayor del que se prestó para obtener mayores reembolsos (Ch. 19).

sobrenadante (supernatant) orina que aparece encima del sedimento cuando se centrifuga; lo drenado antes de que el sedimento sea examinado en el examen microscópico del análisis de orina (Ch. 42).

software (software) equivalente de programa informático (Ch. 11).

software de aplicación (application software) software que realiza una función específica de procesamiento de datos (Ch. 11).

software de reconocimiento de voz (voice recognition software [VRS]) software que traduce comandos de voz y se usa en lugar del mouse y del teclado (Ch. 16).

software de sistema (system software) ver **sistema operativo** (Ch. 11).

solicitud (requisition) formulario de pedido que se envía con una muestra y que especifica las pruebas que se deben realizar; las pruebas más comunes se separan en categorías lógicas con espacio adicional para escribir pedidos especiales (Ch. 38, 39).

solicitud/carta de presentación (application/cover letter) carta que se usa para presentarse y para enviar el curriculum vitae a un posible empleador a fin de obtener una entrevista (Ch. 48).

soluble en agua (water-soluble) relativo a sustancias que son hidrofílicas y, por lo tanto, se disuelven mejor en agua (Ch. 34).

soluble en lípidos (fat-soluble) relativo a sustancias que son hidrofóbicas y, por lo tanto, se disuelven mejor en los lípidos (Ch. 34).

solución salina normal (normal saline) solución de cloruro de sodio (sal) y agua destilada. Tiene la misma presión osmótica que el suero sanguíneo. También se la conoce como solución salina isotónica o fisiológica (Ch. 9).

solvente (solvent) que produce una solución, que se disuelve (Ch. 22).

subjetivo (subjective) síntoma que siente el paciente pero que los demás no pueden observar (Ch. 23).

sublimación (sublimation) redirigir un impulso socialmente inaceptable hacia uno que sea socialmente aceptable (Ch. 4).

subordinado (subordinate) en una organización, persona bajo la dirección (o el mando) de una persona de mayor autoridad (Ch. 45).

suero (serum) parte líquida de la sangre que se obtiene después de que se ha dejado coagular la sangre (Ch. 39, 40).

supercomputadora (supercomputer) la más veloz, grande y cara de las cuatro clases de computadoras que se fabrican actualmente (Ch. 11).

supinación (supination) movimiento del brazo de modo que la palma quede hacia arriba (Ch. 33).

supurante (suppurant) agente que produce formación de pus (Ch. 31).

supurativo (suppurative) que produce la generación de pus o relacionado con ello (Ch. 27).

sustancias radiofarmacéuticas (radiopharmaceuticals) sustancias químicas radioactivas usadas en pruebas de ubicación, tamaño, contorno o función de tejidos, órganos, vasos o líquidos corporales (Ch. 32).

sustituto (surrogate) suplente; alguien que reemplaza a otro (Ch. 8).

sutura (suture) material o hilo quirúrgico; puede describir el acto de coser con hilo y aguja quirúrgicos (Ch. 31).

T

talasemia (thalassemia) anemia hereditaria que puede ser mortal (Ch. 26).

taquicardia sinusal (tachycardia, sinus) latido cardíaco anormalmente rápido superior a 100 latidos/minuto. Tipo de arritmia cardíaca (Ch. 24, 37).

taquipnea (tachypnea) aumento anormal en la frecuencia de la respiración (Ch. 24).

tarjetas de cirugía (surgery cards) referencia escrita para cirugías y procedimientos (Ch. 31).

taxonomía (taxonomy) clasificación de organismos en categorías apropiadas (Ch. 43).

Tay–Sachs (Tay–Sachs) enfermedad congénita que generalmente es mortal (Ch. 26).

teclear (key) ingresar datos mediante teclas en el teclado de la computadora (Ch. 15).

técnica de una sola mano (scoop technique) técnica que usa una sola mano para recoger y tapar una aguja usada únicamente si no hay disponible de manera inmediata un recipiente para objetos filosos; no se manipula la cubierta (tapa) de la aguja de ningún modo; luego se la desecha en el recipiente de objetos filosos más próximo (Ch. 22).

técnicas de entrevista (interview techniques) métodos para promover una mejor comunicación entre el postulante y el entrevistador (Ch. 4).

tecnología de cifrado (encryption technology) convierte la información en un código; se usa para proteger la privacidad y la confidencialidad de las personas en el software informático (Ch. 13).

Tecnólogos Médicos Estadounidenses (AMT) (American Medical Technologists [AMT]) organización médica que acredita a los profesionales de atención médica, incluidos los Asistentes Médicos Matriculados (RMA, por sus siglas en inglés) y los Especialistas Administrativos Médicos Certificados (CMAS, por sus siglas en inglés) (Ch. 1, 47).

teléfonos celulares (cellular telephones) dispositivo portátil de corto alcance usado para comunicación de voz o datos en una red de estaciones base llamadas sitio de celda. El sitio de celda está interconectado a la red telefónica conmutada (Ch. 12).

temperamento (disposition) modo de ser, carácter, personalidad (Ch. 1).

terapia de reemplazo hormonal (TRH) (hormone replacement therapy [HRT]) reemplazo de las hormonas faltantes en el sistema del paciente. En este caso, la TRH se refiere al reemplazo de diferentes niveles de estrógeno y progesterona en mujeres perimenopáusicas y posmenopáusicas (Ch. 26, 39).

Terminología Actual sobre Procedimientos (TAP) (Current Procedural Terminology [CPT]) códigos estándar para procedimientos y servicios. Se usa en la mayoría de los entornos de atención ambulatoria para codificar el formulario de reclamación y es reconocida por la mayoría de las compañías de seguros (Ch. 19).

termófilo (thermophile) resistente a la destrucción por el calor. Característico de algunas bacterias (Ch. 31).

termolábil (thermolabile) afectado fácilmente por el calor (Ch. 22).

termoterapia (thermotherapy) uso del calor para tratar una afección física (Ch. 33).

testamento en vida (living will) documento que permite que una persona tome decisiones relacionadas con el tratamiento de una enfermedad con riesgo de muerte (Ch. 6).

testigo experto (expert witness) persona con conocimientos y habilidades sumamente especializadas en un área en particular que atestigua con respecto a un estándar de atención (Ch. 7).

tiamina (thiamin) vitamina B1 (Ch. 34).

tifus (tifoide) (typhus [typhoid]) enfermedad infecciosa aguda que produce dolor de cabeza intenso, sarpullido, fiebre alta y compromiso neurológico progresivo. Es frecuente en lugares donde las condiciones son insalubres y de hacinamiento (Ch. 3).

timpanostomía (tympanostomy) colocación de un tubo por la membrana timpánica para permitir la ventilación del oído medio; parte del tratamiento de la otitis media (Ch. 27).

tinción de Gram (Gram stain) su nombre proviene de su inventor, Hans Christian Gram, y por lo tanto "Gram" se escribe siempre con mayúscula; tinción más común usada en microbiología para observar las características morfológicas de las bacterias; tinción diferencial que permite la diferenciación entre organismos gramnegativos y grampositivos (Ch. 43).

tinnitus (tinnitus) repiqueteo o zumbido en el oído (Ch. 25).

tira de prueba reactiva (reagent test strip) tira estrecha de plástico en la cual se pegan almohadillas que contienen reactivos; se usa en el examen químico de análisis de orina para detectar, glucosa, bilirrubina, cetonas, densidad urinaria, sangre, pH, urobilinógeno, nitritos y esterasa leucocitaria (Ch. 42).

tira de ritmo (rhythm strip) registro del ECG de una única derivación, generalmente la derivación II, que se usa para determinar el ritmo del latido cardíaco. La arritmia se puede observar más fácilmente en una tira de ritmo porque se prolonga más tiempo, de acuerdo con el pedido del proveedor (Ch. 37).

tirante (taut) estirar o tensar una superficie, como la piel (Ch. 36).

título (titer) medición de la cantidad de anticuerpos presentes contra un antígeno en particular (Ch. 26).

tocoferol (tocopherol) vitamina E (Ch. 34).

toracentesis (thoracentesis) punción quirúrgica de la cavidad torácica para aspirar líquido (Ch. 22).

tormenta de ideas (brainstorming) proceso para desarrollar ideas a través de la interacción sinérgica entre los participantes en un entorno libre de críticas (Ch. 45).

torniquete (tourniquet) dispositivo usado para facilitar la prominencia de la vena (Ch. 40).

toxicidad (toxicity) nivel a partir del cual un fármaco o sustancia química es tóxico o nocivo. Algunas sustancias, como algunos metales, son consideradas tóxicas en cualquier nivel de exposición accidental (Ch. 39).

trabajo en equipo (teamwork) personas que trabajan juntas en forma sinérgica (Ch. 45).

transcriptor (transcriber) dispositivo que permite transformar las grabaciones de voz en documentos transcritos o impresos (Ch. 16).

Transcriptor Médico Certificado (CMT) (Certified Medical Transcriptionist [CMT]) terminación de las dos partes del examen de certificación administrado por la Asociación para la Integridad de la Documentación del Cuidado de la Salud (AHDI, por sus siglas en inglés) (Ch. 16).

transductor (transducer) dispositivo que convierte una forma de energía en otra. Durante un procedimiento de ecografía, el transductor registra los ecos y los convierte en energía eléctrica. La energía se transforma en imágenes digitalizadas que se pueden ver o imprimir. Se pueden tomar fotografías de la imagen (Ch. 32, 37).

transiluminador (transilluminator) instrumento usado para inspeccionar una cavidad o un órgano pasando una luz a través de las paredes (Ch. 28).

transmisible (communicable) contagioso; que puede transmitirse de una persona a otra directa o indirectamente (Ch. 22, 38).

transmisión (transmission) propagación de una enfermedad infecciosa por contacto directo, contacto indirecto, inhalación, ingestión o por transmisión sanguínea (Ch. 22).

transmisión por aire (airborne transmission) propagación de microorganismos causantes de enfermedades por el aire a través de largas distancias (Ch. 22).

transmisión por contacto (contact transmission) diseminación de microorganismos causantes de enfermedades al tocar directa o indirectamente la fuente de la infección o al tocar un objeto o una superficie del ambiente (Ch. 22).

transmisión por gotitas (droplet transmission) método de diseminación de las enfermedades por secreciones respiratorias a través del aire. La diseminación por lo general se limita a 3 pies del paciente infectado (Ch. 22).

transmisión sanguínea (bloodborne) medio de transmisión de una enfermedad infecciosa (como VIH y VHB) a través de la sangre humana (Ch. 22).

trazado (tracing) registro gráfico por lo general de un episodio que cambia con el tiempo y con la actividad eléctrica del corazón (Ch. 37).

triage (triage) proceso para determinar y establecer prioridades en cuanto a las necesidades de los pacientes y el posible beneficio que tendrían al recibir atención médica inmediata. Proviene de la palabra francesa *trier,* que significa "clasificar" (Ch. 2, 9, 12, 13).

tribunal sucesorio (probate court) tribunal que administra sucesiones y valida los testamentos (Ch. 20).

TRICARE (TRICARE) antes llamado Programa Médico y de Salud Civil de los Servicios Uniformados (CHAMPUS, por sus siglas en inglés). TRICARE ofrece HMO, PPO y seguro médico con pago por servicio para dependientes de personal militar en servicio activo y retirado y para dependientes del personal que falleció mientras prestaban servicio (Ch. 17).

tricomoniasis (trichomoniasis) infestación con el parásito *Trichomonas,* que se puede transmitir a través de las relaciones sexuales (Ch. 22, 26).

triglicéridos (triglycerides) forma de lípido del torrente sanguíneo que sirve para almacenar energía (Ch. 44).

trimestre (trimester) tres meses; un tercio del período de gestación del embarazo (Ch. 26).

trinquetes (ratchets) mecanismos de trabado en los mangos de muchos instrumentos quirúrgicos (Ch. 31).

trombocito (thrombocyte) (plaqueta) fragmento celular del megacariocito; cumple un papel importante en la coagulación de la sangre, la hemostasia y la formación de coágulos (Ch. 40, 41).

tuberculosis (TB) (tuberculosis [TB]) enfermedad infecciosa causada por la bacteria *Mycobacterium tuberculosis* (Ch. 44).

tubo de cánula (nasal) (cannula [nasal] tubing) usado para administrar oxígeno (Ch. 36); también, la parte con punta roma de una aguja Bio-Plexus Punctur-Guard® (Ch. 40).

tubos de caldo (broth tubes) tubos llenados con un medio de cultivo líquido llamado caldo que permitirá el crecimiento de determinados microorganismos (Ch. 43).

turbio (turbid) opaco, no claro. Utilizado para describir la orina que es opaca (Ch. 42).

U

ultrasonido (ultrasound) uso de ondas de sonido de alta frecuencia por motivos terapéuticos para generar calor en tejidos profundos (Ch. 33).

unidad (unit) cada parte del nombre (empresa o persona), palabras o números que se indexarán y se codificarán para archivado (Ch. 14).

unidad clave (key unit) primera unidad de indexación del segmento de archivado (Ch. 14).

unidad de cinta (tape drive) dispositivo de almacenamiento de datos que usa cinta magnética como medio de almacenamiento (Ch. 11).

unidad de procesamiento central (CPU) (central processing unit [CPU]) cerebro de la computadora que ejecuta las instrucciones definidas por el software (Ch. 11).

unidad flash (flash drive) dispositivo de almacenamiento de datos en estado sólido (Ch. 11).

unidades de educación continua (UEC) (continuing education units [CEU]) método para obtener puntos a través de una nueva certificación (Ch. 47).

unipolar (unipolar) que tiene o se relaciona con un proceso de un polo (Ch. 37).

urea (urea) producto final principal del metabolismo de las proteínas (Ch. 42).

urgencia (urgency) necesidad de orinar de inmediato (Ch. 30).

urobilinógeno (urobilinogen) compuesto incoloro producido en el intestino después de que las bacterias descomponen la bilirrubina (Ch. 42).

urticaria (urticaria) roncha (Ch. 35).

usual, acostumbrado y razonable (UCR) (usual, customary, and reasonable [UCR]) programa de tarifas que generalmente usan Medicare y algunas compañías aseguradoras. *Usual* se refiere a la tarifa que generalmente cobra un proveedor por determinados procedimientos; *acostumbrado* se basa en la tarifa promedio para un procedimiento específico que cobran todos los proveedores que ejercen la misma especialidad en una región geográfica determinada; *y razonable* se refiere al nivel medio de tarifas que se cobran por ese procedimiento (Ch. 17).

V

vacuna (vaccine) agente farmacológico que puede producir inmunidad activa artificial (Ch. 22).

valle (trough) lo opuesto de "pico", es el punto en el cual el fármaco alcanza su nivel más bajo en el cuerpo. Generalmente ocurre justo antes de administrar la dosis siguiente. En las pruebas de laboratorio, el valle indica al proveedor la influencia más débil que tendría el fármaco en el cuerpo con esa dosis en particular (Ch. 38).

valor de referencia (baseline) medición inicial o conocida con la que se comparan mediciones futuras (Ch. 24, 39); también, línea plana y horizontal que separa las distintas ondas del ciclo del electrocardiograma (ECG) (Ch. 37).

valores críticos (critical values) resultados de una prueba que indican la existencia de una situación con posible riesgo para la vida o sumamente debilitante que se debe informar al proveedor de inmediato (Ch. 42).

valores de referencia (reference values) también llamado valor normal, intervalo normal o intervalo de referencia; intervalo de valores que incluye el 95% de los resultados de pruebas de una población normal sana (Ch. 39).

várices esofágicas (esophageal varices) dilatación tortuosa de la vena esofágica relacionada con cualquier afección que produce la obstrucción del drenaje de las venas esofágicas hacia la vena portal del hígado. Ver cirrosis hepática y alcoholismo (Ch. 32).

vasoconstricción (vasoconstriction) estrechamiento o constricción de los vasos sanguíneos (Ch. 33).

vector (vector) un portador de enfermedad, generalmente un insecto, que es el organismo causante de la enfermedad de personas infectadas a no infectadas (Ch. 22).

velocidad de eritrosedimentación (erythrocyte sedimentation rate) medición de cuánto se asientan los glóbulos rojos en una muestra de sangre en una hora (Ch. 41).

venda (bandage) gasa no estéril u otro material que se aplica sobre un apósito estéril para proteger e inmovilizar un área (Ch. 9, 31).

venopunción (venipuncture) punción en la vena con una aguja para obtener una muestra de sangre (Ch. 40).

verbos de acción (power verbs) palabras indicadoras de acción que se usan para describir sus atributos y sus fortalezas (Ch. 48).

vértigo (vertigo) sensación de pérdida de equilibrio o desvanecimiento; mareos (Ch. 25).

vesicular (vesicular) caracterizado por la presencia de vesículas. Las vesículas son ampollas u otras elevaciones de la piel (Ch. 22, 26).

viable (viable) que puede vivir, crecer y desarrollarse después del nacimiento; generalmente de 24 semanas o más de 1 libra (Ch. 26).

viñeta (bullet point) asterisco o punto seguido de una frase descriptiva que ayuda al lector a identificar puntos importantes con facilidad (Ch. 48).

virología (virology) estudio de los virus (Ch. 39, 43).

virulencia (virulence) potencia relativa de un organismo y grado de patogenicidad (Ch. 22).

virus de Epstein-Barr (VEB) (Epstein–Barr virus [EBV]) se cree que este virus es la causa de la mononucleosis infecciosa y que está involucrado en afecciones como el linfoma de Burkitt africano y el carcinoma nasofaríngeo (Ch. 44).

virus de la inmunodeficiencia humana (VIH) (human immunodeficiency virus [HIV]) virus del SIDA; es un retrovirus que con el tiempo destruye las células del sistema inmunitario (Ch. 22).

viscosidad (viscosity) grado de espesor de un líquido (Ch. 40).

vitíligo (vitiligo) trastorno de la piel caracterizado por manchas blancas claras en diversas áreas del cuerpo (Ch. 25).

volátil (volatile) que se evapora fácilmente (Ch. 31).

X

xeroftalmía (xerophthalmia) membranas mucosas secas y opacas de los ojos (Ch. 34).

Z

ZIP+4 (ZIP+4) código postal estándar que incluye cuatro dígitos adicionales que identifican el área de envío postal. El correo se procesará en forma más eficaz y eficiente con el uso del código ZIP+4 en la dirección (Ch. 15).

Index

Note: Page references in **bold type** refer to boxes, procedures, figures, and tables.

A

E

F

N

Q

R

S

T

Thinking Challenge 2.0
equirements

ft Windows PC:

- perating System: Windows XP w/ Service Pack 2 or Service Pack 3, sta w/ Service Pack 1
- ocessor: Intel Pentium IV 600MHz or higher
- emory: Minimum required by operating system
- reen resolution: 800x600
- 2x CD-ROM drive
- ound card and listening device required for audio features

ion Instructions

- nsert the disc into CD-ROM player. The CTC game should start automatically. If the game does not start, go to step 2.
- rom My Computer, double click the icon for the CD drive. Double click n "CTC 2.exe" file to start the program.
- or more information about how the game is played, see Appendix E.

StudyWare™ to Accompany Delmar's Health Assessment & Physical Examination, Fourth Edition

Minimum System Requirements

- Operating systems: Microsoft Windows 2000 w/SP 4, Windows XP w/SP 2, Windows Vista w/ SP 1
- Processor: Minimum required by Operating System
- Memory: Minimum required by Operating System
- Hard Drive Space: 500 MB
- Screen resolution: 800 x 600 pixels
- CD-ROM drive
- Sound card and listening device required for audio features
- Flash Player 9. The Adobe Flash Player is free, and can be downloaded from http://www.adobe.com/products/flashplayer/

Setup Instructions

1. Insert disc into CD-ROM drive. The StudyWare™ installation program should start automatically. If it does not, go to step 2.
2. From My Computer, double-click the icon for the CD drive.
3. Double-click the *setup.exe* file to start the program.

Technical Support

Telephone: 1-800-648-7450
8:30 A.M.-6:30 P.M. Eastern Time
E-mail: delmar.help@cengage.com

IMPORTANT! READ CAREFULLY: This End User License Agreement ("Agreement") sets forth the conditions by which Cengage Learning will make electronic access to the Cengage Learning-owned licensed content and associated media, software, documentation, printed materials, and electronic documentation contained in this package and/or made available to you via this product (the "Licensed Content"), available to you (the "End User"). BY CLICKING THE "I ACCEPT" BUTTON AND/OR OPENING THIS PACKAGE, YOU ACKNOWLEDGE THAT YOU HAVE READ ALL OF THE TERMS AND CONDITIONS, AND THAT YOU AGREE TO BE BOUND BY ITS TERMS, CONDITIONS, AND ALL APPLICABLE LAWS AND REGULATIONS GOVERNING THE USE OF THE LICENSED CONTENT.

1.0 SCOPE OF LICENSE

1.1 Licensed Content. The Licensed Content may contain portions of modifiable content ("Modifiable Content") and content which may not be modified or otherwise altered by the End User ("Non-Modifiable Content"). For purposes of this Agreement, Modifiable Content and Non-Modifiable Content may be collectively referred to herein as the "Licensed Content." All Licensed Content shall be considered Non-Modifiable Content, unless such Licensed Content is presented to the End User in a modifiable format and it is clearly indicated that modification of the Licensed Content is permitted.

1.2 Subject to the End User's compliance with the terms and conditions of this Agreement, Cengage Learning hereby grants the End User, a nontransferable, nonexclusive, limited right to access and view a single copy of the Licensed Content on a single personal computer system for noncommercial, internal, personal use only. The End User shall not (i) reproduce, copy, modify (except in the case of Modifiable Content), distribute, display, transfer, sublicense, prepare derivative work(s) based on, sell, exchange, barter or transfer, rent, lease, loan, resell, or in any other manner exploit the Licensed Content; (ii) remove, obscure, or alter any notice of Cengage Learning's intellectual property rights present on or in the Licensed Content, including, but not limited to, copyright, trademark, and/or patent notices; or (iii) disassemble, decompile, translate, reverse engineer, or otherwise reduce the Licensed Content.

2.0 TERMINATION

2.1 Cengage Learning may at any time (without prejudice to its other rights or remedies) immediately terminate this Agreement and/or suspend access to some or all of the Licensed Content, in the event that the End User does not comply with any of the terms and conditions of this Agreement. In the event of such termination by Cengage Learning, the End User shall immediately return any and all copies of the Licensed Content to Cengage Learning.

3.0 PROPRIETARY RIGHTS

3.1 The End User acknowledges that Cengage Learning owns all rights, title and interest, including, but not limited to all copyright rights therein, in and to the Licensed Content, and that the End User shall not take any action inconsistent with such ownership. The Licensed Content is protected by U.S., Canadian and other applicable copyright laws and by international treaties, including the Berne Convention and the Universal Copyright Convention. Nothing contained in this Agreement shall be construed as granting the End User any ownership rights in or to the Licensed Content.

3.2 Cengage Learning reserves the right at any time to withdraw from the Licensed Content any item or part of an item for which it no longer retains the right to publish, or which it has reasonable grounds to believe infringes copyright or is defamatory, unlawful, or otherwise objectionable.

4.0 PROTECTION AND SECURITY

4.1 The End User shall use its best efforts and take all reasonable steps to safeguard its copy of the Licensed Content to ensure that no unauthorized reproduction, publication, disclosure, modification, or distribution of the Licensed Content, in whole or in part, is made. To the extent that the End User becomes aware of any such unauthorized use of the Licensed Content, the End User shall immediately notify Cengage Learning. Notification of such violations may be made by sending an e-mail to infringement@cengage.com.

5.0 MISUSE OF THE LICENSED PRODUCT

5.1 In the event that the End User uses the Licensed Content in violation of this Agreement, Cengage Learning shall have the option of electing liquidated damages, which shall include all profits generated by the End User's use of the Licensed Content plus interest computed at the maximum rate permitted by law and all legal fees and other expenses inc Cengage Learning in enforcing its rights, plus penalties.

6.0 FEDERAL GOVERNMENT CLIENTS

6.1 Except as expressly authorized by Cengage Learning, Federal ment clients obtain only the rights specified in this Agreement other rights. The Government acknowledges that (i) all softw related documentation incorporated in the Licensed Content is commercial computer software within the meaning of FAR 27.40 and (2) all other data delivered in whatever form, is limited rig within the meaning of FAR 27.401. The restrictions in this sec acceptable as consistent with the Government's need for softw other data under this Agreement.

7.0 DISCLAIMER OF WARRANTIES AND LIABILITIES

7.1 Although Cengage Learning believes the Licensed Content to able, Cengage Learning does not guarantee or warrant (i) any i tion or materials contained in or produced by the Licensed C (ii) the accuracy, completeness or reliability of the Licensed C or (iii) that the Licensed Content is free from errors or other r defects. THE LICENSED PRODUCT IS PROVIDED "AS IS," OUT ANY WARRANTY OF ANY KIND AND CENGAGE LEA DISCLAIMS ANY AND ALL WARRANTIES, EXPRESSED OR IM INCLUDING, WITHOUT LIMITATION, WARRANTIES OF CHANTABILITY OR FITNESS FOR A PARTICULAR PURPC NO EVENT SHALL CENGAGE LEARNING BE LIABLE FOR RECT, SPECIAL, PUNITIVE OR CONSEQUENTIAL DA INCLUDING FOR LOST PROFITS, LOST DATA, OR OTHERW NO EVENT SHALL CENGAGE LEARNING'S AGGREGATE LIA HEREUNDER, WHETHER ARISING IN CONTRACT, TORT, S LIABILITY OR OTHERWISE, EXCEED THE AMOUNT OF PAID BY THE END USER HEREUNDER FOR THE LICENSE C LICENSED CONTENT.

8.0 GENERAL

8.1 Entire Agreement. This Agreement shall constitute the entire Agr between the Parties and supercedes all prior Agreements and standings oral or written relating to the subject matter hereof.

8.2 Enhancements/Modifications of Licensed Content. From time t and in Cengage Learning's sole discretion, Cengage Learning may the End User of updates, upgrades, enhancements and/or improv to the Licensed Content, and may permit the End User to access a subject to the terms and conditions of this Agreement, such modific upon payment of prices as may be established by Cengage Learnin

8.3 No Export. The End User shall use the Licensed Content solely United States and shall not transfer or export, directly or indirec Licensed Content outside the United States.

8.4 Severability. If any provision of this Agreement is invalid, illegal, or forceable under any applicable statute or rule of law, the provision s deemed omitted to the extent that it is invalid, illegal, or unenforce such a case, the remainder of the Agreement shall be construed in ner as to give greatest effect to the original intention of the parties h

8.5 Waiver. The waiver of any right or failure of either party to exercise respect any right provided in this Agreement in any instance shall deemed to be a waiver of such right in the future or a waiver of an right under this Agreement.

8.6 Choice of Law/Venue. This Agreement shall be interpreted, constru governed by and in accordance with the laws of the State of New York cable to contracts executed and to be wholly preformed therein, w regard to its principles governing conflicts of law. Each party agrees t proceeding arising out of or relating to this Agreement or the bre threatened breach of this Agreement may be commenced and pros in a court in the State and County of New York. Each party consen submits to the nonexclusive personal jurisdiction of any court in th and County of New York in respect of any such proceeding.

8.7 Acknowledgment. By opening this package and/or by accessi Licensed Content on this Web site, THE END USER ACKNOWLE THAT IT HAS READ THIS AGREEMENT, UNDERSTANDS IT, AGREES TO BE BOUND BY ITS TERMS AND CONDITIONS. IF DO NOT ACCEPT THESE TERMS AND CONDITIONS, YOU NOT ACCESS THE LICENSED CONTENT AND RETURN LICENSED PRODUCT TO CENGAGE LEARNING (WITHIN 30 ENDAR DAYS OF THE END USER'S PURCHASE) WITH PROC PAYMENT ACCEPTABLE TO CENGAGE LEARNING, FOR A CR OR A REFUND. Should the End User have any questions/com regarding this Agreement, please contact Cengage Learning at d help@cengage.com.